CANCER NURSING

A Comprehensive Textbook

CANCER NURSING

A Comprehensive Textbook

Susan B. Baird, R.N., M.P.H., M.A.
Director of Nursing
Fox Chase Cancer Center
Philadelphia, and
Editor, *Oncology Nursing Forum*
Philadelphia, Pennsylvania

Ruth McCorkle, Ph.D., F.A.A.N.
American Cancer Society Professor
School of Nursing
University of Pennsylvania
Philadelphia, Pennsylvania

Marcia Grant, D.N.Sc., O.C.N., F.A.A.N.
Associate Research Scientist and Director
Department of Nursing Research and Education
City of Hope National Medical Center
Duarte, California

1991
W. B. SAUNDERS COMPANY
Harcourt Brace Jovanovich, Inc.
Philadelphia   London   Toronto   Montreal   Sydney   Tokyo

W. B. SAUNDERS COMPANY
Harcourt Brace Jovanovich, Inc.

The Curtis Center
Independence Square West
Philadelphia, PA 19106

Library of Congress Cataloging-in-Publication Data

Baird, Susan B.

    Cancer nursing: a comprehensive textbook / Susan B. Baird,
Ruth McCorkle, Marcia Grant.

    p.   cm.

ISBN 0–7216–2698–X

1. Cancer—Nursing.   I. McCorkle, Ruth.   II. Grant,
  Marcia Moeller.   III. Title.

[DNLM: 1. Oncologic Nursing.   WY 156 B163c]

RC266.B334 1991

610.73′698—dc20

DNLM/DLC

for Library of Congress   90-9205
                                     CIP

1991

Editor: Michael Brown
Developmental Editor: Robin Richman
Designer: Joan Wendt
Production Manager: Linda R. Turner
Manuscript Editor: Lee Ann Draud
Illustration Coordinator: Brett MacNaughton
Indexer: Angela Holt
Cover Designer: Ellen Bodner

Cancer Nursing: A Comprehensive Textbook   ISBN 0–7216–2698–X

Last digit is the print number: 9   8   7   6   5   4   3   2   1

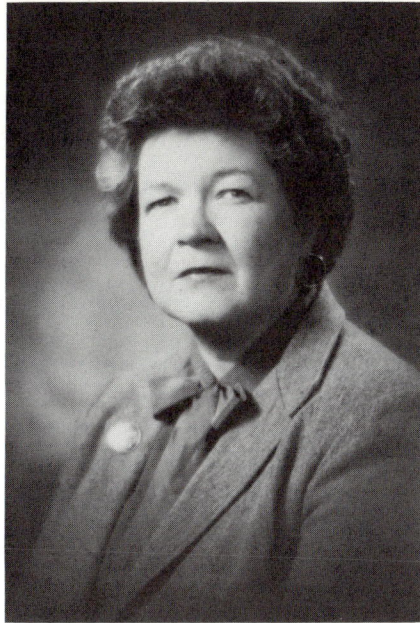

Susan B. Baird, R.N., M.P.H., M.A., is Director of Nursing at Fox Chase Cancer Center, Philadelphia, Pennsylvania and a doctoral student in the History and Sociology of Science at the University of Pennsylvania. She has served as Chief of the Cancer Nursing Service at the Clinical Center, National Institutes of Health and as Associate Director for Cancer Control at the Norris Cotton Cancer Center, Dartmouth-Hitchcock Medical Center, Hanover, New Hampshire. She is an American Cancer Society Doctoral Scholar and the recipient of the 1990 American Cancer Society Distinguished Service Award. She has also served as editor of the *Oncology Nursing Forum,* the official publication of the Oncology Nursing Society, since 1979.

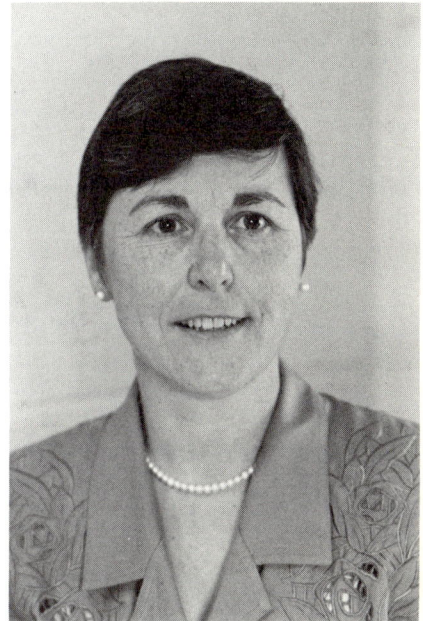

Ruth McCorkle, Ph.D., F.A.A.N., is an American Cancer Society Professor at the University of Pennsylvania's School of Nursing. Her career began as a Clinical Nurse Specialist in Oncology in Iowa. Subsequently, she has established a nationally recognized graduate program in cancer nursing. She is also internationally known for her research with patients with progressive cancer and the measurement of patient and family outcomes to improve the quality of their lives.

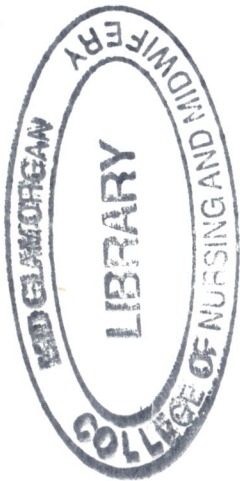

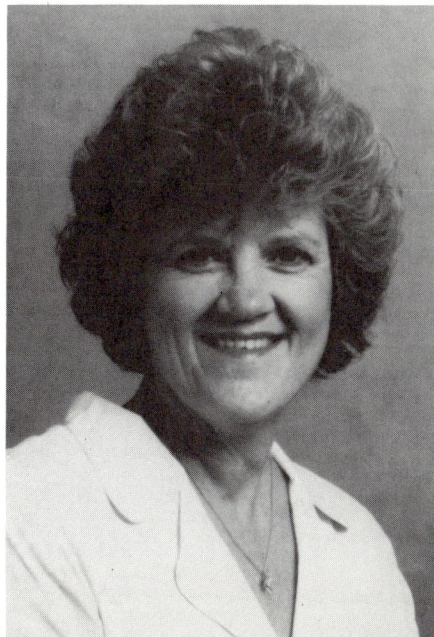

Marcia Grant, D.N.Sc., O.C.N., F.A.A.N., is Director of Nursing Research and Education and Associate Research Scientist at City of Hope National Medical Center in Duarte, California. Her research interests focus on symptom management, and she serves as chairperson of the National Center for Nursing Research's Priority Expert Panel on Symptom Management. She is on the editorial board for *Seminars in Oncology Nursing.* She was an American Cancer Society Doctoral Scholar and the recipient of the 1990 Oncology Nursing Society/Roche Distinguished Service Award.

Elizabeth Abernathy, M.S.N., R.N., O.C.N.
Adjuvant Faculty, Duke University School of Nursing; Clinical Nurse Specialist, Oncology Research, Duke University Medical Center, Durham, North Carolina.
Biologic Response Modifiers

Teresa Ades, B.S.N., R.N., O.C.N.
Coordinator of Nursing Programs, American Cancer Society, Atlanta, Georgia.
Cancer Organizations

Madalon Amenta, B.A., M.N., M.P.H., Dr. P.H.
Associate Professor of Nursing, The Pennsylvania State University, McKeesport Campus, McKeesport, Pennsylvania; Chair, Professional Advisory Committee, Home Health Services of Allegheny County, Pittsburgh, Pennsylvania; Editor of *The Hospice Journal.*
Hospice Services

Sheila B. Baez, M.N., R.N., O.C.N.
Clinical Nurse Specialist Consultant, San Diego, California.
Nursing Management of Persons Treated for Cure: Prototype—Hodgkin's Disease

Judith Baigis-Smith, Ph.D., R.N.
Director, Long-Term Care and Health Promotion, The Johns Hopkins University School of Nursing, Baltimore, Maryland.
Community Assessment: Congruence of Needs and Resources

Susan B. Baird, R.N., M.P.H., M.A.
Director of Nursing, Fox Chase Cancer Center, Philadelphia; Editor, *Oncology Nursing Forum*, Philadelphia, Pennsylvania.
Cancer Nursing as a Specialty

Patricia Benner, Ph.D., R.N., F.A.A.N.
Professor, Department of Physiological Nursing, University of California, San Francisco; Clinical Research and Teaching, University of California, San Francisco; San Francisco Medical Center, San Francisco, California.
Stress and Coping with Cancer

Barbara D. Blumberg, Sc.M.
Adjunct Instructor, University of Texas, Southwestern Medical Center at Dallas, Dallas, Texas; Director of Education, Komen Alliance Clinical Breast Center, Charles A. Sammons Cancer Center, Baylor University Medical Center, Houston, Texas.
The Development and Dissemination of Innovative Resources

Patricia S. Braly, M.D.
Associate Professor and Director, Division of Gynecological Oncology, Department of Reproductive Medicine, University of California San Diego Medical Center, San Diego, California.
Gynecologic Cancers

Jean K. Brown, M.S., R.N.
Doctoral Candidate and Research Consultant, University of Rochester, Rochester, New York.
Role Clarification: Rights and Responsibilities of Oncology Nurses

Nancy Burns, Ph.D., R.N.
Professor and Director, Center for Nursing Research, School of Nursing, University of Texas at Arlington, Arlington, Texas.
Alterations in Body Image

Mary E. Callaghan, M.N., R.N.
Hematology/Oncology/Bone Marrow Transplant Clinical Nurse Specialist, Green Hospital of Scripps Clinic and Research Foundation, La Jolla, California.
Hematopoietic and Immunologic Cancers

Colette Carson, M.N., R.N.
Nursing Consultant, San Diego Regional Cancer Center, San Diego, California; Consultant, Scripps Memorial Hospital Cancer Center, La Jolla, California.
Hematopoietic and Immunologic Cancers

Barrie R. Cassileth, Ph.D.
Associate Professor of Medical Sociology in Medicine, University of Pennsylvania School of Medicine; Director, University of Pennsylvania Cancer Control Program; Director, Psychosocial Programs, and Associate Director for Cancer Control, University of Pennsylvania Cancer Center, Hospital of the University of Pennsylvania, Philadelphia, Pennsylvania.
Questionable Cancer Therapies

Terry Chamorro, M.N., R.N., C.S.
Assistant Clinical Professor, School of Nursing, University of California, Los Angeles; Clinical Nurse Specialist, Gynecologic Oncology, Cedars-Sinai Medical Center and Cedars-Sinai Comprehensive Cancer Center, Los Angeles, California.
Legal Responsibilities of the Nurse

Cynthia Chernecky, M.N., R.N.
Doctoral Candidate in Nursing, Case Western Reserve University, Cleveland, Ohio; Clinical Nurse Specialist in Adult Oncology, Marymount Hospital, Inc., Garfield Heights, Ohio.
Complications of Advanced Disease

Noel J. Chrisman, Ph.D., M.P.H.
Professor, Department of Community Health Care Systems, School of Nursing, University of Washington, Seattle, Washington.
Cultural Systems

Jane C. Clark, M.N., R.N., O.C.N., O.G.N.P.
Clinical Nurse Specialist, Oncology, Emory University Hospital, Atlanta, Georgia.
Cancer Nursing Education Today

Nessa Coyle, M.S., R.N.
Clinical Instructor, Columbia University School of Nursing; Director, Supportive Care Program, Pain Service, Department of Neurology, Memorial Sloan-Kettering Cancer Center, New York, New York.
Alterations in Comfort: Pain

Gregory Curt, M.D.
Clinical Director, National Cancer Institute, National Institutes of Health, Bethesda, Maryland.
Implementation of Clinical Trials

Lesley F. Degner, Ph.D., R.N.
Professor, School of Nursing, University of Manitoba; Clinical Research Associate, St. Boniface General Hospital, Winnipeg, Manitoba, Canada.
Palliative Support

Dorothy J. del Bueno, Ed.D., R.N.
Assistant Dean, School of Nursing, University of Pennsylvania, Philadelphia, Pennsylvania.
Marketing Cancer Nursing

Janet E. DiJuleo, M.S.N., R.N.
Clinical Nursing Coordinator, Oncology Unit, Stanford University Hospital, Stanford, California
Nursing Management of Persons Treated for Cure: Prototype—Hodgkin's Disease

Marylin J. Dodd, Ph.D., R.N., F.A.A.N.
Professor, Department of Physiological Nursing, University of San Francisco; Clinical Associate, The Medical Center at the University of California, San Francisco, California.
Nursing Management of Persons Treated for Cure: Prototype—Hodgkin's Disease

Michele Girard Donehower, M.S.N., N.P.
Adult Nurse Practitioner, University of Maryland Cancer Center, Baltimore, Maryland.
Endocrine Cancers

Marguerite Donoghue, M.S.N., R.N.
Vice President for Research and Regulatory Affairs, Capitol Associates, Inc., Stanton Park, Washington, District of Columbia.
Cancer Legislation

Marilee I. Donovan, Ph.D., R.N.
Associate Hospital Director, Nursing Services, University Hospital, Oregon Health Sciences University, Portland, Oregon.
Issues and Strategies in Professional Education

Karen Hassey Dow, M.S., R.N.
Assistant Professor, MGH Institute of Health Professions; Nurse Specialist, Beth Israel Hospital, Boston, Massachusetts.
Radiation Oncology

Susan Dudas, M.S.N., R.N.
Associate Professor and Acting Associate Dean for Academic Affairs, The University of Illinois at Chicago, Chicago, Illinois.
Alterations in Patient Coping

Karin Dufault, Ph.D., R.N., S.P.
Clinical Assistant Professor, Oregon Health Sciences University School of Nursing, Department of Adult Health and Illness, Portland, Oregon; Administrator, St. Elizabeth Medical Center, Yakima, Washington.
Alterations in Mobility

Graceann Ehlke, D.N.Sc., R.N.
Education and Training, Row Sciences, Rockville, Maryland.
Gastrointestinal Cancers

Barbara A. Farley, M.N. R.N.
Administrative Faculty, Virginia Commonwealth University School of Nursing; Interim Director of Nursing, Medical College of Virginia Hospitals, Richmond, Virginia.
Ambulatory Care Services

Jayne I. Fernsler, D.S.N., R.N.
Associate Professor, Department of Advanced Nursing Science, College of Nursing, University of Delaware, Newark, Delaware.
Developing Strategies for Public Education in Cancer

Sharon Cannell Firsich, M.S., R.N.
Oncology Clinical Nurse Specialist, Providence Medical Center, Portland, Oregon.
Alterations in Mobility

Kathleen M. Foley, M.D.
Professor of Neurology and Pharmacology, Cornell University Medical College; Chief, Pain Service, Department of Neurology, and Attending Neurologist, Memorial Sloan-Kettering Cancer Center, New York, New York.
Alterations in Comfort: Pain

Rosemary C. Ford, B.A., B.S., R.N.
Clinical Practice Coordinator, Nursing Department, Clinical Division, Fred Hutchinson Cancer Research Center, Seattle, Washington.
Bone Marrow Transplantation

Marilyn Frank-Stromborg, Ed.D., R.N., F.A.A.N.
Professor, School of Nursing, Northern Illinois University; Nurse Practitioner, DeKalb County Nursing Home; Nurse Practitioner, DeKalb County Public Health Department, DeKalb, Illinois.
Evaluating Cancer Risk; Cancer Screening and Early Detection

Sara T. Fry, Ph.D., R.N., F.A.A.N.
Associate Professor, Department of Education, Administration, and Health Policy, School of Nursing, University of Maryland, Baltimore, Maryland.
Ethics and Cancer Care

Betty Bierut Gallucci, Ph.D., R.N.
Professor, Department of Physiological Nursing, University of Washington; Staff Appointment, Pathology, Fred Hutchinson Cancer Research Center, Seattle, Washington.
Cancer Biology: Molecular and Cellular Aspects

Barbara Germino, Ph.D., R.N.
Associate Professor, School of Nursing, University of North Carolina at Chapel Hill, Chapel Hill, North Carolina.
Cancer and the Family

Barbara Given, Ph.D., R.N., F.A.A.N.
Professor, College of Nursing, Michigan State University, East Lansing, Michigan.
Compliance and Health Promotion Behaviors

John Godwin, M.D.
Assistant Professor of Medicine, Loyola University Medical School; Attending Physician, and Associate Director, Special Hematology Laboratory, Foster G. McGaw Hospital, Chicago, Illinois.
Blood Component Therapy

Michelle Goodman, M.S., R.N.
Assistant Professor, College of Nursing, Rush University; Oncology Clinical Nurse Specialist and Teacher Practitioner, Section of Medical Oncology, Rush–Presbyterian–St. Luke's Medical Center, Chicago, Illinois.
Delivery of Cancer Chemotherapy

Marcia Grant, D.N.Sc., R.N., O.C.N., F.A.A.N.
Associate Research Scientist and Director, Department of Nursing Research and Education, City of Hope National Medical Center, Duarte, California.
Cancer Nursing as a Specialty; Alterations in Nutrition

Patricia Greene, M.S.N., R.N., F.A.A.N.
Vice President for Nursing, American Cancer Society, Atlanta, Georgia.
Cancer Organizations

Jennifer L. Guy, B.S., R.N.
Administrator, Saint Anthony Regional Oncology Center, Franciscan Health System of Central Ohio, Columbus, Ohio.
Medical Oncology—The Agents

Douglas Haeuber, M.S.N., R.N., O.C.N.
Instructor, School of Nursing, University of Southern Maine, Portland, Maine; Staff R.N., Medical Oncology, Massachusetts General Hospital, Boston, Massachusetts.
Alterations in Protective Mechanisms: Hematopoiesis and Bone Marrow Depression

Gloria A. Hagopian, Ed.D., R.N.
Associate Professor of Oncology Nursing, University of Pennsylvania School of Nursing, Philadelphia, Pennsylvania; Clinician Educator, Department of Radiation Oncology, Hospital of the University of Pennsylvania, Philadelphia, Pennsylvania.
Community Assessment: Congruence of Needs and Resources

Marilyn D. Harris, M.S.N., R.N., F.A.A.N., C.N.A.A.
Executive Director, Visiting Nurse Association of Eastern Montgomery County, Abington Memorial Hospital, Abington, Pennsylvania.
Home Care Services

Cathryn P. Havard, B.A., R.G.N. Dip.N., Onc. Cert.
Former Surgical Manager, Cheltenham General Hospital, Cheltenham, England.
Surgical Oncology

Karen Billars Heusinkveld, Ph.D., R.N.
Associate Professor, School of Nursing, The University of Texas at Arlington, Arlington, Texas.
Preventive Oncology

Laura J. Hilderley, M.S., R.N.
Clinical Nurse Specialist in the private practice of Philip G. Maddock, M.D., Radiation Oncology, Warwick, Rhode Island.
Radiation Oncology

Barbara C. Holmes, M.S.N., R.N., O.C.N.
Oncology Nursing Consultant, San Antonio, Texas
Alterations in Body Image

Linda Edwards Hood, B.S.N., R.N., O.C.N.
Chemotherapy Head Nurse, Hematology/Oncology Ambulatory Clinic, Duke University Medical Center, Durham, North Carolina.
Biologic Response Modifiers

Susan Molloy Hubbard, B.S., R.N.
Director, International Cancer Information Center, and Associate Director, National Cancer Institute, Bethesda, Maryland.
The Biology of Metastases

Anne M. Hughes, M.N., R.N., C.F.N.P.
Assistant Clinical Professor, Department of Physiological Nursing, University of California, San Francisco, California; AIDS/HIV Clinical Nurse Specialist, San Francisco General Hospital, San Francisco, California.
AIDS and the Spectrum of HIV Disease

Robert J. Irwin, Jr., M.D.
Associate Professor of Clinical Surgery, UMD-New Jersey Medical School, Vice Chief, Section of Urology; Chief, Section of Urology, East Orange Veterans Affairs, Medical Center, East Orange, New Jersey.
Genitourinary Cancers

Ryan R. Iwamoto, M.N., R.N., C.S.
Clinical Instructor, Department of Physiological Nursing, School of Nursing, University of Washington; Clinical Instructor, School of Nursing, Seattle University, Seattle, Washington; Instructor, Educational Development and Health Sciences Division, Bellevue Community College, Bellevue, Washington; Clinical Nurse Specialist, Radiation Oncology, Virginia Mason Clinic, Seattle, Washington.
Alterations in Oral Status

Anne Jalowiec, Ph.D., R.N.
Associate Professor, School of Nursing, Loyola University of Chicago, Chicago, Illinois.
Alterations in Patient Coping

Patricia F. Jassak, M.S., R.N., C.S.
Clinical Assistant Professor, Medical/Surgical Nursing, Niehoff School of Nursing, Loyola University; Oncology Clinical Nurse Specialist, Foster G. McGaw Hospital, Loyola University Medical Center, Chicago, Illinois.
Blood Component Therapy

Jean Jenkins, M.S.N., R.N., O.C.N.
Chief, Cancer Nursing Service, National Institutes of Health, Bethesda, Maryland.
Implementation of Clinical Trials

Bonnie Mowinski Jennings, L.T.C., A.N., D.N.Sc.
Intragovernmental Fellow, DHHS National Center for Nursing Research, National Institutes of Health, Bethesda, Maryland.
The Generation of Stress in the Provision of Care

Bonny Johnson, M.S.N., R.N.
Oncology Research Data Manager, University of Connecticut Health Center, Farmington, Connecticut.
Nursing Management of Persons with Recurrent Disease: Prototype—Leukemia

Judith L. Johnson, Ph.D., R.N.
Adjunct Faculty, School of Nursing, University of Minnesota; Nursing Director, Oncology, North Cancer Center, North Memorial Medical Center, Minneapolis, Minnesota.
Helping Families Respond to Cancer

Terri Kirshner, B.S.N., R.N., O.C.N.
Director, Adult Outpatient Clinic, City of Hope National Medical Center, Duarte, California.
Continuity of Care and Discharge Planning

Jennifer M. Kleinbart, B.S.
Former Research Assistant, Cancer Control Program, University of Pennsylvania Cancer Center, Philadelphia, Pennsylvania.
Questionable Cancer Therapies

M. Tish Knobf, M.S.N., R.N.
Assistant Professor, Yale University School of Nursing; Oncology Clinical Nurse Specialist, Ambulatory Service, Yale–New Haven Hospital, New Haven, Connecticut.
Breast Cancer

Ruth L. Krech, M.S.N., R.N.
Clinical Nurse Specialist in Palliative Care, Cleveland Clinic Foundation, Cleveland, Ohio.
Complications of Advanced Disease

Margaret A. Lamb, M.S.N., R.N.
Assistant Professor, Department of Nursing, School of Health and Human Services, University of New Hampshire, Durham, New Hampshire.
Alterations in Sexuality and Sexual Functioning

Cheryl Ann Lane, M.A., R.N., O.C.N.
Consultant, Oncology Nursing, Rockledge, Florida.
Helping Families Respond to Cancer

Patricia J. Larson, D.N.Sc., R.N.
Assistant Professor, Oncology Graduate Program, Department of Physiological Nursing, School of Nursing, University of California, San Francisco, California.
The Generation of Stress in the Provision of Care

Frances Marcus Lewis, Ph.D., R.N.
Professor, School of Nursing, University of Washington; Evaluation Consultant, Cancer Information Service, Fred Hutchinson Cancer Research Center, Seattle, Washington.
Consultation and Collaboration Among Health Care Providers

Marcia C. Liebman, M.S., R.N., O.C.N.
Oncology Clinical Nurse Specialist, Southwood Community Hospital, Norfolk, Massachusetts.
Multimodal Therapy

Julena Lind, M.N., R.N.
Adjunct Assistant Professor, Department of Nursing, University of Southern California; Executive Director, Southern California Cancer Center, Inc., California Medical Center Los Angeles, Los Angeles, California.
Genitourinary Cancers

Ada M. Lindsey, Ph.D., R.N.
Dean and Professor, School of Nursing, University of California, Los Angeles, California.
Lung Cancer

Lance A. Liotta, M.D., Ph.D.
Clinical Professor of Pathology, George Washington University, Washington, District of Columbia; Chief, Laboratory of Pathology, Division of Cancer Biology and Diagnosis, National Cancer Institute, Bethesda, Maryland.
The Biology of Metastases

Alice J. Longman, Ed.D., R.N.
Professor, The University of Arizona College of Nursing, Tucson, Arizona.
Skin Cancers

Catherine Lyons, M.S., R.N.
Adjunct Faculty, School of Nursing, State University of New York at Buffalo; Director of Nursing, Roswell Park Cancer Institute, Buffalo, New York.
The Organization of Cancer Service Settings

Lucy K. Martin, B.S.N., R.N., O.C.N.
Clinical Instructor, City of Hope National Medical Center, Duarte, California.
Gynecologic Cancers

Mary B. Maxwell, Ph.D., R.N., C.M.N.
Adjunct Assistant Professor of Nursing, Department of Adult Health and Illness, School of Nursing, Oregon Health Sciences University; Clinical Nurse Specialist/Nurse Practitioner in Oncology and Director, Nursing Research Program, Veterans Affairs Medical Center, Portland, Oregon.
The Development and Dissemination of Innovative Resources

Mary S. McCabe, B.A., B.S.
Clinical Trials Specialist, EPN 715 Cancer Therapy Evaluation Program, National Cancer Institute, Bethesda, Maryland.
Cancer Legislation

Ruth McCorkle, Ph.D., F.A.A.N.
American Cancer Society Professor, School of Nursing, University of Pennsylvania, Philadelphia, Pennsylvania.
Cancer Nursing as a Specialty

Mary Dee McEvoy, Ph.D., R.N.
Clinical Assistant Professor, School of Nursing, University of Pennsylvania; Clinical Director, Ambulatory Oncology, Hospital of the University of Pennsylvania, Philadelphia, Pennsylvania.
Nursing Management of Persons with Progressive Disease: Prototype—Lung Cancer

Rose F. McGee, Ph.D., R.N.
American Cancer Society Professor of Oncology and Nursing; Professor, Nell Hodgson Woodruff School of Nursing, Emory University, Atlanta, Georgia.
Cancer Nursing Education Today

Diane O. McGivern, Ph.D., F.A.A.N.
Professor and Head, Division of Nursing, New York University, New York, New York.
Introduction to Public Policy

Sue N. McIntire, Ed.D., R.N.
Associate Professor, School of Nursing, Duke University; Associate Professor of Nursing, Duke University Comprehensive Cancer Center, Durham, North Carolina.
Developmental Process

Curtis Mettlin, Ph.D.
Chief of Epidemiologic Research, Roswell Park Memorial Institute, Buffalo, New York.
The Causes of Cancer

Christine Miaskowski, Ph.D., R.N., O.C.N.
Assistant Professor, Department of Physiological Nursing, University of California, San Francisco, California.
Oncologic Emergencies; Documentation of the Nursing Process in Cancer Nursing

Amy L. Mirand, Ph.D.
Research Scientist, Research Institute on Alcoholism, Buffalo, New York; Former Research Scientist, Roswell Park Memorial Institute, Buffalo, New York.
The Causes of Cancer

Darlene W. Mood, Ph.D.
Associate Professor, College of Nursing, Wayne State University; Psychologist, Associate Medical Staff, Departments of Otolaryngology and Psychiatry, Harper Hospital, Detroit, Michigan.
The Diagnosis of Cancer: A Life Transition

Marion E. Morra, M.A.
Associate Clinical Professor, Yale University School of Nursing; Assistant Director, Yale Comprehensive Cancer Center, Yale University School of Medicine, New Haven, Connecticut.
Developing Strategies for Patient Education in Cancer

Lee E. Mortenson, M.S., M.P.A.
Executive Director, Association of Community Cancer Centers, Rockville, Maryland; President and Chief Executive Officer, ELM Services, Inc., Rockville, Maryland.
Understanding Cancer Reimbursement

Shirley A. Murphy, Ph.D., R.N.
Professor, School of Nursing, University of Washington, Seattle, Washington.
Grief and Bereavement

Beverly Nielsen, Ed.D., R.N.
Assistant Professor and American Cancer Society Professor of Oncology Nursing, University of Miami, Miami, Florida.
Documentation of the Nursing Process in Cancer Nursing

Laurel L. Northouse, Ph.D., R.N.
Assistant Professor, College of Nursing, Wayne State University, Detroit, Michigan.
Interpersonal Communication Systems

Peter G. Northouse, Ph.D.
Professor, Department of Communication, Western Michigan University, Kalamazoo, Michigan.
Interpersonal Communication Systems

Denise M. Oleske, Ph.D., R.N.
Assistant Professor, Department of Health Systems Management, and Assistant Professor, Department of Preventive Medicine, Rush University, Chicago, Illinois.
Epidemiologic Principles for Nursing Practice: Assessing the Cancer Problem and Planning Its Control

Sharon J. Olsen, M.S., R.N.
Educator and Consultant, University of Wisconsin Clinical Cancer Center, Cancer Prevention Clinic, Madison, Wisconsin.
Cancer Screening and Early Detection

Geraldine Padilla, Ph.D.
Professor and Associate Dean for Research, University of California Los Angeles School of Nursing, Los Angeles, California.
Continuity of Care and Discharge Planning

Judith A. Paice, M.S., R.N.
Assistant Professor, College of Nursing, Rush University; Practitioner-Teacher, Department of Surgical Nursing, Rush–Presbyterian–St. Luke's Medical Center, Chicago, Illinois.
Issues and Strategies in Professional Education

Carol Ann Parente, M.S.N., R.N., C.R.N.P.
Hospice Coordinator and Adult Nurse Practitioner, Visiting Nurse Association of Eastern Montgomery County, Abington Memorial Hospital, Abington, Pennsylvania.
Home Care Services

Joan A. Piemme, M.N.Ed., R.N., F.A.A.N.
Clinical Nursing Educator, Cancer Nursing Service, National Institutes of Health, Bethesda, Maryland; Policy Analyst for Nursing, National Commission on AIDS, Washington, District of Columbia.
Cancer Legislation

Barbara F. Piper, M.S., R.N.
D.N.Sc. Candidate, Department of Physiological Nursing, University of California, San Francisco School of Nursing, San Francisco, California; Oncology Staff Nurse, Mt. Zion Hospital of the University of California, San Francisco, California.
Alterations in Energy: The Generation of Fatigue

Rosemary Polomano, M.S.N., R.N., C.S.
Oncology/Pain Clinical Nurse Specialist, Hospital of the University of Pennsylvania, Philadelphia, Pennsylvania; Doctoral candidate, School of Nursing, University of Maryland, Baltimore, Maryland.
Nursing Management of Persons with Progressive Disease: Prototype—Lung Cancer

James D. Popkin, M.D.
Clinical Assistant Professor of Medicine, Boston University School of Medicine, Boston, Massachusetts; Active Staff, Norwood Hospital, Norwood, Massachusetts, and Southwood Community Hospital, Norfolk, Massachusetts.
Multimodal Therapy

Jean L. Reese, Ph.D., R.N.
Associate Professor, College of Nursing, University of Iowa, Iowa City, Iowa.
Head and Neck Cancers

Connie R. Robinson, Ph.D., R.N., F.A.A.N.
Associate Professor, Boston College, Boston, Massachusetts.
Central Nervous System Tumors

Mary E. Ropka, Ph.D.
Director, Collaborative Intramural Program, National Center for Nursing Research, National Institutes of Health, Bethesda, Maryland.
Alterations in Nutrition

Sr. Callista Roy, Ph.D., R.N., F.A.A.N.
Professor, Boston College, School of Nursing, Boston, Massachusetts; Neuroscience Nursing Staff Privileges, Beth Israel Hospital, and Beth Israel Center for the Advancement of Nursing Practice, Boston, Massachusetts.
Central Nervous System Tumors

Mary Rubin, M.S.N., R.N.C., C.R.N.P.
Clinical Preceptor and Lecturer, School of Nursing, University of Pennsylvania; Lecturer, Planned Parenthood Federation of America, Ob/Gyn Nurse Practitioner Program in Philadelphia; Codeveloper and faculty member, Nurse Practitioner Colposcopy Training Program in Philadelphia; Gynecologic Oncology Clinical Nursing Specialist, Hospital of the University of Pennsylvania, Philadelphia, Pennsylvania.
Nursing Management of Persons at Risk for Cancer: Prototype—Cervical Intraepithelial Neoplasia

Judith M. Saunders, D.N.Sc., F.A.A.N.
Assistant Research Scientist, Nursing Research and Education, City of Hope National Medical Center, Duarte, California.
Nursing Management of Persons with Disease About Which Little Is Known: Prototype—AIDS

Madeline H. Schmitt, Ph.D., F.A.A.N.
Associate Professor of Nursing, University of Rochester School of Nursing, Rochester, New York.
Social Support, Occupational Stressors, and Health in Cancer Nursing

Jerome Schofferman, M.D.
Assistant Professor, University of California San Francisco School of Medicine, San Francisco, California; Director, Internal Medicine and Chief, Pain Management, Spine Care Medical Group, Daly City, California.
AIDS and the Spectrum of HIV Disease

Roberta P. Scofield, M.S.N., R.N., O.C.N.*
Former Oncology Clinical Nurse Specialist, Southwood Community Hospital, Norfolk, Massachusetts.
Multimodal Therapy

---

*Deceased.

Margaret L. Seager, B.A., R.N.
Clinical Nurse III, University of California and San Francisco Hospitals, San Francisco, California.
Central Nervous System Tumors

Amy Smith-Brassard, M.S., R.N.
Former Associate Professor, University of Vermont School of Nursing, Burlington, Vermont.
Soft Tissue and Bone Sarcomas

Judith A. Spross, M.S., R.N., O.C.N.
Assistant Professor, MGH Institute of Health Professions, Boston, Massachusetts.
Alterations in Protective Mechanisms: Hematopoiesis and Bone Marrow Depression

Stanley K. Stylianos, M.A.
Program Manager, New Outlook, Central Toronto Youth Services, Toronto, Ontario, Canada.
Caring for the Caregiver: A Person-Centered Framework

Anne E. Topping, B.Sc.(Hons.), R.G.N., Onc. Cert.
Senior Lecturer, School of Human and Health Sciences, The Polytechnic of Huddersfield, Queensgate, Huddersfield, England.
Surgical Oncology

Mary L. S. Vachon, Ph.D., R.N.
Associate Professor, Departments of Psychiatry and Behavioral Science, University of Toronto, Toronto, Canada; Research Scientist and Senior Mental Health Consultant, Clarke Institute of Psychiatry, Toronto, Ontario, Canada.
Caring for the Caregiver: A Person-Centered Framework

Connie Henke Yarbro, B.S.N., R.N.
Clinical Associate Professor, School of Medicine, University of Missouri-Columbia, Columbia, Missouri.
The History of Cancer Nursing

Joyce M. Yasko, Ph.D., F.A.A.N.
Professor and Program Director, Graduate Program in Medical Surgical Nursing, University of Pittsburgh; Associate Director, Nursing and Patient Care Services, Pittsburgh Cancer Institute, University of Pittsburgh, Pittsburgh, Pennsylvania.
Role Implementation in Cancer Nursing

Jerome W. Yates, M.D., M.P.H.
Professor of Medicine, State University of New York at Buffalo; Associate Director for Clinical Affairs, Roswell Park Cancer Institute, Buffalo, New York.
The Organization of Cancer Service Settings

Joyce Zerwekh, Ed.D., R.N., C.S.
Assistant Professor, Community Health Care Systems School of Nursing, University of Washington, Seattle, Washington.
Supportive Care of the Dying Patient

Foreword

During the last 50 years, cancer nursing has become a highly specialized and intricate form of practice. As *Cancer Nursing: A Comprehensive Textbook* attests, the activities comprising cancer nursing are many and varied. At one end of the continuum, they consist of selective actions focused on the human needs of individuals living through the life transitions associated with different types of cancer. At the other end, they include collective actions by nurses to influence public policy and legislation supportive of cancer prevention and comprehensive cancer care services for patients and families.

The historical appearance of cancer nursing as specialized practice was associated directly with the explosion of scientific knowledge after World War II and an expansion of biomedical cancer research under the leadership of the National Cancer Institute. Practicing nurses moved into new roles as team members in clinical cancer trials designed to test new medical diagnostic and therapeutic techniques and regimens. Other nurses became specialists in the delivery of services for different types of cancers as they gained knowledge and skill in working with special populations.

Opportunities for education expanded, and many nurses supplemented their strong clinical knowledge with understanding about human behavior derived from the social and behavioral sciences as well as from the humanities. Although many used this knowledge to expand and improve their work as clinical cancer nursing specialists, others moved into research careers to generate systematic knowledge about the effects of the cancer experience on people's lives and to evaluate the effectiveness of specified nursing activities for relieving distress, encouraging interfamilial communications, and promoting healthy adaptations.

The contributors to this comprehensive collection reflect the diversity of knowledge and skill comprising cancer nursing in 1990. The volume as a whole shows the scope of cancer nursing as extensive—ranging from attention to prevention and early detection of cancer to caregiving for those living with progressive malignant diseases, such as lung cancer, and diseases with unpredictable trajectory patterns. As a primary example of the latter category, acquired immunodeficiency syndrome (AIDS) illustrates the range of complex clinical problems that nurses face when working with individuals and families undergoing unclear and uncertain illness transitions.

The organization of the chapters into sections is testimony to the broad range of knowledge required for making effective cancer nursing services available to the appropriate populations. They provide information and direction not only for clinical problems associated with malignant disease but also for implementing multidisciplinary communication and collaboration in the best interests of patients and families receiving services. The editors should be congratulated for bringing into being this valuable resource for nurses.

JEANNE QUINT BENOLIEL, D.N.Sc.
Professor, College of Nursing
Rutgers: The State University of New Jersey (Newark)

Preface

Here, we believe, is the book that educators and students have sought, the resource text that oncology clinical nurse specialists will value, and the ready reference source for the skilled clinician. As each phase of production has been completed, our confidence in the book's value has grown. As editors, we have felt very privileged to have had ongoing access to this tremendous information source and to its authors. Those who have contributed to *Cancer Nursing: A Comprehensive Textbook* have brought to it much of the experience and expertise of cancer nursing as a specialty practice.

Our intent was to encompass the broad spectrum of responsibilities and practice arenas within cancer nursing while incorporating current theory, the latest research, and the most up-to-date clinical practice. Our aim in identifying content, organizing care components, and selecting authors with experience was to promote an integration of medical content, scientific literature, and current nursing approaches into interventions targeted to assist persons at risk for cancer or persons with cancer and their families. We believe that we have achieved our goal.

The many special features of this text were incorporated both to enhance its usefulness and to reflect the current roles and responsibilities of cancer nursing along the disease continuum. The chapters in the "Cancer as an Illness" unit use prototype cancers to illustrate common trajectories of cancer care for persons at risk, for those treated for cure, for those with recurrent disease, and for those with progressive disease. The thorough coverage of treatment modalities, common cancers, and effects of common cancers is augmented by information on communication, education, support, and care delivery systems and settings. Several conceptual frameworks basic to cancer nursing and useful in planning research and care are presented, demonstrating the application of such theory as developmental process, family systems, and cultural systems. Because nurses must become more involved with them, prevention and detection have been given appropriately thorough coverage. The inclusion of information on public policy and legislative issues recognizes that professional nurses are actively involved in defining cancer care services and programs.

We believe the content will serve its readers well regardless of their special interests, knowledge requirements, or experience. The frequent use of tables, figures, and summaries of pertinent research further enhance the text.

There are so many people who should be recognized for their contributions to this book. The authors accomplished their tasks with great vigor within the context of already busy and demanding schedules. Our friends have no idea how much their ongoing support has meant. "How's the book coming?" told us that they cared, and we never got tired of the question. We greatly appreciate the assistance of Michael Brown, Editor in Chief for Nursing Books at W. B. Saunders Company, who believed in the book from its beginnings and has provided tremendous support. Michael's quiet confidence in nurses and in us has been very special. We had wonderful and unending help from the people at W. B. Saunders Company—Robin L. Richman, Lee Ann Draud, Marjory I. Fraser, Linda R. Turner, and many others.

As editors, our backgrounds include advanced cancer nursing knowledge and experience. Our areas of expertise are varied, yet complimentary. Bringing this diversity of interests and experience together was intentional and proved to be an asset. A project of this magnitude demands a belief in its need and value, a confidence that it can be done, and a concerted committment to its successful completion. To begin and complete this project as friends is no small accomplishment. During this project we have each withstood personal and professional changes, and we were truly thankful for each other's presence in our lives. The depth of respect and admiration that we have for each other as individuals and as nursing professionals is profound.

Our common bond throughout has been a deep belief in the care and caring of nurses, a belief that nurses make a difference to patients with cancer; our hope is that this book will aid readers in these efforts.

SUSAN B. BAIRD, R.N., M.P.H., M.A.

RUTH McCORKLE, PH.D., F.A.A.N.

MARCIA GRANT, D.N.SC., O.C.N., F.A.A.N.

Contents

UNIT I
NATURE AND SCOPE OF CANCER NURSING

UNIT II
CONCEPTUAL THEMES BASIC TO CANCER NURSING

xx Contents

CHAPTER 9

Stress and Coping with Cancer 74

CHAPTER 8

Compliance and Health Promotion Behaviors .. 61

CHAPTER 10

Grief and Bereavement 82

UNIT III
CANCER AS A DISEASE

CHAPTER 11

Epidemiologic Principles for Nursing Practice: Assessing the Cancer Problem and Planning Its Control 91

CHAPTER 13

Cancer Biology: Molecular and Cellular Aspects 115

CHAPTER 12

The Causes of Cancer 104

CHAPTER 14

The Biology of Metastases 130

UNIT IV
CLINICAL DETECTION AND SUPPORT

CHAPTER 15

Preventive Oncology 143

UNIT V
CANCER TREATMENT: THERAPIES AND PHYSICAL SUPPORT APPROACHES

UNIT VI
EFFECTS OF COMMON ADULT CANCERS

UNIT VII
CANCER AS AN ILLNESS

UNIT VIII
MAJOR CLINICAL NURSING PROBLEMS

UNIT IX
COMMUNICATION, COLLABORATION, AND EDUCATION

UNIT X
THE DELIVERY OF CANCER CARE SERVICES: RESOURCES AND REFERRAL SYSTEMS

UNIT XI
PROFESSIONAL SUPPORT SYSTEMS

UNIT XII
PUBLIC POLICY AND LEGISLATIVE ISSUES

NATURE AND SCOPE OF CANCER NURSING

CHAPTER 1

Cancer Nursing as a Specialty

MARCIA GRANT
RUTH McCORKLE
SUSAN B. BAIRD

SPECIALIZATION IN NURSING
PHILOSOPHY OF PRACTICE
Components of the Philosophy of Cancer
  Nursing
A Care versus Cure Commitment
The Practice Environment
Nursing's Leadership Potential
INFLUENCING FACTORS
Complexity of Care
Scientific and Technologic Advances

Expanding Knowledge Base
Organization of Cancer Care
Health Care Economics and Policy
Structuring of Groups and Processes
CHALLENGES
Recruitment and Retention of Nurses
Quality of Care
Defining and Promoting Nursing Roles
SUMMARY

SPECIALIZATION IN NURSING

Cancer nursing is a unique nursing specialty. It draws on a knowledge base rich in physiologic, psychological, and social concepts. It encompasses disease that occurs in people of all ages and both sexes. It is concerned with managing the symptoms caused more frequently by the medical treatment than by the disease itself. It spans care settings ranging from health promotion centers to acute care settings, ambulatory care clinics and offices, home care agencies, and hospice arrangements. Care approaches are complicated by the negative stigma that continues to surround cancer and that causes patients to dread the diagnosis and to be uncomfortable talking with others about the disease.

It takes a special kind of nurse to pursue as a career the care of patients with cancer. Cancer nurses are dedicated, intelligent, and caring nurses. It is not uncommon for patients to feel as the following patient felt as she wrote her thanks to the cancer nursing unit staff:

This is the first time that I have ever been in a hospital in my life. It was very hard to come and deal with my leukemia. I had been a picture of good health up to about six weeks ago. I want to acknowledge particularly my nurses for the way they have cared for me and the way they have supported me through the toughest six days of my life. You nurses have made the difference for me during this time. Your commitment to me and this institution has often times inspired me right above the pain I was enduring at the time. You nurses arrived many times like angels to minister to me and take away my pain. Your warm words and kind hearts motivate me to get better so that I can share my life and kind words with others. You are a blessing from God and I know He will reward you for your efforts.

The idea of specialization in nursing is not new, but the recognition of specialization and the definition of its continuation have occurred more recently (American Nurses' Association, 1980; Hamric, 1989). Specialty groups arise from a focus on a specific disease, such as cancer; a specific kind of treatment, such as surgical treatment; or a specific phase of treatment, such as intensive care. Specialization within nursing has evolved because of the extensive and specific body of knowledge necessary to give safe and thorough care to a specific group of patients, such as patients with cancer (Lynaugh & Fairman, 1989).

Content on cancer nursing care has been taught in nursing programs since the early 1900s, but recognition of cancer nursing as a specialty probably began with the education for cancer nursing care sponsored by the Clinical Education Grants Program of the National Cancer Institute (Craytor, 1982). The preparation of nurses through this program led to an increasing number of nurses who considered themselves cancer nursing specialists.

The effort of these specialists was critical in the formation in 1975 of a national organization for cancer nurses, the Oncology Nursing Society. This organization established the specialization and provided support at the national level with national clinical congresses that included sessions on clinical practice, education, and research. (See Chapter 2 for an in-depth development of the history of cancer nursing.)

One of the major activities of the Oncology Nursing Society that has further cemented the specialization of cancer nursing has been the development in 1984 of the Oncology Nursing Certification Corporation. The sole purpose of this corporation is to develop, administer, and evaluate a program for the certification of oncology nurses. The certification examination tests the general oncology nursing knowledge base of the professional nurse. The first examination was offered in 1985 and resulted in 1384 oncology-certified nurses. As of May 1990 there were more than 7300 oncology-certified nurses in the world.

The specialization of cancer nursing is recognized by both the nursing profession and a variety of health care professionals in related fields. In academic settings, recognition of the specialty is evident through the establishment of cancer nursing specialty programs at both the master's and doctoral levels.

Current activity within the specialty of cancer nursing includes the identification and formation of many subspecialty groups. The special interest groups, a recent development within the Oncology Nursing Society, include such diverse subspecialties and interests as bone marrow transplantation, vascular access devices, and advanced research. Thus the specialty continues to grow. Subspecialty areas are being revised continually, depending on influential factors from the clinical arena and the education and research settings.

The specialty can be further described in relation to the philosophy of practice and other factors that continue to influence the shape and nature of cancer nursing.

PHILOSOPHY OF PRACTICE

In helping people through periods of their lives that are so stressful and full of consequence, nurses become involved in the planning and implementing of care as a collective group of professionals and as individuals. Giving and receiving support among nurses and other professionals is essential as patient, family, and professional goals are identified and met. It is very useful for nurses to explicitly identify a philosophy of practice for themselves as individuals and as a collective group and review it periodically to strengthen their practice. A philosophy represents the "ideals" of the nursing staff within a given care environment. Box 1–1 presents an example of a nursing philosophy developed by nurses on an oncology nursing unit at the University of Washington Hospital in Seattle.

Components of the Philosophy of Cancer Nursing

The philosophy of cancer nursing incorporates the importance of collaboration with all members of the health care team, the primacy of the patient and family member as decision maker, and the education and research responsibility of staff within individual health care institutions. It is recommended that the philosophy developed as a collective effort be adopted as a multidisciplinary philosophy by all health care professionals within a specific unit. In this way they can continue to strive for the highest quality of care and for the recognition of patients as human beings with unique needs.

Because patients and families in our society may, generally speaking, have problems coping with the crisis of a cancer diagnosis or the recurrence of cancer, the development of person-centered services is needed to provide assistance with the immediate and long-term consequences of these singular events (Krouse & Krouse, 1984; Benoliel & McCorkle, 1978; Weisman & Worden, 1976–1977). Persons with cancer have a right to know what is happening to them and to participate in the decisions that affect their lives. Further, by virtue of their positions in the health care system, professional nurses can readily assume leadership in developing and implementing services designed explicitly to achieve the goal of personalized patient care. By no means do nurses provide all care needed by patients and families, but nurses are ideally suited by educational background and position to provide coordination of care and problem-focused support services to patients and families undergoing changes in their lives (Benoliel & McCorkle, 1978).

To provide such services, nurses must be able to cope with their own feelings and reactions to cancer and with patients' potential decline, be knowledgeable about the psychosocial impact of these events on family systems and family relationships, be skilled in the use of communication strategies that promote collaboration among the many health care providers likely to be involved, and be clinically competent in the delivery of health services to all members of the family (Tornberg, Burns McGrath, & Quint Benoliel, 1984). To implement such services, nurses must be knowledgeable about the community resources available to assist with different types of family problems. To make these services available on an ongoing basis, nurses must be able to collaborate with one another and have continuing access to a socially supportive system of human relationships. Caplan (1974) believes that persons whose experience of living brings them into frequent contact with emotional crisis and strain are able to function more effectively when they have regular contact with a social network that provides consistent communication, appropriate rewards, and feedback about their performance. In view of this belief, mutual support and consultation among nurses are essential elements in the provision of cancer care to patients and families.

Box 1–1. NURSING PHILOSOPHY OF 8-SOUTH

In accordance with the philosophy of University Hospital and the Department of Nursing services, we, the nursing staff of 8-South, believe that our primary responsibility lies with the patient and with the patient's family. We subscribe to the philosophy of primary nursing in providing for and concerning ourselves with the physical, psychosocial, and spiritual needs of the patient. We acknowledge the special needs of the patient with cancer and are dedicated to the relief of symptoms of cancer and to its treatment, as well as to the promotion of comfort. We uphold the right of patients as individuals to have the opportunity to obtain information about their disease, prognosis, treatment, and available alternatives. We believe that the patient should be the primary participant in the decision-making process. In conjunction with this belief, we believe that all patients have a right to accept or refuse treatment and to receive support for the decisions they make.

We believe that families and individual patients have the need of continual support when their self-images, their social roles, and their functions undergo change. In this way, the patient can live to capacity and die with dignity. Patients and their families must have continual support during periods of adjustment and during times of grief.

We acknowledge the importance of collaboration with other members of the health team within the hospital, clinics, and community. In an effort to provide excellence of care, we have the responsibility to share knowledge, to participate continually in continued education, and to assist and support our colleagues in their research efforts. To this end, it is our intention to be flexible in our approaches and to be receptive to the creative ideas of others. Through an atmosphere of collaboration, we wish to promote an environment of mutual trust, respect, and support for the health providers.

(From McCorkle, R. [1979]. A new beginning: The opening of a multidisciplinary cancer unit. Part I. *Cancer Nursing, 2,* 201–209. Reproduced by permission.)

A Care versus Cure Commitment

Nurses have a long history of concern for the rights of individuals to have access to basic health care resources that promote their health and well-being (Benoliel & McCorkle, 1977; McCorkle, 1980). Current evidence suggests that a major issue for the human community in the 1990s centers on the unbalanced distribution of health care resources between cure- and care-oriented services. The current United States health care system is a reflection of the interplay among several factors. As a result of specialization, it is a system of multiple providers from various professions and occupations. It is a system organized around the primacy of life-saving activity. Differences and priorities in care and in the meaning of caregiving characterize the various professional groups. Among the same professional groups, differences exist in manifest power to influence decisions. Finally, the health care system is not responsive to the rights and responsibilities of professions other than those of medicine (Benoliel, 1972).

In a profound sense, the health care system shows an imbalance in the priorities given to the goals of cure and care. The differences in these goals have been formulated by Benoliel (1976) as follows:

Cure centers on the diagnosis and treatment of disease; in contrast, care is concerned with the welfare and well being of the person. Cure deals with the objective aspects of the case whereas care is concerned with the subject and meaning of the disease experience and the effects of treatment on the person. Cure has many origins and signs and instrumentation "doing to" people. Care has its root in human compassion, respect for the need of the vulnerable and "doing with" people. Although care as a spouse is important, cure is the goal around which the health care system is organized.

Historically, influences on nursing and the social context of practice have affected nurses' perceptions of themselves and the value of their contribution to health care. Nurses have been socialized to believe that cure activities are more important than care activities and take precedence over them on a day-to-day basis. Nurses have also been socialized to believe that they have less to offer the public in medicine in terms of service. In addition, nurses may have low self-esteem and lack self-confidence in many areas of their work, and these attitudes perpetuate a subservient working relationship with physicians. The many different phases of cancer care offer nurses opportunities to initiate and take responsibility for patient care activities, more so than with other diseases. Clearly the majority of patients seen by nurses are hospitalized and require ongoing monitoring and management strategies. It is at these times that nurses can make deliberate shifts in their approaches to patients to respond to their care needs as a priority. Concurrently, nurses will become more comfortable with patients, and their confidence will increase. In addition, their explicit actions will increase the visibility of their role responsibilities for themselves, patients, and other professional caregivers.

Major issues for nurses in the 1990s include action to reverse nurses' invisibility as major contributors to effective health care, to secure identified reimbursement for services rendered by nurses, and to promote the growth of professionalism in nurses through encouragement of effective relationships among all groups of professionals. Nurses must be willing to assume positions of power in the health care system and to use their power as a means of bringing about change in the system. Nurses must assume true leadership for the accountability of the quality of nursing practice and nursing services. Nurses must now move into developing an approach to peer review that focuses on actual practices of nurses and not on what is recorded on the patient care records. Nurses need to assume responsibility for defining practice and behaviors that are important to produce effective patient and family outcomes in the care arena.

The Practice Environment

Regardless of the specialty, the practice environment has to include opportunities to foster the personal growth of nurses new to the specialty to enhance their development. Opportunities for growth must include the development of intellectual inquiry and problem-solving attitudes, the promotion of self-confidence in all participants in the system, and the adoption of excellence in practice as a primary goal. Work environments that emphasize person-centered services facilitate (1) collaboration within nursing and with other professions and occupations toward excellence in service and (2) collective action by nurses to effect changes in the system. Regardless of the setting in which cancer care is delivered, person-centered services should be emphasized.

As person-centered services are established, nurses must also move toward formalizing emerging practices with standards of care. Consumers deserve the protection of practice standards developed and sanctioned by the profession. The Oncology Nursing Society developed its first practice standards in 1979 (American Nurses' Association & Oncology Nursing Society, 1979) and prepared new standards in 1987 to reflect changes in practice (American Nurses' Association & Oncology Nursing Society, 1987). It is also critical to test practice, both as it emerges and after it has been formalized into standards. Nurses must continue to question the tenets of their practice. Changes in the provision of health care services in the 1980s were extensive and broadly based. This baseline of rapid and extensive change provides a ready environment for creative advocacy from nurses. New resources should be conceptualized and implemented. Underserved populations need access to health care programs. Services should be available throughout the person's trajectory of cancer rather than only during times of crisis and at the end of life. Not all people will need care, but cancer nurses must be sensitive to those at high risk for ongoing problems and assist them in securing appropriate resources.

Nursing's Leadership Potential

Nurses have a tremendous potential for leadership in the creation of nursing services that support quality of life for patients with cancer and their families. Nurses, as a collective, must be willing to engage in the politics of negotiation for reallocation of health care resources toward person-centered services and to establish a power base for influencing these decisions at the local, state, and national levels of government and within various organizations offering health care services.

Writing about the need for nursing action in the public arena, Aydelotte (1985) identified five essential attitudes that nurses must develop: (1) respect, trust, and openness in working with other people; (2) recognition of the reality of conflict and confrontation in the process of negotiating competing claims; (3) willingness to learn new language symbols and values in the rapidly changing world; (4) ability to shift leadership styles and response to different situations; and (5) active awareness that all human beings need support and approval. Work in cancer care offers nurses opportunities to develop these essential attitudes and enhances their abilities to work with other professional groups to effect changes in collaboration with management efforts.

Nurses have the potential to influence the redistribution of governmental health resources so that care and cure fall into a more equitable balance than the one that presently exists. This process is dependent on the emergence of nurses as a collective force for change in the policy-making arena (Stevens, 1985). Cancer nurses are becoming more active in the political arena (see Chapters 78 and 82) and can help by representing the public's interest in terms of the need for care-oriented services. Cancer nurses can draw from their practice experience when informing policy makers of the health needs of various vulnerable populations in society. Cancer nurses should seek opportunities to participate in coalitions with lay persons to promote a redistribution of effort in health care. The strides made in oncology nursing as a specialty practice provide a solid foundation for cancer nurses to influence public policy and to lead the way for other specialties in assuming the responsibilities of nurses in the care arena.

INFLUENCING FACTORS

The development of a specialty practice within the health care professions is moved and guided by a variety of influencing factors. Some specialties can trace their emergence to events such as the development of a specific technology. The initial availability of renal dialysis, for example, prompted a need for knowledgeable caregivers—nurses who could both manage chronic yet life-threatening illness and carry out the dialysis procedure. The availability of a specific technology then separated the patient population with renal failure from the general medical-surgical population.

Other specialties emerged more gradually and were based on a growing body of knowledge and care approaches that limited care delivery to a specific population or care setting, such as public or occupational health. A few specialties have formally recognized new or expanded roles for nurses, such as nurse midwives or nurse anesthetists. Yet other specialties have a narrow range of functions, often procedural rather than disease focused, such as operating room nursing or intravenous therapy nursing. Change for these groups focuses on improvement of procedures and techniques. To a certain extent, the growth of oncology nursing is due to a major social investment in a serious health care problem (Lynaugh & Fairman, 1989).

Medical and nursing specialties carve out specific territories or boundaries of disease or care. Once identified, further development occurs with various factors affecting ongoing refinement. Factors commonly identified as influencing cancer nursing as a specialty include the complexity of care, the emergence of scientific and technologic advances, the building of a knowledge base through practice and research, the organization of cancer care within health care facilities, the influence of health care economics and public policy, and the structuring of groups and processes for networking and developing leadership.

Complexity of Care

The care available for patients with cancer is immensely complex. One way to illustrate that complexity and its implications for nurses is to look at the treatment for cancer. Few patients receive only surgery, radiation, or chemotherapy; multimodal treatment is the norm (see Chapter 24). Even within one treatment modality approaches are often complex. Chemotherapy regimens, for example, use combinations of agents. The increased effectiveness of combined agents was first demonstrated in the treatment of advanced Hodgkin's disease (DeVita, Serpick, & Carbone, 1970) and now the use of combinations of agents is commonplace. Although combined modalities have obvious beneficial outcomes, their complexity was an early focus of attention within the specialty and continues to pose challenges for nurses.

First, nurses must understand how each modality affects the others in combined treatments and what modifications are necessary because treatments are being combined; this knowledge is important because of complications that may arise with the disease process or because of the presence of other chronic or acute disease that has its own treatment. To provide care, the nurse must understand each treatment modality. Nurses specializing in one treatment modality must have close communication with nurses working in other modalities to assist in care planning that will promote continuity and ensure safety in care.

Second, because of the specialized body of knowledge within each modality, subspecialties have emerged. Although the separation of medical, surgical, and radiation oncology have been recognized for several years, recent advances in treatment have prompted the emergence of other treatment subspecialties such as bone marrow transplantation and biotherapy. Intensive care support for patients experiencing multisystem failure has influenced both the creation of intensive care units for these patients and the development of oncology critical care as a newer subspecialty.

Finally, nurses interact with a broad variety of providers who are involved in the delivery of complex care. In a multidisciplinary approach to care, nurses learn from and are influenced by the role and contributions other providers make in complex cancer care.

Scientific and Technologic Advances

The delivery of health care has been influenced tremendously by the explosion in health care technology. The application of this technology in cancer care is obvious throughout the disease continuum. Newer detection and monitoring methods such as scans, imaging devices, and tumor markers have influenced the role of nurses who prepare patients for testing, oversee various aspects of detection, monitor outcomes, and assist patients and families in understanding the results and implications of such testing.

The development and testing of new antineoplastic agents and new combinations of existing agents have tremendous impact on the roles of the oncology nurse. Nurses are involved in every aspect of these trials (see Chapter 25) and have gradually assumed increased responsibility. For example, the technologic explosion in delivery and monitoring devices for chemotherapy has allowed care settings to shift. The nurse who once had to master a particular line or pump for chemotherapy infusions on the inpatient unit may now be teaching patients and families to deal with this equipment at home. This is a tremendous responsibility that includes both assessing the abilities of family members to solve problems and to cope with complications that may arise and determining when the patient and family are adequately prepared to assume this role. In addition, experimental or investigational protocols have been extended into a variety of community settings, creating new pressures for nurses who heretofore may not have been involved in any type of clinical research study. This involvement necessitates a redefinition of practice roles.

Merely keeping up with scientific and technologic advances is a challenge. For example, scientific inquiry into immunotherapy and biotherapy has forced cancer nurses to keep their knowledge base about the immune system and related pathophysiologic processes up to date. Because change in these content areas is continual, nurses specializing in cancer care must identify avenues for continued learning.

Many technologic advances result in equipment options. Changing technologies may offer opportunities to influence purchasing decisions. Nurses may be asked, for example, to compare the efficiency of two pumps in terms of the frequency of problems each presents and the nursing time required to correct the problem. Nurses may be asked to consider whether the pump that seems best in the hospital is also best for home use. Nurses may need to assist patients and families in making decisions about product and care alternatives. Manufacturers of equipment and pharmacologic agents also seek information from nurses about their needs and about their experiences with specific products. Many manufacturers of cancer drugs and equipment have oncology nurses as employees for these purposes, and several have product advisory boards through which this information is sought.

Expanding Knowledge Base

Through practice, education, and research a large body of knowledge related to cancer nursing and cancer nursing care has been developed. Because all aspects of cancer care are in a continual state of redefinition and refinement, the body of scientific knowledge that supports cancer nursing practice is also changing and expanding. Nurses entering or practicing in cancer care today need a variety of resources to build their knowledge base initially and then to remain current. In recent years, the cancer nursing literature has proliferated. Numerous texts and journals are readily available. Many nurses have access to computerized databases, such as the National Cancer Institute's Physician Data Query (PDQ) (Deininger, Collins, & Hubbard, 1989). Orientation and staff development programming (Stuckey, 1983), continuing education offerings (Bushy & Kost, 1990; Donaldson et al., 1988), expansion of cancer content in basic education programs (Mooney & Dudas, 1987), and increased availability of graduate preparation in oncology (Hinds, 1989) all reflect a strong educational base for this specialty (see Chapters 64 and 65).

Organization of Cancer Care

Cancer services are organized in various ways, as described in Chapters 67 through 71. The proliferation of service settings has had a positive influence on the refinement of the specialty. The formalization of orientation to these settings, the development and implementation of standards and guidelines of care (American Nurses' Association & Oncology Nursing Society, 1979, 1987; Beck, 1980; Blausey, Barton, & Dicke, 1984; Oncology Nursing Society, 1988, 1990), the beginning definitions of patient acuity (Arenth, 1985) and staffing norms, and the evaluation of care outcomes through quality assurance mechanisms all contribute to creating a structure that facilitates care delivery. Each practice setting offers the nurse a slightly different variation in the provision of care. For example, the nurse new to oncology may find the structure of the inpatient setting supportive. Resources are usually abundant, and the new nurse is assisted by and can learn from the experience of others. A more experienced nurse may prefer the flexibility and autonomy in practice that is usually available through home care. Assessment skills and problem solving abilities are routinely tested, and the veteran nurse can draw on previous experience to develop care approaches for the patient and family.

As experience with different cancer care delivery systems builds, nurses are able to share these experiences and begin to compare care across settings. Policy adjustments, procedure modifications, cost studies, and cross-setting collaboration can result. The cancer che-motherapy and venous access guidelines developed and published by the Oncology Nursing Society (1988, 1990) are examples of the kinds of work that can be accomplished across settings and that result in specific direction for the oncology nurse providing direct care.

Health Care Economics and Policy

Health care economics will probably exert a greater influence on nursing practice than any other single factor. Cancer care providers are well aware that economic concerns frequently affect the availability, accessibility, utilization, and quality of care (see Chapters 78 and 79). The beginnings of the specialty of cancer nursing were marked by the demonstration of how much nurses could do for their patients, how many ways they could address patient concerns. Primarily because of economic considerations, nurses must now find ways to demonstrate how little they can do for patients and still achieve satisfactory ends (Baird & Mortenson, 1990). Comparing care approaches, evaluating delivery systems, and demonstrating cost effectiveness are important areas for practice and research efforts. Efforts in these areas have the potential to substantially influence cancer nursing as a specialty.

Cost-effective care is essential for the viability of cancer programs. To date, an insufficient number of studies have looked at the specifics of staffing, care demands, and delivery systems (Baird, 1989). Although some cost studies have been published, their focus is on the effects of reimbursement mechanisms (Antman, 1989; Horn & Sharkey, 1986; Mortenson, 1989; Mortenson & Baum, 1986) and not on nursing. Important beginning studies on staffing and work load (Mortenson, 1984; Tillman, 1984) need replication and extension. Cost needs to be factored into appropriate nursing research.

It is also reasonable to assume that economic dictates will prompt interest in exploring underdeveloped areas or mechanisms for delivering nursing care such as home care and private practice. In a recent survey of home health professionals, the majority believed that the major influence on home health industry growth is financial coverage (Clinical Homecare, Ltd., 1990). Home infusion, an important component of cancer care, was noted as the fastest growing segment of the home care industry, with a projected growth rate of at least 35 per cent for the next 3 years. The study further noted the underutilization and lack of understanding of home care by consumers. The private practice of nurses is a growing area of interest, but reimbursement is not yet keeping pace with the services nurses can provide. The marketing of cancer nursing has to receive increased attention for its value to be fully realized (see Chapter 66).

Structuring of Groups and Processes

The development of cancer nursing as a specialty has been aided by the overall specialty movement within nursing (Lynaugh & Fairman, 1989) and by specific efforts within cancer care. The American Cancer Society and the Oncology Nursing Society have been vital and continued forces in these efforts (see Chapter 83). In the past decade, the American Cancer Society has strengthened its emphasis on nursing and provided valuable programming and scholarship assistance. As the professional nursing organization for cancer nurses, the Oncology Nursing Society sees its mission as promoting excellence in oncology nursing by promoting professional standards, exchanging information, encouraging specialization, fostering professional development, and maintaining a responsive organizational structure and function (Oncology Nursing Society, 1990). Major efforts affect practice, education, research, and administration activities across the United States and abroad. For example, the development of the Oncology Nursing Certification Corporation and the offering of certification in oncology nursing give nurses a tangible credential in their chosen specialty. Questions now posed to the Oncology Nursing Certification Corporation are whether to develop certification that recognizes advanced preparation in the specialty or in the specific subspecialties.

Both organizations have national and local programs. Perhaps the most valuable yet least easily defined activity made possible through these organizations is the opportunity to build both formal and informal networks for information sharing and program building. Efforts include fostering advanced preparation, developing new care initiatives, and influencing public policy. Networking efforts in nursing have also been developed and formalized in some of the cancer cooperative study groups. These provide for collaboration among nurses working on specific medical research initiatives and have the potential to generate important questions for research.

CHALLENGES

Health care and social trends, both in general and specifically in nursing, exert a tremendous influence on the practice arena. Nurses at all levels and in all settings should be aware of and understand the ramifications of these agents of change. A recent survey of educators, practitioners, and administrators involved with oncology clinical nurse specialists identified trends that they thought would have the greatest influence on the clinical nurse specialist role for the next 10 years. They identified these trends as treatment in alternative settings, increasing acuity and decreasing length of hospital stay, nursing shortage, and reimbursement (Spross, 1990). Although these trends are specific to clinical nurse specialists, they are congruent with trends generally identified in health care and pose a variety of challenges for all cancer nurses wishing to be responsive to change. Some issues that seem especially important are recruiting and retaining nurses within the specialty, monitoring the quality of care delivered to patients, and defining and promoting nursing roles in underserved areas.

Recruitment and Retention of Nurses

Over time, oncology nursing has overcome its stigma among specialty choices—early studies of career preferences of senior students always placed cancer at the bottom (Barckley, 1985). Students exposed to cancer care in their clinical experiences will have witnessed skilled clinicians making vital contributions in patient care. Students should be exposed to the tremendous variety of nursing roles available along the disease continuum. Given the seemingly endless cycle of nursing shortages and the decreased number of young adults choosing nursing as a career, efforts to increase the visibility and satisfactions of cancer nursing must be undertaken. Realistic expectations for orientation must be developed, and opportunities to supplement beginning skills must be ensured.

The recruitment of experienced nurses into cancer care provides a tremendous challenge with stiff competition. Gullatte and Levine (1990) note that retention of skilled nurses should receive as much emphasis as recruitment to avoid high staff turnover and the resultant need for more recruitment. The complexity of care of patients with cancer can benefit from the presence of nurses with a wide variety of backgrounds. The increasing number of older patients with cancer, for example, offers a good opportunity for the geriatric clinician to apply previous skills to a new subpopulation.

Quality of Care

Access to quality care regardless of geographic setting is a commonly cited goal in cancer care and a focus of many funded programs. Nurses frequently express concern about the quality of care that is available and delivered to patients with cancer. Indeed, many of the efforts within the specialty have been undertaken as efforts to improve or ensure the quality of care. Increased complexities of care, variety in the preparation of care providers, the need for continuity across care settings, and cost-containment measures have stimulated efforts to ensure that quality of care remains an important consideration in decision making.

A Delphi study of health care executives reported that adequate quality care for all citizens should be the motivating force behind national health policy (American College of Hospital Administrators, 1987). The executives surveyed in this study also believed that hospitals most likely to succeed in the 1990s would be those most effectively communicating the quality of their care. Although many definitions of quality of care exist, the initiatives of private and regulatory bodies seem to be defining quality of care by both cost containment and efficient utilization of services. It is likely that national initiatives and those within individual facilities will stress quality of care in setting standards. Cancer nurses can make use of opportunities that may arise to participate in setting the definitions, criteria, and measuring approaches used to evaluate quality of care (Baird & Mortenson, 1990).

Defining and Promoting Nursing Roles

Developments within the specialty of cancer nursing have stimulated the creation of a number of roles for nurses. Although the majority of cancer nurses are now employed by hospitals and function in fairly traditional roles, many alternative opportunities offer varied patient populations, work settings, or role functions. More and more cancer care is delivered outside of traditional hospital settings (Sandrik, 1990), and as a result, more cancer nurses will seek and find work in ambulatory care, office practice, and home care.

The modification of position descriptions and procedures for alternative care sites and the development and implementation of standards of care are major nursing challenges. Because fewer nurses may be engaged in these roles or settings in any specific geographic location, mechanisms for effective communication across settings and with other providers are essential to give nurses in new roles the assistance they need. As sufficient numbers of nurses function in newer roles or with specific populations, communication networks evolve. The variety of special interest groups being developed within the Oncology Nursing Society attest to the need for collaboration and communication. These groups can identify areas of need and can move to meet these through educational programming, publishing, and research.

SUMMARY

Cancer nursing offers many varied professional opportunities. Skilled nurses practice in every aspect of care. Although the specialty is fairly young, it is extremely well established in terms of educational opportunities, practice role delineations, delivery of specialized care, research initiatives, and publications. Cancer nursing is an interactive practice well received and respected by other disciplines. As an integral part of the health care system, cancer nursing will be influenced by a variety of factors, with further refinement of the specialty and numerous challenges and rewards.

References

American College of Hospital Administrators. (1987). *Health care in the 1990's: Trends and strategies.* New York: Arthur Anderson & Co.

American Nurses' Association. (1980). *Nursing: A social policy statement.* Kansas City, MO: Author.

American Nurses' Association & Oncology Nursing Society. (1979). *Outcome standards for cancer nursing practice.* Kansas City, MO: American Nurses' Association.

American Nurses' Association & Oncology Nursing Society. (1987). *Standards of oncology nursing practice.* Kansas City, MO: American Nurses' Association.

Antman, L. (1989). Cost effectiveness and reimbursement in patient care. *Seminars in Hematology, 26*(3, Suppl.), 32–45.

Arenth, L. M. (1985). The development and validation of an oncology patient classification system. *Oncology Nursing Forum, 12*(6), 17–22.

Aydelotte, M. K. (1985). Nursing: Societal discontent and profes-

sional change. In R. R. Wieczorke (Ed.), *Power, politics, and policy in nursing* (p. 134). New York: Springer.

Baird, S. B. (1989). More questions than answers. *Oncology Nursing Forum, 16*, 629.

Baird, S. B., & Mortenson, L. E. (1990). Economic concerns in the changing health care delivery system. *Cancer, 65*(3, Suppl.), 766–769.

Barckley, V. (1985). The best of times and the worst of times: Historical reflections from an American Cancer Society national nursing consultant. *Oncology, 12*(1, Suppl.), 16–18.

Beck, J. (1980). The standards as a guide for nursing care plans. *Oncology Nursing Forum, 7*(1), 28–30.

Benoliel, J. Q. (1972). Institutionalized practices of information control. In E. Freidson & J. Lorber (Eds.), *Medical men and their work* (pp. 220–238). Chicago: Aldine-Atherton.

Benoliel, J. Q. (1976). Overview: Care, cure, and the challenge of choice. In A. M. Earle (Ed.), *The nurse as caregiver for the terminal patient and his family* (pp. 9–30). New York: Columbia University Press.

Benoliel, J., & McCorkle, R. (1977, May 10). Ethical consideration in treatment. In *Proceedings of the Second National Conference on Cancer Nursing.* New York: American Cancer Society.

Benoliel J. Q., & McCorkle, R. (1978). A holistic approach to terminal illness. *Cancer Nursing, 1*, 143–149.

Blausey, L. A., Barton, P. J., & Dicke, R. A. (1984). Development of nursing care guidelines: Putting the ONS outcome standards to work. *Oncology Nursing Forum, 11*(1), 54–58.

Bushy, A., & Kost, S. (1990). A model of continuing education for rural oncology nurses. *Oncology Nursing Forum, 17*, 207–211.

Caplan, G. (1974). *Support systems and community mental health.* New York: Behavioral Publications.

Clinical Homecare, Ltd. (1990). *Survey finds consumers lack knowledge of home health care.* Unpublished report from Clinical Homecare, Ltd., Fairfield, NJ.

Craytor, J. (1982). Highlights in education for cancer nursing. *Oncology Nursing Forum, 9*(4), 51–59.

Deininger, H., Collins, J. L., & Hubbard, S. M. (1989). Nurses and PDQ: What's in it for you? *Oncology Nursing Forum, 16*, 547–552.

DeVita, V. T., Serpick, A. A., & Carbone, P. P. (1970). Combination chemotherapy in the treatment of advanced Hodgkin's disease. *Annals of Internal Medicine, 73*, 881–895.

Donaldson, W. S., Glass, E. C., Helmick, F., Ezzone, S., Kellerstraus, B., & Stevenson, B. (1988). Determining continuing education priorities in cancer management for nurses. *Oncology Nursing Forum, 15*, 625–630.

Gullatte, M. M., & Levine, N. M. (1990). Recruitment and retention of oncology nurses. *Oncology Nursing Forum, 17*, 419–423.

Hamric, A. B. (1989). History and overview of the CNS role. In A. B. Hamric & J. A. Spross (Eds.), *The clinical nurse specialist in theory and practice* (2nd ed., pp. 3–18). Philadelphia: W. B. Saunders Co.

Hinds, P. (1989). Survey of graduate programs in cancer nursing. *Oncology Nursing Forum, 16*(6), 881–887.

Horn, S. S. D., & Sharkey, P. D. (1986). A study of patients in cancer-related DRGs. *The Journal of Cancer Program Management, 1*(2), 8–14

Krouse, T. K., & Krouse, J. E. (1984). Careplan for retaining the new nurse. *Nursing Management, 15*(2), 30–33.

Lynaugh, J., & Fairman, J. (1989). Caring for the chronically ill: Historical perspectives. *American Nephrology Nurses' Association Journal, 16*, 192–196.

McCorkle, R. (1980). An ethical dilemma: Information control in cancer care. *Bioethics Quarterly, 2*, 148–158.

Mooney, M., & Dudas, S. (1987). Undergraduate independent study in cancer nursing. *Oncology Nursing Forum, 14*(1), 51–53.

Mortenson L. (1984). Are oncology nurses too expensive? *Oncology Nursing Forum, 11*(1), 14–15.

Mortenson, L. (1989). The cancer care reimbursement constraints. *Oncology Issues: Journal of Cancer Program Management, 4*(3), 8–9.

Mortenson, L. E., & Baum, H. M. (1986). Oncology DRG winners and losers: A second look. *The Journal of Cancer Program Management, 1*(2), 18–28.

Oncology Nursing Society. (1988). *Cancer chemotherapy guidelines* (Modules I–V). Pittsburgh: Author.

Oncology Nursing Society. (1990). *Access device guidelines* (Modules I–III). Pittsburgh: Author.

Sandrik, K. (1990, February 5). Oncology: Who's managing outpatient programs? *Hospitals,* pp. 32–37.

Spross, J. A. (1990). [Delphi survey results. Second national invitational conference on the oncology clinical nurse specialist role.] Unpublished results. Boston.

Stevens, B. J. (1985). Nursing, politics, and policy formulation. In R. R. Wieczorek (Ed.), *Power, politics, and policy in nursing* (pp. 16–21). New York: Springer.

Stuckey, P. A. (1983). Orientation to an oncology unit. *Oncology Nursing Forum, 10*(4), 226–229.

Tillman, M. C. (1984). A comparison of nursing care requirements of patients on general medical surgical units and on an oncology unit in a community hospital. *Oncology Nursing Forum, 11*(4), 42–45.

Tornberg, M. J., Burns McGrath, B., & Quint Benoliel, J. (1984). Oncology transition services: Partnerships of nurses and families. *Cancer Nursing, 7*(2), 131–137.

Weisman, A. D., & Worden, J. W. (1976–1977). The existential plight in cancer: Significance of the first 100 days. *International Journal of Psychiatry in Medicine, 7,* 1–15.

CHAPTER 2

The History of Cancer Nursing

CONNIE HENKE YARBRO

Understanding the emergence of oncology nursing as a specialty provides an appreciation of the tremendous progress made to date and may provide directions on how to achieve still more in the future. Humans knew about and feared cancer for at least 1000 years before Hippocrates, when the Edwin Smith papyrus described what must have been a malignant tumor and advised, "There is no treatment" (Shimkin, 1977). All anyone could offer was supportive care; rational cancer nursing had to await the emergence of rational science.

MILESTONES IN THE HISTORY OF CANCER RESEARCH AND CARE

Eighteenth Century

The eighteenth century has been identified as the Age of Reason in the development of medicine and the biomedical sciences (Shimkin, 1977). Before the eighteenth century, no distinction was made between scientific thought and metaphysical concepts; medicine rested on philosophic thinking (Kardinal & Yarbro, 1979). However, patterns of incidence were emerging. In 1713, Ramazzini noted more cases of lung cancer in nuns when compared with other women. Snuff was associated with cancer, and in 1775 Percivall Pott described scrotal cancer in chimney sweeps. The black bile theory as a cause of cancer was dispelled after more than 1000 years. A rationale for cancer surgery began to develop. The first facility for cancer patients opened in 1740 in Rheims, France, but was moved in 1779 to the outskirts of Rheims because residents were concerned about the contagiousness of cancer (Shimkin, 1977). In 1792, the Middlesex Hospital in London (considered by many to be the first cancer institute) established a cancer ward to study the natural history of cancer and to investigate new methods of treatment.

Nineteenth Century

The nineteenth century marked the modern beginnings of discovery in the biomedical sciences and the development of cancer care facilities.

Facilities

In 1851, the Royal Marsden Hospital was established in London to treat cancer patients exclusively. The New York Cancer Hospital, founded by James M. Sims in 1884, became Memorial Hospital for Treatment of Cancer and Allied Disease in 1899 and is known today as Memorial Sloan-Kettering Cancer Center. In 1898, the New York state legislature appropriated $10,000 for the study of causes, mortality, and treatment of cancer with the establishment of the New York State Pathological Laboratory at the University of Buffalo. In 1911, it became the New York State Institute for the Study of Malignant Diseases and was renamed Roswell Park Memorial Institute in 1946, after its first director. In 1890, what may be considered the first hospice for cancer patients in America was established in New York with the opening of St. Rose's Free Home for Incurable Cancer.

Cancer and Its Treatment

Discoveries of this period provided the foundation for the future refinement of cancer therapy. The introduction of anesthesia in 1846 and antisepsis in 1867 allowed advances in surgery. New surgical approaches for cancer began in the late 1880s and of significance was William S. Halsted's radical mastectomy for breast cancer in 1894. Wilhelm Conrad Roentgen's discovery of x-rays in 1895 was followed by Marie Curie's discovery of radium in 1898. In that same year, Paul Erhlich, considered the founder of modern chemotherapy, was searching for useful agents against cancer

(Shimkin, 1977). The only chemical agent that had been used successfully against cancer was arsenic (Zubrod, 1979).

Nursing Practice

The period of 1890 to 1900 was a time of considerable growth in American nursing. The need for trained nurses became apparent during the Civil War, and the first school of nursing, New England Hospital School of Nursing, opened in Boston in 1872. The number of nursing schools increased rapidly to approximately 400 by 1900. The head nurse was the only graduate nurse on the unit and taught the students who provided the care (Kramer, 1987). Graduate nurses practiced in the hospital, the district, or the home, but home care predominated.

Twentieth Century

The first half of the twentieth century is noted for the use of ionizing radiation in the diagnosis and treatment of cancer and the extension of surgical procedures. The second half of the century is noted for significant progress in systemic chemotherapy, increased understanding of cell biology, and advanced technology that allowed research proliferation.

Early 1900s

At the turn of the century, cancer was considered incurable, and many people thought it was contagious. In one of the first articles in the nursing literature on cancer, Rice (1902) stated, "While cancer has not yet been classed with the transmissible diseases, there are authentic cases where a wife has been infected with cancer by her husband and vice versa." She also noted cancer's prevalence in certain geographic locations, and she designated Buffalo, New York, as "a veritable tropic of cancer." Indeed, the belief that cancer was an infectious disease was so common that some nurses refused to care for patients with the disease (Transmission, 1907). In 1906, C. P. Childe, a British physician, wrote the first book to inform the public about cancer: *The Control of a Scourge* (Ross, 1987). Note that the word *cancer* was not used in the title.

The death rate from cancer was 90 per cent. Although prevention of cancer was not the focus during this period of time, one physician asserted that the development of cancer was due to excessive and faulty nutrition (Scovil, 1915). He recommended exercise, avoidance of coffee and alcohol, and a vegetarian diet with the exception of butter.

The organizational fight against cancer began when the American Association for Cancer Research was established in 1907. In 1913, the American Society for the Control of Cancer, known today as the American Cancer Society (ACS), was established to educate the lay public about cancer. In that same year, the first cancer article aimed at the general public appeared in the *Ladies' Home Journal*. Author Samuel Hopkins

Adams encouraged women to be watchful of themselves and to report any suspicious symptoms (Ross, 1987; Shimkin, 1977). The word *cancer* was rarely printed in newspapers or magazines or discussed openly in society. Women were often too frightened and inhibited to discuss symptoms with their physicians. Despite a high mortality rate from gynecologic and breast cancer (King, 1988), the average time between the discovery by the patient and the seeking of medical advice was 1 year, with longer delays noted for men (Control of Cancer, 1919). In addition, many doctors did not recognize early symptoms. For example, vaginal discharges were not investigated; cancers of the rectum were treated as hemorrhoids; and cancers of the oral cavity were misdiagnosed as syphilis (American Society, 1924). To increase physician awareness, the American Society for the Control of Cancer and the American Medical Association published *Essential Facts about Cancer for the Medical Profession* in 1919 (American Society, 1924).

Cancer nursing in the early 1900s was primarily concerned with bedside care and comfort measures for surgical patients, because surgery was the major treatment method. Most patients presented with advanced cancer and encountered numerous difficulties, yet nurses used ingenuity to address individual problems. One nurse modified a Kelly pad to manage the patient's excessive discharge from the bowels and bladder (New Use, 1916) (Box 2–1). A physician shared with nurses a formula for removing the offensive odor from their hands after changing dressings of patients with inoperable cancers (Cumston, 1900) (Box 2–2). Nurses providing home care also had to improvise and economize. Tucker (1915) reported caring for a patient with pelvic cancer that caused bladder and rectal fistulas. Pads were not thick enough to prevent the bed sheets from getting wet. She improvised by using an air cushion with newspapers underneath and muslin

---

Box 2–1. NEW USE FOR A KELLY PAD

Dear Editor: While nursing a case of cancer, where there was excessive discharge from both bladder and bowels, the patient using cloths and sanitary pads which caused discomfort and chafing, as well as much washing of cloths and bed linen, I thought of trying a Kelly pad. I procured a surgeon's size, which is smaller than the obstetric size, and was more comfortable, relieving the patient's back from pressure. I made pads of cotton batting and cheesecloth, large squares, which I placed inside the pad. When they were wet, they were removed and burned, thus eliminating all washing and keeping the patient dry and comfortable. The results far exceeded my expectations, the patient's suffering and distress being much lessened. The pad could be used in many cases where there is continuous discharge or drainage.
District of Columbia.   **C.E.**

(New use for a Kelly pad [Letter to the editor]. [1916]. *American Journal of Nursing, 16,* 536. Reproduced by permission.)

Box 2–2. FORMULAE USED IN SURGICAL NURSING

On a number of occasions nurses have asked me for formulae to fulfill various indications met with in surgical practice, and I here present at random a few of them that may be of help.

One of the most distressing conditions to meet is a case of inoperable cancer, more particularly on account of the very offensive odor of the secretions, which clings to the hands of those who change the dressings. To remove this odor the following prescription will be found of great value:

Rx Terebene,
Olive oil, equal parts.
Rub freely on the hands and remove
with soap and water.

(Cumston, C. G. [1900]. A new formulae used in surgical nursing. *American Journal of Nursing, 1,* 13–14. Reproduced by permission.)

---

wrapped around the cushion and newspapers. When soiled, only the muslin needed cleaning, which meant a great saving on laundry expenses. As a home nurse, she was provided a budget to carry out her work but was expected to save as much as possible. She recommended that nurses in private work keep an account of everything ordered in case questions were raised about the bills.

1920s

General hospitals often refused to care for patients with chronic diseases, placing a priority on patients with acute conditions. The average hospital stay for all cases was 2 weeks, but cancer patients required terminal care for periods of 4 to 5 months (Eaves & Associates, 1928). The state of Massachusetts, concerned about facilities to care for patients with inoperable cancers, established Pondville Hospital for cancer patients in 1927. For 2 to 3 months after the opening of Pondville, there was no x-ray equipment, the operating room was not ready, and radium had not arrived, but "we showed what good nursing could do" by cleaning up sloughing lesions and reducing infection (Daland, 1969).

Affluent families could afford trained nurses to provide care at home for family members with advanced disease. This demand for nurses often created competition between private duty nursing and hospital nursing for graduates of the nearly 2000 training schools (Lynaugh & Fagin, 1988). Home care of cancer was an important issue, and emphasis began to be placed on the care of patients by public health nurses.

The Boston Community Health Association evaluated the care of 181 cancer patients by nurses of their association, and 628 histories were obtained from surviving relatives (Eaves & Associates, 1928). Approximately 78 per cent of the cancer patients had a hopeless outlook; superstition and misunderstanding by patients and family members prevailed. These attitudes were reinforced by physicians and nurses who practiced deception and concealment that subsequently promoted fear and disgrace. The nursing care required for these patients was demanding and stressful. Nausea and incontinence were major problems, and care focused on surgical dressing changes, enemas, douches, catheter care, nourishment by means of tubes, and pain relief. A home care visit cost $0.85 (Eaves & Associates, 1928); hospital care was $1.50 per day if paid by the patient or $2.50 per day if paid by the city or town (Daland, 1969).

In 1927, the American Society for the Control of Cancer adopted the slogan "Fight Cancer with Knowledge," emphasizing the development of cancer committees within state medical societies to educate physicians (Nursing Advisory Committee, 1948a; Ross, 1987). The attitudes of the medical profession warranted criticism because delays in detection and treatment by approximately 10 per cent of the medical profession were considerable (American Society, 1924–1925). Examples of medical misinformation sound shocking today: a woman with breast cancer was told by her physician to "wait until it begins to bleed and then come back, and I will tell you what to do." Bleeding from a cancerous uterus was ascribed to "a return of menstruation," "rheumatism," or "a cold in the pelvis." Other familiar sayings were, "It is your menopause"; "Don't bother it till it bothers you"; and "Go home and forget it" (American Society, 1924–1925).

In 1928, 158 nurses attended a symposium on cancer at Harvard Cancer Research Hospital (Ross, 1928). Ross (1928) reported that many of the nurses were dissatisfied because speakers gave them no reassurance of positive cures, leaving them with little hope for progress. The literature had little information about nursing care for the cancer patient, but Ross provides some insight regarding patient attitudes and nursing care. Ignorance and superstition contributed to suffering, and many patients spent their earnings on quacks. She reported that excessive use of morphia (morphine) in homebound cancer patients was an unnecessary evil and argued that morphia should only be used to help patients through a special crisis because coal tar products and sedatives can keep patients comfortable (Ross, 1928).

1930s

The convention of considering 5-year end results in cancer as an indication of cure became the basis of clinical statistical consideration (Shimkin, 1977). In the 1930s, fewer than one in five patients were alive 5 years after diagnosis.

In 1931, a physician and a nurse from the Massachusetts State Department of Public Health studied the habits of 387 patients with cancer and 387 patients in a control group (Lombard & McDonald, 1931). Alcohol use and heavy smoking were identified in the cancer group, but no significant difference in food groups eaten by the patients was noted between the two groups. There was also an average 6-month delay in the notification of symptoms to medical authorities in the cancer group. The role of the public health nurse as an important member of the anticancer network was emphasized with regard to patient advocacy, assessment, and follow-up care (Fischel, 1931).

Cancer organizations made considerable progress in the 1930s. The American College of Surgeons established standards for the evaluation of cancer patients. In 1935, the International Union Against Cancer (UICC) was established, and the American Society for the Control of Cancer established the Women's Field Army to educate women about cancer symptoms. Later the Field Army educated both men and women and used lay public volunteers to augment the professional health educators (Nursing Advisory Committee, 1948a; Ross, 1987) (Fig. 2–1). The National Cancer Institute (NCI) was established through an act of Congress on August 5, 1937. In addition, the first course for nurses in radiotherapy began at the Christie Hospital in Manchester, England, in 1938.

Nursing education in the 1930s was in a state of unrest, with movement from an apprentice-type training program to a more formal educational base for practice (Craytor, 1982). Nursing education, which was controlled by hospitals, was not on an equal level with other forms of specialized education. Salaries were low, and nurses worked 12-hour shifts. A proposed scheme of 8-hour shifts was opposed by hospital administrators, who were worried that money would be lost and that other personnel would want an 8-hour schedule (Editorial, 1934).

Cowan (1934), Education Director of Women's Hospital in New York City, published a paper, "Modern Cancer Nursing," that provided some indication of cancer nursing practice in those days. She stressed the importance of nurses' attention to the mental attitude of patients with cancer, including teaching control of pain using mental hygiene measures, personal hygiene measures, and drugs. Nursing care of hemorrhage and strangulation in head and neck cancers was also discussed. Care of the bowels in patients with colon cancer aimed to increase elimination through colonic irrigations with salt solution 1 to 2 times per day.

1940s

One in four patients with cancer was alive 5 years after diagnosis. Chemotherapeutic agents gained recognition. The discovery of the antitumor activity of nitrogen mustard, an agent of the chemical warfare program, was made at Yale by Goodman and colleagues (1946). The first patient treated with it had far

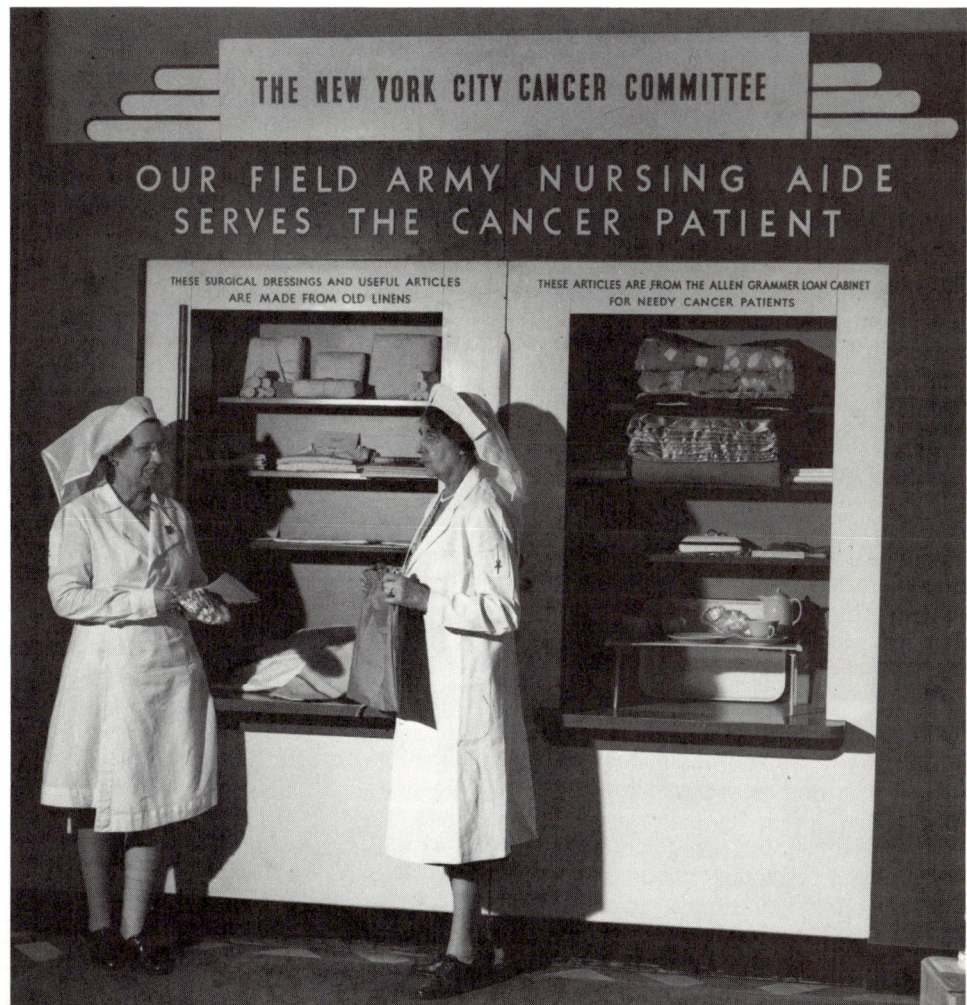

Figure 2–1. As the American Cancer Society expanded its Field Army program, volunteers augmented nurses' efforts. (Courtesy of the American Cancer Society.)

advanced lymphosarcoma. In 1947, Sidney Farber of the Children's Hospital in Boston achieved the first remission in a 10-year-old boy, using the antineoplastic agent aminopterin—an important milestone in the development of chemotherapy. Prevention and early detection was promoted through breast self-examination and development of the Papanicolaou test. In 1944, the American Society for the Control of Cancer became the American Cancer Society and began to emphasize cancer research as well as cancer education.

During the 1940s, the demand increased for nurses to implement new therapies and procedures and to develop resources for World War II. The hospital became the center for health care delivery, but a shortage of nurses existed. Aides and auxiliary workers filled the gap, and practical nursing came into being.

It is probably fair to state that the development of cancer nursing as a specialty had its real beginnings in the decade of the forties, with a primary emphasis on cancer nursing education. This decade was also significant because the first leaders in cancer nursing could be identified.

The Nursing Section of the Cancer Control Branch of the National Cancer Institute was established in 1948. Rosalie Peterson, named Senior Nurse Officer and Chief Public Health Nursing Consultant of the Cancer Control Division, had a significant impact on cancer nursing education. Because of investigations in 1947 that revealed nurses' limited knowledge of cancer, home care, and rehabilitation and their beliefs that cancer was always fatal, Peterson became actively involved in courses on cancer treatment and diagnosis for nursing instructors. She taught cancer care to public health nurses and awarded grants in 1949 to the School of Public Health at the University of Minnesota and the Columbia University Teachers College to enrich the graduate education curriculum (Peterson, 1948, 1956; Peterson & Walker, 1949).

The first university course in cancer nursing specialization was taught by Katherine Nelson in 1947 at Teachers College, Columbia University in New York (Craytor, 1982). The year-long course provided 16 academic credit hours toward a master of arts degree. Anne Ferris, Director of Nursing at Memorial Hospital, initiated the idea for this course and secured a grant of $30,000 from the New York City Committee of the ACS (Craytor, 1982). Elizabeth Walker and Nelliana Best assisted in the teaching, and the clinical practicum was held at Memorial Hospital.

On April 30, 1948, the Nursing Advisory Committee of the American Cancer Society had its first meeting (Table 2–1). Marjorie Schlotterbeck was the first nursing consultant for the ACS, followed by Claire Richmond in 1955, Virginia Barckley in 1962, and Patricia Greene in 1981. The nursing committee made recommendations and advised on projects that were under way and on those that needed to be developed. Responding to an increased emphasis by the ACS on professional education, the nursing committee began work on films, an exhibit, and criteria and standards for scholarships for nurses (Nursing Advisory Committee, 1948a, 1948b). The ACS-sponsored workshops

Table 2–1. MEMBERS OF THE FIRST AMERICAN CANCER SOCIETY NURSING ADVISORY COMMITTEE, 1948

Katherine Nelson, Chair	Columbia University Teachers College, New York
Hedwig Cohen	National Organization of Public Health Nursing
Montrose Williams*	
Fraziska Glienke*	
Irene Carn	League of Nursing Education
Anne Ferris	Memorial Hospital, New York
Ruth Smith*	
Rosalie Peterson	National Cancer Institute
Ethel Chandler*	
Caroline Keller	Memorial Hospital, New York
Marjorie Schlotterbeck	American Cancer Society

*Affiliations unknown.

were launched. A course in cancer control was held at the University of Washington School of Nursing for 25 nurses (Patterson, 1948). Caroline Keller, Director of Nursing, and Margaret Coleman, Director of Nursing Education, both at Memorial Hospital, and Dr. Vera Fry, Dean at New York University established 4- to 6-week oncologic nursing workshops twice a year for registered nurses, who were recruited through ACS state divisions (Co-operating, 1949–1950; Wolf, 1982).

Documentation of cancer nursing practice and care was still minimal in the 1940s, but some insights into care and concerns during that time are available. Hopp (1941) discussed the role of the roentgenologic nurse in cancer treatment and diagnosis, stating that there was "no special routine to follow in caring for these patients and efforts to combat side effects of nausea and vomiting have not been entirely successful." Lemon juice, sour wine sipped slowly, and ginger ale were used for nausea, vomiting, and anorexia. Glienke and Kress (1944b) reported that most cancer deaths occur in the home and that cobra venom was used to control pain. Urea was used to eliminate or decrease odors in malodorous lesions of the breast (Glienke & Kress, 1944a). Cockerill (1948) cited the importance of understanding the fears, reactions, and problems of the individual with cancer.

Home care of patients with cancer was also a concern (Biehusen, 1956; Ferguson, 1948). The Connecticut Division of the ACS developed a cancer nursing reimbursement plan for visiting nurse and public health agencies, allocating $20,000 in 1947 to support nursing services in tumor clinics at $1.50 per hour and nursing visits to the home at $1.00 per visit (Biehusen, 1956). Connecticut was the first state to formally establish a nursing committee in any division of ACS.

1950s

The cobalt 60 unit was developed in the early 1950s, and Best (1950) described the role of the nurse with this new treatment method. In 1955, the NCI developed a national chemotherapy program devoted to testing chemicals that might be effective against cancer. Multimodality treatment approaches replaced single-modality treatment for cancer.

Cancer nursing education continued to improve, and

cancer nursing activities increased tremendously. Hil-kemeyer (1982), who was a consultant in nursing education to the Bureau of Cancer Control, Missouri Division of Health, from 1950 to 1955 and became Director of Nursing for M.D. Anderson Hospital and Tumor Institute, stated, "the 1950's was an era when the nursing profession was concerned about who we were and what we should be doing."

In 1950, Peterson and two other NCI instructors conducted a 3-week institute at the University of Minnesota for 30 nursing instructors from across the country. In 1951, Peterson published a series of articles outlining in-service education for cancer nursing care (Peterson, 1951a, 1951b, 1951c). The following year the NIH funded five pilot studies for education in cancer nursing (Farrell, 1953; Peterson, 1956). The first grant awarded went to Skidmore College for the integration of cancer nursing throughout the basic curriculum. Doris Diller wrote the proposal while taking a research course at Columbia. She and Francis Brady, a fellow faculty member at Skidmore, constructed a test to measure knowledge about cancer among nursing students over 3 successive years (Craytor, 1982; Diller, 1982). Diller received a grant from the NCI to conduct the cancer knowledge investigation in 100 schools (Diller, 1957). Her efforts stimulated interest and emphasized the need for cancer nursing in the basic nursing curriculum.

Cancer nursing education activities flourished during this era. Dr. Rosemary Bouchard, Norma Owens, and Inga Thornblad of the Department of Education at New York University implemented workshops on on-cologic nursing (Craytor, 1982) and collaborated with Memorial Hospital for the Treatment of Cancer and Allied Diseases by offering a year-long cancer nursing internship program for foreign nurses. Hilkemeyer established 5-day institutes on cancer nursing for public health nurses and an in-service education program at Ellis Fischel Cancer Hospital in Columbia, Missouri (Hilkemeyer & Kinney, 1956).

Outside of major centers, a small number of nurses were volunteering for the ACS, reporting on what had been learned about cancer care and cancer nursing. The dedication to volunteer work by these nurses helped spread the word. As Edith Wolf (1982), Associate Director of Nursing Education at Memorial Hospital from 1950 to 1969, stated, "Today, one would receive honoraria for all the hard work but my only thought was to get the information to where it would help those who cared for the patients so their lives would be better."

The ACS nursing committee remained active during the 1950s, with an increased focus on nursing practice and collaboration with the ACS divisions. The ACS published *A Cancer Source Book for Nurses,* and the minutes from the committee's meeting on March 13, 1957, reported that 63 graduate and 263 undergraduate scholarships or fellowships were awarded to nurses by the ACS divisions (Nursing Advisory Committee, 1957). Chairpersons of the ACS Nursing Advisory Committee during the 1950s were Elizabeth Stobo, Vera Fry, and Julia Hereford. In 1958, the committee

surveyed 30 graduate programs; only New York University and Columbia University Teachers College offered advanced programs in cancer nursing and an undergraduate level course. Boston University, University of California at Los Angeles, Teachers College, and New York University were the only schools that identified a faculty member as a cancer nursing specialist (Nursing Advisory Committee, 1958).

While cancer nursing education was moving ahead, the practice arena was encountering unique problems. A nursing shortage existed, and Caroline Keller, Director of Nursing at Memorial Hospital for the Treatment of Cancer and Allied Diseases, decided to go to Argentina to recruit nurses. Through an indirect connection with the Perons and the social reform activity of Evita Peron, women were recruited from the streets to be trained as nurses. Subsequently, Edith Wolf spent 2 years on the monumental task of educating 13 young women in American culture and cancer nursing (Wolf, 1982). At that time, she reported "my mail was heavy, no one outside of Memorial had ever heard of a colostomy irrigation [developed by their chief of gastric surgery] and nurses were clamoring for this information." Wolf provides insights into nursing practice at that time: "Patients were not told they had cancer, we always said tumor or growth" (Wolf, 1982). Meanwhile, Mary Patterson at Memorial Hospital recruited a volunteer pianist and initiated arm exercise classes for mastectomy patients (Higgenbotham, 1957) (Figs. 2–2 and 2–3).

Considerable progress was made in the 1950s in defining cancer nursing. Craytor, in her master's thesis in 1959, defined the well-prepared nurse as a co-worker of the health care team. This work subsequently led to a demonstration project that illustrated the value of a team (physician, nurse, and social worker) to deal with the problems of cancer care (Craytor, 1982). Nelson continued her crusade for cancer nursing. In a letter to Claire Richmond, nursing consultant for ACS, at the renewal of her cancer nursing education grant, Nelson (1959) stated "If we believe that there should be a small number of highly prepared nurse consultants and teachers in cancer nursing, these nurses should be sought out, encouraged to get this preparation and return to their agencies better able to help in the preparation of nurse practitioners in the nursing care of patients with late stage cancer. Cancer nursing is at a crossroads, it either has to be given up as an undesirable thing or it must be looked at critically and really supported."

1960s

Oncology Comes of Age. Cancer statistics improved: one in three individuals was now alive 5 years after diagnosis. The clinical trials program established by NCI led to the development and discovery of other active agents in the 1960s. Skipper and colleagues (1964) established guiding principles in chemotherapy that were related to cellular kinetics. Frei and colleagues (1961) pioneered the first effective combination chemotherapy for treatment of leukemia. Adjuvant

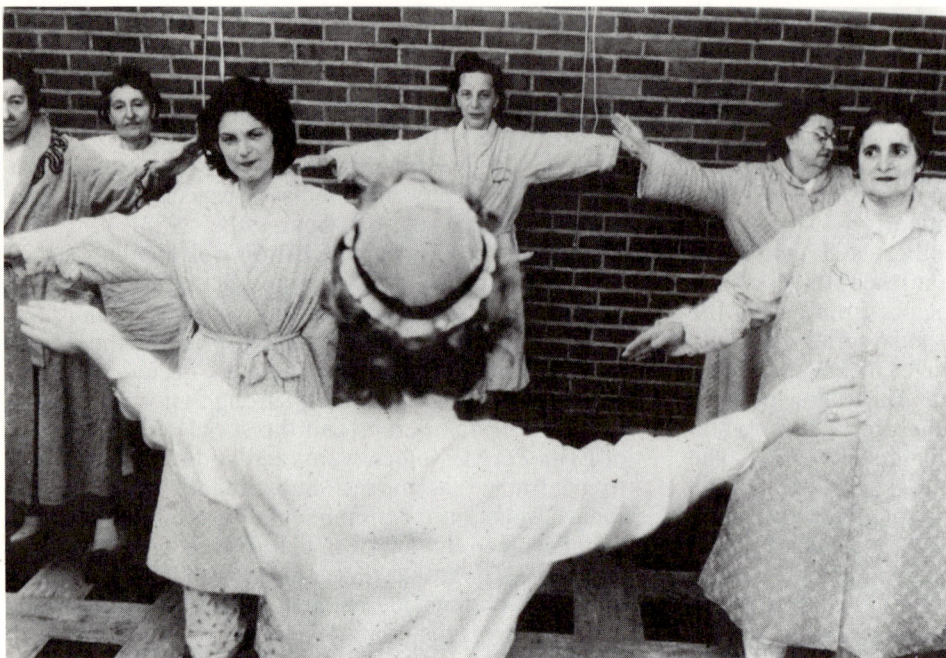

Figure 2–2. An exercise class for mastectomy patients. (Courtesy of the Oncology Nursing Society, historical files.)

chemotherapy, begun in the 1950s, first proved useful in 1965 (Zubrod, 1979). In 1964, the American Society of Clinical Oncology was established to create a forum for the new specialty of medical oncology.

Specialization of Nursing. A distinct growth in nursing specialization paved the road for oncology nursing as a specialty. Coronary care units, surgical intensive care units, dialysis units, burn units, and medical intensive care units necessitated a change in nursing roles to clinical nurse specialists or nurse clinicians (Donahue, 1985) and the need for such specialists (Leone, 1965).

This specialty role was not clear to many. Physician members of the ACS Professional Education Committee wanted to know what defined cancer nursing and how it differed from other nursing. In response, the

ACS nursing committee dropped the term *cancer nursing* in favor of *nursing care of cancer patients* (Nursing Advisory Committee, 1960). However, with a beginning emphasis placed on oncology nursing practice in the later 1960s it was becoming clear what constituted cancer nursing.

The first expanded nursing roles in oncology were those associated with sophisticated clinical trials of new chemotherapeutic agents (Hubbard & Donehower, 1980). Initially, the nurse in a clinical trial team primarily collected patient data for the clinical trial. But gradually the nurse's role changed as patients found the nurse a better source of counsel than an unfamiliar member of the medical house staff or the busy clinical investigator. The clinical investigator found that the research nurse was often a better source of information

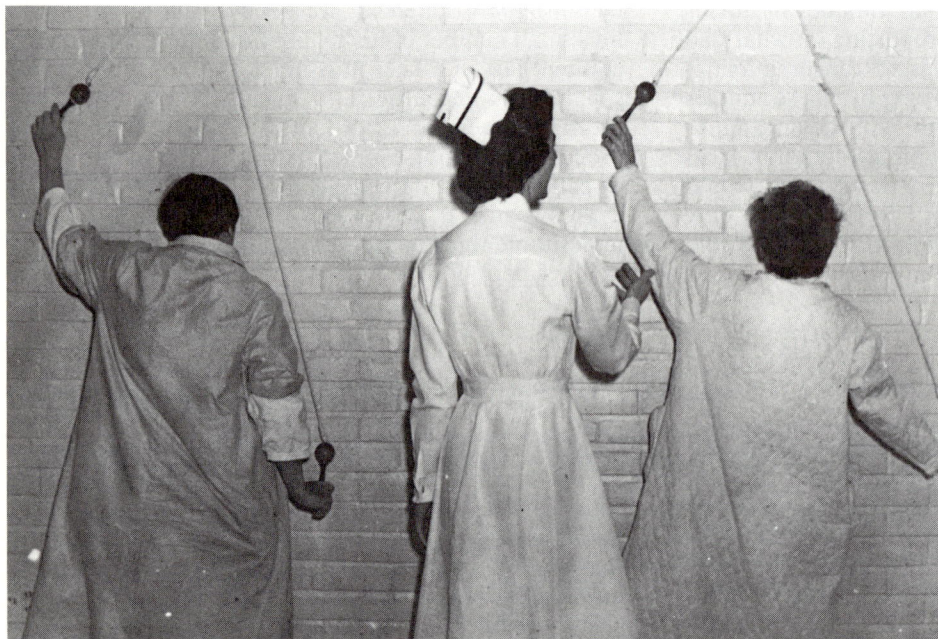

Figure 2–3. Mastectomy patients performing arm exercises. (Courtesy of the Oncology Nursing Society, historical files.)

regarding the subtleties of patient status. Thus before there was an oncology nurse or a medical oncology specialty, a symbiotic relationship grew between two professionals whose special training was acquired on the job (Henke, 1980).

As this symbiosis and interdependence grew, the nursing role was expanded far beyond technical or task-oriented functions. The nurse often became the liaison between the clinical investigator and other services gradually added to the cancer care team (e.g., social work, pastoral care, rehabilitation).

What began as a clinical research team was gradually recognized as a better approach to providing cancer care. Cancer patients as a group began to benefit from this improved system of care, and the oncology nurse became a central figure in the new team approach to cancer care. There were two consequences. As oncologists entered practice in community hospitals, they took with them the team approach and the expanded role for the oncology nurse. Also, as the identity of oncology nursing was formalized, hospital nursing services began to seek out and establish positions for nurses in this emerging specialty (Henke, 1980). One of the first institutions to formally recognize the role of oncology nursing was St. Jude Children's Research Hospital in Memphis by establishing the position of pediatric oncology nurse practitioner in 1969. Andi Wood, Ellen Shanks, Clara Mason, and Shirley Stagner were the first nurses to function in this role (Greene, 1983). They subsequently developed a 3-month fellowship in childhood cancer nursing to share their experiences with other nurses.

The nursing literature expanded concerning nursing care of the patient with cancer. Wolf (1964, 1968) stressed the importance of the role of the nurse in education for patients with cancer, emphasizing the need to teach patients self-care. The ACS published *Care of Your Colostomy: A Source Book of Information* in 1964. There was considerable focus on care of the dying patient (Barckley, 1964, 1967; Kübler-Ross, 1969). The first textbook, edited by Bouchard, *Nursing Care of the Cancer Patient,* was published in 1967. The landmark clinical nursing research study by Quint (1963) identified the psychological needs of women who had breast cancer and were treated with radical mastectomy (Box 2–3). The nurse's role in home care (Hammond, 1964) and the early detection of breast and cervical cancer was also discussed (Lewison, 1965; Leyshon, 1966).

1970s

In 1971, Congress passed the National Cancer Act, the first law by any nation to make the conquest of cancer a national priority. National funding for cancer rose from $233 million in 1971 to $379 million in 1972 and to more than $1 billion over the next 12 years (Ross, 1987). Comprehensive cancer centers expanded from three to 20 centers during the 1970s, and clinical trials began to enter community hospitals by the late 1970s.

Combination drug regimens were used with drugs reconstituted and administered by nurses. The use of scalp vein needles and bolus injections were common practice, and little consideration was given to safety factors for reconstitution and administration.

The management of chemotherapy side effects was a trial and error process. For nausea and vomiting, if one antiemetic did not work, another was tried. Combination antiemetic regimens were unheard of. The development of guidelines for care was just beginning.

Patient education materials were almost nonexistent, which meant that nurses had to spend considerable time on verbal instruction and on developing appropriate patient resources. In addition, considerable time was spent with patients and families in overcoming the myths associated with cancer. Some still thought cancer was contagious and a death sentence with few options available.

Oncology nurses rose to the opportunities at hand, which built on the groundwork that had already been laid. Barckley (1982) summed it up best when she wrote, "The nineteen seventies, when the seeds sown by so many came to a full bloom, were a kind of richness."

Cancer Nursing Education. Nurses were being encouraged to enter the field of cancer nursing, and the future challenges and opportunities for this specialty were emphasized (Hilkemeyer, 1974; Koons, 1976; Leininger, 1977; Marino, 1976; Miller, 1976; Nelson, 1974). The American Cancer Society sponsored a 6-week summer experience for senior nursing students to encourage them to enter cancer nursing (Barckley, 1971). In 1971, the NCI supported a 10-week work-study program in cancer nursing at the NIH Clinical Center in collaboration with the ACS. In 1973, the Division of Cancer Control and Rehabilitation at NCI funded 18 oncology nursing education programs for a 5-year period. These programs developed curricula and materials covering general and specialized aspects of cancer care for continuing education programs and for undergraduate- and graduate-level courses. More than 16,000 nurses were reached through these programs (L. Lunceford, personal communication, April 2, 1982). Graduate education in cancer nursing was also being developed at the University of California at Los Angeles by Anayis Derdiarin and at the University of Washington by Jeanne Quint Benoliel and Ruth McCorkle (Craytor, 1982). In 1979, the NCI funded two post-master's fellowship programs in oncology nursing education at San Jose State University and the University of Alabama.

Cancer Nursing Organizations. In 1973, the ACS sponsored the First National Cancer Nursing Conference in Chicago, the first major cancer conference *for* cancer nurses organized *by* cancer nurses. Lisa Marino, at the University of Chicago and Shirlee Koons, Director of Nursing at the Mountain States Tumor Institute in Boise, coordinated a small meeting after the conference to discuss the idea of a national organization for oncology nurses. The 20 nurses present agreed that an organization was needed. During 1974, Connie Henke, University of Alabama Comprehensive Cancer Center, worked with Marino to establish a communi-

---

Box 2–3. EXPLORATORY INVESTIGATION OF THE PROCESS OF ADJUSTMENT FOLLOWING MASTECTOMY

Principal Investigator: Lulu W. Hassenplug, Dean, School of Nursing, University of California, Los Angeles
Project Director: Jeanne C. Quint, Junior Research Nurse

This 2-year study investigated the process by which a woman adjusts to the loss of a breast because of cancer. Attention was directed toward understanding how women came to terms with two changes precipitated by the surgery: the defeminizing change in body appearance and the decision concerning camouflage and concealment; and the knowledge of having cancer and the impact of an uncertain future. All women admitted to the hospital for breast biopsy were potential subjects. Initial contacts with subjects were made the evening before surgery, and data were collected by participant observation during the hospital stay. Interviews occurred at 2 weeks, 6 weeks, 3 months, 6 months, and between the tenth and eleventh month. Interview guides for the home interviews were based on a combination of previously identified areas of importance and salient events or experiences observed by the nurse fieldworkers during their contacts with the women and their families. Data were obtained from 21 women over an 18-month period. Categories and category relationships were established using the constant comparative method of data analysis. The women ranged in age from 38 to 79 years, with a median of 57. Ten were married; ten were widows, and one was divorced. Six received medical supervision from private physicians, and the others from nonprivate medical services. Death and dying became integral parts of the lives of these women; for all of them, life expectancy was foreshortened. Three patterns of adjustment were found: (1) those who faced an uncertain future with satisfactory wound healing and physical recovery; (2) those who faced an ambiguous future associated with a nonhealing incision or persistent physical discomfort; and (3) those who underwent physical regression and death. Interactional difficulties for the women were associated with complex organizational structure and unspoken death concerns of all participants.

This study was supported by NIH Grant MH 05495 and was conducted under sponsorship of the School of Nursing, University of California, Los Angeles, between September 1, 1961, and August 31, 1963.

---

cations network of oncology nurses. Koons published and distributed the first newsletter in 1974. By January 1975, 400 cancer nurses had been identified. At the same time, Patricia Greene was spearheading a move to identify pediatric oncology nurses. On November 3, 1974, the Association of Pediatric Oncology Nurses came into being, with Greene serving as the first president (Greene, 1983). In May 1975, a nursing session was held at the meetings of the American Society of Clinical Oncology and the American Association for Cancer Research in San Diego, and the decision was made to establish a formal national organization. The initial four officers were Lisa Begg Marino president; Cindi Mantz, vice president; Daryl Maass, secretary; and Connie Henke, treasurer. In July 1975, the Oncology Nursing Society was officially incorporated in the state of Illinois; by the end of the year there were more than 400 members (Yarbro, 1984).

Progress was also being made internationally with cancer nursing. England established its Oncology Nursing Society under the auspices of the Royal College of Nursing, and Switzerland established an oncology nurses interest group within their nursing association in 1978 (Ash, 1983). In the fall of 1978, the first International Cancer Nursing Conference was sponsored by the Royal Marsden Hospital and Nursing Mirror in London. South Africa held its first national cancer nursing conference in 1979.

Cancer Nursing Research. In 1973, Marilyn Oberst from Memorial Sloan-Kettering surveyed a panel of 575 nurses to determine the priorities for clinical research in cancer nursing. The highest priorities were for research on problems related to the side effects of cancer treatment and relief of the physical discomfort experienced by the patient (Oberst, 1978) (Box 2–4).

MacVicar (1975) studied the problems experienced by families after the onset of metastatic disease in the male spouse. Lewis and colleagues (1979) developed a tool to assess the outcomes of cancer patients who received chemotherapy, and McCorkle and Young (1978) developed and tested a symptom distress scale to assess ways in which patients cope or fail to cope with their cancer therapy. The NCI also funded the work of several cancer nurse researchers: Ida Martinson, "Home Care for the Child with Cancer"; Jane Dixon, "Nursing Interventions in Nutrition of Cancer Patients"; Gail Hongladorum, "Community-Based Cancer Nursing Education Program"; and Denise Oleske, "Demonstration Project: Home Nursing for Cancer Patients" (L. Lunceford, personal communication, April 2, 1982).

Cancer Nursing as a Specialty. The rapid growth of oncology nursing was influenced by increased funding for cancer research; medical, scientific, and technologic advances; public interest in cancer; and changes in the nursing profession. Cancer nursing literature increased with the development of two professional journals devoted to cancer nursing: *Oncology Nursing Forum*, official journal of the Oncology Nursing Society, and *Cancer Nursing*. The Oncology Nursing Society grew rapidly to more than 2000 members by 1979, gave national stature to the collective force of nurses involved in cancer care, and provided a forum for the development of cancer nursing activities. One of the major activities was the development of *Outcome Standards for Cancer Nursing Practice* (Oncology Nursing Society, 1979).

1980s

The 1980s witnessed the most significant growth in all aspects of oncology and oncology nursing. Half of

---

Box 2–4. PRIORITIES FOR CANCER NURSING RESEARCH

---

1. Determine effective methods of relieving chemotherapy or radiation induced nausea and vomiting.
2. Study nursing interventions for the relief of pain in individuals with cancer.
3. Establish discharge planning and follow-up programs that effectively mobilize patient, family, and community resources.
4. Identify nursing interventions that assist patients and families in coping with grief and impending death during the preterminal and terminal stages of disease.
5. Find effective ways to prevent or treat stomatitis resulting from chemotherapy.
6. Determine the most effective techniques for venipuncture, maintenance of intravenous lines, and preservation of veins for patients receiving long-term antibiotic or chemotherapy.
7. Delineate modifications in the physical plant, nursing care program, and policy that will promote comfort and dignity for the hospitalized terminally ill individual.
8. Establish effective analgesia protocols for patients with cancer.
9. Develop more effective methods of psychological support for patients and families at various stages of disease and cancer treatment.
10. Clarify the dying patient's rights to make decisions about a health care program and establish more effective mechanisms for the exercise of those rights.

(Adapted from Oberst, M. [1978]. Priorities in cancer nursing research. *Cancer Nursing, 1,* 281–290.)

---

all cancer patients are now cured! Cancer nursing expanded tremendously, with cancer nursing research studies being reported daily. The proliferation of cancer nursing texts and journals has occurred, with the *Journal of the Association of Pediatric Oncology Nursing* and *Seminars in Oncology Nursing* joining the ranks of cancer nursing journals. The number of graduate education programs increased, continuing education programs proliferated, and certification was initiated. The Oncology Nursing Society grew to more than 15,000 members, and its activities were varied and widespread. The accomplishments that took place in the 1980s were abundant.

SUMMARY

The progress made against cancer over the past centuries has been eclipsed by that of the past 15 years. From a cancer nursing perspective, the late 1940s, 1950s, and 1960s were crusades for cancer nursing with major emphasis on education. Very few cancer nurses are aware of what the early cancer nursing leaders contributed; they received very little recognition for their accomplishments. Hilkemeyer (1982) stated, "What many of us did was a real struggle to try to get things accomplished, but if we had never done those initial things we wouldn't be where we are today." In the past few years, information has been collected from some of these leaders about the past; unfortunately, some of them have died, and we are too late to learn what they could share with us. However, we take the legacies they left us and move forward. Cancer nursing history is a record of pioneering, a proud heritage.

References

American Society for the Control of Cancer. (1924). *Essential facts about cancer: A handbook for the medical profession.* New York: Author.

American Society for the Control of Cancer. (Ca. 1924–1925). *Its objects and methods and some of the visible results of its work.* New York: Author.

Ash, C.R. (1983). Cancer nursing: An international perspective. *Oncology Nursing Forum, 10*(2), 69–72.

Barckley, V. (1964). Enough time for good nursing. *Nursing Outlook, 12,* 44–48.

Barckley, V. (1967). Crises in cancer. *American Journal of Nursing, 67,* 278–280.

Barckley, V. (1971). Workstudy program in cancer nursing. *Nursing Outlook, 19,* 328–330.

Barckley, V. (1982). The best of times and the worst of times. *Oncology Nursing Forum, 9,* 54–56.

Best, N. (1950). Radiotherapy and the nurse. *American Journal of Nursing, 50,* 140–143.

Biehusen, I. (1956). Cancer nursing is expensive. *Nursing Outlook, 4,* 438–441.

Bouchard, R. (1967). *Nursing care of the cancer patient.* St. Louis: C.V. Mosby Co.

Cockerill, E.E. (1948). The cancer patient as a person. *Public Health Nursing, 40,* 78–83.

The control of cancer. (1919). *American Journal of Nursing, 19,* 293.

Co-operating in cancer nursing education (1949–1950). Brochure from Memorial Hospital and Department of Nursing Education, New York University.

Cowan, M. (1934). Modern cancer nursing. *Trained Nurse, 92,* 243–255.

Craytor, J.K. (1982). Highlights in education for cancer nursing. *Oncology Nursing Forum, 9,* 51–58.

Cumston, C.G. (1900). A new formulae used in surgical nursing. *American Journal of Nursing, 1,* 13–14.

Daland, E.M. (1969). *Pondville hospital 1927–1969.* Walpole, MA: Massachusetts Department of Public Health.

Diller, D. (1957). *An investigation of learning in ninety-one selected schools of nursing* (3rd rep.). New York: Skidmore College.

Donahue, M.P. (1985). *Nursing, the finest art.* St. Louis: C.V. Mosby Co.

Editorial. (1934). *Trained Nurse, 92,* 278–279.

Eaves, L., & Associates. (1928). Nursing cancer patients in their home. *New England Journal of Medicine, 198,* 240–246.

Farrell, M. (1953). Experimentation in teaching cancer nursing. *Nursing Research, 2,* 41.

Ferguson, M. (1948). The public health nurse and the cancer program. *Public Health Nursing, 40,* 343–346.

Fischel, E. (1931). The public health nurse's responsibility in relation to cancer. *Public Health Nurse, 23,* 334–337.

Frei, E. III, Freireich, E.T., Gehan, E., et al. (1961). Studies of sequential and combination antimetabolite therapy in acute leukemia: 6-mercaptopurine and methotrexate. *Blood, 18,* 431–454.

Glienke, F., & Kress, L.C. (1944a). The cancer patient: Giving bedside care in the home. *American Journal of Nursing, 44,* 434–443.

Glienke, F., & Kress, L.C. (1944b). The cancer patient: Planning for and introducing home care. *American Journal of Nursing, 44,* 351–354.

Goodman, L.S., Wintrobe, M.W., Dameshek, W., Goodman, M.J., Gilman, A., & McLennan, M.T. (1946). Nitrogen mustard therapy. Use of methyl-bis (beta-chloroethyl) amine hydrochloride for Hodgkin's disease, lymphosarcoma, leukemia and certain allied and miscellaneous disorders. *Journal American Medical Association, 132,* 126–132.

Greene, P.E. (1983). The Association of Pediatric Oncology Nurses: The first ten years. *Oncology Nursing Forum, 10,* 59–63.

Hammond, B. (1964). Home care improvisations. *Nursing Outlook, 64,* 49–51.

Henke, C. (1980). Emerging roles of the nurse in oncology. *Seminars in Oncology, 7,* 4–8.

Higgenbotham, S. (1957). Arm exercises after mastectomy. *American Journal of Nursing, 12,* 1573–1574.

Hilkemeyer, R. (1974). Cancer nursing: The state of the art. *Proceedings of the National Conference on Cancer Nursing* (pp. 1–6). New York: American Cancer Society.

Hilkemeyer, R. (1982). A historical perspective in cancer nursing. *Oncology Nursing Forum, 9,* 47–56.

Hilkemeyer, R., & Kinney, H. (1956). Teaching cancer nursing. *Nursing Outlook, 4,* 177–180.

Hopp, M. (1941). Roentgen therapy and the nurse. *American Journal of Nursing, 41,* 431–444.

Hubbard, S.M., & Donehower, M.G. (1980). The nurse in a cancer research setting. *Seminars in Oncology, 7,* 9–17.

Kardinal, C.G., & Yarbro, J.W. (1979). A conceptual history of cancer. *Seminars in Oncology, 6,* 396–408.

King, M. (1988). Volunteerism: Still a tradition in America. *Cancer News,* (Winter), 16–18.

Koons, S.B. (1976). Bicentennial forecast: The future of cancer nursing. *RN, 39,* 23–34.

Kramer, M. (1987). Identity in nursing. *ResMedica* (St. Louis, St. John's Mercy Medical Center) *3,* 3–8.

Kübler-Ross, E. (1969). *On death and dying.* New York: Macmillan Company.

Leininger, M. (1977). Roles and directions in nursing and cancer nursing. *Proceedings of the Second National Conference on Cancer Nursing* (pp. 6–16). New York: American Cancer Society.

Leone, L. (1965). The attack on heart disease, cancer and stroke—Is nursing ready. *American Journal of Nursing, 65,* 68–72.

Lewis, F.M., Firsich, S.C., & Parsell, S. (1979). Clinical tool development for adult chemotherapy patients: Process and content. *Cancer Nursing, 2,* 99–108.

Lewison, E.F. (1965). The nurse's role in early detection of cancer of the breast. *Nursing Forum, 4,* 82–86.

Leyshon, V.N. (1966). Taking cervical smears in the home. *Nursings Times, 62,* 361–362.

Lombard, H., & McDonald, E. (1931). Complete records and control of cancer. *Public Health Nursing, 23,* 532–533.

Lynaugh, J.E., & Fagin, C.M. (1988). Nursing comes of age. *Image, 20,* 184–190.

MacVicar, M. (1975). *The effect of cancer in the male spouses on the family.* Unpublished doctoral dissertation. Ohio State University, Columbus.

Marino, L.B. (1976). Cancer patients: Your special role. *Nursing 76, 6,* 25–29.

McCorkle, R., & Young, K. (1978). Development of a symptom distress scale. *Cancer Nursing, 1,* 373–378.

Miller, S.A. (1976). Is oncology nursing the challenge you are looking for? *Nursing 76, 6,* 70–72.

Nelson, K.R. (1959, March 20). Letter to Claire Richmond, Nursing Committee of American Cancer Society.

Nelson, K.R. (1974). The future in cancer nursing. *Proceedings of the National Conference on Cancer Nursing* (pp. 141–145). New York: American Cancer Society.

New use for a kelly pad [Letter to the Editor]. (1916). *American Journal of Nursing, 16,* 536.

Nursing Advisory Committee minutes. (1948a, April 30). New York: American Cancer Society.

Nursing Advisory Committee minutes. (1948b, October 18). New York: American Cancer Society.

Nursing Advisory Committee minutes. (1957, March 13). New York: American Cancer Society.

Nursing Advisory Committee minutes. (1958, October 20). New York: American Cancer Society.

Nursing Advisory Committee minutes. (1960, October 24). New York: American Cancer Society.

Oberst, M. (1978). Priorities in cancer nursing research. *Cancer Nursing, 1,* 281–290.

Oncology Nursing Society and American Nurses' Association. (1979). *Outcome standards for cancer nursing practice.* Kansas City, MO: American Nurses' Association.

Patterson, L. (1948). Cancer institute. *Public Health Nursing, 40,* 83.

Peterson, R. (1948). Public health nursing in the cancer control program of the U.S. Public Health Service. *Public Health Nursing, 40,* 74–77.

Peterson, R. (1951a). Inservice education in cancer nursing. *Public Health Nursing, 43,* 255–258.

Peterson, R. (1951b). Inservice education in cancer nursing. *Public Health Nursing, 43,* 331–333.

Peterson, R. (1951c). Inservice education in cancer nursing. *Public Health Nursing, 43,* 386–389.

Peterson, R. (1956). Federal grants for education in cancer nursing. *Nursing Outlook, 4,* 103–105.

Peterson, R., & Walker, E. (1949). Integrating nursing service. *Hospitals, 23,* 61.

Quint, J. (1963). Impact of mastectomy. *American Journal of Nursing, 53,* 88–92.

Rice, F. (1902). Tumors. *Trained Nurse, 29,* 89–90.

Ross, E. (1928). How can we help in the control of cancer? *Public Health Nursing, 20,* 13–16.

Ross, W. (1987). *Crusade: The official history of the American Cancer Society.* New York: Arbor House.

Scovil, E.R., (1915). The medical aspects of cancer. *American Journal of Nursing, 15,* 855.

Shimkin, M.B. (1977). *Contrary to nature.* (DHEW Publication No. [NIH] 76–720). Washington DC: U.S. Government Printing Office.

Skipper, H.E., Schabel, F.M., & Wilcox, W.S. (1964). Experimental evaluation of potential anticancer agents. XIII. On the criteria and kinetics associated with the "curability" of experimental leukemia. *Cancer Chemotherapy Reports, 35,* 3–11.

Tatterhall, L.M. (1928). Salaries of public health nurses. *Public Health Nurse, 20,* 244–251.

The transmission and cure of cancer. (1907). *American Journal of Nursing, 7,* 200.

Tucker, L.E. (1915). Needed economies for a long case. *American Journal of Nursing, 15,* 293.

Wolf, E.S. (1964). Where hope comes first. *Nursing Outlook, 12,* 52–54.

Wolf, E.S. (1968). Nurse clinician in a specialty hospital. *Nursing Outlook, 16,* 41.

Yarbro, C.H. (1984). The early days: Four smiles and a post office box. *Oncology Nursing Forum, 11,* 79–85.

Zubrod, C.G. (1979). Milestones in curative chemotherapy. *Seminars in Oncology, 6,* 490–505.

CHAPTER 3

Role Implementation in Cancer Nursing

JOYCE M. YASKO

Cancer nursing, a relatively new area of nursing specialization, has many career opportunities. The development of a career is a lifelong process that requires planning, formulating strategies, and networking. Career development has been described as a process that has four stages. These stages are implementing the roles and functions of a specific career; achieving expertise and competence; expanding the roles and functions to include educating others and consulting; and advancing the practice and status of the career role, engaging in research, and influencing others such as the government and public organizations to develop policies and make decisions that will positively influence the role and function of the oncology nurse (Dalton, Thompson, & Price, 1977). One can set as career goals progression through all four stages of career development, or one can decide to remain at stage 2, 3, or 4 or to return to a former stage after having remained for a period of time at a higher stage. The last option is difficult to carry out, however, because of the expectations of others engaged in the same career. This chapter describes the process of oncology nursing career development and role implementation.

DEVELOPING AND IMPLEMENTING THE ROLE OF THE ONCOLOGY NURSE

Concepts of professionalism that must be introduced early in career development in oncology nursing and maintained throughout are that oncology nurses are responsible for achieving and maintaining competence in their chosen area of nursing specialization; that they are responsible for advancing the practice of oncology nursing; and that they are responsible for advocating oncology nurses and nursing to peers, other health professionals, consumers, and the general public. To implement these concepts in the everyday practice of oncology nursing throughout a career, the oncology nurse must acquire the following:

- a knowledge base in oncology nursing
- a practice base in oncology nursing
- a discipline base in oncology nursing
- a knowledge of the trends and organizational issues that influence or affect oncology nursing

Developing a Knowledge Base in Oncology Nursing

A knowledge base in a specific area of specialization can be acquired through

- formal academic educational programs
- continuing education courses or seminars
- independent study
- mentor-protégé relationships
- government and community resources

Academic Education

Participating in formalized academic educational programs is generally the first step in acquiring a knowledge base in nursing. However, content in oncology nursing is not presented in the majority of undergraduate nursing programs in the United States (Brown, 1983). This absence may be the result of the integrated or medical model approach to nursing education or the inadequate numbers of undergraduate faculty prepared in oncology nursing. Ways that oncology nursing can be taught at the undergraduate level are formalized courses, integrated content, and electives in oncology nursing—all with planned clinical experiences. An elective in oncology nursing may be taken along with the basic curriculum or after graduation. Courses of this nature are a comprehensive foundation for specialization in oncology nursing.

In a survey completed in 1981 by Brown and colleagues, it was learned that only 19 per cent of undergraduate nursing programs included formalized courses, clinical experiences, or both in cancer nursing and that if cancer nursing was included in the curriculum, little time was devoted to this content (Brown, 1983). In a study conducted by Mayer and Yasko (1990), a survey of master's prepared oncology nurses revealed that the number of master's programs in oncology nursing has expanded from 13 in 1981 to 45 in 1988. However, the master's prepared nurses who were functioning in faculty roles had fewer formalized educational courses and less clinical experience than those in clinical nursing specialist and nursing administrator roles. The results of this study further illustrate the fact that students are being taught by teachers who have not had academic preparation in oncology nursing. It is unlikely that the trend of inadequate preparation in oncology nursing will be reversed in the near future. A concentrated effort to remedy this present situation must be made. Providing continuing education courses for nursing educators, developing undergraduate electives in oncology nursing, and influencing undergraduate faculty to include oncology nursing content are but a few of the possible actions that can be taken to remedy the present situation.

Continuing Education

Seminars, courses, and programs of variable length and content are available in most geographic areas. Continuing education programs that meet content and evaluation criteria are reviewed and awarded approval for a specified number of content hours by a provider of continuing education in nursing accredited by a regional accrediting committee of the American Nurses' Association. Continuing education courses should be reviewed to determine whether accreditation has been obtained. This is an essential step to ensure quality.

While attending continuing education programs, participants should identify areas of inadequate knowledge and focus their efforts on obtaining the necessary knowledge and incorporating it in their practice of oncology nursing. A Gaps and Contracts methodology can be utilized to ensure that this occurs. During a continuing education program, the nurse identifies gaps between current practices and what is being presented during the program. At the completion of the program, nurses list the gaps identified in order of importance and develop a contract—written or mental—that includes the methods, resources, and time required to incorporate the newly acquired knowledge into their individual practices or the practices of the oncology nurses working in a specific agency (Donovan, Wolpert, & Yasko, 1981).

Continuing education courses or seminars offer an excellent opportunity to learn from those who have advanced competence in oncology nursing. Continuing education programs in oncology nursing served as the formalized introduction to oncology nursing for the majority of those who call themselves oncology nurses today. History reveals that the first formalized oncology nursing educational courses were continuing education programs. In the mid 1970s when oncology nursing was beginning to organize, the National Cancer Institute (NCI) released a request for proposal to develop oncology nursing educational programs. The proposal was designed to include continuing education programs that provided a foundation in oncology nursing, master's programs that provided advanced preparation in oncology nursing, and a continuing education program that focused on the prevention and early detection of cancer and that taught nurses to utilize early detection skills in their practice of oncology nursing. Academic sites throughout the nation were funded to carry out these efforts. The programs that developed as a result of this NCI effort provided a network of educational resources and prepared nurses to care for persons with cancer.

Participating in independent study is an essential ingredient in obtaining a knowledge base in oncology nursing. A number of written and audiovisual educational resources exist in oncology nursing. Written resources include oncology nursing textbooks; curriculum resources; self-learning modules; educational resources developed by pharmaceutical or medical supply companies; articles in refereed journals; journals devoted entirely to oncology nursing; newsletters sponsored by professional organizations and pharmaceutical companies; and educational resources from the Oncology Nursing Society, the NCI, and the American Cancer Society (ACS).

Developing a resource library is an essential component of independent study. Each person has a limited amount of financial resources to allocate to developing a library; therefore, time should be spent reviewing the available resources before purchases are made. Access to a health center or hospital library is also essential for obtaining journals, textbooks, and other educational resources.

Independent study is essential to achieve and maintain competence in oncology nursing. A knowledge explosion is occurring in cancer research and cancer nursing. Only through consistent, disciplined independent study will a comprehensive knowledge base be achieved and maintained.

Access to a Mentor

A mentor is needed throughout a professional career. A mentor is a professional nurse who has expertise in oncology nursing and who is willing to share that expertise with others—someone who is interested in helping other nurses become the best that they can be. A mentor does not compete but rather takes pleasure in seeing others be and become. Every professional needs a mentor throughout a professional career, a mentor who will give positive and negative feedback; pave the way for opportunities to occur; and offer unconditional support, advice, and counsel. The goal of a mentor-protégé relationship is to help the protégé reach the level of the mentor faster than the mentor and with less difficulty. One outgrows specific mentors but never the need for a mentor.

Mentor-protégé relationships rarely just happen; they must be initiated, developed, and cultivated. Nurses must identify potential mentors who exemplify the kind of oncology nurse that they would like to emulate. They then communicate their perceptions to the would-be mentors; ask if they would be willing to support, teach, and counsel; and then foster the relationship by giving the mentors feedback on how the information provided has been utilized and what outcomes have been achieved. It is important for nurses to acknowledge their mentors as they achieve their goals and to multiply the benefits received by becoming mentors to other nurses who have less knowledge, experience, or both. Becoming mentors to oncology nurses is one of the most effective ways to advance the practice of oncology nursing. This process is both a professional right and a responsibility.

Government and Community Agencies

Government and community agencies are a major source of educational resources and opportunities for the development of a knowledge base. Examples of agencies that produce a variety of written resources, support groups, educational services, and opportunities are the following:

- American Cancer Society: national, state, and local units. The ACS provides continuing education programs and written resources for health professionals, patients and families, and the public. Scholarships for graduate education (master's and doctoral programs) are also available, as are professorships in oncology nursing. A local unit can be contacted for information.
- National Cancer Institute: Cancer centers and cancer information services funded by the NCI are valuable resources. The nearest cancer information center can be reached by calling 1-800-4-CANCER. This service provides information on cancer pathology, prevention, early detection, treatment and rehabilitation, and community resources, as well as information on how to effectively utilize the health care system.
- Cancer centers, university health systems, and community hospitals also provide educational seminars and on-site clinical experiences. Each community also has local resources such as Make Today Count, the Ostomy Association, and others. These resources are usually listed in the telephone directory or are available through the social services depart-

ment of local hospitals. See Chapter 83 for additional information on government and community resources.

The key factors in developing and maintaining a comprehensive knowledge base in oncology nursing are to utilize as many educational resources as possible, capture every teachable moment, learn from those who have gone before, be consistent and thorough, and never stop learning. There is no substitute for a comprehensive knowledge base. Without it one cannot achieve competence as a oncology nurse or enter advanced practice roles. The time, effort, and money expended to develop and maintain a comprehensive knowledge base are sound investments in one's career.

Developing a Practice Base

Nursing is a practice discipline; therefore, bridging the gap between knowledge and practice is essential. Building a practice base can be accomplished by utilizing several methods.

Incorporate what has been learned in the classroom, in independent study, or in other ways in the practice setting. It is not enough just to know; what has been learned must be incorporated and utilized in one's practice of oncology nursing. Only then can patients and families, other oncology nurses, and health professionals benefit from what the nurse has learned. A contract method is often an effective way to facilitate this process. Once practice gaps or deficits have been identified, the deficits must be listed according to their importance and a contract developed that includes a description of the deficit, the reason the deficit received a high priority score, the methods to be utilized to remedy the deficit, the resources needed, and the time needed to convert the practice deficit into a consistent practice pattern. A strategy such as this formalizes the process of changing practice patterns (Donovan, Wolpert, & Yasko, 1981).

Developing mentor-protégé relationships in the practice setting can teach practice skills and patterns as well as a knowledge base. Teaching others the unique role of nursing on the health care team and learning to function as a member of an interdisciplinary health care team are important goals to reach in developing the practice base of nursing. Because members of different disciplines are not educated together, they must learn to function in an interdisciplinary fashion in the practice setting. To be effective in this role, the oncology nurse must have a strong sense of what oncology nursing is and what it is not. In any interdisciplinary interaction, each discipline has clear areas of responsibility and areas in which its responsibilities overlap with those of other disciplines. The oncology nurse must have the ability to negotiate with members of other disciplines so that nursing practice is not diffused and fragmented and oncology nurses do not assume responsibility for practices that should be implemented by one or several of the other disciplines.

Patients and families who are experiencing the diagnosis or treatment of cancer can teach what they have learned to others, especially to the oncology nurses who are caring for them. Patients and families can teach the coping strategies that are necessary to live with a diagnosis of cancer, the patterns of symptoms that are experienced as a result of cancer or cancer treatment, the interventions that are undertaken to manage symptoms related to cancer and cancer treatment, and the effectiveness of community-based resources for cancer care. Listen and hear what they say. Living with cancer can teach those experiencing it things that cannot be learned any other way. Listen and allow them to teach.

Cancer nursing has many areas of clinical practice: radiation therapy; surgical oncology; medical oncology, including chemotherapy and biologic response modifiers; outpatient services; home care; hospice; inpatient hospital care; physician office care; and many more. To have a well-rounded practice base, a variety of clinical experiences are necessary. The oncology nurse should plan to spend several years in each needed area. Experience, coupled with the foundation of a sound knowledge base, is the best teacher. One cannot acquire expertise in a practice discipline without strong clinical experiences that consistently build on one another.

Developing a Discipline Base in Oncology Nursing

To become an advocate for persons with cancer and their families, for oncology nurses, and for nursing, one must acquire a strong nursing discipline base. Strength as a discipline provides status and power that can be utilized to obtain resources to advance the practice of oncology nursing and to improve that which is available to persons with cancer and their families. This can be achieved in several ways.

Becoming aware of the scope of the nurse practice act is important. Reading the act will reveal what the citizens of the state expect of professional nurses. Also, making contact with the state board of nurse examiners who oversee the practice act is a step toward learning the issues and trends that face nurses in each state.

The nurse practice act is a clear statement of the scope of nursing practice that the state legally approves for all persons with the credentials of registered nurse. Most practice acts include assessment; diagnosis; interventions in the form of measures to maintain nutritional status, sleep and rest patterns, comfort, safety, skin cleanliness and integrity, psychological well-being, mobility, and respiratory, cardiac, and renal functions; evaluation of the interventions utilized; health teaching and counseling; coordination of care; and implementation of the plan of treatment prescribed by a licensed physician or dentist. As described by the nurse practice act, the role of nursing is both autonomous and interdependent.

An example of when the nurse practice act or the state board of nursing needs to be consulted is when agencies attempt to fragment nursing practice by making policies that assign certain components of nursing practice such as teaching and counseling to other disciplines. For nursing to be holistic in its approach to caring for the psychological and physiological aspects of care and for actual and potential health care problems, all aspects must be included in the plan of care. It is the nurse's responsibility to coordinate the care by either intervening or referring to others for intervention and seeing that the required interventions are carried out. The practice act and board also should be consulted when nurses are asked to perform new technical procedures that customarily had been carried out by physicians. As the health care system has increased in size and complexity, the scope and responsibility of nursing has also increased. History reveals that simple procedures such as obtaining a blood pressure measurement or initiating an intravenous infusion previously could be done only by a physician. These aspects of care are now incorporated into nursing programs and are accepted aspects of nursing practice. Professional practice is in a constant state of change, and oncology nurses should be in touch with the present status of their scope of practice.

It is important to join professional organizations such as the American Nurses' Association and the state nurses' association, the Oncology Nursing Society and one of its local chapters, and the International Society of Nurses in Cancer Care. Other options are the local unit of the American Cancer Society or the other cancer-related organizations in the immediate geographic area. Most of these organizations also have journals or other literature and professional meetings or seminars that can be used to make contact with other nurses involved in cancer care. Working with other oncology nurses on issues, standards, and problems common to all nurses is an excellent way to increase knowledge about cancer, cancer nursing, and the trends and issues that have an actual or potential impact on oncology nursing; to develop mentor-protégé relationships; and to advance the practice of oncology nursing.

Each nurse should develop a personal philosophy of oncology nursing and a positive concept of the unique and essential role of oncology nurses. A philosophy of nursing is a person's prescribed beliefs about what oncology nursing is and what it is not. It is necessary for an oncology nurse to be in touch with personal beliefs because these beliefs form the foundation of practice. If a nurse believes that oncology nursing is holistic in nature and includes physiologic as well as psychological care but agency policy states that psychological care is to be referred to other disciplines, or if providing psychological care is not rewarded or viewed as important by the nurse's peers or agency, then a conflict will occur between personal beliefs about the practice of oncology nursing and actual practice on a daily basis. These conflicts can cause discomfort, dissatisfaction, and burnout in the work environment. Many researchers have described burnout as unfulfilled job expectations—when what the individual thought a job would be differs from what it actually is (Dolan, 1987; McElroy, 1982); in other words, a person's philosophy of care cannot be fulfilled in the work environment. An exercise that will help to clarify personal beliefs and values is to write a philosophy of oncology nursing by completing the sentence "I believe oncology nursing is. . . ." Once written, the philosophy can be a method of keeping in touch with one's beliefs. A philosophy can be altered or expanded as one's scope of knowledge and experience grows.

Knowing one's beliefs and values about nursing, cancer nursing, and the role of the nurse is essential for consistency in the practice of oncology nursing and appropriate behavior in the advocacy of nursing and nurses' concerns. It is important to determine whether one's philosophy of oncology nursing is compatible with that of one's employing organization, one's supervisor, and one's peers. Nurses should use every teachable moment to explain and illustrate their beliefs and values about oncology nursing and about the care of persons with cancer. These beliefs should be related by words and actions to patients, peers, supervisors, and all those with whom one interacts while engaged in the practice of oncology nursing.

Developing a Knowledge Base in Trends and Issues

The health care system is undergoing rapid and dramatic changes as it converts from a service to a business orientation. Oncology nurses must be aware of economics, reimbursement, and encroachment issues so that proactive problem solving rather than reactive crisis intervention can occur. To keep in touch with current trends and issues, read the health section of magazines such as *Time* and *Newsweek,* the daily newspaper, and the trends and issues sections of professional journals. Belonging to professional organizations also puts one in contact with important issues.

Because the health care system of the future will be driven by governmental regulations, it is important to become active politically. This can be accomplished in several ways:

1. Get to know state and national senators and representatives. Learn their voting record on health-related issues and their health care goals.

2. Inform state and federal senators and representatives about personal beliefs regarding health care needs. Write letters to legislators to describe these beliefs and goals, health care deficits and problems experienced with the present system, and ideas for resolving these deficits or problems.

3. Communicate a willingness to support the proposed beliefs and to identify ways to help the senator or representative be reelected. Contributing to a re-election campaign is an important way to demonstrate support. Oncology nursing can have a great influence on the health care system through political involvement. Refer to Chapters 78 and 82 for more information on the process of becoming politically involved.

PROGRESSING TOWARD ADVANCED PRACTICE

Certification as an Oncology Nurse

Certification is a credential used by the health professions to communicate that a person has the knowledge and experience to care for a specific patient population. The requirement for certification in oncology nursing communicates to the public, patient and family consumers, and other health professionals that specialized knowledge and clinical experience are needed to care safely and effectively for persons with cancer. When a nurse obtains certification via the Oncology Nursing Certification Corporate Examination, it communicates that the nurse has the knowledge and experience to care for persons with cancer and has the privilege of using the OCN (oncology certified nurse) credential. Certification examinations are offered several times each year by the Educational Testing Service of Princeton, New Jersey. Information regarding eligibility criteria and location of testing sites can be obtained by contacting the Oncology Nursing Certification Corporation, 1016 Greentree Road, Pittsburgh, PA 15220-3125.

Advanced Practice

Progressing to the advanced practice of oncology nursing usually occurs as a result of increased knowledge, a sound practice base, and advanced (master's or doctoral level) educational preparation. In addition to providing an advanced knowledge base, a graduate level educational program also provides preparation in the theoretic basis of nursing practice; the trends and issues that have an actual or potential impact on nursing; the process of nursing research; and the theories that influence advanced nursing practice, such as conflict, role, change, stress, learning, organizational management, and system theories. When progressing to the advanced level of practice in oncology nursing, the nurse assumes additional professional responsibilities. These responsibilities include the following:

- Engaging in activities that advance the practice of oncology nursing
- Educating patients, families, health professionals, and the public
- Providing or directing and evaluating the nursing care of persons with cancer and their significant others
- Developing, implementing, and evaluating health care programs
- Developing and implementing a lifelong career in oncology nursing (University of Pittsburgh, 1988; Yasko & Dudjak, 1988).

Advancing the practice of oncology nursing can be achieved in the following manner:

- Implementing change in nursing practice through the utilization of role, conflict, learning, systems, and change theory and the analysis of the structure and function of the organizational system

- Keeping abreast of changing trends and issues and recognizing the impact of these trends and issues on oncology nursing practice
- Developing, implementing, and evaluating standards of care, policies, and procedures that will enhance the nursing care of persons with cancer and the lives of their significant others
- Determining nursing care resources for optimal care based on patient and family needs
- Communicating effectively, verbally or in writing, with interdisciplinary and intradisciplinary health care team members and groups within and outside the employing agency
- Providing consultation for nurses, health professionals, and agency administrators to enhance the care of patients and significant others
- Identifying researchable problems in clinical nursing practice
- Analyzing research studies and implementing valid findings in clinical practice
- Collaborating with others in designing and implementing research investigations
- Writing clinical papers and research studies for publication
- Presenting findings learned through clinical practice or research to audiences of health care professionals
- Facilitating the process of ethical decision making in the practice setting
- Functioning as an advocate to improve the status, power, and autonomy of the consumers of health care

Educating nurses, health professionals, and the public can be achieved by doing the following:

- Identifying the needs of nurses and other health care professionals in the practice setting
- Planning, implementing, and evaluating educational programs for nurses and other health care professionals to facilitate their ability to provide optimal care for patients and significant others
- Serving as a role model for nurses
- Identifying the learning needs of patients, significant others, and the public
- Planning, implementing, and evaluating educational programs and written educational resources for patients, significant others, and the public

Providing, directing, and evaluating optimal nursing care can be achieved by doing the following:

- Assessing and documenting the physical, psychological, and social characteristics of each patient and family
- Evaluating the effect of the pathophysiologic process on the patient and family
- Providing or directing and evaluating the optimal physical care of the patient, managing the symptoms related to the pathology or the management of the pathology, and providing optimal psychological sup-

port and health counseling for the patient and significant others

- Facilitating the achievement and maintenance of optimal life-style patterns such as those of nutritional habits, sleep and rest, coping, elimination, sexual and reproductive activities, comfort, and exercise and mobility
- Effectively teaching the patient and significant others what they should know regarding the pathology, the plan of care, and the plan for self-care
- Coordinating the plan of care to facilitate the effectiveness of the health care system
- Serving as a liaison among acute, ambulatory, and home care through the preparation of patients and significant others for admission to and discharge from health care settings
- Identifying and utilizing appropriate community resources to facilitate care for patients and significant others
- Implementing or directing the implementation of the medical plan of diagnosis and treatment
- Functioning as a advocate for patients and significant others

Developing, implementing, and evaluating health care programs and models or systems of health care delivery in a variety of clinical settings can be achieved by taking the following actions:

- Identifying and documenting the need for the health care program or the model or system of health care delivery
- Developing the program or system within the confines of health care policy or legislation
- Developing and conducting the program or system in a fiscally responsible manner
- Collaborating with others to secure funds for program development
- Marketing the program to the community
- Utilizing the capabilities of computers within the agency and facilitating the development of computer programs to improve patient and family care
- Functioning as an advocate for the employing agency

Developing and implementing a lifelong career in oncology nursing can be achieved by doing the following:

- Continuing to develop and expand clinical, technical, and functional knowledge and skills
- Seeking mentorship for self and providing mentorship for others
- Networking effectively with nurses, health professionals, and consumers
- Developing effective self- and peer evaluation strategies
- Functioning as an advocate for nursing and for advanced nursing practice

The specific advanced practice role that an oncology nurse is implementing determines the emphasis that is placed on the responsibilities associated with advanced practice. It is the rare person who will develop expertise in all areas of advanced nursing practice. It takes the combined efforts of many advanced practice oncology nurses throughout their careers to fulfill the described responsibilities.

Advanced Practice Roles and Responsibilities

As described earlier, careers have four stages of development. Entry into a career includes acquiring the knowledge and skills to function in a safe manner, practicing in the role for a period of time, and being viewed by self and others as displaying expertise in the practice of oncology nursing. Knowing how to assess and to identify needs or problems, being able to set priorities to individualize needs, implementing or directing the implementation of care, and evaluating and determining alternate interventions are part of the second phase of achieving expertise and competence. The oncology nurse at this time also serves as a mentor to other nurses, teaching them what has been learned through experience. This is the advanced practice role of clinician, also described as primary nurse, care manager, nurse practitioner, and private practitioner when the primary focus is the direct care of persons with cancer and their families. This categorization does not mean that a nurse at this stage of career development does not engage in activities associated with advanced practice responsibilities; it means that the focus of the efforts of these nurses who have achieved expertise in oncology nursing is providing or directing the provision of care to persons in their caseload who have cancer. It not only benefits persons with cancer and the family members if these nurses remain at this level of career development, but also it actually benefits oncology nursing as a profession.

The next level of career development is influencing others to provide an advanced level of practice to persons with cancer and their families. This level of career development includes the educators in academic and practice settings; the traditional practice setting administrators as well as the product line managers who are responsible for developing, implementing, and evaluating the oncology program of a particular agency; and the nursing researchers. These individuals, in addition to their functional role, focus on advancing oncology nursing practice through research, publication, and presentation. They are influencing the knowledge base of oncology nursing theory and practice, which has an impact on oncology nursing practice in clinical settings and on the discipline of oncology nursing through efforts exerted in professional and community organizations. These advanced practice oncology nurses focus their efforts on helping the advanced practice clinicians to obtain the knowledge and resources they need to provide the best possible care to persons with cancer and their families.

Oncology nurses can remain at this level of career development throughout their careers, return to the level of advanced practice clinician, or move to the fourth stage of career development: influencing others outside the discipline of oncology nursing to develop policies and provide resources to facilitate the advancement of oncology nursing practice. These oncology nurses become politically involved, sit on boards of various organizations and institutions, develop proposals and white papers, and become advocates for oncology nurses and oncology nursing at every possible opportunity. Again, it does not mean that these nurses are not involved in activities associated with the second and third levels of career development; it means that influencing others is now the focus of their career efforts. Just as with the previously described levels of career development, oncology nurses can remain at the fourth level or can return to the second or third level to focus their efforts.

Strategies for Developing and Maintaining a Career

Regardless of the level of career development that one hopes to achieve, strategies must be learned and utilized. Developing a career is similar to playing a game of chess; one plans strategies, takes risks, takes action based on planned strategies, and has patience to allow the well-planned actions to be realized. The career development strategies discussed are the following:

- Develop and maintain a vision of oncology nursing that is grounded in a personal philosophy of care
- Formulate career goals, both short term and long term
- Maintain a professional image
- Develop professional relationships
- Advocate for the patient population, self, role, employing agency, and oncology nursing

Each nurse should develop and maintain a vision of oncology nursing that is grounded in a personal philosophy of cancer care. What would you like to see oncology nursing become by the end of your career? What will be your unique contribution or contributions to oncology nursing? How central is your vision to the vision of the leadership in this area of specialization? Have you taken into consideration emerging trends and issues that have the potential to influence oncology nursing? Centrality and uniqueness are aspects that generally ensure acceptance of one's ideas and contributions. A vision gives one direction throughout career development. It gives a purpose to work and provides a future to the practice of oncology nursing. It is what keeps the nurse dissatisfied about what is and enthusiastic about what can be.

A vision of what one would like oncology nursing practice to be may or may not be accomplished in the course of a career. To initiate the process of actualizing a personal vision, nurses should set short-term and long-term career goals. These goals should be put in writing and referred to periodically to determine the progress that has been made in reaching them. Goals are rarely reached by a single action or in a short period of time. They take effort, resources, and time to accomplish. They provide short-term direction. As an exercise, nurses can list the goals to be accomplished by the end of their careers and then list 1-yr, 5-yr, and 10-yr goals that will facilitate reaching these career goals. The list should include the necessary resources and the time anticipated to accomplish the goals. These goals are evolving and can be altered during a periodic assessment. Also, the nurse should take time to experience the good feeling that accomplishment of goals brings and recall the accomplishment often to maximize the benefits that can result from experiencing good feelings.

Developing and consistently portraying a professional image is an important component of career development. Nurses must communicate their attitudes, beliefs, and values so that others will learn who they are and what they stand for. There is no substitute for competence, and competence can be achieved only through considerable effort and resource expenditure in creating a professional image. The nurse's communications should be consistent, and sufficient effort should be put forth so that others will perceive this competence and credibility in the implementation of specific roles within oncology nursing. A nurse not only is developing and portraying an image as an oncology nurse but also is functioning as a representative of oncology nursing as a discipline. The perceptions others develop about individual nurses may be generalized to the discipline as a whole.

Considerable time and effort should be devoted to establishing professional relationships throughout the process of career development. Working with other people to achieve goals is a skill worth developing. One quickly learns that goals are usually accomplished through the joint efforts of many people working in concert. Oncology nurses have the opportunity to develop professional relationships with many individuals at a variety of levels. First and foremost, professional relationships must be developed with patients and their significant others. In the process of establishing these relationships, nurses must communicate who they are, their unique role in the health care system, and what the patient and family can expect from engaging in relationships with them. In a recently conducted study, it was learned that within 1 yr of their diagnosis, the majority of persons with cancer could not identify by name a nurse who had ever cared for them (Houts, Yasko, Benham Kahn, Schelzel, & Marconi, 1986). This is an embarrassment to oncology nursing and a situation that must be rectified through consistent communication with patients and families. Patients and families can become effective advocates for oncology nursing by communicating with agency administrators, editors of newspapers, state and federal legislators, and the general public about the worth and value of oncology nursing.

Intradisciplinary or collegial relationships are essential for peer support and for mentor-protégé interactions. Nurses historically have not been socialized to form networks and peer relationships. Open, honest communication about strengths, weaknesses, issues,

needs, and problems will initiate the give-and-take relationships that build strong networks for the sharing of knowledge, skills, resources, and opportunities within as well as outside the employing agency. Nurses need other nurses to learn and to receive support for strategic planning and to expand the status and autonomy of nursing.

Interdisciplinary Relationships

Building interdisciplinary relationships is essential if the health disciplines are to work as a team. Teamwork does not just happen; it is based on trust in, respect for, and dependence on team members and the realization that the whole team is more efficient and effective than any one of its parts. Each discipline has a unique role to play, and it is the responsibility of members of that discipline to communicate to other team members a description of that role so that the expectations of team members will be grounded in reality. Often there are grey areas in which no one has official responsibility but which several team members want to claim as their responsibility; sometimes just the opposite occurs, and no one on the team wants to take responsibility for these grey areas. When this situation occurs, open negotiation with team members should occur so that expectations will be consistent and all responsibilities will be accounted for. Building relationships with members of other disciplines also provides a source of knowledge, support, and acceptance. The greater the amount of interdisciplinary communication and intervention, the greater will become the awareness, understanding, and acceptance of the role and responsibilities of oncology nursing.

Developing relationships with individuals holding administrative positions, such as chief executive officers, fiscal officers, and others within the employing agency, is essential if oncology nurses are to be involved, understood, and allowed to grow and develop. Oncology nurses must take every opportunity to communicate with individuals in administrative roles about the needs of persons with cancer and their families, the resources that are needed to provide an optimal level of care, and the methods to recruit and retain qualified oncology nurses. Oncology nurses can assist the administrative staff in meeting the goals they have set for the employing agency. They should not wait to be invited to participate. Nurses can join together and submit written proposals to develop programs, to decrease the cost of care, to improve the efficiency and effectiveness of care, and to recruit and retain qualified nurses. It is beneficial to develop an attitude of working with administration personnel to accomplish agency goals and to teach them and demonstrate for them how oncology nurses can assist them in the process. This strategy not only will facilitate the acceleration of the power and status of oncology nursing within the agency but also will assist in the process of promoting this attitude in administrators nationally.

Community Relationships

The community and the people it serves must be a focus of communication for oncology nurses. Hearing the needs of the community, facilitating the development of programs to meet these needs, and becoming a valued community resource will provide acceptance, support, and resources when needed. The public must become aware of the role and responsibilities of oncology nurses and must see some evidence of the impact that this profession can make on the community. Prevention, early detection, symptom management, and rehabilitation programs are excellent community resources that can be developed and implemented by oncology nurses through employing agencies or community organizations such as the American Cancer Society. Nurses should develop contacts with the media (radio, television, press) so that cancer programs and oncology nursing will get media attention and publicity. This will greatly facilitate the development of public opinion about nurses and nursing as a discipline.

The opinions expressed by the public about oncology nurses and nursing care also influence legislators on the local, state, and national levels about the worth and value of nursing in the health care system. Legislators also need to be made aware of the strengths and weaknesses of the present health care system through written proposals and verbal communication on how the health care system can be improved. Ways of communicating and developing relationships with legislators are discussed in this chapter as well as in Chapter 82.

SUMMARY

Developing and maintaining meaningful professional relationships ensures consistent career development.

Remember that it is not only what you know but whom you know and who knows you that will open doors of opportunity that otherwise could not be opened.

Advocating for the patient population, for oneself as an oncology nurse, for other oncology nurses, for the oncology programs of one's employing agency, and for oncology nursing as a discipline is an essential ingredient for career development and a responsibility of professional nurses.

References

Brown, J. K. (1983). Survey of cancer nursing education in U.S. schools of nursing. *Oncology Nursing Forum, 10*(4), 82–83.

Dalton, C., Thompson, P., & Price, R. (1977, Summer). *Organizational Dynamics.* AMACOM, A Division of the American Management Associates.

Dolan, N. (1987). The relationship between burnout and job satisfaction in nurses. *Journal of Advanced Nursing, 12*, 3–12.

Donovan, M. L., Wolpert, P., & Yasko, J. (1981). Gaps and contracts: An evaluation strategy. *Nursing Outlook, 29*, 467–471.

Houts, P. S., Yasko, J., Benham Kahn, S., Schelzel, G. W., & Marconi, K. M. (1986). Psychological, social and economic needs of persons with cancer. *Cancer, 58*, 2355–2361.

Mayer, D., & Yasko, J. (1990). *Burnout in oncology administration educators and clinical nursing specialists.* Manuscript submitted for publication.

McElroy, A. (1982). Burnout—a review of the literature with application to cancer nursing. *Cancer Nursing, 5*, 211–217.

University of Pittsburgh. (1988). *Competencies of the graduate of the University of Pennsylvania graduate program in medical-surgical nursing.*

Yasko, J. (1983). Survey of oncology clinical nursing specialists. *Oncology Nursing Forum, 10*(1), 25–30.

Yasko, J., & Dudjak, L. (1988). The emerging role of the oncology clinical nursing specialist. In N. Chaska (Ed.), *The nursing profession.* St. Louis: C. V. Mosby Co.

CONCEPTUAL THEMES BASIC TO CANCER NURSING

Ethics and Cancer Care

SARA T. FRY

The nursing care of the cancer patient necessarily involves questions of ethics. When caring for a patient with terminal cancer, the nurse must confront individual values concerning death, the process of dying, and the allocation of health care resources to someone who will inevitably die. In addition, the nurse must consider the values of the patient, of significant family members, and of other members of the health care team concerning these issues.

The consideration of values in health care falls within the realm of ethics because value orientations usually provide the foundations for our judgments of what is good or right in nursing practice (Veatch & Fry, 1987). In this chapter, traditional nursing values are analyzed for ways that they support a distinctive nursing ethic.

Fundamental ethical principles that apply to all human relationships in general and to nurse-patient relationships in particular provide the framework for this analysis. These principles are defined and discussed in terms of their application to the nursing care of the cancer patient. Potential conflicts among these principles in the assessment, planning, implementation, and evaluation of nursing care to the cancer patient are also discussed.

Finally, the priority of ethical principles within a decision-making framework are presented as one approach to practical ethics in the care of the cancer patient (Jameton, 1984). Although several approaches to decision making can be used to resolve questions of ethics in health care, the value dimensions of nursing and the uniqueness of the nurse-patient relationship must be taken into consideration before using any approach in nursing. It is to these concerns that we now turn.

VALUES IN PATIENT CARE

In the practice of nursing, the nurse makes countless decisions about patient care. Each decision requires the combination of a wide range of facts and a set of values to determine what ought to be done to help the patient meet his or her health needs (Veatch & Fry, 1987). The facts are derived from many sources. Consideration of the facts alone, however, seldom leads to a decision about the morality of a particular nursing intervention. To reach a decision about what is morally right or wrong in nursing practice, the nurse must combine relevant facts with a set of values.

Identifying Moral Values

Some values that we hold are nonmoral in nature; other values are moral. Nonmoral values are usually related to personal preferences, beliefs, or matters of taste (Frankena, 1973). Moral values, in contrast, are those we ascribe to human actions, institutions, or character traits. They have certain distinctive characteristics that set them apart from nonmoral values (Beauchamp, 1982). First, moral values are *ultimate,* meaning that other values cannot, as a rule, override them. Second, they have a *universal* quality that generally applies to everyone. Third, they are *prescriptive* and guide actions rather than merely describe them. Fourth, moral values refer to aspects of human flourishing or have an *other-regarding focus.*

Values that have these characteristics sometimes conflict with one another. Thus any decision made in nursing practice based on a set of values potentially involves a moral conflict (Veatch & Fry, 1987). Nurses must sometimes decide between protecting confidentiality or violating it to provide some good to a patient. At other times, nurses may need to choose whether to protect the patient's self-determined choices or to override these choices to benefit other identified patients. In each situation, the nurse must first identify the values important to the decision and then make a decision based on the priority or importance of one value over the other.

Important Moral Values

The preamble to the American Nurses' Association *Code for Nurses with Interpretive Statements* (hereafter *Code for Nuses*) states that "A code of ethics makes explicit the primary . . . values of the profession" (1985, p. i). This means that any discussion of values related to cancer care would be inadequate without reference to the professional code of ethics and the values that it mentions as fundamental to nursing practice. The primary values contained in the *Code for Nurses* are the values of *respect for persons, advocacy,* and *accountability.*

Respect for Persons

To respect persons is to respect another individual as someone who shares the same human destiny as oneself (Fry, 1987a). To respect self-determined choice is to respect choice as one way for an individual to realize his or her destiny, even though a person may realize this destiny through other means as well. Thus respect for persons is a broader value than respect for autonomy. Respect for autonomy cannot apply to patients who are not capable of acting autonomously. In other words, the nurse must rely on the value of respect for persons rather than respect for autonomy if the patient under care is a young child or is comatose, severely mentally retarded, or mentally ill. It is a fundamental value that supports specific ethical principles such as justice and autonomy.

In the *Code for Nurses,* it is noted that respect for persons is fundamental to all principles of ethics for the nurse. In fact, the first point of the *Code for Nurses* states that "the nurse provides services with respect for human dignity and the uniqueness of the client, unrestricted by considerations of social or economic status, personal attributes, or the nature of health problems" (1985, p. 2). It is fundamental to other values in the code.

Advocacy

A second moral value important to patient care is advocacy. Advocacy is defined as the active support of an important cause (Fry, 1987a) and is often used in a legal context to refer to the defense of basic human rights on behalf of those who cannot speak for themselves. For example, many institutions employ patient advocates who are expected to defend and speak for patients who cannot by virtue of hospitalization or diminished autonomy as a result of illness voice their own concerns or choices or assert their rights. The role of the advocate is, therefore, to assert the patient's choices or desires in the way that a lawyer presents a client's case, pleads for an interpretation of the case, and defends a client's rights in the case.

The value of advocacy has several interpretations in the nursing literature (Fry, 1987a). One interpretation (the rights-protection model) views the nurse as the defender of patients' rights against an impersonal health care system. The nurse informs the patient of his or her rights, makes sure that the patient understands these rights, reports infringements of the patient's rights, and is responsible for ameliorating infringements and preventing further violations of rights.

A second interpretation (the values-based decision model) views the nurse as the person who helps the patient discuss needs, interests, and choices that will be consistent with values, life style, or personal plan of action (Fry, 1987a). The nurse does not impose decisions or values on the patient but helps the patient explore the advantages and disadvantages of available options to make decisions most consistent with personal beliefs and values.

A third interpretation (the respect for persons model) views the patient as possessing certain human characteristics that require respect (Fry, 1987a). The patient's human dignity is respected and advocated regardless of whether the patient is self-determining or autonomous. As advocate, the nurse keeps the basic human values of the patient foremost and acts to protect the patient's human dignity, privacy, and choices (when applicable). When the patient is not self-determining, the nurse advocates the patient's welfare as defined by the patient when he or she was still self-determining or as defined by the surrogate decision maker. When no other person defines the welfare of the patient, the nurse promotes the interests of the patient to the best of his or her nursing ability. In this role, the nurse assumes responsibility for the manner in which the patient's human dignity and other significant human values have been protected during illness and is accountable to society and other members of the nursing profession for the way this important advocate role has been carried out.

This interpretation of advocacy seems to be consistent with the value of respect for persons in the *Code for Nurses.* Indeed, the code describes advocacy as acting so as "to safeguard the client and the public when health care and safety are affected by incompetent, unethical, or illegal practice by any person" (1985, p. 6). This view of advocacy demonstrates the correlative role of accountability as the third value fundamental to nursing practice.

Accountability

The moral value of accountability is defined as answerability for the way one has promoted, protected, and met the health needs of the patient (Fry, 1987b). It means to justify or to "give an account," according to accepted moral standards or norms, of choices and actions that the nurse has made and carried out. It involves a relationship between the nurse and other parties and is contractual. The nurse is an agent who has entered into an agreement to perform services and can be held answerable for performing them according to agreed-on terms.

The terms of *legal accountability* are contained in licensing procedures and state nurse practice acts. The terms of *moral accountability* are contained in the professional code of ethics and other standards of nursing practice in the form of norms set by the members of the profession.

In the *Code for Nurses*, it is noted that accountability means "providing an explanation or rationale" for what has been done in the nursing role (1985, p. 8). It is a very important value of nursing that cannot be superseded by the physician's orders or the employing agency's policies. Thus it seems to be the foundational value on which the values of respect for persons and advocacy find sustenance in nursing. Accountability is the value that helps define the relationships among patient, nurse, and public and is broadly articulated by the professional ethic. As a final point, it sustains the moral dimensions of the nurse-patient relationship and the tradition of nursing, providing both the practice of nursing and the social role of nursing with its necessary historical content.

ETHICAL PRINCIPLES FOR NURSING PRACTICE

The ability to recognize values and conflicts among values in nursing care situations is fundamental to the analysis of ethical issues in cancer nursing care. When used with knowledge of the professional code of ethics, this ability becomes part of the nurse's decision-making framework for specific case situations in cancer care. In using this framework, the nurse appeals to various rules, principles, and even theories to make moral choices or to carry out moral actions (Beauchamp & Childress, 1989). The most important component of this appeal process is the principles that generally serve as moral guides for action or choice. Those principles generally recognized as important to nursing care relationships are (1) beneficence, (2) justice, (3) autonomy, (4) veracity, (5) avoiding killing, and (6) fidelity (Veatch & Fry, 1987).

Beneficence

The principle of beneficence states that "we ought to do good and prevent or avoid doing harm" (Fran-

kena, 1973, p. 45). This principle means that nurses are morally obligated to help others gain what is of benefit to them by reducing risks of harm and are even obligated to provide positive benefits to patients in terms of goods or assets.

The application of this principle in nursing practice often involves making difficult decisions. For example, the nurse is often uncertain whether this obligation means that all the ways in which the patient might be benefited must be considered. The *Code for Nurses* points out that the nurse's primary commitment is to the patient's health, welfare, and safety. This commitment is a substantial one and seems to include a great deal of beneficence! Yet the nurse might not really have the ability to provide *all* benefits to the patient, particularly those related to his or her welfare. Some benefits to patients might simply lie outside the expertise or competency of the nurse.

A second problem in applying this principle is deciding whether the obligation to provide benefit has a higher priority than the obligation to avoid harm. Some ethicists have claimed that the duty to avoid harm is a stronger obligation in health care relationships than the obligation to benefit (Beauchamp & Childress, 1989; Ross, 1939). If the obligation to avoid harm is stronger in nursing, nurses could fulfill the obligation of avoiding harm to patients by simply doing nothing for them. Would we consider this type of nursing care acceptable? I doubt it. However, if the avoidance of harm is balanced by the provision of benefit, then some agreements on the acceptable ranges of benefit and harm should be established.

A third problem with trying to apply this principle in nursing practice concerns the limits of providing benefit to patients (Veatch & Fry, 1987). Is the nurse obliged to provide benefit to patients and neglect his or her own interests and desires? Because the nurse is usually an employee of an institution, to what extent do benefits to the institution take priority over benefits to the patient? Is the nurse also obliged to provide benefits to unidentified patients who might conceivably profit from nursing care services? In other words, some consideration will have to be given to the setting of limits on the obligation to benefit.

These three problems can easily arise in the care of cancer patients when considering the nurse's obligation to do good and to avoid harm.

Justice

Once the principle of beneficence has been considered in patient care, the second question usually concerns the distribution of benefits and burdens among patients (Veatch & Fry, 1987). In considering these types of questions, the nurse appeals to principles of justice in deciding what is a just or fair allocation of resources.

The formal principle of justice claims that equals should be treated equally and those who are unequal should be treated differently according to their needs (Beauchamp & Childress, 1989). Although some theorists advocate the application of other ethical principles in deciding how to distribute resources (for example, to provide the greatest amount of good or benefit or to provide the greatest amount of liberty possible among citizens), other theorists claim that a principle of justice based on resource allocation according to need or equality should be the goal of these decisions (Veatch & Fry, 1987).

It is not possible to provide equal health care goods and resources to everyone, but it is possible to view health care as a good that every citizen should have equal access to, in accordance with need. In a complex health care delivery system with limited resources, as in the United States, this view of resource allocation is about the only socially acceptable one that can be entertained. It tends to treat equals equally and unequals unequally and to provide a means for the just distribution of resources among needy patients.

Autonomy

The third ethical principle important to the nursing care of cancer patients is the principle of autonomy. It claims that individuals are to be permitted personal liberty to determine their own actions according to plans they themselves have chosen (Veatch & Fry, 1987). To respect persons as autonomous individuals is to acknowledge their personal choices.

One of the problems in applying a principle of autonomy to nursing care is that persons appear to be autonomous in varying degrees. No one is perfectly autonomous or capable of choosing a plan without experiencing some internal and external constraints. However, some individuals are capable of being substantially autonomous in making decisions, but the limits of autonomy may be hard to determine.

Applying the principle of autonomy can be very difficult for the nurse who cares for the elderly or those with diminished capability to act autonomously because of debilitating illnesses. Limits to autonomy that arise from organic and psychological factors are basically internal and often require additional health care resources to raise the level of capacity to act autonomously (Veatch & Fry, 1987). When autonomy is limited in this manner, the nurse may need to provide additional explanation of alternative treatments. It may even be necessary to provide financial or physical supports to patients who fall into this category of limited autonomy.

The principle of autonomy may also prove difficult to apply when there is a strong conviction on the part of the nurse or other members of the health care team that respecting self-determined choice is not really in the best interests of the patient and conflicts with the nurse's obligation to provide benefit to the patient. In these situations, the nurse may need to consider the limits of autonomy and the criteria for justified paternalism toward patients. Although paternalism is seldom justified in the care of patients, some situations might warrant overriding a patient's autonomy when the benefits to be received are great and the harms to be avoided are significant (Childress, 1982).

Questions of this type in patient care situations often appear on the agenda of the hospital or institutional ethics committee, although the authority of such committees to make significant decisions related to patient care has been questioned (Ross, 1986). The nurse will surely confront a conflict of values whenever respecting autonomy conflicts with other obligations to the patient that are perceived by the nurse.

Veracity

The principle of veracity is usually defined as the obligation to tell the truth and to avoid lying or deception (Veatch & Fry, 1987). Truthfulness has long been regarded as fundamental to the existence of trust among individuals. In health care relationships, this obligation gains particular significance.

One reason that is often given for truth telling in relationships is that this obligation is part of the respect we owe persons (Beauchamp & Childress, 1989). We respect persons because they are autonomous and thereby have the right to be told the truth and not to be deceived.

Another reason offered for truth telling between patient and nurse, for example, concerns the element of trust that exists in the relationship (Fry, 1987b). Telling the truth is required because *not* to do so will undermine the effectiveness of the nurse's role with the patient and may, in the long run, bring about undesirable consequences for future relationships with patients.

Nurses may withhold information from patients with cancer because they think that these patients, particularly if they are very ill, may not really want to know the truth about their conditions. Yet patients with cancer have consistently maintained that they want to know the full truth about their conditions (Veatch, 1978). As the interpretive statements to the *Code for Nurses* point out, "Truth telling and the process of reaching informed choice underlie the exercise of self-determination, which is basic to respect for persons" (1985, p. 2). The nurse is obligated to respect a principle of veracity in providing nursing care to patients.

Avoiding Killing

In the care of patients with cancer, the problem of taking life arises in a number of contexts but is especially acute in patients wishing to take their own lives; in decisions about ending the lives of terminally ill or suffering patients; and in decisions to terminate treatment, including nutrition and hydration. A principle of avoiding killing can be defined as the obligation to respect the sacredness of human life or, quite simply, the obligation not to take human life (Veatch & Fry, 1987).

Reasons given by health care professionals for killing

in the health care sphere are usually related to mercy. Someone decides that the patient is better off dead (or others would be better off if the patient were dead). Given the nurse's obligation to benefit the patient, *should* the nurse assist in putting a suffering patient out of misery by hastening death in some manner? Is it a role of the nurse to kill the patient, especially when the patient is no longer competent to make such a decision and carry it out? Is there any difference between killing a patient for these reasons and withholding or withdrawing treatments knowing that such action will surely hasten the patient's death (although the patient will live longer under these circumstances than if the nurse killed the patient outright)?

It is claimed by some ethicists that these questions can be answered by applying the principles already discussed (Beauchamp, 1979). In other words, consideration of the principles of beneficence, autonomy, and justice already provide arguments supporting the avoidance of killing patients. However, because of the complex technical aspects of care that nurses give in managing cancer patients, these principles alone do not seem sufficient to govern the potential for killing that always seems to exist in the care of seriously ill patients. Hence, a principle of avoiding killing seems pertinent to the role of the nurse (Veatch & Fry, 1987).

Indeed, the most recent revision of the *Code for Nurses* seems to address these difficult issues when it states, "Nursing care is directed toward the prevention and relief of the suffering commonly associated with the dying process. The nurse may provide interventions to relieve symptoms in the dying client even when the interventions entail substantial risks of hastening death" (1985, p. 4). The code recognizes the potential effects of providing nursing care to a seriously ill patient. It also recognizes the fundamental importance of the principle of avoiding killing by noting that "nurses are morally obligated to respect human existence and . . . therefore must take all reasonable means to protect and preserve human life when there is hope of recovery or reasonable hope of benefit from life-prolonging treatment" (1985, p. 2). Unfortunately, the role of the nurse with the suffering and dying patient is left rather ambiguous by the code. For these reasons, a principle of avoiding killing is important in any ethical framework for the practice of nursing. Killing a patient under any circumstances is simply not an option for the professional nurse.

Is withholding nutrition and hydration from a patient killing? This question undergirds one of the most controversial patient care issues confronting nurses in caring for cancer patients.

Several philosophers (Lynn & Childress, 1983; Paris & Fletcher, 1983) and some legal cases (*In re* Claire C. Conroy, 1983; *In re* Mary Hier, 1984; *In re* Plaza Health and Rehabilitation Center, 1984) have concluded that nutrition and hydration can be withheld on the same grounds as other treatments. Some health care professionals, however, have been reluctant to accept the withholding of nutrition and hydration even when the patient has formally requested that this be done. Some scholars, for example, believe that the

provision of food and fluids is a basic caring function that should always be required in the care of patients (Callahan, 1983). One reason for this view is that the provision of food and fluids is symbolic of our care for the hungry and thirsty among us. However, if patients in terminally ill states do not experience hunger and thirst, does this mean that food and water do not need to be administered? These are difficult questions that cannot be answered easily (Box 4–1).

In a case involving the withdrawal of a nasogastric tube from a terminally ill woman, a New Jersey court ruled that nutrition and hydration could be removed under three conditions (*In re* Conroy, 1985):

1. It is clear that the patient would have refused the treatment.

2. There is some indication that the treatment would only prolong suffering.

3. The burdens clearly and markedly outweigh the benefits.

In many patient care situations, it is not clear that these conditions can be met: the patient might not have expressed definite opinions on the matter; the patient's degree of suffering might not be evident (if the patient is in a coma); and it is often not clear that burdens of treatment really outweigh benefits of continuing treatment. Thus the nurse must resort to the weight and importance of the obligation to avoid killing in nursing practice.

Fidelity

The final ethical principle of importance to the care of the cancer patient is the principle of fidelity, defined

---

Box 4–1. IN RE CONROY, NO. A-108, N.J. SUP. CT., JANUARY 17, 1985.

Claire Conroy was an 84-year-old nursing home resident who received nutrition and hydration by a nasogastric tube. Her nephrew requested that the tube be removed because his aunt was very debilitated and in a near-vegetative state. He said that his aunt would not have wanted to have the tube if she were capable of making this decision. The trial court permitted removal of the tube (*In re Cont’oy,* 188 N.J. Super 523 [Chancery Div. 1983]). The New Jersey Appellate Court reversed this opinion (190 N.J. Super. 435, 464 A 2d 303 App. Div. 1983) and ruled that Conroy's nasogastric tube could not be removed. The New Jersey Supreme Court reversed the appellate court decision on January 17, 1985, ruling that any life-sustaining treatment, including artificial feeding, may be withheld from incompetent nursing home residents in certain circumstances:

1. When there is evidence that the particular patient would have refused treatment.

2. When the decision maker feels that the treatment prolongs the suffering of the patient.

3. When the burdens of continued life with the treatment clearly outweigh any benefits.

The court also required that a New Jersey state ombudsman be notified to consider any decision to remove life-support systems.

as the obligation to remain faithful to one's commitments (Veatch & Fry, 1987). The type of commitments that usually fall within the scope of fidelity are obligations generic to the trust relationship between client and nurse. These obligations are keeping promises, maintaining confidentiality, and caring.

Individuals generally expect that promises will be kept in all human relationships. At least, promises should not be broken unless there is a good reason to do so. The same can be said for maintaining confidentiality, one of the most basic requirements of professional health care ethics.

Exceptions to both obligations are rare but can be made. For example, some persons maintain that it is morally acceptable to break a promise when breaking it would produce more good than would keeping it. Confidences are often broken for the same reasons.

It is also argued that it is morally acceptable to break confidences and promises when the welfare of a third party is jeopardized by the keeping of the confidence or promise. In the *Code for Nurses,* it is stated that the obligation of confidentiality "is not absolute when innocent parties are in direct jeopardy" (1985, p. 4). This reason is usually given for breaking confidentiality and the promise to keep it when child abuse is discovered or when a patient is found to be a carrier of a serious communicable disease (Veatch & Fry, 1987).

Some argue against the breaking of confidences on the basis of potential benefit to other parties. They claim that keeping information confidential is a right independent of the rights of others. Whereas it may be morally acceptable to break promises to provide benefit to others, confidentiality is a basic right of the patient that cannot and should not be foregone for this reason alone.

One way to resolve the ethical commitments to keep confidentiality and keep promises is to ground these obligations in an independent principle of fidelity. Thus to maintain fidelity with the patient, nurses and others should seriously weigh what information can be considered confidential and under what circumstances nurses should be expected to keep promises. Otherwise every instance of breaking promises and confidentiality would also entail a violation of fidelity. The duty to keep one's commitments, in this view, would take on new meaning in the nurse-patient relationship.

The obligation to care for one's patients is also part of the principle of fidelity. Indeed, the caring phenomenon is considered by many to be the central ethic in nursing (Leininger, 1981). When studies are done on the nursing care of cancer patients, caring is consistently mentioned as one of the most important components of cancer nursing care (Fleming et al., 1987; Larson, 1986; Mayer, 1987). Individualized caring, affective behaviors, comforting, trust, and nursing competence have all been mentioned by both nurses and patients as important to caring and feeling cared for. Thus making moral decisions and carrying out moral actions are strongly influenced by the extent to which nurses incorporate a principle of fidelity into their relationships with patients. It is a foundational principle of the professional ethic that often comes in

conflict with other ethical principles considered important in nurse-patient relationships. When conflict occurs, how does the nurse decide on the priority of one principle over another? What guidelines can be offered for balancing all of the ethical principles related to the care of the cancer patient?

A DECISION-MAKING FRAMEWORK FOR A CANCER NURSING ETHIC

Although no single approach to resolving ethical conflicts in nursing practice is ever sufficient for all types of situations and all patients, it may be possible to describe systematically the type of ethical decision making required of the nurse. Toward this end, Jameton has proposed a method for resolving nursing ethics problems that is very helpful in the practice of nursing care (Jameton, 1984). Although not a "recipe" for making ethical decisions related to patient care, it is helpful in demonstrating the steps that are usually taken when making an ethical decision (Table 4–1).

Jameton's method involves six steps:

First, identify the problem. This involves clarifying what is at issue in terms of values, conflicts, and matters of conscience. The nurse should also examine his or her relation to the problem and assess the time parameters for the decision-making process. This latter consideration is very important because some decisions can and should be delayed if the decision does not have to be made immediately.

Second, the nurse should gather additional information. Data that are helpful to acquire during this step are the identities of the main participants in the decision, the wishes of the patient or the surrogate decision maker, and the "story" of the conflict as it has developed.

The third step is to identify all the options that are open to the decision maker, namely, the courses of action, the possible outcomes of these actions, and the potential impacts of outcomes on the various people involved in the decision. The consideration of future decisions that might have to be made is also important to this process.

Fourth, Jameton recommends that the decision maker "think the ethical problem through" (1984). This means considering the basic human values that are important to the individuals involved, the basic human values central to the issues, and the ethical principles that can be brought to bear on the situation. This step is very important and should not be underestimated in consid-

Table 4–1. A DECISION-MAKING FRAMEWORK FOR A NURSING ETHIC

1. Identify the problem.
2. Gather additional data.
3. Identify all the options open to the decision maker.
4. Think the ethical problem through.
5. Make the decision.
6. Act and assess outcomes.

(Adapted from Jameton, A. [1984]. *Nursing practice: The ethical issues.* Englewood Cliffs, NJ: Prentice-Hall, Inc.)

ering the ethical decision-making process. Ethical decision making is necessarily a rational process and requires the careful articulation of values and principles that impinge on a decision.

The fifth step is to make the decision. This means that the decision maker chooses the course of action that best reflects his or her assessment of the previous steps as well as his or her best judgment. It is necessarily individual in that it is made by the decision maker but is also rational in that it reflects a careful process of thought and ethical reasoning.

The sixth step is to act and then to assess the decision and its outcomes. Jameton suggests that actual outcomes should be compared with projected outcomes during the decision-making process. The decision maker should also ask how he or she would improve the process next time and whether this situation can be generalized to future situations having similar characteristics. This is an important consideration and reduces the likelihood that decisions will be made in an ad hoc, situation-dependent framework. Naturally, it would be desirable for our ethical decisions to be generalizable to other patient care situations.

SUMMARY

In the care of the cancer patient, the nurse often confronts difficult ethical questions that involve conflicts of values and principles considered important to the practice of nursing and the provision of patient care. The values of respect for persons, advocacy, and accountability place constraints on the moral acceptability of many nursing decisions and actions. When balanced against the general requirements of ethical principles considered important to all health care relationships, these values assume significant importance in the nurse-patient relationship.

Understanding the nature of values and ethical principles is a fundamental requirement of nursing practice. Several ethical traditions have provided guidelines for the nurse to employ when important human values conflict with one another. The resolution of value conflict is a function of the nurse in providing optimal care for the cancer patient; it sustains the traditions of nursing and the social context for the development of the nursing ethic.

A nursing ethic centered on caring and grounded within the fidelity relationship between nurse and patient is suggested as the foundational ethic for care of the patient with cancer. A decision-making process that allows a full discussion of values and principles important to nursing care decisions is proposed as one means to a practical ethic in nursing. Although no single ethical decision-making framework is adequate for all situations in nursing care, the method offered by Jameton is proposed and described in detail. To the extent that nurses involved in the care of the patient with cancer can implement and evaluate the ethical decision-making process, there is considerable opportunity for the development of a dynamic and progressive professional ethic in cancer nursing.

References

American Nurses' Association. (1985). Code for nurses with interpretative statements. Kansas City: The Association.

Beauchamp, T. L. (1979). A reply to Rachels on active and passive euthanasia. In W. L. Robinson & M. S. Pritchard (Eds.), *Medical responsibility: Paternalism, informed consent, and euthanasia* (pp. 181–194). Clifton, NJ: The Humana Press.

Beauchamp, T. L. (1982). *Philosophical ethics: An introduction to moral philosophy.* New York: McGraw-Hill Book Co.

Beauchamp, T. L., & Childress, J. F. (1989). *Principles of biomedical ethics* (3rd ed.). New York: Oxford University Press.

Callahan, D. (1983). On feeding the dying. *Hastings Center Report, 13*(5), 22.

Childress, J. F. (1982). *Paternalism in health care.* New York: Oxford University Press.

Fleming, C., Scanlon, C., & D'Agostino, N. S. (1987). A study of the comfort needs of patients with advanced cancer. *Cancer Nursing, 10,* 237–243.

Frankena, W. (1973). *Ethics* (2nd ed.). Englewood Cliffs, NJ: Prentice-Hall, Inc.

Fry, S. T. (1987a). Autonomy, advocacy, and accountability: Ethics at the bedside. In M. D. Fowler & J. Levine-Ariff (Eds.), *Ethics at the bedside* (pp. 39–49). Philadelphia: J. B. Lippincott Co.

Fry, S. T. (1987b). Ethics in community health nursing practice. In J. Lancaster & M. Stanhope (Eds.), *Community health nursing: Process and practice for promoting health* (2nd ed., pp. 66–88). St. Louis: C. V. Mosby Co.

In re Claire C. Conroy. Syllabus prepared by the Office of the Clerk, Supreme Court of New Jersey, A-108, September Term 1983.

In re Conroy, No A-108 (N.J. Sup. Ct. Jan. 17, 1985).

In re Mary Hier, 464 N.E. 2d Series 959, Mass. App. 1984.

In re Plaza Health and Rehabilitation Center, Sup. Ct., Onodaga County, New York, Feb. 2, 1984.

Jameton, A. (1984). *Nursing practice: The ethical issues.* Englewood Cliffs, NJ: Prentice-Hall, Inc.

Larson, P. J. (1986). Cancer nurses perceptions of caring. *Cancer Nursing, 9,* 86–91.

Leininger, M. M. (1981). *Caring: An essential human need: Proceedings of the three national caring conferences.* Thorofare, NJ: Slack, Inc.

Lynn, J., & Childress, J. F. (1983). Must patients always be given food and water? *The Hastings Center Report, 13*(5), 17–21.

Mayer, D. K. (1987). Oncology nurses' versus cancer patients' perceptions of nurse caring behaviors: A replication study. *Oncology Nursing Forum, 14,* 48–52.

Paris, J. J., & Fletcher, A. B. (1983). Infant Doe regulations and the absolute requirement to use nourishment and fluids for the dying infant. *Law, Medicine, and Health Care, 11,* 210–213.

Ross, J. W. (1986). *Handbook for hospital ethics committees.* Chicago: American Hospital Publishing.

Ross, W. D. (1939). *The right and the good.* London: Oxford University Press.

Veatch, R. M. (1978). Truth-telling attitudes. In W. T. Reich (Ed.), *Encyclopedia of bioethics* (Vol. 4, pp. 1677–1682). New York: The Free Press.

Veatch, R. M., & Fry, S. T. (1987). *Case studies in nursing ethics.* Philadelphia: J. B. Lippincott Co.

Cancer and the Family

BARBARA GERMINO

In this era of cost containment in health care, cancer care is increasingly being given in outpatient and community settings, and hospitalized patients are being discharged much earlier. Persons with cancer are having to depend on their families and others at home for various kinds of help and support. The experiences of cancer and cancer treatment have significant impact not only on the diagnosed individual but also on the individual's family. Knowledge of how cancer affects family systems is increasingly important to nursing practice because families are much more involved with providing support and care throughout the illness, often over long periods of time. Nurses are central in helping families live with the changes and disruptions cancer and treatment for cancer may cause in their lives.

WHO IS THE PATIENT'S FAMILY?

The patient's family traditionally has been defined in health care literature as those persons related by blood, marriage, or adoption. In many studies of families with children, the mother has been the informant for the entire family, providing a "window" into the family system, but the window provided by the mother's perspective excluded the perspectives of other family members (Feetham, 1984). Studies of families of adults experiencing cancer have largely focused on the spouse; only a few studies have looked at the patient and spouse and fewer still the patient, spouse, and other family members, including adult children.

For purposes of clinical practice, it is most useful to allow patients to define and describe their own families. Those who function as family members may or may not be related to the patient in the traditional sense even though they live in the patient's household. For some people, friends, neighbors, partners, and lovers may be as likely to be considered family as are spouses, children, parents, grandparents, siblings, and other relatives.

THE FAMILY AS A SYSTEM

Structure and Function of Family Systems

Those who function as family are part of a social system in which members have ties to one another, have ongoing interactions with one another, are interdependent, have some common history or frame of reference, and share some goals. Family systems, like other systems, are more than simply the sum of their parts. They are composed of subsystems (e.g., spouses, mother-daughter pairs) of members who have unique ties and relationships. A variety of factors help to shape the rules by which the family system deals with other systems and with events that affect it. The structure of the family (i.e., the members of the system); the relationships among family members; the family's history and past experiences; and the family's culture, religion, and social environment all combine to influence family functioning. Family rules guide the behavior of individual system members as well as the operations of the family unit. The rules may be implicit or explicit; they often relate to issues of communication, for example, who talks to whom about what or what kinds of family issues may be discussed with nonfamily members. Family rules reflect the family's values. Loyalty, privacy, relationships among family members, honesty, and child rearing are all examples of issues around which families often develop rules.

Family System Boundaries

The extent to which family systems are open to outsiders is a reflection of family system boundaries. The nature and extent of a family's relationship with other systems in its environment are governed by its boundaries. The context or environment in which the family lives, then, is not only the physical environment or geographic location but also the other social systems with which the family interacts: extended family, neighborhood, community, and local health care systems are all examples of such systems. Information about family boundaries is crucial to nurses attempting to assist families in dealing with cancer.

THE EFFECTS OF CANCER ON FAMILY SYSTEMS

By definition, a system is an integrated unit, so that experiences associated with a potentially life-threatening illness affect not only the person with the illness but the entire unit and all its members as well. The nature of those effects on individual family members and the family unit are not yet clearly delineated either for types of cancer or for ethnic and socioeconomic groups, but this topic is currently the focus of a number of major nursing research efforts. Evidence from research suggests, however, that families are often primary sources of support and assistance at the time of the cancer diagnosis (Germino & Funk, 1987–1989; Lewis, 1986). In addition, it appears that the family provides a context within which the patient attempts to find meaning in the cancer experience (Lewis, 1986). However, the experience of cancer may be viewed by individuals in the family from very different perspectives, generating different concerns in patients, their partners, and their children both early in the illness and in the advanced stages (Germino, 1984; Germino & Funk, 1987–1989; Gotay, 1984).

THE EFFECTS OF CANCER ON FAMILY COMMUNICATION

Family communication has great importance for the effective care of patients with cancer and their families. Patients and family members have been reported to have difficulty communicating with one another during the time following the diagnosis (Wortman & Dunkel-Schetter, 1979), as evidenced by little or no discussion of emotional concerns (Jamison, Wellisch, & Pasnau, 1978). Family members also have reported difficulties obtaining information from health care and difficulties with the manner in which information is given (Bond, 1982a, 1982b; Irwin & Meier, 1973).

Family members may "protect" one another by not sharing their feelings and concerns, creating tension and what Glaser and Strauss called a "closed awareness context" (Glaser & Strauss, 1965). Patterns of disclosure or sharing of concerns among patients and family members indicate that personal feelings and fears are often not shared. More disclosure may occur in relationships between pairs of family members, particularly married couples. However, gender of the parent and child appear to be related to the extent and kinds of communication between parents and their adult children (Germino, 1984; Germino & Funk, 1987–1989).

Data indicating that family members felt that others in the family, including the patient, did not know what was going on suggest that in the terminal phase of cancer, communications within the family about the illness and about dying may be limited and guarded. Patients and family members are often at different places in their willingness to acknowledge and discuss what is going on with the patient. The least shared communication between family members and patients in hospital settings was in the area of dying or dying-related issues (Krant & Johnston, 1977).

FRAMEWORK FOR CONSIDERING CANCER AND FAMILIES

In discussing cancer and families, it is helpful to look at a few of the factors that may be related to the impact of this kind of illness. The specific kind of cancer diagnosis and treatment, the timing and trajectory of the illness, the personal meaning of experiences for those involved, and the nature of human responses during the cancer experience are all important factors in considering families with cancer (Fig. 5–1).

Impact of Specific Cancer Diagnosis
Body Image Changes

The experience of cancer is shaped to some extent by the particular kind of cancer and its implications

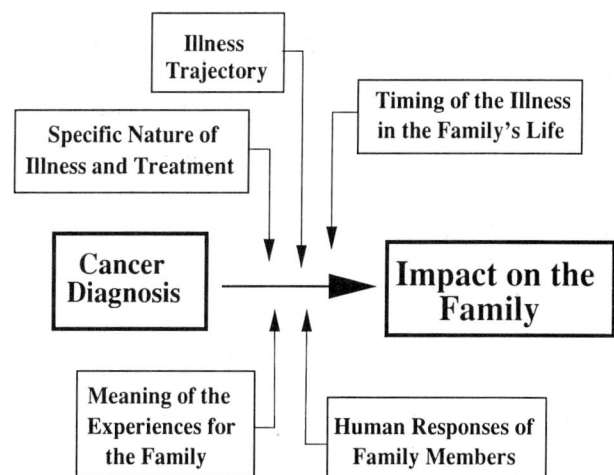

Figure 5–1. The impact of cancer on the family. (Visual design by Larue Coats, Ph.D., Scholarly Support Team, University of North Carolina–Chapel Hill School of Nursing.)

for change. The alteration of one's body or the loss of a body part are significant changes about which much has been written. How persons view their bodies, their selves as persons, and their sexuality are all important issues in the impact of cancer-related physical changes. Studies of self-image and body image in people with cancer have focused primarily on women with mastectomies and hysterectomies and on men and women who have had ostomy surgery (Donahue & Knapp, 1977; Dyck & Sutherland, 1956; Frank-Stromborg & Wright, 1984; Gallagher, 1972). The kinds of surgery that cause visible or symbolic changes in the body have been shown to be related, at least for a time, to negative changes in the patient's self-image and body image, to grief reactions, and to changes in relationships (Woods & Earp, 1978). However, it has become clear that initially devastating physical changes may be integrated into a changed view of oneself, that such changes take time—sometimes years—and that relationships with significant people, especially spouses and partners, can be extremely important and positive as mediators of that impact. The visibility of physical changes may accentuate or minimize the social impact of cancer and the extent to which it affects relationships with others.

Social Impact of Physical Changes

The extent to which physical changes affect important areas of functioning may make a crucial difference in their social impact, both on the person experiencing them and on the family. If the patient has experienced major physical changes, such as loss of a breast or creation of an ostomy, but is still able to carry on functions that are personally important, the impact of the physical changes on relationships may not be as extensive as it is when function is lost. At least one study of women with breast cancer indicated that the women who carried a disproportionate share of household and family responsibilities shifted some of that responsibility to their families and friends during recovery from surgery and during chemotherapy and radiation treatments; within 6 to 12 months after diagnosis, however, the women had returned to their prediagnosis levels of responsibility (Green, 1986). The physical changes of cancer and cancer treatment are significant ones in the cancer experience, but professional caregivers may tend to focus on them sometimes to the exclusion of broader issues that cross diagnostic boundaries. For instance, some evidence suggests that the quality of life for patients with even physically devastating kinds of cancer may at times be low but overall may be perceived by the patient as being quite good in spite of symptom distress and an uncertain future (Cain & Henker, 1978; Frank-Stromborg & Wright, 1984; Germino & Dalton, 1986).

Specific Type of Cancer and Families

Much of the family research has been done with mixed samples of families representing many, often unspecified cancer diagnoses. The emphasis has clearly been less on the specific kind of cancer and treatment than on the impact of the potentially life-threatening group of illnesses that cancer represents. There are some notable exceptions in studies of women with breast cancer and their families.

The family has been described as providing a crucially important context or environment for the woman with breast cancer, the quality of that environment (in this case indicated by tension and conflict) being directly related to the woman's adjustment to her illness over time (Spiegel, Bloom, & Gottheil, 1983). The family's adaptation to breast cancer after the initial diagnostic and early treatment period is characterized by complex feelings. Family members as well as the patient may express a sense of powerlessness in the face of the disease, powerlessness that may be accentuated in situations in which family members do not feel a part of the decision-making process. Ambivalence toward the patient and toward aspects of the treatment experience has been described as a normal response to disruption in family routines and threatened expectations (Lewis, Ellison, & Woods, 1985). Lewis and colleagues describe families experiencing breast cancer as living two lives: the life related to the illness and its contingencies and the life of being a family that must deal with the needs of all its members. Some of the latter needs may conflict with the special care and attention needed by the patient (Lewis et al., 1985).

Families experience periods of uncertainty in living with breast cancer, as do patients. At diagnosis, during remission, and during recurrence (if there is one), uncertainty about the future is a feeling with which family members must learn to continue living.

Timing and Trajectory of Illness

Timing of Cancer in the Family's Life

The timing of a cancer diagnosis in the context of the individual's life and the life of the family is another factor worthy of examination in attempting to understand the potential impact of cancer. In our society, age and stage of life affect how we view and attempt to understand the cancer experience. Cancer is still devastating but may be more "understandable" or more acceptable to us in an elderly person than in a young child, an adolescent, or a younger adult. Cancer may be more difficult for families to accept at particular times of life, for example, at important transitions, such as marriage, the birth of a child, the beginning of a new job, or the beginning of retirement. In these circumstances, the response of those involved may be a sense of the unfairness of it all.

The timing of cancer in a family's life may affect its ultimate impact. Families with young children, for example, must continue to meet the specific developmental needs of those children while trying to incorporate the cancer experience into family life. A newly retired couple planning a life of freedom and travel may find that not only have their plans been put on hold but also their economic future has been jeopardized by catastrophic medical bills. Single parents with only themselves as a source of support could be faced with devastating losses and family disruption.

For families, the timing of cancer is important not only in terms of development but also in terms of other stresses in their lives. For many families, losses of friends and family members, children leaving home, financial difficulties, moving, and other illnesses are occurring along with cancer. Family stress theory (McCubbin & Patterson, 1983) reminds us that an accumulation of stressors can disrupt even the strongest family's ability to continue functioning. Both normative changes and strains can and do often occur simultaneously. Strains often emerge from a particular stressor (e.g., a diagnosis of a potentially life-threatening kind of cancer) and are often difficult or impossible to resolve on a short-term basis. The family's efforts at coping with the situation, for instance, by working extra hours to pay medical expenses, may in themselves add to the stress of a serious illness (McCubbin & Patterson, 1983).

Trajectory of Illness

The trajectory of an illness refers not only to the course of the illness, its "physiologic unfolding over time," but also to the handling or management of the work of the illness and the impact on those involved (Strauss et al., 1984). The trajectory of cancer has many shapes but frequently involves a rapid series of initial events and decisions and a period or periods of uncertainty. With some kinds of cancer, the periods of remission are increasingly longer. We have begun to study the impact of recurrence of cancer after long periods without any signs of disease and find that recurrence may be, from the patient's and family members' perspective, more difficult than the initial diagnosis. Feelings of shock because of the cancer's recurrence, feeling assaulted by the cancer, experiencing uncertainty about the future, and feeling anger and a sense of injustice are examples of patients' and spouses' responses to recurrence. To make matters more difficult, some patients and spouses avoid discussing the possible outcomes of the recurrence with each other, particularly when the outcome may be death (Chekryn, 1984). Because people are living longer with many kinds of cancer, the issues become those of learning to live with a chronic illness. The need to follow families over time both in practice and research becomes clear.

The demands of cancer and cancer treatment as well as the burdens imposed on family caregivers help to shape the trajectory of illness that families must manage. Demands can range from managing physical care needs and role changes required to deal with the illness to coping with emotional demands of family members on each other (Lewis, 1986; Lewis et al., 1985; Stetz, 1987). At least one study has indicated that families able to adapt to such demands with shifting and expanded roles and with effective communication experience less disruption and conflict over time (Vess,

Moreland, & Schwebel, 1985). Spouse caregivers for patients with advanced cancer express difficulty in managing the responsibilities of physical care, which include managing treatment regimens and changes in physical functioning related to the illness (Stetz, 1987). In addition, being a close observer of the spouse's illness is a difficult experience for partners of people who are seriously ill with cancer (Germino, 1984; Krant & Johnston, 1977; Stetz, 1987). Changes in caregivers' health and patterns of living, especially when seen as causing disruption and disorder in their lives, may cause them to have difficulty in adjusting to role changes (Stetz, 1987). Uncertainty—specifically, high levels of unpredictability of the spouse's illness—appears to be important in predicting caregivers' health (Stetz, 1987).

Meaning of the Experience

Personal Meaning of the Cancer Experience

The personal meaning of the cancer experience for those involved is a third major factor in its impact. The personal meaning of the cancer experience is derived over time and clearly may change over time. The individual perceptions of the patient and family members involved—their view of the events related to the cancer, the implications of those events, the changes that evolve during the cancer experience, and the fears and concerns that may emerge—all contribute to the derivation of meaning from the cancer experience.

Uncertainty

Uncertainty characterizes the experience of cancer for many families. The patient's prognosis, the outcomes of the cancer and cancer treatment, the possibility of recurrence, and the unpredictability of future illness contribute to threaten the family's psychological control over the cancer (Lewis, 1986). Uncertainty about the impact of the cancer experience on the family, and on each family member's future, is present in the early period after diagnosis, in the years of living with cancer, in the advanced stages of illness, and at recurrence (American Cancer Society, 1979; Chekryn, 1984; Germino & Funk, 1987–1989; Gotay, 1984; Krant & Johnston, 1977; Lewis, 1986).

Complexity of Meaning for Families

It is in trying to understand the meaning of the cancer experience for families that we see just how complex the impact of cancer can be. Family members, even those living in the same household, may indeed have different perceptions of the situation, different priorities of fear and concern, and different needs (Germino, 1984; Germino & Dalton, 1986; Gotay, 1984; Lewis et al., 1985). For instance, although the initial period after a cancer diagnosis is made has been considered to be one of the most stressful for patients and their families (Northouse, 1984), the nature and timing of that stress may differ for those involved. Women who had mastectomies have reported that the preoperative period was the most stressful (Jamison et al., 1978; Stolar, 1982), whereas their families saw the immediate postoperative period as most stressful for them (Stolar, 1982; Wellisch, 1981) (Box 5–1).

In studies of patients' and adult family members' concerns after cancer diagnosis, all family members shared common concerns about the patient, but each family member also had unique concerns. The patients tended to worry most about physical symptoms (especially fatigue); spouses were most concerned about their own anxiety; and adult children were expending the most energy dealing with existential concerns generated by the threatened loss of a parent (Germino, 1984; Germino & Funk, 1987–1989). Similarly, Gotay found that, both in the early diagnostic and advanced illness periods, patients and spouses shared a fear of cancer and a concern for the patient's emotional upheaval, but their other concerns differed (1984).

Family members' concerns are complex in that they not only reflect particular topics or issues but also have a focus or referent person. In other words, they may focus on themselves in one area and on other family members in other areas. Patients have been reported to be most concerned about their own symptoms, their care and treatment, and their futures. However, they also worry about the futures of their spouses and adult children, their spouses' physical health, and the need to depend on others (Germino, 1984; Germino & Funk, 1987–1989).

Differing perceptions are also reflected in studies of families in which a member had breast cancer. In one study of the perception of demands the cancer imposed, clear differences were evident among family members. The women in this study, for instance, saw the illness as imposing many more demands than the men did (Lewis et al., 1985).

Although we are beginning, through studying family members, to unravel the complexity that is the meaning of cancer to families, we do not yet know very much about how the meaning of cancer relates to a family's responses and functioning, particularly in the ability of the family unit to provide continuing support to patients while continuing to meet other family members' needs and managing family maintenance tasks. The experiences of family members who are caregivers for persons with cancer are important to assess because heavy illness demands over a prolonged period of time may affect their health and well-being. Caregiving may also have positive effects. One study of caregivers whose spouses had advanced cancer indicated that those who saw caring for their ill partners as giving them a sense of purpose in life had a more positive view of their own health (Stetz, 1987).

Family Responses to Cancer

Active Family Responses to Cancer

Finally, the impact of cancer involves human responses to the experience. The impact of cancer on patients and families is not analogous to standing still and being hit by a brick, although there are days when it certainly must feel that way. What is impressive, however, is the resilience of many families, their ability to adapt and to dig deep and find the emotional resources to deal with what must be dealt with. Of course there are exceptions, but initial research and clinical observation seem to be encouraging. Families often respond actively and positively to events that affect them. The human abilities to be hopeful and optimistic, to endure discomfort, to work at keeping life normal in the midst of major disruption, to live with uncertainty, to laugh together, and to grieve for what has been lost and then go on with life are all positive examples of the scope of active human responses to cancer. Many families appear to have significant success in dealing with the disruptions of cancer, maintaining important family functions by shifting roles and responsibilities and by striving to keep as much of family life as normal as possible.

Difficulties Dealing with Cancer

Families who have difficulty dealing with cancer may be those whose perceptions of the illness, ongoing problems, and limited or ineffective resources prevent the system from adapting to the changes and uncer-

---

Box 5–1. RECENT FAMILY STUDIES IN CANCER NURSING

Oberst, M. T., & Scott, D. T. (1988). **Postdischarge distress in surgically treated cancer patients and their spouses.** *Research in Nursing and Health, 11,* 223–233.

Temporal patterns of distress among two groups of nonterminally ill, surgically treated patients with cancer (n = 40) and their spouses (n = 40) during the immediate pre- and postdischarge period were studied. Data about problems encountered and standardized measures of distress (State Anxiety Index, Brief Symptom Index, and Vulnerability Index) were obtained before hospital discharge and at 10, 30, 60, 90, and 180 days after discharge. The intensity of distress experienced by patients and spouses was remarkably similar, although the temporal pattern of occurrence was significantly different. Before discharge, spouse anxiety was significantly higher than that of the patient and was above the norm for hospitalized persons. Spouses were least distressed after 10 days at home but thereafter experienced a rise in vulnerability culminating in observable clinical depression at 90 and 180 days. Peak distress for patients occurred 10 days after discharge as a function of physical symptoms that were unexpected or more severe than anticipated. Patients with ostomies (n = 20) were slower to return to preillness functional levels and had somewhat more psychological distress than nonostomy patients.

tainties the cancer experience may precipitate. Major problems of family functioning and family communication when combined with the potential stressors of a cancer diagnosis may be more disruption than the system can bear. In other situations, an accumulation of stressors has been found to be associated with less family adaptability (Gilliss & Gortner, 1987). The family's resources for all kinds of support and the extent to which family system boundaries are open to outside help may be important in determining how well that family continues to function through stressful cancer-related experiences. Other family response issues that may have an impact on the outcome of cancer experiences for the family include:

1. Emotional strain.
2. The physical demands of caring for the patient.
3. Adverse effects of cancer on life styles, including financial pressures.
4. Lack of availability of health and support services for families.
5. Problems with sexuality and intimacy (Lewis, 1986).

Effect of Responses on the Impact of the Cancer

It is important to view human responses in cancer both as part of the impact of the illness on the family and as themselves affecting what that impact will be. The responses of family members to the demands of illness on emotional, physical, social, spiritual, and financial resources may vary. Roles and relationships within the system may be altered as well. The balance of meeting ongoing family system needs as well as dealing with the demands of cancer, cancer treatment, and the changes they precipitate is a precarious one. Enough energy must be coming into the family system to replenish the tremendous amount of energy that may be expended on dealing with all of these issues.

Although much work remains to be done in studying family responses to cancer, it is reasonable to hypothesize that families, like individuals, can respond effectively to cancer experiences if the nature and quality of major stresses and strains in their functioning allow them the energy and resources to deal with the additional burdens of cancer-related experiences. Research on life events has taught us that individuals can tolerate multiple stressful events and not become ill if support from others is available and is sufficient to buffer that stress (Stetz, 1987). With these issues in mind, the assessment of families and the planning of care that complements and supports the family's ability to respond to the demands of cancer is a challenge for current and future cancer nursing (Box 5–2).

SUMMARY

As cost containment puts people with cancer more and more often in the care of their families, knowledge of family systems under stressful conditions will become increasingly important. Family social systems are

---

Box 5–2. RECENT FAMILY STUDIES IN CANCER NURSING

Northouse, L. L. (1988). **Social support in patients' and husbands' adjustment to breast cancer.** *Nursing Research, 37,* 91–95.

Fifty women with breast cancer who had had mastectomies and their husbands were studied at 3 and 30 days after surgery to determine the nature of the relationship between social support and the adjustment of mastectomy patients and their husbands over time. Psychosocial adjustment was related to both patients' and husbands' levels of social support. Patients and husbands who reported higher levels of social support reported fewer adjustment difficulties at both 3 days and 30 days after surgery. Patients and husbands differed significantly in the levels of support they perceived over time; husbands perceived less support from friends, nurses, and physicians. This study underscores the importance of assessing the support resources of both patients and husbands over time.

---

more than the sum of their parts. They are complex and changing units that are influenced by their structure, their history, their culture, their social environment, and the relationships within the system. Family rules guide the behavior of system members and determine the way the system operates both internally and in its relationships with outsiders. Rules reflect family values and often relate to family communication. Family boundaries govern the nature and extent of the family's relationships with those outside itself. The specific kind of cancer and treatment, the timing and trajectory of the cancer, the personal meaning of experiences for those involved, and the nature of human responses during the cancer experience are important to consider in working to better understand families with cancer.

References

American Cancer Society. (1979). *Report on the social, economic, and psychological needs of cancer patients in California: Major findings and implications.* Oakland, CA: Davison, Inc.

Bond, D. (1982a). Communicating with families of cancer patients 1: The relatives and doctors. *Nursing Times, 78,* 962–965.

Bond, D. (1982b). Communicating with families of cancer patients 2: The nurses. *Nursing Times, 78,* 1027–1029.

Cain, M., & Henke, C. (1978). Living with cancer. *Oncology Nursing Forum, 5,* 4.

Chekryn, J. (1984). Cancer recurrence: Personal meaning, communication, and marital adjustment. *Cancer Nursing, 7,* 491–498.

Donahue, V., & Knapp, R. C. (1977). Sexual rehabilitation of gynecologic cancer patients. *Obstetrics and Gynecology, 49,* 118–121.

Dyck, R., & Sutherland, A. (1956). Adaptation of the spouse and other family members to the colostomy patient. In *The psychological impact of cancer* (American Cancer Society Publication No. 3009-PE). New York: American Cancer Society.

Feetham, S. (1984). Family research: Issues and directions for nursing. In H. H. Werley & J. Fitzpatrick (Eds.), *Annual review of nursing research. Vol. 2.* New York: Springer.

Frank-Stromborg, M., & Wright, P. (1984). Ambulatory cancer

patients' perceptions of the physical and psychosocial changes in their lives since the diagnosis of cancer. *Cancer Nursing, 7,* 117–129.

Gallagher, A. (1972). Body image changes in the patient with a colostomy. *Nursing Clinics of North America, 7,* 669.

Germino, B. (1984). Family members' concerns after cancer diagnosis (Doctoral dissertation, University of Washington, 1984). *Dissertation Abstracts International, 44,* 3358B.

Germino, B., & Dalton, J. (1986). Quality of life in patients with lung cancer. *Oncology Nursing Forum, 13*(Suppl.), 97.

Germino, B., & Funk, S. G. (1987–1989). Development of the family concerns inventory. Grant funded by the National Center for Nursing Research, National Institute of Health, #1R01BR01331-01A1.

Gilliss, C., & Gortner, S. (1987, November). *Family functioning after cardiac surgery.* Paper presented at the National Conference on Family Relations, Atlanta, GA.

Glaser, B., & Strauss, A. (1965). *Awareness of dying.* Chicago: Aldine.

Gotay, C. C. (1984). The experience of cancer during early and advanced stages: The views of patients and their mates. *Social Science, 18,* 605–613.

Green, C. P. (1986). Changes in responsibility in women's families after the diagnosis of cancer. *Health Care for Women International, 7,* 221–239.

Irwin, B., & Meier, J. (1973). Supportive measures for relatives of the fatally ill. *Communicating Nursing Research, 6,* 119–128.

Jamison, K. R., Wellisch, D. K., and Pasnau, R. (1978). Psychosocial aspects of mastectomy: The woman's perspective. *American Journal of Psychiatry, 135,* 432–436.

Krant, M. J., & Johnston, L. (1977). Family members' perceptions of communications in late stage cancer. *International Journal of Psychiatry in Medicine, 8,* 203–216.

Lewis, F. M. (1986). The impact of cancer on the family: A critical analysis of the research literature. *Patient Education and Counseling, 8,* 269–289.

Lewis, F. M., Ellison, E., and Woods, N. F. (1985). The impact of breast cancer on the family. *Seminars in Oncology Nursing, 1,* 206–213.

McCubbin, H., & Patterson, J. (1983). The family stress process: The double ABCX model of family adjustment and adaptation. In H. McCubbin, M. Sussman, & J. Patterson (Eds.), *Advances and developments in family stress theory and research.* New York: Haworth, 1983.

Northouse, L. (1984). The impact of cancer on the family: An overview. *International Journal of Psychiatry in Medicine, 14,* 215–242.

Revenson, T. A., Wollman, C. A., & Felton, B. J. (1983). Social supports as stress buffers for adult cancer patients. *Psychosomatic Medicine, 45,* 321–331.

Spiegel, D., Bloom, J. R., & Gottheil, E. (1983). Family environment as a predictor of adjustment to metastatic breast cancer. *Journal of Psychosocial Oncology, 1,* 30–33.

Stetz, K. M. (1987). Caregiver demands during advanced cancer. *Cancer Nursing, 10,* 260–268.

Stolar, E. (1982). Coping with mastectomy: Issues for social work. *Health and Social Work, 7,* 26–34.

Strauss, A. L., Corbin, J., Fagerhaugh, S., Glaser, B., Maines, D., Suczek, B., & Wiencer, C. (1984). *Chronic illness and the quality of life* (2nd ed.). St. Louis: C. V. Mosby Co.

Vess, J., Moreland, J., & Schwebel, A. (1985). A follow-up study of role functioning and the psychological environment of two families of cancer patients. *Journal of Psychosocial Oncology, 2,* 1–14.

Wellisch, D. K. (1981). Family relationships of the mastectomy patient: Interactions with the spouse and children. *Israel Journal of Medical Science, 17,* 993–996.

Woods, N. F., & Earp, J. (1978). Women with cured breast cancer: A study of mastectomy patients in North Carolina. *Nursing Research, 27,* 279–285.

Wortman, C., & Dunkel-Schetter, G. (1979). Interpersonal relationships and cancer: A theoretical analysis. *Journal of Social Issues, 35,* 120–156.

Cultural Systems

NOEL J. CHRISMAN

Cancer is a disease with fearsome meaning. Many view it as a nearly certain sentence of pain and death. In addition, as a chronic disease, its meaning includes living with these dangers over time. The chronic nature of cancer and cancer's threat to personal integrity tend to involve the family and frequently the community in the illness more than do many other health problems, particularly those that are more self-limited.

All health problems can be considered as part of a cultural system. Any time an individual is sick, cultural meanings are attributed to the sickness (by both patients and clinicians), and members of the patient's social environment are involved. It is particularly important in cancer care, therefore, that the patient's cultural system be taken into account. The meanings and social implications of cancer are such that they become an important component in the need for care, as much as if not more than the traditional biomedical aspects of the disease. In addition, nurses' holistic view of patient care vigorously supports professional attention to the peculiarly human phenomenon of culture.

Concern about providing holistic care to patients that includes professional attention to cultural issues is growing among nurses and other health practitioners. This happy circumstance seems to be the result of a number of different factors. Of primary importance has been the realization, born of the various minority rights movements, that the United States is a pluralistic, multicultural society and not the melting pot it had seemed to be (Gordon, 1964). This realization has meant that practitioners feel less comfortable expecting or demanding that patients conform to behaviors exhibited by the white middle class, from which so many clinicians have come. In addition, our understanding of disease and treatment and patients' responses to them have changed. More can be done with and for the person with cancer now, and this fact has allowed practitioners the freedom to notice the human needs of their patients as well as their biologic needs.

CULTURE

Human cultural needs, however, are not nearly so easily categorized, studied, and treated as are biologic needs. Our biology is roughly consistent across *Homo sapiens;* very little else is so consistent because of cultural differences as well as social and psychological ones. *Culture* can be defined as a learned, shared, and symbolically transmitted design for living (Kluckhohn & Kelly, 1945). Culture provides people with ways to make sense out of life, aiding in imposing meaning on thoughts, behaviors, and events and allowing us to make assumptions about how life is and ought to be led. A key cultural concept that is relevant to patient care is *belief:* a proposition accepted as true (Goodenough, 1963, p. 151). A second essential concept is *value:* a standard by which one's own and others' beliefs and behaviors are evaluated (Williams, 1960, pp. 400–401). Beliefs, values, and other elements of culture differ among societies and frequently among groups. This means that the worlds inhabited by people from different cultures are not the same. Thus the human experience of sickness is viewed differently in different cultures. Herein lies the problem of providing optimal and humanistic care to patients with cancer. What they experience may be more diverse than what might be expected on biologic grounds, even from a disease as complex and multifaceted as cancer.

The value of contemporary treatment approaches to cancer—both the technologic aspects and the human care invested by dedicated clinicians—is their success in prolonging life and increasing comfort during illness. Yet when these treatment approaches are applied without regard for the cultural background of the patient, practitioners run the risk of offering inappropriate and sometimes damaging health care. The possibility of inappropriate health care is related to the mainstream cultural assumptions that are enmeshed in the care itself, the taken-for-granted, common-sense understandings about cancer and its treatment. For example, some mainstream cultural beliefs about cancer are that cancer is only biologic; that chemotherapy, radiation therapy, and surgery are the best treatments; that the nuclear family is the most significant social unit for the patient; and that the use of Laetrile and other unproven treatments constitutes evidence of denial of treatment need. I do not mean to imply that these beliefs are wrong in some global sense. In fact, I believe they are right, and so do many members of other ethnic groups. My point is that they are cultural beliefs and thus are variable across cultures. Although they are not wrong, they are not necessarily right.

CULTURE-SENSITIVE CARE

What is needed in contemporary oncology nursing is a conceptual approach to practice that takes into account the cultural background of patients: we need *culture-sensitive care*. Culture-sensitive care is based on three principles: *knowledge, mutual respect,* and *negotiation* (Chrisman, 1986). *Knowledge* includes information about the patient in his or her cultural context. Nurses need to learn about the cultures of their clients. Frequently, this knowledge is derived from experience and from discussions with patients and family members. However, it is also important to read books and articles about the cultural groups that are part of one's practice. *Mutual respect* is interdependent with knowledge. Respect for the client is much more likely when the nurse has a professional sense of the reasons why the person acts a certain way. Furthermore, client respect for the nurse is vastly increased when it is obvious that the nurse has spent time attempting to learn more about the person and the culture. Finally, *negotiation* depends on knowledge and mutual respect. The desire and ability to modify one's own expectations in return for modifications on the part of the patient are related, in part, to practitioner knowledge about important cultural factors that should be promoted to win patient cooperation and to demonstrate clinician respect for patient opinions.

Ethnocentrism

The issue of the rightness of some beliefs and practices and the wrongness of others is the most significant

barrier to delivering culture-sensitive health care to people from all ethnic backgrounds, because the attitude of being right inhibits the acquisition of knowledge and the development of mutual respect. The anthropologic concept describing this problem is *ethnocentrism:* the belief that one's own cultural ways are the best and the only right ways to believe and behave. Ethnocentrism is an essential characteristic of culture; without it, members of a culture would be less motivated to act like their peers. The fabric of society would be threatened. Ethnocentrism is a problem in health care because not everyone comes from the same ethnic background. Not all cultural beliefs and practices coincide with those of the clinician. Significantly, this lack of congruence may be true even when both practitioner and client share the same ethnic identity. This seemingly odd situation may arise when the practitioner has been so strongly socialized into biomedical culture that previous cultural beliefs are dropped—excluded from the belief repertoire because they are thought to be incorrect—in favor of biomedical beliefs. Thus we must distinguish medical ethnocentrism as the principal barrier to good transcultural health care.

Medical Ethnocentrism

Medical ethnocentrism is a problem in health care because it inhibits practitioner understanding of the patient. Patient beliefs and behaviors that contrast or conflict with what the clinician identifies as expected or appropriate can easily be dismissed as wrong. This judgment carries a great deal of weight. For personal and professional reasons, practitioners want their patients to do as well as they can: to be cured, to live a longer life, or to have a better quality end of life. When seemingly contraindicated behaviors occur, the clinician may become upset; when "irrational" beliefs are expressed, the clinician may react negatively.

Three common ethnocentric reactions are anger, shock, and laughter. When expressed, ethnocentric reactions may induce feelings of lowered self-worth in the patient, the feeling of having done something wrong even though it was logical and appropriate within the patient's own culture. For example, an Asian man told of the embarrassment he was made to feel when he wanted to eat with chopsticks—decidedly outside the norm of his white middle-class hospital environment—even though for him they were the appropriate utensil. Ethnic minority patients whose reference groups have been discriminated against in the past may experience ethnocentric reactions as racism. Patients learn to avoid having to experience these negative self-images by refusing to communicate beliefs or behaviors that they feel are likely to cause negative reactions among caregivers. Therefore, data that could be significant for both the medical care and the transcultural health care of the patient can be lost.

Even unexpressed medical ethnocentrism may reduce the database available to the clinician. Odd or incorrect beliefs may be dismissed and not be assimilated into the clinician's understanding of the patient and the patient's life. This is more likely to occur among physicians than among nurses and social workers because the focus of medicine is much more on the disease than on the whole person. However, the practice of ignoring alternative beliefs because of their lack of fit with the practitioner's own is certainly found among nurses and social workers as well. My students in nursing frequently chastise themselves for missing, and thus not working with, cultural beliefs and practices during the years before they took classes in culture-sensitive care.

Cultural Relativism

The principal antidote to ethnocentrism is *cultural relativism,* the practice of understanding others' behaviors and beliefs in the context of their cultures, not the culture of the practitioner. Cultural relativism, and the concomitant reduction in ethnocentrism, should result in an accepting attitude that supports *working with* a patient's beliefs and behaviors. Although culture-sensitive care ultimately may require negotiating medical and alternative beliefs and practices during the care of a client, the practitioner is obligated to exercise professional judgment to maintain accepted medical and psychosocial practice standards. Culture-sensitive care does not require the adoption of biomedically harmful treatments.

ILLNESS-DISEASE DISTINCTION

Disease

An extremely helpful approach to reducing ethnocentrism is the *illness-disease distinction* (Chrisman, 1985; Fabrega, 1972). This distinction is based on the idea that the same phenomenon may be understood in different ways, depending on whose culture is used as the standard. In this case, the common phenomenon is sickness—the universal human experience of not feeling well. The disease perspective is based on a culture's professional view of sickness. In our culture, *disease* is defined as the "pathological processes of body or mind that are confirmed by scientific biological methods" (Chrisman, 1981, p. 40). Health practitioners' view of sickness as disease underlies contemporary success in treating ill health as a biologic phenomenon. It also underlies much of medical ethnocentrism. That is, the disease perspective is so powerful and convincing to health practitioners that they have a difficult time thinking about sickness in any other way. This difficulty occurs in spite of the fact that all of us were raised to understand sickness with popular, or nonprofessional, perspectives. For example, a native American nurse expressed surprise when she discovered that she had simply discounted, then forgotten, many of the beliefs she had learned among her people.

Illness

The term *illness* refers to "sickness as experienced, described, or explained by the sick individual and/or the family (Chrisman, 1981, p. 40). In contrast with disease, illness is not a less valuable way of understanding sickness; after all, it is what the patient experiences regardless of the way the physician describes it. In fact, people's perceptions of illness frequently change once the doctor has produced a diagnosis, but their *experience* continues to be the experience of illness. And illness is the phenomenon on which people base their treatment decisions (Leventhal, Nerenz, & Steele, 1984).

Illness Variation

Disease, then, is a biomedical way of understanding sickness, and illness is a sociocultural way. Thus illness tends to be much more inclusive of life-style patterns, which is what makes it a useful concept for nurses, who work professionally with people's life styles. In addition, illness becomes a key concept for understanding ethnic and other cultural influences on patient care. Membership in an ethnic group shapes people's illness beliefs in part through the process of childhood socialization. At this time we learn the core of basic understandings about the world.

In my own Anglo-Saxon subculture, I learned about a scientific, physician-oriented approach to sickness, as did others from other ethnic groups. Traditional southern blacks and some of their kin in the North learned about the continuing influence of God in health and illness matters; some learned too that supernatural powers could be manipulated through hexes or "roots," and sickness could result (Snow, 1978). Many Puerto Rican children in New York learned about a complex spirit world that takes notice of and may influence everyday life events (Harwood, 1977). People tend to interpret aspects of life in terms of the perspectives with which they were raised—magical, harmonious, scientific, or some other view—and ultimately these beliefs influence their conceptions of sickness. During adult development, early views can be reinforced by instances of successful treatment of illnesses that were based on these premises, whether by neighborhood lay specialists, folk healers, or physicians. Local group conceptions of sickness also are promoted by the communication patterns among families who have had these experiences.

Illness is related to everyday life through complex worldviews developed and reinforced throughout life. A *worldview* is a set of assumptions, values, and beliefs that are related logically to one another (Jones, 1976). This set colors the way people perceive and experience the world, including the way they experience sickness. The meanings of illness tend to have deep affective roots in people's life styles, including the social relationships through which these meanings are communicated. Thus ethnocentric reactions to unusual or unexpected belief or practice statements can assault a patient's basic sense of self-esteem or social connection with the world. For example, a physician's anger at a Filipino mother who used topically applied camphorated oil on her son's stomach upset her in part because the remedy had been her mother's, and it had always worked to reduce pain.

THE HEALTH SEEKING PROCESS

One way for clinicians to increase their professional attention to the ways sociocultural factors influence their clients' behaviors is to use the health seeking process as a conceptual model (Chrisman, 1977; Chrisman & Kleinman, 1983). This model consists of concepts that describe the natural history of an illness episode: the behaviors that an individual carries out when sick (Fig. 6–1). Although the model was created to describe acute self-limited diseases, the concepts contained in it refer equally well to chronic problems such as cancer. The model serves two purposes: (1) to stimulate attention to each element and thereby to the social and cultural factors that are influencing patient behavior and (2) to show that each element is conceptually related to the others. Thus the clinician is encouraged to attend to related aspects of the illness episode.

Briefly, the elements include (1) symptom definition, the processes involved in applying meaning to the symptoms, the diagnosis or both; (2) treatment action, the suggestions for care of the problem that have been made by self or others, including health practitioners; and (3) adherence, the degree to which treatment advice is carried out. These three elements are closely related to one another in that the patient's view of the illness influences what treatment options will be considered. In addition, the degree to which belief and treatment are congruent influences whether the patient will adhere to any particular treatment suggestion. Two further elements show the ways in which the patient's social environment is integrated with the illness episode. These elements are (4) role shift, the ways in which the patient's life patterns are changed because of the illness; and (5) lay consultation and referral, activities in which family and friends discuss the health problem with the individual.

SYMPTOM DEFINITION

The most important activity during this element of the health seeking process is the application of meaning to the experience of the health problem. It is the process of developing one's sense of the *illness*—although frequently the meanings are strongly affected by what the patient has learned from the health practitioner about the *disease*. The key concept that is part of the symptom definition element is *explanatory model* (Kleinman, 1980, 1982; Kleinman, Eisenberg, & Good, 1978): the patient's description of the onset, cause, pathophysiology, course, and treatment of the health problem. Symptom definition is an ongoing process; people's explanatory models change in response to new information, such as reactions to treatment, comments by health practitioners, comments by family and friends (lay consultants), and knowledge derived from media sources.

Explanatory Model Interview

In cancer nursing, it is essential that the clinician elicit the patient's explanatory model as a matter of routine (Box 6–1). One of the reasons for doing this is simply to demonstrate concern for the patient. Patients appreciate being listened to and believed. More important, however, is that this sociocultural assessment technique provides ongoing data about the condition of the patient. The clinician can tell, through repeated explanatory model assessments, about changes in the patient's beliefs and can perhaps obtain clues that will be useful in evaluating other behaviors.

An explanatory model interview need not be carried out in a stilted fashion. The questions are not particularly different from those normally asked by many clinicians. The key difference is the way the clinician *listens;* that is, the clinician listens for the patient's beliefs, not for the degree to which the patient believes in some standard explanation, such as the practitioner's disease beliefs. Students and experienced clinicians have used questions such as those listed in Box 6–1 with success.

ILLNESS BELIEF SYSTEMS

An explanatory model is an individual instance of belief stated at a particular time. Yet there are correspondences among explanatory models, particularly among people who have been raised in the same cultural context. Oncology nurses, especially in heterogeneous urban areas, are likely to hear a wide variety

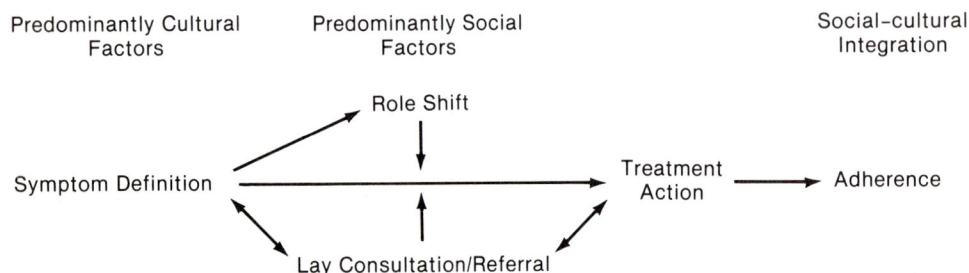

Figure 6–1. Health seeking process. (From Chrisman, N. J. [1977]. The health seeking process: An approach to the natural history of illness. *Culture, Medicine, and Psychiatry, 1,* 351–377. Reproduced by permission.)

Box 6-1. EXPLANATORY MODEL QUESTIONS

1. What do you call your illness?
2. When did it start? What else was going on?
3. What do you think caused it?
4. How does your illness work?
5. How severe is it? How long will it last?
6. What have you been doing to treat the illness?
7. What treatment should you receive now?
8. What do you fear most about your illness?

(Adapted from the work of Kleinman, 1980; Kleinman, Eisenberg, & Good, 1978.)

---

of beliefs in the explanatory models of their cancer patients. One way to conceptualize beliefs so that the variety seems more manageable is to use the idea of an *illness belief system,* which is "a relatively coherent set of ideas regarding what causes illness and its course and treatment" (Chrisman, 1984, p. 158). Illness belief systems focus attention on a series of fundamental beliefs about sickness that occur cross-culturally.

Four illness belief systems are "germ theory," "equilibrium," "God- and spirit-caused illness," and "sorcery and witchcraft." All practitioners have heard germ theory and God-caused explanations, and many have heard equilibrium ideas, so most experienced clinicians will have personal examples to fit within the systems. These systems exist in all areas of the United States. They are distributed differently across ethnic groups. Some groups are more likely to have one cluster of beliefs than another. However, given the amount of cross-communication in current American life, no beliefs are the exclusive province of just one group.

Germ Theory

Germ theory refers to the ways lay people understand the ideas of Western biomedicine. It has a scientific base that includes notions of tumors, abnormal cells, and powerful chemicals. Many lay people, and certainly most cancer patients, acquire a facility with the language of biomedicine and many of the new technologic treatments. The mass media are an important source of such information on a general level; discussions among friends also contribute to people's storehouses of knowledge. People with chronic or life-threatening diseases glean a great deal of information from their health practitioners.

Germ theory beliefs are prevalent in American society across all ethnic groups. Practitioners must be wary, however, of imputing too much knowledge to patients who use the terminology well. Occasionally, language facility obscures beliefs that contrast with medical explanations. For example, a middle-aged nurse who initially espoused a viral explanation for her cancer (germ theory) later disclosed an equilibrium belief, namely, that the fluorocarbons in a spray-on cooking oil had upset the delicate balance of her cells.

Equilibrium

Humoral Pathology

Equilibrium beliefs are distributed broadly throughout the world and thus are diverse in their cultural expressions. The core idea in equilibrium beliefs is that health is promoted by maintaining a balance among significant everyday life elements; illness is the result of an imbalance. The most common beliefs in the United States are those related to *humoral pathology,* the ancient Greek medical system that survived as part of professional medicine until the late nineteenth century (Foster, 1979). The elements of humoral pathology that retain importance today include the presence of two humors—blood and phlegm—and the need for balance among the qualities of hot and cold and wet and dry. Among mainstream whites and others, humoral pathology beliefs are expressed most commonly in regard to colds: one catches a cold by being cold and wet. Phlegm, one of the humors, is related to "slime" reported by black Americans as a substance that builds up in the body as the residue of impurities derived from food (Snow, 1974). One of the ways blood may be related to illness is through its function of cleaning impurities present in the body. If the blood is heavily loaded with impurities, these may erupt as a rash or lesion on the skin.

Hot-Cold System

A particularly significant variant of humoral pathology is the "hot-cold system" found among Mexicans, Puerto Ricans, and other Hispanic Americans (Harwood, 1977; Logan, 1977). In this system, health is to be found in moderation, in the balance of "hot" and "cold" qualities, and in the avoidance of extremes. If an imbalance occurs—too much "hot" or too much "cold"—the excess quality can be treated through the addition of its opposite. For example, the Puerto Ricans studied by Frances Munet de Vilaró believe that cancer is "hot." Thus it should be treated with "cold" remedies. Unfortunately, both radiation therapy and chemotherapy are also considered to be "hot," so biomedical treatment compounds the problem. Munet de Vilaró found that although parents of children with leukemia trusted their physicians enough to agree to treatment, some also gave their children fresh fruits and vegetables at home, both of which are considered to be cold (Munet de Vilaró, 1984).

Harmony

Another significant type of equilibrium system involves the notion of harmony among many elements of the universe. Among native Americans, for example, harmony is a basic principle. People who are sick are believed to have fallen out of harmony. An important reason for visiting a medicine man or woman is to reestablish the essential balance between humans and the universe. Naturally, these healers are required to remain centered themselves. It should not seem odd that some American Indian patients request their own medicine as well as white medicine for treatments. The former establishes the opportunity for recovery; the latter offers the means by which recovery might be accomplished.

God- and Spirit-Caused Beliefs

God- and spirit-caused beliefs are, in various forms, among the most common in the practice of oncology nurses. Some cancer patients feel only a vague sense that they must have done something wrong to deserve their disease. Other patients, however, are more explicit in their attribution of the cause to a supernatural being or force. In this society, God plays a role in the daily lives of millions. Many believe that they can become sick because God may decide to punish them or to test their faith. For some, sickness or other misfortune may be the result of an unknowable part of God's plan (Snow, 1974). Spirit beliefs, however, are encountered less often. Even though belief in the existence of disembodied essences is widespread throughout the world, it is not a part of mainstream American views. For this reason, patients may be hesitant to divulge this belief to a nurse for fear of being laughed at. Beliefs that spirits can cause or cure illness exist to some extent among Hispanics, blacks, Asians, and other ethnic groups in the United States. Spirits may be those of dead ancestors punishing descendants for failing to honor family rules or for lapses in moral behavior. Some Puerto Rican spirits are simply tricksters who cause trouble for sheer enjoyment (Harwood, 1977).

It is essential that the oncology nurse listen sympathetically to statements about the role of the supernatural in a patient's cancer. This attention validates the patient's sense of cultural appropriateness. In addition, clues may be found that signal difficulties in various aspects of the client's life. For example, one black woman mentioned that her wound would not heal because of God's punishment for envy of her sister's wealth. In all cases, if the patient desires, the appropriate religious specialist should be invited to the bedside, or the family should be encouraged to request a home visit. This visit might be from a priest, minister, or *espiritista* (the folk healer who deals with spirits among Puerto Ricans). Some nurses have been reluctant to allow visits by religious practitioners who emphasize the patient's sin as the cause of current medical problems. One strategy for dealing with such people is to establish a collaborative relationship in which it might be possible to negotiate for a softer message on medical grounds.

Sorcery and Witchcraft

Sorcery and witchcraft beliefs as the basis for illness are probably the most difficult to handle. Many Americans simply do not believe that humans can use supernatural power to cause harm to others; this con-

viction is particularly true of rational and scientific health practitioners. Clinicians are at risk for laughing at the idea of sorcery or witchcraft or for inadvertently offending the patient in some other way. For those individuals who do believe in the harm that can come from witchcraft or sorcery, the situation can be extremely frightening. Smith (1972) reported that in a Sicilian-American neighborhood in Buffalo, people would cross the street to avoid one neighbor suspected of being a witch.

Folk Specialists

Most belief systems that include witchcraft or sorcery as a cause of illness also provide practices or practitioners for help. For example, one nurse reported being puzzled when she noticed a native American woman sitting intent at the side of her child in the intensive care unit. The nurse discovered later that this mother believed that her child had been hexed, and she was using her personal power to turn the hex onto the culprit. In many black communities, there are "root doctors" who can remove a hex. Of course, some community members worry that those who can remove a hex may also be able to institute one (Snow, 1974, 1978).

Sensitivity is required of a clinician under these circumstances. It is important to listen in a way that lets patients know that they and their beliefs are valued. In one case, nurses in radiation oncology listened positively to the young black man who was dying. He kept repeating that his ex-wife was probably the cause of his cancer and impending death. The nurses did not understand until much later that they could have intervened psychosocially with the man and his ex-wife, perhaps alleviating some pain and guilt, if they had known about "roots" or hexes. They did listen without overt ethnocentric bias, however. In some cases, the clinician will want to discuss with the family the possibility of consulting with an appropriate community specialist, depending, of course, on the family's desires and finances.

Levels of Cause

The beliefs discussed here only skim the surface of the myriad beliefs available to Americans, who live in an extremely heterogeneous society. It should not be too surprising, then, that people can maintain more than one belief about an illness at the same time. Frequently it is useful to distinguish a patient's belief about the *proximate* cause of illness from the *ultimate* cause. The proximate cause usually describes how the illness works, "the agent (bacteria, virus, twenty-first chromosome) that accounts for the specific condition" (Moore et al., 1980, p. 11). Germ theory or humoral pathology beliefs are likely candidates for proximate cause statements by patients. In contrast, the ultimate cause is seen to be the underlying or "real" reason why the person is sick. Ultimate cause knowledge can answer the ubiquitous questions "Why me? Why now?" that many patients ask. Western biomedicine is poorly equipped to answer these existential questions, but such answers may be central features of the more spiritual or supernatural belief systems.

TREATMENT ACTION

The second element of the health seeking process that is useful for conceptualizing the natural history of an illness episode is treatment action, the kinds of treatment options that exist for the patient. Data for the treatment action element are drawn from explanatory model questions about treatment: What have you been doing for this illness? What expectations do you have for treatment from us (the health care providers)? It is very important to listen openly and positively to these answers (1) so that the patient does not become hesitant to provide unorthodox answers and (2) so that the answers are complete. My experience has been that patients will answer this question with a list of what has been prescribed by a clinician and will overlook (or hide) other practices that are carried out at home. Therefore, the clinician must ask additional questions. Data on treatment provides useful clues about which direction illness beliefs are orienting—toward home- or clinician-suggested treatments.

One should distinguish between the treatment suggestion (e.g., aspirin, antibiotic, or prayer) and the source of the suggestion. Various professional and nonprofessional sources can offer the same treatment suggestion, or the same kind of practitioners can offer quite different types of treatments. Some physicians may suggest unorthodox treatments, such as therapeutic touch or prayer, along with chemotherapy for the patients. More and more nurses who work with the chronically ill are attempting to adopt alternative therapies as their own.

Sources of Treatment Suggestions

The range of treatment sources includes (1) formal health practitioners, such as doctors or nurses; (2) licensed health practitioners, such as pharmacists, midwives, or chiropractors; (3) alternative or native health practitioners, such as herbalists, astrologers, *curanderas* (curers), or spirit mediums; (4) lay consultants; and (5) self (Chrisman & Kleinman, 1983, p. 580). Cancer patients from ethnic groups in which there is a strong folk medical tradition may well turn to practitioners from their own communities. These people are frequently well known and trusted, and their beliefs are likely to be congruent with those of their ethnic clientele. It is important to remember, however, that folk healers are not automatically skilled or respected (Snow, 1978).

Other cancer patients may consult alternative practitioners either because they are upset with the impersonality of orthodox practitioners or because they will turn to any resource for help. In either case, the clinician has a much better opportunity to care for the patient if the patient's activities and beliefs are known than if they have been ignored; ethnocentric reactions or refusal to ask at all will effectively halt communication and therefore the possibility of adequate care.

Alternative practitioners are not always so visible as those associated with cult groups or those who advertise. Some are neighborhood specialists who have gained their expertise through experience and their reputations through word of mouth. In addition, various orthodox and unorthodox churches or sects may be involved in healing (Chrisman & Kleinman, 1983, p. 581). In all these cases, the clinician must ask or listen for this information in a neutral or positive way so that accurate monitoring of patient behavior can take place.

Types of Treatment Suggestions

Types of treatment suggestions also should be listened for and charted. One way to categorize such treatments so that suggestions made by lay people and clinicians may be considered on the same level is the following: (1) activity alterations, such as exercise, bed rest, or sweat baths; (2) application, ingestion, or injection of substances, such as poultices, pills, or shots; (3) verbal or ritual behaviors, such as psychiatric therapy, prayer, or meditation; and (4) physical interventions on the body, such as surgery, cupping (a method of extracting sickness from the body), or massage (Chrisman & Kleinman, 1983, pp. 580–581). A key behavior for the clinician eliciting these sensitive sociocultural data is to respect the patient and to value his or her past decisions whether or not they are the choices the clinician would make.

Although any practitioner or lay person may recommend (or prescribe) any kind of treatment, consistencies have been noted among practitioners and treatments. For example, herbal teas, massage, acupuncture, or martial arts movements are likely to be recommended by practitioners of Chinese medicine; spiritualists are likely to recommend meditation or ritual behaviors; and oncologists are likely to recommend chemotherapy and radiation therapy. When carrying out the assessment, hearing the treatment or the type of healer should be a clue to what to ask next—to elicit beliefs about the cancer and perhaps other potential treatments.

Dual Use

Most of us assume that when a Western physician is involved in the care of the patient, he or she is the only practitioner relevant to the case, which need not be true. When patients maintain both a proximate and an ultimate cause, healers may be chosen to treat each of the causes. This situation is called *dual use* by anthropologists: the simultaneous or nearly simultaneous use of practitioners from two different medical systems (Press, 1969). Dual use is not uncommon among traditional members of some ethnic groups, and the practice is common among Chinese Americans (Hessler, Nolan, Ogbru, & New, 1975). Dual use is an important practice to consider in evaluating possible treatments. Biomedical and folk treatment practices may engender interaction effects, as when herbs and pills contain the same active ingredients (Campbell & Chang, 1973); at times, aspects of the folk treatment may be contraindicated biomedically.

ADHERENCE

Adherence to suggestions is the content of another of the elements of the health seeking process. Adherence in this model is an issue no matter what expertise is possessed by the source of the recommendation. The value in asking about adherence is that the clinician can discover *why* a treatment suggestion was or was not attempted. Adherence is likely to be greater when treatments make sense to the patient; that is, when the treatment is logically coherent with the patient's notion of the cause or pathophysiology of the problem. A second possible factor is the patient's degree of trust in the practitioner (Chrisman & Baker, 1978).

The clinical implication of these two factors, cultural "sense" and trust, is that the clinician can work to increase these features in interactions with patients. Carefully explaining how the illness is conceived by the health care team and thus how the treatment is related is a key behavior. Many clinicians attempt these explanations in their patient teaching, but as will be seen later, the critical first step of asking what the patient thinks may be left out. Second, trust in the judgment of the clinician is enhanced when the patient feels that his or her beliefs have been attended to.

ROLE SHIFT

The role shift element refers to the changes in everyday behavior that the patient has made to accommodate to the illness. Space constraints prevent a complete consideration of this concept; however, a few basic points can be made. Any role behavior changes are the result of overt or covert negotiation with the social environment (Goffman, 1967). Thus members of the patient's social network are involved. Clinicians should pay special attention to the ways in which their own assumptions about how the patient's life "ought" to be led may affect their judgments. For example, a young, twice-married mother of three told an interviewer that she was highly unlikely to follow through on the recommendation of bed rest at home for the next few weeks. She noted that her blue-collar husband would not perform the tasks of a housewife, and she was worried about being divorced and left alone. It is extremely important to investigate fully the social environment in which a patient lives, including beliefs about that environment. Not everyone is accorded the "time-out" that relatively affluent middle-class people enjoy when they are sick. The clinician also should attend to the difficulties created by the patient's being chronically sick. The gracious acceptance of disability may wear thin in some families.

LAY CONSULTATION AND REFERRAL

Lay consultation and referral refers to the constantly occurring discussions that take place among people and their families and friends. This communication process is a significant source of information about what symptoms mean, what to do for particular symptoms, and what type of practitioner to consult for health problems. There are wide variations across ethnic and socioeconomic groups concerning the degree to which lay consultants affect individual decision making. Among some groups, such as Hispanics and Asians, the lay referral network can have a large effect on patient behavior (Freidson, 1970). This situation contrasts strongly with the typical middle-class white patient who is expected to make his or her own decisions with limited advice from lay consultants.

Clinically, data about the role family and friends have played in an illness episode can be discovered by listening carefully to answers to questions already discussed, for example, by noting who has been making treatment suggestions. Additional information may be gathered by finding out who takes care of the patient at home, who has offered referral or diagnostic advice, or who is believed to be supportive emotionally.

Involve the Family

Knowledge of the patient's network of helpers is a major advantage to the clinician who works in the community or who bridges the hospital-community gap. The individuals who already have played a part in the (sometimes recurring) illness episode are the logical first contacts for the nurse who desires to create what might be called a "therapy management group" (Janzen, 1978). Janzen used this term to denote the group of family who took complete charge of their patient family member in Zaire. Perhaps it is useful here in signaling the inclusion of the family, friends, or both in caregiving. Importantly, taking the step of working with the therapy management group means that the original function of this group—to make decisions about patient care—needs to be respected. Nurses are frequently reluctant to give up their control of patients even in outpatient care. The use of this concept requires that the nurse share or even relinquish some or all care responsibilities except as requested by the management group.

SUMMARY

I have been discussing the health seeking process as a framework for understanding patient behavior in its sociocultural context. Accompanying each element, I have made suggestions about how to provide more culture-sensitive care. One useful way to summarize these suggestions is to turn to the third of the three principles—negotiation, the process of reaching agreement through discussions. Negotiation is essential when careful and culturally relativistic monitoring has disclosed a conflict or potential conflict between the patient's beliefs or behaviors and the clinician's expectations of appropriate care. The negotiation process outlined in the following section is designed to aid in solving such cases (Katon & Kleinman, 1981). Just as important, however, is its illustration of the other two culture-sensitive care principles: knowledge and mutual respect.

Negotiation

Negotiation begins with the recognition that negotiation is necessary. This recognition is frequently the result of an open communication link between the nurse and the patient in which the patient feels free to disclose what he or she is doing to engage in self-care. Sometimes nurses discover such conflicts from the family and sometimes only when the patient refuses to comply. An open communication link is the channel through which much knowledge about patient and nurse can be accumulated. The desire to negotiate rather than to make demands for compliance arises in part from mutual respect. Treating the patient as an adult implies that differences can be negotiated. The negotiation process outlined here is useful in dealing with conflict, but it is also a useful process to use during all encounters with clients.

Listen. The patient's perspective—beliefs about the illness, effect of the illness on his or her life, and knowledge and desires about treatment—must be listened to carefully with a culturally relativistic attitude. The explanatory model interview is the common method for eliciting this information. Asking for the patient's perspective provides the clinician with two kinds of information: (1) the beliefs and practices themselves and (2) the extent of patient knowledge about the biomedical perspective and the language and terminology with which he or she is comfortable.

Teach. Using the level of language and terminology with which the patient is comfortable, the clinician makes recommendations for treatment. It is best to phrase this knowledge in terms of one's own experience rather than in more distant, authoritative terms (e.g., "I have found that this treatment provides you with some comfort" versus "This is the correct medical way to treat the problem").

Compare. Nurses should state the prognosis or other outcomes of each of the treatment patterns in the ways they understand them. Sometimes there is not much difference among possible outcomes. For example, a nurse complained that her patient's family wished to take the terminally ill member to Mexico. I pointed out that the outcome—death—was going to be the same whether they remained in cold rainy Seattle or traveled to warm sunny Mexico.

Compromise. Attempt to maximize the contribution

of both biomedicine and folk (or alternative) medicine to a negotiated treatment plan. The key to this process is to remember a basic principle from Hippocrates: do no harm. Folk or alternative treatments should be evaluated from a biomedical point of view. Those practices that are helpful or biomedically neutral (not harmful) should be promoted. Doing so helps patients understand that the clinician is willing to take their perspectives seriously. Practices that are judged to be biomedically harmful should be disapproved of; that is, the patient should be told that more harm than good would come from carrying out that practice. If the patient is unable to give up a practice that the nurse has judged to be biomedically harmful (not simply something odd), and if the nurse is not willing to be involved in unsafe or illegal practices, the patient should be told that ethically the nurse can no longer stay on the case. The nurse can then offer to refer the patient to another nurse specialist.

The negotiation process typifies the nature of culture-sensitive care: respect for the patient, reduction of ethnocentrism, and use of the illness-disease distinction in nursing practice. All of this was summed up long ago by Florence Nightingale: "Nurse the sick, not the sickness."

References

Campbell, T., & Chang, B. (1973). Health care of Chinese in America. *Nursing Outlook, 21,* 245–249.

Chrisman, N. J. (1977). The health seeking process: An approach to the natural history of illness. *Culture, Medicine, and Psychiatry, 1,* 351–377.

Chrisman, N. J. (1981). Nursing in the context of social and cultural systems. In P. H. Mitchell & A. Loustau (Eds.), *Concepts basic to nursing* (3rd ed., pp. 37–52). New York: McGraw-Hill Book Co.

Chrisman, N. J. (1984). Cultural influences on health seeking behavior. In *Proceedings of the Fourth National Conference on Cancer Nursing* (pp. 155–161). New York: American Cancer Society.

Chrisman, N. J. (1985). Alcoholism: Illness or disease? In L. A. Bennett & G. M. Ames (Eds.), *The American experience with alcohol: Contrasting cultural perspectives* (pp. 7–23). New York: Plenum Press.

Chrisman, N. J. (1986). Transcultural care. In D. Zschocke (Ed.), *Mosby's comprehensive review of critical care* (pp. 58–69). St. Louis: C. V. Mosby Co.

Chrisman, N. J., & Baker, R. M. (1978). Exploring the doctor-patient relationship: A sociocultural pilot study in a family practice residency. *Journal of Family Practice, 7,* 713–719.

Chrisman, N. J., & Kleinman, A. (1983). Popular health care, social networks, and cultural meanings: The orientation of medical anthropology. In D. Mechanic (Ed.), *Handbook of health, health care and the health professions* (pp. 569–590). New York: The Free Press.

Fabrega, H. (1972). Medical anthropology. In B. J. Siegel (Ed.), *Biennial review of anthropology, 1971.* Stanford: Stanford University Press.

Foster, G. M. (1979). Humoral traces in United States folk medicine. *Medical Anthropology Newsletter, 10,* 17–20.

Freidson, E. (1970). *Profession of medicine: A study of the sociology of applied knowledge.* New York: Dodd, Mead & Co.

Goffman, E. (1967). *Interaction ritual: Essays on face-to-face behavior.* Garden City, NY: Anchor Books.

Goodenough, W. H. (1963). *Cooperation in change.* New York: Russell Sage Foundation.

Gordon, M. M. (1964). *Assimilation in American life: The role of race, religion, and national origins.* New York: Oxford University Press, Inc.

Harwood, A. (1977). *Rx: Spiritist as needed.* New York: John Wiley & Sons, Inc.

Hessler, R. M., Nolan, R. F., Ogbru, B., & New, P. K. (1975). Intraethnic diversity: Health care of the Chinese-Americans. *Human Organization, 34,* 253–263.

Janzen, J. M. (1978). *The quest for therapy: Medical pluralism in Lower Zaire.* Berkeley: University of California Press.

Jones, W. T. (1976). World-views and Asian medical systems: Some suggestions for further study. In C. Leslie (Ed.), *Asian medical systems* (pp. 383–404). Berkeley: University of California Press.

Katon, W., & Kleinman, A. (1981). Doctor-patient negotiations and other social science strategies in patient care. In L. Eisenberg & A. Kleinman (Eds.), *The relevance of social science for medicine* (pp. 253–379). Dordrecht, Holland: D. Reidel.

Kleinman, A. (1980). *Patients and healers in the context of culture.* Berkeley: University of California Press.

Kleinman, A. (1982). Neurasthenia and depression: A study of somatization and culture in China. *Culture, Medicine, and Psychiatry, 6,* 117–190.

Kleinman, A., Eisenberg, L., & Good, B. (1978). Culture, illness and care: Clinical lessons from anthropological and cross-cultural research. *Annals of Internal Medicine, 88,* 251–258.

Kluckhohn, C. & Kelly, W. H. (1945). The concept of culture. In R. Linton (Ed.), *The science of man in the world crisis.* New York: Octagon.

Leventhal, H., Nerenz, D. R., & Steele, D. J. (1984). Illness representations and coping with health threats. In A. Baum, S. E. Taylor, & J. E. Singer (Eds.), *Handbook of psychology and health (vol. 4).* Hillsdale NJ: L. Erlbaum Associates.

Logan, M. H. (1977). Anthropological research on the hot-cold theory of disease: Some methodological suggestions. *Medical Anthropology, 1*(4), 89–112.

Moore, L. G., Van Arsdale, P. W., Glittenberg, J. E., & Aldrich, R. A. (1980). *The biocultural basis of health: Expanding views of medical anthropology.* St. Louis: C. V. Mosby Co.

Munet de Vilaró, F. (1984). *Coping strategies and adaptation to childhood cancer of Puerto Rican families.* Unpublished doctoral dissertation, University of Washington, Seattle.

Press, I. (1969). Urban illness: Physicians, curers, and dual use in Bogota. *Journal of Health and Social Behavior, 10,* 209–218.

Smith, M. E. (1972). Folk medicine among the Sicilian-Americans of Buffalo, New York. *Urban Anthropology, 1,* 87–106.

Snow, L. F. (1974). Folk medical beliefs and their implications for care of patients. *Annals of Internal Medicine, 81,* 82–96.

Snow, L. F. (1978). Sorcerers, saints, and charlatans: Black folk healers in urban America. *Culture, Medicine, and Psychiatry, 2,* 69–106.

Williams, R. (1960). *American society: A sociological interpretation* (2nd rev ed.). New York: Alfred A. Knopf.

CHAPTER 7

Developmental Process

SUE N. McINTIRE

CANCER NURSING

Nurses care for people of all ages with cancer and need to understand and manage the varied and complex problems that people encounter in living with cancer. Nurses in all professional settings are in a key position to assist patients with cancer. Using concepts from developmental theories is a useful way for nurses to organize the knowledge needed to care for patients with cancer.

The goal of cancer nursing is to help patients and their families use and conserve energy and cope with the problems that accompany the diagnosis of cancer and the application of treatment modalities. Nurses use their knowledge and skills to anticipate, predict, or prevent problems. Cancer as a diagnosis has a devastating psychological impact on a person regardless of age. If nurses understand this profound effect and can relate it to societal developmental tasks, they can anticipate the needs of persons with cancer, provide individualized nursing care, and counsel both patients and families in their responses and management of the disease.

This chapter presents and applies to nursing developmental theories and tasks that are derived from sociologic theories of growth and development. Sections within the chapter review the background of these theories, define developmental tasks, present the major contributions of selected theorists, present examples of developmental tasks, and apply these concepts to cancer nursing.

BACKGROUND

A great deal has been written on the developmental stages of life from birth to 18 years of age. The early literature reflects an emphasis on child development. The focus of this research appears to have changed following World War II from the study of children to the study of adults and, specifically, the beginning of a look at all ages.

The concept of developmental tasks began in the 1930s and early 1940s with the work of Frank, Prescott, Tryon, and Zackery (Havighurst, 1972). The developmental task concept occupies a middle ground between two opposing theories of education: the theory of freedom—that the child will develop best if left as free as possible—and the theory of constraint—that the child must learn to become a worthy, responsible adult through restraints imposed by society. A developmental task is midway between an individual need and a societal demand. For example, major tasks for the adolescent are (1) to find the self as a member of one or more peer groups, (2) to develop skill in relating to the opposite sex, (3) to develop intellectual and work skills, and (4) to develop the social sensitivities of a competent active citizen. It assumes an active learner interacting with an active social environment. Developmental tasks are useful concepts for nurses to relate to human development and behavior and to the problems and processes of cancer nursing.

Living is learning, and growing is learning. One learns to talk, walk, throw a ball, read, bake a cake, get along with peers of the opposite sex, hold down a job, raise children, retire, and manage without a spouse after many years. These are all learning tasks. To understand human development, one must understand learning. The human individual learns throughout life. The path of learning encompasses not one long, slow, uphill climb with something new to learn every day but consists of steep places, when the learning effort is severe, interspersed with plateaus, when one can speed along almost without effort.

In simple societies, the young adult has mastered most of the learning tasks of life. This is not true in modern society, in which changes occur so rapidly that the individual must continually learn to adapt. Living in a modern society includes learning a long series of tasks; learning well brings satisfaction and reward, whereas learning poorly brings unhappiness and social disapproval.

DEVELOPMENTAL TASKS

Developmental tasks may arise from physical maturation; from the pressure of cultural processes on the individual; from the desires, aspirations, and values of the emerging personality; and, in most cases, from combinations of these factors acting together. Havighurst (1972) defines this concept of developmental tasks as follows: "A developmental task is a task which arises at or about a certain period in the life of the individual, successful achievement of which leads to his happiness and to success with later tasks, while failure leads to unhappiness in the individual, disapproval by the society, and difficulty with later tasks."

For example, the developmental tasks of the infant include (1) establishing the self dependent but separate from others, (2) developing a sense of what is alive and what is inanimate in one's environment, (3) developing a feeling for other persons and adjusting to their expectations, (4) developing conceptual abilities and preverbal communication.

In contrast, the developmental tasks of the older adult include (1) deciding where and how to live the remaining years, (2) continuing a close, warm relationship with spouse or significant other, (3) adjusting to living on a retirement income, (4) maintaining a maximal level of health (Murray & Zentner, 1979).

MAJOR THEORISTS
Robert Havighurst

A developmental task, then, is specific learning that an individual needs in terms of the expectations and pressures of the society. These needs and pressures derive from maturing processes in terms of what culture demands of the person at a given age. In his book, *Developmental Tasks and Education* (1972), Havighurst includes a detailed description of the nature of the task; the biologic, psychological, and sociocultural bases of development; and the educational implications and developmental tasks of the growth periods. These developmental tasks do not become complete at any given age but represent an ongoing and unfolding process throughout the individual's life, from tasks occurring in early adulthood through those occurring in later maturity. Individuals learn best those things that are necessary for them to advance from one phase of development to another.

The underlying assumption is that as an individual matures, readiness to learn is decreasingly the product of biologic development and academic pressure and increasingly the product of the developmental tasks required for the performance of evolving social roles. An individual approaching these developmental phases reaches a "readiness to learn" those things necessary to fulfill certain needs. When an individual reaches these respective peaks, a "teachable moment" occurs. The implications for teaching occur when a person has reached a readiness to learn.

The concept of the teachable moment indicates that real learning is based on the perceived need of the learner. Facts can be taught in the abstract, but they are only learned when the learner feels the need to apply them to a personal situation. The teachable moment usually occurs after the learners have gone through the process of identifying a felt need and want additional knowledge or skills to deal with the situation. Regardless of an individual's background, the motivation to learn based on a perceived need is the strongest influence in learning. This concept of the teachable moment is especially relevant to adult education because adults do not have the same peer pressure or the motivation that youth in the classrooms have (Knowles, 1970).

Havighurst proposes reasons why the concepts of developmental tasks and teachable moments are useful. They help to uncover and to state the purposes of education in schools and other learning institutions, thereby helping the individual to achieve certain developmental tasks.

Abraham Maslow

In his earlier work, *Motivation and Personality* (1954), Maslow presented a theory of human motivation and the role of basic need gratification in psychological theory. Maslow describes the chief principle of organization in motivational life as the arrangement of basic needs in a hierarchy of less or greater priority or potency (Fig. 7–1). The chief dynamic principle is the emergence in the healthy person of less potent needs. The physiologic needs when unsatisfied dominate the organism (human being). The concept of need is a basic drive as compared with the societal expectation of developmental tasks. The motivational drive in a person may be a combination of meeting basic needs and becoming socialized to achieve certain tasks. For example, the developmental tasks of adulthood include (1) developing a satisfactory relationship with a mate, (2) achieving a mature sense of social and civic responsibility, (3) continuing to develop in a vocation or profession that provides satisfaction and financial independence, and (4) establishing and developing a family. The motivational drive to succeed and be successful can conflict with the demands of a family of

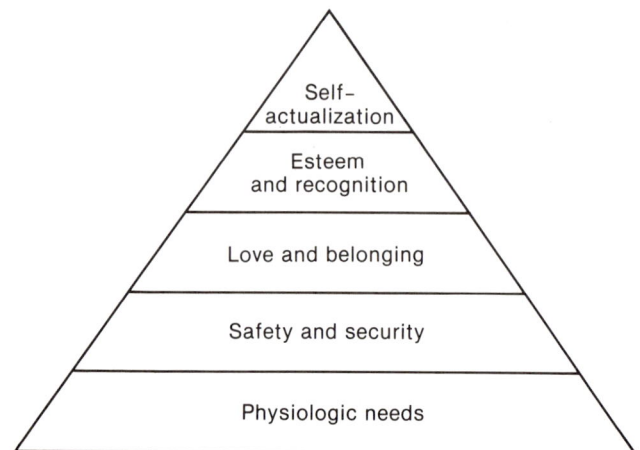

Figure 7–1. Maslow's Need-Priority Model.

Table 7–1. EIGHT AGES OF MAN

	1	2	3	4	5	6	7	8
VIII Maturity								Ego integrity vs. despair
VII Adulthood							Generativity vs. stagnation	
VI Young Adulthood						Intimacy vs. isolation		
V Puberty and Adolescence					Identity vs. role confusion			
IV Latency				Industry vs. Inferiority				
III Locomotor-Genital			Initiative vs. guilt					
II Muscular-Anal		Autonomy vs. shame, doubt						
I Oral Sensory	Basic trust vs. mistrust							

(Adapted from Childhood and Society, 2nd ed., by Erik H. Erikson, by permission of W. W. Norton & Company, Inc. Copyright 1950, © 1963 by W. W. Norton & Company, Inc. Copyright renewed 1978 by Erik H. Erikson.)

school-age or teenage children. Another situation that can create tension is when adults are working hard to achieve but have to reverse roles with their parents when a major illness occurs.

Evelyn Duvall

Duvall further expanded the concept of developmental task and applied it in the field of family life education. The thesis in Duvall's *Marriage and Family Development* (1971, 1977) is that developmental stages can be predicted and identified as the family moves through its life cycle and can be understood in terms of the development of individual family members and of the family as a whole.

Duvall states that the developmental task concept satisfies the search for a frame of reference that deals dynamically with the challenges of human development, keeping responsibility in the hands of the developing persons, yet allowing room for the helping roles that family members, school personnel, and community workers might play.

Erik Erikson

Erikson's influence in this area began in 1950, when he published his first book, *Childhood and Society*. Erikson's work on childhood seems to be better understood and more widely appreciated than his work on adulthood. Levinson (1978) refers to Erikson's work as a historical, sociologic-psychological mode of analysis. Erikson's work is well known and widely used. His major concepts are the Eight Ages of Man, which are presented in Table 7–1.

CANCER NURSING

In cancer nursing textbooks, several investigators have summarized a useful approach to cancer nursing. Donovan and Pierce (1976), Marino (1981), and McIntire and Cioppa (1984) have described the philosophical understanding that they believe a nurse needs to care for patients with cancer. I believe a nurse needs comprehension skills (knowledge), caring skills, com-

Table 7–2. SPECIAL REQUIREMENTS FOR CANCER NURSES

Comprehension
  Knowledge of cancer problem(s)
  Mortality
  Morbidity
  Major treatment modalities
  Knowledge of developmental theories
  Knowledge of specific developmental tasks

Caring
  Nursing role
  Nursing process
  Humanistic care
  Nursing art and skills

Communication
  Visual (seeing)
  Auditory (hearing)
  Kinesthetic (feeling)

Commitment
  Nursing assessment
  Contract with patients or clients
  Nursing follow through and coordination
  Use of developmental tasks

Compassion
  Nursing role
    Physical care
    Emotional care
    Psychosocial care
    Spiritual care

LEVEL III
(full-channel integration)

LEVEL II
(single-channel integration)

LEVEL I
(sensory)

```
                                  ┌──────────────┐
                                  │  Perceiving  │
                                  └──────────────┘
                   ┌─────────────────────┼─────────────────────┐
            ┌──────────────┐      ┌──────────────┐      ┌──────────────┐
            │  Observing   │      │  Listening   │      │   Feeling    │
            └──────────────┘      └──────────────┘      └──────────────┘
                   │                     │                     │
            ┌──────────────┐      ┌──────────────┐      ┌──────────────┐
            │    Seeing    │      │   Hearing    │      │   Touching   │
            └──────────────┘      └──────────────┘      └──────────────┘
                 VISUAL               AUDITORY            KINESTHETIC
```

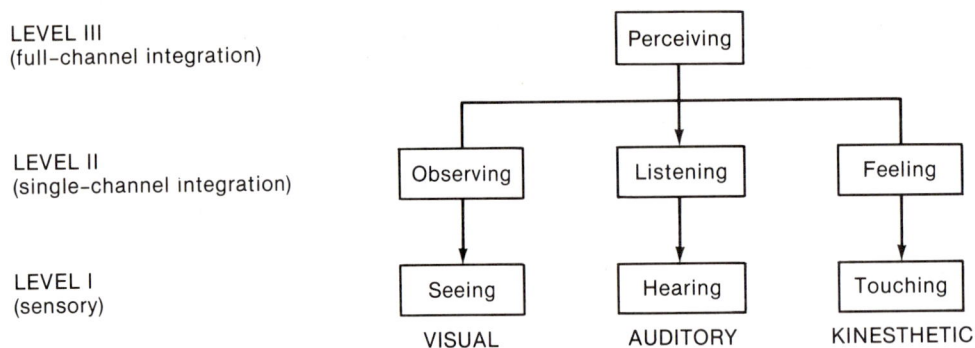

Figure 7–2. Communication levels. (From Bradley, J., & Edinberg, M. [1986]. *Communication in the Nursing Context.* Norwalk, CT: Appleton-Century-Crofts. Reproduced by permission.)

mitment skills, communication skills, and compassion. These major concepts are presented in Table 7–2 and are discussed in the following sections.

MAJOR CONCEPTS

Comprehension. Comprehension in oncology includes (1) knowledge of the cancer problem or problems; (2) mortality, or the actual or projected death rates; (3) morbidity, or the incidence of cancer in specific organ sites; and (4) major treatment modalities of surgery, chemotherapy, immunotherapy, and radiation therapy. Comprehension of knowledge includes knowing and using the developmental tasks.

Caring Skills. Caring skills include one's philosophy of life and death, valuing life, and recognizing individual needs and uniqueness. The nurse brings to the nursing role his or her own unique qualities. The nursing role may consist of the nurse's perception of personal values, society's values, or patients' values and of the health agency or institutional variables.

The nursing process is the organizing framework of the professional nurse for delivering a quality, caring service to people. Care is the nurse seeing and relating to patients as people. The Golden Rule applies here.

Commitment. Commitment refers to a charge or trust, a state of being obligated, and an agreement or pledge to do something in the future. The nurse makes a commitment to the person with cancer for a complete and thorough assessment of the potential or threatened problem. Many nurses today use contracts with their patients. The contract may be verbal or written; the patient should have the opportunity for input. In addition, the nurse demonstrates commitment by coordinating activities such as discharge planning, referrals, home care, and planned telephone or clinic follow-up.

Communication. The literature indicates that Americans spend about 70 per cent of their active hours communicating verbally: listening, speaking, and writing, in that order. Bradley and Edinberg (1986) state that a nurse's effectiveness in communicating with others is certainly one of the most, if not the most, important components of nursing practice. In *Communication in the Nursing Context* (1986), they organize communication into three general categories or channels:

1. Seeing—visual
2. Hearing—auditory
3. Feeling—kinesthetic

These three categories represent major senses that all normal functioning human beings possess to some degree. Within each channel there are different levels of integration (Fig. 7–2). That is, information that is seen, heard, or felt may be reported as it actually was seen, heard, or touched (level I). Information may be reported in terms of observations—what the nurse learned by really listening—or in terms of the nurse's feelings about a patient or client (level II). A third level integrates data from all three channels into the nurse's perceptions about the client (level III).

Compassion. Compassion refers to a consciousness of another's distress together with a desire to alleviate the distress. Oncology nursing demonstrates this attribute in everyday activities for the cancer patient through nursing measures promoting physiologic and psychological comfort.

The nurse's role encompasses the provision of the physical care required; the emotional care of support and counseling; the psychosocial care of the patient and significant others; and the spiritual care, which may also be given by the minister or hospital chaplain.

As individuals grow and develop physically and psychologically, they find themselves facing new demands and expectations from society and the surrounding environment. The ways individuals cope with physical and emotional needs to lead successful and happy lives in their society has been clarified by the concept of developmental tasks. Examples of developmental tasks of early adulthood include (1) accepting self and stabilizing self-concept and body image, (2) becoming established in a vocation or profession, (3) learning to express love responsibly through more than sexual contacts, and (4) deciding to have a family. The nurse uses the concepts of comprehension, commitment, caring, communication, and developmental tasks.

APPLICATION TO NURSING

An example of a patient seen in a southeastern medical center clinic is as follows:

Box 7–1. DEVELOPMENTAL ASSESSMENT GUIDE FOR YOUNG ADULTS WITH CANCER

DIAGNOSIS _____ DATE OF INTERVIEW _____

AGE _____ SEX _____ DATE OF DIAGNOSIS _____

MARITAL STATUS _____ OCCUPATION AND WORK STATUS

TREATMENT _____ _____

OTHER HEALTH PROBLEMS _____ INPATIENT _____

_____ OUTPATIENT _____

PHYSICAL CONCERNS
1. Current physical concerns
2. Adverse effects of disease
3. Side effects of treatment
4. Other

CONCERN ABOUT TREATMENT
1. Treatment itself
2. Side effects
3. Other procedures
4. Other

SATISFACTION WITH HEALTH CARE
1. Hospital/clinic area
2. Physicians
3. Nurses
4. Social Service
5. Lack of continuity of care
6. Getting information
7. Other

FINANCES
1. Medical costs
2. Transportation
3. Other

MOBILITY
1. ADLs
2. Level of disability
3. Work around the house
4. Other

VOCATIONAL
1. Time off from work/school
2. Unemployed due to disease
3. Being treated differently

4. Change in career plans
5. Other

SOCIAL
1. Leisure activity participation
2. Dating pattern changes
3. More solitary activities

SIGNIFICANT RELATIONSHIPS
1. Spouse/significant other
2. Children
3. Siblings
4. Parents
5. Friends
6. Co-workers
7. Communication
8. Other

IMAGE OF SELF
1. Role change
2. Appearance change
3. Self-concept
4. Other

SEXUALITY
1. Sexual activity
2. Changes in sex life
3. Concern over childbearing

LIFE/DEATH CONCERNS
1. Increase in thoughts about dying
2. Faith or religion
3. Other

COPING STRATEGIES

(From Kane, N.E. [1981]. The young adult with cancer: A developmental approach. *Oncology Nursing Forum, 8,* 16–19. Reproduced by permission.)

Mrs. G, a 46-year-old female, was examined for a breast nodule and had a mammogram that revealed an abnormal nodule. She had a surgical biopsy of the lesion as an outpatient. The pathology report was adenocarcinoma of the right breast. She then prepared to enter the hospital for a modified radical mastectomy. Mrs. G is married, with a husband and one daughter about to be married. Her father is 69 years old, a widower since her mother died 8 months ago following a long illness from a stroke. Her father lives alone and has diabetes mellitus, hypertension, and limited vision.

Mrs. G had been helping to care for her mother, and she has continued to help care for her father. She assists him with meal preparation, grocery shopping, and preparing his insulin; she reminds him to take his prescribed medicines and provides transportation. Mrs. G also works at two part-time jobs. She drives a school bus in the mornings and works three evenings a week in a department store. Mrs. G's husband is self-employed in his own business, and she also assists him with his bookkeeping records.

Mrs. G had a modified radical mastectomy with no further evidence of disease. Lymph node tests and body scans were all negative. Mrs. G will return in 3 months for a second follow-up visit.

In considering the developmental tasks of Mrs. G, the nurse can immediately see the need for a thorough assessment and follow-up, perhaps with counseling, support, and teaching regarding her cancer. Mrs. G is completing the middle adulthood developmental tasks and will soon be approaching the later adulthood tasks. Her current developmental tasks include (1) discovering pleasure in generativity and recognition in her work, (2) creating a pleasant, comfortable home appropriate for her values and financial resources, (3) reversing roles with an aging parent, (4) preparing for and accepting the death of a parent, and (5) discovering new satisfactions with her mate. The diagnosis of breast cancer has had an impact on Mrs. G and on her ability to carry out her family responsibilities for a temporary and possibly a permanent period of time. The nurse can use the knowledge of developmental tasks and incorporate the concepts of comprehension, commitment, communication, compassion, and caring skills into coordinating the care and support for Mrs. G.

KANE MODEL

Kane (1981) has proposed a developmental assessment guide (Box 7–1) based on the tasks faced by young adults and Weisman's seven major areas of cancer patients' concerns. These seven areas of predominant concern are health, self-appraisal, work and finances, family and significant relationships, religion, friends and associates, and existential concerns. This approach can help the nurse to make an individual plan for future health and nursing care for Mrs. G and her family.

SUMMARY

A developmental approach is a sound theoretical framework for organizing knowledge and nursing content into an operational approach for the nurse in providing nursing care to patients or clients with cancer. The human developmental framework can enable the nurse to give quality care to patients and to adopt a humanistic approach in a highly technologic medical system environment.

References

Bradley, J., & Edinberg, M. (1986). *Communication in the nursing context.* Norwalk, CT: Appleton-Century-Crofts.

Duvall, E. (1971, 1977). *Family development.* Philadelphia: J. B. Lippincott Co.

Erikson, E. H. (1963). *Childhood and society.* New York: W. W. Norton & Co.

Havighurst, R. (1972). *Developmental tasks and education.* New York: David McKay Co., Inc.

Kane, N. E. (1981). The young adult with cancer: A developmental approach. *Oncology Nursing Forum, 8,* 16–19.

Knowles, M. (1970). *The Modern practice of adult education: Andragogy versus pedagogy.* Boston: Follett Publishing Co.

Levinson, D. (1978). *The seasons of a man's life.* New York: Ballantine Books.

Maslow, A. (1954, 1972). *Motivation and personality.* New York: Harper & Row Publishers, Inc.

McIntire, S. N., & Cioppa, A. (Eds.). (1984). *Cancer nursing: A developmental approach.* New York: John Wiley & Sons, Inc.

Murray, R. B., & Zentner, J. P. (1989). *Nursing Assessment and Health Promotion Through the Life Span,* Englewood Cliffs, N.J., Prentice-Hall.

Valentine, A. (1978). Caring for the young adult with cancer. *Cancer Nursing, 1,* 385–389.

CHAPTER 8

Compliance and Health Promotion Behaviors

BARBARA GIVEN

Individuals can make changes or carry out behaviors in their personal lives to reduce the risks of cancer, facilitate treatment if cancer is diagnosed, and deal with overall health when under treatment for cancer. Little description can be found of how individual responsibility contributes to the effectiveness of cancer prevention and early detection or how compliance behaviors influence the effectiveness of the prescribed treatment when cancer is present. In this chapter a model is presented that can be used to analyze and foster behaviors for health promotion and compliance in clients with cancer.

The model that is outlined is based on the health belief model (Becker, 1984) and on the earlier work of Given and Given (1984). It describes factors related to health-oriented compliance behavior (Fig. 8–1). Three major foci lead to the actual health-oriented compliance behaviors. Although these foci are discussed as if they were discrete variables, they overlap and are better viewed as being interdependent. The first focus in the model is client perceptions; the second is a supportive environment, that is, client-provider and family interactions; and the third is disease and treatment-related variables. Sociodemographic characteristics modify client perceptions and perceived benefits and barriers. Given the interaction of these factors, the client then balances the cost-benefit of the action and makes a decision regarding whether to carry out the prescribed behavior. Whether health promotion or compliance behaviors are actually adopted depends on the client's assessment of the costs and benefits of the behavior. A discussion about compliance related to a therapeutic regimen for clients with cancer is followed by a short discussion of health promoting behaviors.

THE PROBLEM OF COMPLIANCE

Compliance is not generally recognized as being a problem for clients with cancer because of the direct provider involvement in the administration of many dimensions of cancer therapy. It is assumed that clients with cancer are motivated to participate in the prescribed treatment.

Itano and Tanabe found that 33 to 50 per cent of their patients did not follow their therapeutic regimens. Itano and colleagues (1981) found that 21 per cent of 66 adults receiving chemotherapy did not keep scheduled appointments, complete laboratory tests, or appear for prescribed chemotherapy. In contrast to these compliance figures, studies using medical record abstracts and patient self-reports demonstrated that compliance with clinic appointments for chemotherapy may be as high as 98 per cent among adult clients with breast cancer (Cassileth, Zupkis, Sutton-Smith, & March, 1980; Gore, 1978; Taylor, Lichtman, & Wood, 1984). From the results of these studies, one can see that compliance behaviors may be a problem in cancer care.

The issue of client compliance confronts all who practice in cancer nursing. Despite the most progressive, sophisticated, and complex cancer treatments,

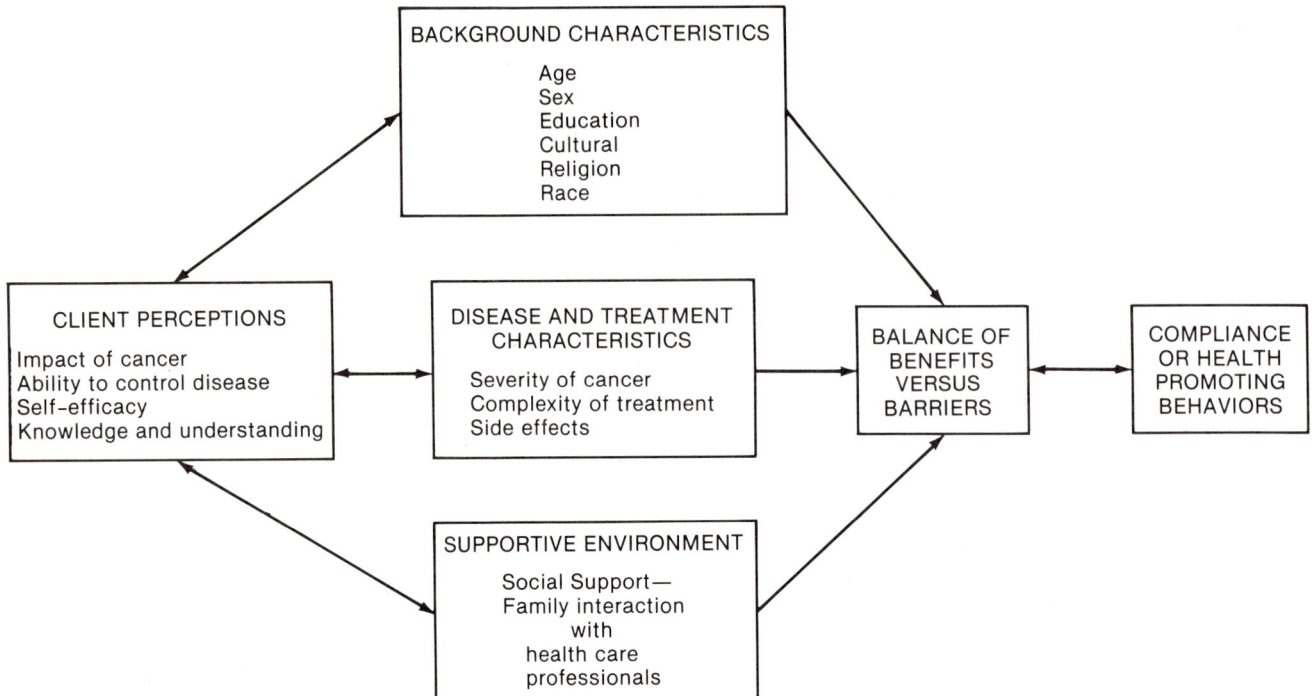

Figure 8-1. Compliance behavior model. (Adapted from Given, B. A., & Given, C. W. [1989]. Compliance among patients with cancer. *Oncology Nursing Forum, 16,* 97-103. Reproduced by permission.)

individuals are ultimately responsible for their own health care practices. All of the advances are to no avail if the prescribed regimen is not followed and if the therapeutic response and desired effectiveness are not reached. The best-designed, randomized protocol effects may be questionable without knowledge of the extent of client compliance. Client compliance with the therapeutic regimen is necessary for cancer control. Early detection, promoting and restoring health, and preventing subsequent recurrence necessitate a partnership among the client, the family, and the health care professionals.

DEFINITION

Compliance can be defined in a positive way to mean "the extent to which a person's behavior such as taking medications, following diets, or instituting lifestyle changes can coincide with medical or health advice" (Hebert, 1977). Compliance is clearly a human response that is aimed at promoting, maintaining, or restoring health. To Given and Given (1984), this definition suggests the importance of health care provider-client partnership, negotiation, and mutual agreement to develop a plan of care. Barofsky's "therapeutic alliance" (Barofsky & Sugarbaker, 1979), Fink's "consensual regimen" (1976), Steckel's "mutual contracting" (1982), and Weintraub's "intelligent noncompliance" (Weintraub, Av, & Lasagna, 1973) are other terms frequently used instead of compliance. These terms also convey the theme of mutual partnership; the client, or consumer, must assume some responsibility and control over the activities directed

toward maintaining health (Bandura, 1982). Compliance using this approach includes entering into and continuing a treatment program, keeping follow-up appointments, making prescribed life-style alterations, and avoiding risk behaviors.

In Figure 8-1 a model that can be used to describe compliance behavior is presented. Compliance behavior evolves from individuals' perceptions of their ability to control the disease, the impact of the disease or treatment on their health, their own skills or ability to carry out what is requested of them, and the perceived efficacy of the treatment. Compliance requires that the individual acquire sufficient information and understanding to facilitate appropriate decision making regarding behaviors required to carry out the therapeutic regimen (Bandura, 1982). The client, in collaboration with the health professionals, helps select the behaviors that support the treatment plan. The client participates as an accountable, responsible, and active partner in the therapeutic plan of care. Age, education, sex, cultural and family values, and a supportive environment influence what the client brings to the therapeutic partnership.

FACTORS INFLUENCING COMPLIANCE

Perceived Impact of Cancer on Health Status

The patient's perception of the impact of cancer on health status needs to be determined. The diagnosis itself may have a major impact and may provoke a fear of pain, death, and disability and may lead to a lack of compliance with the treatment regimen. Clients hold a personal explanation about the disease and about its etiology, course, prognosis, consequences, and responsiveness to treatment (Leventhal, Safer, & Panagis, 1983). The connotation that a client assigns to a cancer diagnosis ultimately influences the ability and action taken to cope with the disease, prognosis, and treatment (Becker, 1984).

The impact of their disease on work, family, social, and leisure activities and the importance of health in relation to other activities may, at times, cause clients to forego initiating or continuing cancer therapy. Some clients are willing to discount future health to maintain their present health status. Mishel (1984) has shown that uncertainty about diagnosis is related to loss of motivation and decreased information seeking and action of cancer patients. Uncertainty may be a deterrent to keeping the client hopeful and actively involved in a plan of care, which could influence compliance behaviors in a negative way.

Perception of a negative health status, such as diagnosis of stage IV breast cancer, may result in decreased health practices (Hallal, 1982). Individuals may decide that the disease is too advanced to be concerned about health. The presence of advanced disease in one breast has been shown to inhibit the employment of early detection practices that might save the remaining breast in patients after breast cancer surgery (Hirshfeld-Bartek, 1982).

Behaviors associated with attaining control of their lives are difficult for clients to accomplish because they involve (1) changing existing habits, (2) modifying normatively prescribed social roles, and (3) redefining and reinterpreting such basic concepts as health and illness. As the treatment and disease cause further disability, major life-style changes may be required. Understanding clients' perceptions and their beliefs about the impact of cancer on their lives and overall health status is important. It is critical that the cancer treatment be integrated into clients' value systems and life styles to preserve the performance of social roles and the maintenance of self-esteem through active participation in the control of the health problems that occur.

Perceived Ability to Control Disease—Efficacy of Treatment

Individuals who undergo therapy for cancer face an uncertain future—one punctuated with periods of relief and periods of loss of control over their lives and their bodies. One approach toward enhancing feelings of control and competency is to increase individuals' cognitive resources by improving their knowledge about the disease and therapeutic regimen. If clients are to complete a long-term regimen of cancer therapy, they need to have realistic perceptions to give them a sense of direction and control over their future health status.

Individuals must perceive the long-term, disruptive, and complex cancer therapy as worth the effort and discomfort for compliance to be sustained. As the course of treatment or disease processes changes, so should the assessment of clients' perceptions related to the efficacy of treatment and ongoing care. The overall perceived benefit of the therapeutic plan on symptoms and disease control should be assessed.

Treatment

Treatment schedules and plans must consider clients' preferences. Clients have to exercise self-responsibility to participate actively in areas in which they *can* make decisions (Dracup & Meleis, 1982). Individuals who have little sense of participation and no control over what is happening to them develop a lack of self-confidence in their ability to participate in and solve problems. Having information about the impact of the diagnosis, treatment, and disease on life style is important to clients' cognitive control, affects clients' perceptions of the situation, and enables them to participate actively and carry out health behaviors (Barofsky, 1984).

Self-Efficacy

The patient's perception of the efficacy of the treatment should be ascertained to determine the sense of hope, expectation, and knowledge of the goals of therapy. The client's perceptions, rather than the actual status of the disease, are what determines and influences compliance behavior. The client's perception of efficacy and long-term effects of *each* dimension of therapy should be determined: chemotherapy, surgery, radiation, immunotherapy, dietary restriction, rehabilitation activities, or other behavioral changes that would be required to carry out the treatment regimen.

Individuals must believe that they have the skills, competence, and ability to do what needs to be done to implement the therapy. Individuals with cancer must acquire the skills and feelings of self-confidence for successful compliance to occur (Bandura, 1977). A patient's perception of efficacy depends on experience with the problem (cancer) and on perceived ability to participate in bringing the disease under control or into remission or cure. Problems posed by cancer and its complex and intense treatment make this feeling of efficacy difficult to maintain. Individuals who seek information and change their behavior patterns to enhance personal control have higher rates of compliance with treatment programs. Self-efficacy reflects an expectation of what the individual believes he or she is competent to do. The client can participate by getting involved with decisions related to the therapeutic regimen, returning for continued treatment, and following prescriptions for home care. Active participation enables clients to fit therapeutic plans into their usual life styles.

By emphasizing the control that clients have, emotional distress can be relieved and problems dealt with more realistically and effectively. Self-esteem and self-efficacy become more of a problem to maintain as uncertainty of the progress of disease and continued complex treatment threaten security, causing disfigurement and loss of identity in social roles due to morbidity and disability. The responsibilities to manage may be overwhelming, especially as the disease progresses or as the exacerbations and remissions continue. Clients need to develop skills for the management of symptoms such as nausea and vomiting, fatigue, or pain and self-regulatory skills to provide control. A program to foster patient involvement and development of self-control skills necessary for early detection of changes, new problems, and need for rehabilitation is essential for the maintenance of a sense of competence and control. This sense fosters the self-image of being effective in self-care.

The clients' abilities to manage or control symptom distress will influence their attitudes toward self and their ability to assume responsibility for compliance with therapeutic care. Clients may want to follow a routine but not have the knowledge, skills, resources, or temperament to undertake therapeutic regimens when they experience difficulties or uncertainties.

Grover, Amsel, and Balshem (1983) suggest that a woman's anxiety and fear about developing a second breast malignancy and the role she can play in early diagnosis affect health-oriented behaviors. Those who changed their health practices and carried out breast self-examination were more highly educated and had learned breast self-examination from the media. Clients' perceptions of their capacities to make changes in their lives were affected by prior experiences but also by a general level of self-esteem and an overall sense of self-control.

In summary, if clients are to maximize their sense of control and cope with the physical and psychosocial effects and disabilities of cancer and multiple phases of cancer therapy, they must believe that cancer has serious consequences and that treatment will have an impact. Further, clients' activity on their own behalf will be maximized if they believe that *their actions* in following the therapy will be beneficial in helping to control the disease, prevent recurrence, or help manage the symptoms. Clients' perceptions that they have the responsibilities and skills to participate in the therapeutic regimen are crucial.

Knowledge about Disease and Treatment

Although no evidence indicates that factual knowledge results in higher compliance behavior, at the very least a basic understanding of the therapeutic regimen, that is, when and how to comply, is a necessary condition (Richardson et al., 1987; Jones, Engstrom, Paul, & Peter, 1983; Bonadonna & Valagussa, 1981). To assume personal responsibility and to be able to make personal choices, a basic knowledge is necessary. Knowledge about symptoms, course of illness and prognosis, extent of illness, likelihood of cure, and complications is relevant information for all clients

with cancer. It is necessary to deal with client knowledge about therapy; the side effects, benefits, and long-term consequences of treatment.

Cassileth and colleagues (1980) reported that clients wanted to have the maximum amount of information and to be able to participate actively in their cancer care. Lum and co-workers (1978) showed that the more information given the client about the disease and therapy and the better the quality of the explanation of the treatment and care regimen, the higher the client's self-esteem and sense of control. In addition, clients who preferred active involvement were more hopeful about the benefits of therapy in overcoming the disease process than were persons who did not actually participate. Uncertainty about illness-related events has been shown to correlate with lack of comprehension among clients (Mishel, Hostetter, King, & Graham, 1984). Uncertainty can be minimized by providing clear information and continuing feedback to the client. This information leads to active compliance behavior.

Richardson and colleagues (1983) and Janis (1982) suggest that information may facilitate compliance. In addition to facts and prognosis about the disease, clients should know what will happen to them during diagnostic tests or treatment. They need to understand how they will feel, what good and bad experiences they might have, and what they can do to cope with the adverse effects they experience.

As information regarding the diagnosis, treatment regimen, and long-term care is shared, activities to achieve desired outcomes can be negotiated. Any effort to provide clients with technical information should be supplemented with efforts to focus on attitudes and perceptions about the regimen that may affect compliance. Clear role responsibilities must be elucidated so that the client can make an informed commitment to needed behaviors that is based on accurate, explicit data (Lucus, 1986).

Individuals need to have information about coping resources, strategies to control symptoms and response, and reassurances. A sense of predictability and control is therefore maximized and should lead to client perceptions of *self-efficacy* to cope with the impending treatments across the trajectory of cancer illness (Boxes 8–1 and 8–2).

According to the model in Figure 8–1, modifying factors, in addition to clients' perceptions, also influence the decision, intent, and actual compliance behavior. These include clients' background characteristics.

MODIFYING FACTORS

Client Background Characteristics

Sociodemographic characteristics such as age, religion, sex, race, socioeconomic status, and educational level are predictors of compliance (Becker, 1984; Haynes, Taylor, & Sackett, 1979). Little evidence of client background information could be found in rela-

Box 8–1. CLIENT ASSESSMENT GUIDE—CANCER COMPLIANCE

PERCEIVED IMPACT OF CANCER ON HEALTH STATUS

1. What is your perception of the impact of cancer on your life?
2. What do you believe the course of the disease will be?
3. How will cancer affect your work?
4. How will cancer affect your family life?
5. How will cancer affect your social and leisure life?
6. How do your think cancer treatment will affect the cancer?
7. What changes will you have to make in your life because of cancer and cancer treatment?

PERCEIVED ABILITY TO CONTROL DISEASE—EFFICACY OF TREATMENT

1. What is the plan of treatment for your cancer?
2. What is the expected outcome of this phase of treatment?
3. What is the benefit of this phase of treatment? How successful do you think therapy will be?
4. What is your role in deciding on treatment?
5. What is your role in carrying out cancer treatment? What help or skills do you need to do that?
6. What do you need to know to help follow the treatment plan?

KNOWLEDGE ABOUT THE DISEASE AND TREATMENT

1. What are the expected signs and symptoms of your disease? side effects of the treatment? complications?
2. What additional information would you like to have?
3. What are the health professionals expecting of you?
4. Do you know how to manage:
   pain?
   nausea and vomiting?
   fatigue?
5. What strategies do you use to cope with cancer and cancer treatment?

SUPPORTIVE ENVIRONMENT

Professionals

1. Are you satisfied with the care you receive from health care professionals?
2. How do health care professionals deal with your expectations about care?
3. Can you share with the health care professionals your concerns?
4. Do you believe the health care professionals are concerned about your well-being?
5. Do you know what they expect of you—your role and responsibility for treatment?

Family and Friends

1. Who assists you when you need someone? Who would help you with important decisions?
2. Who can you talk to when you are upset or distressed?
3. Who provides you with comfort and support for cancer care?
4. What assistance do you find to be unsupportive?
5. How has the support changed during your cancer treatment?
6. What other support would you like to have?

INTENT TO COMPLY

1. What do you see as barriers to following the intended therapeutic plan?
2. Which areas of the plan do you think you can and will follow? Which areas do you think you will not be able to follow?
3. What assistance do you need to follow the plan?

HEALTH PROMOTION ACTIVITIES

1. What health promotion activities do you usually carry out (e.g., diet, exercise, restriction of smoking, stress management)?
2. What practices do you engage in for screening and early detection of cancer?

Box 8–2. STRATEGIES TO ASSIST CLIENTS AND FAMILY COMPLIANCE

IMPACT OF CANCER ON LIFE AND HEALTH

1. Assist client in labeling perceptions and beliefs about health, cancer, and the therapeutic plan.
2. Identify strategies for changing existing life-style patterns.
3. Identify social role changes to be made.
4. Assist client and family in integrating changes caused by cancer and treatment into life style.
5. Assist client and family in dealing with anxiety, depression, or both that are related to cancer diagnosis and treatment.

ABILITY TO CONTROL DISEASE

1. Improve knowledge of disease and therapeutic regimen.
2. Provide information about the intended benefit of the therapeutic plan on disease and symptoms.
3. Assist client and family in participating actively in decisions about the treatment plan.
4. If client and family hold beliefs contrary to the therapeutic plan, help them understand it.
5. Assist clients in acquiring skills to follow therapeutic plan (teach, demonstrate).
6. Identify with client and family their areas of responsibility for cancer care.
7. Encourage the client to be an active partner in control of the disease.
8. Test solutions to find those that best fit the patient's life style and preference.

KNOWLEDGE ABOUT DISEASE AND TREATMENT

1. Provide instructional sessions to obtain needed information for symptom management, signs and symptoms of complications, or evidence of recurrent disease.
2. Assist client in obtaining any psychomotor skills needed to manage equipment related to treatment.
3. Clarify with clients their role in participation in cancer treatment.
4. Ask whether client needs additional information.
5. Provide for future reference written instructions of therapeutic plan.

SUPPORTIVE ENVIRONMENT

1. Assist client in expressing concerns and expectations of assistance from health professionals.
2. Determine congruency between health care professionals and clients on expectations regarding disease and treatment trajectory. Explore reasons behind lack of congruence.
3. Assist client in identifying the type of support desired from family, friends, and other individuals with cancer.
4. Assist client in soliciting and obtaining needed social support.
5. Evaluate with client changes in needed support across treatment trajectory.
6. Enlist the support of family and friends in care.

INTENT TO COMPLY

1. Assist client in identifying specific areas in which compliance is unlikely.
2. Have client identify barriers to compliance behavior.
3. Promote client identifying strategies and support needed to overcome barriers to compliance.
4. Assist client in weighing benefits and barriers to noncompliance and try to overcome those barriers.
5. Validate that client understands what is expected.
6. Assist clients in incorporating the therapeutic plan into their own life styles.

HEALTH PROMOTION

1. Identify client's current health practices.
2. Help client modify health practices and integrate them into life style and cancer treatment.
3. Educate client in early detection practices for cancer (such as breast or testicular self-examination).

---

tionship to cancer. Grover, Amsel, and Balshem (1983) found that breast self-examination practices after mastectomy were positively related to education and inversely related to age. Noncompliance in a pediatric or an adolescent client has a different significance than in an 80-year-old client. Smith, Rosen, Trueworthy, & Lowman (1979) and Tebbe and colleagues (1986) found that 59 per cent of older adolescents with leukemia did not comply with their prescribed dosages of prednisone. Tebbe also found that adolescents may not comply with taking agents that cause embarrassing and socially distasteful side effects.

Cultural attitudes, values, and past experiences are factors that affect compliance behaviors. Negative experiences can preset expectations for further encounters (Lucus, 1986). Few other sociodemographic variables are consistent predictors of compliance behaviors. How developmental stage relates to noncompliance in the cancer client has not been reported in the literature.

Clinical (Disease and Treatment) Characteristics

Illness and treatment variables have not been good predictors of compliance behaviors. Also nonpredictive, as Becker reported (1984), are duration of disease, length of hospital stay, objective severity of disease, and extent of disability. Subjective perception of the severity of disease may relate to compliance. Only complexity of treatment consistently results in lower levels of compliance. Each component of the therapeutic regimen needs to be examined separately. Adherence to radiation treatment, follow-up for reevaluation (Lee, 1983), rehabilitation after extensive surgery, and return for laboratory tests to monitor therapy may also be required. Supportive therapeutic behaviors such as dental hygiene and nutritional therapy are also relevant areas of compliance for cancer clients.

Compliance with oral medications for cancer therapy has received very little attention (Barofsky & Sugarbaker, 1979; Bonadonna & Valagussa, 1981). Given the characteristics of complex cancer treatment, it is important that attention to both antineoplastic and supportive therapy be considered (Richardson et al., 1987). Side effects from treatment regimens are not, however, consistently given as reasons for noncompliance in noncancer populations. Few therapeutic regimens produce effects of the nature and magnitude commonly experienced by cancer clients. Clients, however, may experience profound effects, such as nausea and vomiting, loss of hair, or bone marrow suppression, that result in infection or bleeding (Richardson et al., 1983, 1987). Side effects such as weight loss or hair loss are further problematic because they damage the self-image and are constant reminders of being unwell (Smith, Rosen, Trueworthy, & Lowman, 1979). Visits to the clinic for ongoing treatment over many years and stages of illness serve as an additional reminder of illness. Although some side effects of chemotherapy may be immediate and of short duration, they are frequently intense. The client is constantly confronted with the knowledge that another treatment day is imminent. For clients with cancer, noncompliance is one way of dealing with the lack of personal control that is so threatening (Bonadonna & Valagussa, 1981).

Clients may terminate a therapeutic regimen because of non–life-threatening but pervasive side effects caused by psychological distress or unanticipated disruption of life styles (Lee, 1983; Lucus, 1986; Meyerwitz, Sparks, & Spears, 1979; Smith et al., 1979). Complexity has a negative effect, as individuals cope with the variety of behaviors that are required to follow the regimen, namely, taking medications, changing their diet, changing their activities, and keeping many return appointments. Duration of the regimen is also a major problem for clients if aggressive treatments continue and do not result in disease control.

Different dimensions of treatment requirements may be influenced by different sets of mediating variables because each has its own behavioral demands (Richardson et al., 1987). Gaining compliance requires training in skills, structuring the patient's environment, repetition of information, and reinforcement of behavior (Dunbar, Marshall, & Hovell, 1979; Kasl, 1975). These approaches, however, might be expected to have a stronger impact on compliance with aspects of a regimen that require routine or habitual behaviors, such as daily pill taking; they may have much less effect on irregular demands, such as breast self-examination, arm exercises, or return appointments (Richardson et al., 1987). The changing nature and complexity of the regimen and the extent of adverse effects have major impacts on the perceptions and weighing of the costs and benefits of compliance behavior.

SUPPORTIVE ENVIRONMENT

Health Care Professionals (Nurses and Physicians)

The willingness and ability of the client to follow the selected plan for compliance behavior has much to do with the supportive environment, that is, professional-client interaction and family support. A potent factor in the extent of clients' active involvement in compliance relates to client-provider relationships. Abeldoff, Mellits, and Baumgardner (1981) found that, in addition to side effects, withdrawal from adjuvant therapy for breast cancer was related to unclear and vague physician judgments rather than to a consideration of objective reasons. Health care professionals overestimate the level of compliance (Kasl, 1975; Leventhal et al., 1983). Communication and satisfaction with health care professionals and continuity of care do much to enhance the client's cooperation and the therapeutic partnership that ongoing cancer therapy requires. The client's expectation concerning health care as compared with actual care received is a major factor. Bonadonna and Valagussa (1981) found that physicians often underprescribe chemotherapeutic agents, which alters the effectiveness of therapy.

Researchers suggest that improved client-provider interaction can improve clients' understanding of their disease and treatment (Ley, 1979), their retention of medical information, and their satisfaction with their health (Itano et al., 1981; Korsch, Gozzi, & Francis, 1968). Client satisfaction correlates positively with compliance (Given & Given, 1984; Korsch & Negrete, 1972; Leventhal et al., 1983). Clients must sense provider commitment to the therapeutic regimen and provider support for the myriad problems that may arise during the cancer illness trajectory. An attitude of concern combined with a sense of hope and interest for the client's future well-being affects compliance behaviors.

Abrams (1966) observed that communication patterns of cancer clients *change* during the initial, advanced, and terminal stages of the clinical disease course. Recognition of these changing communication patterns and information needs is important when clients try to follow the therapeutic regimen (Becker, 1984). Changes in the original therapeutic plan and protocol, such as changes in dosage or time of treatment, should be clear to clients. Mutual client–health professional decisions should be fostered. Willingness of the health professionals to support clients psychosocially and physically during adverse reactions and side effects is critical.

Mutual responsibility for care rather than a one-way transfer of information is a prerequisite to the achievement of health promoting behavior. When entering a relationship, role expectations should be clarified. The client enters the therapeutic relationship with preconceived expectations and beliefs about treatment; only when client–health professional expectations are congruent will client satisfaction and responsibility for treatment adherence be increased. Negative experiences can preset expectations for further negative encounters (Lucus, 1986). Responsibility for success can be shared, and mutual trust can be cultivated. In a partnership, noncompliance is not seen as a failure by one of the parties; instead, noncompliance is viewed as the inability to follow the prescribed treatment plan. Both the health care professional and the client assume responsibility for evaluating why the plan cannot be followed and for introducing modifications needed to enhance success. Negotiation, goal setting, argument, and commitment to the development of therapeutic alliance are important for the client's feelings of choice and self-control (Lucus, 1986).

Once nurses recognize their clients' levels of knowledge, perceptions of their health status, perceived benefits of therapy, and perceived social support, they can begin to help clients identify barriers. Strategies can then be developed to resolve problems. Differences in role expectations and outcomes should be resolved at the beginning of the treatment plan and modified over time as the plan is implemented and the illness trajectory changes. Clients are more likely to make a commitment to a clinical treatment plan when health care professionals listen, take time to explain the current medication condition, and care about them as persons.

SOCIAL SUPPORT—FAMILY

Family social support as a reinforcing factor may have a significant influence on patient compliance behaviors (Edwards, 1980). When family members provide rewards, they reinforce the individual's sense of self-worth and being loved, and synergism can occur. Cancer may be responsible for strained and disrupted interpersonal relationships.

Provision of social support (Gore, 1978) is important for maintaining self-esteem and feelings of competence during periods of stress. Social support represents access to intimate others who can offer emotional comfort, assistance, solutions to problems, and reinforcement of the client's sense of self-competency to continue therapy at a time of dependency that results from long-term and intense therapy. Grover and colleagues (1983) found that married women who had had mastectomies were more likely to change and carry out breast self-examination than were those without spouses.

The patient's family and friends play a crucial role in facilitating the patient's ability to make life decisions and to participate actively in care. Family members are a source of rewards as well as transmitters of beliefs and motivaters of patient behavior. A fine line, however, may separate the patient's perception of support and nonsupport (Revenson, Wollman, & Felton, 1983). The notion of support should not be confused with involvement. In their efforts to be supportive, well-meaning families may promote premature dependence for the patient. With the diagnosis and onset of therapy, families and friends attempting to be supportive begin to expend all available energies to assist clients in every dimension of their lives. This smothering and all-consuming attention may threaten the patient's autonomy and self-worth. Family members should be counseled to allocate their energies so that they are available for assistance across the long-term trajectory of the cancer illness.

Social support of a temporary nature may be detrimental to long-term therapy. Clients who find that all support has dissipated when they need it are vulnerable and devastated. Social support is essential when one is adopting and maintaining unfamiliar compliance behaviors. Social support reinforces behavior positively by building up expectations for carrying out appropriate behaviors. Traveling back and forth for treatment, interruptions of employment, and curtailment of domestic and social activities are salient disruptions that may lead to nonsupport from family members.

Clients should be assisted in identifying and labeling the areas in which they need support and then begin to build support. Revenson and colleagues (1983) suggest that those who are not very limited physically can tolerate those who provide support, whereas those who are limited and disabled may resent it. In previous work, Given and Given (1984) identified three types of support: (1) a family member to assist at home with day-to-day activities; (2) a social person (friend, neighbor, or co-worker) with whom the patient can ventilate true feelings; and (3) an individual who has had cancer and understands the experience of having cancer. The third type of support often can be provided from the health care setting. Ongoing social support should be obtained to reduce and manage distress associated with cancer and to reinforce clients as they attempt to solve compliance problems or sustain compliance behaviors.

A match between support needed and support *provided* is important to ongoing success.

COMPLIANCE DECISION

Balance of Barriers versus Benefits

The extent of clients' desires and intentions to actually carry out prescribed compliance behaviors needs to be understood. It is difficult to plan therapeutic care on a long-term basis unless the compliance problems encountered by clients are known and solved. Patterns of compliance behaviors with *each* dimension of the prescribed therapeutic regimen need to be clearly determined. A single question regarding whether one complies cannot determine the full extent of compliance behavior. Only by examining the responses to questions specific to each dimension of the treatment regimen, namely, staying on protocol, follow-up visits, oral medication, maintenance of a diet, or participation in a rehabilitation program, can overall compliance be understood. With medications, for example, compliance may differ depending on the nature of the medication (antibiotics, oral chemotherapy agents, antiemetics, or pain medications). The set of expected compliance behaviors varies from client to client depending on the extent of cancer and the stage of illness.

Weisman and Worden (1980) have demonstrated that problem-solving strategies can be successfully used with clients and can lead to a more realistic appraisal of their illness and therapy. Although clients are asked to identify barriers to each dimension of therapy, they should focus on the primary behaviors to achieve cancer control. Clients require assistance in developing and testing strategies for solving problems and in adapting to the requirements of the prescribed therapy. As they receive support, they then decide on the cost or benefit of that behavior.

As clients discover that following a plan encompassing medications and other therapy interferes with their daily activities, including family, social, and work roles, they then begin to weigh the impositions of such therapy against the benefits of compliance. Some clients discount future health at a higher rate, preferring to maintain their current life style rather than to actively overcome barriers related to their therapy. These clients may choose not to participate in the prescribed cancer therapy. The use of specific, realistic problem-solving steps increases clients' motivational strength, chances of success, and expectancy that one can follow the therapeutic regimen and actively participate in cancer control.

The dimension of barriers to be considered involves cost, inconvenience, change in life style, or interference of therapy with the performance of daily activities. Purchase of special equipment or certain types of food, chemotherapy, and radiation treatment are additional costs. Changes in routines as well as the need to obtain additional social support to continue the treatment on a long-term basis may be barriers.

Complexity, duration, and adverse reactions to the regimen may impede compliance behavior. Treatment-related factors may be major, but clients endure intense responses to therapy across numerous cycles of treatment and continue to participate in the therapy.

Because of their uncertain future, it is often more difficult for clients to plan and to make decisions, especially long-range ones. They cannot always change what life has in store for them. Even though they cannot eliminate the cancer, clients can control how they face problems related to the therapy and disease and know that they will have someone to assist them.

Nurses should demonstrate how the costs associated with carrying out these behaviors can be reduced and help patients see benefits, where possible. Individuals should be made aware that by assuming responsibility for their care, they can participate in the control and management of their disease. In this way, recognition of the problem creates the opportunity for the nurse and client to establish a compliance goal and to identify a set of activities to achieve this goal.

SUMMARY

Activities for achieving compliance goals must be specific, possible, and realistic in view of clients' life styles and the clinical status and stage of their cancers. If individuals internalize their failure, which will lower their self-esteem, they will come to view themselves as being less competent.

In the model presented here, individual perceptions and treatment dimensions, along with family and provider interaction, have been identified as major approaches to improving compliance behavior. Active participation enhances adherence to treatment regimens because it increases the client's sense of control over a dimension of his or her life situation. Nursing activities are designed to assist clients in integrating these perceptions along with desired compliance behaviors into their customary activities. The partnership between provider and client should lead to the achievement of a common goal: the improved effectiveness of cancer therapy and the improved quality of life for clients with cancer.

HEALTH PROMOTION ACTIVITIES FOR CANCER

The same model as outlined in Figure 8–1 with slight variations is appropriate for health promotion for patients with cancer. Health promotion is "health care directed toward growth and improvement in well-being" (Brubaker, 1983).

Definition

Within Brubaker's framework, health promotion is movement toward a positive state of health (Brubaker, 1983). Health promotion is defined by Pender (1982) as "activities directed toward sustaining or increasing the level of well-being, self-actualization, and personal fulfillment of a given individual or group." Consistent with these two definitions, health promotion is defined here as that behavior designed to promote and sustain a sense of well-being. Health promotion as it relates to cancer is used to describe behaviors directed toward health-oriented activity to detect early recurrence and to maintain the overall health status and well-being of the client. Understanding the factors that motivate individuals to take action to protect or promote their overall health is important.

Goal

Health-promoting behavior has as its *goal* the maintenance of current health or movement toward a more desirable level of health. Examples of health promoting behaviors are physical exercise, good nutrition, stress management, and development of a social support system (Pender, 1982). The necessity for client cooperation in cancer care includes, for example, willingness to alter smoking behavior and willingness to engage in regular breast self-examination, to report early symptoms, to carry out regular dental hygiene, and to follow recommended health practices. As the client copes with illness or long-term therapy, it is important to emphasize exercise, stress management, nutrition, and other behaviors that add to an overall sense of well-being.

HEALTH PRACTICES

Health promotion represents an initiative rather than a reaction to existing threats or stimuli. A cognitive model, such as the one outlined in Figure 8–1, can provide the framework for describing health promoting variables as well as compliance behaviors. Individuals' perceptions, modifying variables as well as the balance between barriers and benefits are determinants of health promotion behaviors. Clients diagnosed with cancer may, in fact, be expected to be more vigilant in carrying out health practices. Indeed, certain research suggests that some women with breast cancer do perform breast self-examinations in the unaffected breast, but other studies do not support this finding. Frank-Stromborg and Wright (1984) found that individuals did not alter their life styles after the diagnosis of cancer. Those who take an active role in treatment may also carry out other health promoting behaviors, such as dietary alterations for fiber and fat content or regular exercise. Hirshfeld-Bartek (1982) suggests that women who feel susceptible to cancer recurrence practice breast self-examination.

Nelson's (1986) study of health habits in patients with localized breast cancer reported that these women had positive perceptions of their health. Frank-Stromborg and Wright (1984) also indicate that women with cancer perceived themselves as healthy, practiced health promoting behaviors, and perceived their health status more positively. Reed's study (1983) confirmed that a strong relationship between health habits and health status exists. Health habits appear to improve not only overall health status but also self-esteem, which suggests a relevance for clients with cancer.

Perceived Impact on Health

The perception of risk of recurrence or the need for overall health promoting behaviors may depend on the stage of illness and treatment. Perceived impact of health promotion on overall health and cancer is important. Individuals who feel that they have some control (self-efficacy) over the disease and treatment and that health promotion behaviors may positively affect their overall health may be more likely to carry out these behaviors. Perceived ability to control health will influence the selection and conduct of strategies to initiate and continue the needed practice. For the client with cancer, the perceived ability to control must be strong or else the sense of helplessness, hopelessness, or futility could result in noncompliance.

Perceived Ability to Control

The interaction of desire for control, ability to control, and resultant health behaviors is not well described in the research literature. If individuals are oriented toward health, they will more likely initiate activities to maintain overall health. Perceived health status and ability to detect and control the health risk provides the energy to carry out health promoting behaviors. The difference between perceived benefits and barriers to benefits provides the stimuli for the specific action. Perceived benefits and barriers to health promoting behaviors are central to the model.

Perceived Ability to Carry Out (Self-Efficacy)

Perceived competence may be more obvious in initiating health promoting behavior than in complying with a complex cancer therapeutic regimen. Perceived efficacy would be important to long-term smoking cessation or other such behaviors, for example. Individuals must believe that they can maintain the new behaviors and are more willing to exert an effort to master and sustain the new behavior even though the benefit is long term or not immediately obvious.

Knowledge about Disease and Treatment

Although knowledge of health promoting practices such as breast self-examination does not correlate with frequency of their performance, it is important to increase the amount of knowledge of such practices.

Unwarranted fear and anxiety due to lack of knowledge can delay taking action to solve a problem (Magarey, Todd, & Blizard, 1977). Assessment of skills is important in reinforcing a sense of competence. Confidence in the technique of breast self-examination was found in several studies to correlate with the practice of this technique, namely, Brailey (1986), Edwards (1980), and Mahoney (1977). For example, women must feel confident that they are carrying out the breast self-examination technique correctly and that they would discover an abnormality if one were present. Bandura (1982) emphasized efficacy or confidence in skills as a determining factor in whether an individual will adopt and continue to perform a health behavior.

Supportive Environment

For clients with cancer, the family and therapeutic team often become so involved in the cancer treatment that other health promoting behaviors are not addressed. Nurses should take an active role and impress on the client and family the importance of *general overall* health practices. Modifying forces from health professionals and family support influence the balance of benefits and barriers. Thus if patients believe that health status and prognosis of cancer are good and they also receive support, they may carry out health promoting behaviors. Health promoting behaviors are seldom prescribed for individuals with cancer. Health-oriented behaviors may influence the impact of the cancer treatment on client functioning. Professionals should make recommendations and try to elicit the client's intent and willingness to participate in health promoting behavior. Clients, families, and health care professionals can reinforce the importance of health promotion for the client with cancer.

Compliance Decision

Perceived health status is important in determining the frequency and intensity of health promoting behaviors. For the client with cancer, the threat and fear of recurrence and the lack of response to therapy can reduce the possibility of adopting healthy behavior patterns. It may be more difficult to sustain or initiate health promoting behaviors for those who have cancer. Those who have a perceived risk of cancer may be more likely to carry out behaviors aimed at screening and early detection.

Benefits and barriers are also important to health promoting behaviors. Kegeles and Grady (1982) report that only 18 to 20 per cent of females habitually perform breast self-examination. Of these, many women do not follow the procedure accurately (Hulka, 1979). Age, education, attitudes, and beliefs about cancer are associated with the practice of breast self-examination. Women who are older and less educated and who doubt their ability to detect lumps or do not believe in the *benefit* are less likely to perform breast self-examination.

Barriers have been negatively associated with the frequency of breast self-examination (Champion, 1984; Magarey, Todd, & Blizard, 1977; Trotta, 1980). Persons must assume responsibility for their own health practices for progress to be made toward affecting the morbidity of cancer.

In the screening of 1029 women for breast or pelvic findings, Lane (1983) found that a higher compliance rate in the performance of health promoting practices existed with *diagnostic* mammograms or symptoms of abnormality than with normal screening. Cost was a barrier in asymptomatic women with normal findings, and only symptoms served as stimuli for health promoting behavior.

Benefits may also be difficult to perceive for patients with cancer, but if these patients have a long history of healthy behaviors they are more likely to continue them. They must believe that their actions reduce the threat or improve the chance for longer functioning. The diagnosis and treatment of cancer may be a barrier to health promoting behaviors. Brailey (1986) found that perceived susceptibility to breast cancer, perceived benefits of breast self-examination, previous experience with breast cancer, and confidence in one's skill in breast examinations affected the frequency of breast examinations.

SUMMARY

The model outlined in this chapter applies to compliance and health promoting behavior in clients with cancer. This behavior evolves from the interrelationship of clients' perceptions of the impact of cancer, ability to control the disease, efficacy of treatment, perceived self-efficacy, and knowledge. Background characteristics and family and professional health care support interact with these perceptions to lead to balancing the barriers and benefits of compliance behavior. The single-headed arrows in Figure 8–1 show the influence of the factors on each subsequent factor. The double-headed arrows imply a continuous interaction and feedback mechanism. Based on this weighting, the client decides whether to carry out compliance behaviors. Nurses need to assess the perception of clients as they work in partnership with clients to institute the therapeutic plan across the trajectory of cancer care (see Boxes 8–1 and 8–2 for strategies for clinical practice). Together the partnership can maximize the positive outcomes of cancer care.

References

Abeldoff, M. D., Mellits, E. D., & Baumgardner, R. (1981). Prospective trial of standard vs. low dose cytoxan, methotrexate, 5-FU (CMF) in adjuvant therapy of breast cancer: Assessment of therapeutic efficacy and toxicity. *Proceedings of the American Association of Cancer Research and American Society of Clinical Oncology, 22,* 440.

Abrams, R. D. (1966). The patient with cancer: His changing pattern of communication. *New England Journal of Medicine, 288,* 317–322.

Baer, C. L. (1986). Compliance: The challenge for the future. *Topics in Clinical Nursing, 7*, 77–85.

Bandura, A. (1977). *Social learning theory.* Englewood Cliffs, NJ: Prentice-Hall, Inc.

Bandura, A. (1982). Self-efficacy mechanisms in human agency. *American Psychologist, 37*, 122–147.

Barofsky, I. (1984). Therapeutic compliance and the cancer patient. *Health Education Quarterly, 10* (Special Suppl.), 43–57.

Barofsky, I., & Sugarbaker, P. E. (1979). Determinants of patient nonparticipation in sarcoma clinical trials. *Cancer Clinical Trials, 2*, 237–246.

Barsky, A. J., & Gillum, R. (1974). Diagnosis and management of patient noncompliance. *Journal of the American Medical Association, 228*, 1563–1567.

Basch, C. E., Gold, R. S., McDermott, R. J., & Richardson, C. E. (1983). Confounding variables in the measurement of cancer patient compliance. *Cancer Nursing, 6*, 285–293.

Becker, M. (1984). Health belief model: A decade later. *Health Education Quarterly, 11*, 1–47.

Bonadonna, G., & Valagussa, P. (1981). Dose-response effect of adjuvant chemotherapy in breast cancer. *New England Journal of Medicine, 304*, 10–15.

Brailey, L. J. (1986). Effects of health teaching in the workplace on women's knowledge, beliefs, and practices regarding breast self-examination. *Research in Nursing and Health, 9*, 223–231.

Brubaker, B. (1983). Health promotion: A linguistic analysis. *Advances in Nursing Science, 5*, 1–14.

Bryant, M. J., & Gorton, S. J. (1982). Reporting of common bothersome toxicities of cancer chemotherapy affecting quality of life. In *Proceedings of the Eighteenth Annual Meeting of the American Society of Clinical Oncology, 1*, 68.

Carey, R. W. (1979). Five drug adjunct chemotherapy for breast cancer. *Cancer, 44*, 35–41.

Cassileth, B. R., Zupkis, R. V., Sutton-Smith, K., & March, V. (1980). Informed consent: Why are its goals imperfectly realized? *New England Journal of Medicine, 302*, 896–900.

Champion, V. (1984). Instrument development for health belief construct advances. *Advances in Nursing Sciences, 6*, 73–85.

Clark, S. R. (1986). Compliance and health behaviors. *Topics in Clinical Nursing, 7*, 39–46.

Davidson, S. B. (1986). Using compliance research in clinical practice. *Topics in Clinical Nursing, 7*, 65–76.

Dennis, K. E. (1987). Dimensions of client control. *Nursing Research, 36*, 151–156.

Dracup, K. A., & Meleis, A. I. (1982). Compliance: An interactionist approach. *Nursing Research, 31*, 31–36.

Dropkin, M. J. (1979). Compliance in postoperative head and neck patients. *Cancer Nursing, 5*, 379–384.

Dunbar, J. M., Marshall, G. D., & Hovell, M. F. (1979). Behavioral strategies for improving compliance. In R. B. Haynes, D. W. Taylor, & D. L. Sackett, (Eds.), *Compliance in health care.* Baltimore: Johns Hopkins University Press.

Edwards, V. (1980). Changing breast self-examination behavior. *Nursing Research, 29*, 301–306.

Feldman, J. G., Carter, A. C., & Nicostri, A. D. (1981). Breast self-examination, relationship to stage of breast cancer at diagnosis. *Cancer, 47*, 2740–2745.

Fernsler, J. (1986). A comparison of patient and nurse perceptions of patients' self-care deficits associated with cancer chemotherapy. *Cancer Nursing, 9*, 50–57.

Fink, D. L. (1976). Tailoring in the consensual regimen. In D. Sackett & R. Haynes (Eds.), *Compliance with therapeutic regimen* (pp. 110–118). Baltimore: Johns Hopkins University Press.

Frank-Stromborg, M., & Wright, P. (1984). Ambulatory cancer patients perception of the physical and psychological changes in their lives since the diagnosis of cancer. *Cancer Nursing, 7*, 117–129.

Friedenbergs, I., Gordon, W., Hibbard, M., Levine, L., Wolf, C., & Diller, L. (1982). Psycho-social aspect of living with cancer. *International Journal of Psychiatric Medicine, 11*, 303–329.

German, P. S., Klein, L. E., McPhee, S. J., & Smith, C. R. (1982). Knowledge of and compliance with drug regimens in the elderly. *Journal of American Geriatric Society, 30*, 568–571.

Given, B. A., & Given, C. W. (1984). Creating a climate for compliance. *Cancer Nursing, 7*, 139–147.

Given, B. A., & Given C. W. (1989). Compliance among patients with cancer. *Oncology Nursing Forum, 16*, 97–103.

Glass, A., Wieand, H. S., Fisher, B., Redmond, C., Lerner, H., Wolter, J., Shibata, H., Plotkin, D., Foster, R., Margolese, R., & Wolmark, N. (1981). Acute toxicity during adjuvant chemotherapy for breast cancer. *Cancer Treatment Reports, 65*, 363–376.

Gore, S. (1978). The effect of social support in moderating the health consequences of unemployment. *Journal of Health and Social Behavior, 19*, 157.

Green, J. A. (1983). Compliance and cancer chemotherapy. *British Medical Journal, 287*, 778.

Greenwald, H. P., Becker, S. W., & Nevitt, M. C. (1978). Delay and noncompliance in cancer detection: A behavioral perspective for health planners. *Milbank Memorial Fund Quarterly, 56*, 212–231.

Grover, P., Amsel, Z., & Balshem, B. (1983). Breast self-examination post mastectomy: Empirical findings and their implications. In *Progress in cancer control* (pp. 293–303). New York: Alan R. Liss, Inc.

Hahn, D. M., Schimpff, S. C., Fortner, C. L., Smyth, A. C., Young, V. M., & Wiernick, P. H. (1978). Infection in acute leukemia patients receiving oral nonabsorbable antibiotics. *Antimicrobial Agents Chemotherapy, 13*, 958–964.

Hallal, J. C. (1982). The relationship of health beliefs, health locus of control, and self concept to the practice of breast self-examination in adult women. *Nursing Research, 31*, 137–142.

Haynes, B. R., Taylor, D. W., & Sackett, D. L. (1979). *Compliance in health care.* Baltimore: Johns Hopkins University Press.

Hebert, D. (1977). The assessment of the clinical significance of noncompliance with prescribed schedules of irradiation. *Journal of Radiation Oncology and Biological Physiology, 2*, 763–772.

Hirshfeld-Bartek, J. (1982). Health beliefs and influence on breast self examination practices in women with breast cancer. *Oncology Nursing Forum, 9*, 77–81.

Hoagland, A. C., Morrow, G. R., Bennett, J. M., & Carnrike, C. L. M. (1983). Oncologists' views of cancer patient noncompliance. *American Journal of Clinical Oncology (CCT), 6*, 239–244.

Holzman, D., & Celentano, D. (1983). Breast self-examination competency. *American Journal of Public Health, 73*, 1324–1325.

Hulka, B. S. (1979). Patient-clinician interactions and compliance. In R. B. Haynes, D. W. Taylor, & D. L. Sackett (Eds.), *Compliance in health care.* Baltimore: Johns Hopkins University Press.

Itano, J., Tanabe, P., & Lum, J. (1983). Compliance and noncompliance. In *Advances in cancer control: Cancer patients* (pp. 483–495). New York: Alan R. Liss, Inc.

Itano, J., Tanabe, P., Lum, J., Lamkin, L., Rizzo, E., Wieland, M., & Sato, P. (1981). Compliance and noncompliance in cancer patients. In *Advances in cancer control: Research and development* (pp. 483–495). New York: Alan R. Liss, Inc.

Janis, I. L. (1982). *Counseling on personal decisions: Theory and research on short term helping relationships:* New Haven, CT: Yale University Press.

Jennings, B. M., & Muhlenkamp, A. F. (1981). Systematic misperception: Oncology patients' self-reported affective states and their caregivers' perceptions. *Cancer Nursing, 4*, 485–489.

Jones, W. L., Engstrom, P. F., Paul, A., & Peter, R. (1983). Important gaps in patients' knowledge prior to chemotherapy. In *Progress in cancer control IV: Research in the cancer center* (pp. 391–400). New York: Alan R. Liss, Inc.

Kasl, S. V. (1975). Issues in patient adherence to health care regimens. *Journal of Human Stress, 1*, 5–17.

Kegeles, S. S., & Grady, K. E. (1982). BSE versus dogmatism. *American Journal of Public Health, 72*, 406.

Kesselring, A., Lindsey, A. M., Dodd, M. J., & Lovejoy, N. C. (1986). Social network and support perceived by Swiss cancer patients. *Cancer Nursing, 9*, 156–163.

Klopovich, P. M., & Trueworthy, R. C. (1985). Adherence to chemotherapy regimens among children with cancer. *Topics in Clinical Nursing, 7*, 19–25.

Korsch, B., Gozzi, E., & Francis, V. (1968). Gaps in doctor patient communication. *Pediatrics, 42*, 855–871.

Korsch, B., & Negrete, V. (1972). Doctor patient communication. *Scientific American, 227(2)*, 66–74.

Lane, D. S. (1983). Compliance with referrals from a cancer-screening project. *The Journal of Family Practice, 17*, 811–817.

Laszlo, J., & Lucas, V. S. (1981). Emesis as a critical problem in chemotherapy (Editorial). *New England Journal of Medicine, 305*, 948–949.

Lauer, P., Murphy, S. P., & Powers, M. J. (1982). Learning needs of cancer patients: A comparison of nurse and patient perceptions. *Nursing Research, 31,* 11–16.

Lee, Y-TN. (1983). Adjuvant chemotherapy (CMF) for breast carcinoma: Patient compliance and total dose received. *American Journal of Clinical Oncology (CCT), 6,* 25–30.

Leventhal, H., Safer, M. A., & Panagis, D. M. (1983). The impact of communications on the self-regulation of health beliefs, decisions, and behavior. *Health Education Quarterly, 10,* 3–29.

Levy, S. M. (1981). Compliance in cancer patients: Major research needs. Bethesda, MD: National Cancer Institute.

Levy, S. M. (1982). Biobehavioral interventions in behavioral medicine: An overview. *Cancer, 50,* 1936.

Lewis, C., Linet, M. S., & Abeloff, M. D. (1983). Compliance with cancer therapy by patients and physicians. *American Journal of Medicine, 74,* 673–678.

Ley, P. (1979). Improving clinical communication. In J. Dokborne (Ed.), *Research in psychology and medicine, Vol. 2* (pp. 221–229). London: Academic Press.

Lucus, C. M. (1986). Compliance and illness responses. *Topics in Clinical Nursing, 7,* 47–56.

Lum, J., Chase, M., Cole, S., Johnson, A., Johnson, J., & Link, M. (1978). Nursing care of oncology patients receiving chemotherapy. *Nursing Research, 27,* 340–346.

Magarey, C. J., Todd, P. B., & Blizard, P. J. (1977). Psychosocial factors influencing delay and breast self-examination in women with symptoms of breast cancer. *Social Science and Medicine, 11,* 229–232.

Mahoney, L. J. (1977). Early diagnosis of breast cancer. The breast self-examination problem. *Canadian Family Physician, 23,* 481–483.

Marecki, M. (1981). Need priorities of adrenalectomy patients as perceived by patients, nurses, and physicians. *Journal of Obstetric, Gynecologic, and Neonatal Nursing, 10,* 379–383.

Mettlin, C., Reese, P., & Murphy, G. P. (1980). Care-seeking behavior among positive screenees. *Preventive Medicine, 9,* 518–524.

Meyerwitz, B. E., Sparks, F. C., & Spears, I. K. (1979). Adjuvant chemotherapy for breast carcinoma: Psychological implications. *Cancer, 43,* 1613–1618.

Mishel, M. (1981). The measurement of uncertainty in illness. *Research in Nursing and Health, 30,* 258–263.

Mishel, M., Hostetter, T., King, B., & Graham, V. (1984). Predictors of psychosocial adjustment in patients newly diagnosed with gynecological cancer. *Cancer Nursing, 7,* 291–299.

Murfin, G. D., & Wagstaff, D. A. (1983). Cancer prevention/detection behavior by the public: Lessons from three surveys. In *Progress in cancer control IV: Research in the cancer center* (pp. 103–112). New York: Alan R. Liss, Inc.

Nelson, J. P. (1986). *Health habits and self-esteem of postmastectomy patients.* Thesis paper, Intercollegiate Center for Nursing Education, Spokane, WA.

Padrick, K. P. (1986). Compliance: Myths and motivators. *Topics in Clinical Nursing, 7,* 17–22.

Patterson, P. (1981). *Cancer patients and informed consent.* Unpublished master's thesis, California State University, Los Angeles, CA.

Pender, N. J. (1982). *Health promotion in nursing practice.* Norwalk, CT: Appleton-Century-Crofts.

Reed, W. L. (1983). Physical health status as a consequence of health practices. *Journal of Community Health, 308,* 393–395.

Revenson, T. A., Wollman, B. A., & Felton, B. J. (1983). Social supports as stress buffers for adult cancer patients. *Psychosomatic Medicine, 45,* 321–331.

Richardson, J. L., Johnson, C. A., Selser, J., Evans, L. A., Kishbaugh, C., & Levine, A. M. (1983). Compliance with chemotherapy: Theoretical basis and intervention design. *Progress in cancer control IV: Research in the cancer center* (pp. 379–390). New York: Alan R. Liss, Inc.

Richardson, J. L., Marks, G., Graham, J. W., Chan, K. K., Johnson, C. A., & Levine, A. M. (1987). *Assessment of compliance with cancer therapy: Conceptual and methodological issues.* Grant No. RO1 CA 31151, University of Southern California, Los Angeles, CA.

Smith, S. D., Rosen, D., Trueworthy, R. C., & Lowman, J. T. (1979). A reliable method for evaluating drug compliance in children with cancer. *Cancer, 43,* 169–173.

Steckel, S. B. (1982). Predicting, measuring, implementing and following-up on patient compliance. *Nursing Clinics of North America, 17,* 493–495.

Taylor, S. E., Lichtman, J. W., & Wood, J. V. (1984). Attributions, beliefs about control, and adjustment of breast cancer. *Journal of Personality and Social Psychology, 46,* 489–502.

Taylor, S. E., Lichtman, R. R., & Wood, J. V. (1984). Compliance with chemotherapy among breast cancer patients. *Health Psychology, 3,* 553–562.

Tebbe, C. K., Cummings, K. M., Zevon, M. A., Smith, L. A., Richards, M., & Mallon, J. (1986). Compliance of pediatric and adolescent cancer patients. *Cancer, 58,* 1179–1184.

Trotta, P. (1980). Breast self-examination: Factors influencing compliance. *Oncology Nursing Forum, 7,* 13–17.

Weintraub, M., Av, W. Y. W., & Lasagna, L. (1973). Compliance as a determinant of serum digoxin concentration. *Journal of the American Medical Association, 224,* 481–485.

Weisman, A., & Worden, W. (1980). *Psychological screening and intervention with cancer patients.* Bethesda, MD: National Cancer Institute.

Westfall, U. E. (1986). Methods for assessing compliance. *Topics in Clinical Nursing, 7*(4), 23–30.

Wilcox, P. M., Fetting, J. S., Nettesheim, K. M., & Abeloff, M. D. (1982). Anticipatory vomiting in women receiving cyclophospadmide, methotrexate, and 5-FU (CMF) adjuvant chemotherapy for breast carcinoma. *Cancer Treatment Research, 66*(8), 1–4.

Worden, J. K., Costanza, M. C., Foster, R. S., Lang, S. P., & Tidd, C. A. (1983). Content and context in health education: Persuading women to perform breast self-examination. *Preventive Medicine, 12,* 331–339.

Wortman, C. B., & Dunkel-Schetter, C. (1979). Interpersonal relationships and cancer: A theoretical analysis. *Journal of Social Issues, 35,* 120–155.

Zapka, J. G., & Mamon, J. A. (1982). Integration of theory, practitioner standards, literature findings and baseline data: A case study in planning breast self-examination education. *Health Education Quarterly, 9,* 330–356.

CHAPTER 9

Stress and Coping with Cancer

PATRICIA BENNER

COPING WITH WHAT AND TO WHAT END?
A TRANSACTIONAL DEFINITION OF STRESS
    AND COPING
STIGMA AND PERSONAL RESPONSIBILITY

The Caretaker's Response
LIFE STAGE AND THE ILLNESS CONTEXT
COPING WITH DEATH AND DYING
Family Coping and Coping with Caregiving

COPING WITH WHAT AND TO WHAT END?

The person with cancer must obtain an accurate diagnosis and effective treatment, confront the cultural meanings and stigma associated with cancer, and face the prospect of a life-threatening illness (Benner & Wrubel, 1989; Taylor, 1977). Cancer is stressful because it confronts the patient with strategic issues related to getting appropriate help and solving many problems related to diagnosis and treatment. Diagnosis and treatment present the individual with myriad questions and strategic decisions, which make it difficult for families to evaluate the options for enlightened and efficacious health care. Cancer is also stressful because it confronts the person with significance issues such as loss, pain, suffering, fear of death, economic threats, and anxiety. This chapter argues that the first step in assisting patients and families in coping with the stress of cancer and cancer treatment is to address the question from the patient-family perspective: "Coping with what, and to what end?" Answering this question requires attending to both problem-solving issues regarding diagnosis and treatment (strategic issues) and significance issues.

A TRANSACTIONAL DEFINITION OF STRESS AND COPING

Stress is defined as "the disruption of meanings, understanding and smooth functioning so that harm, loss or challenge are experienced, and sorrow, interpretation or new skill acquisition is required" (Benner & Wrubel, 1989). This definition draws on the work of Lazarus and his colleagues (Lazarus, 1966, 1968, 1981, 1985; Lazarus & Cohen, 1977; Lazarus & Folkman, 1984; Lazarus & Launier, 1978). It is a transactional definition of stress, meaning that the person shapes the situation and the situation shapes the person. A transaction implies more than just an interaction. Transaction implies the generation of possibilities and constraints in a specific situation. A transactional definition of stress avoids the confusion of considering stress as a stimulus or as a response and attends to the person in the situation.

Lazarus's theory of stress and coping posits that stress involves both the person and the situation. Stress results when the person's perceptual grasp or appraisal of his or her situation taxes or exceeds adaptive capacities. Thus any transaction between a person and a situation that creates harm, threat, loss, or challenge that taxes the person's adaptive capacities is considered stressful. Coping is anything the person does to change the situation or the way the person feels or thinks about the situation (Lazarus & Folkman, 1984).

Coping cannot be understood adequately when it is separated from the stressful transaction; therefore, context-free lists of "good coping" and "bad coping" such as those suggested in the work of Weisman (1979) are misleading because such lists ignore the resources, demands, constraints, and interpersonal concerns *in* the situation. One never copes with cancer in general but rather with the many different problems, phases, and meanings of cancer over time (Mages & Mendelsohn, 1979). Although it is possible to think of idealized versions of "flexible, reality-based" coping as preferable, as do theorists such as Haan (1977), Vailiant (1977), and Weisman (1979), these terms can be misleading in actual clinical situations, because what counts as flexible and realistic depends on the person-situation transaction. For example, Weisman's advice to "avoid avoidance" works well when it refers to a patient's attention to possible warning signs or diagnostic clues, but it may be misguided when it refers to a patient's attempt to gain respite or perspective during a difficult treatment regimen. Effectiveness or adaptiveness can only be assessed in relation to the person's concerns, notions of good, situational demands, resources, and constraints.

The treatment settings, stages, and demands of cancer care are different and create different coping demands. Different kinds of cancer typically follow different treatment and illness patterns, each creating distinct coping demands (Parker, 1981). Thus the questions that must always be asked when studying stress and coping are What are the demands of the situation?

What are the person's concerns? What is the content of the stress? What coping options are available to the person? From a transactional perspective, stress and coping processes are linked; thus coping cannot be construed as an antidote to stress because the available coping options are linked to the person's understanding of the stressful transaction (Benner & Wrubel, 1989; Lazarus, 1985; Lazarus & Folkman, 1984).

When considering coping, it helps to make a distinction between illness and disease (Benner & Wrubel, 1989; Kleinman, 1988). Disease is what occurs at the tissue or cellular level, and illness is the human experience of loss or dysfunction. As Benner and Wrubel (1989) note:

We posit that stress cannot be "cured," not only because, short of miracles, there is no cure for disasters, calamities and tragedies, but also because, in the phenomenological view of the person, there is no way to step outside of one's own history. . . . A person with cancer who has a remission beyond the five-year mark may be judged to be cured of the disease, but the experience of having had the disease will inform the rest of that person's life. One might feel strengthened by the experience and feel that having survived cancer, one can handle easily the more mundane upsets of daily life. Or, one might feel vulnerable because of the close brush with death, and smaller contretemps would be understood as confirmation of the precariousness of existence. In fact, there is a whole range of diverse ways in which the experience of surviving a life-threatening illness could constitute a person. The only experience which is not a possibility is that one could view the world in exactly the same way as before. One can be rid of the disease, but not of the experience of the disease. (p.61)

Context-free lists of "good" and "bad" coping cannot address the questions of coping with what, to what end, and under what circumstances. The astute nurse clinician can strengthen coping resources and strategies by listening systematically to the actual concerns of the patient and family and augmenting individual and family coping and caring practices. What are the meanings, concerns, and practices that are disrupted? Typically the nurse is given access to the daily issues surrounding care of the body and coping with daily activities, caring practices, family rituals, and routines. Understanding these particular issues along with the general issues confronting persons with cancer provides the nurse with the basis for strengthening individual family coping practices and reducing the stress associated with cancer. The following general stress and coping issues related to the experience of cancer are discussed: stigma and personal responsibility, life stage and illness situation, death and dying, and family coping and coping with caregiving.

STIGMA AND PERSONAL RESPONSIBILITY

The person whose diagnosis is cancer may be stigmatized and may have to confront a set of subtle, unwarranted prejudices that assign ultimate responsibility for the disease to the afflicted individual. This stance is common with any illness in Western culture, which stresses autonomy and individualism, but it seems to be even more prevalent in illnesses such as cancer in which the causes and cures are so uncertain (Benner & Wrubel, 1989; Sontag, 1979). Larson (Larson, Benner, & Koetters, 1990) conducted an interview with a young woman newly diagnosed with Hodgkin's disease who depicts poignantly the additional burden of self-blame or recrimination that many cancer patients face:

I've always taken good care of myself and my body, especially health wise. You know, I've been a vegetarian for over 10 years, but a careful one. And I've been very health conscious—no drugs, no cigarette smoke, no coffee, caffeine, soda, anything. . . . Cancer is something I'm just starting to identify with because that's a difficult word, because I guess it's associated with like toxins, and I just never did any of those carcinogenic things. . . . I'm kind of angry at the stuff that I read where people say that it was your fault that you got it. You know, I wonder, and I've thought about it, but you know could it be because I was under stress or unhappy or depressed or had a difficult year, and it could be, but I would rather think that it is not. Because I look around at my friends, and they're all having struggles and they're all having concerns about their careers, and they're under stress from school, and I just don't think that it was my fault. So that's how I'm choosing to look at it right now.

This study participant describes the searching and pain caused by thinking that she had full responsibility for all of her actions, thoughts, and feelings and that wrong actions, thoughts, and feelings can "cause" illness. This alienated view suggests that the person possesses and controls feelings as if they were raw material or resources to be managed (Benner & Wrubel, 1989). Ultimately such a view results in a blindness to the limits of personal control. Blaming the victim by overestimating the victim's capabilities and responsibilities is an extreme "mind over matter" or "thinking makes it so" position. This practice of blaming the victim is particularly common in a society in which it is believed that the individual has ultimate control over and responsibility for any personal event and in which the effects of social and environmental forces such as air pollution, food additives, and early introduction to cigarette smoking are overlooked or underestimated (Bellah, Madsen, Sullivan, Swidler, & Tipton, 1985; Benner & Wrubel, 1989).

The patient may discover causal links between disease and exposure to toxic wastes at work or in the environment and feel betrayed and victimized. In the case of the patient who may have had carcinogenic habits (e.g., smoking and heavy alcohol use or exposure to known carcinogens), acknowledging possible responsibility for cancer may cause great remorse or may bring some clarity to an otherwise unexplainable, capricious event. The patient may prefer a sense of known cause and effect to the uncertainty and lack of control that accompanies coping with an unexplained cause. Caretakers—professional or lay—are not immune to these cultural meanings and may inflict more blame and social burden on the person with cancer because they may link a moral entitlement to care to the individual's personal responsibility to prevent illness. This is the dark side of extreme individualism and must be combatted if we are to avoid blaming the victim and to create healing environments and communities for cancer patients. This issue of responsibility is indeed complex in an era of antismoking campaigns and pressure for taking increasing responsibility for one's health and for creating a "healthist body" (Lowenberg, 1989; Scheper-Hughes & Lock, 1987).

The Caretaker's Response

Patients' coping may be strongly influenced by the caretakers' understanding of the illness and ability to cope with the threat of cancer. Some people involved with the patient (including health care workers) may seek to assign personal responsibility for the disease to the cancer patient as a way of warding off the threat of contracting cancer themselves. The young woman quoted previously (Larson et al., 1990) had a very troubling disagreement with her mother because her mother believed that persons defined as patients had to accept responsibility for developing their diseases:

My mother feels that it is somehow my fault, so that's kind of strange because it is very important for me not to feel that way. She doesn't feel that I am to blame necessarily, but she is of a different belief than I am right now. And it is hard because I did kind of come from that belief, that somehow, if you got sick, you have to take some sort of responsibility for that. . . . [One of the difficult things this week] has been when I was arguing with my mother about the two different ways that we saw why I am sick.

Finding the source of the responsibility within the afflicted person may give an illusion of control or an illusion that the world is just, predictable, and completely interpretable (the "just world hypothesis" in social psychology; see Rubin & Peplau, 1975). Blaming the patient may give those who are free from disease a sense of immunity but may provoke feelings of helplessness, guilt, loss of control, or victimization in the patient. Because of the danger of blaming the victim and of placing moral entitlements on receiving care (e.g., one must have lived a healthy life style to merit care), nurses, family members, and other health care workers should be mindful of their own methods of coping with the threat of disease. A consumer warning label should be placed on all stress management approaches that make patients feel that they must manage all distress and be totally in control of their feelings. The goal of being responsible for a "fighting spirit" or a positive attitude as a prerequisite for health and recovery can place an insurmountable burden on the patient during some of the more distressing times of the illness. Thus any stress management approach that requires one to step outside one's own history may only increase the sense of alienation and distress. Eventually the goal is not to step outside one's history but rather to come to terms with it. This argument has been stated elsewhere (Benner & Wrubel, 1989):

A purely veridical, rational view of "good coping" held by ideal models of mental health breaks down when they are used to consider extreme situations. Mastery, control, rationality and autonomy without regard to situation and relationships tend to be the cultural ideals underlying most versions of "ideal" coping or ideal mental health. Mastery, autonomy, and rationality were not real options in the Concentration Camps. When a committed couple must weather an extreme illness of a partner or parents must face a devastating illness of their child, autonomy, mastery, control, and rationality are not the salient issues. In the extreme situation, the person *in* the situation must be studied, and an ideal and its concomitant deficit or pathology, is of little use. (p. 84)

The cultural metaphors and treatments of cancer fit in with a technologic understanding of the self as raw material to be shaped, mastered, and dominated by the self (Benner & Wrubel, 1989). Control is the major term in this mechanistic, technologic self-understanding. Self-control and control of the disease are the major themes of the cancer patient and the health care workers. But the fear of loss of control is never very far away because this self-understanding believes that the self must be managed and the "body" must be controlled by the "mind." Patients may lose their sense of trust in and integrity of their bodies with the diagnosis of cancer and the experience of invasive treatments. It is easy for both patient and health care worker to lose sight of the body's capacity for healing and recovery. A recovered sense of body integrity is required for the patient to recover from the "illness" of cancer as well as from the disease. The Simonton method of counseling patients is aimed at restoring a sense of control, integrity, and possibility, although Simonton and Matthews-Simonton (1981) openly acknowledge that their strategies seem highly beneficial to some but detrimental to others. The nurse is in a unique position to support the patient through whatever increase in hope, reduction in tension, and restoration of function seems to work and to inhibit the placement of total responsibility for a cure on the patient. When a patient feels that "feelings" are life threatening or at least damaging, it is extremely difficult to acknowledge and work through the normal feelings of discouragement that accompany a difficult disease and treatment regimen. The young woman quoted previously (Larson et al., 1990) describes working through an acceptance of feelings:

I started thinking that because I was depressed that I really got caught up in being depressed . . . but now I'm starting to pull back a little bit and realize that I don't have to find out all the answers, that everybody else also thinks about these things. Just because I'm sick, doesn't mean I'm the only one that gets depressed or the only one that thinks about these things. That took the focus off of me, that I can be like that sometimes and not be like that, just as other people are in their wellness.

As this young woman describes, it is easy to lose a sense of legitimacy for feelings. Trying to "manage" all feelings can intensify rather than dampen them. Ascribing a life-threatening or a healing role to emotions can further confuse the everyday issues of living and can make it difficult to feel well, whole, or normal.

The rationale for stress reduction is sometimes based on the erroneous belief that stress, coping, or personality style is the precipitant or cause of cancer. The psychosocial epidemiology of cancer is an extremely difficult field of research because it is fraught with post-hoc analyses and overinterpretations (Benner & Wrubel, 1989; Sontag, 1979). The major theoretic perspectives for investigating links between cancer and personality or stress have been psychodynamic (Bahnson, 1980, 1981) or have involved life change or loss of important relationships (Greer & Morris, 1975; Grissom, Weiner, & Weiner, 1975; Grossarth-Maticek, 1980; Schonfield, 1972; Smith et al., 1984) and life-style and coping patterns (Fox, 1978; Kissen & Rao, 1969). Each of these theoretic perspectives has been reviewed and critiqued (Benner & Wrubel, 1989). None of these psychosocial causes has been clearly demonstrated, and none of the causal theories is clearly related to the issue of cure or regression of the tumor as a result of altered stress and coping responses (Cassileth, Lusk, Miller, Brown, & Miller, 1985).

The impact of stress and coping on tumor progression is extremely difficult to determine. Creating a healing environment and decreasing negative feelings of despair, panic, and fear are valuable in and of themselves, however. The goal is to offer patients various options for stress reduction, respite, and recreation as beneficial in their own right, not to insist that they "control" their body's responses to "cure" themselves. Tension reduction and pleasant feelings may well strengthen one's immunity or place one's body in the best condition for healing, but in any case they are desirable and good in themselves. The patient is placed in an untenable position if he or she is told that all negative feelings are dangerous or that "control of emotions" is essential to recovery. This stance has the undesirable consequence of making it even more difficult to work through negative feelings and gain access to hopeful, positive emotions.

Each person comes to the experience of cancer with his or her own history of coping with threat, loss, or harm. It can be an added burden to have emotions singled out as being the cure or the problem. The starting point must be an understanding of the lived experience of hope, possibility, threat, loss, or harm (i.e., the content of emotions). The person's own coping strategies, sources of support, and caring practices form the basis for offering comfort measures and stress management strategies and for augmenting personal and family caring practices. Having heard and understood the patient's and family's concerns (coping with what and to what end?) and having assessed the family coping resources and caring practices, the nurse can then teach the person and family about the available health care resources, the predictable treatment demands, and the management of symptoms (strategic problem-solving issues). When it is appropriate, the nurse can also attend to significance issues (personal and family concerns, meanings, and practices). Illness, pain, disfigurement, and threat of death can cause alienation and a rupture in meanings that separates the one suffering from significant others. Alienation and meaninglessness are the positions most bereft of coping options (Benner & Wrubel, 1989). Caring practices and coping strategies help to bridge the gulf and reunite patients with their significant others and their concerns.

LIFE STAGE AND THE ILLNESS CONTEXT

Understanding the life stage and the illness context is an essential coping resource and caring practice. Illness never occurs in a vacuum. It interrupts plans, threatens futures, and disrupts usual relationships. To understand coping, one must consider the person's situation as defined by current resources, constraints and demands, history, growth and development, and family stage. For example, older people typically respond to cancer with more equanimity than younger people (Mages & Mendelsohn, 1979). Family stage also shapes the demands of the illness because the implications for the person with a young family and for the person with adult children are quite different.

Cancer can present a threat to work security. A study conducted by the California Division of the American Cancer Society (1976) reported that 90 per cent of the cancer patients surveyed were employed full- or part-time; however, of the 29 per cent who were no longer with their pre-illness employer, 40 per cent stated that they had left for reasons related to their cancer. Many of the respondents believed that they had experienced work discrimination as a result of their cancer. Disruption of work in addition to the demands of a serious illness can add considerably to the coping demands of the illness. Extreme caution should be taken in advising cancer patients about whether to continue their jobs during treatment programs. For many, work is a major coping resource (Benner, 1984) and may provide a sense of self-worth and control and offer a valuable distraction from the demands of the illness. Health care professionals should take care that the patient does not give up working unnecessarily and thus create new coping demands (e.g., decreased financial security, role loss, decrease in self-esteem, separation from supportive others, and inactivity).

A major illness can severely deplete family finances because of the cost of treatment, loss of work, and altered care needs. The patient's financial situation deserves special attention because the treatment can result in a great financial burden. Cohen and Cordoba (1983) point out that patients may feel trapped in their jobs because they would lose their insurance and insurability if they transferred to a new job. Early referral to social workers who can assist with insurance and financial planning can ease the burden and ensure future access to financial assistance.

The illness trajectory may be divided roughly into the prediagnostic and diagnostic phase, the treatment selection phase, the treatment phase, and the remission or recovery phase or, alternatively, the terminal phase. As Mages and Mendelsohn point out (1979), the coping demands and issues for each phase differ. The patient's and family's usual coping patterns may work well for one phase but not so well for another. For example, vigilant copers who seek as much information as possible may fare better during the prediagnostic and treatment selection and treatment phases but find it difficult to reduce their vigilance to a normal level during the remission or recovery phase and actually become hypervigilant and excessively worried about recurrence. Assessing and understanding coping issues at different phases of the illness improves the nurse's ability to assess the patient's and family's needs at any given time. For example, patients, families, and physicians may persist in the "curative intent" phase of treatment past the time of reasonable possibility for recovery, which only stretches the patient's and family's tolerance for suffering; all may feel ill at ease, not knowing when or how to redefine the situation to one of palliation and preparation for dying. Patients and families can be coached to explore their options. This transition is illustrated in the exemplar by Welsh later in the chapter.

When the decision is clear and mutually held by health care workers, family, and patient, the patient may feel a great sense of relief and be able to prepare to die rather than continue to fight a losing battle. Note that the change from "fighting a very difficult battle where little or no signs of hope are seen" to "preparing for dying as comfortably as possible" raises very different coping possibilities. This transition is often difficult to make and may require the most astute communication skills, because the desire for survival is so great or because the desire for survival is different for the patient and the significant others. Furthermore, understandings about the potential for recovery can vary considerably among health care workers, patients, and families.

COPING WITH DEATH AND DYING

The diagnosis of cancer raises the possibility of death. How one copes with death is determined by personal, historical, and cultural possibilities. Death and dying are sources of threat and even cultural embarrassment to a technologic society that seeks to control life and death. Death interrupts the cultural theme of constant progress and the promise of technologic breakthroughs that prevent or ward off death. Consequently the North American cultural discourse on death and dying has been strained, if not rendered taboo. It is no small cultural achievement that during the last 20 years Americans have begun to develop the capacity to talk about death and dying. Death and dying are no longer culturally taboo subjects. However, much of the discourse on death and dying has been framed in terms of stage theory (Kübler-Ross, 1969), with a description of the person moving through the stages of denial, shock, bargaining, and finally acceptance. Stage theory increasingly has been called into question (Benner & Wrubel, 1989; Kestenbaum & Costa, 1977; Kleinman, 1988; Parker, 1981).

Kestenbaum and Costa (1977) point out that although the paradoxical quest for "healthy dying" as a

consumer demand for a death experience that exceeds ordinary life may at first appear to glamorize death, the end result may be trivialization or a sense of defeat and failure. As Gordon Stuart, a 33-year-old writer dying of cancer points out to his hospice physician (Kleinman, 1988), stage theory inadequately captures the change and issues surrounding dying:

Gordon: I am dying now, aren't I?
Hadley: Yes, you are.
Gordon: I can look into my garden and see sunshine. I know that next week, maybe tomorrow it will be shining just as brightly, just as beautifully, but I won't be part of it. I will no longer be here. Do you know, can you imagine what it—it feels like to make that statement and know that it is true for you that you are dying?
Hadley: I think I can, but I'm not sure.
Gordon: All that nonsense that's written about stages of dying as if there were complete transitions—rooms that you enter, walk through, then leave behind for good. What rot. The anger, the shock, the unbelievableness, the grief—they are part of each day. And in no particular order, either. Who says you work your way eventually to acceptance—I don't accept it! Today I can't accept it. Yesterday I did partly. Saturday I was there: kind of in a trance, waiting ready to die. But not now. Today it is the fear all over again. I don't want to die. I'm only thirty-three; I've got my whole life to live. I can't be cut off now. It isn't just. Why me? Why now? You don't have to answer. I'm just in a lousy mood right now. You get maudlin and morally weak waiting for the end. I'm usually pretty good aren't I? Only sometimes something young and scared breaks out. Otherwise, I become like an old man, preparing myself—but over weeks, not years. (p. 147)

Such a quest is not new. Taylor's *The Rule and Exercises of Holy Dying,* originally written in 1665, has been reprinted (1977). However, the modern version of the death awareness movement's search for a revival of the significance of the dying person as a consumer movement may focus on the psychological experience without having a social and cultural context for attending to the meaning issues. "Why" questions are no longer considered productive or accessible and are replaced with "how" questions. Consumers may be left with vague expectations of having a "self-actualizing" experience in dying that exceeds their experience in ordinary living. This instrumental take-over, making a goal of further self-development in dying, can be excessively demanding for the patient and can take what comfort may be left in the mystery, finiteness, and kinship out of the human experience of death. Patients and families may be poorly prepared for the uncontrollable aspects of a terminal illness, unprepared for the delirium and loss of bodily control that may occur as part of dying. It is unclear what the expert might reasonably prescribe for a "healthy" death and under what circumstances such prescriptions would provide comfort and help for the dying because meanings and expectations around death and dying vary, as does the actual experience of dying. What the nurse can promise is astute comfort care, and pain management along with coaching, presencing, and helping patients maintain their concerns and relationships as much as possible. The term *presencing* is used to convey being with and being available to listen (Benner & Wrubel, 1989).

Family Coping and Coping with Caregiving

Families (*family* is used broadly here to include any significant others) of cancer patients are confronted with a world-changing threat or loss and may experience distress equal to or even more than the person with cancer. Glaser and Strauss (1968) point out that the patient may be fully absorbed in the situation and may have adapted to decreased capacity and well-being, whereas it may be difficult for the ones standing alongside to see the patient in any terms but those of comparative loss. This is not to say that caregivers do not constrict their expectations and understanding of the patient, just that the process may proceed at a different pace from that of the patient's because caregivers do not share the same physical reality.

One of the most enabling coping capacities is that of responding to the possibilities inherent in the actual lived situation (Benner & Wrubel, 1989). Thus a patient and family may come to have expectations centered around a pain-free hour or around planning a feasible pleasurable experience. Nurses learn from patients and families over time a range of "situated possibilities" within the bounds of an illness experience and may be effective coaches to patients and families in expanding their sense of situated possibility (Benner, 1985).

Caregivers, whether professionals or family members, can become overextended and experience fatigue, irritability, resentment, and impatience. Supportive care structures must be provided for family members early so that respite and rest can sustain the caregiver. Weisman (1981) notes that the caregiver who is overwhelmed and extremely fatigued may show signs of abhorrence and avoidance. This reaction is a signal for respite rather than guilt and further demands. Well-timed coaching about the signs of burnout and exhaustion can help the family member be receptive to seeking support when needed. Timing is crucial because family members' concerns and fears are often best alleviated by being present and involved in the care of the loved one, and many warnings of self-protection can actually undermine family meanings and coping. Continuity of care allows for the shoring up of family caring practices, along with well-timed assistance with respite when the situation warrants.

Nurse Patrice Welsh gives a condensed, vibrant version of the rewards and demands of caring for a person with cancer over time (1988). Her account leaves out much detail but provides a kaleidoscopic glimpse of the range of care and coping demands and rewards involved in caring for patients and families. Her account illustrates the existence of a community of caregivers and patients who provide support and encouragement for the most difficult challenges of a serious illness.

We love to hear and tell James Steel stories. He epitomizes so much of what the Oncology Clinic people are and do and try to be. For example, I remember Jim's early encounters with physicians in the clinic:

Jim: "I'm not through talking with him. Why did he walk out? Get Dr. Keller back here for me!"

This was about two months after his diagnosis; he was in the clinic to see the doctor. Jim spoke clearly of his urgent need that the system and the people pay close attention to him.

Jim was thirty-five years old, a Ph.D. in biology, first-year medical student with leiomyosarcoma.

Jim: "When Dr. Keller first came into my room in the hospital he was direct, brusque almost, . . . but he said there are drugs and we can make a difference." And so we began to deal with and struggle against this cancer. Jim had lots going for him and good support. I met and started teaching Janet, his wife. She mastered easily the sterile dressing change and central line heparinization. Our week of work gave the three of us building time. Their relationship was solid, but his life threatening disease and the invasive treatments caused many fears. Jim and Janet were not sure of the questions, but mainly they just needed someone who could assure them that they and that we were doing the most and the best we could.

Janet was quiet but we were bonded. I didn't see her often because she worked and most of the time Jim came alone to the clinic. Of course their four children, Jason, Kelley, Sally and Lynn, also accompanied him at intervals. We really liked to see them in person because we knew so much about them. There is the family starting the first fish tank story . . . I can hear him tell it. Or how his youngest, Lynn, didn't want to go near him at first when his hair fell out—he shaved his head just as so many do because the process is so irritating and the days of hair everywhere is just awful. But in a week or so Lynn became his defender at the preschool when the other children would react to her dad's appearance. One afternoon, several months later we had to hurry him out of the clinic because he was invited to go with her class on their walk and ice cream outing—he was so proud!

Usually once a month his mother and dad would drive eight hours to spend a treatment day in the clinic with him. His brother, John, came from West Texas in his jeans and boots, and that was a fine day for both of them. They reminisced and laughed and even four hours into the DTIC when vomiting came, John stayed and sat with Jim.

We tried all the anti-nausea drug regimens, talked him into counseling and relaxation therapy, did his chemo as an outpatient, as an in-patient, at home, and again as an outpatient. The chemotherapy regimens were tough!

His anatomy lab stories were interspersed with his recognition that he couldn't keep up; so he dropped out of medical school "on leave." Being in school was hard, but not being in school was even worse. His medical school classmates still included him at times, but his whole schedule now was his illness. The days he felt well, he was so bored. I talked with him for months about this problem. Finally he took a job at a nearby duplicating office. Working like this—it was too hard.

The family moved to a bigger apartment, the children passed the chicken pox one to the other, he tried all the anti-nausea drug regimens we had, he suffered through drug reactions and one hospitalization with sepsis, but he completed ten courses of chemo. He was in the clinic those ten months about three times a week.

One of the wonderful things about the clinic is that the patients have the opportunity to become their own community. One day he passed us on his way to Mary's room carrying a pint of Texas' finest ice cream and the latest supermarket scandal sheet. Mary and Bob were clinic friends. She was a small, elderly black woman with lung cancer. It was important to him to be at her funeral the next year; as it was for several of us, staff and patients to go together.

Jim was back in medical school and only had to come in for follow up evaluations every couple of months. But he was still a regular. He'd come by to check on his friends, meet new patients, help us with our Christmas decorations, and just update us on his life. The re-evaluation times were tense. Waiting for the CT results—no evidence of disease—until just before the end of the school year when we knew things were changing because he started having some abdominal symptoms.

In June, another biopsy and a new chemo. A compassionate protocol from the NCI. No vomiting this time, but the recurrent disease perspective, weight loss, diarrhea, constipation, and a change in primary physicians because Dr. Keller changed jobs within the University. Another change in chemo and Jim said: "I brought you this book about foods and cancer. I'm going to try it."

Each time we'd see him there were the old problems to assess but new ones as well. New and different medicines for symptoms until the scans confirmed what we already knew. He was to change hospitals so he could be considered for investigational Stage I and Stage II therapy. He was back with Dr. Keller. Changing hospitals was not easy. There were problems with his central line, the system functioned differently, and just—he was new there. He continued to come to see us and then when he was hospitalized he'd call, Dr. Keller would call, and we would go to see him. Jim: "It'll be all right!" There wasn't any hands on nursing that I could do—I was an outsider in that hospital, but I could keep talking with him and with Janet. One afternoon in his hospital room I sensed his parents wished I hadn't spoken; but I needed to be honest and real with him just as we had been all along. When he asked me about his therapy choices I answered directly: "Maybe no chemo or the less toxic chemo is a good choice at this point; and you can go home with chemo and with your N.G. tube." I went back to my office and called Janet, she talked about the children and herself and Jim's approaching death—she was O.K. In about a week he was home—hospital bed, N.G. suction, I.V. pain meds, and oxygen. I checked on them by phone and went by once to visit and once because they called with a tube problem. Jim was wonderful at home, so different from his hospitalized days and such a part of his family. Admiring Kelley in her new special dress for her sixth grade graduation: Jim: "Kelley you look so pretty! Lynn stop pounding on the piano! Janet don't forget the camera."

There are mornings when I choose my Jim Steel coffee mug: "Those of real character take their coffee black" and head for the clinic knowing that the real world awaits.

Welsh's account illustrates much of the theory presented in this chapter. It is a successful coping story for the family, for Jim, and for Welsh. Jim was allowed to live as a central member of his family until he died. The difficult transition between curative intent and comfort care was made at the right time for Jim and Janet. Welsh leaves out the details of her actual coaching and nursing care but gives us a glimpse of the best of a caring practice. It is clear that she had a deep understanding of the coping issues and demands as they changed. She moved easily and appropriately from strategic to significance issues. She listened and understood Jim's story and the family's story and was strengthened by it. When confronted with such a

narrative that explores the question Coping with what? the impossibility of coping prescriptions is clarified.

References

Bahnson, C. B. (1980). Stress and cancer: The state of the art, Part 1. *Psychomatics, 21*, 975–988.

Bahnson, C. B. (1981). Stress and cancer: The state of the art, Part 2. *Psychomatics, 22*, 207–220.

Bellah, R. N., Madsen, R., Sullivan, W. M., Swidler, A., & Tipton, S. M. (1985). *Habits of the Heart.* Berkeley, CA: University of California Press.

Benner, P. (1984). *Stress and satisfaction on the job.* New York: Praeger Scientific Press.

Benner, P: (1985). The oncology clinical nursing specialist: An expert coach. *Oncology Nursing Forum, 12*, 40–44.

Benner, P., Roskies, E., & Lazarus, R. S.: (1980). Stress and coping under extreme conditions. In J. E. Dimsdale (Ed.), *Survivors, victims, and perpetrators: Essays on the Nazi Holocaust.* Washington, DC: Hemisphere.

Benner, P., & Wrubel, J. (1989). *The primacy of caring.* Menlo Park, CA: Addison-Wesley Publishing Co., Inc.

Cassileth, B. R., Lusk, E. J., Miller, D. S., Brown, L. L., & Miller, C. (1985). Psychosocial correlates of survival in advanced malignant disease. *The New England Journal of Medicine, 312*, 1551–1555.

Cohen, J., & Cordoba, C. (1983). Psychologic, social and economic aspects of cancer. *Surgery Annual, 15*, 160.

Feldman, F. L. (1976). *Work and cancer health histories—A study of the experiences of recovered patients.* Oakland, CA: American Cancer Society, California Division.

Fox, B. H. (1978). Premorbid psychological factors as related to cancer incidence. *Journal of Behavioral Medicine, 1*, 45–133.

Glaser, B. G. & Strauss, A. L. (1968). *Time for dying.* Chicago: Aldine.

Greer, S., & Morris, T. (1975). Psychological attributes of women who develop breast cancer: A controlled study. *Journal of Psychosomatic Research, 19*, 147–153.

Grissom, J. J., Weiner, B. J., & Weiner, E. A. (1975). Psychological correlates of cancer. *Journal of Clinical Psychology, 45*, 113.

Grossarth-Maticek, R. (1980). Psychological predictors of cancer and internal diseases: An overview. *Psychotherapeutic Psychosomatics, 33*, 122–128.

Haan, N: (1977). *Coping and defending: Processes of self-environment organization.* New York: Academic Press.

Kestenbaum, R., & Costa, P. T. (1977). Psychological perspectives on death. In M. R. Rosenzweig & L. W. Porter (Eds.), *Annual Review of Psychology* (pp. 225–250). Palo Alto, CA: Annual Reviews, Inc.

Kissen, D. & Rao, L. G. S. (1969). Steroid excretion patterns and personality in lung cancer. *Annals of the New York Academy of Science, 164*, 476–482.

Kleinman, A. (1988). *The illness narratives.* New York: Basic Books.

Kübler-Ross, E. (1969). *On death and dying.* New York: Macmillan Co.

Larson, P., Benner, P., & Koetters, T. (1990). [A clinical ethnography of two cancer trajectories]. Unpublished Study Sponsored by the Oncology Nursing Society.

Lazarus, R. S. (1966). *Psychological stress and the coping process.* New York: McGraw-Hill Book Co.

Lazarus, R. S. (1968). Emotions and adaptation: Conceptual and empirical relations. In W. J. Arnold (Ed.), *Nebraska symposium on motivation.* Lincoln: University of Nebraska Press.

Lazarus, R. S. (1981). The stress and coping paradigm. In C. Eisdorfer, D. Cohen, A. Kleinman, & P. Maxim (Eds.), *Models for clinical psychopathology.* Hanover, NH: University Press of New England.

Lazarus, R. S. (1985). The trivialization of distress. In J. C. Rosen & L. J. Solomon (Eds.), *Preventing health risk behaviors and promoting coping with illness. Vol. I.* Hanover, NH: University Press of New England.

Lazarus, R. S., & Cohen, J. B. (1977). Environmental stress. In I. Altman & J. F. Wohlwill (Eds.), *Human behavior and the envi-*

ronment: Current theory and research. New York: Plenum Publishing Corp.

Lazarus, R. S., & Folkman, S. (1984). *Stress, appraisal, and coping.* New York: Springer Publishing Co., Inc.

Lazarus, R. S. & Launier, R. (1978). Stress-related transactions between person and environment. In L. A. Pervin & M. Lewis (Eds.), *Perspectives in interactional psychology.* New York: Plenum Publishing Corp.

Lowenberg, J. (1989). *Caring and responsibility.* Philadelphia: University of Pennsylvania Press.

Mages, N. L., & Mendelsohn, G. A. (1979). Effects of cancer on patients' lives: A personological approach. In G. C. Stone, F. Cohen, & N. E. Adler, *Health psychology: A handbook* (pp. 255–284). San Francisco: Jossey-Bass.

Parker, J. (1981). *Cancer passage: Continuity and discontinuity in terminal illness.* Unpublished doctoral dissertation, Monash University, Australia.

Rubin, Z., & Peplau, L. A. (1975). Who believes in a just world? *Journal of Social Issues, 31*(3), 65–88.

Scheper-Hughes, N., & Lock, M. M. The mindful body: A prolegomenon to future work in medical anthropology. *Medical Anthropology Quarterly, 1,* 6.

Schonfield, J. (1972). Psychological factors related to delayed return to an earlier life-style in successfully treated cancer patients. *Journal of Psychosomatic Research, 16,* 44–46.

Simonton, O. C., & Matthews-Simonton, S. (1981). Cancer and stress: Counselling the cancer patient. *The Medical Journal of Australia, 1,* 679–683.

Smith, C. K., Harrison, S. D., Ashworth, C., Montano, D., Davis, A., & Fefer, A. (1984). Life change and the onset of cancer in identical twins. *Journal of Psychosomatic Research, 28,* 525–532.

Sontag, S. (1979). *Illness as metaphor.* New York: Vintage Books.

Taylor, C. (1985). *Philosophical papers, vols. I–II.* Cambridge: Cambridge University Press.

Taylor, J. (1977). *The rules and exercises of holy dying.* New York: Arno Press. (Original work published 1665).

Vaillant, G. E. (1977). *Adaptation to life.* Boston: Little, Brown & Co., Inc.

Weisman, A. D. (1979). *Coping with cancer.* New York: McGraw-Hill Book Co.

Weisman, A. D. (1981). Understanding the cancer patient: The syndrome of caregiver's plight. *Psychiatry, 44,* 161–168.

Welsh, P. N. (1988, February). *Oncology clinical practice: A patient remembered.* Paper presented at a conference at Hermann Hospital, Houston, TX.

CHAPTER 10

Grief and Bereavement

SHIRLEY A. MURPHY

Grief and bereavement are consistent themes in cancer nursing. Grief is experienced by the terminally ill patient, the family, and the caregivers—both lay and professional. Bereavement is influenced by many contextual factors, including recognition of "survivorship" by the family and professional nurses.

The terms *grief* and *bereavement* are often used interchangeably; they are not synonymous, however (Murphy, 1983). Grief is an *intrapersonal, affective* response to any loss. Grief is characterized by sadness, despair, anxiety, and conflict and may precipitate disruptions in physiologic, cognitive, and interpersonal functioning. Understanding the complexity of the process of grief is an important goal in cancer nursing. For example, grief is experienced repeatedly by cancer patients as they cope with loss of hair resulting from chemotherapy, loss of body parts, and anticipated loss of valued relationships. Grief is an important component of the bereavement process because so much emotional energy is involved in the search for meaning and in the resolution of incremental losses and the ultimate loss—death.

Bereavement, a broader construct, can be viewed as a major life transition that is both socioculturally and personally defined. From a sociocultural perspective, bereavement norms regarding mourning rituals and behavior vary according to culture and to one's status in it. From a personal perspective, bereavement is characterized by ongoing change and adjustment in role behavior, social interactions, socioeconomic status, and other factors.

To clarify the differences between grief and bereavement: grief is a subjective response to an objective loss, whereas bereavement is the period after death in which numerous stressful concerns unfold for the survivors over a lengthy period of time. This chapter focuses on the bereavement process, with special applications to cancer nursing. Several chapters in this volume address grief associated with other cancer losses (see, for example, Chapters 14, 28, 52, 57, 60, 68 to 71, and 74 to 77).

Of interest to both clinicians and researchers is the process of change and adjustment that occurs between the death of the loved one and the assimilation or accommodation to loss of the survivors. Several investigators have identified individual "developmental tasks" associated with grieving (Freud, 1917; Parkes & Weiss, 1983; Worden, 1982), but less attention has been given to the many complex factors associated with bereavement. This chapter proposes a transition framework as a vehicle to discuss factors that explain human responses to the death of a valued other. *Transition* is defined as a significant life change that produces lasting effects (George, 1980) or a change that necessitates the abandonment of one set of assumptions and the development of a new set to enable the individual to cope with loss (Parkes, 1971).

GRIEF AND BEREAVEMENT THEMES FROM PUBLISHED LITERATURE

A review of the grief and bereavement literature revealed four major conceptual themes: grief as an introspective response to loss, grief as a normal or pathologic response, grief as a series of stages, and death as a crisis-producing response. Each of these themes provides a historical account of our present understanding of grief and bereavement.

Grief as an Introspective Response to Loss

The predominant theme that emerged from the literature can be described as an introspective or psychodynamic response discussed by Freud in his classic paper, "Mourning and Melancholia," published in 1917. Viewed introspectively, grief is a normal process and involves four essential tasks: (1) to accept the reality of loss, (2) to experience the pain of grief, (3) to adjust to an environment in which the deceased is missing, and (4) to form new relationships. These tasks are measured by self-report and grief inventories (Parkes, 1972; Sanders, Mauger, & Strong, 1979). Questions regarding attachment, loss, and adjustment to a new environment are usually included in the bereavement home visit and telephone follow-up protocols that are used in health care agencies.

Grief as Normal or Pathologic

A second conceptual theme noted was that the grief response can be either normal or pathologic. Lindemann (1944) differentiated among typical, atypical, and delayed grief responses in his treatment of survivors and bereaved victims of a supper club fire. He suggested that atypical and delayed grief responses were pathologic but that the course of atypical grief could be reversed with early detection and intervention. Similarly, Engel (1961) believed some grief responses were abnormal and should be viewed as illnesses.

Conceptualizing grief as normal or pathologic has generated a number of hypotheses that involve mortality; grief intensity specification and its measurement; and relationships between loss-related depressions and immune response, and immune response and infectious disease or psychosomatic illness (Bartrop et al, 1977; Bugen, 1977; Schleiter, Keller, Camerino, Thornton, & Stein, 1983; Stroebe, Stroebe, Gergen, & Gergen, 1981–1982). Clinicians also attempt to assess whether grief seems typical or atypical and make referrals based on their judgments.

Grief as a Series of Stages

A third theme was the stage approach, advanced most prominently by Kübler-Ross (1969). This model posits that individuals go through a series of five predictable stages and that recovery is the outcome. The stages are denial, anger, bargaining, depression, and resolution. Both theoretic weaknesses and lack of empiric support for stage models of grief have fostered a movement away from this approach in research. The model has been both overused and misused in clinical practice.

Death as a Crisis-Producing Response

A fourth theme noted was that death produces a crisis (Raphael, 1979–1980; Rubin, 1977, 1981; Williams, Lee, & Polak, 1976). Viewed from this perspective, the death of a valued person affects the day-to-day physiologic, cognitive, and behavioral role func-

tioning of bereaved survivors. However, this initial overwhelming disequilibrium can be altered by crisis intervention. Persons are said to return to precrisis stability, attain higher levels of functioning and personal growth, or experience a more lasting deficit state. A promising construct—anticipatory grief—emerged from this perspective and has had widespread clinical application. Critical reviews of the bereavement literature suggest that crisis theory may also be an inadequate conceptualization because current thinking is that bereavement should be viewed as a *lengthy process* of adjustment that may take several years (Parkes & Weiss, 1983; Silver & Wortman, 1980; Silverman, 1986).

The four perspectives are similar in that they imply change and adaptation. However, one criticism is that they emphasize the grief process and exclude other factors, such as age and gender of both the bereaved and deceased, mode of death, and potentially mediating influences. A second criticism is that a conceptual theme may be stated early in a publication but not referred to again; in other words, there appears to be no connection between the conceptual theme cited and the work being reported. In summary, current conceptualizations of grief and bereavement are not useful in and of themselves because they exclude important factors affecting bereavement and because they are difficult to apply clinically.

RECONCEPTUALIZATION: BEREAVEMENT AS A MAJOR LIFE TRANSITION

Definitions and Assumptions of Transition

George (1980) defines transitions as changes that are lasting in their effects, and Parkes states that transitions imply "change that necessitates the abandonment of one set of assumptions and the development of a fresh set to enable the individual to cope with the new altered life space" (1971, p. 103).

Crucial to understanding the concept of transition are the following: (1) assumptions or structures of meaning enable an individual to understand the world and to interpret personal experiences in it; (2) assumptions shape behavior; (3) events, especially uncontrollable and unpredictable ones such as death, challenge or change assumptions, undermine meanings of the world and the individual's place in it, and lead to perceptions of stress; (4) change encompasses not only external circumstances but also, and more important, self-perceptions; and (5) stresses associated with loss require the passage of time to cope with the change and to incorporate role and identity changes, and these stresses require several kinds of support (Parkes, 1971; Pearlin & Schooler, 1978; Raphael, 1978; Schlossberg, 1981; Wethington & Kessler, 1986). The assumptions of transition are exemplified in a study on cancer bereavement conducted by McCorkle (1988). Widows and widowers were asked to (1) describe their relationships with their spouses before and after the spouse became ill; (2) share their beliefs about whether illness and death could have been prevented; (3) describe major changes in their lives brought about by their spouse's death, such as adjustment to single parenthood; and (4) discuss their transition to a new identity.

Dimensions and Scope of Transitions

According to Schlossberg (1981), three dimensions are essential in predicting the success or failure (the fourth dimension) of transitions and in assisting individuals through transitions. These dimensions, shown in Figure 10–1, are the nature of an event and the significance of its meaning to the individual involved, the attributes of the individual, and the resources and support that were available and used. Factors associated with an event and its meaning to the individual include the anticipation, type, timing, onset, and duration of the event and the perception of the impact of the event on relationships, routines, assumptions, and roles. Factors associated with the individual include age, gender, ethnicity, state of health, psychosocial competence, socioeconomic status, value orientation, and previous experience with a similar transition. Factors associated with resources and supports include the composition of the social network

and the resources or options available. Adaptation depends on one's perceptions and one's resource-deficit balance. These factors have also been identified as central to the stress-coping health outcome process (Andrews, Tennant, Hewson, & Vaillant, 1978; Caplan, 1981; Houser, 1981; Hyman & Woog, 1982).

An advantage of Schlossberg's dimensions is that they can be adapted to any transition for clinical and research purposes. In bereavement transitions, additional examples of event dimension factors that are not shown in Figure 10–1 but that have been inversely related to bereavement recovery are mode of death (Lindemann, 1944; Parkes & Weiss, 1983; Rubin, 1982; Sanders, 1982–1983); type of death, for example, sudden death versus death following illness (Parkes, 1972; Parkes & Weiss, 1983; Silver & Wortman, 1980); number of deaths (e.g., multiple deaths) (Lindemann, 1944); witnessing deaths of loved ones and being a survivor of the same event (Lindemann, 1944), and relationship to deceased (Horowitz et al., 1984; Murphy, 1983; Parkes & Weiss, 1983; Sanders, 1979–1980). Examples of factors in the individual attribute dimension that are said to affect bereavement outcome are age, gender, and socioeconomic status (Parkes & Weiss, 1983; Vachon et al., 1982). Examples of variables in the mediating processes dimension that affect bereavement recovery are perceptions of social support

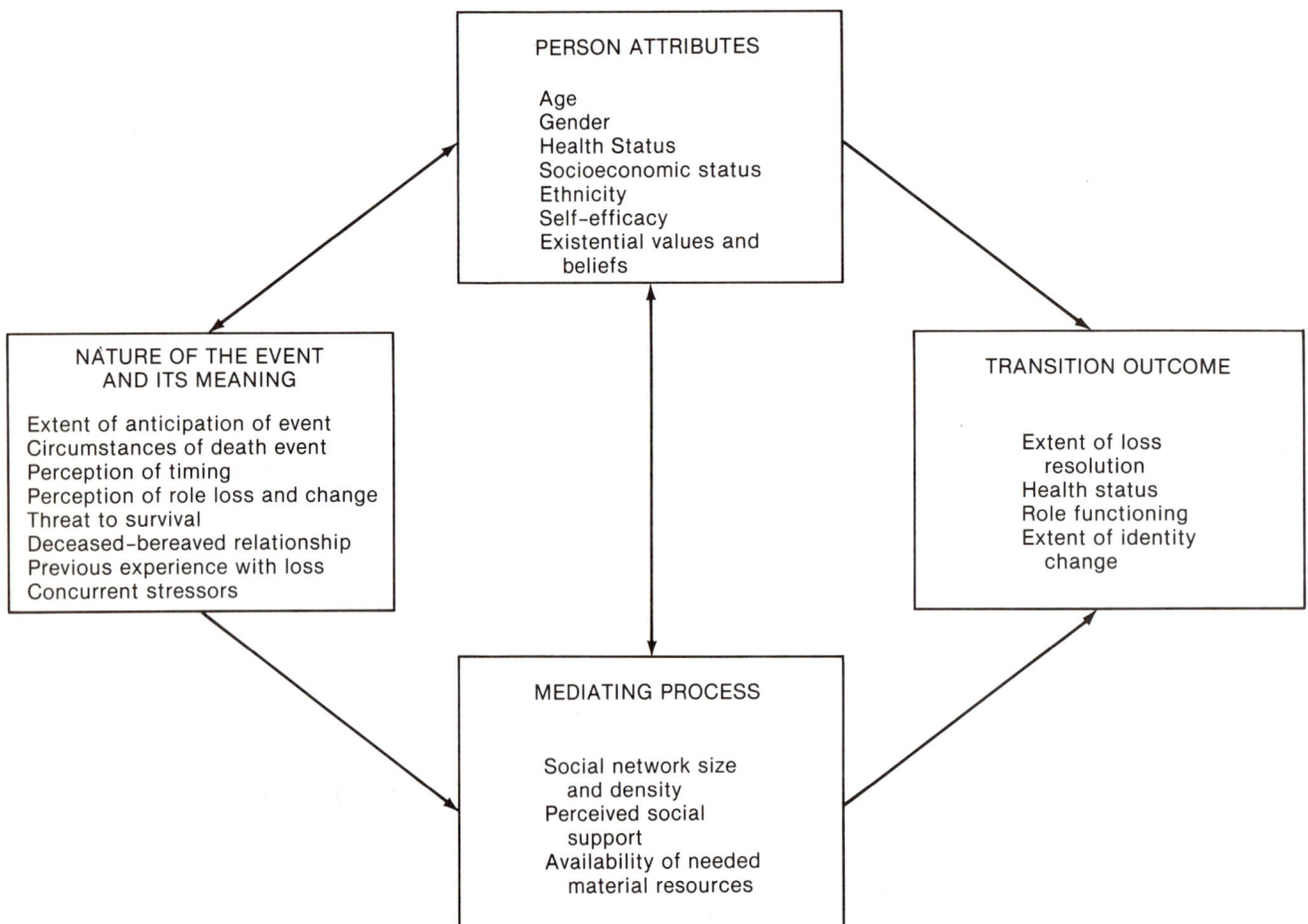

Figure 10–1. Bereavement transition conceptual framework.

(Silverman, 1986; Vachon et al., 1982), size and density of support network (Horowitz et al., 1984; Murphy, 1983), and reference group contacts (Silverman, 1986; Vachon et al., 1982) (see Fig. 10–1).

Marris (1982), Parkes and Weiss (1983), and Silverman (1986) have used findings from longitudinal studies of widowhood to further our understanding of bereavement as a major life transition. Of particular importance is the suggestion that it takes a year or more to resolve the loss emotionally and intellectually and to construct a new view of the self and the world. An additional 2 to 3 years are needed to consolidate the new self-image. These observations have implications for health professionals who intervene on behalf of bereaved family members. For example, a transitions perspective would be helpful to a cancer nurse in deciding which supportive interventions would be most helpful and at what point in the transition. Similarly, McCorkle (1988) tested relationships among several factors shown in Figure 10–1. For example, she was interested in learning how cancer diagnosis, treatment, and length of illness (event factors) affected family roles, assistance with care (mediating factors), and the spouses' grief responses and health status (transition outcome). An abstract of McCorkle's study is shown in Box 10–1.

To exemplify the use of a transition framework specific to cancer nursing, two factors have been selected from each dimension to demonstrate their use in clinical practice, research, and theory development. The factors selected for illustration are circumstances of the death event, bereaved-deceased relationship, gender of the bereaved, self-efficacy, perceived social support, availability of needed material resources, health status, and extent of identity change.

Transition Dimension 1: The Event and Its Meaning to the Individual

Circumstances of the Death Event

One of the most stressful realities faced by family members of cancer patients is the uncontrollability and unpredictability of their loved one's death. Glaser and Strauss (1968) identified five trajectories or patterns of decline associated with the dying process: (1) sudden and unexpected death, (2) unexpected quick death but not expected to die, (3) unexpected quick death, but expected to die, (4) expected quick death, and (5) lingering death. In the third trajectory, in which one is expected to die but one dies more quickly than expected, grief is predicted to be more intense and prolonged because the expectations of family members differ from the actual occurrence of death (Bugen, 1977). This situation frequently occurs with those diagnosed with pancreatic cancer. Survivors may feel cheated or become angry with health professionals for not anticipating the death event.

Another trajectory that causes a great deal of stress is the expected quick death that does not occur. In this death trajectory, the patient improves significantly, and the family no longer anticipates and plans for death. However, uncertainty regarding the changed status, hope, ambivalence, and disbelief have to be dealt with. I served as a consultant to a hospice staff who had a patient who was expected to die quickly. Family members thought their relative was near death and disposed of all the man's personal belongings. A few weeks later the patient's condition improved significantly. The patient's physician suggested the hospice staff begin discharge planning. A member of the nursing staff shared the discharge decision with the patient's family. The family perceived the situation as an acute crisis. One hospice nurse was designated to coordinate the discharge planning for the patient because of the extreme sensitivity required. The nurse began by exploring the patient's feelings about his change in health status and what this change meant to him. The same process was then undertaken with close family members. Then the patient was asked to share his thoughts and feelings with close family members. After both patient and family were able to explore together the previous disposal of belongings, what led to this action, and how the situation had been resolved, discharge details were worked out.

Research that includes circumstances surrounding the death event has shown its relationship to loss resolution, a component of the bereavement transition outcome. In general, the more unexpected the circumstances of death, the more intense and prolonged the grief process (Murphy, 1983; Weisman, 1973). As Figure 10–1 indicates, these variables affect and are affected by person attributes of the bereaved.

The Bereaved-Deceased Relationship

Some past bereavement studies have examined widows' perceptions of the nature of the marital relationship (e.g., "good," "ambivalent," "unhappy") (Parkes, 1972; Sanders, 1979–1980, 1982–1983; Vachon et al., 1982). However, Bugen (1977) was the first to develop a testable model of grief outcomes based on the closeness of the bereaved-deceased relationship and the bereaved person's belief of preventability. According to Bugen, preventability is the *single most influential factor* in predicting both the intensity and duration of grief. (Even though Bugen published a testable model of the role of preventability in predicting grief in 1977, no empirical tests of hypotheses derived from the model could be found.)

According to Bugen, grief responses can be predicted by two factors: centrality, or degree of closeness or importance, of the relationship between the deceased and the bereaved, and beliefs about whether the death could have been prevented (Table 10–1). Centrality of the relationship between the bereaved and the deceased was defined by Bugen at one extreme as referring to a person (1) without whom life is meaningless or senseless, (2) whose love is experienced as being a needed element in one's own life, (3) to whom the survivor had become behaviorally committed through daily activities, or (4) whose very existence

---

Box 10–1. SPOUSE BEREAVEMENT

McCorkle, R. (1988). **A prospective and concurrent study of spouse bereavement (Final Report–NR01626).** Bethesda, MD: National Institutes of Health.

Spouse bereavement is a complex process that involves intense personal pain. Although it has been recognized as a major public health problem, little is known about the impact illness has on spouses prior to patient's death. The overall purpose of this study was to compare data obtained from spouses before patients' death with data obtained after death. The aim was to document the impact of the illness and death on the survivors' health, their relationship with others, and the subsequent changes in their roles and activities. Prospective data were collected at approximately 6-week intervals 2 months after the cancer diagnosis and continued for a period of 6 months. Concurrent data were obtained 6 weeks after the death of the patient and continued for 25 months after death. Using a combination of standardized instruments and semistructured interviews, data were obtained from spouses on symptoms, health perceptions, personal and family relationships, grief responses, utilization of services, evaluation of health professionals' support, and identity transition characteristics. One hundred spouses were entered in the study. Patients diagnosed with lung cancer were randomly assigned to three different nursing interventions: a specialized oncology home care program, a standard home care program, or an office care program. Analysis consisted of comparing mean scores on prospective and concurrent variables in repeated measures using univariate and multivariate analyses of variance. Our findings indicated that spouses experienced similar patterns of symptoms and decreased health perceptions before and after the death. The major difference in the patterns among the groups was the quickened recovery of the group who received care from master's-prepared clinical nurse specialists in oncology. We attributed this improved pattern to the nursing intervention of home care provided by specialized oncology nurses.

---

serves as a reminder and symbol for one's hopes and beliefs. Peripherality of relationship was defined at the other extreme as referring to a person (1) whose presence is both felt and respected but whose loss is not viewed or experienced as irreplaceable or (2) on whose behavior or presence rewards and pleasures are not contingent. A belief of preventability was defined at one extreme as (1) a *general belief* that the factors contributing to the death may have been sufficiently controlled so that death might have been avoided or (2) a *specific belief* of survivors that they themselves contributed to the death either directly or indirectly. The belief of unpreventability at the other extreme refers to the conviction that (1) nothing could have been done by any mortal to divert the forces contributing to the death or (2) everything was done to divert the forces contributing to the death. Attributions of unpreventability are demonstrated by attributions to God, fate, inevitability, luck, or misfortune.

As Table 10–1 shows, centrality and preventability interact to produce one of four predictable grief states. If bereaved persons perceive their relationship with the deceased as central and if they believe the death was preventable, an intense and prolonged grieving process would be expected. If the relationship is perceived as central but the death was believed to be unpreventable, an intense but brief grief response is predicted. With a peripheral relationship, the expected response is mild in intensity, with the duration contingent on the belief of preventability. If the belief of preventability of the death predominates, the duration of the grief is predicted to be more prolonged than if the belief of unpreventability is present. The outcomes—"mild," "intense," "brief," and "prolonged"—were not defined by Bugen, nor did he test the model empirically. In cancer, as in other illnesses and also in sudden death, the central relationship part of the model may be the easiest to understand. Beliefs of preventability, however, may be a very complex and sensitive issue. Some persons believe cancer is completely out of an individual's control (Wortman, 1983). In contrast, more people are becoming increasingly aware of early detection strategies; if these strategies are not used, some individuals would perceive death from cancer as preventable.

Transition Dimension 2: Personal Attributes

Gender of the Bereaved

Widowers have been shown to be at greater health risk than widows during the first 6 months of bereavement, whereas health risks increase for widows during the second year of bereavement, suggesting gender may affect assimilation of loss (Shubin, 1978; Stroebe & Stroebe, 1983). Similarly, studies involving bereaved parents have shown that mothers and fathers have had different relationships with their deceased children and have responded differently to environmental cues following a child's death. For example, mothers may not be able to tolerate cooking the deceased child's favorite food but may share their problem with other bereaved

Table 10–1. INTERACTION OF CLOSENESS OF RELATIONSHIP AND PERCEPTION OF PREVENTABILITY OF DEATH AS PREDICTORS OF GRIEF

	Preventable	Unpreventable
Central Relationship	Intense and prolonged	Intense and brief
Peripheral Relationship	Mild and prolonged	Mild and brief

(Data from Bugen, L. [1977]. Human grief: A model for prediction and intervention. *American Journal of Orthopsychiatry, 47,* 196–206.)

mothers. In contrast, fathers may work longer hours and may share their grief with no one (Rando, 1984; Schatz, 1986). Because of gender and role socialization, parents are said to grieve differently and are not necessarily supportive of each other, which may eventually cause conflict in the marital relationship (Rando, 1986; Rubin, 1982; Schatz, 1986).

Self-Efficacy

A major intrapersonal resource may be one's ability to effect outcomes. Self-efficacy theory (Bandura, 1977) is based on the premise that expectations have a profound effect on behavior. Bandura describes two components of expectation. First, an *outcome expectation* is defined as a person's estimate that a given behavior will lead to a certain outcome. Next, an *efficacy expectation* is the conviction that one can successfully initiate and execute the behavior required to produce the desired outcome. Thus whether a person tries to cope and how long the person persists in coping depend on the belief or expectation the person has at the outset. Self-efficacy has not been measured in many bereavement studies. However, several bereavement studies suggest that many persons report feeling overwhelmed and helpless, at least temporarily. For example, Shubin (1978), in a review of studies of cancer widows, reported that they felt more angry, stigmatized, and helpless than women whose husbands died of cardiovascular disease.

In addition to their importance as research factors, personal attributes are essential sources of information in clinical practice. For example, it is suggested that the more similar individuals are regarding socioeconomic status and similarity of circumstances of loss, the more likely it is that they will participate regularly in support groups (Silverman, 1986).

Transition Dimension 3: Mediating Processes

Perceived Social Support

Despite its appearance in hundreds of studies in the past decade, much remains to be learned about social support (Kessler, McLeod, & Wethington, 1983; Thoits, 1986). Some of the areas most in need of research are the analysis of helpful and unhelpful transactions between bereaved persons and supportive others (Davidowitz & Myrick, 1984), the costs and benefits of being a primary support person (Kessler, McLeod, & Wethington, 1983), and the timing of support (Parkes & Weiss, 1983). Studies by Dunkel-Schetter (1984), Dunkel-Schetter and Wortman (1982), Peters-Golden (1982), and Wortman (1983), are examples of relevant knowledge development in cancer populations accomplished by examining social support as a mediating process.

Support network factors have also been shown to differentiate "at risk" status in those who are bereaved

---

Box 10–2. PREDICTORS AND CORRELATES OF ADAPTATION TO CONJUGAL BEREAVEMENT

Vachon, M., Rogers, J., Lyall, W. A., Lancee, W. J., Sheldon, A. R., & Freeman, S. J. (1982). **Predictions and correlates of adaptation to conjugal bereavement.** *American Journal of Psychiatry, 139,* 998–1002.

Vachon and her colleagues interviewed 162 widows at 1, 6, 12, and 24 months after the deaths of their husbands. They wanted to learn which of the following categories of factors were related to highest distress levels: demographic profiles, predeath factors, social support, the role of religion, and additional problems. They reported that social support variables were the most important in explaining early (1-month) bereavement distress. Data at 24 months' bereavement identified three distinct distress patterns among percentages of the sample: (1) no high distress at any time (30 per cent), (2) an initial high distress level that gradually returned to normal (41 per cent), and (3) continuation of high distress levels at the end of 2 years (28 per cent). Those in the last group had multiple indicators of distress in early (1-month) bereavement that included poor functioning, role dissatisfaction, dissatisfaction with available help, and continued sense of husband's presence. The investigators concluded that they were able to predict 2-year postdeath distress levels with 86 per cent accuracy using ten early adjustment factors identified 1 month after the death of a spouse.

---

following both a cancer death and a death from another cause. Box 10–2 illustrates an example.

Availability of Needed Material Resources

Hospice programs offer opportunities for anticipatory guidance and an immediate plan for bereavement aftercare, which is based on risk assessments of bereaved family members at several points in time. Referral of widowers and widows to support groups, transportation networks, and chore services provides vital linkages with bereaved who are psychologically vulnerable, physically disadvantaged, or both. Examples of other community resources are legal and financial services (Rando, 1984).

Transition Dimension 4: Outcome

Health Status

The health status of bereaved persons has been measured in several ways: perceptions of health (McCorkle, 1988), mental health (McCorkle, 1988; Parkes, 1972; Parkes & Weiss, 1983; Sanders, 1982–1983), and general health (Vachon et al., 1982) and long-term effects of mental distress on immune function (Schleifer et al., 1983). All of these perspectives have added to our knowledge that bereavement is associated with negative effects on health status. More longitudinal studies are needed, however.

Extent of Identity Change

Identity change is a basic assumption of transition: major life changes affect self-perceptions and identity. Parkes and Weiss (1983) suggest that identity change is one of the most difficult transitions to achieve. Ways to operationalize identity change in research studies are limited. In studies involving widows, the widows are sometimes asked about new relationships and about how long they continue to wear their wedding rings. This area of research is still emerging. For example, studies that compare identity change processes between widows and widowers have not been conducted.

SUMMARY

Bereavement can be regarded as a significant life transition that requires adjustment and change over a lengthy period of time. Bereavement is the most stressful of life events, the least prepared for, and the hardest to accept: in Western cultures, it is a passage not always eased by mourning customs and extended family networks, because these have all but disappeared (Blauner, 1966). Knowledge of the bereavement transition is limited because of the emphasis on the grief process and because of the methodological limitations of some studies, such as relying on small samples without control groups and cross-sectional data. Both grief and bereavement are central constructs in cancer nursing.

This chapter proposed a transition framework as an organizing framework to advance empirical research, theory development, and clinical practice regarding bereaved populations. Although the merit of this approach is not yet known, it is appealing for nursing science because it focuses on process, it suggests that multiple factors are central to the bereavement recovery process, and it is organized by dimensions. Factors within each dimension can be included or excluded, depending on relevance.

REFERENCES

Andrews, G., Tennant, C., Hewson, D. M., & Vaillant, G. E. (1978). Life event stress, social support, coping style and risk of psychological impairment. *Journal of Nervous and Mental Disease, 166,* 307–316.

Bandura, A. (1977). Self-efficacy: Toward a unifying theory of behavioral change. *Psychological Review, 84,* 191–215.

Bartrop, R. W., Luckhurst, E., Lazarus, L., Kilch, L. G., & Penny, R. (1977). Depressed lymphocyte function after bereavement. *Lancet, 1,* 834–836.

Blauner, G. (1966). Death and social structure. *Psychiatry, 29,* 378–394.

Bugen, L. (1977). Human grief: A model for prediction and intervention. *American Journal of Orthopsychiatry, 47,* 196–206.

Caplan G. (1981). Mastery of stress: Psychological aspects. *American Journal of Psychiatry, 138,* 413–420.

Davidowitz, M., & Myrick, R. D. (1984). Responding to the bereaved: An analysis of "helping" statements. *Research Record, 1,* 35–42.

Dunkel-Schetter, C. (1984). Social support in cancer: Findings based on patient interviews and their implications. *Journal of Social Issues, 40,* 77–98.

Dunkel-Schetter, C., & Wortman, C. (1982). The interpersonal dynamics of cancer: Problems in social relationships and their impact on the patient. In H. S. Friedman & M. R. DiMalteo (Eds.), *Interpersonal issues in health care.* New York: Academic Press.

Engel, G. L. (1961). Is grief a disease? A challenge for medical research. *Psychosomatic Medicine, 23,* 18–22.

Freud, S. (1968). Mourning and melancholia. In W. Gaylin (Ed.), *The meaning of despair.* New York: Science House. (Originally published 1917).

George, L. K. (1980). *Role transitions in later life.* Monterey, CA: Brooks/Cole.

Glaser, B. G., & Strauss, A. L. (1968). *Time for dying.* Chicago: Aldine.

Horowitz, M. J., Weiss, D. S., Kaltreider, N., Kruprick, J., Marmar, C., Wilner, N., & DeWitt, K. (1984). Reactions to the death of a parent. *Journal of Nervous and Mental Disease, 172,* 383–392.

House, J. (1981). *Work stress and social support.* Reading, MA: Addison-Wesley Publishing Co., Inc.

Hyman, R., & Woog, P. (1982). Stressful life events and illness onset: A review of critical variables. *Research in Nursing and Health, 5,* 155–163.

Kessler, R. C., McLeod, J. D., & Wethington, E. (1983). The costs of caring: A perspective on the relationship between sex and psychological distress. In I. G. Sarason & B. R. Sarason (Eds.), *Social support: Theory, research and applications.* The Hague: Martinus.

Kübler-Ross, E. (1969). *On death and dying.* New York: Macmillan.

Lindemann, E. (1944). Symptomatology and management of acute grief. *American Journal of Psychiatry, 101,* 141–148.

Marris, P. (1982). Attachment and society. In C. M. Parkes & J. Stevenson-Hinde (Eds.), *The place of attachment in human behavior.* New York: Basic Books.

McCorkle, R. (1988). *A prospective and concurrent study of spouse bereavement* (Final Report—NRO1626). Bethesda, MD: National Institute of Health.

Murphy, S. A. (1983). Theoretical perspectives on bereavement. In P. L. Chinn (Ed.), *Advances in nursing theory development* (pp. 191–206). Rockville, MD: Aspen Systems Corp.

Parkes, C. M. (1971). Psychosocial transitions: A field for study. *Social Science and Medicine, 5,* 101–115.

Parkes, C. M. (1972). *Bereavement: Studies of grief in adult life.* New York: International Universities Press.

Parkes, C. M., & Weiss, R. S. (1983). *Recovery from bereavement.* New York: Basic Books.

Pearlin, L. I., & Schooler, C. (1978). The structure of coping. *Journal of Health and Social Behavior, 19,* 2–21.

Peters-Golden, H. (1982). Breast cancer: Varied perceptions of social support in the illness experience. *Social Science and Medicine, 16,* 483–491.

Rando, T. A. (1984). *Grief, dying, and death.* Champaign, IL: Research Press.

Rando, T. A. (1986). *Parental loss of a child.* Champaign, IL: Research Press.

Raphael, B. (1977). Preventive intervention with the recently bereaved. *Archives of General Psychiatry, 34,* 1450–1454.

Raphael, B. (1979–1980). A primary prevention action programme: Psychiatric involvement following a major rail disaster. *Omega, 10,* 211–226.

Rubin, L. R. (1982). Children in automobile accidents: The effects on the family (Final report). Washington, DC: U.S. Department of Transportation.

Rubin, S. (1977). *Bereavement and vulnerability: A study of mothers of sudden infant death syndrome children.* Unpublished doctoral dissertation, Boston University, Boston, MA.

Rubin, S. (1981). A two-track model of bereavement: Theory and application in research. *American Journal of Orthopsychiatry, 51,* 101–109.

Sanders, C. (1979–1980). A comparison of adult bereavement in the death of a spouse, child, and parent. *Omega, 10,* 303–321.

Sanders, C. (1982–1983). Effects of sudden vs. chronic illness death in bereavement outcome. *Omega, 13,* 227–241.

Sanders, C. M. (1989). Grief: The mourning after. New York: John Wiley & Sons, Inc.

Schatz, W. (1986). *Grief of fathers.* In T. A. Rando (Ed.), *Parental loss of a child.* Champaign, IL: Research Press.

Schleifer, S. J., Keller, S. E., Camerino, M., Thornton, J. L., & Stein, M. (1983). Suppression of lymphocyte stimulation following bereavement. *Journal of the American Medical Association, 250,* 374–377.

Schlossberg, N. K. (1981). A model for analyzing human adaptation to transition. *The Counseling Psychologist, 9,* 2–18.

Shubin, S. (1978). Cancer widows—a special challenge. *Nursing '78, 8,* 56–60.

Silver, R., & Wortman, C. (1980). Coping with undesirable life events. In J. Garber & M. Seligman (Eds.), *Human helplessness: Theory and application* (pp. 279–341). New York: Academic Press.

Silverman, P. R. (1986). *Widow to widow.* New York: Springer.

Stroebe, M., & Stroebe, W. (1983). Who suffers more? Sex differences in health risks of the widowed. *Psychological Bulletin, 93,* 279–301.

Stroebe, M., Stroebe, W., Gergen, K., & Gergen, M. (1981–1982). The broken heart: Reality or myth? *Omega, 12,* 87–106.

Thoits, P. (1986). Social support as coping assistance. *Journal of Consulting and Clinical Psychology, 54,* 416–423.

Vachon, M., Rogers, J., Lyall, W. A., Lancee, W. J., Sheldon, A. R., & Freeman, S. J. (1982). Predictors and correlates of adaptation to conjugal bereavement. *American Journal of Psychiatry, 139,* 998–1002.

Weisman, A. (1973). Coping with untimely death. *Psychiatry, 36,* 366–379.

Wethington, E., & Kessler, R. C. (1986). Perceived support, received support, and adjustment to stressful life events. *Journal of Health and Social Behavior, 27,* 78–89.

Williams, W., Lee, J., & Polak, P. (1976). Crisis intervention: Effects of crisis intervention on family survivors of sudden death situations. *Community Mental Health Journal, 12,* 128–136.

Worden, J. W. (1982). *Grief counseling and grief therapy: A handbook for the mental health practitioner.* New York: Springer Publishing Co., Inc.

Wortman, C. (1983, April). *Social support and the cancer patient—conceptual and methodologic issues.* Paper presented at the American Cancer Society Workshop Conference: Methodology in Behavioral and Psychosocial Cancer Research. St. Petersburg Beach, FL.

CANCER AS A DISEASE

Epidemiologic Principles for Nursing Practice: Assessing the Cancer Problem and Planning Its Control

DENISE M. OLESKE

CLASSIFICATION SYSTEMS
DATA SOURCES FOR EPIDEMIOLOGIC RESEARCH
Decennial Census
The National Death Index
The SEER Program
Cancer Registry
Population Surveys
The Behavioral Risk Factor Surveillance System
CANCER OCCURRENCE
Person
    Age
    Sex and Race

Life Style
    Genetic Predisposition
Place
Time
ANALYTIC EPIDEMIOLOGIC METHODS
Cross-Sectional Study
Prospective Study
Retrospective Study
Randomized Clinical Trial
CAUSALITY
SUMMARY

The increased life expectancy of the United States population is one indicator of the health of the nation. However, this phenomenon raises new challenges—namely, the increased likelihood of health problems associated with an aging society and problems stemming from technology and associated life styles that in themselves may promote chronic diseases such as cancer. Epidemiology is the study of the distribution and determinants of disease in a population. In addition, its methods assist in the identification of factors associated with the development of cancer. This chapter discusses the application of epidemiologic principles relevant to nursing practice that aid in understanding the cancer problem and guide in the formulation of approaches to control it.

CLASSIFICATION SYSTEMS

Because *cancer* is a term that represents a process common to a very heterogeneous group of diseases, it is particularly important to be able to distinguish cases and classify them according to their type. Epidemiology

has been in the forefront in stimulating efforts to improve the definition and classification of cancer. Currently, cancers are typically classified at diagnosis by anatomic site, cell type, and stage. The most widely used scheme for classifying cancers according to anatomic site is contained in the publication *The International Classification of Diseases*, 9th revision (ICD-9). Each anatomic site is assigned a four-digit code, the first three digits indicating the general anatomic site and the fourth digit designating a subsite. Table 11–1 contains a list of the ICDs associated with neoplasia. Among the most common coding systems for histologic classification is the *Systematized Nomenclature of Pathology* (SNOP). The procedures generally followed for staging of a cancer are those described by the American Joint Committee for Cancer Staging and End-Results Reporting. Cancer stage may be based on clinical findings alone or include the observations made during a surgical procedure with the results of histopathologic studies. For some cancers, additional laboratory information may be important in classification—for example, karyotyping in leukemia. The more exactly a neoplasm may be defined, the more precisely

Table 11–1. TABULAR LIST OF MAJOR HEADINGS FOR NEOPLASIA IN ICD-9

Category of Malignant Neoplasm	ICD-9 Codes
Lip, oral cavity, and pharynx	140–149
Digestive organs and peritoneum	150–159
Respiratory and intrathoracic organs	160–165
Connective tissue, skin, and breast	170–175
Genitourinary organs	179–189
Other, unspecified sites	190–199
Lymphatic and hematopoietic tissue	200–208
In situ	230–234

ICD-9, *International Classification of Diseases*, 9th Rev. (U. S. Department of Health and Human Services, 1989.)

cancer epidemiologists may be able to identify its associated risk and prognostic factors.

DATA SOURCES FOR EPIDEMIOLOGIC RESEARCH

Data for epidemiologic research in cancer may be obtained either through existing systems or through the collection of primary data in surveys or other types of studies. A number of resources useful to persons conducting epidemiologic studies are available. Those commonly utilized in cancer epidemiology studies are described in the following sections.

Decennial Census

Each decade the Bureau of the Census seeks to count each person in the United States, according to "usual place of residence." In attempting to derive specific information about the population, a core set of questions is asked about each person within the housing unit contacted, and from a subset of these units a more detailed questionnaire is administered. The items covered on the core set are the following: name, household relationship, sex, race, age, marital status, Hispanic origin, and some characteristics of housing. Information on ancestry, previous residence, occupation, poverty status, and education are obtained from a sample. Data from the census are useful for constructing a demographic profile of the community of interest as well as serving as the denominator in calculating population-based rates for descriptive epidemiologic measures.

The National Death Index

Mortality information is useful for a variety of reasons in epidemiologic studies, including monitoring of vital status and outcomes of participants in prospective studies and in clinical trials. A central source of death record information called the National Death Index (NDI) is maintained by the National Center for Health Statistics (NCHS), and this index can assist investigators in these efforts (Patterson & Bilgrad, 1986). To use this service, the investigator needs to complete an application form ensuring that the data are for health research and provisions are made for maintaining confidentiality. Data files containing subjects' names and pertinent identification criteria are forwarded to the NDI, where the names are sought in the NDI's file. Computer reports returned may contain some false matches, thus requiring that death certificates be obtained from a state Vital Records Division to confirm the information received. The cost of the computerized service is nominal, and turn-around time for handling requests is short.

The SEER Program

The principal source of national estimates of cancer incidence for the United States is the SEER Program (Surveillance, Epidemiology, and End Results). Ten regional areas participate in this program and collect detailed information on the incidence and mortality of malignant neoplasms. The areas involved in the SEER program are Metropolitan Atlanta; Metropolitan Detroit; San Francisco-Oakland SMSA; the Seattle–Puget Sound area; the entire states of Connecticut, Hawaii, Iowa, New Mexico, and Utah, and the Commonwealth of Puerto Rico. The information collected for each cancer case includes demographic characteristics of the patient, anatomic site, histologic cell type, extent of disease at the time of diagnosis, treatment data, and vital status over time (Pollack, 1984). From an epidemiologic perspective, the national cancer incidence data from the SEER program help identify demographic groups with exceptionally high or low risk of developing cancer. Population-based site-specific mortality and survival data also are accumulated in this program. From these data, etiologic hypotheses and prognostic indicators can be generated, and programs geared to those target groups for cancer prevention and early detection can be developed. And, because SEER serves as a population-based surveillance system, the effects of cancer control measures may be evaluated.

Cancer Registry

A cancer registry is one means of gathering data about the disease process and treatment efforts. It comprises the listing of cancer patients and the administrative system by which this listing is maintained and updated. The registry maintains only those data that are not likely to change: demographic characteristics (age at diagnosis of cancer, race, and sex), tumor characteristics at diagnosis (site, histology, stage), and general type of treatment. Most registries in the United States are hospital based and have a service-oriented focus. Registries began with the intent of being a type of medical audit system to ensure quality care for cancer patients by recording information on the treatment process. Hospitals participating in the American College of Surgeons (ACS) cancer registry program are required to collect information on the histologic diagnosis obtained before treatment. In addition, registries are required to query physicians each year regarding the vital status of each treated patient, thereby promoting the continued follow-up of patients after the initiation of treatment. For epidemiologic purposes, the hospital tumor registry is a useful source for the identification of incident cases in a retrospective (case-control) study. It is necessary, however, to be cautious in the use of cancer registries in instances in which more than one hospital serves a geographic area. In these circumstances, patients may be listed in more than one registry because of second opinions, transfers for therapy resources, changes of physician, and so forth.

Population Surveys

The National Health Survey was enacted through congressional legislation in 1956 to obtain periodic information about the health status and health needs of the United States population. This activity is carried

Table 11–2. ESTIMATES OF THE PERCENTAGE OF THE POPULATION WITH SELECTED BEHAVIOR AND KNOWLEDGE FROM THE NATIONAL HEALTH INTERVIEW SURVEY QUESTIONNAIRE ON HEALTH PROMOTION AND DISEASE PREVENTION, UNITED STATES, 1985

Health Behaviors or Knowledge Reported	All Ages	18–29 Years	30–44 Years	45–64 Years	65 Years and Over
Interval since last Papanicolaou smear (women only):					
<1 year	46	60	50	38	25
1–2 years	27	22	31	30	25
3 + years	20	6	17	18	35
Never	7	13	1	4	15
Interval since last breast examination by doctor or other health professional (women only):					
<1 year	50	60	52	45	39
1–2 years	28	22	31	30	24
3 + years	15	6	14	20	23
Never	8	11	2	5	14
The chances of getting bladder cancer from cigarette smoking:					
Increases	35	41	34	33	31
Does not increase	25	29	29	21	14
Don't know/no opinion	40	30	37	45	55
The chances of getting lung cancer from cigarette smoking:					
Increases	94	96	95	93	87
Does not increase	2	1	1	2	2
Don't know/no opinion	5	3	3	5	11

(From Thornberry, O. T., Wilson, R. W., & Golden, P. M. [1986]. Health promotion data for the 1990 objectives: Estimates from the National Health Interview Survey of Health Promotion and Disease Prevention, U. S., 1985. *Advance data from vital and health statistics* [No. 126]. [DHHS Publication No. [PMS] 86-1250]. Hyattsville, MD: U. S. Public Health Service.)

Table 11–3. AGE-ADJUSTED DEATH RATES AND PERCENTAGE OF TOTAL DEATHS FOR THE 15 LEADING CAUSES OF DEATH, UNITED STATES, 1985

Cause of Death	Rate per 100,000	Total Deaths (Per Cent)
All Causes	873.9	100.0
Specific causes:		
1 Heart diseases	323.0	37.0
2 Malignant neoplasms, including neoplasms of lymphatic and hematopoietic tissues	193.3	22.1
3 Cerebrovascular diseases	64.1	7.3
4 Accidents and adverse effects	39.1	4.5
Motor vehicle accidents	19.2	—
All other accidents and adverse effects	19.2	—
5 Chronic obstructive pulmonary disease and allied conditions	31.3	3.6
6 Pneumonia and influenza	28.3	3.2
7 Diabetes mellitus	15.5	1.8
8 Suicide	12.3	1.4
9 Chronic liver disease and cirrhosis	11.2	1.3
10 Atherosclerosis	10.0	1.1
11 Nephritis, nephrotic syndrome, and nephrosis	8.9	1.0
12 Homicide and legal intervention	8.3	1.0
13 Certain conditions originating in the perinatal period	8.1	0.9
14 Septicemia	7.2	0.8
15 Congenital anomalies	5.4	0.6
All other causes	107.8	12.3

(From National Center for Health Statistics. [1987]. *Advance report of final mortality statistics, 1985. Monthly Vital Statistics Report,* 36 [5] Supplement. [DHHS Publication No. [PHS] 87-1120]. Hyattsville, MD: U. S. Public Health Service.)

out through the NCHS. Random samples of households are selected for the Health Interview Survey, in which questions are asked on acute and chronic conditions; activity limitations; and visits to a hospital, doctor, or dentist. Through the Health Examination Survey, random samples for the population are selected for a complete physical examination, which includes laboratory testing as well as electrocardiograms and pulmonary function testing. The National Health and Nutrition Examination Survey (NHANES), conducted from 1971 to 1975, represents the first time that inter-

Table 11–4. AGE-SPECIFIC DEATH RATES FOR MALIGNANT NEOPLASMS PER 100,000 POPULATION, UNITED STATES, SELECTED YEARS, 1950 THROUGH 1984

Age	1950	1960	1970	1980	1982	1984
All ages, age-adjusted	124.4	125.8	129.9	132.8	132.5	133.5
All ages, crude	139.8	149.2	162.8	183.9	187.2	191.8
<1	8.7	7.2	4.7	3.2	3.7	3.1
1–4	11.7	10.9	7.5	4.5	4.6	4.0
5–14	6.7	6.8	6.0	4.3	4.1	3.6
15–24	8.6	8.3	8.3	6.3	5.9	5.5
25–34	20.0	19.5	16.5	13.7	13.2	13.0
35–44	62.7	59.7	59.5	48.6	46.2	46.6
45–54	175.1	177.0	182.5	180.0	176.0	170.5
55–64	392.9	396.8	423.0	436.1	439.7	448.4
65–74	692.5	713.9	754.2	817.9	824.9	835.1
75–84	1153.3	1127.4	1168.0	1232.3	1238.7	1272.3
≥85	1451.0	1450.0	1417.3	1594.6	1598.6	1604.0

(Data from Breslow & Cumberland, 1988.)

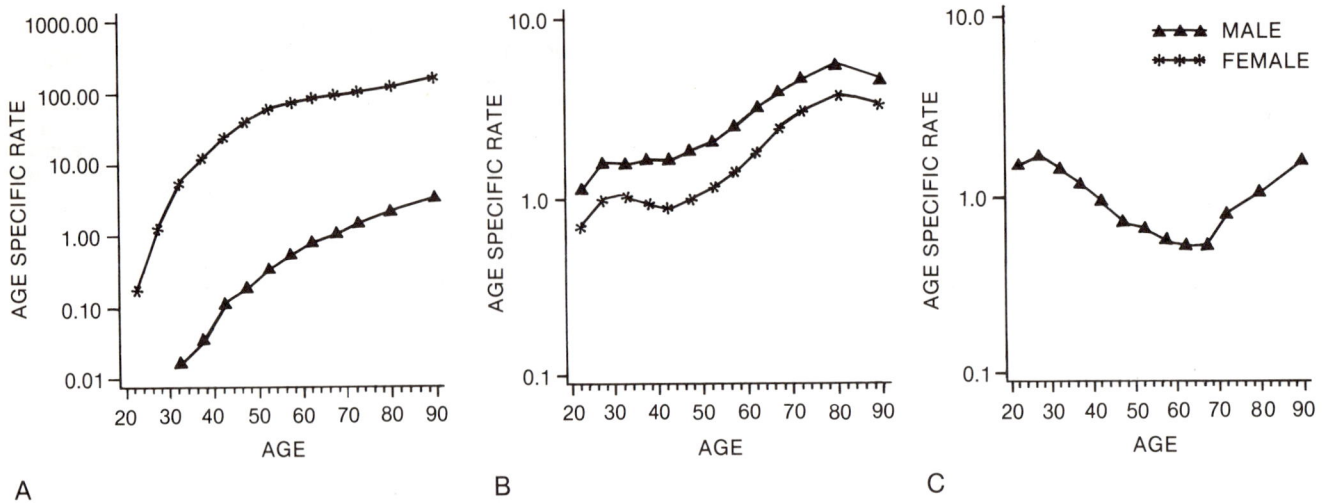

Figure 11–1. Cancer mortality among the white population, 1950–1980, by state economic area. *A*, Breast. *B*, Hodgkin's disease. *C*, Testis. (From Pickle, L. W., Mason, T. J., Howard, N., Hoover, R., & Fraumeni, J. F., Jr. [1987]. *Atlas of U.S. cancer mortality* [DHHS Publication No. NIH 87-2900]. Washington, DC: U.S. Government Printing Office.)

view and physical examination data were linked. In a random sample of the population, a detailed medical history was obtained and a dietary questionnaire was administered; in addition, the patient underwent a standardized medical examination in which blood and urine specimens were taken to obtain nutrient levels. These survey results provide prevalence information on the rates of illness and health problems of the United States population by geographic region.

In addition to periodic surveys of the health of the United States population, the NCHS also periodically surveys hospitals, skilled care facilities, and home care agencies to obtain information on utilization rates and personnel. Among persons diagnosed as having cancer, hospitalization rates and length of stay are declining in all age groups and for most cancer types (National Center for Health Statistics [NCHS], 1986, 1988).

Changes in the financing of health care and the shift to the delivery of services in nonhospital settings have stimulated these trends. In 1987, the average length of stay for cancer patients was 8.0 days. The length of stay for cancer patients increases with age, with persons aged 65 years and over experiencing an average length of hospital stay of 9.3 days. Data on the rates of health care utilization are important prevalence measures and may be used to represent levels of realized access to health care in an area. They may also assist in the planning of facilities and personnel for delivering health care.

In 1985, as part of the Health Interview Survey questionnaire, the topic of health promotion and dis-

Table 11–5. DEATH RATES* FOR MALIGNANT NEOPLASM OF BREAST AMONG ILLINOIS WOMEN, BY RACE AND AGE, 1969–1971 AND 1979–1981

Age Group	All Races 1979–81	All Races 1969–71	White 1979–81	White 1969–71	All Other 1979–81	All Other 1969–71
All ages, age adjusted†	29.1	29.7	29.1	29.9	28.3	27.0
All ages, crude	33.3	31.6	35.7	33.6	21.8	19.4
Under 15 yr	—	—	—	—	—	—
15–24 yr	‡	‡	‡	‡	‡	‡
25–34 yr	3.7	4.3	3.6	4.0	4.3	5.8
35–44 yr	17.2	22.2	16.6	22.0	20.3	23.4
45–54 yr	50.4	54.8	49.5	54.3	55.6	58.4
55–64 yr	82.8	86.1	83.2	87.8	79.9	69.2
65–74 yr	117.7	107.7	120.4	109.0	93.7	93.0
75–84 yr	144.1	140.5	144.3	141.8	142.2	119.6
85 yr and over	191.8	173.4	192.6	176.6	181.2	130.6

*Rates per 100,000 women in specified groups.
†Age-adjusted by the direct method to the total 1970 population of Illinois.
‡Rate not calculated, fewer than 10 deaths.
(Data from Office of Planning, Illinois Department of Public Health, 1985.)

Table 11–6. SUMMARY OF INCIDENCE AND MORTALITY RATES AND 5-YEAR SURVIVAL FOR MAJOR CANCER SITES BY RACE

Site or Type	Incidence* Black	Incidence* White	Mortality† Black	Mortality† White	Survival‡ Black	Survival‡ White
Esophagus	2.9	11.5	2.6	9.2	5	3
Stomach	8.0	13.8	5.8	10.0	14	15§
Rectum	15.0	11.7	3.5	3.5§	49	37
Pancreas	8.9	13.6	8.6	11.0	3	3§
Larynx	4.6	6.6	1.3	2.5	67	59
Lung (men)	81.0	119.0	70.7	91.4	13	10
Breast	85.6	71.9	26.6	26.3§	75	63
Cervix	8.8	20.2	3.2	8.8	68	63
Corpus uteri	25.1	13.4	2.0	2.9	88	57
Prostate	75.1	121.3	21.0	43.9	69	59
Bladder	15.4	8.6	3.9	3.8§	74	50
Multiple myeloma	3.4	7.9	2.4	5.0	24	27§

*Incidence is given in number of cases per 100,000 persons for 1978–1981, age-adjusted to the 1970 United States population.
†Mortality is given in number of deaths per 100,000 persons for 1978–1981, age-adjusted to the 1970 United States population.
‡Survival figures are for 1973–1981.
§Black-white differences are not significant at the 0.05 level.
(From Greenwald, P., & Sondik, E. J. [1986]. *Cancer control objectives for the nation.* NCI monograph No. 2, NIH Publication No. 86-2880.)

Rate per 100,000

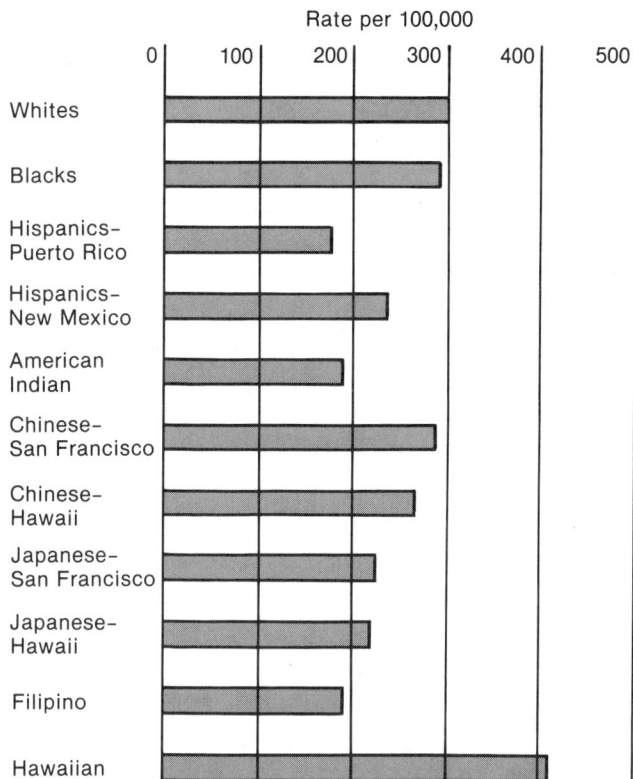

Figure 11–2. Average annual age-adjusted cancer incidence in females for all sites, SEER Program, 1973–1977. (From Bureau of Health Professions. [1985]. *Health status of minorities and low income groups* [DHHS Publication No. HRS-P-DV-85-1]. Washington, DC: U.S. Government Printing Office.)

ease prevention was covered. The survey included questions on general health (including nutrition), stress, high blood pressure, injury control, exercise, smoking, alcohol consumption, dental care, and occupational safety and health (Thornberry, Wilson, & Golden, 1986). Selected survey results are displayed in Table 11–2. These data indicate that persons aged 65 years and over are less knowledgeable about the relationship of cigarette smoking to either cancer of the lung or cancer of the bladder. More than one third of the women in this age group have not had recent screening for mammary or uterine cancer. From an epidemiologic perspective, the survey results are useful for monitoring progress toward achieving the 1990 health objectives for the nation. Health professionals conducting community-based assessments are likely to find these national normative data useful when comparing the results of their surveys. The comparison would help in identifying specific health knowledge and health behaviors that may need improvement in their local areas.

The Behavioral Risk Factor Surveillance System

The Behavioral Risk Factor Surveillance System (BRFSS) was started by the Centers for Disease Control (CDC) in 1984 for the purpose of rapidly obtaining

continuous information on the prevalence rates of personal behaviors associated with the leading causes of death in the United States (Centers for Disease Control [CDC], 1985). The personal behaviors monitored include current smoking status, alcohol consumption, hypertension and compliance with treatment, seat belt use, physical activity and being overweight, obtaining Papanicolaou smears, routine mammograms, and stool testing for blood. Within the 30 states participating in the system, approximately 100 adults per month are selected for interview by random digit dialing. In contrast to the Health Interview Survey, this system is designed to yield valid estimates at the state level of selected behavioral risk factors over time so that trends in selected behaviors can be monitored. For example, this system has identified that people from both Indiana and New York are lagging behind those from the other states in cessation of smoking, with 32.2 and 31.4 per cent, respectively, of their adult populations being current smokers, compared with the average prevalence of 26.3 per cent among other reporting states. This database is also useful for states in estimating the impact of intervention programs for changing behavior patterns associated with the development of cancer.

CANCER OCCURRENCE

Today cancer is the second leading cause of death in the United States, accounting for about one fifth of

Rate per 100,000

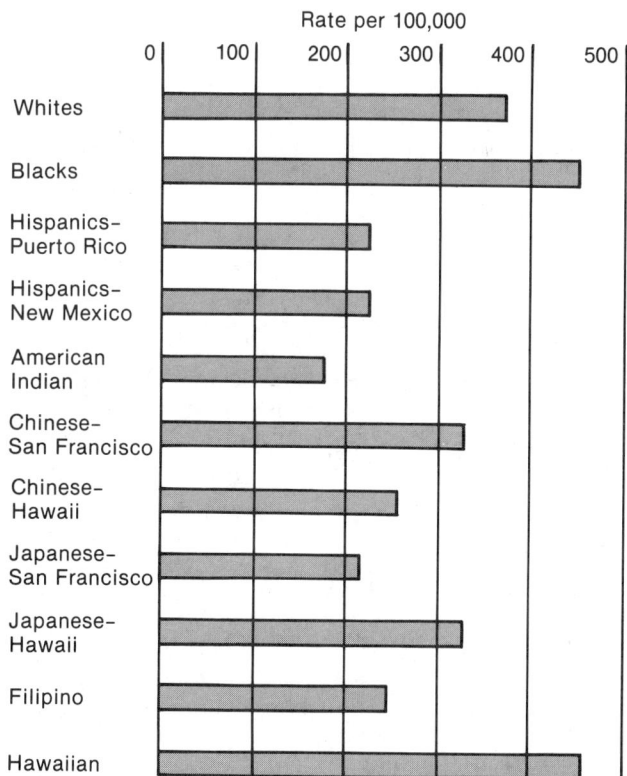

Figure 11–3. Average annual age-adjusted cancer incidence in males for all sites, SEER Program, 1973–1977. (From Bureau of Health Professions. [1985]. *Health status of minorities and low income groups* [DHHS Publication No. HRS-P-DV-85-1]. Washington, DC: U.S. Government Printing Office.)

all deaths (Table 11–3). Using data sources, such as those previously mentioned, nurses may compile descriptive statistics to assess the nature and magnitude of the cancer problem in their own communities. The most common descriptive measures used in cancer epidemiology are rates—namely, incidence, mortality, and prevalence rates. These measures may be used simultaneously to assess the cancer problem in a population by addressing the questions: In whom does it occur (person)? Where does it occur (place)? When does it occur (time)? Examples of the use of rates as descriptive measures in assessing the cancer problem follow.

Person

Age

For most types of cancer, incidence and mortality rates increase dramatically with increasing age (Table 11–4). This means that both the risk of developing cancer and the risk of dying from it increase as people get older. In addition, each cancer type has a unique age pattern with respect to the onset and mortality associated with it. Figure 11–1A–C displays the age-specific mortality patterns associated with cancers of the breast, cancer of the testis, and Hodgkin's disease to illustrate these concepts. Examination of rates can also be employed to generate etiologic hypotheses. For example, using data from Illinois, the age-adjusted breast cancer mortality rates for whites is higher than for nonwhites (Table 11–5). However, in examining the age-specific rates further, the rates among nonwhites exceed those for whites in the under-55-years-old age group, a finding consistent with national data (Horm, Asire, Young, & Pollack, 1984). Changes in life-style practices may be responsible for the reversals in the white and nonwhite breast cancer mortality rates, and these should promote interest in developing epidemiologic studies to identify the etiologic mechanisms that might account for this change. These data also emphasize the importance of including nonwhite women (particularly black women, who often represent more than 95 per cent of the nonwhite figures) in programs aimed at reducing the morbidity and mortality from breast cancer.

Sex and Race

Historically, there have been marked differences in cancer incidence, mortality, and survival between the sexes and among the races. The overall age-adjusted incidence and mortality from cancer are generally higher among men than among women for all races. Variations by race are apparent when examining specific cancer types (Table 11–6). Of concern is the fact that death rates among blacks are increasing faster than among whites for cancers of the lung, prostate, esophagus, breast, colon and rectum, and pancreas. In addition, high incidence rates among Hawaiians and Chinese in San Francisco in both men and women

suggest the need for additional studies with respect to the cultural factors that influence these rates (Figs. 11–2 and 11–3).

Life Style

Over the years, a long list of individual life-style factors have been found to be associated with various types of cancers. Table 11–7 summarizes these and their estimated contributions to the current cancer mortality rates. From these data, it is estimated that 80 per cent of the total cancer mortality may be due to life-style factors. Therefore, most, if not all, of the cancer mortality may be preventable. Descriptive statistics, as available through vital registration systems and cancer registries, contain limited information on specific risk factors. Analytic studies are used for this purpose. However, descriptive statistics may be used to monitor a community's progress toward the reduction of cancer mortality presumed to be linked with certain life styles.

Genetic Predisposition

Genetic factors by themselves are thought to be responsible for only a small percentage of types of cancer. An understanding of the mechanisms for heritable cancers is gained from examining the patterns of cancer occurrence in certain high-risk populations such as those with familial polyposis (colon cancer), dysplastic nevus syndrome (malignant melanoma), and albinos (basal cell carcinoma). In addition, the identification of a single case of any of these conditions should signal the nurse to have the parents, siblings, and possibly children of the patient's family also be examined and counseled regarding their high risk.

Place

Definitions of place considered in cancer epidemiology are those areas defined by latitude and longitude. Analyses commonly focus on comparison of geopolitical units (urban-rural; intercountry, and so forth) and physical units (areas of different soil types, elevations, water sources). Examination of disease rates by some unit of place is useful in developing hypotheses concerning the cause of the disease under investigation. Research on the role of diet in cancer had been

Table 11–7. ESTIMATES OF CANCER MORTALITY ASSOCIATED WITH LIFE-STYLE FACTORS

Life-style Factor	Percentage of All Cancer Deaths and Estimate of Mortality (Range)
Tobacco	30 (25–40)
Alcohol	3 (2–4)
Diet	35 (10–70)
Reproductive and sexual behavior	7 (1–13)
Occupation	4 (2–8)
Medicines and medicinal products	1 (0.5–3)

(Data from Doll & Peto, 1981.)

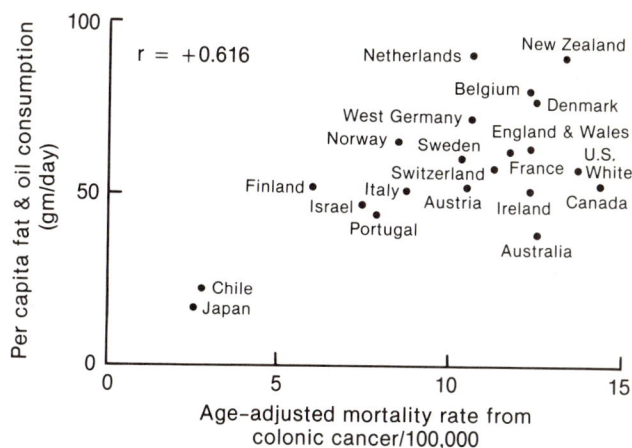

Figure 11–4. Age-adjusted mortality rate from colon cancer (per 100,000 people) by per capita fat and oil consumption. (From Wynder, E. L. [1975]. The epidemiology of large bowel cancer. *Cancer Research, 35,* 3388–3394. Reproduced by permission.)

Table 11–8. AGE-ADJUSTED (1970 UNITED STATES STANDARD) CANCER MORTALITY RATES PER 100,000 FOR CHICAGO AND SEER URBAN AREAS FOR ALL CANCER SITES BY RACE AND SEX

Race Sex	Chicago 1978–1981	Atlanta 1978–1981	Detroit 1978–1981	San Francisco–Oakland 1978–1981	Seattle–Puget Sound 1978–1981
White man	236.1	215.9	224.0	217.0	202.4
White woman	149.0	125.3	138.8	149.6	135.7
Black man*	305.9	281.2	285.8	303.3	—
Black woman*	150.0	140.0	158.1	153.7	—

SEER, Surveillance Epidemiology and End Results Program, National Cancer Institute.

*Chicago rates are for all races other than white, but this category is over 90 per cent black.

(Data from Horn, Asire, Young, & Pollock, 1984.)

stimulated by studies of intercountry comparisons of mortality rates from colon cancer. From these comparisons, it was observed that developing nations had substantially lower colon cancer mortality than industrialized nations. Associations between environment and disease can be further explored descriptively using an ecologic approach whereby disease rates are correlated with exposure levels of groups rather than individuals. Figure 11–4 illustrates this methodology, showing the strong positive relationship between colon cancer mortality and levels of fat consumption in the population. Observations generated from such studies further support the statement that certain dietary components, such as fats, are related to cancer in humans.

Place is useful not only in identifying etiologic factors associated with personal life style or cultural practices, but also in exploring associations whereby some natural features of the environment or contamination of the environment by human action represent a carcinogenic threat to human populations.

Finally, from a service delivery perspective, examination of rates by some unit of place has implications for planning for resource utilization. For example, an examination of SEER urban areas reveals differentials among nonwhite groups for overall cancer mortality (Table 11–8). Although this pattern may be linked to life-style differences among blacks in urban areas, such data may also suggest differential utilization of health care, implying that the areas with the highest cancer mortality may have the greatest need to increase their efforts in the delivery of health care services for cancer prevention, detection, and treatment to those population groups.

Time

Variations in cancer incidence rates over time indicate changes in the prevalence of known or suspected etiologic factors that give rise to the observed rates or progress in controlling or treating the disease. Between 1973 and 1981, the total age-adjusted cancer incidence rate increased from 317.5 to 342.6 per 100,000 population. Differential mortality rates between the sexes over time for the various types have also been apparent (Table 11–9). The largest increase is found to occur in lung cancer, with women experiencing a 35.7 per cent rise in mortality. Among men, the increase was 19.6 per cent. This phenomenon offsets gains in survival

Table 11–9. AGE-ADJUSTED DEATH RATES (PER 100,000 POPULATION) FOR MALIGNANT NEOPLASMS, BY RACE AND COLOR, UNITED STATES, SELECTED YEARS FROM 1950 TO 1980

Year	Total Both Sexes	Men	Women	White Both Sexes	Men	Women	Nonwhite Both Sexes	Men	Women
1980	132.8	165.5	109.2	129.6	160.5	107.7	158.2	209.0	120.2
1970	129.9	157.4	108.8	127.8	154.3	107.6	148.3	185.3	117.6
1960	125.8	143.0	111.2	124.2	141.6	109.5	139.3	154.8	125.0
1950	125.4	130.8	120.8	124.7	130.9	119.4	128.6	125.8	131.0

(From Bureau of Health Professions. [1985]. *Health status of minorities and low income groups.* [DHHS Publication No. (HRSA) HRS-P-DV-P5-1]. Washington, DC: U. S. Government Printing Office.)

achieved for cancer of other sites, such as the decrease of 18.5 per cent in mortality from cancer of the uterine cervix and of 14.5 per cent in mortality from endometrial cancer in women, and the declines of approximately 20 per cent—or more—in stomach cancer and lip cancer for both sexes. White and nonwhite differentials in mortality from cancer over time are also noted (see Table 11–9). The steep increase in mortality among nonwhites is attributable to the higher cancer incidence rates and lower survival among blacks, particularly among black males.

In summary, mortality rates, prevalence rates, and incidence rates, when available, can be used to rank order the specific cancer types occurring in a community, and they therefore serve as a guide for targeting cancer control interventions and evaluating the effects of these over time.

ANALYTIC EPIDEMIOLOGIC METHODS

Etiologic hypotheses are generated with descriptive epidemiologic methods. These hypotheses are then tested with analytic epidemiologic methods. In addition, analytic studies are utilized for refining knowledge of risk factors. Most cancer epidemiologic studies use an observational design as the analytic approach. The primary purpose of observational studies is to identify which exposures are associated with the cancer type under investigation. Design types that are classified as observational include cross-sectional studies (surveys), prospective studies (concurrent or historical), and retrospective studies (case-controlled). The major distinguishing feature among these design types is the time element—that is, when the exposure occurred relative to the disease outcome at the time the study is being conducted. Intervention studies may also be utilized to test etiologic hypotheses. Generally, the purpose of experimental epidemiologic studies is to determine if intervention, aimed at eliminating or modifying a risk factor, prevents disease.

Cross-Sectional Study

In a *cross-sectional study*, the relationship between diseases and the variables of interest are examined as they exist in the group at one specific time. Data pertaining to the presence or absence of disease and the presence or absence of exposure factors are obtained from each member of the study population or from a representative sample. Measures of effect in a cross-sectional study are prevalence rates and odds ratios (computed in the same manner as for a prospective study). The surveys conducted by the NCHS are examples of cross-sectional designs.

Prospective Study

A *prospective study* (concurrent study) consists of observing over time a group of volunteers (cohort)

Table 11–10. INCIDENCE OF LUNG CANCER FIRST DIAGNOSED IN 1968–1972 BY VITAMIN A INDEX, MEN AGED 45–54 YEARS

Lung Cancer	Vitamin A Index	
	≥5	<5
Yes	4	4
No	1805	686
Total	1809	690

(Data from Bjelke, 1975.)

who are initially free of the disease under investigation. This group is heterogeneous with respect to the exposure factor or factors that are of interest. The incidence of the disease subsequently identified in the cohort can be directly related to various exposure levels. Cohorts may also be assembled to represent a group that existed at some point in the past whose membership may be reconstructed. This design is acceptable exposure if the factors and disease outcomes of interest were adequately documented or are accessible through other sources during the time period of interest. This type of prospective study is termed *historical prospective* and is possible in large, "stable" populations such as clients in a Health Maintenance Organization (HMO), employees of an industry, or students from a certain school. Although a prospective study can determine if the risk factor under investigation precedes the disease, it requires a long period of time to conduct and a large number of participants to obtain a sufficient number of people with the outcome variables of interest for analysis.

A number of important prospective studies in cancer epidemiology have been conducted. Examples of cohorts used and the relationships are: (1) concurrent: American Cancer Society Cancer Prevention Studies: volunteers (family history, surgical procedures, smoking, alcohol consumption, diet, drug usage, and occupations and occupational exposures) (Garfinkel, 1985); (2) historical prospective: steelworkers' cohort (coke oven emissions and lung cancer) (Rockett & Redmond, 1985); medical specialists (occupational radiation exposure and leukemia) (Seltser & Sartwell, 1965).

In a prospective study, the degree of the relationship between exposure to a factor and a disease is measured by either the relative risk (RR) or the odds ratio (OR). Mathematically, the RR is defined as follows:

$$RR = \frac{\text{Incidence rate in exposed}}{\text{Incidence rate in nonexposed}}$$

Substituting in data from Table 11–10, the RR of lung cancer associated with a high vitamin A index (≥5) for the 45- to 54-year-old age group is

$$RR = 4/1809 \div 4/690 = 0.38$$

With a baseline value of 1, indicating no difference in the disease incidence rates of the exposed and nonexposed, the RR of 0.38 obtained may be interpreted to mean that those with a high vitamin A index are at lower risk of having disease. In this situation, the exposure of interest is said to be "protective."

The OR for a prospective study is defined as the

Box 11–1. SMOKING AND CARCINOMA IN SITU OF THE UTERINE CERVIX

A case-control study was conducted by Lyon and colleagues (1983) to investigate the relationship between cigarette smoking and carcinoma in situ of the uterine cervix. Cases were residents of the metropolitan area of Utah identified through the Utah Cancer Registry (a population-based registry) and were all histologically diagnosed between 1975 and 1977 as having squamous cell carcinoma in situ of the cervix. Controls were selected from the same geographic area using random digit dialing and were frequency matched to obtain an approximately equal number of cases and controls in each county and age category. Through personal interviews of the cases and controls, information was obtained concerning pregnancy, sexual behavior, types of birth control, use of alcohol and tobacco, previous illness, and demographics. The relationship between exposure to selected risk factors and in situ carcinoma of the uterine cervix was evaluated using crude and adjusted odds ratios. Even after adjusting for the confounding effects of age, lifetime number of sex partners, and other well-established risk factors, cases were 3.5 times more likely to have been smokers than controls.

Table 11–11. COMPUTATION OF AN ODDS RATIO IN A RETROSPECTIVE STUDY

Exposure Status	Disease Status	
	Disease	No Disease
Exposed	a	b
Not Exposed	c	d

$$\text{Odds Ratio (OR)} = \frac{a}{c} \div \frac{b}{d} = \frac{ad}{bc}$$

ratio of the odds of the disease among the exposed to the odds of disease among those without the exposure. Using the data from Table 11–10, the computation of the OR is mathematically represented as $4/1805 \div 4/686 = 0.38$. Thus it can be seen that the OR is a close approximation of the RR and yields a similar conclusion, that is, that lung cancer is less likely to occur among those with a high vitamin A index.

The major disadvantages of a prospective study are the cost and effort associated with a study that is long term and large scale. Loss of participants in follow-up and death occurring from causes other than the disease being investigated are other limitations. Thus this study

design is not employed unless an association that is consistently detected in cross-sectional or case-control studies needs to be confirmed.

Retrospective Study

A retrospective (or case-control) study compares the prevalence of a risk (exposure) factor among persons with the disease under investigation to that observed in a control group without the disease. An important design consideration is that both cases and controls must be representative of some defined population base. This may be achieved by either selecting all known incident cases of a disease within a certain time period or electing a sample of them. Controls may be selected either through a random sample from the same population group from which the cases arose or through some matching strategy (e.g., pairwise, frequency, or group matching).

The retrospective approach is commonly used in cancer epidemiology because it can be implemented quickly to test etiologic hypotheses, even with a small

Table 11–12. COMPUTATION OF THE ODDS RATIO (OR) IN A RETROSPECTIVE STUDY OF SMOKING AND CARCINOMA IN SITU OF THE UTERINE CERVIX

Age Group	Smoking Status	Cases	Controls	Crude OR[a]	Adjusted OR* (90 per cent CI)[b]
20–29	Yes	41	6	28.0	17 (6.5, 44)
	No	13	53		
30–39	Yes	66	25	5.9	3.1 (1.8, 5.5)
	No	37	83		
40+	Yes	23	14	2.8	1.6 (0.7, 3.7)
	No	37	62		
Total	Yes	130	45 ⎫	6.6	3.5 (2.3, 5.2)
	No	87	198 ⎭		

$$\text{OR (20–29)} = \frac{41 \times 53}{13 \times 6} = 28.0$$

$$\text{OR (30–39)} = \frac{66 \times 83}{37 \times 25} = 5.9$$

$$\text{OR (40 +)} = \frac{23 \times 62}{37 \times 14} = 2.8$$

[a]OR = Odds ratio
[b]CI = Confidence interval
*Adjusted for lifetime number of sex partners and religion.
(From Lyon, J. L., Gardner, M. D., West, D. W., Stanish, W. M., & Herbertson, R. M. [1983]. Smoking and carcinoma *in situ* of the uterine cervix. *American Journal of Public Health, 73*, 558–562. Reproduced by permission.)

number of cases. Some examples of retrospective studies investigating the role between cancer and previous exposure to carcinogenic substances are exemplified in the work of Herbst, Ulfelder, & Poskanzer, (1963) (diethylstilbestrol and vaginal adenocarcinoma); Lowengart and colleagues (1987) (fathers with occupational exposure to chlorinated solvents after birth of child and risk of leukemia in their children); and Doll and Hill (1952) (cigarette smoking and lung cancer). Box 11–1 contains an abstract illustrating the features of a retrospective study.

The primary measure of the degree of the relationship between exposure and disease in a retrospective study is the OR because incidence rates cannot be derived from a retrospective study. As demonstrated earlier, the OR is an approximation of the relative risk, and hence it is sometimes referred to as the estimated relative risk in retrospective studies. The OR derived from a retrospective study represents the likelihood of exposure among the cases relative to the likelihood of exposure among the controls. An OR = 1 is the reference level, with values of the OR > 1 indicating that cases were more likely to have the exposure (risk factor) than the controls. An OR < 1 indicates that the factor under investigation exerts a protective effect among the case groups. The OR is a descriptive measure of the strength of the association between a risk factor and a disease, which may be statistically evaluated to determine if the OR derived represents a significant effect. It is a measure that can be used to compare the risk factor–disease relationships regardless of whether the study was cross-sectional, prospective, or retrospective. Table 11–11 illustrates how the crude OR is derived from a retrospective study for two variables (a 2 × 2 table). The OR may be "adjusted"—that is, weighted—to control for the effect of confounding variables. A confounding variable is one that is associated with both the exposure and the disease. When it is present, it is unequally distributed among the exposed and the unexposed such that it distorts the apparent magnitude of risk. In Table 11–12 crude and adjusted ORs are displayed to represent the likelihood of in situ cancer of the uterine cervix developing from cigarette smoking among three age groups. Adjustment for confounding decreased the values of the ORs. In addition, the confidence interval (CI) can be computed for an OR to evaluate the reliability of this measure. This interval relates the range in which the true OR is thought to be within a specified level of confidence (usually 95%). The wider the range, the more imprecise the OR is. A CI whose limits contain 1 indicates that the OR is not statistically significantly different from the reference level (e.g., OR = 1.6; 95% CI of 0.7 and 3.7). When the lower limit of the CI is higher than 1, the OR is elevated statistically significantly (e.g., OR = 17; 95% CI of 6.5 and 44). When the upper limit of the CI is lower than 1, the OR is significantly less than the reference level.

Although retrospective studies have more advantages, several sources of bias may be encountered that may lead to either an artificial increase or a decrease in the OR obtained. Because information on previous exposure is typically obtained by self-report, recall bias is a major limitation of this design. Bias may also arise in the selection of cases or controls. For example, a hospital control series might yield an overestimate of exposure if the exposure under investigation is associated with hospitalization. This was identified as a limitation of early retrospective studies of smoking and lung cancer, with the result that the effect of cigarette smoking was initially underestimated because cigarette smoking is associated with many diseases whose courses are likely to lead to hospitalization, such as chronic obstructive pulmonary disease. To eliminate this problem, the selection of hospital controls from patients with a wide variety of diagnoses or from the population at large should be considered.

Randomized Clinical Trial

A randomized clinical trial is an experiment involving human volunteers that determines which intervention is superior among various alternatives. The features of this design type are randomization, control, and manipulation. This design is also prospective in nature as the entire study group is followed over time and monitored for the occurrence of the outcomes of interest. In cancer epidemiology, the intervention usually consists of the modification of host characteristics (e.g., chemoprevention), life-style changes (e.g., diet modification), or screening (e.g., mammography) to prevent the disease. The treatment efficacy can be evaluated through a variety of approaches, including conventional statistical methods, measures of effect used in prospective studies, and life-table analysis. If the hypothesized effect is demonstrated, additional evidence is garnered for the causal relationship between a risk factor and the disease under investigation. Sources of bias in this study design include that generated when withdrawal from participation or loss to follow-up occurs. Bias emerging from the documentation of the study outcomes may be minimized by "blinding" the participant and the observer as to the participant's study group assignment. Box 11–2 contains an abstract describing a clinical trial to evaluate the efficacy of screening by mammography in the reduction of breast cancer mortality. Illustrated in Table 11–13 are completed clinical trials which were conducted to evaluate the efficacy of chemoprevention for human cancers. Often the objective of chemoprevention trials is to achieve regression of the precursor lesions associated with the occurrence of a cancer type in the risk group. However, chemoprevention is also being evaluated to prevent tumor recurrence.

In a clinical trial, *survival analysis* is often employed to help judge the efficacy of an intervention. Survival analysis is a technique for estimating and comparing the probability that a particular outcome will occur (e.g., development of a cancer, or death) in various treatment groups, and hence, for evaluating their efficacy. Survival analyses may also be used to identify which disease and host characteristics influence the

---

Box 11–2. REDUCTION IN MORTALITY FROM BREAST CANCER AFTER MASS SCREENING WITH MAMMOGRAPHY

A randomized controlled clinical trial was conducted in two counties in Sweden to investigate the efficacy of mass screening by mammography in reducing breast cancer mortality (Tabar et al., 1985). Within the counties, 19 blocks were selected that represented socioeconomic homogeneity. The populations of the blocks were divided into units of roughly equal size and randomly assigned either to receive screening every 2 or 3 years depending on their age or to a control group in which screening was not offered. Women over the age of 40 in each block entered the study at the same time, having been sent individual letters inviting them to participate before the start of each screening round. A total of 162,981 women entered the study and were followed for an average of 6 years. At the end of the study, the relative risk (RR) of dying from breast cancer was significantly reduced in the group screened with mammography (RR = 0.69, 95% CI: 0.51, 0.92). The relative risk of developing a stage II or more advanced breast cancer in the screened group was also significantly reduced (RR = 0.75, 95% CI: 0.65, 0.87). This study demonstrates that early detection utilizing mammography is effective in reducing mortality from breast cancer.

---

probability that the outcome being monitored will occur. These characteristics are called *prognostic factors*. Johnston-Early and co-workers (1980) utilized this technique to examine the relationship of smoking cessation on survival in a group of persons with small cell lung cancer, all treated with the same protocol. These investigators found that those who quit smoking either before or at the time of diagnosis had a significantly greater median survival time than those who continued to smoke (Fig. 11–5). The implication of this survival analysis is that cigarette smoking is a prognostic factor—that is, it is associated with a lower probability of survival among those with lung cancer. Thus, even at the time of diagnosis of a cancer it is not too late to advise the patient to stop smoking. Knowledge of expected probability of survival can serve as a guide for health professionals in making realistic short-term and long-term plans for cancer patients. Clues concerning disease causation may also be generated from knowledge of prognostic factors. For example, the marked differences in survival between premenopausal and postmenopausal women treated with chemotherapy observed in several countries led to epidemiologic studies, which subsequently identified different risk factor relationships for the two types of breast cancer (Helmrich et al., 1983; Lubin et al., 1985). The SEER program publishes results of survival analyses for various cancer types by cancer stage, treatment modality, race, and sex (see Table 11–6). Nurses should refer to the results of such data to aid in the formulation of realistic long- and short-term goals for cancer patients.

CAUSALITY

Generally, hypotheses concerning a risk factor are generated from clinical or field observations or descriptive statistics, or both. An association between a risk factor and a disease is not declared by the scientific community without rigorous and extensive evaluation of the relationship. For this pupose, cross-sectional, case-controlled and prospective studies, laboratory investigations, and clinical trials are conducted. The results from these studies are then examined to determine if evidence for causality exists. The criteria used to evidence causality are (1) strength of association—the larger the value of a measure of the effect (relative risk, odds ratio, attributable risk, correlation or regression coefficient), the higher the likelihood of a causal relationship; (2) dose-response relationship—increasing levels of an exposure factor result in a correspond-

Table 11–13. COMPLETED RANDOMIZED CLINICAL TRIALS OF CHEMOPREVENTION

Target Site or Organ; Target or Risk Group	Inhibitory Agent	Response*	Reference
Bladder			
Recurrence of bladder tumors	Etretinate	No difference (73 patients)	Pederson et al., 1984.
Recurrence of bladder tumors	Etretinate	11/15 vs. 4/15 CR† + PR ($P < 0.01$)	Alfthan et al., 1983.
Breast			
Mammary dysplasia	Alpha-tocopherol	No difference (128 patients)	London et al., 1985.
Colon			
Familial polyposis	Ascorbic acid	Reduction of polyp area in treated group (49 patients) ($P < 0.03$)	Bussey et al., 1982.
Lung			
Bronchial metaplasia	Etretinate	Metaplasia reduced in treated group (40 patients) ($P < 0.05$)	Misset et al., 1986.
Oral cavity			
Leukoplakia	Isotretinoin (p.o.)	10/14 vs. 1/2 CR + PR ($P = 0.0049$)	Hong et al., 1985.
Skin			
Actinic keratosis	Transretinoic acid (topical)	24/60 CR	Bollag & Ott, 1975.

*In those cases in which response or number of cases was not clear from the report, a qualitative statement is provided. The numbers refer to the number of patients except where noted.

†CR, complete remission; PR, partial remission.

(Data in part from Bertram, J. S., Kolonel, L. N., & Meyskens, F. L. J. [1987]. Rational strategies for the prevention of cancer. *Cancer Research, 47*, 3012–3031.)

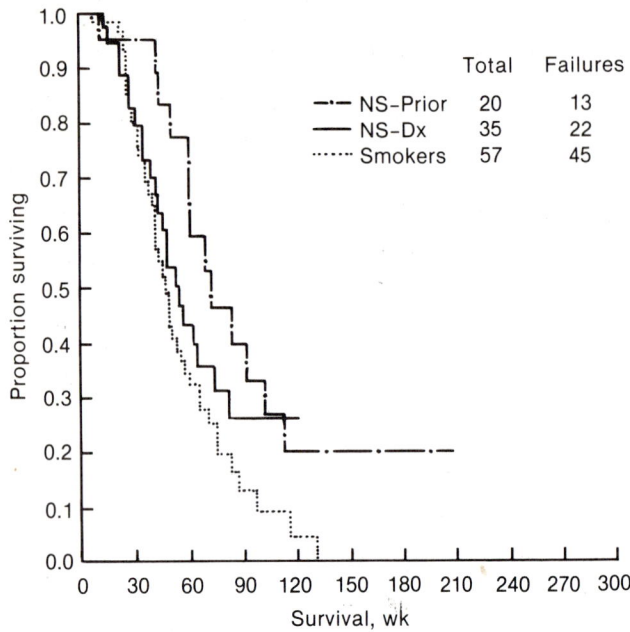

Figure 11–5. Survival analysis of 112 individuals meeting the National Cancer Institute–Veterans Administration Medical Oncology Branch small-cell lung cancer treatment protocol. *NS-Prior*, Nonsmokers prior to diagnosis; *NS-Dx*, stopped smoking prior to diagnosis. (From Johnston-Early, A. et al. [1980]. Smoking abstinence and small cell lung cancer survival. *Journal of the American Medical Association, 244*, 2175–2179. Copyright 1980, American Medical Association.)

ing rise in disease occurrence (Fig. 11–6); (3) detection of the association in other populations and using different study methods and designs; (4) temporality—the factor must precede the disease, allowing for any period of induction and latency; (5) specificity—the degree to which a specific causal factor is related to or produces a single disease; and (6) coherence—biologic support exists for the relationship between a risk factor and disease (e.g., pathology studies, laboratory experiments), including how disease progression differs in those with continued exposure versus those whose exposure is discontinued. In addition, the relationship between a risk factor and a disease must be found to be statistically significant, but only after ruling out the effects of bias and confounding variables. The relationship between cigarette smoking and lung cancer is said to be causal, having met all the foregoing criteria (U.S. Department of Health and Human Services, 1982). However, the relationship between dietary factors and human cancer is still being investigated. To provide accurate information on cancer prevention to patients and families or to the lay community, the oncology nurse should be able to interpret the scientific literature in terms of the evidence it contains to support a causal relationship between the disease of concern and the risk factors thought to be associated with it.

SUMMARY

Cancer epidemiology goes beyond identification of risk factors and studies of causes. For nurses, it provides (1) a framework for assessing the needs of a community, (2) data to guide in the formulation of short-term and long-term goals for cancer patients, and (3) a means for the evaluation of interventions aimed at the control of cancer.

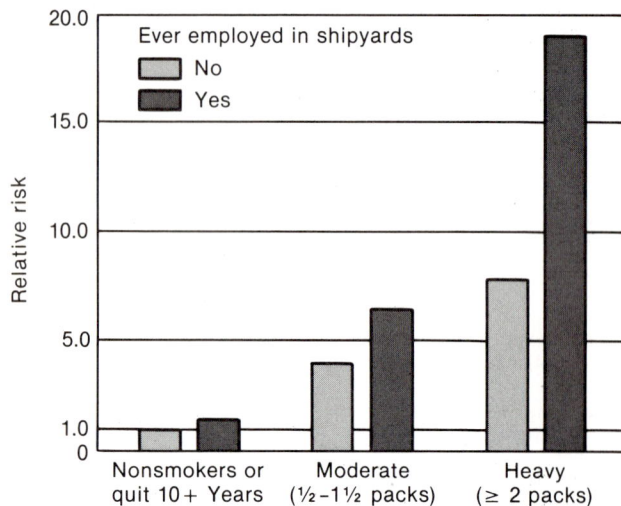

Figure 11–6. Case-control study of lung cancer among shipyard workers, by smoking status. (From Blot, W. J., Harrington, M., Toledo, A., Hoover, R., Heath, C. W., & Fraumeni, J. F., Jr. [1978]. Lung cancer after employment in shipyards during World War II. *New England Journal of Medicine, 299*, 620–624. Reproduced by permission of the *New England Journal of Medicine*.)

References

Alfthan, O., Tarkkanen, J., Grohn, P., Heinonen, E., Pyrhonen, S., and Saila, K. (1983). Tigason (etretinate) in prevention of recurrence of superficial bladder tumors: a double-blind study. *European Urology, 9*, 6–9.

Bertram, J. S., Kolonel, L. N., & Meyskens, F. L. J. (1987). Rational strategies for the chemoprevention of cancer. *Cancer Research, 47*, 3012–3031.

Blot, W. J., Harrington, M., Toledo, A., Hoover, R., Heath, C. W., & Fraumeni, J. F., Jr. (1978). Lung cancer after employment in shipyards during World War II. *New England Journal of Medicine, 299*, 620–624.

Bjelke, E. (1975). Dietary Vitamin A and human lung cancer. *International Journal of Cancer, 15*, 561–565.

Bollag, W., & Ott, F. (1975). Vitamin A acid in benign and malignant epithelial tumors of the skin. *Acta Dermatovenereologica, 74*(Suppl.):163–166.

Breslow, L., & Cumberland, W. G. (1988). Progress and objectives in cancer control. *Journal of the American Medical Association, 259,* 1690–1694.

Bureau of Health Professions. (1985). *Health status of minorities and low income groups.* (DHHS Publication No. [HRSA] HRS-P-DV-85-1) Washington, DC, U.S. Government Printing Office.

Bussey, H. J. R., DeCosse, J. J., Deschner, E. E., Eyers, A. A., Lesser, M. L., Morson, B. C., Ritchie, S. M., Thomson, J. P. S., & Wadsworth, J. A. (1982). A randomized trial of ascorbic acid in polyposis coli. *Cancer, 50,* 1434–1439.

Centers for Disease Control. (1985). Behavioral risk factor surveillance in selected states. *Journal of the American Medical Association, 256,* 697–698.

Doll, R., & Hill, A. B. (1952). A study of the aetiology of carcinoma of the lung. *British Medical Journal, 1,* 1451–1455.

Doll, R., & Peto, R. (1977). Mortality among doctors in different occupations. *British Medical Journal, 1,* 1433–1436.

Doll, R., & Peto R. (1981). The causes of cancer: Quantitative estimates of available risk of cancer in the United States today. *Journal of the National Cancer Institute, 66,* 1191–1308.

Garfinkel, L. (1985). Selection, follow-up, and analysis in the American Cancer Society prospective studies. *National Cancer Institute Monograph, 67,* 49–52.

Greenwald, P., & Sondik, E. J. (1986). Cancer control objectives for the nation. NCI Monograph No. 2, NIH Publication No. 86-2880.

Helmrich, S. P., Shapiro, S., Rosenberg, L., Kaufman, D. W., Slone, D., Bain, C., Miettinen, O. S., Stolley, P. D., Rosenshein, N. B., Knapp, R. C., Leavitt, T., Schottenfeld, D., Engle, R. L., & Levy, M. (1983). Risk factors for breast cancer. *American Journal of Epidemiology, 117,* 35–45.

Herbst, A. L., Ulfelder, H., & Poskanzer, D. C. (1963). Adenocarcinoma of the vagina: Association of maternal stilbestrol therapy with tumor appearance in young women. *New England Journal of Medicine, 284,* 878–881.

Hong, W. J., Itri, L., Endicott, J., Bell, R., Vaughan, C., Doos, W., Gunter, P., & Strong, S. (1985). The effectiveness of 13-cis retinoic acid in the treatment of premalignant lesions in oral cavity. *Proceedings of the American Society of Clinical Oncologists, 4,* 906.

Horm, J. W., Asire, A. J., Young, J. L., Jr., & Pollack, E. S., eds. (1984). *SEER Program: Cancer incidence and mortality in the United States, 1973–81* (NIH Publication No. 85-1837). Bethesda, MD, National Cancer Institute.

Johnston-Early, A., Cohen, M. H., Minna, J. D., Paxton, L. M., Fossieck, B. E., Ihde, D. C., Bunn, P. A., Matthews, M. J., & Makuch, R. (1980). Smoking abstinence and small cell lung cancer survival. *Journal of the American Medical Association, 244,* 2175–2179.

London, R. S., Sundaram, G. S., Murphy, L., Manimekalai, S., Reynolds, M., & Goldstein, J. (1985). The effect of vitamin E on mammary dysplasia: A double-blind study. *Obstetrics and Gynecology, 65,* 104–106.

Lowengart, R. A., Peters, J. M., Cicioni, C., Buckely, J., Bernstein, L., Preston-Martin, S., & Rappaport, E. (1987). Childhood leukemia and parents' occupational and home exposures. *Journal of the National Cancer Institute, 79,* 39–46.

Lyon, J. L., Gardner, M. D., West, D. W., Stanish, W. M., & Herbertson, R. M. (1983). Smoking and carcinoma *in situ* of the uterine cervix. *American Journal of Public Health, 73,* 558–562.

Lubin, F., Ruder, A. M., Wax, Y., & Modan, B. (1985). Overweight and changes in weight throughout adult life in breast cancer etiology. *American Journal of Epidemiology, 122,* 579–588.

Misset, J. L., Mathie, G., Santelli, G., Gouveia, J., Homasson, J. P., Sudve, N. C., & Gaget, H. (1986). Regression of bronchial epidermoid metaplasia in heavy smokers with etretinate treatment. *Cancer Detection and Prevention, 9,* 167–170.

National Center for Health Statistics. (1986). 1985 summary: National Hospital Discharge Survey. *Advance data from vital and health statistics* (No. 127) (DHHS Publication No. [PHS] 86-1250). Hyattsville, MD, U.S. Public Health Service.

National Center for Health Statistics. (1987). Advance report of final mortality statistics, 1985. *Monthly Vital Statistics Report, 36*(5) Supplement. (DHHS Publication No. [PHS] 87-1120). Hyattsville, MD, U.S. Public Health Service.

National Center for Health Statistics. (1988). 1987 Summary: National Hospital Discharge Survey. *Advance data from vital and health statistics* (No. 159 [Rev]). (DHHS Publication No. [PHS] 88-1250). Hyattsville, MD, U.S. Public Health Service.

Office of Planning, Illinois Department of Public Health. (1985). *Mortality from breast cancer among Illinois women, 1969–71 and 1979–81: A vital statistics special report.* Springfield, IL: Author.

Patterson, B. H., & Bilgrad, R. (1986). Use of the National Death Index in cancer studies. *Journal of the National Cancer Institute, 77,* 877–881.

Pederson, H., Wolf, H., Jensen, S. K., Lund, F., Hansen, E., Olsen, P. R., & Sorenson, B. L. (1984). Administration of a retinoid as prophylaxis of recurrent non-invasive bladder tumors. *Scandinavian Journal of Urology and Nephrology, 18,* 121–123.

Pickle, L. W., Mason, T. J., Howard, N., Hoover, R., & Fraumeni, J. F., Jr. (1987). *Atlas of U.S. cancer mortality.* (DHHS Publication No. [NIH] 87-2900). Washington, DC, U.S. Government Printing Office.

Pollack, E. S. (1984). Tracking cancer trends: Incidence and survival. *Hospital Practice, 19,* 99–116.

Rockette, H. E., & Redmond, C. K. (1985). Selection, follow-up and analysis in the Coke Oven Study. *National Cancer Institute Monograph, 67,* 89–94.

Seltser, R., & Sartwell, P. E. (1965). The influence of occupational exposure to radiation on the mortality of American radiologists and other medical specialists. *American Journal of Epidemiology, 81,* 2–22.

Tabar, L., Gad, A., Holmberg, L. H., Ljungquist, U., Fagerberg, C. J. G., Baldetorp, O., Lundstrom, B., & Manson, J. C. (1985). Reduction in mortality from breast cancer after mass screening with mammography. *Lancet, 1,* 829–832.

Thornberry, O. T., Wilson, R. W., & Golden, P. M. (1986). Health promotion data for the 1990 objectives: Estimates from the National Health Interview Survey of Health Promotion and Disease Prevention, U.S., 1985. *Advance data from vital and health statistics* (No. 126) (DHHS Publication No. [PMS] 86-1250). Hyattsville, MD, U.S. Public Health Service.

U.S. Department of Health and Human Services, Public Health Service. (1982). *The health consequences of smoking–cancer.* (NIH Publication No. DHHS [PHS] 82-50179). Washington, DC, U.S. Government Printing Office.

U.S. Department of Health and Human Services. Public Health Service. (1989). *International Classification of Diseases, 9th Rev., Clinical Modification.* DHHS Pub. No. (PMS) 89-1260, Washington, DC, U.S. Government Printing Office.

Wynder, E. L. (1975). The epidemiology of large bowel cancer. *Cancer Research, 35,* 3388–3394.

CHAPTER 12

The Causes of Cancer

CURTIS METTLIN
AMY L. MIRAND

Cancer in some form occurs in virtually every higher organism. It has been recorded as a human malady since early history, and archaeologic evidence suggests it afflicted humans throughout prehistory. In modern times cancer is observed in every geographic region and culture and occurs in varying form and intensity in every subgroup of age, sex, and race. Although some persons would view cancer as an antagonist or aberration of nature, its nearly universal occurrence as a biologic phenomenon suggests that cancer is among the most common processes of nature. As such, scientists believe that we can understand cancer using the same kinds of tools we use to understand other natural phenomena—that by observation and reason, we can identify the cause of cancer and, as a result, possibly learn to prevent or modify its occurrence or natural course.

This ultimate goal, however, has proved elusive. Understanding fully the processes by which the cell is stimulated to seemingly unregulated growth, loses its inhibition to grow in the presence of other cells and tissues, and ceases its harmonious contribution to the functioning of the organism remains only partly understood. The term for this fundamental process is *carcinogenesis*. *Etiology* refers to study of the causes that initiate the process of carcinogenesis. Carcinogenesis and etiologic research practically are sciences in their own right with a unique body of theory and specialized terminology. A glossary of some of that terminology is presented in Table 12–1.

Understanding the natural history of cancer has important implications for health care professionals. It can help their role as a public health agent in educating the public on risk reduction and disease prevention. Better knowledge of the principles of cause and prevention also may permit the specialist in cancer to better contribute to public policy in matters relating to cancer risk, such as environmental protection, workplace safety, and safe use of medicines and medical procedures. Finally, understanding more clearly the processes of cancer cause and prevention may better enable the health care provider to advise patients and their families on how they can understand and reduce their risk of cancer.

HISTORICAL PERSPECTIVE

The study of carcinogenesis has many historical landmarks. These have been reviewed by Shimkin (1977). Holleb and Randers-Pehrson (1987) have collated the original reports of researchers and observers in a text termed *Classics in Oncology*. Both of these works should be required reading for students of the history of cancer research. It suffices for our purposes simply to note a few of the events that these authors and others have seen in retrospect as important in the history of cancer research.

The first phase of this history has numerous examples of astute clinical observations linking some form of cancer with a suspected causative factor. Ramazzini of Padua, Italy, reported in 1713 that breast cancer occurred more frequently among nuns, and we now recognize nulliparity as a risk factor for this disease. In 1775, the English surgeon Percivall Pott described

Table 12–1. GLOSSARY OF TERMS USED IN CARCINOGENESIS RESEARCH

Antioncogene: Gene having the ability to regulate growth and inhibit carcinogenesis

Analytical Epidemiology: Hypothesis-testing investigative method used to study the association between the dependent variable, disease, and possible causative variables in a defined human population

Carcinogenesis: Process resulting in abnormal cell expression characteristic of malignant transformation, including loss of both contact inhibition and mitotic inhibition

Descriptive Epidemiology: Hypothesis-generating research method used to characterize a study population with respect to demographics, general exposures, behaviors, and health status

Etiology: Study of all factors preceding development of disease

Genome: The diploid set of chromosomes that contributes a complete group of hereditary factors

Genotoxin: Chemical, physical, or biologic factor capable of damaging the genome

Initiation: The early-stage process of cellular transformation induced by an agent that causes irreversible molecular alteration of the genetic component of the cell

Latency: Quiescent interval between initiation and the cellular proliferation characteristic of cancer

Mutagen: Chemical, physical, or biologic factor that induces genetic mutations

Oncogene: Gene that is capable of causing malignant transformation of cells

Promotion: Later stage process of carcinogenesis involving the enhancement of the expression of previously initiated genetic alteration

Synergy: Enhancement of the effects of multiple carcinogens or promoters resulting from their combined occurrence

Vectors: Factors or situations that lead to exposure to potential disease causes

the common occurrence of scrotal cancer among chimneysweeps as resulting from their chronic exposure to soot. Harting and Hesse investigated the high frequency of respiratory diseases among miners in the Black Forest regions. Their careful investigation and classification of causes of death clearly linked the occurrence of lung cancer with the mining environment. Ludwig Rehn observed an epidemic of bladder cancer among workers in the aniline dye industry, and his 1895 observations are considered an important event in the development of modern industrial hygiene.

Although the importance of clinical observation in identifying potential sources of risk continues in present-day medicine, other important lines of inquiry have developed in parallel. The movement of cancer research into the laboratory was accelerated by the development of methodologies that enabled the transplantation of tumors from one animal or species to another and by Yamagiwa and Ichikawa's observation (1918) that cancer could be induced in the ear of the rabbit by repeated application of coal tar. The ability to observe important living malignant processes in a setting other than the whole animal was made possible by the development of systems for observing malignant transformation of cells in culture and for studying mutagenesis in the bacteria assay developed by Ames and colleagues (1973).

The systematic inquiries of epidemiologists and statisticians have also been important. Early classics in this field include Rigoni-Stern's analyses of late eighteenth-century deaths in Verona showing breast cancer to be five times more common in nuns than among other women. Modern classics include Wynder and Graham's case-controlled study (1950) strongly linking lung cancer to cigarette smoking and the several studies conducted by Selikoff and associates linking mesothelioma and lung cancer to occupational asbestos exposure (Selikoff, Hammond, & Churg, 1964, 1968; Selikoff, Churg & Hammond, 1965; Selikoff, Hammond, & Seidman, 1973).

In addition to the efforts of individual investigators, some credit for progress in this field must be given to the public health officials who have developed the modern systems of cancer reporting and registration, which permit monitoring of disease trends by characteristics of time, person, and place. The first large-scale cancer registry in the United States was established in Connecticut in 1935, and national surveys of the occurrence of cancer were undertaken by the National Cancer Institute in 1937 and 1947.

MODERN CARCINOGENESIS RESEARCH

Although in the early history of carcinogenesis research investigative tools were few and relatively simple, in the modern era a large number of disciplines and investigative approaches are involved. Most research on cancer cause and prevention, however, can be classified according to whether it is conducted on cells or molecule constituents, whole animals, or human populations (the level of observation). The first two types of research are typically experimental, whereas the last is usually observational. Each has advantages and disadvantages, and each has made unique contributions to our current understanding of carcinogenesis.

Levels of Observation

Cellular-Molecular

The most fundamental level of understanding carcinogenesis is at the cellular or, even more accurately, the molecular level. Although the typical clinical presentation of cancer is as a mass or as disseminated disease, we know that it is possible for such extensive growths to originate from a single malignant cell. For example, it is possible to induce leukemia in a mouse experimentally by the injection of a single leukemic cell (Furth & Kahn, 1937). In naturally occurring cancers, the cancer cell is not acquired exogenously but arises intrinsically from the transformation of a normal cell to a cancer cell. Something affects the normal cell to cause it eventually to express two traits which are basic to cancer: unregulated growth and loss of function.

In the normal cell, both the pattern of growth and the nature of cell function are genetically regulated, and a significant aspect of carcinogenesis is the alteration of specific genes regulating growth and function. The genes themselves are the unique sequences occurring within the DNA making up the genome. Modern techniques of molecular biology have made it possible to describe, locate, and reproduce the specific biochemical sequences that constitute individual genes. By these means, at least 30 genes have been identified, which, when activated, result in the malignant transformation of a cell (Vahde Woude & Gilden, 1985). These transformed genes are known collectively as *oncogenes*. Genes that have yet not been transformed to their oncogenic state are called *proto-oncogenes*. The change in the gene that leads to malignant transformation may be the result of one of many different processes, including environmental insult by chemicals, viruses, or radiation. It also is possible to inherit an oncogene that is incomplete or altered.

Just as some genes are capable of initiating cancer, others appear to have the ability to regulate growth and inhibit carcinogenesis by their mere presence. These regulatory genes are called *antioncogenes*. It has been shown that some instances of retinoblastoma, a pediatric intraocular tumor, result from the absence or mutation of a specific antioncogene (Lee et al., 1987). It is possible that several other types of cancer are related to this particular antioncogene and that many other oncogenes and antioncogenes remain to be discovered.

The discovery of oncogenes represents a major advance in carcinogenesis research. This knowledge combined with many other pieces of information about the nature and function of the cell and its components provides an understanding of basic events of cancer. However, understanding an event does not necessarily lead to the ability to predict its occurrence or modify the ultimate course of events. Baltimore (1987) has described some of the limitations relating to the discovery of oncogenes on the cancer problem. The number of genes that may be involved in human cancer are several, and the number of ways by which they may be activated or inactivated is large. Preventive measures cannot yet be precisely targeted to specific genes or pathways of genetic transformation. The potential of using knowledge of oncogenes to diagnose cancer or to identify persons who harbor exceptional susceptibility to cancer by virtue of their genetic makeup may be the most immediate application of these technologies.

Animal Models

The fundamental processes of cancer may occur within the cell, but the actual pathologic condition always involves the entire living organism. The progressive development of cancer after the required alteration has occurred in the genome can be highly variable. The tumor cell may be recognized and destroyed by surrounding cells, the proliferation of the tumor cell may be accelerated or retarded, and the growing tumor may have a greater or lesser malignant character. In addition, the impact of potential sources of damage to the genome may be greatly influenced by the natural defenses of the organism. Host immunity to viruses and the ability to metabolize chemical carcinogens are both examples of the body's interfering with processes that theoretically would result in cancer. Because of these and many other similarly complex processes, it always has been important that carcinogenesis be studied in vivo.

For obvious ethical reasons, however, the opportunities to conduct carcinogenesis experiments on humans are very limited. Because of the grave health threat cancer can pose, it is not acceptable to induce and observe cancer in human subjects the same way one might study the common cold. To carry out experimental carcinogenesis in whole living organisms, researchers have developed a number of models of human cancer in lower mammals. The rat and mouse are often used, and most common human cancers can be induced in similar form in rodents. In addition to being able to produce analogous cancers in test animals, use of small species with a brief natural life span allows the researcher to study large populations economically in relatively short periods of time. Also, it is possible to control in the experimental animal factors that would be uncontrollable in human populations. For example, animals can be selected by their pedigrees to be particularly susceptible to induction of a given tumor type. An even more special example is the use of so-called nude mice, a mutant strain having no immunologic competence, to conduct types of experiments with which an immunologic response would otherwise interfere (Giovanella, Yim, Stehlin, & Williams, 1972).

In spite of the important things that can be learned about human cancer from animal models, some caution must be used in extrapolating findings from one species to another. There are few, if any, biologic universals. That which is true for one type of organism may not be true for another. For example, certain dyes that are carcinogenic to humans do not cause cancer in rodents. Alcohol and asbestos both cause cancer in humans but not in test animals. The dosage levels used in animal experimentation typically are far greater than those humans experience, and extrapolation from levels of risk observed in the laboratory to those actually encountered in the environment often is difficult. Finally, the controlled experimental situation does not duplicate the complex environment in which human populations exist. All of the interactions or antagonisms among multiple sources of risk that occur in real life are impossible to simulate in the laboratory.

Human Population Research

Although the risks of experimental carcinogenesis research are too great to justify exposure of human populations, it is possible to identify "natural experiments," which can tell us much about the processes of cancer causation in populations. These natural experiments occur when some segment of a population is exposed to risk while another is not. For example, the influence of an industrial hazard may be evaluated by studying the disease experience of persons who worked directly with the hazard compared with those who did not. Similarly, the effects of a habit of living, such as a dietary practice or cigarette smoking, may be studied by comparing groups that have the habit compared with those who do not. Another approach is to study populations whose exposures change. Changes in the disease experience of migrating populations as they move from one region and culture to another or changes in the risk of disease within a region as the environment or habits of the population change are both common research topics. The roles of nonexperimental epidemiologic research designs in cancer research were discussed in Chapter 11, and the strengths and weaknesses of these methods have been examined in detail elsewhere (Mettlin, 1988).

The characterization of epidemiology as a nonexperimental approach to cancer cause and prevention research is no longer as accurate as it once may have been. The discovery of possible mechanisms of cancer inhibitors in the diet or of synthetic origin has given rise to the concept of *chemoprevention* and the possibility that clinical trials of potential preventive agents may be conducted. Such trials truly are experimental in nature and are closely modeled on the principles of the clinical trial (see Chapter 25). They also are similar to the large-scale intervention trials that have been conducted in the field of cardiovascular disease prevention and control. Such trials are difficult because they can require that large populations be studied over a long period of time. Their high cost will likely ensure that prevention trials will be undertaken only selectively, after other research methods have suggested a high likelihood of effectiveness for the intervention to be studied.

The distinction between research at the cellular-molecular level and human population research also may be becoming less clear than it traditionally has been. A new level of inquiry is emerging that links the expertise of the laboratory investigator with that of the epidemiologist. These hybrid approaches, known as molecular or biochemical epidemiology, use modern biochemical techniques to study the distribution of changes in the human genome across populations. For example, Stitch and Rosin (1983) have studied abnormalities suggestive of genotoxic damage in the cells obtained from the mouths of persons with different smoking and alcohol consumption habits. From such research it may be possible to obtain valid biologic markers of an individual person's susceptibility to cancer, and this might allow preventive measures to be tailored to the person's unique risk status.

Multistep Carcinogenesis

Initiation, Promotion, and Latency

The starting point of cancer development may be the mutation or damage of the genome, but the progression from that origin is not simple. It is not usually the actual cell in which the malignant transformation has occurred that expresses the disorganized pattern of growth characteristic of cancer. Cancer growth may not occur until many generations of descendants from the affected cell have passed. For example, the atomic bomb explosions in Japan represented an exposure to carcinogenic radiation that occurred at a single point in time and which was not repeated. The excesses of leukemia and other cancers, however, did not occur until several years after the radiation exposure, long after the exposed cells and tissues had been replaced by new growth. The quiescent period during which the "memory" of the carcinogenic event is maintained across reproduction by cellular division but during which time the traits of cancer are not expressed is called *latency* (Pitot, 1985).

It follows from the ability of cancer to remain latent for long periods that events other than the initial damage to the genetic makeup of the cell may be necessary for the full development of cancer. That carcinogenesis may involve multiple steps has been shown repeatedly in laboratory experiments. Berenblum (1941) theorized that carcinogenesis is a two-step process. The first step, in which the cell is transformed so that it or its progeny are capable of behaving as cancer, is termed *initiation*. The second event, that which causes initiated cells to begin the unregulated proliferation leading to tumor formation, is termed *promotion*.

Many carcinogens are known to be complete carcinogens, capable of both initiating and promoting the development of cancer. Some agents appear, however, only to be capable of promotion. Croton oil, for example, does not cause skin tumors when applied to mouse skin, but when it is applied to the skin after application of the initiator benz(a)pyrene, more tumors occur more rapidly than are observed with benz(a)pyrene alone. Initiators may be of chemical, physical, or biologic origin. They act by causing irreversible damage to the molecular structure of the genetic component of the cell. In contrast, promoters influence the expression of the genetic code but may not alter the genetic code itself. Thus promoters may not have the irreversible effects of initiators, tending to influence the expression of cancer only at the time of their presence.

The two-step model of carcinogenesis has many implications for human cancer. It may explain why persons can be exposed to a number of different known carcinogens in the environment without any of them immediately, or ever, resulting in cancer. The exposure to an initiator alone may not set into motion the events required for cancer to develop. Multistage carcinogenesis also has important implications for cancer prevention. It suggests that many, if not all, people by the time they reach a certain age bear cells for which the first stage of carcinogenesis already has occurred. Because these changes are irreversible, avoidance of further exposure to initiators may not be as beneficial as avoidance of promoters. It is likely that many of the factors regarded as sources of human cancer risk are promoters rather than complete carcinogens. Alcohol, hormones, and dietary fat all are agents that do not act as carcinogens in the experimental setting but that do appear to promote the occurrence of cancer in human populations.

The Importance of Dose

The evidence on the differences between initiators and promoters suggests clearly that not all sources of cancer risk exert their effects in the same way. It also is known from experimental data that there is a wide range of potency for different agents in initiating or promoting cancer. The weakest known carcinogen requires a dose a million times greater than the most powerful carcinogen to achieve the same biologic effect (Ames, 1983a). An example of a very potent carcinogen is *aflatoxin*, a toxin produced by a mold found on stored agricultural products. A weak carcinogen may be saccharin, its potency being so low that there is uncertainty about whether it truly is carcinogenic in humans.

This broad range of carcinogenic potency is another means by which we may explain how the human species is able to survive in an environment in which some exposure to carcinogens is certain. Some levels of risk to which humans are exposed are so low that they probably never lead to cancer in the normal life span. This knowledge of the importance of dose can have important implications for efforts to control environmental exposure to carcinogens, with strong carcinogens potentially deserving greater attention than weak ones.

Anticarcinogens and Inhibitors

Until relatively recently, the focus of prevention and carcinogenesis research has been on discovery and control of carcinogens and promoters, those substances and exposures that increase cancer risk. Within the last decade, however, there has been strong interest in the discovery and evaluation of substances, natural and synthetic, that have protective effects. Researchers have identified a small number of these substances called anticarcinogens or inhibitors, but the number that eventually may be discovered may equal or exceed the number of carcinogens and promoters in the environment. These discoveries would provide yet another explanation for the natural defenses against cancer, and, if some agents are proved safe and effective in clinical use, provide additional tools to practice prevention in populations at risk for cancer.

An anticarcinogen exerts its effect by preventing cancer initiation, and inhibitors operate in the later stage, suppressing the expression of pathology. The search for these protective factors has focused mainly on natural substances occurring in the human diet. Of these, the anticarcinogenic antioxidants and the inhibiting vitamin A compounds are most studied. Ames (1983b) theorizes that antioxidants in the diet act as defense mechanisms against the oxygen radicals, which are major contributors to DNA damage. Examples of antioxidants in the diet include vitamin E, beta-carotene, selenium, glutathione, and ascorbic acid (vitamin

C). In addition to those naturally occurring in the diet, some antioxidants are added to the diet in the form of preservatives commonly used in foods, such as butylated hydroxytoluene (BHT) and butylated hydroxyanisole (BHA), to extend their shelf life.

Animal experiments have shown that supplementation of the diet with vitamin A or its synthetic analogues, all of which are termed retinoids, inhibits chemically induced cancers (Saffiotti, Monte Santo, Sellakuman, & Borg, 1967). These effects are observed for a number of different tumors of epithelial tissue induced by a number of different chemical carcinogens. Epidemiologic studies have supported the concept that vitamin A may inhibit carcinogenesis. Interview studies have shown that lung cancer patients report less frequent consumption of food sources of vitamin A in comparison to healthy control subjects (Mettlin, Graham, & Swanson, 1979). Similar effects have been reported for bladder and breast cancers. Serum studies have shown that persons with lower levels of serum beta-carotene, the precursor form of vitamin A, experience greater risk of cancer (Menkes et al., 1986). Much more needs to be learned about the fundamental processes involved, but the evidence to date has motivated researchers to conduct trials of different forms of vitamin A and its precursors to determine whether so-called chemoprevention of cancer can be done in a safe and effective manner.

Types of Carcinogens

The agents and materials in the human environment that are capable of acting as carcinogens can be categorized as physical, chemical, or biologic. Physical factors known to play a role in carcinogenesis include ultraviolet radiation from sunlight, ionizing radiation, and inhaled or embedded particles and fibers. Other physical forces under investigation for which the data are less convincing include microwave radiation and electromagnetic fields. Chemical carcinogens include compounds found in nature as well as those developed synthetically for commercial and medical uses. The biologic factors that generated the greatest interest are the several viruses now linked to different cancers.

Ultraviolet Radiation

Skin cancer is the most common of all cancers, and its high incidence in regions of high sunlight exposure and among workers in outdoor occupations provides epidemiologic evidence of a cause and effect association. The association has been defined more clearly as involving ultraviolet radiation (UVR) on the basis of animal experimentation. The association is dose dependent; therefore, protective measures that reduce exposure to sunlight reduce risk. Skin pigmentation is a natural defense to UVR damage, and the human cell appears to have mechanisms to repair UVR-induced damage to the DNA. This repair capability is not present among persons with the inherited disease xeroderma pigmentosum, who have hypersensitivity to sunlight and high risk of developing skin cancers, including melanoma.

Microwave Radiation and Electromagnetic Fields

Microwave radiation is employed as a means of electronic communication and rapid food preparation. The energy of microwave radiation is too low to affect chemical bonds or cause DNA damage, and this form of radiation is not likely to be carcinogenic (Shore, 1988).

Large numbers of persons are exposed to electromagnetic fields (EMFs) from household electrical wiring, appliances, electrical transmission lines, and electrical production. Although there are known biologic effects of EMFs, the effects are not clearly carcinogenic. Savitz and Calle (1987) have found childhood leukemia to be weakly associated with living close to high-voltage electrical transmission lines. Persons in occupations involving high exposure to EMFs, such as power linemen and electronic engineers, have been surveyed with respect to cancer risk, and the data do suggest some greater leukemia risk. These studies, however, are methodologically very weak because of the inability to measure accurately long-term exposure to EMFs. Whether there is significant risk to human populations is an unresolved research issue.

Ionizing Radiation

The cancer risks of ionizing radiation are well documented. Even in the early days of experimentation with x-rays and radium, the risks of skin cancer and leukemia were suspected. Early radiologists experienced higher rates of death from leukemia, and the workers who painted radium on watch dials to give them luminescence suffered high rates of osteosarcoma. Much of our knowledge about the effects of ionizing radiation on humans comes from careful investigations of the populations of Hiroshima and Nagasaki, who survived the blast effects of the only two nuclear weapons ever used in warfare.

In studies just mentioned, it was possible to study the effects of dose according to distance from the blast epicenter and to examine the interactions of age and sex with exposure. Follow-up studies have shown that excesses of leukemia, multiple myeloma, and cancers of the lung, female breast, stomach, colon, esophagus, and urinary tract all were attributable to the radiation exposure (Preston, Kato, Kopecky, & Fujita, 1987). Greater rates for solid tumors occurred among women than among men, and persons who were young at time of blast were apparently more sensitive to the radiation than those who were older.

Persons exposed occupationally before the dangers were appreciated and the large atomic bomb–exposed populations all represent examples of high exposure to radiation. Some segments of the United States population continue to have high levels of exposure to radiation. Uranium miners are an example, as are persons receiving radiation therapy. There also has

been a recognition that many homes can harbor high levels of radon gas, the result of seepage of the gases from the rock formations on which the homes are built (Council on Scientific Affairs, 1987). Most populations, however, are exposed to much lower doses of radiation, principally from medical x-rays, naturally occurring radiation, nuclear power production, past atmospheric weapons tests, and other minor sources.

Shore (1988) has estimated the distribution by source of the ionizing radiation to which the United States population is exposed annually. Table 12–2 shows that, for the average person in the population, the largest single source of radiation is medical diagnostic procedures followed closely in rank by natural sources. Other sources are one twentieth to one thousandth as significant as contributors to risk. All sources considered, Shore estimates that between 0.5 and 3.5 per cent of all cancer deaths in the United States are the result of radiation exposure. The risk associated with radiation from diagnostic medical procedures should be weighed relative to the health benefits derived from these procedures. This assessment has been done in the case of mammography, for example, with the analyses suggesting that the risks of not detecting breast cancer far exceed the risks of the screening procedure (American Cancer Society, 1980).

Particles and Fibers

A form of physical carcinogen different from radiation is that of solid bodies embedded in tissue. Asbestos is the most significant such carcinogen, with higher rates of lung cancer and mesothelioma found among workers involved with the mining, manufacturing, or installation of asbestos products (Selikoff, Churg, & Hammond, 1965; Selikoff, Hammond, & Churg, 1964, 1968; Selikoff, Hammond, & Seidman, 1973). The mechanisms of particulate carcinogenesis are not well understood. Animal studies have shown that films such as cellophane implanted subcutaneously in the rat cause the formation of tumor where tissue meets film (Oppenheimer, Oppenheimer, & Stout, 1948). Pulverizing the material and implanting it seems to have no tumorigenic effect, suggesting that the mechanism is physical rather than chemical. Perforating the film reduces the tumorigenic effect. It is possible that asbestos particles act in the same manner, with the

Table 12–2. ANNUAL EXPOSURES TO IONIZING RADIATION FOR THE UNITED STATES POPULATION

Source	Dose (mrem/yr), Total Population
Medical diagnostic procedures	90
Natural background (cosmic, terrestrial, and internal)	80
Atmospheric weapons tests	5
Nuclear power plants (nearby residents)	<0.1
Television sets	0.5
Airline travel	0.5

(Adapted from Shore, R. E. [1988]. Electromagnetic radiations and cancer: Cause and prevention. *Cancer, 62,* 1747–1754. Reproduced by permission of J. B. Lippincott Co.)

surface of the fiber interfering with normal patterns of cellular growth and proliferation. The fibers, to the extent that they perforate the cell's protective membrane, might also act as conduits for other carcinogens to enter the cell.

Chemicals

Chemical carcinogens may act as initiators, promoters, or both. The potential of certain chemicals to initiate carcinogenesis is believed to arise from their ability to affect the chemical bonding within the cellular DNA, causing the deletion of segments or the inclusion of disruptive genetic information. It is known that the host organism can influence significantly the course of chemical carcinogenesis by metabolizing substances to more or less carcinogenic forms and by repairing or failing to repair the DNA damage (Miller, 1978).

Chemical carcinogens can be identified by a variety of laboratory test procedures, including short-term assays such as the Ames test, which detects mutagenicity, and whole animal assays. With new chemicals continually being discovered, these laboratory testing procedures can help protect the public against exposure to new carcinogenic substances. In spite of the importance of these test systems, most of our knowledge about chemicals carcinogenic to humans comes from studies of chemicals in the workplace. Table 12–3 lists the chemicals known to be carcinogenic to humans that have been determined from occupational studies. Other chemicals are suspected of being human carcinogens from laboratory and other studies, and the International Agency for Research on Cancer (IARC) has identified chemicals requiring special attention because of their potential carcinogenicity in humans (International Agency for Research on Cancer (IARC), 1982; Tomatis et al., 1978).

Viruses

The first viral cause of cancer to be identified was Rous's discovery of a virus associated with sarcomas in chickens. Although discoveries of, among others, feline and mouse leukemia viruses followed, the identification of human cancer viruses was slower in coming. Burkitt's lymphoma, a tumor found mainly in subtropical Africa, eventually was found to be associated with the Epstein-Barr virus. Liver cancer, common in underdeveloped regions, was linked to hepatitis B virus. Viruses are believed to be capable of inducing cancer by their ability to integrate segments of genetic information into the human chromosome.

Modern techniques of molecular biology have made the detection of new classes of viruses possible. Perhaps of greatest public health significance are retroviruses. The retrovirus human T-cell leukemia virus is associated with a leukemia found predominantly in Japan (Hinuma et al., 1982) and the Caribbean (Blattner et al., 1982). A related retrovirus, now known as human immunodeficiency virus, is the means of transmission of AIDS and also is responsible for the occurrence of the associated cancer, Kaposi's sarcoma. The human papillomavirus is yet another virus suspected of playing an important role in human cancer (cervical cancer) (Zur Hause, De Villiers, & Gissman, 1981).

Vectors of Exposure

Laboratory investigations have identified a wide range of potential carcinogens and possible mechanisms of carcinogenesis, but that information does not necessarily reflect the true nature of cancer as a public health phenomenon. Many laboratory carcinogens are not usually encountered in the environment, and the infinitely variable mix of harmful materials to which a

Table 12–3. CHEMICAL AGENTS EXHIBITING A CARCINOGENIC RISK TO HUMANS IN ASSOCIATION WITH OCCUPATION

Chemical Process or Industry	Associated Neoplasm
Acrylonitrile	Lung, colon, prostate
Arsenic	Lung
Asbestos	Lung, mesothelioma, gastrointestinal tract(?)
Auramine manufacture	Bladder
Aromatic amines (aminobiphenyl, benzidine, 2-naphthylamine, 4-nitrobiphenyl)	Bladder
Benzene	Leukemia
Beryllium and its compounds	Lung
Bis (chloromethyl) ether	Lung
Boot and shoe manufacture and repair	Nasal carcinoma
Cadmium and its compounds	Lung, prostate(?)
Chromium and some of its compounds	Lung
Furniture manufacture (hardwood)	Nasal carcinoma
Hematite mining (underground)	Lung
Isopropyl alcohol manufacture	Cancer of paranasal sinuses
Nickel refining	Lung, nasal sinuses
Phenoxyacetic acids and herbicides	Soft tissue sarcoma
Rubber industry (certain occupations)	Leukemia, bladder
Soots, tars, and oils	Skin, lung, bladder, gastrointestinal tract
Vinyl chloride	Liver (angiosarcoma)

(Adapted from Pitot, H. C. [1985]. Principles of cancer biology: Chemical carcinogenesis. In V. T. De Vita, S. Hellman, & S. A. Rosenberg [Eds.], *Cancer: Principles and practice of oncology* [2nd ed., pp. 79–99]. Philadelphia: J. B. Lippincott Co. Reproduced by permission.)

population may be exposed cannot be recreated in the laboratory setting. To better describe the causes of cancer in human populations, it is necessary to shift focus from the underlying biologic mechanisms to the circumstances and situations that expose persons to carcinogens or promoters. These situations or circumstances are known to epidemiologists as *vectors of exposure*.

It is possible to prevent or control disease, without knowing the fundamental processes involved, by controlling vectors of exposure. A classic example is Snow's discovery of the transmission of cholera via the nineteenth-century London water system many years before the organism causing the disease was identified. A more recent example is the knowledge that cigarette smoking is the vector for lung cancer even though the specific carcinogens in tobacco smoke that lead to the disease have not been completely delineated.

The vectors of human cancer risk can be classified broadly into those of inherited, life-style, or environmental nature. Of these, the life-style and environmental vectors of risk are believed to offer the greatest opportunities for prevention because an inherited susceptibility to cancer currently cannot be modified. Life style is the constellation of habits and behaviors customary to a person or population. Diet, tobacco and alcohol use, sexual conduct, and childbearing patterns are all culturally influenced aspects of life style. Environmental vectors include exposures to natural and artificial radiation as well as chemicals and biologic agents in the air, water, or workplace. Generally speaking, life-style risks are those to which persons subject themselves by their own acts, whereas environmental risks are experienced involuntarily.

The relative significance of these different vectors of exposure is an important question because it helps define how people may best reduce their risks of cancer and it also indicates what kinds of governmental, industrial, or other public actions might be beneficial. Doll and Peto (1981) have calculated estimates of the proportions of cancer that are attributable to different vectors of exposure. The public's opinion may be that air and water pollution, toxic dumpsites, and carcinogens in the workplace are the greatest hazards, but the figures in Table 12–4 suggest that the most important sources of cancer risk in the United States are of life-style origin, namely, smoking and diet. Some of the evidence for each of these vectors of exposure will be reviewed. The roles of tobacco, diet, and sexual and reproductive practices, although they are among the most important vectors, are discussed only briefly here because they are examined in detail in Chapter 15.

Tobacco

The role of tobacco in cancer causation is perhaps the best understood aspect of the cancer problem. Lung cancer is the leading cause of cancer deaths in men and women in the United States, and an estimated 85 per cent of all lung cancer is attributable to cigarette smoking (United States Public Health Service [USPHS], 1982). Cigarette use also contributes to the occurrence of cancers of the mouth, larynx, esophagus, bladder, kidney, uterine cervix, and pancreas.

Diet

Although our knowledge of the role of diet in cancer causation and prevention is less certain than that for tobacco, the overall importance of diet may ultimately prove to be greater. This importance, in part, is because the effects of smoking are mainly on the respiratory organs, but the effects of diet can potentially cause cancer in every organ system. The evidence for dietary factors comes from multiple sources. Many differences in cancer rates between groups or regions are correlated with differences in dietary practices. Similarly, trends in diets across time have been linked to trends in the risk for certain cancers. Persons with cancer report histories of dietary practices that differ from those of comparable persons who did not develop the disease. In addition, laboratory experiments have shown that tumor growth in animals may be affected by many different kinds of dietary manipulation.

Reproductive and Sexual Behavior

Nulliparity is a risk factor for breast cancer, as is delayed age of first pregnancy (MacMahon, Cole, & Brown, 1973). Pregnancy is related to risk of developing cancers with estrogen sensitivity, suggesting that the effect is the result of the influence of pregnancy on the production and distribution of endogenous hormones. Multiple sex partners and early age of first intercourse are established risk factors for cervical cancer (LaVecchia et al., 1986).

Occupation

In addition to the chemical risks listed in Table 12–3, work environments can involve exposure to ionizing and UVR as well as to a variety of fibers and dusts. Asbestos is the most common occupational carcinogen because asbestos products were, at one time, used so commonly in different construction and industrial applications. Lung cancer is the most common tumor linked to occupational exposures, but cancers of virtually every type have been linked to different carcin-

Table 12–4. PROPORTIONS OF CANCER DEATHS ATTRIBUTED TO VARIOUS FACTORS

Factors or Class of Factors	Percentage of All Cancer Deaths	
	Best Estimate	Range of Reasonable Estimates
Tobacco	30	25–40
Diet	35	10–70
Reproductive and sexual behavior	7	1–13
Occupation	4	2–8
Pollution	2	<1–5
Medicines and medical procedures	1	0.5–3

(Data from Doll & Peto, 1981.)

ogens found in the workplace. The problem is not necessarily an industrial problem. Farmers are exposed to pesticides, herbicides, and animal populations that may harbor viruses. Despite extensive data on occupational risks, Doll and Peto (1981) estimate the proportion of cancers attributable to occupational exposures is small relative to some of the other factors they considered.

Pollution

The natural environment is a vector of exposure to a number of different chemical contaminants (Swanson, 1988). Air pollution originates from motor vehicles, manufacturing, and power generation, among other sources. "Indoor air pollution" results from home heating, tobacco use, and sometimes seepage of natural gases. Water supplies are contaminated by known carcinogens from manufacturing, by leakage from hazardous dumpsites, and by the byproducts of mining, agriculture, and forestry work. Chlorination of water supplies to control microorganisms also is known to lead to the formation of chemical byproducts with carcinogenic potential (Wilkins & Comstock, 1981).

Although it is possible to detect the presence of carcinogens throughout our natural environment, there is little evidence that any significant portion of the cancer burden in the United States results from ambient pollutants. This is, perhaps, because the dose of carcinogens to which the population is exposed is so low. Ames (1983b) has estimated, for example, that it is necessary to breathe severely polluted air for 2 weeks to inhale the amount of particulate matter inhaled by smoking just a single cigarette. On the other hand, it is possible that part of the risk of environmental pollution is overlooked because the entire population is exposed to some level of risk and, lacking a point of reference for the nonexposed, the true effect cannot be gauged.

Medicines and Medical Procedures

As noted earlier, medical x-rays are a major vector of exposure to ionizing radiation, and several drugs and chemical used in medicine have carcinogenic potential. Table 12–5 lists a number of carcinogens used in medicine. The estrogens are perhaps the most significant of this list because of the numbers of women who have been exposed through use of oral contraceptives or replacement estrogens taken at menopause. Oral contraceptive use has not been shown to significantly increase the risk for breast cancer and may, in fact, reduce risk for ovarian cancer (Center for Disease Control Cancer and Steroid Hormone Study, 1983; Newhouse, Pearson, Fullerton, Bosen, & Shannon, 1977). Replacement estrogens, in contrast, have been linked to endometrial cancer (Hulka, 1980). At one time diethylstilbestrol (DES) was prescribed to prevent miscarriage. Women exposed in utero were later shown to be at high risk for developing vaginal cancers (Herbst, Ulfelder, & Poskanzer, 1971). Some antineo-

plastic drugs have proved to have carcinogenic potential, and medical practice often involves balancing a small future risk against greater, immediate benefit.

Types of Prevention

Primary, Secondary, and Tertiary Prevention

Given the complexity of cancer causes, no single intervention aimed at preventing cancer can be expected to address the problem completely. Cancer prevention requires multidisciplinary approaches carried out at different levels. Cancer prevention has been divided into three stages according to the stage of the natural history of the disease. *Primary* prevention refers to efforts to block the cancer during carcinogenesis, before initiation or no later than the promotion stage. Regulation of carcinogens, cessation of smoking, and dietary change all are primary prevention measures. *Secondary* prevention efforts are undertaken after the onset of pathology but before signs and symptoms are present. Screening to detect unsuspected cancers at a time when their treatment may be most effective is the most common form of secondary prevention. *Tertiary* prevention hardly seems like prevention at all because it comes after the disease has been discovered. Nevertheless, important interventions even at this late stage may prevent the most serious consequences of the disease. Prompt appropriate treatment and rehabilitation are both examples of tertiary interventions.

Universal, Selective, and Indicated Prevention

Another way to classify levels of preventive intervention is by their target (Gordon, 1983). Some preventive measures are suitable for *universal* application. Interventions from which virtually all persons might benefit include avoidance of tobacco use, proper nutrition, and control of environmental carcinogens. Other preventive measures may be prescribed on a *selective* basis. Some groups have unique types of exposure to risk that warrant special measures for the entire group. Examples of these include workplace safety measures, cervical cancer screening for sexually active young women, or breast cancer screening for middle-aged and older women. Finally, some preventive measure can be applied only on an *as indicated* basis. Examples of these include early detection guidelines for persons with a history of cancer or special measures for patients with diagnosed precursor lesions, such as colorectal polyps or dysplastic nevi, which place them at increased risk.

FUTURE DIRECTIONS

Research on the causes of cancer has progressed greatly. Much of this progress is attributable to the melding of clinical, laboratory, and public health per-

Table 12–5. CHEMICAL AGENTS EXHIBITING A CARCINOGENIC RISK TO HUMANS IN ASSOCIATION WITH MEDICAL THERAPY AND DIAGNOSIS

Chemical or Drug	Associated Neoplasm
Alkylating agents (cyclophosphamide, melphalan)	Bladder, leukemia
Inorganic arsenicals	Skin, liver
Azathioprine (immunosuppressive drug)	Lymphoma, reticulum cell sarcoma, skin, Kaposi's sarcoma(?)
Chlornaphazine	Bladder
Chloramphenicol	Leukemia
Diethylstilbestrol	Vagina (clear cell carcinoma)
Estrogens	
Premenopausal	Liver cell adenoma
Postmenopausal	Endometrium
Methoxypsoralen with UV light (PUVA)	Skin
Oxymetholone	Liver
Phenacetin	Renal pelvis (carcinoma)
Phenytoin	Lymphoma, neuroblastoma
Thorium dioxide in dextran (Thorotrast)	Liver (angiosarcoma)

(Adapted from Pitot, H. C. [1985]. Principles of cancer biology: Chemical carcinogenesis. In V. T. De Vita, S. Hellman, & S. A. Rosenberg [Eds.], *Cancer: Principles and practice of oncology* [2nd ed., pp. 79–99]. Philadelphia: J. B. Lippincott Co. Reproduced by permission.)

spectives. The future course of research and development in cancer prevention may further reflect this trend toward multidisciplinary efforts. In addition, based on present understanding of fundamental processes, future efforts may tend more toward development of practical interventions. This may be particularly true with respect to the development of chemopreventive interventions. Until such clinical interventions are proved safe and effective, traditional reliance on early detection and avoidance of exposure to carcinogens will remain the most effective tools of prevention at our disposal.

References

American Cancer Society. (1980). Guidelines for the cancer related checkup: Recommendations and rationale. *CA:A Cancer Journal for Clinicians, 30,* 4–50.

Ames, B. N. (1983a). The detection of environmental mutagens and potential carcinogens. *Cancer, 53,* 2034–2039.

Ames, B. N., (1983b). Dietary carcinogens and anticarcinogens. Oxygen radicals and degenerative diseases. *Science, 221,* 1256–1264.

Ames, B. N., Durston, W. E., Yamasaki, E., & Lee, F. D. (1973). Carcinogens as mutagens: A simple test system combining liver homogenates for activation and bacteria for detection. *Proceedings of the National Academy of Sciences, U.S.A., 70,* 2281–2285.

Baltimore, D. (1987). The impact of the discovery of oncogenes on cancer mortality rates will come slowly. *Cancer, 59,* 1985–1986.

Berenblum, I. (1941). The mechanism of carcinogenesis: A study of the significance of cocarcinogenic action and related phenomena. *Cancer Research, 1,* 807–814.

Blattner, W. A., Kalyanaraman, V. S., Robert-Guroff, M., Lister, T. A., Galton, D. A. G., Sarin, P. S., Crawford, M. H., Catovsky, D., Greaves, M., & Gallo, R. C. (1982). The human type-C retrovirus, HTLV, in blacks from the Caribbean region, and relationship to adult T-cell leukemia/lymphoma. *International Journal of Cancer, 30,* 257–264.

Centers for Disease Control Cancer and Steroid Hormone Study. (1983). Oral contraceptive use and the risk of ovarian cancer. *Journal of the American Medical Association, 249,* 1596–1599.

Council on Scientific Affairs. (1987). Radon in homes. *Journal of the American Medical Association, 258,* 668–672.

Doll, R., & Peto, R. (1981). The causes of cancer. *Journal of the National Cancer Institute, 66,* 1191–1308.

Furth, J., & Kahn, M. C. (1937). The transmission of leukemia of mice with a single cell. *American Journal of Cancer, 31,* 276–282.

Giovanella, B. C., Yim, S. O., Stehlin, J. S., & Williams, L. J., Jr. (1972). Development of invasive tumor in the "nude" mouse after injection of cultural human melanoma cells. *Journal of the National Cancer Institute, 48,* 1531–1533.

Gordon, R. S., Jr. (1983). An operational classification of disease prevention. *Public Health Reports, 98,* 107–109.

Herbst, A. L., Ulfelder, H., & Poskanzer, D. C. (1971). Adenocarcinoma of the vagina: Association of maternal stilbestrol therapy with tumor appearance in young women. *New England Journal of Medicine, 284,* 878–881.

Hinuma, Y., Komoda, H., Chosa, T., Konda, T., Kohakura, M., Tanenaka, T., Kikuchi, M., Ichimuru, M., Yunoki, K., Sato, I., Matsuo, R., Takiuchi, Y., Uchino, H., & Hanaoka, X. (1982). Antibodies to adult T-cell leukemia-virus associated antigen (ATLA) in sera from patients with ATL and controls in Japan; a nation-wide sero-epidemiologic study. *International Journal of Cancer, 29,* 631–635.

Holleb, A. I., & Randers-Pehrson, M. B. (Eds.). (1987). *Classics in oncology.* New York: American Cancer Society.

Hulka, B. (1980). Effect of exogenous estrogen in postmenopausal women: The epidemiologic evidence. *Obstetrical and Gynecological Survey, 35,* 389–399.

International Agency of Research on Cancer. (1982). *Chemicals, industrial processes and industries associated with cancer in humans.* (IARC Monographs, Supplement 4). Lyon: International Agency for Research on Cancer.

La Vecchia, C., Franceschi, S., Decarli, A., Fasoli, M., Gentile, A., Parazzini, F., & Regallo, M. (1986). Sexual factors, venereal diseases, and the risk of intraepithelial and invasive cervical neoplasia. *Cancer, 58,* 935–941.

Lee, W. H., Bookstein, R., Hong, F., Young, L.-J., Shew J.-Y., & Lee, E. Y.-H. P. (1987). Human retinoblastoma susceptibility gene: Cloning, identification, and sequence. *Science, 235,* 1394–1399.

MacMahon, B., Cole, P., & Brown, J. (1973). Etiology of human breast cancer: A review. *Journal of the National Cancer Institute, 50,* 21–42.

Menkes, M. S., Comstock, G. W., Vuilleumier, J. P., Helsing, K. S., Rider, A. A., & Brookmeyer, R. (1986). Serum beta-carotene, vitamins A and E, selenium, and the risk of lung cancer. *New England Journal of Medicine, 315,* 1250–1254.

Mettlin, C. (1988). Descriptive and analytical epidemiology: Bridges to cancer control. *Cancer, 62,* 1680–1687.

Mettlin, C., Graham, S., & Swanson, M. (1979). Vitamin A and lung cancer. *Journal of the National Cancer Institute, 62,* 1435–1438.

Miller, E. C. (1978). Some current perspectives on chemical carcinogenesis in humans and experimental animals: Presidential address. *Cancer Research, 38,* 1479–1496.

Newhouse, M. L., Pearson, R. M., Fullerton, S. M., Bosen, E. A. M., & Shannon, H. (1977). A case control study of carcinoma of the ovary. *British Journal of Preventive and Social Medicine, 31,* 148–153.

Oppenheimer, B. S., Oppenheimer, E. T., & Stout, A. P. (1948). Sarcomas induced in rats by implanting cellophane. *Proceedings of the Society of Experimental and Biological Medicine, 67,* 33–34.

Pitot, H. C. (1985). Principles of cancer biology: Chemical carcinogenesis. In V. T. DeVita, S. Hellman, & S. A. Rosenberg (Eds.), *Cancer: Principles and practice of oncology* (2nd ed., pp. 79–99). Philadelphia: J. B. Lippincott Co.

Preston, D. L., Kato, H., Kopecky, K. J., & Fujita, S. (1987). Studies of the mortality of A-bomb survivors, 8. Cancer mortality, 1950–1982. *Radiation Research, 111,* 151–178.

Saffiotti, U., Montesano, R., Sellakuman, A. R., & Borg, S. A. (1967). Experimental cancer of the lung. Inhibition by vitamin A of the induction of tracheobroncial squamous metaplasia and squamous cell tumors. *Cancer, 20,* 857–864.

Savitz, D. A., & Calle, E. E. (1987). Leukemia and occupational exposure to electromagnetic fields: Review of epidemiologic surveys. *Journal of Occupational Medicine, 29,* 47–51.

Selikoff, I. J., Churg, J., & Hammond, E. C. (1965). Relationship between exposure to asbestos and mesothelioma. *New England Journal of Medicine, 272,* 560–565.

Selikoff, I. J., Hammond, E. C., & Churg, J. (1964). Asbestos exposure and neoplasia. *Journal of the American Medical Association, 143,* 329–336.

Selikoff, I. J., Hammond, E. C., & Churg, J. (1968). Asbestos exposure, smoking, and neoplasia. *Journal of the American Medical Associaion, 204,* 106–112.

Selikoff, I. J., Hammond, E. C., & Seidman, H. (1973). Cancer risk of insulation workers in the United States. In: International Agency for Research on Cancer. *Biological effects of asbestos* (pp. 209–216). Lyon: Author.

Shimkin, M. B. (1977). Some historical landmarks in cancer epidemiology. *Contrary to nature.* (DHEW Publication No. [NIH] 76-720, pp. 60–74). Washington, DC, U.S. Department of Health, Education, and Welfare, Public Health Service. National Institute of Health.

Shore, R. E. (1988). Electromagnetic radiations and cancer: Cause and prevention. *Cancer, 62,* 1747–1754.

Stitch, H. F., & Rosin, M. P. (1983). Quantitating the synergistic effect of smoking and alcohol consumption with the micronucleus test on human buccal mucosa cells. *International Journal of Cancer, 31,* 305–308.

Swanson, G. M. (1988). Cancer prevention in the workplace, and natural environment: A review of etiology, research design, and methods of risk detection. *Cancer, 62,* 1725–1746.

Tomatis, L., Agthe, C., Bartsch, H., Huff, J., Montesano, R., Saracci, R., Walker, E., & Wilbourn, J. (1978). Evaluation of the carcinogenicity of chemicals: A review of the monograph program of the International Agency for Research on Cancer. *Cancer Research, 38,* 877–885.

United States Public Health Service (1982). *The health consequences of smoking. A report of the Surgeon General of the Public Health Service, U.S. Department of Health and Human Services, Office on Smoking and Health.* Washington, DC: U.S. Government Printing Office.

Vahde Woude, G. F., & Gilden, R. V. (1985). Principles of cancer biology: molecular biology. In V. T. DeVita, S. Hellman & S. A. Rosenberg (Eds.). *Cancer: Principles and practice of oncology* (2nd ed., pp. 23–47). Philadelphia: J. B. Lippincott Co.

Wilkins, J. R., & Comstock, G. W. (1981). Source of drinking water at home and site-specific cancer incidence in Washington County, Maryland. *American Journal of Epidemiology, 114,* 178–190.

Wynder, E. L., & Graham, E. A. (1950). Tobacco smoking as possible etiologic factor in brochogenic carcinoma: Study of six-hundred and eighty-four proved cases. *Journal of the American Medical Association, 143,* 329–336.

Yamagiwa, K., & Ichikawa, K. (1918). Experimental study of the pathogenesis of carcinoma. *Journal of Cancer Research, 3,* 1–29.

zur Hausen, H., DeVilliers, E. M., & Gissmann, L. (1981). Papillomavirus infections and human genital cancer. *Gynecologic Oncology, 12,* s124–s128.

CHAPTER 13

Cancer Biology: Molecular and Cellular Aspects

BETTY BIERUT GALLUCCI

This chapter focuses on cancer as a disease of cells—in particular, a disease of cellular differentiation. Some historical aspects of the molecular biology of cancer cells are highlighted to provide a perspective, to place recent developments in an context of previous accomplishments, and to illustrate that trends and fads also exist in scientific research. Clinical examples are often given after the basic biologic discussion as a bridge from the laboratory to the clinical arenas.

AN OVERVIEW

Often an understanding of the disease known as cancer begins with defining the word. Pitot (1986) distinguishes between *cancer* and *neoplasm*, referring to the clinical entity as a cancer and using neoplasm (or neoplasia) to emphasize the basic biologic processes underlying the disease. Pitot's definition, a modification of Ewing's, is as follows: "A neoplasm is a heritably altered, relatively autonomous growth of tissue" (Pitot, 1986).

This physiologic definition proposed by Pitot emphasizes the concepts of tissue, autonomy, and growth. Autonomy implies that some normal regulatory controls over cell growth and division are lacking. The term *relatively* is included because cancer cells are not completely independent of all regulatory processes. If they were, such tumors as breast and prostate cancers would not respond to hormonal therapies.

Other definitions emphasize, or imply, that *cellular* abnormalities are crucial to the definition of neoplasia. This is not surprising because the basic building block of all tissue is the cell. Bonfiglio and Terry (1983) defined cancer as "a disease of the cell in which the normal mechanisms of control of growth and proliferation are disturbed. This results in distinctive morphologic alterations of the cell and aberrations of tissue patterns." These morphologic differences and aberrations (in which the cells in the malignant tissue appear immature or less differentiated) are clues for the pathologist, who helps determine the presence or absence of a malignancy.

Clinically, the ability of a malignant cell to invade the surrounding tissue and to metastasize (i.e., to migrate and proliferate at a site distant from the primary tumor) are cellular characteristics of utmost importance. When tumor cells invade the surrounding tissue and outgrow their blood supply, cell death and tissue necrosis occur. Then infected and draining lesions form. Surgery, radiation, and chemotherapy used separately or in combination often are able to control most primary tumors and local invasion, but not the metastatic lesions. Many patients die from metastases rather than from their primary disease.

Although there are several definitions of cancer and neoplasia, selecting the most appropriate definition will depend ultimately on the individual person's framework. One useful perspective is to define cancer or neoplasia as a process. In this way, the conceptualization is broad enough to include all the aspects of this disease as studied both in the clinical and in the laboratory setting.

The Natural History of Cancer

Some well-known phenomena can help us understand that cancer is a process—not one event or one alteration, but a series of events. A classification system based on distinguishing cytologic and histologic features of a malignant growth was established by 1900 (Rather, 1978). However, even with these established features, tissue alterations were discovered that could not be placed into either normal or neoplastic categories. Instead these intermediate lesions were considered to represent the sequential changes leading from the normal cell and tissue structure to the neoplastic ones. These forms included metaplasia, dysplasia, and carcinoma in situ (Fig. 13–1). This purported sequence helped to emphasize that the development of cancer has a natural history and that the clinical manifestations are often the final stages in a series of events (Correa, 1982; Goldfarb, 1983).

Studies of metastases provide a second example of cancer as a process. Metastasis is possible because cancer cells invade the blood vessels, withstand the natural immune mechanisms while traveling in the vessels, attach to capillary walls, enter tissue, and grow

in the new milieu of the metastatic site. Each of these steps listed and perhaps a dozen others may involve genetic changes in the cell. Indicators of genetic changes include the formation of new clones of malignant cells, the activation of new enzymes, and the expression of new molecules on the cell surface and the loss of others (see Chapter 14, Fig. 14–1). Because most primary cancers can now be controlled by current therapies, understanding of the steps involved in metastasis should lead to better or more effective lifesaving therapies (Fidler & Hart, 1982; Hart, 1986; Sukumar, Carney, & Barbacid, 1988; Wolberg, 1983).

Current knowledge of cancer as a clinical phenomenon is based on results of investigations ranging from the biochemical to the cellular and continues to the level of multiple physiologic interactions in the whole individual. This very brief outline of the pathology of cancer and metastasis illustrates the complexity of the processes involved. Currently our understanding is evolving at so rapid a rate that it is difficult for any

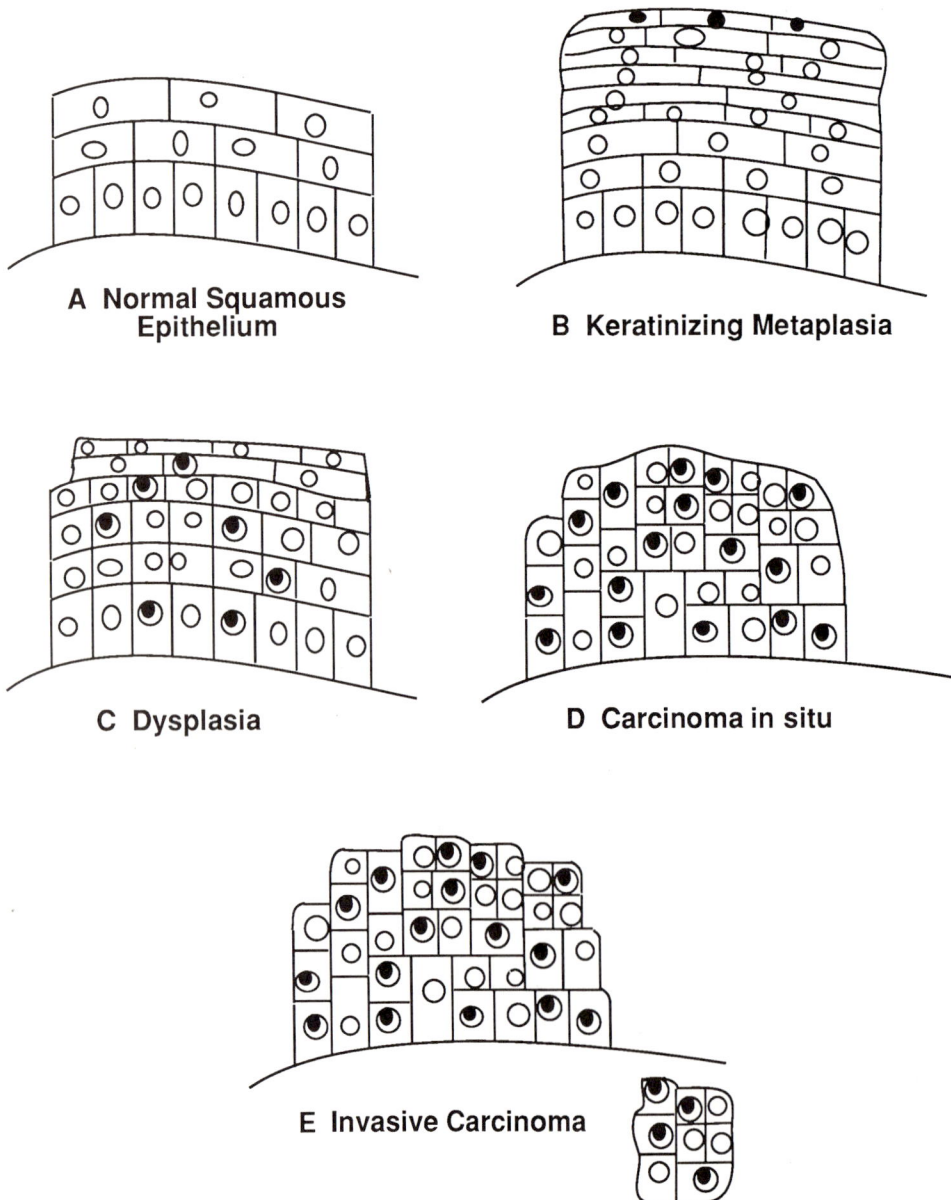

A Normal Squamous Epithelium

B Keratinizing Metaplasia

C Dysplasia

D Carcinoma in situ

E Invasive Carcinoma

Figure 13–1. The lesions that are presumably antecedent to invasive carcinoma: metaplasia, dysplasia, carcinoma in situ. A, Normal endocervical epithelial differentiation, from a columnar basal cell to a flat, mature surface cell. B, Metaplasia: normal epithelium replaced by a keratinizing epithelium that is typical of skin and areas of irritation. C, Dysplasia: some atypical cells, but the surface is flattened and contains mature cells. D, Carcinoma in situ: total loss of differentiation with many atypical and dividing cells. E, Invasive carcinoma: malignant cells can be found beneath the basal lamina in the connective tissue.

one individual to keep pace with all the new developments.

CANCER: A DISEASE OF CELL DIFFERENTIATION

In normal growth and development, a cell becomes more specialized or *committed* to a particular line of development, and it acquires specific new characteristics. *Differentiation* is the process that results in readily observable changes in cellular characteristics. These changes are irreversible, self-perpetuating, and passed on to the daughter cells. Because most cells contain the entire genome, differentiation is the result of expression of certain genes and the repression of others (Alberts et al., 1983; Ruddon, 1981; Watson, Hopkins, Roberts, Steitz, & Weiner, 1987).

Differentiated cells are mature cells that perform the functions of the particular tissues which they comprise. In the adult, *undifferentiated cells* (not totally committed) are known as pluripotent cells, precursor cells, or *stem cells*. Cells with the least amount of differentiation are found in the embryo. The fertilized egg is a totipotent cell and undergoes primary differentiation. As a cell becomes more differentiated, its potential becomes more restricted (Fig. 13–2). Totally differentiated cells often lose their ability to replicate, implying that the fate of the mature cell is death. Examples of fully differentiated cells are red blood cells, neurons, muscle cells, and helper T lymphocytes (Alberts et al., 1983; Ruddon, 1981; Watson et al., 1987).

The most obvious reason why cancer is considered an altered differentiation state is that many neoplasms resemble undifferentiated tissue. For instance, both neoplastic and embryonic cells often are rapidly dividing, are motile, and have similar markers on their cell surfaces, such as carcinoembryonic antigen. Conversely, the most differentiated cells generally have lost their ability to divide.

One way of visualizing the differentiation process is to consider the development of a red blood cell in the adult (see Fig. 13–2). The stem cell resides in the bone marrow. This stem cell (pluripotent stem cell) has the capability to generate cell lines that will form any one of the blood cells (i.e., red blood cells as well as many of the white blood cells). As differentiation proceeds, some of the daughter cells of this stem cell acquire the cytologic characteristics of the mature cell and they become committed (terminal differentiation) to a particular cell line. These cytologic features may be identified by a variety of cytologic and biochemical characteristics. The mature red blood cell will be anucleated, will be packed with hemoglobin, and will circulate in the blood (Alberts et al., 1983; Greaves, 1986; Ruddon, 1981; Sachs, 1987; Watson et al., 1987).

Neoplasia can develop at any point in the process of differentiation. A cancer of the cell line leading directly to the red blood cell (at the point of terminal differentiation) is a erythroleukemia, a rare leukemia (Fig. 13–3). An example of a leukemia occurring in the cells at an earlier stage of differentiation is acute myelogenous leukemia (see Fig. 13–3). In this disease, the cell possesses staining characteristics and markers of an immature cell. During the natural history of many cancers, as the malignant cells grow and divide, they often lose more and more of their mature characteristics. In the natural history of erythroleukemia, this shift to a less differentiated cell type appears as a myeloblastic leukemia phase of the disease (Greaves, 1986; Oishi, 1983; Ruddon, 1981; Sachs, 1987).

Knowledge of differentiation prompts the obvious question: does induction of differentiation reduce the ability of malignant cells to divide? In the mouse erythroleukemia model, the addition of dimethylsulfoxide (DMSO) (as well as other chemicals such as retinoic acid) is capable of inducing some differentiation. While the leukemic cells are exposed to DMSO, the cells take on characteristics of a more mature cell (Pitot, 1986). So far this treatment approach in mice has increased their survival times but has not led to cure. However, in this experimental model, it remains unclear whether the increase in survival time could be attributed either to the process of differentiation or to an enhancement of the immune system's ability to kill the leukemic cells (Pitot, 1986; Ruddon, 1981).

To establish which of these two mechanisms was

TOTIPOTENT CELL
(Fertilized Ovum)

↓

Primary Differentiation

↓

MULTIPOTENT CELL

↓

ONE OF SEVERAL
EMBRYONIC LAYERS

↓

Intermediate Differentiation

↓

PLURIPOTENT CELL OR STEM CELL
(Colony-Forming Unit in Bone Marrow)

↓

Commitment

↓

UNIPOTENT CELL
(Colony-Forming Unit-Erythoid)

↓

Terminal Differentiation

↓

MATURE OR DIFFERENTIATED CELL
(Red Blood Cell)

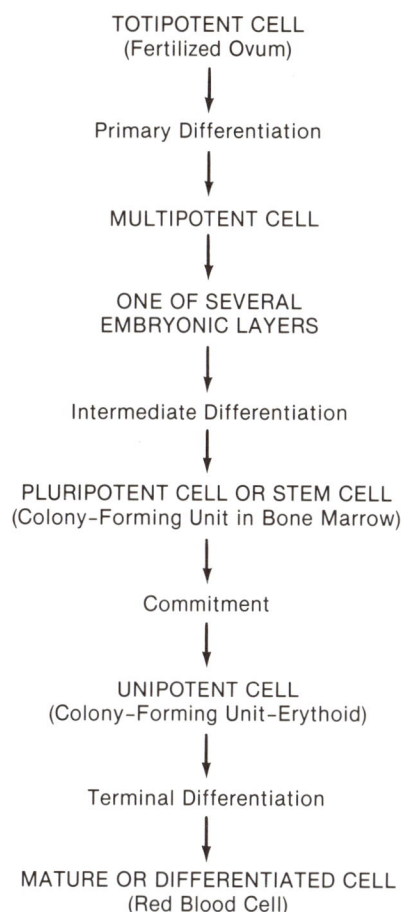

Figure 13–2. An example of how differentiation results in the production of red blood cells. Differentiation occurs many times in the life history of a cell. Each step in differentiation further limits the potential of the cell. The most differentiated cell is one that cannot divide and is destined to die.

PLURIPOTENT CELL

HEMOPOIETIC
STEM CELL
(ACUTE MYELOID LEUKEMIA)

LYMPHOPOIETIC
STEM CELL

CFU
ERYTHROCYTES
(ERYTHROCYTIC LEUKEMIA)

CFU
GRANULOCYTES

CFU
MONOCYTES

CFU
MEGAKARYOCYTES

MATURE RBC

NEUTROPHILS, BASOPHILS,
EOSINOPHILS

MONOCYTES

PLATELETS

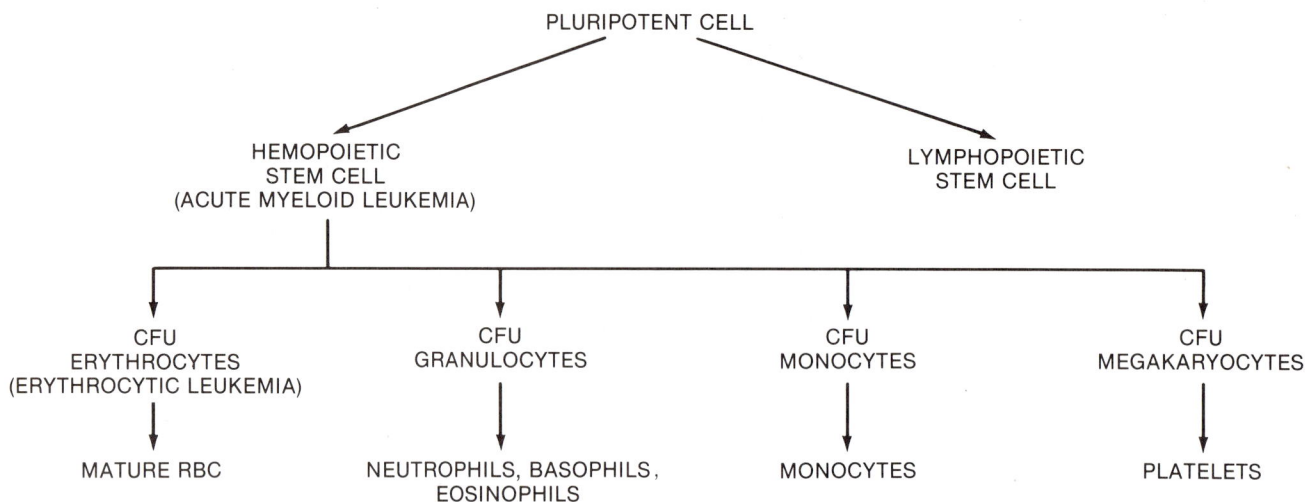

Figure 13–3. An expansion of Figure 13–2. An outline of differentiation in a hemopoietic cell line. The differentiation stages are noted in which erythrocytic leukemia and acute myeloid leukemia occur. *CFU*, colony-forming units; *RBC*, red blood cell.

operating, Jimenez and Yunis (1987) extracted differentiation factors from the tissue of adult rats. Then they placed myeloid leukemic cells in a diffusion chamber implanted in the rat and exposed the cells to the differentiation factors. Thus the leukemic cells were exposed to the body fluids of the animal yet were recoverable. After being in the body for 48 hours, the cells in the diffusion chamber were removed and examined. Ninety-four per cent of the exposed leukemic cells were differentiated and had stopped dividing. The control cells not exposed to the differentiation agents did not differentiate and continued to divide (Jimenez & Yunis, 1987). So, it appears that the induction of differentiation led to a decrease in the ability of the leukemic cells to divide and destruction by the immune system could be ruled out. Currently some of these differentiation agents are being tested in human clinical trials (Pitot, 1986; Ruddon, 1981).

CLASSIFICATION OF TUMORS

The definitive diagnosis of cancer is made by the pathologist after examining cells and tissues obtained at biopsy or from cytologic procedures. Classification of the tumor type is based on tissue and cellular staining. Differences in cytoplasmic and nuclear staining distinguish one cell type from another and identify their stages of differentiation. A malignant neoplasm, for instance, is classified as a *carcinoma* if the tissue of the tumor origin is epithelium; as an *adenocarcinoma* if the tissue of origin has both epithelial and glandular components; and as a *sarcoma* if the tissue of origin is connective tissue. (For a list of selected characteristics of benign and malignant tumor types and a simple classification system, see Tables 13–1 and 13–2.) Classification of the tumor type is imperative before decisions can be made about the type of treatment that is appropriate (Bonfiglio & Terry, 1983).

In addition to classifying the neoplasm, often a grade will be given to the tumor. The grade of the tumor is based on how well differentiated the tissue or the cells appear. A grade of 1 is given to a neoplasm that is well differentiated (that is, one that appears similar to the adult tissue from which it arose). The highest grade of 4 is given to a neoplasm that appears so undifferentiated (anaplastic) that it is difficult to identify the tissue of origin. For many tumors, the higher the grade or the less differentiated the tumor is, the poorer the prognosis (Bonfiglio & Terry, 1983).

Determination of grades between the two extremes of well differentiated and poorly differentiated tumor is difficult. Subjectivity and experience of the decision maker plays a role. Currently pathologic reports tend to emphasize the description of the tumor and not the assignment of a numerical grade. New advances in laboratory medicine, such as the development of flow cytometry, which can automatically characterize the DNA content of thousands of cells at one time and estimate the number of dividing cells, may lead to better prognostic indicators than the grade of the tumors.

PHENOTYPIC CHARACTERISTICS OF MALIGNANT AND TRANSFORMED CELLS

At this point the question might be asked, What features of a malignant cell distinguish it from a normal cell? And how are these characteristics studied? The characteristic features of the cell—known as its *phenotype*—are the result of the expression of hereditary information (Alberts et al., 1983, p. 6). The phenotype of an individual person is described by hair, skin, and eye coloring and other physical features. The cell's phenotype is determined by histologic and cytologic techniques: the quality and type of cytoplasmic and nuclear staining, the presence of mitosis, the number of nucleolar bodies, and the membrane characteristics. The malignant cell is usually basophilic, has a high nuclear-to-cytoplasmic ratio, and has multiple nucleoli (Bonfiglio & Terry, 1983; Goldfarb, 1983). The hered-

Table 13–1. SOME EXAMPLES OF THE DIFFERENCES BETWEEN BENIGN AND MALIGNANT TUMORS

Property	Benign Tumors	Malignant Tumors
Growth	Slow expansile	Invasive
Differentiation	Fully differentiated	Immature, not differentiated
Metastasis	Absent	Present
Cytoplasm	Normal, uniform	Irregular in size and shape, pleomorphic
	Regular in size and shape	Basophilic
Nucleus	DNA content euploid	DNA content euploid to aneuploid
	Infrequent mitosis	Frequent mitosis
		Many nucleoli
Paraneoplastic syndromes	Absent	Present in many cases; for example, anorexia, cachexia

itary information of the organism or the cell, on the other hand, is the *genotype* (Alberts et al., 1983).

Cell Culture and Transformation

It would seem profitable to study cell differentiation, the generation of the cell's phenotype, and carcinogenesis in isolation from the influence of all the other supporting structures of the host, as in cell cultures. However, malignant tissue from actual patients is not always available, nor is it the best experimental system. Studies of normal cells that have been transformed have led to insights into the process of neoplasia and the ability to distinguish critical events in oncogenesis separate from the nutritional and hormonal status of the host. Ultimately many of the characteristics of the neoplastic phenotype will be attributed to changes in the genome (Pardee, 1982).

As early as the 1920s, when modern biochemistry was emerging, neoplastic cells were removed from the animal or the patient and brought to the laboratory, where attempts were made to cultivate them (in vitro cell culture studies). These neoplastic cells then were examined with respect to their phenotypic properties. Attempts were also made to sequence the changes characteristic of the neoplastic process. However, these cells already had a long "malignant history" (Alberts et al., 1983; Pardee, 1982; Pitot, 1986; Ruddon, 1981; Watson et al., 1987).

To overcome these problems, and in an attempt to study the earliest stages of oncogenesis, normal cells were established in culture (cell lines) and then exposed to carcinogens (chemicals, viruses, or radiation). These cultured cells subsequently developed characteristics of malignant cells; this process was termed *transformation*. Because these cells are not derived from a tumor in an human or an animal, they are termed transformed rather than malignant cells (Box 13–1) (Alberts et al., 1983; Pardee, 1982; Pitot, 1986; Ruddon, 1981; Watson et al., 1987).

Methodological problems also exist when studying carcinogenesis and the neoplastic phenotype via transformation. Criteria were established to help ensure that what was happening in culture (in vitro) was similar to the neoplastic process in vivo. One of the main criteria is the ability of transformed cells to establish a tumor in an appropriate animal model. The putatively transformed cells are injected into an animal, and if a tumor results, then transformation is said to have occurred. However, this definitive experiment is not always done because of the expense and time commitment. Thus some of the reported examples of phenotypic changes may not be exclusively associated with neoplastic phenotype but rather are correlated with normal cell division (Alberts et al., 1983; Pardee, 1982; Pitot, 1986; Ruddon, 1981; Watson et al., 1987).

Characteristics of Transformed Cells

The physically obvious features of size, shape, and orientation, and the growth characteristics of trans-

Table 13–2. SELECTED EXAMPLES OF BENIGN AND MALIGNANT TUMORS

Tissue of Origin	Benign Tumors	Malignant Tumors
Epithelial		
Glandular	Adenoma	Adenocarcinoma
Epithelial	Polyp, papilloma	Carcinoma
Connective		
Bone	Osteoma	Osteosarcoma
Fibrous	Fibroma	Fibrosarcoma
Fat	Lipoma	Liposarcoma
Smooth muscle	Leiomyoma	Leiomyosarcoma
Striated muscle	Rhabdomyoma	Rhabdomyosarcoma
Hematopoietic		
Erythrocytes		Erythroleukemia
Lymphocytes		Lymphocytic leukemia
Lymphatic tissue		Malignant lymphoma, Hodgkin's disease
Plasma cell		Multiple myeloma
Pigmented cells	Nevus	Melanoma
Neural	Neuroma	Glioblastoma

Normal cells transferred from the animal into tissue culture undergo only a fixed number of divisions. For instance, skin cells will undergo approximately 50 to 100 divisions before the culture dies out.

From a *culture* of normal cells, some cells arise that can undergo repeated divisions. Once this process becomes established the culture is called a *cell line*. Even though this cell line is *immortal*, it does not have other biologic characteristics of a true malignancy. One of the easiest cell lines to establish in culture is the fibroblast. Much of the original transformation work was done on fibroblasts even though tumors of this cell type are very rare in humans (Alberts et al., 1983; Pardee, 1982; Pitot, 1986; Ruddon, 1981; Watson et al., 1987).

Transformed cells are cells derived from established cell lines and are essentially immortal (i.e., they can undergo repeated cell divisions). These lines can be kept in culture for years without dying if the proper culture conditions are maintained. They also have cytoplasmic and nuclear characteristics of malignant cells (Alberts et al., 1983; Pardee, 1982; Pitot, 1986; Ruddon, 1981; Watson et al., 1987).

formed cells, distinguish them from normal cell lines (Fig. 13–4; see also Chapter 14, Fig. 14–1). Transformed cells in culture have basophilic cytoplasm, irregular cellular outlines, and large nuclei that contain multiple nucleoli. Mitotic figures are more numerous in transformed cell lines than in a normal cell line. In addition, transformed cells differ from normal cells in such important characteristics as mobility and growth requirements (Alberts et al., 1983; Pardee, 1982; Pitot, 1986; Ruddon, 1981; Watson et al., 1987).

The Cell Surface

The study of the cytoplasmic membrane adds an important dimension in the study of transformation because (1) loss of contact inhibition is linked to changes in the cell surface; (2) establishment of metastatic deposits depends on the ability of the tumor cells

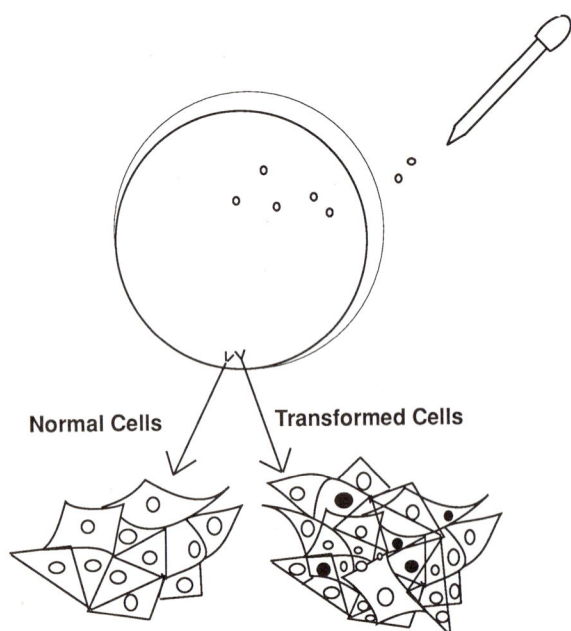

Figure 13–4. A schematic representation of normal cells in culture and transformed cells in culture. Cells are deposited onto a Petri dish containing suitable growth media. Normal cells exhibit contact inhibition. Transformed cells are more diverse with respect to their cytoplasmic and nuclear characteristics; they can form multilayers, and they lack contact inhibition.

to invade and move; (3) hormones and growth factors often act at the surface, and tumor cells often lose the ability to be regulated by these factors; and (4) it is at the surface that the immune system will or will not recognize the cell as altered (Nicolson & Poste, 1974; Pitot, 1986; Ruddon, 1981).

The cytoplasmic membrane is the interface between the cell and the extracellular medium. It consists of lipids (phospholipids), proteins, and carbohydrates bound to either the lipid or the protein components. The bilipid layer of the membrane is capable of movement. Molecules in the membrane can move or rearrange themselves. Tumor cells have a greater fluidity, perhaps owing to changes in the lipid composition. This property of malignant cells may in the future be exploited by the packaging of chemotheraputic agents into liposomes. These liposomes (spheres with an outer lipid layer and an internal core of drugs) are more readily taken up by the malignant cell membrane than by the normal cell membrane. Thus the malignant cells would receive a greater dosage of the chemotherapeutic agent than normal cells (Nicolson & Poste, 1974; Pardee, 1982; Ruddon, 1981).

The plasma membrane proteins are involved in transport of metabolites, as receptors, and in enzymatic activity. Some of the proteins are located at the surface, others span the whole bilipid leaflet layer, and some of these integral membrane proteins are linked to the cytoplasmic skeletal structures (see Chapter 14, Fig. 14–1). These skeletal structures, such as microtubules and microfilaments, give structure, shape, and rigidity to the cell. Some proteins serve as receptors for hormones, growth factors, and antibodies (Nicolson & Poste, 1974; Pardee, 1982; Pitot, 1986; Ruddon, 1981). It is estimated that a single cell could have 100,000 or more specific membrane receptors (Pardee, 1982).

Proteins can transport ions and metabolites across the osmotic barrier of the cytoplasic membrane. Transformed cells often have higher transport activities than normal cells; for instance, some sugars and amino acids are transported into the cell at a faster rate. Higher transport activities in turn may alter the ratios of cyclic nucleotides in the cytoplasm. These nucleotides serve as intracellular messages altering the metabolic state of the cells and perhaps DNA synthesis. If transformed cells are treated in vitro with protease inhibitors, their surface properties temporarily revert towards a normal phenotype (Pardee, 1982; Pitot, 1986; Ruddon, 1981; Watson et al., 1987).

The cell surfaces of transformed cells will often contain new antigens not present in the normal cell type. Some of these antigens are called tumor-associated antigens in animal models; in human cells they are oncofetal antigens, viral antigens, or tumor-associated molecules. Two examples of oncofetal antigens used in monitoring patients are carcinoembryonic antigen and alpha-fetoprotein. Other antigens, or surface molecules, are absent in transformed cells. It has been proposed that the loss or shedding of tumor antigens or antigen-antibody complexes might form blocking factors and prevent the immune cells or molecules from attaching to malignant cells (Nicolson & Poste, 1974; Pitot, 1986; Ruddon, 1981; Watson et al., 1987).

Cytoplasmic Structures

Much has been written about the differences in the cytoplasmic structures and metabolic processes of transformed cells and their normal counterparts. In addition, as in the case of the cytoplasmic membrane, it is not clear at this point which changes are a result of transformation and which initiate transformation. To ask the question in another way, at which stage of oncogenesis do these events occur? With our increased understanding of oncogenes, the sequence of cytoplasmic and nuclear events is being unraveled.

The mitochondrial changes and the intermediary metabolism of glucose were among the first cellular systems to be investigated, starting with Warburg's work in the 1920s and 1930s. Warburg developed an elaborate hypothesis of carcinogenesis based on the observation that malignant cells utilized anaerobic glycolysis to a greater extent than normal cells (i.e., malignant cells consumed less oxygen and produced more lactic acid than normal cells). Warburg proposed that carcinogens poisoned the mitochondria, allowing the more primitive cells (those with fewer mitochondria) to survive. Mitochondria generate adenosine triphosphate (ATP) via oxidative phosphorylation. Because the more primitive cells could survive in oxygen-poor environments, Warburg contended that it was from this population that malignant cells arose (Pardee, 1982; Pitot, 1986; Watson et al., 1987). His observations still stand today. However, the present theoretical framework is very different. Currently the interpretation would be that tumor cells survive in oxygen-poor environments because of oncogenesis rather than the lack of oxygen being the initiator. It must be remembered that during Warburg's time it was not known which molecules in the cell were the repository of genetic information, and therefore his reasoning was logical. With the rapid increase in knowledge of oncogenesis today, how many current ideas will be rejected even 5 years from now?

Warburg's hypothesis is given here as an example of cytoplasmic changes in transformation. But for every cytoplasmic structure and metabolic pathway, a similar story holds:

1. When the phenomenon is first investigated it seems to hold for all the cases investigated. As more experiments are done, exceptions are found, owing to the extreme heterogeneity of neoplasms.

2. It is difficult to determine which alterations in the cytoplasm and cell membrane are primary and which are secondary events in transformation.

Contact Inhibition

Normal cell lines in culture exhibit a property known as contact inhibition. That is, when a cell line is plated onto a Petri dish, the cells will keep growing and dividing until the bottom of the dish is covered with cells, and then division stops. This monolayer of cells will orient themselves with respect to one another. Transformed cells, on the other hand, do not stop dividing. Instead, they move over and pile on top of one another until a multilayered culture is formed (see Fig. 13–4). This lack of contact inhibition is thought to be the result of two independent properties of the cell, mobility and replication (Pardee, 1982; Pitot, 1986; Ruddon, 1981; Watson et al., 1987).

First, transformed cells are more mobile and do not adhere to other cells as well as do normal cells. This property is linked to changes in the plasma membrane of the transformed cell as well as to alteration in the cytoplasmic skeletal elements. Normal cells, however, will form tight junctions and other areas of close contact with cells of their own type.

Second, as already noted, transformed cells do not stop dividing and therefore grow to a high density in culture. Because contact inhibition may be the result of either property, the term *density-dependent inhibition of growth* is now considered the more precise term. This ability to grow in conditions unfavorable to normal cell lines often signals when transformation has occurred.

Growth Requirements

The environment provided for the cell cultures determines the success of establishing cell lines. As knowledge of the conditions necessary for cell growth has accumulated, more and different types of cell lines have become cultured. The first lines that were established were mainly those of fibroblasts (cells from the connective tissue), and most of the experiments on transformation used these cell lines (Pardee, 1982; Pitot, 1986; Ruddon, 1981; Watson et al., 1987). The conditions necessary for epithelial lines have now been identified (Fusenig et al., 1982; Montesano et al., 1980). This means that understanding of epithelial transformation can begin, and the results will, it is hoped, be applicable to human tumors. Most human tumors are epithelial tumors—carcinomas—rather than sarcomas.

Most cell lines require a rigid substrate on which to grow; this requirement is known as substrate dependency. Fibroblasts, for example, can proliferate in plastic Petri dishes. Other cell lines, particularly those derived from epithelial tissue, require that the surface of the Petri dish be conditioned. Sometimes a layer of "feeder cells" is first plated onto the Petri dish, which allows the more fastidious cells to grow in culture. Transformed cells often do not have this requirement; in fact, they can grow in soft agar (Pardee, 1982; Pitot, 1986; Ruddon, 1981; Watson et al., 1987). In one study, the ability to induce a tumor in an animal was associated, 94 per cent of the time, with the ability to grow in soft agar (Montesano et al., 1977).

Adequate nutrients are also necessary for cell growth to occur. Besides the usual requirements, such as an energy source, normal cell lines require the addition of serum to the nutrient bath. Fetal calf serum, which is often added to the medium, contains many complex substances, among which are polypeptide growth factors, pituitary hormones, insulin, epidermal growth factor, vitamins, minerals, and a variety of other substances, some of which have not been characterized. These substances must be present to stimulate and support cell replication. Transformed cells often can be grown in culture in the absence of serum or in the presence of reduced amounts of serum (Pardee, 1982; Pitot, 1986; Ruddon, 1981; Watson et al., 1987).

Autocrine Growth Factors

The process by which transformed cells became autonomous of growth factors present in serum was conceptualized as autocrine secretion. This hypothesis came into prominence because it linked the new data generated by oncogene research and the molecular biology studies of transformation and growth factors (Kahn & Graf, 1986; Sachs, 1987; Sporn & Roberts, 1985; Waterfield, 1986).

In normal cells, binding of growth factors to membrane receptors initiates a cascade of metabolic events that ultimately leads to cell division. Three mechanisms have been proposed to explain the transduction of the signal from the surface membrane to cytoplasmic and nuclear molecules. The first is the activation of protein kinases, which generate cyclic nucleotides such as cyclic adenosine monophosphate (cAMP) and cyclic guanosine monophosphate (cGMP). The second involves endocytosis (engulfing and incorporation) of the complexed hormone and receptor. The third mechanism involves the influx into the cytoplasm of small ions such as calcium and magnesium. These mechanisms then often act at the genetic level, perhaps regulating DNA synthesis and stimulating mitosis (Alberts et al., 1983; Watson et al., 1987).

Malignant and transformed cells are known to have surface receptors for growth factors as well as the ability to release growth factors. This discovery led to the hypothesis of autostimulation (Fig. 13–5). A variety of mechanisms were proposed by which malignant cells could become independent of growth factors, and there is some evidence for all of them. These mechanisms include the following:

1. Manufacture by the transformed cell of its own growth factors.
2. Reduction in the amount of growth factor necessary for division.
3. Alteration of the growth factor receptor, as by
   a. increase in the number of receptors
   b. increase in the receptor affinity for the growth factor
   c. production of a defective receptor that will signal the cytoplasmic events without first binding to a growth factor.
4. Alteration of the receptor signaling pathway (second messenger). (Kahn & Graf, 1986; Sporn & Roberts, 1985; Waterfield, 1986; Watson et al., 1987).

Sporn and Roberts (1985) have broadened the concept of autocrine growth factors to embrace both positive and negative factors. Type b transforming growth factor (TGF-b) is a potent inhibitor of division in many cells, including normal, neoplastic, fibroblastic, and epithelial. For instance, when confluent monkey kidney cells produce TGF-b, cells in the culture stop dividing. Perhaps this is an example of a growth inhibitory substance. (In other systems, however, TGF-b has stimulated cell division. It appears that the relationship is not a simple one and that ultimately the effect of TGF-b will be the result of the concentration of several growth factors.) Sporn and Roberts (1985) then explain the independence from growth factors in neoplasia as either a result of positive autocrine stimulation or a release from the inhibitory control (Kimchi, Wang, Weinberg, Cheifetz, & Massague, 1988; Sporn & Roberts, 1985; Waterfield, 1986).

GENETIC CHANGES IN CANCER CELLS

Cancer is recognized and diagnosed by the phenotypic, functional, and growth requirement changes in cells. However, the evidence is strong that these phenotypic alterations, and other changes, result from a change in the genetic information of the cell. One of the simplest lines of evidence is that daughter cells of malignant cells inherit the malignant phenotype. Human malignant cells transplanted into a "permissive" animal (an animal that will not reject the transplanted cells, such as the nude mouse) will grow and divide and continue to exhibit their malignant characteristics.

In broad terms, there are three major methods for studying the genome of the organism. The first is descriptive, that is, studying the inheritance patterns from one generation to the next, such as in family inheritance studies. This method involves classic mendelian genetics. The second method consists of basic descriptive biologic studies of the chromosomes, which investigate the genes involved in growth and differentiation of the cell, mutations, and epigenetic phenomena. The third type of evidence is experimental, in which specific single gene changes are induced and the development of a malignancy occurs. Therefore, genetic changes are studied from multiple perspectives, including familial, epidemiologic, chromosomal, and oncogenic. All of these areas of research give a slightly different perspective on the linkage of genetic changes with malignancy.

What is exciting about current scientific develop-

A

Cell C

Growth
Factor

Growth
Factor
Receptor

Division

Cell D

Cell D

Cell D

Cell D

B

Cell D

Growth
Factor

Growth
Factor
Receptor

Division

Cell D

Cell D

Cell D

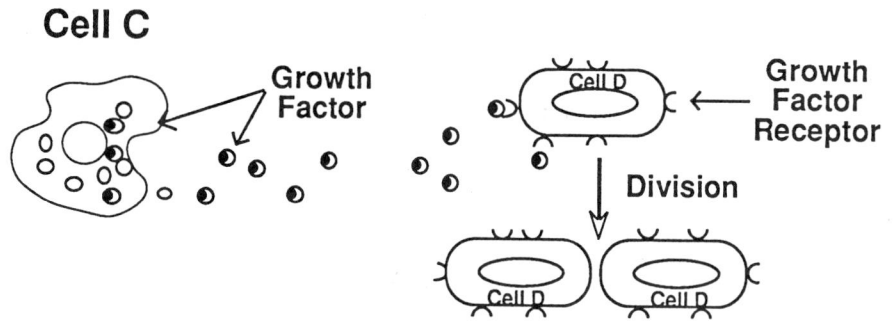

Figure 13–5. *A,* In normal tissues, growth factors are produced by one cell type (cell C) that stimulates division in another cell type (cell D). *B,* In autostimulation, the same cell type produces both the growth factor and the growth factor receptor.

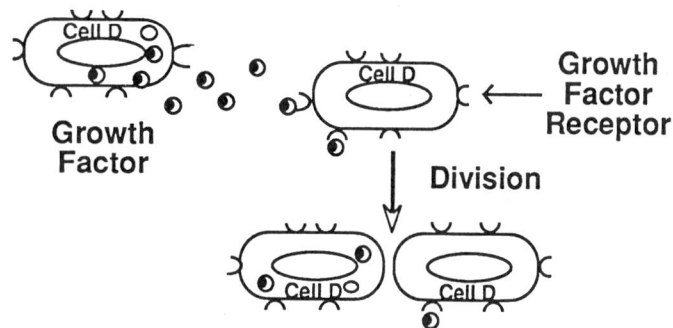

ments is the convergence of these various lines of evidence into a more coherent picture. Familial disorders are being linked to specific chromosomal defects, chromosomal defects to oncogenes and antioncogenes, and these genes, in turn, to the molecular events that occur in carcinogenesis (Leppert et al., 1987). Thus the evidence garnered in one field is being extended and confirmed by entirely different lines of research.

Hereditary Cancers

"Cancer families" were described as early as 1913 (Warthin, 1913). In these extremely rare families, cancer is inherited in an autosomal dominant fashion. In familial polyposis coli (FPC), family members have a very high risk of developing colon cancer (Anderson, 1982; Cannon-Albright, Skolnick, Bishop, Lee, & Burt, 1988; Heim & Metelman, 1987; Meisner, 1983; Vogelstein et al., 1988). The probability of developing colon cancer is 80 per cent by the time the person reaches the age of 40 years unless preventive treatment is initiated. Two other examples are Gardner's syndrome and basal cell nevus syndrome. It is critical that members of families with these diseases be followed, that they be examined periodically, and that prophylactic surgery or therapy be initiated before an advanced malignancy develops (Anderson, 1982; Meisner, 1983).

Other families appear to have an increased risk of cancer, but the inheritence pattern is suggestive of a strong familial tendency rather than a simple autosomal dominancy. One example of this type is premenopausal breast cancer. Daughters of mothers with bilateral premenopausal breast disease have close to a 50 per cent probability of developing the disease themselves (Anderson, 1982). Other examples include Bloom's syndrome, Fanconi's anemia, and xeroderma pigmentosum. In xeroderma pigmentosum, the gene that repairs DNA damage created by ultraviolet light is defective. This syndrome is an example of how a gene defect interacts with environmental factors, such as sun exposure, to increase the risk for cancer. Individuals with xeroderma pigmentosum have an increased risk for developing basal and squamous cell cancers of the skin (Anderson, 1982; Meisner, 1983; Pitot, 1986).

Characteristic patterns in families with increased risk for the development of cancer include the following:

1. Diagnosis of the cancer in these families occurs at an earlier age than in the general population (for example, premenopausal versus postmenopausal breast cancer). In addition, a diagnosis of colon cancer in the patient's thirties is indictive of a familial tendency, because the incidence of this cancer rises dramatically in the forties for the general population.

2. For the individual family member, there is increased risk of having a primary cancer in both sites in bilateral tissues such as the breast. In organs such as the gut there is an increased risk for having multiple primary sites.

3. In some of the hereditary cancer syndromes, there is a higher incidence of second primaries in other

organs. In familial polyposis coli, an increased incidence occurs for breast and endometrial cancer (Anderson, 1982; Meisner, 1983).

Chromosomal Studies: Congenital and Noncongenital

As early as 1914, chromosomal abnormalities of tumor cells have been known. At that time Boveri put forth the hypothesis that chromosomal abnormalities were involved in the transition of the cell from normal to malignant (Heim & Mitelman, 1987; Pitot, 1986). Modern studies of karyotypic changes with malignancy had to wait for technical developments in the study of mammalian chromosomes (cytogenetic studies). Not until 1956 was the correct chromosomal number for humans reported by Tjio and Levan (Heim & Mitelman, 1987).

The association of malignant conditions with congenital chromosomal syndromes also advanced the hypothesis that genomic changes may be involved in the development of tumors. For example, persons with Down's syndrome are at an increased risk for developing leukemia, and people with Klinefelter's syndrome (XXY karyotype) have an increased risk of developing breast cancer (Alberts et al., 1983; Meisner, 1983).

The first specific karyotypic change found to be associated with a malignancy was the description of the Philadelphia chromosome in patients with chronic myeloid leukemia, by Nowell and Hungerford (1960). However, not until 1973 was the exact chromosomal aberration responsible for the Philadelphia chromosome described (Rowley, 1973). This finding was the result of better imagining techniques (banding techniques) that enabled abnormalities within the chromosome itself to be visualized. Up to this time, only very large aberrations in the chromosomes and changes in absolute numbers of chromosomes were identifiable (Heim & Mitelman, 1987).

The Philadelphia chromosome results from the translocation of material from chromosome 22 to the long part of the arm of chromosome 9. This is represented by the abbreviation t(9;22). During the natural history of chronic myeloid leukemia, other chromosomal changes occur. These other chromosomal changes are secondary aberrations, associated with the progression of the disease from its chronic phase to its accelerated and blast phases. As the tumor progresses in the patient, these secondary chromosomal aberrations probably give the new clone of cells growth advantages, resulting in a new clinical phase. In the blast phase, on the average, three additional chromosomal changes can be identified in addition to the Philadelphia chromosome (Heim & Mitelman, 1987; Kurzrock, Gutterman, & Talpaz, 1988).

Oncogenes have been localized to the sites of translocation in the Philadelphia chromosome (chromosomes 9 and 22). The human oncogene similar to the mouse oncogene, Abelson murine leukemia virus oncogene *(c-abl)*, is located in the area of the break in chromosome 9; the human homologue, simian sarcoma virus *(c-sis)*, is located at the break of chromosome 22. The evidence is accumulating that the alteration in chromosome 9 is the important pathogenic event in leukemogenesis. When the gene from the break in chromosome 9 is positioned at the breakpoint in chromosome 22, a new hybrid gene is formed (Heim & Mitelman, 1987; Kurzrock et al., 1988).

Chronic myelogenous leukemia is one of the best known cancers in terms of cytogenetic changes that have been studied. In general, knowledge of cytogenetics is more advanced for the leukemias and lymphomas, and, in comparison, very little is known about the solid tumors. Approximately 20 different chromosomal structural abnormalities have been described for the seven subtypes of acute nonlymphocytic leukemia. In Burkitt's lymphoma, translocation between chromosomes 8 and 14 occurs in 75 to 85 per cent of all patients, including those with the African and nonendemic tumor types (Heim & Mitelman, 1987).

The cytogenic changes in solid tumors appear to be more complex and numerous than those in the leukemias and lymphomas. This may be due to the advanced nature of the solid tumor when studied. Often studies were done on metastatic lesions or cells isolated from effusions. But even with these types of tumors, there are nonrandom chromosomal abnormalities (which means the changes can be identified and studied); and the more advanced the tumor, the more numerous the cytogenetic abnormalities (Heim & Mitelman, 1987).

Oncogenic Studies: Studies at the Single Gene Level

In general three main types of genes are involved in the development of the malignant phenotype (Klein & Klein, 1985). The first type is the oncogene, which actively induces the development of a tumor or transformation in cell culture. The second type is the antioncogene, the loss or the inactivity of which permits the development of a tumor. Most of the evidence for these genes derives from the study of heritable forms of cancer, such as retinoblastoma. The third type is the modulating genes that are involved in the modification of tumor-host interactions and therefore involved in tumor progression. Because single genes cannot be visualized even by the most sensitive chromosomal banding techniques, transformation studies are used to detect the presence of a gene or an altered form of the gene (Heim & Mitelman, 1987; Kahn & Graf, 1986; Klein & Klein, 1985; Nowell, 1988; Pitot, 1986; Teich, 1986; Watson et al., 1987).

Oncogenes

Oncogenes are studied by introducing a gene into cells growing in culture and noting whether the cells then undergo transformation. The genes causing the transformation can be obtained from two sources, tumor viruses or malignant cells. More than 30 oncogenes have been identified and have provided a great deal of evidence that the critical event in carcinogenesis is a genetic change (Table 13–3).

Oncogenes were first studied in the retroviruses. These viruses can induce the formation of multiple tumors in infected animals and transform cells in culture. The genetic material of retroviruses is RNA, and once inside a cell the viral RNA is used as a template to form viral DNA. The viral DNA can then induce the formation of more viral particles or become incorporated into the host's genetic material and remain latent. While studying the genes of these viruses, it became possible to separate the gene that caused transformation from the viral genes. The oncogene could by itself induce transformation, and the viral genes without the oncogene could produce infective viral particles (Klein & Klein, 1985; Nowell, 1988; Pitot, 1986; Teich, 1986).

In 1976 Stehelin, Varmus, Bishop, and Vogt discovered that viral oncogenes were very similar, if not identical, to normal cellular genes. These cellular genes were termed *cellular oncogenes (c-onc)* or proto-oncogenes. It appears that at some point in its evolutionary history, the retrovirus captured the cellular oncogene and incorporated it into viral genome. The oncogene, it was thought, conferred an advantage to the virus, and therefore the oncogene was conserved in the viral genome and could be found in the infected cell.

Cellular oncogenes were found in every species that has been studied. Indeed, the structure of cellular oncogenes has been found to be similar no matter where found, from mammalian cells to yeast cells to fruit fly cells. This evolutionary conservation means that these genes are very important and probably serve an essential function in the cell. Cellular oncogenes are likely to be the regulators of normal proliferation and differentiation during embryogenesis, growth, and wound healing. In this sense, the term oncogene does not adequately describe the function of these genes but rather describes how they were first investigated (Heim & Mitelman, 1987; Kahn & Graf, 1986; Nowell, 1988; Teich, 1986; Watson et al., 1987).

The other method used to study or "see" oncogenes is termed *transfection*. In this technique, DNA from malignant cells, either human or experimentally induced tumors, is introduced into normal cultured cells.

Some of these recipient cells will then undergo transformation and acquire a malignant phenotype (Bar-Sagi & Feramisco, 1986; Gebhardt & Foulkes, 1986; Hanafusa, 1986; Watson, Tooze, & Kurtz, 1983). The gene that caused the transformation is then cloned and analyzed. Murray and colleagues (1981) and Krontiris and Cooper (1981) reported that DNA from bladder cancer induced transformation. Later this gene turned out to be the homologue of the viral oncogene *ras* (murine sarcoma virus).

How do oncogenes differ from their normal cellular counterparts—that is, if they do? Theoretically, two major mechanisms can be responsible for the activation of oncogenes. The first involves the *regulation* of the gene and the second the *alteration of the structure* of the gene itself. Oncogenes, like all other genes, are regulated, and the decoupling of the regulation of the oncogene could result in overexpression of the gene. This probably occurs in the *c-myc* gene in Burkitt's lymphoma, in which there appears to be a physical uncoupling of the gene from its regulator. Another process, called *gene amplification*, occurs when multiple copies of the gene are made; this could also lead to overexpression of the oncogene. For some oncogenes, it appears that a mutation (structural change) has occurred. Therefore, the oncogene differs from its normal counterpart by one or more DNA bases. This seems to be the case with the *ras* oncogene. In addition, major structural changes are seen in other oncogenes such as the *abl* gene in chronic myeloid leukemia (Heim & Mitelman, 1987; Kahn & Graf, 1986; Klein & Klein, 1985; Nowell, 1988; Pitot, 1986; Teich, 1986; Watson et al., 1987).

However, it is likely that activation of the oncogene in a cell is *necessary* but *not sufficient* to trigger the development of a malignant phenotype. One of the requirements needed to induce transformation or a malignancy is the activation of the oncogene in a particular cell type. In addition, the cell probably must be in a particular state of differentiation, otherwise activation will be of no consequence. Because carcinogenesis involves multiple steps, a particular oncogene probably is responsible for only one of several necessary genetic changes (Heim & Mitelman, 1987; Kahn & Graf, 1986; Klein & Klein, 1985; Nowell, 1988; Pitot, 1986; Teich, 1986; Watson et al., 1987).

How do oncogenes contribute to carcinogenesis? The answer to this question cannot be stated satisfactorily at this time. The function of the cellular (normal) oncogenes is not adequately understood, so that the role of oncogenes can only be hypothesized. What is known is that (1) families of oncogenes exist, and the actions of one family will be different from those of the others; (2) growth factors, receptors for growth factors, the transduction of the growth factor signal, and inhibition of the growth factor signals are all major candidates for the primary mechanisms of carcinogenesis; (3) carcinogenesis may involve the sequential activation of oncogenes—that is, the activation of more than one oncogene may be necessary to induce a malignancy; and (4) many oncogenes are located at chromosomal breakpoints (Kahn & Graf, 1986; Schlessinger, 1986; Schwab, 1986).

Table 13–3. EXAMPLES OF ONCOGENES, THEIR ORIGINS, AND THE CHROMOSOME(S) ON WHICH THEY ARE LOCATED

Oncogene	Origin*	Chromosome(s)
abl	Abelson murine leukemia	9
erbB	Avian erythroblastosis	7
fms	Feline sarcoma	5
met	Human osteosarcoma	3
myc	Avian myelocytomatosis	8
L-myc	Human lung carcinoma	1
N-myc	Human neuroblastoma	2
ras	Murine sarcoma (several types)	6, 11, 12
N-ras	Human neuroblastoma	1
sis	Simian sarcoma	22

*Virally induced tumor or the tumor in which the oncogene was discovered.

For instance, the oncogene *v-src* (Rous sarcoma virus) codes for a tyrosine kinase. A tyrosine kinase is found at the epidermal growth factor receptor and is involved in the transmission of the signal resulting from the binding of the factor to its receptor. In turn, epidermal growth factor is a powerful mitogen for fibroblasts in culture. This type of evidence suggests that an altered cellular oncogene results in a disturbed pathway for growth signals, which then results in uncontrolled cellular division (Kahn & Graf, 1986; Schlessinger, 1986; Schwab, 1986). Five of the oncogenes of the *ras* family (which codes for serine-threonine or tryosine kinase) were found to be efficient in inducing the metastatic phenotype (Egan et al., 1987; Marshall, 1986). These genes—*mos, raf, src, fes,* and *fms*—were introduced into a fibroblast cell line, and the resulting transformed cells were then injected into nude mice. Metastatic lesions arose in the lungs (Egan et al., 1987).

The viral oncogene *erbB* is a mutation of the gene coding for the epidermal growth factor receptor, and the *v-fms* (from the feline sarcoma virus) codes for an altered receptor to macrophage colony-stimulating factor. The *sis* oncogene of simian sarcoma virus codes for the β chain of platelet-derived growth factor, which also is a potent mitogen of fibroblasts (Heldin & Westermark, 1986). In this case, the *sis* oncogene may allow the cells to produce their own growth factor, and this results in autocrine stimulation. The function of other oncogenes, however, is not known, but new studies are being published weekly (Heldin & Westermark, 1986).

Antioncogenes

Antioncogenes have also been termed *recessive cancer genes* and *tumor suppressor genes*. They were first discovered in hereditary cancers, notably in hereditary retinoblastoma. The significant cytogenetic change appears to be the loss (deletion) of a gene from each of a pair of chromosomes. In hereditary retinoblastoma the deletion occurs in both copies of chromosomes 13. (Up to this point in the discussion of cytogenetics the focus was on only one gene in one of the chromosomes of a pair.) The term antioncogene does not imply that this gene inhibits an oncogene, because the functional role of antioncogenes is not yet known. Even less is known about the gene products of the antioncogenes than about those of the oncogenes. Antioncogenes involve gene deletion or inactivation, as compared with oncogenes, which are involved in gene activation (Friend, Dryja, & Weinberg, 1988; Knudson, 1985; Wyke & Green, 1986).

In hereditary retinoblastoma, both copies of the antioncogene (both alleles) are absent; therefore, the development of this malignant tumor in genetic terminology is named recessive. The existence of only one of the antioncogenes would prevent the tumor. (That is, the antitumor state of the cell is the dominant state.) Knudson first hypothesized this in 1971 with his two-step model of carcinogenesis (Knudson, 1983, 1985, 1987).

In the Knudson model, the first step in carcinogenesis in persons with hereditary cancer occurred in the germ line of cells. Therefore, this defect is present in all the cells of the body at birth. The second step (the second mutation, or second deletion) then occurs in the somatic cell, and only when this second genetic change occurs does the malignant phenotype develop in the cell and in each of the daughter cells. Because the first genetic change is present in all cells of the body, there is a greater likelihood for multiple primaries. In nonhereditary cancers, both genetic changes must occur in the somatic cells, so these cancers appear later in life in comparison to the hereditary forms, and there is less chance for multiple primaries to occur (Knudson, 1972, 1983, 1985, 1987).

Chromosomal deletions were detected in kidney carcinoma, small-cell lung cancer, meningioma, retinoblastoma, and familial polyposis coli. It may be that the loss of antioncogenes is more important in carcinogenesis than it is in leukemogenesis. Evidence for the deletion of the retinoblastoma gene has also been detected in small-cell lung cancer but not in other types of lung cancers (Harbour et al., 1988). Both retinoblastoma and small-cell lung cancer are derived from cells of neuroendocrine origin. Perhaps similar patterns of genetic changes, whether involving oncogenes or antioncogenes, will be identified with related groups of cancers. This will then change the current view of cancer as consisting of hundreds of different diseases to one of groups of cancers with similar genetic and molecular pathogenesis.

Transgenic Mice or Gene Studies at the Whole Organism Level

As discussed earlier, studies of transformation have certain advantages over the study of carcinogenesis in animals. Yet the question always arises, Are studies of cells in culture relevant to carcinogenesis in animals or humans? The development of transgenic mice is a bridge between these two types of experimental orientations.

Transgenic mice are defined as "mice in which the genome of each cell contains specific DNA sequences that were introduced experimentally during early embryogenesis" (Hanahan, 1986, p. 348). Genes, such as oncogenes, are injected into the pronuclei of fertilized eggs of mice. Usually the pronucleus of the male (sperm) is used because this pronucleus is larger than the female pronucleus. The injected gene integrates into the egg genome. The eggs then are implanted into a pseudopregnant mouse, and approximately 20 per cent of the mice born will express the injected oncogene (Fig. 13–6). The second and third generations of these mice may also inherit the injected gene, if the oncogene was incorporated into the germ line cells (eggs and sperm). Therefore, clones of animals can be developed that express the oncogene(s) of interest (Hanahan, 1986).

The oncogenes that are transferred can be either the "natural" oncogene with its normal regulatory com-

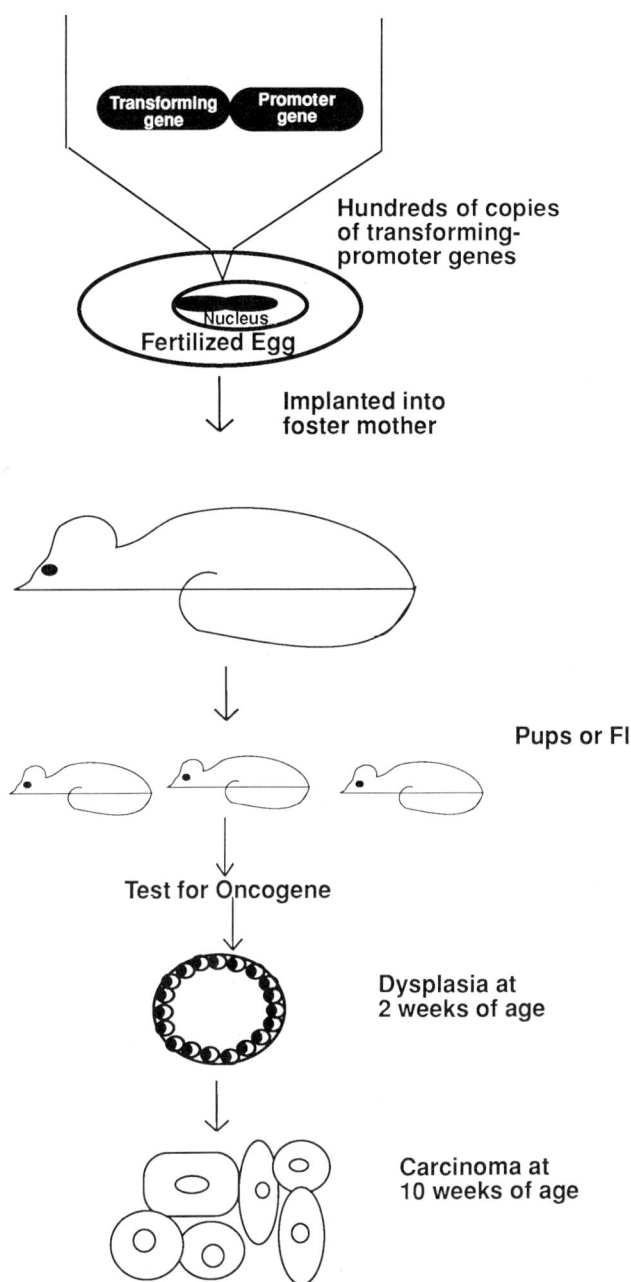

Figure 13–6. In transgenic mice, hundreds of copies of the transforming gene fused to the promoter gene are introduced into the nucleus of the fertilized egg. The fertilized egg is implanted into a pseudopregnant female. A few of the first generation of progeny will contain the oncogene, which then leads to the development of a malignancy.

ponent attached or a hybrid or recombinant oncogene. In the hybrid form, the oncogene is fused to a regulatory component of an unrelated gene (enhancer component). The fusion enhances the potential of the oncogene to be expressed in a specific tissue (Hanahan, 1986).

In one experiment, Ornitz, Hammer, Messing, Palmiter, and Brinster (1987) linked the early genes of the SV-40 virus with the rat elastase gene (enhancer component). The early genes of the simian virus 40 contain the T-antigen genes, which transform cultured cells, reduce contact inhibition, and reduce the serum growth factor requirements (Ornitz et al., 1987). The regulatory component of the rat elastase gene ensures that the acinar (exocrine) cells of the pancreas express the T-antigen genes or oncogenes. Elastase is one of the proteins that is normally produced and released by the acinar cells of the pancreas (Ornitz et al., 1987).

In the resulting strains of mice that expressed the T-antigen gene, the animals who reached 3 months of age developed pancreatic cancer. The natural stages of development of this tumor were followed. The newborn mice had hyperplastic pancreatic acini by the time they were 2 weeks old. At 10 weeks the mice had pancreatic tumor masses. Death from pancreatic cancer occurred between 10 and 23 weeks of age. Metastatic lesions rarely occurred, but seeding of tumor cells into the peritoneal cavity was fairly common (Ornitz et al., 1987).

These investigators demonstrated that, early in life, the acinar cells expressed the T-antigen gene and that the architecture of the tissue was reasonably normal. This was interpreted as the preneoplastic state. When the tumor nodules start to develop, the acinar cells no longer manufacture those proteins that signify a mature or differentiated state and the amount of T-antigen RNA production increased. At this same time, the chromosome numbers in the tumor cells become aneuploid (aneuploidy occurs when the cell has an abnormal number of chromosomes. The number is not a multiple of the haploid or diploid number. An example of aneuploidy occurs when a human cell contains 31 or 61 chromosomes). These investigators suggested that the chromosomal loss results in an alteration of the regulation of growth (Ornitz et al., 1987). The loss may be similar to the loss of antioncogenes in retinoblastoma. The deregulation of growth confers a growth advantage, and numerous tumor nodules are formed in the pancreas.

This experiment exemplifies the current state of the art in understanding the molecular events in the development of tumors. The investigators started with a known gene, then induced its expression in an animal. What resulted in the offspring is a tumor that develops through all the pathologic stages found in human tumors—from hyperplasia to frank carcinoma, from euploid to aneuploid cells. This elegant animal model may help to shed some light on the development of pancreatic tumors, which for humans has a very poor prognosis.

The knowledge of oncogenes, however, has not been translated as quickly into clinical applications. This is probably owing to a lack of understanding of the normal events in differentiation. Probably the first benefits from oncogene research will result in new and better diagnostic tests. For instance, the protein coded by the Philadelphia chromosome is unique and is not manufactured by normal cells. If techniques are developed to identify this as truly a cancer marker (that is, this protein is not made by any normal tissue or in other diseases), the diagnosis of chronic myeloid leukemia will be made easier. Identification of the other unique proteins produced in the different stages of neoplastic progression eventually might lead to new therapeutic approaches for the treatment of cancer. If these therapies are directed at true differences between cancer cells and normal cells, toxicities of cancer therapy might be reduced and the patient would receive the ultimate benefit, a better quality of life.

SUMMARY

Present knowledge of cancer as an abnormality of differentiation is derived from various disciplines and methods (biochemical, histologic, karyotypic). Not all the "facts" from each of these methodologies have been reconciled with one another. Because the molecular biology methods that are currently being used to study cancer are new, large gaps still exist in our knowledge. Currently it is impossible to distinguish all the events between the initiation of carcinogenesis and the development of the metastatic lesion. However, the pace of our understanding of the events of carcinogenesis has quickened at an unprecented rate in the past 10 years. In the same 10 years the hybridoma technique, which made possible the manufacture of monoclonal antibodies, has led to new therapies, which are currently being tested in clinical trials.

References

Alberts, B., Bray, D., Lewis, J., Raff, M., Roberts, K., & Watson, J. D. (1983). *Molecular biology of the cell.* New York: Garland Publishing, Inc.

Anderson, D. E. (1982). Familial predisposition. In D. Schottenfeld & J. Fraumeni (Eds.), *Cancer epidemiology and prevention* (pp. 483–493). Philadelphia: W. B. Saunders Co.

Bar-Sagi, D., & Feramisco, J. R. (1986). Induction of membrane ruffling and fluid-phase pinocytosis in quiescent fibroblast by *ras* protein. *Science, 233,* 1061–1068.

Bonfiglio, T. A., & Terry, R. (1983). The pathology of cancer. In P. Rubin (Ed.), *Clinical oncology: A multidisciplinary approach* (6th ed., pp. 20–29). New York: American Cancer Society.

Cannon-Albright, L. A., Skolnick, M. H., Bishop, T., Lee, R. G., & Burt, R. W. (1988). Common inheritance of susceptibility to colonic adenomatous polyps and associated colorectal cancers. *New England Journal of Medicine,* 319:533–537.

Correa, P. (1982). Morphology and natural history of precursor lesions. In D. Schottenfeld & J. F. Fraumeni (Eds.), *Cancer epidemiology and prevention* (pp. 90–118). Philadelphia: W. B. Saunders Co.

Egan, S. E., Wright, J. A., Jarolim, L., Yanagihara, K., Bassin, R. H., & Greenberg, A. H. (1987). Transformation by oncogenes encoding protein kinases induces the metastatic phenotype. *Science, 238,* 202–205.

Fidler, I. J., & Hart, I. R. (1982). Principles of cancer biology: Biology of cancer metastasis. In V. T. DeVita, S. Hellman, & S. A. Rosenberg (Eds.), *Cancer: Principles and practice of oncology* (pp. 80–92). Philadelphia: J. B. Lippincott Co.

Friend, S. H., Dryja, T. P., & Weinberg, R. A. (1988). Oncogenes and tumor-suppressing genes. *New England Journal of Medicine, 318,* 618–622.

Fusenig, N. E., Breitkreutz, D., Dzarlieva, R. T., Boukamp, P., Herzmann, E., Bohnert, A., Pohlman, J., Rausch, C., Schutz, S., & Hornung, J. (1982). Epidermal cell differentiation and malignant transformation in culture. *Cancer Forum, 6,* 209–240.

Gebhardt, A., & Foulkes, J. G. (1986). Transformation by the *v-abl* oncogene. In P. Kahn & T. Graf (Eds.), *Oncogenes and growth control* (pp. 114–119). New York: Springer-Verlag, Inc.

Goldfarb, S. (1983). Pathology of neoplasia. In S. B. Kahn, R. R.

Love, C. Sherman, & R. Chakrovorty (Eds.), *Concepts in cancer medicine* (pp. 127–142). New York: Grune & Stratton, Inc.

Greaves, M. F. (1986). Biology of human leukaemia. In L. M. Franks & N. M. Teich (Eds.), *Introduction to the cellular and molecular biology of cancer* (pp. 40–62). Oxford: Oxford University Press.

Hanafusa, H. (1986). Activation of the *c-src* gene. In P. Kahn & T. Graf (Eds.), *Oncogenes and growth control* (pp. 100–105). New York: Springer-Verlag, Inc.

Hanahan, D. (1986). Oncogenesis in transgenic mice. In P. Kahn & T. Graf (Eds.), *Oncogenes and growth control* (pp. 349–363). New York: Springer-Verlag, Inc.

Harbour, J. W., Lai, S.-L., Whang-Peng, J., Gazdar, A. F., Minna, J. D., & Kaye, F. J. (1988). Abnormalities in structure and expression of the human retinoblastoma gene in SCLC. *Science, 241,* 353–356.

Hart, I. R. (1986). The spread of tumors. In L. M. Franks, & N. M. Teich (Eds.), *Introduction to the cellular and molecular biology of cancer* (pp. 27–39). Oxford: Oxford University Press.

Heim, S., & Mitelman, F. (1987). *Cancer cytogenetics* (p. 309). New York: Alan R. Liss, Inc.

Heldin, C. H., & Westermark, B. (1986). Role of PDGF-like growth factors in autocrine stimulation of growth of normal and transformed cells. In P. Kahn & T. Graf (Eds.), *Oncogenes and growth control* (pp. 43–50). New York: Springer-Verlag, Inc.

Jimenez, J. J., & Yunis, A. A. (1987). Tumor cell rejection through terminal cell differentiation. *Science, 238,* 1278–1280.

Kahn, P., & Graf, T. (Eds.). (1986). Malignant transformation as a multistep process. In *Oncogenes and growth control* (pp. 292–293). New York: Springer-Verlag, Inc.

Kimchi, A., Wang, X.-F., Weinberg, R. A., Cheifetz, S., & Massagué, J. (1988). Absence of TGF-B receptors and growth inhibitory responses in retinoblastoma cells. *Science, 240,* 196–198.

Klein, G., & Klein, E. (1985). Evolution of tumours and the impact of molecular oncology. *Nature, 315,* 190–195.

Knudson, A. G. (1977). Genetic predisposition to cancer. In H. H. Hiatt, J. D. Watson, & J. A. Wisten (Eds.), *Origins of human cancer. Book A. Incidence of cancer in humans* (pp. 45–54). Cold Spring Harbor, NY: Cold Spring Harbor Laboratory.

Knudson, A. G. (1983). Hereditary cancers of man. *Cancer Investigation, 1,* 187–193.

Knudson, A. G., Jr. (1985). Hereditary cancer, oncogenes and antioncogenes. *Cancer Research, 45,* 1437–1442.

Knudson, A. G., Jr. (1987). A two-mutation model for human cancer. In G. Klein (Ed.), *Advances in viral oncology* (Vol. 7, pp. 1–17). New York: Raven Press.

Krontiris, T. G., & Cooper, G. M. (1981). Transforming activity of human tumor DNA's. *Proceedings of the National Academy of Sciences USA, 78,* 1181–1184.

Kurzrock, R., Gutterman, J. U., & Talpaz, M. (1988). The molecular genetics of Philadelphia chromosome–positive leukemias. *New England Journal of Medicine, 319,* 990–998.

Leppert, M., Dobbs, M., Scambler, P., O'Connell, P., Nakamura, Y., Stauffer, D., Woodward, S., Burt, R., Hughes, J., Gardner, E., Lathrop, M., Wasmuth, J., Lalouel, J.-M., & White, R. (1987). The gene for familial polyposis coli maps to the long arm of chromosome 5. *Science, 238,* 1411–1413.

Marshall, C. J. (1986). The *ras* gene family. In P. Kahn & T. Graf (Eds.), *Oncogenes and growth control* (pp. 192–199). New York: Springer-Verlag, Inc.

Meisner, L. F. (1983). Genetic factors in human cancer. In S. B. Kahn, R. R. Love, C. Sherman, R. Chakrovorty (Eds.), *Concepts in cancer medicine* (pp. 165–176). New York: Grune & Stratton, Inc.

Montesano, R., Bannifkov, G., Drevon, C., Kuroki, T., Saint Vincent, S., & Tomatis, L. (1980). Neoplastic transformation of rat liver epithelial cells in culture. *Annals of the New York Academy of Sciences, 349,* 323–331.

Montesano, R., Drevon, C., Kuroki, T., Saint Vincent, L., Handleman, S., Sanford, K. K., DeFeo, D., & Weinstein, I. B. (1977). Test for malignant transformation of rat liver cells in culture: Cytology, growth in soft agar, and production of plasminogen activator. *Journal of the National Cancer Institute, 59,* 1651.

Murray, M. J., Shilo, B. Z., Shih, C., Cowing, D., Hsu, H. W., & Weinberg, R. A. (1981). Three different human tumor cell lines contain different oncogenes. *Cell, 25,* 355–361.

Nicolson, G. L., & Poste, G. (1974). The cancer cell: Dynamic aspects and modifications in cell-surface organization parts 1 and 2. *New England Journal of Medicine, 295*, 197–203, 253–258.

Nowell, P. C. (1988). Molecular events in tumor development. *New England Journal of Medicine, 319*, 575–577.

Nowell, P. C., & Hungerford, D. (1960). A minute chromosome in human granulocytic leukemia. *Science, 132*:1497.

Oishi, N. (1983). The leukemias. In S. G. Kahn, R. R. Love, C. Sherman, & R. Chakrovorty (Eds.), *Concepts in cancer medicine* (pp. 597–617). New York: Grune & Stratton, Inc.

Ornitz, D. M., Hammer, R. E., Messing, A., Palmiter, R. D., & Brinster, R. L. (1987). Pancreatic neoplasia induced by SV40 T-antigen expression in acinar cells of transgenic mice. *Science, 238*, 188–193.

Pardee, A. B. (1982). Principles of cancer biology: Cell biology and biochemistry of cancer. In V. T. DeVita, S. Hellman, & S. A. Rosenberg (Eds.), *Cancer: Principles and practice of oncology* (pp. 59–72). Philadelphia: J. B. Lippincott Co.

Pitot, H. C. (1986). *Fundamentals of oncology*, (3rd ed., p. 532). New York: Marcel Dekker, Inc.

Rather, L. J. (1978). *The genesis of cancer: A study in the history of ideas* (p. 262). Baltimore: Johns Hopkins University Press.

Rowley, J. D. (1973). A new consistent chromosomal abnormality in chronic myelogenous leukaemia identified by quinacrine fluorescence and Giemsa staining. *Nature, 243*, 290–293.

Ruddon, R. W. (1981). *Cancer biology* (p. 344). New York: Oxford University Press.

Sachs, L. (1987). The molecular control of blood cell development. *Science, 238*, 1374–1379.

Schlessinger, J. (1986). Regulation of cell growth by the EGF receptor. In P. Kahn & T. Graf (Eds.), *Oncogenes and growth control* (pp. 77–84). New York: Springer-Verlag, Inc.

Schwab, M. (1986). Amplification of proto-oncogenes and tumor progression. In P. Kahn & T. Graf (Eds.), *Oncogenes and growth control* (pp. 332–339). New York: Springer-Verlag, Inc.

Sporn, M. B., & Roberts, A. B. (1985). Autocrine growth factors and cancer. *Nature, 313*, 745–747.

Stehelin, D., Varmus, H. E., Bishop, J. M., & Vogt, P. K. (1976). DNA related to the transforming genes(s) of avian sarcoma viruses is present in normal avian DNA. *Nature, 260*, 170–173.

Sukumar, S., Carney, W. P., & Barbacid, M. (1988). Independent molecular pathways in initiation and loss of hormone responsiveness of breast carcinoma. *Science, 240*, 524–526.

Teich, N. M. (1986). Oncogenes and cancer. In L. M. Franks & N. M. Teich (Eds.), *Introduction to the cellular and molecular biology of cancer* (pp. 200–228). Oxford: Oxford University Press.

Vogelstein, B., Fearon, E. R., Hamilton, S. R., Kern, S. E., Preisinger, A. C., Leppert, M., Nakamura, Y., White, R., Smits, A. M. M., & Bos, J. L. (1988). Genetic alterations during colorectal-tumor development. *New England Journal of Medicine, 319*, 525–532.

Warthin, A. S. (1913). Heredity with reference to carcinoma: As shown by the study of the cases examined in the pathological laboratory of the University of Michigan, 1895–1913. *Archives of Internal Medicine, 12*, 546.

Waterfield, M. D. (1986). The role of growth factors in cancer. In L. M. Franks & N. M. Teich (Eds.), *Introduction to the cellular and molecular biology of cancer* (pp. 27–39). Oxford: Oxford University Press.

Watson, J. D., Tooze, J., & Kurtz, D. T. (1983). *Recombinant DNA: A short course* (p. 260). New York: Scientific American Books, W. H. Freeman and Co.

Watson, J. D., Hopkins, N. H., Roberts, J. W., Steitz, J. A., & Weiner, A. M. (1987). *Molecular biology of the gene: Vol. II. Specialized aspects* (4th ed., pp. 747–1163). Menlo Park, CA: The Benjamin/Cummings Publishing Company, Inc.

Wolberg, W. H. (1983). Metastasis. In S. B. Kahn, R. R. Love, C. Sherman, & R. R. Chakrovorty (Eds.), *Concepts in cancer medicine* (pp. 149–156). New York: Grune & Stratton, Inc.

Wyke, J. A., & Green, A. R. (1986). Suppression of the neoplastic phenotype. In P. Kahn & T. Graf (Eds.), *Oncogenes and growth control* (pp. 341–345). New York: Springer-Verlag, Inc.

CHAPTER 14

The Biology of Metastases

SUSAN MOLLOY HUBBARD
LANCE A. LIOTTA

All neoplasms are characterized by a certain degree of autonomy from the host and are detrimental inasmuch as they compete for the nutrients and space required by normal cells. However, because the cells of benign tumors remain encased within a capsular membrane, tissues are generally damaged only when the mass grows large enough to damage vital tissues. Malignant cells are not encapsulated and are characterized by the ability to invade and destroy normal tissues even when microscopic in size. This ability to metastasize is the principal functional characteristic that makes an abnormal cell malignant.

How cancer cells form metastases is one of the most important questions in tumor biology. Current statistics now indicate that existing programs using surgery, radiation, and chemotherapy alone and in combination cure approximately 50 per cent of all patients who develop cancer (Division of Cancer Prevention and Control, 1986). The vast majority of persons who are not cured die from the direct effects of metastases or from complications associated with their treatment. Occult dissemination is often present at diagnosis in these patients and is widespread before evidence of metastases becomes clinically apparent. Although it is generally appreciated that certain tumors have unique patterns of dissemination, it is not possible to predict the metastatic potential of an individual tumor. Even tumors of identical size and histologic type can demonstrate markedly different metastatic patterns.

The development of a metastasis is a dynamic process that occurs as a complex cascade of events whose outcome hinges on anatomic factors, various forces in the host microenvironment, and intrinsic tumor cell properties (Bishop, 1987; Fidler & Balch, 1987; Frost & Fidler, 1986; Lapis, Liotta, & Rabson, 1986; Liotta, 1987, 1989; Liotta & Hart, 1982; Nicolson & Milas,

1984; Schirrmacher, 1985; Sugarbaker, 1981; Weiss, 1976; Welch, Bhuyan, & Liotta, 1986). Disseminated tumor cells that cannot complete all of the steps in the metastatic cascade are eliminated by host defenses. Experimental evidence indicates that less than 0.01 per cent of cancer cells that disseminate actually become established as metastases (Fidler, 1987; Fidler, Gersten, & Riggs, 1977; Liotta, Kleinerman, & Saidel, 1974; Weiss, 1983). Those that do have survived a series of potentially lethal interactions and, therefore, represent a select subpopulation of cells with unique biologic properties that are not shared by all cells within the tumor mass.

Recent advances in molecular and cell biology have led to the identification of biologic properties that influence tumor cell invasion, dissemination, and metastasis formation in experimental systems. These data have provided a theoretical framework for the existence of active cellular and biochemical mechanisms of metastasis. Experimental data on how these mechanisms operate are providing much-needed information on the fundamental properties that enable cells to invade and metastasize. The elucidation of the properties that endow cancer cells with metastatic potential is the principal focus of current research in this area.

CELLULAR PROPERTIES THAT INFLUENCE INVASION AND METASTASIS

Cell Surface Membrane Determinants

Certain intrinsic physicochemical properties appear to be cellular determinants of metastatic potential. Comparisons of normal cells, embryonic cells, and metastatic tumor cells in experimental models have implicated a number of cell surface factors as partial determinants. A key component of the cell surface membrane structure is its lipid bilayer, which allows membrane proteins to move freely. Cell membrane proteins, particularly glycoproteins, function as enzymes, transporters, antigens, and cell membrane receptors (Hakomori, 1973; Hynes, 1987; Liotta & Hart, 1982; Nicolson, 1987; Nicolson & Milas, 1984; Nicolson, Robbins, & Winkelnake, 1975; Poste, 1977). The controlled distribution of these cell surface proteins is a key feature of normal differentiated cells. A cytoskeletal apparatus, comprising membrane-associated microtubules and microfilaments, regulates the distribution of cell surface proteins in the lipid bilayer and holds them in patterns that are recognized by receptors on other cells. A wide variety of cellular feedback mechanisms and recognition systems are mediated by molecules on the cell's surface that either interact with or bind to molecules on adjacent cells. Alterations in the cell surface, depicted in Figure 14–1 and discussed in Chapter 13, are known to develop during neoplastic transformation and are thought to contribute to loss of growth control, increased cell motility, altered patterns of cell recognition, diminished cell cohesion, and the development of cellular and biochemical properties that enable tumor cells to overcome mechanical barriers to invasion.

Cell-to-cell communication is an important factor in growth control. When normal mammalian cells are grown in culture, they migrate away from the center of the colony in an orderly radial pattern until continued cell contact is made; then forward motion abruptly ceases (Abercrombie, 1975). This phenomenon, known as *contact inhibition of movement*, is a feedback mechanism that serves to regulate normal cell growth and to suppress tissue invasion. Other mechanisms, also discussed in Chapter 13, regulate parameters such as adhesive specificity, density-dependent growth inhibition, anchorage-dependent growth, and cell orientation, which enable normal cells to organize into functional tissues. Defects in these feedback mechanisms are thought to contribute to the invasive behavior demonstrated by metastatic cancer cells, a key cellular determinant of metastatic potential.

Although tumor growth may be promoted by loss of the cell's ability to regulate growth, it may also be enhanced by autocrine stimulation (discussed in detail in Chapter 13). Autocrine (self-stimulatory) growth involves the secretion of and response to endogenously produced polypeptides that serve as growth hormones by a cell (Anzano, Roberts, Smith, Sporn, & DeLarco, 1983; Bishop, 1987; Todaro, Fryling, & DeLarco, 1980). Autocrine growth is mediated by receptors on the cell's surface. The action of autocrine growth factors depends, therefore, on the presence of functional receptors on the surface of the cells that produce

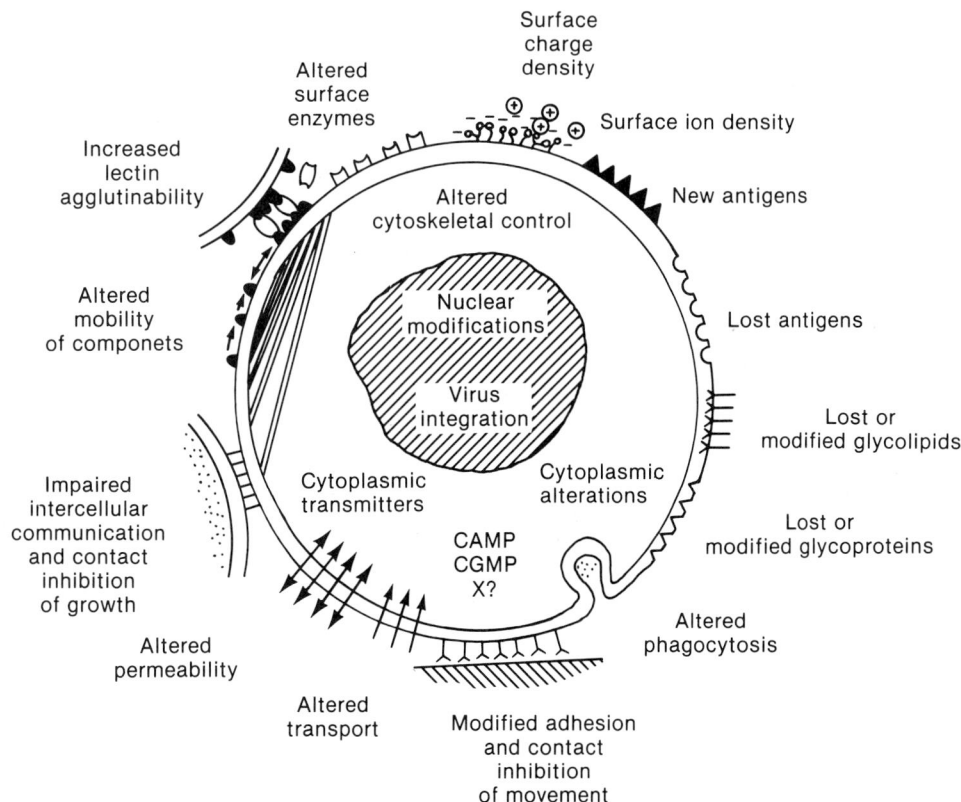

Figure 14–1. Alterations in cell surface properties that contribute to tumor cell invasion and metastasis. The interaction of tumor cells with their environment is mediated by cell surface constituents. A wide variety of cellular feedback mechanisms and recognition systems are mediated by molecules on the cell surface. Alterations in the cell surface contribute to loss of growth control, increased cell motility, altered patterns of cell recognition, diminished cell cohesion, and development of cellular and biochemical properties that enable tumor cells to overcome mechanical barriers to invasion and metastasis.

the growth factor as well as on the availability of the growth-stimulating polypeptide. Autocrine growth factor expression appears directly or indirectly linked to changes in cellular genes (proto-oncogenes) that cause neoplastic growth when damaged or activated (Bishop, 1987). The endogenous production of excessive amounts of growth factors and the expression of functional receptors for these growth factors on the cell's surface represent an active and important, although incompletely understood, mechanism for escaping from normal exogenous growth controls.

Invasion

Local invasion of the normal stroma by tumor cells is a prerequisite for metastasis and represents the first step in the metastatic cascade. In its earliest stages, local invasion may occur as a function of direct tumor extension. At some point, however, cells or clumps of cells become detached from the primary tumor and infiltrate the surrounding interstitial spaces. Among the mechanisms believed to play a role in local invasion by neoplastic cells are the generation of mechanical pressure by the tumor growth, decreased cell-to-cell cohesion, increased cell motility, and the release of chemotactic substances and matrix-degrading enzymes by neoplastic cells and host inflammatory cells (Day, Mylrs, Stansly, Garattini, & Lewis, 1977; Fidler, Gersten, & Hart, 1978; Hart, 1981; Liotta & Hart, 1982; Mareel & Calmman, 1984). Physical and biochemical properties that facilitate the invasion of normal stroma also enable tumor cells to penetrate lymphatic channels and blood vessels, promoting their dissemination to distant sites (Fig. 14–2). Once the cells are arrested in the capillary bed of a target organ, these invasive properties enable tumor cells to extravasate from the vasculature and infiltrate the perivascular stroma and the parenchyma of a target organ.

During invasion and metastasis formation, tumor cells perform various physiologic functions for which there are normal counterparts. Normal cells exhibit a variety of behavioral characteristics during embryogenesis that closely resemble invasion and metastasis. However, embryonic cells are regulated by genetic programs that limit these behaviors to those required for the development of organ systems that have normal functional relationships with other tissues. In the mature adult, only special cells, such as leukocytes, remain endowed with the ability to infiltrate tissues that are normally not freely permeable to cell migration. These facts suggest that the capacity for invasive behavior is encoded in the genome but is not generally expressed in the mature organisms except under special conditions. Neoplastic transformation may represent such a circumstance.

Angiogenesis

Tumor growth is limited by the ability of nutrients and waste products to diffuse into and out of the mass efficiently. Experiments have demonstrated that tumor implants cannot grow more than a few millimeters in diameter without developing new blood vessels to sustain them (Folkman, Merler, Abernathy, & Williams, 1971). Experiments on the induction of blood vessel growth into the cornea, a structure that does not normally have a vasculature, revealed that tumors do not form their own blood vessels. Tumor cells secrete a diffusible substance called angiogenin or tumor angiogenesis factor (TAF) that causes the host to make blood vessels for them (Folkman, 1981; Folkman et al., 1971; Folkman & Tyler, 1977; Furcht, 1986). Tumor implants placed in the cornea induce the continual ingrowth of blood vessels from the cornea into the implant (Folkman & Tyler, 1977). Invasion of newly formed blood vessels is facilitated by the fact that the walls of capillary sprouts are often defective and offer little resistance to infiltration.

Before vascularization, tumors generally are unable to shed cells into the circulation and have a lower probability of metastasizing than tumors in which vascularization has occurred. In experimental systems, malignant cells are found only in the effluent of implanted tumors after tumor vascularization has taken place (Liotta et al., 1974). As the tumor becomes vascularized, the number of cells released into the circulation increases. In fact, in experimental systems, the rate of release can be mathematically related to the number of pulmonary metastases that develop (Liotta, Saidel, & Kleinerman, 1976). The rate of hematogenous spread is also correlated with tumor vascularity in clinical situations. Small cell carcinoma of the lung, prostate carcinoma, and undifferentiated carcinoma of the thyroid gland, which all arise in highly vascular capillary beds, frequently develop early and lead to widespread blood-borne dissemination to highly vascular organs such as the bone marrow, lung, and brain.

The growth of metastasis is also dependent on the development of a vascular supply. Therefore, tumor angiogenesis also is critical at the end of the metastatic cascade. However, it may be possible for small populations of tumor to remain in an avascular phase for

PRIMARY TUMOR

METASTASES

Circulating tumor cells

Invasion   Intravasation

Extravasation

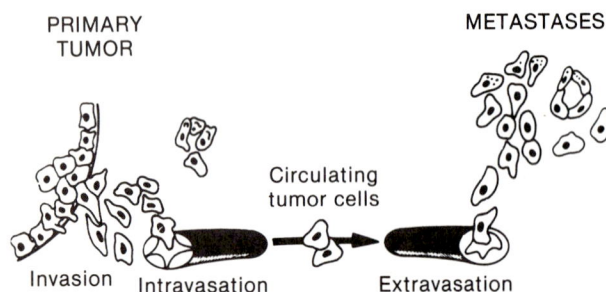

Figure 14–2. Multistep metastatic cascade. Following transition from in situ to invasive carcinoma, tumor cells infiltrate normal stroma and gain access to host blood vessels and lymphatics. Tumor cells enter the blood stream directly (or indirectly via lymphatic-hematogenous communications) and are carried to a distant site, where they arrest in a vascular bed, extravasate, infiltrate normal stroma, and initiate a metastatic colony. Continued growth of the metastases requires angiogenesis and escape from host defenses.

prolonged periods, a phenomenon that may partially explain dormant metastases (Folkman & Tyler, 1977). Immunologic defenses that keep tumor growth in check or dependence on exogenous hormones or autocrine growth factors, or both, may also play important roles in tumor dormancy (Schirrmacher, 1985). These concepts are discussed in greater detail in Chapter 13.

BIOCHEMICAL MECHANISMS OF INVASION AND METASTASIS

Interactions with the Extracellular Matrix

The mammalian organism is composed of a series of tissue compartments separated from each other by two types of extracellular matrix: interstitial stroma and basement membranes (Hay, 1982; Vracko, 1974). The interstitial stroma contains blood vessels, lymphatics, and nerves that support the parenchymal cells of organs. Parenchymal cells are attached to a basement membrane, which, in turn, is anchored to the interstitial stroma.

The molecular composition of each extracellular matrix is tissue specific. Each unique set of matrix components identifies the tissue of origin and reflects the organization and physical properties of the tissue (Vracko, 1974). Collagens are the major structural elements in the matrices. More than 10 collagenous proteins are known and each differs chemically, genetically, and immunologically. The interstitial collagens (types I, II, and III) are present in fibrous structures (types I and III) and cartilage (type II) and form tightly ordered fibrils. Other types of collagen (types IV and V) are arranged in nonfibrous structures.

Extracellular matrix exists as a dense latticework composed of collagens and elastin that is embedded in a visoelastic ground substance composed of glycoproteins and proteoglycan (a modified glycoprotein that forms a hydrated filler substance between collagen fibers). This meshwork forms a three-dimensional supporting scaffold that isolates tissue compartments, mediates cell attachment, determines tissue architecture, and serves as a mechanical barrier to invasion. The spacing, orientation, and charge of matrix components influence the filtration of soluble macromolecules through the matrix. Regulatory signals are transmitted from matrix components through specific cell surface receptors. These receptors enable matrix components to exert chemical and mechanical influences on the shape and biochemistry of the cell and play an important role in cell morphology, mitogenesis, and cytodifferentiation (Hay, 1982; Liotta, 1987, 1989; Vracko, 1974; Wicha, Liotta, Garbisa, & Kidwell, 1980).

Basement membranes contain three major components: type IV collagen, laminin, and a specific proteoglycan (Hay, 1982; Vracko, 1974; Wicha et al., 1980). These molecules bind together to form homogeneous sheets that resist physical penetration of cells. Sheets of basement membrane form the interface between the parenchymal cells of organs and the interstitial connective tissue. Normal epithelial cells are thought to require a basement membrane for anchorage and growth (Hay, 1982; Kleinman, Klebe, & Martin, 1981; Vracko, 1974; Wicha et al., 1980). Three layers of basement membrane have been identified: the lamina lucida, a lucid zone that exists just below the cell membrane of the basal cells or the endothelial cells that interface with basement membrane; the lamina densa, a network of randomly oriented fibrils; and the reticular layer, a network of anchoring fibrils that blend into the collagen fibers of the underlying connective tissue.

Basement Membrane Loss in Invasive Carcinoma

Tumor cell interaction with the extracellular matrix occurs at multiple stages in the metastatic cascade (Barsky, Siegal, Jannotta, & Liotta, 1983; Forster, Talbot, & Critshley, 1984; Kleinman et al., 1981; Liotta, 1986, 1987, 1989; Liotta, Abe, Gehron, & Martin, 1979; Liotta, Guirguis, & Schiffmann, 1986; Liotta & Hart, 1982; Liotta, Kleinerman, Catanzara, & Rynbrandt, 1977; Liotta et al., 1974; Liotta, Mandler, Murano, et al., 1986; Liotta, Rao, & Barsky, 1983; Liotta, Rao, & Wewer, 1986; Liotta, Saidel, & Kleinerman, 1976; Liotta & Schiffmann, 1988; Liotta, Thorgeirsson, & Garbisa, 1982). During the transition from in situ to invasive carcinoma, changes in the organization, distribution, and quantity of the epithelial basement membrane occur as tumor cells penetrate the membrane and enter the underlying interstitial stroma. During intravasation and extravasation, tumor cells must also penetrate the vascular subendothelial basement membrane. Following extravasation from the circulation, tumor cells must traverse the perivascular interstitial stroma to establish a metastatic focus in the parenchyma of a target organ.

Although proliferative disorders of the breast are all characterized by disorganization of the normal epithelial stromal architecture, benign disorders are always characterized by a continuous basement membrane separating the epithelium from the stroma (Kleinman et al., 1981). In contrast, invasive breast carcinomas consistently exhibit defective extracellular basement membrane with zones of loss surrounding the invading tumor cells (Barsky et al., 1983; Liotta, Rao, & Weaver, 1986; Siegel et al., 1981). The basement membrane is also markedly defective adjacent to metastatic cells, lymph nodes, and organs. This phenomenon occurs in all types of carcinomas. Invasive bowel carcinoma, both primary and metastatic, exhibits loss of basement membranes. Moreover, the extent of basement membrane loss has been correlated with an increased incidence of metastases and a poor 5-year survival (Forster et al., 1984).

Invasion of the Extracellular Matrix: A Three-Step Process

A sequence of biochemical events occurs during tumor cell invasion of the extracellular matrix (Barsky et al., 1983; Kalebic, Garbisa, Glaser, & Liotta, 1983; Liotta, 1986, 1987, 1989; Liotta & Hart, 1982; Liotta & Schiffmann, 1988; Liotta et al., 1974, 1977, 1979, 1983; Liotta, Guirguis, et al., 1986; Liotta, Mandler, et al., 1986; Liotta, Rao, et al., 1986; Liotta, Saidel, et al., 1976; Liotta, Thorgeirsson, et al., 1982; Terranova, Heyanen, & Martin, 1986; Terranova, Williams, & Liotta, 1984; Terranova, Liotta, Russo, & Martin, 1982; Terranova, Rao, & Kalebic, 1983; Thorgeirsson, Turpeenniemi-Hujanin, & Liotta, 1985; Vlodavsky, Fuks, Bar-Ner, Ariav, & Schirrmacher, 1983). This process, which occurs in three phases, is depicted in Figure 14–3. The first step is tumor cell attachment via cell surface receptors that bind to specific attachment factors in the matrix, such as laminin and fibronectin. The anchored tumor cell then either secretes hydrolytic enzymes or induces host cells to secrete enzymes that degrade the matrix in a highly localized region close to the tumor cell surface, where the amount of active enzyme outbalances the natural protease inhibitors present in the serum and in the matrix itself. In blood vessels, the release of these enzymes induces the active retraction of the endothelial cells that cover the basement membrane and exposes naked basement membrane, to which the tumor cell attaches itself and into which it dissolves. The third step requires tumor cell locomotion into the degraded matrix. During this phase, the pseudopodia of tumor cells attached to blood vessel walls traverse the basement membrane, allowing the cells to extravasate from the vasculature into the interstitial stroma. Continued invasion of the matrix occurs by cyclic repetition of these steps. Directional migration of tumor cells invading the extracellular matrix is influenced by chemotactic factors derived from the serum, organ parenchyma, or the matrix itself and from autocrine motility factors. Thus it appears that tumor cells that disseminate hematogenously are a select subpopulation of cells that have the ability to degrade vascular basement membranes.

The fate of arrested tumor cells also differs according to the mechanism and location of lodgment (Fig. 14–4) (Liotta, 1989). Tumor cells adherent to the surface of venule or capillary endothelium rapidly induce the active retraction of endothelial cells (in 1 to 4 hrs). This allows the tumor cell to attach to the exposed basement membrane. Once attachment occurs, the adjacent endothelial cells extend over the tumor cell and separate it from the blood stream. Local dissolution of the basement membrane is then observed in association with a tumor cell pseudopodium traversing the basement membrane. This step is soon followed by complete extravasation of the tumor cell.

Endothelial retraction does not occur after arterial arrest (see Fig. 14–4). Intra-arterial tumor cells can actually proliferate and expand as colonies. As the tumor colonies enlarge, they become covered by a host endothelial surface that lacks a basement membrane. Once the tumor colony fills the arteriole, mechanical damage to the endothelium occurs, and this damage exposes the basement membrane. Tumor cells at the periphery of the interarterial colony then invade through the basement membrane and the elastic lamina of the capillary-arteriole wall to gain an extravascular position.

Attachment Factors

A major mechanism by which cells attach to the extracellular matrix is through matrix component glycoproteins, which serve as attachment factors (see Fig. 14–3) (Liotta, 1986, 1987, 1989; Yamada et al., 1985). These attachment factors form a bridge between the tumor cell surface and other structural components of

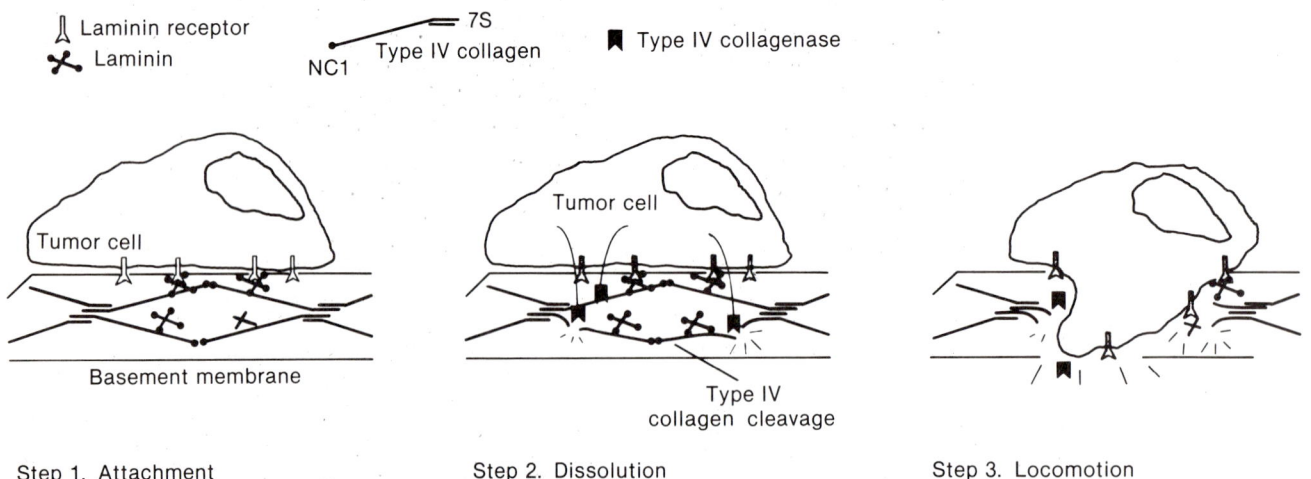

Figure 14–3. Three-step hypothesis of tumor cell invasion of the extracellular matrix. Schematic diagram of tumor cell invasion of the basement membrane, a homogeneous matrix that resists physical penetration of cells. Step 1 is tumor cell attachment to the matrix. Surface receptors on the tumor cell (in this case, laminin receptors) bind to components of the basement membrane (laminin) in the extracellular matrix. Step 2 is local degradation of the matrix by tumor cell proteases. The anchored tumor cell either secretes hydrolytic enzymes (shown here as type IV collagenase) or induces host cells to secrete proteolytic enzymes that degrade the matrix in a highly localized region close to the tumor cell surface. Step 3 is the migration of the tumor cell through the degraded basement membrane. During this phase, pseudopodia of the tumor cell traverse the basement membrane, enabling the cell to extravasate from the blood vessel into the interstitial stroma.

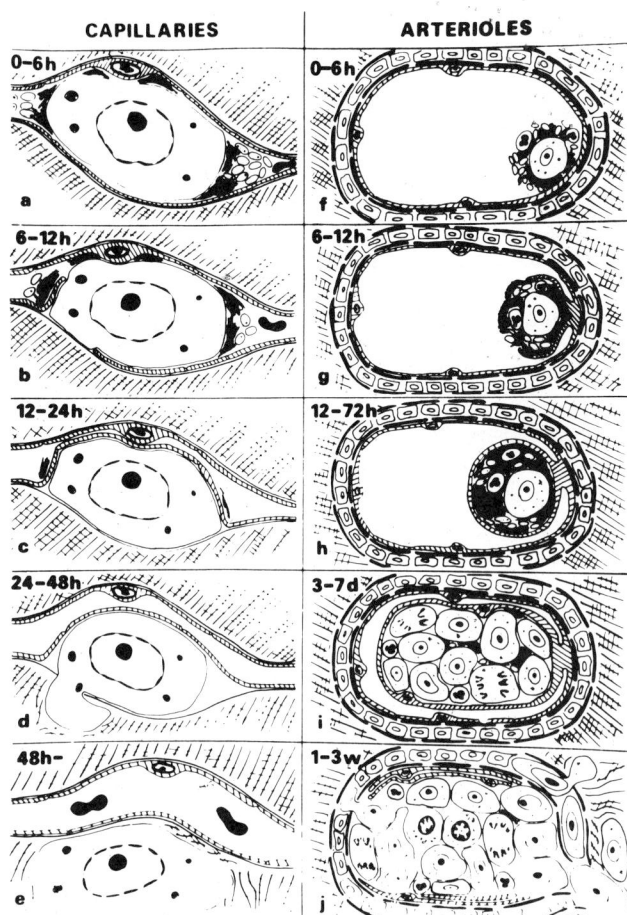

Figure 14–4. Extravasation of tumor cells. Steps during hematogenous extravasation of tumor cells differ, depending on whether the tumor cells arrest in capillaries or venules *(left panels)* versus arterioles *(right panels)*. In the capillaries, tumor cells, coated with platelets and fibrin, adhere loosely to the endothelial *(EN)* surface *(A)*, causing the endothelial cells to retract *(B)* and exposing the underlying basement membrane *(BM) (small arrow)*. Tumor cells attached to the exposed basement membrane are covered by endothelial cells *(C)* and separated from the blood stream. After a period of time, local dissolution of the basement membrane occurs and is followed by protrusion of tumor cell pseudopodia *(D–E)* and ultimately by extravasation of the whole tumor cell. Arteriole arrest of tumor cells is also associated with fibrin and platelets *(F)*, but it does not induce endothelial retraction. Instead, the surrounding endothelium covers the tumor cell emboli and expands as the colony grows *(G–I)*. After 2 to 3 weeks, the tumor colony disrupts the endothelium and exposes the basement membrane *(J)*. Invasion of the arteriole wall follows.

the matrix, such as collagen. Attachment factors may be synthesized by the cell that is attaching itself to the matrix, or the cell may utilize attachment factors already present in the matrix.

Although metastatic tumor cells undoubtedly use a variety of attachment mechanisms to interact with the extracellular matrix, in vitro assays developed for evaluating biochemical events that occur during attachment have revealed that type IV collagen and laminin are the matrix components that block cell migration. Laminin is a large, complex glycoprotein that is a major constituent of all basement membranes. It has a distinctive cruciform shape that enables it to bind to multiple matrix components and to play a key role in cell attachment to basement membrane (Barsky, Rao, Hyams, & Liotta, 1984; Barsky, Rao, Williams, & Liotta, 1984; Barsky, Siegal, Tannotta, & Liotta, 1983; Charonis, Tsilibary, Yurchenco, & Furthmayr, 1985; Charpin et al., 1986; Forster et al., 1984; Liotta, 1986, 1987, 1989; Liotta et al., 1983; Liotta, Rao, & Wewer, 1986; Rao, Barsky, Terranova, & Liotta, 1983; Terranova et al., 1982, 1983, 1984, 1986; Thorgeirsson et al., 1985). Highly metastatic cells show a distinct preference for attachment to laminin (Barsky, Rao, Hyams, et al., 1984; Hand, Thor, Schlam, Rao, & Liotta, 1985; Kalebic et al., 1983; Liotta et al., 1982; Yamada et al., 1985). Laminin is also chemotactic for certain tumor cells and promotes cell growth (Vlodavsky, Fuks, Bar-Ner, Ariav, & Schirrmacher, 1983).

Laminin receptors appear to be altered in human carcinomas (Barsky, Rao, Hyams, & Liotta, 1984; Barsky et al., 1983; Charpin et al., 1986; Forster et al., 1984; Liotta, 1986, 1987, 1989; Terranova et al., 1982, 1983, 1984, 1986; Yamada et al., 1985). Breast and colon cancer tissue contains high levels of unoccupied laminin receptors (Barsky, Rao, Hyams, et al., 1984; Yamada et al., 1985). It is postulated that the membrane vesicles on the cell surface of tumor cells are rich in laminin receptors, which facilitates their attachment to basement membrane (Terranova et al., 1986). In animal models, tumor cells selected for the ability to attach to basement membrane via laminin demonstrate a tenfold increase in hematogenous metastases (Liotta et al., 1983). Preincubation of tumor cells with laminin also increases hematogenous metastases, whereas treating the cells with the receptor-binding fragment of laminin markedly inhibits or abolishes metastases from hematogenously introduced tumor cells (Liotta et al., 1983).

Proteolytic Enzymes

Cellular proteinases exert destructive effects on the extracellular matrix and have long appeared to play a role in tumor invasion and metastasis (Roblin, 1981; Strauli, 1980; Thorgeirsson et al., 1985). Those that are most commonly associated with metastatic potential include collagenases, plasminogen activators, and lysosomal enzymes. Proteolytic enzymes secreted by tumor cells are thought to play an important role in the degradation of collagens, which abound in the perivascular basement membrane area and the adjacent connective tissues. Tumor cells can either release collagenases—enzymes that can preferentially digest collagen—or secrete collagenolytic substances in latent forms that are converted to active collagenase by lysosomal proteases such as plasmin. Collagenases that degrade interstitial collagen (types I, II, and III) have been identified by a number of investigators. However, type IV collagen, the structural element of the vascular basement membrane, is resistant to classic collagenase. A type IV–specific collagenase that is augmented in many highly metastatic tumor cells has been identified (Garbisa et al., 1987). Expression of this collagenase can be induced in rodent cells by transfecting them with the *ras* oncogene. (See Chapter 13 for more information on oncogene-induced expression of gene products and transfection.) These data provide support for the hypothesis that metastatic phenotypes can be induced by the activation of certain oncogenes and establish a biochemical link between the amplification of type IV collagenase production and the induction of the metastatic phenotype. Whether the increased metastatic potential is caused by the introduction of new genetic information or by augmented expression of genes that have been activated during malignant transformation is unknown at present.

A number of other proteases that are bound to or released from the cell surface appear to facilitate tumor invasion through proteolysis. One of the hydrolytic enzymes that is augmented in tumor cells and appears to play a role in invasive behavior is plasminogen activator (Roblin, 1981; Strauli, 1980; Thorgeirsson et al., 1985). Plasminogen activator converts the serum proenzyme plasminogen into the protease plasmin, which can hydrolyze a variety of proteins. Plasmin formation plays a role in the degradation of local connective tissue in a variety of normal processes, such as ovulation. It is believed that proteolysis mediated by plasminogen activator makes an important contribution to the degradation of the extracellular matrix during tumor cell invasion. A functional role that has been proposed for plasminogen activator is to allow tumor cells to escape the fibrin meshwork associated with tumor emboli. Other enzymes, such as cathepsin B, appear to play a role in the detachment of tumor cells from the primary tumor. Yet another cathepsin degrades proteoglycan, another important component of the capillary basement membrane and the perivascular connective tissue.

Locomotion

Like leukocytes, tumor cells possess the organelles necessary for locomotion and can actively migrate through tissues (Coman, 1953; Easty & Easty, 1976; Hart, 1981; Hynes, 1981; Liotta & Hart, 1982; Mareel, 1983; Mareel & Calman, 1984; Roos, Dingemans, van de Pavert, & van den Bergh-Weerman, 1977). Active migration of normal cells also occurs during embryogenesis, although most differentiated cells generally have lost this capacity under normal conditions. The motility of tumor cells is increased by a relative lack of cohesiveness in comparison to normal cells. Pseudopodia, cytoplasmic processes formed by microfilament bundles located in the cellular cytoskeleton, enable cells to migrate by diapedesis (the process by which leukocytes pass through unruptured vessel walls into the tissues). Proteins on the surface of these cytoplasmic processes contain receptors for specific substrates. Cell motility occurs as attachments with these substrates are made and broken (Raz & Geiger, 1982). Local factors in the host microenvironment influence migratory behaviors by stimulating directional locomotion (chemotaxis). For example, it has been shown that cells move preferentially along continuous gradients of adhesiveness (Carter, 1967) and toward regions of neutral pH (Weiss & Scott, 1963).

The movement of neoplastic cells through cellular and connective tissue as well as other biologic barriers may well be influenced by chemotactic factors. Studies on in vitro chemotaxis of tumor cells indicate that various compounds stimulate directional migration, much the way chemotactic mechanisms act as a beacon to migrating leukocytes (Hayashi, Yoshida, Ozaki, & Vshijima, 1970; McCarthy, Basera, Palm, Sas, & Furcht, 1985). It is also known that tumor cells can influence the motility of normal cells in a number of instances, frequently to the benefit of the tumor. Tumor cells produce antileukotactic factors, chemotactic factors for the endothelial cells that are responsible for the formation of new blood vessels, and chemoattractants for fibroblasts (Liotta, 1989).

However, although host-derived chemoattractants undoubtedly contribute to the directional tumor cell migration, their actions do not sufficiently explain the initiation of tumor cell locomotion or the sustained migration of highly invasive tumor cells. A search for active mechanisms of tumor migration has led to the identification of a new class of proteins that are endogenously produced and profoundly stimulate the intrinsic motility of tumor cells (Guirguis, Margulies, Taraboletti, Schiffman, & Liotta, 1987; Liotta, Guirguis, & Schiffman, 1986; Liotta, Mandler, et al., 1986; Liotta & Schiffman, 1988). These "autocrine motility factors" stimulate both random and directional tumor cell motility without affecting leukocyte migration. They exert a recruiting effect on adjacent tumor cells, which enables them to move into normal tissues under their own power (Fig. 14–5).

When human breast cancer cells have been exposed to autocrine motility factor (AMF) on a filter, the cells extended pseudopodia through the pores of the filter and began to migrate through the pores (Guirguis et al., 1987). Moreover, an anti-AMF antibody that has been developed inhibits pseudopodia protrusion and, in turn, cell motility. Besides setting the cell in motion, pseudopodia contain receptors that act as the cell's eyes, guiding it to its destination. One of these receptors binds to the laminin in the basement membrane. AMF-induced pseudopodia in human breast cancer cells have a twentyfold increase in laminin receptors as found in the plasma membrane of unstimulated cells (Guirguis et al., 1987). This increase in laminin receptors facilitates attachment of tumor cells to the basement membrane.

Like autocrine growth factors, the action of autocrine motility factors is dependent on the presence of functional receptors on the tumor cell surface as well as on the production and secretion of a motility stimulating protein. It is unclear at present whether the production of autocrine motility factor is the result of oncogene activation. Oncogenes can activate genes that produce the proteins and enzymes that cause cell migration via pseudopodia, followed by attachment and penetration of the basement membrane.

RESTING CELL **EXPLORATORY PSEUDOPODIA** **CHOICE OF DIRECTION**

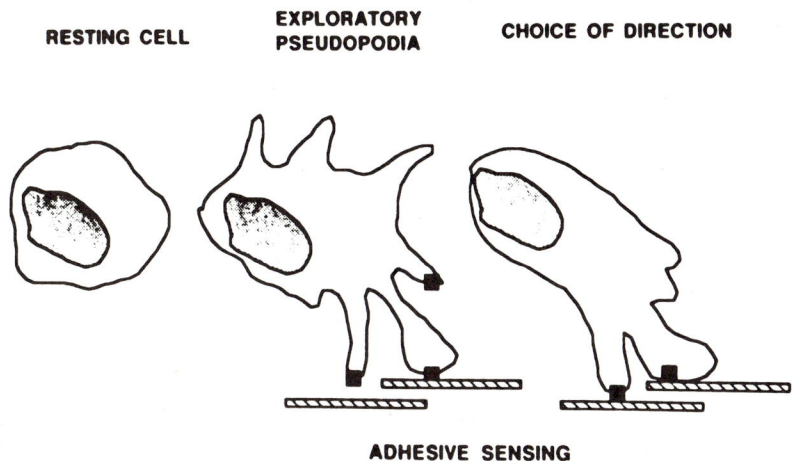

ADHESIVE SENSING

Figure 14–5. Stepwise generation of a motile response. Autocrine motility factors, which stimulate intrinsic motility, induce the formation of exploratory pseudopodia that serve as sensory organs that locate directional stimuli. Pseudopodial proteins are enriched with matrix receptors and provide the propulsive traction for locomotion.

PATTERNS OF DISSEMINATION

Three basic patterns of metastases exist: direct extension, lymphatic dissemination, and hematogenous spread. However, these mechanisms are not mutually exclusive. The body contains numerous microscopic anatomic connections that permit free passage of tumor cells, facilitating metastatic spread by more than one route. In fact, tumor cell dissemination via one mechanism often facilitates metastasis through others.

Direct Extension

Rapid proliferation of cells within a tumor mass can create intratumoral pressures that force finger-like projections of tumor cells directly into normal tissues in much the same way plants force their roots through soil. Anatomic routes of direct tumor extension involve infiltration of interstitial spaces, coelomic and epithelial cavities (serosal seeding), and cerebrospinal spaces. Until the 1970s, tumor invasion and metastases were thought to be passive, produced by enlarging tumors that compressed and destroyed host tissues. However, simple growth pressure does not account for the differences in invasive behavior between rapidly growing benign and malignant tumors. Breast fibroadenomas and uterine leiomyomas often generate significant growth pressure but never invade or metastasize. Mechanical pressure alone cannot explain how the tumor cells traverse cellular and connective tissue as well as other mechanical barriers, nor the discontinuous invasion of tumor cells frequently identified on serial histologic sectioning. Furthermore, experimental data from in vitro invasion assays have clearly demonstrated that pressure alone is not sufficient for invasion (Gabbert, 1985; Mareel, 1983). Mechanical forces appear to assist invasion rather than serve as the primary mechanism of tissue invasion.

Lymphatic Metastasis

Involvement of the regional lymph nodes draining a cancer is the first clinical sign of metastasis. For the most part, sites of nodal metastases are easily explained by anatomic and mechanical considerations. However, much about the mechanisms that enhance and control lymphatic spread is incompletely understood. There is considerable evidence that the immune system has both inhibitory and stimulatory effects on tumor growth, and these effects can be manifested simultaneously (Fidler, 1979). The increased incidence of virulent cancers in immunosuppressed patients suggests that some tumors develop and metastasize more readily when the immune system is suppressed (Krueger, Tallent, Richie, & Johnson, 1985). However, data from animal studies suggest that an activated immune system can significantly enhance the development of metastases by selecting out weakly antigenic cell lines, leading to the proliferation of tumor cells that the host's immune system does not recognize as foreign. The lack of antigenicity may enable tumor cells to evade macrophages and other elements of the cell-mediated immune system in the circulation. Factors that determine whether a stimulatory or an inhibitory response will predominate are not known for certain but may involve the properties that are specific to a particular tumor antigen, the mode of presentation, and the initial site of interaction with host immune cells.

Tumors generally lack a well-formed lymphatic network. Communication between tumor cells and lymphatic channels occurs only at the tumor periphery and not within the tumor mass. Tumor cells entering the lymphatic drainage are carried to regional lymph nodes, where they lodge in the large lymphatics of the subcapsular sinus. Initially, regional lymph nodes may exert a barrier effect, impeding the dissemination of tumor cells into the lymphatic system. Nonspecific host defenses, such as macrophages and natural killer cells, play an important role in the elimination of circulating tumor cells and in the destruction of micrometastases. At some point in the metastatic cascade, lymph nodes lose their ability to filter and destroy tumor cells. Numerous physiologic and immunologic factors have been implicated, but the basic mechanisms responsible for this loss are not as yet completely elucidated. Factors such as the intensity and duration of challenge by tumor cells also appear to play a role in the development of nodal involvement. Although tumor-specific antigens have been identified in animal models, it remains unclear whether similar antigens play a role in human tumors (Frost & Kerbel, 1983; Hanna & Key, 1982).

Experimental data reveal that within 10 to 60 minutes after tumor cells arrest in a lymph node, a significant fraction of the tumor cells detach and enter the efferent lymphatics (Fisher & Fisher, 1966). These tumor cells eventually end up in the regional or systemic venous drainage owing to the existence of numerous lymphatic-hematogenous communications. As a result, regional lymph nodes do not function as true mechanical barriers to tumor dissemination, and it is likely that lymphatic and hematogenous dissemination occur in parallel.

Hematogenous Metastasis

Hematogenous dissemination is a complex process that requires tumor cells to penetrate and leave blood vessels to disseminate to distant organs. However, data from experimental systems indicate that vascularized tumors probably shed malignant cells constantly as they grow, often releasing millions of cells without producing metastases (Fidler, 1970; Fidler et al., 1978; Liotta et al., 1974; Weiss, 1983). Thus the mere presence of tumor cells in the blood stream does not predict metastasis. Circulating tumor cells are detectable in patients who are curable with surgical removal of the tumor (Griffiths, McKinna, Rowbotham, Tsolakidis, & Salisbury, 1973; Salsbury, 1975). To establish a metastasis, circulating tumor cells must be able to evade host defenses, survive mechanical trauma in the blood stream, and lodge in the venous or capillary bed of the target organ (Cady et al., 1976; Lindberg, 1972; Shah, Cendron, & Farr, 1976). Circulating tumor cells utilize a variety of means to lodge in the vessels of the target organ, where they will initiate metastatic colonies. Approximately 80 per cent of the tumor cells circulate as single cells and attach directly to the intact endothelial surface or to preexisting regions of exposed subendothelial basement membrane (Liotta, 1987). Emboli of circulating tumor cells or tumor cells aggregated with leukocytes, fibrin, or platelets can directly embolize in the precapillary venules by mechanical impaction. The formation of a fibrin-platelet complex is thought to protect tumor cells within the emboli from host defenses and to facilitate successful attachment to the vascular epithelium. Having become arrested in a blood vessel, a tumor cell must then actively invade the vascular wall and interstitial stroma to invade the parenchyma of the target organ and must possess the ability to grow in a foreign "soil." Cancer cells that simply become attached to blood vessel surfaces never establish metastases in distant parenchyma, although they may shed additional tumor emboli into the circulation if they survive and grow on the endothelial surface. As noted earlier, growth in the target organ parenchyma requires the development of a vascular network and continued evasion of host immune and nonimmune defenses.

Size and Metastatic Potential

The metastatic potential of many common solid epithelial tumors is statistically related to the size of the primary tumor (Sugarbaker, 1981). Metastases generally do not develop until the primary tumor reaches approximately 1 cm^3 in size (10^9 cells) (Weiss, 1983). Although the reasons for this are not completely clear, it is possible that more aggressive tumor cells evolve in larger tumors. Larger tumors may also provide a greater antigenic burden that favors the survival of disseminated cells. In breast cancer, if the tumor is less than 1 cm in diameter, less than 25 per cent of the patients will have axillary metastases. If the tumor is greater than 3 cm in diameter, 50 per cent of the patients will have lymph node metastases. Once the tumor reaches 5 cm, 80 per cent of the patients have axillary metastases (Sugarbaker, 1981). Mesenteric metastases from colorectal carcinomas also are related to tumor size. Tumors less than 3 cm in diameter have a 22 per cent incidence of metastases. If the tumor is 5 to 7 cm in diameter, the incidence of metastases rises to 53 per cent (Sugarbaker, 1981). Tumor size is also a predictive factor in melanoma. For melanomas that are less than 1.5 mm in thickness, the risk of regional lymph node metastases is 7 per cent. If the primary tumor is greater than or equal to 1.5 mm, the risk for regional lymph node metastases rises to 23 per cent (Balch, Soong, & Murad, 1979). Transitional carcinoma of the bladder, carcinoma of the stomach, and squamous carcinoma of the lung all show a relationship between size and probability of metastases (Sugarbaker, 1981).

Anatomic Location

The distribution of metastases also varies with the anatomic location of the primary tumor (Liotta, 1989) (Table 14–1). The most frequent location of distant metastasis in many types of cancer appears to be the first capillary bed encountered by the circulating cells (Schirrmacher, 1985; Sugarbaker, 1981). Although all blood eventually passes through the heart and lungs, the shunting of tumor cells through different vascular pathways predisposes certain organs to develop hematogenous metastasis. For example, tumor cells in the systemic venous system spread to the lungs, whereas cancers disseminating via the portal vein frequently spread to the liver, and those arising in the lung spread to a variety of organs via the arterial system. In addition, the vertebral vein system (Batson's plexus) that drains blood from the pelvis to the base of the skull communicates with the venous circulation at many different levels and plays an important role in determining metastases from the penis, prostate, breast, and other sites. A series of illustrative examples follows:

1. Sarcomas arising in the extremities metastasize primarily to the lungs as tumor cells enter the venous drainage and are carried into the inferior vena cava, right heart, and the lungs via the pulmonary artery.

Table 14–1. INCIDENCE OF METASTASES AT AUTOPSY (PER CENT)

Primary Tumor	Site of Metastases			
	Lung	*Colon*	*Breast*	Melanoma
Liver	30–50	50–60	40–60	58–70
Lung	20–40	25–40	60–80	66–80
Bone	30–45	5–10	50–90	30–48
Brain	15–43	0–1	15–30	40–55
Adrenal	17–38	14	38–54	40–47
Pituitary	0–2	0–1	20	18
Ovary	0–2	14	15–30	10–15
Kidney	16–23	8	13	31–35
Spleen	9	5	17	31

2. Lung cancer disseminates widely to multiple organs, including the brain, as tumor cells have direct access to the general arterial circulation via the pulmonary vein and left ventricle.

3. Colorectal carcinomas tend to develop hepatic metastases as tumor cells enter the mesenteric lymphatics and portal venous system and are carried to the liver.

4. Testicular tumors metastasize via the lymphatics to nodes in the periaortic area and then, by lymphatic-hematogenous communications, enter the subclavian veins, where they go to the right heart and the lungs.

5. Prostate cancer metastasizes primarily (90 per cent) to vertebral bone via Batson's plexus of paravertebral veins. Tumor cells entering the prostatic plexus of veins are carried to the veins about the sacrum, ilium, and lumbar spine.

6. Tumors arising in the head and neck metastasize most frequently to regions drained by the local lymphatics.

7. Ovarian cancer spreads to the peritoneal surfaces, the posterior gutters, and the diaphragm, remaining confined to the abdominal cavity for prolonged periods. Hepatic metastases generally occur late, usually by direct invasion from omental implants or by mesenteric venous emboli derived from omental implants.

8. Breast cancer often metastasizes to vertebral bone. The mammary venous drainage can communicate with Batson's plexus of paravertebral veins, carrying tumor cells to the clavicles, intercostal veins, head of the humerus, cervical vertebrae, and transverse cranial sinuses (Liotta, 1989; Schirrmacher, 1985; Sugarbaker, 1981).

Organ Tropism for Metastases

The location of metastases does not always correlate with patterns of blood flow and the locations of capillary beds. An explanation for why some tumors preferentially metastasize to specific organs was first set forth by Paget (1873). He hypothesized that metastases to a particular organ were the result of properties of the tumor cell (the "seed") or the organ (the "soil"). Autopsy statistics and modern research models have shown that both the seed and the soil are important. Although 50 to 60 per cent of metastatic sites can be explained by the circulatory anatomy, many cannot be predicted on the basis of anatomic considerations

alone. Examples of "organ tropism" include ocular melanoma, which frequently metastasizes to the liver, and clear cell kidney carcinomas, which often spread to bone and the thyroid. A number of theoretical mechanisms have been developed to explain organ tropism (Liotta, 1987; Shah et al., 1976; Sugarbaker, 1981). These mechanisms include preferential growth in specific organs due to local growth factors or hormones that are present in the target organ, preferential adherence to the endothelial surface of certain target organs, and the presence of chemotactic factors that diffuse from the target organ and cause circulating tumor cells to extravasate from the vasculature and aggregate in the target organ. Clear evidence exists that tumor cells contain organ-specific receptors that can discriminate between various vascular beds and cause preferential "homing" to certain organs. These data suggest that organ tropism is genetically determined. Indeed, experimental evidence indicates that the metastatic potential of individual tumor cells in a primary tumor is quite variable and that different patterns of preferential metastasis exist among the cells in an individual tumor (Fidler & Balch, 1987; Fidler et al., 1977, 1978; Fidler & Hart, 1982; Fidler & Nicolson, 1976; Nicolson, 1978, 1984, 1987; Poste, 1986).

BIOLOGIC HETEROGENEITY

Biologic heterogeneity is an important concept in tumor biology, which is basic to the pathogenesis of metastasis as well as the inherent problems associated with the treatment of metastatic disease. Even tumors that arise from a single transformed cell are thought to contain a heterogeneous population of abnormal cells by the time that they are detectable. The generation of biologic heterogeneity in tumors and tumor metastases is attributable to genetic instability that is either inherent in malignant cells, or acquired during tumor growth (Fialkow, 1979; Fidler & Balch, 1987; Fidler et al., 1977, 1978; Fidler & Hart, 1982; Fidler & Nicolson, 1976; Foulds, 1975; Frost & Fidler, 1986; Nicolson, 1978, 1984, 1987; Nowell, 1976, 1986; Poste, 1986). Genetic instability predisposes them to undergo spontaneous somatic mutations at random intervals, which produce permanent and irreversible changes in cellular DNA that are inherited by all the cell's progeny. Phenotypic changes also contribute to biologic heterogeneity. Genotypic and phenotypic variations are clinically manifested by heterogeneity with regard to growth rates, karyotypic abnormalities, cell surface

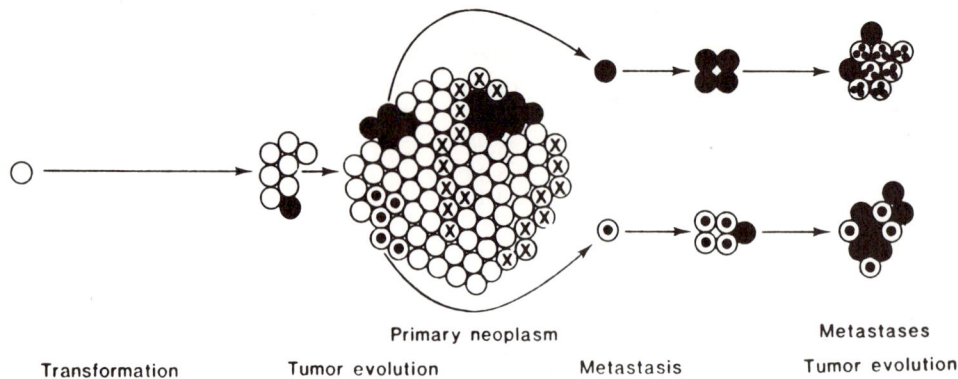

Figure 14–6. The origin of biologic heterogeneity in a tumor and its metastases. Many tumors are unicellular in origin but are composed of a biologically heterogeneous population of cells by the time they are detectable. The generation of cellular diversity within a tumor is attributable to genetic instability that either is inherent in malignant cells or is acquired during tumor growth. Highly malignant cell clones that are capable of metastasis are thought to arise during this process. Metastases may arise from different progenitor cells within a heterogeneous parent tumor, which leads to tumor cell heterogeneity within and among metastases.

receptors, marker enzymes, a variety of cellular and biochemical properties, and responsiveness to radiotherapy and chemotherapy. Highly malignant subpopulations are thought to arise spontaneously as a result of these changes. The emergence of clones that are resistant to therapy is also attributed to genotypic and phenotypic changes. The heterogeneity of a tumor with regard to metastatic potential has been demonstrated in experimental systems and widely confirmed. These studies have also confirmed that genotypic and phenotypic diversity develop in metastases as well as in primary tumors and are potential sources of continual tumor progression (Fig. 14–6).

SUMMARY

The mechanisms thought to play a role in tumor invasion and metastases have progressed from a simple passive mechanical explanation to a highly complex cascade of active biochemical and cellular factors. In parallel with these developments, a revolution has occurred in our understanding of the roles of tumor heterogeneity and the activation of cellular genes as modulators of metastases. Oncogenes activating genes that produce proteins and enzymes can confer unique cellular and biochemical properties on tumor cells that enable them to metastasize. Research on the pathogenesis of metastasis is being conducted in an attempt to identify cellular and biochemical properties that are uniquely augmented in metastatic cells, such as matrix-degrading enzymes and cell surface receptors, which can be used as targets for more effective diagnostic and therapeutic tools.

References

Abercrombie, M. (1975). The contact behavior of invading cells. In *Cellular membranes and tumor cell behavior.* 28th Annual Symposium on Fundamental Cancer Research (pp. 21–37). Baltimore: Williams & Wilkins.

Anzano, M. A., Roberts, A. B., Smith, J. M., Sporn, M. B., & DeLarco, J. E. (1983). Sarcoma growth factor from conditioned medium of virally transformed cells is composed of both types of transforming growth factors. *Proceedings of the National Academy of Sciences USA, 80,* 6264–6268.

Balch, C. M., Soong, S., & Murad, T. (1979). A multifactorial analysis of melanoma. II. Prognostic factors of clinical stage I disease. *Surgery 86;* 343–347.

Barsky, S. H., Rao, C. N., Hyams, D., & Liotta, L. A. (1984). Characterization of a laminin receptor from human breast tissue. *Breast Cancer Research and Treatment, 4,* 181–188.

Barsky, S. H., Rao, C. N., Williams, J. E., & Liotta, L. A. (1984). Domains of laminin which alter metastases in a murine model. *Journal of Clinical Investigation, 74,* 843–848.

Barsky, S. H., Siegal, G. P., Jannotta, F., & Liotta, L. A. (1983). Loss of basement membrane components by invasive tumors but not their benign counterparts. *Laboratory Investigation, 49,* 140–148.

Bishop, J. M. (1987). The molecular genetics of cancer. *Science, 235,* 305–311.

Cady, B., Sedgwick, C., Meissner, W. A., Bookwalter, J. R., Romagosa, V., & Werber, J. (1976). Changing clinical, pathologic, therapeutic, and survival patterns in differentiated thyroid carcinoma. *Annals of Surgery, 184,* 541.

Carter, S. B. (1967). Haptotaxis and the mechanism of cell motility. *Nature, 213,* 256–261.

Charonis, A. S., Tsilibary, T. S., Yurchenco, P. D., & Furthmayr, H. (1985). Binding of laminin to type IV collagen: A morphological study. *Journal of Cell Biology, 100,* 1848–1853.

Charpin, C., Lissitzky, J. C., Jacquemier, J., Lavaut, M. N., Kopp, F., Pourreau-Schneider, N., Martin, P. M., & Toga, M. (1986). Immunohistochemical detection of laminin in 98 human breast carcinomas: A light and electron microscopic study. *Human Pathology, 17,* 355–365.

Coman, D. R. (1953). Mechanisms responsible for the origin and distribution of blood-borne metastases. *Cancer Research, 13,* 397–405.

Day, S. B., Myers, W. P., Stansly, P., Garattini, S., & Lewis, M. G. (Eds.). (1977). *Cancer invasion and metastasis: Biologic mechanism and therapy.* New York: Raven Press.

Division of Cancer Prevention and Control. (1986). P. Greenwald & E. Sondik (Eds.), *Cancer control objectives for the nation: 1985–2000. NCI Monographs 2,* 1–105.

Easty, G. C., & Easty, D. M. (1976). Mechanisms of tumor invasion. In T. Symington & R. L. Carter (Eds.), *Scientific foundations of oncology,* (pp. 167–172). Chicago: Year Book Medical Publishers.

Fialkow, P. J. (1979). Clonal origin of human tumors. *Annual Review of Medicine, 30,* 135–176.

Fidler, I. J. (1970). Metastasis: Quantitative analysis of distribution and fate of tumor emboli labeled with ^{125}I-5-iodo-2'-deoxyuridine. *Journal of the National Cancer Institute, 45,* 773–782.

Fidler, I. J. (1974). Immune stimulation-inhibition of experimental cancer metastasis. *Cancer Research, 34,* 491–498.

Fidler, I. J., & Balch, C. M. (1987). The biology of cancer metastasis and implications for therapy. *Current Problems in Surgery, 24,* 129–209.

Fidler, I. J., Gersten, D. M., & Hart, I. R. (1978). The biology of cancer invasion and metastasis. *Advances in Cancer Research, 28,* 149–160.

Fidler, I. J., Gersten, D. M., & Riggs, C. W. (1977). Quantitative analysis of tumor-host interaction and the outcome of experimental metastasis. In S. B. Day, (pp. 277–304). W. P. Myers, P. Stansly, S. Garattini, M. G. Lewis (Eds.), *Cancer invasion and metastasis: Biological mechanisms and therapy.* New York: Raven Press.

Fidler, I. J., & Hart, I. R. (1982). Biologic diversity in metastatic neoplasms: Origins and implications. *Science, 217,* 998–1003.

Fidler, I. J., & Nicolson, G. L. (1976). Organ selectivity for implantation, survival and growth of B-16 melanoma variant tumor lines. *Journal of the National Cancer Institute, 57,* 1199–1202.

Fisher, B., & Fisher, E. R. (1966). The relationship of hematogenous and lymphatic tumor cell dissemination. *Surgery, Gynecology, & Obstetrics, 122,* 791–798.

Folkman, J. (1981). Tumor angiogenesis. *Cancer Biology Reviews, 2,* 175–199.

Folkman, J., Merler, E., Abernathy, C., & Williams, G. (1971). Isolation of a tumor factor responsible for angiogenesis. *Journal of Experimental Medicine, 133,* 275.

Folkman, J., & Tyler, K. (1977). Tumor angiogenesis: its possible role in metastasis and invasion. In S. B. Day, W. P. Myers, P. Stansly, S. Garattini, & M. G. Lewis (Eds.), *Cancer invasion and metastasis: biological mechanisms and therapy.* (pp. 95–104). New York: Raven Press.

Forster, S. J., Talbot, I. C., & Critshley, D. R. (1984). Laminin and fibronectin in rectal adenocarcinoma: Relationship to tumor grade, stage and metastasis. *British Journal of Cancer, 50,* 51–61.

Foulds, L. (1975). *Neoplastic development.* New York: Academic Press.

Frost, P., & Fidler, I. J. (1986). Biology of metastasis. *Cancer, 58,* 550–553.

Frost, P., & Kerbel, R. S. (1983). Immunology of metastasis. Can the immune response cope with tumor dissemination? *Cancer and Metastasis Reviews, 2,* 375–378.

Furcht, L. T. (1986). Critical factors controlling angiogenesis: Cell products, cell matrix, growth factors. *Laboratory Investigation, 55,* 505.

Gabbert, H. (1985). Mechanisms of tumor invasion: Evidence from in vivo observations. *Cancer and Metastasis Reviews, 4,* 283–310.

Garbisa, S., Pozzatti, R., Muschel, R. J., Saffiotti, U., Ballin, M., Goldfarb, R. H., Khoury, G., & Liotta, L. A. (1987). Secretion of type IV collagenolytic protease and metastatic phenotype: Induction by transfection with *c-Ha-ras* but not *c-Ha-ras* plus *AD2-E1A*[1]. *Cancer Research, 47,* 1523–1528.

Griffiths, J. D., McKinna, J. A., Rowbotham, H. D., Tsolakidis, P., & Salsbury, A. J. (1973). Carcinoma of the colon and rectum: Circulating malignant cells and five-year survival. *Cancer, 31,* 226.

Guirguis, R., Margulies, I., Taraboletti, G., Schiffmann, E., & Liotta, L. (1987). Cytokine-induced pseudopodial protrusion is coupled to tumour cell migration. *Nature, 329,* 261–263.

Hakomori, S. I. (1973). Glycolipids of tumor cell membrane. *Advances in Cancer Research, 18,* 265–315.

Hand, P. H., Thor, A., Schlom, J., Rao, C. N., & Liotta, L. A. (1985). Expression of laminin receptor in normal and carcinomatous human tissues as defined by a monoclonal antibody. *Cancer Research, 45,* 2713–2719.

Hanna, M. G., & Key, M. E. (1982). Immunotherapy of metastases enhances subsequent chemotherapy. *Science, 217,* 367–369.

Hart, I. R. (1981). Mechanisms of tumor cell invasion. *Cancer Biology Review, 2,* 29–58.

Hay, E. D. (1982). *Cell biology of extracellular matrix.* New York: Plenum Press.

Hayashi, H., Yoshida, K., Ozaki, T., & Ushijima, M. K. (1970). Chemotactic factor associated with invasion of cancer cells. *Nature, 226,* 174–175.

Hynes, R. O. (1981). Relationships between fibronectin and the cytoskeleton. In G. Poste, & G. L. Nicolson (Eds.), *Cytoskeleton elements and plasma membrane organization: Cell surface reviews* (Vol. 7, pp. 97–139). Amsterdam: Elsevier-Biomedical Press.

Hynes, R. O. (1987). Integrins: A family of cell surface receptors. *Cell, 48,* 549–554.

Kalebic, T., Garbisa, S., Glaser, B., & Liotta, L. A. (1983). Basement membrane collagen: Degradation by migrating endothelial cells. *Science, 221,* 281–283.

Kleinman, H. K., Klebe, R. J., & Martin, G. R. (1981). Role of collagenous matrices in the adhesion and growth of cells. *Journal of Cell Biology, 88,* 473–482.

Krueger, T. C., Tallent, M. B., Richie, R. E., & Johnson, H. K. (1985). Neoplasia in immunosuppressed renal transplant patients: A 20-year experience. *Southern Medical Journal, 78,* 501–506.

Lapis, K., Liotta, L. A., Rabson, A. S. (Eds.). (1986). *Biochemistry and molecular genetics of cancer metastasis.* The Hague: Martinus Nijhoff.

Lindberg, R. (1972). Distribution of cervical lymph node metastases from squamous cell carcinoma of the upper respiratory and digestive tracts. *Cancer, 29,* 1446–1449.

Liotta, L. A. (1986). Tumor invasion and metastases—role of the extracellular matrix: Rhoads Memorial Award Lecture. *Cancer Research, 46,* 1.

Liotta, L. A. (1987). Overview of the biology of cancer invasion and metastases. In S. A. Rosenberg (Ed.), *Surgical treatment of metastatic cancer* (pp. 1–36). Philadelphia: J. B. Lippincott Co.

Liotta, L. (1989). Biology of metastasis. In W. N. Kelley (Ed.), *Textbook of internal medicine* (pp. 1148–1152). Philadelphia: J. B. Lippincott Co.

Liotta, L. A., & Hart, I. R. (Eds.). (1982). *Tumor invasion and metastasis.* The Hague: Martinus Nijhoff.

Liotta, L. A., Abe, S., Gehron, P., & Martin, G. R. (1979). Preferential digestion of basement membrane collagen by an enzyme derived from a metastatic murine tumor. *Proceedings of the National Academy of Sciences USA, 76,* 2268–2276.

Liotta, L. A., Guirguis, R. A., & Schifmann, E. (1986). Tumor autocrine motility factor. In *Cancer metastasis: Experimental and clinical strategies* (pp. 17–22). New York: Alan Liss, Inc.

Liotta, L. A., Kleinerman, J., Catanzara, P., & Rynbrandt, D. (1977). Degradation of basement membrane by murine tumor cells. *Journal of the National Cancer Institute, 58,* 1427–1439.

Liotta, L. A., Kleinerman, J., Saidel, G. M. (1974). Quantitative relationships of intravascular tumor cells, tumor vessels, and pulmonary metastases following tumor implantation. *Cancer Research, 34,* 997.

Liotta, L. A., Mandler, R., Murano, G., Katz, D. A., Gordon, R. K., Chiang, P. K., & Schiffmann, E. (1986). Tumor cell autocrine motility factor. *Proceedings of the National Academy of Sciences USA, 83,* 3302–3306.

Liotta, L. A., Rao, C. N., & Barsky, S. H. (1983). Tumor invasion and the extracellular matrix. *Laboratory Investigation, 49,* 636–649.

Liotta, L. A., Rao, C. N., & Wewer, U. M. (1986). Biochemical interactions of tumor cells with the basement membrane. *Annual Review of Biochemistry, 55,* 1037–1057.

Liotta, L. A., Saidel, G., & Kleinerman, J. (1976). Stochastic model of metastases formation. *Biometrics, 32,* 535–550.

Liotta, L. A., & Schiffmann, E. (1988). Autocrine motility factors. In V. T. DeVita, S. A. Hellman, & S. A. Rosenberg (Eds.), *Important advances in oncology* (pp. 17–30). Philadelphia: J. B. Lippincott Co.

Liotta, L. A., Thorgeirsson, U. P., & Garbisa, S. (1982). Role of collagenases in tumor cell invasion. *Cancer and Metastasis Reviews, 1,* 277–288.

Mareel, M. M. (1983). Invasion in vitro: Methods of analysis. *Cancer and Metastasis Reviews, 2,* 201–219.

Mareel, M. M., & Calman, K. C. (Eds.). (1984). *Invasion: Experimental and clinical implications.* Oxford: Oxford University Press.

McCarthy, J. B., Basera, M. L., Palm, S. L., Sas, D. F., & Furcht, L. T. (1985). Stimulation of haptotaxis and migration of tumor cells by serum spreading factors. *Cancer Metastasis Reviews, 4,* 125–152.

Nicolson, G. L. (1978). Experimental tumor metastasis: Characteristics and organ specificity. *Bioscience, 28,* 441–447.

Nicolson, G. L. (1984). Generation of phenotypic diversity and progression in metastatic tumors. *Cancer Metastasis Reviews, 3,* 25–42.

Nicolson, G. L. (1987). Tumor cell instability, diversification, and progression to the metastatic phenotype: From oncogene to oncofetal expression. *Cancer Research, 47,* 1473–1487.

Nicolson, G. L., & Milas, L. (Eds.). (1984) *Cancer invasion and metastasis: Biologic and therapeutic aspects.* New York: Raven Press.

Nicolson, G. L., Robbins, J. G., & Winkelhake, J. L. (1975). Tumor surfaces and metastasis: Dynamic changes in neoplastic membrane structure and their relationship to tumor spread. In *Cellular membranes and tumor cell behavior* (pp. 82–123). 28th Annual Symposium on Fundamental Cancer Research. Baltimore: Williams & Wilkins.

Nowell, P. C. (1976). The clonal evolution of tumor cell populations. *Science, 194,* 23–28.

Nowell, P. C. (1986). Mechanisms of tumor progression. *Cancer Research, 46,* 2203–2207.

Paget, J. (1863). *Lectures on surgical pathology.* London: Longman, Brown, Green, and Longmans.

Poste, G. (1986). Pathogenesis of metastatic disease: Implications for current therapy and for the development of new therapeutic strategies. *Cancer Treatment Reports, 70,* 183–198.

Poste, G. (1977). The cell surface and metastasis. In S. B. Day, W. P. Myers, P. Stansly, S. Garattini, & M. G. Lewis (Eds.), *Cancer invasion and metastasis: Biologic mechanism and therapy* (pp. 163–174). New York: Raven Press.

Rao, C. N., Barsky, S. H., Terranova, V. P., & Liotta, L. A. (1983). Isolation of a tumor cell laminin receptor. *Biochemical and Biophysical Research Communications, 111,* 804–808.

Raz, A., & Geiger, B. (1982). Altered organization of cell-substrate contacts and membrane-associated cytoskeleton in tumor cell variants exhibiting different metastatic capabilities. *Cancer Research, 42,* 5183–5190.

Roblin, R. (1981). Contributions of secreted tumor cell products to metastasis. *Cancer Biology Reviews, 2,* 59–92.

Roos, E., Dingemans, K. P., van de Pavert, I. V., & van den Bergh-Weerman, M. (1977). Invasion of lymphosarcoma cells into the perfused mouse liver. *Journal of the National Cancer Institute, 58,* 399–407.

Salsbury, A. J. (1975). The significance of the circulating cancer cell. *Cancer Treatment Reviews, 2,* 55.

Schirrmacher, V. (1985). Cancer metastasis: Experimental approaches, theoretical concepts, and impacts for treatment strategies. *Advances in Cancer Research, 43,* 1–73.

Shah, J. T., Cendon, R. A., & Farr, H. W. (1976). Carcinoma of the oral cavity. Factors affecting treatment failure at the primary site and neck. *American Journal of Surgery, 132,* 504.

Siegal, G. P., Barsky, S. H., Terranova, V. P., & Liotta, L. A. (1981). Stages of neoplastic transformation of human breast tissue as monitored by dissolution of basement membrane components. *Invasion and Metastases, 1,* 54–70.

Strauli, P. (1980). Proteinases and tumor invasion. In P. Strauli, A. J. Barrett, & A. Bauci (Eds.), *Proteinases and tumor invasion* (pp. 215–222). New York: Raven Press.

Sugarbaker, E. V. (1981). Patterns of metastasis in human malignancies. *Cancer Biology Reviews, 2,* 235–278.

Terranova, V. P., Hujanen, E. S., & Martin, G. R. (1986). Basement membrane and the invasive activity of metastic tumor cells. *Journal of the National Cancer Institute, 77,* 311–316.

Terranova, V. P., Liotta, L. A., Russo, R. G., & Martin, G. R. (1982). Role of laminin in the attachment and metastasis of murine tumor cells. *Cancer Research, 42,* 2265–2273.

Terranova, V. P., Rao, C. N., & Kalebic, T. (1983). Laminin receptor on human breast carcinoma cells. *Proceedings of the National Academy of Sciences, USA, 80,* 444–451.

Terranova, V. P., Williams, J. E., & Liotta, L. A. (1984). Modulation of the metastatic activity of melanoma cells by laminin and fibronectin. *Science, 226,* 982–984.

Thorgeirsson, U. P., Turpeenniemi-Hujanen, T., & Liotta, L. A. (1985). Cancer cells, components of basement membranes, and proteolytic enzymes. *International Review of Experimental Pathology, 27,* 203–234.

Todaro, G. J., Fryling, C., & De Larco, J. E. (1980). Transforming growth factors produced by certain human tumor cells: Polypeptides that interact with epidermal growth factor receptors. *Proceedings of the National Academy of Sciences, USA, 77,* 5258.

Vlodavsky, I., Fuks, Z., Bar-Ner, M., Ariav, Y., & Schirrmacher, V. (1983). Lymphoma cell-mediated degradation of sulfated proteoglycans in the subendothelial extracellular matrix: relationship to tumor cell metastasis. *Cancer Research, 43,* 2704–2711.

Vracko, R. (1974). Basal lamina scaffold-anatomy and significance for maintenance of orderly tissue structures. *American Journal of Pathology, 77,* 313.

Weiss, L. (1976). Biophysical aspects of the metastatic cascade. In L. Weiss (Ed.), *Fundamental aspects of metastasis.* New York: Elsevier.

Weiss, L. (1983). Random and non-random processes in metastasis and metastatic inefficiency. *Invasion and Metastases, 3,* 193–207.

Weiss, L., & Ward, P. M. (1983). Cell detachment and metastasis. *Cancer Metastasis Reviews, 2,* 111–123.

Weiss, P., & Scott, B. (1963). Polarization on cell locomotion in vitro. *Proceedings of the National Academy of Sciences, USA, 50,* 330–336.

Welch, D. R., Bhuyan, B. K., & Liotta, L. A. (Eds.). (1986). *Cancer metastasis: Experimental and clinical strategies.* New York: Alan R. Liss, Inc.

Wicha, M. S., Liotta, L. A., Garbisa, S., & Kidwell, W. R. (1980). Basement membrane collagen requirements for attachment and growth of mammary epithelium. *Experimental Cell Research, 124,* 181–190.

Yamada, K. M., Akiyam, S. K., Hasegawa, T., Humphries, M. J., Kennedy, D. W., Nagata, K., Urushihara, H., Olden, K., & Chen, W. T. (1985). Recent advances in research on fibronectin and other cell attachment factors. *Journal of Cell Biochemistry, 28,* 79–97.

CLINICAL DETECTION AND SUPPORT

CHAPTER 15

Preventive Oncology

KAREN BILLARS HEUSINKVELD

In 1990, approximately 1,040,000 Americans will be diagnosed with cancer. Nonmelanoma skin cancer and carcinoma in situ have not been included in these statistics. The incidence of nonmelanoma skin cancer adds an additional 500,000 cases. In 1990, approximately 510,000 individuals will die of these cancers (American Cancer Society, 1990). Cancer will surpass heart disease as the number one cause of death by the year 2000 (Greenwald & Sondek, 1986). Certainty is growing about which agents start the abnormal process leading to cancer. Recent evidence leads to the inescapable conclusions that cancer is not entirely inevitable and that individual life styles may influence its occurrence. Life-style habits of tobacco use, diet and nutrition, and sexual practices have been found to influence the frequency of cancer (American Cancer Society, 1990). Years of research will be necessary to find the exact role of each of these behaviors in cancer onset and prevention.

Cancer prevention attempts to interrupt the complex causal pathway of initiation and promotion that leads to the transformation of normal cells into cancer cells. *Initiation* is the exposure to agents that results in the alteration of DNA and is irreversible. DNA alteration causes the cell to be sensitized to the second phase of development—*promotion*—which is a multistage process and occurs over a prolonged period of time (Miller & Miller, 1981). Agents that promote the growth of

cells that have mutated proliferate so that these cells increase more rapidly than the neighboring unmutated cells in the same tissue (Resenberger, 1984). Persistent exposure to carcinogens may result in cancer. Carcinogens are thought to be mostly exogenous and are related to environmental and life-style factors.

Avoidance of tobacco is the best-known method of cancer prevention. The deleterious effects of cigarette smoking are well known. The American Cancer Society states that cigarette smoking is responsible for 75 to 85 per cent of lung cancer cases and accounts for approximately 30 per cent of all cancer deaths (1990). Epidemiologic studies have shown that cigarette smoking is responsible for many more than 300,000 deaths annually in the United States. Cigarette smoking is an addictive behavior; consequently, cancer prevention involves encouraging individuals who are nonsmokers not to start. Individuals who do smoke must be encouraged to quit (U.S. Department of Health and Human Services [USDHHS], 1988).

Nutritional factors are important in cancer prevention. Evidence suggests that individuals might reduce the risk of cancer by avoiding obesity; cutting down on total fat intake; increasing intake of high-fiber foods; increasing intake of foods rich in vitamins A and C; including cruciferous vegetables in the diet; eating only moderate amounts of salt-cured, smoked, and nitrite-cured foods; and drinking only moderate amounts of alcohol if it is consumed at all (American Cancer Society, 1984).

Sexual practices have a relationship to cancer of the uterine cervix (Brinton & Fraumeni, 1986). Factors such as early age at first intercourse, multiplicity of sexual partners, male penile or prostate cancer, and sexually transmitted papilloma virus have been found to increase the risk of uterine cervical cancer (Brinton & Fraumeni, 1986; Cramer, 1982).

During the past 15 to 20 years, progress in cancer research has resulted in an impressive information base related to cancer prevention. A national commitment to cancer prevention is reflected in the National Cancer Institute's goal of reducing cancer mortality by 50 per cent by the year 2000 (Greenwald & Sondek, 1986). A substantial part of the solution to the cancer problem at the present time lies within the grasp and responsibility of each individual. The current trend and growing sensitivity of the public to cancer prevention has awakened in oncology nursing a new commitment to educate the public concerning risk factors and guidelines. Cancer nurses must help individuals redefine their life goals and expectations and learn to manage new health and self-care practices, thereby helping them to become more active participants in their own health care. Nurses represent an extraordinary potential for expanding health education in cancer prevention in all realms of health care. Nurses work with clients and families in all stages of health and illness and in a variety of health care settings, including hospitals, clinics, industry, and schools within rural, urban, and inner-city communities. Nurses can make a difference.

To promote compliance with guidelines for cancer prevention effectively, oncology nurses must develop approaches that address individual and group needs. They must provide information on self-protective actions to increase the proportion of individuals who consistently, rationally, and freely take action to prevent illness. A full understanding of the factors involved in individuals taking action is a prerequisite for the planning or revision of any cancer prevention educational programs.

FRAMEWORKS FOR PREVENTION

The relatively low levels of public participation in preventive health behaviors and screening for cancer have been extensively documented. The belief that the problem of prevention is mainly a failure of the health professional to communicate pertinent factual information to the public about the condition has been discounted for some time. Almost 30 years ago, Hochbaum noted that ample evidence "points to the conclusion that while information is often one of several necessary conditions for rational behavior, it is rarely sufficient to produce it" (1960, p. 13).

Many frameworks for health education for a variety of health problems and situations have been developed and evaluated. By careful consideration of behavioral and attitudinal factors, nurses can have an impact by promoting compliance with prevention guidelines. The health belief model and the PRECEDE model, a discussion of which follows, may be helpful in health education efforts.

Health Belief Model

The health belief model may have considerable value in explaining and predicting an individual's cancer prevention behavior. The model holds that individuals who exhibit the appropriate combination of beliefs will take action to prevent and detect illness in the absence of symptoms. It hypothesizes that for an individual to take any action or engage in any health behavior, minimal levels of relevant health motivation and knowledge must be present.

The individual's readiness to be concerned about the particular health issue and to comply with recommended behavior is determined by a perceived susceptibility to the possible illness and a perception of the probable severity of the illness. If the individual believes in both the likelihood of personal susceptibility to the disease and the likelihood that the consequences of the disease will be serious, he or she must then evaluate the benefits or barriers to the health action.

Benefits as defined in the health belief model are beliefs in the efficacy of the health behavior or effectiveness of the health action in relation to the illness; *barriers* are the physical, financial, and psychological costs of engaging in that behavior. To take the health action, the individual must perceive that the benefits outweigh the barriers (Fig. 15–1).

Specifically, the health belief model (Becker & Rosenstock, 1975) contains the following elements:

1. Individual Perceptions: The individual's subjective state of readiness to take action, which is determined by both perceived likelihood of *susceptibility* to the particular illness and perceptions of the probable *severity* of the consequences (organic and social) of contracting the disease.

2. Modifying Factors: A cue to action, which must occur to trigger the appropriate health behavior; this stimulus can be either internal (e.g., symptoms) or external (e.g., interpersonal interactions, mass media communications).

3. Likelihood of Action: The individual's evaluation of the advocated health behavior in terms of its feasibility and efficaciousness (i.e., an estimate of the action's potential *benefits* in reducing susceptibility or severity) weigh against perceptions of physical, psychological, financial, and other costs or *barriers* involved in the proposed action. (p. 25)

This approach to health behavior relates the perceived susceptibility and severity of the particular illness to the health action the individual will take. Perceived susceptibility or perceived likelihood of occurrence are known to vary widely among individuals. At one extreme are individuals who deny any possibility of contracting a particular illness, and at the other extreme are individuals who feel a real danger of

INDIVIDUAL PERCEPTIONS   MODIFYING FACTORS   LIKELIHOOD OF ACTION

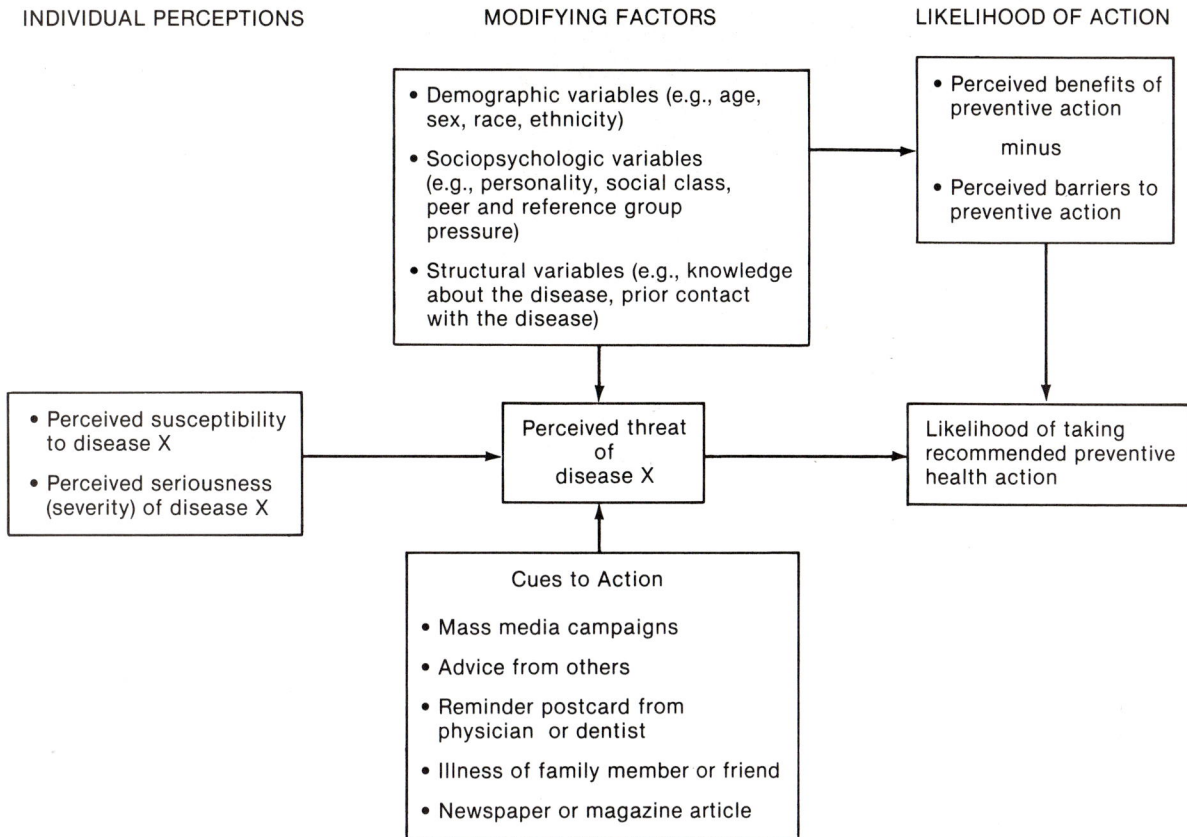

Figure 15–1. The health belief model as predictor of preventive health behavior. (From Becker, M. H., Drachman, R. H., & Kirscht, J. P. [1975]. A field experiment to evaluate various outcomes to continuity of physician care. *American Journal of Public Health, 64*, 1062–1070. Reproduced by permission.)

contracting a particular illness. Perceived seriousness of a given illness varies among individuals; it may be seen in terms of a reduction in physical or mental functioning for long periods of time, a permanent disability, or a cause of death. Perceived seriousness of a condition may have even broader or more complex implications, such as effects on career, family life, and social relationships. A smoker's perception of the risk of getting cancer from smoking may influence a decision to quit.

A health action directed toward cancer prevention and early detection can lower the individual's perceived susceptibility to cancer and reduce the perceived severity of the illness. According to the model, the expectation of success of the health action for an individual in a particular situation is a function of the perceived benefits of taking the action minus the effects of the barriers that inhibit taking the action. Barriers for an individual may be expressed in terms of physical, psychological, sociologic, and economic costs. The health benefits of quitting smoking must outweigh the relaxation and stress reduction associated with smoking.

The cue to action makes the individual become conscious of feelings and begin thinking about how to deal with the threat of cancer. Thus the likelihood of taking action is predicted to be predicated on the individual's belief that the comparable benefits of the protective action outweigh the inconvenience, discom-

fort, or undesired consequences of taking that action. Motivation as a necessary condition for action is assumed in the health belief model and is operationalized as the psychological state of readiness to take specific action and as the extent to which a particular health action is believed to be beneficial in reducing the threat (Rosenstock, 1966).

Taking a specific action is a function of the individual's evaluation of several sets of factors, including the individual's assessment of susceptibility to a given disease and the individual's evaluation of the severity of the condition. Perceived threat in the model is the individual's estimation of the chances of the condition worsening if health advice is not followed. Modifying factors, including sociodemographic and structural characteristics and cues to action, such as media and advice from others, are included in the model. The specific combination of these factors for an individual results in an increased or decreased probability that the recommended health action will be undertaken.

PRECEDE Model

The PRECEDE model, designated by Green and colleagues (1980), is a framework that nurses may find useful in cancer prevention education programs in community settings. The basic tenet of the model is that health behavior is a voluntary behavior and the reason for a behavior change must be understood by those whose behavior is in question.

The framework PRECEDE (which stands for *predisposing, reinforcing*, and *enabling causes* in *educational diagnosis* and *evaluation*) asks what behavior precedes each health benefit and what causes precede each health behavior. PRECEDE utilizes a deductive approach that starts with the final consequences and works back to the original causes. The PRECEDE model directs the initial attention to outcomes rather than to inputs and encourages the asking of "why" questions before the asking of "how" questions. By beginning with the final outcome, one determines what must precede that outcome by determining what causes that outcome. The factors important to an outcome must be diagnosed before interventions are designed. If this is not done, the interventions may be based on guesswork and run a greater risk of being misdirected and ineffective.

The PRECEDE model identifies seven phases (Fig. 15–2). Phase 1–epidemiologic diagnosis—delineates the extent, distribution, and causes of a health problem in a population. Quality of life is assessed by looking at some of the social problems and concerns of the people in the population. The demands of social prob-

lems in a given community are good barometers of the community's quality of life. Phase 2—social diagnosis—identifies the specific high priority health problems that appear to be contributing to the social problems. Available data and data generated by appropriate investigations for vital indicators and dimensions of the health problem are used. Phase 3—behavioral diagnosis—delineates the specific health behaviors that appear to be linked to the health problem. Preventive actions, utilization, consumption patterns, compliance, self-care, economics, genetics, and environment are assessed in this phase. These behaviors and dimensions are identified specifically and are carefully ranked.

Phase 4—educational diagnosis—requires the sorting and categorizing of predisposing, enabling, and reinforcing factors that have a direct impact on the health problem. Predisposing factors are attitudes, beliefs, and perceptions that facilitate or hinder health behaviors. Enabling factors are barriers such as limited facilities, lack of income or health insurance, and inadequate personnel or community resources. The skills and knowledge required for a desired behavior to occur are also enabling factors. Reinforcing factors are those related to feedback from others concerning health behaviors. The feedback may either encourage or discourage the behavioral change. In phase 5—

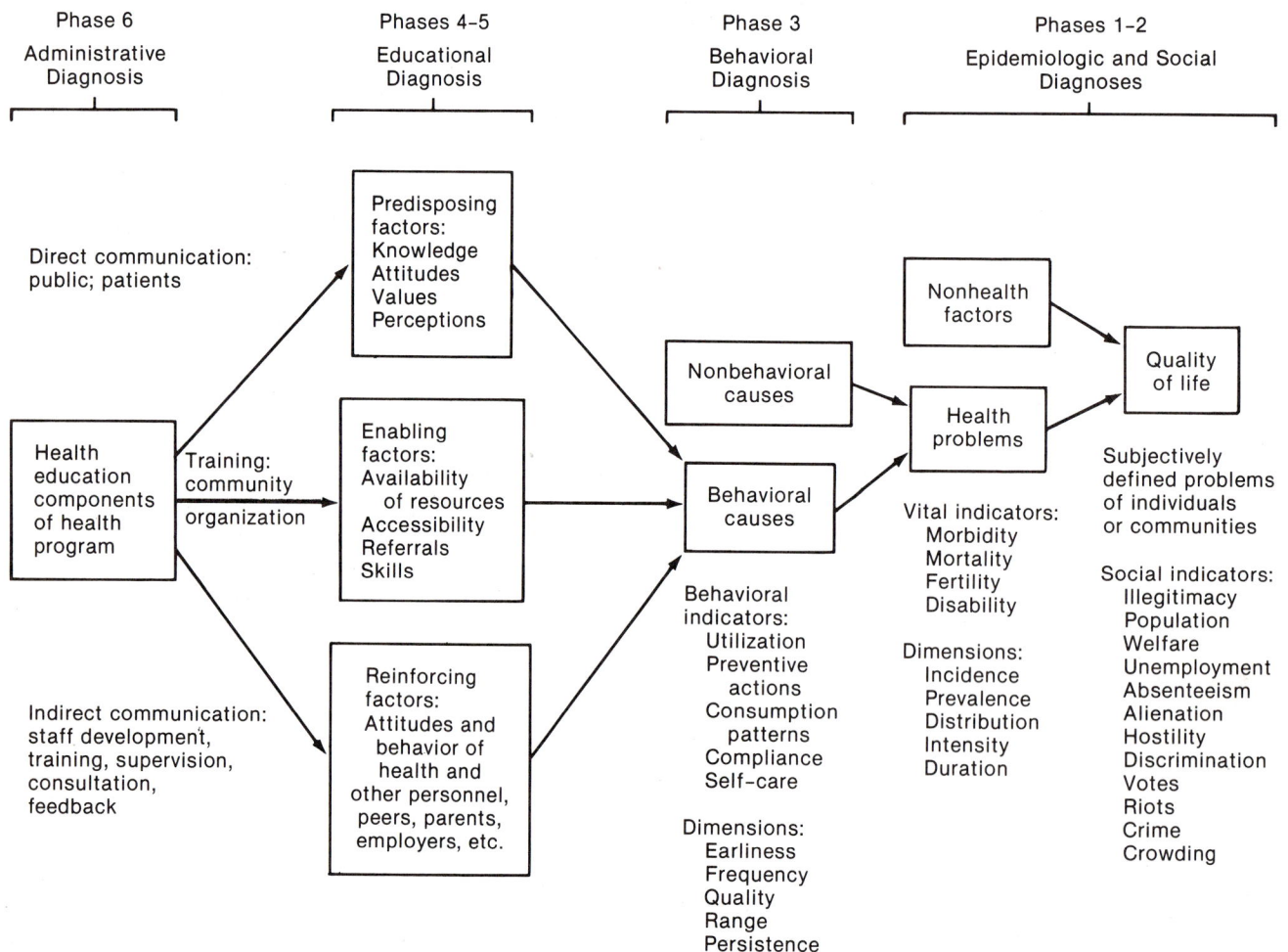

Figure 15–2. PRECEDE framework. (From Green, L. W., Kreuter, M. W., Deeds, M. W., & Partridge, K. B. [1980]. *Health education planning. A diagnostic approach.* Palo Alto, CA: Mayfield Publishing Co. Reproduced by permission.)

prioritizing—the relative importance of each of the factors and available resources is determined. These factors are the focus of the intervention.

Phase 6—administrative diagnosis—is the actual development and implementation of a program. Based on knowledge of limitations of resources, time constraints, and abilities, the appropriate educational interventions are determined. Administrative problems and resources are assessed. Phase 7—evaluation—is not a phase unto itself but is considered an integral and continuous part of the entire framework. It begins with clearly stated program and behavioral objectives in the diagnostic phases and ends with evaluation of long-range goals of improved quality of life and social benefits.

PRECEDE requires epidemiologic, social-survey, and demographic data for the identification of major social and health problems in a group. Those problems that are important enough to the group to be targets of the cancer prevention education program are the focus of health education.

TOBACCO USE

The accumulation of data relating cigarette smoking to serious illness has accelerated at a rapid pace. Thousands of studies have documented that smoking causes lung cancer, bladder and stomach cancers, chronic obstructive lung disease, heart disease, and complications of pregnancy (Gritz, 1988; USDHHS, 1988). As early as 1958, a classic epidemiologic study on smoking and death rates showed a high degree of association between cigarette smoking and the total death rate (Hammond & Horns, 1958).

The link between smoking and cancer has been firmly established (USDHHS, 1987). Smoking is the single largest preventable cause of premature death and disability as well as the major cause of cancer mortality, accounting for 30 per cent of all cancer deaths in the United States (USDHHS, 1987). Furthermore, the 1988 United States surgeon general's report concluded that cigarettes and other forms of tobacco are addictive and that nicotine is the drug that causes the addiction (USDHHS, 1988).

Smoking and tobacco use constitute the single most serious public health problem in our society today. Smoking is implicated in more than 320,000 deaths per year, and the economic burden to society is tremendous. The cost of smoking to the economy is estimated to be $65 billion per year. This amounts to $2.17 in lost productivity and treatment of smoking-related diseases for each pack of cigarettes sold (U.S. Congress, 1985).

More than 50 million Americans continue to smoke cigarettes, and the use of other forms of tobacco is increasing. The death rate from cancer for male cigarette smokers is more than double the rate for nonsmokers, and the death rate for female smokers is 67 per cent higher than that for nonsmokers. The higher cancer rate for men reflects the fact that in the past,

more men than women smoked and smoked more heavily. The gap between male and female smoking has been narrowing in recent years (American Cancer Society, 1988). The reported smoking rate for blacks has exceeded that for whites, and the reported rate of quitting has been less for blacks than for whites (Novotny, Warner, Kendrick, & Remington, 1988; USDHHS, 1987).

In the last 15 years, the percentage of adults who report being regular smokers has been declining steadily (USDHHS, 1983). The percentage for white males dropped from 51.3 per cent in 1965 to 37.1 per cent in 1980; the percentage for white females during this same period declined from 34.5 per cent to 30.0 per cent. Among black adults, a similar pattern is seen: for males, a decline from 59.6 per cent to 44.9 per cent; for females, a decline from 32.7 per cent to 30.6 per cent.

The average smoker appears to be smoking more heavily: the mean of 20.0 cigarettes per day in 1970 has risen to 21.7 cigarettes per day in 1980. Although males continue to smoke a greater average number of cigarettes per day than do females, the increase in mean number of cigarettes smoked daily was slightly greater for females than for males. The heaviest daily consumption is observed in middle-aged groups (35 to 65 years). A greater mean increase from 1970 to 1980 was observed among women aged 35 to 64 years (USDHHS, 1983).

Surveys have repeatedly shown that blue-collar workers are more likely than white-collar workers to smoke cigarettes (USDHHS, 1985). Overall, the smoking rate for blue-collar men (47.1 per cent) exceeds that of white-collar men (33.0 per cent). The same pattern holds for women, with the smoking rate of blue-collar women (38.1 per cent) exceeding that of white-collar women (31.9 per cent). Among women, the white-collar–blue-collar difference exists only for the younger age group (20 to 44 years); for older women (45 to 65 years), virtually no difference in smoking prevalence is evident between the two categories of workers (USDHHHS, 1985).

In 1984 more than 22 million people in the United States used smokeless tobacco (USDHHS, 1986). Teenagers are using smokeless tobacco, and this early addiction could ensure exposure for many years. There is evidence that the incidence of oral cancer among users of smokeless tobacco is increasing (Squire, 1984). The involuntary inhalation of tobacco smoke—passive smoking—has recently received widespread attention. The concern to protect nonsmokers from the annoyances and the adverse health effects of exposure to the cigarette smoke of others has resulted in pressure to limit smoking in public places. Evidence is growing that passive or involuntary smoking causes an increase in health problems (USDHHS, 1982).

Challenge for Cancer Prevention Efforts

Fortunately the risk of smoking-related cancers can be reduced, even for those who have been smoking for many years. Cessation of smoking reduces the excess risk of lung cancer. And over a period of a decade, the risk of lung cancer morbidity for an individual who ceases to smoke gradually approaches that of a lifelong nonsmoker (USDHHS, 1982).

Smoking has been given a high priority in the national cancer control effort (Cullen, 1986). The goal of the National Cancer Institute, the American Cancer Institute, and the American Cancer Society is to decrease the incidence of cancer that is caused or related to smoking and to decrease the use of tobacco products. Public awareness of the dangers of smoking and tobacco use is at an all-time high. Although most smokers would like to quit, more than 50 million Americans continue to smoke. Ex-smokers describe their main reasons for quitting as relating to serious health concerns. The most successful programs for adolescents are those that emphasize the social and immediate consequences of smoking rather than the long-term health consequences.

Individuals who are at high risk for tobacco-related cancers need to be identified, and intervention studies to reduce smoking must follow. High-risk target groups include heavy smokers; minorities, particularly blacks and Hispanics; women; and youth. These groups are at greater risk and may be more difficult to reach with present interventions. All of these groups will require interventions that use PRECEDE and health belief model frameworks, which emphasize specific needs and concerns.

Proven strategies to reduce smoking are not available. It is believed that the vast majority of ex-smokers (now about 40 million) stopped without the use of an organized smoking cessation program. They were able to quit smoking by using self-help resources, informal social supports, and media information on smoking (USDHHS, 1982).

This experience of past smokers points to the desirability of effective self-help programs in smoking cessation. Such programs would appeal to many who are unlikely to be reached by organized cessation clinics. Programs that involve the mass media and programs with single informational contacts have been effective. The self-help approaches may include brief advice on or encouragement for quitting. Information campaigns to keep the public aware of smoking and tobacco-related issues are necessary.

Having smoking cessation interventions become part of the smoker's natural environment may address the issue of smokers who prefer to stop without the aid of a formal program. When prevention and intervention efforts are woven into the smoker's daily life (workplace, health care setting, school, and media to which the smoker is exposed), they may prove to be more effective and cost effective (Ockene, 1984).

Nurses, more than any other health professionals, are in positions to promote effective health behaviors for cancer prevention within the general population and for those individuals who are at high risk for cancer. Because nurses practice in various settings and have contact with numerous clients, families, and significant others, they can be powerful agents for bringing about smoking cessation. Whether at a hospital, clinic, private office, industry, or school, nurses have an opportunity to affect the smoking habits of the American public. The integration of smoking cessation interventions in the health care setting takes advantage of existing services and of a natural setting. Given that a large percentage of smokers have contact with a health care setting, it is appropriate for the nurse to provide interventions.

In spite of the fact that nurses have a good understanding of the risks of smoking and are aware of their role as health behavior models for the community, the percentage of nurses who smoke has been reported as higher than the rate for the general population (Murry, Swan, & Matter, 1983; Scholes, 1982). In the United States, a greater percentage of physicians and dentists who smoked have quit compared with the percentage of nurses (Scholes, 1982). Given the surgeon general's directive for a smoke-free environment, nurses have a responsibility to be nonsmokers so that they are able to direct and participate in teaching and counseling clients and the public about the harmful effects of smoking. The American Cancer Society and the Oncology Nursing Society have encouraged nurses to quit and to participate in antismoking activities.

Frameworks for Smoking Cessation

Health Belief Model

Quitting smoking requires a major change in health behavior, and the health belief model provides a framework that the nurse can use to help individuals achieve that goal (Becker, Drachman, & Kirscht, 1975). According to the model, the smoker's perceived susceptibility to cancer or other illness and perception of the severity of that cancer or illness is important. The individual who smokes must believe that he or she is susceptible and that the condition is serious.

To help increase the smoker's perceived susceptibility to cancer, the latest information on smoking and cancer needs to be available as well as information on the high mortality of smoking-related cancers. If the smoker believes that he or she is susceptible and that the condition is serious, then the benefits or barriers to the health action must be evaluated.

The benefits of quitting smoking must be made known to the smoker (smoking-related cancers can be reduced, money will be saved, tobacco smell will be eliminated, risk to family members will be lessened). The benefits must outweigh the barriers (losing relaxation effect, gaining weight, experiencing withdrawal symptoms) before the smoker will take the health action and quit. A cue to action, either external, such as from interpersonal communications or the mass media, or internal, such as from coughing and experiencing difficulty breathing, must occur to make the smoker consciously aware of the problem and of the dangers of smoking behavior.

As the nurse is working with individual smokers or with smokers in high-risk groups to help them quit smoking, the components in the health belief model may help focus time and energy on effective interventions. Because the majority of ex-smokers stopped smoking by using self-help resources and not organized programs, a model that requires individuals to evaluate several sets of factors and to make a decision regarding quitting smoking may be effective.

PRECEDE Model

PRECEDE may be used as a framework for health education (Green, Kreuter, Deeds, & Partridge, 1980) because quitting smoking is a voluntary health behavior. Phase 1—epidemiologic diagnosis—and phase 2—social diagnosis—require that the nurse determine whether smoking is a problem of concern for the population targeted and then determine incidence and mortality rates of smoking-related cancers for that population. Identification of individuals in the population who are at high risk for smoking-related cancers as well as for behaviors that contribute to smoking would be included as phase 3, in which health behaviors are linked to health problems.

Phase 4—educational diagnosis—includes determining the predisposing, enabling, and reinforcing factors that contribute to smoking. Predisposing factors can be explored by questions such as What does the target group of smokers know about smoking and cancer? Do they believe that they have a problem? Is smoking part of the culture? Do they think that quitting smoking will help? Enabling factors include determining whether the smokers have the resources available to obtain current information on the dangers of smoking. Reinforcing factors can be determined by questions such as Do the smokers have family and peer support for quitting smoking? Are other health professionals willing to reinforce quitting smoking? Phase 5—prioritizing—requires determining those factors that appear to have the greatest impact on smoking. Phase 6—administrative diagnosis—requires the determination of the health education components for either a self-help program or a structured health program for smoking cessation.

Tobacco Use Summary

Nurses can have a significant impact on smoking cessation in the United States through their involvement in individual and group programs that identify smokers, advise them of the health risks of smoking, personalize their reasons for cessation, and provide and discuss self-help materials. Table 15–1 summarizes factors associated with smoking cessation that nurses may use in programs.

In a larger sense, the nurse role includes political involvement and influencing public policy. Political involvement at the local level includes working for the right of nonsmokers to be protected from possible effects of passive smoking or working on antismoking programs in communities and schools. On the state

Table 15–1. FACTORS ASSOCIATED WITH SUCCESSFUL SMOKING CESSATION

Motivational Factors
Desire to overcome minor smoking-related symptoms (coughing, wheezing, shortness of breath)
Expectation of improved future health
Sense of personal vulnerability to risk
Desire to increase self-mastery and self-esteem
Expectation of many quitting benefits—health, freedom, social and economic advantages
Expectation of success
Expectation that benefits will outweigh difficulties
Support and encouragement from family (especially spouse), friends, work associates

Effective Quitting Skills
Quitting abruptly instead of tapering off
Using a variety of coping methods for withdrawal symptoms, such as deep breathing, positive thinking, and specific cigarette substitutes
Using a variety of methods to remain off cigarettes, such as avoiding temptations to smoke, finding alternative ways to relax and cope with stress (such as hobbies or exercise), using substitute self-rewards to counteract sense of loss and prevent relapse
Taking a long-range, problem-solving approach

Social Supports and Psychosocial Assets
Personalized and medical quit-smoking advice and support
Encouragement, inspiration, and advice from ex-smokers
Good psychosocial resources (such as education and income)

Smoking Habit Factors
Lower smoking rate and nicotine intake and dependence
Less reliance on cigarettes for regulation of negative affect
Past success in quitting for 6 months or more
Good stress management skills

(From Orleans, C. T. [1985]. Understanding and promoting smoking cessation: Overview and guidelines for physical intervention. *Annual Review of Medicine, 36,* 51–61. Reproduced by permission of the *Annual Review of Medicine,* vol. 36. © 1985 by Annual Reviews, Inc.)

and national level, nurses must work for restrictions on cigarette and smokeless tobacco advertising, mandatory display of warning labels, taxation of cigarettes and smokeless tobacco products, and government actions to stop tobacco subsidies.

General efforts by nurses to reduce smoking include (1) encouraging smoking prevention programs for preteens and young teenagers in the schools because cigarette smoking in the United States today is a habit that is usually established by the age of 16; (2) supporting smokers who wish to quit; (3) supporting legislation and policies in public places, at work, at school, and in the home that benefit nonsmokers; (4) writing letters to editors of local papers on issues related to smoking tobacco products; (5) speaking at clubs and organizations concerning smoking and cessation options; (6) communicating with editors and publishers of magazines and publications to articulate concerns about cigarette advertising; and (7) discouraging cigarette company sponsorship of sporting, fashion, and arts events and educational and medical programs.

Cigarette smoking is currently the single most preventable cause of illness and death in America. The time has come for nurses to act on what they know about smoking and cancer.

NUTRITION

The potential role of nutrition in the etiology and prevention of cancer has gained considerable attention in the last two decades. Doll and Peto (1981) provided a wide range of estimates (10 to 70 per cent) for the proportion of deaths from cancer that are related to various dietary factors. They concluded that dietary modification might eventually result in a 35 per cent reduction in mortality from cancer in the United States.

The Committee on Diet, Nutrition, and Cancer of the National Research Council concluded that cancers of most major sites are influenced by dietary patterns. They found that the differences in the rates at which various cancers occur in different human populations are often correlated with differences in diet (National Research Council, 1982). The evidence for fat as a cause of human cancer is sufficient to recommend a reduction in dietary intake of both saturated and unsaturated fats. Studies of human populations indicate that high fiber consumption may offer protection from some cancers.

There are many ways in which diet may be an etiologic factor in human cancers and may influence cancer risk. Diet may have special consequences for the alimentary tract, whose tissues are in direct contact with ingested food. The most consistent dietary correlate for cancers of the upper alimentary tract (oral cavity, oropharynx, pharynx, esophagus, and upper larynx) is the large consumption of alcohol. Stomach and colon cancer have been associated with nitrites, and primary liver cancer has been shown to be associated with aflatoxin. Cancers of the colon have been associated with diets high in fat andd low in fiber (Armstrong, McMichael, & Maclennan, 1982).

The recognition that breast cancer is highly correlated with consumption of fat was first recognized in the late 1960s (Lear, 1966). Additional evidence suggests that a diet high in fat is a factor in the etiology of human breast cancer and can explain much of the present geographic variation in the incidence of breast cancer (Armstrong et al., 1982). Endometrial cancer has been associated with obesity (Armstrong, 1977).

Challenge for Cancer Prevention Efforts

The various dietary factors that have been associated with human cancers are by no means certain. In some cases only a class of foods can be listed because the chemical or chemicals responsible for its effect are uncertain. The National Research Council, the National Cancer Institute, and the American Cancer Society have suggested lowering total fat intake to less than 30 per cent of total calories; consuming no more than one to two drinks of alcohol per day, if at all; consuming very small amounts of smoked and cured foods; and increasing consumption to 20 to 30 grams per day of vegetables (green and yellow, carotene-rich, and cruciferous), citrus fruits, whole-grain products, and other foods containing fiber (American Cancer Society, 1984; National Cancer Institute, 1984; National Research Council, 1982).

Even though current knowledge concerning dietary intake and cancer is not certain, the evidence is sufficient to conclude that dietary patterns may influence carcinogenesis and that cancer risk may be lowered by dietary modifications. With the available data on diet and cancer, nurses can play a vital role in helping individuals and groups to modify their dietary patterns.

Frameworks for Nutrition Counseling

Health Belief Model

The health belief model can be used by nurses (Becker et al., 1975). To increase the individual's or group's perceived susceptibility to cancer because of diet, the evidence on diet and cancer must be made available to them. The individual must believe that he or she is susceptible to cancer because of dietary factors and that the cancer would be serious. When the individual has these beliefs, he or she must then evaluate the benefits or barriers to the dietary change. The benefits of changing one's diet must be made known to the individual, for example, that diet-related cancers can be reduced and overall health can be improved. The benefits must outweigh the barriers (e.g., food likes, cultural significance of foods) before the individual will modify dietary behaviors. A cue to action, such as an interpersonal communication or a mass media message, must occur to make the individual consciously aware of the problem and of the possible dangers of dietary intake. As the nurse is working with the individual or group to help reduce the intake of some foods and increase the intake of others, the components of the health belief model may help to focus effective interventions.

PRECEDE Model

Modifying dietary intake is a voluntary health problem that nurses may address by using the PRECEDE framework (Green et al., 1980). Phase 1—epidemiologic diagnosis—and phase 2—social diagnosis—will require the nurse to determine whether diet is a problem for the targeted group and then determine incidence and mortality from dietary-related cancers for that group. Identification of individuals in the population who may be at risk and any behaviors that contribute to dietary intake would be included in Phase 3—behavioral diagnosis.

Phase 4—educational diagnosis—would include determining the predisposing, enabling, and reinforcing factors contributing to the diet. Questions that explore predisposing factors include What do the individuals know about diet and cancer? Do they believe they have a problem? Do they have eating habits specific to their culture? Do they believe diet can affect cancer incidence? Enabling factors are addressed by questions such as Do the individuals have the skills necessary to modify their dietary intake? Are food products whose

Table 15–2. DIET, NUTRITION, AND CANCER

Total Caloric Intake
- Animal studies show reduction decreases incidence of cancer.
- Human studies do not show clear evidence.

Fats and Lipids
- Evidence suggests a causal relationship between high fat intake and cancer occurrence.

Protein
- High protein may be associated with increased risk of cancer.
- No firm conclusion on the effect of protein.

Carbohydrates
- Limited and inconclusive data.

Dietary Fiber
- Specific components of fiber, not total amount of fiber, exert a protective effect against colorectal cancer.

Alcoholic Beverages
- Excessive beer drinking has been associated with increased risk of colorectal cancer.
- Excessive alcohol consumption and cigarette smoking act synergistically to increase risk of cancers of mouth, larynx, esophagus, and respiratory tract.

Vitamins
- Vitamin A: evidence suggests foods rich in carotenes or vitamin A are associated with reduced risk of cancer.
- Vitamin C: limited evidence that the consumption of vitamin C–containing foods lowers risk of cancer of the stomach and esophagus.
- Vitamin E: no conclusion can be drawn.
- Vitamin B: no conclusion can be drawn.

Fruits and Vegetables
- Carotene-rich vegetables (dark green and deep yellow): frequent consumption is associated with lower incidence of cancer.
- Vegetables of the *Brassica* genus (cabbage, broccoli, cauliflower, and Brussels sprouts): frequent consumption is associated with lower incidence of cancer.

(Adapted from Palmer, [1986]. Dietary considerations for risk reduction. *Cancer, 58,* 1949–1933. Reproduced by permission.)

consumption should be increased available and easily accessible? Reinforcing factors can be determined by asking, Do the individuals have family and peer support for dietary modifications? Are health professionals available and willing to reinforce the modifications? By supplying answers to the previous questions, the nurse can determine the health education components for formal or informal programs.

Nutrition Summary

No specific dietary advice can be given that will guarantee the prevention of any specific human cancer. However, as more and more evidence suggests the association between nutrition and cancer, dietary changes may be desirable. Practical recommendations for inclusion in nutrition–cancer prevention programs are to avoid obesity; to cut down on total fat intake; to eat more foods that are high in fiber; to eat foods rich in vitamins A and C; to increase intake of cruciferous vegetables; to consume only moderate amounts of alcohol; and to decrease consumption of salt-cured, smoked, and nitrate-treated foods (Table 15–2). The nurse's role in this area of cancer prevention will become more critical as dietary evidence continues to be studied. Nurses will counsel individuals and groups to help them determine specific risks and protection measures.

SEXUAL BEHAVIORS

Uterine cervical cancer is the most common gynecologic cancer. Deaths from cancer of the uterine cervix represent approximately 1.5 per cent of all cancer deaths in the United States (American Cancer Society, 1988). Through the use of cytologic screening, the frequency of early diagnosis of cervical cancer has increased. Subsequently, the number of women with more advanced stage II and stage III invasive cancer has decreased significantly.

No single causative agent has been found for cervical cancer. In fact, research has shown a multifactorial origin (Table 15–3). Carcinoma of the cervix appears to be a sexually transmitted disease. As a result, the sexual habits of women and their male partners appear to be important risk factors (Cramer, 1982).

Two strong risk factors for cervical cancer are early age at first intercourse and multiple sexual partners (Brinton & Fraumeni, 1986; Cramer, 1982). Women who had sexual relations before the age of 20 have approximately twice the risk of developing cervical cancer of women who initiated sexual relations at a later age. Women who have multiple sexual partners have approximately two to three times the risk for cervical cancer of women who have one partner (Cramer, 1982). Early age of first coitus as a risk factor for cervical cancer may result from the susceptibility of the adolescent cervix. The association of multiple sexual partners with cervical cancer suggests a viral factor as the cause (Cramer, 1982).

The male sexual partner has been shown to have an influence in cervical cancer (Cramer, 1982; Hulka, 1982; Skegg, Corwin, Paul, & Doll, 1982). Male circumcision, which previously had been considered a predisposing factor in cervical cancer, has decreased in importance. There are reports of marital clusters of cervical cancer in which two or more wives of the same men developed cervical cancer. There is also an increased incidence of cervical cancer in wives whose husbands had prostate or penile carcinoma (Brinton & Fraumeni, 1986).

Sexually transmitted infectious agents, particularly the papilloma virus, are suspect in cervical cancer. Human papilloma virus is widespread in both males

Table 15–3. SEXUAL BEHAVIORS AND THEIR ASSOCIATION WITH CERVICAL CANCER

Factor	Association
Early age at first coitus	Strong
Multiple sexual partners	Strong
Age at menarche or menopause	None
Character of menses	None
Multiple pregnancies	Questionable
Use of oral contraceptives	Questionable
Circumcision of partner	Questionable
Female or male sexually transmitted viral infections	Strong
Use of barrier contraceptives	Moderate

(Adapted from Cramer, D. W. [1982]. Uterine cervix. In D. Schottenfeld & J. F. Fraumeni [Eds.], *Cancer epidemiology and prevention* [pp. 881–900]. Philadelphia: W. B. Saunders Co. Reproduced by permission.)

and females and is found in approximately 70 per cent of cervical cancers (Brinton & Fraumeni, 1986). Herpes simplex virus II was thought to have an association with cervical carcinoma, but the evidence no longer supports this association. The role the male partner plays in cervical cancer has not been assessed fully, but it is an important factor in the disease.

Challenge for Sexual Behaviors

Preventive measures for cervical cancer can be accomplished through modifications in sexual behaviors. Young teenagers may be an important target group for counseling. Both males and females must be informed of the cancer risk advantages of delaying sexual relations until they reach maturity (Cramer, 1982). Barrier contraception through the use of condoms should be encouraged if abstinence is not an acceptable alternative. Women and men with multiple sexual partners also should use barrier contraceptives.

Maintaining good genital hygiene is important. Genital sores and discharge or odor must be assessed and treated. In addition, all women should have an annual Papanicolaou smear.

Frameworks for Sexual Behaviors

Health Belief Model

Current knowledge concerning sexual practices and cervical cancer suggests that behavior modification may be necessary for some women. Nurses can use the health belief model (Becker et al., 1975) to help women decrease the risk of cervical cancer. To increase women's perceived susceptibility to cervical cancer, evidence regarding risk factors for cervical cancer should be stressed. The seriousness of cervical cancer should also be emphasized.

When a woman believes that she is susceptible to cervical cancer because of her sexual practices, she must then evaluate the benefits or barriers to a modification of sexual behavior. The benefits of this modification must be made known to the woman (e.g., risk of cervical cancer can be reduced). The benefits must outweigh the barriers before the woman will modify her sexual practices. Barriers might include cultural or religious beliefs against condom use or peer pressure against abstinence. A cue to action, as either an interpersonal communication or a mass media message, must occur to make the woman consciously aware of the problem and of the possible dangers of her sexual practices.

PRECEDE Model

Modification of sexual practices is a health problem that may be addressed by using the PRECEDE framework (Green et al., 1980). Phase 1—epidemiologic diagnosis—and phase 2—social diagnosis—require that the nurse determine the concern about cervical cancer for the targeted group and the incidence of and mortality from cervical cancers for that group. Phase 3—behavioral diagnosis—would include identification of women in the population who may be at risk for cervical cancer.

Phase 4—educational diagnosis—would include determining the predisposing, enabling, and reinforcing factors contributing to sexual practices associated with increased cancer risk. Questions to determine predisposing factors would include What do the individuals know about sexual practices and cervical cancer? Do they believe they have a problem? Do they have cultural sexual practices that place them at risk? Do they believe changing sexual habits can affect cervical cancer incidence? Enabling factors are addressed by questions such as Do the individuals have the skills necessary to modify their sexual practices? Are condoms and protective devices available? Questions to assess the reinforcing factors are Do the women have family, especially a mother, and peer support for modification of sexual practices? Are health professionals available and willing to reinforce the modifications?

Sexual Behaviors Summary

Sexual factors are beginning to be seen as a very important aspect of any cancer prevention program. The sensitivity of discussing sexual behaviors with all cultures and age groups may have resulted in a lack of attention to this area. Abstinence and the use of barrier contraceptives are recommended as appropriate preventive behaviors and must be stressed. As more evidence is found that associates certain sexual practices with uterine cervical cancer, the nurse will play an even greater role in this area of cancer prevention. Many individuals and groups may feel more comfortable discussing sexual practices with nurses than with other health professionals.

COMMUNITY-BASED PROGRAMS

Nurses who have cancer prevention information and health education framework knowledge can promote effective strategies for cancer prevention in their communities and specifically for those who are at high risk for cancer. The oncology nurses in a community can develop and implement projects for cancer prevention. The nutrition and cancer educational health fair in metropolitan Minneapolis–St. Paul, Minnesota, may be useful as a model for these activities (Post-White, Herzan, Drew, & Anglin, 1989). To increase public awareness of cancer risks and benefits of certain cancer prevention dietary behaviors, oncology nurses designed and implemented a health fair at seven locations. Oncology nurses staffed the booths and presented assessments and information on diet and cancer according to the American Cancer Society guidelines. Two weeks after the health fair, postcard surveys were sent to 200 participants. Ninety-five per cent found the assessment helpful in evaluating their diet, and 80 per cent made dietary changes in the 2 weeks following the health fair.

All nurses need to be cancer prevention nurses. Nurses who are not always thought of as cancer nurses are critical to the overall community cancer prevention efforts. School nurses, occupational health nurses, nurses in private physicians' offices, nurses in ambulatory care, and health department nurses are of prime importance to community cancer prevention programs.

At this time, a comprehensive program for cancer prevention education among nurses does not exist. Nurses may receive information on cancer prevention during their formal academic preparation, at conferences and workshops, or through the literature. Therefore, health education in cancer prevention for nurses is in its infancy and must be addressed. A conscious effort must be made to reach all nurses in the community.

To ensure that nurses have and use cancer prevention information in their practices, a nurse workgroup can be established in each community. The workgroup would include nurse leaders from a variety of practice areas (hospitals, schools, health departments, physician offices, industry, ambulatory clinics, and private practice) in the community. A group of nurses whose special clinical practice is oncology should be the initiators of the workgroup. They would invite nurse leaders in various practice settings in the community to meet and discuss issues and possible strategies.

The workgroup would plan for dissemination of cancer prevention information to all nurses. This dissemination could be done formally, through established nursing groups, or informally, through the workplace. Nurses in the local workgroup would know the nurses in practice settings similar to their own and would know the strengths, needs, and concerns of these nurses.

Because the workgroup nurses will represent a variety of health care settings in the community, they will know not only the needs for nurse education but also the health needs of the community for cancer prevention. The workgroup would plan for dissemination of cancer prevention information to all nurses and help nurses with health education strategies and evaluation. Workgroup planning for cancer prevention may be done in conjunction with cancer screening and detection education. By using the community-based nurse workgroup process, the commitment to cancer prevention would be strengthened.

SUMMARY

Cancer prevention efforts by nurses are feasible and practical but have not been emphasized in the war against cancer. We now have an opportunity to influence cancer morbidity and mortality by looking at agents in our life styles and in our environment that may cause cancer. The best defense against cancer is limiting exposure to known carcinogens and making appropriate life-style changes. Decreasing the number

of people who use tobacco products, helping people change questionable dietary patterns, and educating people concerning sexual practices are cancer prevention goals that every nurse must address. Nurses have an exceedingly important role in cancer prevention and must take leadership roles in helping themselves, individuals, groups, and communities change behaviors. If we are willing to use the knowledge we now have about how to prevent cancer, we will be well on the road to eliminating cancer.

References

American Cancer Society. (1984). Nutrition and cancer: Cause and prevention. New York: American Cancer Society.
American Cancer Society. (1990). Cancer facts and figures. Atlanta: American Cancer Society.
Armstrong, B. K. (1977). The role of diet in human carcinogenesis with special reference to endometrial cancer. In H. H. Hiat, J. D. Watson, & J. A. Winsten (Eds.), Origins of human cancer (pp. 557–565). New York: Cold Spring Harbor Laboratory.
Armstrong, B. K., McMichael, A. J., & Maclennan, R. (1982). Diet. In D. Schottenfeld and J. F. Fraumeni (Eds.), Cancer epidemiology and prevention (pp. 419–433). Philadelphia: W. B. Saunders Co.
Becker, M. H., Drachman, R. H., & Kirscht, J. P. (1975). A field experiment to evaluate various outcomes to continuity of physician care. American Journal of Public Health, 64, 1062–1070.
Becker, M. H., & Rosenstock, I. M. (1975). Socio-psychological research on determinants of prevention health behavior. In The behavioral sciences and prevention medicine: Opportunities and dilemmas (The Fogarty International Center Series on the Teaching of Preventive Medicine), 4. Bethesda, MD: National Cancer Institute.
Brinton, L. A., & Fraumeni, J. F. (1986). Epidemiology in uterine cervical cancer. Journal of Chronic Disease, 39, 1051–1065.
Cramer, D. W. (1982). Uterine cervix. In D. Schottenfeld & J. F. Fraumeni (Eds.), Cancer epidemiology and prevention (pp. 881–900). Philadelphia: W. B. Saunders Co.
Cullen, J. W. (1986). A rationale for health promotion in cancer control. Preventive Medicine, 15, 442–450.
Doll, R., & Peto, R. (1981). The causes of cancer: Quantitative estimates of avoidable risks of cancer in the United States today. Journal of the National Cancer Institute, 66, 1192–1308.
Green, L. W., Kreuter, M. W., Deeds, M. W., & Partridge, K. B. (1980). Health education planning. A diagnostic approach. Palo Alto, CA: Mayfield Publishing Co.
Greenwald, P., & Sondek, E. (Eds.). (1986). Cancer control objectives for the nation. National Cancer Institute Monograph, 1985–2000.
Gritz, E. R. (1988). Cigarette smoking: The need for action by health professionals. CA: A Cancer Journal for Clinicians, 38, 194–212.
Hammond, E. C., & Horn, D. (1958). Smoking and death rates: Report on forty-four months of follow up of 187,783 men. JAMA, 166, 1294–1308.
Hochbaum, G. M. (1960). Modern theories of communication. Children, 7, 13–18.
Hulka, B. (1982). Risk factors for cervical cancer. Chronic Disease, 35, 311.
Lea, A. J. (1966). Dietary factors associated with death rates for certain neoplasms in man. Lancet, 1, 332–333.
Miller, C. E., & Miller, J. A. (1981). Mechanism of chemical carcinogenesis. Cancer, 47, 1055–1064.
Murry, M., Swan, A. V., & Matter, N. (1983). The task of nursing and the risk of smoking. Journal of Advanced Nursing, 8, 131–138.
National Cancer Institute. (1984). Diet, nutrition, and cancer prevention (85–2711). Washington, DC: National Cancer Institute.
National Research Council Committee on Diet, Nutrition, and Cancer. (1982). Diet, nutrition, and cancer. Washington, DC:

National Research Council. Novotny, T. E., Warner, K. E., Kendrick, J. S., & Remington, P. L. (1988). Smoking by blacks and whites: Socioeconomic and demographic differences. *American Journal of Public Health, 78,* 1187–1189.

Ockene, J. K. (1984). Toward a smoke free society. *American Journal of Public Health, 74,* 1198–1208.

Orleans, C. T. (1985). Understanding and promoting smoking cessation: Overview and guidelines for physician intervention. *Annual Review of Medicine, 36,* 51–61.

Palmer, S. (1986). Dietary considerations for risk reduction. *Cancer, 58,* 1949–1953.

Post-White, J., Herzan, D., Drew, D., and Anglin, M. A. (1989). Nutrition and cancer: Educating the public through a health fair. *Oncology Nursing Forum, 16,* 115–118.

Resenberger, B. (1984). Cancer: The new synthesis. *Science, 9,* 28–39.

Rosenstock, I. M. (1966). Why people use health services. *Milbank Memorial Fund Quarterly, 44,* 94–127.

Scholes, M. E. (1982). Smoking and nurses. *Health Bulletin, 40,* 77–80.

Skegg, D., Corwin, P., Paul, C., & Doll, R. (1982). Importance of the male factor in cancer of the cervix. *Lancet, 2,* 581–583.

Squire, C. A. (1984). Smokeless tobacco and oral cancer: A cause for concern? *CA: A Cancer Journal for Clinicians, 34,* 242–247.

U.S. Congress, Office of Technology Assessment. (1985). *Smoking related deaths and financial costs.* Office of Technology Assessment Staff Memorandum. Washington, DC.

U.S. Department of Health and Human Services. (1982). *The health consequences of smoking. A report of the surgeon general* (DHHS Publication No. 82-50179). Washington, DC: U.S. Government Printing Office.

U.S. Department of Health and Human Services. (1983). *The health consequences of smoking: Cardiovascular disease. A report of the surgeon general* (DHHS Publication No. 84-50204). Washington, DC: U.S. Government Printing Office.

U.S. Department of Health and Human Services. (1985). *The health consequences of smoking: Cancer and chronic lung disease in the workplace. A report of the surgeon general* (DHHS Publication No. 85-50207). Washington, DC: U.S. Government Printing Office.

U.S. Department of Health and Human Services. (1986). *The health consequences of using smokeless tobacco. A report of the advisory committee to the surgeon general* (DHHS Publication No. 86-2874). Washington, DC: U.S. Government Printing Office.

U.S. Department of Health and Human Services. (1987). *Smoking tobacco, and health: A fact book.* Rockville, MD: Office of Smoking and Health.

U.S. Department of Health and Human Services. (1988). *The health consequences of smoking: Nicotine addiction. A report of the surgeon general* (DHHS Publication No. 88-273-672-0). Washington, DC: U.S. Government Printing Office.

CHAPTER 16

Evaluating Cancer Risk

MARILYN FRANK-STROMBORG

DEFINITION OF TERMS

Many terms are used in discussing the risks for developing cancer. *Risk* is the potential realization of unwanted consequences of an event; it is the probability of injury or death. Both the probability of occurrence of an event and the magnitude of its consequence are involved (Rowe, 1986, p. 4). *Risk factor* is an element of personal behavior or genetic makeup or an exposure to a known cancer-causing agent that increases a person's chances of developing a particular form of cancer (White, 1986, p. 184). Hazard is another term that is frequently used in discussions of cancer risk. *Hazard* implies the existence of some threat, whereas risk implies both the existence of a threat and the potential for its occurrence. An example of a hazard is vinyl chloride; its toxicity in terms of amount of exposure and incidence of cancer is documented. However, until vinyl chloride has pathway to humans or to the environment, it poses no risk.

Because living itself involves risks, there is no such thing as a zero-risk situation, only ones that involve involuntary and voluntary risks. For instance, although risks are involved in crossing streets, eating calorie-rich desserts, and adding extra automobile driving time to a daily routine, most people routinely undertake one or more of these activities because the benefits outweigh the risks or because the risks (an accident or obesity) are so minimal. Smoking is a classic example of a *voluntary risk*, in which 30 per cent of the American population participate, whereas air pollution is an example of an *involuntary risk* (Ernster, 1987; Stokes, 1987).

Risk factors play a significant part in any discussion of cancer causation and prevention. Alcohol consumption, smoking, and typical American diet practices are all personal risk factors (voluntary risks) that have been linked to cancer mortality. Elimination of smoking would reduce lung cancer deaths by an estimated 83 per cent, modification of the Western diet could reduce cancer mortality by 30 per cent, and elimination of alcohol consumption could cut approximately 5 per cent of cancer deaths in the United States (Costanza, Frederick, Green, & Patterson, 1986; Newell & Vogel, 1987). Air pollution (involuntary risk) that disturbs the stratospheric ozone layer may significantly increase the solar ultraviolet radiation that reaches the earth, thereby causing an increase in skin cancer of 60 per cent or more in the twenty-first century (Sternburg, 1983).

There are many *classifications of risk factors,* including those by Senie (1986), who classifies them into exogenous factors (environmental and life-style) and endogenous factors (host factors); Burack and Drelichman (1982), who classify risk factors into three categories: (1) genetic and familial, (2) personal, or (3) group; and Ash and colleagues (1982), who divide risk factors into behavioral-environmental factors (controlled or minimized by the individual or society) and host factors (individuals' physical attributes and inherited characteristics). Although occupational exposures have been studied intensively, the proportion of cancers attributable to exposures in the workplace has been estimated to be only 6 per cent, whereas the proportion attributable to life-style factors may be more than 80 per cent (Senie, 1986). Risk factors may be individual or group attributes. A *high-risk group* is one that shares risk factors due to its members' common genetic makeup, socioeconomic status, habits, occupation, geographic location, medical treatments, culture, or race or ethnic background (Table 16–1 lists examples of high-risk groups in each of these categories). Because black Americans have the highest incidence and mortality rates for all cancers combined among the major racial and ethnic groups in the United States, they are an example of a high-risk group (National Cancer Institute, 1986). In contrast, Mormons are an example of a low-risk group, with cancer mortality and incidence rates significantly below the average rate experienced by the U.S. white population in the United States (Enstrom & Kanim, 1983).

IDENTIFICATION AND QUANTIFICATION OF RISK FACTORS

For some activities, risk is not difficult to determine. It is possible to estimate accurately the risks of accidental death due to driving a car or riding a bicycle because historical statistical data are available and because demonstrating the causal connection between injury and these types of activities is not very difficult. Determination of the causes of cancer is much more complex. Cancer appears to be characterized by a latency of onset, making it difficult to determine reliably a direct cause-and-effect relationship between exposure and incidence (Baeck & Eisenberg, 1985). The fact that the development of cancer is thought to be a multistage process further complicates attempts to identify the causes of cancer. Other barriers to the determination of risk factors are that (1) it is difficult to determine many individual risk factors for cancer because they tend to be multiple and interactive; (2) an individual risk factor may have multiple consequences; and (3) if little evidence exists on the connection between risk behavior and a specific pathologic process, the causal relationship may be unclear (Hirschman & Leventhal, 1983).

When a substance is suspected of directly or indirectly causing cancer, human epidemiologic studies or animal studies are utilized to determine whether the substance is a carcinogen and whether it poses a risk to humans. The study by Rinsky and colleagues (1987) is an example of an epidemiologic study to determine quantitatively the association between a suspected carcinogen and the development of cancer. This study examined the association between benzene exposure and leukemia by looking at the mortality rate of a cohort of rubber workers who were exposed to benzene. A typical animal study to determine risk is the long-term inhalation assays in rodents to determine the carcinogenic potential of formaldehyde (Squire & Cameron, 1984). The National Research Council details four steps in carcinogenic risk assessment.

Hazard Identification. Evidence of potential carcinogenic risk from environmental chemicals derives from four sources: epidemiologic studies of human populations, bioassay of animals, short-term tests for genotoxicity or cell transformation, and chemical structure relationships to known carcinogens. They are designed to answer questions such as Is this substance a carcinogen? What type of carcinogen is it? What is the nature and strength of the evidence supporting this evaluation? (Robbins, 1978).

Dose Response Assessment. This relationship is the estimation of the potency of a chemical substance that is measured by evaluating the relationship between administered or received dose and incidence of cancer. This step almost always involves high-to-low dose extrapolation and frequently involves extrapolation from experimental animals to humans.

The dose-response relationship *quantitatively* defines the role of the dose of a chemical in evoking a biologic response. In the absence of the chemical, no response is seen. As the chemical is introduced into the system, the response is initiated at the threshold dose and increases in intensity as the dose is raised. Ultimately a dose is reached beyond which no further increase in response is observed (Snyder, 1984).

Exposure Assessment. For each potential route of exposure, an effort must be made to evaluate the frequency, magnitude, and duration of an exposure event and the number and susceptibility of people affected.

Risk Assessment. This measurement involves combining the information on dose-response with that on exposure to derive estimates of the probability that the hazards associated with a substance or activity will be realized under the conditions of exposure experienced by the population group of interest (Baeck & Eisenberg, 1985, pp. 672–673; Rodricks & Tardiff, 1984, pp. 9–10).

Table 16–1. EXAMPLE OF CATEGORIZATIONS OF HIGH-RISK GROUPS

Category	Example	Resultant Cancer
Genetic	Xeroderma pigmentosum	Skin
	Familial polyposis	Colon
Geographic	Transkei, Africa	Esophageal
	Japan	Gastric
	Sections of India	Oral
Socioeconomic	High socioeconomic status in U.S.	Breast
	Low socioeconomic status in U.S.	Cervical
Habits	Smoking	Lung cancer
	Chewing betel	Oral
Iatrogenic	Diethylstilbestrol	Vaginal
Occupational	Individuals who work with vinyl chloride	Angiosarcoma of the liver

(From Clemmesen, J. [1987]. Parameters for identification of high-risk groups. In H. Nieburgs [Ed.], *Prevention and detection of cancer. Part I. Prevention. Vol. 2. Etiology* [pp. 1513–1516]. New York: Marcel Dekker, Inc.)

Individual Risk Factors

Once a substance (or a habit, occupation, or geographic location) is identified as a risk factor, the task for the health professional is to determine the *individual's* risk factors and assist that individual in reducing the risks. Existing evidence suggests that (1) individuals at risk for cancer are often unaware of their risk; (2) health professionals may not be familiar with those factors associated with the highest cancer risk; and (3) methods to reduce cancer risk have been underapplied because of lack of knowledge, funds, or motivation among patients and health professionals. The traditional health history and physical examination is one method of obtaining the individual's cancer-risk profile. Specialized cancer-risk assessment forms have been developed that concentrate on the known risk factors for specific cancer sites. Examples of risk factors from a typical cancer-risk assessment form follow (Faulkenberry, 1983):

Breast:
_____ Family history of breast cancer
_____ No children or first birth after age 30
_____ Obesity
_____ High dietary fat intake
_____ Personal history of ovarian or endometrial cancer
_____ Early menarche or late menopause

Another approach that has been advocated for *identifying* and *quantifying* an individual's risk factors is the Health Hazard Appraisal (HHA) or Health Risk Appraisal (HRA). Dr. Lewis C. Robbins is generally credited with developing the HRA. His work on cervical cancer and heart disease prevention during the late 1940s led him to the idea of keeping a record of a patient's health hazards to use as a guide to encouraging preventive efforts and then to the creation of a simple health hazard chart that could give the medical examination a more prospective orientation (Schoenbach, 1987; Stokes, 1987). The HHA is a simple approach to estimating personal risk (i.e., an individual's chance for developing cancer) and providing the basis for practical advice to persons wishing to reduce that risk. By explaining risk factors to people in terms of their chances of dying in the next 10 years, the health professional is describing the risk in terms the individual can understand easily. The actual risk factor value is derived by comparing the mortality rate for an individual associated with a specific behavior or characteristic (e.g., a cigarette smoker) with the mortality rate for an individual who does not have this behavior or characteristic (a nonsmoker of the same age, sex, and race) (Ross, 1981). An HHA can be achieved by a simple hand computation or a computerized appraisal. At present, more than 52 different instruments are available (Healthfinder, 1985). Sample questions from the HHA are the following:

How often do you examine your breasts for lumps? (women only)

_____ monthly
_____ once every few months
_____ rarely or never

Did your mother, sister, or daughter have breast cancer? (women only)

_____ Yes
_____ No
_____ Not sure
_____ Not applicable

It must be noted that HRAs have been criticized in the literature in terms of the reliability of the approach (Sacks, Krushat, & Newman, 1980) and the validity of HRA risk scores (Schoenbach, 1987). However, Schoenbach acknowledges that "HHA, as a vehicle for what might be termed 'prospective health assessment,' potentially has a number of very desirable qualities for health professionals: preventive orientation, systemic approach, ability to emphasize modifiable factors, and grounding in current scientific knowledge" (1987, p. 410). Preliminary studies document that changes in behavior do occur as a result of HHA programs.

In summary, the nurse has several options for obtaining a history that will delineate persons at high risk for cancer from life-style habits, occupational exposure, or family history ("at-risk" asymptomatic individuals). Identifying risk factors is important because preventive teaching cannot occur unless the risks are known by both the at risk individual and the health professional. Those individuals who are at risk for cancer can be targeted for screening, more intensive follow-up, and behavior modification. The approaches that can be used are as follows:

1. A standard health questionnaire; the clinician can probe for more information when indicated.
2. A health screening flow sheet that indicates risk factors and behaviors most important to consider in preventing disease and maintaining good health.
3. A customized history questionnaire (self-administered or used as an interview tool) that is designed to elicit risk factors for cancer and is usually site specific.
4. Computerized questionnaires that ensure standardization of medical records, provide a comprehensive history, are time effective, and yield a concise and legible printout (Burack & Drelichman, 1982).

Regardless of the approach taken, no one method should be seen as an end in itself. The most important element in risk identification is the rapport established between the nurse and the individual so that questions are understood and complete information is obtained. Above all, the results of risk identification must be translated into sound practical advice that the individual can follow. The effort that the nurse expends to identify the major risk factors for cancer is the first step in managing those risks successfully.

ASSESSING INDIVIDUAL RISK THROUGH IDENTIFYING PREDISPOSING FACTORS OR SUSCEPTIBILITIES

Individuals can be described according to an infinite number of variables. The variables that have been evaluated in studies to determine cancer risks range from increasing age to past occupations. Recognition is increasing that the identification of high-risk individuals or groups provides a key to the ultimate reduction of cancer incidence and mortality through opportunities for surveillance, early detection and treatment, etiologic research, and preventive measures. The delineation of high-risk individuals or groups may come from clinical studies, animal and laboratory studies, or epidemiologic studies. It is clear that advances will be needed in risk identification before a major impact can be made on clinical and public health practices (Fraumeni, 1975b).

Age

Cancer is predominantly a disease of middle and old age; this finding is graphically depicted in Figure 16–1. Cancer occurs most frequently between the ages of 60 and 65 (Page & Asire, 1985). However, the incidence rate for the majority of cancers increases continually after the first decade of life; the older a person becomes, the more likely he or she is to develop cancer. After 85 to 90 years of age, both incidence and mortality from all forms of cancer decline for both white males and females. The probability that a 65-year-old man will develop cancer in the next 5 years is 1 in 14, compared with 1 in 700 for a 25 year old. The incidence rate for all sites of cancer combined rises

steadily throughout life until it peaks at 2308 per 100,000 in persons aged 85 years and older (Birdsell, 1986).

The types of cancers seen in aging men and women differ considerably from those found in younger individuals. The classification of *elderly* is defined as individuals older than 65 years of age. Cancer of the breast, colon, and lung are *less aggressive* in the elderly than in the young, whereas cancer of the prostate and thyroid, leukemias, and melanoma are *more aggressive* in the elderly than in the young. Cancer of the vulva and chronic lymphocytic leukemia characteristically occur in the elderly. When the median age for the occurrence of the most common kinds of cancer is examined, the effect of age becomes readily apparent: the median age for breast cancer is 60; the median age for lung cancer is 65; and the median age for colon and prostate cancer is 70. The three leading cancer sites for aging men are lung, prostate, and colon-rectum; for aging women they are breast, lung, and colon-rectum (Silverberg & Lubera, 1987). Cancers of the stomach, colon, rectum, prostate, and breast account for more than 50 per cent of the invasive carcinomas in patients older than 60. Table 16–2 details the mortality figures for the most common cancers among different age groups.

The importance of these facts is underscored by the demographic changes that are occurring in the United States. Nearly 23 million Americans are older than 65, and they represent 11 per cent of the population

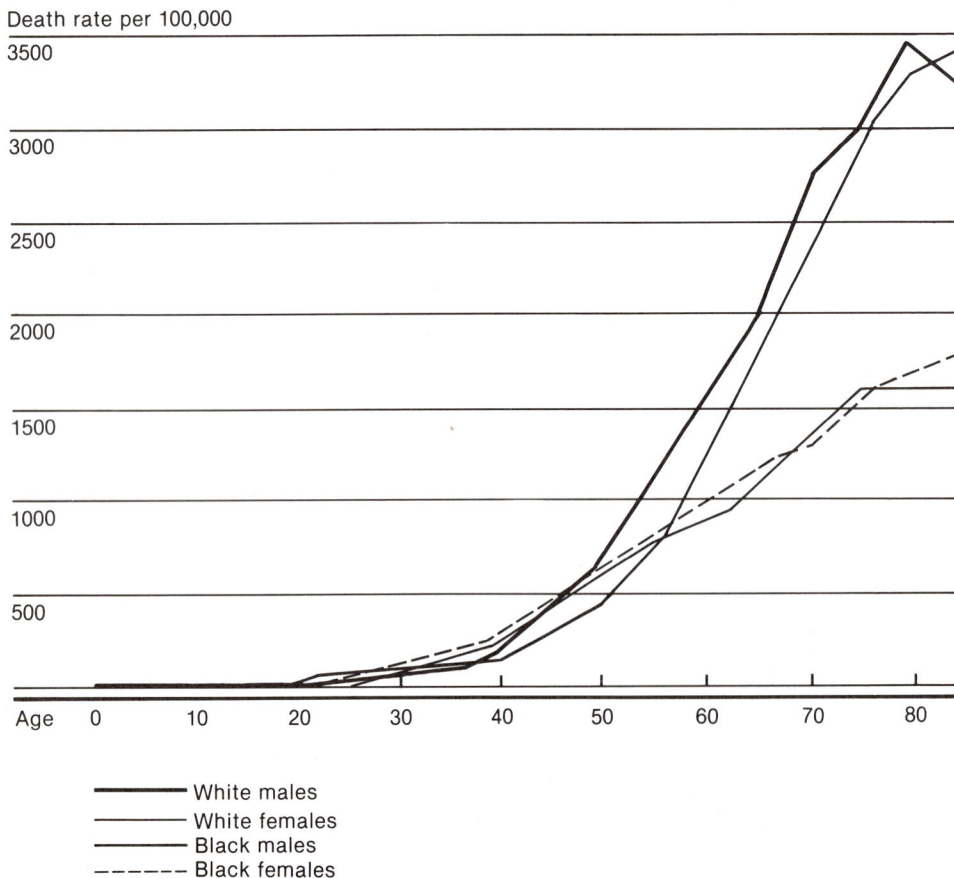

Death rate per 100,000

Figure 16–1. Average annual age-specific cancer incidence per 100,000 U.S. population by race and sex, all sites combined, 1973–1977. (From Surveillance of Epidemiology and End Results Program.)

White males
White females
Black males
Black females

Table 16–2A. MORTALITY FOR THE FIVE LEADING CANCER SITES FOR MALES BY AGE GROUP, UNITED STATES—1986

All Ages	Under 15	15–34	35–54	55–74	75+
All Cancer 250,559	*All Cancer* 1033	*All Cancer* 4171	*All Cancer* 25,581	*All Cancer* 137,927	*All Cancer* 81,825
Lung 85,057	Leukemia 383	Leukemia 771	Lung 8819	Lung 54,050	Lung 21,999
Colon and rectum 27,469	Brain and CNS 244	Skin 483	Colon and rectum 2206	Colon and rectum 14,532	Prostate 15,888
Prostate 27,262	Non-Hodgkin's lymphomas 103	Non-Hodgkin's lymphomas 477	Skin 1308	Prostate 11,066	Colon and rectum 10,530
Pancreas 11,403	Bone 46	Brain and CNS 459	Non-Hodgkin's lymphomas 1305	Pancreas 6673	Pancreas 3571
Leukemia 9565	Connective tissue 37	Hodgkin's disease 300	Brain and CNS 1251	Stomach 4445	Bladder 3376

CNS, central nervous system.
(From Vital Statistics of the United States, 1986.)

Table 16–2B. MORTALITY FOR THE FIVE LEADING CANCER SITES FOR FEMALES BY AGE GROUP, UNITED STATES—1986

All Ages	Under 15	15–34	35–54	55–74	75+
All Cancer 218,817	*All Cancer* 798	*All Cancer* 3548	*All Cancer* 27,210	*All Cancer* 107,681	*All Cancer* 79,556
Breast 40,539	Leukemia 284	Breast 668	Breast 8391	Lung 25,153	Colon and rectum 14,231
Lung 40,465	Brain and CNS 198	Leukemia 472	Lung 4967	Breast 20,166	Breast 11,308
Colon and rectum 28,347	Connective tissue 40	Uterus 368	Colon and rectum 1948	Colon and rectum 11,993	Lung 10,230
Pancreas 12,055	Kidney 36	Brain and CNS 325	Uterus 1798	Ovary 6563	Pancreas 5506
Ovary 11,903	Bone 34	Non-Hodgkin's lymphomas 215	Ovary 1688	Pancreas 5784	Ovary 3510

CNS, central nervous system.
(From Vital Statistics of the United States, 1986.)

(Ouslander & Beck, 1982). The elderly population will double to nearly 50 million by the year 2030, but those older than 75 will increase more rapidly, with the number older than 85 expected to triple (Somers, 1978). As we progress into the twenty-first century, a greater proportion of our society will be older than 65 years of age. This development has important implications for nurses. It is essential that nurses use any contact with the elderly to educate them about early cancer detection and to determine individual risk factors and perform physical assessments if appropriate. Furthermore, the elderly should be educated about the need for regular physical examinations to detect cancer in the early stages rather than after symptoms have occurred. Also they should be educated in techniques that can help in the early detection of cancer, for example, performing breast self-examinations, inspecting the skin under dentures, and reporting changes in skin lesions.

Gender

Sex differences in risk for cancer are commonly observed for most cancers. Some of the observed sex differences are explainable because they are related to different occupations and life styles. The causes of other sex differences in rates for such cancers as thyroid and kidney cancer and Hodgkin's disease are unknown. Sexual factors, pregnancy, or both are thought to contribute substantially to the pathogenesis of a large group of cancers (e.g., breast, uterus, ovary, cervix, penis) (Henderson, Gerkins, & Pike, 1975). The causes of cancer of the prostate and testis are at present unknown. Comparing the worldwide incidence of cancer among men and women indicates that cancer is generally less common among women. The risk factors for cancer of the breast, uterus, ovary, cervix, and penis are discussed in the following sections.

Breast Cancer

Breast cancer is the most common form of cancer (after skin cancer) among American women and accounts for more deaths among them than any other type. The average woman is estimated to have a 9 per cent chance (one in 11) of developing breast cancer during her lifetime. The cumulative probability of breast cancer over the fifth or sixth decades of life

Table 16–3. KNOWN OR SUSPECTED RISK FACTORS FOR BREAST CANCER

Risk Factor	Explanation	May Reduce Risk
Age	Rate increases sharply after age 30 and continues to rise. Two thirds of all breast cancers occur in women older than 50 years.	
Family History	Risk increased twofold if mother or sister had it, sixfold if both had breast cancer.	
Previous Breast Cancer	After cancer in one breast, woman has between 3 and 6 per cent risk of second cancer.	
Reproductive History	Women with no children or first child after age 30 have a risk 3 times greater than women who have first child before age 18.	Have children before age 30.
Breast Disease	If lesions proliferate, risk is 1.9 times that for women with no proliferative lesions. If atypical hyperplasia is present, risk increased to 5.3 times normal. Positive family history of women with atypical hyperplasia increases risk to 11 times normal.	
Estrogens and Oral Contraceptives	Debate about risk with oral contraceptives. May act as tumor promoters, especially in women older than age 35, or may promote previously transformed cells, rather than acting as a carcinogen and initiating the transforming event. Debate about increased risk with use of replacement estrogens, particularly long-term users.	Unless medically indicated, avoid long-term replacement estrogens.
Menstrual History	Early onset of menstruation and late menopause may increase risk. Menopause induced by removal of ovaries before age 40 reduces risk.	
Socioeconomic Status	Higher socioeconomic status appears to be related to higher risk.	
Nutrition	High dietary fat intake contributes to increased risk.	Reduce fat intake to 25 to 30 per cent total calories. Some oils, monosaturates, medium-chain fatty acids, or omega-3 fatty acids lack tumor-promoting effects.
Race	Caucasian women have the highest risk.	

(Data from Berg, 1984; Cancer and Steroid Hormone Study, 1986; Carbone, 1983; Henderson, Gerkins, & Pike, 1975; Kleinberg, 1987; Longman & Burhring, 1987; Page & Asire, 1985; Winder & Rose, 1984; Wynder, Rose, & Cohen, 1986.)

(approximately 1.5 per cent and 1.8 per cent, respectively, or 3.3 per cent for the entire 20-year span) is a one in 30 risk (Love, 1987). Certain factors may increase or decrease this "average" risk of breast cancer. However, 70 to 80 per cent of all women with breast cancer have *no known* risk factors. The longitudinal study by Seidman and co-workers (1985) of 570,000 white American women found that when they considered known risk factors* alone or in combination, the risk factors explained only 21 per cent of the breast cancer risk among women aged 30 to 54 and 29 per cent of the risk among women aged 55 to 84: "We have not appreciably increased our ability to identify substantial numbers of truly 'high-risk' women. From the point of view of the clinician, *all women should be treated as being at appreciable risk for breast cancer*" (p. 311).

Berg (1984) supports the Seidman study's statement by saying ". . . for health maintenance, every woman with breast tissue must be considered at high risk for breast cancer, whatever that implies at her particular age" (p. 590). Bulbrook and colleagues (1986) conducted a prospective study of 15,000 women and found that there was a *small subset* of women who were at high risk for the development of breast cancer. Women who are nulliparous or have a first child at or after 28 years of age have a high proportion of their blood E_2 (estradiol) not bound to protein or a low concentration

of sex hormone–binding globulin, and have high-risk Wolfe grades on mammograms appear to be at considerable risk for breast cancer. However, a combination of classic, endocrinologic, and radiologic risk factors *failed to identify 70 per cent of the potential breast cancer cases.*

To date, no one factor or combination of factors has been found that can predict the occurrence of breast cancer in any one individual, although major risk factors have been identified. When asking about major risk factors, the nurse should remember that, regardless of the responses, all women should be considered at risk for this cancer. Table 16–3 gives the known or suspected risk factors for breast cancer.

Cervical Cancer

An estimated 46,500 new invasive cases of uterine cancer will be reported in 1991, which will include 13,500 cases of cancer of the cervix and 33,000 cases of cancer of the endometrium of the uterus (Cancer Facts and Figures, 1990). For the past three decades, the incidence and mortality of invasive cancer of the cervix have been declining steadily. In terms of the epidemiology of this cancer, major differences exist among the races and ethnic groups. The incidence in the United States is almost two and one-half times higher in black women than in white women, and the mortality is almost three times higher in blacks. However, native American women have a higher incidence of cervix uteri cancer than do black women (National Cancer Institute, 1986).

The factors considered to increase risk include cer-

---

*Risk factors: history of breast cancer, history of breast surgery, Jewish, late menopause, early menarche, never married, first birth at 30 years of age, college graduate, daily alcohol consumption, 10 per cent or more above average weight for height and age.

tain genital infections, chemical carcinogens, life-style habits, and number of male sexual partners. Although the literature reports multiple risk factors for cervical cancer, most authorities in the field feel it is a venereally transmitted disease. "The epidemiologic evidence that the determinant(s) of cervix cancer is related to sexual experience is fairly conclusive and implicates a venereally transmitted biological agent tentatively identified as the human papilloma virus" (Shanmugaratnam, 1985, p. 442). Researchers believe that most cervical cancers have a fairly long detectable preclinical phase, and the identification of in situ cancers followed by adequate therapy has been shown to reduce the incidence of invasive cancer and cervix cancer mortality. Observations on the natural history of cancer in situ reveal that it takes at least 10 years to develop into invasive cancer and that cervical dysplasia takes even longer (Schneiderman, 1981). Table 16–4 lists all the known or suspected risk factors for cervical cancer. When asking women about these risk factors during the health history, the nurse should remember that the *three major risks* for cervical cancer are multiple sex partners, early age of first intercourse, and human papilloma viral infections.

Endometrial Cancer

The risk of endometrial cancer is clearly age related; the disease usually strikes women 55 to 69 years old.

The median age for diagnosis in white women is 61, and in black women it is 64 (Dunn, 1981). Other than the doubts about estrogen replacement therapy, little controversy exists about the majority of risk factors (Table 16–5). Evidence that estrogen replacement therapy is an important cause of endometrial cancer has been derived from two main sources: studies of trends in endometrial cancer incidence in the United States and case-controlled studies.

Estrogen therapy was introduced in the United States in the 1930s, and estrogens were suspected of contributing to the development of endometrial carcinoma early on (Schlaff & Rosenshein, 1985). The hormone estrogen was popular with menopausal women because it helped to control menopausal symptoms such as hot flashes or thinning of the vaginal lining, which caused painful sexual intercourse. From 1963 to 1973 the sale of estrogens as replacement therapy (e.g., Premarin) rose fourfold, and a rise in the incidence of endometrial cancer was noted by researchers beginning in 1969. The use of estrogens for the treatment of menopausal symptoms increased until around 1975, when it began to decrease after reports appeared that associated estrogen use with endometrial cancer.

It is now believed that estrogens are not carcinogenic but are promoters in the process of malignancy. Because the risk of endometrial cancer was found to rise with increasing duration of use and with increasing

Table 16–4. KNOWN OR SUSPECTED RISK FACTORS FOR UTERINE CERVICAL CANCER

Risk Factor	Explanation	May Reduce Risk
Genital Infections		
Human papillomaviruses	Strong relationship between genital warts and precancerous lesions.	Treatment of infections and frequent surveillance. Barrier methods of birth control (condoms).
Herpes simplex virus II (HSV II)	Women with genital HSV II infections are at greater risk of developing precancerous lesions.	Barrier methods of birth control (condoms).
Multiple Sexual Partners	May relate to high protein content of sperm in some men. Risk may be due to immunosuppressive effects or chronic immune stimulation of sperm of different partners.	Limit number of sexual partners.
Immunosuppression	Persons with multiple medical conditions (e.g., cancer, scleroderma) that cause suppression of the immune system and transplant surgery patients are at increased risk.	
Type of Contraception Used	Use of barrier methods of contraception (condom or diaphragm) associated with low risk; oral contraceptives increase risk.	Barrier methods, especially if multiple sexual partners.
Smoking by the Female(?)	One study found female smokers who were monogamous had a risk 7 times that of nonsmoking women of developing precancerous lesions.	Stop smoking.
Characteristics of Male Sexual Partner	Penile warts and cancer; multiple sexual partners; sexual intercourse with prostitutes; previous wives with precancerous or invasive cervical cancer.	
Racial and Religious Group Membership	Religious differences noted—Jews, Mormons, and Seventh-Day Adventists have low risk. Related to low prevalence of divorce, use of barrier methods, and intercourse confined to marriage. High incidence in Latin America.	
Coital Factors(?)		
Douching frequently; poor hygiene; intercourse during menses	Douching may relate to use of coal tar derivatives in douching solution. Orthodox Jews who abstain during menses rarely develop invasive cervical cancer.	

(Data from Hendershot, 1983; Henderson, Gerkins, & Pike, 1975; Lovejoy, 1987; Page & Asire, 1985; Shanmugaratnam, 1985.) The reader is referred to Lovejoy (1987) for an excellent in-depth discussion of the risk factors for cervical cancer.

Table 16–5. MAJOR RISK FACTORS FOR CORPUS UTERI CANCER

Risk Factor	Explanation	May Reduce Risk
Estrogen Replacement Therapy	Prolonged, continuous exposure of the endometrium to estrogen stimulation increases risk to 6 to 7 times for postmenopausal women. Risk increases with duration of use and dosage of replacement estrogens. Women who have taken conjugated estrogen for 1 or more years remain at increased risk for at least 10 years after they discontinue use.	Cyclic progestogen therapy with estrogen therapy reduces risk.
Obesity	Obese women (30% more than normal weight for height) are twice as likely to develop endometrial cancer. Risk increases with increasing weight. Obese women, particularly after menopause, have higher levels of estrogens in blood. Tallness, coupled with obesity, also increases risk.	Maintain ideal body weight.
Fertility	Women who have four or more children are 1.3 times as likely to develop endometrial cancer.	
Conditions Associated with Continuous Estrogenic Status	Polycystic ovary syndrome (Stein-Leventhal), thecagranulosa cell tumors, infertility secondary to failure of the ovulatory mechanism.	Treatment of medical condition.
High Socioeconomic Status	More affluent women use replacement estrogens more frequently than less affluent women.	
Birth Control Pills	Women who use "sequential" birth control pills have double the risk of endometrial cancer as women who use other forms of birth control. Sequential pills have been removed from the American market. Women who use combination pills (estrogen and progesterone in each pill) for at least 1 year have one half the risk of endometrial cancer as women who do not use this form of birth control. Decreased risk persisted for at least 10 years after discontinuing use and was most notable in nulliparous women.	Avoidance of sequential birth control pills.
Late Natural Menopause *Turner's Syndrome(?)* *Family History of Endometrial Cancer*		

(Data from Dunn, 1981; Henderson, Gerkins, & Pike, 1975; Lynch & Lynch, 1978; Page & Asire, 1985; Rubin & Peterson, 1985; Schlaff & Rosenshein, 1985; Shapiro, Kelly, Rosenberg, Kaufman, Helmrich, Rosenshein, Lewis, Knapp, Stolley, & Schottenfeld, 1985; Vessey, 1985.)

dose, it is suggested that the therapy be of as short a duration and at as low a dose as possible (Vessey, 1985). There is clinical evidence that periodic administration of a progestin (cyclic progestogen therapy) will protect postmenopausal women who are receiving estrogen replacement therapy from developing endometrial cancer.

Ovarian Cancer

As with endometrial cancer, age is a significant risk factor; maximum risk is in the 50- to 59-year-old group, with a mean age of 59.5 and a median of 60 (Earhart, 1983). The specific incidence rates for ovarian cancer show a steady rise with age up to the age of 80, when the rate begins to drop off slightly. According to the third National Cancer Survey, an estimated one of every 70 newborn girls (1.4 per cent) will develop cancer of the ovary. Although ovarian cancer ranks second in incidence among gynecologic cancers, it causes more deaths than any other cancer of the female reproductive system because ovarian tumors are difficult to diagnose; at initial diagnosis, approximately 60 to 70 per cent have already reached stage III or IV (Barber, 1986). The incidence varies with race and ethnic origin. In the United States, the rate for white women is higher than that for nonwhites. Native American women have the lowest rate of ovarian cancer of all American women.

Childbearing appears to be the most important known factor in preventing ovarian cancer, suggesting that hormones may play an important role in the development of this cancer. The use of oral contraceptives, which create a hormonal balance similar to that of pregnancy (suppression of ovulation), has been found to decrease the risk of epithelial ovarian cancer (Cancer and Steroid Hormone Study, 1987). Ovarian cancer is also increasing in Western countries in which number of children born to successive generations of women is decreasing. Table 16–6 lists the known or suspected risk factors for ovarian cancer.

Cancer of the Penis

Cancer of the penis occurs most frequently in areas of the world in which circumcision is not practiced and penile hygiene is poor. For instance, cancer of the penis is common in East Africa and Bali and is 100 times more common in Jamaica than in Israel (Cook-Mozaffari, 1985; Gray, 1985). In Israel circumcision is religiously prescribed for all males. Some authorities feel that circumcision will prevent this cancer, but in Third World countries the risk of infection and septicemia from the procedure may offset the benefits. At one time, smegma (the secretion that is under the male prepuce in uncircumcised men) was believed to be the etiologic factor in the development of this cancer. Now there is evidence that a sexually transmitted infection

Table 16–6. KNOWN OR SUSPECTED RISK FACTORS FOR OVARIAN CANCER

Risk Factor	Explanation	May Reduce Risk
Lack of Childbearing	Several pregnancies confer more protection than one pregnancy. Women who have had a child are half as likely to get ovarian cancer as nulliparous women. Pregnancy suppresses ovulation. "Incessant" ovulation increases risk. Delayed childbearing may also increase the risk of ovarian cancer.	Having children at a young age.
History of Breast Cancer	Twice the expected risk of developing ovarian cancer. Women who have had ovarian cancer are three to four times more likely to develop breast cancer.	
Type of Birth Control Utilized	*Decreased risk* with use of oral contraceptives; protective effect evident for women who used oral contraceptives for as little as 3 to 6 months; protective effect continued for 15 years after use ended.	Use of oral contraceptives.
Exposure to Asbestos and Talc	Conflicting data on risk of ovarian cancer and talc. Stronger evidence on risk of asbestos and ovarian cancer.	
High Socioeconomic Status and Living in a Western Country	May relate to high-fat diet or a small number or absence of children.	
Irradiation of Pelvic Organs (also mentioned in the literature)		

(Data from Barber, 1986; Cancer and Steroid Hormone Study, 1987; Earhart, 1983; Page & Asire, 1985; Rawson, 1978; Rubin & Peterson, 1985; Schlaff & Rosenshein, 1985.)

is a cause of cancer of the penis. Specifically, researchers report an association between human papillomavirus infection and cancer of the penis.

Racial or Ethnic Origin

Many variations exist in cancer incidence and mortality among various racial and ethnic groups. Variations may reflect environmental factors, life-style practices, and genetic susceptibilities and may provide important clues for epidemiologic investigation. "Although the racial and ethnic differentials for most cancers appear to be largely modulated by environmental influence, genetic factors appear to contribute to some high rates (e.g., nasopharyngeal cancer among Chinese and gallbladder cancer among American Indians and certain Hispanic groups) and some low rates (e.g., testicular cancer and Ewing's sarcoma among blacks in Africa and the United States)" (Fraumeni, 1982, p. 96). Skin cancer exemplifies the factor of genetic susceptibility because ethnic variations correspond to the degree of protective skin pigmentation. Table 16–7 lists cancer incidence information about racial and ethnic groups in the United States.

A study of different populations (a multinational approach) has value in helping to determine the causes of cancer. In 1944 Kennaway was the first to observe that the high incidence of primary cancer of the liver among blacks in Africa was not found in blacks in the United States. He hypothesized that the cause of the liver cancer was an extrinsic factor or factors rather than one that was racially related. Oettle in 1964 pointed out the concentration of primary liver cancer in regions of high humidity, where *Aspergillus flavus* growth is favored. Scientists now know that aflatoxin, a lactone derivative of *Aspergillus* that grows on peanuts and grains, is the most potent carcinogen known for rats. The normal practices of food and grain storage in parts of Africa and the Far East lead to heavy contamination of grains and peanuts with aflatoxin (a fungi). Thus the initial study of the differences in incidence of primary liver cancer in blacks in Africa and the United States generated the hypothesis that race was not the causative factor and that there existed an extrinsic factor or factors that needed to be identified.

Another study that illustrates the benefit of utilizing a multinational approach is Rose, Boyar, and Wynder's investigation into the mortality rates for cancer of the breast, ovary, prostate, and colon in 26 to 30 countries (1986). They found positive correlations between the four cancer mortality rates and caloric intake from animal sources but negative correlations between mortality rates and vegetable-derived calories. Thus the study suggests that animal fat and not energy is the major dietary influence on cancer risk for breast, ovary, prostate, and colon cancers. Table 16–8 gives the highest and the lowest international cancer incidence rates.

Congenital and Genetic Disorders

The genetic basis for many human cancers has been demonstrated convincingly by retrospective studies, comparisons of twins, and pedigree analyses. More than 200 genetic or familial disorders are associated with a high risk of cancer development (Meadows & Li, 1983). Cancer genes induce cancer in the majority of affected individuals and are specific for a limited number of neoplasms.

In the last decade, profound advances have occurred in the field of genetics as it relates to the study of human cancer genes. One group of cancer genes that has been identified is that of human cancer susceptibility genes, which appear to be "suppressor" or "regulatory" genes for cancer development. Benedict (1987) reports that the retinoblastoma gene (Rb) has

Table 16–7. CANCER INCIDENCE IN DIFFERENT ETHNIC OR RACIAL GROUPS

Racial or Ethnic Group	Cancers Unique to Group
Black Americans	*Highest incidence* rates for esophagus, colon, larynx, lung (male), multiple myeloma, pancreas, prostate, female breast (women under age 40). Highest incidence rate for all cancers combined. Overall cancer rate: Male = 487.9 per 100,000, 1978–1981 Female = 290.3 per 100,000, 1978–1981
Native Americans	*Highest incidence* rate for cancers of the cervix uteri. Native Americans have stomach cancer rate twice as high as that for whites. Male native American men have highest rate for gallbladder cancer in the world and lowest rate of lung cancer in the world. *Lowest incidence* rates for cancers of the bladder, colon, rectum, larynx, male and female lung, female breast, corpus uteri, pancreas, ovary. Overall cancer rate: Male = 172.3 per 100,000, 1978–1981 Female = 155.5 per 100,000, 1978–1981
Native Hawaiians	*Highest incidence* rates for cancers of the female breast, ovary, corpus uteri, stomach, and lung (female). *Highest incidence rate* of breast cancer in the world. Overall cancer rate: Male = 390.9 per 100,000 Female = 336.5 per 100,000
Japanese-Americans	*Highest incidence* rates for rectal cancer, colon and rectum combined. *Lowest incidence* for cervix uteri and multiple myeloma. Stomach cancer rate is twice as high as that for whites. Overall cancer rate: Male = 300.4 per 100,000, Hawaii Female = 225.5 per 100,000, San Francisco
Hispanics	*Lowest rate* for cancer of esophagus. Overall cancer rate: Male = 279.8 per 100,000, New Mexico Male = 245.2 per 100,000, Puerto Rico Female = 218.4 per 100,000, New Mexico Female = 181.3 per 100,000, Puerto Rico

(Data from Cancer Facts and Figures for Minority Americans, 1986; Clemmesen, 1987; Cook-Mozaffari, 1985; Enstrom & Kanim, 1983; National Cancer Institute, 1986; Page & Asire, 1985.)

been isolated in laboratories and is the first human cancer susceptibility gene ever cloned:

The retinoblastoma (Rb) gene is the prototype of "suppressor" or "regulatory" genes and predisposes to the formation not only of retinoblastoma, the most common ocular tumor of childhood, but also is responsible for osteosarcoma, a bone tumor, as well as likely other tumor types of different tissue origin. Over 90 per cent of individuals who carry the Rb gene develop tumors. Therefore the gene is highly penetrant.

It is hoped that DNA clones from the Rb gene can be used to identify either prenatally or postnatally those individuals who carry this potent cancer susceptibility gene.

"Genetic changes may involve one or more gene mutations, gross chromosomal abnormalities, or no change in DNA structure, but rather changes in gene transcription involving dedifferentiation and altered growth properties resulting from expression of embryonic genes which had been repressed in early development" (Meisner, 1983, p. 165). Genetic factors are typically considered in three groups:

Chromosomal

Individuals in this group are marked by a genetic imbalance because entire lengths of genetic material are absent or present in excess (Mulvihill, 1975). In chronic myelocytic leukemia, 70 to 90 per cent of patients have the Philadelphia chromosome (chromosome 22), which is considered a chromosomal marker of the disease.

Single-Gene Locus

Ataxia-telangiectasia is an example of an autosomal recessive disease caused by a chromosomal translocation that leads to lymphoid neoplasms. Of the known single-gene traits in humans, 9 per cent have neoplastic or preneoplastic manifestations or complications. Fanconi's anemia, Bloom's syndrome, Kostmann's infantile genetic agranulocytosis, and glutathione reductase deficiency represent gross defects of DNA associated with malignancy (Mulvihill, 1975).

Polygenic

In a polygenic disease, many genes, rather than a single gene, interact with the environment to cause the condition. The increased risks observed for siblings or other relatives of patients with cancer of the stomach, breast, large intestine, uterus, and lung are attributed to a polygenic influence.

Table 16–8. INTERNATIONAL RANGE OF INCIDENCE FOR COMMON CANCERS

Site of Origin of Cancer	High-Incidence Area	Low-Incidence Area
Skin (chiefly nonmelanoma)	Australia, Queensland	India, Bombay
Esophagus	Iran, northeast section	Nigeria
Lung and bronchus	England	Nigeria
Stomach	Japan	Uganda
Cervix uteri	Colombia	Israel
Prostate	United States	Japan
Liver	Mozambique	England
Breast	Canada, British Columbia	Israel
Colon	United States, Connecticut	Nigeria
Corpus uteri	United States, California	Japan
Buccal cavity	India, Bombay	Denmark
Rectum	Denmark	Nigeria
Bladder	United States, Connecticut	Japan
Ovary	Denmark	Japan
Nasopharynx	Singapore	England
Pancreas	New Zealand	India, Bombay
Larynx	Brazil, São Paulo	Japan
Pharynx	India, Bombay	Denmark
Penis	Parts of Uganda	Israel

(Modified from Doll, R., & Peto, R. [1981]. *The causes of cancer.* New York: Oxford University Press.)

Table 16–9 details the genetic conditions that are associated with increased cancer risk.

Familial Susceptibility

Some families show an unusually excessive incidence of cancers of all types, usually adenocarcinoma of the colon, endometrium, or breast. These families are termed *cancer families*. Depending on the family history, the risks of developing breast cancer or colon cancer may be twentyfold to thirtyfold greater than normal in persons from cancer families. In cancer families there is (1) an increased frequency of multiple primary malignancies; (2) a tendency for the same type of neoplasm to develop in a single site or tissue system, a tendency for a single histologic type to occur in various sites or organs, or a tendency for different types to occur in an organ system (Anderson, 1975); (3) an early age of onset of cancer; and (4) an autosomal dominant transmission of susceptibility to adenocarcinomas. In general, more than 20 per cent of members of cancer families develop cancer at an earlier age than that of the general population. The average age of onset of cancer in members of these families may be several years or decades earlier than the average age at onset of the same cancer in the general

population. The characteristics of tumor specificity, multiple sites of tumor development, and early average age of onset thus serve to distinguish between familial occurrences having genetic causation and those arising from environmental exposure (Anderson, 1975).

In some familial cancers, a genetic marker has been found that will identify asymptomatic persons at risk of cancer in the future. Renal cell carcinoma is one such example of a familial cancer with a genetic marker. Researchers have found a translocation between chromosomes 3 and 8 in somatic cells that is transmitted in an autosomal dominant pattern. By age 60, up to 90 per cent of carriers of the translocation were considered likely to develop renal cancer as compared with no elevated risk for family members with normal chromosome patterns (Meadow & Li, 1983).

Lynch and associates at Creighton University have been pioneers in the identification of cancer-prone families. In their study of a cancer-prone family— Family "G"—a subject originally investigated in 1895, they found more than 650 blood relatives, 95 of whom developed malignant neoplasms; of the 95, 13 developed primary malignant neoplasms (14 per cent). They also found cancer involving specific anatomic sites occurring in cancer-prone lines of the family but a paucity or complete absence of cancer occurring in

Table 16–9. GENETIC CONDITIONS ASSOCIATED WITH INCREASED CANCER RISK

Genetic Condition	Associated Cancer
Familial polyposis coli (dominant inheritance)	Colon carcinoma
Gardner's syndrome (dominant inheritance)	Colon carcinoma, osteomas
Peutz-Jeghers syndrome (dominant inheritance)	Gastrointestinal carcinoma
Familial Wilms's tumor (dominant inheritance)	Wilms's tumor
Cancer family syndrome (dominant inheritance)	Mostly adenocarcinoma of colon, endometrium
Familial retinoblastoma (dominant inheritance)	Retinoblastoma
Ataxia telangiectasia (dominant inheritance)	Lymphoid neoplasm
Fanconi's anemia (recessive inheritance)	Acute myelomonocytic leukemia, hepatoma
Xeroderma pigmentosum (recessive inheritance)	Basal and squamous cell cancer of skin
Retinoblastoma, bilateral	Sarcoma
Multiple lipomatosis	Skin cancer
Hereditary pancreatitis	Carcinoma of pancreas
Familial, juvenile, and neonatal cirrhosis	Hepatocellular carcinoma
Familial hydronephrosis	Congenital sarcoma of kidney
Fibrocystic pulmonary dysplasia	Bronchial adenocarcinoma
Albinism (recessive inheritance)	Skin cancer
Polycythemia vera	Acute myelocytic leukemia
Dyskeratosis congenita	Leukoplakia with squamous cell carcinoma
Torre's syndrome	Diverse gastrointestinal and urogenital cancers
Klinefelter's syndrome	Breast cancer risk approaches the risk in normal women and is approximately 66 times the risk in normal men
Gonadal dysgenesis	Gonadal malignancy—risk is 25 per cent
Turner's syndrome	Tumors of neural crest origin and brain and pituitary tumors. Endometrial cancer but only with prolonged estrogen therapy
Cryptorchidism	Testicular cancer
Glutathione reductase deficiency	Leukemia
Kostmann's syndrome (infantile genetic agranulocytosis)	Acute monocytic leukemia
Bloom's syndrome (recessive inheritance)	Acute nonlymphocytic leukemia, gastrointestinal tumors
Neurofibromatosis or von Recklinghausen's disease (dominant inheritance)	Neurologic sarcomas, gliomas, Wilms's tumor, rhabdomyosarcoma, myeloid leukemia
Nevoid basal cell carcinoma syndrome (dominant inheritance)	Medulloblastoma, basal cell carcinomas, ovarian fibrosarcoma
Down's syndrome	Acute leukemia—risk increased 11 times in children with Down's syndrome
XY gonadal dysgenesis (sex-linked recessive, a male-limited dominant)	Gonadoblastoma, dysgerminoma
Mixed gonadal dysgenesis	Gonadoblastoma
Testicular feminization (sex-linked recessive)	Gonadoblastoma

(Data from Anderson, 1975; Meadows & Li, 1983, pp. 17–24; Meisner, 1983, pp. 167, 168, 169; Mulvihill, 1975, p. 21; Rawson, 1978.)

other branches of this kindred. The mode of transmission was consistent with an autosomal dominant inherited factor (Lynch & Krush, 1971; Lynch, Lynch, Harris, Lynch, & Guirgis, 1978). They have found the same type of transmission with endometrial cancer in other cancer-prone families (Lynch & Lynch, 1978).

Immune Deficiency Diseases, Acquired Diseases, and Medicinal Drugs

Data from both animal and human experiments indicate immunodeficiency predisposes to cancer. It is well known that organ transplant patients (e.g., those receiving renal transplants) who receive immunosuppressive drugs have a higher incidence of cancer. Non-Hodgkin's lymphoma, the most common type of cancer in these patients, occurs 32 times more often among them than in the general population (Meisner, 1983). Kersey and Spector (1975) note that cancers not only develop more frequently in patients with drug-induced immunodeficiencies than in age-matched control populations but also have shorter latency periods than expected. A significant proportion of patients develop cancer in the months and years following transplantation, and the bulk of the cancers are lymphoreticular, with an especially high incidence of de novo brain tumors.

In children with primary immunodeficiency syndrome (as opposed to drug-induced immunosuppressive states), the incidence of cancer is nearly 100 times the expected incidence of certain kinds of tumors (Sondel, 1983). Most primary immunodeficiency disorders are genetically determined, either as X-linked or autosomal recessive traits. Some functional defects of the immune system include Wiskott-Aldrich syndrome, X-linked lymphoproliferative syndrome, severe combined immune deficiency of infancy, ataxia-telangiectasia, and IgM deficiency. Solid lymphoreticular malignancies predominate in children with primary immunodeficiency syndromes but are uncommon in children generally. The system that is defective in all the previously named diseases is the primary site for most malignancies—the lymphoid system. Few children with primary immunodeficiency diseases live to adulthood because they die at an early age of cancer or infections.

Many acquired diseases are known or believed to predispose the individual to cancer. Templeton points out that the predisposition may be because (1) the acquired disease predisposes the individual to the cancer, (2) the cancer predisposes the individual to the acquired disease, (3) the treatment for the acquired disease actually causes the cancer, (4) the acquired disease exposes the individual to the health care system and thus to diagnosis, (5) an unknown third factor causes both the acquired disease and the cancer, and (6) the acquired disease and the cancer are phases of the same process (1975). Table 16–10 lists acquired diseases and drugs linked with cancer. The reader

should remember that the connection among many of the diseases and drugs and cancer is tentative and not conclusive at this time.

A study of cancer incidence in hypertensive patients by Buck and Donner (1987) points out the difficulty in determining if the disease (hypertension) caused the cancer or the cancer caused the disease. Their study reached a tentative conclusion that the causal direction is from cancer to hypertension rather than the reverse. The study observations "are more consistent with the hypothesis that certain sites of cancer are capable of producing hormones that raise blood pressure, than with the hypothesis that hypertension is directly or indirectly a cause of cancer" (Buck & Donner, 1987).

The use of prescription and over-the-counter medications is universal in our society. It is not unusual for individuals to consume the same drugs for months or years. Surprisingly, medicines do not appear to be a common cause of cancer. It is believed that medicinal agents account for only about 1 to 2 per cent of all cancers (Fraumeni, 1982). Some classes of drugs have been found to have varying but strong degrees of carcinogenic potential (e.g., cytotoxic agents). Alkylating agents appear to have the strongest potential for carcinogenic activity of all the cytotoxic agents. The risks of using alkylating agents, especially melphalan, cyclophosphamide, and chlorambucil, may be acceptable when treating conditions with a poor prognosis, such as metastatic cancer, but for conditions with a favorable long-term prognosis the benefits have to be weighed against the risks. One alkylating agent, chlornaphazine, was found to be so hazardous (development of bladder tumors) that its use was abandoned. In contrast, analgesics as a class of drugs are not considered carcinogenic unless they contain phenacetin.

Generally, drugs are tested in laboratory situations before release to the public, using long-term tests, short-term tests, or both. Unfortunately, it is not yet possible to use data from long-term or short-term tests to make a quantitative evaluation of human risk, which presents a significant problem in assessing drugs (Skegg, 1985). Because of this problem, clinical and epidemiologic observations of humans taking the medications become essential. Skegg (1985) pointed out that they may offer the only means for detecting carcinogenic risks of drugs that have not been tested adequately in laboratories. Sometimes it is fairly easy to detect clinically that a drug is a carcinogen because the resultant cancer is rare (e.g., hemangioendothelioma of the liver caused by Thorotrast); in other instances, the link between the cancer and the drug is impossible to determine. For that reason, cohort studies and case-controlled studies (epidemiologic methods) are used to provide the quantitative information about the use of a drug and the development of a cancer. Record linkage is a newer method that is being proposed to establish the carcinogenic risks of drugs. In this method, records of prescriptions dispensed to people are linked with records of their subsequent morbidity and mortality. Record linkage requires both a large population (minimum of 500,000 people) and time to reach conclusions.

Table 16-10. ACQUIRED DISEASES AND DRUGS USED TO TREAT DISEASES THAT HAVE BEEN IMPLICATED AS PREDISPOSING TO CANCER

Disease and Drug	Cancer
1. INFECTIOUS STATES*	
a. Viral	
Herpes group organisms	
Human papillomavirus	Cervix, penis
Epstein-Barr virus	Lymphoma
Hepatitis B	Liver
Mumps orchitis	Testes
b. Bacterial	
Fistula	
Osteomyelitis	Skin, soft tissue
Urethra	Skin
Phagedenic ulcers	Skin
Syphilis	Tongue
Tuberculosis	Lung
c. Plasmodial	
Malaria	Lymphoma
d. Parasitic	
Schistosomiasis	
Schistosoma haematobium	Bladder
Schistosoma mansoni	Lymphoma
Clonorchis sinensis	Biliary tract
Intestinal parasites	Lymphoma
2. NONINFECTIOUS INFLAMMATORY STATES*	
Gastritis	Stomach
Crohn's disease	Intestine
Ulcerative colitis	Colon, bile ducts
Adult celiac disease	Intestine, lymphoma
Cirrhosis	Liver
Pulmonary fibrosis	Lung
(e.g., pneumoconiosis, hematite lung, scleroderma, sarcoid)	
Hashimoto's disease	Lymphoma of thyroid
Sjögren's syndrome	Lymphoma
Pancreatitis	Pancreas
3. ENDOCRINE STATES*	
Diabetes	Pancreas
Thyrotoxicosis	Breast
Cystic mastopathy	Breast
Prostatic hyperplasia	Prostate
Stein-Leventhal syndrome	Uterus
4. NUTRITIONAL DISORDERS*	
Iron excess	Liver
Iron deficiency	Pharynx, esophagus
Iodine deficiency	Thyroid
Vitamin A deficiency	Colon, other
Vitamin B deficiency	Liver
Alcoholism	Esophagus, oropharynx, larynx, liver, pancreas
Obesity	Breast, uterus
5. TRAUMA*	
Calculi	
Urinary stones	Renal, pelvis
Gallstones	Gallbladder
Burns (thermal, caustic)	Skin
	Esophagus
6. POSTOPERATIVE STATES*	
Immune interference	
Appendectomy	(?)
Tonsillectomy	Hodgkin's disease
Thymectomy	(?)
Transplantation	Lymphoma
Radical mastectomy	Lymphangiosarcoma
7. BENIGN PROLIFERATIONS*	
Polyps (adenomatous)	Colon
Nevi	Melanoma
Hydatidiform mole	Choriocarcinoma
Enchondroma	Chondrosarcoma
Paget's disease of bone	Bone

Table continued on following page

Table 16–10. ACQUIRED DISEASES AND DRUGS USED TO TREAT DISEASES THAT HAVE BEEN IMPLICATED AS PREDISPOSING TO CANCER *Continued*

Disease and Drug	Cancer
8. OTHER DISORDERS*	
Myeloproliferative states	Leukemia
Pernicious anemia	Leukemia, stomach
Heroin addiction	Hodgkin's disease
Pharyngeal pouch	Pharynx
Bladder diverticulum	Bladder
9. MEDICAL TREATMENTS†	
Replacement estrogens in postmenopausal women	Endometrial, breast(?)
Use of diethylstilbestrol during pregnancy	Adenocarcinoma of the vagina in female offspring
Use of stilbestrol and other estrogens in first trimester of pregnancy	Cancer of the testis in male offspring(?)
Use of contraceptive steroids	Liver
	Breast(?)
	Cervical cancer—carcinoma in situ and dysplasia
Use of immunosuppressive drugs in transplant patients (e.g., azathioprine, corticosteroids)	Non-Hodgkin's lymphoma
Use of rauwolfia alkaloids (reserpine therapy)	Breast
Use of chlornaphazine (Erysan) for polycythemia	Urinary bladder
Use of phenacetin	Urinary bladder
Androgenic-anabolic steroids used in aplastic anemia and body building	Hepatocellular carcinoma
Arsenic medicines containing inorganic arsenic compounds	Skin
Iron dextran	Site of injection
Methoxypsoralens used with ultraviolet radiation for psoriasis (PUVA)	Skin
Oxymetholone	Liver
Radioisotopes:	
Phosphorus (^{32}P) used with polycythemia vera	Acute leukemia
Radium, mesothorium used to treat bone tuberculosis	Osteosarcoma
Radioiodine used to treat thyroid cancer	Leukemia
Thorium oxide (Thorotrast)	Hemangioendothelioma of liver
Cytotoxic Drugs:	
Use of MOPP regimen (mechlorethamine hydrochloride [Mustargen], vincristine sulfate [Oncovin], prednisone, procarbazine) for Hodgkin's disease.	Acute myelomonocytic leukemia
Use of melphalan in multiple myeloma (alkylating)	Acute myelomonocytic leukemia
Use of chlorambucil (alkylating)	Bladder
Use of methyl CCNU (semustine) for stomach, colon, rectum cancer	Leukemia
Use of cyclophosphamide for multiple myeloma (alkylating)	Bladder, acute myelomonocytic leukemia
Myleran (alkylating)	Marrow
Treosulfan (alkylating)	Marrow
Cytotoxic drugs classified as "probably carcinogenic"—sufficient evidence for carcinogenicity found in animals:	
Doxorubicin (Adriamycin)(antibiotic)	
BCNU (carmustine)—(nitrosourea)	
CCNU (lomustine)—(nitrosourea)	
Dacarbazine	
Nitrogen mustard (alkylating)	
Procarbazine	
Thiotepa (alkylating)	
Uracil mustard (alkylating)	
Drugs classified as "probably carcinogenic" in humans based on sufficient evidence of carcinogenicity in animals:	
Metronidazole (antiprotozoal)	
Phenazopyridine (urinary tract analgesic)	
Propylthiouracil (antithyroid)	
Drugs under investigation:	
Cimetidine—reduces gastric acidity; needs more study	Gastric cancer(?)
Diazepam—tranquilizer, unlikely carcinogen	Breast cancer(?)
Phenytoin (Dilantin)(?)	Lymphoma
Chloramphenicol(?)	Leukemia
Amphetamine(?)	Hodgkin's disease

*From Templeton, A. C. (1975). Acquired diseases. In J. Fraumeni (Ed.), *Persons at high risk of cancer* (pp. 70–72). New York: Academic Press. Reproduced by permission.

†Drug information from Bryan, 1983; Clemmesen, 1987; Hoover & Fraumeni, 1975; Lewison, 1978; Page & Asire, 1985; Pike, 1985; Skegg, 1985, Vessey, 1985.

Precancerous Lesions

A *precancerous lesion* may be defined as a "morphologically altered tissue in which cancer is more likely to occur than in its apparently normal counterpart" (Wood, Heffez, & Sawyer, 1985). If left alone, precancerous lesions will progress to invasive cancer. The time between the identification of the precancerous lesion and the development of invasive cancer is extremely variable and differs with the organ involved. In the uterine cervix and breast, the process at present is estimated at 10 years or more. In other organ systems (e.g., urinary bladder, stomach), the period is much longer. The majority of precancerous lesions are not identifiable by clinical examination alone and require microscopic examination to determine nuclear and mitotic abnormalities and abnormal patterns of growth. The following is a list of the precancerous lesions of multiple organ system:

Uterine Cervix

Two types of lesions are identified as precancerous; dysplasia and carcinoma in situ. Dysplasia refers to lesions involving less than the full thickness of the epithelium; carcinoma in situ refers to lesions involving the full thickness. Dysplasias are subdivided into very mild, mild, moderate, and severe, depending on the extent of involvement of the epithelium. In a different classification system (cervical intraepithelial neoplasia nomenclature), three types of lesions are described: atypical cells involving (1) less than one third of the epithelium (CIN1), (2) one third to two thirds of the epithelium (CIN2), and (3) the full-thickness of the epithelium (CIN3) (Lovejoy, 1987, p. 2).

Oral

Precancerous lesions of the oral cavity consist of the (1) leukoplakia, a painless white patch; (2) erythroplakia, a red patch; and (3) erythroleukoplakia, which is known as a speckled leukoplakia or speckled erythroplakia. These oral precancerous lesions are epithelial in origin and will become carcinomas if they progress to frank malignancy (Wood et al., 1985).

Vagina

Three precancerous lesions have been identified for the vagina: (1) carcinoma in situ (squamous type), which tends to produce early metastases; (2) adenosis of the vagina, which may occur with and without diethylstilbestrol exposure; and (3) postradiation carcinoma in situ (epidermoid type), which may appear 1 or more years after treatment for cancer of the cervix and progress to invasive cancer in a short period of time (Koss, 1975).

Endometrium

A form of endometrial hyperplasia also termed *endometrial carcinoma in situ* or *adenomatous hyperplasia* is considered a precancerous lesion and has been shown to progress to endometrial carcinoma.

Breast

Lobular carcinoma in situ (lobular CIS) has been cited as a precancerous lesion and is diagnosed by microscopic examination of the specimen. Some clincians prefer the term *atypical lobular hyperplasia* It arises within the end parts of the lobule. Lobular CIS is characterized by clusters of anaplastic small cells of high nuclear grade that lie within lobules. For a woman with lobular CIS, the risk of developing homolateral breast cancer is approximately 70 per cent in 24 years, and the chance of developing carcinoma of the opposite breast is approximately 40 per cent (Harris, Hellman, Canellos, & Fisher, 1985; Koss, 1975). This precancerous lesion has a tendency to involve both breasts, either synchronously or asynchronously. Lobular carcinoma of the breast seems to require years before progressing to invasive carcinoma, and some lesions never progress to cancer.

Skin

Precancerous lesions of the skin are (1) actinic (solar) keratosis, which consists of dysplasias of the upper layers of the epidermis that are squamous cell, white, scaly, keratotic lesions; (2) Bowen's disease (squamous cell), which is a dysplasia of the basal layer of the dermis that is considered a carcinoma in situ; the lesions are flat, reddish, scaly patches with superficial erosions (Sherman, 1983); (3) arsenical keratosis; (4) Queyrat's erythroplasia, which occurs on the penis and is identical to carcinoma in situ of the skin; lesions are raised, red, and velvet in appearance (Haynes, Mead, & Goldwyn, 1985); and (5) extramammary Paget's disease, which can affect any part of the skin in which epidermis and sweat glands coexist.

Bladder

Nonpapillary carcinoma in situ is a noninvasive precancerous lesion, but it has a high potential for subsequent invasion. The rate of recurrent cancer and the rate of progression to invasive carcinoma of the bladder are approximately 80 per cent over a period of 5 years (Koss, 1975). Carcinoma in situ is often found in close proximity to other bladder tumors. It is more common in men than in women and is associated with irritative symptoms ("interstitial cystitis"). It is multifocal and diffuse and reflects the potential for the entire urothelial surface to undergo exposure to potential carcinogens (Richie, Shipley, & Yagoda, 1985).

Colon

Strong evidence suggests that adenomatous polyps are a precursor of colorectal cancer. Sugarbaker, Gunderson, and Wittes (1985) list several arguments for an adenomatous polyp-to-cancer transition, including the following:

1. Patients who are kept polyp free remain cancer free.

2. Incidence of cancer increases as number of polyps increases.

3. The peak age at which polyps are diagnosed precedes that for cancer by about approximately 5 years.

4. A similar distribution of polyps and cancer occurs within the large bowel. Not all colon polyps undergo malignant transformation, but the more polyps allowed to grow for a longer time to larger size, the greater the chance that cancer will develop from them. Table 16–11 and Box 16–1 show recommended screening for colorectal cancer for low- and high-risk individuals.

Life Style

Social factors pertaining to personal habits or life styles are important determinants of cancer. Research data support the estimate that life style and environmental factors are related to the development of roughly 90 per cent of cancer incidence and therefore support the widely accepted conclusion that, in principle, most cancer is preventable (De Vita, 1985; Greenwald & Sondik, 1986). Fraumeni (1982) reports that

These estimates are derived from the substantial international variation in cancer incidence, in which rates for the lowest risk countries are subtracted from the rates prevailing in the United States. The resulting difference is attributed to extrinsic causes, and the lowest risk is assumed to represent the baseline level for tumors that may be difficult or impossible to avoid. (p. 87)

The wide international variation of cancer incidence has suggested that the bulk of human cancer is related to environmental and life-style factors and is not an inevitable consequence of the aging process.

Life-style factors are defined as behaviors over which the individual has some control, such as tobacco use, diet, alcohol consumption, exposure to the sun, sexual behavior patterns, and maladaptive psychological responses. The specific roles of these life-style factors in the development of cancer are detailed as follows.

Alcohol Consumption

Alcohol contributes to an estimated 2 to 4 per cent of all cancer deaths. High alcohol consumption has been associated with cancer of the buccal cavity, pharynx, larynx, esophagus, liver, large bowel, and breast (Greenwald & Sondik, 1986). A weak correlation exists between alcohol abuse and pancreatic cancer. Because people tend to drink and smoke at the same time, it is difficult to evaluate the role of alcohol consumption alone. Drinking and smoking together undoubtedly have a synergistic, or combined, effect and do contribute to the high incidence of some cancers (Meisner, 1983). For heavy drinkers who do not smoke, the risks of cancer appear only slightly elevated, so the effects are strongly dependent on smoking habits (Fraumeni, 1982). Alcohol use and the development of cancer have been observed internationally. The combination of excessive alcohol ingestion and smoking markedly increases the risks of oral and laryngeal cancer in both sexes compared with the effect of either of these habits alone or of their absence (Pitot, 1985). It has been observed that poor nutrition may contribute to the effects of alcohol by not providing protective nutrients. In parts of China and Africa, there is a link between esophageal cancer and use of "home brews" (*samshu,* a Chinese rice wine combined with grain alcohol; *aragi,* a Sudanese distillate made from dates).

Tobacco Use

Cigarette smoking has been identified as the single most important source of preventable morbidity and

Table 16–11. RECOMMENDED SCREENING FOR COLORECTAL CANCER FOR BOTH LOW-RISK AND HIGH-RISK INDIVIDUALS

Risk Factor	Risk of Developing Colorectal Cancer	Recommended Screening
Asymptomatic persons not at high risk		Annual digital rectal examination from age 40; annual fecal occult blood test from age 50; and sigmoidoscopy beginning at age 50 to be repeated every 3 to 5 years after two consecutive annual normal examinations (see Box 16–1 for research study related to screening)
Family history of familial polyposis coli or Gardner's syndrome	Approaches 110% by 40 years of age	Biannual screening with fecal occult blood tests beginning at age 10 years, with annual flexible sigmoidoscopy beginning by age 15 years: at age 45 years, screening frequency may be relaxed if patient is asymptomatic
Cancer family syndrome	Risk in first-degree relative approaches 50%	Periodic colonoscopy beginning in the third decade of life, recommended every 3 years, and annual fecal occult blood testing
History of one or two first-degree relatives with colorectal cancer	Twofold to threefold increase in risk for colorectal cancer	Yearly fecal occult blood testing and periodic flexible sigmoidoscopy beginning at age 40 years
History of ulcerative colitis	After 30 years' duration, overall cumulative risk is 50%	Biannual screening colonoscopy beginning after 8 years of disease with frequency increased to annually after 15 years of disease
History of colorectal cancer or adenomatous polyps	Additional carcinomas found in 4 to 5% of patients with colorectal cancer	Periodic colonoscopic examination along with annual fecal occult blood testing for follow-up of all patients who have had either a cancer or a polyp detected
History of endometrial, ovarian, or breast cancer	Twofold increase in risk for colorectal cancer	Periodic screening sigmoidoscopy and annual fecal occult blood testing

Data from DeCosse, 1988; Selby & Friedman, 1989; Vessey, 1985.

Box 16–1. SCREENING AND RESCREENING FOR COLORECTAL CANCER

This randomized, experimental, control group study was conducted in Sweden with individuals between 60 and 64 years of age. The 27,700 participants were divided into a test and a control group. The test group members were asked to test their stool using the Hemoccult II slides twice over a 3-day period and again after 16 to 22 months. The majority of people in the test group participated in the initial 3-day testing and again 16 to 22 months later, 66 per cent and 58 per cent, respectively. In addition, the test group was divided into two subgroups. In one group the Hemoccult II fecal occult blood testing slides were rehydrated on the first screening, and in the other group they were not rehydrated before the slides were treated and read. All Hemoccult II slides were rehydrated in the second screening that took place 16 to 22 months later. Two results were obtained from this experiment: (1) rehydration of the Hemoccult II test is strongly indicated, and (2) screening with Hemoccult II slides is an effective way to detect colorectal cancers in the early stages. These results are supported by the fact that the number of diagnosed cancers in the first screening was significantly larger ($p>0.01$) in the rehydrated group compared with the unhydrated group, 50 and 24 cancers, respectively. Also significantly more cancers (61) were found in the test group than were found by chance in the control group (20).

(From Kewenter, J., Bjork, S., Haglind, E., Smith, L., Svanvik, J., & Ahren, C. [1988]. Screening and rescreening for colorectal cancer. A controlled trial of fecal occult blood testing in 27,700 subjects. *Cancer, 62,* 645–651.)

---

premature mortality. The weight of evidence linking tobacco use to cancer is so uniformly persuasive that the surgeon general of the United States has stated that "Cigarette smoking is the chief, single, avoidable cause of death in our society and the most important public health issue of our time" (Fielding, 1985, p. 491). Smoking, especially cigarette smoking, contributes to an estimated 25 to 35 per cent of all cancer deaths in men and 5 to 10 per cent in women (Fraumeni, 1982); an estimated 85 to 90 per cent of the lung cancer cases in the United States annually are the direct result of tobacco smoking (Pitot, 1985). It has also been estimated that an average of 5.5 minutes of life is lost for each cigarette smoked. For a 25-year-old man who smokes one pack per day (20 cigarettes), the reduction averages 4.6 years; for a man of the same age who smokes two packs per day (40 cigarettes), 8.3 years of expected longevity are lost (Fielding, 1985). The following additional facts are known about tobacco use:

1. Individuals who smoke filtered, low-tar cigarettes have a lower lung cancer risk than individuals who smoke nonfiltered, high-tar cigarettes.

2. Smoking prevalence rates for blacks are higher than for all other racial groups.

3. Smoking prevalence is high among blue-collar workers and the unemployed; prevalence of smoking decreases among men as income increases.

4. Rates for lung cancer are rising more sharply in women than in men.

5. Occupational exposures to carcinogens in conjunction with smoking multiply the risk of cancer. Asbestos workers who smoke have four to five times the risk of lung cancer as other smokers and more than 50 times the risk of those who neither smoke nor are exposed to asbestos (Greenwald & Sondik, 1986).

6. Smokers who have quit for 15 or more years have a lung cancer mortality rate between one and two times that of nonsmokers.

Tobacco use is a major cause of cancers of the larynx, oral cavity, lung, and esophagus and is also linked with increased incidence of cancers of the bladder, pancreas, and kidney. Noncancerous conditions attributable to tobacco use include coronary heart disease, peripheral arterial occlusive disease, cerebrovascular disease, chronic obstructive lung disease, peptic ulcer disease, and strokes (Abbott, Yin, Reed, & Yano, 1986; Fielding, 1985).

New evidence indicates that the risk of disease from inhalation of tobacco smoke is not limited to others who merely inhale the smoke in room air. *Involuntary smoking* refers to the exposure of nonsmokers to smoke, especially in contained environments such as homes, offices, restaurants, and airplanes. Environmental tobacco smoke is a combination of sidestream smoke and that fraction of mainstream smoke exhaled and therefore not retained by the smoker. Research has demonstrated the presence of carcinogens and other toxins in *both* sidestream and mainstream smoke and has shown that both act as carcinogens in bioassay systems (Stern, 1987). Humble, Samet, and Pathak (1987) found that nonsmokers (who had never smoked) married to smokers had an approximate twofold increased risk of lung cancer, and this risk increased with the duration of exposure to a smoking spouse. These findings are consistent with other reports of elevated risk for lung cancer and possibly other cancers among nonsmokers who live with a spouse who smokes (Matsukura, Taminato, Kitans, et al., 1984). See Box 16–2.

Smokeless tobacco is increasingly becoming a public health problem because it substantially increases the user's risk of oral cancer. The risk of cancers of the cheek and gum is increased nearly fiftyfold in long-term snuff users (snuff dipping is the practice of holding a cud of finely ground tobacco in the cheek). The prevalence of smokeless tobacco use among male adolescents that has been reported from regional and state surveys indicates usage rates as high as 30 to 40 per cent in some junior and senior high schools. Approximately 2 per cent of females of all ages have used smokeless tobacco in the last year ("Smokeless tobacco," 1987). Three classes of carcingogens have been identified in smokeless tobacco products: N-nitrosamines, polonium-210, and polynuclear aromatic hydrocarbons. These carcinogens are found in snuff at

Box 16–2. EFFECTS OF SPOUSE CIGARETTE SMOKING
ON LUNG CANCER INCIDENCE

The researchers collected data on spouses' tobacco smoking habits and on-the-job exposure to asbestos in this population-based case-controlled study of lung cancer patients in New Mexico. Of the 724 eligible cases selected for the study, interviews were completed with 641 (88.5 per cent). Nine hundred forty-four controls were selected for this study, and 784 (83.1 per cent) were interviewed. The cases selected for study were Hispanic and non-Hispanic residents of New Mexico who were less than 85 years of age at the diagnosis of primary lung cancer. No effect of spouse cigarette smoking was found in this study among current or former smokers. However, never smokers married to smokers had an approximate twofold increased risk of lung cancer. "Lung cancer risk in never smokers also increased with duration of exposure to a smoking spouse, but not with increasing number of cigarettes smoked per day by the spouse." The researchers comment that the findings of their study are similar to those of other studies that report elevated risk for lung cancer among never smokers living with a spouse who smokes cigarettes.

(From Humble, C., Samet, J., & Pathak, D. [1987]. Marriage to a smoker and lung cancer risk. *American Journal of Public Health, 77,* 598–602.)

"alarmingly high" concentrations when compared with those found in other consumer products (Stockwell, 1986).

Psychosocial Variables

Epidemiologic studies examining the empirical relationship between emotional, behavioral, and personality factors and cancer risk are rare. However, several studies have found that self-reports of depression and lack of social support had long-range, predictive value for increased cancer incidence. Grossarth-Maticek, Frentzel-Beyme, and Becker (1984) interviewed 1353 people in 1966 and again in 1976 and found that persons reporting feelings of hopelessness showed a steadily increasing risk ratio for cancer, depending on the intensity of this reaction. "A gradual increase of cancer became evident more than 3 years after an event causing unresolved depression and hopelessness of more than 1 year's duration" (p. 201). Other diseases did not show the same consistent pattern. Animal studies using an analogue of human passivity or "helplessness" have shown increased tumor growth in the acute, helpless condition (Levy, Herberman, Maluish, Schlien, & Lippman, 1985). This area of investigation merits further attention and research (Wellisch & Yager, 1984).

Diet

Poor dietary practices, including inadequate intake of fiber and important micronutrients, are thought by some scientists to be as significant as tobacco smoking in causing cancer. About 27 per cent of all cancer deaths are caused by lung cancer, the vast majority caused by smoking. Another 30 per cent of all cancer deaths are due to cancer of the colon-rectum, breast, and prostate. For these three cancers, dietary practices are implicated as risk factors. The consensus of investigators is that as much as 25 to 35 per cent of cancer mortality is related to dietary factors (Greenwald & Sondik, 1986). Estimates of risk from diet range from 10 to 70 per cent. These estimates are based on a large number of studies, although the exact magnitude of the association and the biologic mechanisms involved are uncertain. As Weinhouse (1986) points out, much of the information on the relationship between diet and development of cancer is inferential. Although convincing associations have been found between cancer and dietary practices throughout the world, association is not necessarily equatable with causation.

The delineation of dietary risk factors is not simple. Creasey (1985, p. 6) details some of the reasons, including the following:

1. Carcinogenesis is a multistage process that takes a long time to complete; initiating events may have occurred decades before the cancer appears.

2. Conclusions from dietary surveys involving individuals who have cancer are misleading because the disease changes dietary habits.

3. Prospective studies are rare, and blind–double-blind experiments used in typical clinical trials are impossible to perform.

4. The elevated incidence of a cancer may be the result of two or more factors in combination rather than one alone.

5. The type of role played by dietary factors may affect the ease with which an association can be demonstrated.

Research into the etiology and prevention of cancer has been an important branch of research for several decades. In the course of this research, epidemiologists have reported large differences in cancer incidence and mortality among countries and have suggested that these differences are largely due to environmental factors. Some leading scientists and national advisory bodies have proposed that dietary patterns are among the important environmental determinants of human cancer (Birdsell, 1986, p. 284). Cancer patterns in migrating populations provide further compelling data. Japanese in Japan have a tenfold higher mortality rate from stomach cancer than do Americans in the United States, but Japanese who have migrated to Hawaii or the United States mainland and their succeeding generations have progressively lowered mortality rates for stomach cancer.

Dietary factors are associated with cancers of the gastrointestinal tract (esophagus, stomach, colon, rectum, pancreas, and liver) and some sex- and hormone-specific sites (breast, prostate, ovaries, and endometrium). The dietary components that have been implicated in the development of cancer are summarized in Table 16–12. Table 16–13 lists the National Institutes of Health's suggestions on how to increase fiber and reduce fat in the daily diet.

Table 16–12. DIETARY COMPONENTS AND THEIR KNOWN OR SUSPECTED RELATIONSHIP TO CANCER

Dietary Component	Anatomic Site Affected	Mechanism	Discussion	Year 2000 Dietary Objectives
Fat	Breast, colon, endometrium, and prostate cancers associated with diets high in fat.	May act as a promoter: exact mechanism unknown.	Dietary polyunsaturated vegetable oils promote tumorigenesis in animals, saturated fats and polyunsaturated fish oils either have little effect or are inhibitory. Total fat intake accounts for 40% of total calories in U.S. diet compared with only 20% in Japanese diet.	Per capita daily consumption of fat will decrease from 40 to 25% or less of total calories.
Fiber	Colon cancer associated with diets low in fiber.	Production of short-chain fatty acids (products of fiber fermentation), regulation of energy intake, dilution of colonic contents, and absorption of bile acids decreases production of mutagens in stool.	No consistent thread of evidence through either human or experimental data that confers an unequivocally protective role on fiber in general or some specific fiber or fiber component in particular (Kritchevsky, 1986). Inverse association between eating vegetables and occurrence of colon cancers. U.S. diet includes only 15 to 20 g of fiber a day: 25 to 30 g a day is recommended.	Per capita consumption of fiber from grains, fruits, and vegetables will increase from 8 to 12 g per day to 20 to 30 g per day.
Vitamin C (ascorbic acid)	Inverse association between fresh fruit/vegetable consumption and stomach and esophagus cancer.	Animal studies show vitamin C can inhibit formation of carcinogenic *N*-nitroso compounds from ingested nitrates. Ascorbic acid plays key role in maintenance of immune system.		
Vitamin E		Blocks formation of carcinogenic nitroso compounds. Laboratory studies show may inhibit tumorigenesis.	No evidence that megadoses protect individuals against cancer. Vitamin E, a fat-soluble vitamin, is potentially toxic in high doses.	
Vitamin A*	Inverse association between dietary vitamin A or carotenoids and cancers of the oral cavity, urinary bladder, pharynx, larynx, and lung.	Carotenoids have a potent antioxidant effect and reduce cancer risk by preventing tissue damage due to oxidation. Retinoids have potent hormone-like effects on cell growth and differentiation: in vitro studies show they can reverse keratinization and other premalignant changes.	Fat-soluble, stored in liver, and toxic in high doses.	
Selenium	Inverse correlation between selenium intake and cancer, specifically of the head and neck.	May be mediated through an increase in the activity of the selenium-dependent enzyme glutathione peroxidase.	Selenium in high doses is toxic.	
Cured, Pickled, and Smoked Foods	Inverse relationship between pickled, cured, and smoked foods and stomach cancer.	Formation of nitrosamines occurs in vitro during curing processes and has been demonstrated to occur in animals in vivo. Evidence of carcinogenicity of nitrosamines is not conclusive.	Nitrates and nitrites are used as preservatives in many foods as curing agents. Smoking and pickling foods produce higher levels of polycyclic aromatic hydrocarbons and *N*-nitroso compounds. Cyclic aromatic hydrocarbons are mutagenic, carcinogenic, or both. Fish and beef cooked at high temperatures produced mutagenic activity from the breakdown products of proteins and amino acids. Formed only with temperatures of 250° C or greater.	Minimize consumption of foods preserved by salt curing (including salt pickling or smoking). Avoid frying and high-temperature cooking.
Protein	Dietary protein associated with breast, endometrium, prostate, colon, rectum, pancreas, and kidney cancers.	Laboratory studies with animals have demonstrated carcinogenesis can be suppressed by a dietary level of protein at or below the minimum required for optimal growth. Chemically induced carcinogenesis seems to be enhanced as protein intake is increased up to 2 or 3 times the normal requirement.	Because there is a strong correlation between intake of fat and protein in the Western diet, it is difficult to separate protein from fat as an independent cancer risk factor.	

*Carotenoids are provitamins or natural precursors of vitamin A. *Retinoids,* or preformed vitamin A, occur only in foods of animal origin.
(Data from *Cancer prevention research summary,* 1985; Carroll, Braden, Bell, & Kalamegham, 1986; DeVita, 1985; Greenwald, 1985; Greenwald, Sondik, & Lynch, 1986; Hennekens, Mayrent, & Willett, 1986; Kritchevsky, 1986; Newell, 1985; Page & Asire, 1985; Palmer, 1986.)

Table 16–13. SUGGESTIONS TO INCREASE FIBER AND REDUCE FAT IN THE DAILY DIET

To *increase* dietary fiber, select the following:	Select the following *less* often:
1. Bakery products such as bran muffins, whole-wheat crackers, rye, bagels, and pumpernickel	1. Refined bakery and snack foods such as croissants, chips, and pastries
2. Breakfast cereals such as shredded wheat, whole-grain or whole-wheat flake cereals	
3. Foods made with whole-grain flours such as waffles and pancakes	
4. All fruits and vegetables with the skins on	
5. All dried peas and beans	

To *decrease* fat, select the following:	Select the following *less* often:
1. Lower fat, poultry, fish, and meat (water-packed canned fish, chicken, and turkey)	1. Tuna packed in oil, poultry with skin, duck, and goose
2. Beef, veal, lamb, and pork cuts trimmed of all fat and no visible fat in meat	2. Luncheon meats
3. Low-fat or skim milk dairy products (mozzarella, ricotta, sherbet, low-fat yogurt)	3. Beef, veal, lamb, and pork with fat and marbling
4. Peas and beans	4. Nuts and seeds
5. "Diet" and low-fat salad dressings and low-fat margarine	5. Full-fat dairy products (butter, sweet cream, sour cream)
6. Prepare food by baking, oven broiling, boiling, stewing, poaching, stir frying, simmering, and steaming	6. Hard cheeses, full-fat soft cheeses such as cream cheese, and ice cream
	7. Mayonnaise, gravies, butter sauces over vegetables, and salad oils
	8. Preparing food by deep-fat frying: adding cream or butter to vegetables
	9. Snack and bakery foods such as doughnuts, pies, cakes, cookies, brownies, chips, granola, and croissants

(From U.S. Department of Health and Human Services. [1985]. *Diet, nutrition and cancer prevention: A guide to food choices* [NIH Publication No. 85–2711]. Washington, DC: U.S. Government Printing Office). This is an excellent publication for lay people that offers practical advice on following a cancer-prevention diet.

Radiation

Ionizing radiation is believed to account for approximately 3 per cent of all cancers. Recognition of the carcinogenic effects of ionizing radiation came soon after the discovery of roentgen rays in 1895. However, the awareness that low to moderate exposures to ionizing radiation could cause cancer has come about largely in the last 30 years (Shore, 1984). The mechanism for causing cancer is that radiation removes electrons from atoms and changes the molecular structures of cells, which may ultimately cause cancer to develop. The genetic DNA in the cell nucleus is believed to be the critical target for radiation-induced damage (Page & Asire, 1985). Radiation sources are quite varied: natural background, medical and dental procedures, occupational exposures, weapons tests, industrial uses and products (e.g., nuclear power plants), and miscellaneous (e.g., television sets, airline travel cosmic radiation, radiation from brick and masonry buildings).

Much of our information on the long-term effects of radiation and dose-response relationships comes from studies of atomic bomb survivors of Hiroshima and Nagasaki. Leukemia was the first radiation-related malignant condition identified among the survivors, followed by thyroid carcinomas a decade later; still later, breast cancer was detected. Late atomic bomb radiation effects include cancers of the lung, stomach, colon, and multiple myeloma. Among survivors, excessive mortality from cancer excluding leukemia was reported beginning around 1960, 15 years after exposure, among persons whose doses were estimated at more than 100 rads.

Two of the more common sources of radiation are from the natural background and from medical and dental procedures.

Natural Background. Background radiation is the single greatest source of exposure, and little can be done to avoid exposure to it. Radon is becoming a public health concern in some areas because of its presence in ground and building materials. Cosmic irradiation varies by roughly a factor of two based on the altitude at which one lives; people living at higher altitudes receive more exposure. Likewise, exposure varies with latitude; people living closer to the equator receive more exposure ("The dark side," 1986). Sunlight (ultraviolet radiation) is regarded as the probable factor in the pathogenesis of skin cancer and of primary melanoma of the skin of white persons. The National Academy of Sciences has stated that for "a Caucasian population living at 40 degrees latitude (Philadelphia) no less than 40 per cent of the melanomas and 80 per cent of the squamous and basal cell carcinomas are caused by ultraviolet radiation" (Joblon, 1975).

Medical and Dental Procedures. The single largest manufactured source of radiation exposure comes from medical and dental diagnostic procedures. It has been estimated that about 65 per cent of the population receives one or more radiographs each year (Shore, 1984). Some of the first evidence that radiation causes cancer came from studies of patients who received radiation therapy before 1954 for ankylosing spondylitis. These patients suffered a substantially increased risk of leukemia, aplastic anemia, and cancer. Women treated with radiation in the 1930s to induce an artificial menopause also had an excess risk of leukemia. Between 1935 and 1954, fluoroscopy was used to monitor treatment of patients with tuberculosis. Ten to 15 years later, these women who had undergone fluoroscopy had a high incidence of breast cancer. Before 1950, therapeutic or prophylactic radiotherapy of the thymus was done to shrink the thymus. Physicians at that time believed an enlarged thymus interfered with respiration. Other children received tonsilar, thyroid, and facial irradiation for noncancerous conditions of the head and neck (Clifton, 1983). An elevated risk of thyroid cancer and leukemia has been found in this population.

The weight of scientific evidence supports the idea that in utero radiation exposure does increase the risks of childhood cancers. This was first reported in the 1950s, and available data suggest that the fetus may be especially sensitive to the carcinogenic effect of low doses of radiation.

Occupational Exposures

Occupational exposure to carcinogens is thought to be responsible for 4 to 6 per cent of cancer mortality in industrialized countries. However, this estimate is a generalization for the entire population, and those specific groups at high levels of exposure suffer a much greater risk (Greenwald & Sondik, 1986). Observations about the relationships of occupation and cancer date back to 1472 with the first publication by Ulrich Ellenbog concerning an occupational disease. He described the irritating effects of the fumes of lead and mercury experienced by goldsmiths (Schottenfeld & Haas, 1978). In 1713 Ramazzini described the high incidence of mammary cancer in nuns and attributed it to their celibate life. A classic study was done by Percivall Pott in 1775 when he observed that cancer of the scrotum was common among chimney sweeps. Pott's study is considered the first clinical report of occupational chemical carcinogenesis. Over the years other researchers have made observations about work exposures and the increasing risk of cancer.

The goals related to occupational exposures of the National Cancer Institute's Year 2000 include the goal that workers be informed routinely of life-style behaviors that interact with factors in the work environment to increase risks for cancer. The synergistic relationship of asbestos and cigarette smoking is well known. The observed increased risk of cancer found in some occupations may arise from mixed chemical and physical exposures or from the interaction of occupational and nonoccupational factors. Other Year 2000 goals include having at least 25 per cent of the workers able to state the occupational health and safety risks they are exposed to and the potential consequences; seeing that at least 70 per cent of health care providers include questions about occupational exposures on the medical history and know how to interpret the information given to them; and ensuring that all firms with more than 500 employees have a plan of hazard control for everything associated with suspected carcinogens.

The growth of the chemical industry has resulted in more and more workers being exposed to possibly carcinogenic substances. In 1940, approximately 1 billion pounds of synthetic organic chemicals were produced in the United States. By 1965, this quantity had increased nearly a hundredfold, and it now exceeds 300 billion pounds a year (Houk, 1982). The rate of synthesis of organic chemicals in 1977 was about 6000 new compounds each week. Approximately 1500 pounds of synthetic chemicals are manufactured per person per year in the United States (Bryan, 1983). The majority of known occupational carcinogens were identified from the mid-1960s to the early 1970s. The International Agency for Research on Cancer (IARC), an agency of the World Health Organization, has assigned individual chemicals, chemical groups, industrial processes, and occupational exposures to one of three categories of risk: group 1 for casually associated chemicals, group 2 for chemicals considered probably carcinogenic, and group 2A for chemicals with the highest carcinogenic risk to humans. Chemicals that the IARC considers carcinogenic for humans (group 2A) are the following (Greenwald & Sondik, 1986):

1. 4-Aminobiphenyl
2. Arsenic and arsenic compounds
3. Asbestos
4. Benzene
5. Benzidine
6. *N, N*-Bis(2-chloroethyl)-2-naphthylamine (chlornaphazine)
7. Bis(chloromethyl) ether and technical-grade chloromethyl methyl ether
8. Chromium and certain chromium compounds
9. Diethylstilbestrol
10. Melphalan
11. Mustard gas
12. 2-Naphthylamine
13. Soots, tars, and oils
14. Vinyl chloride

Table 16–14 lists occupations carrying an increased risk of cancer. There are many difficulties in determining a cause and effect relationship between occupational exposures and incidence of cancer:

1. Many workers do not know which substances might be hazardous or whether their working environment contains hazardous substances.
2. Workers change jobs and positions and forget about previous exposures in former occupations.
3. Job titles do not correspond to actual exposures.
4. Most cancers have an incubation period of 10 to 20 years or more (Sharp, Eskenazi, Callas, & Smith, 1986).
5. Patterns of exposure in different groups of workers who are exposed to a common agent differ greatly.
6. There is considerable variability in latency in individual cases, reflecting intensity and duration of exposure.
7. In our society, occupations are closely related to social class. Social class is closely linked with personal habits, aspects of life style that include patterns of nutrition, and nonoccupational environmental factors. Soft-coal miners have an increased risk of cancer of the stomach, but when the effects of social class are evaluated, the occupational association is reduced (Cole & Goldman, 1975).

Organic agents, especially the aromatic hydrocarbons, have been the most thoroughly studied occupational carcinogens. Aromatic amines have been implicated since 1895 as bladder carcinogens. Rehn, a German surgeon, published his observations on bladder cancer among dye workers. Subsequent studies over the next 50 years identified benzidine, 1-naphthylamine, and 2-naphthylamine as the primary agents. In 1981, the National Institute for Occupational Safety and Health initiated a study to determine the risk of bladder cancer in a cohort of chemical workers exposed to aromatic amines, specifically B-naphthylamine. It found that the incidence of bladder cancer increased with the duration of employment (Weinhouse, 1986). Workers with 5 or fewer years of employment had an increased risk of 0.4 per cent, and those with greater than 20 years' exposure had an increased risk of 30 per cent. There were also racial differences; the cancer

Table 16–14. OCCUPATIONS CARRYING AN INCREASED RISK OF CANCER

Industry	Occupation	Site	Reported or Suspected Causative Agent
(a) Occupations recognized to present an increased risk of cancer, causally related to the occupation.			
Agriculture, forestry, and fishing	Vineyard workers using arsenical insecticides	Lung, skin	Arsenic
Extractive	Arsenic mining	Lung, skin	Arsenic
	Iron-ore mining	Lung	Causative agent not identified
	Asbestos mining	Lung, pleural and peritoneal mesothelioma	Asbestos
	Uranium mining	Lung	Radon
Asbestos production industry	Insulated material production (pipes, sheeting, textile, clothes, masks, asbestos cement manufacts)	Lung, pleural and peritoneal mesothelioma	Asbestos
Petroleum industry	Wax pressmen	Scrotum	Polycyclic hydrocarbons
Metal industry	Copper smelting	Lung	Arsenic
	Chromate producing	Lung	Chromium
	Chromium plating	Lung	Chromium
	Ferrochromium producing	Lung	Chromium
	Steel production	Lung	Benzo(a)pyrene
	Nickel refining	Nasal sinuses, lung	Nickel
Shipbuilding, motor vehicles, and transport	Shipyard and dockyard workers	Lung, pleural and peritoneal mesothelioma	Asbestos
Chemical industry	BCME and CMME products and users	Lung (oat cell carcinoma)	BCME, CMME
	Vinyl chloride producers	Liver angiosarcoma	Vinyl chloride monomer
	Isopropyl alcohol manufacturing (strong acid process) workers	Paranasal sinuses	Causative agent not identified
	Pigment chromate producing	Lung	Chromium
	Dye manufacturers and users	Bladder	Benzidine, 2-naphthylamine, 4-aminodiphenyl
	Auramine manufacture	Bladder	Auramine (together with the other aromatic amines used in the process)
Pesticides and herbicides pro-duction industry	Arsenical insecticide production and packaging	Lung	Arsenic
Gas industry	Coke plant workers	Lung	Benzo(a)pyrene
	Gas workers	Lung, bladder, scrotum	Coal carbonization products, β-naphthylamine
	Gas-retort house workers	Bladder	α/β-naphthylamine
Rubber industry	Rubber manufacture	Lymphatic and hematopoietic system (leukemia)	Benzene
		Bladder	Aromatic amines
	Calendering, tire curing, tire building	Lymphatic and hematopoietic system (leukemia)	Benzene
	Millers, mixers	Bladder	Aromatic amines
	Synthetic latex producers, tire curing, calender operatives, reclaimers, cable makers	Bladder	Aromatic amines
Construction industry	Insulators and pipe coverers	Lung, pleural, and peritoneal mesothelioma	Asbestos
Leather industry	Boot and shoe manufacturers, repairers	Nose, marrow (leukemia)	Leather dust, benzene
Wood pulp and paper industry	Furniture and cabinet makers	Nose (adenocarcinoma)	Wood dust
Other	Roofers, asphalt workers	Lung	BAP
(b) Occupations reported to present an increased risk of cancer but for which the assessment of the causal relation with the occupation is not definitive			
Agriculture, forestry and fishing	Fishermen	Skin, lip	Pitch, ultraviolet radiation
	Farmers	Lymphatic and hematopoietic system (leukemia, lymphoma)	Undefined
	Basal bark sprayers	Lymphatic and hematopoietic system (lymphoma), soft tissue sarcomas	Phenoxyacetic acids, chlorophenols (presumably contaminated with PCDF, PCDD, and polychlorinated benzodioxins)
	Railway embankment sprayers	Lymphatic and hematopoietic system (lymphoma), lung cancer	Phenoxyacetic acids, amitrol, monuron, durion
	Pesticide appliers	Lung	Hexachlorocyclohexane combined and other pesticides
Extractive	Zinc-lead mining	Lung	Radiation
	Coal	Stomach	Coal dust
	Talc	Lung, pleura	Talc (contaminated with asbestos?)
Asbestos production industry	Insulation material production (pipes, sheeting, textiles, clothes, masks, asbestos cement manufacts)	Larynx, gastrointestinal tract	Asbestos
Petroleum industry	Oil refining	Esophagus, stomach, lung	Polycyclic hydrocarbons
	Boilermakers, painters, welders, oilfield workers	Lung	Polycyclic hydrocarbons
	Petrochemical plant workers	Brain, stomach	Polycyclic hydrocarbons
	Petroleum refining	Marrow (leukemia)	Benzene
Metal industry	Aluminium production	Lung	Benzo(a)pyrene
	Beryllium refining	Lung	Beryllium
	Smelters	Respiratory and digestive system	Lead
	Nickel refining	Larynx	Nickel
	Battery plant workers, cadmium alloy producers, electroplating workers	Prostate, kidney	Cadmium
	Cadmium smelters	Prostate, lung	Cadmium

Table 16–14. OCCUPATIONS CARRYING AN INCREASED RISK OF CANCER *Continued*

Industry	Occupation	Site	Reported or Suspected Causative Agent
Shipbuilding, motor vehicles, and transport	Filling station, bus and truck drivers, operators of excavating machines	Marrow (leukemia)	Petroleum products and combustion residues containing benzene
	Haulers	Lung	Polycyclic aromatic hydrocarbons
	Shipyard and dockyard workers	Larynx, digestive system	Asbestos
Chemical industry	Acrylonitrile production	Lung, colon	Acrylonitrile
	Vinylidene chloride producers	Lung	Vinylidene chloride (mixed exposure to VC and acrylonitrile)
	Isopropyl alcohol manufacturing (strong acid process) workers	Larynx	Undefined
	Polychloroprene producers	Lung	Chloroprene
	Dimethylsulfate producers	Lung	Dimethylsulfate
	Epichlorohydrin producers	Lung, lymphatic and hematopoietic system (leukemia)	Epichlorohydrin
	Ethylene oxide producers	Lymphatic and hematopoietic system (leukemia), stomach	Ethylene oxide
	Ethylene dibromide producers	Digestive system	Ethylene dibromide
	Flame retardant and plasticizer users	Skin (melanoma)	Polychlorinated biphenyls
	Styrene and polystyrene producers	Lymphatic and hematopoietic system (leukemia)	Styrene
	Ortho- and *para*-toluidine producers	Bladder	*Ortho/para*-toluidine
	Benzoylchloride producers	Lung	Benzoylchloride
	Magenta producers	Bladder	Aniline, *o*-toluidine
Pesticides and herbicides pro-duction industry	Tetrachlorodibenzodioxin producers and those exposed after accidents	Lung, stomach	DCDD and TCDD dichlorodibenzodioxin, trichlorodibenzodioxin
Rubber industry	Rubber manufacturing	Lymphopoietic system, stomach, brain, pancreas	Undefined
	Processors, composers, cementing synthetic plant	Stomach	Undefined
	General service	Lymphatic and hematopoietic system (leukemia), lymphatic and hemopoietic tissue	Undefined
	Synthetic latex producers and tire curing	Lung	Undefined
	Calender operatives and reclaimers	Prostate, lung	Undefined
	Compounding, mixing, and calendering	Prostate	Undefined
	Styrene butadiene rubber producers	Lymphatic and hematopoietic system (lymphomas)	Styrene
	Pliofilm producers	Lymphatic and hematopoietic system (leukemia)	Benzene
	Rubber compounding, extruding, milling	Stomach	Undefined
	Tire assembly	Skin	Mineral extender oil
		Brain	Undefined
Construction industry	Insulators and pipe coverers	Larynx, gastrointestinal tract	Asbestos
Printing industry	Rotogravure workers, binders	Marrow (leukemia)	Benzene
	Printing pressmen	Buccal cavity, rectum, pancreas, lung, prostate, kidney	Oil mist, solvents, dyes, cadmium, lead
	Newspaper pressmen	Buccal cavity	Oil mist, solvents, dyes, cadmium, lead
	Commercial pressmen	Pancreas, rectum	Oil mist, solvents, dyes, cadmium, lead
	Compositors	Multiple myeloma	Solvents
	Machine room workers	Lung	Oil mist
Leather industry	Tanners and processors	Bladder, nasal, lung	Leather dust, other chemicals, chromium
	Leather workers, unspecified	Nose, larynx, lung, bladder, lymphatic and hematopoietic system (lymphomas)	Undefined
	Boot and shoe manufacturers and repairers	Buccal cavity	Undefined
	Other leather goods manufacturers	Marrow (leukemia)	Benzene
Textile industry	Cotton and wool workers	Mouth, pharynx	Cotton and wool dust
Wood pulp and paper industry	Lumbermen and sawmill workers	Nose, Hodgkin's lymphoma	Wood dust, chlorophenols
	Pulp and papermill workers	Lymphopoietic tissue	Undefined
	Carpenters, joiners	Nose, Hodgkin's lymphomas	Wood dust, solvents
	Wood workers, unspecified		Undefined
Other	Radium dial workers	Breast	Radon
	Laundry and dry cleaners	Lung, skin, cervix uteri	Tritetrachloroethylene and carbon tetrachloride
	Roofers, asphalt workers	Mouth, pharynx, larynx, esophagus, stomach	Benzo(a)pyrene, other pitch volatile agents

(From Simonato, L., & Saracci, R. [1983]. Cancer: Occupational. *Encyclopedia of occupational health and safety* [3rd rev. ed., pp. 369–375]. Geneva: International Labor Organisation. Copyright 1983, International Labor Organisation, Geneva. Reproduced by permission.)

occurred 15 years earlier in black workers. The average latency period between exposure and development of the cancer was 16 years for blacks and 22 years for whites (Report of the Task Force, 1981).

Although many of the occupations listed in Table 16–14 historically have been male dominated, this picture is rapidly changing with the influx of women into the work force. In 1981, 42.3 per cent of the United States work force was female, representing nearly 47 million women, compared with 38 per cent in 1973 (Stellman & Stellman, 1983). The proportion of women working outside the home continues to rise. There are a number of female-dominated occupations that pose potential health hazards. Many women are exposed to ionizing radiation in their jobs as nurses, dental health service workers, health technologists and technicians, and hairdressers. For instance, hairdressers are exposed to hair dyes, vinyl chloride spray-can propellants, and asbestos from hair dryers. Table 16–15 lists selected female-dominated occupations that expose those who work in them to known or suspected carcinogens.

Environmental Exposures

It has been estimated that pollution accounts for at least 1 to 5 per cent of all cancer deaths. Although

environmental pollution has received a tremendous amount of media attention, research has not demonstrated a strong link between air or water pollution and cancer. Since the 1930s, Congress has enacted a number of laws and established a number of federal agencies to control carcinogens in the environment and in the food and water supply (Pitot, 1983). Some of the federal laws that Congress passed to control toxic and carcinogenic environmental substances are the following:

1. The Food, Drug, and Cosmetic Act (1938, 1960)
2. The Clean Air Act (1970)
3. The Federal Water Pollution Control Act amendments of 1972
4. The Occupational Safety and Health Act (1970)
5. The Federal Environmental Pesticide Control Act (1972)
6. The Atomic Energy Act (amended in 1974)
7. Safe Drinking Water Act (1974)
8. The Toxic Substances Control Act (1976)
9. The National Environmental Policy Act (1978)

Air pollution is defined by the United States government as air that contains six pollutants: carbon monoxide; sulfur dioxide; nitrogen dioxide; particulate matter; gaseous hydrocarbons; and photochemical oxidants such as ozone. There is little evidence that any of these pollutants are carcinogenic. The main class of

Table 16–15. POTENTIAL OCCUPATIONAL HEALTH HAZARDS IN SELECTED WOMEN'S OCCUPATIONS

Occupation	Women Employed (in thousands)	Known or Suspected Cancer Risk Factors
Health care professions (e.g., nurses, nursing aides, dental assistants, and lab workers)	3268	Sterilizing agents and disinfectants (ethylene oxide, ultraviolet light) Anesthetic gases (halothane) Ionizing radiation Radioisotopes Cancer drugs, carcinogenic chemicals Hepatitis B
Clothing and textile workers	1109	Benzidine-type dyes Asbestos Formaldehyde finishes (BCME) Flame retardants (TRIS)
Laundry workers	219	Dry cleaning solvents (TCE, perchloroethylene) Contaminant asbestos dust
Meat wrappers and cutters	46	Wrap decomposition fumes (vinyl chloride, polyvinylchloride, hydrogen chloride, carbon monoxide)
Hairdressers and cosmetologists	483	Hair dyes Asbestos from dryers Ultraviolet light Solvents Vinyl chloride spray-can propellants
Artists and craftspersons	250	Arsenic and alloys Beryllium, cadmium, and chromium Nickel oxides and carbonyl Asbestos Wood dust and glues Cleaning solvents: "benzine" (petroleum distillates), carbon tetrachloride, trichloroethylene, formaldehyde Vinyl chloride, polyvinylchloride Dyes and pigments
Agricultural workers	509	Organochlorine pesticides: aldrin, dieldrin, endrin, chlordecone (Kepone), methoxychlor, mirex, DDT, lindane, chlordane, heptachlor, and toxaphene Arsenic pesticides and herbicides Phenoxy herbicides: 2,4-D, 2, 4, 5-T ("Agent Orange")
Electrical machinery manufacturers	1000	Polychlorinated biphenyls, trichloroethylene, cadmium, and other metals

BCME, bis chlormethyl ether: TRIS, tris(hydroxymethyl) aminomethane: TCE, trichloroethylene.
(From Stellman, J., & Stellman, S. [1983]. Occupational lung disease and cancer risk in women. *Occupational Health Nursing, 31* (11), 40–46. Reproduced by permission.)

chemically identified carcinogens found in the air is polycyclic aromatic hydrocarbons (Pike, Gordon, Henderson, Menck, & Soo Hoo, 1975). There is conflicting evidence about the effect of benzo[a]pyrene or B[a]P (a combustion product) on risk of cancer. Measurement of B[a]P concentrates is used as an indicator of polycyclic aromatic hydrocarbons. Pike and colleagues (1975) suggest that in the United States 10 ng/m^3 B[a]P in the air can be equated with the effect of smoking one cigarette per day.

The concern over the association between organic contaminants in drinking water and increased rates of human cancer led to research to investigate the levels of organic contaminants in water and to estimate the potential risk they raised for incidence of human cancer (Crump & Guess, 1986). Chlorinated surface water usually contains traces of chloroform, bromoform, bromodichloromethane, and dibromochloromethane. These four substances are called *trihalomethanes*, and they are formed when chlorine used to purify drinking water reacts with organic compounds in water. Many case-controlled studies have investigated the association between chlorinated water and the incidence of cancer and have reported that rectal, bladder, and colon cancer risks with drinking chlorinated water are about 1.1. to 2.0 times higher than the risk of drinking unchlorinated water. The association between chlorination and cancer found in these studies is weak by traditional epidemiologic standards (Crump & Guess, 1986). A major problem with these studies is separating confounding risks associated with other environmental factors from the weak association found between drinking chlorinated water and cancer. In addition, low levels of nitrates, arsenic, and radon have not been found to pose a hazard to humans (Meisner, 1983).

It must be remembered that occupational carcinogens are seldom restricted to the workplace; they are often transported to the more general environment. Frequently they are transported via water. Contamination of the water sources of the United States with pesticides, industrial solvents, and other industrial chemicals such as polychlorinated biphenyls (PCBs) is becoming a serious national problem. The Safe Water Drinking Act requires that the Environmental Protection Agency publish a list of suspected carcinogenic substances found in drinking water and then establish maximum contaminant levels (Pitot, 1983).

A substance in the environment that has necessitated governmental intervention is asbestos. Asbestos was used as a spray-on material in the construction of school ceilings, primarily during the 1950s through the early 1970s, because of its acoustic, fire-proofing, and decorative qualities. It was also used in insulating materials for pipes, boilers, and structural beams in schools. Because of the potential long-term hazards of exposure to asbestos, Congress passed legislation (the Asbestos School Hazard Abatement Act of 1984) that appropriated $50 million in 1984 and authorized the expenditure of $50 to $100 million per year during the next 6 years, in loans and grants from the Environmental Protection Agency, to assist local school districts with asbestos removal. The urgency of removing asbestos from public schools is based on research that found that workers employed in asbestos factories from 1941 to 1945 and exposed to asbestos for *merely* a month had a clear excess risk of cancer. With longer direct exposure (e.g., 2 months, 3 months, 6 months) the cancer risk became greater. Moreover, with very brief direct exposure, increased cancer risk was found only after 25 years (Seidman, Lilis, & Selikoff, 1978).

SITE-SPECIFIC CANCER RISK FACTORS

The risks for the individual (and groups) have been discussed in the previous section. The totality of our existence (past, present, and future activities and exposures) determines our risks for cancer. Another method of analyzing risk is to look at the specific risks for *each* anatomic site. The method combines all the predisposing factors and susceptibilities that are discussed in the previous section. For instance, the risk factors for skin cancer include factors from the areas of environment, occupation, life style, and congenital or genetic disorders.

The "review of systems" of the traditional medical history questionnaire is an excellent vehicle for asking about specific risk factors for each anatomic site. Again, using the skin system as an example, the nurse could ask questions about long-term sunbathing; occupational exposures to arsenic or coal tar; genetic conditions (e.g., xeroderma pigmentosum); previous medical exposure to radiation or treatment for precancerous lesions (actinic keratosis); and family history of skin cancers. Although a systems review requires a thorough knowledge of the site-specific risk factors, it is worth the effort because it can yield important information and trigger the individual's memory to reveal forgotten exposures, symptoms, or activities.

It is not uncommon for health care professionals to use self-administered site-specific risk assessment forms. These self-administered forms are cost effective, reduce the time of professional involvement in conducting a risk assessment, and can be scanned rapidly to identify positive responses that may merit further discussion. Table 16–16 lists the significant site-specific risk factors for the most commonly occurring cancers and the recommended action to reduce the risk. Also included in this table are the early signs and symptoms of each site-specific cancer. These are included because the early signs and symptoms of cancer may be the nurse's first indication of the need to explore the existence of related risk factors.

NURSING RESPONSIBILITIES

This chapter has focused on the individual risk factors that predispose to the development of cancer (e.g., life style, family history, occupation). It has been argued that information about risk factors can be obtained during the initial interview (health history interview). Many opportunities are available to the nurse for conducting the risk assessment. When a

Text continued on page 185

Table 16-16. SITE-SPECIFIC RISK FACTORS FOR CANCER

Anatomic Location	Risk Factors	Discussion	Actions to Reduce Risk	Early Signs and Symptoms
Lung	Cigarette smoking	*Cigarette smoking:* Estimated to cause 85% of lung cancer. People who smoke 2 or more packs/day have a death rate 15 to 20 times greater than that of nonsmokers.	Stop smoking or do not start smoking.	1. Cough—at first nonproductive, with time productive 2. Discomfort in chest 3. Rust streaked or purulent sputum 4. Hemoptysis 5. Pneumonitis that persists longer than 2 weeks despite antibiotic therapy 6. Dyspnea 7. Hoarseness 8. Loss of weight
	Male	Male to female ratio is now 3:1. Data suggest cigarette smoking will become number one cancer killer of American women in 1980s.[1]		
	Black male	Black males have highest incidence rates in U.S.		
	Asbestos	Exposure to airborne asbestos is largest cancer threat in workplace. Mesothelioma (cancer of lining of chest cavity) is due to exposure to asbestos. Risk increases if worker smokes.	Follow government guidelines for reducing asbestos exposures in occupational setting. Do not smoke. Follow government guidelines for recommended medical surveillance. (A)	
	Occupational exposure to arsenic, chromium, nickel, ionizing radiation, chloromethyl ethers, coal products, mustard gas, vinyl chloride	Uranium miners and hard rock miners have elevated risks of lung cancer due to inhalation of radon daughters.[2] Copper smelter workers and welders have increased risk of lung cancer.[3]	Follow government guidelines for reducing exposures to high-risk materials in the workplace setting and guidelines for recommended medical surveillance. (B)	
	Passive smoking		Avoid environments that are smoked filled. Participate in political action to legislate smoke-free environments.	
Colon and Rectum	Older than 40 years of age	Twofold increase in each decade, peaks at age 75.		*Right colonic lesions:* anemia, gastrointestinal tract bleeding, vague pain characterized as dull and annoying, weight loss, and anorexia.
	Associated diseases: ulcerative colitis	Dysplastic mucosal changes in the colon occur with ulcerative colitis.[4] Colorectal risk is 5 to 11 times higher than that of an individual who does not have the disease.	Medical surveillance following American Cancer Society's (ACS) guidelines for high-risk individuals. See Table 16–11.	*Left colonic lesions:* change in bowel habits and increased use of laxatives, decrease in caliber of stools, bright red blood coating surface of stools, "gas" pain.
	Crohn's disease (granulomatous colitis)		Medical surveillance following ACS guidelines for high-risk individuals. See Table 16–11.	*Rectal tumors:* gross blood per rectum, tenesmus, sense of incomplete evacuation, change in bowel habits. Rectal pain is late manifestation.
	Family syndromes: Familial polyposis syndrome (adenomatous polyps)	Autosomal dominant condition, most frequent genetic polyposis disorder. If colon not removed, can develop colon cancer from 20 years of age on. Death from colon cancer approaches 100% by age 55.	Medical surveillance following ACS guidelines for high-risk individuals. See Table 16–11.	*Sigmoid lesions:* gross blood per rectum.
	Family syndromes: Peutz-Jeghers syndrome[5]	Autosomal dominant condition with gastrointestinal polyps and mucocutaneous pigmentation.	Medical surveillance following ACS guidelines for high-risk individuals. See Table 16–11.	
	Family syndromes: Turcot's syndrome	Autosomal dominant condition with gastrointestinal polyps. Tumors of the central nervous system with adenomatous and villous colonic polyps.	Medical surveillance following ACS guidelines for high-risk individuals. See Table 16–11.	
	Family syndromes: Gardner's syndrome[6]	Polyposis syndrome. Multiple polyposis with soft tissue and bone tumors.	Medical surveillance following ACS guidelines for high-risk individuals. See Table 16–11.	
	Colorectal adenomas		Removal of polyps.	
	Previous history of colorectal cancer		Medical surveillance following ACS guidelines for high-risk individuals. See Table 16–11.	
	Family history of colorectal cancer	Family members have risk 3 to 4 times general population.		
	Female genital cancer or breast cancer			
	Cancer family syndrome	High frequency of colon cancer, often at multiple sites.	Medical surveillance following ACS guidelines for high-risk individuals. See Table 16–11.	
	High dietary intake of fats	Diets high in fruits and vegetables appear to protect against colorectal cancers.	Reduce daily fat intake to 25% or less of total calories, increase fiber from grains, fruits, and vegetables to 20 to 30 g per day. See Table 16–13 for specific suggestions.	

Table 16–16. SITE-SPECIFIC RISK FACTORS FOR CANCER *Continued*

Anatomic Location	Risk Factors	Discussion	Actions to Reduce Risk	Early Signs and Symptoms
Oral	Oral use of tobacco, finely powdered as snuff, leaf form for chewing	Major risk factor in development of oral cancers. Estimated 22 million users in the United States, many of whom are young. Epidemiologic data from India found use of chewing tobacco (mixed with nut of the betel palm, betel leaf, and slaked lime) was major etiologic factor in high incidence of oral cancer. Constitutes around 20% of all cancers in India, and India has highest rates of mouth and throat cancers in the world.[7]	Stop chewing tobacco or do not start.	Painless ulcer, induration of oral mucosa; white spot or bright red area in mouth; a "sore" in mouth or on lips, foul breath; swelling in the mouth; difficulty chewing, swallowing, or speaking.
	Male	Ratio of male to female is 4:1. No major change in incidence of head and neck cancer over past three decades in either male or female population.[8]		
	Older than 40 years Cigarette and pipe smoking	Pipe smokers tend to develop lip cancers, whereas cigarette smokers develop throat cancers. Heavy smokers (more than 1 pack/day) have sixfold increase in risk of oral cancers over nonsmokers.[9]	Do not start smoking cigarettes or pipes: stop both habits.	
	Heavy alcohol consumption and heavy smoking	Smoking and drinking have a synergistic effect. Individuals who drink at least 1.5 oz of alcohol and smoke 40 or more cigarettes/day have fifteenfold increase in risk of oral and throat cancer. Estimated that 75% of cancers of mouth and pharynx in U.S. men due to tobacco and alcohol use.	Moderate intake of alcohol and smoking cessation. Moderate alcohol intake is two or fewer drinks a day.	
	Chronic irritation from broken or decayed teeth	May lead to premalignant lesions from constant irritation.	Daily dental hygiene and repair of broken or decayed teeth.	
	Long-term exposure to the sun for lip cancer found in farmers, ranchers, sailors		Use of sun-screen products on lips and face of individuals who are constantly exposed to the sun.	
	Premalignant lesions: leukoplakia, erythroplakia, erythroleukoplakia		Dental referral and treatment, usually removal of the lesion.	
	General dietary deficiencies	May relate to heavy use of alcohol and smoking in individuals with oral cancer and resultant malnutrition found in alcohol abusers.		
Liver	Infection by hepatitis B-virus followed by chronic carrier state	Major determinant of hepatocellular carcinoma. In China, South East Asia, and Africa high rate of infection with virus and incidence of primary liver cancer.	Immunization with hepatitis B vaccines. Recommend vaccine for high-risk groups in the United States: health care personnel, dialysis patients, drug addicts, homosexuals, and contacts with acute cases.[10]	Weakness, anorexia, weight loss, anemia, pain in right hypochondrium or epigastrium, abdominal fullness or bloating, nausea, vomiting, epigastric fullness. Late signs and symptoms are palpable tender liver with nodules, ascites, edema, jaundice, signs and symptoms of portal hypertension.
	Alcohol consumption	Alcohol use is linked with cirrhosis, and cirrhosis is linked with liver cancer. Sixty to 90% of liver cancer occurs in association with cirrhosis.	Moderate to light use of alcohol. Moderate alcohol use is two or fewer drinks a day.	
	Exposure to arsenic, anabolic steroids, thorium oxide (Thorotrast), and vinyl chloride associated with hepatic angiosarcomas	Thorium oxide (Thorotrast) not used now as contrast agent in diagnostic imaging: vinyl chloride occupational exposure is federally controlled now that carcinogenic potential of vinyl chloride is known.		
	Diet of grain or peanuts contaminated with aflatoxins	Infection of food supply with aflatoxins is factor in Africa and Asia, but in the United States the Food and Drug Administration controls the amount of this potent carcinogen allowed in peanut butter.	Improved food handling and storage in Third World countries will reduce incidence of primary liver cancer.	
	Uncooked infected fish	Cholangiocellular carcinoma associated with clonorchiasis occurs when infected fish is eaten raw.	Avoidance of raw fish, e.g., sushi.	
	Oral contraceptives		A contraindication for taking oral contraceptives is known liver disease or abnormal liver function.	

Table continued on following page

Table 16—16. SITE-SPECIFIC RISK FACTORS FOR CANCER *Continued*

Anatomic Location	Risk Factors	Discussion	Actions to Reduce Risk	Early Signs and Symptoms

Prostate	Black male	Highest-incidence group in the world: incidence and mortality among black males are almost twice those of whites.[11]		1. Small asymptomatic nodule on rectal examination
				  a. firm or stony consistency
				  b. earliest palpable change
				  c. probability of being neoplastic in about 50% of cases
				2. Frequency of urination—common symptom
				3. Nocturia—common symptom
				4. Difficulty starting stream
				5. Dysuria
				6. Hematuria
				7. Urinary retention

	Increased numbers of sexual partners and high frequency of previous venereal disease	These risk factors are controversial.[12]		
	Men older than 65 years of age	Average age of prostate cancer patient is 73 years of age.		
	May be associated with dietary fat intake. Cancer of the prostate has been linked with the consumption of animal fat and protein among several ethnic groups in Hawaii.[13]		See recommendations for reducing fat in diet (Table 16–13).	
Testis	Atrophic cryptorchid testes (undescended testes)	Twelve per cent of all testicular neoplasms arise in cryptorchid testes: risk of cancer is increased about fourteenfold with maldescent of the testicle.	Instruction of testicular self-examination (TSE). See Figure 16–2 for TSE instructions.	1. Painless, hard, freely movable mass that is either smooth or uneven in the scrotum 2. History of trauma in scrotum 3. Gynecomastia and pigmentation of nipples (choriocarcinoma) 4. Hydrocele 5. Heaviness in scrotum, lower abdomen, and groin 6. Sensation of discomfort and increase in testicular sensitivity 7. Painless swelling 8. Dull ache in scrotum
	Rare genetic abnormalities associated with testicular cancer	Klinefelter's syndrome, hermaphroditism, Turner's syndrome, gonadal aplasia, hypospadias.		
	Men aged 20 to 34			
	Literature reports increased maternal weight immediately before the index pregnancy associated with an increasing risk of cancer of the testis.[14] This is an obscure risk factor.			
	Hormone administration, stilbestrol, and other estrogens during the first trimester of pregnancy found to be associated with an increased risk of cancer.[15]			
Bladder	Cigarette smoking	Bladder cancer occurs 2 to 3 times more often in smokers than in nonsmokers. Smoking is estimated to be responsible for about 40% of bladder cancers in men and 29% in women. Considered the most important known risk factor.	Smoking cessation	1. Hematuria is the most common presenting symptom that may occur intermittently or persist throughout the entire voiding. 2. Bladder irritability—frequency, urgency, dysuria 3. Difficulty in urination 4. Persistent lower urinary tract infection
	Male to female ratio is 3:1.			
	Infection with schistosomiasis, a parasitic disease that is common in Third World countries.[16]			
	Individuals employed in the dyestuffs, rubber, and leather industries. Also painters, chemical workers, printers, metal workers, hairdressers, textile workers, mechanics, and truck drivers.	Workers in dyestuff industry are exposed to aromatic amines; chemicals of this class are potent bladder carcinogens.		
Skin Cancer (nonmelanoma)	Caucasians who are fair skinned, red-headed with freckles, and live in sunny climates			
	Long-term exposure to nonionizing ultraviolet radiation	Need to avoid unnecessary ultraviolet light exposure from artificial sources, such as sunlamps and tanning booths. Ultraviolet radiation emitted by tanning beds can cause sunburn, premature aging of skin, and adds to total amount of ultraviolet radiation individual receives in lifetime.	Use of sunscreens (sun protection factor of 15 or greater and sunscreen that blocks both ultraviolet A and ultraviolet B) when in the sun: avoidance of excessive amounts of sun.	
	Ultraviolet radiation			
	Arsenical drugs applied to the skin	Medicines containing inorganic arsenic compounds have generally been abandoned in many countries.[17]	Use of arsenic compounds on the skin is not recommended.	
	Psoriasis patients treated with psoralens and ultraviolet radiation (PUVA)	Sufficient evidence from epidemiologic studies that PUVA therapy is carcinogenic in humans.		
	Premalignant lesions—actinic keratosis, arsenical keratosis, Bowen's disease, leukoplakia			

182

Table 16–16. SITE-SPECIFIC RISK FACTORS FOR CANCER *Continued*

Anatomic Location	Risk Factors	Discussion	Actions to Reduce Risk	Early Signs and Symptoms
	Genetic conditions—xeroderma pigmentosum, albinism, multiple basal cell carcinoma			
	Epidermodysplasia verruciformis—rare disorder in which papillomaviruses cause widespread skin lesions.[18]	Squamous cell cancer occurs more frequently in individuals with this disorder.		
	Occupations involving the following chemicals: arsenicals, pesticides, polycyclic aromatic hydrocarbons, coal tar and pitch, soot, liquid tar and paraffin, oils and petroleum		Follow recommended federal guidelines to reduce exposure to the skin. (B)	
	Ionizing radiation used in medical and dental procedures	This risk has decreased substantially among health professionals and occupations involving ionizing radiation because of the reduced exposures, decreased radiation doses, and knowledge of relationship between skin cancer and radiation.		
Melanoma	Caucasians with light-colored eyes and light complexions who are easily burned		Use of sunscreen (sun protection factor of 15 or greater) when in the sun, avoidance of excessive amounts of sun, keep skin covered when out in the sun, avoidance of sun from around 11 A.M. to 2 P.M. Use sunscreen that blocks out both ultraviolet A and ultraviolet B.	
	Genetic condition: xeroderma pigmentosum		Same risk-reducing actions as under Caucasians.	
	People who had severe sunburns, especially in childhood through their early teens to twenties.[19]		Same risk-reducing actions as under Caucasians.	
	Living near the equator		Same risk-reducing actions as under Caucasians.	
	Family history of melanoma		Same risk-reducing actions as under Caucasians.	
	People who work outdoors or are habitually in the sun			
	Precursor lesions: dysplastic nevus and congenital melanocytic nevus	Dysplastic nevi may be familial or sporadic and may be an autosomal dominant trait. Overall, people with dysplastic nevi have a lifetime risk for malignant melanoma of 5 to 10% compared with a risk of about 0.7% for the general population.[20] Dysplastic nevi have irregular outlines: may contain variations of tan, brown, red, and black: and are usually larger than common nevi, from 6 mm to 15 mm.	Follow-up and monitoring by physician every 6 months or more; high-risk patients shown skin self-assessment techniques and told to monitor themselves closely during pregnancy and puberty (hormonal changes); report all changing lesions as soon as possible. (C)	

(A) *Asbestos Exposure: What It Means, What to Do.* National Cancer Institute Publication #89–1594. Office of Cancer Communications, Building 31, Room 10A24, Bethesda, MD 20892.

(B) U.S. Department of Labor, Occupational Safety and Health Administration, Washington, DC: booklets on health hazards of materials in the workplace and protective measures employers and employees can take. Examples of booklets are *Health Hazards of Chromate Pigments and Paints: Hexavalent Chromium* and *Health Hazards of Inorganic Arsenic.*

(C) Excellent patient education materials on skin self-inspection and monitoring dysplastic nevi are *About Dysplastic Nevi,* National Cancer Institute, Office of Cancer Communications, Bethesda, MD 20892: Josten, D., *Guidelines for Families with Dysplastic Nevus Syndrome,* Cancer Prevention Program, Wisconsin Clinical Cancer Center, 1300 University Avenue—7C, Medical Science Center, Madison, WI 53706: Lawler, P. (1989). Be sun sensible: Steps toward safety in the sun. *Oncology Nursing Forum, 16,* 424–427.

[1] Weinhouse, 1986: Jett, Cortese, & Fontana, 1983.
[2] Ouslander & Beck, 1982.
[3] Stern, 1987.
[4] Lynch & Krush, 1971.
[5] Fenoglio-Preiser & Hutter, 1985.
[6] Stromborg, Krafka, Gale, & Porter, 1986.
[7] Spitz, 1983.
[8] Meisner, 1983.
[9] Ouslander & Beck, 1982.
[10] Senie, 1986.
[11] Huben & Murphy, 1986.
[12] Palmer, 1986.
[13] Ouslander & Beck, 1982.
[14] Perez, Fair, Ihde, & Labrie, 1985.
[15] Perez, Fair, Ihde, & Labrie, 1985.
[16] Gray, 1985.
[17] Silverberg & Lubera, 1987.
[18] Kleinberg, 1987.
[19] Finley, 1986.
[20] Friedman, Rigel, & Kopf, 1985.

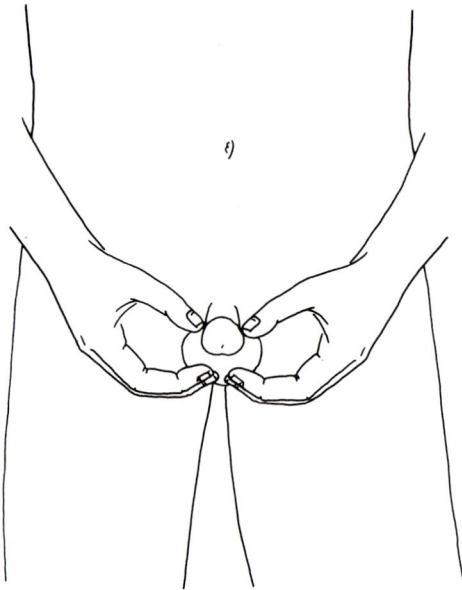

How to examine your testes

The best time to examine your testes is right after a hot bath or shower. The heat causes the testicle to descend and the scrotal skin to relax, making it easier to find anything unusual.

Each testicle should be examined with the fingers of both hands. Place your index and middle fingers on the underside of the testicle and your thumb on the top. Gently roll your testicle between your thumb and fingers, feeling for a small lump. If you do find anything abnormal, chances are it will be at the front or side of your testicle.

It's that simple. The next time you take a shower or bath, do TSE. Then make it a regular health habit. It's no bother—and it could save your life. If you do find anything unusual, see your doctor without delay.

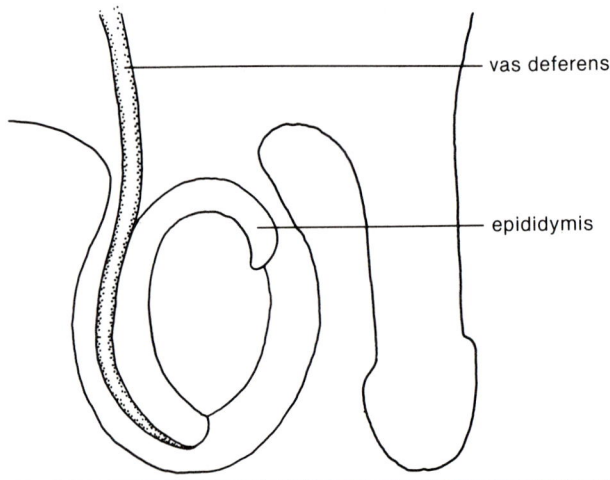

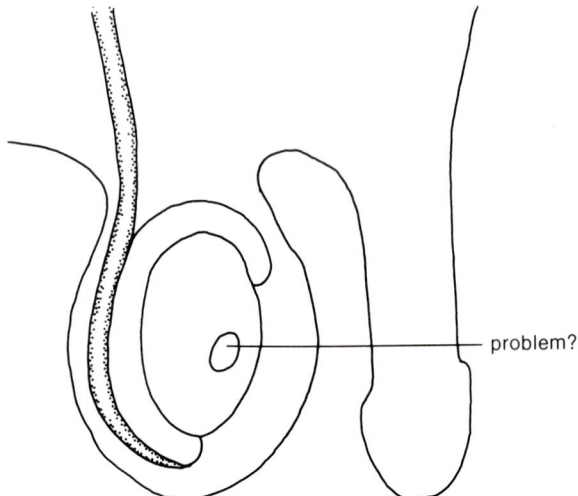

vas deferens

epididymis

If you have a teenage son, pass this pamphlet on to him. Get him started early on the good health habit of TSE.

problem?

Figure 16–2. How to examine your testes. (From American Cancer Society, Iowa Division, Inc., West Des Moines, IA 50265-0710. Reproduced by permission.)

patient is hospitalized, the risk assessment can be done over time rather than in one session. Risk assessments can also be obtained over a series of appointments for patients in ambulatory care settings. It is also possible to combine self-administered questionnaires with an interview to follow up on positive risk factors or suspicious signs and symptoms. Many settings are experimenting with the use of computers with user-friendly programs that enable clients who can read to enter directly their own risk information into the computer.

Taking the time to query a client about risk factors for cancer serves multiple purposes. It establishes baseline data on cancer risks that can then be monitored for changes; it generates a problem list; and it allows for plans and follow-up to be designed. The risk assessment information frequently provides an educational opportunity for the nurse to explore the individual's knowledge about risk factors in general and personal risk factors in particular. Although it is acknowledged that many risk factors are beyond the individual's control, this chapter has shown clearly that life-style practices, which are under a person's control, are responsible for the majority of cancers. Obtaining a risk profile enables the nurse to design a care plan that includes primary and secondary prevention activities that are tailored to the individual. A rational program of primary prevention requires knowledge of the causes, risk factors, or antecedents of the disease (Shannugaratnam, 1985). A thorough history may reveal long-forgotten or ignored risk factors. As previously pointed out, individuals cannot attempt to control occupational, environmental, and life-style risks if they are unaware of them. The effort expended to identify the major risk factors for cancer is the first step in successfully managing those risks.

After obtaining the risk-oriented health histories, the nurse should inform individuals about their cancer-related risks, provide informational resources, and counsel them about specific behavioral changes that they can make to modify the cancer risks (Sternberg, 1983). The general goal of cancer education should be to provide information to the individual about cancer risks, to teach skills to prevent cancer, and to communicate an attitude to actively fight cancer. Identification of cancer risks also enables the nurse to involve the person in setting goals for risk modification.

It is not practical to obtain a complete occupational history in every risk assessment interview. In clients for whom the nurse does *not* suspect an occupational disease, a brief statement concerning current job titles, job tasks, and employer may be sufficient. Medical records should routinely contain the two occupations persons have held the longest and the materials with which they worked or to which they were exposed in these occupations. If there is any indication that the problem may be work related, a complete occupational history should be taken (Levy & Wegman, 1981).

Physical problems that should raise a suspicion that occupational factors may be a factor in disease are respiratory disease, skin disorders, hearing impairment, and back and joint symptoms. If there is doubt about the advisability of obtaining a complete occupational history, the nurse is encouraged to confer with the physician or other key members of the health team. A *complete* occupational history includes the following (Levy & Wegman, 1981, pp. 126–127):

1. Description of all jobs since completion of education, including summer and part-time jobs.
2. Exposures at work, including biologic, chemical, and physical exposures.
3. Timing of symptoms to help determine whether the symptoms are work related.
4. Nonwork exposure and other factors, such as smoking, alcohol, and hobbies.
5. Epidemiology of symptoms or illness among other workers.

When counseling individuals about risk factors, nurses must be aware that the nurse serves as a role model. Research has documented that the public perceives health professionals to be role models and is influenced by the behaviors they observe in health professionals. A study at Johns Hopkins University Hospital found that the attitudes of some nurses may indirectly encourage patients to smoke ("Nurses' Smoking Habits," 1987). A University of Minnesota survey showed that people feel safer about smoking when they see health professionals smoke.

It is vital that the purpose of a risk assessment not be forgotten. It is *not* designed to generate paperwork or be another "task" assigned to nursing. The risk assessment is for the specific purposes of constructing a database and planning interventions with the client that are designed to reduce the identified risks of cancer. Another very important purpose of risk assessments is in terms of case finding. *Case finding* is the identification of individuals at higher than average risk for cancer who would profit from interventions (formal or informal) to change risk behavior, learn self-examination skills, and participate in early cancer detection programs (Van Parijs & Eckhardt, 1984). Whether it is a computer printout or a hand-checked list, the cancer risk profile provides the nurse and other health care professionals with valuable data for teaching clients about their cancer risk factors (White, 1986).

It can also be an effective patient motivator; it may help the individual make personal health choices that will minimize his risk of cancer, and it may encourage individuals to perform self-examinations (Fig. 16–2) and have cancer screening checkups to detect any early signs of cancer, especially when the risk factors are outside the individual's control.

References

Abbott, R., Yin, Y., Reed, D., & Yano, K. (1986). Risk of stroke in male cigarette smokers. *New England Journal of Medicine, 315,* 717–720.

American Cancer Society. (1985). *Cancer management network. Breast cancer module.* Boston: American Cancer Society, Massachusetts Division, Inc.

Anderson, D. (1975). Familial susceptibility. In J. Fraumeni (Ed.), *Persons at high risk of cancer. An approach to cancer etiology and control* (pp. 39–54). New York: Academic Press.

Ash, C., Oberst, M., Stalker, M., Park, D., Avellanet, C., & Glasel, M. (1982). *Cancer prevention. A course for nurse practitioners.* New York: Memorial Sloan-Kettering Cancer Center, Division of Nursing.

Baeck, M. L., & Eisenberg, M. (1985). Carcinogenic risk assessment: Concepts and issues. *Maryland Medical Journal, 34,* 672–674.

Barber, H. (1986). Ovarian cancer. *CA: A Cancer Journal for Clinicians, 36,* 149–183.

Benedict, W. (1987). Hereditary factors. Human cancer susceptibility genes. *Proceedings of the Second National Conference on Cancer Prevention and Detection.* New York: American Cancer Society.

Berg, J. (1984). Clinical implications of risk factors for breast cancer. *Cancer, 53,* 589–591.

Birdsell, J. (1986). Cancer in the aged. In D. Welch-McCaffrey (Ed.), *Nursing considerations in geriatric oncology.* Columbus, OH: Adria Laboratories.

Borden, E., Steeves, R., & Hogan, T. (1983). Infectious carcinogenesis: Viruses and human neoplasia. In S. B. Kahn, R. Love, C. Sherman, & R. Chakravorty (Eds.), *Concepts in cancer medicine* (pp. 89–100). New York: Grune & Stratton, Inc.

Bryan, G. (1983). Chemical carcinogenesis in human subjects. In S. B. Kahn, R. Love, C. Sherman, & R. Chakravorty (Eds.), *Concepts in cancer medicine* (pp. 45–66). New York: Grune & Stratton, Inc.

Buck, C., & Donner, A. (1987). Cancer incidence in hypertensives. *Cancer, 59,* 1386–1390.

Bulbrook, R. D., Hayward, J. L., Wang, D. Y., Thomas, B., Clark, G., Allen, D., & Moore, J. (1986). Identification of women at high risk of breast cancer. *Breast Cancer Research and Treatment, 7*(Suppl.), 7–10.

Burack, R. C., & Drelichman, A. (1982). *Risk assessment through the patient interview: A model emphasizing cancer prevention (Module IX).* Detroit: Wayne State University School of Nursing.

Cady, B., Macdonald, J., & Gunderson, L. (1985). Cancer of the hepatobiliary system. In V. DeVita, S. Hellman, & S. Rosenberg (Eds.), *Cancer. Principles and practice of oncology* (2nd ed., pp. 741–770). Philadelphia: J. B. Lippincott Co.

Cancer and Steroid Hormone Study. Centers for Disease Control, Atlanta, and the National Institute of Child Health and Human Development, Bethesda, MD. (1986). Oral-contraceptive use and the risk of breast cancer. *New England Journal of Medicine, 315,* 405–411.

Cancer and Steroid Hormone Study of the Centers for Disease Control and the National Institute of Child Health and Human Development. (1987). The reduction in risk of ovarian cancer associated with oral-contraceptive use, *New England Journal of Medicine, 316,* 650–655.

Cancer Facts and Figures, 1990. (1990). Atlanta: American Cancer Society.

Cancer Facts and Figures for Minority Americans, 1986. (1986). New York: American Cancer Society.

Carbone, P. (1983). Breast cancer. In S. B. Kahn, R. Love, C. Sherman, & R. Chakravorty (Eds.), *Concepts in cancer medicine* (pp. 401–416). New York: Grune & Stratton, Inc.

Carroll, K., Braden, L., Bell, J., & Kalamegham, R. (1986). Fat and cancer. *Cancer, 58,* 1818–1825.

Clemmesen, J. (1987). Parameters for identification of high-risk groups. In H. Nieburgs (Ed.), *Prevention and detection of cancer. Part I. Prevention. Vol. 2. Etiology* (pp. 1513–1516). New York: Marcel Dekker, Inc.

Clifton, K. (1983). Ionizing radiation carcinogenesis in man. In S. B. Kahn, R. Love, C. Sherman, & R. Chakravorty (Eds.), *Concepts in cancer medicine* (pp. 67–88). New York: Grune & Stratton, Inc.

Cole, P., & Goldman, M. (1975). Occupation. In J. Fraumeni (Ed.), *Persons at high risk of cancer. An approach to cancer etiology and control* (pp. 167–184). New York: Academic Press.

Cook-Mozaffari, P. (1985). The geography of cancer. In M. P. Vessey & M. Gray (Eds.), *Cancer risks and prevention* (pp. 15–43). Oxford: Oxford University Press.

Costanza, M., Frederick, L., Green, H., & Patterson, W. B. (1986). Cancer prevention and detection. Strategies for practice. In *Cancer manual* (7th ed. pp. 14–35). Boston: American Cancer Society, Massachusetts Division, Inc.

Creasey, W. (1985). *Diet and cancer.* Philadelphia: Lea & Febiger.

Crump, K., & Guess, H. (1986). Drinking water and cancer. Review of recent epidemiological findings and assessment of risks. *Annual Review of Public Health, 7,* 339–357.

"The Dark Side of Cancer." (1986, June 9). *Newsweek,* pp. 60–64.

Davies, J. N. P. (1975). Overview: Geographic opportunities and demographic leads. In J. Fraumeni (Ed.), *Persons at high risk of cancer. An approach to cancer etiology and control* (pp. 373–381). New York: Academic Press.

DeCosse, J. (1988). Early cancer detection. Colorectal cancer. *Cancer, 62,* 1787–1790.

DeVita, V. (1985). Cancer as a preventable disease. *Maryland Medical Journal, 34,* 41–43.

Dunn, L. (1981). Endometrial cancer increasing but highly curable. *Diagnosis, 3,* 39–50.

Earhart, R. (1983). Cancer of the ovary. In S. B. Kahn, R. Love, C. Sherman, & R. Chakravorty (Eds.), *Concepts in cancer medicine* (pp 483–491). New York: Grune & Stratton, Inc.

Enstrom, J., & Kanim, L. (1983). Populations at low risk. In G. Newell (Ed.), *Cancer prevention in clinical medicine* (pp. 49–78). New York: Raven Press.

Ernster, V. (1987). Trends in tobacco use and cancer risk. *Proceedings of the Second National Conference on Cancer Prevention and Detection.* New York: American Cancer Society.

Faulkenberry, J. (1983). Cancer prevention and detection: Risk assessment. The medical history. *Cancer Nursing, 7,* 388–401.

Fenoglio-Preiser, C., & Hutter, R. (1985). Colorectal polyps: Pathologic diagnosis and clinical significance. *CA: A Cancer Journal for Clinicians, 35,* 322–344.

Fielding, J. (1985). Smoking: Health effects and control. *New England Journal of Medicine, 313,* 491–498.

Finley, C. (1986). Malignant melanoma: A primary care perspective. *Nurse Practitioner, 1,* 18–38.

Fraumeni, J. (1975a). Epidemiologic approaches to cancer etiology. In J. Fraumeni (Ed.), *Persons at high risk of cancer. An approach to cancer etiology and control* (pp. 85–100). New York: Academic Press.

Fraumeni, J. (1975b). Preface. In J. Fraumeni (Ed.), *Persons at high risk of cancer. An approach to cancer etiology and control* (p. xvi). New York: Academic Press.

Fraumeni, J. (1982). Epidemiological approaches to cancer etiology. In L. Breslow, J. Fielding, & L. Lave (Eds.), *Annual Review of Public Health, 3,* 85–100.

Friedman, R., Rigel, K., & Kopf, F. (1985). Early detection of malignant melanoma: The role of physician examination and self-examination of the skin. *CA: A Cancer Journal For Clinicians, 35,* 130–151.

Gray, N. (1985). Cancer risks and cancer prevention in the third world. In M. P. Vessey & M. Gray (Eds.), *Cancer risks and prevention* (pp. 269–299). Oxford: Oxford University Press.

Greenwald, P. (1985). Diet and cancer prevention. *Maryland Medical Journal, 34,* 44–49.

Greenwald, P., & Sondik, E. (Eds.). (1986). *Cancer control objectives for the nation: 1985–2000.* (NIH Publication No. 86-2880). Washington, DC: U.S. Government Printing Office.

Greenwald, P., Sondik, E., & Lynch, B. (1986). Diet and chemoprevention in NCI's research strategy to achieve national cancer control objectives. *Annual Review of Public Health, 7,* 267–291.

Grossarth-Maticek, R., Frentzel-Beyme, R., & Becker, N. (1984). Cancer risks associated with life events and conflict solution. *Cancer Detection and Prevention, 7,* 201–209.

Harris, J., Hellman, S., Canellos, G., & Fisher, B. (1985). Cancer of the breast. In V. DeVita, S. Hellman, & S. Rosenberg (Eds.), *Cancer. Principles and practice of oncology* (2nd ed., pp. 1119–1178). Philadelphia: J. B. Lippincott Co.

Haynes, H., Mead, K., & Goldwyn, R. (1985). Cancers of the skin. In V. DeVita, S. Hellman, & S. Rosenberg (Eds.), *Cancer. Principles and practice of oncology* (2nd ed., pp. 1343–1370). Philadelphia: J. B. Lippincott Co.

Healthfinder. (1985). National Health Information Clearinghouse. Office of Disease Prevention and Health Promotion. Washington, DC: US Department of Health and Human Services.

Hendershot, G. (1983). Coitus-related cervical cancer risk factors: Trends and differentials in racial and religious groups. *American Journal of Public Health, 73,* 299–301.

Henderson, B., Gerkins, V., & Pike, M. (1975). Sexual factors and pregnancy. In J. Fraumeni (Ed.), *Persons at high risk of cancer. An approach to cancer etiology and control* (p. xx). New York: Academic Press.

Hennekens, C., Mayrent, S., & Willett, W. (1986). Vitamin A, carotenoids, and retinoids. *Cancer, 58*, 1837–1841.

Hirschman, R., & Leventhal, H. (1983). The behavioral science of cancer prevention. In S. B. Kahn, R. Love, C. Sherman, & R. Chakravorty (Eds.), *Concepts in cancer medicine* (pp. 229–240). New York: Grune & Stratton, Inc.

Hoover, R., & Fraumeni, J. (1975). Drugs. In J. Fraumeni (Ed.), *Persons at high risk of cancer. An approach to cancer etiology and control* (pp. 185–199). New York: Academic Press.

Houk, V. (1982). Determining the impacts on human health attributable to hazardous waste sites. In F. Long & G. Schweitzer (Eds.), *Risk assessment at hazardous waste sites* (pp. 21–31). Washington, DC: American Chemical Society.

Huben, R., & Murphy, G. (1986). Prostate cancer: An update. *CA: A Cancer Journal for Clinicians, 36*, 274–292.

Humble, C., Samet, J., & Pathak, D. (1987). Marriage to a smoker and lung cancer risk. *American Journal of Public Health, 77*, 598–602.

Jablon, S. (1975). Radiation. In J. Fraumeni (Ed.), *Persons at high risk of cancer. An approach to cancer etiology and control* (pp. 151–165). New York: Academic Press.

Jett, J., Cortese, D., & Fontana, R. (1983). Lung cancer: Current concepts and prospects. *CA: A Cancer Journal for Clinicians, 33*, 74–97.

Kennaway, E. L. (1944). Cancer of the liver in the Negro in Africa and America. *Cancer Research, 4*, 571.

Kersey, J., & Spector, B. (1975). Immune deficiency disease. In J. Fraumeni (Ed.), *Persons at high risk of cancer. An approach to cancer etiology and control* (pp. 55–67). New York: Academic Press.

Kewenter, J., Bjork, S., Haglind, E., Smith, L., Svanik, J., & Ahren, C. (1988). Screening and rescreening for colorectal cancer. A controlled trial of fecal occult blood testing in 27,700 subjects. *Cancer, 62*, 645–651.

Kinlen, L. J. (1985). Infections and immune impairment. In M. P. Vessey & M. Gray (Eds.), *Cancer risks and prevention* (pp. 149–165). Oxford: Oxford University Press.

Kleinberg, D. (1987). Prolactin and breast cancer. *New England Journal of Medicine, 316*, 269–270.

Knight, K., Fiedling, J., & Battista, R. (1989). Occult blood screening for colorectal cancer. *Journal of the American Medical Association, 261*, 587–593.

Koss, L. (1975). Precancerous lesions. In J. Fraumeni (Ed.), *Persons at high risk of cancer. An approach to cancer etiology and control* (pp. 85–102). New York: Academic Press.

Kritchevsky, D. (1986). Diet, nutrition, and cancer. *Cancer, 58*, 1830–1836.

Levy, B., & Wegman, D. (1981). Environmental and occupational hazards. In L. Schneiderman (Ed.), *The practice of preventive health care* (pp. 124–155). Menlo Park, CA: Addison-Wesley Publishing Co., Inc.

Levy, S., Herberman, R., Maluish, A., Schlien, B., & Lippman, M. (1985). Prognostic risk assessment in primary breast cancer by behavioral and immunological parameters. *Health Psychology, 4*, 99–113.

Lewison, E. (1978). Use of hormones and human tumorigenesis. In H. Nieburgs (Ed.), *Prevention and detection of cancer. Part I. Prevention. Vol. 1. Etiology* (pp. 609–616). New York: Marcel Dekker, Inc.

Longman, S., & Buehring, G (1987). Oral contraceptives and breast cancer. *Cancer, 59*, 281–287.

Love, R. (1987). The risk of breast cancer in American women. *Journal of the American Medical Association, 257*, 1470.

Lovejoy, N. (1987). Precancerous lesions of the cervix. Personal risk factors. *Cancer Nursing, 10*, 2–14.

Lynch, H. & Krush, A. (1971). Cancer family "G" revisited: 1895–1970. *Cancer, 27*, 1505–1511.

Lynch, H., & Lynch, P. (1978). Constitutional factors and endometrial carcinoma. In H. Nieburgs (Ed.), *Prevention and detection of cancer. Part I. Prevention. Vol. 2. Etiology* (pp. 2105–2117). New York: Marcel Dekker, Inc.

Lynch, P., Lynch, H., Harris, R., Lynch, J., & Guirgis, H. (1978).

Heritable colon cancer and solitary adenomatous polyps. In H. Nieburgs (Ed.), *Prevention and detection of cancer. Part I. Prevention. Vol. 2. Etiology* (pp. 1573–1589). New York: Marcel Dekker, Inc.

Matheny, R., & Symmonds, R. (1986). The incidence of colon carcinoma complicating ulcerative colitis. *Surgical Clinics of North America, 66*, 801–806.

Matsukura, S., Taminato, T., Kitano, N., Seino, Y., Hamada, H., Uchihashi, M., Nakajima, H., & Hirata, Y. (1984). Effects of environmental tobacco smoke on urinary cotinine excretion in nonsmokers. *New England Journal of Medicine, 311*, 828–832.

Meadows, A., & Li, F. (1983). The practicing etiologist. In G. Newell (Ed.), *Cancer prevention in clinical medicine* (pp. 19–32). New York: Raven Press.

Meisner, L. (1983). Genetic factors in human cancer. In S. B. Kahn, R. Love, C. Sherman, & R. Chakravorty (Eds.), *Concepts in cancer medicine* (pp. 165–176). New York: Grune & Stratton, Inc.

Million, R., Cassisi, N., & Wittes, R. (1985). In V. DeVita, S. Hellman, & S. Rosenberg (Eds.), *Cancer. Principles and practice of oncology* (2nd ed., pp. 407–506). Philadelphia: J. B. Lippincott Co.

Muir, C. S. (1986). Value of a multinational approach in determining the causation of cancer. *Yale Journal of Biology and Medicine, 59*, 485–496.

Mulvihill, J. (1975). Congenital and genetic diseases. In J. Fraumeni (Ed.), *Persons at high risk of cancer. An approach to cancer etiology and control* (pp. 3–37). New York: Academic Press.

National Cancer Institute. (1986). *Cancer among blacks and other minorities: Statistical profile* (NIH Publication No. 86-2785). Washington, DC: U.S. Government Printing Office.

Newell, G. (1985). Epidemiology of cancer. In V. DeVita, S. Hellman, & S. Rosenberg (Eds.), *Cancer. Principles and practice of oncology* (2nd ed, pp. 151–182). Philadelphia: J. B. Lippincott Co.

Newell, G., & Vogel, V. (1987). Personal risk factors: what do they mean? *Proceedings of the Second National Conference on Cancer Prevention and Detection.* New York: American Cancer Society.

"Nurses' Smoking Habits and Attitudes Influence Patients." (1987). *Cancer Nursing Letter, 1*(12), 4–5.

Oettle, A. G. (1964). Cancer in Africa, especially in regions south of the Sahara. *Journal of the National Cancer Institute, 33*, 383–439.

Ouslander, J., & Beck, J. (1982). Defining the health problems of the elderly. In L. Breslow, J. Fielding, & L. Lave (Eds.), *Annual Review of Public Health, 3*, 55–84.

Page, H., & Asire, A. (1985). *Cancer rates and risks* (3rd ed.) (NIH Publication No. 85-691). Washington, DC: U.S. Government Printing Office.

Palmer, S. (1985). Diet, nutrition, and cancer. *Progress in Food and Nutrition, 9*, 283–341.

Palmer, S. (1986). Dietary considerations for risk reduction. *Cancer, 58*, 1949–1953.

Perez, C., Fair, W., Ihde, D., & Labrie, F. (1985). Cancer of the prostate. In V. DeVita, S. Hellman, & S. Rosenberg (Eds.), *Cancer. Principles and practice of oncology* (2nd ed., pp. 929–964). Philadelphia: J. B. Lippincott Co.

Pike, M., Gordon, R., Henderson, B., Menck, H., & Soo Hoo, J. (1975). Air pollution. In J. Fraumeni (Ed.), *Persons at high risk of cancer. An approach to cancer etiology and control* (pp. 225–239). New York: Academic Press.

Pike, M. C. (1985). Endogenous hormones. In M. P. Vessey & M. Gray (Eds.), *Cancer risks and prevention* (pp. 195–210). Oxford: Oxford University Press.

Pitot, H. (1983). Evaluation of the toxic and carcinogenic risk of environmental chemicals to human beings: Scientific, legal, and risk-benefit considerations. In S. B. Kahn, R. Love, C. Sherman, & R. Chakravorty (Eds.), *Concepts in cancer medicine* (pp. 101–118). New York: Grune & Stratton, Inc.

Pitot, H. (1985). Principles of cancer biology: Chemical carcinogenesis. In V. DeVita, S. Hellman, & S. Rosenberg (Eds.), *Cancer. Principles and practice of oncology* (2nd ed., pp. 79–112). Philadelphia: J. B. Lippincott Co.

Porter, I. (1982). Control of hereditary disorders. In L. Breslow, J.

Fielding, & L. Lave (Eds.), *Annual Review of Public Health, 3,* 277–319.

Rawson, R. (1978). Identification of tumor susceptibility of individuals at high risk for the development of cancer. In H. Nieburgs (Ed.), *Prevention and detection of cancer. Part I. Prevention. Vol. 2. Etiology* (pp. 1493–1512). New York: Marcel Dekker, Inc.

Report of the Task Force on Cancer and the Aged, Nursing Subcommittee. (1981). *Report on cancer and the aged.* Oakland, CA: American Cancer Society, California Division, Inc.

Richie, J., Shipley, W., & Yagoda, A. (1985). Cancer of the bladder. In V. DeVita, S. Hellman, & S. Rosenberg (Eds.), *Cancer. Principles and practice of oncology* (2nd ed., pp. 915–928). Philadelphia: J. B. Lippincott Co.

Rinsky, R., Smith, A., Hornung, R., Filloon, T., Young, R., Okun, A., & Landrigan, P. (1987). Benzene and leukemia. An epidemiologic risk assessment. *New England Journal of Medicine, 316,* 1044–1050.

Robbins, L. (1978). Evaluation of risk factors in cancer prevention. In H. Nieburgs (Ed.), *Prevention and detection of cancer. Part I. Prevention. Vol. 2. Etiology* (pp. 2099–2143). New York: Marcel Dekker, Inc.

Rodricks, J., & Tardiff, R. (1984). Conceptual basis for risk assessment. In J. Rodricks & R. Tardiff (Eds.), *Assessment and management of chemical risks* (pp. 1–12). ACS Symposium Series. Washington, DC: American Chemical Society.

Rose, D., Boyar, A., & Wynder, E. (1986). International comparisons of mortality rates for cancer of the breast, ovary, prostate, and colon, and per capita food consumption. *Cancer, 58,* 2363–2371.

Ross, C. (1981). Health hazard appraisal. In L. Schneiderman (Ed.), *The practice of preventive health care* (pp. 26–36). Menlo Park, CA: Addison-Wesley Publishing Co., Inc.

Rowe, W. (1986). Identification of risk. In A. Brigger (Ed.), *Risk and reason: Risk assessment in relation to environmental mutagens and carcinogens* (pp. 3–22). New York: Alan R. Liss.

Rubin, G., & Peterson, H. (1985). Researchers can now investigate long-term effects of OCs on cancer. *Contraceptive Technology Update, 6,* 7–12.

Sacks, J., Krushat, M., & Newman, J. (1980). Reliability of the health hazard appraisal. *American Journal of Public Health, 70,* 730–732.

Saracci, R. (1985). Occupation. In M. P. Vessey & M. Gray (Eds.), *Cancer risks and prevention* (pp. 99–118). Oxford: Oxford University Press.

Schlaff, W. B., & Rosenshein, N. B. (1985). Estrogens and endometrial cancer. *Maryland Medical Journal, 34,* 57–62.

Schneiderman, L. (1981). Screening, case finding and prevention. In L. Schneiderman (Ed.), *The practice of preventive health care* (pp. 1–25). Menlo Park, CA: Addison-Wesley Publishing Co., Inc.

Schoenbach, V. (1987). Appraising health risk appraisal. *American Journal of Public Health, 77,* 409–411.

Schottenfeld, D., & Haas, J. (1978). The workplace as a cause of cancer. *Clinical Bulletin, 8,* 54–60, 107–119.

Schulte, P., Ringen, K., Hemstreet, G., Altekruse, E. B., Gullen, W. H., Patton, M. G., Alsbrook, W. C., Jr., Crosby, J. H., West, S. S., & Witherington, R. (1985). Risk assessment of a cohort exposed to aromatic amines. *Journal of Occupational Medicine, 27,* 115–121.

Seidman, H., Lilis, R., & Selikoff, I. (1978). Short-term asbestos exposure and delayed cancer risk. In H. Nieburgs (Ed.), *Prevention and detection of cancer. Part I. Prevention. Vol. 2. Etiology* (pp. 943–949). New York: Marcel Dekker, Inc.

Seidman, H., Mushinski, M., Gelb, S., & Silverberg, E (1985). Probabilities of eventually developing or dying of cancer—United States, 1985. *CA: A Cancer Journal for Clinicians, 35,* 36–56.

Seidman, H., Stellman, S., & Mushinski, M. (1982). A different perspective on breast cancer risk factors: Some implications of nonattributable risk. *CA: A Journal for Clinicians, 32,* 301–311.

Selby, J., & Friedman, G (1989). Sigmoidoscopy in the periodic health examination of asymptomatic adults. *Journal of the American Medical Association, 26,* 595–601.

Senie, R. (1986). Assessment of carcinogenesis through epidemiologic and environmental investigations. *Seminars in Oncology Nursing, 2,* 154–160.

Shanmugaratnam, K. (1985). Prevention and early detection of cancer. *Cancer Detection and Prevention, 8,* 431–445.

Shapiro, S., Kelly, J., Rosenberg, L. Kaufman, D., Helmrich, S., Rosenshein, N., Lewis, J., Knapp, R., Stolley, P., & Schottenfeld, D. (1985). Risk of localized and widespread endometrial cancer in relation to recent and discontinued use of conjugated estrogens. *New England Journal of Medicine, 313,* 969–972.

Sharp, D., Eskenazi, B., Callas, P., & Smith, A. (1986). Delayed health hazards of pesticide exposure. *Annual Review of Public Health, 7,* 441–471.

Sherman, C. (1983). Skin cancer. In S. B. Kahn, R. Love, C. Sherman, & R. Chakravorty (Eds.), *Concepts in cancer medicine* (pp. 557–563). New York: Grune & Stratton, Inc.

Shore, R. (1984). Radiation induced cancer: Risk assessment and prevention. *Cancer Detection and Prevention, 7,* 181–190.

Silverberg, E., & Lubera, J. (1987). Cancer statistics, 1987. *CA: A Cancer Journal for Clinicians, 37,* 2–19, 20–25.

Skegg, D. (1985). Other drugs. In M. P. Vessey & M. Gray (Eds.), *Cancer risks and prevention* (pp. 211–230). Oxford: Oxford University Press.

"Smokeless tobacco use in rural Alaska." (1987). *Journal of the American Medical Association, 257,* 1816–1865.

Snyder, R. (1984). Basic concepts of the dose-response relationship. In J. Rodricks & R. Tardiff (Eds.), *Assessment and management of chemical risks* (pp. 37–55). ACS Symposium Series. Washington, DC: American Chemical Society.

Somers, A. R. (1978). The high cost of care for the elderly: Diagnosis, prognosis, and some suggestions for therapy. *Journal of Health Politics Law, 3,* 163–180.

Sondel, P. (1983). The immunology of cancer. In S. B. Kahn, R. Love, C. Sherman, & R. Chakravorty (Eds.), *Concepts in cancer medicine* (pp. 187–200). New York: Grune & Stratton, Inc.

Spitz, M. (1983). The role of the primary care physician in cancer prevention. In G. Newell (Ed.), *Cancer prevention in clinical medicine* (pp. 231–245). New York: Raven Press.

Squier, C. (1984). Smokeless tobacco and oral cancer: A cause for concern? *CA: A Cancer Journal for Clinicians, 34,* 242–247.

Squire, R., & Cameron, L. (1984). An analysis of potential cardiogenic risk from formaldehyde. *Regulatory Toxicology and Pharmacology, 4,* 107–129.

Stellman, J., & Stellman, S. (1983). Occupational lung disease and cancer risk in women. *Occupational Health Nursing, 31*(11), 40–46.

Stern, J. (1987, February). Surgeon general's report cites risks of "involuntary smoking." *Oncology Times.*

Stern, R. M. (1983). Assessment of risk of lung cancer for welders. *Archives of Environmental Health, 38,* 148–155.

Sternburg, J. K. (1983). Identification and management of risk factors for cancer. In S. B. Kahn, R. Love, C. Sherman, & R. Chakravorty (Eds.), *Concepts in cancer medicine* (pp. 241–253). New York: Grune & Stratton, Inc.

Stockwell, S. (1986, July). Snuff found to contain high concentrations of carcinogens. *Oncology Times,* p. 44.

Stokes, J. (1987). The methods of clinical prevention. In H. Vanderschmidt, D. Koch-Weser, & P. Woodbury (Eds.), *Handbook of clinical prevention* (pp. 29–58). Baltimore: Williams & Wilkins.

Stromborg, M., Krafka, B., Gale, D., & Porter, N. (1986). Carcinogens: Are some risks acceptable? *American Journal of Nursing, 86,* 814–817.

Sugarbaker, P., Gunderson, L., & Wittes, R. (1985). Colorectal cancer. In V. DeVita, S. Hellman, & S. Rosenberg (Eds.), *Cancer. Principles and practice of oncology* (2nd ed, pp. 795–884). Philadelphia: J. B. Lippincott Co.

Templeton, A. C. (1975). Acquired diseases. In J. Fraumeni (Ed.), *Persons at high risk of cancer. An approach to cancer etiology and control* (pp. 69–84). New York: Academic Press.

U.S. Department of Health and Human Services. (1985). *Cancer prevention research summary—nutrition* (NIH Publication No. 85-2616). Bethesda, MD: National Cancer Institute.

Van Parijs, L. J., & Eckhardt, S. (1984). Public education in primary and secondary cancer prevention. *Hygiene, 3,* 16–28.

Vessey, M. (1985). Exogenous hormones. In M. P. Vessey & M. Gray (Eds.), *Cancer risks and prevention* (pp. 166–194). Oxford: Oxford University Press.

Weinhouse, S. (1986). Keynote address: The role of diet and nutrition in cancer. *Cancer, 58,* 1791–1794.

Weiss, W. (1983). Lung cancer. In S. B. Kahn, R. Love, C. Sherman,

& R. Chakravorty (Eds.), *Concepts in cancer medicine* (pp. 417–435). New York: Grune & Stratton, Inc.

Wellisch, D., & Yager, J. (1984). *Is there a cancer-prone personality?* Professional Education Publication (No. 3338-PE). New York: American Cancer Society.

White, L. (1986). Cancer risk assessment. *Seminars in Oncology Nursing, 2*, 184–190.

Wood, N., Heffez, L., & Sawyer, D. (1985). Oral precancerous lesions and conditions. Chicago: American Cancer Society, Illinois Division, Oral Cancer Subcommittee.

Wynder, E., & Rose, D. (1984). Diet and breast cancer. *Hospital Practice, 19*, 73–88.

Wynder, E., Rose, D., & Cohen, L. (1986). Diet and breast cancer in causation and therapy. *Cancer, 58*, 1804–1813.

CHAPTER 17

Cancer Screening and Early Detection

SHARON J. OLSEN
MARILYN FRANK-STROMBORG

The National Cancer Institute (NCI), Division of Cancer Prevention and Control, in its *Cancer Control Objectives for the Nation: 1985–2000* directs health care providers to "inform patients of the value of cancer screening and recommend utilization of efficacious screening procedures" (1986, p. 31). The extent to which nurses today can and do become actively involved in cancer screening is increasingly broad and complicated. Nurses aid in case finding, inform clients of guidelines and frequencies for selective screening examinations, and counsel and educate clients about how to recognize cancer signs and symptoms and how to perform self-examination techniques. They are instrumental in developing and organizing community efforts for cancer control and frequently reinforce client teaching previously received from other health care providers. Nurses provide anticipatory guidance regarding cancer prevention and screening as they work with expectant and young families with genetic and life-style predispositions for cancer. And they participate in health education in schools and community groups providing risk factor assessment and health education.

The Oncology Nursing Society recognizes the importance of cancer screening and early detection in cancer nursing. In 1987 this society developed the *Standards of Oncology Nursing Practice* (American Nurses Association and Oncology Nursing Society [ANA-ONC], 1987) and in 1989, the Education Committee of the Oncology Nursing Society updated and published two documents, which also incorporate cancer screening and detection: *Standards of Oncology Nursing Education: Generalist and Advanced Practice* (Oncology Nursing Society [ONS], 1989b) and *Standards of Oncology Education: Patient/Family and Public* (ONS, 1989a). All three publications recommend population-specific cancer screening and early detection guidelines for practice and education.

The fourth standard of oncology nursing practice states that "the oncology nurse develops an outcome-oriented care plan that is individualized and holistic. This plan is based on nursing diagnoses and incorporates preventive . . . actions" (ANA-ONS, 1987, p. 9). Examples of currently published nursing diagnoses relevant to screening and early detection include "knowledge deficit related to prevention and early detection of lung cancer . . . colon cancer . . . breast cancer" (p. 23). Five client outcome criteria have been specified for the fourth standard (ANA-ONS, 1987, p. 11):

The client

1. Recognizes factors that place an individual at risk and may lead to cancer, such as the use of tobacco, improper nutrition, immunosuppressive agents, aging, and exposure to carcinogens.

2. Is able to identify specific high-risk behaviors, health-promoting activities (such as smoking cessation), and early detection methods (such as breast self-examination, oral self-examination, and self-testing for guaiac).

3. Describes cancer warning signals.

4. Identifies a plan for seeking health care assistance whenever any alteration in health status occurs.

5. Describes applicable cancer self-detection measures.

This chapter focuses on cancer screening and the early detection of cancer. Its aim is to provide a firm foundation from which to understand and adapt screening and early cancer detection issues and practices in clinical settings unique to the practicing nurse clinician.

DEFINITIONS

Screening and Early Detection

The term *screening* is frequently used synonymously with "early detection" or "secondary prevention." For *screening* and *early detection,* finding cancer while it is still localized and curable is the common goal; however, there is an important distinction between them. *Early detection* refers to an attempt to diagnose cancer in a curable stage, whereas cancer *screening* is just one of the strategies used to achieve this goal (Miller, 1986b). According to the American Cancer Society ". . . early detection ideally should be a continuous day-by-day process of self-observation and heightened awareness. It implies a degree of individual responsibility for self-care together with ready access to medical facilities for diagnosis and treatment. It means paying attention to symptoms and seeking prompt help should anything unusual be detected. Cancer *screening,* on the other hand, must be done intermittently or periodically by a health care professional" (Miller, 1986b, p. 16). Screening for cancer involves the use of examinations and tests to search for and identify disease in asymptomatic persons (Eddy, 1985, 1986; Hakama, 1986). A person is considered asymptomatic if he or she is not aware of any signs or symptoms of cancer (Eddy, 1985). In some cases, cancer can be detected in a premalignant state (e.g., leukoplakia of the mouth, dysplasia of the cervix, and adenomas of the colon). More commonly, a lesion has already developed into a cancer by the time it is discovered (e.g., breast cancer). There are three implicit assumptions underlying screening for most cancers: that the tests are capable of detecting cancers before the appearance of signs or symptoms; that these tests will find a greater proportion of cancers in early stages; that persons with cancers detected through screening will have higher survival rates and tend to live longer after diagnosis and treatment (Eddy, 1986).

Mass Screening

Mass screening involves the general population. Some suggest it is generally neither practical nor justified (Love, Leventhal, Hughes, & Fryback, 1984) primarily because of the rarity of cancer. Very large populations and large numbers of health care practitioners must be mobilized and issues such as long-term compliance, cost of test versus benefit offered, and untoward morbidity (perhaps even mortality) from tests with low sensitivity and specificity make such testing prohibitive. As an example, Ekelund, Carlsson, and Janzon (1985) extrapolated from a pilot study in Malmo, Sweden, designed to ascertain the potential of mass screening with Hemoccult testing in the prevention of death from colorectal cancer. They calculated that to prove a 25 per cent reduction in mortality from colorectal cancer, 319,000 persons would need to be followed for at least 5 years, assuming a 60 per cent compliance rate, which was achieved during their pilot study.

Selective Screening

Selective screening is targeted at persons with risk factors that predict for high disease prevalence—that is, high-risk groups. Selective screening involves surveillance and is the attentive follow-up of persons at risk for cancer with the intent to detect any premalignant or malignant condition early (Patterson, 1986). Underlying selective screening is the presumption that no matter how carefully designed a screening program may be, it will have finite resources and, therefore, the yield and subsequently the cost-benefit ratio of such efforts will be greater when targeted to high-risk persons.

Risk factors may be divided into the following categories: age, symptoms, signs, historical risk factors, and environmental and occupational risk factors. It is possible and desirable to target select populations at risk. For instance, it is known that the incidence of cancer of the prostate rises eight times between the ages of 45 and 54 years, whereas for the testis, the incidence remains the same. Lung cancer almost triples, and colon cancer more than doubles for the same age group. Historical risk factors, such as family history of breast cancer, polyposis coli, or maternal use of diethylstilbestrol (DES) during gestation; personal risk factors, such as ulcerative colitis, undescended testes, and leukoplakia; and exposure to environmental and occupational carcinogens all influence the risk factor pattern for any particular person.

Carriers of certain cancer genes (e.g., ataxia-telangiectasia) and certain members of cancer families can have an unusually high risk of developing specific cancers, often at unusually early ages. In some of these individuals, precursor states, such as dysplastic nevus syndrome, can identify genetic predisposition to cancer and can lead to appropriate measures for disease prevention and early detection (Li, 1986). Frank-Stromborg has detailed for the reader risk factors associated with specific cancers in Chapter 16. The NCI lists the following as high-risk persons: those with a strong family history of cancer of the breast, ovaries, and colon, or melanoma; adolescent boys and young men (testicular cancer); and those exposed to known environmental or occupational carcinogens (National Cancer Institute, 1986).

Case Finding

Case finding is "the detection of disease by means of tests or procedures that are undertaken by health workers on clients who are consulting for unrelated symptoms. (This means that the 'case finder' is responsible for the investigation and follow-up of high-risk persons identified in this way)" (Canadian Task Force on the Periodic Health Examination, 1979, p. 1203). Love and colleagues (1984) suggest that a skin examination checking for early melanomas, testes examination, and breast examination are inexpensive and worthwhile in the general population. Mammography, sigmoidoscopy, and stool occult blood tests, on the other hand, are more costly and of benefit only in select populations.

Cancer Control

According to NCI's Division of Cancer Prevention and Control (1986), cancer control consists of two components: screening and communication. This group suggests that screening be aimed at cancer detection in large populations, including symptomatic and asymptomatic individuals. Communication involves educating the public and, in particular, those persons at risk, about cancer and cancer prevention, and motivating them to indulge in behaviors that are associated with lowered risk for cancer.

IMPORTANT FEATURES OF TESTS USED IN SCREENING

The critical features of screening tests have been detailed in various degrees of depth and importance by many authors (Eddy, 1986; Frame, 1986; Hakama, 1986; Love et al., 1984; Patterson, 1986). Love and associates (1984) suggest that there are two aspects of screening tests that should be of concern to the clinician: application in the clinical setting and issues generic to the test themselves.

Application of Screening Tests in the Clinical Setting

To enhance compliance and utilization, particularly regarding tests that need regular follow-up (e.g., mammography, triannual sigmoidoscopy, and self-exami-

nation), tests must be comfortable and acceptable to the client. Tests should be convenient, preferably readily available during medical visits, and of low cost. Long-term side effects should be rare, given that large populations of individuals may be screened.

Issues Generic to Screening Tests

The test itself should be be able to detect cancer before the onset of signs and symptoms. Herein lies the importance of sensitivity, specificity, and the predictive value of a test. *Sensitivity* is the percentage of persons with cancer who have positive screening tests. *Specificity* is the percentage of persons without cancer who have negative screening tests. The *predictive value* of a positive test is the percentage of persons with a positive screening test who actually have cancer. To calculate the sensitivity, specificity, or predictive value for any screening test, see Table 17–1.

No perfect test exists at present. Generally, the more sensitive a test is, the less specific it will be, and a balance must be struck between the two indices of sensitivity and specificity (Patterson, 1986). In tests with less than 100 per cent *sensitivity*, a proportion of *preclinical* cancers will not be diagnosed at screening. Sensitivity has been estimated to range from 60 to 99 per cent for Papanicolaou smears (Love & Camilli, 1981) and is approximately 69 per cent for digital rectal examinations for prostate cancer.

In tests with less than 100 per cent *specificity*, false positives will be expected. Tests with low specificity not only overwhelm diagnostic services and result in prohibitive follow-up costs but also expose individuals to the risks of unnecessary diagnostic work-ups, resulting in potentially substantial physical and psychological morbidity and possible mortality (Love & Camilli, 1981; Love et al., 1984). Specificity has been estimated at 99 per cent for Papanicolaou tests (Love & Camilli, 1981) and at 89 per cent for digital rectal examinations for prostate cancer. False-positive test results occur in about 1.5 per cent of mammograms and 1 to 3 per cent of Hemoccult tests (Eddy, 1985).

Table 17–1. CALCULATION OF SENSITIVITY, SPECIFICITY, AND PREDICTIVE VALUES OF SCREENING TESTS

	Preclinical Disease Status		
	Present	*Absent*	*Totals*
Screen positive	A	B	SP
Screen negative	C	D	SN
	DP	DN	

A = True positive   Sensitivity $= \dfrac{A}{DP}$
B = False positive
C = False negative   Specificity $= \dfrac{D}{DN}$
D = True negative
SP = Patients screen positive
SN = Patients screen negative   Predictive value
DP = Patients with disease   of positive test $= \dfrac{A}{SP}$
DN = Patients without disease

(From Love, R. R., Leventhal, H., Hughes, B. S., & Fryback, D. G. [1984]. Critical concepts in cancer screening. *Cancer Prevention for Clinicians: Course Test.* Cancer Prevention Program, University of Wisconsin Clinical Cancer Center, Board of Regents of the University of Wisconsin System, II–10. Reproduced by permission.)

Up to 10 per cent of chest radiographs for lung cancer can produce false-positive results (Eddy, 1985).

The predictive value of screening tests depends on the prevalence of the disease in the population screened. The lower the prevalence, the lower the predictive value (Patterson, 1986).

Love and associates (1984) caution that sensitivity and specificity can vary from setting to setting. Potential factors that can influence these indices include improper application of the test, poor technique, suboptimal laboratory practice, and clinical expertise. Nurses and nurse practitioners, specifically, can have a substantial impact on the accuracy of such screening techniques as the Papanicolaou smear, digital rectal examination for prostate cancer, and physical breast examination.

GUIDELINES FOR SCREENING

Decisions regarding who to screen, when, and at what intervals continue to be controversial. The NCI, the American Cancer Society (ACS), and the Canadian National Task Force have set forth varying recommendations. This lack of general agreement has had a disconcerting effect on the screening efforts of practitioners. Screening recommendations often vary from clinical practice to clinical practice and even among cancer prevention centers.

American Cancer Society

In general, the most well known are the guidelines offered by the ACS (Miller, 1986b), but the Society itself warns that its guidelines are "not rules" and apply to only individuals without symptoms. Until further conclusive experimental data, cost-benefit, cost-efficacy, and more complete mortality data are available (Love et al., 1984), agreement on screening will remain uncertain. The current recommendations for screening by the ACS are presented in Table 17–2.

Canadian Task Force

The Canadian Task Force on the Periodic Health Examination was established in September 1976, to recommend a plan for a lifetime program of periodic health assessments for all persons living in Canada. Clinicians and scientists sought to recommend an age- and sex-specific lifetime health care plan. Their recommendations resulted in a national health protection package comprising various detection methods (such as blood pressure measurement and tests for occult blood in the stool) and interventions (such as immunization and counseling). The recommendations of the Task Force were to be regarded as minimal standards, clearly recognizing persons who were at special risk would require more than the recommended inverventions. The Task Force also recognized that continuing research would necessitate periodic modification of the

disease-specific recommendations and that new ones would be added to maintain state-of-the-art recommendations.

In judging whether a specific condition should be considered in a periodic health examination, three aspects were studied: (1) the current burden of mortality, morbidity, and suffering caused by the condition; (2) the validity and acceptability of the method used to prevent or identify risk or the early asymptomatic stage of the condition; and (3) the recommendations that should be carried out during case finding rather than as screening techniques; that is, they should be performed when the person is seen for unrelated symptoms rather than for a specific prevention purpose. Current recommendations from the Canadian Task Force (1979, 1982; Goldbloom & Battesta, 1986; Spitzer, 1984) are presented in Table 17–3.

National Cancer Institute

In 1987 the NCI published its "working guidelines" for early cancer detection (Miller, 1986b). The guidelines were based on currently available statistical and clinical information and are subject to change as additional data become available. Accordingly, "every effort has been made to develop guidelines which all relevant medical organizations could support and promote" (p. 1). They are intended to aid health care practitioners and patients in the selection of the best available early detection procedures. Table 17–4 sets forth the NCI guidelines and documents the rationale associated with each guideline.

BENEFITS AND RISKS OF SCREENING

Screening asymptomatic adults for cancer can be a valuable health activity but, as noted earlier, it also has risks and associated costs. The benefits of cancer screening include improved prognosis for some cases but not for all; the possibility of less pain, disfigurement, and disability; the need for less radical treatment to cure some cases detected early; reassurance for those with negative test results; resource savings in terms of less treatment expense if less radical treatment is appropriate and lesser costs for management of patients who, without early screening, otherwise would have died, as the costs for cancer can often be substantial (Chamberlain, 1983; Eddy, 1986; Miller, 1986a).

Risks may be direct, such as radiation or perforation, or indirect, such as false-positive test results (Eddy, 1985; Miller, 1986a). Eddy (1985) suggests that perforation rates in rigid or flexible sigmoidoscopy can range from 1 per 1000 to 1 per 50,000. Perforation from colonoscopy can range from 1 per 87 to 1 per 250. The danger is that symptoms following a false-negative screen will be ignored, resulting in postponement of the normal date of diagnosis and thus a poorer prognosis. In addition, more complex and costly investiga-

Table 17–2. GUIDELINES FOR CANCER-RELATED CHECK-UPS: AMERICAN CANCER SOCIETY (ASYMPTOMATIC POPULATIONS)

Risk Factors for Types of Cancer	Age (years)	
	20–39	*40 and Older*
General Cancer-Related Check-up	Every 3 years. Should include health counseling (such as tips on stopping cigarette smoking) and examinations for cancers of the thyroid, testes, prostate, oral cavity, ovaries, skin, and lymph nodes. Some people are at higher risk for certain cancers and may need to be tested more frequently.	Every year.
Breast Cancer Older age, family history in mother or sisters, precancerous condition on breast biopsy, first child born after age 30, obesity, never had children.	Physical breast examination every 3 years; self-examination monthly; one baseline mammogram between ages 35 and 39.	Physical breast examination every year; self-examination monthly; mammogram every year after age 50, every 1–2 years between ages 40 and 49.
Bladder Cancer, Urinary Tract Smoking, exposure to chemical carcinogens, personal history of bladder cancer.	No recommendations.	No recommendations.
Cervical Cancer Early age at first intercourse, multiple sexual partners, smoking, human papillomavirus infection (condyloma or warts).	Annual Papanicolaou test and pelvic examination for all women who are or have been sexually active, or who have reached the age of 18. After three or more consecutive normal annual examinations, the Papanicolaou test may be performed less frequently at the discretion of the physician.	
Colorectal Cancer Colorectal polyp(s), family history of colorectal cancer(s), inflammatory bowel disease, diet high in fat and low in fiber.	No recommendations.	Digital rectal examination for men and women aged 40 and over; stool blood test for men and women aged 50 and over annually; sigmoidoscopy for men and women beginning at age 50 every 3–5 years based on the advice of the physician.
Endometrial Cancer Obesity, prolonged use of unopposed postmenopausal estrogens, hypertension, diabetes.	No recommendations.	Endometrial biopsy for women at menopause and for women at high risk (history of infertility, obesity, failure to ovulate, abnormal uterine bleeding, estrogen therapy).
Lung Cancer Voluntary smoking and involuntary smoke inhalation; occupational exposures such as to asbestos.	No recommendations.	No recommendations.
Oral Cancer Smoking and alcohol use, use of smokeless tobacco.	Oral examination for men and women annually.	Oral examination for men and women annually.
Prostate Cancer None.	No recommendations.	Digital examination for men over 40 annually.
Skin Cancer Fair skin, sun exposure, severe sunburn in childhood, familial conditions such as dysplastic nevus syndrome.	Skin examination for men and women over 20 every 3 years.	Skin examination for men and women over 40 annually.

(Modified from American Cancer Society. [1988]. *The health professional and cancer prevention and detection* [Brochure No. 3372-PE]. New York: American Cancer Society; Fink, D. J. [1987, November]. *Change in checkup guidelines for cervical cancer detection* [Memo]. New York: American Cancer Society; Miller, D. G. [1986]. Cancer prevention: steps you can take. In A. I. Holleb [Ed.], *The American Cancer Society cancer book* [pp. 27–28]. Garden City, NY: Doubleday & Co. Reproduced by permission.)

tions and diagnostic procedures may be necessary. A longer and perhaps more emotionally and financially costly period of observation may be inevitable if the screening test is capable of detecting presymptomatic cases. Finally, longer periods of morbidity for patients in whom prognosis is unaltered and the risk of overtreatment of borderline abnormalities cannot be minimized.

Substantial psychological and monetary costs can be associated with the risks of screening. Direct costs include the physician or clinic charge for the visit; direct costs of the test or examination, including proc-

essing and interpretation; morbidity and mortality from the test itself; and the dollar cost of diagnostic evaluation of persons with false-positive screening tests. Indirect costs include those incurred while going for the screening test (e.g., time lost from work, babysitting, automobile gasoline, parking fees) and the nonfinancial costs of inconvenience, anxiety, discomfort, and psychological stress if early screening incurs no prolonged survival benefit (Eddy, 1985; Love et al., 1984). Pain cannot be underestimated as a substantial direct cost of, for example, endometrial tissue biopsy. Eddy (1985) suggests that the pain associated with this

Table 17–3. GUIDELINES FOR SCREENING FOR CANCER, CANADIAN NATIONAL TASK FORCE

Condition, Age	Maneuver	Recommendation*
Breast Cancer		
40–49	Annual physical breast examination	C
50–59	Annual mammography and physical breast examination	A
≥60	Annual mammography and physical breast examination	B
≤40	Teach breast self-examination	C
Cervical Cancer		
18–35; sexually active	Annual Papanicolaou smear	B (based on 1976 recommendations
>35–60; sexually active	Papanicolaou smear every 5 years	
35+; high risk	Women whose contact with the health care system is through venereal disease clinics or penal institutions should not be discouraged from having smears more frequently than every 5 years if they request them.	
>60	If a women has had repeated satisfactory smears without significant atypia, she may stop having Papanicolaou smears.	
Colorectal Cancer		
<40; with NO known risk factors	No routine recommendations	C
>40; with NO known risk factors	No routine recommendations; however, evidence does not warrant stopping the use of fecal occult blood testing or sigmoidoscopy where it already exists.	C
People with two or more first-degree relatives with colorectal cancer	Periodic colonoscopy (beginning at age 40 years)	C
People with one first-degree relative with colorectal cancer detected after age 40	Fecal occult blood testing and sigmoidoscopy (beginning at age 40)	C
Women with a history of endometrial, ovarian, or breast cancer	Periodic signoidoscopy	C
People with a history of colorectal cancer, adenomatous polyps, or ulcerative colitis of 10-years' duration	Periodic colonoscopy	
Family members of patients with familial polyposis	Periodic sigmoidoscopy at an early age, followed by periodic colonoscopy after age 30	
Prostate Cancer	Digital palpation per rectum	C
Testis Cancer	Clinical examination of testes	C
Bladder Cancer	Cytologic urine analysis for high-risk groups: workers occupationally exposed to bladder carcinogens, smokers. Frequency based on clinical judgment.	D for general population; B for high-risk groups
Hodgkin's Disease	Physical examination and x-ray studies	C
Oral Cancer	Visual examination of males and all smokers annually beginning at age 65.	C
Skin Cancer Including Melanoma	Counseling to reduce exposure and foster use of sunscreens and periodic skin examination at appropriate intervals on the basis of clinical judgment.	D for general population; B for high-risk groups

* A There is good evidence to support the recommendation that the condition be specifically considered in a periodic health examination.

B There is fair evidence to support the recommendation that the condition be specifically considered in a periodic health examination.

C There is poor evidence regarding the inclusion of the condition in a periodic health examination, and recommendations may be made on other grounds.

D There is fair evidence to support the recommendation that the condition be excluded from consideration in a periodic health examination.

(Modified from Canadian Task Force. [1979, November 3]. The periodic health examination. *Canadian Medical Association Journal, 121,* 1195, 1206–1246; Canadian Task Force on Cervical Cancer Screening Programs. [1982, October 1]. Cervical cancer screening programs: summary of the 1982 Canadian task force report. *Canadian Medical Association Journal, 127,* 581–589; Canadian Task Force. [1986, April 1]. The periodic health examination 2. 1985 update. *Canadian Medical Association Journal, 134,* 724; Canadian Task Force on the Periodic Health Examination. [1989, August 1]. The periodic health examination: 2. 1989 update. *Canadian Medical Association Journal, 141,* 209–216. Reprinted with permission of the Health Services Directorate, Health Services and Promotion Branch, Department of National Health and Welfare and the *Canadian Medical Association Journal.*)

Table 17–4. WORKING GUIDELINES FOR EARLY CANCER DETECTION, NATIONAL CANCER INSTITUTE

Guidelines	Bases for Guidelines
Breast Cancer	
Physicians should encourage their female patients to do monthly breast self-examination.	• Breast cancer is the most frequent cancer in women and is second only to lung cancer as the leading cause of death from cancer.
Physicians are encouraged to do clinical breast examinations on all female patients in whom they are doing a periodic examination.	• Early stage breast cancer has an excellent survival rate (90%).
Beginning at the age of 40, a mammogram should be encouraged for the patient every 1 to 2 years until the age of 50, after which it should become annual.	• Mammography and physical examination are proven methods of detecting early breast cancer.
In women with a personal history of cancer, mammography should be encouraged on an annual basis.	• Mortality has been reduced in randomized screening trials using mammography and physical examination.
Cervical Cancer	
All women who are or have been sexually active, or who have reached age 18 years, should have an annual Papanicolaou test and pelvic examination. After a woman has had three or more consecutive satisfactory normal annual examinations, the Papanicolaou test may be performed less frequently at the discretion of her physician.	• The Papanicolaou test has been proved to decrease mortality. • The general recommendation has been changed back to yearly because of the change in sexual practices and recent observations on papillomavirus.
Colorectal Cancer	
A rectal examination should be included as a part of the periodic health examination.	• Colorectal cancer is the second leading cause of death from cancer. The majority of patients have advanced disease at diagnosis.
At the age of 50, annual fecal occult blood testing and a sigmoidoscopy every 3 to 5 years should be done.	• Removal of premalignant lesions whose natural history leads to cancer will decrease incidence and eventual mortality.
The physician should identify, for special surveillance, high-risk patients, including those with a strong family history of colon cancer, or with a personal history of polyps, colon cancer, or inflammatory bowel disease.	• Early testing of asymptomatic patients results in the detection of adenomatous polyps, increased numbers of early stage cancers, and decreased numbers of advanced stage cancers.
Oral Cancer	
Oral examination, including palpation of the tongue, floor of the mouth, salivary glands, and lymph nodes of the neck should be performed as part of the periodic health examination.	• Cancers of the oral cavity and pharynx are a major cause of death from cancer in the United States.
Special attention should be given to those at high risk owing to tobacco and alcohol use.	• This is a region of the body that is generally accessible to examination by the patient, the dentist, and the physician.
	• Oral cancer occurs predominantly in patients who smoke cigarettes or chew tobacco or consume considerable amounts of alcohol.
	• An oral examination looking for leukoplakia and early cancer should be a part of every periodic health examination in a dentist's or physician's office without additional cost.
	• The routine examination of symptomatic and asymptomatic patients results in the detection of earlier stage cancers.
	• Treatment outcome is better in patients with early stage disease.
Prostate Cancer	
Annual digital rectal examination of the prostate should be performed on all men over 40 years of age.	• Prostate cancer is a significant health problem for men in terms of both morbidity and mortality.
More specific education and training should be given to physicians in the detection of prostate cancer.	• With the advancing age of the United States population, the overall impact of prostate cancer on the national health will increase.
	• Despite improved understanding of the biologic potential of prostate cancer as it relates to histologic grade and tumor volume, the need to treat or diagnose a given case of prostate cancer cannot be proved at this time. It follows, then, that rigorous statistical validation or cost effectiveness of any current screening test as a matter of national rather than personal health policy cannot be accomplished at this time.
	• It is clear that disease-free survival is increased in patients treated for localized versus advanced prostate cancer (length and lead times biases notwithstanding).
	• Until we can predict the biologic potential of a given tumor, attempts to decrease morbidity and mortality from prostate cancer require a uniform screening method for earlier detection of disease.
	• Given the imperfections of every available method, routine annual digital rectal examination for men over 40 years of age appears to be the most reasonable screening test for prostate cancer with regard to overall efficiency, noninvasiveness, morbidity, availability, and cost.
	• A continued search for more precise methods for the early detection of curable *and* biologically active prostate cancer is warranted.
Skin Cancer (Melanoma)	
Based on the recommendation of the American Academy of Dermatology, all persons should be encouraged to examine their skin thoroughly on a regular basis.	• Melanoma in the United States makes up 2% of all malignancies and 1% of cancer deaths (slightly more than for cancer of the cervix). The incidence has increased more rapidly than that for any other cancer in recent years.
Primary care physicians should be encouraged to examine the skin as part of the periodic health examination.	• Education of the public and physicians has resulted in earlier detection, improved survival, and stabilization of mortality in other countries.
Further public and professional education should be promoted on the early detection of skin cancers and in particular malignant melanoma.	• The examinations are a part of usual medical practice and have no cost implications.
Testes Cancer	
Periodic (monthly) testicular self-examination should be encouraged.	• This is a rare disease in an organ that is readily accessible to examination by the individual person.
Routine palpation of the testicles by a physician during physical examination should be carried out as part of the health examination.	• Although germ cell testicular tumor is relatively uncommon, it is a significant cause of cancer-related morbidity and mortality in young men.
	• Testis cancer has uniformly high virulence.
	• Testis cancer is very responsive to therapy.
	• The morbidity and cost to achieve cure is lower for low stage and low volume of disease compared to advanced disease.
	• Treatment failures are more often associated with bulky late-stage disease.
	• Diagnosis by simple palpation, which is noninvasive, inexpensive, and nonmorbid, should be easily taught to health professionals and to the male population with a high positive predictive value.

(Modified from Early Detection Branch, Division of Cancer Prevention and Control [1987, December 17]. *Working guidelines for early cancer detection: rationale and supporting evidence to decrease mortality.* Bethesda, MD: National Cancer Institute.)

Note: As of April 1990, no changes have been made in these guidelines, per telephone conversation with Charles R. Smart, M.D., Chief of the Early Detection Branch, Division of Cancer Prevention and Control, National Cancer Institute, Bethesda, MD.

procedure will be mild for 70 per cent of women but moderate to severe for the majority of nulliparous women.

THE POTENTIAL FOR SCREENING TO REDUCE CANCER MORTALITY

Ideally, screening should reduce mortality. It is generally agreed that the strongest evidence is provided by randomized, controlled, clinical trials using mortality as an end point. Evidence from studies that are controlled but not randomized, such as case-control studies and those with historical controls, is generally weaker but still useful. The mere fact that a screening procedure is capable of detecting a cancer does not by itself mean that screening will reduce mortality. However, if there is evidence that therapy is more efficacious when delivered to cancers in early stages, then evidence that a screening procedure is able to detect a cancer early suggests, but does not prove conclusively, that screening reduces mortality (Division of Cancer Prevention and Control, 1986).

The Division of Cancer Prevention and Control of the NCI (1986) has divided the effectiveness of screening for specific cancers into three categories:

1. Cancers and screening techniques for which there is general agreement that screening reduces mortality;

2. Cancers and screening techniques for which there is general agreement that screening does not appreciably reduce mortality;

3. Cancers and screening techniques for which there is no general consensus that screening reduces mortality, either because of a lack of information or because of different interpretations of the existing information.

Table 17–5 summarizes the Division's findings.

The best results currently available from screening trials indicate that screening can potentially reduce mortality from breast cancer by about 30 per cent, colon and rectal cancers by about 60 per cent, cervical cancer by about 90 per cent, melanoma (through public awareness of early detection) by 20 per cent, and oral cancer in high-risk persons by 20 per cent (Early Detection Branch Division of Cancer Prevention and Control, 1987; Eddy, 1986). Few data are available to estimate the effect of screening on mortality from cancers of the stomach, esophagus, bladder, or liver; however, Eddy (1986) predicts that if only a 10 per cent reduction were possible, the potential value of early detection would be that a screening program in 1977 could have saved about 750 million person-years of life throughout the world, and by the year 2000 almost 1000 million person-years of productive life could be saved for each year of screening.

DEVELOPING SCREENING PROGRAMS

A rapid increase in the number of screening programs initiated in primary, secondary, and tertiary care settings is occurring today. Increasingly, nurses are becoming more actively involved in the development,

Table 17–5. EFFECTIVENESS OF SCREENING TO REDUCE CANCER MORTALITY

Category 1: Screening Effective

Screening women over the age of 50 years for breast cancer with a combination of mammography and physical breast examination by a health care professional.

Screening for cervical cancer by Papanicolaou smears at least once every 3 years for women aged 20 to 70.

Category 2: Screening Ineffective

Lung cancer screening with chest radiographs and sputum cytology.

Category 3: Screening Impact Uncertain

Breast self-examination.*

Digital rectal examination.*

Annual oral examination.*

Monthly testicular self-examination.*

Periodic medical examination or self-examination for melanoma.*

Annual physical examination and mammography for women under 50 years.

Periodic combined digital rectal and sigmoidoscopy.†

Periodic screening for bladder cancer.*

Endometrial aspiration for endometrial cancer and pelvic examination for ovarian and uterine cancer.*

Use of endoscopy in esophageal and gastric cancers.‡

Serum marker assays.§

---

*The lack of controlled clinical trials prevents the estimation of impact on cancer mortality for this screening activity.

†Randomized, controlled clinical trials have been done but methodologic problems limit the results. In reviewing all the evidence, no general agreement was reached to signify that screening definitely reduced mortality.

‡No consensus was reached that screening for these two cancers would be appropriate in the United States.

§For the present, and for a variety of reasons, all assays have failed to be useful as screening techniques.

(From Division of Cancer Prevention and Control [1986]. Screening. In P. Greenwald & E. Sondik [Eds.], *Cancer control objectives for the nation: 1985–2000*. NCI Monograph, NIH Publication 86–2880. Bethesda, MD: National Institute of Health.)

implementation, and ongoing operation of these programs. It is clear that the use of a screening test as part of an office visit does not constitute a screening program (Prorok & Connor, 1986). Several authors (Eddy, 1986; Love & Olsen, 1984; Prorok & Connor, 1986) have provided suggestions and guidelines for the development of comprehensive and well-designed screening programs. According to Prorok and Connor (1986), a screening program depends on the organizational entity, the specialized facility dedicated to carrying out a screening protocol, and the personnel to ensure that it is followed. It includes an outreach or recruitment program for a target population or populations; the necessary equipment and personnel to perform, evaluate, and monitor the quality control of the screening tests; and sufficient resources to follow up positive and suspicious results with appropriate action.

Eddy (1986) emphasizes that the following conditions should be considered when developing a screening program:

1. A formal analysis should be performed to estimate the effectiveness, risks, and costs of screening the selected populations.

2. The screening program should be planned as part of an integrated and holistic health care program.

3. Screening should be limited to circumstances in which the principles of screening are adhered to.

4. Screening should be applied selectively to those persons most likely to benefit.

5. The risks as well as the expected benefits of screening should be explained to the prospective subjects. The risks include any possible complications of the examination procedures and the possibility of false-positive and false-negative test results.

6. The program should be organized to ensure high-quality examinations and to minimize costs.

7. Facilities should be available to follow, diagnose, and treat people who have positive results on examination.

8. Records should be kept to monitor the program's quality and success.

Love and Olsen (1985) specify a prescriptive framework for organizing and integrating cancer prevention strategies into clinical practice. Four goals for a comprehensive screening and early detection program that relies on interdependent and complementary clinical practice between nursing and medicine are described. The first goal is to designate specific staff responsibilities. Initially, this requires staff agreement on a philosophy of client care and designation of the policies of the practice. A philosophy that is receptive to and promotes self-care encourages clients to take control of their own health and provides them with open access to health care information and education in specialized skills. Designated staff responsibilities may vary from program to program but should be limited only by practitioner competence and creativity or organizational necessity.

Development of a medical records system to facilitate staff work is the second goal. A detailed database for each client permits in-depth and accurate analysis of risk factors, planning of personalized and comprehensive screening and health education, and facilitates regular follow-up. The third goal entails the definition of specific screening and detection behaviors and attitudes for both clients and staff. Consensus must be reached regarding which screening tests and frequency guidelines will be regularly monitored and promoted by the practice. Health education protocols and educational media must be agreed on. The goals of ancillary, nursing, and medical staff must all be directed toward these common goals to present a holistic and unified clinical practice milieu committed to the importance of primary prevention, cancer screening, and early detection. Finally, the fourth goal emphasizes staff education. Love and Olsen (1985) suggest that commitment to a practice-wide continuing education system that legitimizes and promotes personal as well as professional education is mandatory for personal growth, continued job satisfaction, and the delivery of up-to-date and high-quality client care.

PUBLIC ATTITUDES AND SCREENING PRACTICES

Between February and April 1985, the NCI and the United States Food and Drug Administration (Office of Cancer Communications [OCC], 1987) conducted the second (Wave II) of a two-part telephone survey designed to assess the change in public knowledge, attitudes, and practices related to cancer prevention and risk since their first survey (Wave I) in June 1983. The findings of the Wave II survey were based on responses from 1898 interviews. In general, the survey takers found that much of the public remains inadequately informed about cancer. People in 1985 were not aware that the chances of being cured of cancer were better then than ever before, nor were they any more aware that they could actively take steps to reduce personal cancer risk. Respondents did, however, report a small but statistically significant increase in the number of activities that they believed they could do to reduce their risk of cancer. These included exercising, making changes in food choices, stopping smoking, limiting alcohol consumption, and altering work and medical practices and life style. Of particular importance to screening, 19.7 per cent of respondents indicated that they could have more checkups or tests, whereas 10.3 per cent indicated they could do more self-examinations.

However, when asked what they actually had done to decrease the chances of getting cancer, only 14.7 per cent indicated they had had more checkups or tests, and only 6.4 per cent had done more self-examinations. There is evidence that only 15 to 20 per cent of American women have regular Papanicolaou testing (Fink, 1987), and for women between the ages of 50 and 70 years, only 45 per cent have annual physical breast examination and 15 per cent have annual mammograms (NCI, 1986).

Celentano, Shapiro, and Weisman (1982) studied factors that distinguished elderly women (aged 65 years or older) from younger women in cancer screening participation. The proportion of women reporting "ever" having had any test to detect cancer was approximately 80 per cent for women aged 18 to 64 years, 67 per cent for women aged 65 to 74, and 50 per cent for women 75 or older. The major factor relating to lower rates of experience in cancer detection seemed to be type of provider utilized. Younger women were more likely to report seeing an obstetrician-gynecologist, whereas women aged 55 years or older were more likely to identify a family physician or general practitioner as the regular medical care provider.

Clearly the challenge exists for nurses not only to enhance the knowledge base of the general public regarding screening examinations but also to bridge the gap between beliefs and practices through psychosocial and educational research. The influence of mass media on public education is an area ripe for research. According to the Wave II report, the most frequent source of cancer prevention information for both blacks and the general population was television (66.4 and 75.3 per cent, respectively), followed by magazines (44.6 per cent) for blacks, and newspapers (63.1 per cent) for the general public (OCC, 1987).

FACTORS INFLUENCING SCREENING AND EARLY DETECTION

Delay

Early detection refers to the application of screening and diagnostic tests that allow presumptive diagnoses of various cancers in asymptomatic persons (Shanmugaratnam, 1985). The process of cancer diagnosis involves the recognition of a complaint by the individual, its evaluation by a health care professional, and confirmation by laboratory tests or procedures (e.g., endoscopy). Herein lies the problem with early detection of cancer: the person with the physical complaint has to be the one to bring himself or herself to the health care professional. It is not uncommon, once symptoms appear, for people to delay months before seeking medical attention.

For instance, the average delay between the time a man first notices a testicular lump and the date treatment actually begins is 6 months (Swanson, 1987). Young men usually delay seeking evaluation of minor symptoms (e.g., a slightly enlarged testis or a "lump" on the testis) because of lack of knowledge about the early signs and symptoms of testicular cancer (Carlin, 1986). The widespread lack of knowledge about testicular cancer is underscored by Blesch (1986). She took a random sample of 233 professional men and found that although 61.2 per cent were aware of testicular cancer, 4 in 9 men reporting a personal history of undescended testis (a significant risk factor) had not heard of it. In general, for all cancers, research documents that two thirds of patients who were found to have cancer delayed reporting their problems by more than 1 month, and 25 per cent delayed by more than 6 months (Kahn, 1983).

Knowledge of Early Warning Signs

Publishing "Cancer's Seven Warning Signals" was an attempt by the ACS to educate the American public to the early signs and symptoms that merit the attention of a health professional. Rovinski (1980) points out that laypeople frequently turn to a socially authoritative source on health matters before "bothering" their work-ladened and time-restricted doctor. Thus family members and acquaintances often consult a nurse as an informal preliminary expert in weighing the advisability of calling the physician when they are confronted with a new physical sign or symptom. Unfortunately, Rovinski found that only two registered nurses of the 91 she interviewed could recall all seven of the cancer warning signs, indicating that an inability to remember what the signs are is not an uncommon phenomenon among this group of health professionals, let alone the general public.

Surveys by the ACS have also shown general lack of knowledge about the seven cardinal early warning signs among the public. For instance, in 1966, 76 per cent of persons surveyed correctly identified "a change in a wart or mole" as a warning signal; in 1978 the percentage had dropped to 68 per cent identifying this sign as a signal meriting medical attention (Fraser, 1982). A 1982 survey by the ACS on attitudes toward cancer of the colon and rectum found that most people did not associate blood in the stool with cancer and still fewer associated it with colon or rectal cancer ("Cancer of the colon," 1983). Racial and socioeco-nomic differences exist on knowledge of cancer's warning signals. A 1979 ACS survey found that urban black Americans tend to be less knowledgeable than white Americans about cancer warning signals; in fact half as many black Americans as white Americans recognized five or more of cancer warning signals (Subcommittee on Cancer in the Economically Disadvantaged, 1986). A similar study in 1985 found that Hispanic-Americans were not adequately aware of most of the warning signals of cancer or of ways to reduce cancer risk ("A study of Hispanics' attitudes," 1985).

Individual Personality Characteristics

There are many other reasons why people do not seek early detection, including individual characteristics that may facilitate or impede early detection. Kelly (1983) identified several barriers to effective communication about primary and secondary prevention of cancer that the person may possess. Primary prevention is defined as the "identification and control by appropriate interventions of those environmental and host factors that influence the occurrence of cancer and its progression to clinical disease," whereas secondary prevention involves early detection of cancer so that prompt treatment will arrest it (Newell, 1986). The traits that Kelly identified as barriers are as follows:

1. Low self-esteem. Persons with low self-esteem suffer from a distortion of perception that can lead them to misinterpret the cancer information they are given.

2. Denial. Denial of the possibility of getting cancer can prevent the person from seeking early detection examinations or from conducting self-examination procedures.

3. Fear. While people are in an acute stage of fear, they will absorb little information. If they have a family history of cancer, their fear of the disease may be so intense that they do not hear, nor are they receptive to, messages urging them to attend a cancer detection clinic or have a suspicious complaint investigated; alternatively, they may fear their complaint will be viewed as hypochondriacal.

4. Embarrassment. Embarrassment can stem from multiple causes, including embarrassment about having a physical examination or about returning and "bothering" the physician when a symptom does not resolve.

Evans, Love, Meyerowitz, Leventhal, & Nerenz (1985) studied 78 people who were from families in which the incidence of cancer was higher than normal to determine characteristics of those persons who actively sought the services provided by a Cancer Prevention Clinic. They found that prior involvement in cancer prevention activities, interest in cancer-specific information, and level of perceived susceptibility to cancer all contributed significantly to active participation in the clinic. Mettlin and Cummings (1983) studied the 5879 persons who visited Roswell Park's Prevention-Detection Clinic during its first three years of operation in the early 1980s and found the majority were female, white, and middle-class by socioeconomic status. The overwhelming majority (95 per cent) of people who attended reported that their decision to attend the clinic was influenced by their belief in the value of regular medical checkups, motivated in part by the fact that a relative had had cancer (78 per cent), the examination was free (56 per cent), or they had a personal physical problem (54 per cent). Although many individual characteristics play a part in seeking or not seeking early detection services, a belief in the value of prevention would appear to be a facilitator.

Confidence

A review of the literature on early detection of colon and rectal cancer reveals other factors that play a part in the success or failure of early detection programs. For instance, surveys document that the American public not only lacks confidence in early detection of colon and rectal cancer but also holds many misconceptions about the disease. The disease is seen as a male problem, the people believe that colorectal cancer is a crippling disease, and they generally believe that when a colorectal cancer is discovered, its growth is fairly well advanced and survival chances are poor ("Cancer of the colon," 1983).

Attitudes

Farrands, Hardcastle, Chamberlain, & Moss (1984) found that participants in a colorectal screening program were more likely to have positive attitudes toward preventive health practices, were better informed about serious illnesses, and were more optimistic and less frightened about cancer. They also found that more women than men accepted the Hemoccult blood test, and the participation rate in people over the age of 65 years was lower than the rate in younger people. The observation that women and individuals in younger age groups are more likely to participate in colorectal screening was also found in a study by Box and colleagues (1984). The observed sex differences in levels of participation reported by Foster and co-workers (1978) and by Farrands and colleagues (1984) are consistent with other researcher's results that more health preventive behavior is shown by women (Lallemand, Vakil, Pearson, & Box, 1984). It has been suggested that women are socialized to be more compliant and are accustomed to seeking health care services (Bostock, Jacobson, & Seymour, 1982).

Age

It has also been demonstrated that participation in cancer screening programs decreases with age (Farrands, Griffiths, & Britton, 1981; Levy, 1983; Morrow, Way, Hoagland, & Cooper, 1982). In general, a poor response in the over-70 age group is predictable. A delay is also noted among the elderly when suspicious symptoms arise. Studies show that older women are more likely to delay contacting a physician once a suspicious breast symptom has been noted (Levy, 1983). Box and colleagues (1984) have suggested that older patients may delay because the suspicious symptoms or signs are obscured by competing health problems or appear insignificant in comparison to other, more painful or disabling conditions.

With increasing age it has been reported that individuals accept poor health more readily, believing that it is to be expected. If poor health is expected then it may not seem useful to the individual to have this confirmed by a test (Farrands et al., 1984, p. 23).

It must also be remembered that the elderly persons encountered today were educated in an era without health education or emphasis on early detection. Barriers to early detection include gender differences (women are more likely to engage in early detection programs than men) and increasing age (persons over 65 years of age are less likely to engage in early detection programs than younger people).

Socioeconomic Status, Ethnicity, and Access to Care

Higher income and accessibility of care emerge as significant factors in determining utilization of early detection services from the literature on primary prevention of cancer in ethnic and poor populations (McCuskey & Morrow, 1980). Wilkinson and Wilson (1983) found that the greatest proportion of users of a cancer information service were women, from the higher social classes, and 20 to 39 years of age. Socioeconomic status (i.e., higher income) has been shown to have major ramifications on health resources, including accessibility, availability, utilization, quality, and continuity of health services, including state-of-the-art cancer screening, detection, treatment, and rehabilitation (Baquet & Rengen, 1985).

All the studies comparing whites and blacks document the fact that black patients are more likely to delay seeking medical attention when confronted with suspicious symptoms (Adams & Kerner, 1982; Bassett & Krieger, 1986; Gregorio, Cummings, & Michalek, 1983; Satariano, Belle, & Swanson, 1986). In general, black Americans delay from 3 to 7 months or more before seeking cancer detection and treatment. This affects the stage at diagnosis as well as the prognosis for treatment response. Specifically, the study by Gregorio and colleagues (1983) found that fewer than 40 per cent of white breast cancer cases remained untreated 6 months or longer after initial symptom recognition, compared with 52 per cent of black American breast cancer patients.

As discussed previously, black Americans tend to know less about cancer than whites, although the differences vary depending on specific cancers and screening and diagnostic tests. National surveys have found that blacks tend to underestimate the prevalence of cancer, tend to be more pessimistic than whites about their chances for survival should they get cancer, and are less likely to believe that early detection makes a difference or that existing treatments are effective.

Lack of knowledge and pessimism about cancer are not limited to a single racial group. A comprehensive national survey conducted by the ACS in 1985 found that, in comparison with the general population, Hispanics (1) believe to a lesser degree that early detection increases the chances of cure, (2) were less aware of the warning signals and specific cancer tests, and (3) were somewhat more fearful of developing cancer. Other barriers to early detection of cancer found in the survey and unique to this group were that Spanish was the language spoken by 63 per cent of the people at home, the majority had a clear preference for information in Spanish, one third had no medical insurance, and the majority were most comfortable with Spanish-speaking male physicians ("A study of Hispanics' attitudes," 1985). Belonging to a minority group would appear to be a significant barrier to early cancer detection owing to knowledge deficits and pessimism about the disease as well as language barriers to obtaining cancer information.

Although lack of knowledge among ethnic groups does contribute to delay in early detection of cancer, it is believed that socioeconomic status also plays a significant role. A dramatic illustration of the *interaction* between race and socioeconomic status was shown in a study by Freeman (1981) conducted at Harlem Hospital in New York City. Freeman noted that half of the 165 consecutive cases of breast cancer seen at Harlem Hospital were incurable at the time of the patient's admission; all of the Harlem patients were black and poor. The 5-year cure rate was 20 per cent, compared with 65 per cent in white American women (Freeman, 1981).

In studies that have considered SES and ethnic differences together (based on black/white comparison), controlling for SES greatly reduces (and sometimes nearly eliminates) the apparent mortality and incidence disparities between ethnic groups. This suggests that ethnic differences in cancer are largely secondary to socio-economic factors and associated processes (Subcommittee on Cancer, 1986, p. 9).

It is estimated that at least 50 per cent of the survival differential (seen in ethnic groups) is due to late diagnosis in the economically disadvantaged. This suggests a major role for early detection programs and improved access to treatment for the poor. It is postulated that social class (socioeconomic status) influences access to health care as well as early detection behaviors, thereby accounting for the differences in survival seen between ethnic groups and whites, as well as the differences between lower and upper socioeconomic status whites (Butler, King, & White, 1983; Denniston, 1981).

Further evidence of the role of socioeconomic status on early detection is shown in a study at the University of Iowa Hospital. The relationship of survival to economic status was studied on patients admitted from 1940 to 1969 for 39 different kinds of cancer. Results showed that indigent patients (patients receiving public aid, and who were nearly all white Americans) had poorer chances of survival. Because indigent as well as nonindigent groups of patients were treated in a uniform way by the same clinical team, quality of care was not a factor affecting the outcome. Because low socioeconomic status often adversely affects knowledge, attitudes, and behaviors, poor Americans are frequently seen with more advanced and therefore less localized disease at diagnosis. The poor in the United States frequently have a fatalism born of powerlessness. They tend to think in terms of the present rather than to be concerned with the future. "The reality of their situation places a high priority on sheer survival. Thus the struggle of living from day to day precludes concern about future health problems. In the case of cancer, this reality often makes early detection highly improbable" (Subcommittee on Cancer, 1986, p. 8). See Boxes 17–1 and 17–2 for two research studies that illustrate the barriers to early detection of breast cancer.

Health Belief Model Variables

Many researchers have used the health belief model to try to explain screening behaviors with varying degrees of success (McCusker & Morrow, 1980). In their study of 581 people who were offered a fecal occult blood test, Macrea and colleagues (1984) found the following:

1. Real and perceived susceptibility to colorectal cancer was positively related to acceptance of the Hemoccult kit.

2. Perceived barriers to taking the Hemoccult kit ("Embarrassing to test bowel action with the Hemoccult test" and "It would cause worry to test bowel action") contributed significantly to explaining differences between compliers and noncompliers.

Lack of perceived individual need to participate in early detection programs for colorectal cancer has been reported by others (Silman & Mitchell, 1984; Spector, Applegate, Olmstead, DiVasto, & Skipper, 1981). Spector and associates found in their study of 202 clinic patients that nonvolunteers were more likely to deny that they could have cancer (lack of perceived susceptibility to the disease) and objected to specific aspects of the early detection programs, such as sampling stool (perceived barriers). Two variables that have been shown to be barriers to early detection of cancer are the person's feeling that he or she could not get the disease (low susceptibility) and the perception that the difficulties in doing the early detection procedures are formidable (high barriers).

SELF-EXAMINATION TECHNIQUES

The self-examination techniques that are utilized in early detection of cancer are breast self-examination (BSE), testicular self-examination (TSE), self-administered Hemoccult testing, and oral self-examination. Hemoccult testing is designed to detect occult blood in the stool, and oral self-examination has been rec-

---

Box 17–1. BREAST SCREENING: COMPARING THOSE INVITED AND THOSE WHO REFUSE THE INVITATION

Two medical group practices in England invited all women in their practices (n = 2768) who were 50 to 70 years of age to undergo breast screening. Interviews were conducted with a random sample of the women who accepted the invitation (acceptors), those who declined the invitation (rejectors), and those who heard about breast screening and referred themselves. A random sample of 100 women from the first two groups and 50 from the last group was chosen and those women interviewed about personal and social characteristics, previous health behavior, and beliefs about cancer. The following results were reported:

1. Self-referred women were younger, belonged to higher socioeconomic classes, and more likely to be employed outside the home than acceptors and rejectors.
2. Self-referred women had a more extensive history of previous health-seeking behaviors than either the acceptors or rejectors.
3. Self-referred women reported more family and personal histories of breast disease and breast cancer than the acceptors or the rejectors.
4. Self-referred women had the strongest beliefs in the value of early detection of breast cancer.

The authors make the point that "the very high level of confidence in the value of early treatment found among the self-referred suggests that such confidence is an important element in prompting self-referral" (p. 22).

(Data from Hobbs, P., Smith, A., George, W., & Bellwood, R. [1980]. Acceptors and rejectors of an invitation to undergo breast screening compared with those who referred themselves. *Journal of Epidemiology and Community Health, 34,* 19–22.)

---

ommended for persons at risk for oral lesions (e.g., heavy smokers, those with a history of leukoplakia or erythroplakia). Breast self-examination, and self-administered Hemoccult testing have received the most intensive investigation and questioning, whereas there is a dearth of information or research on TSE and oral self-examination. Because breast and colorectal cancer are two of the leading causes of cancer deaths in the United States, subsequent discussion of self-examination techniques will focus primarily on BSE and self-administered Hemoccult testing.

Breast Self-Examination

The Breast Self-Examination Debate

For many years BSE has been advocated for all women as a screening technique for detecting breast cancers in the early clinical stage and thereby reducing mortality. It has been argued that BSE should be taught in connection with yearly physical examinations or other health-related encounters. There are two major arguments for encouraging BSE.

1. Research has documented that between 85 to 90 per cent of all breast cancers are discovered by women themselves (Carlile & Hadaway, 1985).

2. The National Institutes of Health–American Cancer Society Breast Cancer Detection Demonstration Projects reported that 17 per cent of the breast cancers were detected during intervals between visits (termed interval cancers) (Foster, Costanza, & Worden, 1985). Higher percentages of interval cancers have been reported by Tabar and colleagues (1985), who found that 20 to 25 per cent of breast cancers were detected in the interval between annual mammograms or clinical breast examinations, or both.

Breast self-examination was believed to be a cost-effective early detection method because it required no special equipment, needed no appointment with a health professional, and could be done in the privacy of a woman's home at her convenience. A series of Gallup surveys conducted for the ACS over the last decade have indicated a steady increase in women's awareness of BSE; it is now nearly universal at 95 per cent (Van Parijs, & Eckhardt, 1984). However, even though most women have heard of BSE, only 15 to 40 per cent are reported to perform it monthly (O'Malley & Fletcher, 1987).

More recently, there has been increasing debate about the merit of BSE. A recurring criticism is the

---

Box 17–2. WOMEN WHO DECLINE BREAST SCREENING

A random sample of 125 women who had been invited but declined an invitation to attend a breast screening clinic in Britain were interviewed. Their ages ranged from 45 to 64 years of age. When compared to women who attended the clinic: (1) they were of a lower socioeconomic class than the middle-class women who sought out breast screening, (2) they had a low record of using preventive facilities, (3) they had a limited knowledge about breast cancer, (4) the prospect of breast screening caused profound anxieties in those women who declined to attend the breast screening clinic. The authors point out that "most of the attributes of women who declined the invitation are not subject to rapid modification" (p. 281).

(Data from Maclean, U., Sinfield, D., Kleinn, S., & Harnden, B. [1984]. Women who decline breast screening. *Journal of Epidemiology and Community Health, 38,* 278–283.)

lack of prospective randomized controlled trials to establish the effectiveness of BSE in reducing breast cancer mortality (Diem & Rose, 1985; Frank & Mai, 1985). Studies measuring the effectiveness of treatment after screening by BSE have been retrospective or descriptive in design (Table 17–6). Most retrospective BSE data have been from women who have developed breast cancer, raising questions of recall bias.

The most recent and widely quoted study to support the argument that regular BSE does improve survival was done by Foster and colleagues (1978), in which they investigated the relationship of BSE to survival in 1004 newly diagnosed breast cancer patients. Survival at 5 years was 75 per cent for women who had practiced BSE versus 57 per cent for those who had not. Furthermore, they found that 90 per cent of the women who performed BSE detected their own breast cancers, and 50 per cent of the lesions were less than 2 cm in diameter when diagnosed. In contrast, 54 per cent of the women who never examined themselves discovered their cancers accidentally, and 23 per cent were less than 2 cm in diameter. Love (1985) points out that the improvement in survival may be illusory:

Absolute survival may not be improved but survival may appear lengthened by advancing the time of diagnosis (lead time bias). A second bias that may negate the apparent benefits from BSE is that patients with slower growing tumors and a more favorable prognosis more frequently find their cancers by BSE (length bias sampling). (p. 10)

Risks of Breast Self-Examination

Although it is rare to see any discussion of the risks of performing BSE, Frank and Mai (1985) argue that this self-examination technique does pose some potential risks to women.

1. Some women experience considerable anxiety when they examine their bodies for cancer.

Table 17–6. DESCRIPTIVE STUDIES OF THE EFFECTIVENESS OF TREATMENT FOLLOWING SCREENING BY BREAST SELF-EXAMINATION (BSE)

| | | | Tumor Size and Nodal Involvement by BSE Practice | | | | Tumor Stage by Detection Method | | | |
| | | | *BSE Performance* | | *Tumor Size, Mean or % <2 cm* | *No Nodal Involvement, %* | *Stage or Tumor Size by Detection Method* | | *BSE Detection/ ACC* Ratio* | *Significance Stage by Detection Method* |
Source, year	*Data*	No.	*Frequency*	%			*Method*	%		
Foster et al, 1978	Vermont Breast Cancer Network, 1975–1977	335	1/mo <1/mo NE	25 28 47	1.97 cm 2.47 cm 3.59 cm	60 57 43	NA*		NA	NA
Greenwald et al, 1978	Regional Breast Cancer Program, Northeastern New York & Western Massachusetts, 1975–1977	293	Yes No	28 72	NA	NA	Pathologic stage 0, 1 BSE ACC	22 17	1.29	NS*
Smith et al, 1980	Cancer Surveillance System, Seattle, 1977	230	>2/yr ≤2/yr	61 39	23% 22%	NA	Pathologic stage 0, 1 BSE > 2/yr BSE ≤ 2/yr	59 58	NA	NA
Senie et al, 1981	Memorial Sloan-Kettering Cancer Center, 1976–1978	1216	1/mo <1/mo orNE*	29 71	47% 43%	64 58	NA		NA	NS†
Huguley and Brown, 1981	Georgia Cancer Management Network, 1975–1979	2092	1/mo <1/mo NE	34 33 33	47%‡ 37%‡	57‡ 41	Pathologic stage 0, 1 BSE ACC	27 22	1.23	NA
Feldman et al, 1981	Brooklyn Breast Cancer Demonstration Network, 1975–1979	996	1/mo <1/mo Rarely NE	19 22 26 33	56%‡ 39%§	53 54 42 38	NA		NA	NA
Tamburini et al, 1981	Istituto Nationale Tumori, Milan, Italy, 1978–1979	500	1/mo <1/mo NE	11 24 65	37%‡ 21%‡	59‡ 49	NA		NA	NA
Gould-Martin et al, 1982	Los Angeles County Cancer Surveillance Program, 1976–1977	274	≥6/yr <6/yr NE	43 22 35	NA	59‡ 64	In situ or localized BSE ACC	52 59	0.89	NA
Hislop et al, 1984	British Columbia Cancer Registry, 1980–1982	416	1/mo <1/mo NE	54 18 28	21%* 14%	85‡ 78	NA		NA	NA
Owen et al, 1985	Oklahoma Hospitals Breast Cancer Control Network, 1975–1977	2063	NA		NA	NA	In situ or localized BSE ACC	58 52	1.12	NA
Smith and Burns, 1985	Iowa SEER, 1980–1982	365	≥2/yr <2/yr	56 44	NA	NA	In situ or localized BSE ACC	59 50	1.18	NS

*ACC indicates accidental patient detection; NA, not available; NS, not significant; NE, never.
†Nonsignificance noted but data not presented.
‡Monthly and less than monthly BSE categories combined.
§Rarely and never BSE categories combined.
(From O'Malley, M., & Fletcher, S. [1987]. Screening for breast cancer with breast self-examination. *Journal of the American Medical Association, 257,* 2197–2203. Copyright 1987, American Medical Association.)

2. There are potential risks of false reassurance (false-negative results) from BSE when a woman finds nothing. The sensitivity of BSE (the ability to detect a cancerous lump present in breast tissue) has been estimated to be 26 per cent, compared with an estimated sensitivity of 75 per cent for the combination of mammography and clinical breast examination (these estimates are from the Breast Cancer Detection Demonstration Project data) (O'Malley & Fletcher, 1987).

3. False-positive results are expensive, are time consuming, and result in unnecessary medical tests. A Finnish study found that in 56,177 women aged 20 to 80 years who were taught BSE, 750 women came to medical attention with breast symptoms in the first year and 300 in the second year of the study. Gastrin (1980) found a 99 per cent likelihood that a breast abnormality found by BSE was benign (predictive value for cancer of BSE in this study was 12 per cent). The results of another large-scale study in England indicated that only 43 cancers were identified from a total of 717 self-referrals (of 14,827 women), giving a predictive value for a positive BSE finding of 6 per cent (Holliday, Roebuck, & Doyle, 1983).

Because the evidence that BSE's accuracy (sensitivity and specificity) "appears to be considerably inferior to that of the combination of clinical breast examination and mammography," the United States Preventive Services Task Force makes no recommendation about the inclusion or exclusion of teaching BSE during the periodic health examination (1987, p. 2196). This task force (1987) also states that it endorses the following World Health Organization statement about BSE.

There is insufficient evidence that BSE as applied to date is effective in reducing mortality from breast cancer. Therefore BSE screening programmes are not at present recommended as public health policy, although there is equally insufficient evidence to change them where they already exist. (p. 2196)

Until there is definitive evidence on the long-term benefits or lack of long-term benefits of BSE, nurses should continue teaching this self-examination practice. Many researchers suggest that BSE will contribute to earlier detection of breast cancer and thereby will save lives. Although no proof exists that periodic BSE reduces mortality due to breast cancer, there is evidence to support this theory. Foster and colleagues (1985) caution that the degree of certainty that may be possible with randomized controlled trials would likely not be worth the cost of such studies with this approach. They make the point that prospective randomized studies do not provide 100 per cent certainty and are costly and time consuming, as well as being difficult to control for all extraneous variables. For instance, it would be impossible to control for information sharing that could occur through television, radio, and the printed media.

Research in Breast Self-Examination

The literature is replete with studies investigating the characteristics of women who practice and do not practice BSE. In general, women more likely to engage in BSE practice are younger, are better educated, are oriented toward prevention, have higher perceived vulnerability to breast cancer, and have been shown how to perform BSE by a health professional (Adams & Kerner, 1982; Hirshfield-Bartek, 1982; Bennett, Lawrence, Fleischman, Gifford, & Slack, 1983; Cole & Goman, 1984; Hallal, 1982; Kahn, 1984; Kegeles, 1985; Massey, 1986; McCusker & Morrow, 1980; Perez, Fair, Ihde, & Labrie, 1985). Nurses need to be cognizant of these characteristics when instructing women in this technique. A woman who does not believe in the value of early detection of cancer or who thinks that her chances of developing cancer are remote may not practice BSE. Thus teaching BSE should include a discussion of these attitudes as well as efforts to (1) promote the benefits of the early detection of breast cancer and (2) point out the research documenting that all women over the age of 35 in the United States should consider themselves at risk for breast cancer (Seidman, Stellman, & Mushinski, 1982).

Figure 17–1 is the United States National Institutes of Health (NIH)–recommended technique for BSE. All BSE instruction should include an opportunity for the woman to repeat the demonstration under the supervision of the nurse or health care professional doing the teaching. This gives the health professional the opportunity to increase the woman's confidence in her ability to do BSE as well as correct any mistakes in technique. Several different educational approaches have been used to improve BSE practice.

Group Approaches. Kegeles and Grady (1982) suggested that group procedures could improve knowledge, specific skills, and perhaps the quality of BSE but that it was uncertain whether they increased BSE frequency. Other evaluations of group approaches included 6-month follow-ups. However, whether performance would be sustained after 6 months was unclear. Marty, McDermott, and Gold (1983) and Boyle, Michalek, Bersani, Nemoto, and Mettlin (1981) exemplify the BSE research on the group approach. Marty and associates (1983) randomly assigned 219 female college students to one of three groups. One group was given ACS pamphlets on BSE, one group was exposed to discussions by a facilitator who covered breast disease and models of BSE, and one group was assigned to a program containing the features of modeling with the addition of guided practice. The group exposed to modeling and guided practice had more positive attitudes about the benefits of BSE than the other two groups ($P < 0.01$) and a higher practice frequency on follow-up ($P < 0.05$).

Wilkes's approach (1983) was two tiered. The first part was presented to nurses and included didactic (lecture) and psychomotor practice. At the end of the experience, nurses could become certified instructors in BSE. The intent was to have the nurses become active teachers in BSE programs to lay women and their partners. The second portion was a model for programs presented in the community to lay audiences. This program included lectures, pamphlets, and breast models for practicing on. At the 3-month follow-up they found the following:

Breast Self-Examination

Breast self-examination (BSE) should be done once a month so that you become familiar with the usual appearance and feel of your breasts. Familiarity makes it easier to notice any changes in the breast from one month to another. Early discovery of a change from what is "normal" is the main idea behind BSE. The outlook is much better if you detect cancer in an early stage.

If you menstruate, the best time to do BSE is 2 or 3 days after your period ends, when your breasts are least likely to be tender or swollen. If you no longer menstruate, pick a particular day, such as the first day of the month, to remind yourself it is time to do BSE.

Some women do the next part of the exam in the shower because fingers glide over soapy skin, making it easy to concentrate on the texture underneath.

Here is one way to do BSE:

1. Stand before a mirror. Inspect both breasts for anything unusual such as any discharge from the nipples or puckering, dimpling, or scaling of the skin.

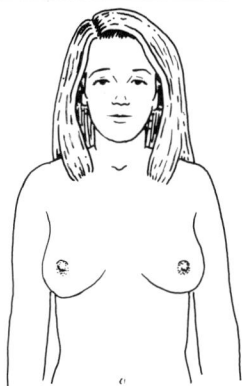

The next two steps are designed to emphasize any change in the shape or contour of your breasts. As you do them, you should be able to feel your chest muscles tighten.

2. Watching closely in the mirror, clasp your hands behind your head and press your hands forward.

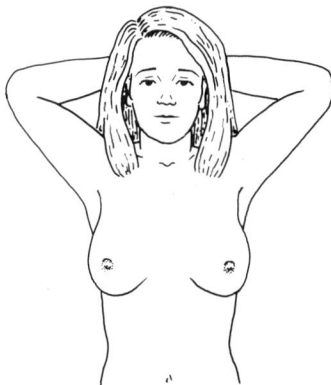

3. Next, press your hands firmly on your hips and bow slightly toward your mirror as you pull your shoulders and elbows forward.

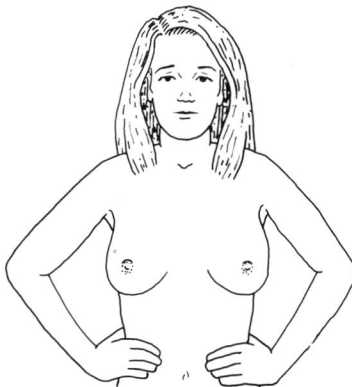

4. Raise your left arm. Use three or four fingers of your right hand to explore your left breast firmly, carefully, and thoroughly. Beginning at the outer edge, press the flat part of your fingers in small circles, moving the circles slowly around the breast. Gradually work toward the nipple. Be sure to cover the entire breast. Pay special attention to the area between the breast and the underarm, including the underarm itself. Feel for any unusual lump or mass under the skin.

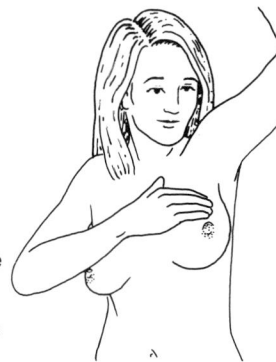

5. Gently squeeze the nipple and look for a discharge. (If you have any discharge during the month—whether or not it is during BSE—see your doctor.) Repeat steps 4 and 5 on your right breast.

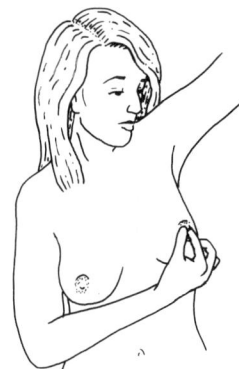

6. Steps 4 and 5 should be repeated lying down. Lie flat on your back with your left arm over your head and a pillow or folded towel under your left shoulder. This position flattens the breast and makes it easier to examine. Use the same circular motion described earlier. Repeat the exam on your right breast.

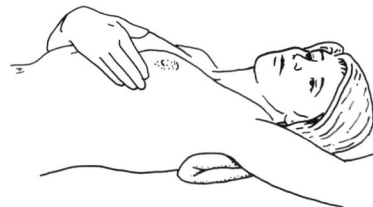

Figure 17–1. Recommendations for conducting breast self-examination. (From National Institutes of Health. [1983]. *Breast cancer: We're making progress every day* [USDHHS Publication No. NIH 83–2409]. Bethesda, MD: National Cancer Institute.)

1. In a sample of 110 nurses, 97 per cent reported practicing BSE 3 months after instruction, with 85 per cent doing so at least monthly.

2. In a sample of 305 lay people, 82 per cent reported regular practice, with 87 per cent reporting at least monthly practice. However, at the 6-month follow-up, fewer than 25 per cent of the certified nurses had taught BSE. The reasons for lack of participation were not enough time, lack of confidence, never being asked, and not feeling comfortable in front of groups.

Wilkes writes that nurses who take the course in the future should be told that it is expected that they will promote and teach BSE to others.

Individual Approaches. Kegeles and Grady (1982) reviewed the literature related to individual approaches to teaching BSE. They report that this method appeared successful in attracting both low users of health services and women at high risk for cancer. As with the group approach, the individual approach has attempted to increase the frequency of BSE with some success up to 6 months' duration (Kegeles, 1985). Three studies typify the individual approach. Shamian and Edgar (1987) designed a quasi-experimental, one-group pretest-posttest study to determine the role of nurses as agents for change in teaching BSE. Data were collected from 223 women who had been exposed to a predetermined educational program (posters, charts, group session) and one-to-one teaching by nurse-clinicians. Their findings, based on a pretest, posttest, and 6-month follow-up, concluded that nurses influenced positively the factual and proficiency knowledge base of clients as well as the frequency of BSE practice. At the pretest, 13 per cent of the women were regular practitioners and at the 6-month follow-up after the educational intervention, 52 per cent of the women were regular practitioners. Although nurses have the potential to positively influence women to practice BSE, Sawyer (1986) found in her study that few hospital-based nurses were asking female patients about BSE. Furthermore, she found that fewer than one fourth of them taught correct BSE technique to hospitalized patients. She makes the point that nurses are missing opportunities to provide this valuable health promotion information to their clients.

The research by Hall and colleagues (1980) is representative of individual training using models. Twenty female volunteers were given a pretest and two posttests that consisted of an examination of both breasts of each of six women with known palpable benign breast lesions. The 20 volunteers received a training session on silicone models. Hall and colleagues found that "proficiency in examination of natural breast tissue can be dramatically increased following a brief training procedure incorporating realistic simulated breasts with graduated lumps" (p. 412). The training session resulted in increased confidence in the examination skill as well as an increased frequency of reported false-positive results. Although the increase in false-positive findings is a problem that needs to be addressed, the increase in confidence in women's BSE skills is highly desirable. The only intraindividual characteristics that have consistently differentiated frequent and less-fre-

quent practitioners of BSE are knowledge of how it should be done and confidence in one's BSE ability (Kegeles, 1985).

Whereas the definitive research on the impact of BSE on survival still needs to be done, nurses are urged to use every opportunity both during work and in the community to encourage and educate women in BSE. Even though, as this review has shown, there are risks and significant questions to be answered about BSE, it would appear that it is better to err on the side of overcaution than to abandon the practice entirely.

Self-Administered Hemoccult Testing

Colorectal cancer incidence and mortality among men and women in the United States are second only to those of lung cancer. However, the same concerns that are raised about BSE are raised about Hemoccult (blood in stool) testing. Does early detection of colorectal cancer through Hemoccult testing result in a decrease in mortality from that disease? At present, a large-scale randomized prospective study is being conducted in Minnesota to answer this question. Over 45,000 volunteers have been assigned to one of the following three groups:

1. Screened for occult blood every other year.
2. Screened annually for occult blood.
3. Not screened at all (control group).

The study is now 12 years old and represents the only true prospective randomized controlled study on this topic in the United States (Minnesota study aimed at finding final answer, 1987). It is important to note that the use of a parallel control group should eventually permit assessment of cancer outcome relatively free of lead time, length, and selection biases. According to Simon (1985, p. 829), Gilbertson (the principal investigator of the Minnesota study) has acknowledged that until the results of this study are known, "there is no proof of the merit of hemoccult examination in improving the prognosis for people with colorectal cancer."

The original guaiac test depended on the reaction between a colorless dye (gum guaiac) and hemoglobin in the presence of hydrogen peroxide to yield a blue color. This test resulted in a high number of both false-positive and false-negative results (Alquist, McGill, & Schwartz, 1984). At present, most of the tests are done with guaiac-impregnated cards that have the advantage of permitting some storage before they are tested. In the Hemoccult test gum guaiac is impregnated in a test paper, and hydrogen peroxide is provided in a developer solution. The resultant phenolic oxidation of guaiac in the presence of blood yields a blue color (Simon, 1985). However, there are still problems with false-positive and false negative results, including the following:

1. False-negative results can be due to the ingestion of an oxidizing agent such as ascorbic acid or to a delay of more than 5 days in developing the test.

2. The test appears to be more sensitive for cancer

than for adenoma because the false-negative rate is higher for adenoma (Winawer, 1983).

3. The reaction is not specific for human hemoglobin, and contamination can occur with dietary vegetable peroxidases and meat, causing false-positive results.

4. Aspirin, iron, and cimetidine can give false-positive reaction.

5. Research indicates that these tests do not detect the portion of hemoglobin that is converted to porphyrins in the gut (Alquist et al., 1984).

6. Rehydration of slides increases the possibility of false-positive results (Simon, 1985). (See Chapter 15 for an in-depth research study on the value of rehydration of fecal occult blood slides.)

Numerous causes for false-negative tests exist, including the fact that not all tumors cause bleeding, occult blood may not be uniformly distributed in the feces, and the test simply does not detect fecal blood losses of less than 20 ml/day. Simon (1985) writes that at least 33 per cent and perhaps 50 per cent of colorectal cancers in a screened population can be missed. Thus the sensitivity of occult blood testing (the proportion of diseased subjects who have a positive result) is low, probably only in the 50 to 65 per cent range.

Compliance is another significant problem in any discussion of early detection of colorectal cancer. Reported compliance rates based on literature reviews vary tremendously. Morrow and colleagues (1982) report compliance rates between 30 and 80 per cent, Box and associates (1984) between 27 and 42 per cent in asymptomatic people and 92.5 per cent in symptomatic patients, and Simon (1985) a low of 15 per cent to a high of 98 per cent, with most in the 50 to 70 per cent range. Three studies that most carefully document compliance with Hemoccult test reported compliance rates ranging from 22 per cent to less than 30 per cent (Elwood, Erickson, & Lieberman, 1978; Morrow et al., 1982; Winchester et al., 1980).

The Third International Symposium on Colorectal Cancer held in 1983 issued recommendations for obtaining fecal occult blood tests; these are provided in Box 17–3. Other recommendations designed to decrease false-negative and false-positive results include (1) women should not be tested during or immediately following a menstrual period (Rakel, 1983), and some clinicians recommend that people should eat plenty of fruits and vegetables and moderate amounts of fiber-containing foods to stimulate colorectal lesions to bleed (Leffall, 1981). To date the value of a high-residue diet during the 3 days of testing has never been validated (Simon, 1985). Several new tests designed to remedy problems encountered with the widely used Hemoccult tests are available commercially.

1. *HemoQuant.* HemoQuant is a quantitative test that measures human blood loss with a high degree of sensitivity and specificity and is designed to enhance clinical validity. The advantages of this test are that (1) it is unaffected by stool hydration and storage, dietary peroxidases (which reduce false-positive results), iron, and ascorbic acid; (2) it detects both upper and lower gastrointestinal bleeding with equal sensitiv-

ity (Simon, 1985); (3) it does not require dietary prescription and thus it may result in higher compliance rates (Winawer, Schottenfeld, & Sherlock, 1985). A disadvantage is that it requires greater stool sampling than present tests do.

2. *Immunochemical Detection.* A test developed by Songster and colleagues (1980) is reported to detect human hemoglobin and not be affected by animal heme, drugs, or foodstuffs. This test eliminates dietary and chemical restrictions placed on people who participate. The researchers report that the smear is stable for up to 30 days; however, there is a 24- to 48-hour delay between receiving and interpreting the test. It is technically very simple and may enhance specificity (Winawer et al., 1985).

3. *Immunochemical Test* (using blood serum). Louvard from the Pasteur Institute in Paris has developed a simple, inexpensive immunochemical blood test that relies on the determination of the blood level of villin. Villin is a protein found mainly in the absorptive cells of the small and large intestines, as well as in the duct cells of the pancreas and biliary system and the cells of kidney proximal tubules. Cells of other organs contain little to no villin. Preliminary data show that false-positive results do not exceed 10 per cent and false-negative results are as high as 50 per cent. If the ratio of false-negative results is reduced, this test could become a major tool for the diagnosis of colorectal cancer (Dorozynski, 1987).

Fecal occult blood testing has not been proved to reduce mortality; however, it is anticipated that the prospective, randomized study being conducted in Minnesota will provide the definitive answer in the near future. The present method of obtaining fecal occult blood (Hemoccult slides) has low sensitivity and requires dietary and drug restrictions to avoid false-positive and false-negative results. For screening and early detection, it is most important to avoid false-negative findings; thus tests with high sensitivity are desired. Low compliance rates have been reported in a majority of large-scale screening programs, and compliance has been shown to decrease with age. Many of the issues raised about BSE are also raised with self-administered occult blood testing. Until definitive answers are known, nurses are urged to use every professional encounter to educate and motivate people over the age of 40 years (or earlier if they have known risk factors) to participate in colorectal screening for cancer.

Because compliance decreases with advancing age, special education and motivation efforts need to be directed toward elderly persons who live alone.

Testicular Self-Examination

Although cancer of the testes accounts for only about 1 per cent of all male cancers, it is the most common type of cancer in men between 20 and 36 years of age. Two groups of men have a greater risk of developing testicular cancer: those whose testes have not descended into the scrotum and those whose testes de-

Box 17–3. RECOMMENDATIONS ON PERFORMING A FECAL OCCULT BLOOD TEST FROM THE THIRD INTERNATIONAL SYMPOSIUM ON COLORECTAL CANCER, 1983

1. The patient should avoid rare red meat and high peroxidase foods for three days *before* and during testing. High peroxidase foods include broccoli, turnip, rare red meat, cauliflower, parsnip, cabbage, potato, and cantalope. These foods can give a false-positive reaction.
2. Vitamin C, iron tablets, and nonsteroidal anti-inflammatory drugs should be avoided. Vitamin C will give a false-negative reaction.
3. The delay between preparation and laboratory testing should not exceed 6 days.
4. Slides should *not* be rehydrated. Rehydrating the stool samples by adding a drop of water to them induces false-positive reactions.
5. Two samples of each of three consecutive stools should be tested (*six smears*). Increasing the number of samples tested from each stool will make up for the nonuniform distribution of blood in stools, especially from left-sided lesions. The sample size must be sufficient to produce a detectable blue color; patients must be instructed to cover the whole test slide with fecal material.
6. *Important:* A single positive smear should be considered a positive test and lead to the recommended work-up, even in the absence of dietary restrictions. Having the patient repeat the slide testing is not recommended.

(Data from Gnauck, R., MacRae, F., & Fleisher, M. [1984]. How to perform a fecal occult blood test. *CA: A Cancer Journal for Clinicians, 34,* 130–133.)

scended after the age of 6. Testicular cancer is 10 to 40 times more likely to develop in these men (National Cancer Institute, 1985).

Ten years ago, testicular cancer was often fatal because it spread rapidly to vital organs, particularly the lungs. Recent advances in treatment have made cancer of the testes one of the most curable cancers, especially if detected and treated promptly.

The most common symptom of testicular cancer is a painless scrotal mass. Mild testicular pain, a dull ache, and dragging sensation in the lower abdomen, groin, or scrotum are other symptoms of testicular cancer (Ganong & Markovitz, 1987). Benign conditions that can be confused with testicular tumors include hydrocele, varicocele, spermatocele, torsion, and hematoma (Reno, 1988). Although never evaluated systematically as a screening or early detection method, it is generally thought that regular testicular self-examination (TSE) will provide the opportunity for early diagnosis of testicular cancer.

Studva (1983) suggests professional clinical testicular examination be performed in the following manner. The client should be examined in both the supine and the standing positions. In the supine position, suspected varicocele can be ruled out because this entity will collapse when the client is lying down with the scrotum elevated. The firmness and weight of a testicular tumor can be evaluated best in the upright position. Orderly examination of the intrascrotal contents is recommended. If the client has symptoms, the uninvolved testis should be examined first to serve as a baseline. The testes should be carefully palpated between the thumb and first two fingers. Generally, the glands are fairly uniform in size and consistency and move freely. Any area of induration, nodularity, or irregularity should be considered a tumor until proved otherwise. The epididymis and the spermatic cord should be palpated along their entire course.

Nine studies have investigated knowledge about testicular cancer and practice of TSE. The findings of these studies are summarized in Table 17–7. In general, it continues to be true that most men are not knowledgeable about testicular cancer or TSE, nor do they regularly practice this skill. Ganong and Markovitz (1987) suggest that lack of knowledge may be the consequence of (1) a general denial among young men that they are "at risk" for any health problem, (2) failure to actively seek out information about personal health care or to have regular checkups in this age group, or (3) lack of awareness about testicular cancer by health care providers or their hesitation to discuss this potentially embarrassing subject with their male clients. Reasons cited by subjects for not practicing TSE included forgetfulness, not remembering the proper technique, not feeling it was necessary to do it at their age, not concerned about getting cancer at this time, and too busy (Reno, 1988; Rovinski, 1980).

Nurses can help to decrease the current testicular cancer and TSE information gap that exists among young men. First and foremost, nurses' personal knowledge deficits must be filled. Then creative approaches to educating these men need to be investigated. Integrating men's health issues into school health curricula needs further exploration, as does reaching the young man through health fairs. The effectiveness of educating late grade school and junior high school boys (boys who are most likely to have required health examinations for school) about TSE also needs to be examined. Finally, the influence of regular TSE on testicular cancer mortality has not been investigated and clearly needs further study if monthly self-examination technique for all men is to be recommended, given that only about 1 per cent of the population will develop this disease.

DIAGNOSTIC TECHNIQUES

The early detection of cancer is the attempt to diagnose cancer in its earliest, most treatable stage.

Table 17–7. STUDIES OF MEN'S KNOWLEDGE OF TESTICULAR CANCER AND TSE

Reference	Sample	Methodology	Findings
Conklin et al. (1978)	90 randomly chosen college men (ages 18–23).	Interview developed by the researchers.	75% had never heard of TC; none knew how to do TSE; 75% said they would probably do TSE.
Cummings, Lampone, Mettlin, & Potes, (1983)	266 male students (ages 17–41); convenience sample drawn from health courses.	Questionnaire; investigated knowledge.	42% knew age at greatest risk; 52% did not know any symptoms; 16% had heard of TSE but only 33% of these had done TSE; 88% interested in learning TSE.
Goldenring & Purtell (1984)	147 male college athletes (ages 18–23).	Interviews during physical examination; Investigated knowledge and practice.	12.9% knew TC was most common in their age group; 9.5% had been taught TSE; 6.1% had done TSE.
Ostwald & Rothenberger (1985)	577 male high school and college students.	Questionnaire developed by researchers was given to men who viewed a slide tape on TSE; investigated knowledge and practice.	61% had heard of TC; 54% had no information about TSE; 14% did TSE regularly; 75% of a follow-up group did TSE after instruction.
Thornhill et al. (1986)	395 Irish men (ages 21–65), selected because they had more education and were from higher SES groups.	Mailed questionnaire to 500 men (395 responded).	32% unaware of TSE; 87% did not know high-risk ages; 72% did not know any symptoms; 8% knew of TSE; 5% did TSE regularly; 90% wanted more information.
Blesch (1986)	Random sample of 129 men drawn from a group of 3300 professional men employed in a telecommunications firm.	Mailed questionnaire developed by the researcher sent to 233 men; investigated practice, knowledge, and relationship of health beliefs to TSE and TC.	61% had heard of TC; 31% knew of TSE; 9.5% practiced TSE; 96% said lack of knowledge was a barrier to doing TSE.
Ganong & Markovitz (1987)	A convenience sample of 64 male college students (ages 18–36).	Survey-questionnaire investigated knowledge and intention to do TSE.	18% had heard of TSE; 5% had done TSE; 49 of 50 who never heard of TSE wanted to learn about it; exposure to brief printed information increased intentions to perform TSE this week and this month ($P<0.001$).
Reno (1988)	Convenience sample of 126 male college students.	Questionnaire measured knowledge and beliefs about TSE and TC.	12 reported TSE practice, and of these 41% practiced monthly; 87% of the 114 who did not practice TSE had not heard of TSE; 88.9% reported that if given TSE information, they would practice TSE.
Rudolph & MacEwen-Quinn (1988)	Convenience sample of 64 male college students (ages 17–24).	Modified Blesch's questionnaire; assessed TSE practice before and after video tape and didactic program.	Before education, 22% claimed TSE practice; 8 weeks after intervention there was no significant increase in TC knowledge, but 39 of the initial 61 who never practiced TSE did so after the education session.

TC, Testicular cancer; TSE, testicular self-examination; SES, socioeconomic status.
(Modified with permission from Ganong, L. H., & Markovitz, J. [1987]. Young men's knowledge of testicular cancer and behavioral intentions toward testicular self-exam. *Patient Education & Counseling, 9,* 253.)

Clearly screening is an important strategy for achieving this goal. However, certain diagnostic techniques must also be employed to rule out or confirm the actual presence of a cancer. The following section details the nurse's role in diagnosis.

Obtaining the History

Frequently the first contact a person has with the health care system is with a nurse. The nurse establishes the tone of future interactions and obtains the initial health history. When obtaining the health history, it is important to inquire into risk factors for cancer that are related to the chief complaint. It is not uncommon for people to supply vague, nondescriptive complaints in the hope that the physician will find nothing wrong. They may in fact have very specific signs and symptoms that they consciously withhold from the health professional, particularly if they are frightened. Therefore, when taking a health history, the nurse needs to carefully question the person about any early signs, symptoms, and risk factors for cancer specifically related to the chief complaint as well as other cancer-related risk factors.

Elements of the history that are important aids to the clinician include the family, social, occupational, and past medical histories (Kahn, 1983). A complete sexual history also provides important information. For instance, women at risk for cancer of the reproductive organs can be identified when a thorough and complete gynecologic and sexual history has been obtained. Because early age of first intercourse, multiple sexual partners, and a history of human papillomavirus (HPV) infection are key risk factors for cervical cancer, it is important that the nurse include questions about these areas. Chapter 16 details the known risk factors and early signs and symptoms for individual cancers.

Elements of a Complete History

The history should contain questions that will enable the nurse to identify known risk factors for cancer. Identification of risk factors is essential for effective client education as well as for alerting the other health professionals about potential problem areas. "Risk factors also form the basis for a hypothesis about what might be wrong with the patient even before details of the history of the present illness completely unfold" (Kahn, 1983, p. 270).

Family History. A family history should include information about acute and chronic illnesses of blood relatives and exact causes of deaths. Cancer should be specifically inquired about, including asking about the presence of "tumors" and "growths."

Social History. Significant risk factors for cancer include tobacco, alcohol, and drug use. If the client has any of these habits, the length of use, amounts, complications from use of the substance, side effects, and attempts to quit should be detailed. Sexual history should include the number of partners, type of sexual protection commonly used (such as barrier methods), history of venereal disease, specifically condyloma and herpes simplex, abnormal Papanicolaou smears, and follow-up. A residential history should be obtained, and exposure to environmental pollutants in these residences determined. Military experience and known military exposures (e.g., to Agent Orange) should also be inquired about of both men and women. An occupational history is frequently included in the social history and includes asking about the person's lifetime area of employment, work locations, work materials used in the occupational setting, illness of other workers, carcinogenic exposures if known, and required safety procedures or equipment to avoid exposures. A history of hobbies or leisure-time activities and toxic materials to which the client may have been exposed while working on hobbies should be also obtained.

Past Health History. Ideally, the following information should be obtained: all prior acute and chronic illnesses and their treatments; past x-ray treatments, including treatments for acne, swollen tonsils, and enlarged thymus (a practice abandoned in the 1950s); maternal use of diethylstilbestrol (DES); blood transfusions; past surgeries; all prior medications (including birth control pills); vitamins, over-the-counter drugs; relevant dietary practices and, if appropriate, a history of obesity; reproductive history, including mensus and menopause history.

When obtaining the history, questions should be phrased in a manner that will ensure the client will understand. Shortridge and McLain (1979) suggest that, when asking about the review of systems for the urinary system,

. . . rather than asking "Do you have any hesitance?" ask

instead a more specific symptoms-oriented question such as "Do you have to wait for your stream to begin?" or "Does your stream stop while you still have the urge to void/urinate?" Such phrasing is more apt to uncover subtle symptoms of obstruction otherwise overlooked.

It is important to remember that cultural beliefs influence not only health practices but also perceptions of what merits medical attention. For instance, a man who believes or has been told by friends that a growing feeling of heaviness in his scrotum is a sign of increasing virility will not perceive this symptom to merit medical attention. Nurses must make a conscious effort to acquaint themselves with the folk beliefs and health practices of different cultural groups, particularly those with whom they come into contact. Open-ended questions during the health assessment encourage the client to express his or her health beliefs; in addition, the nurse may be able to identify myths and misconceptions relating to the chief complaint and present illness. One method of encouraging sharing of culturally determined health beliefs is to open a discussion with the statement, "Many people believe that . . ." Frequently people are reticent to share their health beliefs with health professionals because they are afraid they will be laughed at, so the nurse should avoid value judgments. By openly identifying and acknowledging that a health belief is held by many people, the nurse makes it easier for the client to admit he or she also believes these statements to be true. Once misconceptions are identified, the nurse has a professional and moral obligation to alter false opinions that will prevent early detection of cancer and facilitate corrective education. However, as with any effective teaching, it should take place when the learner is receptive.

Physical Examination and Diagnostic Testing

The process of history taking and physical examination leads to formulation of a differential diagnosis by the physician. It is at this point that laboratory and radiologic tests designed to aid in the determination of a correct diagnosis are ordered. Table 17–8 lists the sensitivity and specificity of commonly used approaches to the diagnosis of cancer. Some diagnostic testing can be done during the physical examination (e.g., the Papanicolaou smear). However, most testing necessary to confirm the diagnosis of cancer requires the person to return to the health care setting for additional testing. Table 17–9 lists the physical assessment and diagnostic tests for each anatomic site used to confirm cancer. Although this table includes many recommended physical assessment techniques, the reader is referred to any standard physical assessment textbook for a more comprehensive discussion and to Tables 17–2, 17–3, and 17–4 for the recommended screening frequencies. The anatomic system(s) to which the chief complaint and present illness refer should be examined meticulously, as should common sites of metastasis. The physical examination should be thorough and include all four of the cardinal techniques of physical

Table 17–8. TESTS IN THE DIAGNOSIS OF CANCER

Test	Diagnosis	Staging	Sensitivity	Specificity	PV
I Routine blood or urine studies (complete blood count, urine, multiphasic biochemical screen)	+	−	Fair-good	Fair-poor	Low
II Routine x-ray studies (chest, intravenous pyelogram, upper and lower gastrointestinal series, mammogram) (only chest radiograph is used in staging)	+	− to +	Good-excellent	Good	Medium
III Special x-ray or imaging and endoscopic studies (ultrasonography, computed tomography, lymphangiography, angiography)	+	+	Good-excellent	Good	High
IV Radionuclide scanning (liver, bone, gallium)	−	+	Good	Poor	Low
V Biochemical markers (acid phosphatase, beta chorionic gonadotropin, alpha ± = fetoprotein, carcinoembryonic antigen)	+ to −	+	Good-excellent	Good-excellent	High

PV, Predictive value in diagnosis of symptomatic patients.

+, Useful; −, not useful; ±, may be useful selectively.

(From Kahn, S. B. [1983]. Cancer diagnosis. In S. Kahn, R. Love, C. Sherman, & R. Chakravorty [Eds.], *Concepts in cancer medicine* [pp. 267–287]. New York: Grune & Stratton, Inc. Reproduced by permission.)

assessment: inspection, palpation, percussion, and auscultation. Cancer is diagnosed using appropriate combinations of the following: cytologic methods, biochemical tests, radiographic techniques, clinical examination, and endoscopy.

NURSING RESPONSIBILITIES

Early detection of cancer is a complex issue that involves many separate decisions on the part of both the consumer and the health professional. On the one hand, health care professionals must actively strive to integrate cancer screening and detection into their day-to-day clinical practices. On the other hand, it is incumbent on the individual to make a conscious decision to seek the services of a health professional for a cancer detection examination or test or to report a suspicious symptom. The suspicious sign or symptom may have been discovered through the decision to engage in a cancer detection self-examination technique (e.g., BSE, TSE), or it may have been discovered accidentally. Once the person has contacted a health professional, the health professional in turn must judge how extensive the history, physical examination, and laboratory tests will be. If a suspicious symptom or finding is present, a tentative hypothesis about its cause is formulated.

The previous discussion has clearly shown that there is tremendous variation in who decides to practice cancer detection self-examination techniques, who decides to seek the services of health care professionals for early detection of cancer, and what diagnostic tests can be used in the detection of cancer. The task of the nursing profession is to continue to identify the barriers

to early detection that occur in persons and groups and to design, implement, and evaluate interventions that will assist in removing or decreasing these barriers. For example, research has shown that the elderly have significant delay in reporting the signs and symptoms of cancer owing to transportation difficulties, lack of financial resources, assumptions that the signs and symptoms are part of the normal aging process, and reluctance to undergo cancer treatments. Designing inexpensive early detection programs for the elderly in which the screeners go out into the community is one method to decrease barriers created by transportation needs and lack of financial resources. These programs could be offered in Golden Age Clubs, nursing homes, residential centers for the elderly, food gathering centers, and day care centers for the elderly.

The nurse needs to recognize that the barriers to early detection differ in geographic location and with different racial, ethnic, religious, and socioeconomic groups. What works with one group of people in one part of the country may not work equally well somewhere else. Thus it is essential that the nurse be familiar with the research on the barriers to early detection found in the groups he or she works with the most.

Nurses need to consider using creative as well as cost effective, nontraditional approaches when designing cancer early detection programs. For instance, the church is the focal point of the political and social activities in the typical black community, and most black churches have a health-oriented guild within the church structure. Early detection programs could be held in these churches using nurses and other health care professionals who are church members. This community-based approach has been used in the past with other diseases commonly found in black Americans

Table 17-9. CANCER DETECTION: PHYSICAL EXAMINATION AND DIAGNOSTIC TESTING

Site	Physical Examination	Diagnostic Testing
Cervical Cancer ("ACS modified guideline," 1987; Perez, Knapp, Disaia, & Young, 1985; Smith, Clarke-Pearson, & Creasman, 1985).	**Vagina:** Evaluate consistency of cervix, check for presence of papilloma, Bartholin's cysts, unusual vaginal discharge and tissue friability; evaluate depth of vaginal fornices; check size, position, and mobility of uterus; evaluate color, discharge, and presence of any lesions. **Rectum:** Evaluate elasticity and softness of parametrium; evaluate Douglas' pouch (retro-uterine pouch)—normally not palpable; evaluate consistency and shape of cervix; evaluate size, position, and mobility of uterus.	**Papanicolaou smear:** Cytologic examination of exfoliated cervical cells; sample taken from transition zone, ectocervix, and endocervix. **Colposcopy:** The vagina and cervix are washed with acetic acid to highlight abnormal tissue and then examined with magnifying instrument; colposcopy is done following an abnormal Papanicolaou smear or the presence of cervical lesions; a directed biopsy may be done if abnormal tissue is found. **Conization:** A cone-shaped excision is made of the abnormal areas of the cervix. **Biopsy:** In the presence of gross lesions, multiple punch biopsies are taken.
Endometrial Cancer	**Vagina:** Palpate vagina, sub-uretheral areas, and meatus to detect metastases. **Rectum:** Palpate cul-de-sac of Douglas, noting consistency and thickening; palpate rectum for extension of neoplasm.	**Endometrial biopsy:** Use a Novack curette or less widely used Gravlee jet washer to obtain specimens. **Suction curettage:** Tissue is obtained from endometrial cavity. **Fractional dilatation and curettage (D & C):** This is done if endometrial pathology is suspected. **Colposcopy:** Colposcopy is used for directed biopsies of abnormal sites in the vagina.
Vaginal Cancer	**Inspect** vulva and palpate vagina, noting areas of induration; note vaginal bands and cervical structural changes; rotate speculum to visualize entire vagina (vividly red focal areas should arouse suspicion).	
Ovarian Cancer (Khan, Slack, & Cosgrove, 1985; Sargris, 1983; Young, Knapp, Fules, & Disaia, 1985)	**Inspect** for skin signs of abdominal distention, contour for distention, masses (generalized or symmetrical or asymmetrical), bulging flanks. **Palpate** for masses and tenderness. **Percussion:** Solid tumor is dull to percussion and fluid wave will be dull to percussion. **Bimanual pelvic examination:** Palpate adenexa for masses; any enlargement in a premenarchal or postmenopausal woman should be evaluated; solid, bilateral, or fixed masses greater than 10 cm should raise suspicion of malignancy; palpate cul-de-sac via rectovaginal examination (nodularity in cul-de-sac is suspect).	**Ultrasound:** Used in prestaging assessment of suspected ovarian cancer and preoperatively to assess degree of tumor extension in pelvic, abdominal, and retroperitoneal regions; high level of accuracy in detecting tumors. **Lymphangiography:** For prestaging evaluation of women known or suspected to have ovarian cancer. **Computed tomography:** Computed tomography (CT) provides additional diagnostic and staging information.
Breast Cancer (Carlile & Hadaway, 1985; Paulus, 1987)	**Inspection:** Sitting with arms at the side, sitting with arms elevated, sitting with pectoral muscle contraction, sitting bending forward. **Palpation:** Inspect breasts with patient in sitting and supine positions with superficial palpation for thickening and temperature changes, and with deeper palpation for lesions; palpate with patient in sitting position for women with pendulous breasts and women with present or past complaints of breast masses; supine: have women lie in left and right lateral decubitus positions to check for lesions between ribs. **Examine** nipples for discharge and fix discharge for cytologic examination.	**Film-screen mammography or xeromammography:** These methods detect noninvasive or invasive cancers smaller than 0.5 cm. **Galactography:** Used in evaluation of nipple discharge; detects papillomas; water-soluble contrast medium is injected into duct. **Pneumocystography:** Mammography is performed after removal of fluid and introduction of air into a breast cyst; this is definitive in the detection of intracystic tumors.
Stomach Cancer (Macdonald, Cohn, & Gunderson, 1985; Thompson, 1985)	**Abdominal examination:** Inspect contour for ascites, peristaltic waves (which move from left to right), pallor of mucous membranes indicating anemia, jaundice. **Palpate abdomen:** Check painless mass in epigastrium (cancer of stomach is palpable to left of midline). Nodular liver may indicate metastasis to liver; ovarian mass (Krukenberg tumors) may indicate metastasis to ovaries; check for umbilical metastasis. **Percussion of abdomen:** Check for dullness, ascites, fluid wave, shifting dullness, puddle test done for small amounts of fluid in the abdomen; palpate nodes in supraclavicular region (Virchow's node is usually on the left) and axillary region. **Rectal examination:** Palpate cul-de-sac for metastasis. **Skin:** Inspect skin for acanthosis nigricans (suggests cancer of the stomach). Acanthosis nigricans is brown to black pigmentation of the skin.	**Double-contrast barium studies:** Reported to miss 8 to 10% of gastric cancers; combination of air and barium enables radiologist to better visualize colonic mucosa. **Fiberoptic endoscopy:** Supplemented by biopsy and cytology techniques, this is judged to be superior to barium examination; sensitivity reported to be 100% and specificity is 99%. **Gastric biopsy:** Take specimens from suspected lesions or ulcers; diagnostic accuracy as high as 96%. **Cytology:** Obtain specimens of gastric walls using brushing technique, gastric washings, or endoscopic jet wash technique. Accuracy rates are reported to be over 90%.

Table 17-9. CANCER DETECTION: PHYSICAL EXAMINATION AND DIAGNOSTIC TESTING *Continued*

Site	Physical Examination	Diagnostic Testing
Liver Cancer (Cody, Macdonald, & Gunderson, 1985)	**Abdomen:** Inspect for masses, signs of portal hypertension, jaundice; palpate liver—note tenderness and surface consistency (hard, nodular, irregular masses or masses adjacent to the liver are suspicious for cancer); percuss liver borders, fist percussion of liver for tenderness, percuss for fluid; palpate extremities for edema. **Respiratory tract:** Impairment of air entry in right basal segments may be heard in cancer of the liver; check for restriction of diaphragmatic movement on the right side with a friction rub in cancer of the liver. **Skin:** Inspect for signs suggesting cirrhosis—e.g., spider angiomas, palmar erythemia, gynecomastia in males, sparse axillary, pubic, and pectoral hair in men.	**Serum alkaline phosphatase:** This enzyme is elevated in 70 to 80% of patients with hepatic metastases. **Alpha-fetoprotein (AFP) assay:** This is useful in diagnosis and follow-up of people with hepatocellular carcinoma; AFP strongly associated with hepatocellular carcinoma; reports suggest that 75 to 90% of people with primary hepatic cancer have levels above the normal values of 20 to 40 ng/ml. **Posteranterior and lateral chest x-ray films:** These depict the shape of diaphragm. **Radionuclide liver scanning:** This demonstrates whether the liver has an abnormality consistent with hepatoma. **Biopsy:** Biopsy may be considered to establish a tissue diagnosis.
Lung Cancer (Grant, 1985; Menna, Higgins, & Glatstein, 1985)	**Palpation:** Palpate supraclavicular region for lymphadenopathy; palpate liver for nodularity, indicating metastatic spread. **Wheeze:** Any unilateral wheeze merits further evaluation.	**PA (posteroanterior) chest x-ray film:** PA and lateral films should be obtained if a lesion is seen on PA film; conventional and computed tomography also are done in presence of peripheral opacity. **Cytology:** Examination of 3-day pooled sputum has identified cancer in persons with normal chest radiographs. **Flexible fiberoptic bronchoscopy:** This technique provides a visual examination of the interior of the bronchi and, when used with bronchial washings, the combined technique gives an overall accuracy of 79% with a false-positive rate of 0.8%. **Transthoracic fine needle aspiration biopsy:** This new procedure is done under fluoroscopic guidance and can diagnose intrapulmonary and solitary pulmonary nodules; research shows low false-positive and false-negative results.
Colorectal Cancer (Boyle, Michatek, Bersani, Nemoto, & Mettlin, 1981; Sugarbaker, Gunderson, & Wittes, 1985; Thompson, 1987)	**Rectum:** Palpate entire circumference of anorectal segment for masses and ask patient to strain while examining, palpate Blumer's rectal shelf, check for occult blood in stool. **Abdomen:** Inspect contour for distention or masses, use light palpation for subcutaneous nodules or signs of metastatic cancer (enlarged nodular liver, bilateral ovarian tumors, umbilical metastases); percuss for ascites, distention, or areas of dullness indicating masses.	**Fecal occult blood testing:** The patient collects stool samples for 3 days using Hemoccult slides; these slides are designed to detect blood in the stool when a chemical is applied. **Barium enema x-ray studies:** Barium plus air contrast is recommended over single-contrast technique because the latter can miss up to 40% of polypoid lesions and 20% of carcinomas; reports suggest that barium and air contrast technique can detect 92% of cancers. **Proctosigmoidoscopy:** This technique finds lesions low in rectum; approximately 55% of colon cancers occur within 25 cm of anal verge. **Flexible sigmoidoscopy:** Physician can see 50 to 60 cm of colon, and biopsy and polyp removal can be performed. Nearly two thirds of cancers seen with this instrument. **Colonoscopy:** If barium enema shows lesions, additional lesions are often found at colonoscopy; can provide specimens for cytologic examination (biopsy, brushing, or washing); polypectomy can also be done; entire colon can be visualized. **Biopsy:** Definitive diagnosis can be made.
Skin Cancer (Finley, 1986)	**Inspection:** Entire skin. Note size, shape, color, surface, location, sensations, and surrounding skin of any lesions; note development of any itchiness or irritation. **Malignant melanoma:** inspect back above the waist; head, scalp, and neck; finger and toe webs and soles of feet in deeply pigmented people; the skin between the border of mucous membranes and body orifices; fingernails. Any pigmented nevus that grows rapidly, ulcerates, bleeds or becomes infected should be considered a possible melanoma. Persons with dysplastic nevus syndrome and high-risk characteristics should be examined routinely (see Chapter 15 for specific recommendations).	

Table continued on following page

Table 17–9. CANCER DETECTION: PHYSICAL EXAMINATION AND DIAGNOSTIC TESTING *Continued*

Site	Physical Examination	Diagnostic Testing
Thyroid Cancer (Brennan & Macdonald, 1985)	**Inspect:** Inspect neck, especially on swallowing, for mass or asymmetry; palpate cervical lymph nodes, salivary glands, and thyroid gland, (noting size, contour, symmetry, consistency); masses should be evaluated for firmness, fixation irregularity, or pain; indirect laryngoscopy should be done.	**Biopsy:** Biopsy of the thyroid nodule is the only unequivocal diagnostic tool; percutaneous needle biopsy can provide tissue for histologic analysis; fine-needle aspiration is used to obtain tissue for cytologic examination. **Ultrasonography:** Ultrasonography is used to distinguish benign from malignant thyroid lesions. **Thyroid scintigram:** This is useful in demonstrating size, shape, and position of lesions detected clinically; with both ultrasound and radionuclide methods, tumors of 0.5 cm can be detected.
Testicular Cancer (Einhorn, Donohue, Peckham, Williams, & Loehrer, 1985; Hogan, 1983)	**Palpation:** Palpate the scrotum and testicles with both hands while patient stands; note size, shape, consistency, tenderness, and weight of testicles; weight differential between testicles is a clue to malignancy—tumor will feel weighty. Testicle feels neither hard nor soft—it has a somewhat rubbery consistency; surface should be smooth and free of lumps except for the ductus deferens; common sites for tumors are on the testicular anterior and lateral surfaces; check for hydrocele. **Transillumination:** When scrotum is transilluminated, tumors do not permit passage of light, but cysts do; palpate abdomen to check for retroperitoneal lymph node involvement; metastatic nodes usually lie at the level of, or slightly caudal to, the umbilicus; palpate supraclavicular node area for evidence of metastasis.	**Ultrasonography:** This technique is reported to distinguish a solid mass from a cystic mass and to be able to show whether the mass involves testis or epididymis or both. **Serum markers (AFP and beta-human chorionic gonadotropin):** When measured together one or the other will be positive 85% of the time in men with testicular cancer; not sufficiently sensitive to be relied on alone and not used in early detection. Definitive diagnosis is by removal of testes and pathologic analysis.
Prostate Cancer ("New prostate cancer detection group," 1987; Perez, Fair, Ihde, & Labrie, 1985)	**Rectal examination:** With patient in knee-chest position, evaluate anal sphincter (which is relaxed in prostate cancer); when palpating prostate, note size, median furrow, surface, shape, consistency, mobility, and sensitivity; cancer is usually a nontender, palpable hard nodule on posterior surface; palpable lymph nodes in groin and supraclavicular region suggest metastasis.	**Digital rectal examination:** Earliest stage detectable by rectal examination is Stage B disease; However, digital rectal examination is judged to be the best method of early detection. **Needle biopsy:** Needle biopsy is the standard method to diagnose tumor in United States; aspiration biopsy is the preferred method in Europe. **Transrectal Ultrasonography:** This method currently is in testing state to assess its value in early detection; it is useful in detecting tumor invasion through the prostatic capsule (anteriorly).
Bladder Cancer (Cetrin, 1983; Richie, Shipley, & Yagoda, 1985)	Tumor may be palpated suprapubically; bladder can be best felt by rectal or vaginal palpation under anesthesia.	**Urinary cytology:** This test may lead to presumptive diagnosis of bladder cancer. **Cytoscopy:** Cytoscopic examination and transurethral biopsy confirm the diagnosis. **Ultrasonography:** This technique is used in staging to assess invasion of the bladder wall by cancer.
Detection of Cancer in General (Van Der Werf, 1987)		**Water-suppressed nuclear magnetic resonance (NMR) spectroscopy:** Blood test should be done when lipoprotein widths are measured. Differences will be noted between persons with benign and malignant tumors, and in persons with tumors and without tumors. This method is in the investigative stage.

(e.g., sickle cell anemia, hypertension) and has proved to be effective in involving the "hard to reach" person.

From 1985 to 1987, the ONS conducted a series of 2-day regional cancer prevention–early detection workshops for black American nurses. These workshops were funded by the NCI for the following purposes:

1. Increasing the knowledge and skill level of black American nurses in primary and secondary prevention of cancer.

2. Increasing their level of community-based participation in activities related to primary and secondary prevention of cancer.

3. Fostering positive attitudes toward cancer prevention and early detection.

The results from the workshops clearly indicate that nurses brought about significant changes in attitudes toward the early detection and prevention of cancer, increased the level of participation of the workshop participants in community-based activities, and resulted in increased cancer-related knowledge and skills (Frank-Stromberg, Johnson, & McCorkle, 1987). A partial list of the nontraditional settings and cancer-related activities implemented by workshop participants is given in Box 17–4.

Compliance, a significant issue in any discussion of cancer self-examination practices, is another area that merits further attention and research. Nurses can increase compliance by addressing the issue in a forth-

Box 17–4. EXAMPLES OF NONTRADITIONAL SETTINGS AND CANCER-RELATED ACTIVITIES OF NURSES PARTICIPATING IN NCI-SPONSORED BLACK NURSES REGIONAL CANCER PREVENTION–EARLY DETECTION WORKSHOPS FROM 1985 to 1987

1. Implemented screening programs in food pantries and feeding centers.
2. Organized church-sponsored educational and screening programs through the nursing guild.
3. Organized a multistate church program that designated one month "Cancer in Black Americans." The month was filled with educational programs as well as screening programs.
4. Organized cancer-related programs in local schools, Parent-Teacher Organizations, family planning, and Parents-Too-Soon programs.
5. Designed health fairs which included cancer-related activities in collaboration with local black sororities.
6. Contacted black political organizations in the community and designed and implemented community education programs that focused on educating the community about cancer and the importance of early detection. The program was designed to use block volunteers who would go door-to-door.
7. Offered cancer-oriented educational and screening programs in work settings with the cooperation of the local unions and site management.
8. Contacted local veterans groups and offered cancer-related programs to the membership.
9. Designed and implemented both educational and screening programs in low-income housing. Programs focused on the elderly in these settings and offered transportation to the program.
10. Offered special cancer screening programs during the evening and on weekends at local store-front free health clinic.
11. Designed and implemented a hospital-based multimedia educational approach (posters, slide-tape programs, announcements over loudspeakers, newspaper articles, TV spots) focusing on early detection of cancer in black Americans. These programs were targeted to hospital employees, hospital patients, and their families.

right manner. When teaching self-examination techniques, the nurse needs to spend time understanding how people feel about the technique, what barriers prevent them from practicing it, what is needed to help them practice it, and what benefits they feel are inherent in the procedure. These areas need to be discussed *with* the person learning the technique, and consumer (rather than health professional)-generated solutions should be encouraged.

Nurses need to keep abreast of new research findings documenting whether cancer self-examination techniques (e.g., BSE, Hemoccult testing, TSE) make a difference in decreasing cancer mortality. Currently, there are no definitive answers to this question; however, it is recommended that self-examination techniques be taught to high-risk persons (Chapter 16 details high-risk persons or groups).

The health history can be used as a vehicle for identifying high-risk individuals. When appropriate, nurses with physical assessment skills can use these skills to conduct an examination designed for early cancer detection. All nurses with physical assessment skills can be involved in community-based programs designed to detect cancer in the early stages as well as provide education on cancer self-examination techniques. As has been demonstrated from the NCI-funded black nurses' regional workshops, nurses can carry out cost-effective early detection programs in both traditional and nontraditional settings and attract people typically difficult to reach. The importance of offering programs in nontraditional settings is shown by the research on participation in early detection programs; nonparticipants are less educated, have lower incomes, and are older than participants (Van Parijs & Eckhardt, 1984). Because these demographic variables are associated with higher risk for various cancers, lack of participation presents a serious challenge to cancer education.

A final example of using nursing to offer early cancer detection programs is found in a report on cancer nurses in action ("Nurse helps promote screening services," 1987). Screening clinics in a small rural hospital were set up on a monthly basis and included mammary and cervical, skin, male genitourinary, oral, head and neck, and colorectal cancers. These clinics were coordinated by a nurse with special training in early cancer detection physical assessment techniques. This nurse formulated risk assessments, taught cancer self-examination techniques, and conducted site-specific physical examinations.

References

Adams, M., & Kerner, J. (1982). Evaluation of promotional strategies to solve the problem of underutilization of a breast examination/education center in a New York City Black community. *Issues in Cancer Screening and Communications, 83,* 151–161.

Alquist, D., McGill, D., & Schwartz, S. (1984). HemoQuant: A new quantitative assay for fecal hemoglobin. *Annals of Internal Medicine, 101,* 297–309.

American Nurses Association and Oncology Nursing Society. (1987). *Standards of oncology nursing practice.* Kansas City, MO: American Nurses' Association.

A study of Hispanics' attitudes concerning cancer and cancer prevention (1985). Unpublished manuscript prepared for the American Cancer Society, Atlanta, GA, by Clark, Martire, and Bartolomeo, Inc.

Baquet, C., & Ringen, K. (1985). Cancer control in blacks: Epidemiology and NCI program plans. In L. Mortenson, P. Engstrom, & P. Anderson (Eds.), *Advances in cancer control: Health care financing and research.* New York: Alan Liss, Inc.

Bassett, M., & Krieger, N. (1986). Social class and black-white differences in breast cancer survival. *American Journal of Public Health, 76,* 1400–1403.

Bennett, S., Lawrence, R., Fleischmann, S., Gifford, C., & Slack, W. (1983). *Journal of the American Medical Association, 249,* 488–491.

Blesch, K. (1986). Health beliefs about testicular cancer and self-examination among professional men. *Oncology Nursing Forum, 13,* 29–33.

Bostock, Y., Jacobson, B., & Seymour, L. (1982). Ad-man's bull's eye—researcher's blank. *Times Health Services.*

Box, V., Nichols, S., Lailemand, R., Pearson, P., & Vakil, P. (1984). Haemoccult compliance rates and reasons for non-compliance. *Public Health, London, 98,* 16–25.

Boyle, M., Michalek, A., Bersani, G., Nemoto, T., & Mettlin, C. (1981). Effectiveness of a community program to promote early breast cancer detection. *Journal of Surgical Oncology, 18,* 183–188.

Brennan, M., & Macdonald, J. (1985). Cancer of the endocrine system. In V. DeVita, S. Hellman, & S. Rosenberg (Eds.), *Cancer: Principles and practice of oncology* (2nd ed., pp. 1179–1241). Philadelphia: J. B. Lippincott Co.

Butler, L., King, G., & White, J. (1983). Communications strategies, cancer information and black populations: An analysis of longitudinal data. In *Progress in cancer control IV: Research in the cancer control* (pp. 171–182). New York: Alan Liss, Inc.

Cady, B., Macdonald, J., & Gunderson, L. (1985). Cancer of the hepatobiliary system. In V. DeVita, S. Hellman, & S. Rosenberg (Eds.), *Cancer: Principles and practice of oncology* (2nd ed., pp. 741–770). Philadelphia: J. B. Lippincott Co.

Canadian Task Force. (1982). Cervical cancer screening programs summary of the 1982 Canadian task force report. *Canadian Medical Association Journal, 127,* 581–588.

Canadian Task Force on the Periodic Health Examination. (1979). The periodic health examination. *Canadian Medical Association Journal, 121,* 1193–1248.

Cancer of the colon and rectum: Summary of a public attitude survey (1983). *CA: A Cancer Journal for Clinicians, 33,* 359–365.

Carlile, T., & Hadaway, E. (1985). Screening for breast cancer. In B. A. Stoll (Ed.), *Screening and monitoring of cancer* (pp. 135–152). New York: John Wiley & Sons, Inc.

Celentano, D. D., Shapiro, S., & Weisman, C. S. (1982). Cancer preventive screening behavior among elderly women. *Preventive Medicine, 11,* 454–463.

Chamberlain, J. (1983). Screening for cancer. *Journal of Applied Medicine, 9,* 11–15.

Citrin, D. (1983). Bladder cancer. In S. Kahn, R. Love, C. Sherman, & R. Chakravorty (Eds.), *Concepts in cancer medicine* (pp. 493–502). New York: Grune & Stratton, Inc.

Cole, C., & Goman, L. (1984). Breast self-examination: Practices and attitudes of registered nurses. *Oncology Nursing Forum, 11*(5), 37–41.

Conklin, M., Klint, K., Morway, A., Sawyer, J. R., & Shepard, R. (1978). Should health teaching include self-examination of the testes? *American Journal of Nursing, 78,* 2073–2074.

Cummings, K. M., Lampone, D., Mettlin, C., & Potes, J. (1983). What young men know about testicular cancer. *Preventive Medicine, 12,* 326–330.

Diem, G., & Rose, D. (1985). Has breast self-examination had a fair trial? *The New York State Journal of Medicine, 85,* 479–480.

Division of Cancer Prevention and Control (1986). Screening. In P. Greenwald & E. Sondik (Eds.), *Cancer control objectives for the nation: 1985–2000.* NCI Monograph, NIH Publication 86–2880. Bethesda, MD: National Institutes of Health.

Dorozynski, A. (1987). Test for early detection of colorectal cancer under development. *Oncology & Biotechnology News, 1*(2), 3.

Early Detection Branch Division of Cancer Prevention and Control (1987, December 27). *Working guidelines for early cancer detection rationale and supporting evidence to decrease mortality.* Bethesda, MD: National Cancer Institute.

Eddy, D. A. (1985). Screening for cancer in adults. *CIBA Foundation Symposium 110,* 88–109.

Eddy, D. M. (1986). Secondary prevention of cancer: An overview. *Bulletin of the World Health Organization, 64,* 421–429.

Einhorn, L., Donohue, J., Peckham, M., Williams, S., & Loehrer, P. (1985). Cancer of the testes. In V. DeVita, S. Hellman, & S. Rosenberg (Eds.). *Cancer: Principles and practice of oncology* (2nd ed., pp. 979–1011). Philadelphia: J. B. Lippincott Co.

Ekelund, G., Carlsson, U., & Janzon, L. (1985). The feasibility of large scale population screening. *British Journal of Surgery, 72,* (Suppl.), 571–572.

Elwood, T., Erickson, A., & Lieberman, S. (1978). Comparative educational approaches to screening for colorectal cancer. *American Journal of Public Health, 68,* 135–138.

Evans, A., Love, R., Meyerowitz, B., Leventhal, H., & Nerenz,

D. (1985). Factors associated with active participation in a cancer prevention clinic. *Preventive Medicine, 14,* 358–371.

Farrands, P. A., Griffiths, R. L., & Britton, D. C. (1981). The Frome experiment—value of screening for colorectal cancer. *Lancet, 1,* 1231–1232.

Farrands, P. A., Hardcastle, J., Chamberlain, J., & Moss, S. (1984). Factors affecting compliance with screening for colorectal cancer. *Community Medicine, 6,* 12–19.

Feldman, J. G., Carter, A. C., Nicastri, A. D., & Hostat, S. T. (1981). Breast self-examination, relationship to stage of breast cancer at diagnosis. *Cancer, 47,* 2740–2745.

Fink, D. J. (1987, November). Change in checkup guidelines for cervical cancer detection. New York: American Cancer Society Memo.

Finley, C. (1986). Malignant melanoma: A primary care perspective. *Nurse Practitioner, 11,* 18–38.

Foster, R., Costanza, M., and Worden, J. (1985). The current status of research in breast self-examination. *The New York State Journal of Medicine, 85,* 480–482.

Foster, R. S., Lang, S. P., Costanza, M. C., Worden, J. K., Haines, C. R., & Yates, J. W. (1978). Breast self-examination and breast cancer stage. *New England Journal of Medicine, 299,* 265–270.

Frame, P. S. (1986). A critical review of adult health maintenance. Part 3: Prevention of cancer. *The Journal of Family Practice, 22,* 511–520.

Frank, J., & Mai, V. (1985). Breast self-examination in young women: More harm than good? *Lancet, 2,* 654–657.

Frank-Stromborg, M., Johnson, J., & McCorkle, R. (1987). A program model for nurses involved with cancer education of black Americans. *Journal of Cancer Education, 2,* 145–151.

Fraser, M. (1982). The role of the nurse in the prevention and early detection of malignant melanoma. *Cancer Nursing, 5,* 351–360.

Freeman, H. (1981). *Cancer mortality: A socio-economic phenomenon.* American Cancer Society's Twenty-Third Science Writers' Seminar. New York: American Cancer Society.

Ganong, L. H., & Markovitz, J. (1987). Young men's knowledge of testicular cancer and behavioral intentions toward testicular self-exam. *Patient Education and Counseling, 9,* 251–261.

Gastrin, G. (1980). Program to encourage self-examination for breast cancer. *British Medical Journal, 2,* 193.

Goldbloom, R., Battista, R. N. (1986). The periodic health examination. *Canadian Medical Association Journal, 135,* 721–729.

Goldenring, J. M., & Purtell, E. (1984). Knowledge of testicular cancer risk and need for self-examination in college students: A call for equal time for men in teaching or early cancer detection techniques. *Pediatrics, 74,* 1093–1096.

Gould-Martin, K., Paganini-Hill, A., Casagrande, C., Mack, T., & Ross, R. K. (1982). Behavioral and biological determinants of surgical stage of breast cancer. *Preventive Medicine, 11,* 429–440.

Grant, I. (1985). Screening for lung cancer. In B. A. Stoll (Ed.), *Screening and monitoring cancer* (pp. 119–133). New York, John Wiley & Sons, Inc.

Greenwald, P., Nasca, P. C., Lawrence, C. E., Horton, J., McGarrah, M. S., Gabrielle, T., & Carlton, K. (1978). *New England Journal of Medicine, 299,* 271–273.

Gregorio, D., Cummings, M., & Michalek, A. (1983). Delay, stage of disease, and survival among white and black women with breast cancer. *American Journal of Public Health, 73,* 590–593.

Guinan, P., Sharifi, R., & Bush, I. (1984, January). Prostate cancer: Tips toward earlier detection. *Your Patient & Cancer,* 37–42.

Hakama, M. (1986). Scientific basis of screening in early detection. *Cancer Detection and Prevention, 9,* 139–143.

Hall, D., Adams, C., Stein, G., & Stephenson, H., Goldstein, M., & Pennypacker, H. (1980). Improved detection of human breast lesions following experimental training. *Cancer, 46,* 408–414.

Hallal, J. (1982). The relationship of health beliefs, health locus of control, and self-concept to the practice of breast self-examination in adult women. *Nursing Research, 31,* 137–142.

Hirschfield-Bartek, J. (1982). Health beliefs and their influence on breast self-examination practices in women with breast cancer. *Oncology Nursing Forum, 9,* 77–81.

Hislop, T. G., Coldman, A. J., & Skippen, D. H. (1984). Breast self-examination: Importance of technique in early diagnosis. *Canadian Medical Association Journal, 131,* 1349–1352.

Hogan, T. (1983). Testicular germ cell cancers. In S. Kahn, R. Love, C. Sherman, & R. Chakravorty (Eds.), *Concepts in cancer medicine* (pp. 513–525). New York: Grune & Stratton, Inc.

Holliday, H., Roebuck, E. J., & Doyle, P. J. (1983). Initial results from a programme of BSE. *Clinical Oncology, 9,* 11–16.

Huguley, C. N., & Brown, R. L. (1981). The value of breast self-examination. *Cancer, 47,* 989–995.

Khan, O., & McCready, V. R. (1985). Isotope imaging in staging and monitoring. In B. A. Stoll (Ed.), *Screening and monitoring cancer* (pp. 31–46). New York: John Wiley & Sons, Inc.

Khan, O., Slack, N., & Cosgrove, D. (1985). Ultrasound imaging in staging and monitoring. In B. A. Stoll (Ed.), *Screening and monitoring cancer* (pp. 79–94). New York: John Wiley & Sons, Inc.

Kahn, S. B. (1983). Cancer diagnosis. In S. B. Kahn, R. Love, C. Sherman, & R. Chakravorty (Eds.), *Concepts in cancer medicine* (pp. 267–283). New York: Grune & Stratton, Inc.

Kegeles, S. S. (1985). Education for breast self-examination: Why, who, what and how? *Preventive Medicine, 14,* 702–720.

Kegeles, S. S., & Grady, K. E. (1982). Behavioral dimensions in cancer control. In D. Schottenfeld & J. G. Fraumeni (Eds.), *Cancer epidemiology and prevention* (pp. 1049–1063). Philadelphia: W. B. Saunders Co.

Kelly, P. (1983). Counseling persons who have family histories of cancer. In G. R. Newell (Ed.), *Cancer prevention in clinical medicine* (pp. 147–164). New York: Raven Press.

Lailemand, R., Vakil, P., Pearson, P., & Box, V. (1984). Screening for asymptomatic bowel cancer in general practice. *British Medical Journal, 288,* 31–33.

Leffall, L. (1981). *Early diagnosis of colorectal cancer.* New York: American Cancer Society Publication, No. 3311–PE.

Levy, S. (1983). The aging cancer patient: Behavioral research issues. In R. Yancik (Ed.), *Perspectives on prevention and treatment of cancer in the elderly* (pp. 239–247). New York: Raven Press.

Li, F. P. (1986). Genetic and familial cancer: Opportunities for prevention and early detection. *Cancer Detection and Prevention, 9,* 41–45.

Love, R. (1985). *Screening for cancer: Controversies and guidelines for clinical medicine.* Kalamazoo, MI: Upjohn Company (8509 PTV146291).

Love, R. R., & Camilli, A. E. (1981). The value of screening. *Cancer, 48,* 489–494.

Love, R. R., Leventhal, H., Hughes, B. S., & Fryback, D. G. (1984). *Cancer prevention for clinicians, course text.* Madison, WI: Board of Regents of the University of Wisconsin System.

Love, R. R., & Olsen, S. J. (1985). An agenda for cancer prevention in nursing practice. *Cancer Nursing, 8,* 329–338.

Macdonald, J., Cohn, I., & Gunderson, L. (1985). Cancer of the stomach. In V. DeVita, S. Hellman, & S. Rosenberg (Eds.), *Cancer principles and practice of oncology* (2nd ed., pp. 659–690). Philadelphia: J. B. Lippincott Co.

Macrea, F., Hill, D., St. John, J., Ambikatathy, A., Garner, J., & Ballarat General Practitioner Research Group. (1984). Predicting colon cancer screening behavior from health beliefs. *Preventive Medicine, 13,* 115–126.

Marty, P., McDermott, R., & Gold, R. (1983). An assessment of three alternative formats for promoting breast self-examination. *Cancer Nursing, 6,* 207–211.

Massey, E. (1986). Perceived susceptibility to breast cancer and practice of breast self-examination. *Nursing Research, 35,* 183–185.

McCusker, J., & Morrow, G. (1980). Factors related to the use of cancer early detection techniques. *Preventive Medicine, 9,* 388–397.

Mettlin, C., & Cummings, K. M. (1983). Experience with a cancer prevention-detection clinic. In G. R. Newell (Ed.), *Cancer prevention in clinical medicine* (pp. 131–146). New York: Raven Press.

Miller, A. B. (1986). Screening for cancer: Issues and future directions. *Journal of Chronic Diseases, 39,* 1067–1077.

Miller, D. G. (1986). Cancer prevention: Steps you can take. In A. I. Holleb (Ed.), *The American Cancer Society Cancer Book* (pp. 15–40). Garden City, NY: Doubleday & Co.

Minna, J., Higgins, G., & Glatstein, E. (1985). Cancer of the lung. In V. DeVita, S. Hellman, & S. Rosenberg (Eds.), *Cancer: Principles and practice of oncology* (2nd ed., pp. 507–598). Philadelphia: J. B. Lippincott Co.

Minnesota study aimed at finding final answer on hemoccult screening (1987). *Cancer Letter, 13*(30), 4–6.

Morrow, G., Way, J., Hoagland, A., & Cooper, R. (1982). Patient compliance with self-directed hemocult testing. *Preventive Medicine, 11,* 512–520.

National Cancer Institute (1985). *Testicular Self-Examination.* Bethesda, MD: U.S. Department of Health and Human Services, Public Health Service, National Institutes of Health, NIH Publication No. 86–2636.

Newell, G. R. (1980). Overview of cancer prevention. *Cancer Bulletin, 32,* 128–129.

Office of Cancer Communications (1987, July). *Technical report, cancer prevention awareness survey, Wave II.* Bethesda, MD: National Cancer Institute, National Institutes of Health, NIH Publication No. 87-2907.

O'Malley, M., & Fletcher, S. (1987). Screening for breast cancer with breast self-examination. A critical review. *Journal of the American Medical Association, 257,* 2196–2203.

Oncology Nursing Society (1989a). *Standards of oncology education, patient/family and public.* Pittsburgh: Author.

Oncology Nursing Society (1989b). *Standards of oncology nursing education, generalist and advanced practice levels.* Pittsburgh: Author.

Ostwald, S. K., & Rothenberger, J. (1985). Development of a testicular self-examination program for college men. *Journal of the Association of Community Hospitals, 33,* 234–239.

Owen, W. L., Hoge, A. F., Asal, N. R., Anderson, P. S., Owne, A. S., & Cucchiara, A. J. (1985). Self-examination of the breast: Use and effectiveness. *Southern Medical Journal, 78,* 1170–1173.

Patterson, W. B. (1986). Screening for colorectal cancer in asymptomatic patients. In G. Steele & R. R. Osteen (Eds.), *Colorectal cancer: Current concepts in diagnosis and treatment* (pp. 138–152). New York: Marcel Dekker, Inc.

Paulus, D. (1987). Imaging in breast cancer. *Cancer, 37,* 133–150.

Perez, C., Fair, W., Ihde, D., & Labrie, F. (1985). Cancer of the prostate. In V. DeVita, S. Hellman, & S. Rosenberg (Eds.). *Cancer: Principles and practice of oncology* (2nd ed., pp. 929–964). Philadelphia: J. B. Lippincott Co.

Perez, C., Knapp, R., DiSaia, P., & Young, R. (1985). Gynecologic tumors. In V. DeVita, S. Hellman, & S. Rosenberg (Eds.), *Cancer: Principles and practice of oncology* (2nd ed., pp. 1013–1081). Philadelphia: J. B. Lippincott Co.

Prorok, P. C., & Connor, R. J. (1986). Screening for the early detection of cancer. *Cancer Investigation, 4,* 225–238.

Rakel, R. (1983, December). A clinician's guide: Tips on fecal occult blood testing. *Your Patient and Cancer, 3*(12), p. 23.

Reno, D. R. (1988). Men's knowledge and health beliefs about testicular cancer and testicular self-examination. *Cancer Nursing, 11,* 112–117.

Richie, J., Shipley, W., & Yagoda, A. (1985). Cancer of the bladder. In V. DeVita, S. Hellman, & S. Rosenberg (Eds.), *Cancer: Principles and practice of oncology* (2nd ed., pp. 915–928). Philadelphia: J. B. Lippincott Co.

Rovinski, C. (1980). Nurses and cancer's seven warning signals. *Cancer Nursing, 3,* 53–55.

Rudolph, V. N., & MacEwen-Quinn, K. L. (1988). The practice of TSE among college men: Effectiveness of an educational program. *Oncology Nursing Forum, 15*(1), 49–58.

Sargis, N. (1983). Detecting ovarian cancer: A challenge for nursing assessment. *Oncology Nursing Forum, 10*(2), 48–52.

Satariano, W., Belle, S., & Swanson, M. (1986). The severity of breast cancer at diagnosis: A comparison of age and extent of disease in black and white women. *American Journal of Public Health, 76,* 779–782.

Sawyer, P. (1986). Breast self-examination: Hospital based nurses aren't assessing their clients. *Oncology Nursing Forum, 13*(5), 44–48.

Seidman, H., Stellman, S. D., & Mushinski, M. H. (1982). A different perspective on breast cancer risk factors: Some implications of the nonattributable risk. *Cancer, 32,* 301–313.

Senie, R. T., Rosen, P. P., Lesser, M. L., & Kinne, D. W. (1981). Breast self-examination and medical examination related to breast cancer stage. *American Journal of Public Health, 71,* 583–590.

Shamian, J., & Edgar, L. (1987). Nurses as agents for change in teaching breast self-examination. *Public Health Nursing, 4*(1), 29–34.

Shanmugaratnam, K. (1985). Prevention and early detection of cancer. *Cancer Detection and Prevention, 8,* 431–445.

Shortridge, L., & McLain, B. (1979). Primary care and prostate cancer. *The Nurse Practitioner, 4,* 25.

Silman, A., & Mitchell, P. (1984). Attitudes of non-participants in an occupational based programme of screening for colorectal cancer. *Community Medicine, 6,* 8–11.

Simon, J. (1985). Occult blood screening for colorectal carcinoma: A critical review. *Gastroenterology, 88,* 820–837.

Smith, E. B., Clarke-Pearson, D., & Creasman, W. (1985). Screening for cervical cancer. In B. A. Stoll (Ed.), *Screening and monitoring cancer* (pp. 153–165). New York: John Wiley & Sons, Inc.

Smith, E. M., Francis, A. M., & Polissar, L. (1980). The effect of breast self-exam practices and physician examinations on extent of disease at diagnosis. *Preventive Medicine, 9,* 409–417.

Songster, C. L., Barrows, G. H., & Jarrett, D. D. (1980). Immunochemical detection of human fecal occult blood. In S. J. Winawer, D. Schottenfeld, & P. Sherlock (Eds.), *Colorectal cancer: Prevention, epidemiology, and screening* (pp. 193–204). New York: Raven Press.

Spector, M., Applegate, W., Olmstead, S., DiVasto, P., & Skipper, B. (1981). Assessment of attitudes toward mass screening for colorectal cancer in a Veterans Administration hospital. *American Journal of Surgery, 145,* 89–93.

Spitzer, W. O. (1984). The periodic health examination. *Canadian Medical Association Journal, 130,* 1276–1292.

Staff. ACS modifies guidelines for Pap test frequency: Physician discretion. (1987, November 27). *Cancer Letter,* p. 6.

Staff. New prostate cancer detection group to study potential of ultrasound. (1987, March 6). *Cancer Letter,* p. 4.

Staff. Nurse helps promote screening services at community hospital. (1987, March). *Cancer Nursing Letter,* p. 5.

Studva, K. V. (1983, December). Cancer prevention and detection: Testicular cancer. *Cancer Nursing, 6,* 468–485.

Subcommittee on Cancer in the Economically Disadvantaged (1986). *Cancer in the economically disadvantaged. A special report.* New York: American Cancer Society.

Sugarbaker, P., Gunderson, L., & Wittes, R. (1985). Colorectal cancer. In V. DeVita, S. Hellman, & S. Rosenberg (Eds.), *Cancer: Principles and practice of oncology* (2nd ed., pp. 795–884). Philadelphia: J. B. Lippincott Co.

Swanson, D. (1987). Why you should conscientiously promote testicular self-examination. *Consultant, 27,* 142–147.

Tabar, L., Fagerberg, C. J. G., & Gad, A., Holmberg, H. L., & Thomas, B. A. (1985). Reduction in mortality from breast cancer after screening with mammography. *Lancet, 1,* 829–832.

Tamburini, M., Massara, G., Bertario, L., Re, A., & Dipietro, S. (1981). Usefulness of breast self-examination for an early detection of breast cancer. Results of a study on 500 breast cancer patients and 652 controls. *Tumori, 67,* 219–224.

Thompson, H. (1985). Screening for stomach cancer. In B. A. Stoll (Ed.), *Screening and monitoring cancer* (pp. 167–193). New York: John Wiley & Sons, Inc.

Thompson, W. (1987). Imaging strategies for tumors of the gastrointestinal system. *Cancer, 37,* 165–185.

Thornhill, J. A., Conroy, R. M., Kelly, D. B., Walsh, A., Fennelly, J. J., & Fitzpatrick, J. M. (1986). Public awareness of testicular cancer and the value of self-examination. *British Journal of Medicine, 293,* 480–481.

U.S. Preventive Services Task Force. (1987). Recommendations for breast cancer screening. *Journal of the American Medical Association, 257,* 2196.

Van Der Werf, M. (1987). New diagnostic technique for cancer to enter clinical trials. *Oncology and Biotechnology News, 1*(3), 18.

Van Parijs, L. G., & Eckhardt, S. (1984). Public education in primary and secondary cancer prevention. *Hygie, 3,* 16–28.

Wilkes, B. (1983). The development of a two-tier BSE educational program. In *Progress in cancer control III: A regional approach* (pp. 127–131). New York: Alan Liss, Inc.

Wilkinson, G., & Wilson, J. (1983). An evaluation of demographic differences in the utilization of a cancer information service. *Social Science Medicine, 17,* 169–175.

Winawer, S. J. (1983). Detection and diagnosis of colorectal cancer. *Cancer, 51,* 2519–2524.

Winawer, S. J., Schottenfeld, D., & Sherlock, P. (1985). Screening for colorectal cancer: The issues. *Gastroenterology, 88,* 841–844.

Winchester, D. P., Schull, J. H., Scanlon, E. F., et al. (1980). A mass screening program for colorectal cancer using chemical testing for occult blood in the stool. *Cancer, 45,* 2955–2958.

Young, R., Knapp, R., Fuks, Z., & DiSaia, P. (1985). Cancer of the ovary. In V. DeVita, S. Hellman, & S. Rosenberg (Eds.), *Cancer: Principles and practice of oncology* (2nd ed., pp. 1083–1117) Philadelphia: J. B. Lippincott Co.

CHAPTER 18

The Diagnosis of Cancer: A Life Transition

DARLENE W. MOOD

A MODEL OF THE CANCER EXPERIENCE

In most cultures, the word *cancer* carries with it a threatening and frightening connotation (Holland, 1982; Krant, 1976; Lierman, 1988; Weisman, 1979a). Although each individual may have a personal meaning for cancer, the cross-culturally shared meaning with its many negative features affects the way people react when confronted with a cancer experience. This includes not only the persons who are patients or their families, but also the many health professionals with whom they interact and the larger network of persons who constitute the world in which they live. Basic human relationships are significantly altered: communication barriers may arise between spouses, parents and children may become dishonest with one another, health providers may avoid discussing certain topics with the client, employers may become fearful and lose confidence in their formerly valued employee. The personal discovery that one has cancer often involves major and dramatic shifts in peoples' lives. This chapter examines the transition that occurs when a person without cancer experiences the first signs and symptoms and then reaches the stage of formal diagnosis of cancer. This chapter also addresses the psychosocial effects of that transition as well as some factors that facilitate or serve as barriers to making the transition. Finally, the nursing implications of the transition and associated factors are discussed.

Several models have been proposed in the psychosocial oncology literature to describe the cancer experience (Giacquinta, 1977; Weisman, 1979b). One very practical model, shown in Figure 18–1, was first proposed by Holland (1982) and later elaborated on by Saunders and McCorkle (1985). In this model, the patient experiencing some symptoms seeks medical consultation and then goes through a series of tests and evaluations, which result in a cancer diagnosis. This is the first transition. At this point, depending on the site and stage of the disease, a curative treatment attempt is made. In the most satisfactory of outcomes, the cancer is completely responsive to the treatment, and the patient never experiences a recurrence and is cured (course A). However, there are two other possible outcomes after the curative attempt. In the first (course B), the cancer is initially or partially responsive to the treatment but later recurs or spreads to other parts of the body, or both. The duration of the response could be very brief and limited (e.g., days or weeks) or it could last for many years. The other outcome after the curative attempts is no response (course C). Both clinical courses B and C generally follow a trajectory of progressive disease and then death. These final steps also constitute course D. In this clinical course, no curative attempt is ever made, and the disease progresses to death.

Each of the arrows in Figure 18–1 could be considered a transition stage in the cancer experience. This chapter focuses on the first of these transitions, namely, the transition that takes the individual from being a person without cancer through a personal discovery that "I do have cancer" (a formal cancer diagnosis). This transition has three phases: becoming aware of the first signs and symptoms, obtaining a formal diagnosis, and planning for treatment. The entire transition may be accomplished in several weeks, or it may take months or years to complete, depending on a great number of personal and situational factors.

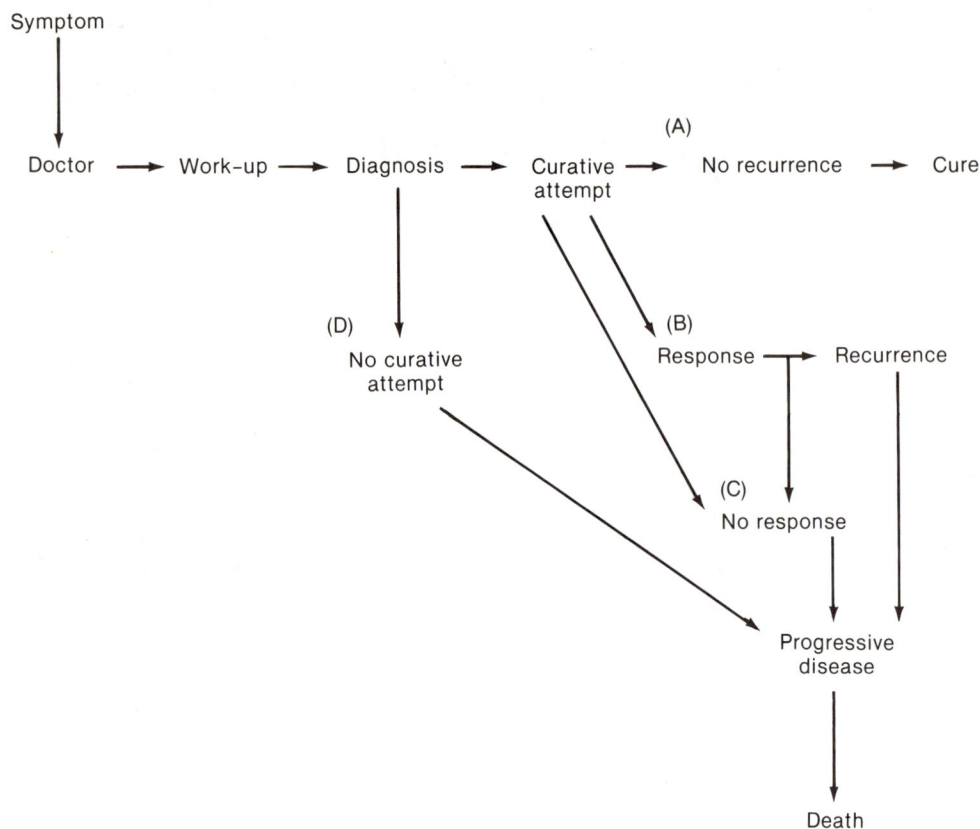

Figure 18–1. Possible clinical courses of cancer. (From Holland, J. [1982]. Psychologic aspects of cancer. In J. Holland & E. Frei III [eds.], *Cancer medicine*. Philadelphia: Lea & Febiger. Reproduced by permission.)

THE FIRST SIGNS

Biologically, the change from being cancer free to having a cancerous condition is a very slow process occurring silently within the individual person's physical structure. It is not known with certainty what causes the abnormal cells to develop and multiply. Diet, environmental contamination, life-style choices, stress, and heredity have all been implicated in carcinogenesis. It has been proposed, in fact, that abnormal cells capable of producing a cancer are produced regularly in the body, but that the body's alert immune system monitors for these abnormal cells and destroys them before they become a cancer (Le Shan, 1966; Simonton, Matthews-Simonton, & Creighton, 1978). Within this theoretical framework, then, the occurrence of cancer represents a failure of the body's immune system to function effectively. Psychological as well as physical triggers of this process have been proposed (Borysenko, 1982; Le Shan, 1966; Thomas & Greenstreet, 1973). The avoidance of cancer, in turn, is achieved in part through the physical and perhaps psychological maintenance of the effectively functioning immune system (Simonton et al., 1978).

Whatever the causes of cancer are, the biologic shift that occurs is believed to differ significantly from the psychosocial transition. Although the cancer cells usually divide and grow undetected over a long period of time, the person is unaware of those processes until some event brings it to sudden awareness.

What are some of the events that people experience that catapult them from the belief that they are cancer-free to the suspicion and discovery that they have cancer? The most sudden shift is the self-detection of an obvious sign or symptom. For example, a woman is showering and she finds a lump in her breast that she does not recall having felt before; a man faces the mirror shaving and notices an unevenness between the two sides of his neck; a person notes blood in the urine or feces. These common first signs trigger an awareness that something may be wrong and generally place the person in a state of hyperalertness that eventually will lead to some action. The rapidity of each individual's response will depend on many factors.

Other signs and symptoms commonly are first detected by the person but are not so obvious in their association with cancer, for example, a persistent cough or sore throat, or shortness of breath. Sometimes a cut or bruise that just will not heal, as it would have in the past, is noticed first. The appearance of, or changes in the appearance of, skin moles may be an initially unrecognized sign. Changes in bladder or bowel habits may be attributed to many different causes. Although pain frequently is difficult to ignore, rarely would cancer be considered as the first explanation. Extreme fatigue likewise may be the initial sign noticed. These less obvious manifestations are often overlooked as the individual waits for them to disappear. However, when these events are signals of cancer, they persist; eventually, the person becomes aware of the potential threat and enters the already mentioned state of hyperalertness likely to lead at some point to action.

A final possible situation occurs when a person with no known signs and symptoms of cancer, often in apparent good health, enters the health care system for a routine examination or acute care of an unrelated health problem. In the course of examination, something occurs that makes the health provider suspicious. This may be the unusual results of a blood test or an x-ray study, or it may be the discovery of a sign that had not been detected by the patient or client. Such discoveries may lead to further testing that, even before the physician has shared the findings with the person, may raise anxieties because the testing is recognized as extraordinary.

Therefore, it is clear that although people may detect the first signs of cancer themselves or discover the suspicious signs of cancer during a totally unrelated interaction with the health care system, the discovery is virtually always an unexpected event. It catches the person off guard and generally unprepared to cope with its meaning and threat.

RESPONDING TO THE THREAT

Conventional wisdom would dictate that, given a sign or symptom that suggests the possibility of cancer or a persistent symptom that will not go away, the person involved would seek medical advice and diagnosis. In fact, how the person responds to these first signs will depend on many factors. During this early phase of cancer detection, people struggle to make sense of the symptoms they are experiencing. Often these initial symptoms are ambiguous, and symptom meaning can consist of highly speculative attributions about the underlying cause. Mechanic (1972) suggested that symptom attributions generally are loosely constructed hypotheses or hunches until clinical confirmation is made. It is not uncommon for people to attribute their initial symptoms to minor illnesses (Comaroff & Maguire, 1981). People tend to normalize their symptoms within the context of everyday life experience (Chrisman & Kleinman, 1986).

Eventually symptoms come to interfere with daily activities of living or otherwise cause the person to seek care from a primary health provider. Zola's research (1973) documented that symptoms that persisted beyond an expected time frame and that interfered with vocational or daily activities often guided the decision to seek health care.

Other factors affect the person's responses to first signs: *personal characteristics*, such as age and gender; *financial issues*, such as income and insurance; *psychological makeup*, including coping resources and typical coping patterns; *social considerations*, such as family structure, social network and support, and work status; and the person's configuration of *knowledge, experience, and attitudes,* including awareness of the implications of the symptoms, valuing the importance of early diagnosis, previous experience with the health care system, spiritual orientation including religious

beliefs and practices and personal existential philosophy, and beliefs about or experiences with cancer. Any of the factors can either facilitate or impede the person's response to the initial alerting event signaling the possibility of cancer. The speed or delay in seeking diagnosis and treatment has been referred to as *lag time* (Weisman, 1979a; Worden & Weisman, 1975) and is further divided into (1) the period of time between the alerting event and the first health provider contact, referred to as *patient delay*; and (2) the time between the first health provider contact and the initiation of treatment, or *diagnostic delay* (Marshall & Funch, 1986).

Personal Characteristics

Characteristics such as age, gender, ethnic background, and level of education are associated with people's response to a threatening health or illness signal. For example, younger and middle-aged persons are more likely to use prevention and detection services in the absence of symptoms (National Center for Health Statistics [NCHS], 1986). This may be a function of the fact that screening programs generally are directed toward women in their reproductive years (Given & Given, 1989). Young adults have longer periods of patient delay than older persons. This response may be attributable to less awareness of the significance of the symptoms, disbelief or denial of susceptibility or that something serious could be wrong, less adequate insurance, and less time. As a group, middle-aged persons have the shortest lag times. Lierman (1988) reported that the women in her sample who sought medical attention for their symptoms of breast cancer quickly (less than 4 weeks) were significantly younger (59.8 years) than those who delayed a year or more (71.8 years). The data on patient delay among the elderly are less clear. Older persons spend more time interacting with the health care system in response to a greater number of somatic complaints. This can result in shorter lag times, especially if there is a personal history of cancer (Mettlin, Reese, & Murphy, 1980). As all subjects in Lierman's study were at least 50 years old and would be considered "older" in the general population, her finding that 60 per cent of the women had short or intermediate delay times is consistent with the description that older persons have shorter lag times. It has been noted, however, that older persons tend to practice fewer cancer detection behaviors (Holmes & Hearne, 1981) and fail to seek specific cancer examinations on the assumption that their interactions with providers for other health problems are sufficient to identify signs of cancer (Given & Given, 1989). Also, cancer symptoms in the elderly can easily be confused with signs of normal aging (Frank-Stromborg, 1986). These observations may explain why elderly persons are found to have more advanced disease at the time of diagnosis (Holmes & Hearne, 1981). Delay may be extended also if the elderly person has less education and limited financial resources and insurance benefits (Funch, 1985). Thus age does appear to be a significant factor in lag time, but the relationship is complex and nonlinear.

Gender is another significant factor in determining a person's response to signs of illness. Verbrugge (1979a, 1982) points out that, in general, women are more likely than men to seek medical attention, but their health problems are likely to be of a less serious or life-threatening nature. Women use more prevention and detection services (NCHS, 1986), perhaps because cancer screening programs are more likely to be directed toward them (Given & Given, 1989). Men have more serious chronic health conditions, a higher incidence of injuries, more long-term disability, and ultimately a shorter life span. Because women are more likely to utilize the health care system, they might be expected to seek treatment more promptly than men. However, in one examination of women's health care practices and cancer, McCorkle (1989) reported that women showed significant delays in seeking treatment for a variety of cancer symptoms. For example, between 20 and 35 per cent of women who discovered a lump in their breasts waited months or even more than a year to seek treatment. These findings are consistent with those reported by Funch (1985), Funch and Francis (1982), and Lierman (1988). Among colorectal cancer patients of both genders, the sexes differed in both patient delay and diagnostic delay (Marshall & Funch, 1986). In both components of lag time, delay was longer for women. A variety of explanations for these differences have been proposed, and Lierman (1988) expressed particular concern over the fact that many of the causes of delay were a function of health providers' differential response to women's symptoms rather than to delays caused by the women themselves. Even women who sought prompt medical attention did not necessarily receive prompt diagnosis and treatment.

McCorkle (1989) also summarized the controversial findings in studies of women's practice of breast self-examination (BSE). She concluded that there is some tendency for women who practice BSE to delay seeking treatment on discovery of a symptom. This might suggest that the practice of BSE, at least for these women, is motivated more by fear than by a positive attitude of self-care. In addition, McCorkle noted that further delays may be related to age, education, physical stature, and past experience with breast cancer.

Education also is a factor in the promptness with which people respond to their initial symptoms. Persons with less education are more likely to delay seeking treatment (Funch, 1985; Germino & McCorkle, 1985). Ethnicity has also been associated with differences in response to warning signs. Degree of trust in the health care system often is a key factor in determining whether persons will seek out standard medical care or choose to try folk cures. Nonwhite persons are more likely to delay than are whites. Blacks tend to be more fatalistic than whites, believing more cancer myths, and being less likely to believe that early detection makes a difference (EVAXX, 1981; National Cancer Institute, 1986; U.S. Department of Health and Human Services [USDHHS], 1986). Other findings, however, attribute these apparent racial or ethnic differences to poverty (American Cancer Society [ACS], 1989).

Financial Considerations

Financial resources are clearly a significant factor affecting persons' response to their cancer symptoms (Houts et al., 1985). Persons from lower socioeconomic classes tend to have significantly longer delays in seeking diagnosis (Hackett, Cassem, & Raker, 1973; Lewis & Bloom, 1978–79). An American Cancer Society (ACS) report on cancer in the poor (1989) concluded that economically disadvantaged Americans have severely limited access to health care and health insurance, and they obtain care only at great personal sacrifice. Furthermore, the care they receive is often inadequate, insensitive, and at times irrelevant to their needs. Thus the poor face many barriers to responding to their cancer symptoms, and they sometimes appear to believe that the outcomes are not worth the effort required.

People need not be poverty stricken, however, to feel constraints in their cancer health care. For example, the relatively high cost of a mammogram has been reported to be one reason for not using this valuable detection procedure (Crooks & Jones, 1989). Whether the person has health insurance is another important consideration. Uninsured persons are likely to delay seeking diagnosis and treatment. Even with health insurance, out-of-pocket expenses for transportation, meals away from home, hotel costs during outpatient care in a distant city, and other costs not covered by insurance are a serious burden to families on limited incomes, especially for single-parent families and the elderly on fixed incomes. Loss of time from work poses an additional financial problem. These threats of financial burden are likely to lead to delay in seeking medical attention, especially if the symptoms are not painful or visible. Financial resources clearly become a direct factor in the decision to take advantage of some of the latest but most expensive diagnostic procedures or to obtain more complex cancer treatment, such as bone marrow transplants.

Psychological Makeup

When people suddenly recognize that a symptom may be a possible indicator of cancer, their response will be influenced by their complex psychological makeup. Although the literature on the role of psychosocial factors in predicting the onset of cancer is growing (Cunningham, 1985; Fox, 1983; Greer & Morris, 1975; Morris & Greer, 1980; Stams & Steggles, 1987), few investigators have discussed these factors in association with delay in seeking diagnosis or treatment (Levy, 1985). People tend to respond to the threat of cancer in much the same way they have responded to other crises in their lives (Holland, 1976; Worden & Weisman, 1975). Generally, persons who have used denial as a major coping mechanism can be expected to delay longer in seeking treatment (Greer, 1974; Magarey, Todd, & Blizard, 1977), although these findings are not undisputed. Delay may also be a function of the unwillingness of individuals to become dependent on their health providers or family (Hammerschlag, Fisher, De Cosser, & Kaplan, 1964). Weisman points out that delay may be consistent with a "trait of independent self-reliance" just as well as "fearful procrastination" (1979a, p. 15). This mixture of coping strategies may explain why some investigators have found no differences between deniers and acceptors in their length of delay in seeking treatment (Watson, Greer, Blake, & Sharpnell, 1984). Intellectualization, isolation, guilt, anxiety, and depression also have been associated with delay in seeking diagnosis and treatment (Gold, 1964; Krant, 1981; Magarey et al., 1977). Fear of the diagnosis of cancer, of the treatment modalities, and of pain or disfigurement have all been implicated in delay (Crooks & Jones, 1989; Gold, 1964). Fear also may explain why some women engage is self-detection behaviors but delay seeking diagnosis when they find a possible symptom (McCorkle, 1989). Assessing psychological factors associated with delay is very difficult because the subjects needed for a prospective study of this topic are unknown until they enter the health care system. By this time, they will have gone through a number of steps in their decision making that may alter their psychological state and interfere with their ability to accurately reproduce their feelings at the time of the discovery of symptoms.

Social Considerations

Family dynamics, marital status, social support and work status are among the social factors believed to be associated with response to warning signs of cancer. Married women who discover a breast lump become concerned about their spouses' reaction to the lump or to the loss of the breast; mothers worry about how their children will react (Lambert & Lambert, 1979; Verbrugge, 1979b). Family members, reluctant to see their elderly family member subjected to aggressive therapies for cancer, may delay seeking diagnosis (Given & Given, 1989).

Members of a person's social network can play a major role in reducing delay. Wool (1986), in her study that compared women with breast lumps who delayed longer than 3 months (extreme deniers) with women who sought medical attention more promptly, observed that the deniers were significantly more likely to see the doctor only if encouraged to do so by a relative or friend. Yet family members may inadvertently support delaying behavior because they are more likely to share common values and characteristics. Salloway and Dillon (1973) found that persons with more *friends* in their social networks were less likely to delay seeking health care then persons with large *family* networks. Giacquinta (1977) has described in detail the family's stresses and concerns when a member has cancer. Some

of these problems may contribute to patient delay in seeking health care.

Knowledge, Experience, and Attitudes

A person experiencing a signaling event must have the knowledge that a lump in the breast or a wound that does not heal has meaning that should not be overlooked. To this end, agencies such as the National Cancer Institute (NCI) and the ACS invest large sums of money and effort into public education. Research has shown that increasing people's understanding of the importance of screening and detection can also increase their likelihood of their partaking in them (Crooks & Jones, 1989; Kegeles, 1969). Nonetheless, many persons remain unaware of many of the publicized danger signs, with elderly persons who are at greater risk being even less knowledgeable than the population as a whole (Weinrich & Weinrich, 1986). Many women, for example, remain uneducated regarding BSE despite having at least occasional Papanicolaou smears. Only about 15 per cent of women aged 50 years old and older obtain recommended annual mammograms (Crooks & Jones, 1989). Thus lack of knowledge continues to be a serious source of delay in seeking medical attention for a signaling event.

Knowledge, however, is never enough in and of itself. Knowing is not always accompanied by the desirable health behavior. Among women who have been taught BSE, few carry out this easy practice regularly, although it has repeatedly been shown to be associated with the discovery of tumors at an earlier stage. There is also some question of whether women who report performing BSE are actually following the recommended procedures accurately. Nurses may be even less likely than women in general to practice BSE on a regular basis. This may be an act of denial, related to nurses' expressed fears of cancer therapies (Mood, Brenner, & Richardson, 1985). Women who do practice BSE know the possible meaning of a breast lump, but those who have more knowledge regarding breast cancer are sometimes *more* likely to delay seeking medical treatment (Owens, Duffy, & Ashcroft, 1985). Similarly, it was found that when women detected lumps in their breast by BSE, they were more likely to delay (Gould-Martin, Paganini-Hill, Casagrande, Mack, & Ross, 1982). Thus it would seem that some knowledge can interact with other factors to become another source of delay.

Beliefs and attitudes can affect a person's responses to many aspects of life. These include individual spiritual beliefs, which may be religious but may also derive from a personal existential philosophy. Some evidence exists that religiosity—measured by the extent to which a person affiliates with a religious group, engages in religious activities, and reports that religious experiences influence beliefs about life and death—is associated with significantly less fear of death (Mood & Van Fossen, 1983; Wendt, 1989). Reducing fear and inspiring hope (Miller, 1985) may be one important way of reducing delay in seeking health care when confronted by threatening symptoms. Although beliefs held by some religious groups deter their followers from seeking health care, most mainstream religions in the United States support prompt and active intervention.

Beliefs specifically related to health may also affect people's health behaviors. In particular, their belief in their susceptibility to illness or its potential seriousness are among the factors that influence the decision to seek medical advice (Cox, 1982; Kegeles, 1969; Rosenstock, 1974).

One important factor that influences beliefs and attitudes is past experience with the health care system (Holland, 1982). Persons who have had limited experience may have an idealized image of the system—a "Dr. Marcus Welby syndrome"—which may lead them to seek medical assistance more readily but perhaps more naively. If men and women with prior experience judge that they have received good health care in the past and they feel a sense of trust in their care providers, they may be inclined to contact them more rapidly. If, on the other hand, their experience has been one of poor communication, fear, painful interventions without adequate preparation or explanation, or a sense of anonymity within a large uncaring system, they are less likely to seek help promptly.

Even more influential in persons' decisions to seek care than their general experience with health care systems is their experience with, and resulting attitudes and beliefs about, cancer. Many persons still believe that a cancer diagnosis is a death sentence (Holland, 1982; Krant, 1976). To the extent they recognize that their signaling event is a cancer risk sign, they may be afraid of confirming their worst fears. Fear of cancer treatment, when thought of as mutilating surgery or cancer-producing radiation, or even as treatments causing nausea and hair loss, can be as intense as the fear of cancer itself (Holland, 1976; Leis & Pilnik, 1974; Vettese, 1976). Furthermore, persons who have experienced the death of a family member or close friend from cancer are more likely to delay seeking diagnosis of a possible cancer symptom even if they regularly engage in cancer detection behavior (Funch, 1985; Hackett et al., 1973). However, experience may interact with age to reverse this trend because older persons with a personal history of cancer seek medical care more promptly (Mettlin et al., 1980).

Thus it is clear that knowledge is important, but it is not always enough to ensure prompt action in the face of symptoms. Experience also is important and interacts with knowledge to form beliefs and attitudes that may help or hinder the person's motivation to take action. When knowledge or experience or both lead to a fearful reaction, the result may be patient delay.

Other Factors

A variety of other factors have been shown to be related to the person's decision to take prompt action or to delay seeking treatment. One factor that generally hastens a decision to act is the severity of any symptoms. Pain is a major motivator to seeking treatment. Symptom distress heightens the person's awareness of the possible seriousness of the condition and tends to interfere with the use of denial (Germino & McCorkle, 1985). It should be noted, however, that even extreme symptoms can be seen in some deniers. For example, a woman with a draining lesion in the breast delayed seeking medical attention for 7 years and finally did so only when another, more serious condition made it necessary (Lierman, 1988). Her beliefs and attitudes were such that although she knew the potential seriousness of her symptoms from the start, and although her mother had died of breast cancer, she chose to close her eyes to the situation and delay professional care.

Stage of disease has also been associated with the speed with which treatment is sought, although the relationship is not a clear one. Advanced disease is generally associated with greater symptom distress, which is more likely to lead to prompt seeking of treatment. On the other hand, as shown earlier, women who practice BSE and seek prompt treatment are significantly more likely to have early stage breast cancer (Crooks & Jones, 1989; Funch, 1985; McCorkle, 1989).

Some physical characteristics may also be important. For example, Funch (1985) found that women with large breasts delayed seeking care longer than women with small breasts. Funch offered no explanation of this finding, so that it is unclear whether women with large breasts were more embarrassed or self-conscious about their breast size, or whether it was perhaps a more general issue of weight. Whatever the specific dynamics are, Funch's findings suggest that body image may affect health care decisions.

In summary, then, it is clear that people can become aware of the first signs of cancer in a variety of ways. They may discover an obvious symptom; they may experience a sign or symptom that is not immediately obvious but which, over time, is clearly different from their past experience; or the first signs may be found by a health care provider in the course of providing unrelated health care or routine checkups. In whatever manner the first signs become known to the person, there is an experience of sudden awareness that opens a door to the personal discovery of a new life role; that is, the transition from being a person without cancer to being a person with cancer, or at least suspected cancer. The transition is not really complete until a formal diagnosis and treatment plan are obtained. Individual responses to this first step in the transition vary widely, with some persons moving quickly to seek diagnosis and treatment and others delaying in taking health care action. Many factors, both internal and external to the person, have been shown to be related to that critical decision. What is not known at this time is the relative importance of these factors and whether these findings, many of which are based on studies of women, are similar for men. It is also unclear which factors would have the greatest impact on altering attitudes, behaviors, and outcomes if systematic nursing interventions were planned to facilitate such changes.

THE DIAGNOSIS

The many factors that propel or impede individual responses to the first signs of cancer have been reviewed. If those signs are obvious, the degree of certainty regarding the diagnosis may be high even before the person obtains a formal diagnosis. More often, however, the signs are equivocal. For example, most breast lumps are benign. Similarly, virtually any sign or symptom of cancer could also be a sign or symptom of something else. Therefore, the real impact of this first transition comes with a formal diagnosis. The conditions under which the diagnosis is made and then shared with the patient can have a significant effect on patients' reactions, the meanings they ascribe to their diagnosis, their ability to cope with this new dimension in their lives, and their later behavior. Therefore, the diagnosis of cancer will be considered from the perspectives of the both professionals who make and give the diagnosis and the persons (i.e., patients and family) who receive the diagnosis.

Giving the Diagnosis: Professional Attitudes and Actions

In the United States, the prevailing practice among health professionals in the field of oncology is to provide patients with an accurate description of their diagnosis and treatment plans. However, this is a relatively new phenomenon that began in the late 1960s. A survey of physicians conducted in 1961 reported that 90 per cent said they did not disclose a cancer diagnosis to the patient (Novack et al., 1979; Oken, 1961). By 1977, physicians' attitudes and behavior regarding disclosure had changed dramatically, with 97 per cent reporting that it was better to inform patients of their cancer diagnoses, treatment options, and realistic expectations for outcomes (Israel, 1978; Novack et al., 1979). However, as Holland (1976) points out, physicians must deal with their own feelings about cancer when faced with the decision of what to tell their patients. Many times, these practitioners have not resolved their own fears and anxieties, resulting in behavior that is sometimes overly protective and paternalistic or sometimes overly blunt and cold. Therefore, although a very high proportion of physicians now favor disclosing accurate diagnostic and treatment information to their patients, their actual behavior in practice may reflect a much more limited change in approach from earlier years.

Nurses also show some discrepancy between their attitudes and practices with respect to sharing information with patients. Nurses who were asked about their attitudes and experiences with dying patients consistently expressed a belief in openness and honesty with all patients as long as the patients were mentally competent (Castles & Murray, 1979). When asked about their behavior, however, many nurses described practices that were not consistent with their stated belief. They offered many different reasons—for example, "there's a policy here against it," "the patients don't want to hear about that stuff," "I don't really have enough time for that." In a secondary linguistic analysis of these nurses' responses, it was found that in every one of the 40 interviews evaluated, the nurses were more likely to substitute the pronoun *it* for terms such as *cancer, tumor*, and *death* than for less negative terms such as *nursing care* or *temperature* (Mood, 1980). This highly consistent finding was interpreted as an unconscious linguistic mechanism that allowed the nurses to avoid the use of unpleasant words while continuing to discuss the topic. These findings have since been replicated in a study of staff nurses, half of whom worked in oncology units (Mood et al., 1985). The oncology nurses were just as likely to manifest linguistic signs of avoidance and denial as were the general medical or surgical nurses.

The high disclosure rates reported by American physicians are not typical of the disclosure practices in other parts of the world. In Great Britain and Europe, as well as the eastern world, many physicians continue to adhere to the practice of withholding the cancer diagnosis from patients (Israel, 1978), sometimes causing bitter disputes among international colleagues. This nondisclosure practice continues even though as long ago as 1959, Aitken-Swan and Easson reported that 66 per cent of a sample of 231 British patients with various early stage curable cancers approved of having been given an accurate diagnosis. Remembering that this study was conducted at a time and place in which disclosure was virtually unheard of, the fact that only 12 per cent of the patients said they would have preferred not to have been told was quite amazing. The remaining 22 per cent were neutral in their opinions. Patients who were contacted a second time more than a year later tended to adhere to their original reaction, with a high proportion of the patients continuing to approve of the disclosure practice.

An interesting observation reported by Aitken-Swan and Easson (1959) is that one of the negative consequences of nondisclosure, especially to early stage cancer patients, is that the general public never learns that cancer is a curable disease. If the experience of the general public is that all persons with cancer die (because persons with curable cancers never had their diseases labeled as such), the belief that people always die of cancer is reinforced. Patients in the Aitken-Swan and Easson study reported that friends and relatives would not believe them when they shared their diagnoses and favorable prognoses.

Thus the giving of a cancer diagnosis is an important step. It involves physicians, nurses, and other health care providers coming to grips with their own beliefs regarding cancer and death and how these may be affecting their disclosure practices. The speed, clarity, and care with which the diagnosis is made, the attitudes and behaviors of the health care providers during the diagnostic work-up period, and the manner in which the diagnosis is finally given have a major impact on the patient, the family and friends, and even the public at large.

Receiving the Diagnosis: Patients' and Families' Responses

Despite the more open disclosure practices of American physicians and broad programs of public education to increase the awareness of cancer as curable or avoidable by life-style changes such as stopping smoking and watching the diet, cancer is still more dreaded than any of the other major life-threatening illnesses. Krant (1976) suggests that this fear is due to the fact that people associate cancer not only with likely death but also with protracted pain and disability. Cancer "is equated with a withering away of life's essential elements, and is associated with foul smells, feelings of dirtiness, hopeless irrevocability, severe and relentless pain, and eventual death after weeks and months of this suffering" (p. 270).

Although very little research has addressed the question of people's reactions to a diagnosis of cancer, the many anecdotal reports and articles based on clinical experience paint a grim picture of shock, disbelief, fear, depression, sadness, and hopelessness (Krant, 1981). Fear and panic are the most common initial reactions at this time (Novotny, Hyland, Coyne, Travis, & Pruyner, 1984). The response to the cancer diagnosis has been described as similar to grief reactions often seen in the face of disaster or great threatened losses (Holland, 1976, 1986). This seems to be especially true when surgery is the recommended treatment, perhaps because of the threat of mutilation (Vettese, 1976). Loss of self-determination or of a sense of control can also accompany the intense emotional reactions (Fountain, 1985; Vettese, 1976), which in turn can lead to withdrawal, anxiety, and agitation (Giacquinta, 1977).

In one descriptive study of patients' reactions to their cancer diagnoses, Weisman and Worden (1976–1977) summarized the experience of 120 patients in the first 100 days after their diagnosis. They describe this time frame as the period of "existential plight in cancer." *Existential plight* consists of two substages: *impact distress* (the initial immediate response to the diagnosis) and *existential plight proper* (the first 3 to 4 months after diagnosis, which often includes patients' completion of primary treatment). During these 120 days, patients in Weisman and Worden's study completed a series of questionnaires and interviews, including standardized and investigator-developed instruments. Patients' responses indicated that this is a period of great emotional impact. However, the intensity and duration of the initial distress varied widely—from brief and transient discomfort to extreme and continuing anxiety, depression, anger, and desperation. These investigators noted that it was sometimes difficult to detect the level of distress from overt signs, an observation substantiated by other reports (Box 18–1) (Jamison, Wellisch, & Pasnau, 1978; Maguire, 1975, 1985).

Box 18–1. CANCER AS CRISIS: THE CRITICAL ELEMENTS OF ADJUSTMENT

This study examined the course and duration of the crisis inherent in the diagnosis and treatment of cancer in women. Three groups of female patients, breast cancer, gynecologic cancer, and breast biopsy patients, were compared on the variables of depression and body image. The women were assessed prior to surgery and at one- and two-month intervals to determine whether their crisis had been resolved within the normal six-month framework. An additional follow-up was made after 20 months to evaluate any long-term effects of the diagnosis of cancer or its treatment. Results of the study revealed that only breast biopsy and mastectomy patients adapted appropriately and were able to resolve their crises. In examining the gynecologic cancer patients, initial feelings of depression and body image continued to worsen even at 20 months after surgery. Implications for nursing practice are discussed, and suggestions for future research are presented.

(Data from Krouse, H. J., & Krouse, J. H. [1982]. Cancer as crisis: The critical elements of adjustment. *Nursing Research*, 31:96–101.)

During the initial period after diagnosis, Weisman and Worden found that patients' concerns focused more on existential issues of life and death than on any other of the areas assessed, including patients' health, work and finances, religion, self, and relationships with family and friends. Earlier, Benoliel (Quint, 1963) had made a similar observation of the primacy of existential concerns among women following mastectomy. In later studies, she and her colleagues (McCorkle & Benoliel, 1983) again reported findings consistent with Weisman and Worden's description.

Although it is not unusual, then, to observe extreme emotional reactions as the first response to a cancer diagnosis, it is nonetheless important to assess the nature of the patient's response carefully. Holland (1982) recommends that an assessment of psychological and social resources be included as part of the medical history because the initial reactions are often predictive of later adjustment (Graydon, 1988; Morris, Greer, & White, 1979; Northouse, 1984; Weisman & Worden, 1976–1977) and can identify those persons at risk and in greatest need of psychosocial intervention (Weisman, Worden, & Sobel, 1980; Worden, 1983). Such assessments must be done with caution, however. Although a large proportion of patients retrospectively describe the diagnostic period as the most stressful of their entire cancer experience (Jamison et al., 1978), many did not or could not share their feelings with either family members or health professionals at the time (Jamison et al., 1978; Maguire, 1975, 1985). This may be an example of what Lazarus (1979, November) refers to as "positive denial," a coping strategy persons use to delay dealing consciously with the threat of a situation to be able to get through the situation. When newly diagnosed cancer patients appraise the diagnosis as demanding more coping abilities than they feel they can muster, positive denial allows them some time to gather their resources and reappraise the situation as more manageable. During the time they are using positive denial effectively, patients are not likely to be able to report the distress because they cannot allow themselves to think about it, in much the same way as persons who perform heroic deeds block out thoughts of danger so that they can carry out their acts of bravery. Later, upon reflection, cancer patients, like heroes, are able to provide a retrospective report of their intense distress, as seen in the studies noted earlier by Jamison and colleagues (1978) and Maguire (1975, 1985). This may explain why some investigators observe low levels of distress in the responses to questionnaires from newly diagnosed patients, contrary to expectations (Edlund & Sneed, 1989; Mood & Bickes, 1989). It suggests that the timing of assessments may be an important factor in the findings obtained. Age appears to be another important factor affecting this assessment as well, with younger persons (under 50 years old) showing more psychological distress than older persons (over 70 years) (Edlund & Sneed, 1989).

Another common reaction at the time of diagnosis is the fear of abandonment (Fountain, 1985); patients often fear that they will lose the love and support of their family and friends. In turn, these "significant others" are frequently at a loss as to how to communicate effectively. Fears of discussing sensitive issues are common and can sometimes lead to a "conspiracy of silence" (Weisman & Hackett, 1961). Emotional reactions, physical symptoms, and treatment demands can disrupt the intimacy of the family and a couple's sexual relationship. Because of the significant impact of the cancer diagnosis on the persons closest to the patient, cancer is often described as a disease of the family system (Giacquinta, 1977; Lewandowski & Jones, 1988; Marino, 1981; Northouse, 1984, 1989; Weisman, 1979a; Woods, Lewis, & Ellison, 1989). Oncology nursing in particular often defines the family unit rather than the individual patient as the client. This is a critical distinction because the responses of the patient's significant others are critical to the patient's own response (Litman, 1974). As family system theory would suggest, when one family member makes a significant life transition, each of the other members must make his or her own parallel transition. Studies of the reactions of family members to the patient's cancer diagnosis are limited (Gotay, 1984; Northouse, 1984, 1989). It has been reported that the family's concerns during this initial phase focus on providing support for the patient, on being assured that the patient is receiving the best possible care, and on gathering information to better understand what is happening (Dyck & Wright, 1985; Lewandowski & Jones, 1988). Often it is the family who is the first to be informed of the cancer diagnosis, and not uncommonly their initial reaction is to want to withhold the information from the patient. Holland (1976) suggests that this is a response to the family's own inability to accept the diagnosis. However, by the time the diagnosis is shared with the patient, the family has had some time to adjust to the initial shock.

Family members share the existential concerns of the patients as well as their own concerns about how their lives will change with the illness and possible death of the patient (Giacquinta, 1977; Northouse, 1989). This experience can precipitate many dysfunctional family dynamics. Family members have some painful issues of their own to resolve. They need to find the time to support the ill member, take on added role responsibilities that the ill member is unable to fulfill, and still maintain their own life roles. They may experience emotions they find unacceptable. For example, they may feel relieved that they are not the one with the illness. They may resent some aspects of the patient's past behavior that they perceive to be a cause of the cancer (e.g., smoking). They may also experience anger toward the ill person for becoming ill and altering their lives. These are feelings that they will have difficulty acknowledging or sharing and will often need assistance to resolve. If the patient is a child, siblings will feel abandoned as parents spend long hours away from home and are not physically or emotionally able to meet their needs. Thus the impact of the cancer diagnosis is more far-reaching than the reactions of the patient alone.

Although reports in the literature clearly communicate the devastating emotional impact of a cancer diagnosis on the patient and family, some evidence suggests that, at times, there are positive reactions as well. First, as described earlier, Weisman and Worden's study (1976–1977) of patients' reactions during the first 100 days after diagnosis indicated that a significant proportion (50 to 60 per cent) of patients adjust well to their diagnosis and cope effectively without intervention. Investigators who have examined patients' reactions to cancer have found that many persons report positive coping strategies, such as taking firm action and finding something favorable about the situation (Gotay, 1984), maintaining optimism about the future and meaning in their lives (Mages et al., 1981), and having an active determination to recover (Hughes, 1982). It has also been proposed that denial may have a beneficial effect, at least for a period of time, in assisting persons to cope effectively with a threatening situation (Forester, Kornfeld, & Fleiss, 1978; Lazarus, 1979; Watson et al., 1984). Frank-Stromborg and her associates (Stromborg, Wright, Segella, & Diekmann, 1984) reported that 27 per cent of the responses provided by 340 ambulatory cancer patients who were asked to recall their feelings after receiving their cancer diagnosis were classified as reflecting positive attitudes (e.g., "I decided to make the best of it" and "I decided to conquer the cancer"). In a later instrument development study, a sample of 441 ambulatory cancer patients in active treatment responded to a 36 item questionnaire assessing their reactions to their cancer diagnosis (Frank-Stromborg, 1989). The questionnaire contained both negative and positive items. Respondents readily endorsed the positive as well as negative items.

Thus it appears that responses to a diagnosis of cancer can be positive as well as negative. This raises some interesting questions which will need to be addressed in future research:

1. Are reports of devastating emotional reactions exaggerated, perhaps by observers' bias; that is, do professionals who expect patients to be devastated by a cancer diagnosis merely see what they expect to see? Alternatively, are the apparent positive reactions now being reported actually a form of denial that can be reported only retrospectively as emotionally traumatic?

2. Are attitudes toward cancer changing with greater openness and more public education and media attention? Will patients no longer receive reactions of disbelief when they share their cancer diagnosis and favorable prognosis with family and friends?

3. Do health care providers continue to give "mixed messages" to patients and family about the appropriateness of sharing feelings?

Oncology nursing research may be able to provide answers to these questions by accurately assessing patients' reactions over time and by identifying some of the factors that predict or explain those reactions.

The Meaning of the Diagnosis

There is increasing evidence that the human experience of receiving a diagnosis of cancer elicits a wide array of personal and social meanings. The process of seeking clinical confirmation for symptoms of a cancer diagnosis is characterized by a series of ambiguous situations. People are often unprepared for several aspects of the experience, including the urgency that surrounds the diagnostic work-up, the new experience of being hospitalized and subjected to a series of diagnostic tests, and the eventual disclosure of the life-threatening diagnosis.

During the clinical diagnostic period, people may have limited access to information about their health condition. Many clinicians are guarded about the information they disclose until a substantive diagnosis is established. An alternative approach is to keep patients informed of the ongoing nature of the diagnostic experience. This approach would allow health professionals to minimize the uncertainty that is generated by a deficiency in information.

Building explanatory models of cancer during the early phase centers on the process of transforming clinical knowledge into personal terms. People may search for the cause of their cancer. They may struggle with the question, "Why me?" It is an effort both the patient and the family members engage in as each tries to understand what he or she is experiencing. Answers are sought to the questions of why this is happening to this person at this time. This search for meaning may represent a basic spiritual need (Highfield & Cason, 1983; Sodestrom & Martinson, 1987). Thus seeking the meaning of a cancer diagnosis represents a normal human response. It is an effort to find hope and purpose, sometimes through prayer (Miller, 1985; Sodestrom & Martinson, 1987). Within a nursing conceptual framework, patients and their families are exercising their self-care abilities (Hanucharurnkul, 1989; Orem, 1985).

The search for meaning has also been described as

an attempt to use cognitive resources to gain intellectual mastery over the emotional reactions to the cancer process (Giacquinta, 1977; Lewandowski & Jones, 1988). People may formulate beliefs about how the illness works as a disease process, and they may gather information to estimate the severity of the illness condition. For family members, this search for meaning may also include an effort to reassure themselves that they are not subject to the same sources of vulnerability and therefore at great risk for developing cancer themselves. The meaning people ascribe to their diagnoses may even affect their bodies' response to their disease and treatment (Simonton et al., 1978).

Personal Meaning

Cognitive reappraisals are a key component of peoples' personal construction of the illness experience. Reappraisals lead to an interpretive change in personal meaning. When a person is confronted with illness, he or she must evolve and develop new "meaning" to understand and give order or coherence to life. This is often a period of profound reorganization of personal goals and priorities. Cognitive reappraisals also demonstrate the person's resilience to adapt to the adverse situation and the ability to construe some personal benefit from a tragic situation. Specifically, these reappraisals allow the person to assign positive meanings to the situation. Reappraisals such as "take things day by day," "appreciate each day to its fullest," and "there must be some purpose to this" are generated to redefine the situation so that some of its threatening aspects can be diminished. Another reappraisal strategy is for people to make social comparisons of their own situation with that of others who are living through similar experiences (Taylor, 1983). When a person takes notice that another patient with a similar diagnosis is not doing so well, *downward comparison* is used to enhance the first person's self-esteem. In contrast, an *upward comparison* allows the individual to emulate as a positive role model someone who is perceived as coping effectively.

Social Meaning

A number of social implications occur with the confirmation of the cancer diagnosis. As the person integrates a set of personal meanings about the experience, a self-identity evolves within a social environment. Additional meanings are derived from social transactions with others. One of the most difficult social interactions that occurs is the disclosure of the diagnosis to family and friends. It is not uncommon for the person to want to protect significant others from the devastating news. Giacquinta (1977) points out that this information may be shared prematurely, before the patient and the immediate family have had adequate opportunity to process the information and their initial reactions themselves. It is difficult, under these circumstances, to derive the support and sense of courage that can come when the social sharing is timed more appropriately.

Causal Attributions

Causal attributions are defined as naive perceptions or common-sense explanations for events or experiences (Frieze & Bar-Tal, 1978). A growing body of research argues that people search for reasons why important and unexpected events happen. Such searching is carried out by persons attempting to understand their own life situations or by larger groups within society. The latter is sometimes called *research* and has resulted in causal attributions for cancer such as "smoking causes cancer" and "breast cancer is hereditary." The reasons we identify, both individually and collectively, are interpreted by each person, influencing the way the event is perceived. Causal search may be a necessary prerequisite for the full interpretation of the emotions linked to important events such as a diagnosis of cancer (Weiner, 1979). Additionally, expectations for the future are determined by the causal attributions of past events.

When people ask "Why me?" they are attempting to ascribe a cause to an event or an experience. Events that are considered stressful, those that are not expected, or situations in which the goal is not attained tend to prompt causal thinking. Taylor (1983) has proposed that one part of the coping process involves finding meaning in an event, such as a cancer diagnosis, and this search can involve a search for a cause.

Causal search, however, was not found to be related to adjustment in a sample of 78 women with breast cancer who were interviewed about 2 years after their operations (Taylor, Lichtman, & Wood, 1984). The responses about causal thinking were prompted by a question asking subjects to share their hunches or theories about how they got their cancer. The time causal thinking occurred in relation to diagnosis and how controllable they thought the cancer was were also determined, as were the patients' psychological and overall adjustments. Patients were also asked to rate their agreement with 22 potential causes listed on a questionnaire.

Although 95 per cent of subjects eventually ascribed a cause, few patients (28 per cent) reported making attributions at the time of diagnosis, with 71 per cent indicating that causal thinking was not important at that time. During recovery and at the time of the study, 41 per cent believed causal thinking was important.

Adjustment scores were evaluated for the groups who constructed causes and those who did not, as well as for groups who thought causal search was important and those who did not. No differences were found between groups. Adjustment was generally unrelated to the specific causes either from the interview or from the attributional questionnaire. It was argued that, for a continuing threat such as cancer, it may be more important to treat it than to wonder why it occurred. No attempt was made to relate these findings to variables such as patient delay (Taylor et al., 1984).

Gotay (1984) also found that neither the process of causal search nor the specific attribution was related to adjustment. She interviewed 42 early-stage gyneco-logic patients within 2 weeks of their cancer diagnosis and 31 advanced-stage gynecologic or breast patients who had been diagnosed from several months to 10 years before the interview. Subjects were asked if they had ever asked "Why me?" with respect to cancer and, if so, what answer they reached. A structured attributional measure was also used, which asked subjects to assign a percentage of blame to four factors: "yourself; the kind of person you are," "things you have done," "the environment and other people," and "chance."

In response to the open-ended question, 26 early-stage and 16 advanced-stage patients indicated they had asked "Why me?". "Chance" was the most common response of early-stage subjects, and "God's will" was identified most commonly by advanced-stage patients. Chance was also the most common attribution in the structured survey, with 64 per cent of early-stage patients and 56 per cent of advanced-stage subjects choosing that response. It is interesting to note that all patients, including the 42 per cent who either had not asked "Why me?" or had asked it and failed to answer it, chose an attribution on the structured questionnaire. Gotay (1984) reached a somewhat different conclusion than Taylor and colleagues (1984). She interpreted her findings to mean that patients may avoid making connections between cancer and its perceived causes because of the frightening nature of the disease. This interpretation is supported in a study of patients with cancers of the head and neck who were significantly less willing to endorse items reflecting personal responsibility for their cancer than similarly worded items that addressed their health in general. The cancer-specific items may have been more threatening (Mood & Parzuchowski, 1986).

Thus whereas the search for meaning has been described as a universal response to a cancer diagnosis, the specific focus on causal attributions is not, especially at the time of diagnosis. Only 28 per cent of patients in the study by Taylor and associates (1984) and 62 per cent of the early-stage patients in the Gotay study (1984) reported making such inferences early in their cancer experience. Furthermore, whether or not they attempted such attribution and regardless of the causes they identified, no relationship was found between these factors and various measures of coping and adjustment.

In summary, then, the diagnostic stage of the transition to becoming a person with cancer is a difficult and emotional one for all persons involved. Physicians, nurses, and other health professionals struggle with issues of how best to carry out the complicated diagnostic work-up, balancing the desire to avoid unnecessary anxiety for patients with the patient's right to a fair and accurate description of what is being done. Patients and their families, during the diagnostic work-up period, struggle with the uncertainties and ambiguities of what is readily recognized as an unusual process. If they are aware that a cancer diagnosis is the probable or even likely outcome of this process, they have already begun the period of existential plight, with its intense concern for life and death matters.

With the completion of the diagnostic work-up, the

professionals confront the challenge of disclosing the cancer diagnosis to the patient and family. This can raise many anxieties in the professional, who has often learned to cope with these feelings by suppressing them. In the process, many professionals develop styles of talking to patients that involve little feeling or empathy. Patients and their families, in turn, often are unable to show or communicate their intense emotional reactions, which are the signs of the initial impact of the diagnosis.

Although most patients experience an initial reaction of shock, fear, and anxiety, many find the actual diagnosis to be a relief from the previous uncertainty. Knowing what they face, they are now able to draw on their personal and social resources as they reappraise their situation. In their search for meaning, they find strengths in themselves and those around them as well as challenges in the experience. At this point, they are ready to complete the transition by entering the last stage and making plans for their treatment.

Planning for Treatment

With the firm establishment of the cancer diagnosis, the planning for treatment begins. If patients have been given a clear understanding of their condition while being encouraged to maintain hope, the initial reaction of shock, fear, and desperation can give way to a sense of optimism at this time (Holland, 1982). Most patients understand that the first course of treatment offers the best chance for cure or durable remission. Any sense of "fighting spirit" or determination to "beat the cancer" can be seen most prominently at this time.

The three major treatment options are surgery, chemotherapy, and radiation therapy. These methods may be used alone, concurrently or sequentially, or in combination with other forms of therapy such as immunotherapy. Some evidence suggests that both individual and group psychotherapy or counseling and various types of other nonmedical interventions may also be beneficial when used in combination with the traditional medical interventions (Bellert, 1989; Cousins, 1979; Mast, Meyers, & Urbanski, 1987; Siegel, 1986; Simonton et al., 1978). Whatever therapeutic regimen is planned, however, the most critical factors in patient care at this time are keeping them informed and actively participating in their own care and helping them to cope with the demands of the disease and its treatment (Mood & Bickes, 1989). Helping patients to understand that they have treatment alternatives and to evaluate the risk-benefit ratios of those alternatives is important. Personal, nonmedical factors will need to be weighed against survival statistics and physical side effects in determining the relative risks and benefits (Valanis & Rumpler, 1985). For example, body image may be the critical variable in a woman's decision to elect lumpectomy with radiation therapy over mastectomy for the treatment of her early-stage breast cancer.

Treatment planning is also a time when patients' readiness to cooperate and endure even pain and discomfort are at their highest point (Holland, 1982). It is an especially suitable time for patient teaching and preparation for self-care, before the side effects of treatment, the adjustment demands of the disease, and the recurring anxieties about living and dying return. At this point, persons who just days or weeks ago had no awareness of the silent biologic changes taking place in their bodies have now made the critical life transition through the personal discovery of themselves as a *person with cancer*.

NURSING IMPLICATIONS

Nursing's role in facilitating this first critical transition in the cancer experience is carried out at three levels: *direct care* to persons involved in making this transition; *indirect care* to other clients through patient education and cancer risk assessment; and *self-care* in the recognition, assessment, and resolution of the nurse's own unhealthy or negative attitudes in working and living with cancer.

Direct Client Care

The first opportunity to provide direct patient care occurs when the person with symptoms comes to the health care system. The initial stage of the diagnostic process often involves a series of clinical assessments and laboratory procedures. This battery of tests can be quite complex and frightening to the patient and the family. Ambiguity and uncertainty are high. One of the important interventions the nurse can provide at this time is to review the diagnostic test battery with the patient and family, describing each of the procedures to be followed, the time demands each procedure will require, the order in which the procedures will be done, any special preparation the patient needs to make in advance of the procedures, the discomforts that might accompany any of the tests, and any self-care measures or suggestions that might facilitate the patient's adjustment to the experience. Unless it is contraindicated, the purpose of each test and what information will be gained by the test should also be given. Providing an opportunity for patients to preview the laboratories where large unfamiliar equipment is to be used is very helpful. This can be accomplished either by a visit to the laboratory or through visual aids. Also, it has repeatedly been demonstrated that information on sensation (i.e., descriptions of what patients can expect to experience through the senses of sight, hearing, smell, taste, and touch) is an important and beneficial element in preparatory information (Johnson & Leventhal, 1974; Johnson, Rice, Fuller, & Endress, 1978). Preparatory information can help familiarize the patient with what to expect and reduce the *fear of the unknown* (Mood, Cook, & Chadwell, 1988). It can also assist patients and family members to recognize that fear is a normal reaction to the threatening experiences they are having.

Encouraging a family member or friend to participate in preparatory information sessions can have many benefits. First of all, it sets a model for collaboration between patient and significant others that encourages communication and coping with the demands of the experience. It also allows the nurse to meet other important persons in the patient's life and gain greater insight into the patient's level of coping and available resources. Finally, because the increased anxiety typically experienced at this time is likely to reduce the patient's ability to assimilate the information, it is helpful to have someone close to the patient also hear what is said. This associate can then assist the patient in reviewing, recalling, and applying the content as needed through the complex set of procedures. Preparatory information provided by the nurse is helpful even if it is a review of information already given by other members of the professional team. Again, most likely because of disruptions in the patient's cognitive functioning, a good deal of information is lost on first hearing. A review by the nurse can significantly increase the amount of information the patient recalls (Dodd & Mood, 1981). Recommendations for oncology nurses preparing educational programs for newly diagnosed patients have been provided in the literature (Anderson, 1989; Derdiarian, 1987a, 1987b; Mood et al., 1988).

The period of the diagnostic work-up is especially delicate psychologically. The nurse, as well as the other members of the professional team, must strike a balance between honesty on the one hand and premature diagnosis on the other. When a cancer diagnosis is in doubt, it does not serve the client well to emphasize that particular possibility. At the other extreme, when cancer is a virtual certainty and the diagnostic battery is being run to determine the exact nature of the disease or the extent of spread, then refusing to mention cancer serves no useful purpose for the client. Nurses can assist with clarifying information about treatment alternatives and treatment expectations. Persons with cancer should be allowed to participate in the choices and decisions regarding the treatment of their illness and how it will affect their lives and the lives of their families (McCorkle & Germino, 1984; Valanis & Rumpler, 1985). Assisting the client to maintain a sense of optimism and hopefulness is essential under any circumstance. This is sometimes best achieved by responding to the client's spiritual needs (Highfield & Cason, 1983; Miller, 1985; Sodestrom & Martinson, 1987).

Once the patient and family receive the formal diagnosis, the nurse can play a major role in assisting them to respond effectively to this crisis. This often involves listening carefully to the patients' and family members' perceptions of what their needs are. It has been shown repeatedly that these needs are not always what the nurse thinks they are (Dyck & Wright, 1985; Larson, 1987; Young-Brockepp, 1982). Giacquinta (1977) identifies five goals for nursing intervention during this stage: fostering *hope* to meet the hurdle of despair, fostering *cohesion* in response to a sense of isolation, fostering *security* against the feelings of vulnerability, fostering *courage* to deal with the crisis first

within the family and then with others outside the immediate circle, and fostering *problem-solving skills* to cope with the sense of helplessness. Treating the family as the client will give the patient the benefit of a supportive environment at home, where most of the patient's day-to-day living will occur (Litman, 1974), in addition to the hospital, clinic, or other treatment facility where the professional team provides care.

Indirect Patient Care

In addition to the nursing care provided directly to patients and their families as they begin their cancer experience, nurses in many different settings can indirectly assist with the first transition in a number of ways. First of all, nurses play an active role in public education regarding health promotion and cancer prevention. As patient educators, nurses teach all kinds of persons in all kinds of settings about life-style choices and life-style changes that can reduce cancer risks and improve health in general. Early diagnosis is a major point to be made in this context. The fact that cancer can be a curable disease is an important message. Nurses also teach the various self-examination techniques for both men and women, such as testicular or breast self-examination (BSE). Introducing more men and women to the use of these easy practices, developing teaching strategies that communicate the simplicity of their use in addition to their importance, and helping persons who do practice the techniques to understand the importance of taking action immediately on finding any suspicious sign or symptom are nursing actions that could have a major impact on what stage some cancers are in at the time of diagnosis. Nurses are in a position to provide cancer education programs in occupational and community settings (Crooks & Jones, 1989; Frank-Stromborg, 1988). School nurses teaching these techniques to high school—or even junior high school—boys and girls could produce future generations of adults for whom these cancer detection practices are as common as brushing the teeth.

In addition to general public education, nurses can use their interactions with the clients they see for other purposes as opportunities for cancer risk assessment. The one-to-one interaction in the nurse-client contact is a superior basis for discussing life-style changes and planning individualized programs that may be suitable for that particular client. For example, determining a woman's willingness and ability to do BSE cannot easily be achieved across a stage when addressing an audience; it can be approached more readily when providing maternity care or administering a flu shot.

Especially important in the one-to-one contacts that nurses have with clients is the cancer risk assessment and the identification of factors that might predict who is likely to delay seeking diagnosis if symptoms do appear. The woman with a family history of breast cancer needs more careful assessment and education regarding her increased risk. Obese persons need to know that they increase their risk of cancer in addition to their other health risks by not decreasing their fat intake. However, the nurse also needs to be aware that overweight persons may also be at greater risk for delay in seeking health care advice when symptoms occur if they are generally embarrassed or self-conscious about their bodies. Similarly, people with a fierce sense of individualism may be as likely to delay seeking care as the denier or the fearful procrastinator (Weisman, 1979a). Nurses who identify clients who might fit any of these patterns can be alert to signs of concern, or they can take a more aggressive stance in alerting the client to the dangers of delay. Through assessment of cancer risk and assessment of risk for delay, nurses can indirectly promote their clients' initial transitions should they have to confront the cancer experience.

Professional Self-Care

The third level at which nurses can help their clients is through self-assessment and resolution of their own fears and negative attitudes toward cancer. Nurses are, after all, members of the society at large and as such, carry with them many of the culturally shared values and attitudes. Often, negative attitudes can go unrecognized because they are shared by so many people around them. In a study of nurses' attitudes toward death, the nurses often mentioned cancer and projected how they might handle the situation if they themselves had cancer (Mood et al., 1985). It was clear that, like the public at large, many nurses shared the belief that a cancer diagnosis is a death sentence; that it would be one of the worst possible ways to die; and that if they were so unfortunate as to have cancer themselves, they would forego any therapy and let "nature take its course." Nurses employed on oncology units were as likely to express these negative attitudes toward cancer as their nononcology colleagues. It must be asked what effect these attitudes may have on the care these nurses provide to their patients. Can the nurse who is so fearful of cancer discuss cancer openly with a patient? Does the nurse use linguistic devices of avoidance and inadvertently communicate high levels of anxiety to patients? At present, these questions have not been adequately studied. However, it is likely that the nurse who is fearful of cancer, its treatment, and its sequelae will not be able to provide the best nursing care.

The solution to this problem lies in its recognition. Taking an introspective approach and assessing one's own feelings and attitudes about cancer is the important first step. No one has to maintain a false professional demeanor in the privacy of his or her own thoughts. It is a measure of professionalism to engage in self-assessment. If areas needing attention are recognized, seeking the information, peer support, or counseling necessary to resolve the fears and apprehensions will lead to a transition for the nurse, and the end result will be a person who can provide optimal oncology nursing care for clients at any stage of the cancer experience.

References

Aitken-Swan, J., & Easson, E. (1959). Reactions of cancer patients on being told their diagnosis. *British Medical Journal, 1,* 779–783.

American Cancer Society. (1989). A summary of the American Cancer Society report to the nation: Cancer in the poor. *CA: Cancer Journal for Clinicians, 39,* 263–265.

Anderson, J. L. (1989). The nurse's role in cancer rehabilitation: Review of the literature. *Cancer Nursing, 12,* 85–94.

Bellert, J. L. (1989). A therapeutic approach in oncology nursing. *Cancer Nursing, 12,* 65–70.

Borysenko, J. Z. (1982). Behavioral-physiological factors in the development and management of cancer. *General Hospital Psychiatry, 4,* 69–74.

Castles, M. R., & Murray, R. (1979). *Dying in an institution.* New York: Appleton-Century-Crofts.

Chrisman, N. J., & Kleinman, A. (1980). Health beliefs and practices. In S. Thernstrom, A. Orlov, & O. Handlin, (Eds.), *Harvard encyclopedia of American ethinic groups.* Cambridge: Harvard University Press.

Comaroff, J., & Maguire, P. (1981). Ambiguity and the search for meaning: Childhood leukemia in the modern clinical context. *Social Science and Medicine, 15,* 115–123.

Cox, C. (1982). Interaction model of client health behavior: Theoretical prescription for nursing. *Advances in Nursing Science, 5*(1), 41–56.

Crooks, C. E., & Jones, S. D. (1989). Educating women about the importance of breast screenings: The nurse's role. *Cancer Nursing, 12,* 161–164.

Cousins, N. (1979). *Anatomy of an illness as perceived by the patient.* New York: W. W. Norton.

Cunningham, A. J. (1985). The influence of mind on cancer. *Canadian Psychology, 26,* 13–29.

Derdiarian, A. (1987a). Informational needs of recently diagnosed cancer patients: A theoretical framework. Part I. *Cancer Nursing, 10,* 107–115.

Derdiarian, A. (1987b). Informational needs of recently diagnosed cancer patients: Method and description. Part II. *Cancer Nursing, 10,* 156–163.

Dodd, M. J., & Mood, D. W. (1981). Chemotherapy: Helping patients to know the drugs they are receiving and their possible side effects. *Cancer Nursing, 4,* 311–318.

Dyck, S., & Wright, K. (1985). Family perceptions: The role of the nurse throughout an adult's cancer experience. *Oncology Nursing Forum, 12,* 53–56.

Edlund, B., & Sneed, N. V. (1989). Emotional responses to the diagnosis of cancer: Age-related comparisons. *Oncology Nursing Forum, 16,* 691–697.

EVAXX, Inc. (1981). *A study of black Americans' attitudes toward cancer and cancer tests.* New York: American Cancer Society.

Forester, B. M., Kornfeld, D. S., & Fleiss, J. (1978). Psychiatric aspects of radiotherapy. *American Journal of Psychiatry, 135,* 960–963.

Fountain, M. J. (1985). Psychosocial support for the person experiencing cancer. *Orthopedic Nursing, 4,* 33–35.

Fox, B. H. (1983). Current theory of psychogenic effects on cancer incidence and prognosis. *Journal of Psychosocial Oncology, 1,* 17–31.

Frank-Stromborg, M. (1986). The role of the nurse in early detection of cancer: Population 66 years of age and older. *Oncology Nursing Forum, 13,* 107–115.

Frank-Stromborg, M. (1988). Nursing's role in cancer prevention and detection: Vital contributions to attainment of the Year 2000 goals. *Cancer, 62,* 1833–1838.

Frank-Stromborg, M. (1989). Reaction to the diagnosis of cancer questionnaire (RDCQ): Development and psychometric evaluation. *Nursing Research, 38,* 364–369.

Frieze, I., & Bar-Tal, D. (1978). Attribution theory: Past and present. In I. H. Frieze, D. Bar-Tal, & J. S. Carroll (Eds.), *New approaches to social problems.* San Francisco: Jossey-Bass Publishers.

Funch, D. P. (1985). The role of patient delay in the evaluation of breast self-examination. *Journal of Psychosocial Oncology, 2*(3), 31–39.

Funch, D. P., & Francis, A. M. (1982). Issues in the early detection and rehabilitation of breast cancer patients. In C. Mettlin & G. P. Murphy (Eds.), *Issues in cancer screening and communications* (pp. 219–229). New York: Alan R. Liss, Inc.

Germino, B., & McCorkle, R. (1985). Acknowledged awareness of life-threatening illness. *International Journal of Nursing Studies, 22*, 33–44.

Giacquinta, B. (1977). Helping families face the crisis of cancer. *American Journal of Nursing, 77*, 1585–1588.

Given, B., & Given, C. W. (1989). Cancer nursing for the elderly: A target for research. *Cancer Nursing, 12*, 71–77.

Gold, M. A. (1964). Causes of patient delay in diseases of the breast. *Cancer, 17*, 564–577.

Gotay, C. C. (1984). The experience of cancer during early and advanced stages: The views of patients and their mates. *Social Science and Medicine, 18*, 605–613.

Gould-Martin, K., Paganini-Hill, A., Casagrande, C., Mack, T., & Ross, R. K. (1982). Behavioral and biological determinants of surgical stage of breast cancer. *Preventive Medicine, 11*, 429–440.

Graydon, J. E. (1988). Factors that predict patients' functioning following treatment for cancer. *International Journal of Nursing Studies, 25*, 117–124.

Greer, S. (1974). Psychological aspects: Delays in the diagnosis of breast cancer. *Proceedings of the Royal Society of Medicine, 67*, 470–479.

Greer, S., & Morris, T. (1975). Psychological attributes of women who develop breast cancer: A controlled study. *Journal of Psychosomatic Research, 19*, 147–153.

Hackett, T. P., Cassem, N. H., & Raker, J. W. (1973). Patient delay in cancer. *New England Journal of Medicine, 289*, 14–20.

Hammerschlag, C. A., Fisher, S., De Cosser, F., & Kaplan, E. (1964). Breast symptoms and patient delay: Psychological variables involved. *Cancer, 17*, 1480–1485.

Hanucharurnkul, S. (1989). Predictors of self-care in cancer patients receiving radiotherapy. *Cancer Nursing, 12*, 21–27.

Highfield, M. F., & Cason, C. (1983). Spiritual needs of patients: Are they recognized? *Cancer Nursing, 6*, 187–192.

Holland, J. C. (1976). Coping with cancer: A challenge to the behavioral sciences. In J. W. Cullen, B. H. Fox, & R. N. Isom (Eds.), *Cancer: The behavioral dimensions*. New York: Raven Press.

Holland, J. C. (1982). Psychologic aspects of cancer. In J. C. Holland & E. Frei III (Eds.), *Cancer medicine* (pp. 1175–1184). Philadelphia: Lea & Febiger.

Holland, J. C. (1986). Doctors should be aware of patients' emotional responses to cancer. *Oncology Times, 8*(4), 1.

Holmes, F., & Hearne, E. (1981). Cancer stage-to-age relationships: Implications for cancer screening in the elderly. *Journal of the American Geriatric Society, 19*, 55–57.

Houts, P. S., Harvey, H. A., Simmonds, M. A., Marshall, M., Gottlieb, R., Lipton, A., Martin, B. A., Dixon, R. H., Gelman, E. S., & Valdevia, D. (1985). Characteristics of patients at risk for financial burden because of cancer and its treatment. *Journal of Psychosocial Oncology, 3*(2), 15–22.

Hughes, J. (1982). Emotional reactions to the diagnosis and treatment of early breast cancer. *Journal of Psychosomatic Research, 26*, 277–281.

Israel, L. (1978). *Conquering cancer*. New York: Random House.

Jamison, J. R., Wellisch, D. K., & Pasnau, R. P. (1978). Psychological aspects of mastectomy. I. The woman's perspective. *American Journal of Psychiatry, 135*, 432–436.

Johnson, J. E., & Leventhal, H. (1974). Effects of accurate expectations and behavioral instructions on reactions during a noxious medical examination. *Journal of Personality and Social Psychology, 29*, 710–718.

Johnson, J. E., Rice, V. H., Fuller, S. S., & Endress, M. P. (1978). Sensory information instruction in a coping strategy and recovery from surgery. *Research in Nursing and Health, 1*, 4–17.

Kegeles, S. S. (1969). A field experimental attempt to change beliefs and behavior of women in an urban ghetto. *Journal of Health and Social Behavior, 10*, 115–124.

Krant, M. J. (1976). Problems of the physician in presenting the patient with the diagnosis. In J. W. Cullen, B. H. Fox, & R. N. Isom (Eds.), *Cancer: The behavioral dimensions* (pp. 269–274). New York: Raven Press.

Krant, M. J. (1981). Psychosocial impact of gynecological cancer. *Cancer, 48*, 608–612.

Lambert, V. A., & Lambert, C. E. (1979). *The impact of physical illness*. Englewood Cliffs, NJ: Prentice-Hall, Inc.

Larson, P. J. (1987). Comparison of cancer patients' and professional nurses' perceptions of important nurse caring behaviors. *Heart and Lung, 16*, 187–192.

Lazarus, R. S. (1979, November). Positive denial: The case for not facing reality. *Psychology Today*, pp. 44–60.

Leis, H., & Pilnik, S. (1974). Breast cancer: A therapeutic dilemma. *AORN Journal, 19*, 813–820.

LeShan, L. (1966). An emotional life history associated with neoplastic disease. *Annals of the New York Academy of Science, 125*, 780–795.

Levy, S. M. (1985). *Behavior and cancer: Lifestyle and psychosocial factors in the initiation and progression of cancer*. San Francisco: Jossey-Bass.

Lewandowski, W., & Jones S. L. (1988). The family with cancer. *Cancer Nursing, 11*, 313–321.

Lewis, F. M., & Bloom, J. R. (1978–1979). Psychosocial adjustment to breast cancer: A review of selected literature. *International Journal of Psychiatry in Medicine, 9*, 1–17.

Lierman, L. M. (1988). Discovery of breast changes: Women's responses and nursing implications. *Cancer Nursing, 11*, 352–361.

Litman, T. J. (1974). The family as a basic unit in health and medical care: A social-behavioral overview. *Social Science and Medicine, 8*, 495–519.

Magarey, C. J., Todd, P. B., & Blizard, P. J. (1977). Psychosocial factors influencing delay and breast self-examination in women with symptoms of breast cancer. *Social Science and Medicine, 11*, 229–232.

Mages, N. L., Castro, J. R., Fobair, P., Hall, J., Harrison, I., Mendelsohn, G., & Wolfson, A. (1981). Patterns of psychosocial response to cancer: Can effective adaptation be predicted? *International Journal of Radiation Oncology Biology Physics, 7*, 385–392.

Maguire, P. G. (1975). The psychological and social consequences of breast cancer. *Nursing Mirror, 140*, 54–57.

Maguire, P. (1985). The psychological impact of cancer. *British Journal of Hospital Medicine, 34*, 100–103.

Marino, L. (1981). *Cancer nursing*. St. Louis: C. V. Mosby Co.

Marshall, J. R., & Funch, D. P. (1986). Gender and illness behavior among colorectal cancer patients. *Women and Health, 11*, 67–82.

Mast, D., Meyers, J., & Urbanski, A. (1987). Relaxation techniques: A self-learning module for nurses: Unit I. *Cancer Nursing, 10*, 141–147.

McCorkle, R. (1989). Women and cancer. In R. Tiffany (Ed.), *Oncology for nurses and health care professionals* (2nd ed., Vol. 2, pp. 281–292). London: Harper & Row, Publishers.

McCorkle, R., & Benoliel, J. Q. (1983). Symptom distress, current concerns, and mood disturbance after diagnosis of life-threatening disease. *Social Science and Medicine, 17*, 431–438.

McCorkle, R., & Germino, B. (1984). What nurses need to know about home care. *Oncology Nursing Forum, 12*, 63–69.

Mechanic, D. (1972). Social psychological factors affecting the presentation of bodily complaints. *New England Journal of Medicine, 286*, 1132–1139.

Mettlin, C., Reese, P., & Murphy, G. P. (1980). Care-seeking behavior among positive screenees. *Preventive Medicine, 9*, 518–524.

Miller, J. F. (1985). Inspiring hope. *American Journal of Nursing, 85*, 22–25.

Mood, D. W. (1980). Linguistic indicators of attitudes toward death and dying: A measure of denial? In M. A. Simpson (Ed.), *Psycholinguistics in clinical practice* (pp. 260–291). New York: Irvington Press.

Mood, D. W., & Bickes, J. T. (1989). Strategies to enhance self-care in radiation therapy. *Oncology Nursing Forum, 16*(Suppl.), 143.

Mood, D. W., Brenner, P. S., & Richardson, C. (1985). *Linguistic indicators of nurses' attitudes toward aging and dying*. Paper presented at the Eighth Annual Research Symposium, Sigma Theta Tau, Ann Arbor, MI.

Mood, D. W., Cook, C. A., & Chadwell, D. K. (1988). Increasing patients' knowledge of radiation therapy. *International Journal of Radiation Oncology Biology Physics, 15*, 989–993.

Mood, D. W., & Parzuchowski, J. (1986). Health and illness versions of the Multidimensional Health Locus of Control scales. Proceedings of the Great Lakes Oncology Nursing Conference, Lansing, MI.

Mood, D. W., & Van Fossen, M. (1983). *Assessment of children's development of the concept of death.* Annual report, Nursing Research Emphasis Grant, Wayne State University, Detroit, MI.

Morris, T., & Greer, S. (1980). A "Type C" for cancer? Low trait anxiety in the pathogenesis of breast cancer [Abstract 102]. *Cancer Detection and Prevention, 3,* 114.

Morris, T., Greer, S., & White, P. (1977). Psychological and social adjustment to mastectomy. *Cancer, 40,* 2381–2387.

National Cancer Institute. (1986). *Cancer among blacks and other minorities: Statistical profile* (NIH Publication No. 86–2785). Bethesda, MD: National Institutes of Health.

National Center for Health Statistics. (1986). Use of selected preventive care procedures, United States, 1982. *Vital and health statistics,* Series 10, #157 (U.S. Department of Health and Human Services, Publication No. (PHS) 86-1585. Public Health Service). Washington, DC: U.S. Government Printing Office.

Northouse, L. (1984). The impact of cancer on the family: An overview. *International Journal of Psychiatry in Medicine, 14,* 215–242.

Northouse, L. (1989). A longitudinal study of the adjustment of patients and husbands to breast cancer. *Oncology Nursing Forum, 16,* 511–516.

Novack, D. H., Plumer, R., Smith, R. L., Ochitill, H., Morrow, G. R., & Bennett, J. M. (1979). Changes in physicians' attitudes toward telling the cancer patient. *Journal of the American Medical Association, 241,* 897–900.

Novotny, E., Hyland, J., Coyne, L., Travis, J., & Pruyner, H. (1984). Factors affecting adjustment to cancer. *Bulletin of the Menninger Clinic, 48,* 318–328.

Oken, D. (1961). What to tell cancer patients: A study of medical attitudes. *Journal of the American Medical Association, 175,* 1120–1128.

Orem, D. E. (Ed.). (1985). *Nursing: Concepts of practice* (3rd ed.). New York: McGraw Hill Book Co.

Owens, R. G., Duffy, J. E., & Ashcroft, J. J. (1985). Women's response to detection of breast lumps: A British study. *Health Education Journal, 44,* 69–70.

Quint, J. C. (1963). The impact of mastectomy. *American Journal of Nursing, 63,* 88–92.

Rosenstock, J. M. (1974). Historical origins of the Health Belief Model. *Health Education Monographs, 2,* 328–335.

Salloway, J. C., & Dillon, P. B. (1973). A comparison of family networks and friend networks in health care utilization. *Journal of Community Family Studies, 4,* 131–141.

Saunders, J. M., & McCorkle, R. (1985). Models of care for persons with progressive cancer. *Nursing Clinics of North America, 20,* 365–377.

Siegel, B. S. (1986). *Love, medicine, and miracles.* New York: Harper & Row Publishers, Inc.

Simonton, O. C., Matthews-Simonton, S., & Creighton, J. L. (1978). *Getting well again.* New York: Bantam Books.

Sodestrom, K. E., & Martinson, I. M. (1987). Patients' spiritual coping strategies: A study of nurse and patient perspectives. *Oncology Nursing Forum, 14,* 41–46.

Stams, H. J., & Steggles, S. (1987). Predicting the onset or progression of cancer from psychological characteristics: Psychometric and theoretical issues. *Journal of Psychosocial Oncology, 5(2),* 35–46.

Stromborg, M., Wright, P., Segalla, M., & Diekmann, J. (1984). Psychological impact of the cancer diagnosis. *Oncology Nursing Forum, 11,* 16–22.

Taylor, S. E. (1983, November). Adjustment to threatening events: A theory of cognitive adaptation. *American Psychologist,* pp. 1161–1173.

Taylor, S. E., Lichtman, R. R., & Wood, J. V. (1984). Attributions, beliefs about control, and adjustment to breast cancer. *Journal of Personality and Social Psychology, 46,* 489–502.

Thomas, C. B., & Greenstreet, R. L. (1973). Psychobiological characteristics in youth as predictors of five disease states: suicide, mental illness, hypertension, coronary heart disease and tumor. *Johns Hopkins Medical Journal, 132,* 16–43.

U.S. Department of Health and Human Services. (1986). *Report of the Secretary's task force on black and minority health.* Vol IV. Cancer. Washington, DC: U.S. Government Publications Office.

Valanis, B. G., & Rumpler, C. H. (1985). Helping women to choose breast cancer treatment alternatives. *Cancer Nursing, 8,* 167–175.

Verbrugge, L. M. (1979a). Female illness rates and illness behavior: Testing hypotheses about sex differences in health. *Women and Health, 4,* 61–79.

Verbrugge, L. M. (1979b). Marital status and health. *Marriage and Family, 41,* 267–285.

Verbrugge, L. M. (1982). Sex differentials in health. *Public Health Report, 97,* 417–437.

Vettese, J. M. (1976). Problems of the patient confronting the diagnosis of cancer. In J. W. Cullen, B. H. Fox, & R. N. Isom (Eds.), *Cancer: The behavioral dimensions* (pp. 275–280). New York: Raven Press.

Watson, M., Greer, S., Blake, S., & Sharpnell, K. (1984). Reaction to a diagnosis of breast cancer: Relationship between denial, delay, and rates of psychological morbidity. *Cancer, 53,* 2008–2012.

Weiner, B. (1979). A theory of motivation for some classroom experiences. *Journal of Educational Psychology, 71,* 3–25.

Weinrich, S. P., & Weinrich, M. C. (1986). Cancer knowledge among elderly individuals. *Cancer Nursing, 9,* 301–307.

Weisman, A. D. (1979a). *Coping with cancer.* New York: McGraw-Hill Book Co.

Weisman, A. D. (1979b). A model for psychosocial phasing in cancer. *General Hospital Psychiatry, 1,* 187–195.

Weisman, A. D., & Hackett, T. (1961). Predilection to death. *Psychosomatic Medicine, 23,* 232.

Weisman, A. D., & Worden, J. W. (1976–1977). The existential plight in cancer: Significance of the first 100 days. *International Journal of Psychiatry in Medicine, 7,* 1–15.

Weisman, A. D., Worden, J. W., & Sobel, H. J. (1980). *Psychosocial screening and intervention with cancer patients: Final report of the Omega Project (CA 19797).* Bethesda, MD: National Cancer Institute.

Wendt, P. (1989). *Ethnicity, parental anxiety, and religiosity: Their relationship to children's death concept development and death anxiety.* Unpublished master's thesis, Wayne State University, College of Nursing, Detroit, MI.

Woods, N. F., Lewis, F. M., & Ellison, E. S. (1989). Living with cancer: Family experiences. *Cancer Nursing, 12,* 28–33.

Wool, M. S. (1986). Extreme denial in breast cancer patients and capacity for object relations. *Psychotherapy and Psychosomatics, 46,* 196–204.

Worden, J. W. (1983). Psychosocial screening of cancer patients. *Journal of Psychosocial Oncology, 1(4),* 1–10.

Worden, J. W., & Weisman, A. D. (1975). Psychosocial components of lagtime in cancer diagnosis. *Journal of Psychosomatic Research, 19,* 69–79.

Young-Brockapp, D. (1982). Cancer patients' perceptions of five psychosocial needs. *Oncology Nursing Forum, 9,* 31–35.

Zola, I. K. (1973). Pathways to the doctor—from person to patient. *Social Science and Medicine, 7,* 677–689.

CANCER TREATMENT: THERAPIES AND PHYSICAL SUPPORT APPROACHES

CHAPTER *19*

Surgical Oncology

CATHRYN P. HAVARD
ANNE E. TOPPING

A HISTORICAL PERSPECTIVE

Malignant disease in humans has been traced back to the ancient Egyptians and beyond. A skull in the Duckworth Library in Cambridge, England, showing widespread cancerous disease is estimated to be nearly 5000 years old. The famous papyrus discovered by Edwin Smith in the tomb in Luxor contains extracts referring to tumors of the breast and limbs.

The writings of the Hippocratic era certainly recognized the disease, although in those times people believed that cancer was caused by one of the four humors of the body. The concept of humors was derived from the ancient Greek belief that everything can be described by the four universal elements—fire, air, wind, and earth—and by the four qualities of hot, cold, moist, and dry. These elements and qualities were assigned to four humors: blood, phlegm, yellow bile and black bile, the last being the cause of cancer. Treatment for tumors was primarily surgery, lancing, or bloodletting, which would release the collection of humor causing the cancer (Denton, 1988).

Hippocrates also realized that fundamentally he was unable to treat the disease and cautioned against interfering with hidden cancers within body cavities. However, many of his disciples experimented with surgical techniques, particularly on breast and limbs. The basic principles were to purge the black humors and then totally excise the affected part, cauterizing vessels as necessary. These principles in essence were adhered to for the next thousand years, until the seventeenth century saw the beginning of experimental medicine.

Gradually, the humoral theories were replaced by more scientific hypotheses as discoveries were made about anatomy, the lymphatic system, and the circulatory system. The concept that cancer was a manifestation of a constitutional disease became replaced by the idea that it had a more local origin. John Hunter, father of scientific surgery, believed that cancer was local disease but was also aware that it could appear in other parts of the body. He believed that "coagulated lymph" was a cause of cancer and that cancers were nourished by the vessels of the organism. These beliefs formed the basis of his practice of removing local lymph nodes when possible and ligating vessels that supplied the tumor. Hunter's "Lectures on the Principles of Surgery," published in 1835, had a profound effect on both contemporary and subsequent medical and surgical thinking. A report and questionnaire published in 1802 posed a series of questions for investigating the nature and cure of cancer, which are just as relevant today, even in the light of modern theories and new knowledge (Gallucci, 1985).

Descriptions of early surgical techniques for excising breast tumors make harrowing reading. Lorenz Heister, in his "General System of Surgery," published in 1743, advocated the piercing of large tumors by needles carrying thick string. By pulling on these, the mass could be elevated away from the chest wall and then cut off cleanly with a long knife. The knowledge that such procedures were carried out without anesthesia and with little analgesia makes the suffering of the patients awful to contemplate. It was not until 1846 that sulfurous ether was first used by Morton in the United States, and chloroform was used by Simpson in Edinburgh a year later. This, combined with Pasteur's work on the causes of sepsis and Lister's antiseptic techniques, allowed great advances to be made in all branches of surgery.

Yet surgery was often performed at a great cost, because mortality figures were appallingly high, largely as a result of infection. Hospitals were far from safe places at that time, and nursing services were rudimentary in most areas. Not until the early twentieth century did the situation begin to improve. The admonishment of Florence Nightingale that, "Hospitals should do the patient no harm" was not a reality until well into the twentieth century.

However, the past four decades have seen great developments in every field of medical science, all of which have facilitated the advance of cancer surgery. Sophisticated techniques in radiology and whole body scanning allow noninvasive assessment of the extent of disease and accurate planning of surgical procedures. Tumor classification systems and a better understanding of the physiology, biochemistry, and molecular biology of the cell suggest new and more effective approaches to treatment. Developments in anesthesia, antibiotic therapy, and critical care technology have enabled surgical resections to exceed anatomic boundaries not dreamed of by the early pioneer surgeons (Westbury, 1988).

For all this, surgery alone can effect a cure only when malignant disease is confined to its primary site. It is increasingly used, therefore, in conjunction with other treatment methods as part of a multidisciplinary approach to cancer therapy. Moreover, there is an increasing recognition that it is not enough to remove the cancer without making every attempt to repair defects and restore function. Unless the patient is able to fully live the life that has—it is hoped—been extended by heroic surgery and rehabilitation efforts, treatment cannot be regarded as truly successful.

Nurses form an important part of the multidisciplinary team providing care and support at all stages of a patient's course of treatment. In the same way that medical knowledge has progressed from its "dark ages" to its present level of sophistication, so has nursing developed to meet the challenge of caring for cancer patients. Specialist nursing skills such as those utilized in the operating room and critical care unit are vital in the perioperative period, but, increasingly, it is the role of the nurse in the rehabilitation of patients to their maximum potential that is essential for a successful outcome to surgery.

THE SCOPE OF CANCER SURGERY

Developments in complementary fields of medicine and patient care have increased the scope of surgery. Advances in critical care, nutritional support, anesthesia, pain management, and antibiotic coverage have all helped improve the potential outcome from surgery. Technical advances in bioengineering and developments in cardiovascular and reconstructive surgery have also made valuable contributions to extend the possibilities of oncologic surgery. The long-term implications of extensive surgery in terms of adaptation, along with developments such as the end-to-end anastomosis (EEA) stapling device, have meant that the outcomes of cancer surgery can be less disfiguring even though equally successful in controlling the disease (Priestman & Fielding, 1987).

Increasingly, it is becoming the norm for surgery to be used in combination with other treatment methods. Optimal management for both cure and palliation necessitates individualized treatment regimens with input from all members of the multidisciplinary team. Another influence that has promoted multimodality treatment has been the general acceptance of the concept that a tumor is not confined to the primary site at diagnosis, and that micrometastases will be more than likely to have disseminated (McKenna, 1986; Szopa, 1987; White, 1978).

The shift in emphasis away from single-modality treatment has not detracted from the significant and expanding role of surgery in the management of the patient with malignant disease. Table 19–1 gives examples of the variety of interventions currently in use within cancer care.

Table 19–1. SURGICAL APPROACHES TO CANCER CARE

Intervention	Example
Diagnosis	Breast biopsy
Staging	Staging laparotomy
	Second-look laparotomy
Treatment of primary tumor	Curative resection (abdominal perineal resection)
Reconstruction, rehabilitation	Breast reconstruction
	Continent urostomy or ileostomy
Palliative	Endocrine ablation
	Pericardial window
Adjuvant	Para-aortic node dissection
	Hickman line insertion
Complications of other methods	Excision of bowel stricture
	Excision of radionecrotic tissue
Resection of metastases	Partial hepatectomy
	Pulmonary resection
Cytoreductive	Abdominal soft tissue sarcomas
	Ovarian peritoneal carcinoma
Emergencies	Obstruction
	Hemorrhage
Cancer prevention	Colectomy (familial polyposis)
	Orchidopexy (testicular tumors)

DIAGNOSIS

A cancer diagnosis may be suspected from physical examination or from radiologic examination. Confirmation, however, needs to be established from a sample of tissue. A number of methods can be used to obtain a tissue specimen, but careful selection of an appropriate method cannot be overemphasized. The ideal biopsy technique is one that is the least invasive, least expensive, most convenient, easiest to perform, and revealing of enough information to understand the diagnosis (Ames, 1986). A number of techniques may be used; these are described in greater detail in Table 19–2.

STAGING

Staging is undertaken to establish stage and extent of disease. A diagnostic laparotomy may be performed before radical surgery to ascertain whether occult metastases are present, which may affect the ultimate extent of resection. Alternatively, the laparotomy may be used to obtain tissue specimens and as a basis for treatment planning. In Hodgkin's disease, this often includes exploratory laparotomy, splenectomy, liver biopsy, retroperitoneal node biopsy, and the placement of metal clips on organs to denote the borders for future radiotherapy treatment (Szopa, 1987).

A second-look procedure may be performed to confirm the absence or presence of disease after other treatments. This is sometimes adopted in the treatment plan of patients with ovarian tumors (Gilbertson & Wangensteen, 1964).

Staging laporotomies are becoming less common with the widespread availability of advanced diagnostic procedures, laboratory tests, and assessment of tumor markers as a means to evaluate response to treatment (Barber, 1986).

Table 19–2. SURGICAL BIOPSY TECHNIQUES

Technique	Method	Example
Incisional	Removal of small portion of tissue, performed under a general or local anesthetic	Punch or shave biopsy
Excision	Removal of complete tumor with little or no margin of surrounding tissue	Lump biopsy
Needle	Aspiration of fluid or actual tissue	Aspiration of breast lump
Exfoliative	Direct smear or scrape or examination of shed cells	Papanicolaou smear
Endoscopy	Removal of tissue from normally inaccessible sites using a rigid or fiberoptic instrument	Laryngoscopy Cystoscopy Bronchoscopy

TREATMENT OF PRIMARY TUMOR

Surgery is the dominant treatment method in primarily curative approaches to disease. More cancers are cured by surgery than by all other forms of cancer treatment, although success in terms of cure depends on the biology of the particular cancer in question—that is, its tendency to metastasize via the blood stream. Skin cancers (excluding melanoma), differentiated thyroid cancer, and early tumors of the rectum and colon are typical examples of cancers for which excellent prospects of cure can be achieved through excision of local and regional disease.

RECONSTRUCTIVE OR REHABILITATIVE SURGERY

Radical surgical resections can result in defects that cannot be repaired satisfactorily by simple wound closure. Complicating these technical difficulties is the effect radical surgery can have on the quality of life of the cancer patient. Traditionally, reconstructive surgery was often delayed to allow the patient to be monitored for recurrence of the disease. Early reconstruction is now often performed and preferred. Early breast reconstruction may assist psychological recovery and reduce psychiatric morbidity related to the negative effects on body image associated with mastectomy (d'Angelo & Gorrell, 1989; Larson & McMurtrey, 1983; Maguire, Tait, Brooke, Thomas, & Sellwood, 1980). Formation of a continent ileostomy or urostomy may allow the patient to gain greater control and freedom than traditional ostomy surgery (Cumming, Worth, & Woodhouse, 1987).

PALLIATIVE TREATMENT

Surgery may be the appropriate treatment method for those patients whose disease makes life at least difficult and at worst intolerable. The decision to use palliative surgery is often a difficult one. In such cases, the multidisciplinary approach allows risks and benefits to be assessed within the wider context of the client's overall treatment. There are a number of indications for palliative surgery; these include measures to provide functional improvement, symptomatic relief, and ablation of endocrine production. Some of the common oncologic problems are identified in Table 19–3 with their potential surgical interventions.

ADJUVANT SURGERY

Surgical techniques are increasingly being used in the overall management of the oncology patient. A number of malignant conditions and treatment regimens require surgical intervention to make effective treatment possible. These range from relatively minor techniques to provide long-term vascular access to

Table 19–3. COMMON ONCOLOGIC PROBLEMS AND SURGICAL INTERVENTIONS

Problem	Site of Cancer	Surgery
Secondary bone tumors causing pain	Breast Prostate	Oophorectomy Orchidectomy Adrenalectomy Hypophysectomy
Gastrointestinal obstruction	Stomach Small bowel Colon and rectum Soft tissue (sarcomas) Ovary	Esophagojejunostomy Enteroenterostomy Dysfunctioning colostomy
Nutritional deficit	Eosophagus	Feeding gastrostomy or jejunostomy Insertion of endoesophageal tube Dilatation and bougienage
Airway obstruction	Larynx Thyroid	Formation of tracheostomy
Vesicovaginal fistulae	Cervix, vagina, or bladder	Formation of ileal conduit
Rectovaginal fistulae	Rectum Cervix or vagina	Formation of colostomy
Fungating lesions	Breast Soft tissue (sarcomas)	Mastectomy Limb amputation
Biliary obstruction	Pancreas	Choledochojejunostomy
Renal failure	Bladder or prostate	Insertion of ureteric stent Ileal conduit formation

more extensive surgical excision before or following other treatment methods. Table 19–4 gives examples of surgical interventions that are utilized in this way.

COMPLICATIONS OF OTHER TREATMENT METHODS

Surgery may be deemed appropriate to treat the complications of other treatment methods used in oncology. Radiotherapy and chemotherapy may lead to the development of a new malignancy or to a benign condition that behaves in a malignant fashion. Table 19–5 gives examples of such complications and possible surgical approaches to provide symptomatic relief.

Table 19–4. ADJUVANT SURGICAL TECHNIQUES

Purpose	Examples
Vascular access	Central venous access catheter Implanted vascular access device Limb perfusion Intra-arterial chemotherapy
Radiotherapy	Radioactive implants Intracavity or interstitial
Ventricular access	Reservoir insertion for instillation of central nervous system chemotherapy and to monitor cerebrospinal fluid Central nervous system instillation of pain medication
Peritoneal access	Catheter insertion for interperitoneal chemotherapy
Removal of residual tumor	Para-aortic node dissection after chemotherapy

Table 19–5. COMPLICATIONS OF OTHER TREATMENT METHODS

Method	Complication	Surgical Intervention
Radiotherapy	Skin necrosis	Excision, grafting, and skin flap coverage
	Proctitis or colitis fistulae	Resection and anastomosis with or without ostomy formation
	Bladder contraction	Ileal loop diversion
	Ureteral stricture	Ureteral dilatation Stent insertion
	Bone necrosis	Debridement
	Bone fracture	Internal fixation
Chemotherapy	Tissue necrosis from extravasation	Excision, grafting, and skin coverage Possibly amputation
	Intestinal inflammation and perforation	Laparotomy and resection

RESECTION OF METASTASES

In selected cases there is a place for resection of isolated metastases. This is usually performed when cure will be effected and when the cancer is controlled at the primary site. The psychological as well as physical status of the patient before surgery is an important consideration. Other factors that influence the decision to intervene surgically are the nature of the tumor, the disease-free interval, and the tumor doubling time. Isolated metastases in the bone, liver, lung, and brain have been resected with success (Beattie, 1984; Fortner, 1984).

CYTOREDUCTIVE SURGERY

The place for this type of surgery is controversial. In theory, cytoreductive surgery should be beneficial in reducing tumor cell mass to a level that will render chemotherapy, immunotherapy, and host defenses more effective (Blythe & Wahl, 1964; McKenna & McKenna, 1986).

SURGERY FOR ONCOLOGIC EMERGENCIES

The decision to intervene surgically in oncologic emergencies is often highly controversial and something of an ethical dilemma. Whatever the procedure, the end result should optimally relieve symptoms and improve the quality of the patient's life. The adoption of a nonintervention stance may in some instances be a more humane approach and one that deserves careful consideration.

Advances in chemotherapy and radiotherapy have greatly improved the outlook in many cancers. Preoperative radiotherapy can result in widespread fibrosis and adhesions, which make salvage surgery technically difficult. The side effects from some chemotherapeutic agents (e.g., bleomycin) may present problems to the anesthesiologist and pulmonary complications for the patient. Steroids and radiotherapy can seriously interfere with healing processes.

Malignant disease does unfortunately produce life-threatening conditions such as airway obstruction, which demands immediate surgical relief. Gastrointestinal tumors can cause perforation, leading to acute peritonitis or obstruction, which may necessitate surgery. Skeletal metastases can create oncologic emergencies such as vertebral collapse, leading to cord compression. Pathologic fractures of long bones may require internal fixation to facilitate rehabilitation.

PROPHYLACTIC SURGERY

In the area of cancer prevention there are certain clinical settings in which the use of surgery can be effective. Some epithelial cancers evolve from a premalignant phase and even when they actually become malignant remain locally confined within the epithelial layer. The efficacy of surgery in cancer prevention can be seen in the management of cervical cancer. This condition can be readily detected through simple cytologic screening, and limited surgical excision or laser or cryotherapy techniques can effectively reduce spread of the disease.

Surgery is also used in the management of certain familial diseases. In the case of familial polyposis coli, colectomy may be advocated to prevent colonic cancer. Breast cancer is another malignant disease with a strong familial link. Approximately 9 per cent of women with breast cancer demonstrate hereditary causation. Certain women with a very high risk may become candidates for prophylactic mastectomy as a treatment alternative to surveillance. (Fitzsimmons, Conway, Madsen, Lappe, & Coody, 1989).

THE SURGICAL EXPERIENCE: IMPLICATIONS FOR THE PATIENT AND FOR NURSING MANAGEMENT

To provide optimal perioperative care for the patient undergoing surgery for malignant disease, nursing care needs to be based on psychosocial as well as biologic factors. Technical expertise and effective physiologic monitoring play important roles.

Cancer care requires innovative strategies so that patients' needs are met. Managing pain, meeting nutritional requirements, and attending to wound care often present real problems for the surgeon, nurse, and patient. Pain control for the postoperative cancer patient can be often made more difficult by the prior experience of severe preoperative pain requiring opiate analgesia. While making preoperative assessment, the nurse may have the opportunity to identify coping strategies that can be used effectively in the postoperative period by the patient. Pain-relieving measures such as epidural analgesia and patient-administered analgesia are being used increasingly in cancer care to reduce the negative aspects of surgical pain (Finch,

1989). For the nurse, these approaches require continuous patient observation, support, and education to ensure patient safety.

Wound management in the cancer patient can present many problems. Healing rate and progression can be severely hindered by a patient's nutritional status, immunologic response, age, drug therapy, and prior exposure to radiotherapy. Bacterial contamination can also have serious implications in terms of healing and management. Care of all wounds should be directed toward providing the ideal microenvironment to effect successful healing. Nursing care should be appropriate and supported by research-based rationale. Many preparations and dressings are available for wound care. Products come with varying claims, and nurses must recognize that they have a responsibility to their patients to evaluate and investigate thoroughly all products before using them in the clinical setting (Pritchard & David, 1988).

The psychological and social influences that contribute to human well-being are significant considerations for the oncology surgical nurse. Considerable investigation of surgery-related anxiety and stress has been conducted, and the patient's need for information has been pinpointed as a highly significant factor in reducing perioperative anxiety (Boore, 1978; Hayward, 1978; Wilson-Barnett, 1978, 1981). A number of studies conducted in various settings have demonstrated the effectiveness of nursing measures designed to reduce anxiety when correlated to biochemical indices of physiologic stress (Boore, 1978; Foster, 1974).

Immune system activity does appear to play a role in the body's resistance to cancer. In certain types of malignant disease, it is possible to identify antibodies to the patient's tumor in his or her serum in vitro. Experimental data suggest that, in certain cases, these antibodies are undetectable in the presence of malignant disease. However, after surgery, a significant and rapid rise in antibody titers in serum appears, and this rise is considered to be a defense mechanism to destroy accessible blood-borne tumor cells (Moore, 1979). From this evidence it could be concluded that optimal immune system functioning may influence later development of metastases.

A more controversial proposal is the one that suggests that the patient's psychological status is associated with occurrence and progression of cancer. Studies in which persons were interviewed while awaiting biopsy results indicate that personality can be an accurate predictor of disease (Muslin, 1983; Schmale & Iker, 1961). Feelings of hopelessness and helplessness have been associated with malignant disease, and strategies that promote hope may increase immune activity and produce a reduction in abnormal cells (Zee, 1979). However, the lack of solid prospective research does at present limit our knowledge of how psychological factors may influence recurrence of disease (Denton & Baum, 1983).

The site-specific aspects of the care required by oncology patients are addressed in other parts of this book. The general implications of surgery and potential nursing interventions are presented in Tables 19–6 and

Table 19–6. PREOPERATIVE CARE

Patient Needs	Nursing Implications or Interventions
Care Relating to Diagnosis and Biopsy	
Preparation for procedure	Have knowledge of and initiate appropriate preparation (e.g., bowel preparation, skin preparation, positioning)
Information and learning	Identify and provide appropriate information
	Use written and verbal material to assist in reinforcement
Emotional support	Promote a nurse-client relationship that encourages patient to voice fears and anxieties
	Provide information
	If appropriate, involve family or significant others so they can be supported and supportive
Care Relating to Surgical Intervention	
Specific preparation	Have knowledge and initiate appropriate preparation
	Take nursing history, which should include patient profile and assessment of baseline physiologic parameters
Physical comfort	Assessment of needs or deficits (e.g., skin integrity, nutritional status, mobility, fluid balance, pain assessment)
	Implement care to maintain and prevent complications of surgery
Self-care	Assess patient's abilities and deficiencies and implement care to fulfill patient's needs
	Encourage patient involvement in care planning.
Emotional support	Promote discussion to explore fears and anxieties
	Explore understandings and perceptions of disease and planned surgical procedure
	Explore implications of the disease to the patient and the anticipated outcome from the surgery
	Assess if patient is realistic
	Provide written and verbal information according to client's needs
	Involve family or significant others in discussions if appropriate
Information and learning	Teach skills to promote expectation shaping and postoperative recovery (e.g., deep breathing exercises)
	Explain use of equipment (e.g., anti-emboli stockings)
	When possible allow patient to see or handle equipment to be used postoperatively
	Explain operation and expected status after surgery

19–7 in a sequential manner from diagnosis to rehabilitation. The points illustrated in tabular form should be interpreted as guidelines.

REHABILITATION AND SUPPORTIVE CARE

Whether surgery has been major or minor, all patients will require supportive care and a period of rehabilitation. The diagnosis and treatment of malignancy assaults many facets of a person's identity. It usually produces feelings of vulnerability and a heightened awareness of the patient's own mortality. It must not be assumed that because a person's cancer is considered "minor" in medical terms, it will not produce extreme reactions of fear, anxiety, or depression. Similarly, a person with an aggressive tumor requiring radical therapy may genuinely demonstrate a stoical acceptance and not require the degree of overt support that health care professionals may regard as necessary. Obviously, the question is one of individual assessment, and it is the primary responsibility of the nurse in the period after physical recovery from surgery to discover the particular needs of the persons being cared for.

However, it is possible to make some assumptions about the needs and problems that patients may have after different kinds of surgical intervention. It is beyond the scope of this chapter to address all the possible consequences of surgery to different areas of the body. Our aim, therefore, is to identify some of the ways in which patients may be affected both physically and psychologically by surgery and the role

of the nurse in providing supportive care and facilitating successful rehabilitation.

ALTERED FUNCTIONING

After surgery, all patients will experience a degree of alteration in their normal bodily functions and in their ability to care for themselves. This may be a transient event due to the effects of anesthesia, for example, being unable to pass urine or requiring the assistance of the nurse to wash or get out of bed. For some patients—those who have undergone radical surgery for bladder or bowel cancer, for example—changes in the process of elimination may be permanent, and they will require intensive supportive care to enable them to learn physical care and adapt to a urinary or fecal stoma.

Any period of illness or psychological stress may affect libido or potency in any person, even those without cancer. However, for those who undergo radical surgery of the abdomen or pelvis, sexual activities may be profoundly affected by both anatomic changes and profound changes in self-esteem and body image. For some patients, this may be a small price to pay for what they hope will be a prolonged life with freedom from distressing symptoms, but others may find it quite unacceptable and never successfully adapt and adjust to their altered state. Their problems may not be primarily sexual but related more to feelings of social isolation, stigma, and depression (Devlin, Plant, & Griffin, 1971; Jones, Breckman, & Hendry, 1980; Maguire et al., 1980; Tait, 1988).

Table 19–7. POSTOPERATIVE CARE

Patient Needs	Nursing Implications or Interventions
Care Relating to Diagnosis and Biopsy	
Specific care relating to procedure	Have understanding of procedure and implement appropriate care (e.g., wound and dressing care, positioning, medication) Assess patient's status and recovery, including physiologic status Observe for complications
Emotional support	Provide suitable environment for discussion of results Provide support for patient and significant others Refer to appropriate resource agencies (e.g., support programs, self-help groups, counselors)
Maintenance of physiologic status and prevention of complications	Monitor important parameters (e.g., shock, hemorrhage, wound dehiscence, infection)
Physical comfort	Monitor efficacy of pain control and implement alteration if necessary Give assistance with positioning and movement Encourage activity and rest as needed Provide adequate nutrition and supplement if appropriate Assist with elimination, ensuring patient privacy and hygiene needs are met Monitor fluid and electrolyte balance Monitor wound healing and provide skilled wound management
Self-care	Assess deficiencies in self-care abilities and implement care to fulfill needs
Information and learning	Provide information regarding specific problems or complications of the procedure Teach use of equipment and dressings if required Provide support, information, and reinforcement for future treatment plan Provide information and planned teaching to assist patient to adapt to altered function, physical status, etc. Involve family or significant others and provide information and teaching where appropriate
Emotional support	Facilitate opportunities for client to explore feelings and responses to altered health status Organize appropriate support agencies in liaison with client and family Provide information as required Provide environment for privacy and interaction when necessary

BODY IMAGE CONSEQUENCES

A person's body image, which may be defined . mental picture of one's body, the way in which the body appears to the self" (Wood, 1978)—often undergoes a severe assault as a consequence of cancer surgery. It is important that the nurse be aware of the nature of this assault to effectively assist the patient in coping with it. Body image forms a part of the whole concept of "self." This concept is discussed more fully in Chapter 51, but for the purposes of this chapter, a useful description is provided by Schain (1980), who identifies four components:

1. The body self (functional or esthetic self)
2. The interpersonal self (how the person responds and is responded to by others)
3. The achieving self (individual goals and aspirations)
4. The identification self (individual ethics, values, beliefs, and behaviors)

Using this framework, it can easily be seen how all these aspects of self can be disrupted in both the short term and long term by surgery. Individual reactions to this assault on the self vary enormously but may include denial, hostility, anxiety, depression, or even apparent unconcern. Attempts to quantify the extent of disfigurement felt by patients have not been wholly successful. However, one study (Dropkin, Malgady, Scott, Oberst, & Strong, 1983), summarized in Box 19–1, attempts to rate disfigurement and dysfunction caused by head and neck surgery. Further work in this area may provide health care professionals with a framework to identify those persons most at risk for developing psychological disturbance. It is important that the nurse be able to demonstrate respect for the patient's reactions and a readiness to help. The increasing tendency to enlist the patient as an active member in planning and to a degree controlling his or her care may prove helpful in minimizing the negative aspects of hospitalization and submission to surgery.

FACILITATING ADAPTATION AND REHABILITATION

Patients undergoing minor surgery may require little assistance to adapt to the diagnosis of cancer and current and subsequent treatment. Preoperative information and the provision of information at the right time is useful in allaying fears and anxieties. However, patients undergoing radical therapy resulting in permanent changes require a great deal more supportive care and need to adopt major adaptive strategies.

A useful model is that proposed by Wright (1960) for persons who have suffered mutilating injuries or extensive disabilities. The general principles include the following:

1. Changing value systems to give less emphasis to physical characteristics as measures of worth.
2. Confining the effects of the disability so that other noninvolved parts of the body are not also devalued.

Text continued on page 244

Box 19–1. DISFIGUREMENT IN HEAD AND NECK PATIENTS

STUDY

Dropkin, M. J., Malgady, R. G., Scott, D. W., Oberst, M. T., & Strong, E. W. (1983, Sept./Oct.). **Scaling of disfigurement and dysfunction in postoperative head and neck patients.** *Head and Neck Surgery, 6,* 559–570.

SAMPLE

100 registered nurses employed at a large urban cancer center. Age range, 22 to 60 years; median, 29 years.

MEASURES

Photographs were prepared of 11 surgical defects superimposed on either the same male or female "normal" face and typed descriptions of eight dysfunctions. All the nurses were asked to judge the severity of all possible combinations: 55 male and 55 female pairs of disfigurement; and 28 pairs of male and 28 female pairs of dysfunctions. Statistical analysis based on the "law of comparative judgments" was used to ensure that nurses' judgments were transitive and consistent.

FINDINGS

Results indicated that a separate rating scale existed for disfigurement and dysfunction. Two important characteristics emerged associated with the severely rated disfigurements, namely procedures involving the mandible and removal of soft tissue and bone from the central portion of the face. Aphonia was considered the most severe dysfunction.

LIMITATIONS

The nurses were all employed at a specialist cancer center and could hold similar attitudes and beliefs with respect to head and neck disfigurement and dysfunction. This study looked at nurses' rating of disfigurement and dysfunction and therefore has limited value as far as patients' responses are concerned.

Box 19–2. POSTDISCHARGE DISTRESS IN SURGICAL CANCER PATIENTS

STUDY

Oberst, M. T., & Scott, D. W. (1988). **Postdischarge distress in surgically treated cancer patients and their spouses.** *Research in Nursing and Health, 11,* 223–233.

SAMPLE

40 patient-spouse dyads (N = 80); 31 men and nine women in the patient group. All were recently diagnosed as having bowel or urinary system cancer. Mean age of patient group 59.9 years, spouse group 54.4 years. Half the patient group had a permanent ostomy (N = 20).

MEASURES

Brief Symptom Inventory (BSI); State Trait Anxiety Inventory; Vulnerability Scale; and semistructured interviews following a COPE format at 10, 30, 60, 90, and 180 days after discharge.

FINDINGS

Minimal variation between patients and spouses in intensity of distress. Results suggest that the crisis of initial cancer treatment is not resolved, even when the prognosis is favorable, until 3 to 6 months after discharge. The majority of spouses displayed a degree of anger, frustration, or fatigue at 2 months after discharge, and at 90 and 180 days had raised BSI scores.

LIMITATIONS

Small study of patient-spouse pairs with similar diagnosis, who received care at the same urban cancer center; therefore, it is difficult to draw parallels with patients with cancer at other sites. The patient group was predominantly male and therefore gender differences could have affected results. The majority of respondents were middle or upper class with annual incomes above the national average.

Table 19–8. SOME GENERAL PHYSICAL AND PSYCHOLOGICAL CONSEQUENCES FROM CANCER

Site or Purpose of Surgery	Altered Functions	Body Image Consequences	Adaptation Strategies and Sources of Help
Head and neck	Swallowing secretions Eating and drinking Talking and communicating Dietary habits Maintenance of adequate hydration and nutrition Sexuality: kissing, lovemaking positions. Relationships with significant others and at work	Depends on extent of surgery (i.e., if defects are permanent or temporary) Any change is permanently visible to public view	Planned teaching to facilitate self-care Involvement of physiotherapist, speech therapist, dietitian Advice on prosthetics Information about self-help groups
Breast	If surgery is radical: Reduced mobility of arm on affected side Potential problem of lymphedema Paresthesia General: Sexuality: loss of major erogenous zone, inhibition with partner Change in dressing style Depression: short-term and long-term	Major effect on most women Permanent change in body contour Physical sensation of loss Reduced physical sensation	Opportunity to discuss surgical options (e.g., breast reconstruction) Physiotherapy to regain maximum mobility Discussion of feelings about self and relationships with others Involvement of significant other Suggestions for strategies for lovemaking Advice on prosthesis and clothing Early identification of psychological morbidity Planned teaching to prevent injury to arm on affected side
Bowel or bladder	Following radical surgery with stoma formation: Normal elimination patterns with voluntary control Maintenance of adequate hydration and nutrition Dietary habits Social isolation (if patient feels stigmatized or lacks confidence) Sexuality: loss of self esteem; feelings of disgust because of stoma; practical difficulties of lovemaking due to appliances or altered anatomy; impotence or sensory impairment (depends on type of surgery and individual variations) Relationships with others (e.g., whether to tell colleagues at work) Special arrangements when traveling, visiting friends, etc. Interference with life style, hobbies, etc. Change in skin integrity	Major and permanent change in body contour, although "concealed" from public view In men, genitalia left externally intact, but may be dysfunctional	Planned teaching to facilitate self-care Discussion of feelings about self and relationships with others Discussion of actual or potential sexual problems; alternative lovemaking; prosthesis and reconstructive surgery for impotence Advice on availability of ostomy supplies and home care arrangements Advice on diet, clothing, travel, etc. Referral to voluntary services, self-help groups (e.g., United Ostomy Association) Planned teaching to educate patient about skin care and skin integrity
Pelvis (uterus, ovaries, vulva, vagina)	Depending on type of surgery: Menstruation Hormonal changes—treatment-induced menopause Altered internal or external anatomy Potential complications of surgery, other treatments, recurrence (e.g., fistulae, fungating lesions, impaired healing, discharge) Sexuality: loss of femininity; fear of partner's reaction; loss of childbearing ability	May be no external change other than scarring but may produce profound feelings of "loss of womanliness" Radical surgery (e.g., pelvic exenteration) may result in stoma formation and grossly altered genital anatomy Overt wound lesions with or without offensive odor may result in distress, feelings of uncleanliness, and withdrawal	Discussion of feelings about self and relationships with others Advice on hormone replacement therapy if appropriate Discussion of actual and potential sexual problems Planned teaching to facilitate self-care Imaginative wound management strategies to contain or disguise odor and effluent and education to promote individual control and self-care. Information regarding support agencies
Limb surgery with or without amputation	Reduced mobility if lower limb; consequences for self-care in hygiene, dressing, mobility, etc. Restriction of whole range of normal living activities Potentially may affect employment prospects Potential difficulties in relationships with others, particularly the very young and elderly Management of stump	Major change with external implications: Physical sensation of loss	Physiotherapy to regain maximum mobility Occupational therapy to facilitate adaptation to new ways of performing activities of daily living Involvement of family in care at home Referral to social service agencies for assistance with house adaptation, employment, etc. Early referral for prosthesis fitting Planned teaching to promote self-care of stump or wound and develop ways of dealing with phantom pain
Devices used for supplemental nutrition (e.g., intravenous or enteral) Devices to provide access for chemotherapy or pain control	Eating and drinking Dietary habits Maintenance of adequate hydration and nutrition Sexuality: fear that physical closeness may result in displacement Management of device Life-style restrictions (e.g., travel, participation in games)	May not be apparent externally but profound feelings of loss may be experienced Maintenance of weight may affect self-image	Planned teaching to encourage self-care by patient or care by significant other Advice and details of agencies for supplies of equipment, dietary constituents, etc. Provision of written and verbal information to supplement teaching of device management Discussion of ways device can be secured to allow close contact and lovemaking

3. Coming to view altered physical factors or functions as an asset rather than a liability. For example, viewing a stoma as useful in allowing social activity because of freedom from incontinence or frequent visits to the bathroom, rather than feeling stigmatized because there has been a change in a normal elimination pattern.

The nurse can be of enormous assistance in helping patients to "work through" their feelings about how they perceive themselves and what problems they anticipate in the future. Watson (1983) found that patients who had received counseling interventions demonstrated positive alterations in self-concept and self-esteem compared with subjects who were not counseled. Improvement in independence, self-care abilities, and feelings about self were maintained 1 month after discharge from the hospital. Denton and Baum (1983) confirmed the efficacy of counseling for women undergoing mastectomy for breast cancer. Similarly, their results indicate a positive short-term effect. The long-term effects for cancer patients who experience counseling initiatives have not yet been fully evaluated.

Patients may require counseling, advice, training, and support from many different sources to achieve successful rehabilitation. In the hospital, a whole range of services and personnel are available, and the patient may undergo a rigorous program tailored to individual needs. However, the process of rehabilitation extends well beyond the period of hospitalization, and plans must be made to ensure that progress is maintained beyond discharge. Here the nurse's main function is to act as a coordinator for continuity of care at home and, when appropriate, to provide information about voluntary services and self-help groups that may be useful. Such facilities will vary from area to area, and it is essential that hospital-based nurses are aware of outside agencies and their functions.

Spouses, family members, and significant others also are exposed to the stresses and strains that the diagnosis of cancer and resulting treatment can bring. They may also have the added stress of providing physical care as well as emotional support. Box 19–2 outlines a study (Oberst & Scott, 1988) that has identified and quantified the distress encountered by patients and their spouses in the early postdischarge period.

It is not possible to detail here all the consequences of all types of cancer surgery. Table 19–8 attempts to summarize some of the major physical and psychological effects of surgery in different areas of the body. Most, if not all, of these will be discussed in greater length in subsequent chapters.

SUMMARY

It is our hope that this chapter has demonstrated the complexities of modern cancer surgery and the wide-ranging implications for the patients, their significant others, and health care professionals. It was our intention to propose that quality patient care can only be delivered when that care is a reflection of planning, when it is based on sound knowledge and expertise, and when it is constantly reappraised by the assessment of patients' needs.

However, it is our belief, based on our experience, that the ultimate goal of successful adaptation to the surgical experience can only be achieved by the promotion of a patient-centered philosophy of care, education, and support to achieve optimum self-care and control.

References

Ames, F. C. (1986). In R. J. McKenna & G. P. Murphy (Eds.), *Fundamentals of surgical oncology* (pp. 40–55). New York: Macmillan Publishing Co.

Barber, H. R. K. (1986). In R. J. McKenna & G. P. Murphy (Eds.), *Fundamentals of surgical oncology* (pp. 763–773). New York: Macmillan Publishing Co.

Beattie, E. J. (1984). Surgical treatment of pulmonary metastases. *Cancer, 54*, 2729–2731.

Blythe, J. G., & Wahl, T. P. (1964). Debulking surgery: Does it increase the quality of survival? *Gynecologic Oncology, 14*, 396.

Boore, J. (1978). *Prescription for recovery*. London: Royal College of Nursing.

Cumming, J., Worth, P. H. L., & Woodhouse, C. R. J. (1987). The choice of suprapubic continent catheterisable urinary stoma. *British Journal of Urology, 60*, 227–230.

d'Angelo, T. M., & Gorrell, C. R. (1989). Breast reconstruction using tissue expanders. *Oncology Nursing Forum, 16*(1), 23–27.

Denton, S., (1988). Cancer: History, myths and attitudes. In V. Tschudin (Ed.), *Nursing the patient with cancer* (pp. 1–9). London: Prentice Hall.

Denton, S., & Baum, M. (1983). Psychosocial aspects of breast cancer. In R. Margolese (Ed.), *Breast cancer: Update in clinical oncology* (pp. 173–185). Edinburgh: Churchill Livingstone.

Devlin, H. B., Plant, J. A., & Griffin, M. (1971). Aftermath of surgery for anorectal cancer. *British Medical Journal, 3*, 413–418.

Dropkin, M. J., Malgady, R. G., Scott, D. W., Oberst, M. T., & Strong, E. W. (1983). Scaling of disfigurement and dysfunction in postoperative head and neck patients. *Head and Neck Surgery, 6*, 559–570.

Finch, M. (1989). Continuous pain relief. *Nursing Times, 26*(85), 30–31.

Fitzsimmons, M. L., Conway, T. A., Madsen, N., Lappe, J. M., & Coody, D. (1989). Hereditary cancer syndromes: Nursing's role in identification and education. *Oncology Nursing Forum, 16*(1), 87–94.

Fortner, J. M. (1984). Multivariate analysis of a personal series of 247 consecutive patients with liver metastases from colorectal cancer. *Annals of Surgery, 199*, 306–316.

Foster, S. B. (1974). An adrenal measure for evaluating nursing effectiveness. *Nursing Research, 23*, 118–124.

Galluci, B. B. (1985). Selected concepts of cancer as a disease: From the Greeks to 1900. *Oncology Nursing Forum, 12*(4), 67–71.

Gilbertson, V. A., & Wangensteen, O. H. (1964). A summary of 13 years with the second look program. *Surgery, Gynecology, and Obstetrics, 114*, 438.

Hayward, J. (1978). Preoperative factors affecting postoperative recovery. In *Proceedings of the Nursing Mirror International Cancer Conference*. London: Nursing Mirror.

Jones, M. A., Breckman, B., & Hendry, W. F. (1980). Life with an ileal conduit: Results of questionnaire surveys of patients and urological surgeons. *British Journal of Urology, 52*, 21–25.

Larson, D. L., & McMurtrey, M. J. (1983). Chest wall resection and reconstruction in breast cancer patients. *Current controversies in breast cancer*. New York: Raven Press.

Maguire, P., Tait, A., Brooke, M., Thomas, C., & Sellwood, R. (1980). The effect of counselling on the psychiatric morbidity associated with mastectomy. *British Medical Journal, 281*, 1454–1456.

McKenna, R. J., Jr., & McKenna, R. J. (1986). Overview of surgical oncology. In R. J. McKenna & G. P. Murphy (Eds.), *Fundamen-*

tals of surgical oncology (pp. 3–13). New York: Macmillan Publishing Co.

Moore, M. (1979). Tumor immunology. In J. Irvine (Ed.), *Medical immunology*. Edinburgh: Teviot Scientific Publications.

Muslin, H. L., Gyarfas, K., & Pieper, W. J. (1966). Separation experience and cancer of the breast. *Annual New York Academy of Science Journal, 125*, 802–806.

Oberst, M. T., & Scott, D. W. (1988). Postdischarge distress in surgically treated cancer patients and their spouses. *Research in Nursing and Health, 11*, 223–233.

Priestman, T. J., & Fielding, J. W. L. (1987). Colorectal cancer. *Cancer Care*, 10–13.

Pritchard, A. P., & David, J. A. (Eds.) (1988). *The Royal Marsden manual of clinical nursing procedures* (2nd ed., pp 423–425). London: Harper & Row.

Schain, W. S. (1980). Body self, sexual functioning, self esteem & cancer care. In J. M. Viath (Ed.), *Body image, self esteem & sexuality* (pp. 12–19). New York: S. Karger.

Schmale, A. H., & Iker, H. P. (1961). The effect of hopelessness and the development of cancer. *Psychosomatic Medicine, 28*, 714–721.

Szopa, T. J. (1987). In C. R. Ziegfield, (Ed.), *Core curriculum for oncology nurses* (pp. 199–206). Philadelphia: W. B. Saunders Co.

Tait, A. (1988). Whole or partial breast loss: The threat to womanhood. In M. Salter (Ed.), *Altered body image: The nurse's role* (167–177). New York: John Wiley & Sons.

Watson, P. G. (1983). The effects of short term postoperative counseling on cancer/ostomy patients. *Cancer Nursing, 6*, 21–29.

Westbury, G. (1988). Surgical oncology. In P. Pritchard (Ed.), *Oncology for nurses and health care professionals* (2nd ed., Vol I., pp. 203–222). New York: Harper & Row.

White, H. (1978). Surgical oncology. In R. Tiffany (Ed.), *Oncology for nurses and health care professionals* (Vol. I, pp. 169–186). London: George Allen & Unwin.

Wilson-Barnett, J. (1978). Patients' emotional responses to barium x-rays. *Journal of Advanced Nursing, 3*, 37–46.

Wilson-Barnett, J. (1981). Assessment of recovery with special reference to a study with postoperative cardiac patients. *Journal of Advanced Nursing, 6*, 435–445.

Wood, N. (1978). *Human sexuality in health and illness*. St. Louis: C. V. Mosby Co.

Wright, B. (1960). *Physical disability—a psychological approach*. New York: Harper & Row.

Zee, H. (1979). Stress and cancer. *Journal of the Medical Association of Georgia, 68*, 845–847.

CHAPTER 20

Radiation Oncology

LAURA J. HILDERLEY
KAREN HASSEY DOW

Radiation therapy is the use of high-energy, ionizing radiation or x-rays to treat diseases. Although it is used primarily in the treatment of cancer, radiation has also been used to treat benign disorders such as desmoid tumors and hyperthyroidism. Twenty years ago, statistics indicated that half of those persons with cancer were treated with radiation therapy and the majority of these were being treated palliatively. Today, with the shift toward earlier detection of cancer, the development of more sophisticated radiation therapy techniques, the improvement in our knowledge and understanding of multimodal therapy, and the development of newer methods of cancer therapy (biologic response modifiers), radiation is used in treatment of 60 per cent or more of individuals with cancer.

As the science of radiation oncology has evolved, so too has the role of health providers in the delivery of this treatment. Radiation oncologists, physicists, and technologists have long been involved in the discipline of radiation oncology. The oncology nurse's presence has been a more recent development. Since the early 1970s, the role of the oncology nurse in radiation

therapy has grown in its dimensions from primarily an assistant or task-oriented function to a patient management and interdisciplinary role with broad responsibilities (Hilderley, 1980). One study by Grant, Dodd, Hilderley, & Patterson (1984), which surveyed 1088 radiation therapy facilities, indicated that 179 of 414 respondents employed one or more nurses. Although a repeat study has not been done, personal observation (requests for consultation on the nursing role in radiation from either nurses new to the role or physicians or administrators interested in employing nurses) indicates that there is a steady upward trend in the number of nurses employed in radiation oncology. In 1990, the Oncology Nursing Society established Special Interest Groups (SIGs), and the radiation oncology nursing SIG was one of the first and largest to be officially recognized.

As the number of nurses has increased, so too has the scope of their contribution to patient care. Box 20–1 summarizes the study by Grant and colleagues (1984).

This chapter provides an overview of radiation ther-

Box 20–1. RADIATION ONCOLOGY NURSING ROLE

STUDY

Grant M., Dodd, M., Hilderley, L., & Patterson, P. (1984). **Radiation oncology nurses' role: A national survey.** *Oncology Nursing Forum Supplement: Proceedings of the Tenth Annual Congress, 11*(2), 107.

SAMPLE

414 institutions with radiation oncology departments from throughout the United States (respondents from a total of 1088 institutions on the mailing list).

METHODOLOGY

A 133-item questionnaire in four parts: (1) description of the facility, (2) description of department personnel, (3) demographic information about the nurse, and (4) specific functions of the nurse. 110 functions were listed in part 4, and these were further defined as to (a) person primarily responsible for that function, (b) whether nurse assumes this function if others are not available, (c) nurse's priority for the function, and (d) nurse's willingness to perform function.

FINDINGS

Number of institutions with no nurse: 235
Number of institutions with one nurse: 146
Number of institutions with more than one nurse: 33
Number of nurses increased with size of institution
Lines of authority in general were tied to radiation oncology department; however, as number of nurses increases, ties with nursing department increase
Average age of nurse: 35 yr

Educational preparation:	nonbaccalaureate	55%
	baccalaureate	23%
	graduate	9%
	vocational (LPN)	13%
Job satisfaction:	not at all	0%
	a little satisfied	2%
	somewhat satisfied	20%
	very satisfied	75%
Functions with highest priority ratings:	side-effect management	
	patient counseling	
	teaching patient before treatment	
	dietary counseling	
	nursing assessment	

Functions for which the nurse was responsible, but rated as low priority and was unwilling to perform:
  assisting physician with examination
  teaching radiation therapy technology students
  conducting collaborative research

---

apy, with a discussion of the scientific concepts of radiation physics and tumor biology that underlie treatment, and a discussion of the critical role nurses play in supporting patients, managing side effects, and improving quality of life for patients undergoing this cancer treatment.

PRINCIPLES OF RADIATION PHYSICS

The therapeutic goal of radiation oncology is to deliver a precise dose of ionizing radiation to a specific tumor volume while sparing the surrounding healthy tissue (Rubin, 1983). Ideally, this procedure will result in eradication of tumor, repair of healthy tissue, and a reasonably high quality of life for the patient.

Radiation treatment is based on several physical and biologic principles. When subjected to ionizing radiation, the living organism responds in a generally predictable manner. Irradiated cells are either destroyed or rendered incapable of reproduction.

All living matter is composed of molecules, the basis of which is the atom. An atom consists of two parts: a nucleus containing protons with a positive charge and neutrons with no charge; and the shell or shells composed of electrons (with negative charge) that circle in orbit around the nucleus. Figure 20–1 illustrates the structure of stable and radioactive atoms. In a stable atom, the number of negative electrons equals the

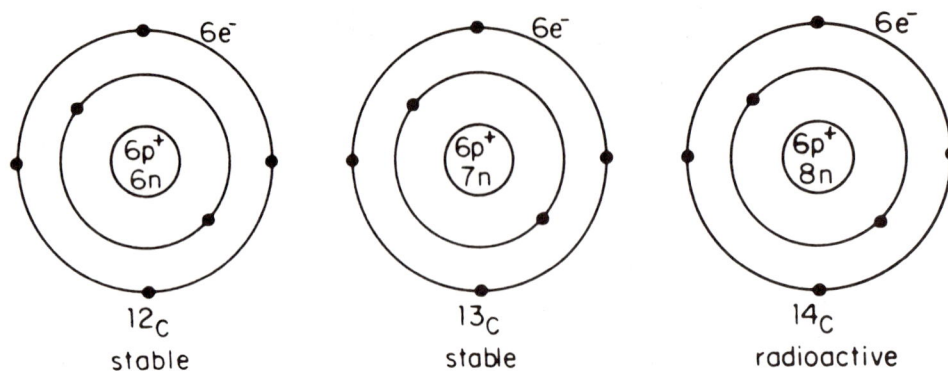

Figure 20–1. Composition of atoms of matter: in the stable atom, electrons are equal to the number of protons. Nuclides with the same number of protons but different number of neutrons are called isotopes. (Reprinted with permission from Shapiro, J. [1981]. *Radiation protection: A guide for scientists and physicians* [2nd ed.]. Cambridge, MA: Harvard University Press. Reproduced by permission.)

number of positive protons in the nucleus; this balance between protons and electrons maintains the stability of the atom. Ionizing radiation disrupts the atom's stability by displacing electrons (ejecting them from their orbital position) and triggering a process of physical and chemical change that leads ultimately to cell injury or death.

Ionizing radiation is part of the electromagnetic spectrum, whose scale ranges from radio and microwaves of very long length at one end of the spectrum to ionizing radiation of relatively short wavelength at the opposite end of the spectrum. The penetrating power of ionizing radiation depends on the energy of that radiation and the composition of the tissue being traversed. Thus radiotherapy equipment of varying energies is needed to meet particular needs (Tables 20–1 and 20–2).

Tissue density is a major factor in the effectiveness of ionizing radiation. As the radiation penetrates body tissue, interactions occur and energy is released. Linear energy transfer (LET) is the rate at which energy is deposited per unit distance. The significance of LET is seen in the degree of cell damage that occurs when ionizing events are closely spaced as opposed to the degree of damage in those that are more widely separated. This difference in cell damage as influenced by LET is known as the relative biologic effectiveness or RBE (Griffin, 1987).

PRINCIPLES OF RADIOBIOLOGY

Target Theory

The exact mechanism of cell killing or cell damage by ionizing radiation has been the subject of research for many years. The actual mechanism by which radiation energy causes biologic damage is a highly complex sequence of events with a time scale of from 1×10^{-16} seconds to many years (Boaz, 1975). *Target theory*

Table 20–1. TELETHERAPY EQUIPMENT AND ITS USE

Equipment	Emission	Beam Characteristics and Radiobiologic Effects	Clinical Application, Advantages, Disadvantages
Kilovoltage 40–150 kV	X-rays	Superficial, limited range, poor skin tolerance	Skin cancers or other very superficial lesions, if electrons are not available
Orthovoltage 150–1000 kV	X-rays	Deep penetration, high skin dose, high bone absorption	Limited, owing to poor skin tolerance and potential for bone necrosis
Cesium-137 radioisotope (600 kV)	gamma rays	Large source size with large penumbra	Long half-life; low energy and output; used in head and neck treatment
Megavoltage or Supervoltage Cobalt-60 1.25–2 MeV	gamma rays	Deeply penetrating; skin-sparing due to maximum dose build-up beneath the skin; produces penumbra area at edge of beam that receives less dose	Deep-seated tumors; ease of mechanical operation Slower dose-rate (longer treatment time) as source decays
Linear Accelerators 4–20 MeV	photons	Deeply penetrating; skin-sparing; increased versatility and precision of dose distribution	Deep-seated tumors; large field capability; complex electronics with tendency for "down-time"
6–30 MeV	Electrons (optional)	Electrons give maximum dose on skin and a few centimeters beneath, falling off rapidly thereafter	Skin lesions, chest wall recurrence, superficial nodes
Betatron 10–30 MeV	Electrons	High-velocity electrons with deep penetration	High dose rate with shorter treatment time; limited field size; bulky equipment; low dose rate photons
18–40 MeV	X-rays	High-energy photons	

(From Hassey, K., Hilderley, L. [in press]. *Nursing perspectives in radiation oncology.* Albany, NY: Delmar Publishers, Inc. Reproduced by permission.)

Table 20–2. HIGH LINEAR ENERGY TRANSFER (LET) AND HEAVY CHARGED PARTICLE BEAMS

Energy Source	Beam Characteristics and Radiobiologic Effects	Use in Clinical Trials
Fast Neutrons 16–50 MeV deuterons	Fixed field size and beam position; wide penumbra; absorbed dose decreases exponentially with depth; low OER; RBE is higher with small dose increments	Advanced cancers of the head and neck, pelvis, gliomas, and melanoma; esophageal cancer and osteosarcomas
Protons and Helium Ions 600 MeV	Precise dose distribution with ability to deliver very high tumor dose with sparing of adjacent normal tissues; RBE and OER similar to those obtained with gamma and photon sources	Pituitary tumors, chondrosarcoma, cordoma; abdominal and pelvic tumors; soft-tissue sarcomas; head and neck tumors
Negative Pi-Mesons 40–70 MeV	Absorbed dose increases slowly with depth, then rises sharply; lower OER; enhanced RBE	Head and neck tumors, brain, prostate, pancreas; skin metastases

OER, Oxygen enhancement ratio; RBE, relative biologic effectiveness.
(From Hassey, K., Hilderley, L. [in press]. *Nursing perspectives in radiation oncology.* Albany, NY: Delmar Publishers, Inc. Reproduced by permission.)

proposes that radiation damage is the result of both direct and indirect hits (Travis, 1975; Withers & Peters, 1980). A *direct hit* refers to damage to DNA, the critical target. Results of a direct hit are (1) change or loss of a base (thymine, adenine, guanine, or cytosine), (2) breakage of the hydrogen bond between the two chains of the DNA molecule, (3) breaks in one or both chains of the DNA molecule, and (4) cross-linking of the chains after breakage.

An *indirect hit* refers to the ionization of water, the medium surrounding the molecular structures within the cell. Ionizing radiation absorbed by water molecules initiates a series of chemical interactions, the most important of which is production of the hydroxyl radical, OH·. This free radical is now available to combine with others, forming new and potentially cytotoxic agents. Because water is the predominant substance in any tissue, the likelihood that indirect hits and resulting cell injury will occur is greater than that for direct damage to the DNA structure. Box 20–2 illustrates the sequence of events in the ionization of water by radiation.

The Four Rs of Radiobiology

Radiation effect at the cellular level is a function of the cell's response to the damaging effects of ionization. Although the goal of treatment is to destroy tumor tissue, healthy tissue must be preserved. Fractionation of dose is based upon the following four Rs of radiobiology: repair, repopulation, redistribution, and reoxygenation.

Repair

The dose should allow repair of sublethal damage. Between daily treatment fractions, the normal tissue is able to repair radiation injury, whereas tumor cells are less likely to be able to do so.

Repopulation

Repopulation of normal cells through mitosis after repair of radiation injury allows continued proliferation of normal tissue. Tumor cells are less likely to undergo mitosis because of inability to repair sublethal damage.

Redistribution

Ionizing radiation is believed to be most effective during the mitotic stage of the cell cycle. With each successive dose of radiation, more cells are likely to be in actual mitosis through cycle delay, therefore increasing the effectiveness of each dose. Normal cells are much less likely to be delayed or redistributed in their cycle than tumor cells.

Reoxygenation

Well-oxygenated cells are more sensitive to radiation effect than hypoxic cells. Protracted fractionation of dose allows reoxygenation and therefore enhances radiosensitivity of tumor cells, which may have been hypoxic.

Biologic Response to Radiation

Response to radiation occurs at the cellular level, triggering a sequence of biologic events that result in tissue injury, destruction, or ultimate repair. Some of the earliest work in radiobiology was that of Bergonie and Tribondeau (1959), who theorized that radiosensitivity is directly related to the reproductive capacity of a cell. This theory was based on their experiments on rat testes, in which they successfully destroyed the germ cells, leaving the interstitial and supporting cells of the seminiferous tubules intact.

Radiosensitivity

Radiosensitivity refers to the degree and speed of response to radiation of any given tissue, whether tumor or normal healthy tissue. Within the cell cycle, radiosensitivity also varies, and, according to Hall (1978), (1) cells are most sensitive at or close to mitosis; (2) resistance is usually greatest in the latter part of the S phase; (3) if G_1 has an appreciable length, a resistant period is evident early in G_1, followed by a sensitive period toward the end of G_1; and (4) the G_2 phase is usually sensitive, perhaps as sensitive as the M phase, to radiation.

Radiosensitivity varies with the type of tumor as well as with its size and location. Some malignant

---

Box 20–2. IONIZATION OF WATER MOLECULES

Water, which constitutes 80 per cent of the mammalian cell content, undergoes a series of chemical reactions when exposed to ionizing radiation. In the following, water (HOH) is converted to hydrogen peroxide (H_2O_2).

The final products of the ionization of water molecules (HOH) by radiation are an ion pair (H^+, OH^-) and free radicals (H·, OH·), which are capable of damaging the cell. The ionization of water is shown in the following steps:

$$HOH \xrightarrow{\text{Radiation}} HOH^+ + e^-$$

The free electron (e^-) is then captured by another available water molecule and, as shown in the next step, forms the second ion:

$$HOH + e^- \longrightarrow HOH^-$$

Because the two ions (HOH^+, HOH^-) produced by these reactions are unstable, rapid breakdown occurs (in the presence of other normal water molecules), forming yet another ion and a free radical as follows:

$$HOH^+ \longrightarrow H^+ + OH·$$

$$HOH^- \longrightarrow OH^- + H·$$

Although the resulting ion pair (H^+, OH^-) have some potential for cellular damage through chemical reactions, they are more likely to recombine and form water (HOH). The free radicals (H·, OH·) are extremely reactive, and they too may simply recombine to form water. However, free radicals appear to be more likely to undergo chemical interactions with other free radicals, forming cytotoxic agents, as shown in this reaction:

$$OH· + OH· \longrightarrow H_2O_2 \text{ (hydrogen peroxide)}$$

Free radicals that result from the interaction of radiation with water are capable of triggering a variety of chemical reactions within the cell and are therefore believed to be a major factor in the production of damage in the cell.

(From Groenwald, S. [1987]. *Cancer Nursing: Principles and Practice* [p. 329]. Boston: Jones and Bartlett Publishers, Inc. Reproduced by permission.)

---

lesions generally classified as radiosensitive include seminoma, acute lymphocytic leukemia, Hodgkin's disease, and lymphomas. Among the more radioresistant tumors are squamous cell carcinomas, ovarian tumors, soft-tissue sarcomas, and gliomas (Rubin, 1983).

Similarly, normal tissues and organs can be classified according to degree of radiosensitivity, based on parenchymal hypoplasia. Lymphoid organs, bone marrow, gonads, skin, and mucous membranes are highly radiosensitive. Those organs and tissues categorized as having a low degree of radiosensitivity (relatively radioresistant) include mature bone and cartilage, liver, thyroid gland, muscle, brain, and spinal cord.

Radiocurability

Radiocurability is a term used to describe the ability to eradicate tumor at the local or regional site. Unfortunately, radiosensitivity does not necessarily equate with radiocurability. Some of the most radiosensitive tumors are also among the most anaplastic and undifferentiated (metastasizing early and rapidly) and thus are not radiocurable.

RADIATION TECHNIQUES

Two means of delivering radiation therapy are used: teletherapy and brachytherapy. Teletherapy makes use of a machine (such as a linear accelerator) to deliver ionizing radiation from outside the body. Brachytherapy involves placement of a radioactive source within or close to the tissue to be treated, such as the interstitial or intracavitary techniques used in the treatment of breast and gynecologic cancers.

Teletherapy

Teletherapy (from *tele*, Greek prefix meaning at a distance) is external radiation treatment given with a machine or source at some distance from the target site. Early machines had a kilovoltage in the range of 40 to 150 kV and produced x-rays with minimal penetration because of their low energy. Between 1920 and 1940, orthovoltage equipment, with a range of 180- to 250-kV energy, was introduced, providing the capability to treat much more deeply seated tumors. Healthy tissues were not spared, however, and poor skin tolerance combined with late bone necrosis limited the therapeutic value of orthovoltage equipment.

Nuclear research in the era of World War II led to technology that helped to develop radioactive sources for therapeutic use. In the early 1940s, radiation therapy entered the supervoltage era. Atomic reactors made Cobalt-60 a more readily available source, and the betatron and linear accelerator were developed. The betatron was the first generator of supervoltage x-rays used therapeutically, and this machine was favored for its ability to produce high energy at a relatively low cost. There were disadvantages, however, including the low intensity of the beam and the physical massiveness of the equipment required to produce the x-rays. Cobalt-60 was first used in a teletherapy unit in

1951. Cobalt machines became the standard source for deep therapy and were utilized in most radiotherapy treatment centers. Their major advantage is the relative simplicity of the equipment, which requires minimal maintenance (time and cost) and is highly reliable.

The linear accelerator (Linac) evolved out of the electronics era of the 1960s and 1970s and is widely used today. An example of a linear accelerator is shown in Figure 20–2. These highly sophisticated machines operate on the principle of rapid acceleration of electrons in a vacuum. As the electrons strike a metal target such as tungsten, photons are produced. Photons are the equivalent of gamma rays and x-rays, differing only in their means of production. Some linear accelerators are dual purpose, capable of emitting either electrons or photons. If electrons are used, the metal target is removed from the path of the accelerated electrons, allowing them to emerge from a narrow window in the vacuum tube, targeted directly at the treatment site. Table 20–1 lists low LET standard teletherapy equipment, types of emissions, beam characteristics, and clinical applications as well as limitations.

High LET and Heavy Charged Particle Beams

Megavoltage teletherapy equipment, as described previously, is the most common means of delivering radiation therapy. In some situations, a distinct therapeutic advantage can be gained through the use of heavy charged particle beams or high linear energy transfer (LET) radiations (Griffin, 1987). Characteristics of high LET and heavy charged particle beams are described in Table 20–2. The two major advantages to these sources of ionizing radiations are (1) deposition of large doses of radiation in small volumes of tissue, with sparing of surrounding normal tissue (by proton beams, heavy ions, and negative pi mesons); and (2) biologic advantages, including more effective killing of hypoxic cells and decreased fluctuation in radiosensitivity throughout the cell cycle (by fast neutrons, heavy ions, and pi mesons) (Griffin, 1987; Parker, 1976).

The physical and biologic advantages of high LET and heavy charged particle beams are offset somewhat by the complexity and costs of the equipment and

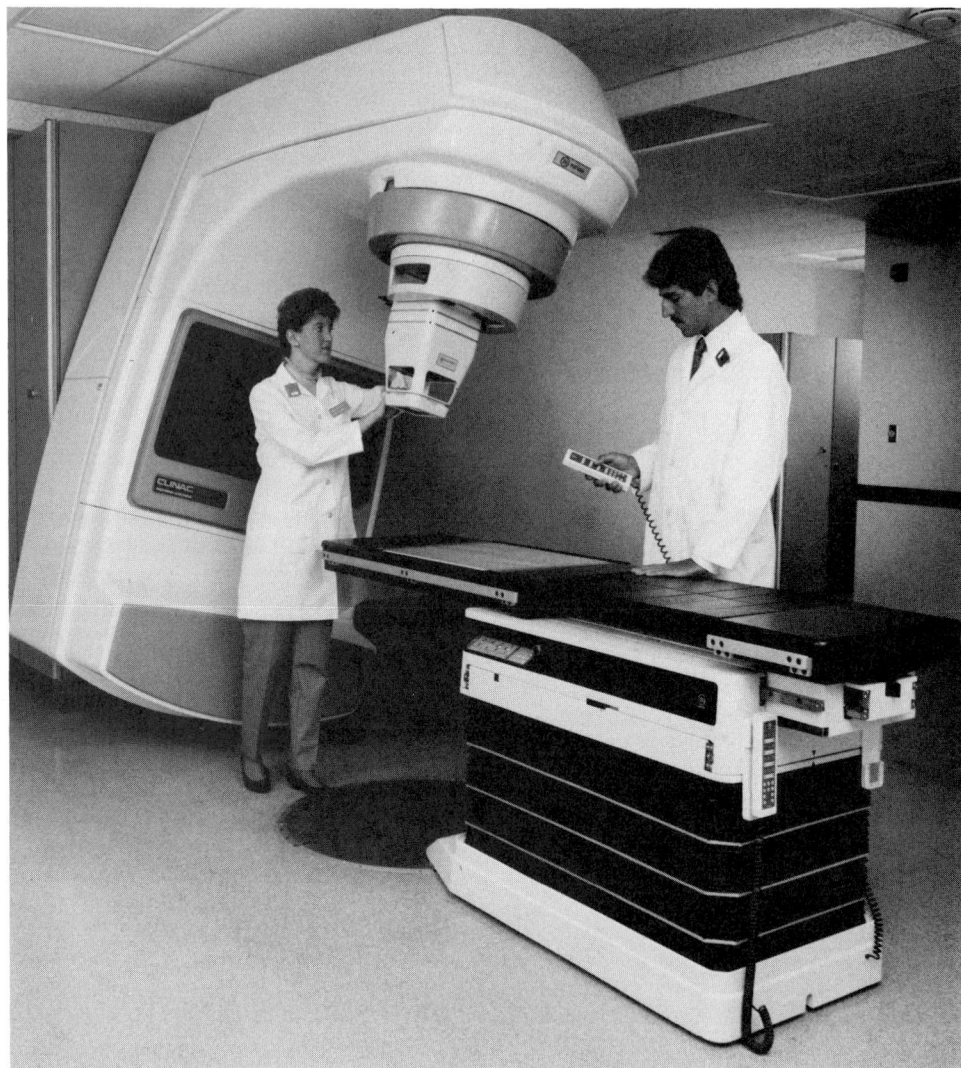

Figure 20–2. A Varian Clinac 2100-C linear accelerator with x-ray energies ranging from 6 to 18 Mv and electron beams from 4 to 20 MeV. (Varian Associates, Inc., Palo Alto, CA. Reproduced by permission.)

facilities required. However, it is generally agreed (Griffin, 1987; Parker, 1976) that despite slow accumulation of data, the sparsity of population groups in any given tumor category, and the complexity and cost of equipment, research into the clinical application of high LET and charged particle beam therapy should continue and expand.

GOALS OF RADIATION THERAPY IN CANCER MANAGEMENT

Radiation therapy has multiple applications in cancer treatment. It may be given (1) with curative intent; (2) to help control local disease; (3) as an adjuvant to surgery, chemotherapy, or biologic therapy; and (4) as palliative treatment. Radiation dosage terminology is listed in Table 20–3.

Curative radiation therapy generally refers to a situation in which this modality is the primary treatment, as in treating skin cancers or early-stage breast, laryngeal, or prostate cancers (Hussey, 1980; Marks & Sessions, 1987; Million, Cassisi, & Wittes, 1985; Perez, 1987). Generally, if radiation is the primary treatment, extensive surgery can be avoided, thus sparing the patient from the significant physical and psychological side effects of radical surgery. When the intent is curative and radiation is the primary method being used, the treatment course is generally longer and the

Table 20–3. RADIATION DOSAGE TERMINOLOGY

In 1985 the International Commission on Radiation Units and Measurements (ICRU) designated several new terms related to radiation dose. Medical and nursing literature began to reflect these changes in the late 1980s. Therefore, for clarity, both the old and the new terms are listed here.

Becquerel (Bq): Unit of measure for the amount of activity of a radioactive nuclide in a particular energy state. One becquerel equals one nuclear disintegration per second. The becquerel replaces the former unit designation *curie*. (1 Bq $\approx 2.7 \times 10^{-11}$ Ci)

Curie (Ci): Unit of measure formerly used to describe the rate of nuclear disintegration of a radioactive source. This unit is now called a becquerel (Bq). (1 Ci = 3.7×10^{10} Bq)

Gray (Gy): Unit of radiation dose (one joule per kilogram). Measure of the energy deposited by radiation in an absorbing medium. The gray has replaced the term *rad*. 1 gray equals 100 cGy equals 100 rad. (1 rad equals 1 cGy)

Rad (r): Acronym for *rad*iation *a*bsorbed *d*ose. One rad equals an energy absorption of 100 ergs per gram of absorber. In 1985, the term gray (Gy) became the official term for radiation absorbed dose, replacing the rad. One gray equals 100 rad, and 1 cGy equals 1 rad.

Rem: Acronym for *r*oentgen *e*quivalent—*m*an, the term used to measure the dose equivalent of ionizing radiation when considering radiation safety and radiation protection rather than therapeutic radiation dose. Dose in rem equals dose in rad × quality factor (QF). The QF has a different value for different radiations. Rem has been replaced by the term *sievert* (Sv). (1 rem = 0.01 Sv)

Roentgen (R): Unit of exposure to ionizing radiation: refers to the ability of X-rays to ionize air.

Sievert (Sv): The unit of dose equivalent of ionizing radiation is equivalent to one joule per kilogram. The Sv has replaced the term *rem* and is used in radiation protection and radiation safety when quantifying occupational exposure. (1 Sv = 100 rem)

dose is higher than in a palliative situation. Curative doses of 45 to 70 grays (Gy) given over 6 to 8 weeks are usual. For example, when radiation is combined with minimal surgery (lumpectomy) in the woman with early-stage breast cancer, the intent is cure and doses range between 50 and 65 Gy (Harris, Hellman, Canellos, & Fisher, 1985; Levitt & Perez, 1987; Wang, 1988; Wilson, 1989).

Radiation therapy is also used to *control* local disease and is often combined with chemotherapy and surgery in achieving local and regional control. For example, control of locally advanced breast cancer and head and neck cancer is greatly enhanced by combining radiotherapy with adjuvant chemotherapy (Hellman, 1985). Radiation is unquestionably effective in control of microscopic nodal disease (Richter, Share, & Goodman, 1985).

Adjuvant therapy is given to enhance or assist the primary method of treatment. For example, radiation is used in an adjuvant manner when it is given preoperatively for early colorectal cancers (Hellman, 1985). In this instance, the purpose of the radiation is to sterilize microscopic disease beyond the surgical margins, to reduce tumor bulk, to reduce the likelihood of residual tumor cell implants, and to avoid the need for regional lymphadenectomy. A second example of the use of adjuvant radiotherapy is in treating sanctuary sites (central nervous system) in patients with acute lymphocytic leukemia, whose primary treatment is chemotherapy (Hellman, 1985). Radiation facilitates transfer of the chemotherapeutic agent across the blood-brain barrier, which is composed of the perivascular glial membrane and vascular endothelium.

Approximately one half of all patients treated with radiation therapy are treated for *palliation* of symptoms. Treatment to sites of bone metastases is very effective in relieving pain as well as in restoring mobility in some situations. Pain attributable to pressure or obstruction of a hollow viscus by bulky lesions can also be palliated with radiotherapy. Other situations requiring palliation include bleeding, necrosis, ulceration, superior vena caval (SVC) syndrome, central nervous system metastases, and functional obstruction (respiratory, gastrointestinal, genitourinary). When radiation treatment is needed in an emergency situation (SVC syndrome, spinal cord compression, bronchial obstruction, hemorrhage), it is generally given with palliative intent as well.

Principles of palliative treatment include use of a short, sometimes intensive course of treatment to achieve a rapid result. Treatment is generally completed in 1 or 2 weeks, and it may be discontinued if palliation has been achieved before the prescribed course is completed. This is especially important if quality of life is diminished or disturbed more by the daily travel to the treatment facility than by the symptoms being palliated. The nurse has an important role in observing the patient's response and communicating with the radiotherapist regarding the patient's total situation.

STEPS TO DELIVERY OF RADIATION THERAPY

Consultation

The patient's initial visit to the radiation therapy facility is for consultation, assessment, and discussion of the role of radiation in his or her treatment. A family member or significant other should be encouraged to accompany the patient to help provide information as well as to reinforce information given by the caregivers. During this visit, a complete history is taken, a physical examination is performed, and a plan of radiation is described. Diagnostic studies and pathology reports may be reviewed before the consultation, and they may also be presented for discussion at a multidisciplinary tumor conference.

Ideally, the radiation therapy nurse meets with the patient on the consultation visit. In addition to performing a nursing assessment, the nurse may begin the physical orientation to the radiation facility, initiate patient and family education about the proposed treatment and potential side effects, and provide both physical and emotional support as needed. By establishing contact on this first visit, the nurse becomes a resource for both the patient and the staff in providing continuity throughout treatment and follow-up.

Treatment Planning

Before radiation treatments can be started, a series of steps are taken to define the treatment target, ensure the accuracy of daily set-ups, and protect healthy tissues from radiation injury. The radiation technologist, physics staff members, and radiotherapist are involved in a process termed *simulation*.

In simulation the target volume is localized and defined by using x-rays, scans, and physical landmarks. The patient is positioned exactly as he or she will be positioned for the actual treatment, using coordinate points on the body to ensure alignment. This process takes place using a simulator machine, which mimics the physical characteristics of the teletherapy machine but does not deliver ionizing radiation. Figure 20–3 illustrates an example of a treatment simulator.

Immobilization devices such as casts (or other molded materials), head-holders, or restraints may be needed to ensure accurate positioning. Need for such devices is determined during simulation, and the appropriate devices are prepared.

Skin markings are needed to define the target or portal. During simulation, ink marks are placed to indicate the area of treatment as well as to mark the coordinate points as a guide to proper positioning. These markings may be left in place for a period of days until accuracy of positioning has been verified. At a later point, permanent tattoos are placed to identify the field and coordinate points, at which time the ink markings may be removed. Tattoos are very tiny, discrete, permanent dots that are barely visible to the casual observer.

Lead blocks are often needed to help shape the radiation beam and block radiation from reaching organs and tissues adjacent to the tumor site. A radiation beam is rectangular, and its size can be adjusted by adjusting the collimater on the machine. However, because treatment portals are not always rectangular in shape, lead blocks must be prepared for positioning between the beam source and the patient to block areas within the beam that are not to be treated.

Computerized treatment plans based on measurements and radiographs taken during simulation as well as on beam characteristics are now a routine part of treatment planning. These computer-generated plans help to determine the final treatment prescription, which includes description of the treatment field or fields, total dose, daily dose fraction, and elapsed time.

RADIATION TREATMENTS

When simulation and treatment planning are complete, the patient begins a course of therapy, which ranges from 2 to 8 weeks, with the average course lasting 5 weeks. Treatments are given on a daily basis, 5 days per week. Altered fractionation regimens (such as two treatments per day, fewer than five treatments per week, or single hemibody treatments of very large doses) may be employed in special situations. Two treatments per day (separated by at least 4 hours) may be used for a particularly radioresistant tumor. Severely debilitated patients or those with transportation problems may be treated three or four times per week. Widespread bony metastasis can be effectively treated with a single dose of 500 cGy to the upper, middle, or lower hemibody. The reader is referred to Dudjak (in press) for details of treatment with altered fractionation and nursing implications.

Treatment Process

Teletherapy treatments take only a few minutes of actual radiation exposure and require approximately 10 min in the treatment room altogether. Most of this time is spent in positioning the patient and the machine, then repositioning the beam to a second, third, or fourth angle to treat each prescribed field. For example, treatment of the uterus or prostate is generally done utilizing the four-field box technique, which employs anterior, posterior, and two lateral fields. Some treatments are more complex, requiring multiple angles or changing the patient's position (for example, supine to prone), and therefore take longer to complete. Others are very simple set-ups in which only a single field is utilized and the treatment is completed in a few minutes.

Periodic beam films (also called check films or portal films) are taken to ensure the accuracy of the set-up. A beam film is a radiograph taken through the treatment beam that is then compared to the original simulation films to evaluate positioning and technique.

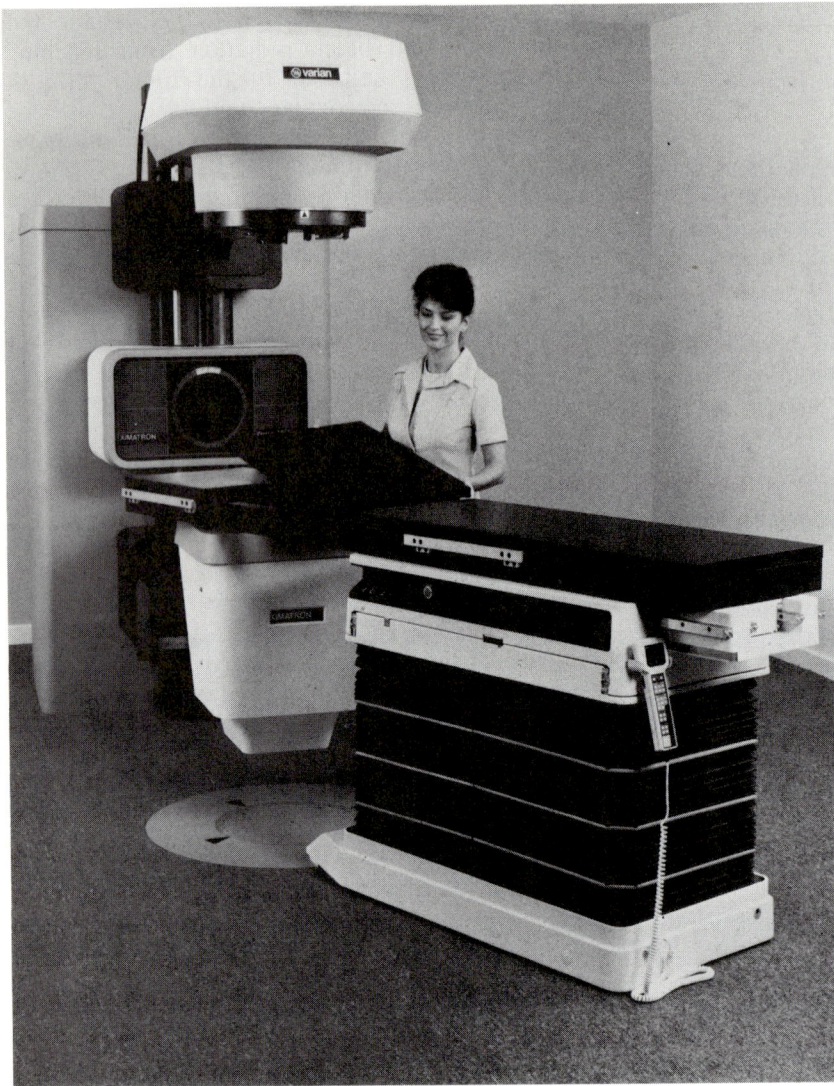

Figure 20–3. A Varian Ximatron™ C-Series radiation therapy simulator. (Varian Associates, Inc., Palo Alto, CA. Reproduced by permission.)

This process takes a few extra minutes on the treatment table, and patients mistakenly think that this film will show changes such as tumor shrinkage. Careful explanation of the process and its purpose is important.

Treatment machines are very large and may be somewhat noisy, but patients can be assured that there is no pain or sensation of any kind during the treatment. People expect to feel heat, tingling, or some other sensation, but this does not happen. Some discomfort may result from positioning or from lying on a very firm table, however. An example of a linear accelerator is shown in Figure 20–2.

Treatments are given by the registered radiation technologist, who has an important role both in patient care and in the technical delivery of the prescribed treatment. Technologists see the patient daily (the nurse and radiation therapist may not) and can therefore monitor any alterations in either physical or emotional status. Patients are then referred to the nurse or physician for management of problems. In the absence of radiation therapy nursing staff, the technologist is typically responsible for nursing procedures.

During a course of treatment, the patient is usually seen and examined by the radiotherapist or the nurse (or both) at least once per week. This status check (on-therapy review) serves to monitor the progress of treatment, to assess reactions, and to offer supportive physical and emotional interventions. It is vital that patients and their families understand the importance of completing the prescribed course of therapy. Nurses are frequently in a pivotal position in which they can effectively support the patients throughout a lengthy treatment course, thus helping to ensure compliance and completion.

Patients can expect to be weighed each week during therapy and to have a complete blood count (CBC) and platelet count obtained weekly as well.

In some treatment centers, radiation therapy patients are also seen and assessed by other members of the cancer care team on a regular basis. Social workers, dietitians, physical therapists, dentists, and psychologists are valuable resource persons. In addition to working with individual patients, these professionals also are participants in conferences that are held to review patient progress.

The Posttreatment Period

When a course of treatment has been completed, the radiation therapy patient is again examined by the radiation oncologist and the nurse. The appropriate physical examination is followed by review of posttreatment instructions and discussion of changes that can be expected in the coming weeks. The radiation oncology nurse has primary responsibility for patient education and side-effects management, often maintaining close telephone contact with the patient after a course of treatment. Referrals to the appropriate community agencies are made, and in addition the nurse serves as a consultant on radiation patient care to nurses in these agencies as well as to those in the hospital.

Most radiation oncologists follow the treated patient with periodic checkups for varying periods of time. Particularly if radiation is the primary treatment (early breast, head and neck, and skin cancers), the radiation oncologist may remain as the patient's primary cancer physician.

Posttreatment evaluation varies in scope from a physical examination to multiple radiographic studies. Patients are eager for concrete evidence that their cancer is either gone or greatly reduced in size. Obviously, this cannot always be assessed, because treatment may have been either prophylactic or adjuvant, in which case there was no measurable tumor in the first place. When a definable tumor mass has been treated, an obvious change, shrinkage, and improvement in symptoms may occur even during the course of therapy. Conversely, it may take weeks or months after treatment for tumor shrinkage to be measurable. These are frustrating times for the patient, during which nursing support and patient education continue to be important.

SIDE EFFECTS AND THEIR MANAGEMENT

Radiation therapy is local treatment delivered to those structures located within the target volume. Most treatment fields encompass a limited volume or area of the body, with the exception of total body irradiation (TBI), used before bone marrow transplantation or hemibody treatment for extensive bone metastases. Most side effects of radiation therapy are confined to those tissues and organs within the path of the radiation beam. Onset, severity, and duration of reactions can be correlated with the cell renewal characteristics of the target tissue, total dose, fractionation, concomitant therapies, nutritional status, and volume of tissue irradiated.

Side effects, which occur during a course of treatment and up to 6 months afterward, are considered acute reactions. Those that occur or persist after 6 months are categorized as late or chronic effects. Acute radiation reactions develop as a result of radiation effect on cell renewal tissues of the skin and mucous membranes. The mucosa of the oropharynx, small intestine, rectum, bladder, and vagina is often affected and produces some of the more severe reactions seen. Size and number of doses (fractionation) and the length of course (protraction) are the factors that influence the severity of acute side effects (Hellman, 1985). Acute effects usually resolve fairly quickly when treatment is completed as the rate of new cell proliferation returns to normal and cell destruction ends.

Late or chronic effects of ionizing radiation—which persist or occur 6 months or more after treatment—are frequently unrelated to the occurrence or severity of acute reactions. Late effects appear to be closely related to *total* dose of radiation and *size* of dose fraction. In contrast to acute reactions, the damage seen in late effects is thought to be related to injury to stromal vasculature or to endothelial cells rather than solely to the cell renewal system. In addition to specific organ damage (blindness, transection of the spinal cord), such late effects as necrosis, ulceration, and fibrosis may be seen. Table 20–4 lists major site-specific early and late effects of radiation therapy.

Management of radiation-induced side effects is a primary function of the nurse. The concept of *local treatment–local effect* is very important in planning and providing nursing care. Most side effects can be predicted, and patients can, therefore, be prepared with appropriate self-care behaviors. Knowledge of what to expect and when to expect it usually helps to reduce anxiety, particularly in the patient who has preconceived ideas about radiation therapy. Most patients benefit as much from learning what *will not* happen as what to anticipate.

Common Acute Side Effects of Radiation Therapy: Symptom Management

Skin Reactions

Regardless of body site, radiation must penetrate skin to reach its target within the body. Skin reaction varies from very mild erythema to moist desquamation, and some patients exhibit no skin changes at all. Various systems have been used to categorize skin reactions (Hilderley, 1983), and each treatment facility devises a method of skin care that seems most effective in minimizing both discomfort and any permanent skin changes.

Some of the basic principles of care include the following:

1. Avoid friction, pressure, and thermal extremes.
2. Cleanse treated site gently, using mild soap.
3. Avoid using any skin care products other than those recommended by the radiation oncologist or nurse.

An example of skin care instructions for the patient is shown in Table 20–5. When reactions become very intense, with moist desquamation (owing to high dose, surface treatment, enhancement by concomitant medications), special procedures may be needed. These measures might include daily flushing and cleansing followed by application of topical agents or dressings,

Table 20–4. MAJOR ACUTE AND CHRONIC SIDE EFFECTS OF RADIATION THERAPY

Site	Acute Effect	Chronic Effect
Skin	Erythema (3000–4000 cGy); dry desquamation, moist desquamation (4500–6000 cGy)	Fibrosis, atrophy, telangiectasia, permanent darkening of skin
Oral cavity	Change and loss of taste, dryness, mucositis (3000–4000 cGy)	Permanent xerostomia, permanent taste alterations, dental caries
Esophagus	Pain, esophagitis	Fibrosis
Stomach	Nausea and vomiting (125 cGy)	Obstruction, ulceration, fibrosis
Intestines	Diarrhea (2000 + 3000 cGy)	Malabsorption strictures, necrosis (6000–7000 cGy)
Kidney		Radiation nephritis
Bladder	Cystitis (3000 cGy)	Fibrosis, contracted bladder (6500–7000 cGy)
Bone marrow	↓ White blood cells and platelets	May be chronic anemia especially with combined modality treatment
Respiratory system	Pneumonitis (2500–3000 cGy)	Fibrosis
Cardiovascular system	Rare reports of pericarditis, myocarditis	Fibrosis
Central nervous system	Edema and inflammation	Infarction, occlusion, necrosis
Brain and spinal cord		
Peripheral nerves		
Eyes		Cataracts
Bone and cartilage (child)		Growth disturbances if growth plate of bone is in field (2000–3000 cGy)
Gonads		
Spermatogonia	↓ Sperm count after 90–120 days; temporary sterility (100–300 cGy)	
Ovary	Sterility (500–1000 cGy) depends on age	

(From Strohl, R. [1988]. The nursing role in radiation oncology: Symptom management of acute and chronic reactions. *Oncology Nursing Forum, 15*[4], 431. Reprinted by permission.)

or both. Occlusive dressings should not be used because they tend to inhibit healing. Moisture- and vapor-permeable dressings help to promote healing. A study in which moisture- and vapor-permeable dressings were

Table 20–5. SKIN CARE DURING RADIATION

Skin over the area where you are receiving radiation therapy needs to be treated with gentle care. During your course of radiation treatment, please follow these guidelines:

KEEP THE TREATED AREA DRY AND FREE FROM IRRITATION

• Do not wash the treated area until the technologist tells you to. This may not be until 2 or 3 days after the start of treatments.

• Do not remove the lines or ink marks that have been placed on your skin until the technologist or doctor tells you to.

• When permitted, wash the treated skin gently, using a mild soap, and rinse well before patting dry. Always use warm or cool water, *not* hot water.

• Do not apply any lotions, creams, alcohol, aftershave, perfume, deodorants, or other preparations in the treated area.

• Heating pads and hot-water bottles should not be used on treated skin.

• Avoid friction, that is, avoid clothing that is tight or may rub over the treated skin such as tight shirt collars, ties, undergarments, belts, and so forth.

• Men should use an electric razor if they are receiving treatment to the face or neck area. Do not use aftershave.

• If treated skin becomes reddened or tender, you may apply a thin layer of vitamin A and D ointment. Be sure to tell us when this happens. If further irritation develops, we will give you special instructions or medications for skin care.

• Protect the treatment area from exposure to direct sunlight. While you are receiving a course of therapy, do not sunbathe or spend more than a few minutes in the bright sun if the treated area is exposed. We will give you special instructions about future sun exposure when you finish your course of treatment.

(Reproduced by permission from Philip G. Maddock and Laura Hilderley, Radiation Oncology, Warwick, Rhode Island.)

compared with standard dressings for radiation skin reactions is described in Box 20–3. Care must be taken to avoid placing tape on irradiated skin, because each time it is removed, the skin beneath is further traumatized.

Some of the topical agents currently used for brisk erythema and moist desquamation include vitamin A and D ointment, suspensions or ointments containing petrolatum, aloe, or lanolin, and silver sulfadiazine.

Most radiation skin reactions heal very well when appropriate care is taken. A severe reaction that includes moist desquamation may result in increased pigmentation of that skin.

Alopecia

When the head is irradiated, alopecia (either partial or complete) will occur. Doses between 30 and 35 Gy cause temporary hair loss, with regrowth starting approximately 1 month after treatment. Rate of regrowth varies, but most patients will have a reasonable regrowth in 6 to 9 months. At higher doses (40 Gy and above) to the scalp, alopecia is usually permanent.

Radiation-induced alopecia is not preventable. However, care of the hair and scalp is important in minimizing skin reaction. Use of a mild shampoo, followed by thorough rinsing and gentle towel drying, is recommended. Patients should avoid hair dryers, curling devices, chemicals (for coloring or curling), and even vigorous brushing of the hair. Any of these will hasten the inevitable hair loss but, more important, will likely enhance skin reaction on the scalp. Areas particularly susceptible to erythema and desquamation include the forehead and periauricular tissues. Care of the scalp follows general guidelines for skin care. In addition, patients will want to purchase a wig or use hats, turbans, or scarves. Protection of the scalp from sum-

Box 20–3. TESTING MOISTURE VAPOR PERMEABLE DRESSINGS

Shell, J., Stanutz, F., & Grimm, J. (1986). **Comparison of moisture vapor permeable (MVP) dressings to conventional dressings for management of radiation skin reactions.** *Oncology Nursing Forum, 13*(1), 11–16.

A prospective randomized pilot study was conducted to compare conventional hydrous lanolin gauze dressings to a moist technique using MVP dressings for patients with moderate to severe radiation skin reactions. Twenty-one eligible patients were entered into the study; however, wound complications in five of these patients necessitated excluding them from the study. Of the 16 remaining patients, eight had been entered into each arm of the study.

Results of the study:
1. Ranges of healing times were comparable (5 to 54 days for MVP group, 6 to 52 days for conventional dressing group).
2. Average healing time (19 days for MVP group, 24 days for conventional dressing group). Difference between the two groups was not considered statistically significant.
3. All patients experienced brief but severe discomfort corresponding with the period of greatest desquamation.
4. Discomfort lessened when dressings were reapplied; period of relief was brief in hydrous lanolin group.

Additional beneficial effects found in use of MVP dressings include the following:
1. MVP dressing does not act as a bolus (bolus material increases skin dose).
2. MVP dressing does not require frequent (daily) removal.
3. MVP dressing requires no protective covering.

Disadvantages of MVP dressings include some difficulty in keeping them in place on contoured areas or areas with skin folds, and occlusive properties can lead to maceration of the skin.

The investigators conclude that MVP dressings are potentially suitable for use as standard dressing material when caring for moderate to severe radiation skin reactions. A larger comparative study is recommended.

---

mer sun, as well as protection from heat loss via the bare scalp in winter, should be part of patient education content.

Mucositis

Mucosa of the respiratory, digestive, and genitourinary tracts is sensitive to radiation. Mucous membrane undergoes continuous proliferation and when cell renewal cannot keep up with cell loss as a result of radiation exposure, mucositis occurs.

Intraoral and pharyngeal reactions include xerostomia, taste alterations, mucosal erythema, and mucositis. Severity is dose related, with onset of symptoms occurring at doses of 20 to 25 Gy. Oral care includes use of a soft toothbrush and frequent rinsing with water, saline solution, or nonalcohol-containing oral care preparations. Elixir of benadryl and water in a 1-ounce to 1-quart solution makes a mild, soothing rinse. Inspection of the oral cavity and assessment for candidiasis should be done regularly. Nystatin (Mycostatin) (tablets or suspensions) or ketoconazole tablets can be prescribed for candidiasis.

Dental consultation before treatment is essential for patients who will be having treatments to the oral cavity. Salivary changes can lead to late radiation caries, particularly after high doses to the mouth or oral cavity. Dental prophylaxis, fluoride treatments, and coverage with antibiotics before any dental extractions or other oral surgery procedures are recommended after treatment.

Esophagitis

Esophagitis can occur when the chest is irradiated. Onset of symptoms is usually marked by a sensation of "a lump in the throat" or an object stuck in the esophagus. This can be due to edema or to spasm of the esophageal musculature, triggered by the presence of food attempting to pass the irritated mucosa. Within a few days, true esophagitis with dysphagia develops, and the patient experiences pain, particularly when attempting to eat.

Antacids and mild anesthetic agents may be helpful in relieving symptoms; however, until treatment is completed and healing takes place, the discomfort remains.

Dietary adjustments are necessary when intraoral or esophageal mucositis occurs. Protein and calorie requirements may be met with the use of liquid food supplements and soft foods. In addition, the diet should be bland to avoid further local irritation (Iwamoto, in press).

Nausea and Vomiting

Treatment to the abdomen, particularly to large fields, can cause nausea and vomiting. Patients receiving spinal irradiation (especially to the thoracic and lumbar vertebrae) may also have nausea, and occasionally patients will experience nausea after lower abdominal or pelvic field radiation. Nausea and vomiting are not, however, an inevitable side effect of radiation therapy. Even when treatment is expected to produce these distressing symptoms, reaction can be minimized or prevented with the use of antiemetics. The prescribed medication should be taken before treatment and repeated as necessary. In addition, a light diet should be consumed before treatment and for several hours afterward.

Patients experiencing nausea and vomiting related to radiation therapy treatments need support and encouragement (as well as antiemetics), emphasizing that these distressing symptoms often will decrease as treatments proceed. The new patient may have an element of anxiety, which enhances the potential for radiation-induced nausea. It is not unusual for nausea to either disappear or decrease in severity as the treatment course progresses. The body somehow adjusts to the treatment, the patient relaxes, and nausea is no longer significant.

Diarrhea

Patients at risk for radiation-induced diarrhea include those receiving treatment to the abdomen or pelvis. Changes in the epithelial layer of the small bowel are related to the highly proliferative nature of the cells of the columnar epithelium. Normal cell loss coupled with radiation-induced cell injury results in flattening or loss of the villi. This in turn decreases the absorptive surface area of the intestine, leading to diarrhea. Cramping, increased flatus, and a feeling of distention sometimes accompany diarrhea.

The diarrhea is usually dose related and occurs after doses of 18 to 30 Gy. Patients with previous abdominal surgery, colitis, ileitis, or other bowel disorders are more likely to develop radiation-related diarrhea, and symptoms develop at a lower dose. Diarrhea is usually controlled with dietary modification (low-residue diet) and various antidiarrheal medications. When treatments are completed, several weeks to months may elapse before the intestinal lining recovers and returns to normal function. During this recovery period, it is especially important that the patient maintain a low-residue diet, adding other foods back into the diet on a very gradual basis. For some patients, certain foods (such as corn, legumes, or milk products) may no longer be tolerated by the irradiated bowel.

Nursing management of diarrhea requires frequent patient assessment and reinforcement of dietary and medication instructions. As with any dietary adjustments, it is important to include the person responsible for meal preparation in the teaching plan.

Fatigue

Fatigue is a common occurrence in the person receiving radiation therapy (Aistars, 1987; Piper, Lindsey, & Dodd, 1987). Although it is true that many patients are able to perform their normal daily activities in addition to coming for treatment each day, most will report feeling fatigued as the treatment course progresses.

Theories presented to explain the occurrence of fatigue include (1) increased metabolic rate, (2) the presence of toxic breakdown products as a result of cell injury or death, (3) energy expenditure required for tissue repair, and (4) the tiring effects of travel to and from the radiation facility on a daily basis.

Patients should be told they may experience fatigue as treatment progresses; if not forewarned, they may become concerned that their fatigue is an indication of tumor progression. They may also fail to respond to the need for increased rest, thinking that to do so means giving in to the disease itself. Many patients are able to carry out all normal daily activities (including work) throughout a course of treatment; others are unable to perform their usual daily tasks.

Although it is anticipated that volume of tissue irradiated will influence degree of fatigue, other variables can cause fatigue as well, such as recent surgery, low hemoglobin level, travel time or distance, length of treatment course, and total dose of radiation. Haylock and Hart (1979) reported on a study of 30 patients who were surveyed on a daily basis throughout their course of treatment. In addition to noting a significant increase in fatigue level over the course of treatment, a strong correlation was seen between certain physical symptoms and fatigue level, supporting the belief that the cause of radiation fatigue is physiologic rather than psychological.

Nursing interventions for the patient experiencing radiation-related fatigue include monitoring blood counts, nutritional assessment and support, education regarding the need for increased rest and sleep, and emotional support and encouragement throughout this difficult period. Assurance that fatigue is a common and temporary side effect may be the most helpful nursing intervention of all.

Discussion of this point has dealt primarily with the principles of radiobiology, physics, treatment planning, and treatment with *teletherapy*. Nursing care as presented thus far also is specific to the patient receiving teletherapy.

A second method of treatment utilizes radioactive sources in the technique known as *brachytherapy*. This method of treatment is based on somewhat different principles of radiation biology and has very different implications for nursing because of the need for radiation safety and protection.

BRACHYTHERAPY

Brachytherapy is the form of internal radiation therapy in which a radioactive isotope is used for surface, interstitial, or intracavitary application. Brachytherapy techniques provide for a high dose of radiation to be delivered to the treated tumor volume and a rapid fall-off in radiation dose in adjacent normal tissues.

Brachytherapy techniques may be used as the sole method for delivering radiation therapy dose. In most instances, however, this therapy is combined with external beam radiation (teletherapy) to improve local control of disease, preserve vital function, and spare normal surrounding tissues from damage. Historically, brachytherapy techniques were first developed for gynecologic cancer in the early 1900s (Grigg, 1965). The Fletcher-Suit applicator was developed during the fifth decade for intracavitary implantation of radium-226. Since then, multiple radioactive sources have been used for intracavitary, interstitial, and surface application. Today, implantation techniques are used for cancers of the breast, head and neck, lung, liver, colon, bladder, prostate, and brain. Table 20–6 lists the various ways in which radioactive implants are used for various cancers.

Table 20–6. APPLICATIONS OF BRACHYTHERAPY

Type of Application	Disease	Radioisotopes Used
Sealed Sources		
Intracavitary	Cervical cancer	Radium-226, cesium-137
	Uterine cancer	Radium-226, cesium-137
Interstitial	Breast cancer	Iridium-192
	Prostate cancer	Iodine-125, gold-198
	Head and neck cancer	Iridium-192, cesium-137
Surface	Choroid cancer	Iodine-125
	Pterygium	Strontium-90
Unsealed Sources		
Oral	Hyperthyroidism	Iodine-131
Intravenous	Polycythemia vera	Phosphorus-32
Intrapleural	Mesothelioma	Phosphorus-32
	Malignant pleural effusion	Gold-198
Intraperitoneal	Ovarian cancer	Phosphorus-32

Radiobiology of Brachytherapy

The radiobiologic principles of repair, repopulation, redistribution, and reoxygenation have different implications when radiation is given *continuously* in brachytherapy as opposed to being *fractionated* in external beam radiation.

Repair

Brachytherapy provides for a continuous low-dose rate of radiation. Sublethal damage accumulation decreases at a low-dose rate. Thus repair of cells in the radiated volume is less likely after continuous low-dose radiation.

Redistribution and Repopulation

After one fractionated dose of radiation, irradiated cells redistribute and are blocked in late G_2 phase. With continuous low-dose rate radiation, a greater percentage of cells are blocked in G_2 and are damaged by the radiation. Cellular proliferation can occur during low-dose rate radiation. However, when these new cells cycle and progress to the G_2 phase, they will be blocked and damaged by the radiation.

Redistribution of a significant proportion of the cell population into G_2 can result in a net sensitization effect. The repopulation of the tumor during continuous low-dose rate radiation results in cells that progress to late G_2, are blocked in their progression through the cell cycle, and are likely to be destroyed by the radiation. Thus repair, repopulation, and redistribution augment the radiation effect in low-dose rate brachytherapy.

Reoxygenation

With a dose of radiation delivered continuously at a low rate, there is a decreased requirement for oxygen to eradicate the tumor. Thus brachytherapy techniques may be more effective in treating anoxic tumors than techniques using conventional, fractionated external beam radiation (Glicksman, 1987; Hall, 1978).

Properties of Radioactive Isotopes

As discussed earlier in this chapter, an atom is unstable when the balance between protons and neutrons is unequal (see Fig. 20–1). Nuclides with the same number of protons but different number of neutrons are called isotopes. Some isotopes are radioactive and occur naturally, such as radium-226; others are produced artificially in atomic reactors by bombarding stable elements with neutrons. Examples of artificially produced isotopes are cobalt-60 and phosphorus-32.

Modes of Radioactive Emission and Decay

The process in which an unstable isotope transforms to a stable one is known as radioactive decay or disintegration. Decay products are alpha and beta particles and gamma rays. The rate of decay is constant, as the number of atoms that disintegrate per unit of time is proportional to the number of radioactive atoms.

Alpha Particle Decay

An unstable nucleus may eject an alpha particle that consists of two protons and two neutrons. Alpha particles are very heavy and have a charge of +2. They have high LET, and when they travel through matter, they lose energy at a very fast rate by colliding with electrons in their path. Because of their high LET, alpha particles cannot penetrate more than 0.04 mm into tissue. One of the first radioactive sources used was radium-226. One of the byproducts of radium decay was radon gas, an alpha emitter. When radon gas is inhaled, it causes damage to the lung. Thus radioactive isotopes that emit only alpha particles are not used in brachytherapy.

Beta Particle Decay

Beta particles are moderate- to high-speed electrons with a charge of −1 that are emitted by atoms when they release energy. Kinetic energies of beta particles range from a few thousand to several million volts. Beta particles, like alpha particles, have high kinetic energy and high LET, so that their range of penetration in tissue is limited to the outer layers of skin. Phosphorus-32 and strontium-90 are two examples of pure beta emitters used in brachytherapy.

Gamma Radiation

Radioactive sources may also decay by emitting excess energy in the form of gamma rays. Gamma rays are electromagnetic radiation emitted as packets of energy called photons. Gamma rays and beta particles are often ejected together from nuclei of atoms. Gamma rays travel at the speed of light. Because of their penetrating power, gamma emitters (cesium-137, gold-198, iodine-131, radium-226) constitute the greatest number of radioisotopes used in brachytherapy.

Mechanism of Radiation Injury

Alpha and beta particles and gamma rays produce damage by transferring energy to living matter. They ionize molecules in cells to cause physical and chemical changes that affect the biologic processes responsible for reproduction. Irradiated cells are either destroyed or rendered incapable of reproduction.

The extent of radiation injury depends primarily on the type of energy transfer. Energy transfer may be either directly or indirectly ionizing. Alpha and beta particles are directly ionizing radiations. Because they are electrically charged, they produce ionization at small intervals along their paths through collision.

Gamma rays are indirectly ionizing. Unlike charged particles, they have no electrical charge. Energy loss does not occur until gamma rays interact with an atom, an electron, or a nucleus in their path. Gamma rays then transfer energy to directly ionizing particles such as electrons. Electrons are ionized, liberated from the atom, and proceed to ionize other particles in their path. The net result is that indirectly ionizing gamma rays transfer energy to directly ionizing particles deep in tissue, more penetrating than what directly ionizing particles can reach from outside the atom. As noted earlier, because gamma emitters possess the greatest capacity to produce damage deep in tissue, they are the most useful in brachytherapy. However, they also present the greatest hazard to care providers. Table 20–7 lists commonly used radioisotopes in brachytherapy and their physical properties.

Other Radioactive Properties

Sealed or Unsealed Sources. Radioactive sources may be either sealed or unsealed. A sealed radioactive source is one in which the radioactive isotope is contained within an outer sheath of material such as platinum. An unsealed source is contained in a colloidal suspension and placed in direct contact with tissues.

Half-life. The half-life of a radioactive isotope refers to the time it takes for it to decay to 50 per cent of its

activity. Half-lives vary among the elements, and range from several days (gold-198) to more than 1600 years (radium-226). A particular radioisotope is selected for either temporary or permanent use on the basis of its half-life. For example, gold-198 has a half-life of less than 3 days and can be inserted permanently. Cesium-137 has a half-life of 30 years and is thus used as a temporary implant (see Table 20–7).

General Nursing Care Guidelines

Nursing care may differ slightly depending on the type of radioactive isotope used, whether it is a sealed or unsealed source, and whether it is a temporary or permanent implant. Knowledge of the specific properties of radioisotopes and the way they are used helps nurses to provide safe care (Hassey, 1985).

Sealed, temporary sources include radium-226, cesium-137, and iridium-192. Because they are sealed sources, they do not present a potential contamination problem. Owing to their long half-lives, these sources are inserted into body tissue or cavities for a specified time period and are then removed. Afterloading techniques have been developed in which the empty applicator is inserted during the operative procedure, but the radioactive source is not loaded until the patient returns to the hospital room. The standard use of afterloading techniques and equipment has helped to reduce exposure. Nursing care should be preplanned so that as much direct care as possible is provided during this period before loading the source. Once the implant is loaded, time spent in the room should be minimized and distance maximized.

Patients with radioactive implants must have a private room with private bath. Some institutions have specially designed radiation precaution rooms with built-in lead shields lining the walls of the room. Others have an automatic remote control device in the patient's room so that sources of high activity can be inserted by remote control for short periods of time (Leung, 1984). In institutions that are not equipped with these rooms, the radiation safety officer may designate rooms that are suitable for patients with radioactive implants. These are usually located at the ends of halls or corridors where there may be less chance of exposure to occupants of adjacent rooms (National Council on Radiation Protection and Measurements [NCRP], 1974).

Dose limits for the public are 500 millirems (5 mSv) per year (see Table 20–3) (NCRP, 1987). Therefore, each visitor should be limited to approximately one-half hour per day. A distance of at least 6 feet is to be maintained between the visitors and the source of radiation. Pregnant women and children under the age of 18 are prohibited from visiting.

A pair of long-handled forceps and a lead container should be present in the patient's room. In the extremely unusual—but still potential—event that a source becomes dislodged from the patient, forceps must be used to retrieve the source, which should then be placed in the lead container. The radioactive source

Table 20–7. RADIOISOTOPES AND THEIR PROPERTIES

Radioisotope	Symbol	Half-Life	Type of Emission
Cesium-137	^{137}Cs	30 yr	Beta, gamma
Gold-198	^{198}Au	2.7 days	Beta, gamma
Iodine-125	^{125}I	60 days	Beta, gamma
Iodine-131	^{131}I	8 days	Beta, gamma
Iridium-192	^{192}Ir	74.4 days	Beta, gamma
Phosphorus-32	^{32}P	14.3 days	Beta
Radium-226	^{226}Ra	1620 yr	Alpha, gamma
Strontium-90	^{90}Sr	28.1 yr	Beta

(From National Council on Radiation Protection and Measurements. [1972]. NCRP Report #40. *Protection against radiation from brachytherapy sources.* Washington, DC: Author. Reproduced by permission.)

should never be touched with bare hands. The radiation therapist and radiation safety officer should be notified immediately in the event of a dislodged source or applicator (Bucholtz, 1987; Hassey, 1985).

The removal of sealed sources does not present a contamination hazard. However, all linens and dressings should be kept in the patient's room during the course of the implant to ensure safe disposal of the radioisotope used (in case of dislodgment, for example). Linen and dressings can be disposed of in the usual manner once the source is removed and accounted for.

Sealed, permanent implants such as gold-198 and iodine-125 seeds have a short half-life so they may be inserted permanently into tissues, such as the prostate. Because these sources decay rapidly, patients may be discharged home within a few days after implantation. However, radiation dose levels must be less than 30 millicuries (111×10^7 Bq) of activity before patients may be discharged from the hospital (NCRP, 1974).

An unsealed source is in a colloidal suspension and placed in direct contact with tissues. Unsealed sources may be administered orally (iodine-131 for hyperthyroidism); intravenously (phosphorus-32 for polycythemia vera); intrapleurally (phosphorus-32 for lung cancer); or intraperitoneally (phosphorus-32 for ovarian cancer).

Use of unsealed sources, such as iodine-131 in the treatment of hyperthyroidism, requires special precautions because it presents a potential contamination hazard. As iodine-131 is systemically administered, the isotope is excreted in feces, urine, vomitus, saliva, sweat, and other body fluids. One half of the radioactive iodine is excreted in the first 2 days. During this time, rubber gloves should be worn while providing direct care. Patients must flush the toilet several times after each bowel movement or urination (Wood, 1985).

Because linen and patient gowns may be contaminated, they must be kept in separate isolation bags. Other articles in the room, such as telephone, call light, and floors, must be covered with plastic. Disposable plastic or paper products should be used for dietary trays and utensils (NCRP, 1974).

Standards for Radiation Safety

Federal regulations mandate that maximum permissible dose for whole body occupational exposure is 5000 millirem (50 mSv) per year, or 3000 millirem (30 mSv) in a 3-month period (NCRP, 1973). Standards are based on risk-versus-benefit criteria and take into account factors such as age, occupational versus non-occupational exposure limits, and critical organ exposure. The recommendations on limits of exposure to radiation therapy are listed in Table 20–8.

Because many nurses who care for patients with implants are of childbearing age, the recommendation that allows dose accumulation of up to 3000 millirem (30 mSv) in a 3-month period does not apply to them. Maximum permissible dose for women of reproductive capacity is 1250 millirem (12.5 mSv) per quarter, equal

Table 20–8. RECOMMENDATIONS ON LIMITS FOR EXPOSURE TO IONIZING RADIATION

	Dose
Occupational exposure (annual)	
Effective dose equivalent limit	5.0 rem/yr
Dose equivalent limits for tissues and organs:	
Lenses of eyes	15.0 rem/yr
All others (red bone marrow, breasts, lungs, gonads, skin, and extremities)	50.0 rem/yr
Guidance: Cumulative exposure	1 rem × age in yr
Public exposure (annual)	
Effective dose equivalent limit	0.1 rem/yr
Effective dose equivalent limit, infrequent exposure	0.5 rem/yr
Education and training exposures	
Effective dose equivalent limit	0.1 rem/yr
Dose equivalent limit for lens of eye, skin, and extremities	5.0 rem/yr
Embryo-fetus exposures	
Total dose equivalent limit	0.5 rem/yr
Dose equivalent limit in a month	0.05 rem/yr
Negligible individual risk level (annual)	
Effective dose equivalent per source or practice	0.001 rem/yr

(From National Council on Radiation Protection and Measurements. [1987]. NCRP Report #91. *Recommendations on limits for exposure to ionizing radiation.* Bethesda, MD: Author. Reproduced by permission.)

to 5000 millirem (50 mSv) a year delivered at an even rate. Under these conditions, the dose to an embryo during the critical first 2 months of organogenesis would normally be less than 1 rem (0.01 Sv) (NCRP, 1977). However, it is recommended that a nurse who is pregnant should not care for patients with implants.

Regardless of maximum limits, occupational exposure should be "as low as reasonably achievable" or ALARA. In practice, nurses working with patients treated with brachytherapy receive less than 100 millirem (1 mSv) or 2 per cent of the maximum permissible dose limit per year. Dose levels in this range can be achieved through close monitoring by the radiation safety officer, supervision by the radiation therapist, and careful adherence and observation by nursing staff.

Principles of Time, Distance, and Shielding

The way in which nurses can keep radiation exposure limits as low as reasonably achievable is to follow three key principles of time, distance, and shielding.

Time

The longer the time of exposure, the greater the amount of absorbed radiation. Minimum exposure time must be stressed because no one can feel the presence of radiation or any physical discomfort to remind them to limit their exposure (i.e., working) times. Generally, nurses are limited to one-half hour per shift of direct time with the patient (Hassey, 1987).

Distance

Radiation exposure and distance are inversely related. That is, the intensity of radiation decreases as the square of the distance from the source increases. The following rule can be used to calculate exposure: amount of radiation exposure at 1 m from the radioactive source × distance squared = the amount of radiation exposure at any distance from the source × distance squared.

Shielding

The type of shielding device used in brachytherapy depends on the type of particle or gamma ray. The maximum thickness that particles can penetrate is called the range. Owing to their short range in tissue, alpha particles cannot penetrate the outermost layers of skin. A thin sheet of paper is sufficient to stop alpha particles. Alpha particles, therefore, are not an external hazard.

Most beta particles are not external hazards because they cannot penetrate the outermost layer of skin. For example, the range in tissue of phosphorus-32 is 0.8 cm.

Gamma rays are indirectly ionizing and a percentage of gamma rays can pass through any shield. The percentage of radiation that can penetrate decreases as the thickness of the shield increases. The effectiveness of shielding for gamma rays is expressed in terms of half-value layers. A half-value layer is the thickness required for a shield to reduce the intensity of gamma rays by a factor of 2 (Noz & Maguire, 1979; Shapiro, 1981).

Personnel Monitoring Devices

Personnel monitoring devices, which are required by law, offer a measure of radiation safety and protection. Devices do not protect the individual from radiation but only provide a record of exposure. Monitoring is done in several ways and depends on the type and level of radiation exposure and the cost and reliability of the monitoring device. Records of exposure are kept by the radiation safety officer.

Nurses must always wear a monitoring device when caring for patients with implants. Several types of monitoring devices or detectors are used for personnel and environmental monitoring. These include the nuclear emulsion monitor or film badge, the thermoluminescent dosimeter detector (TLD) or ring badge, and the pocket ion-chamber dosimeter. Monitoring devices are intended to provide an accurate record of *occupational* exposure and should not be worn outside the hospital (Khan, 1984; Noz & Maguire, 1979; Shapiro, 1981).

The film badge is the most widely used personnel monitor because it is accurate, reliable, and inexpensive to use. A film badge should not be shared. The film consists of a photographic emulsion mounted in a plastic holder. It provides a measure of whole body exposure. The film darkens in proportion to exposure to radiation. A film badge must be changed every month owing to fading of the film.

The TLDs are used for personnel monitoring in the same way as film badges. Owing to their small size, TLDs are especially useful for monitoring doses of radiation to the hand, hence the term *ring badge*. They contain a thermoluminescent powder such as lithium fluoride. Electrons in the lithium are raised to an excited state when exposed to the radioactive source. The excited energy appears in the form of visible light, and the amount of light is proportional to the energy absorbed by the radiation. The major disadvantage of TLDs is that a permanent record of exposure cannot be kept.

Pocket ion-chamber dosimeters are shaped like pens and are attached to clothing. These ionization chambers must be charged before use. Exposure of the chamber to radiation results in loss of the charge proportional to the amount of radiation exposure. These self-reading monitors provide immediate information on the person's amount of exposure. The nurse records the reading on the pocket ion-chamber before entering the patient's room, wears the device while in the room, and then records a reading when leaving the patient's room. As with TLDs, once readings are taken and values recorded, it is not possible to double-check the information on exposure.

The Geiger-Mueller counter (G-M counter) is used for surveying a patient's room. Survey meters are not used for personnel monitoring because they do not measure exposure or dose rate. The device responds to the presence of ionizing particles by producing electrical pulses that are triggered by the transfer of energy of the radioisotope to electrons in the G-M counter. The G-M counter is the most popular of survey meters owing to its ease of operation, sensitivity, and reliability.

Summary of Brachytherapy

Safety and protection are essential in providing care for patients with radioactive implants. Radiation safety and protection require basic knowledge of the physical properties of the radioisotopes and application of the principles of time, distance, and shielding. Close collaboration among the radiation safety officer, the radiation therapist, and the nursing staff must be established and maintained.

FUTURE TRENDS IN RADIATION ONCOLOGY

Intraoperative Radiation

In an attempt to deliver a high dose of radiation directly to the tumor bed without damaging normal structures in the beam pathway, the method of treatment called *intraoperative radiation therapy* (IORT) has been explored. The technique is in use in several centers in the United States and in other countries as well (Kinsella & Sindelar, 1985; Smith, in press).

Intraoperative radiation therapy is accomplished by surgically exposing the tumor-bearing organ, excising the diseased portion, and then delivering a single high dose of radiation directly to the tumor bed. Radiation is delivered via a conventional teletherapy machine through a specially constructed adapter, which is placed in very close proximity to the opened surgical site. All of this takes place with the fully anesthetized and surgically exposed patient being monitored by the surgical team. Because noninvolved organs such as the intestine can be packed out of the pathway of the radiation beam, little or no radiation effect is seen except in the target site. Thus side effects are virtually nonexistent despite the high treatment dose. After the radiation dose has been delivered, the incision is closed and the patient is transferred to the recovery unit.

Intraoperative radiation therapy takes place either in the operative suite, with a dedicated therapy machine, or in the radiation therapy department. Treatment given in any other locale outside the surgical suite requires elaborate planning and preparation, because the fully anesthetized patient must be transported through the hospital corridors.

Most IORT is given prophylactically after surgical removal of bulk disease or as adjuvant therapy in locally advanced carcinomas, such as colorectal, gastric, pancreatic, and soft-tissue sarcomas (Kinsella & Sindelar, 1985). Once the patient recovers from surgery, a further course of external beam therapy is usually given.

Hyperthermia

Heat is known to be cytotoxic, and when it is applied at temperatures high enough to produce cell death, this effect is seen in normal as well as tumor tissues. Heat is not selective; therefore, it is not useful as a single agent in cancer treatment. The use of controlled hyperthermia *combined* with radiation therapy has been shown to achieve tumor cell killing without excess toxicity to normal tissues.

Several factors combine to produce the desired biologic effect of hyperthermia plus radiation therapy:

1. Hyperthermia is known to be most effective during the S phase of the cell cycle, when radiation is *least effective*.
2. Hypoxic cells that are generally radioresistant are heat sensitive.
3. Heat inhibits repair of radiation injury (Valdagni, Fei-Fei, & Kapp, 1988).

Thus three of the four Rs of radiobiology are enhanced by the addition of hyperthermia to radiation therapy.

Hyperthermia is administered by several techniques, the choice of technique usually depending on the volume of tissue to be heated. Standard techniques include the use of ultrasound, microwaves, immersion in a heated bath, perfusion, and interstitial probe implants (Bahman & Perez, 1985; Guy & Chou, 1983).

Nurses caring for patients receiving hyperthermia therapy may have multiple responsibilities, including surgical assistance with probe implantation, monitoring treatment tolerance, and assessing posttreatment response for research protocols. However, primary nursing interventions are focused on provision of patient and family education, emotional support, and symptom management (Wojtas, in press).

Chemical Modifiers of Radiation Effect

Radiosensitizers and radioprotectors are chemical compounds used to modify the effect of radiation on cells and tissues. Since the early 1970s, clinical trials using a variety of compounds have been under way (Hellman, 1985; Wasserman & Kligerman, 1987). The rationale for the use of radiosensitizers is based on the knowledge that many tumors have hypoxic portions that are highly radioresistant (oxygen effect). Chemical radiosensitizers are drugs that take the place of oxygen in hypoxic cells in order to enhance radiation effectiveness. Compounds in current use include SR-2508, RO-03-8799, metronidazole, misonidazole, and desmethylmisonidazole.

Pyrimidine analogues (BUdR, IUdR) are also useful as radiosensitizers. These substances are very readily incorporated into DNA and subsequently inhibit the repair of sublethal damage (Fowler, 1985; Hellman, 1985; Phillips, 1981). Perfluorocarbons are a third group of chemical modifiers that absorb high amounts of oxygen when exposed to hyperbaric conditions, then release oxygen when environmental oxygen is low. These compounds, therefore, serve as an oxygen transport vehicle bringing oxygen to hypoxic tumors and enhancing the radiation effect. Thiol depletors such as diethyl maleate (DEM) and butionine sulphoximine (BSO) act to deplete intracellular glutathione (GSH) prior to irradiation. The presence of GSH tends to protect against radiation damage and decreases the radiosensitivity of tumor cells. When used in combination with radiosensitizing agents, thiol depletors have enhanced tumor response in the laboratory setting (Fowler, 1985; Phillips, 1981; Wasserman & Kligerman, 1987).

Protection of normal tissue while enhancing tumor radiosensitivity is a therapeutic challenge. Compounds that serve as radioprotectors must be selective to the healthy tissue to obtain the desired results. Sulfhydryl compounds are the major group of radioprotectors currently under investigation and are described as scavengers in their affinity for the products of irradiated water (Wasserman & Kligerman, 1987). Repair of the critical molecules damaged by ionization is facilitated by donation of a hydrogen atom from the sulfhydryl compound. The radioprotective compound WR 2721 (a cystamine analogue) is the subject of numerous investigations (Fowler, 1985).

Whenever therapies are combined to produce

greater cytotoxicity, side effects are also increased. In addition, radiosensitizers characteristically have their own specific side effects of neurotoxicity and affect both the central and peripheral nervous systems. Prominent among these effects are peripheral neuropathy, somnolence, confusion, and transient coma. Gastrointestinal effects (nausea and vomiting) are also frequently seen (Noll, in press).

Patient and family education in preparation for treatment with chemical modifiers is essential. Nurses have a pivotal role in providing this information, assisting the patient and family to cope with the physical and emotional effects of treatment; they also assist in providing symptom management (Noll, in press).

SUMMARY

Radiation therapy, whether used alone as the primary treatment of cancer or combined in a multimodality approach, has a major role in oncology. Patients today may have options for treatment in which they are given a choice between surgery or radiation therapy (early breast and laryngeal cancers) when either option has equal probability of cure or local control. Others may not have the same choice, but are referred for radiation treatment because of its known palliative effects in advanced disease. Nurses caring for oncology patients in all settings have a responsibility to assist the patient and family by providing accurate information about radiation therapy. The science of radiation oncology has been presented here as background for the science and art of oncology nursing intervention in care of the person receiving irradiation.

References

Aistars, J. (1987). Fatigue in the cancer patient: A conceptual approach to a clinical problem. *Oncology Nursing Forum, 14*(6), 25–30.

Bahman, E., & Perez, C. (1985). Interstitial thermoradiotherapy: An overview. *Endocurietherapy/Hyperthermia Oncology, 1*, 35–40.

Bergonie, J., & Tribondeau, L. (1959). Interpretation of some results of radiotherapy and an attempt at determining a logical technique of treatment. *Radiation Research, 2*, 587.

Boaz, J. W. (1975). The time scale in radiobiology. In O. F. Nygaard, H. I. Adler, & W. K. Sinclair (Eds.), *Radiation research: Proceedings of the 5th International Congress of Radiation Research* (p. 9). New York: Academic Press.

Bucholtz, J. (1987). Radiation therapy. In C. Ziegfeld (Ed.), *Core curriculum for oncology nursing* (pp. 207–224). Philadelphia: W.B. Saunders.

Dudjak, L. (in press). Alterations in fractionation. In K. Hassey & L. Hilderley (Eds.), *Nursing perspectives in radiation oncology*. Albany, NY: Delmar Publishers Inc.

Fowler, J. F. (1985). Chemical modifiers of radiosensitivity—theory and reality: A review. *International Journal of Radiation Oncology, Biology, Physics, 11*, 665–674.

Glicksman, A. (1987). Radiobiologic basis of brachytherapy. *Seminars in Oncology Nursing, 3*, 3–6.

Grant, M., Dodd, M., Hilderley, L., & Patterson, P. (1984). Radiation oncology nurses' role: A national survey. *Oncology Nursing Forum Supplement: Proceedings of the Ninth Annual Congress, 11*(2), 107.

Griffin, T. W. (1987). High linear energy transfer and heavy charged particles. In C. A. Perez & L. W. Brady (Eds.), *Principles and practice of radiation oncology* (pp. 298–309). Philadelphia: J. B. Lippincott Co.

Grigg, E. R. N. (1965). *The trail of the invisible light*. Springfield, IL: Charles C Thomas Publisher.

Guy, A., & Chou, C. K. (1983). Physical aspects of localized heating by radiowaves and microwaves. In F. Storm (Ed.), *Hyperthermia in cancer therapy* (pp. 279–304). Boston: G. K. Hall.

Hall, E. (1978). *Radiobiology for the radiologist* (2nd ed.). Philadelphia: Harper & Row Publishers, Inc.

Harris, J. R., Hellman, S., Canellos, G. P., & Fisher, B. (1985). Cancer of the breast. In V. T. DeVita, S. Hellman, & S. A. Rosenberg (Eds.), *Cancer: Principles and practice of oncology* (Vol. 2, 2nd ed., pp. 1119–1178). Philadelphia: J. B. Lippincott Co.

Hassey, K. (1985). Demystifying care of patients with radioactive implants. *American Journal of Nursing, 85*, 788–792.

Hassey, K. (1987). Principles of radiation safety and protection. *Seminars in Oncology Nursing, 3*, 23–29.

Haylock, P. J., & Hart, L. K. (1979). Fatigue in patients receiving localized radiation. *Cancer Nursing, 2*, 461–467.

Hellman, S. (1985). Principles of radiation therapy. In V. T. DeVita, S. Hellman, & S. A. Rosenberg (Eds.), *Cancer: Principles and practice of oncology* (Vol. 1, 2nd ed., pp. 227–255). Philadelphia: J. B. Lippincott Co.

Hilderley, L. (1980). The role of the nurse in radiation oncology. *Seminars in Oncology, 7*:39–47.

Hilderley, L. (1983). Skin care in radiation therapy: A review of the literature. *Oncology Nursing Forum, 10*(1), 51–56.

Hussey, D. H. (1980). Carcinoma of the prostate. In G. H. Fletcher (Ed.), *Textbook of radiotherapy* (3rd ed., pp. 894–914). Philadelphia: Lea & Febiger.

Iwamoto, R. (in press). Nutritional alterations in persons receiving radiation therapy. In K. Hassey & L. Hilderley (Eds.), *Nursing perspectives in radiation oncology*. Albany, NY: Delmar Publishers, Inc.

Khan, F. M. (1984). *The physics of radiation therapy*. Baltimore: Williams & Wilkins.

Kinsella, T. J., & Sindelar, W. F. (1985). Newer methods of cancer treatment: Intraoperative radiotherapy. In V. T. DeVita, S. Hellman, & S. A. Rosenberg (Eds.), *Cancer: Principles and practice of oncology* (2nd ed, pp. 2293–2304). Philadelphia: J. B. Lippincott Co.

Leung, P. (1984). Experience with remote afterloading technique in intracavitary therapy. *International Journal of Radiation Oncology Biology Physics, 10*, 157–162.

Levitt, S. H., & Perez, C. A. (1987). Breast cancer. In C. A. Perez & L. W. Brady (Eds.), *Principles and practice of radiation oncology* (pp. 730–792). Philadelphia: J. B. Lippincott Co.

Marks, J. E., & Sessions D. G. (1987). Carcinoma of the larynx. In C. A. Perez & L. W. Brady (Eds.), *Principles and practice of radiation oncology* (pp. 598–618). Philadelphia: J. B. Lippincott Co.

Million, R. R., Cassisi, N. J., & Wittes, R. E. (1985). Cancer of the head and neck. In V. T. DeVita, S. Hellman, & S. A. Rosenberg (Eds.), *Cancer: Principles and practice of oncology* (Vol. 1, 2nd ed., pp. 407–506). Philadelphia: J. B. Lippincott Co.

National Council on Radiation Protection and Measurements. (1972). NCRP Report #40. *Protection against radiation from brachytherapy sources*. Washington, DC: Author.

National Council on Radiation Protection and Measurements. (1973). NCRP Report #37. *Precautions in the management of patients who have received therapeutic amounts of radionuclides*. Washington, DC: Author.

National Council on Radiation Protection and Measurements. (1974). NCRP Report #39. *Basic radiation protection criteria*. Washington, DC: Author.

National Council on Radiation Protection & Measurements. (1977). NCRP Report #53. *Review of NCRP radiation dose limit for embryo and fetus in occupationally-exposed women*. Washington, DC: Author.

National Council on Radiation Protection and Measurements. (1987). NCRP Report #91. *Recommendations on limits for exposure to ionizing radiation*. Bethesda, MD: Author.

Noll, L. (in press). Chemical modifiers of radiation therapy. In K. Hassey & L. Hilderley (Eds.), *Nursing perspectives in radiation oncology*. Albany, NY: Delmar Publishers, Inc.

Noz, M., & Maguire, G. (1979). *Radiation protection in the radiologic and health sciences*. Philadelphia: Lea & Febiger.

Parker, G. (1976). Particle radiation therapy. In *Proceedings of the American Cancer Society National Conference on Radiation Oncology* (pp. 802–805). New York: American Cancer Society.

Perez, C. A. (1987). Carcinoma of the prostate. In C. A. Perez & L. W. Brady (Eds.), *Principles and practice of radiation oncology* (pp. 867–898). Philadelphia: J. B. Lippincott Co.

Phillips, T. L. (1981). Sensitizers and protectors. *Seminars in Oncology, 8,* 65–82.

Piper, B. F., Lindsey, A. M., & Dodd, M. J. (1987). Fatigue mechanisms in cancer patients: Developing nursing theory. *Oncology Nursing Forum, 14*(6), 17–23.

Richter, M. P., Share, F. S., & Goodman, R. L. (1985). Principles of radiation therapy. In P. Calabresi, P. S. Schein, & S. A. Rosenberg (Eds.), *Medical oncology: Basic principles and clinical management of cancer* (pp. 280–291). New York: Macmillan Publishing Co.

Rubin, P. (1983). *Clinical oncology: A multidisciplinary approach* (6th ed.). New York: American Cancer Society.

Shapiro, J. (1981). *Radiation protection: A guide for scientists and physicians* (2nd ed.). Cambridge, MA: Harvard University Press.

Shell, J., Stanutz, F., & Grimm, J. (1986). Comparison of moisture vapor permeable (MVP) dressings to conventional dressings for management of radiation skin reactions. *Oncology Nursing Forum, 13*(1), 11–16.

Smith, R. (in press). Intraoperative radiation therapy. In K. Hassey & L. Hilderley (Eds.), *Nursing perspectives in radiation oncology*. Albany, NY: Delmar Publishers, Inc.

Strohl, R. A. (1988). The nursing role in radiation oncology: Symptom management of acute and chronic reactions. *Oncology Nursing Forum, 15*(4), 429–434.

Travis, E. (1975). *Primer of medical radiobiology*. Chicago: Year Book Medical Publishers.

Valdagni, R., Fei-Fei, L., & Kapp, D. (1988). Important prognostic factors influencing outcome of combined radiation and hyperthermia. *International Journal of Radiation Oncology, Biology, Physics, 15,* 959–972.

Wang, C. C. (1988). Cancer of the breast. In C. C. Wang (Ed.), *Clinical radiation oncology: Indications, techniques and results* (pp. 180–195). Littleton, MA: PSG Publishing Company.

Wasserman, T. H., & Kligerman, M. (1987). Chemical modifiers of radiation effect. In C. A. Perez & L. W. Brady (Eds.), *Principles and practice of radiation oncology* (pp. 360–376). Philadelphia: J. B. Lippincott Co.

Wilson, J. F. (1989). The breast. In W. T. Moss & J. D. Cox (Eds.), *Radiation oncology: Rationale, technique, results* (6th ed., pp. 312–350). St. Louis: C. V. Mosby Co.

Withers, H. R., & Peters, L. J. (1980). Biologic aspects of radiotherapy. In G. H. Fletcher (Ed.), *Textbook of radiotherapy* (3rd ed., pp. 103–180). Philadelphia: Lea & Febiger.

Wojtas, F. (in press). Hyperthermia and radiation therapy. In K. Hassey & L. Hilderley (Eds.), *Nursing perspectives in radiation oncology*. Albany, NY: Delmar Publishers, Inc.

Wood, H. (1985). Radiation therapy implants. In B. L. Johnson & J. Gross (Eds.), *Handbook of oncology nursing* (pp. 567–589). New York: John Wiley & Sons.

CHAPTER 21

Medical Oncology—The Agents

JENNIFER L. GUY

HISTORICAL PERSPECTIVES
DRUG DEVELOPMENT
HOW ANTINEOPLASTICS WORK
PRINCIPLES OF CHEMOTHERAPY
  ADMINISTRATION
CLASSIFICATION OF ANTINEOPLASTICS
Alkylating Agents

Plant Alkaloids
Antitumor Antibiotics
Antimetabolites
Miscellaneous Antineoplastics
HORMONALLY ACTIVE AGENTS
BIOLOGIC ANTINEOPLASTICS
NEW HORIZONS

Medical oncology focuses on the systemic management of malignant disease by the use of antineoplastic medications, commonly referred to as *chemotherapy*. Chemotherapy is "the treatment of disease by chemical agents; first applied to the use of chemicals that attack the causative organisms unfavorably but do not harm the patient" (*Dorland's Illustrated Medical Dictionary*, 1981). Chemotherapy administered to patients for the management of confined or disseminated malignant disease is the focus of this discussion.

Today many diseases are curable with chemotherapy. Prolonged disease-free intervals and increased survival times have been documented with chemotherapeutic intervention for a number of tumors. For other tumors, chemotherapy can help to control pain and ease suffering (Table 21–1).

The clinical management of medical oncology patients is based on an understanding of the principles of chemotherapeutic intervention and of the host factors that determine the choice of drugs, dose, route, and schedule, as well as knowledge of the agents and their acute and delayed toxicities.

HISTORICAL PERSPECTIVES

The concept of using chemicals to treat malignant disease dates to the sixteenth century, when heavy metals were used systemically to treat cancers. They were mostly ineffective and extremely toxic, and thus they were discarded until the resurgence of the use of arsenic in 1865 in the treatment of chronic leukemias (Burchenal, 1977). Today heavy metals such as cis-diamminedichloroplatinum (cisplatin) are a mainstay in the treatment of solid tumors.

Chemotherapy evolved from the unlikely province of chemical warfare. During World War I, soldiers were observed to suffer severe bone marrow suppression, aplasia, and death after exposure to sulfur mustard gas. World War II fostered the recognition of the therapeutic application of alkylating agents to the treatment of malignancy (Gilman & Phillips, 1946; Zubrod, 1979). Nitrogen mustard was the first antineoplastic drug to undergo clinical trials; it was shown to produce significant therapeutic effect in patients with tumors of the lymphoid organs (Gilman, 1963; Gilman & Phillips, 1946). Folic acid antagonists were shown to be effective in acute leukemia in children by Farber and colleagues (1948) (Box 21–1). Thioguanine and mercaptopurine were synthesized and were found to produce remissions in antifolate-resistant acute leukemia (Burchenal, 1977).

In the 1950s, antibiotics were resurrected as antineoplastics. During this decade, asparaginase was isolated from *Escherichia coli*, paving the way for the use of enzymes in cancer treatment.

Rosenberg and co-workers demonstrated the effect of platinum coordinate complexes in the 1960s, initially in bacteria, then in lymphosarcoma and solid tumors (Rosenberg, Van Camp, & Krigas, 1965; Rosenberg, Van Camp, Trosko, & Mansour, 1969). In the late

Table 21–1. IMPACT OF CHEMOTHERAPY IN MALIGNANT DISEASE

Curable	Improved Survival
Choriocarcinoma	Small-cell carcinoma of the lung
Acute lymphoblastic leukemia (children)	Ovarian carcinoma
Embryonal rhabdomyosarcoma	Breast carcinoma
Wilms' tumor	Osteosarcoma
Diffuse histiocytic lymphoma	Multiple myeloma
Germinal testicular carcinoma	Chronic leukemia (lymphocytic and myelogenous)
Burkitt's lymphoma	
Hodgkin's disease	Non-Hodgkin's lymphoma
Ewing's sarcoma	Soft-tissue sarcomas
Acute myelogenous leukemia	Neuroblastoma

(Data from DeVita, 1985, and Skeel, 1982.)

The author thanks Dr. Jerry T. Guy for his support and advice in the preparation of this manuscript, Nancy Cohen for her assistance with literature review, and Donna Shrout and Jay Kelley for assistance in the preparation of this chapter.

Box 21–1. AN EARLY CHEMOTHERAPY STUDY

STUDY

Farber, S., Diamond, L. K., Mercer, R. D., Sylvester, R. F., & Wolfe, J. A. (1948). **Temporary remissions in acute leukemia in children produced by folic acid antagonist, 4-aminopteroyl-glutamic acid (aminopterin).** *New England Journal of Medicine, 238,* 787–793.

SAMPLE

Sixteen children with acute leukemia, many of whom were moribund at the onset of therapy. Five case reports are detailed, all with bone marrow confirmation of acute leukemia.

TREATMENT

Aminopterin was administered at a dose of 0.5 to 1.0 mg IM daily for variable periods of time in the cases detailed. Some subjects concomitantly received liver extract and folic acid in an attempt to prevent toxicity.

RESULTS

Ten of the 16 children responded to treatment with aminopterin as evaluated by improvement in peripheral blood counts, bone marrow blast counts, splenomegaly, hepatomegaly, and lymphadenopathy, and improvement in performance status. Six patients failed to respond. Remissions were temporary. Toxicity included stomatitis with early ulceration, which was reversible.

CONCLUSIONS

Aminopterin induces temporary remissions in children with acute leukemia, but produces "significant" toxicity, which "may make continued use of the drug impossible." The authors state "these studies justify the search for other antagonists to folic acid which are less toxic and may be even more powerful."

LIMITATIONS

Variable amounts of aminopterin were administered for variable periods of time. In an attempt to control toxicity, liver extract and folic acid were administered to some subjects. No distinction is made between acute lymphoblastic and acute myelogenous leukemia. Limitations of the study emanate from technologies extant at the time the investigation was undertaken.

SIGNIFICANCE

This study documented the efficacy of antimetabolites in hematologic malignancies. Performance status was carefully assessed; improvement in performance status was a parameter of response. This study employed the concept of "rescue" of normal cells, albeit primitive, from the effects of antimetabolites. Toxicity was evaluated critically and considered prohibitive by the authors. The study lends insight into the evolution of clinical investigations and discoveries in cancer chemotherapy.

1960s and early 1970s, multidrug chemotherapy regimens were found to improve remission rates without inducing undue toxicity. The use of chemotherapy in combination with other methods of cancer treatment also came into clinical practice in this decade (see Chapter 24).

The 1970s and 1980s were dedicated to the synthesis and clinical testing of available agents, alone and in combination, and the continued screening and synthesis of new agents. The antineoplastic effects of biologic response modifiers have been identified in this decade and are currently under investigation to define their role in oncologic therapeutics (see Chapter 23).

The current armamentarium of antineoplastics consists of more than 50 agents used as treatment for a broad spectrum of diseases collectively known as cancer. Pharmacologic considerations (doses, routes, schedule), disease variables (biologic behavior, primary site, stage, histology), and patient factors (age, organ system function) result in multiple permutations and combinations of therapeutic interventions, some yet to be studied.

Identification of antineoplastic activity → Acquisition of active compounds → Screening for potential in human tumors →

→ Formulation of a preparation for clinical use → Toxicology testing and LD_{10} determination → FDA Investigational New Drug Application

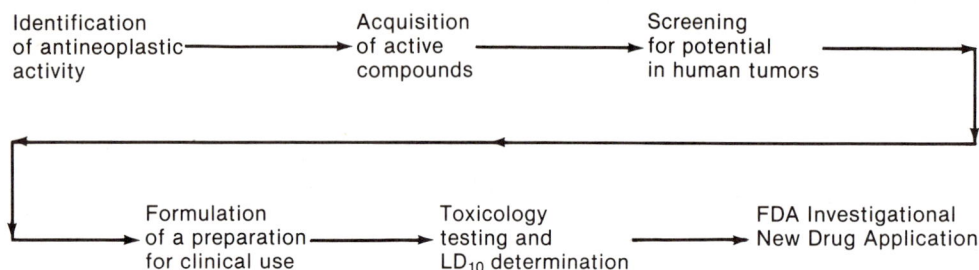

Figure 21–1. Preclinical development of antineoplastics. LD_{10}, lethal dose in 10 per cent of mice tested; FDA, Food and Drug Administration.

DRUG DEVELOPMENT

The identification of compounds with antitumor activity and their subsequent development into clinically useful and available agents began in the 1930s with Shear's efforts at the National Cancer Institute (NCI) (Zubrod, 1984). In 1955, at the direction of the United States Congress, the NCI established the Cancer Chemotherapy National Service Center (CCNSC) and a national drug development program was initiated.

The first step in drug development is the recognition of potential antineoplastic effect and synthesis of the active compound. Agents are then screened, using in vitro and in vivo tumor panels. Currently, the NCI alone screens over 15,000 compounds a year (DeVita, 1985).

Once an agent has shown antineoplastic activity in the screening process, it must be produced and synthesized in a clinically usable formulation, a challenge sometimes insurmountable despite positive tumor screens. Preclinical toxicology testing of active compounds is accomplished in mouse models to establish the lethal dose; a reproducible lethal dose in 10 per cent of the rodents (LD_{10}) is accepted for initial human use. Because some clinically significant toxic effects of antineoplastics have not been consistent between rodent and human systems, further evaluation is accomplished in dogs, with which better correlation has been shown. This phase of preclinical testing includes pathologic examination of the tissue to define the mechanisms of toxicities. The progress of a new agent through preclinical testing is summarized in Figure 21–1. DeVita (1985) reports that 1 in 40,000 compounds screened is ultimately useful.

HOW ANTINEOPLASTICS WORK

Malignant tumors are characterized by cell division, which is no longer controlled as it is in normal tissue.

Loss of contact inhibition of continued replication is a well-known characteristic of malignant cells. However, cancer cells continue to move through the cell cycle, progressing from a resting state (G_0) through mitosis (M). A malignant tumor is composed of millions of cells with various proportions of cells distributed through the five phases of the cell cycle at any one time. The proportion of cells actively dividing at any given time constitutes the growth fraction of the tumor. The time required for a malignant tumor to increase cell number by 100 per cent is referred to as the doubling time. Cell cycle time refers to the time required for a single cell to progress through the cell cycle and reproduce itself (Schackney, 1985).

Antineoplastic lethality depends on halting cellular biochemical functions that allow cell replication. The higher the proportion of dividing cells or the shorter the time it takes for the cell to divide, the more likely it is that chemotherapy will induce tumor regression. Table 21–2 classifies common tumors according to their cell cycle time and compares them with the division rates of normal tissues (See-Lasley & Ignoffo, 1981; Schackney, 1985). Normal cells with shorter cycle times are most often adversely affected by chemotherapy.

Table 21–3 delineates the phases of the cell cycle and their duration, cellular activities, and sensitivity to chemotherapy. The resting phase of the cell cycle (G_0) is highly variable in duration. The higher the proportion of cells in this phase, the longer the doubling time will be. Phases G_1, S, and G_2 are preparatory to mitosis, which occurs in the M phase. After the mitotic phase, normal cells then differentiate, whereas malignant cells reenter G_0 and eventually continue to divide. Newer approaches to chemotherapy focus on agents that potentiate cellular differentiation (Cheson, Jasperse, Chun, & Friedman, 1986).

Antineoplastics may be classified according to the point in the cell cycle at which they exert their effect. Agents that are lethal only if the cell is dividing (i.e., in G_1, S, G_2, and M) are cell cycle specific. If the drug is effective only on resting cells (G_0), it is cycle non-

Table 21–2. COMPARATIVE CELL CYCLE TIMES

	Short	Intermediate	Long
Doubling time			
Cell cycle time	Hours to days	Weeks	Months
Normal cell	Gastrointestinal mucosa	Skin	Liver
	Mucous membrane	Hair follicles	Kidney
	Bone marrow		
Malignancies	Burkitt's lymphoma	Small-cell lung cancer	Breast cancer
	Germ-cell tumors	Hodgkin's disease	Colon cancer
	Acute myelogenous leukemia	Non-Hodgkin's lymphoma	Lung cancer (non-small-cell)

(Data from See-Lasley & Ignoffo, 1981, and Schackney, 1985.)

Table 21–3. PHASES OF THE CELL CYCLE

Antineoplastic Sensitivity	Phase	Cellular Events	Duration
±	→G_0	Resting (cells not committed to cell division)	Highly variable
+	G_1	RNA and protein synthesis (enzymes produced that are necessary for DNA synthesis)	18–30 hr
+	S	DNA synthesis	18–20 hr
+	G_2	RNA, protein synthesis (specialized)	2–10 hr
+	←M	Mitosis (cell division)	0.5–1 hr
±	Differentiation	Permanently nondividing cells that will die, resulting in expected cell loss	

specific. If lethality is restricted to cells in a specific phase of the cell cycle, the agent is considered to be phase specific. Recruitment refers to motivating cells to leave G_0 and enter the growth phases of the cell cycle, in which they are susceptible to cell cycle–specific and phase-specific agents (Dorr & Fritz, 1980; Schackney, 1985). This may be accomplished by rapid reduction in the dividing cell population, which mobilizes nondividing cells into an active growth phase (Schackney, 1985).

Theoretically, cell cycle–specific agents will be most effective in tumors with a short cell cycle time and high growth fraction (*fast growing tumor*). Alternatively, tumors with a high percentage of cells in G_0, or a long cell cycle time, will experience greater lethality from cell cycle–nonspecific agents. Many antineoplastics act on both resting and cycling cells and are classified as cell cycle specific and phase nonspecific. Antineoplastic effect may also be demonstrated in more than one phase of the cell cycle (Table 21–4).

Scheduling and punctual administration are imperative to obtain the desired effects on the cell cycle. Continuous infusion of a chemotherapeutic agent is based on exposing cells to the agents as they enter the phase of the cycle during which the agent exerts its effect. Agents designed to enhance cell synchronization or recruitment must be administered at times consistent with data on the cell cycle time to effect cell kill (Schackney, 1985). The newer regimens for the treatment of non-Hodgkin's lymphoma (M-BACOD, PRO-MACE-MOPP) involve administration of nonmyelosuppressive agents on day 14, the time when the cells

Table 21–4. EFFECT OF ANTINEOPLASTICS ON CELL CYCLE PHASES*

Cell Cycle Phase	Antineoplastics Active in this Phase
G_0	Nitrosoureas, alkylating agents
G_1	Enzymes, steroids, hormones, antibiotics, alkylating agents
S	Antimetabolites, hydroxyurea
G_2	Antibiotics, antimetabolites
M	Plant alkaloids

*Major effect of each class is in the designated phase of the cell cycle. Alkylating agents, nitrosoureas, and many antitumor antibiotics are also active throughout the cell cycle.

recruited into an active growth phase by the rapid cytoreduction accomplished with day 1 therapy, are in phases G_1 through M.

Tumor burden at the onset of chemotherapy has prognostic implications for its success in eradicating the tumor. Antineoplastics induce cell kill by first order kinetics (i.e., the same proportion of cells are killed with each subsequent exposure to the lethal agent). The absolute number of cells killed by a second exposure to a lethal drug is smaller than the number killed with the first exposure, assuming a constant fraction of actively dividing cells. However, as tumor burden increases, the rate of growth slows, decreasing the number of cells in active division. Sensitivity to cycle-specific agents then decreases (Dorr & Fritz, 1980; Schackney, 1985).

In 1979, Goldie and Coldman described a model of spontaneous tumor cell mutations, demonstrating that a mass of fewer than one million cells may contain clones with variable antineoplastic sensitivity. This hypothesis explains why curability of a small tumor cannot always be ensured despite treatment. The earliest possible institution of chemotherapy may minimize the development of resistant clones and increase curability. Alternating different, non–cross-resistant agents and regimens is aimed at killing resistant clones. The Goldie-Coldman hypothesis explains the variation of response that can be observed among identically treated patients with tumors of the same primary site, stage, and histologic features (Schackney, 1985). Additional mechanisms of tumor cell resistance have been described: amplification of genetic control, development of alternate metabolic pathways allowing cell survival, and antineoplastic alteration of cellular ploidy that increases genetic instability and mutation rate (Schackney, 1985). For example, gene amplification has been documented to produce resistance to methotrexate. Tumor cells previously exposed to prolonged low doses of methotrexate (2.5 mg weekly for 3 years) have been shown to expand the genetic sequence that controls the production of dihydrofolate reductase (Trent, Buick, Olson, Horns, & Schimke, 1984). Thus increasing amounts of this enzyme are produced that are no longer inhibited by standard doses of methotrexate.

Box 21–2. AN EARLY COMBINATION CHEMOTHERAPY STUDY

STUDY

DeVita, V. T., Serpick, A. A., and Carbone, P. P. (1970). **Combination chemotherapy in the treatment of advanced Hodgkin's disease.** *Annals of Internal Medicine, 73,* 881–895.

SAMPLE

Forty-four patients with histologically confirmed Hodgkin's disease, Stages III and IV, who had no more than one prior dose of single-agent chemotherapy, or who had relapsed after primary radiation therapy; 20 women; 23 men; mean age 31 years (range, 12 to 69 years); 8 Stage III; 35 Stage IV. One patient was not evaluable.

TREATMENT

Thirty-two patients were treated with vincristine, 1.4 mg/m² IV on days 1 and 8; nitrogen mustard, 6 mg/m² IV, days 1 and 8; procarbazine, 100 mg/m² PO, days 1 through 14; prednisone, 40 mg/m² PO, days 1 through 14 during the first and fourth courses only. Twelve patients had cyclophosphamide substituted for nitrogen mustard at a dose of 650 mg/m² IV on days 1 and 8. Cycles were repeated at 28-day intervals. Dose adjustments for subsequent courses were made by sliding scale titrated to blood counts on day 29. Patients were evaluated after six courses of therapy.

RESULTS

Two patients died after their initial course of treatment both as a result of rapid necrosis of tumor. Thirty-five patients (81 per cent) achieved a complete remission; 6 patients responded to treatment but failed to attain a complete remission. Survival time was markedly increased for patients attaining a complete remission. Toxicity included leukopenia, thrombocytopenia, anemia, neurotoxicity, nausea, vomiting, and alopecia. All of these were tolerable and reversible.

SIGNIFICANCE

This study documented that combinations of antineoplastics could be administered without undue toxicity and could induce significant, durable responses. DeVita and co-workers also found that prolonged therapy (6 months) was efficacious in inducing remission, as opposed to the standard approach (at that time) of declaring treatment failures after 4 to 6 weeks of chemotherapy.

PRINCIPLES OF CHEMOTHERAPY ADMINISTRATION

Chemotherapy may be administered as a single agent, such as busulfan used to lower the white blood cell count in the chronic phase of chronic myelogenous leukemia. Hydroxyurea alone may then be administered to control leukocytosis and splenomegaly in the accelerated phase. Busulfan may be used in high doses in preparation for bone marrow transplant.

Combinations of antineoplastic agents are more effective than single agents in tumors that are responsive (i.e., sensitive) to multiple agents. The basic principle of combination chemotherapy regimens is to simultaneously administer multiple drugs that do not have overlapping toxicities. The classic example of this principle is the MOPP regimen (mechlorethamine [Mustargen], vincristine [Oncovin], procarbazine, and prednisone) for the treatment of Hodgkin's disease (Box 21–2) (DeVita, Serpick, & Carbone, 1970). To circumvent the problem of drug resistance, alternation of regimens may be used, such as the alternation of MOPP with doxorubicin (Adriamycin), bleomycin, vinblastine (Velban), and dacarbazine (ABVD) in

Hodgkin's disease (Bonadonna, Valagussa, & Santoro, 1986). Alternating non-cross-resistant agents improves cell death rate by affecting clones resistant to the alternate agents.

Chemotherapy may be administered as the primary curative modality, an example of which is the platinum, vinblastine (Velban), and bleomycin (PVB) regimen in the treatment of testicular cancer (Einhorn, 1981) or the MOPP regimen in the treatment of Hodgkin's disease (De Vita et al., 1970). In childhood lymphoblastic leukemia, chemotherapy is the primary curative modality.

Control of malignant disease may be accomplished with chemotherapy when improved survival can be demonstrated. Doxorubicin-containing regimens, hormonal chemotherapy, alkylating agents, and the cyclophosphamide, methotrexate, and 5-fluorouracil (CMF) regimen are effective in controlling breast cancer. In multiple myeloma, vincristine, melphalan, cyclophosphamide, and prednisone (VMCP) and vincristine, carmustine (BCNU), doxorubicin (Adriamycin), and prednisone (VBAP) induce remission, can result in remarkable pain relief, and prolong life.

Palliation may be accomplished with chemotherapy.

Box 21–3. AN EXAMPLE OF ADJUVANT CHEMOTHERAPY

STUDY

Bonadonna, G., Brusamolino, E., Valagussa, P., Rossi, A., Brugnatelli, L., Brambilla, C., DeLena, M., Tancini, G., Bajetta, E., Musumeci, R., & Veronesi, U. (1976). **Combination chemotherapy as an adjuvant treatment in operable breast cancer.** *New England Journal of Medicine, 294,* 405–410.

SAMPLE

Three hundred ninety-one women with primary breast cancer. All patients had conventional or extended radical mastectomy for potentially curable disease. Only patients with T1a through T2b and one or more histologically positive axillary lymph nodes without distant metastases (M0) were included. Patients with fixed primary tumors (T3B1-T4) and clinically obvious nodal disease (N2-N3) were excluded.

EXPERIMENTAL DESIGN

Patients were stratified by age, number of positive axillary nodes, and type of mastectomy and were randomized to receive 12 cycles of chemotherapy or no further treatment after mastectomy. The cyclophosphamide, methotrexate, and 5-fluorouracil (CMF) regimen was used: cyclophosphamide, 100 mg/m² orally on days 1 through 14; methotrexate, 40 mg/m² IV on days 1 and 8; 5-fluorouracil, 600 mg/m² IV on days 1 and 8. Cycles were repeated at 28-day intervals. Women over 65 years of age were treated at reduced doses. Dose decreases were made for toxicity; no dose escalations were allowed in the absence of toxicity. Both the treatment and the control groups were monitored with serial laboratory and radiographic studies to detect recurrence (local, regional, or distant), the end point of the study. Three hundred eighty-six patients were evaluable, 179 in the control group and 207 in the treatment group.

RESULTS

After 27 months of study, 24 per cent of patients in the control group and 5.3 per cent in the treatment group had relapsed (P<10⁻⁴). Relapse was more frequent in patients with greater than four positive nodes (40.7 per cent in the control group compared to 8.8 per cent in the treatment group). Recurrence occurred at distant sites in 81.5 per cent of the relapsing patients. Both premenopausal and postmenopausal patients benefited from CMF in terms of relapse-free interval. Toxicity was acceptable and consisted of myelosuppression, variable degrees of alopecia, oral mucositis, conjunctivitis, cystitis, and amenorrhea.

SIGNIFICANCE

Bonadonna and colleagues demonstrated a statistically significant reduction in recurrence rate in women treated with prolonged (12 cycles) combination chemotherapy (CMF) following radical mastectomy for primary breast cancer with nodal metastases. Adjuvant combination chemotherapy improved disease-free interval irrespective of menopausal status. Toxicity of chemotherapy resulted in a decrement in performance status in fewer than approximately 10 per cent of the patients.

LIMITATIONS

At the time of publication the major limitation of this study was the short follow-up time, 27 months from the initiation of the study. Thus, the impact of improved disease-free interval on the rate of survival could not be determined. However, by 1990, it has become clear that a prolonged disease-free interval affects survival. In addition, the primary surgical procedure was extended or conventional radical mastectomy; thus, extrapolation to lesser surgical procedures must be done cautiously.

Hydroxyurea may produce a decrease in splenomegaly and splenic pain in chronic myelogenous leukemia (CML). Chemotherapy may produce dramatic pain relief in multiple myeloma and in breast cancer.

As an adjunct to curative surgical resection, chemotherapy has been shown to improve the disease-free interval and survival in breast cancer. The success of adjuvant chemotherapy depends on effective agents used in patients with minimal tumor burden (Box 21–3). Studies in colon cancer document that improvement in the disease-free interval and survival may also be accomplished in this malignancy with the use of chemotherapy as an adjunct to surgery (Friedman & Hamilton, 1988; Moertel et al., 1990).

Chemotherapy may be employed preoperatively in an attempt to convert nonresectable disease to resectable disease. Preoperative chemotherapy, sometimes referred to as neoadjuvant therapy, is currently being studied in bladder and breast cancer (Scher, Yagoda, & Herr, 1988).

CLASSIFICATION OF ANTINEOPLASTICS

Cancer chemotherapy agents are classified into several categories on the basis of their mechanism of action, derivation, and chemical structure. Although agents may be assigned to a given group, individual agents may exhibit properties that overlap with other classes. A discussion of the five main classes is presented next with clinically important agents emphasized within each class. Table 21–5 presents a more comprehensive alphabetical listing of commercially available contemporary antineoplastics and also provides data on availability, storage and stability, route of administration, and acute and delayed toxicity.

Alkylating Agents

Alkylating agents, the oldest class of antineoplastics, act by substituting an alkyl group ($R-CH_2-CH_2$) for a hydrogen atom in organic compounds. The ultimate effect is an abnormal cross linking of DNA base pairs that results in cell death or mutation by altering the decoding and replication process. The mutagenic property of alkylating agents is potentially carcinogenic. Six chemical classes of alkylating agents are known (Table 21–6).

Alkylating agents are most active in the G_0 or resting cell; they are non-cell cycle specific. The oral alkylators (cyclophosphamide, chlorambucil, melphalan, busulfan) are frequently administered as single agents on a daily schedule, with breaks in therapy being titrated to bone marrow suppression. High-dose intermittent use may take place with busulfan in chronic myelogenous leukemia and with chlorambucil, melphalan, and cyclophosphamide in myeloma.

Cyclophosphamide may be administered intravenously at high doses (0.5 to 1.5 g/m^2) repeated at 3- or 4-week intervals. This route is used in combination regimens in the treatment of both solid tumors and hematologic malignancies. Ultra high dose cyclophosphamide (greater than or equal to 2 g/m^2) may be used in preparation for bone marrow transplantation (see Chapter 27). Intravenous cyclophosphamide can produce a syndrome of inappropriate secretion of antidiuretic hormone (SIADH), an oncologic emergency (see Chapter 57). Cyclophosphamide is metabolized to its active form in the liver and excreted via the kidneys. Hemorrhagic cystitis may result from both oral and intravenous administration owing to its excretion in the urine.

The most important clinical role for mechlorethamine (nitrogen mustard) is in the treatment of Hodgkin's disease in the MOPP regimen (De Vita et al., 1970) and its variants. Mechlorethamine may be used for intracavitary instillation to control malignant

pleural and pericardial effusions. It may also be applied topically in mycosis fungoides and skin cancers. If extravasation occurs, nitrogen mustard causes severe tissue necrosis. Treatment of extravasation is detailed in Chapter 22. Mechlorethamine is unstable when reconstituted and must be administered promptly (Duagin, 1982).

Thiotepa is a sulfur-containing compound enjoying a resurgence of use in breast cancer and intravesicularly in early bladder cancer (see Chapter 22). Thiotepa is the only clinically important agent in this chemical class.

Busulfan has its primary effect on cells of the granulocytic series and thus is used in chronic myelogenous leukemia; it has not proved useful in acute myelogenous leukemia. Unique to busulfan is its ability to produce an abrupt, marked bone marrow hypoplasia, which may progress to aplasia, an effect also seen less frequently with chlorambucil. Ultra high-dose busulfan (4 mg/kg/day for 4 days) may be used in preparation for bone marrow transplantation; seizures have been reported with doses this high (Hartmann et al., 1986).

Dacarbazine must be transformed to its active metabolite in the liver. It may be administered as a high-dose bolus or at lower doses on sequential days; a short continuous infusion may increase the exposure of cells in G_0 phase. Dacarbazine is active in melanoma, sarcomas, and Hodgkin's disease. It can be hepatotoxic, the clinical manifestations of which must be differentiated from hepatic metastases (Sutherland & Krementz, 1981).

Unlike the other alkylators, nitrosoureas are lipid soluble and cross the blood-brain barrier. They are useful in the treatment of primary brain tumors. Nitrosoureas are non-cross-resistant with other alkylators; their effect is on the G_0 (resting) phase of the cell cycle. The nitrosoureas produce delayed bone marrow suppression (5 to 6 weeks after administration) owing to the half-lives of their active metabolites. The investigational drug methyl-CCNU is active in colorectal cancer; however, it has been associated with the development of acute myelogenous leukemia (Boice et al., 1983).

Streptozocin is a unique natural product with specificity for pancreatic exocrine cells. Its primary use is in the treatment of islet cell carcinoma of the pancreas; it may be effective in other endocrine malignancies. Hypoglycemia is an acute complication of therapy; chronically, glucose intolerances can occur, requiring the use of insulin or oral diabetic agents. Blood and urine sugar levels must be evaluated frequently. Streptozocin is excreted renally and is nephrotoxic. Renal tubular acidosis may occur, identified by electrolyte imbalances preceded by proteinuria.

Use of the platinum complexes, the first inorganic compounds employed in human malignancy, had almost been abandoned when diuresis was found to be effective in preventing their nephrotoxicity. These complexes are classed as alkylators; however, their inhibition of DNA synthesis takes place by a different mechanism than that of classic alkylators. Cisplatin persists in tissues for months, and thus toxicities mimic

Text continued on page 282

Table 21–5. DRUG DATA

Drug and Availability*	Storage and Stability	Administration	Toxicity—Acute	Toxicity—Delayed
AMINOGLUTETHIMIDE (Cytadren) Tablets: 250 mg	Room temperature	PO	Drowsiness (40%); skin rash (17–20%); dizziness (14%); nausea and anorexia (10–13%); ataxia (10%); vomiting (3–10%); pruritus (5%); fever (5%); headache (5%); orthostatic hypotension (3%); myalgia (3%); tachycardia (2.5%)	Hypothyroidism (occasional); virilization (occasional); hepatotoxicity: elevated liver function test results, cholestatic jaundice (rare); myelosuppression (rare)
ASPARAGINASE (Elspar); Injection: 10,000 IU vial *Erwinia* asparaginase (Porton asparaginase) INVESTIGATIONAL Injection: 10,000 IU vial	Unreconstituted: Refrigeration Elspar: Reconstituted: Refrigeration, 8 hr Diluted: Refrigeration, 8 hr Erwinia: Reconstituted: Room temperature, 20 days; refrigeration, 20 days Diluted: Diluted to a concentration of 35 IU/ml: room temperature, 4 days; refrigeration, 4 days	Intra-arterial, IVP, IV infusion, IM	Nausea (30%); vomiting (30%); anorexia (30%); hypersensitivity reactions (20–35%); anaphylaxis after one to four doses (3.3%), after five or more doses (32%); hyperglycemia	Myelosuppression: leukopenia (100%) (nadir day 4 to 7), thrombocytopenia (30%) (nadir day 5 to 10); hepatotoxicity: fatty metamorphosis (42–87%), elevated liver function test results (50%); hypercholesterolemia (85%); neurotoxicity: personality changes (66%), somnolence, lethargy (33%), confusion (10%); clotting disorders (60%); azotemia (30%); proteinuria (15%); pancreatitis (5%)
BLEOMYCIN (Blenoxane) Injection: 15 units/ampule	Unreconstituted: refrigeration Reconstituted: Room temperature, 14 days; refrigeration, 28 days Diluted: Room temperature, 24 hours in D_5W, 0.9% NaCl, or D_5W containing heparin, 100 to 1000 units/ml	Intra-arterial, intrapleural, IVP, IV infusion, SC, IM	Fever and chills (30%); hypersensitivity reaction (20–50%); nausea and vomiting (15%); anorexia and weight loss (common); anaphylaxis (rare)	Pulmonary toxicity (10–40%): pneumonitis (8%), fibrosis (1%); dermatologic toxicity (25–50%): hyperpigmentation (25%), skin peeling (10%), nail banding (10%), alopecia (50%); stomatitis (15%); ulceration (10%); radiation recall (occasional)
BUSULFAN (Myleran) Tablets: 2 mg	Room temperature	PO	Hypersensitivity reaction (rare); nausea and vomiting (rare); diarrhea (rare)	Myelosuppression: leukopenia (100%) (nadir day 7), thrombocytopenia (70%) (nadir day 11 to 30, recovery day 24 to 54); hyperpigmentation (5–10%); pulmonary toxicity: interstitial fibrosis (2.5–11.5%); hyperuricemia; cataract formation (rare); gonadal suppression: amenorrhea, azoospermia, gynecomastia (rare); alopecia (rare)
CARBOPLATIN (CBDCA) Injection: 150-mg vial	Unreconstituted: Refrigeration, 1 year Reconstituted: Refrigeration, 24 hr; room temperature, 24 hr Diluted: Refrigeration, 24 hr; room temperature, 24 hr Other: Light sensitive	Intraperitoneal, intra-arterial, IV infusion	Nausea and vomiting	Myelosuppression: leukopenia, thrombocytopenia, erythrosuppression; ototoxicity; renal failure (reversible); hyperuricemia
CARMUSTINE (BCNU, BiCNU) Injection: 100-mg vial	Unreconstituted: Refrigeration, 2 yr Reconstituted: Room temperature, 6 hr; refrigeration, 24 hr Diluted: Refrigeration, 48 hr when diluted in 500 ml 0.9% NaCl or D_5W Other: Light sensitive	MD: Intra-arterial, topical Oncology RN: IV infusion	Nausea and vomiting (80%); facial flushing (frequent); vein irritation (frequent)	Myelosuppression: leukopenia (100%) (nadir 5 to 6 weeks), thrombocytopenia (100%) (nadir 4 to 5 weeks); hepatotoxicity: mild changes in liver function tests (26%), bilirubinemia (5–25%); nephrotoxicity: elevated BUN (10%), renal failure or interstitial nephritis (9%); pulmonary toxicity: interstitial fibrosis (1.3–30%); pigmentation at injection site (occasional); neurotoxicity with intra-arterial administration (4–31%)

Table continued on following page

273

Table 21–5. DRUG DATA *Continued*

Drug and Availability*	Storage and Stability	Administration	Toxicity—Acute	Toxicity—Delayed
CHLORAMBUCIL (Leukeran) Tablets: 2 mg	Room temperature Light sensitive	PO	Nausea and vomiting (10%); hypersensitivity reactions (rare)	Myelosuppression: leukopenia (100%) (nadir day 14 to 20, recovery day 28 to 42), thrombocytopenia (100%) (nadir day 10 to 14, recovery day 21); hepatotoxicity (rare): elevated SGOT and alkaline phosphatase levels, cholestatic hepatitis; alopecia (occasional); exfoliative dermatitis (rare); interstitial pneumonitis and fibrosis (rare); hyperuricemia
CISPLATIN (Platinol, CACP, DDP) Injection: 10-mg and 50-mg vials	Unreconstituted: Room temperature, 2 yr Reconstituted: Room temperature, 20 hr Diluted: Room temperature, 20 hr Other: Do not refrigerate after reconstitution as the drug may precipitate; light sensitive	Intra-arterial, intraperitoneal, IVP, IV infusion	Nausea and vomiting (100%); seizures (9%); hypersensitivity reactions (1–20%)	Myelosuppression: leukopenia (36%) (nadir day 18 to 23, recovery day 39), thrombocytopenia (5%) (nadir day 14, recovery day 21), anemia (25–30%); hemolytic anemia (rare); nephrotoxicity; elevated creatinine level (40%), elevated BUN (30%), acute tubular necrosis (25%); ototoxicity (30%): tinnitus (9%), deafness (6%); hyperuricemia (30%); neurotoxicity, peripheral neuritis (6%); hyperpigmentation (occasional)
CYCLOPHOSPHAMIDE (Cytoxan) Injection: 100-mg, 200-mg, 500-mg, 1-g, and 2-g vials Tablets: 25 mg and 50 mg	Tablets: Room temperature Unreconstituted: Room temperature Reconstituted: Room temperature, 24 hr; refrigeration, 6 days Diluted: Room temperature, 24 hr	Intraperitoneal, intrapleural, PO, IVP, IV infusion	Nausea and vomiting (50–90%, dose dependent); anorexia; diarrhea; stomatitis	Myelosuppression: leukopenia (100%) (nadir day 8 to 15, recovery day 17 to 28), thrombocytopenia (20%) (nadir day 10 to 14, recovery day 21); reversible alopecia (50%); gonadal suppression (10–33%); SIADH (20%); hemorrhagic cystitis (7–12%); cardiotoxicity; hemolytic anemia; pulmonary toxicity (rare): interstitial fibrosis; hyperuricemia; radiation recall (occasional); nail changes (frequent)
CYTARABINE (Cytosar-U, ARA-C, cytosine arabinoside) Injection: 100-mg and 500-mg vials	Unreconstituted: Controlled room temperature (15° C to 30° C) Reconstituted: Controlled room temperature, 48 hr; do not refrigerate solution after reconstitution Diluted: Room temperature, 8 days	Intrathecal, intraperitoneal, IVP, IV infusion, IM, SC	Nausea and vomiting (15–20%); diarrhea (20–25%); fever and chills (10–20%); skin rash (20%); anaphylaxis (rare)	Myelosuppression: leukopenia (100%) (first nadir day 7 to 9, recovery day 12; second nadir day 15 to 24, recovery day 34), thrombocytopenia (100%) (nadir day 12 to 15, recovery day 25), anemia, megaloblastosis; hepatotoxicity: elevated liver function tests (30–50%); stomatitis (30–50%); hyperuricemia; reversible alopecia (occasional)
DACARBAZINE (DTIC-Dome, DTIC, imidazole carboxamide) Injection: 100-mg and 200-mg vials	Unreconstituted: Refrigeration Reconstituted: Room temperature, 8 hr; refrigeration, 72 hr Diluted: Room temperature, 8 hr; refrigeration, 24 hr Other: Light sensitive	Intra-arterial, IVP, IV infusion	Nausea and vomiting (90%), anorexia (90%); vein irritation; anaphylaxis (rare); facial flushing (occasionally); paresthesias	Myelosuppression: leukopenia (30–50%), thrombocytopenia (30–50%) (nadir day 10 to 14, recovery day 24), anemia; flu-like syndrome of fever, malaise, and myalgia; alopecia; skin rash; hepatotoxicity, elevated liver enzymes (50%); vein thrombosis, necrosis (rare)

Table 21–5. DRUG DATA *Continued*

Drug and Availability*	Storage and Stability	Administration	Toxicity—Acute	Toxicity—Delayed
DACTINOMYCIN (Actinomycin D, Cosmegen) Injection: 0.5-mg vial	Unreconstituted: Room temperature Reconstituted: Use immediately Other: Light sensitive	Isolated perfusion, IVP, IV infusion	Nausea and vomiting, mild (80%), moderate to severe (20%); drug fever; anaphylaxis (rare)	Myelosuppression: leukopenia (55%), thrombocytopenia (47%), anemia (50%) (nadir day 14 to 21, recovery day 21 to 28); dermatologic reactions: follicular acne (80–90%), erythema, desquamation, hyperpigmentation (occasional), rash, reversible alopecia (47%); inflammation and ulceration of oral and GI mucosa (5–30%); diarrhea (3–5%); radiation recall (common); gonadal suppression: amenorrhea, azoospermia
DAUNORUBICIN (Cerubidine, DNR, daunomycin, rubidomycin) Injection: 20-mg vial	Unreconstituted: Room temperature Reconstituted: Room temperature, 24 hr; refrigeration, 48 hr Diluted: Room temperature, 24 hr Other: Light sensitive	IVP, IV infusion	Nausea and vomiting (50%); fever and chills (33%); local irritation (occasional)	Myelosuppression: leukopenia (90%) (nadir day 8 to 10, recovery day 21), thrombocytopenia (90%) (nadir day 4 to 15, recovery day 15 to 21); alopecia (90%); phlebitis (30%); diarrhea (25%); gonadal suppression: azoospermia (25%), amenorrhea (40%); stomatitis (15%); skin rash (6%); cardiotoxicity: arrhythmias (30%), CHF (2–5%), cardiomyopathy (1%); hyperuricemia; radiation recall reaction; nail changes (occasional)
DIETHYLSTILBESTROL (DES, stilbestrol) Tablets: 0.1 mg, 0.25 mg, 0.5 mg, 1 mg, and 5 mg (regular or enteric-coated) Other: Also available as cream, lotion, powder, or suppositories Diethystilbestrol diphosphate (Stilphostrol, fosfestrol) Tablets: 50 mg Injection: 250 mg/5 ml ampules	Tablets: Room temperature Injection: Room temperature Diluted: Room temperature, 24 hr Other: Light sensitive Protect from freezing	PO, IM, IV infusion, topical, and intravaginal	Diarrhea (12%); nausea (9%); anorexia (3%); vomiting (2%); headache (1%); glucose intolerance	Gynecomastia (80%), breast tenderness (69%); elevated liver function test results (37%); fluid retention (18%); thromboembolic disorders (18%), thrombophlebitis (7%), pulmonary emboli (5%); skin pigment changes (3%); lassitude (3%), mental depression (2%); hypercalcemia (10%)
DOXORUBICIN (ADR, Adriamycin) Injection: 10-mg and 50-mg vials	Unreconstituted: Room temperature Reconstituted: Room temperature, 24 hr; refrigeration, 48 hr Diluted: Room temperature, 24 hr; refrigeration, 48 hr Other: Light sensitive	Intra-arterial, intraperitoneal, IVP, IV infusion, intravesicular	Nausea and vomiting (45%); cardiotoxicity: ECG changes and arrhythmias (33%); lacrimation (25%); phlebitis (5–10%); fever and chills (5%); anaphylaxis (rare); local skin reactions (3%)	Myelosuppression: leukopenia (100%) (nadir day 10 to 14, recovery day 21), thrombocytopenia (30–40%) (nadir day 14, recovery day 21 to 24), anemia (nadir day 14, recovery day 21); reversible alopecia (85–100%); stomatitis (75%); cardiotoxicity: CHF (1–31%, cumulative dose dependent); radiation recall reaction; hyperuricemia; gonadal suppression: amenorrhea, azoospermia; hyperpigmentation (10%); nail changes
ESTRAMUSTINE (Emcyt) Capsules: 140 mg	Refrigerate Light sensitive	PO	Nausea (16%); diarrhea (13%); gastrointestinal upset (12%); hypertension; glucose intolerance	Gynecomastia (76%), breast tenderness (71%); hepatotoxicity: elevated liver function test results (38%); fluid retention (20%); hypercalcemia

Table continued on following page

Table 21–5. DRUG DATA *Continued*

Drug and Availability*	Storage and Stability	Administration	Toxicity—Acute	Toxicity—Delayed
ETOPOSIDE (VePesid, VP-16-213) Injection: 50 mg/2.5-ml vial, 100 mg/5-ml vial Capsules: 50 mg	Capsules: Room temperature Injection: Unreconstituted: Room temperature Diluted: Room temperature for either 96 hr (0.2 mg/ml) or 48 hr (0.4 mg/ml)	IV infusion, PO	Nausea and vomiting (31%); diarrhea (13%); anorexia (13%); anaphylactic-like reactions (2%); hypotension (2%); stomatitis (1%)	Myelosuppression: leukopenia (60%) (nadir day 7 to 14, recovery day 20), thrombocytopenia (28%) (nadir day 9 to 16, recovery day 20); alopecia (20%); hepatotoxicity (3%); CNS toxicity (somnolence and fatigue) (3%); peripheral neuropathy (paresthesias) (0.7%)
FLOXURIDINE (FUDR) Injection: 500-mg vial	Unreconstituted: Room temperature Reconstituted: Refrigerated, 14 days Diluted: Room temperature, 24 hr	Intra-arterial, IV infusion	Gastrointestinal toxicity: gastritis (60%), abdominal pain (30%), diarrhea (15%), nausea and vomiting, anorexia; stomatitis (56%); erythema at injection site; fever; CNS toxicity: lethargy, malaise, weakness	Hepatotoxicity, elevated liver function test results (54%), hepatitis (23%); gastrointestinal ulceration (8%); myelosuppression: leukopenia (57%) (nadir day 21, recovery day 30), thrombocytopenia, anemia; alopecia; skin rash (10%), photosensitivity, hyperpigmentation
FLUOROURACIL (5-FU, 5-fluorouracil) Injection: 500 mg/10-ml vial (Fluorouracil, Adrucil) Topicals: 1% cream and 1% solution (Fluoroplex); 2% and 5% solutions, and 5% cream (Efudex)	Undiluted: Room temperature Diluted: Room temperature, 36 hr Other: Do not refrigerate or freeze; light sensitive	PO, IVP, IV infusion, topical	Nausea and vomiting (20% with weekly schedule, 50–90% with high-dose schedule); anorexia (30–50%); cardiotoxicity (ECG changes) (1.7%)	Myelosuppression: leukopenia (100%) (nadir day 9 to 14, recovery day 21 to 25), thrombocytopenia (nadir day 7 to 17, recovery day 30); oral and gastrointestinal ulceration (4–8%, weekly; 60–75%, high-dose); diarrhea (5%, weekly; 30–80%, high-dose); alopecia (5–10%, weekly; 5–50%, high-dose); excessive lacrimation (30%); dermatologic reactions: scaling (10–20%), rash (5%), hyperpigmentation (frequent); radiation recall (frequent); cerebellar ataxia (5%); gonadal suppression: amenorrhea, azoospermia; nail changes (occasional)
FLUOXYMESTERONE (Halotestin) Tablets: 2 mg, 5 mg, and 10 mg	Room temperature Protect from light	PO	Nausea (30–40%); headache; anaphylaxis (rare)	Virilization (56%); fluid retention and electrolyte imbalance (50%); hypercalcemia (10%); hepatotoxicity (9%); elevated liver function test results, cholestatic jaundice, hepatic neoplasms, peliosis hepatis; menstrual irregularities, gynecomastia
GOSERELIN ACETATE (Zoladex) Injection: Device 3.6 mg sustained release/28 days	Room temperature	SC	Pain at injection site	Hot flashes (62%), sexual dysfunction (21%), decreased erections (18%), lower urinary tract symptoms (13%), lethargy (8%), pain flare (8% in first 30 days of treatment), edema (7%), rash (6%), diaphoresis (6%), CHF (5%), anorexia (5%), dizziness (5%), insomnia (5%), nausea (5%), hypertension, acute MI, chest pain, CVA, arrhythmia, peripheral vascular symptoms (1–5%), anxiety, depression, headache (1–5%), constipation, diarrhea, vomiting, ulcer (1–5%), anemia (1–5%), gout, hyperuricemia, weight gain (1–5%), chills, fever (1–5%), urinary obstruction, UTI (1–5%), breast swelling, tenderness (1–5%)

Table 21–5. DRUG DATA *Continued*

Drug and Availability*	Storage and Stability	Administration	Toxicity—Acute	Toxicity—Delayed
HYDROXYUREA (Hydrea) Capsules: 500 mg Injection: 2-g vial, INVESTIGATIONAL	Capsules: Room temperature Unreconstituted: Room temperature Reconstituted: Refrigeration, 72 hr	IVP, IV infusion, PO	Nausea and vomiting (25%); dermatologic reactions (20%): rash, facial erythema (occasional), pruritus; diarrhea (10%); constipation; anorexia	Myelosuppression (nadir day 7, recovery day 14 to 21): leukopenia (70%), thrombocytopenia (20%), anemia (34%), megaloblastosis (90%); reversible alopecia (frequent); neurologic disturbances: headache, dizziness, disorientation, hallucinations, convulsions; stomatitis (occasional); hyperuricemia; nail changes (occasional); radiation recall reaction (frequent); drug fever; gonadal suppression: amenorrhea, azoospermia
IFOSFAMIDE (Isophosphamide) Injection: 1-g and 3-g vials	Unreconstituted: Room temperature Reconstituted: Room temperature, 7 days; refrigeration, 6 weeks Diluted: Diluted to a concentration between 0.6 mg/ml and 16 mg/ml: room temperature, 7 days; refrigeration, 6 weeks Other: Will liquefy at temperatures above 35° C	IVP, IV infusion	Nausea and vomiting (10–15%); hematuria, gross and microscopic (50%)	Myelosuppression: leukopenia (12%) (nadir day 10, recovery day 18), thrombocytopenia (6%); hemorrhagic cystitis (29%), acute tubular necrosis (high doses); reversible alopecia (50%); neurotoxicity at high doses (10%), lethargy, convulsions; hepatic enzyme elevations
INTERFERON-αA-2a (IFN-αA, I Roferon-AFLA) Injection: 3 MU/1-ml and 18 MU/3-ml vials	Refrigeration Do not freeze Room temperature, 24 hr	IV, IM, SC Intraperitoneal	Fever (98%); fatigue (89%); myalgias (73%); headache (71%); chills (64%); anorexia (46%); nausea (32%), diarrhea (29%); vomiting (10%); hypotension (6%)	Myelosuppression: leukopenia (69%) (nadir day 22), thrombocytopenia (42%) (nadir day 17), neutropenia (58%); hepatotoxicity: SGOT (78%), alkaline phosphatase (48%), LDH (47%), bilirubin (31%); nephrotoxicity: proteinuria (25%), elevated uric acid (15%), elevated serum creatinine (10%), elevated BUN (10%); hypocalcemia (51%); elevated FBS (39%); elevated serum phosphorus (17%); dizziness (21%); confusion (10%); paresthesias (6%); numbness (6%); lethargy (3%); edema (3%); hypertension (<3%); chest pain (<3%); arrhythmias (<3%); skin rash (18%); dryness or inflammation of the oropharynx (16%); dry skin or pruritus (13%); partial alopecia (8%); weight loss (14%); change in taste (13%); diaphoresis (8%); transient impotence (6%); arthralgia (5%); inflammation at injection site (rare)
INTERFERON-α A-2b (IFN-α2; IFN-2; 2-interferon, Intron A) Injection: 3-MU, 5-MU, 10-MU, and 25-MU vials	Unreconstituted: Refrigeration, 24 months Reconstituted: Refrigeration, 30 days; room temperature, 24 hr	IV, IM, SC Intraperitoneal	"Flu-like" symptoms: fever, chills, fatigue, malaise, tachycardia, myalgias, and headache (98%); nausea (46%); vomiting (29%); hypotension (14%); hypertension (3%); diarrhea (27%)	Myelosuppression: leukopenia (18%), thrombocytopenia (18%), granulocytopenia (20%), anemia (4%); hepatotoxicity: elevated SGOT and SGPT (10%), elevated alkaline phosphatase (6%), elevated lactic dehydrogenase (3%); elevated BUN (1%); CNS effects: somnolence (14%), confusion (12%), coma (rare); arrhythmia or tachycardia (3%); skin rash (12%)

Table continued on following page

Table 21–5. DRUG DATA *Continued*

Drug and Availability*	Storage and Stability	Administration	Toxicity—Acute	Toxicity—Delayed
LEUCOVORIN (leucovorin calcium, folinic acid, citrovorum factor, Wellcovorin, 5-formyl-tetrahydrofolate) Tablets: 5 mg and 25 mg Injection: 3-mg/1 ml ampule; 50-mg vial; 5 mg/1 ml, 1-ml and 5-ml ampules	Tablets: Room temperature Unreconstituted: Room temperature Reconstituted: Preserved, 7 days; unpreserved, use immediately (or within 8 hr) Diluted: 24 hr Other: Light sensitive; protect from freezing	IM, PO, IVP, IV infusion	Hypersensitivity reactions (rare)	None reported; delayed toxicities of stomatitis, mucositis, diarrhea occur from use in combination with antimetabolites
LEUPROLIDE (leuprolide acetate, Lupron, Lupron depot) Injection: 5 mg/ml and 14 mg/2.8-ml vials	Refrigerate until dispensed Store unrefrigerated solution below 30° C Protect vial from light—store vial in carton until use	SC, IM (depot only)	Vasomotor hot flashes (40–70%); increased bone pain (10%); myalgia (<3%); renal disturbances: hematuria, dysuria, flank pain, polyuria, increased BUN and serum creatinine (<3%); CNS disturbances: dizziness (6%), pain (5%), headache (5%), paresthesia (3%); blurred vision, lethargy, insomnia, memory disorder, sour taste, numbness (<3%); gastrointestinal: anorexia (2%), constipation (3%), nausea and vomiting (5%); erythema, ecchymosis, and irritation at the injection site (occasional)	Impotence and decreased libido (frequent); gynecomastia or breast tenderness (3%); amenorrhea or vaginal bleeding (occasional); testicular atrophy (<3%); cardiovascular: peripheral edema (8%), congestive heart failure (1%), thrombophlebitis, phlebitis, or pulmonary embolus (1%); respiratory effects: difficulty in breathing, pleural rub, worsening of pulmonary fibrosis (rare); decreased hematocrit and hemoglobin (<3%); asthenia (<3%); fatigue (<3%); fever (<3%); facial swelling (<3%); rash (<3%); hives (<3%); hair loss (<3%); itching (<3%)
LOMUSTINE (CCNU, CeeNU) Capsules: 10 mg, 40 mg, and 100 mg	Room temperature Avoid storage temperature above 40° C	PO	Nausea and vomiting (90%); anorexia	Myelosuppression: leukopenia (65%) (nadir day 42, recovery day 49 to 56), thrombocytopenia (90%) (nadir day 28, recovery day 35 to 42), anemia (nadir 4 to 7 weeks); hepatotoxicity: elevated transaminase levels (35%); stomatitis (frequent); alopecia; pulmonary fibrosis; renal toxicity
MECHLORETHAMINE (nitrogen mustard, HN$_2$, Mustargen) Injection: 10-mg vial	Unreconstituted: Room temperature Reconstituted: Use immediately (within 1 hr) Other: Less stable in neutral or alkaline solutions	Intracavitary, intralesional, IVP, topical	Nausea and vomiting (95%); fever and chills (30–40%); diarrhea (10%); anorexia; weakness; headache; skin rash (occasional); metallic taste; phlebitis; anaphylaxis (rare); stomatitis (frequent)	Myelosuppression: leukopenia (100%) (nadir day 10, recovery day 21 to 28), thrombocytopenia (100%) (nadir day 10, recovery day 21 to 28); gonadal suppression: amenorrhea (79%), azoospermia (88%); alopecia (75%); hyperuricemia
MEDROXYPROGES-TERONE ACETATE (Provera, Amen, Curretab) Injection: 100 mg/ml, 5-ml vials; 400 mg/ml, 2.5-ml and 10-ml vials; 400 mg/1-ml syringes (Depo-Provera) Tablets: 2.5 mg and 10 mg	Injection: Room temperature; protect from freezing Tablets: Room temperature	IM, PO	Sterile abscesses (30%); nausea (10–20%); glucose intolerance (7%); local pain at injection site; anorexia; CNS toxicity: headache, dizziness, fatigue, insomnia, somnolence, nervousness	Fluid retention (30%), cushingoid facies (26%), weight gain (25%); hypercalcemia (10%); rash (7%); thromboembolic disorders; menstrual irregularities; alopecia; photosensitivity; skin pigment changes; hepatotoxicity: jaundice, elevated liver function tests; breast tenderness, galactorrhea; depression
MEGESTROL ACETATE (Megace, Pallace) Tablets: 20 mg and 40 mg	Room temperature	PO	None reported	Weight gain (10–20%); fluid retention (10–20%)

Table 21–5. DRUG DATA *Continued*

Drug and Availability*	Storage and Stability	Administration	Toxicity—Acute	Toxicity—Delayed
MELPHALAN (PAM, L-PAM, phenylalanine mustard, L-sarcolysin, Alkeran) Tablets: 2 mg Injection: 100-mg vial, INVESTIGATIONAL	Tablets: Room temperataure Injection: Unreconstituted: Room temperature below 25° C, or refrigeration Reconstituted: Room temperature, 15 to 30 min Diluted: Room temperature, 15 to 30 min Other: Light sensitive	Regional perfusion, IV, PO	Nausea and vomiting (high dose: 30%; divided doses: 10%); diarrhea (10%); hypersensitivity reactions (2.4%)	Myelosuppression: leukopenia (65%) (nadir day 21 to 25, recovery day 28 to 42), thrombocytopenia (75%) (nadir day 21 to 25, recovery day 28 to 42), anemia (75%) (nadir day 8 to 10, recovery day 42 to 50); alopecia (4%); stomatitis (1%); pulmonary pneumonitis and fibrosis (rare); skin rash; hyperuricemia; gonadal suppression: amenorrhea, azoospermia; nail changes (occasional)
MERCAPTOPURINE (6-mercaptopurine, 6MP, Purinethol) Tablets: 50 mg Injection: 500-mg vial, INVESTIGATIONAL	Tablets: Room temperature Injection: Unreconstituted: Room temperature Reconstituted: Room temperature, 21 days Diluted: Room temperature, 3 days Other: Light sensitive	IVP, IV infusion, PO	Nausea and vomiting (25%); anorexia (25%); drug fever (5%); diarrhea	Myelosuppression: leukopenia (nadir day 14, recovery day 21, thrombocytopenia (nadir day 14, recovery day 21), anemia; hepatotoxicity: cholestatic jaundice (33%), elevated transaminases (15%), hepatic necrosis (rare); skin rash (5–10%); stomatitis (rare); depressed cellular immunity; radiation recall (occasional); pulmonary interstitial fibrosis (rare); gonadal suppression: amenorrhea, azoospermia
METHOTREXATE (MTX, amethopterin, Mexate) Tablets: 2.5 mg Injection: Preserved and preservative-free: 5 mg/2-ml, 50 mg/2-ml, 100 mg/4-ml, and 200 mg/8-ml vials Powder for injection: Preservative-free: 20-mg, 50-mg, 100-mg, and 250-mg vials INVESTIGATIONAL FORMS: Powder for injection (preservative free): 50-mg and 1-g vials Tablet: 50 mg	Tablets: Room temperature Injections: Room temperature Unreconstituted: Room temperature Reconstituted: Room temperature, 7 days Diluted: Room temperature, 7 days	Intra-arterial, intrathecal, IVP, IV infusion, PO, IM	Nausea and vomiting (low-dose, 10%; high-dose, 65%); hypersensitivity reactions (10%); diarrhea (5–10%)	Myelosuppression: leukopenia (30%) (first nadir day 4 to 7, recovery day 7 to 13; second nadir day 12 to 21, recovery day 15 to 29), thrombocytopenia (30%) (nadir day 5 to 7, recovery day 15 to 27), anemia (nadir day 6 to 13); stomatitis (10–40%); hepatotoxicity: elevated transaminase levels (20%), periportal fibrosis (27%), cirrhosis (19%); conjunctivitis (14%); skin rash (10% with high doses); alopecia (5–10%); gastrointestinal ulceration (5%); renal failure (5% with high doses); pneumonitis (1%); hyperpigmentation (occasional); radiation recall (frequent); depressed cellular immunity; hyperuricemia; gonadal suppression: amenorrhea, azoospermia
MITOMYCIN (mitomycin-C, MTC, MMC, Mutamycin) Injection: 5-mg and 20-mg vials	Unreconstituted: Room temperature Reconstituted: Room temperature, 7 days; refrigeration, 14 days Diluted: In D₅W, 3 hr; in 0.9% NaCl, 12 hr; in sodium lactate, 24 hr (solution concentration, 20–40 μg/ml) Other: Light sensitive	Intra-arterial, intravesicular, IVP, IV infusion	Nausea and vomiting (75%); diarrhea (20%); anorexia (14%); fever (14%)	Myelosuppression: leukopenia (50%) (nadir day 25, recovery day 32 to 39), thrombocytopenia (40%) (nadir day 28, recovery day 42 to 49), anemia (3%); stomatitis (20%); pulmonary toxicity (5–12%): dyspnea with nonproductive cough, pulmonary infiltrates; skin rash (5–10%); nephrotoxicity (1–10%): elevated BUN and serum creatinine (2%), glomerular sclerosis; hemolytic uremic syndrome; general debilitation; cardiotoxicity: CHF; nail banding (rare)

Table continued on following page

Table 21–5. DRUG DATA *Continued*

Drug and Availability*	Storage and Stability	Administration	Toxicity—Acute	Toxicity—Delayed
MITOTANE (o,p'-DDD, Lysodren) Tablets: 500 mg	Room temperature Light sensitive	PO	Nausea (80%); vomiting (80%); diarrhea (80%); anorexia (80%); skin rash (15%); visual disturbances (3%)	Hypouricemia (100%); hyperlipoproteinemia (55%); CNS effects (40%): decreased memory (50%), lethargy and somnolence (25%), dizziness or vertigo (15%), mental depression; arthralgia (19%); gynecomastia (17%); leukopenia (7%)
MITOXANTRONE (DHAD, dihydroxyanthracenedione dihydrochloride, Novantrone) Injection: 10 mg/5-ml, 20 mg/10-ml, and 30 mg/15-ml ampules	Undiluted: Room temperature Diluted: Room temperature, 48 hr Other: Storage under refrigeration may cause formation of a precipitate, which will redissolve on warming to room temperature	IV infusion	Nausea (31%); vomiting (19%); drug fever (42%)	Myelosuppression: leukopenia (50%) (nadir day 10 to 12, recovery day 21), anemia (17%), thrombocytopenia (12%) (nadir day 8 to 16, recovery day 21); elevated liver function tests (33%); mucositis (25%); alopecia (20%); diarrhea (10%); cardiotoxicity
PLICAMYCIN (Mithracin) Injection: 2.5-mg vial	Unreconstituted: Refrigeration Reconstituted: Room temperature, use immediately Diluted: Room temperature, 4 to 6 hr	IV infusion	Nausea and vomiting (90%); fever (15–83%); facial flushing (3%); diarrhea (2%); anorexia	Myelosuppression (nadir day 5 to 10, recovery day 10 to 18): thrombocytopenia, leukopenia (6%); hepatotoxicity: elevated enzyme levels (90%), necrosis; dermatologic reactions (33%): facial blushing, thickening of facial features; nephrotoxicity: proteinuria (20–40%), elevated BUN and serum creatinine (20–40%), tubular necrosis (20%); stomatitis (15%); nervousness, irritability (6–75%); bleeding syndrome (5–12%); hypocalcemia; metallic taste; reversible alopecia
PREDNISONE Tablets: 1 mg, 2.5 mg, 5 mg, 10 mg, 20 mg, 25 mg, and 50 mg Syrup: 5 mg/5 ml	Room temperature	PO	Gastrointestinal distress	HPA axis suppression: Cushing's disease (depression, moon facies, truncal obesity, striae, bruises, muscle weakness); fluid and electrolyte disturbances; increased appetite; impaired wound healing; masked signs of infection; decreased glucose tolerance; mental disturbances ranging from euphoria to psychoses; acne; osteoporosis
PROCARBAZINE (Matulane) Capsules: 50 mg	Room temperature Protect from moisture	PO	Nausea and vomiting (75–95%); anorexia (75%); diarrhea (10%); hypersensitivity reactions; skin rash (5%); urticaria (5%); pneumonitis (rare)	Myelosuppression: leukopenia (100%) (nadir day 25 to 36, recovery day 36 to 50), thrombocytopenia (100%) (nadir day 21, recovery day 28), anemia (5%); alopecia (18%); CNS depression (10%); stomatitis (6–10%); peripheral neuropathy (5%); interstitial pneumonitis and fibrosis (rare); gonadal suppression: amenorrhea, azoospermia

Table 21–5. DRUG DATA *Continued*

Drug and Availability*	Storage and Stability	Administration	Toxicity—Acute	Toxicity—Delayed
STREPTOZOCIN (STZ, Zanosar) Injection: 1-g vial	Unreconstituted: Refrigeration Reconstituted: Refrigeration, 96 hr; room temperature, 48 hr Diluted: Refrigeration, 96 hr; room temperature, 48 hr Other: Protect from light	Intra-arterial, IVP, IV infusion	Nausea and vomiting (90%); diarrhea; glucose intolerance (6–60%); local necrosis (occasional)	Nephrotoxicity (65%): proteinuria (50–73%), tubular necrosis (30–40%); hypophosphatemia (25%); azotemia; glycosuria (80%); renal tubular acidosis (25%); hepatotoxicity: elevated liver function tests (67%), hypoalbuminemia, jaundice; myelosuppression: anemia (20%), leukopenia (5%) (nadir day 14, recovery day 21), thrombocytopenia (5%) (nadir day 14, recovery day 21)
TAMOXIFEN (Nolvadex) Tablets: 10 mg	Room temperature Protect from light and heat	PO	Nausea and vomiting (10–20%); hot flashes (25%); headache	Myelosuppression: leukopenia, transient (10%) (nadir day 10), thrombocytopenia, transient (10%) (nadir day 12), anemia (26%); lethargy (26%); bone and tumor pain (20%); sodium and fluid retention (80–90%); skin rash (4%); menstrual irregularities (2%); hypercalcemia (2%); hypercoagulability
TESTOLACTONE (Teslac) Injection: 500-mg vial Tablets: 50 mg	Injection: Room temperature; protect from freezing Tablets: Room temperature	PO, IM	Nausea and vomiting (30–40%); diarrhea (8%); anorexia; increased blood pressure	Sodium and fluid retention (50%); hypercalcemia (10%); paresthesias; skin rash; glossitis; alopecia; nail growth disturbance; hepatotoxicity: jaundice
THIOGUANINE (6-TG, 6-thioguanine) Tablets: 40 mg Injection: 75-mg vial, INVESTIGATIONAL	Tablets: Room temperature Injection: Unreconstituted: Refrigeration Reconstituted: Refrigeration, 24 hr Diluted: Room temperature, 24 hr; refrigeration, 24 hr	IV, PO	Nausea and vomiting (16%); anorexia; stomatitis; diarrhea; rash	Myelosuppression: leukopenia (100%) (nadir day 14 to 28), thrombocytopenia (100%) (nadir day 14, recovery day 21), anemia; hepatotoxicity: elevated liver function tests (11%), cholestatic jaundice (6%); veno-occlusive disease; hyperuricemia; decreased vibrational sensitivity; unsteady gait; gonadal suppression: amenorrhea, azoospermia
THIO-TEPA (Triethylenethiophosphoramide, TSPA, TESPA) Injection: 15-mg vial	Unreconstituted: Refrigeration Reconstituted: Refrigeration, 5 days Diluted: Room temperature, 24 hr	Intravesicular, intra-arterial, intratumor, intrathecal, intracavitary, ophthalmic; IVP, IV infusion, topical	Local pain (10–20%); nausea and vomiting (10–15%); anorexia; stomatitis; dizziness; tightness of throat; hypersensitivity reactions (rare): hives, skin rash, anaphylaxis	Myelosuppression: thrombocytopenia (80%), anemia (50%) (nadir day 14, recovery day 28), leukopenia (40%); hyperuricemia; alopecia (occasional); gonadal suppression: amenorrhea, azoospermia; hyperpigmentation (occasional)
VINBLASTINE (VLB, Velban) Injection: 10-mg vial Tablets: 5 mg, INVESTIGATIONAL	Tablets: Refrigeration Injection: Unreconstituted: Refrigeration Reconstituted: refrigeration, 30 days Diluted: Room temperature, 24 hr Other: Light sensitive	IVP, IV infusion, PO	Nausea and vomiting (20%); anorexia (20%); headache; paresthesias (10%); jaw pain (10%); diarrhea or constipation (20%); fever; local necrosis (occasional)	Myelosuppression (nadir day 5 to 9, recovery day 14 to 21): leukopenia (100%) (nadir day 5 to 10, recovery day 12 to 24), thrombocytopenia (100%), anemia (50%) (nadir day 10, recovery day 17); neurotoxicity (10–20%): peripheral neuritis, numbness, areflexia (10%); depression; convulsions; dermatologic effects: phototoxicity, dermatitis, reversible alopecia (occasional); stomatitis (frequent); hyperuricemia; gonadal suppression: amenorrhea, azoospermia

Table continued on following page

Table 21–5. DRUG DATA *Continued*

Drug and Availability*	Storage and Stability	Administration	Toxicity—Acute	Toxicity—Delayed
VINCRISTINE (Oncovin, VCR) Injection: 1 mg/1-ml, 2 mg/2-ml, and 5 mg/5-ml vials	Undiluted: Refrigeration Diluted: Room temperature, 24 hr; refrigeration, 24 hr	IVP, IV infusion	Nausea (6%); jaw pain; fever; local vein irritation (occasional)	Peripheral neuritis (100%); areflexia (50–100%); reversible alopecia (90%); bowel dysfunction (33%); paralytic ileus (5–10%); myelosuppression (nadir day 4 to 5, recovery day 7), leukopenia (5%); stomatitis (frequent); SIADH (rare); hyperuricemia; gonadal suppression: amenorrhea, azoospermia

This information is adapted from Grant Medical Center (1987). *Chemotherapy: A data compendium.* It is intended to provide a reference to specific agents, addressing drug names, availability, storage and stability, administration, and toxicity.

PO, oral; IVP, intravenous push; IV, intravenous; IM, intramuscular; D₅W, 5% dextrose in water; SC, subcutaneous; BUN, blood urea nitrogen; SGOT, serum glutamic-oxaloacetic transaminase; SIADH, syndrome of inappropriate secretion of antidiuretic hormone; CHF, congestive heart failure; CNS, central nervous system; ECG, electrocardiogram; LDH, lactic dehydrogenase; FBS, fasting blood sugar; SGPT, serum glutamic-pyruvate transaminase; HPA, hypothalamic-pituitary-adrenal axis; MU, million units; CSF, cerebrospinal fluid; MI, myocardial infarction; CVA, cardiovascular accident; UTI, urinary tract infection.

*Explanation and interpretation of format is as follows, using aminoglutethimide as an example:

Aminoglutethimide is also known as Cytadren (drugs may have more than one generic name), and is available in 250-mg tablets. It may be stored at room temperature. Administration is by mouth. Acute toxicities include drowsiness, occurring in 40% of patients receiving it. Delayed toxicities include hypothyroidism, which occurs occasionally.

The information relative to stability and toxicity has been compiled from a variety of sources; in this changing field of medical oncology, data are subject to constant change. The reader should update them with current sources.

those of heavy metal poisoning: nephrotoxicity, peripheral neuropathy, seizures, ototoxicity, and anemia. Concomitant administration of fluids and maintenance of adequate urinary output during, and immediately after, administration is imperative to avoid renal damage. The peripheral neuropathy associated with cisplatin is cumulative and may worsen after the drug is discontinued. Hypomagnesemia and hypocalcemia may occur from renal tubular damage; oral and intravenous supplementation may be utilized (Gonzalez & Villasanta, 1982; McCauley, Begent, Phillips, & Newlands, 1982). Concomitant administration of intravenous magnesium may prevent this toxicity. Less frequently, hypophosphatemia, hypokalemia, and other manifestations of renal tubular damage (Fanconi's syndrome–like picture) may occur and require dietary supplements.

The platinum complexes have rendered nonseminomatous testicular cancer curable and have prolonged survival in other tumors. Cisplatin is used in many solid tumors; its use is currently being extended to non-Hodgkin's lymphomas. Clinically active analogues

have been synthesized. Carboplatinum and iproplatinum are being studied and may be less emetogenic, nephrotoxic, and neurotoxic but of equal efficacy (Rose & Schurig, 1985).

The selection of alkylators for clinical use must consider the patient's hepatic function (biotransformation), renal function (excretion), bone marrow reserves (myelosuppression), and inherent alkylator sensitivity of the tumor. Because of the mutagenic, teratogenic, and carcinogenic capabilities of alkylators, patient age and childbearing capability should also be considered (Kyle, 1982).

Plant Alkaloids

The plant alkaloids are so named because they are extracted from foliage. Clinically efficacious agents are listed in Table 21–7.

The vinca alkaloids are extracted from the periwinkle plant (*Vinca rosea*). These cell cycle–specific, phase-specific compounds arrest mitosis (M); in addition,

Table 21–6. CHEMICAL CLASSES OF ALKYLATING AGENTS

Class	Agents	Clinical Use
Mustard derivatives	Mechlorethamine Cyclophosphamide Chlorambucil Melphalan Ifosfamide	Hodgkin's disease, non-Hodgkin's lymphoma, chronic leukemias, acute lymphocytic leukemia, myeloma, cancers of breast, ovary, skin, lung
Ethylenimines	Thiotepa	Breast, bladder cancers (intravesicular)
Alkyl sulfonates	Busulfan	Chronic myelogenous leukemia
Triazenes	Dacarbazine derivatives	Melanoma, Hodgkin's disease, sarcoma
Nitrosoureas	BCNU, CCNU, methyl-CCNU* Streptozocin	Myeloma, Hodgkin's disease, non-Hodgkin's lymphoma, melanoma, gastric cancer
Metal salts	Carboplatinum Cisplatin	Lung, testis, ovary, head and neck, colon cancers

*Investigational.

Table 21–7. PLANT ALKALOIDS

Class	Agents	Clinical Use
Vinca alkaloids	Vincristine Vinblastine	Acute leukemia, Hodgkin's disease, non-Hodgkin's lymphoma, myeloma, Burkitt's lymphoma, breast cancer, Wilms' tumor, testicular cancer, myeloma
Podophyllotoxins	Etoposide VM-26*	Non-Hodgkin's lymphoma, acute myelogenous leukemia, acute lymphoblastic leukemia, testicular and lung cancers

*Investigational.

they also inhibit DNA synthesis (S) and RNA synthesis (G_2). Although they are chemically similar, vincristine and vinblastine are non-cross-resistant and exhibit a difference in spectrum of efficacy and toxicity.

Both vincristine and vinblastine are administered intravenously and are vesicants (see Chapter 22). Continuous infusions of these agents are being investigated to determine if increasing exposure to increasing numbers of cells in the M phase will increase tumor cell kill (Guy et al., in press; Yap et al., 1980). Because they are vesicants, administration via a central line is recommended. Neurotoxicity, manifested acutely as constipation, urinary retention, and jaw pain (the latter uncommon), occurs with both drugs but is more prevalent with vincristine. Peripheral neuritis occurs with cumulative doses; its onset is heralded by paresthesias of the fingers and toes, which can progress to generalized sensorimotor weakness. This neuropathy generally is reversible and disappears once the drug is discontinued but may take months to abate. Bone marrow suppression and gastrointestinal toxicity (nausea, vomiting, mucositis) are more frequent with vinblastine.

Podophyllotoxins, derived from the May apple plant, act in the M phase to inhibit mitosis and in the G_2 phase to inhibit entry into the M phase. These cycle- and phase-specific agents can also act in the late G_2 and S phases, similar to the vinca extracts. Etoposide is effective in testicular cancer and lung cancer (small-cell and non-small-cell); recently its use has expanded to the hematologic malignancies. Intravenous administration may be associated with significant hypotension, necessitating monitoring of blood pressure. Slowing the infusion rate prevents clinically significant hypotensive events. An oral form of etoposide has recently been marketed; hypotension does not occur with oral administration.

The podophyllotoxins are extensively protein bound. Hemolytic anemia has been reported. Monitoring of serial hemoglobin levels, urine occult blood, and Coombs' test may identify this uncommon reaction (Habibi et al., 1982).

The plant alkaloids are metabolized hepatically and excreted by both the liver and the kidney. Because they are natural products, allergic reactions are known to occur, including anaphylaxis.

Antitumor Antibiotics

Species of the soil fungus *Streptomyces* produce natural products with antineoplastic activity called antitumor antibiotics (Table 21–8).

The anthracyclines act in multiple phases of the cell cycle and are considered cell cycle specific, phase nonspecific. Their action on DNA (intercalation) interferes with DNA synthesis and DNA-directed production of RNA and DNA. The anthracyclines are biotransformed to their active metabolites in the liver; they exhibit tissue binding and a prolonged half-life. Excretion is primarily hepatic. Pretherapy liver dysfunction may preclude their use or mandate dose reductions. Anthracyclines are vesicants and are administered intravenously. Treatment of anthracycline extravasation remains under investigation (see Chapter 22). Traditionally, the anthracycline antibiotics have been administered on an intermittent bolus schedule; however, weekly low-dose administration of doxorubicin has been shown to have equal efficacy with less toxicity (cardiac, gastrointestinal, alopecia) in some tumors (Legha et al., 1982; Weiss & Manthel, 1977).

The cardiotoxicity of the anthracyclines is dose limiting. The mechanism is a direct effect on the myocardium, resulting in left ventricular hypertrophy and a clinical cardiomyopathy, which may be manifested as congestive heart failure (Unverferth et al., 1981). For doxorubicin, the incidence is 10 per cent at doses in excess of 550 mg/m². Research is ongoing to find agents that protect the myocardium; continuous infusions may decrease the incidence of anthracycline-induced cardiotoxicity (Legha et al., 1982). Monitoring is accomplished with baseline and serial electrocardiograms (ECGs) and measurements of left ventricular function (resting and stress multigated analysis, echocardiography); endomyocardial biopsy may be useful in selected patients (Bristow, Lopez, Mason, Billingham, & Winchester, 1982). Acute cardiotoxicities are manifested as transient ECG changes and arrhythmias, which usually occur in patients with preexisting heart disease; rarely, acute pericarditis may occur (Bristow et al., 1982; Kaszyk, 1986).

Because anthracyclines act in all phases of cell growth, they exhibit toxicities in multiple organ systems: gastrointestinal, mucosal, hair follicles, bone marrow, gonads. Their derivation from microbes predisposes to allergic reactions, which range from local cutaneous reactions to anaphylaxis. The local cutaneous reactions must be differentiated from frank extravasation.

The anthracyclines, particularly doxorubicin, are a mainstay of chemotherapy in both hematologic malignancies and solid tumors. During the last decade, efforts have been directed at the production of analogues with equivalent efficacy but less toxicity (Crossley, 1984). Mitoxantrone, recently approved by the United States Food and Drug Administration (FDA), induces significantly less toxicity (nausea, vomiting, alopecia) than doxorubicin, but the incidence of cardiotoxicity is nearly equivalent to that of doxoru-

Table 21–8. ANTIBIOTICS

Class	Agent	Clinical Use
Anthracyclines	Doxorubicin Daunomycin Mitoxantrone	Acute leukemia, Hodgkin's disease, non-Hodgkin's lymphoma, chronic lymphocytic leukemia, breast cancer, sarcoma, ovarian and lung cancers, hepatoma
Chromomycins	Dactinomycin Plicamycin	Melanoma, sarcoma, testicular cancer, choriocarcinoma, malignant hypercalcemia
Miscellaneous	Mitomycin	Colonic, rectal, gastric cancers, pancreatic adenocarcinomas, testicular, breast, cervical cancers, cloacogenic, vulvar, head and neck, bladder cancers (intravesicular), lung cancer
	Bleomycin	Hodgkin's disease, non-Hodgkin's lymphoma, melanoma, cervical, anal, head and neck cancers

bicin at equipotent doses. Mitoxantrone turns the urine blue and the serum green (Crossley, 1984).

The chromomycins act by the same mechanisms as the anthracyclines; they are cycle specific, phase nonspecific. Their chemical structure is markedly different, and they do not induce cardiotoxicity. Both available chromomycins are administered intravenously and may be associated with local and systemic allergic reactions; skin necrosis occurs with extravasation. Dactinomycin is useful in melanomas, gastrointestinal tumors, germ cell tumors, sarcoma, and lung cancer. Plicamycin is most commonly utilized in a low-dose schedule by intravenous infusion for the control of malignancy-associated hypercalcemia. Chronic administration in this situation results in bone marrow suppression and may exacerbate the myelosuppressive effect of agents given for control of the underlying malignancy. A thickening of facial features and renal and hepatotoxicity occur with chronic use for hypercalcemic control (Dorr & Fritz, 1980). Plicamycin is rarely used for its direct antitumor effects because of its significant toxicities at tumoricidal doses.

Mitomycin C must be biotransformed to an active alkylating agent. Interestingly, alkylator-resistant tumors are often sensitive to mitomycin, whereas mitomycin-resistant cells rarely are sensitive to other alkylating agents. Blue in solution, mitomycin is administered intravenously and is a known vesicant without accepted antidote. Bone marrow suppression is dose limiting and cumulative. Excretion is via the bile and kidney; a selective effect may occur on the glomerulus, resulting in renal failure. Hemolytic uremic syndrome, manifested by rising creatinine levels, elevated results of liver function tests, hemolytic anemia, and thrombocytopenia, has been described with prolonged repetitive mitomycin C administration. This syndrome is often fatal. Plasmapheresis may be used in its control (Doll & Weiss, 1985; Verway, Boven, van der Meulen, & Pinedo, 1984). Mitomycin C is used in adenocarcinomas of the gastrointestinal tract, breast cancer, and non-small-cell lung cancer.

Unlike the other antibiotics, bleomycin exerts its best effect on slowly proliferating cells, phase specifically, in G_1 (RNA and protein synthesis) and M (mitosis). It may also induce scission of the DNA strand. Agents that act by intercalation appear to potentiate its cytotoxicity; experimentally, bleomycin has been used to synchronize cells into the G_2 and S phases for attack by other phase-specific antineoplastics.

Myelosuppression from bleomycin is mild. Allergic reactions, including anaphylaxis, constitute its most clinically significant toxicity. Temperatures over 38.5° C (101° F) and chills occur acutely and may be controlled by the administration of antipyretics. Because bleomycin is concentrated in the keratin, palmar and plantar erythema, hyperpigmentation, and nail changes occur. Pulmonary fibrosis, developing from a dose-related pneumonitis, may be heralded by the development of rales and dyspnea. Pulmonary infiltrates appear on chest radiographs (Ginsberg & Comis, 1982; Seipp, 1985). Bleomycin is not a vesicant. Its primary route of administration is intravenous; topical preparations may be used in cutaneous malignancies. Intracavitary administration may control malignant effusions. The affinity of this agent for squamous epithelium has fostered its use in the treatment of tumors of this origin (cervical, head and neck, vulvular cancers, melanoma) and in Hodgkin's disease and non-Hodgkin's lymphoma.

Antimetabolites

This group exerts its effect by interrupting cellular metabolic function. These agents are structurally similar to intracellular substances; the cell incorporates them into essential sites of cellular metabolism and then is unable to continue to divide. Antimetabolites are classified by the compounds with which they interfere (Table 21–9).

Antimetabolites are phase specific in the S phase. They are most effective in tumors with a high growth fraction. The first documented cure of a malignant tumor by chemotherapy occurred with methotrexate in 1956 (Li, 1979).

Methotrexate binds the enzyme dihydrofolate reductase (DHR), making it unavailable for the conversion of folic acid to tetrahydrofolic acid, which is required for DNA, RNA, and protein synthesis; cellular growth is stopped. Because only minuscule amounts of DHR are required, sufficient amounts of methotrexate must be administered to bind all the DHR.

The inhibition of production of tetrahydrofolic acid (calcium leucovorin, folinic acid) also occurs in normal cells and thus prohibits their proliferation. Cells of the gastrointestinal mucosa and bone marrow are most commonly affected, producing mucositis of the oral

Table 21–9. ANTIMETABOLITES

Class	Agents	Clinical Use
Folic acid antagonist	Methotrexate	Acute lymphoblastic leukemia, non-Hodgkin's lymphoma, breast cancer, sarcoma, head and neck and colon cancers, choriocarcinoma, testicular and bladder cancers
Pyrimidine antagonist	5-Fluorouracil Floxuridine Cytarabine 5-Azacytidine*	Acute leukemia, chronic leukemia, and colonic, gastric, esophageal, pancreatic, pulmonary, cloacogenic, breast, and skin cancers
Purine antagonist	6-Mercaptopurine 6-Thioguanine	Acute leukemia

*Investigational.

cavity and gastrointestinal tract and bone marrow depression.

To maximize the antimetabolic effect in tumor cells without undue toxicity, variability in cell cycle times between malignant and normal cells and differential mechanisms of transport into the cells between methotrexate and tetrahydrofolate can be used to maximize the tumoricidal effects of methotrexate. Administration of high, potentially lethal doses of methotrexate may be followed by a carefully timed administration of calcium leucovorin. Ideally, methotrexate will block the production of tetrahydrofolic acid in tumor cells more rapidly than in normal cells; the subsequent administration of calcium leucovorin will then allow its differential incorporation into normal cells, allowing them to continue with normal cellular function. The result should be maximal tumor cell kill with minimal toxicity to the patient. Carefully timed administration of methotrexate and leucovorin rescue are imperative. If oral forms of calcium leucovorin are prescribed, the patient must be carefully observed for interference with its absorption (vomiting, malabsorption). If gastrointestinal absorption is compromised, parenteral administration is indicated. Serum methotrexate levels should be monitored to guide the duration and dose of leucovorin rescue. High (greater than 0.5 g/m²) and intermediate (100 mg/m²) doses of methotrexate with leucovorin rescue are used in osteogenic sarcoma, non-Hodgkin's lymphoma, head and neck tumors, soft tissue sarcomas, and breast cancer.

Methotrexate is also administered orally and intramuscularly. Intrathecal administration is useful in the prevention of leptomeningeal leukemia and in the treatment of leptomeningeal carcinomatosis (see Chapter 22). Unlike the other pyrimidine analogues, methotrexate does not require biotransformation. Its excretion is primarily renal. Renal dysfunction may exacerbate its toxicities or require reduced doses. Methotrexate precipitates in the kidney at pH of less than 5; urine alkalinization (with sodium bicarbonate, Diamox) may be utilized. Methotrexate is highly protein bound and accumulates in third-space fluids. It is bound to drugs such as salicylates, sulfonamides, tetracycline, and probenecid. Protein-bound methotrexate is released slowly, resulting in delayed toxicities. Methotrexate may be hepatotoxic, as manifested by mild elevations in liver function test results; continued administration may result in cirrhosis (Perry, 1982). Resistance to methotrexate can occur by gene amplification (Trent et al., 1984).

The pyrimidine antagonists act as irreversible enzyme inhibitors. 5-Fluorouracil (5-FU) inhibits thymidylate synthetase, which is essential for DNA synthesis. 5-Fluorouracil is metabolized in the liver to its active component after intravenous administration. Bolus and continuous infusion schedules are repeated at weekly or monthly intervals. Interest in the use of 5-FU has been piqued by constant low-dose infusion to provide an uninterrupted inhibition of thymidylate synthetase in cells advancing to the S phase (O'Connell, 1987).

The toxicities of 5-FU result from action on rapidly dividing cells with high growth fraction (bone marrow, gastrointestinal mucosa). Skin toxicity, manifested as photosensitivity, palmar and plantar erythema, and hyperpigmentation, may occur. 5-Fluorouracil may be used topically in the treatment of skin cancers. Somnolence, ataxia, and pyramidal tract signs also may be seen. These generally revert with discontinuation of the drug; persistence demands evaluation for an alternative cause (brain stem metastases, cerebrovascular accident). Floxuridine also inhibits thymidylate synthetase. It is most often used for the treatment of hepatic metastases from colorectal carcinoma. Prolonged administration may induce a chemical hepatitis in addition to the toxicities commonly seen with 5-FU (Skeel, 1982).

Cytarabine is a pyrimidine antagonist that blocks the action of DNA polymerases. It is phase specific and is most effective by continuous infusion. Cytarabine is a mainstay in the induction of remission in acute myelogenous leukemia, in which it may be used in standard doses (200 mg/m²/24 hr) or high doses (3 to 6 g/m²/day). Cytarabine may also be administered intrathecally for the control of leukemic and nonleukemic leptomeningeal carcinomatosis. Intrathecal administration is required to achieve cerebrospinal fluid concentrations that are tumoricidal. Maintenance regimens in acute myelogenous leukemia utilize intermittent subcutaneous administration. Cytarabine crosses the blood-brain barrier; the high-dose regimens are associated with higher central nervous system (CNS) concentration and thus increased frequency of CNS toxicity. Pellagra-like symptoms (diarrhea, dementia, dermatitis), conjunctivitis, cerebellar signs, seizures, and hepatic dysfunction may occur at both standard and high doses, but their incidence increases with increasing dose.

Azacytidine, an investigational inhibitor of pyrimidine metabolism, exerts its action and toxicity through mechanisms similar to those of cytarabine; however, its instability in solution limits its clinical utility, which is currently restricted to the treatment of acute myelogenous leukemia. Rhabdomyolysis has been associated with its use (Cline & Haskell, 1980).

6-Mercaptopurine (6-MP) and thioguanine (6-TG) compete with purines in the leukemic cell. Xanthine oxidase is required for the degradation of 6-MP; concomitant administration of allopurinol requires dose reduction. Both purine antagonists require biotransformation to their active components; 6-MP and 6-TG are excreted renally. The available oral forms are mildly emetogenic; intravenous preparations are available investigationally. Myelosuppression is common with both agents and represents their dose-limiting toxicity. Cholestatic jaundice may occur; progression to hepatic necrosis has been reported with 6-MP (Perry, 1982). Cross resistance occurs between the two drugs. 6-Mercaptopurine is active in the treatment of acute myelogenous leukemia and in combination with methotrexate in maintenance regimens for acute lymphoblastic leukemia. Thioguanine is most valuable in acute myelogenous leukemia (Dorr & Fritz, 1980).

Miscellaneous Antineoplastics

A few agents with clinical utility exist today whose mechanism of action is poorly defined or unique (Table 21–10). Procarbazine, an oral agent, inhibits monoamine oxidase and, therefore, exhibits the clinical effects of other monoamine oxidase inhibitors. Procarbazine's primary role is in the treatment of Hodgkin's disease in the well-known MOPP regimen (DeVita et al., 1970).

The toxicities of procarbazine include myelosuppression, allergic skin rashes, pleuropulmonary reactions with occasional pneumonitis and fibrosis, and hemolytic anemias with formation of Heinz bodies in erythrocytes (Cline & Haskell, 1980). Ataxia, orthostatic hypotension, urticaria, and neuropathies may occur. Because procarbazine inhibits monoamine oxidase, concomitant administration of tricyclic antidepressants, sympathomimetics, or foods high in tyramine (aged cheese, chocolate, Chianti wine, dark beer) may result in hypertensive episodes. Similarly, procarbazine may yield a disulfiram-like reaction with the concomitant ingestion of alcohol, including medications containing alcohol (e.g., cough syrup, cold preparations).

Hydroxyurea inhibits ribonucleotide reductase, phase specifically (S). It is used in chronic leukemia and as emergency therapy for rapid lysis of blasts in patients with acute leukemia (both myelogenous and lymphocytic) who have blast levels that interfere with circulatory function. In the latter situation, simultaneous administration of allopurinol is indicated to prevent the development of tumor lysis syndrome (see Chapter 57) (Hughes, 1987). Hydroxyurea may be used palliatively to decrease splenic size in advanced myelofibrosis and chronic myelogenous leukemia. It is non-cross-resistant with busulfan. Toxicities include bone marrow depression, predominantly of the leukocytes; thrombocytopenia is less common. However, patients with massive splenomegaly may exhibit pronounced thrombocytopenia before and during therapy, owing to splenic sequestration of platelets. Skin reactions (hyperpigmentation, scaly atrophy, nail changes) and erythema and swelling of the hands and face may occur. Alopecia is possible. Neurologic disturbances, including headaches, dizziness, disorientation, hallucinations, and seizures, have been reported. An investigational parenteral preparation is available.

Mitotane, a derivative of the insecticide DDT, has a single antineoplastic indication: malignant carcinoma of the adrenal gland. Mitotane binds to the mitochondria in the cells of the adrenal cortex, preventing the conversion of cholesterol to steroids. Spironolactone potentiates its activity and should not be administered concomitantly. The onset of action after oral daily administration of mitotane may not be clinically detectable for 2 to 3 months after initiation of therapy.

The toxic manifestations of mitotane include nausea, vomiting, diarrhea, anorexia, orthostatic hypotension, and skin rashes. Visual disturbances, decreased memory, lethargy, somnolence, dizziness, vertigo, and mental depression occur because mitotane's lipid solubility allows it to cross the blood-brain barrier. Adrenal insufficiency should be anticipated. Patients experiencing trauma, infections, or shock must be treated with supplemental steroids; mitotane should be discontinued during this period.

Asparaginase is an enzyme that acts by destruction of extracellular supplies of L-asparaginine, resulting in the death of tumor cells that lack the ability to produce this essential amino acid. Asparaginase may block some cells in G_1 or S, but it is generally considered

Table 21–10. MISCELLANEOUS AGENTS

Class	Agents	Clinical Use
Monoamine oxidase inhibitor	Procarbazine	Hodgkin's disease
		Brain tumors
		Lung cancer
Ribonucleotide reductase inhibitor	Hydroxyurea	Chronic myelogenous leukemia
		Acute myelogenous leukemia
		Acute lymphoblastic leukemia
Adrenocortical steroid inhibitor	Mitotane	Adrenocortical cancer
Enzyme	L-Asparaginase	Acute lymphoblastic leukemia
Adenosine deaminase inhibitor	Pentostatin*	Hairy cell leukemia

*Investigational.

Table 21–11. HORMONALLY ACTIVE AGENTS

Class	Agents	Clinical Use
Estrogens	DES Estradiols Estramustine*	Breast cancer Prostate cancer
Progestins	Megestrol acetate Medroxyprogesterone Hydroxyprogesterone caproate	Breast cancer Endometrial cancer Renal cell cancer
Androgens	Fluoxymesterone Oxymetholone Testolactone Testosterone	Breast cancer Myelodysplasia ("preleukemia")
Antiestrogens	Tamoxifen	Breast cancer Endometrial cancer
Antiandrogens	Flutamide	Prostate cancer
LHRH blockers	Leuprolide Goserelin acetate	Breast cancer (Osbourne, 1989) Prostate cancer
Steroids	Prednisone Dexamethasone	Hodgkin's disease, non-Hodgkin's lymphoma, myeloma, breast cancer, acute leukemia, chronic leukemia
Steroid blockers	Aminoglutethimide Mitotane	Breast cancer, prostate cancer, adrenal cortex cancer

LHRH, Luteinizing hormone-releasing hormone; DES, diethylstilbestrol.
*DES conjugated to mechlorethamine.

cell-cycle phase nonspecific. Asparaginase is extracted from *E. coli;* anaphylaxis is the most dangerous toxicity. Pretreatment skin tests should be administered and test doses should be given; in the event of hypersensitivity reactions, desensitization regimens must be administered before a therapeutic dose. Skin testing should be repeated when doses occur after long separations in time. Asparaginase has also been isolated from *Erwinia.* Allergic intolerance to the *E. coli* preparation may require using the *Erwinia* preparation, which is available investigationally from the NCI. The enzymatic nature of asparaginase results in some unique toxicities; hypercholesterolemia, hyperglycemia, decreased synthesis of clotting factors, and neurotoxicity manifested as personality changes, somnolence, lethargy, and confusion may occur. Azotemia and proteinuria may develop; rarely, pancreatitis has been reported. Asparaginase has its current role in the treatment of acute lymphoblastic leukemia and is incorporated into most induction regimens.

HORMONALLY ACTIVE AGENTS

Many tumors arise from hormonally active tissues; manipulations of the hormonal milieu are used to inhibit their growth. Hormonal manipulations are based on the observation that tumor cells contain surface receptors for specific hormones, which are then transported intracellularly and are required for cell growth. Antineoplastic hormonal manipulations include obliterating host production of the required hormone; blocking the hormone receptors with competing agents; and substituting chemically similar agents for the active hormone, which cannot be utilized by the tumor cell. Hormonal cancer chemotherapeutics are summarized in Table 21–11.

Adrenocorticosteroids have direct antineoplastic effects in hematologic malignancies. Agents that block the production of adrenocorticosteroids are also used in the treatment of hormonally active cancers. Because aminoglutethimide induces a medical adrenalectomy, cortisone must be administered simultaneously. The reader is referred to endocrinology texts for in-depth discussion of the hormones; their toxicities do not differ substantially when used in the treatment of malignant disease.

BIOLOGIC ANTINEOPLASTICS

Biologic response modifiers in cancer therapy entered clinical trials in the 1980s (Abernathey, 1987). Their definitive role is yet to be determined. It is anticipated that biotherapy will be combined with antineoplastic treatment in the management of malignant disease. Biologicals may be utilized to effect the differentiation of cancer cells, making them more sensitive to antineoplastics. Monoclonal antibodies may be conjugated to available antineoplastics, creating immunoconjugates that can direct the antineoplastic agent to the malignant cell. Other biologicals, such as tumor necrosis factor, may be directly cytotoxic and thus may be considered antineoplastic. Chapter 23 discusses the biologic response modifiers and their roles in cancer therapy.

NEW HORIZONS

The 1980s saw the initiation of investigations into alternative delivery mechanisms of chemotherapy. High-dose chemotherapy with autologous bone marrow transplantation (see Chapter 27), regional chemotherapy—such as arterial infusions in the treatment of liver metastasis and brain tumors and limb perfusions in the

Table 21–12. COMMON ORGAN SYSTEM TOXICITIES OF ANTINEOPLASTICS*

Organ System	Toxicity	Class of Agent					
		AA	PA	A	AM	M	H
Gastrointestinal (Coons, Leventhal, Love, & Larson, 1987; Conrad, 1986; Dorr & Fritz, 1980; Mitchell & Schein, 1982)	Nausea, vomiting (Duigon, 1986; Needleman, 1987; Sallan & Cronin, 1985; See-Lasley & Ignoffo; 1981)	1–4	1–2	3	2	3–4	1
	Diarrhea	1	1	1	2–3	1	1
	Constipation	1	2	1	1	1	1
	Mucositis	1–2	1	2	3–4	1	1
Hepatotoxicity	↑ LFT results	1	1	1	2	1	1
	Cholestatic jaundice	1	1	2	2	1	1
	Hepatitis	1	1	1	2	1	1
Bone marrow (Grant Medical Center, 1987; Hoagland, 1982)	Leukopenia	4	4	4	4	1–4	1
	Thrombocytopenia	2–3	1–4	2–3	2	1–4	1
Cutaneous (Doll & Weiss, 1985; Duagin, 1982; Lovejoy, 1979; Parker, 1987; Weiss, 1982)	Rash	1	1	2–3	2–3	2–3	1
	Nail changes	1	1	1–2	2	1	1
	Hyperpigmentation	1	1	1–2	1–3	1	1
	Radiation recall	1	1	2	2	1	1
	Alopecia (Dean, Salmon, & Griffith, 1979; O'Brian, Zelson, Schwartz, & Pearson, 1970; Parker, 1987; Seipp, 1985)	1–4	1	1–4	1–4	1	1
Pulmonary (Buzdar et al., 1980; Ginsberg & Comis, 1982; Wickham, 1986)	Allergic pneumonitis	1	1	1	2	2	1
	Pulmonary fibrosis	1–2	1	1–2	1	1	1
Genitourinary (Lydon, 1986; Schilsky, 1982; Verway et al., 1984)	Kidney (Schilsky, 1982)	2–4	1	1	2	1	1
	Bladder	1	1	1	1	1	1
Cardiac (Kaszyk, 1986; Myers et al., 1983; Unverferth et al., 1981; Von Hoff, Rosenczweiz & Piccart, 1982)	Myocardial damage	1	1	2	1	1	1
	Electrocardiographic changes	1	1	2	1	1	1
Neurologic (Conrad, 1986; Holden & Felde, 1987; Kaplan & Wiernik, 1982; Lopez & Agrwal, 1984)	Central nervous system	1	1	1	2	2	1
	Peripheral nerves	1	2	1	2	1	1
Reproductive (Chapman, 1982; Grant Medical Center, 1987)	Gondal function	2–3	?	1–3	?	1–2	1–4

*Based on reported incidence and the likelihood of occurrence in general medical oncology practice.

↑, increased; LFT, liver function test; AA, alkylating agents; PA, plant alkaloids; A, antibiotics; AM, antimetabolites; M, miscellaneous; H, hormones.

1, Rare; incidence range, 0–19%.
2, Occasional; incidence range, 20–49%.
3, Common; incidence range, 50–75%.
4, Frequent; incidence range, greater than 75%.
?, Requires further definition.
When ranges are given, there is marked variability among drugs, doses, and routes.

treatment of melanoma—are currently under investigation. Clonogenic assays, or tumor stem cell assays, have been developed that require incubating fresh tumor cells with antineoplastic agents in vitro to determine effective agents for use in vivo. Clonogenic assays are expected to be refined, allowing improved selection of effective chemotherapy in individual patients.

Additional approaches to combined therapy such as hyperthermia and perioperative (neoadjuvant) chemotherapy will doubtlessly be explored through the end of the century (Berger, 1986; Scher et al., 1988). Hyperthermia is used to increase the core temperature of the tumor before treatment with radiation therapy or chemotherapy, in an effort to enhance cell kill. Perioperative or neoadjuvant chemotherapy is administered preoperatively, during, or immediately after the surgical procedures (Scher et al., 1988).

Other agents, such as hematoporphyrin esters combined with light, may prove directly cytotoxic and have a role in defining surgical margins, in detecting recurrent disease, and in palliation (Ball, 1987). Minimizing the toxicities of antineoplastics by general or selective protection of target organs is an evolving area of investigation (Table 21–12) (Chapman, 1982; Myers et al., 1983).

Advances in the application of currently available antineoplastics will be based on improved understanding of tumor kinetics allowing efficacious selection, dosing, and scheduling (DeVita, 1985; DeVita, Hellman, & Rosenberg, 1988). Under study is the simultaneous administration of noncytotoxic agents to potentiate antineoplastic effect (e.g., calcium leucovorin + 5-FU) (O'Connell, 1987).

New strategies will be developed to enhance the mechanisms of cell death (Berger, 1986). Methods to manipulate oncogene expression to improve antineoplastic sensitivity will be identified (Vesell, 1985). Improved knowledge about the mechanisms of resistance will allow the development of non-cross-resistant agents and regimens (Berger, 1986; DeVita, 1985).

Chemotherapy is a mainstay of cancer treatment. It is a continually and constantly changing modality whose role is well established in some malignancies and evolutionary in others. As the predominant systemic therapy for malignant disease, chemotherapy will continue to play a major role in oncologic therapeutics (see Table 21–5).

References

Abernathey, E. (1987). Biotherapy: An introductory overview. *Oncology Nursing Forum Supplement, 14*(6), 13–15.

Ball, K. (1987). Photodynamic therapy of malignant tumors. *Today's OR Nurse, 9*(6), 9–15.

Berger, N. (1986). Cancer chemotherapy: New strategies for success. *Journal of Clinical Investigation, 78*, 1131–1135.

Boice, J. D., Greene, M. H., Killen, J. Y., Ellenberg, S. S., Keechn, R. J., McFadden, E., Chen, T. T., & Fraumeni, J. F. (1983). Leukemia and preleukemia after adjuvant treatment of gastrointestinal cancer with semustine (methyl-CCNU). *New England Journal of Medicine, 309*, 1079–1084.

Bonadonna, G., Brusamolino, E., Valagussa, P., Rossi, A., Brugnatelli, L., Brambilla, C., DeLena, M., Tancini, G., Bajetta, E., Musumeci, R., & Veronesi, U. (1976). Combination chemotherapy as an adjuvant treatment in operable breast cancer. *New England Journal of Medicine, 294*, 405–410.

Bonadonna, G., Valagussa, P., & Santoro, A. (1986). Alternating non-cross resistant combination chemotherapy or MOPP in Stage IV Hodgkin's disease. *Annals of Internal Medicine, 104*, 739–746.

Bristow, M. R., Lopez, M. B., Mason, J. W., Billingham, M. E., & Winchester, M. A. (1982). Efficacy and cost of cardiac monitoring in patients receiving doxorubicin. *Cancer, 45*, 236–244.

Burchenal, J. H. (1977). The historical development of cancer chemotherapy. *Seminars in Oncology, 4*, 135–148.

Buzdar, A. U., Legha, S. S., Luna, M. A., Tashima, C. K., Hortobagyi, G. N., & Blumenschein, G. R. (1980). Pulmonary toxicity of mitomycin. *Cancer, 50*, 32–41.

Chapman, R. M. (1982). Effect of cytotoxic therapy on sexuality and gonadal function. *Seminars in Oncology, 9*, 84–94.

Cheson, B. D., Jasperse, D. M., Chun, H. G., & Friedman, M. A. (1986). Differentiating agents in the treatment of human malignancies. *Cancer Treatment Reviews, 13*, 129–145.

Cline, M. J., & Haskell, C. M. (1980). *Cancer chemotherapy.* Philadelphia: W. B. Saunders Co.

Conrad, K. J. (1986). Cerebellar toxicities associated with cytosine arabinoside: A nursing perspective. *Oncology Nursing Forum, 13*(5), 57–59.

Coons, H. L., Leventhal, D. R., Love, R. R., & Larson, S. (1987). Anticipatory nausea and emotional distress in patients receiving cisplatin-based chemotherapy. *Oncology Nursing Forum, 14*(3), 31–35.

Crossley, R. J. (1984). Clinical safety and tolerance of mitoxantrone. *Seminars in Oncology, 9*(1), 84–94.

Dean, J. C., Salmon, S. E., & Griffith, K. S. (1979). Prevention of doxorubicin-induced hair loss with scalp hypothermia. *New England Journal of Medicine, 301*, 1427–1429.

DeVita, V. T., Jr. (1985). Principles of chemotherapy. In V. T. DeVita, S. Hellman, & S. A. Rosenberg (Eds.), *Cancer: Principles and practice in oncology* (2nd ed., pp. 257–285). Philadelphia: J. B. Lippincott Co.

DeVita, V. T., Hellman, S., & Rosenberg, S. A. (1988). *Important advances in oncology 1988.* Philadelphia: J. B. Lippincott Co.

DeVita, V. T., Jr., Serpick, A. A., & Carbone, P. P. (1970). Combination chemotherapy in the treatment of advanced Hodgkin's disease. *Annals of Internal Medicine, 73*, 881–895.

Doll, D. C., & Weiss, R. B. (1985). Hemolytic anemia associated with antineoplastic agents. *Cancer Treatment Reports, 69*, 777–782.

Dorland's illustrated medical dictionary (26th Ed.) (1981). Philadelphia: W. B. Saunders Co.

Dorr, R. T., & Fritz, W. L. (1980). *Cancer chemotherapy handbook.* New York: Elsevier Science Publishing Co.

Duagin, W. G. (1982). Clinical toxicity of chemotherapeutic agents: Dermatologic toxicity. *Seminars in Oncology, 9*, 14–22.

Duigon, A. (1986). Anticipatory nausea and vomiting associated with cancer chemotherapy. *Oncology Nursing Forum, 13*(1), 35–40.

Einhorn, L. H. (1981). Testicular cancer as a model for curable neoplasm. The Richard and Linda Rosenthal Foundation Award lecture. *Cancer Research, 41*, 3275–3280.

Farber, S., Diamond, L. K., Mercer, R. D., Sylvester, R. F., & Wolfe, J. A. (1948). Temporary remissions in acute leukemia in children produced by folic acid antagonist, 4-aminopteroyl-glutamic acid (aminopterin). *New England Journal of Medicine, 238*, 787–792.

Friedman, M., & Hamilton, J. M. (1988). Progress in adjuvant therapy of large bowel cancer. In V. T. DeVita, S. Hellman, & S. A. Rosenberg (Eds.), *Important advances in oncology* (pp. 273–296). Philadelphia: J. B. Lippincott Co.

Gilman, A. (1963). The initial clinical trial of nitrogen mustard. *American Journal of Surgery, 105*, 574–578.

Gilman, A., & Phillips, F. J. (1946). The biological actions of therapeutic applications of b-chloroethyl amines and sulfides. *Science, 103*, 409–415.

Ginsberg, S. J., & Comis, R. L. (1982). The pulmonary toxicity of antineoplastic agents. *Seminars in Oncology, 9*, 34–51.

Goldie, J. H., & Coldman, A. J. (1979). A mathematical model for relating the drug sensitivity of tumors to their spontaneous mutation rate. *Cancer Treatment Reports, 63*, 1727–1733.

Gonzalez, C., & Villasanta, U. (1982). Life-threatening hypocalcemia and hypomagnesemia associated with cisplatin chemotherapy. *Obstetrics and Gynecology, 59*, 732–734.

Grant Medical Center (1987). *Chemotherapy: A data compendium.* Columbus: Author.

Guy, J. T., Fleming, T., Pollock, T. W., Rivkin, S. E., Pugh, R. P., Saiers, J. H., Hynes, H. E., & Boyd, J. F. (in press). 5-Day vinblastine infusion for pancreatic adenocarcinoma, a phase II Southwest Oncology Group study. *Investigational New Drugs.*

Habibi, B., Lopez, M., Serdaru, M., Baumelou, A., Vonlanthen, M. D., Marteau, R., & Salmon, C. (1982). Immune hemolytic anemia and renal failure due to teniposide. *New England Journal of Medicine, 306*, 1091–1093.

Hartmann, O., Benhamoa, F., Beanjean, F., Pico, J. L., Kalifa, C., Patte, C., Flamant, F., & Lemerle, J. (1986). High-dose busulfan and cyclophosphamide with autologous bone marrow transplantation support in advanced malignancies in children: A phase II study. *Journal of Clinical Oncology, 4*, 1804–1810.

Hoagland, H. C. (1982). Hematologic complications of cancer chemotherapy. *Seminars in Oncology, 9*, 95–102.

Holden, S., & Felde, G. (1987). Nursing care of patients experiencing cis-platin related peripheral neuropathy. *Oncology Nursing Forum, 14*(1), 13–19.

Hughes, C. (1987). Tumor lysis syndrome: A serious complication of chemotherapy. Implications for the I.V. nurse. *National Intravenous Therapy Association, 10*(2), 112–114.

Kaplan, R. S., & Wiernik, P. H. (1982). Neurotoxicity of antineoplastic drugs. *Seminars in Oncology, 9*, 103–130.

Kaszyk, L. K. (1986). Cardiac toxicity associated with cancer therapy. *Oncology Nursing Forum, 13*(4), 81–88.

Kyle, R. A. (1982). Second malignancies associated with chemotherapeutic agents. *Seminars in Oncology, 9*, 131–142.

Legha, S. S., Benjamin, R. S., Mackay, B., Ewer, M., Wallace, S., Valdivieso, M., Rasmussen, S. L., Blumenschein, G. R., & Freireich, E. J. (1982). Reduction of doxorubicin cardiotoxicity by prolonged continuous intravenous infusion. *Annals of Internal Medicine, 96*, 133–139.

Li, M. C. (1979). The historical background of successful chemotherapy for advanced gestational trophoblastic tumors. *American Journal of Obstetrics and Gynecology, 135*, 266–272.

Lopez, J. A., and Agrwal, R. P. (1984). Letter: Acute cerebellar toxicity after high-dose cytarabines associated with CNS accumulation of its metabolite, uracil arabinoside. *Cancer Treatment Reports, 68*, 1309–1310.

Lovejoy, N. C. (1979). Preventing hair loss during Adriamycin therapy. *Cancer Nursing, 2*, 117–121.

Lydon, J. (1986). Nephrotoxicity of cancer treatment. *Oncology Nursing Forum, 3*(2), 68–77.

McCauley, V. M., Begent, R. H. J., Phillips, M. E., & Newlands,

E. S. (1982). Prophylaxis against hypomagnesemia induced by cis-platinum combination chemotherapy. *Cancer Chemotherapy and Pharmacology, 9,* 179–181.

Mitchell, E., & Schein, P. S. (1982). Gastrointestinal toxicity of chemotherapeutic agents. *Seminars in Oncology, 9,* 52–64.

Moertel, C. G., Fleming, T. R., MacDonald, J. S., Haller, D. G., Laurie, J. A., Goodman, P. J., Ungerleider, J. J., Emerson, W.A., Tormey, D. C., Glick, J. H., Veeder, M. H., & Mailliard, J. A. (1990). Levamisole and fluorouracil for adjuvant therapy of resected colon carcinoma. *New England Journal of Medicine, 322,* 352–358.

Myers, C., Bonow, R., Palmeri, S., Jenkins, J., Corden, B., Locker, G., Doroshow, J., & Epstein, S. (1983). A randomized controlled trial assessing the prevention of doxorubicin cardiomyopathy by N-acetylcysteine. *Seminars in Oncology, 10,* 53–55.

Needleman, R. (1987). Chemotherapy—an overview of nausea and vomiting in the cancer patient: Etiology and management of serious complications of chemotherapy. *American Association of Occupational Health Nursing Journal, 35,* 179–182.

O'Brian, R., Zelson, J. H., Schwartz, A. D., & Pearson, H. A. (1970). Scalp tourniquet to lessen alopecia after vincristine. *New England Journal of Medicine, 283,* 1469.

O'Connell, M. J. (1987). Antipyrimidines: 5-fluorouracil and 5-fluoro-2'-deoxyuridine. In J. J. Lokich (Ed.), *Cancer chemotherapy by infusion* (pp. 117–122). Chicago: Precept Press, Inc.

Osbourne, C. K. (1989). Breast cancer. In R. Wittes, (Ed.), *Oncologic therapeutics* (pp. 201–211). Philadelphia: J. B. Lippincott Co.

Parker, R. (1987). The effectiveness of scalp hypothermia in preventing cyclophosphamide-induced alopecia. *Oncology Nursing Forum, 14*(6), 49–53.

Perry, M. C. (1982). Hepatotoxicity of chemotherapeutic agents. *Seminars in Oncology, 9,* 65–74.

Rose, W. C., & Schurig, J. E. (1985). Preclinical antitumor and toxicologic profile of carboplatinum. *Cancer Treatment Reviews, 12*(Suppl. A), 1–19.

Rosenberg, B., Van Camp, L., & Krigas, T. (1965). Inhibition of cell division in *Escherichia coli* by electrolysis products from an electrode. *Nature, 205,* 698–699.

Rosenberg, B., Van Camp, L., Trosko, J. E., & Mansour, V. H. (1969). Platinum compounds: A new class of potent antitumor agents. *Nature, 222,* 385–386.

Sallan, S. E., & Cronin, C. M. (1985). Nausea and vomiting. In V. T. DeVita, Jr., S. Hellman, & S. A. Rosenberg (Eds.), *Cancer: Principles and practice in oncology* (2nd ed., pp. 2008–2013). Philadelphia: J. B. Lippincott Co.

Schackney, S. E. (1985). Cell kinetics and cancer chemotherapy. In P. Calabresi, P. S. Schein, & S. A. Rosenberg (Eds.), *Medical oncology: Basic principles and clinical management of cancer* (pp. 41–60). New York: Macmillan.

Scher, H. I., Yagoda, A., & Herr, H. W. (1988). Neoadjuvant M-VAC (methotrexate, vinblastine, doxorubicin, and cis-platin) effect on primary bladder lesion. *Journal of Urology, 139,* 470–474.

Schilsky, R. L. (1982). Renal and metabolic toxicities of cancer chemotherapy. *Seminars in Oncology, 9,* 75–83.

See-Lasley, K., & Ignoffo, R. J. (1981). *Manual of oncology therapeutics.* St. Louis: C. V. Mosby Co.

Seipp, C. A. (1985). Hair Loss. In V. T. DeVita, Jr., S. Hellman, & S. A. Rosenberg (Eds.), *Cancer: Principles and practice in oncology* (2nd ed., pp. 2007–2008). Philadelphia: J. B. Lippincott Co.

Skeel, R. T. (1982). *Manual of cancer chemotherapy.* Boston: Little, Brown, & Co., Inc.

Sutherland, C. M., Krementz, E. T. (1981). Hepatotoxicity of DTIC. *Cancer Treatment Reports, 65,* 321–322.

Trent, J. M., Buick, R. N., Olson, S., Horns, R. C., Jr., & Schimke, R. T. (1984). Cytologic evidence for gene amplification in methotrexate-resistant cells obtained from a patient with ovarian adenocarcinoma. *Journal of Clinical Oncology, 2,* 8–15.

Unverferth, D. V., Magonen, R. D., Unverferth, B. P., Tallay, R. L., Balcerzak, S. P., & Baba, N. (1981). Human myocardial morphologic and functional changes in the first 24 hours after doxorubicin administration. *Cancer Treatment Reports, 65,* 1033–1097.

Verway, J., Boven, E., van der Meulen, J., & Pinedo, H. M. (1984). Recovery from mitomycin C–induced hemolytic uremic syndrome: A case report. *Cancer, 54,* 2878–2881.

Vesell, E. S. (1985). Genetic host factors: Determinants of drug response [letter to the editor]. *New England Journal of Medicine, 313,* 261–262.

Von Hoff, D. D., Rosencweiz, M., & Piccart, M. (1982). The cardiotoxicity of anticancer agents. *Seminars in Oncology, 9,* 23–33.

Weiss, A. J., & Manthel, R. W. (1977). Experiences with the use of Adriamycin in combination with other anticancer agents using a weekly schedule with particular reference to lack of cardiac toxicity. *Cancer, 40,* 2046–2052.

Weiss, R. B. (1982). Hypersensitivity reactions to cancer chemotherapy. *Seminars in Oncology, 9,* 5–13.

Wickham, R. (1986). Pulmonary toxicity secondary to cancer treatment. *Oncology Nursing Forum, 13*(5), 69–76.

Yap, H. Y., Blumenschein, G. R., Kanting, M. J., Hortabagyi, G. N., Tashima, C. K., & Loo, T. L. (1980). Vinblastine given as a continuous 5-day infusion in the treatment of refractory breast cancer. *Cancer Treatment Reports, 64,* 279–283.

Zubrod, C. G. (1979). Historic milestones in curative chemotherapy. *Seminars in Oncology, 6,* 490–505.

Zubrod, C. G. (1984). Origins and development of chemotherapy research at the National Cancer Institute. *Cancer Treatment Reports, 68,* 9–19.

CHAPTER 22

Delivery of Cancer Chemotherapy

MICHELLE GOODMAN

At no other time in the history of medical oncology have the schedule, method, and route of administration of chemotherapy been so varied. Although most drugs are given systemically, regional drug therapy is also gaining prominence. Currently, antineoplastic agents are being administered directly into the peritoneal cavity to treat metastases of ovarian carcinoma and colon cancer; into the bladder intravesically to treat early bladder cancer; into the central nervous system to treat meningeal carcinomatosis; and into the arterial system for more direct organ or limb perfusion, which may be the treatment for metastatic colon cancer to the liver or osteogenic sarcoma.

The clinician who administers chemotherapy should have a thorough knowledge of the drugs; their modes of administration, distribution, and elimination; and the technical skills of venipuncture and management of vascular access devices (VADs).

This chapter discusses issues pertinent to chemotherapy administration. These issues include determining the qualifications of the clinician who administers chemotherapy, safe handling of chemotherapy, prevention and management of extravasation of vesicant agents, VADs, and systemic and regional drug delivery.

CHEMOTHERAPY ADMINISTRATION

Professional Qualifications

Chemotherapy drugs are administered to patients in a variety of health care settings, including the hospital, the outpatient facility, and the home. To ensure optimal quality of care and patient safety, antineoplastic agents are administered by professional nurses who have received specialized training in chemotherapy administration.

The basic design of such an educational program varies depending on the setting and the ability of the facility to provide clinical experience. The educational guidelines provided by the Oncology Nursing Society (1988) include three major components:

1. The core didactic element includes the science of cancer chemotherapy and the pathophysiology of side effects.

2. The clinical applications component includes nursing and medical management of the side effects of chemotherapy and methods of drug delivery. Such information is learned by a variety of teaching methods, including audiovisual techniques; reviews of current literature, with an emphasis on research verification of approaches to patient care; and lectures.

3. The clinical practicum includes the application of knowledge and skills gained in the core and clinical applications to direct patient care situations. Under the guidance of a skilled clinician, the nurse gains expertise and confidence in drug administration and ability to anticipate and manage side effects and other complications of therapy. To maintain skill and a high level of expertise, the nurse administers these drugs on a regular basis. Venipuncture skills are evaluated yearly in accordance with institutional policies and procedures. Because the field of medical oncology and methods of drug delivery are ever changing, provisions for continued educational experiences are mandatory to promote expert and safe patient care.

Preparation and Handling of Antineoplastic Agents

With more than 500,000 patients receiving antineoplastic agents for cancer treatment, it is estimated that

291

thousands of health care employees (e.g., pharmacists, nurses, physicians, housekeeping and maintenance personnel) are potentially at risk for adverse health effects from exposure to these drugs. Although exposure levels during preparation, administration, and disposal are much lower than the pharmacologic doses received by the patient, the health care workers' exposure can be additive over many years (Sotaniemi, Sutinen, Arranto et al., 1983). In addition, there is no known maximal safe level of exposure below which there is no risk. It is believed that the extent of health risk to employees who handle antineoplastic drugs is a combination of exposure time, amount and method of exposure, and class of drug. The main routes of exposure are inhalation of drug aerosols or droplets, absorption through the skin and mucous membranes either during preparation and handling or during exposure to the patient's body fluids and linens, and ingestion through contact with contaminated food or cigarettes.

The potential hazards of chemotherapy exposure are many and varied when health care personnel do not follow recommendations for safe handling of these drugs. Physical complaints such as skin, mucous membrane, and eye irritation; lightheadedness; facial flushing; hair loss; nausea; and headache may be experienced (Anderson, Puckett, Dana, et al., 1982; Ladik, Stoehr, & Maurer, 1980; Neal, Wadden, & Chiou, 1983).

Experimental studies have shown that many antineoplastic drugs are carcinogenic, mutagenic, and teratogenic. It has been established further that without proper protection and safe workplace practices when patients are tested, there is an increase of mutagenic activity in the urine and chromosomal damage in health care workers who handle these drugs (Hirst, Tse, Mills, et al., 1984; Nguyen, Theiss, & Matney, 1982; Waksvik, Klepp, & Brogger, 1981). It is not known whether these measures are valid indicators of occupational hazards of antineoplastics. Until more direct measures are available and affordable, all persons who come in contact with these drugs should employ proper precautions to minimize exposure. This is especially true for the woman who is planning a pregnancy, is pregnant, or is breast feeding. The potential reproductive risk to health workers, male or female, and to a developing fetus is indeterminable at this time. Research concerning this issue is inconclusive. Selevan and colleagues (1985) analyzed the incidence of spontaneous abortions among Finnish nurses and reported a statistically significant association between fetal loss and possible exposure to antineoplastics during the first trimester. Although the study suggests a causal relationship, it does not establish one.

A study by Rogers and Emmett (1987) found that the association between exposure to antineoplastic agents during pregnancy and spontaneous abortion was statistically significant, with a risk factor of 2.5 for those handling antineoplastic agents without the use of personal protective equipment (Box 22–1).

Current evidence suggests that if appropriate safety measures are employed, potential health hazards will be minimized (National Study Commission, 1987; Oncology Nursing Society, 1989). The Occupational Safety and Health Administration recommendations and the Oncology Nursing Society's cancer chemotherapy guidelines are offered as standards to be incorporated into institutional policies and procedures and are summarized in Table 22–1 (Oncology Nursing Society, 1988, 1989; U.S. Department of Labor, 1986).

The nurse is often the central figure in establishing appropriate policies and procedures for chemotherapy drug administration. Applying the aforementioned recommendations and guidelines to one's practice setting requires that the nurse remain informed of current issues in drug handling safety and establish a means of sharing that knowledge with other members of the health care team (Gullo, 1988; Miller, 1988).

Chemotherapy Administration: The Setting

Chemotherapy is administered in various physical settings, including the ambulatory setting, outpatient clinic, physician's private office, hospital setting, and patient's home. The majority of chemotherapy drugs are given to individuals who are well enough to be at home and to be physically capable of traveling to a physician's office or an outpatient clinic to receive the treatment. The advent of both prospective payment systems and cost-containment plans has shifted the emphasis of treatment to the outpatient setting, making it imperative that outpatient facilities be designed to accommodate most, if not all, patients requiring routine chemotherapy.

The drug administration area may range from the surface of a physician's desk to a more elaborate, specifically designated drug treatment area. Whatever the setting, certain precautions must be taken to ensure a safe environment for the patient and the health care worker. Emergency drugs and resuscitation equipment, including suction tubes and oxygen tanks, should be available and in good working order. Emergency drugs may be needed to take care of fluid overload, heart attack, or respiratory distress as a result of aspiration or anaphylaxis (Table 22–2). Policies and procedures for the management of such complications should be known to all concerned. An extravasation kit should also be available in the event that a vesicant agent is infiltrated. Up-to-date procedures for the management of extravasation for particular vesicant agents should be included in each kit (Table 22–3).

To ensure a safe work environment, a physician should be available in the event of unforeseen complications of therapy. A physician should be present especially when patients are receiving blood, lengthy infusions, or agents that are under investigation.

Concerning the physical environment, reclining chairs (for more lengthy infusions), venipuncture chairs with armrests, and movable overhead lighting provide optimal conditions for venipuncture. A call light or similar mechanism should be available and within easy reach of the patient.

Box 22–1. IS HANDLING CHEMOTHERAPY A POTENTIAL OCCUPATIONAL HAZARD?

STUDY

Rogers, B., & Emmett, E. A. (1987). **Handling antineoplastic agents: Urine mutagenicity in nurses.** *Image: Journal of Nursing Scholarship, 3,* 108–113.

SAMPLE

Fifty-nine nurses who handle chemotherapy (exposed subjects) and 64 community health nurses (unexposed subjects) were invited to participate. All subjects were expected to work a minimum of 3 consecutive days, take time off for 2 consecutive days, and be free from cancer. The exposed subjects were required to have prepared or administered antineoplastic agents during the exposure period. The mean ages of the exposed and unexposed groups were 34 and 44 years, respectively. Exposed subjects worked in hospital oncology units (32 per cent), ambulatory oncology clinics (48 per cent), or private oncology physician offices (20 per cent). Almost all comparison subjects worked in community health agencies and schools. A similar number in each group smoked cigarettes and drank alcohol. Ninety-seven per cent were white, and all were female.

MEASURES

A cross-sectional design was used in which interview data and urine sample analyses were compared from exposed and unexposed nurses. The questionnaires were administered by trained interviewers. The demographic information requested in the questionnaires concerned occupation, current health status, medication, alcohol consumption, smoking, pregnancy history, reproductive outcomes (live births, still births, spontaneous abortions, congenital malformations), and work practices, which included the use of personal protective equipment (PPE), the number and type of antineoplastic agents handled, and the duration of exposure.

FINDINGS

Work Practices of Exposed Nurses

- Five nurses (8 per cent) used masks; 8 nurses (13 per cent) used protective clothing some of the time; 12 nurses (20 per cent), only 2 of whom worked in private oncologists' offices, used gloves most of the time while handling the drugs.
- No subjects used ventilatory hoods during drug preparation.
- Subjects who worked in clinics or private oncologists' offices were significantly more likely to prepare the drugs, and they also worked more consecutive days.
- Seventy-four per cent of exposed nurses who worked in hospital oncology units gave fewer than 12 doses of antineoplastic agents per week; sixty-eight per cent of oncology clinic nurses and 75 per cent of oncology office-based nurses gave an average of at least 33 doses per week.
- Nurses working in private oncologists' offices are more likely to be exposed to the antineoplastic agents through duration and quantity of exposure and are less likely to use protective measures.

• Urine Mutagenicity Analyses

- Thirty-six of 59 (61 per cent) of exposed nurses had positive urine mutagenicity. Eleven of 64 (17 per cent) of unexposed nurses had positive urine mutagenicity.

• Health Status Questionnaire

- Hair loss, headaches, abdominal pain, and skin rash were reported significantly more frequently in the exposed group.
- A total of 233 pregnancy events were reported. There was a significantly higher proportion of untoward pregnancy outcomes (13/31), including 12 spontaneous abortions and 1 congenital malformation, reported for pregnancies during which antineoplastic drugs were handled, as compared with pregnancies in which there was no exposure (47/202).
- No association was found with smoking, age, medication usage, illness, x-ray exposure, or use of birth control pills during pregnancy.

LIMITATIONS

- Because of small numbers in each cell, actual relationships among variables could not be ascertained and therefore caution should be taken when interpreting the significance of findings.
- Pregnancy history and physical complaints are subject to the individual's accuracy of recall.
- There was no validation of hospital records to determine accuracy of the nurses' recall of pregnancy events.
- Findings demonstrate that risk exists for exposed nurses who do not use PPE but do not demonstrate that there is no risk for nurses who do use PPE.
- The incidence of untoward outcomes of pregnancy in older women in the general population should be considered a factor in the interpretation of findings.

Table 22–1. GUIDELINES FOR SAFE HANDLING AND DISPOSAL OF ANTINEOPLASTIC AGENTS

A. Drug Preparation
1. All antineoplastic drugs should be prepared by specially trained individuals in a centralized area to minimize interruptions and risk of contamination.
2. Drugs are prepared in a class II biologic safety cabinet (vertical laminar air-flow hood) with vents to the outside, if possible. The blower is left on 24 hours a day, 7 days a week. The hood is serviced regularly according to the manufacturer's recommendations.
3. Eating, drinking, smoking, and applying cosmetics in the drug preparation area are prohibited.
4. The work surface is covered with a plastic absorbent pad to minimize contamination. This pad is changed immediately in the event of contamination and at the completion of drug preparation each day or shift.
5. The prescribed drug is prepared using aseptic technique according to the physician's order, other pharmaceutic resources, or both.
6. Disposable surgical latex unpowdered gloves are used when handling the drugs. Gloves should be changed hourly or immediately if torn or punctured.
7. A disposable long-sleeved gown made of lint-free fabric with knitted cuffs and a closed front is worn during drug preparation.
8. A thermoplastic (Plexiglas) face shield or goggles and a powered air-purifying respirator should be used if a biologic safety cabinet is not available.
9. Because exposure can result when connecting and disconnecting intravenous (IV) tubing, when injecting the drug into the IV line, when removing air from the syringe or infusion line, and when leakage occurs at the tubing, syringe, or stopcock connection, priming of all IV tubing is carried out under the protection of the hood.
10. Other measures to guard against drug leakage during drug preparation include venting the vial and using large-bore needles, Luer-Lock fittings, and sterile gauze or sponge around the neck of the vial during needle withdrawal. Aerosolization may also be minimized by attaching an aerosol protection device (CytoGuard, Bristol-Myers) to the vial of drug before adding the diluent.
11. Once reconstituted, the drug is labeled according to institutional policies and procedures; the label should include the drug's vesicant properties and antineoplastic drug warning.
12. Antineoplastic drugs are transported in an impervious packing material and are marked with a distinctive warning label.
13. Personnel responsible for drug transport are knowledgeable of procedures to be followed in the event of drug spillage.
B. Drug Administration
1. Chemotherapeutic agents are administered by registered professional nurses who have been specially trained and designated as qualified according to specific institutional policies and procedures.
2. Before administering the drugs, the nurse ensures that informed consent has been given and clarifies any misconceptions the patient might have regarding the drugs and their side effects.
3. Appropriate laboratory results are evaluated and found to be within acceptable levels (e.g., complete blood count, renal and liver function).
4. Measures to minimize side effects of the drugs are carried out before drug administration (e.g., hydration, antiemetics and antianxiety agents, and patient comfort).
5. An appropriate route for drug administration is ensured according to the physician's order.
6. Personal protective equipment is worn, including disposable latex surgical gloves and a disposable gown made of a lint-free, low-permeability fabric with a closed front, long sleeves, and elastic or knit closed cuffs (optional).
7. The work surface is protected with a disposable absorbent pad.
8. The drug or drugs are administered according to established institutional policies and procedures.
9. Documentation of drug administration, including any adverse reaction, is made in the patient's medical record.
10. A mechanism for identification of patients receiving antineoplastic agents is established for the 48-hour period following drug dispensing.
11. Disposable surgical unpowdered latex gloves and a disposable gown are worn when handling body secretions such as blood, vomitus, or excreta from patients who received chemotherapy drugs within the previous 48 hours.
12. In the event of accidental exposure, remove contaminated gloves or gown immediately and discard according to official procedures.
13. Wash the contaminated skin with soap and water.
14. Flood an eye that is accidentally exposed to chemotherapy with water or isotonic eye wash for at least 5 minutes.
15. Obtain a medical evaluation as soon as possible after exposure and document the incident according to institutional policies and procedures.
C. Drug Disposal
1. Regardless of the setting (hospital, ambulatory care, or home), all equipment and unused drugs are treated as hazardous and are disposed of according to the institution's policies and procedures.
2. All contaminated equipment including needles are disposed of intact to prevent aerosolization, leaks, and spills.
3. All contaminated materials used in drug preparation are disposed of in a leak-proof, puncture-proof container with a distinctive warning label and are placed in a sealable 4-mil polyethylene or 2-mil polypropylene bag with appropriate labeling.
4. Linen contaminated with bodily secretions of patients who have received chemotherapy within the previous 48 hours is placed in a specially marked laundry bag, which is then placed in an impervious bag that is marked with a distinctive warning label.
5. In the event of a spill, personnel should don double surgical latex unpowdered gloves; eye protection; and a disposable gown made of a lint-free, low-permeability fabric with a closed front, long sleeves, and elastic or knit closed cuffs.
6. Small amounts of liquids are cleaned up with gauze pads, whereas larger spills (more than 5 ml) are cleaned up with absorbent pads.
7. Small amounts of solids or spills involving powder are cleaned up with damp cloths or absorbent gauze pads.
8. The spill area is cleaned three times with a detergent followed by clean water.
9. Broken glassware and disposable contaminated materials are placed in a leak-proof, puncture-proof container and then placed in a sealable 4-mil polyethylene or 2-mil polypropylene bag and marked with a distinctive warning label.
10. Contaminated reusable items are washed by specially trained personnel wearing double surgical unpowdered latex gloves.
11. The spill should be documented according to established institutional policies and procedures.

(Data from Oncology Nursing Society, 1988; Sotaniemi, Sutinen, Arranto, Sutinen, Sotaniemi, Lehtola, & Pelkonen, 1983; U.S. Department of Labor, 1986.)

When patients are treated in a central drug treatment area, privacy can be difficult to create. Room dividers, either stationary or portable, can be useful. Persons who are weakened from disease or physically ill from treatment are more comfortably treated in an individ-ual examination room. For patients who require aggressive antiemetic therapy and hydration, a private room with a hospital bed and bathroom is ideal.

In some situations, it may be advantageous to have additional materials to help comfort patients or simply

Table 22–2. EMERGENCY DRUGS AND EQUIPMENT*

Drugs	Strength	Volume
Epinephrine 1:1000 (1 mg/ml)	1:10,000	10 ml
Anhydrous theophylline	400 mg	100 ml
Diphenhydramine	50 mg	1 ml
Hydrocortisone	2 ml	100 ml
Dopamine (200 mg)	800 µg	250 ml
Levarterenol bitartrate	2 mg	500 ml
Sodium bicarbonate	8.4%	50 mEq/50 ml
Furosemide	40 mg	4 ml
Diazepam	10 mg	2 ml
Lidocaine	100 mg	5 ml
Naloxone hydrochloride	0.1–0.4 mg	5 ml
Nitroglycerine (sublingual)	0.15 mg	

Equipment
Suction machine with catheters
Oxygen tank with nasal and face mask
Ambu bag with adult-child face mask
Syringes and needles
Standard resuscitation equipment

*Check daily and restock as necessary.

to help them pass the time. Television, individual relaxation tapes or music cassettes with ear phones, and reading materials are useful.

Chemotherapy Administration: Preparing the Patient and Family

The ideal situation for teaching the patient and family is attained through the collaborative efforts of the medical oncologist, pharmacist, and oncology clinical nurse specialist. The patient should understand that it is normal to feel overwhelmed with information and that opportunities exist for reinforcement of the

Table 22–3. EXTRAVASATION KIT: ITEMS AND QUANTITIES*

Needles: 18 gauge (2)
         25 gauge (2)
         filter needle (1)
Tape: 1 inch paper
Telfa pads: 4 × 4 in (4)
Sterile gauze dressing 4 × 4 in (2)
Alcohol wipes (4)
Syringes: tuberculin
         3 ml
         5 ml
         10 ml
         20 ml
Local anesthetic: ethyl chloride
Diluent: sterile saline: 10 ml (1) preservative free
       sterile water: 10 ml (1)
Steroid cream: 1% topical lotion (optional)
Antidotes: 10% sodium thiosulfate (10 ml)
         hydrocortisone solution (100-mg vial)
         dexamethasone: 4 mg/ml
         hyaluronidase (150 U) (in refrigerator)
         dimethyl sulfoxide (50–100%) topical
Latex gloves
Hot pack
Cold pack
Policy and procedure for extravasation management
Extravasation record (see Table 22–8)

*Restock kit after each use. Kit should be available wherever vesicant drugs are being administered.

verbal and written information in the form of drug information cards or similar patient teaching aids. Although the physician has the responsibility of obtaining informed consent, the nurse is usually the member of the team who, during conversations with patient and family, is able to clarify the goals of treatment, restate side effects, and reassure the patient that all efforts will be made to minimize the complications of therapy.

Written or oral consent for treatment is mandatory whether the patient is receiving standard therapy or therapy of an investigational or research nature (Miller, 1980). The only difference in principle between standard and investigational therapy is that a signature is required for the latter. The purpose of this signature is to demonstrate the individual's understanding of the proposed therapy and voluntary agreement to participate in the investigational study. Informed consent is an important factor in patient compliance and adherence to the treatment regimen. Although most patients are highly motivated to receive therapy, being informed about the side effects and expected outcome will increase their cooperation with the prevention and management of the complications of therapy. Full disclosure of information concerning the patient's disease and treatment is rarely useful and is likely to increase the patient's difficulty with decision making. In a study of 144 patients, Penman and colleagues found that 41 per cent of patients beginning chemotherapy were less than eager for details of the treatment (Penman, Holland, Bahna, et al., 1984). Their primary reasons for agreeing to participate in a research study were trust in the physician and belief that the treatment would help them.

Although the patient requires enough information to make a decision regarding therapy, the opportunity to ask additional questions and acquire more information may help the patient feel informed and comfortable with the decision. Five major points should be addressed concerning a patient's consent for treatment:

1. What are the possibilities of treatment-related risks and side effects, both early and delayed?

2. What are the expected benefits of therapy and goals of treatment, and how will the success or failure of the therapy be measured?

3. Is the treatment program research oriented? If so, the patient should be aware of this fact. Likewise, if any other therapy is known to be better, the individual should be offered such therapy. If another kind of therapy has been proved to be better for the individual, he or she is not eligible to participate in the research study.

4. Are there alternate forms of therapy for which the patient would be eligible? Such options are often confusing and should be explained in a straightforward manner.

5. Is the patient aware of the right to refuse therapy or to withdraw from the treatment program at any time?

Written information is not generally identified as a primary factor in a patient's decision-making process (Penman et al., 1984). However, written information may serve to supplement verbal information and to help family members, especially those who are not present during the verbal exchange, understand the goals of therapy.

MODES OF ADMINISTRATION

There are two fundamental methods of antineoplastic drug administration: *systemic* and *regional*. The purpose of systemic drug administration is to kill tumor cells from presumed or proven metastatic disease. The goal of systemic chemotherapy is to reach a sufficient drug concentration to achieve a therapeutic cytotoxic effect without causing excessive toxicity to normal tissues. The goals of regional chemotherapy are to deliver the drug or drugs directly into the blood vessel supplying the tumor or cavity in which the tumor is isolated. Regional therapy often permits higher doses of the drug to be delivered to the area of the tumor. Because less of the drug reaches the systemic circulation, toxicities tend to be less severe.

Systemic chemotherapy may be given orally, intravenously, subcutaneously, or intramuscularly. The dose and schedule of drug administration are determined by the effect of the drugs on both normal and neoplastic tissues. The dose is usually increased gradually until the optimal tolerable dose is reached. The major limitations of the use of systemic chemotherapy are its short-term and long-term complications.

Pretreatment Considerations

Before attempting venous access and drug delivery, it is important to consider the following:

1. If the patient is receiving chemotherapy for the first time, make sure he or she has received adequate instruction regarding the treatment plan and that the patient feels sufficiently informed.

2. If treatment is of an investigational nature, verify that an informed consent form has been signed before initiating therapy.

3. Check the drug dosage against the physician's order. The order should include the patient's name, name of drug or drugs, frequency of administration, and, if appropriate, rate of administration. Most drug doses are based on a calculation of milligrams per kilogram or on body surface area (m^2). Body surface area is usually based on a calculation of the individual's ideal body weight and height. Obesity, ascites, or other factors such as the loss of a limb are important considerations in dose adjustment. Consider whether the dose and route of administration seem appropriate for the patient.

4. Check the patient's most recent laboratory test results. The complete blood count (CBC) including the platelet count should be within normal limits or within the limits specified in the research protocol. A dose modification or treatment delay may be needed if the CBC is below normal limits.

5. If the white blood cell count (WBC) is low, calculate the absolute granulocyte count (AGC) to determine the patient's ability to fight infection. The AGC is computed by multiplying the percentages of neutrophils and bands by the total WBC. When the AGC is less than 1200 cells/mm^3, treatment with myelosuppressive agents is generally not recommended. An AGC of less than 1000 cells/mm^3 is associated with a more severe risk for infection.

6. Consider the way each drug is metabolized and eliminated. If there is any clinical or laboratory evidence of organ dysfunction (e.g., liver or kidney), the pharmacokinetics or pharmacodynamics of the drug may be hindered, leading to excessive toxicity. Dose reductions or treatment delays may be warranted.

7. Consider any pretreatment antiemetics, hydration, or measures to minimize hair loss.

8. Check to see that emergency equipment, including materials to manage an allergic reaction or extravasation, is available. If a vesicant is being injected, review the policy and procedure on management of an extravasation. Be prepared to manage an allergic or anaphylactic reaction should one occur.

9. Ensure adequate lighting and patient comfort. A call light or similar method of communication should be available if the patient is left unattended or is receiving an infusion.

10. Review the patient's medication history, including over-the-counter drugs. Be alert to drug incompatibilities, drug interactions, and additive toxicities.

Intravenous Drug Administration

Chemotherapy may be given intravenously (1) through the direct push method, also known as the two-syringe technique; (2) through the side port of a freely running intravenous (IV) line; (3) as a mini-infusion; or (4) as a continuous infusion over several hours or days. The method of IV drug delivery is often dictated by the vesicant properties of the drugs; their potential to cause vein irritation; their potential for immediate or delayed complications, such as allergic reactions, hypertension, or hypotension; and the logistics of the specific treatment protocol. In general, the majority of vesicants and nonvesicants are given by the direct push method. The decision to administer a vesicant by the side-arm technique is dependent on whether the patient requires the intravenous infusion for another purpose; for example, for hydration, antiemetics, or antibiotics. The two-syringe technique is the preferred method of administering vesicant agents in that it permits precise and direct control of fluid into the vein without drug back-up in the IV tubing. Briskness of blood return and appreciation of any pressure changes (resistance) in the vein are most easily perceived with the two-syringe method. Using the side-arm technique for additional dilution for vesicant agents is unnecessary because the drugs are already optimally diluted according to the package directions. Although either method of drug delivery is considered safe, it is a misconception that the side-arm technique is safer than the two-syringe technique. By way of clarification, the drug—vesicant or nonvesicant—would never be injected directly into a peripheral vein without first flushing with normal saline to ensure adequate blood flow and venous integrity.

Administering the drug as a short-term infusion is generally reserved for agents that produce untoward symptoms or complications when given by the direct push method. For example, etoposide (Vp-16–213, VePesid) and teniposide (VM-26, Vumon) are given over 30 to 60 minutes to prevent hypotension; carmustine (BCNU) is given over 1 to 2 hours to minimize perivenous irritation and discomfort; higher doses of cisplatin (Platinol) and cyclophosphamide (Cytoxan, Neosar, Endoxan) are commonly given as infusions over 4 to 6 hours and 1 to 2 hours, respectively, to minimize nausea and vomiting as well as urinary tract toxicity.

Continuous infusion therapy has gained prominence as a means of overcoming cytokinetic resistance and thereby enhancing tumor response and minimizing toxicities. Prolonged exposure of cancer cells to the drugs may be beneficial because cell cycle times vary and are generally measured in days. An additional benefit of continuous infusion therapy is that the intracellular levels of the drugs may be maximized by prolonged exposure to low extracellular concentrations of the drug. In addition, the transport mechanisms of the cell membrane are enhanced by the saturation process provided by continuous infusion therapy (Carlson & Sikic, 1983). Toxicities may be minimized because continuous infusion of chemotherapy avoids the peak plasma levels achieved by bolus administration. For example, a decreased incidence of cardiac toxicity has been reported with continuous infusion of doxorubicin (Brenner, Grosh, Noone, et al., 1984; Legha, Benjamin, MacKay, et al., 1982; Torti, Bristow, Howes, et al., 1983; Von Hoff, Layard, Basa, et al., 1979). In the case of 5-fluorouracil, a higher total dose of the drug can be given without enhanced toxicities (myelosuppression and diarrhea) and without loss of antitumor activity if the drug is infused over 4 to 5 days rather than given as a daily bolus injection (Lokich, Bothe, Fine, et al., 1981).

Vein Selection and Cannulation

Only persons knowledgeable and trained in venipuncture and chemotherapy administration should administer intravenous chemotherapy. If the patient has a preexisting peripheral IV line, nonvesicant agents may be administered through this line provided there are no signs or symptoms of phlebitis and the blood return is adequate. If the blood return is absent or sluggish or if the IV line has been in place for longer than 24 hours, a new line should be established. If the patient is receiving a vesicant agent and has a preexisting peripheral IV line in place, it is safe to use it provided blood return is adequate and venous irritation or phlebitis is absent. This practice is especially prudent when the patient has small, fragile veins. If any doubt exists as to the integrity of the vein, a new IV line should be established before injecting the drug. The following is a list of some issues to consider in vein selection and cannulation.

1. Selecting the proper site for venipuncture should begin with a careful, systematic assessment of all available arm veins. Extra time spent selecting the proper vein usually results in successful venous access, whereas a hurried approach can result in inadequate venous distention, vein collapse, and repeated needle insertions. Full visibility of the arms unencumbered by constricting jewelry or clothing aids in determining venous access, as does good lighting and a firm surface on which to place the arm.

2. All equipment required to achieve venipuncture and secure the line should be assembled before attempting venipuncture. Because this step requires the handling of chemotherapy drugs, in particular, the removal of Luer-Lock caps from the syringes containing the drugs, the nurse should put on any personal protective equipment at this time. In some institutions nurses do not wear gowns to administer chemotherapy, preferring instead to wear a lab coat or uniform. Most experienced clinicians are confident in their ability to handle the drugs during administration and feel gowns are unnecessary. Nurses who are less experienced and handle or administer chemotherapy infrequently are advised to wear gowns (Miller, 1988). Wearing gloves is unquestionably a minimal precaution, which should be taken during equipment assembly and venipuncture.

3. During vein selection, the nurse should avoid venipuncture in any arm with possible or proven compromised circulation (e.g., phlebitis, lymphedema due to tumor invasion or axillary dissection, and prior trauma to veins such as drug extravasation). The risk for drug extravasation is increased when drugs are infused into an arm with evidence of superior vena cava syndrome or compromised circulation or into phlebitic veins that are inflamed and irritated.

4. To preserve venous integrity over time, the nurse should begin distally and alternate venipuncture sites, if possible. In general, veins of the dorsum of the hand are preferred because they are easy to visualize and stabilize. However, the favored site for the administration of vesicant agents is the forearm because this area has more underlying muscle and tissue to protect vital nerves and provide tissue coverage if necessary in the event of surgical management of an extravasation. If no obvious vein is found in the forearm, the dorsum of the hand is a good second choice, followed by the wrist area. A large vein on the dorsum of the hand is preferred to a small vein in the forearm. The antecubital fossa is generally avoided for vesicant drug administration. If the drug infiltrates into this area, the signs and symptoms are difficult to detect early. Consequently, severe structural and functional problems can occur, with damage to nerves and tendons in and around the antecubital area. With the advent of numerous VADs, it is no longer reasonable or safe to resort to administering vesicant agents in the area of the antecubital fossa.

5. If an obvious site for venipuncture is not apparent by observation or palpation following the use of traditional methods of venous distention (tourniquet, vein

percussion, heat), a colleague should be consulted before attempting venipuncture. Also, seek assistance after two unsuccessful attempts to secure adequate venous access. Consider whether the patient should have a VAD placed before receiving the drug.

6. A cannula should be selected that is appropriate for both the length of the therapy and the patient's available veins. A 25- or 23-gauge scalp vein needle (butterfly) is ideal for direct push (two-syringe technique) or short-term infusions (30 to 60 minutes). A plastic thin-walled catheter is appropriate for more lengthy infusions such as for blood components or hydration regimens that last 2 to 3 hours (Knobf & Fischer, 1989). The site is sterilized by a 1-minute alcohol rub or a povidine-iodine and alcohol rub. To avoid contaminating the area, do not repalpate before venipuncture. Once the scalp vein needle enters the vein and blood return is obvious, release the tourniquet and attach a syringe of saline to the tubing. Tape the phalanges of the needle securely without obstructing the entrance of the needle. Aspirate the air from the tubing and flush the catheter with 7 to 10 ml of saline to ensure that the needle has not punctured the vein. Palpate the site gently and observe for swelling or any evidence of infiltration. If the needle rests securely in the vein with a brisk, full blood return and no evidence of infiltration, the chemotherapy is injected slowly to prevent undue pressure on the vein wall. Check for blood return after every 1 to 2 ml of solution is administered. Flush the vein with 3 to 5 ml of saline between agents and with 5 to 7 ml of saline before removing the needle.

7. If the drug is to be given via the side arm of a freely running IV line, any dressing hindering visualization of the site should be removed. The size of the needle attached to the syringe must be smaller than the size of the needle in the patient's vein to permit the IV solution to drip while the drug is being injected. Otherwise fluid backs up in the tubing and makes this method of drug delivery no different from straight push using the two-syringe technique. Ensure a blood return by lowering the infusion bag or by aspirating blood into the tubing.

8. When injecting a vesicant into the side arm of a peripheral IV line, the line should not be infusing with the aid of an infusion pump because of the increased potential for extravasation and the impossibility of quickly reversing the direction of drug flow in the event of a possible extravasation.

9. If a drug in combination is known to be associated with rapid onset of nausea and vomiting (e.g., high-dose cyclophosphamide or cisplatin), it is generally administered last. If a vesicant is to be given along with an infusion, it should be given first in anticipation of perivenous irritation from movement during the time of the infusion. The order of administration of drugs (vesicant first or last) has not been shown to have any bearing on long-term venous integrity or risk of extravasation. Regardless of the order of the drugs, the line should be flushed with saline before changing drugs and at the end of the treatment.

10. The entire course of the vein should be visible during the injection and infusion. Observe for any evidence of vein irritation. The patient is encouraged to report any feelings of pain, itching, or burning during the treatment.

11. A vesicant agent should not be injected distal to a previous puncture site.

12. Vesicant agents should not be infused as a mini-infusion or continuous infusion into a peripheral vein. Regardless of its dilution, the drug has the potential to cause tissue destruction if infiltration occurs. Given the ease of insertion of the numerous short-term and long-term VADs, infusing a vesicant agent into a peripheral vein places the patient at unnecessary risk for drug extravasation and tissue damage. If an infusion of a vesicant is required to achieve the optimum therapeutic result, a central venous access line, as a tunneled, a nontunneled, or an implanted device, should be inserted before initiating therapy (see "Vascular Access Devices").

Management of an Extravasation

Extravasation may be defined as the extrusion or passage of caustic fluid, in this case vesicant chemotherapeutic agents, from a vein into the surrounding subcutaneous tissues (Jameson & O'Donnell, 1983). Once this occurs, tissue damage of varying degrees ensues. The actual clinical course of tissue destruction is variable depending on the drug itself, the concentration, the amount extravasated, and the specific measures utilized to manage the infiltration. The tissue damage may appear initially to be minimal owing to the indolent course of most extravasations. Gradually, after 3 to 5 days, the area appears obviously inflamed and is painful to the touch, providing evidence of cellular destruction. After 12 to 14 days, the actual extent of damage is usually evident with frank ulceration, demarcation, and eschar formation (Montrose, 1987). The damage to underlying structures (tendons and nerves) may lead to functional impairment. Infection and cellulitis can result in progressive tissue damage and limb dysfunction. Table 22–4 lists the antineoplastic agents according to their vesicant or irritant properties.

The reported incidence of inadvertent chemotherapy extravasation ranges from 0.45 to 5 per cent of all toxic reactions to chemotherapy (Ignoffo & Friedman, 1980; Larson, 1982; Laughlin, Landeen, & Habal, 1979). Differences in occurrence may be related to inexperience or lack of knowledge of the signs and symptoms of extravasation. Current recommendations are that these drugs be administered according to established policies and procedures by persons who are specially trained in chemotherapy drug administration. The factors that affect the risk of extravasation are (1) the skill of the practitioner, (2) the condition of the vein, (3) the drug administration technique, (4) the order of vesicant administration, (5) the site of venous access, and (6) the use of a preexisting IV line. Table 22–5 summarizes strategies that are effective in the prevention of extravasation.

The management of an extravasation is dependent

Table 22–4. VESICANTS AND IRRITANTS

VESICANT AGENTS: Capable of producing a blister and gradual tissue destruction with necrosis if extravasated
Commercial
Epirubicin hydrochloride (Pharmorubicin)
Dactinomycin (Cosmegen, Actinomycin, ACT-D)
Doxorubicin (Adriamycin, Rubex)
Mitomycin (Mutamycin, Mitomycin-C)
Mechlorethamine (Mustargen, nitrogen mustard)
Vinblastine (Velban, Velsar)
Vincristine (Oncovin, Vincasar)
Daunorubicin hydrochloride (Cerubidine, Daunomycin)

Investigational
Amsacrine (M-AMSA)
Bisantrene
Maytansine
Vindesine (Eldisine)
Pyrazofurin (Pyrazomycin)

IRRITANT AGENTS: Capable of producing perivenous pain at the site of injection or along the vein during injection or infusion
Commercial
Etoposide (VP-16-213, VePesid)
Carmustine (BCNU)
Streptozocin (Zanosar, Streptozotocin)
Plicamycin (Mithracin, Mithramycin)
Dacarbazine (DTIC-Dome, DTIC)
Teniposide (VM-26)

Investigational
Mitoguazone (Methyl-GAG)

largely on the drug infiltrated and on whether an antidote exists to inactivate the infiltrated drug. For most vesicant agents, no such antidote exists: for extravasations of these agents, it may be advisable to do nothing more than apply ice locally for symptomatic relief. Currently two antidotes are recommended by manufacturers as treatment for inadvertent drug extravasation: sodium thiosulfate for mechlorethamine (nitrogen mustard) infiltration and hyaluronidase for vinblastine and vincristine infiltration (Table 22–6). Table 22–7 includes local treatment for vesicant infiltration.

The signs and symptoms of extravasation can be subtle. Pain, stinging, or burning can occur, but these are not always present. Resistance to flow, swelling, or diffuse induration may occur but may be less evident in an individual who is obese or dehydrated. The absence of blood return can indicate that the needle bevel is against the vein wall or that the needle is not in the vein. The presence of blood return does not guarantee that an infiltration has not occurred because the needle may have extended partially through the posterior wall of the vein, allowing for a subtle leakage of the vesicant.

How, then, does one determine whether the drug has actually infiltrated? Even a slight change in the appearance of the tissue surrounding the insertion site is ample reason to restart the injection in another vein. However, in the absence of tissue swelling, a complaint of pain, stinging, or burning or a change in the quality of the blood return is highly suspect and warrants further investigation. The first step is to stop the injection of the vesicant and immediately aspirate the contents of the tubing. Then a syringe of saline is attached to the tubing, and the line is flushed to test the patency of the vein. After an adequate amount of fluid (20 to 30 ml) has been injected without evidence of swelling and a blood return is ensured, the vesicant may again be injected. If the patient subsequently complains of pain or burning, the injection should be stopped despite the absence of any other signs of extravasation (absence of blood return or frank swelling).

The procedure for management of an extravasation of a vesicant agent depends on the drug infiltrated and the recommendations of current research concerning appropriate management. In general, the decision to leave the needle in place depends on whether an antidote is available or whether any fluid can be aspirated from the site. If fluid cannot be aspirated or no antidote exists, the needle should be removed. The following describes basic guidelines for management of a known or presumed extravasation:

1. Stop the administration of the drug (note amount remaining in syringe); estimate amount infiltrated.

2. Exchange the syringe of chemotherapy for an empty 20-ml syringe.

3. Attempt to aspirate any residual drug and blood in the intravenous tubing (up to 20 ml).

4. Note the amount aspirated.

5. Remove the needle if no antidote is available; otherwise stabilize the syringe and prepare the antidote.

6. Instill the intravenous antidote via the existing needle or cannula if indicated (see Table 22–6).

7. Remove the needle, being careful not to apply undue pressure to the site.

8. If unable to aspirate the vesicant drug from the tubing, remove the needle. Apply ethyl chloride locally to numb the site. Inject the antidote subcutaneously into the area using a 25-gauge needle. Multiple (3 to 4) injections may be necessary, depending on the extent of drug infiltration.

9. Remove the needle and apply a bandage without applying pressure to the site. Immobilize the extravasation site, and elevate the arm for 3 days. Observe regularly for pain, erythema, and induration.

10. Notify physician.

11. Consider plastic surgery consultation if pain persists after 72 hours.

12. Document the occurrence in the patient's chart, and complete the extravasation record (Table 22–8).

13. Include a photograph of the site in the patient's record once an extravasation occurs, and take a photograph regularly with each visit to document progress.

Most extravasations of vesicant agents resolve spontaneously, especially if only a small amount of the drug is infiltrated (less than 0.5 ml). However, if a large amount (5 to 7 ml) has infiltrated, extensive tissue damage can be expected, and surgical intervention may be warranted. Surgical excision is generally indicated if pain persists after 3 to 7 days (Larson, 1982). The use of fluorescein aids in the identification of devitalized tissues, and surgery results in removal of all necrotic tissue. A biologic covering, usually a pigskin graft, is applied initially because of the potential for

Table 22–5. EXTRAVASATION OF VESICANT ANTINEOPLASTIC AGENTS: PREVENTIVE STRATEGIES

Risk Factor	Preventive Strategy	Rationale
Skill of the Practitioner	Chemotherapy administration only done by registered nurses who are specifically trained and supervised.	Procedures for management of extravasation vary according to the drug infiltrated. Certain drugs (streptozocin or BCNU) may cause a burning sensation during infusion, which is normal. However, it is abnormal and indicative of a problem if burning occurs during infusion of drugs such as doxorubicin and mitomycin.
	No attempts by practitioner to do procedures beyond his or her expertise. Practitioners are skillful in venipuncture. Practitioners are knowledgeable of the signs and symptoms of extravasation and drug therapy. Practice is based on institutional policies and procedures that are routinely updated to meet the changing standards and methods of practice.	Procedures change rapidly. Techniques need to be learned and mastered before assuming responsibility for administration of chemotherapy. The definition of customary care in the community helps dictate standard of practice.
Condition of the Veins • Small fragile veins • Access limited owing to axillary surgery, vein thrombosis, prior extravasation • Long-term drug therapy • Multiple vein punctures	Use conventional methods for venous distention such as heat and percussion. Assess all available arm veins. Assess veins in a methodical fashion, taking time to select the most appropriate vein. If practitioners do not feel confident in their ability to cannulate a person's veins successfully, they should seek the assistance of a colleague. After attempting one or two injections without success, the practitioner should seek the assistance of a colleague before trying again. A patient who consistently needs two or more attempts to secure venous access should be considered a candidate for a VAD. The time to place a VAD is before an extravasation, not after.	Risk of vesicant drug seepage exists with repeated venipuncture. Multiple vein injections lead to thrombosis and limited availability. Before the advent of vascular access devices (VADs), multiple venous injections to administer a drug might have been accepted as the only method of drug administration. This is no longer the case. Instead, treatment should be delayed until a VAD can be placed. Most VADs can be used immediately or within 24 to 48 hours, so delay in drug therapy is not usually an issue.
Drug Administration Technique	Vesicant agents are never given as continuous infusions into a peripheral vein.	The risk of infiltration of a vesicant from a peripheral vein infusion is great owing to the following: 1. Blood return is not assessed frequently. 2. The longer the infusion, the greater the possibility of needle dislodgment. 3. The patient can move the extremity, which could dislodge the intravenous (IV) cannula. 4. Even a small amount of vesicant can cause tissue damage. 5. Infiltration can be subtle and difficult to detect until a large volume has infiltrated. 6. The patient may be sedated from an antiemetic and be unable to report sensations associated with extravasation. 7. The pump forces drug into the tissues.
	If peripheral line is on a controlled infusion pump, disconnect pump before injection of chemotherapy. When a vesicant is to be given as a continuous infusion, the drug should be infused via an externally based central venous catheter whenever possible.	When an implanted port already exists, the patient is taught to check the needle three times a day to ensure placement during continuous infusion of a vesicant. The incidence of vesicant drug extravasation from ports used for continuous infusion is well documented and presents a risk to be avoided, if possible.
	Vesicant agents are most commonly administered using the two-syringe technique or through the side port of a free-flowing peripheral intravenous line.	The two-syringe technique allows for proper assessment of blood flow and resistance in the vein. A scalp vein needle causes minimal vein irritation.

Table 22–5. EXTRAVASATION OF VESICANT ANTINEOPLASTIC AGENTS: PREVENTIVE STRATEGIES *Continued*

Risk Factor	Preventive Strategy	Rationale
	Two-Syringe Technique 1. Select an appropriate vein. 2. Begin a new intravenous line using a scalp vein needle (25 or 23 gauge). 3. Access vein using a single approach. 4. Flush line with 8 to 10 ml of saline. Assess for brisk, full blood return and any evidence of infiltration. Check for swelling at the site, redness or pain, and lack of blood return. 5. Once access is assured, switch to syringe of chemotherapy. 6. Dilute drugs according to the package insert. 7. Inject drugs slowly and with minimal resistance. 8. Assess for blood return every 1 to 2 ml of infusion. 9. Irrigate with 3–5 ml of saline between each drug and 8–10 ml at the completion of the infusion of the drug or drugs.	A subtle leak can be caused by accidentally piercing the vein before accessing it; avoid searching for a vein with repeated approaches. Increasing the dilution increases the time it takes to administer the drug, thus increasing risk of infiltration. The speed of the injection is determined by the resistance in the vein. Resistance will vary depending on the size of the needle used.
	Side-arm Technique 1. Ensure proper venous access site. The IV fluid should be additive free. 2. Cannula used to access the vein should be at least a 20 gauge to ensure an adequate blood return and fluid flow. 3. Secure cannula but do not obstruct entrance site. 4. Pinch off tubing and assess for blood return. 5. Test the vein with 50 to 100 ml to ensure an adequate and swift drip of infusion. 6. With IV fluid continuing to drip, slowly inject vesicant into IV line. 7. Do not allow vesicant to flow backwards. 8. Do not pinch off tubing except to assess for blood return. 9. Assess for blood return every 1 to 2 ml of injection. 10. Flush scalp vein needle with saline at the completion of injection.	The main rationale for the side-arm technique is the added dilution of the drug by the continuous drip of the IV fluid. Common pitfalls: 1. Not using a large enough cannula for a brisk infusion of infusate. 2. Vesicant backs up into IV line. 3. Intravenous line has to be pinched off to inject vesicant, which defeats the purpose. 4. Clinician tends to take eyes off of the site of drug infusion to watch fluid drip more than with two-syringe technique.
Order of Vesicant Drug Administration *Note:* Sequencing is probably unimportant. The most critical issue is adequately testing the vein with saline (8–10 ml) before administering any drug (vesicant or nonvesicant).	Give vesicant first. Give vesicant between two nonvesicants. Give vesicant last.	Vascular integrity decreases over time. Practitioner's assessment skills are most acute initially. Patient may be more sedated from antiemetic and less able to report changes in sensation at infusion site as time goes on. Chemotherapy is irritating to the veins. Nonvesicants are presumed to be less irritating than vesicants. Because venous spasm occurs early during the injection, it is less likely to be confused with pain of extravasation if vesicant is given last. It is assumed that because the vein tolerated the nonvesicants, it will also tolerate the vesicant.
Site of Venous Access Choosing the best vein	VADs, including tunneled catheters, implanted ports, and nontunneled central venous catheters, are indicated when patients have small, frail veins and are in need of long-term indefinite chemotherapy, continuous infusion of vesicant drugs, or both. Although a VAD is a good way to prevent extravasation, it is not indicated just because someone is receiving a vesicant drug.	VADs are important options for patients with poor venous access. Externally based catheters are ideal for continuous infusion of vesicant chemotherapeutic agents because the risk of extravasation is very minimal. Expert technique and a knowledgeable clinician are the most cost-effective and safe means of administering vesicant drugs.

Table continued on following page

Table 22–5. EXTRAVASATION OF VESICANT ANTINEOPLASTIC AGENTS: PREVENTIVE STRATEGIES *Continued*

Risk Factor	Preventive Strategy	Rationale
	Peripheral access is optimal in the large veins of the forearm, especially the posterior basilic vein. After these, the metacarpal veins of the dorsum of the hand are easy to access and stabilize. The veins over the wrist are risky because of potential damage to tendons and nerves should extravasation occur. *Note:* A large straight vein over the dorsum of the hand is preferable to a smaller vein of the forearm.	Veins in the forearm are large and adequately supported by surrounding tissue. Adequate tissue exists around veins to provide coverage and promote healing should a problem occur.
	The antecubital fossa is to be avoided for vesicant drug administration. If the antecubital fossa appears to be the only vein available for access, the patient needs an access device. Hold chemotherapy—insert VAD.	The area is dense with tendons and nerves. Seepage of a vesicant can be subtle and go unnoticed. Damage here can result in loss of structure and function. Risking extravasation and subsequent tissue damage is not worth the temptation to give "just one more treatment" before considering other options. There is no evidence that delaying chemotherapy for 24 hours in selected cases is detrimental to the overall outcome.
	Avoid administering chemotherapy in lower extremities.	Risk for thrombosis is increased when chemotherapy is given in lower extremities.
Using a Preexisting IV Line	Do not use a preexisting peripheral intravenous line if any of the following are true: 1. The IV cannula was placed more than 12 hours earlier. 2. The site is reddened, swollen, or sore, or there is evidence of infiltration. 3. The site is over or around the wrist. 4. Evidence of blood return is sluggish or absent. 5. The IV fluid runs erratically and the IV seems positional. If the IV fluid runs freely; the blood return is brisk and consistent; and the site is without redness, pain, or swelling, then there is no reason to inflict unnecessary pain by injecting the patient again.	It is unreasonable to disregard the potential for a perfectly adequate venous access line because it was not started by the person administering the vesicant drug. Our ability to assess the vein and evidence of blood return should be adequate to ensure the practitioner of an adequate and safe venous access.
	Prior dressings must be carefully removed over the cannula insertion site to fully visualize the vein during injection of the vesicant agent.	Dressings and tape can severely impede both visually and tactilely an assessment for an extravasation.

infection. The area may need additional mechanical or surgical debridement. If the wound appears clean after 2 to 3 days, a skin graft may be applied (Larson, 1985). Provided the excision is adequate, surgical intervention results in immediate pain relief and provides appropriate wound coverage to permit healing. Surgery does not generally interrupt the patient's chemotherapy schedule. In most situations, chemotherapy can be resumed 7 to 10 days following surgery (Larson, 1985).

Additional research is needed to delineate methods for the management of extravasation of vesicant antineoplastic agents. No single antidote is useful for all drugs, and many of the currently recommended therapies are based on anecdotal findings and limited experimental data. Recommendations given in the product brochure or findings from animal or clinical experiments should be followed. When these are absent, it may be in the patient's best interest to institute no local therapy beyond cooling, immobilization, and elevation of the extremity.

Mechlorethamine. Mechlorethamine (nitrogen mustard) is a severe vesicant that rapidly destroys local tissues once extravasated. Animal studies have demonstrated the need for rapid treatment of mechlorethamine extravasations (within minutes) to prevent tissue damage (Dorr, Soble, & Alberts, 1988). Sodium thiosulfate, 5 to 6 ml (1:6 molar), is divided equally and given through the existing IV line and subcutaneously into the infiltrated area. Sodium thiosulfate effectively binds with and inactivates the nitrogen mustard (Owen, 1980). Only one instillation of sodium thiosulfate is necessary. Ulceration may occur up to 2 weeks after the extravasation. If pain is severe after 7 days, the site should be evaluated for surgical excision.

Plant Alkaloids. As a group, the plant alkaloids are weakly toxic to tissues if infiltrated. Extravasation of these drugs generally causes local pain and induration. Cellulitis, phlebitis, and local inflammation may be evident over 3 to 5 days. Minor infiltration usually resolves after 5 to 6 weeks without ulceration. However, the area may remain tender and the vein thrombosed for months. In rare situations, tissue damage

Table 22–6. EXTRAVASATION MANAGEMENT: KNOWN ANTIDOTES AND LOCAL TREATMENT

Drug	Antidote	Antidote Preparation	Method of Administration
Mechlorethamine (nitrogen mustard)	Isotonic sodium thiosulfate (1 gm/10 ml)	Mix of 4 ml of 10% sodium thiosulfate with 6 ml sterile water for injection (1:6 molar solution results)	1. For each mg of drug extravasated, inject 5 ml intravenously through the existing line and subcutaneously into the extravasated site.* 2. Only a single course of sodium thiosulfate is recommended. 3. Apply cold compresses. 4. Elevate the extremity. *Note:* Initiate treatment immediately and liberally.
Vinblastine (Velban) Vincristine (Oncovin)	Hyaluronidase (150 U/ml)	Add 1 to 3 ml U.S.P. sodium chloride to vial of hyaluronidase	1. Inject 1 to 3 ml of hyaluronidase solution (150 U) into needle or catheter or inject subcutaneously into site. 2. Gently apply a heat pack to site for 1 hour. 3. Elevate the extremity.

*If subcutaneous injections are needed, a topical anesthetic such as ice or ethyl chloride may be applied to the site immediately before injection.

may proceed to necrosis, with the amount of ulceration and infection depending on the concentration of the drug and the amount infiltrated. Vincristine, vinblastine, and vindesine are usually given by intravenous injection and are considered potential vesicants. If infiltration occurs, hyaluronidase (150 U/ml), 1 to 6 ml injected subcutaneously into the extravasated site, plus heat, appears to enhance the absorption and systemic dispersion of the extravasated drug. Should extravasation occur from other plant alkaloids (etoposide or teniposide), the same procedure can be used to minimize local tissue changes even though they are likely to be minor. In contrast, the use of steroids, cooling, or both as local therapy for plant alkaloid infiltrations appears to worsen tissue destruction and should be avoided (Dorr & Alberts, 1985).

Table 22–7. EXTRAVASATION MANAGEMENT: LOCAL TREATMENT

Drug	Local Treatment	Method of Administration
Anthracycline antibiotics Doxorubicin (Adriamycin, Rubex) Daunomycin	Hydrocortisone solution (100-mg vial)	1. Press diluent stopper into vial to reconstitute. 2. Inject 1 ml (5 mg) hydrocortisone through the indwelling intravenous (IV) line or, in the absence of a blood return, remove IV line and inject hydrocortisone in a radical fashion into site. 3. Do not repeat dosing. 4. Apply sterile bandage. 5. Apply cold pack every 2 to 3 hours for 24 hours (on 50 minutes, off 10 minutes).
	OR DMSO (50–100%) (topical)	OR 1. Soak a sterile gauze or cotton ball in DMSO solution. 2. Apply solution to site, allowing it to become saturated. 3. Allow site to air dry. 4. Apply a sterile bandage. 5. Apply cold pack as above. 6. Repeat every 4 hours for 7 to 10 days.
Mitomycin C Mutamycin	DMSO (50–100%) (topical)	1. Soak a sterile gauze or cotton ball in DMSO solution. 2. Saturate site with DMSO immediately after infiltration. 3. Allow site to air dry. 4. Apply a sterile bandage. 5. Apply ice pack for symptomatic relief only. 6. A single application of DMSO may be sufficient.
	OR Sodium thiosulfate (1 gm/10 ml); mix 4 ml of 10% sodium thiosulfate with 6 ml sterile water for injection.	OR 1. Inject 3 to 5 ml intravenously through the existing line or subcutaneously into the extravasated site. 2. Cover with a sterile bandage. 3. Apply ice pack for symptomatic relief only. 4. Elevate extremity.

DMSO, dimethyl sulfoxide.

Table 22–8. CHEMOTHERAPY DRUG EXTRAVASATION RECORD

Date_____
Time_____

Patient_____ Risk Factors_____
Drug_____ Dilution mg/mL_____
Method of Administration: Two-syringe technique IV push _____
                          Side-arm _____
                          VAD: Port _____
                          Type of needle _____
                          Other: _____

Amount infiltrated_____ Amount aspirated_____
Size of infiltration (note size in cm)

Location of Extravasation
Hand: Dorsal Surface   *Arm:* Ventral Surface

hand_____	rt_____	lt_____	forearm_____	rt_____	lt_____
forearm_____	rt_____	lt_____	wrist_____	rt_____	lt_____
wrist_____	rt_____	lt_____	ac fossa_____	rt_____	lt_____

VAD: Describe_____
other_____ Photograph yes_____ no_____

Process Documentation:
S: (Patient Symptoms)_____

O: (Clinical Signs)_____

A: (Assessment) suspected extravasation_____definite extravasation _____
P: (Plan of care)_____Physician notified: Date_____Time_____Initials_____

Follow-up (document with serial photographs):_____

Anthracyclines (Daunomycin and Doxorubicin). When considering the anthracyclines doxorubicin and daunorubicin, it is important to note that currently no known antidotes are available to inactivate these drugs. The majority of research concerning the management of local tissue toxicity concerns doxorubicin, a commonly used antineoplastic agent. There are two distinctly different local skin reactions to doxorubicin injection: a benign skin reaction called *flare* and a severe ulceration and necrosis due to infiltration of the drug. The flare reaction is characterized by a local erythematous streaking and inflammation that persists up to 30 minutes after the drug infusion. The redness and induration are usually accompanied by itching along the course of the vein. This reaction occurs infrequently (3 per cent of cases) and does not preclude subsequent use of the drug (Vogelzang, 1979). The occurrence of the flare reaction may be related to injecting doxorubicin too rapidly or injecting the drug into a small vein. The flare reaction may also be influenced by the practice of injecting doxorubicin after dexamethasone, which is commonly used as an antiemetic. By giving the doxorubicin first, a 4- to 5-ml saline flush next, and the dexamethasone last, the incidence of flare may be reduced. If flare occurs under any circumstance, the first step is to determine that the local redness is not due to a frank extravasation. By flushing liberally with 10 to 20 ml of saline, the symptoms generally resolve, permitting the continued slow injection of the doxorubicin and eliminating the need to re-stick the patient. Local therapy with antihistamines is unnecessary because the flare reaction resolves spontaneously 20 to 30 minutes after the injection.

A severe ulceration is another local skin reaction caused by the infiltration of an anthracycline into the subcutaneous tissues. The exact mechanism of anthracycline-induced tissue damage is not known but may be related to a process called *endocytosis*. Once the anthracycline-DNA complex is formed, the cell dies, releasing the anthracycline unchanged and free to attach itself to a neighboring cell. The drug itself persists and accounts for the indolent and progressive nature of the tissue damage (Averbuch, Gaudiano, & Koch, 1986). Alternately, the anthracycline may be reduced to a free radical that can cause cellular membrane damage. Fluorometric examination following extravasation shows the persistence of doxorubicin in cell nuclei for 1 to 8 weeks following injection (Desai & Teres, 1982; Luedke, Kennedy, & Rietschel, 1979). Whatever the exact mechanism may be, clinical and histologic studies have demonstrated that major changes in tissues occur within 3 days of extravasation and persist up to 12 weeks or longer (Coleman, Walker, & Didolkar, 1983).

Using various animal models, a variety of pharmacologic approaches have been evaluated to treat doxorubicin and daunorubicin extravasations (Averbuch et al., 1986; Coleman et al., 1983; Luedke et al., 1979). Although animal studies have demonstrated encouraging findings, applications to clinical situations have not produced similar results, probably because of differences in tissue composition, drug concentrations, volume infiltrated, and time elapsed between infiltration and treatment.

One commonly proposed therapy for doxorubicin extravasation has been local injection of a corticosteroid such as hydrocortisone. Theoretically, the action of a corticosteroid stabilizes the cell membrane, thereby inhibiting the uptake of doxorubicin (Dorr, Alberts, & Chen, 1980). In addition, it acts as an anti-inflammatory agent. However, histologic examination of these doxorubicin lesions fails to demonstrate an inflammatory response, making hydrocortisone less likely to be of benefit (Cox, 1984; Luedke et al., 1979). Although the injection of low-dose hydrocortisone (25 to 50 mg) locally into the extravasation site has been recommended (Barlock, Howser, & Hubbard, 1979; Okano, Ohnuma, Efemidis, et al., 1983; Oncology Nursing Society, 1988), not all studies have reported significant benefit from the use of steroids (Bowers & Lynch, 1978; Cox, 1984; Dorr et al., 1980).

Local instillation of sodium bicarbonate (5 ml of 8.4 per cent solution) through the existing IV line has been recommended as a means of raising the local pH and thereby disrupting cellular uptake, DNA binding, and subsequent damage by doxorubicin (Bartowski-Dodds & Daniels, 1980). Other studies report no benefit from the use of sodium bicarbonate as a local antidote to doxorubicin extravasation (Barr & Sertic, 1981; Dorr, 1987). Likewise sodium bicarbonate is known to cause severe tissue necrosis in higher doses (Gaze, 1978; Jackson & Robinson, 1976). Dimethyl sulfoxide (DMSO) and alpha-tocopherol are two free radical scavengers that have been tested as potential antidotes to doxorubicin extravasation. Svingen and colleagues (1981) reported that a combination of DMSO and alpha-tocopherol applied topically for 48 hours following doxorubicin infiltration significantly reduced the mean ulcer size in rats. Although some investigators have confirmed these positive effects of topical DMSO (Desai & Teres, 1982; Okano et al., 1983), the findings are inconsistent. Dorr and Alberts (1983) found that neither intradermal nor topical DMSO with or without alpha-tocopherol administered up to 7 days reduced doxorubicin-induced skin ulcerations. In fact, some investigators have concluded that the intradermal or subcutaneous use of DMSO-containing solutions is contraindicated owing to their increased ulcerogenic effect (Dorr & Alberts, 1983; Smith, Hadidian, & Mason, 1967). Likewise, Harwood and Bachur (1987) found no difference in terms of lesion severity between topical DMSO for 7 days and no treatment at all. In addition, time until healing appeared to be lengthened by DMSO application. However, when used in the clinical situation, Oliver and Schwarz (1983) described three cases in which topical DMSO appeared to lessen doxorubicin ulceration. It is important to note that in this study the exact benefit of DMSO is difficult to interpret because patients were also treated with 2 to 5 ml of 8.4 per cent sodium bicarbonate and ice packs.

A true antidote inactivates or renders a substance nontoxic, usually by changing its chemical composition. DHM_3 is a radical dimer that reacts with doxorubicin in vitro to produce an inactive anthracycline metabolite that has potential for clinical application. DHM_3 has been shown in animal experiments to be an effective antidote for doxorubicin-induced skin necrosis when administered within 60 minutes of infiltration (Averbuch et al., 1986).

Another local therapy commonly recommended for doxorubicin extravasation is the immediate application of ice for 20 to 60 minutes four to six times a day (Dorr, Alberts, & Stone, 1985; Harwood & Bachur, 1987; Larson, 1982). Cold causes a vasoconstriction that limits concentration of the drug to the infiltrated site. Decreasing the temperature locally also reduces the metabolic rate and mitotic activity of the cells. Larson (1982, 1985) recommends applying ice to the site of extravasation for 20 minutes four times a day for 3 days. The limb is elevated, and the site is observed closely. Using this treatment, 89 per cent of patients (N = 175) required no further therapy following extravasation (Larson, 1985). The remainder required surgical intervention. The major indication for wide excision of all tissues that appear abnormal is pain. Delaying surgery for 3 to 5 days allows for a clear definition of the extent of tissue destruction and a delineation of which lesions are likely to resolve on their own and which require surgical intervention (Coleman et al., 1983; Larson, 1982).

In summary, no effective local antidote is currently available to treat anthracycline extravasation. Although topical DMSO or local infiltration of low-dose hydrocortisone may lessen the local reaction in some situations, the application of ice appears to be the most useful local measure to minimize tissue destruction in the event of an anthracycline extravasation.

Mitomycin. Mitomycin is a severe vesicant that is capable of producing extensive local damage if infiltrated. In addition, mitomycin has been noted to produce delayed ulcerations distant from the injection site (Argenta & Manders, 1983; Johnston-Early & Cohen, 1981; Wood & Ellerhorst-Ryan, 1984). A commonly proposed local therapy for mitomycin extravasation is 1:6 molar sodium thiosulfate (R. Ignoffo, personal communication, 1987; Ignoffo & Friedman, 1980). Injecting the 3 to 5 ml of sodium thiosulfate in a pincushion fashion or singly through the existing intravenous line may effectively inactivate the infiltrated mitomycin.

Dorr, Soble, Liddie, and Keller (1986) tested numerous local pharmacologic interventions for their ability to reduce mitomycin extravasation in mice (Box 22–2). Among the agents tested and found to be ineffective were hyaluronidase, fumaric acid, hydrocortisone, heparin, isoproterenol, and vitamin E. Neither topical cooling nor topical heating was found to be effective. Sodium thiosulfate was noted to be somewhat effective in treating small lesions but not larger lesions. Of note is the finding that immediate application of topical DMSO (100 per cent) appears to protect against mitomycin tissue damage in the mouse. The mechanism of the protective effect of topical DMSO is not known. Initially it was felt that DMSO might enhance the systemic uptake of the mitomycin from the tissues, but this was found not to be the case. It is more likely that DMSO somehow interferes with the destructive alkylating reaction between the mitomycin and cellular target sites (Dorr et al., 1986).

Vascular Access Devices

The most common avenue for antineoplastic drug delivery is an intravenous one. Vascular access devices

---

Box 22–2. DMSO FOR MITOMYCIN EXTRAVASATION

STUDY

Dorr, R. T., Soble, M. J., Liddie, J. D., Keller, S. H. (1986). **Mitomycin C skin toxicity studies in mice: Reduced ulceration and altered pharmacokinetics with topical dimethyl sulfoxide.** *Journal of Clinical Oncology, 4,* 1399–1404.

PURPOSE

To compare the biologic effects of different local treatment approaches on mitomycin C (MMC) skin ulcerations in a standardized mouse model.

SAMPLE

Hair over the dorsal area was removed from adult BA1B/c female mice, using a topical depilatory lotion.

MEASURES

The mice were injected with two MMC drug doses: 0.025 and 0.075 mg. Local treatment included topical dimethyl sulfoxide, heat, cold, hyaluronidase, heparin, diphenhydramine, isoproterenol, hydrocortisone, fumaric acid, superoxide dismutase, catalase, vitamin E, lidocaine, *N*-acetylcysteine, and sodium thiosulfate.

Skin lesions were measured daily by a single observer using a micrometer caliper. Skin induration, erythema, and ulceration were noted. Statistical analyses of the different local treatments involved an initial analysis of variance and a multiple range test. Summary pharmacokinetic data for different groups were compared using the Student's T test. Samples of skin and plasma were obtained, and skin and plasma MMC pharmacokinetic studies and drug binding studies were performed.

FINDINGS

- Consistent skin ulcers were apparent within 1 to 5 days of intradermal MMC.
- DMSO was beneficial only when applied immediately after intradermal MMC injection. DMSO applied at 1, 4, 12, 24, and 48 hours after intradermal MMC did not significantly reduce skin ulceration.
- Neither local heating nor cooling of the mouse skin reduced MMC-induced skin ulcers.
- .33 mol/L sodium thiosulfate demonstrated significant protection from MMC-induced ulceration.
- No treatment benefits were seen with fumaric acid, hydrocortisone, heparin, isoproterenol, hyaluronidase, or vitamin E.
- Diphenhydramine, lidocaine, catalase, and superoxide dismutase increased MMC skin ulcers in mice.
- Topical DMSO alters the disposition of intradermal MMC in skin, which results in retention of the unchanged drug in the skin. Its therapeutic effect may be due to reduced reactivity of MMC with target cellular nucleophiles.

LIMITATIONS

- These findings need to be replicated in similar animal models, specifically in the pig model.
- The findings cannot be applied directly to the human clinical situation because of the experimental nature of the study.
- The therapeutic effects of DMSO are limited to the immediate postextravasation period and would not be useful for the occasional delayed MMC extravasation or for those lesions that appear distant from the drug treatment site.

(VADs) have evolved over the past 15 or more years and are currently designed to enable a patient to safely receive chemotherapy, ease the discomfort of intravenous drug delivery and blood sampling, facilitate blood component therapy and continuous infusion therapy of vesicant and nonvesicant agents in the inpatient or outpatient setting, and permit multiple drug and fluid therapies to be given concurrently or alternately with the chemotherapy.

The nurse is commonly in a position to recommend the insertion of a VAD. Factors to consider include the frequency of venous access, length of treatment, type of treatment, mode of administration, venous integrity, and patient preference. Table 22–9 lists the basic criteria to use to identify a patient as a potential candidate for a VAD (Goodman & Wickham, 1984; Miller, 1982).

When a patient requires only short-term continuous or intermittent administration of chemotherapy, fluids, or blood components, a percutaneous, nontunneled catheter is usually preferred. Central catheters such as the Cook (Cook, Inc.) are inserted via the subclavian vein by a physician, whereas the single-lumen peripheral nontunneled catheter such as the Per-Q-Cath

Table 22–9. PATIENT ASSESSMENT CRITERIA FOR VASCULAR ACCESS DEVICES

Frequency of Venous Access
Type of Treatment
Mode of Administration
Venous Integrity
Patient Preference

Low Priority	High Priority
Infrequent venous access	Frequent venous access
Short-term therapy	Long-term, indefinite treatment
Intermittent single injections	Continuous infusion of chemotherapy
Nonvesicant or nonirritating drugs	Home infusion of chemotherapy
No previous intravenous therapy	Vesicant or irritating drugs
Both extremities available	Venous thrombosis or sclerosis due to previous intravenous therapy
Venous access with two or fewer venipunctures	Venous access limited to one extremity
Patient does not prefer vascular access device	Prior tissue damage due to extravasation
	Multiple (>2) venipunctures to secure venous access
	Patient prefers vascular access device

(Adapted with permission from Goodman, M., & Wickham, R. [1984]. Venous access devices: An overview. *Oncology Nursing Forum, 11* [5], 17.)

(Gesco International) or Intrasil (Baxter Healthcare) is inserted by a physician or a specially trained nurse (Lawson, Bottino, & McCredie, 1979). A transparent dressing is placed over the exit site that allows the extension tubing to extend beyond the dressing for easy access. These catheters require daily irrigation with heparin and meticulous sterile technique during dressing changes. Because they are not tunneled, theoretically they carry a higher risk for infection. With proper care and maintenance, the incidence of infection is low and similar to that for the percutaneous tunneled catheters (Slater, Goldfarb, & Jacob, 1985). If a catheter-related infection is suspected, the nontunneled catheter can be replaced by an over-the-wire technique.

The percutaneously placed silicone tunneled catheters are intended for long-term indefinite use. They are usually placed on the anterior chest and tunneled beneath the skin to rest in the cephalic, internal, or external jugular or the subclavian vein (Fig. 22–1). The tip of the catheter rests near the entrance to the right atrium. When the patient is experiencing a superior vena cava syndrome, subclavian vein thrombosis, severe radiation changes, or tumor invasion of the chest and underlying tissues, it may be more appropriate to place the catheter into the saphenous vein with the tip resting in the inferior vena cava. The exit site is either on the lower abdomen or in the groin. This alternate placement site is generally associated with more difficulty in drawing blood but is an excellent alternative for long-term vascular access in these patients.

All tunneled catheters have a Dacron cuff, which serves a dual purpose. After about 2 weeks, fibroblasts form around the cuff, securing the catheter in place

and theoretically minimizing the risk of bacterial invasion around the catheter. To further minimize the incidence of infection, especially in the bone marrow transplantation population, an infection-control device called a Vitacuff (Vitaphore Corp.) may be placed around the catheter at the time of insertion. This attachable subcutaneous cuff is composed of a collagen impregnated with silver ions. The collagen induces tissue ingrowth, which stabilizes the catheter. The broad-spectrum antimicrobial activity of the silver ions acts as an additional barrier to organisms migrating into the subcutaneous catheter tract (Flowers et al., 1989).

These catheters are available as single-lumen, double-lumen, and triple-lumen designs (Fig. 22–2). The medical care needs of the individual patient dictate which catheter is most appropriate. These catheters are primarily indicated for patients who require frequent vascular access for blood sampling and chemotherapy administration. Tunneled catheters are the VAD of choice for continuous infusions of a vesicant agent, especially when it is administered by an ambulatory infusion pump on an outpatient basis. The patient can be taught to disconnect the pump and flush the catheter once the therapy is complete.

Disadvantages of the tunneled catheters are that they are costly, they require exit-site care and frequent flushings, and they may lead to body image changes. Immediately after placement, an occlusive dressing is placed over the exit site, which remains in place for 24 to 48 hours. After this time the dressing is changed using a sterile technique, and a transparent dressing is placed over the exit site and is changed every week or as necessary. After 2 weeks, a dressing is no longer required, provided the patient is not immunocompromised. However, most patients prefer to wear a dressing of some type or an adhesive bandage over the exit site to stabilize and secure the catheter in place. The catheter should always be taped to the patient to prevent its being inadvertently pulled out.

The tunneled catheter is irrigated every other day or once a week with 3 to 5 ml of heparinized saline solution (100 to 500 units of heparin/ml). The cap is changed once a week or once a month, depending on how often the catheter is irrigated. If the patient is using a Groshong catheter (C. R. Bard), the care needs vary slightly (Fig. 22–3). This single- or double-lumen catheter has a pressure-release valve that prevents blood from backing up into the catheter unless suction is exerted by a syringe to withdraw blood. Therefore, the catheter does not need to be irrigated with heparin, nor is a clamp required at any time. Indeed, to clamp the catheter could damage it. The Groshong catheter is flushed once a week with 5 ml of saline when not being used and with 20 ml after drawing blood. The Groshong is ideal for the elderly patient who is marginally capable of caring for a VAD but requires short-term or long-term continuous infusion of a vesicant agent. The exit-site care and catheter flushing can be provided weekly by a visiting nurse or a trip to the physician's office.

Implanted ports are primarily used for intravenous

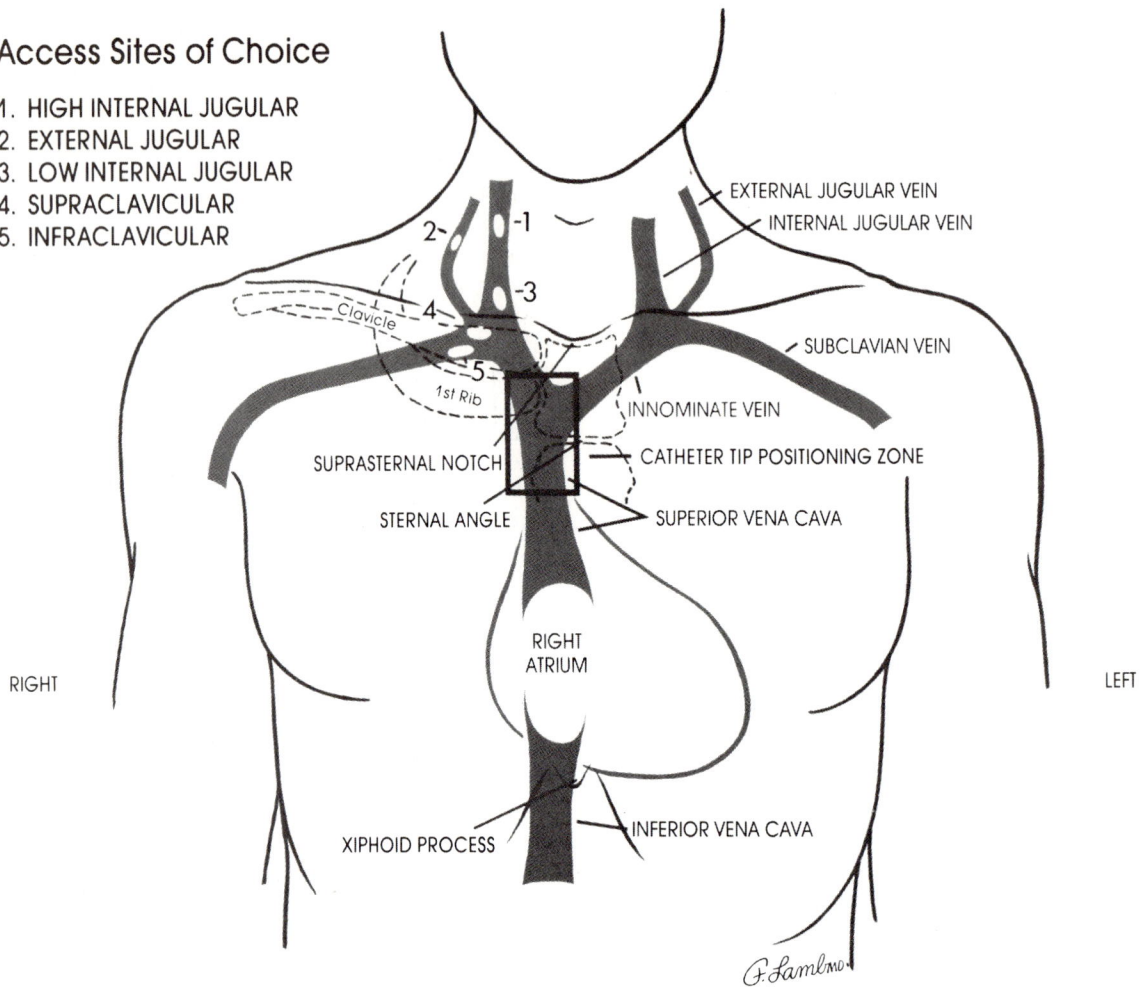

Access Sites of Choice

1. HIGH INTERNAL JUGULAR
2. EXTERNAL JUGULAR
3. LOW INTERNAL JUGULAR
4. SUPRACLAVICULAR
5. INFRACLAVICULAR

EXTERNAL JUGULAR VEIN

INTERNAL JUGULAR VEIN

SUBCLAVIAN VEIN

INNOMINATE VEIN

CATHETER TIP POSITIONING ZONE

SUPERIOR VENA CAVA

Clavicle

1st Rib

SUPRASTERNAL NOTCH

STERNAL ANGLE

RIGHT ATRIUM

RIGHT

LEFT

XIPHOID PROCESS

INFERIOR VENA CAVA

Figure 22–1. Anatomic location of vascular access catheters. (Courtesy of Cook, Inc., Bloomington, IN.)

therapy but can be used to administer drugs in the arteries (Niederhuber, Ensminger, & Gyves, 1982) and into the peritoneum (Pfeifle, Howell, & Markman, 1984). There are numerous types of implanted ports on the market. The Hickman subcutaneous port (Fig. 22–4); the Port-A-Cath (Fig. 22–5); Infusaid MicroPort (Fig. 22–6); and Norport-LS (Fig. 22–7); and the Hickman and Groshong ports (Fig. 22–8), are but a few examples of front-entrance ports. An example of a side-entrance port is the Norport-SP (Fig. 22–9).

The implanted ports are made of various materials,

including plastic, stainless steel, and titanium. The port septum consists of a dense silicone that is capable of withstanding 1000 to 2000 needle injections. A specially designed deflected point (Huber) needle is used to gain access to these ports and is designed to prevent damage to the septum with repeated injections. Figure 22–10 depicts the cross section of a port with the Huber point needle in place. The optimal placement for implanted ports used for vascular access is on the

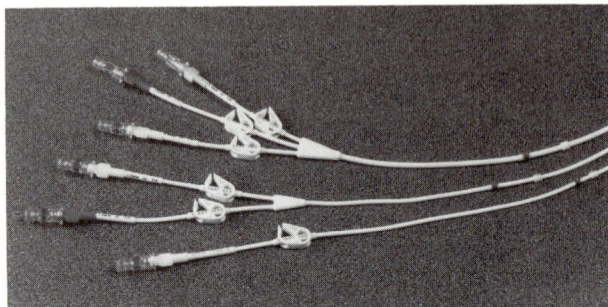

Figure 22–2. Single-lumen, double-lumen, and triple-lumen Hickman catheters (C. R. Bard, Inc.), with VitaCuff (Vitaphore Corp.). (Photographs courtesy of Davol Inc.)

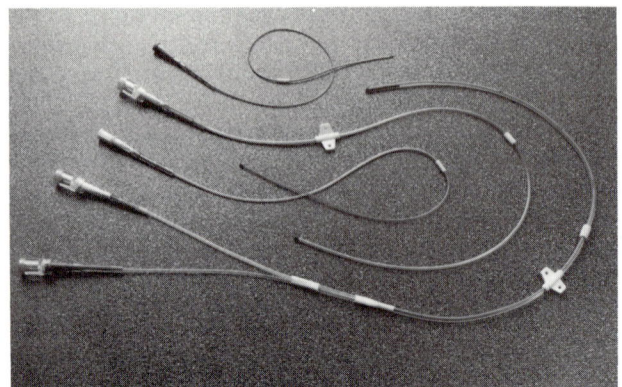

Figure 22–3. Single-lumen and double-lumen Groshong catheters (C. R. Bard, Inc.). (Photographs courtesy of Davol Inc.)

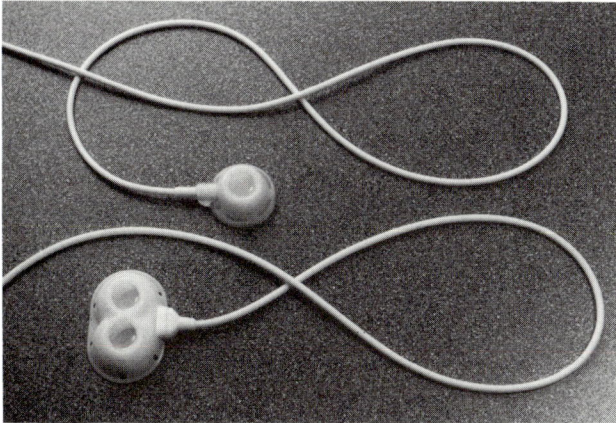

Figure 22–4. Single-lumen and double-lumen ports (MRI). (Photographs courtesy of Davol Inc.)

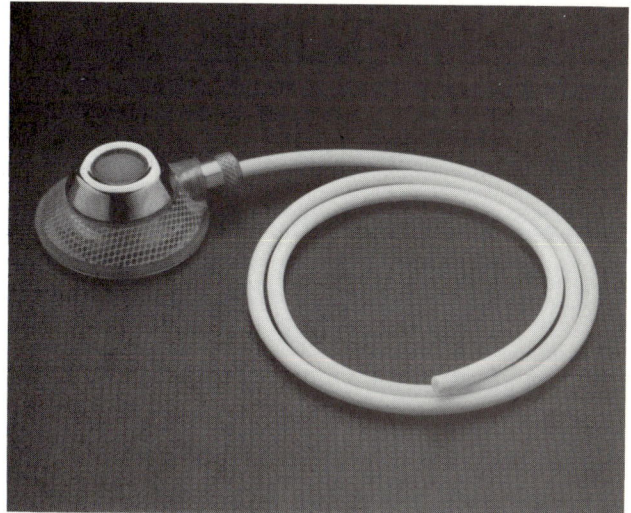

Figure 22–7. Norport-LS vascular access port. (Courtesy of Norfolk Medical Products, Inc., Skokie, IL.)

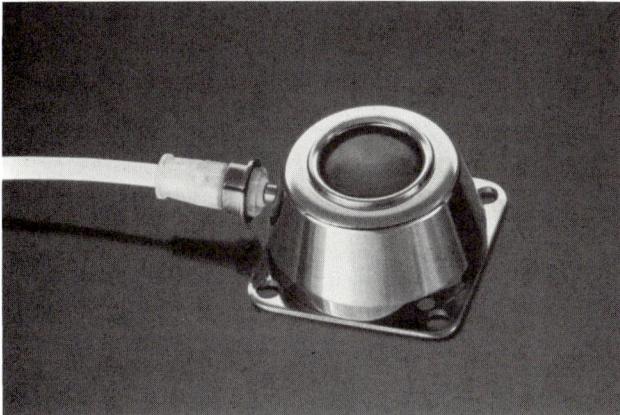

Figure 22–5. Port-A-Cath® catheter. (Courtesy of Pharmacia Deltec Inc., St. Paul, MN.)

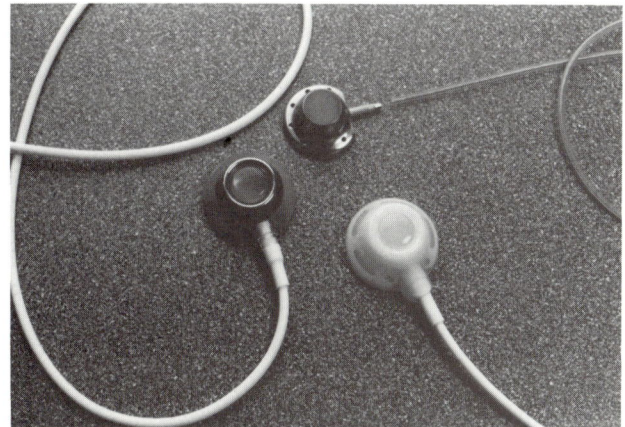

Figure 22–8. Hickman (C. R. Bard, Inc.) and Groshong (C. R. Bard, Inc.) single-lumen ports. (Photographs courtesy of Davol Inc.)

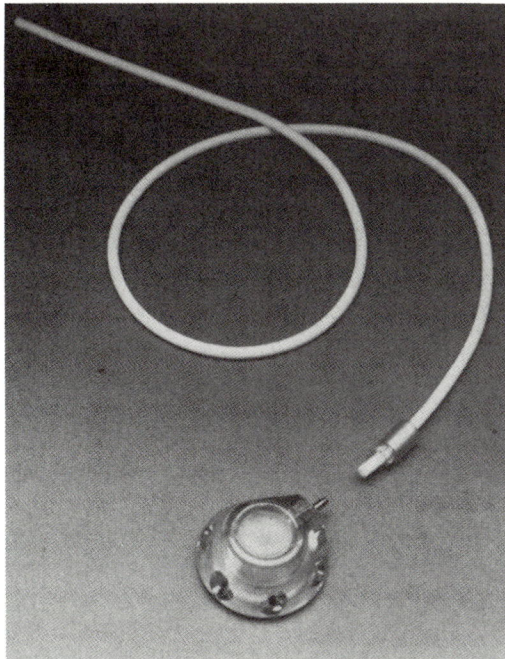

Figure 22–6. Infusaid MicroPort. (Courtesy of Shiley Infusaid, Inc., Norwood, MA.)

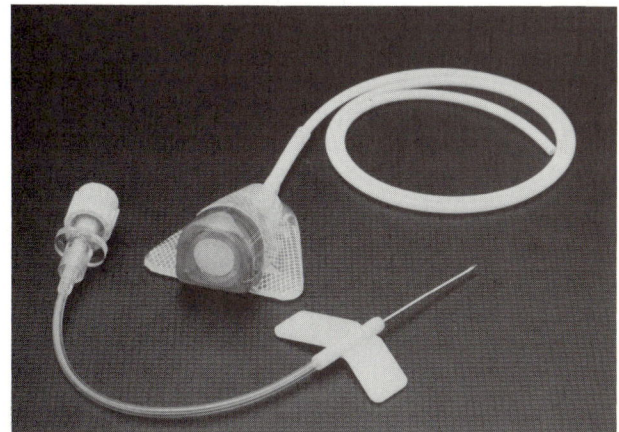

Figure 22–9. Norport-SP: a side-entrance port. (Courtesy of Norfolk Medical Products, Inc., Skokie, IL.)

Accessing The System

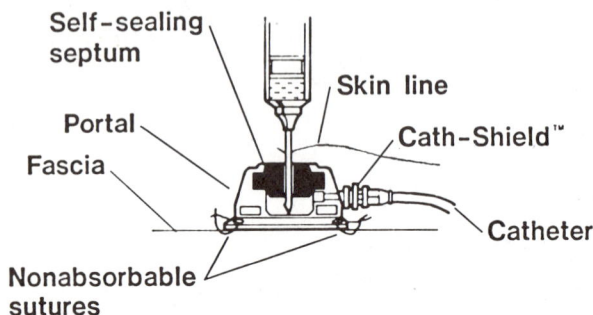

Figure 22–10. Port-A-Cath® cross section with Huber point needle in place. (Courtesy of Pharmacia Deltec Inc., St. Paul, MN.)

Labels in figure: Self-sealing septum; Portal; Fascia; Nonabsorbable sutures; Skin line; Cath-Shield™; Catheter

upper chest at the midclavicular line rather than laterally on the pectoral muscle, where normal arm movement can increase the risk of needle dislodgment (Wickham, 1988). The catheter is tunneled a short distance and then placed into a large vein, usually the subclavian. Similar to the tunneled catheters, these ports can be placed in the groin with the catheter resting in the iliac or femoral vein for patients in whom anterior chest placement is contraindicated. These ports can remain in place indefinitely and can be used for drawing blood and for administering blood products, total parenteral nutrition, and chemotherapy. Because of the risk of needle dislodgment and drug extravasation, these ports are not recommended for long-term infusions of vesicant drugs on an outpatient basis. If a continuous infusion of a vesicant into a port is necessary because of prior circumstances, it is advisable to admit the patient into the hospital during the infusion so that proper needle placement can be assured and documented every 8 hours.

Vascular access ports are ideal for patients who have poor veins or who require frequent venous access such as weekly injections of doxorubicin. To enter the port, the site is sterilized with a povidone-iodine solution, alcohol, or both. A Huber point needle is inserted transdermally through the septum until it meets the back of the port. Proper needle placement is assured with the presence of a blood return. However, it is not uncommon for a blood return to be absent. If a blood return is not obtained, the port can be irrigated with 20 to 30 ml of saline. In the absence of tissue swelling, proper needle placement is assured. If neither irrigation nor aspiration is possible, the catheter may be clotted. Forceful irrigation should be avoided because the catheter may burst. In the majority of cases, the inability to irrigate or aspirate occurs because the needle is malpositioned in the septum itself. Simply advancing the needle farther through the septum generally solves the problem. If the catheter is clotted, however, the procedure for declotting ports is identical to the procedure for declotting tunneled or nontunneled devices (Table 22–10). In the event that there is swelling at the site or pain during the infusion of fluids, the port and catheter should be further evaluated by

Table 22–10. MANAGEMENT OF A CLOTTED VAD*

1. Obtain urokinase for catheter clearance.†
2. Reconstitute to 5000 IU of urokinase per milliliter.
3. Withdraw 1 ml of urokinase in a tuberculin syringe.
4. Using sterile technique and proper clamping procedures, disconnect cap from catheter or port tubing.
5. Connect syringe of 1 ml urokinase and slowly inject an amount equal in volume to that of the catheter.
6. Remove syringe.
7. Connect 5-ml syringe; wait 5 to 10 minutes.
8. Attempt to aspirate to remove clot.
9. If successful, slowly irrigate catheter or port with 10 to 20 ml of saline, then flush with a heparin saline solution per routine.
10. If there is no blood return, wait 30 to 60 minutes before trying to aspirate.
11. Repeat steps 1 to 10 if unable to clear catheter.

*Procedure is the same for tunneled, nontunneled, and implanted devices.
†Urokinase (Abbokinase Open-Cath).
Streptokinase-streptodornase (Varidase).

injecting a radiopaque substance through them and viewing them under fluoroscopy.

Oral Drug Administration

Oral antineoplastic agents are generally considered convenient to administer, economical, and usually less toxic than drugs given intravenously. However, oral ingestion of antineoplastics means that the drugs' availability and concentration are potentially erratic and incomplete for drugs that are poorly soluble; slowly absorbed; unstable; or extensively metabolized by the liver, which is especially a problem in situations of questionable liver or renal function. Oral chemotherapy requires careful patient teaching to ensure compliance and minimize toxicity. Table 22–11 lists the most common orally administered antineoplastic agents, their doses and schedules, side effects, and pharmacokinetics (Cancer Chemotherapeutic Agents, 1984; Dorr & Fritz, 1980; Hubbard, 1985). Additional information about these medications is included in Chapter 21. Patients are given written instructions concerning their medications and are encouraged to learn the names of their medications and to keep a record of all the prescription medications they are taking including their schedule and toxicities. In addition, they are cautioned to check with their physician or nurse before taking any nonprescription medications. Because of the nature of antineoplastics and their toxicities, it is advisable to prescribe only enough medication for a single-treatment course to avoid an accidental overdose.

Regional Drug Delivery

The inability to achieve sufficient concentration of the drug at the tumor site without undue toxicity to normal tissues is considered a major factor in the failure of systemic chemotherapy to adequately control disease. Theoretically, regional drug delivery can enhance the dose-response curve by increasing the con-

Table 22–11. ORAL ANTINEOPLASTIC AGENTS

Drug and Disease Indications	Dose and Schedule	Side Effects: Acute or Delayed	Pharmacokinetics	Comments
Cyclophosphamide (Cytoxan, Endoxan) Breast cancer Multiple myeloma Small-cell lung cancer	Tab: 50-mg Dose: 1–5 mg/kg/day 60–120 mg/m² Adjust dose in presence of renal dysfunction	Nadir: 7–14 days Bone marrow suppression (BMS) Anorexia, nausea, and vomiting Alopecia Hemorrhagic cystitis with gross or microscopic hematuria Amenorrhea Sterility	Activated in the liver Oral absorption in 1 hour 30% of drug excreted unchanged in urine	Vigorous hydration (3 L/day). Encourage frequent voiding to prevent hemorrhagic cystitis (a sterile inflammation of the urinary bladder). If patient complains of burning on urination or bladder incontinence, urinalysis may reveal occult blood. Control by withdrawal of the drug and hydration. May take pills in divided doses early in the day and with meals or all at one time. Better tolerated with cold foods. Barbiturates and other inducers of hepatic microsomal enzymes may enhance toxicity, e.g., cimetidine. Allopurinol may enhance BMS.
Chlorambucil (Leukeran) Leukemia Hodgkin's disease Breast cancer Ovarian cancer	Tab: 2-mg white Dose: 4–8 mg/m²/day × 3–6 weeks 16 mg/m²/week every 4 weeks	Nadir: 7–10 days Severe BMS Slight nausea and vomiting Occasional dermatitis Abnormal liver function Pulmonary fibrosis with prolonged use Second malignancy Sterility	Hepatic metabolism to active compound Renal excretion of 50% of unchanged drug	Good oral absorption. Concomitant barbiturate administration may enhance toxicity. Marrow suppression may be prolonged.
Busulfan (Myleran) Leukemia	Tab: 2-mg white Dose: 4–12 mg/day; for several weeks.	Nadir: 10–30 days delayed marrow recovery Potentially teratogenic Pulmonary fibrosis with long-term use Dermatologic hyperpigmentation Gynecomastia Amenorrhea	Well absorbed Extensive hepatic metabolism to inactive compounds Renal excretion	Bone marrow recovery may be delayed; therefore caution is advised with long-term use. Hydration and allopurinol may be indicated to prevent hyperuricemia. Total cumulative dose: 600 mg. Long-term daily administration is not recommended owing to the risk of second malignancies with chronic alkylating agents.
6-Thioguanine Leukemia	Tab: 40 mg: green/yellow Dose: 80–100 mg/m² Reduce dose if stomatitis occurs	Nadir: 7–28 days Stomatitis Diarrhea Hepatotoxicity	Variable, incomplete absorption Hepatic metabolism Renal excretion	Administer on an empty stomach. Does not require dose reduction when used in conjunction with allopurinol.
6-Mercaptopurine (6 MP) Leukemia	Tab: 50 mg Dose: 80–100 mg/m²/day Titrate dose based on blood counts Reduce dose in presence of hepatic or renal dysfunction	Nadir: 10–14 days Nausea, vomiting Mucositis Diarrhea Drug fever Intrahepatic cholestasis Pulmonary toxicity with prolonged use	Incomplete oral absorption Hepatic inactivation Renal excretion 10% unchanged in 24 hours	Protect pills from light. Administer as single dose on an empty stomach. Increased toxicity with allopurinol (reduce dose by one third to one fourth of the original dose). Administer with caution to patients on sodium warfarin (Coumadin). Monitor liver function tests.

Table continued on following page

Table 22–11. ORAL ANTINEOPLASTIC AGENTS *Continued*

Drug and Disease Indications	Dose and Schedule	Side Effects: Acute or Delayed	Pharmacokinetics	Comments
Hexamethylmelamine Lung cancer Ovarian cancer Lymphomas	Cap: 50–100-mg cream-colored (in 4 divided doses) Dose: 240–320 mg/m²/day	Nadir: 21–28 days Acute liver toxicity is dose limiting; nausea and vomiting are dose-related Mild BMS Abdominal cramping Diarrhea Peripheral neuropathies Agitation, confusion	Variable absorption Rapid metabolism Urine excretion 90% in 72 hours	Pyridoxine 50 mg/day may decrease neuropathy. Take with food, prophylactic antiemetics. May worsen vincristine-related peripheral neuropathy.
L-phenylanine mustard (melphalan, alkeran) Multiple myeloma Ovarian cancer Breast cancer	Tab: 2-mg white Dose: 0.1–0.15 mg/kg/day × 2–3 weeks Reduce dose with hepatic or renal impairment	Nadir: 10–18 days Nausea and vomiting usually mild Dermatitis Pulmonary fibrosis Long-term therapy can result in acute leukemia	Hepatic metabolism Renal excretion 20–35% (10% unchanged) 20–50% excreted in feces within 6 days	Protect pills from sunlight. Take on an empty stomach. BMS may be cumulative in older patients.
Semustine (MeCCNU) (not currently available)	Cap: 100 mg: black/brown 50 mg: brown 10 mg: white Dose: 100–150 mg/m²/day q 6–20 weeks	Nadir: 28–42 days Severe cumulative BMS Hepatotoxicity Alopecia Severe nausea and vomiting 5–8 hours after dosing Second malignancy	Well-absorbed Rapid hepatic metabolism Crosses into cerebrospinal fluid (CSF)	Refrigerate: take on an empty stomach, just before bedtime. Pretreat with aggressive antiemetic regimen.
Lomustine (CCNU) Brain cancer Lymphomas	Cap: 100 mg: green/green 40 mg: green/purple 10 mg: purple Dose: 100–130 mg/m² q 6–8 weeks	Nadir: 28–42 days Severe cumulative BMS Nausea and vomiting 4–6 hours after dosing Anorexia Alopecia Stomatitis Hepatotoxicity	Absorbed rapidly (<60 minutes) Hepatic metabolism Renal excretion of 50% in 24 hours and 75% in 96 hours Crosses into CSF	Dispense one dose at a time to prevent accidental overdose. Take on an empty stomach just before bedtime. Pretreat with aggressive antiemetics. Protect pills from heat and humidity.
Hydroxyurea (Hydrea) Chronic myelocytic leukemia Melanoma Head and neck cancer	Cap: 500 mg Dose: 80 mg/kg/day every third day 750–1000 mg/m²/day × 5 Decrease dose in presence of renal dysfunction Store in tight container in a cool environment	Nadir: 13–17 days Acute nausea and vomiting Chronic and severe anemia Neurologic seizures and hallucinations Dermatitis Dysuria Azotemia	Well-absorbed Hepatic metabolism Renal excretion of 80% of compound in 12 hours Crosses into CSF	Concomitant radiation, and/or 5-FU, or both, may enhance neurotoxicity. Dysuria and renal impairment may occur. Consider pretreatment with allopurinol.
VP-16-213 (etoposide, VePesid) Lung cancer Testicular cancer	Cap: 50 mg Dose: 2 × the intravenous dose or 100–200 mg/m²/day over 3–5 days every 3–4 weeks.	Nadir: 7–14 days (white blood cell count) Nausea and vomiting: 9–16 days (platelets) Alopecia Bone marrow suppression is dose limiting	Renal and hepatic metabolism Incomplete and variable absorption	Nausea is mild though can be more severe with oral route than with intravenous route.
Procarbazine (Matulane) Hodgkin's disease	50-mg capsules Dose: 100 mg/m²/day × 14 days every 4 weeks; reduce dose in presence of hepatic or renal dysfunction	Nadir: 4 weeks Bone marrow suppression, nausea, vomiting, and diarrhea gradually subside; flu-like syndrome, paresthesias, neuropathies, dizziness, and ataxia	Well absorbed from the gastrointestinal tract Metabolized in the liver with a biologic half-life of about 1 hr 70% of the drug is eliminated by 24 hr in the urine, 5% appears as unchanged drug	Drug and food interactions can occur. Central nervous system (CNS) depression can occur with concomitant administration of procarbazine and CNS depressants. Hypertensive crisis can occur when procarbazine is administered with certain antidepressants (tricyclics and monoamine oxidase inhibitors) and tyramine-rich foods. Severe nausea and vomiting can occur if taken with ethanol, mixed drinks, and beer.

Table 22–11. ORAL ANTINEOPLASTIC AGENTS *Continued*

Drug and Disease Indications	Dose and Schedule	Side Effects: Acute or Delayed	Pharmacokinetics	Comments
Methotrexate Squamous cell carcinoma Lung cancer	Tab: 2.5 mg Dose: 2.5–10 mg/day PO or 15–30 mg/day PO × 5 days every 1–3 weeks	Nadir: 7–10 days Nausea and anorexia can occur; stomatitis and ulcerations can occur and are dose limiting.	Serum half-life is 2–4 hr Excreted by the kidneys	Dose is reduced with renal impairment; dosing on an empty stomach may enhance bioavailability. Excretion may be impaired in patients with simultaneous administration or weak acids such as salicylates or vitamin C; oral dosing is generally well tolerated. Avoid administration of methotrexate with ketoprotein or probenecid because toxicity of methotrexate may be enhanced.

centration of the drug at the tumor site and at the same time lower systemic drug exposure, thereby improving the therapeutic index (Keizer & Pinedo, 1985). Drugs most effective by this route are those with a high total body clearance and those that are rapidly bound or inactivated after one pass through the region. The site of delivery, whether in a cavity such as the peritoneum or in the central nervous system, should have a low exchange rate so that systemic absorption is minimal (Collins, 1984). The drug or drugs must be active in their administered form.

The most common methods of regional drug delivery include intra-arterial, intraperitoneal, intrathecal or intraventricular, and intravesical bladder chemotherapy. With the development of implantable pumps, ports, and catheters, such therapies are now more technically feasible.

Intra-arterial Chemotherapy

Intra-arterial drugs are administered through a catheter that rests in the vessel supplying the tumor. Intra-

arterial chemotherapy has been used for osteogenic sarcoma, bladder carcinoma, head and neck carcinoma, cervical carcinoma, melanoma, brain tumors, primary hepatoma, and metastatic disease of the liver. Angiography is employed to demonstrate the blood supply to a particular tumor-bearing area. The artery or vein is then cannulated either during surgery or percutaneously, under radiologic control. Anticoagulation measures are especially important to prevent clotting of the vessel before and during catheterization in patients undergoing infusions that last several days. Patency of the catheter lumen is maintained by continuous pump infusion or intermittent heparinization (Carrasco, Wallace, & Charnsangavej, 1985; Wallace, Carrasco, & Charnsangavej, 1984).

There are basically three methods of arterial catheterization: (1) external rigid, (2) implanted ports, and (3) implanted pumps. The first method involves angiographic placement of a rather stiff catheter for arterial perfusion that lasts minutes to hours. The area is immobilized during the treatment, and the site is

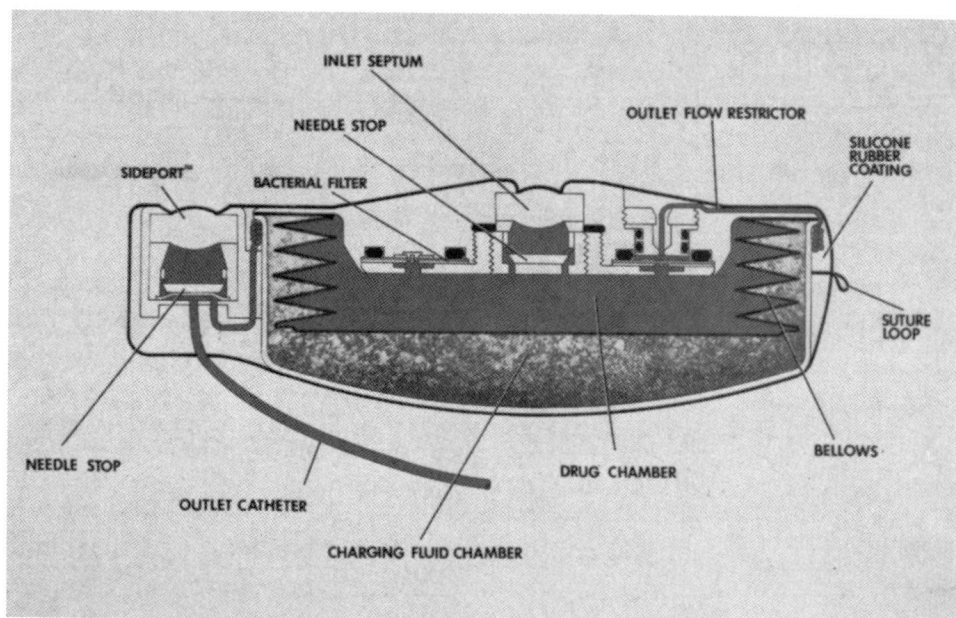

Figure 22–11. Infusaid model 400 implantable pump, internal view. (Courtesy of Shiley Infusaid, Inc., Norwood, MA.)

Table 22–12. PROCEDURE FOR FILLING THE INFUSAID PUMP

Equipment:
- 50-ml syringe (remove plunger)
- 50-ml syringe filled with chemotherapy or saline and heparin 50,000 U (total volume always equal to 50 ml)
- 1½-inch 22-gauge Huber point needle (curved) with connecting tubing or 1½-inch 22-gauge straight needle with a three-way stopcock
- Povidone-iodine swabs (3)
- Alcohol wipes (3)
- Adhesive bandage
- Sterile gloves

1. Prepare a sterile field containing sterile equipment.
2. Palpate pump: attempt to locate septum.
3. Cleanse area over pump with alcohol and povidone-iodine swabs three times using a circular motion.
4. Don sterile gloves. Place Huber point needle on a three-way stopcock and attach 50-ml syringe. Turn stopcock to off OR attach needle to tubing and attach 50-ml syringe to the tubing. Clamp tubing. Relocate septum. Insert the needle perpendicular to the septum. The needle will puncture the septum and meet the needle stop. Open stopcock or clamp and observe fluid rising in the syringe as the pump empties.
5. Once fluid has stopped rising in the syringe, note amount and disconnect syringe from stopcock or tubing. The needle will be open to air, but air will not enter the pump because it is pressurized. Discard pump fluid properly as one would chemotherapy.
6. Connect the syringe filled with chemotherapy or saline to the stopcock or tubing. While maintaining the needle in the pump, inject contents of the syringe.
7. Check for correct placement (fluid will rise in syringe when pressure is released from plunger).
8. Once completed, remove the syringe and needle while stabilizing the pump. Apply an adhesive bandage.
9. Calculate the rate of flow by subtracting the amount left in the syringe at the time of emptying from 50 ml and divide by the total number of days since the pump was filled. This will reveal the ml/day and ensure that the patient is receiving the appropriate dose of the drug as planned. Most pumps will infuse between 1.5 and 2.5 ml/day (consult individual manufacturer's insert). Temperature elevation and the use of less than 50,000 U of heparin in 50 ml of solution will increase the speed of the pump.

assessed regularly for bleeding. The catheter is removed after therapy, and pressure is applied to the site. In the second method, a more flexible (silicone) catheter is surgically placed into the artery, sutured to the skin, or connected to an implanted port for long-term access. These catheters are irrigated regularly to maintain patency. The external catheter is irrigated daily, and the implanted port is irrigated once a week with heparinized saline. Each of these catheters or devices can be connected to an infusion pump for protracted intra-arterial infusion chemotherapy. The third method involves surgical placement of a catheter that is connected to a totally implanted infusion pump (the Infusaid 400 or the Medtronics pump; Fig. 22–11). This pump is filled with chemotherapy or saline, and it constantly infuses the involved organ—usually the liver via the hepatic artery. The pumps are refilled by percutaneous injection approximately every one to two weeks (Table 22–12). The toxicities of intra-arterial drug therapy relate to the region perfused (Ensminger, 1984) (Table 22–13). Although systemic toxicities may also be present, they are often minimal.

Table 22–13. INTRA-ARTERIAL CHEMOTHERAPY TOXICITIES AS RELATED TO REGION AND ORGAN INFUSED

Brain
Retinal damage or blindness in eye from a direct infusion
Brain necrosis
Ischemia due to vascular damage or emboli
Dermatitis over forehead

Head and Neck
Mucositis
Dermatitis
Ulceration or abscess formation

Liver
Hepatitis
Gastritis
Sclerosing cholangitis

Pelvis
Cystitis
Proctitis
Mucositis or dermatitis
Myelosuppression

Extremity
Dermatitis or ulceration
Myositis or neuritis
Ischemia claudication of vasculitis or thrombosis

(Adapted with permission from Ensminger, W. D. [1984]. Management, complications, and evaluation of intraarterial infusions. In S. B. Howell [Ed.], *Intraarterial and Intra-cavitary cancer chemotherapy* [p. 37]. Boston: Martinus Nijhoff Publishers.)

Intraperitoneal Chemotherapy

Intraperitoneal chemotherapy plays a role in the treatment of ovarian carcinoma, gastrointestinal malignancies, and metastatic disease of the liver (Markman, 1984; Speyer, 1985). By administering the chemotherapy directly into the abdominal cavity, higher drug concentrations at the tumor site can be achieved. The majority of abdominal cavity fluid is absorbed and detoxified in the portal circulation after one pass through the liver. Because most of the drugs are either metabolized or detoxified in the liver, toxicities are less than when the drugs are given systemically. Cisplatin, a drug commonly used for intraperitoneal perfusion, concentrates in the liver and the kidneys once absorbed. Therefore, a sodium thiosulfate infusion may be given systemically to prevent toxicity. Table 22–14 lists the side effects of the major drugs used for intraperitoneal chemotherapy (Swenson & Eriksson, 1986).

Patient acceptance of this therapy is a major concern with this method of drug delivery. Routinely, the

Figure 22–12. Placement of Tenckhoff catheter for administration of intraperitoneal chemotherapy. (From DeVita, V. T., & Hellman, S. [Eds.]. [1985]. *Cancer: Principles and practice of oncology* [2nd ed., p. 1102]. Philadelphia: J. B. Lippincott Co. Reproduced by permission.)

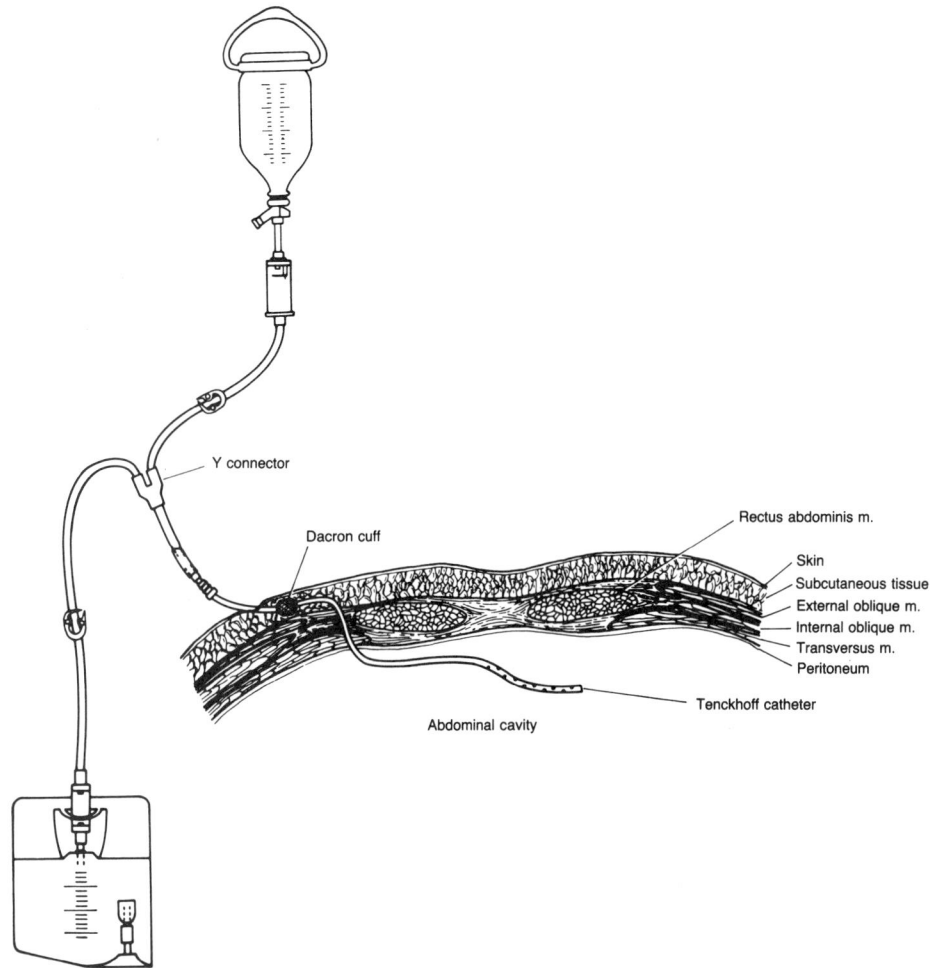

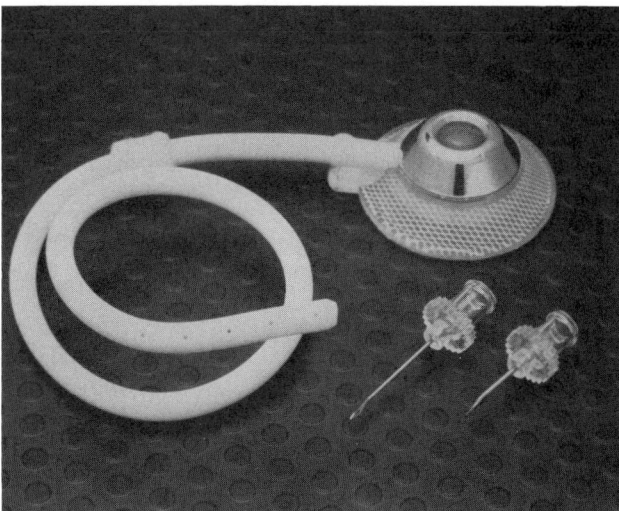

Y connector

Dacron cuff

Rectus abdominis m.

Skin

Subcutaneous tissue

External oblique m.

Internal oblique m.

Transversus m.

Peritoneum

Tenckhoff catheter

Abdominal cavity

Figure 22–13. Norport-PT peritoneal access port. (Courtesy of Norfolk Medical Products, Inc., Skokie, IL.)

Table 22–14. TOXIC EFFECTS OF INTRAPERITONEAL CHEMOTHERAPY

Agent	Myelosuppression	Abdominal Pain	Nausea and Vomiting	Nephrotoxicity	Mucositis	Other
Cisplatin	+*	0	†	+	0	Prolonged nausea and fatigue
Carboplatin	†	0	+	+	0	Thrombocytopenia and anemia can be severe
Doxorubicin	+	†	+	0	0	Utility limited owing to intense abdominal pain
5-Fluorouracil	+	+	+	0	+	Alopecia, diarrhea
Cytosine arabinoside	+*	0	+*	0	0	—
Melphalan	+	0	+	0	0	—
Methotrexate	+	+*	+*	0	+*	Diarrhea
Etoposide	+	+	0	0	0	Alopecia
Biologic response modifiers						
Interferon	+*	+	+	0	0	Fever (high)

0 = absent, + = present, * = mild, † = severe.
(Adapted with permission from Swenson, K. K., & Eriksson, T. H. [1986]. Nursing management of intra-peritoneal chemotherapy. *Oncology Nursing Forum, 13*[5], 33–39.)

Table 22–15. INTRAVESICAL THERAPY FOR SUPERFICIAL BLADDER CANCER

Drug	Dose	Schedule	Dwell Time	Toxicities
Thio-TEPA (15-mg vials)	30–60 mg (1 mg/ml) Reconstitute vial with 1.5 ml sterile water, further dilute to 1 mg/ml with sterile water Contains no preservative Discard unused portion	4×/week for 1 week OR Weekly doses for prophylaxis: weekly doses followed by monthly doses	½–2 hours	Because thio-TEPA is absorbed systemically, myelosuppression and thrombocytopenia may occur. Bladder contracture and chemical cystitis may occur.
Mitomycin C (Mutamycin) (5-mg and 20-mg vials)	20–60 mg (1 mg/ml) Reconstitute with sterile water Store at room temperature (stable for 7 days) Stable for 14 days if refrigerated Protect from light	Weekly for 8–10 weeks	1–2 hours	Rare systemic absorption may occur. Most common side effect is bladder irritation. Contact dermatitis as evidenced by palmar rash is preventable by washing hands and perineum after the treatment. Dysuria and frequency may occur.
Doxorubicin (Adriamycin) (10-mg and 50-mg vials)	40–80 mg (2 mg/ml) Reconstitute with normal saline or sterile water	Every 3–4 weeks	2 hours	Systemic absorption is minimal. Urgency and chemical cystitis may require discontinuation. Urinary tract infections may require antibiotics. Hematuria rarely occurs. Dysuria and bladder spasms may occur. Hypotension, bronchospasm may occur.
Teniposide (VM-26) Investigational (10 mg in 5 ml)	50 mg diluted in 30–100 ml of normal saline Store at room temperature Stable for 4 hours when diluted in normal saline	Biweekly	1–2 hours	Minimal systemic absorption may occur. Chemical cystitis may occur.
Bacille Calmette-Guérin (BCG) immunotherapy	120–699 mg in 50 ml normal saline; solution should not contain any preservative or bacteriostatic agents	Weekly for 6 weeks Usually given in combination with intradermal BCG	2 hours	Systemic absorption occurs and is manifested by fever, chills, anorexia, and malaise; abnormal liver function tests may occur. Dysuria and frequency are common. Hematuria may occur. Severe cystitis may occur.

(Data from Torti & Lum, 1984.)

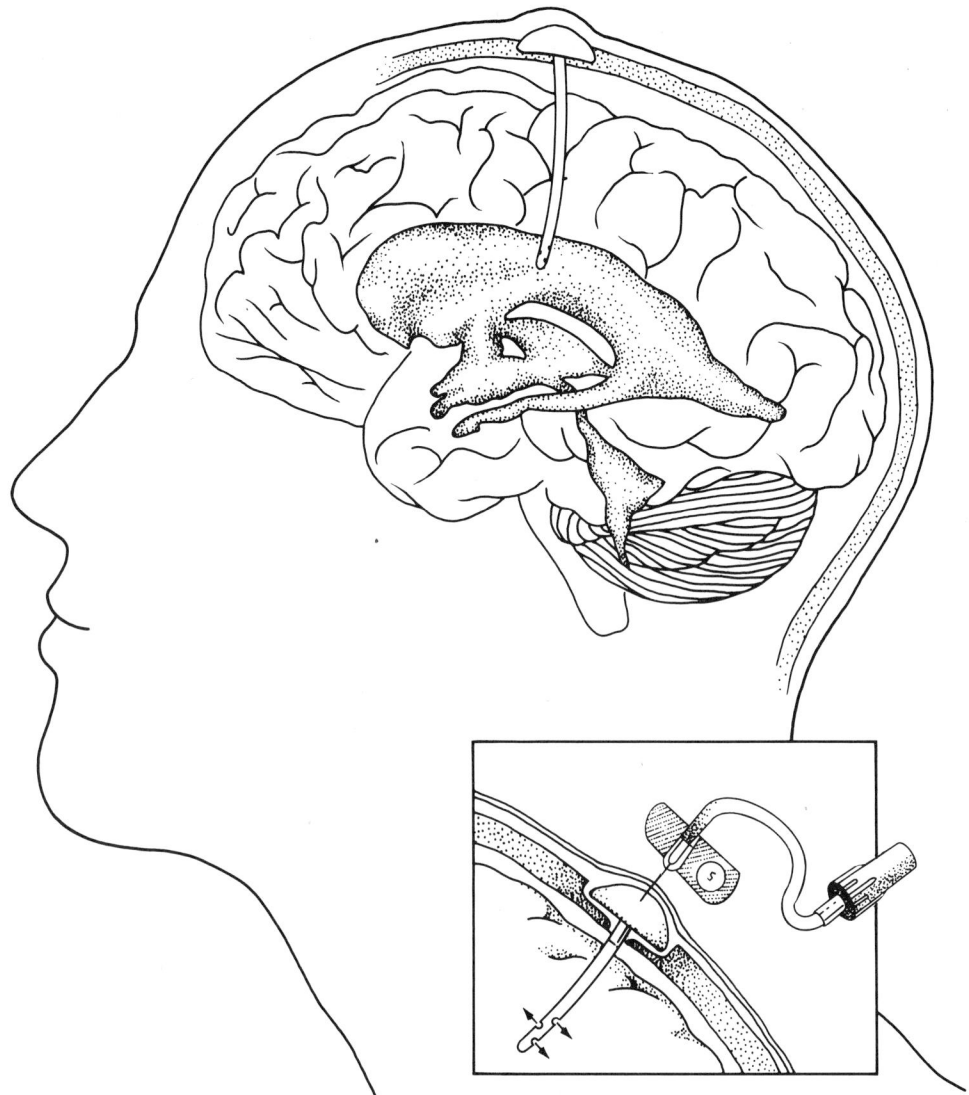

Figure 22–14. Ommaya reservoir. (Drawing by Pamela Townsend.)

Tenckhoff catheter has been used to maintain long-term access to the abdominal cavity to deliver fluid and chemotherapy (Fig. 22–12). The catheter is secured by two Dacron cuffs to prevent dislodgment. Because the catheter exits from the abdomen, it may be uncomfortable, and thus low patient acceptability is common owing to the maintenance required and the body image changes. Sterile technique including a mask is used whenever the catheter is manipulated for chemotherapy or irrigations (Jenkins, 1985). The Hickman- and Groshong-type catheters are also being used for intraperitoneal chemotherapy and are more comfortable and easily tolerated by patients. An alternate method of drug delivery includes the use of the totally implanted port (Fig. 22–13). The port is generally placed over the lower rib cage in the midclavicular line, which provides support for the port during cannulation. Patient acceptance of these ports is generally very good because they are completely implanted, require little maintenance, and do not significantly alter body image.

The port or catheter is accessed using the sterile technique previously described. The chemotherapy is infused in 1 to 2 liters of fluid to ensure adequate drug distribution. The fluid is usually allowed to dwell in the abdomen for 1 to 4 hours, after which it is drained by gravity through the catheter or port. Some protocols do not drain the fluid at all. Fibrous ingrowth can occur around the catheter or the port, creating a one-way valve effect that prevents drainage. This problem occurs in about 30 per cent of patients regardless of the type of access device (Lucas, 1984; Markman, Howell, & Lucas, 1984). The one-way effect occurs whether the catheter is irrigated routinely with saline, heparin, or dextran. Although the patient may be uncomfortable temporarily from abdominal distention, the one-way catheter presents no real problem because the dialysate is gradually absorbed. Occasionally the catheter can be irrigated vigorously to release a fibrin clot.

Intravesical Bladder Chemotherapy

The purpose of intravesical bladder chemotherapy is to allow a high concentration of the drug to come in contact with the urothelium over a relatively long period of time (Torti & Lum, 1984). A significant proportion (50 to 70 per cent) of patients with superficial (stage 0 or stage A) transitional cell carcinoma

Table 22–16. INTRAVENTRICULAR CHEMOTHERAPY USE OF THE OMMAYA RESERVOIR

The Ommaya reservoir has a catheter that rests in the lateral ventricle. The general uses of the reservoir include the following:
  Sample cerebrospinal fluid (CSF)
  Monitor CSF pressure
  Administer analgesics into the CSF
  Administer antibiotics into the CSF
  Administer chemotherapy into the CSF

Equipment:
  Sterile gloves
  Povidone-iodine swabs (3)
  Alcohol wipes (3)
  Shave or preparation kit (optional)
  23-gauge scalp vein needle
  Premixed drugs (preservative free)
  Equipment for specimen collection:
    3-ml syringe(s)
    Collection tubes
    Requisitions

1. Assemble equipment; prepare a sterile field.
2. Position patient in a semirecumbent position. Support head with pillow.
3. Examine reservoir for any signs or symptoms of infection. Palpate disc to locate center.
4. Cleanse area over disc in a circular motion with povidone-iodine swabs (three times). Allow to dry for 2 minutes.
5. Repeat the procedure in no. 4, using alcohol.
6. Using a sterile procedure, puncture the disc perpendicularly with a 23-gauge scalp vein needle. Normally, CSF is clear and colorless as it rises into the tubing. Attach collection syringe.
7. Two to 3 ml of CSF is obtained and set aside to flush the reservoir after drug instillation.
8. Obtain CSF specimens for cytologic or microbiologic studies and set aside. Slowly aspirating the CSF into a syringe is not contraindicated but may cause the reservoir catheter to become clogged. If this occurs, flush to clear and continue collection.
9. Attach syringe of medicine and inject drug slowly over 5 to 10 minutes. Barbotaging is not necessary, provided sufficient solvent is used, e.g., methotrexate 1 mg/ml. (Barbotaging is recommended with concentrations of methotrexate of 2.5 mg/ml.)
10. Follow medicine with 2 to 3 ml of CSF flush.
11. Remove needle, gently compress reservoir, and apply adhesive bandage.

of the bladder have recurrent disease following traditional therapy (Garnick, Maxwell, Gibbs, & Richer, 1984). Intravesical bladder chemotherapy is intended to destroy any viable cancer cells in the bladder, thereby preventing recurrence of the cancer and the need for cystectomy. The drugs most commonly used to treat superficial bladder cancer are listed and discussed in Table 22–15 (Torti & Lum, 1984). Benefits of this therapy include minimal systemic toxiciticies and preservation of urinary and sexual function. In general, the drug is instilled via a urinary catheter into the bladder and retained for about 1 to 3 hours. The patient changes position about every 15 minutes to ensure optimal bladder exposure. The common side effects of intravesical chemotherapy include dysuria, frequency of urination, hematuria, and bladder spasms. If the drug is allowed to dwell longer than the prescribed time, the patient can experience excessive exfoliation of the bladder epithelium and cystitis.

Intraventricular and Intrathecal Chemotherapy

Meningeal carcinomatosis is characterized by a diffuse seeding of the surface layers of the brain and spinal cord by tumor. Metastasis to the leptomeninges is often manifested by obstruction of the cerebrospinal fluid pathways and invasion of the nerves within the subarachnoid space, which produces cranial nerve and lower motor neuron dysfunction (Wujcik, 1983). The cancers most commonly associated with meningeal metastasis include breast cancer, lung cancer, gastroin-

testinal carcinoma, leukemia, and lymphoma. The central nervous system is considered a sanctuary for tumor cells because most systemically administered antineoplastic drugs do not cross the blood-brain barrier in sufficient concentrations to be therapeutic. Therefore, intrathecal or intraventricular drug administration provides an amount of drug that is essential to treat presumed or proven leptomeningeal metastases.

Intrathecal drug administration involves the insertion of a needle into the lumbar region and the injection of the drug through the dura and the arachnoid into the subarachnoid space. Regardless of positioning, the lumbar puncture technique does not ensure cisternal and ventricular distribution of the drug. In fact, ineffective treatment of meningeal leukemia or carcinomatosis has been related to inadequate drug concentration and distribution into the ventricles.

The large production of cerebrospinal fluid from the ventricles and its outflow generate a pressure that probably inhibits ascent of the drug to the ventricles following lumbar puncture (Rieselbach, Dichior, & Freireich, 1962). The Ommaya reservoir is a small, Silastic dome-shaped disc with an extension catheter that is surgically implanted through the cranium into a lateral ventricle. Figure 22–14 demonstrates the placement of the reservoir and flow of cerebrospinal fluid. Once placement is verified by radiograph, the scalp-flap covering is sutured into place. Twenty-four to 48 hours is generally allowed before gaining access to the reservoir. One of the benefits of an intraventricular reservoir is that the patient is spared the pain and discomfort of repeated lumbar punctures. Injecting drugs directly into the ventricles ensures more consistent drug concentrations and distribution. Table 22–16 describes the procedure for utilizing the Ommaya reservoir.

The drugs used for intrathecal therapy should contain no preservatives and may be mixed in Elliott's B solution, preservative-free saline, or the patient's own cerebrospinal fluid. The drug is mixed in 10 to 12 ml of diluent and injected over 5 to 10 minutes to ensure distribution and to minimize acute meningeal irritation. Patients are instructed to remain supine or semirecumbent for 20 to 30 minutes. Acute complications include headache, nausea, vomiting, fever, and nuchal rigidity, which usually subside in 48 to 72 hours.

SUMMARY

Over the years, the administration of antineoplastic agents has become the responsibility of the oncology nurse. This responsibility has become more than the actual task of drug delivery and is fast becoming an opportunity for nurses to influence patient care outcomes. It is an opportunity to influence decisions regarding care delivery and to teach patients and their families about the treatment and about how they can minimize the toxicities of the treatment and remain active participants in their own care. The responsibility also exists for the nurse to design and conduct research with other members of the health care team, specifically in the areas of safe handling of antineoplastics, extravasation management, and various issues concerning the management of VADs.

References

Anderson, R. W., Puckett, W. H., Dana, W. J., Nguyen, T. V., Theiss, J. C., & Mathey, T. S. (1982). Risk of handling injectable antineoplastic agents. *American Journal Hospital Pharmacy, 39,* 1881–1887.

Argenta, L. C., & Manders, E. K. (1983). Mitomycin-C extravasation injuries. *Cancer, 51,* 1080.

Averbuch, S. D., Gaudiano, G., & Koch, T. H. (1986). Doxorubicin induced skin necrosis in the swine model: Protection with a novel radical dimer. *Journal of Clinical Oncology, 4,* 88–94.

Barlock, A., Howser, D., & Hubbard, S. (1979). Nursing management of adriamycin extravasation. *American Journal of Nursing, 79,* 94–96.

Barr, R. D., & Sertic, J. (1981). Soft tissue necrosis induced by extravasated cancer chemotherapeutic agents: A study of active intervention. *British Journal of Cancer, 44,* 267–269.

Bartowski-Dodds, L., & Daniels, J. R. (1980). Use of sodium bicarbonate as a means of ameliorating doxorubicin-induced dermal necrosis in rats. *Cancer Chemotherapy and Pharmacology, 4,* 179–181.

Bowers, D. G., & Lynch, J. B. (1978). Adriamycin extravasation. *Plastic and Reconstructive Surgery, 61,* 86–92.

Brenner, D. E., Grosh, W. W., Noone, R., & Greco, F. A. (1984). Human plasma pharmacokinetics of doxorubicin: Comparison of bolus and infusional administration. *Cancer Treatment Symposia, 3,* 77–83.

Cancer Chemotherapeutic Agents. (1984). Pharmacists sub-committee and consultants of the American Cancer Society. Oakland, CA: American Cancer Society, California Division, Inc.

Carlson, R. W., & Sikic, B. I. (1983). Continuous infusion or bolus injection in cancer chemotherapy. *Annals of Internal Medicine, 99,* 823–833.

Carrasco, C., Wallace, S., & Charnsangavej, C. (1985, Summer). Intra-arterial embolization and infusion of neoplasms. *Current Concepts in Oncology,* pp. 15–22.

Coleman, J. J., Walker, A. P., & Didolkar, M. S. (1983). Treatment of adriamycin induced skin ulcers: A prospective controlled study. *Journal of Surgical Oncology, 22,* 129–135.

Collins, J. M. (1984). Pharmacologic rationale for regional drug delivery. *Journal of Clinical Oncology, 2,* 498–503.

Cox, R.F. (1984). Managing skin damage induced by doxorubicin hydrochloride and daunorubicin hydrochloride. *American Journal of Hospital Pharmacy, 41,* 2410–2414.

Desai, M. H., & Teres, D. (1982). Prevention of doxorubicin induced skin ulcers in the rat and pig with dimethyl-sulfoxide (DMSO). *Cancer Treatment Reports, 66,* 1371–1374.

DeVita, V. T., & Hellman, S. (Eds.). (1985). *Principles and practice of oncology* (2nd ed.). Philadelphia: J. B. Lippincott Co.

Dorr, R. T. (1987). Personal communication.

Dorr, R. T., & Alberts, D. S. (1983). Failure of DMSO and vitamin E to prevent doxorubicin skin ulceration in the mouse. *Cancer Treatment Reports, 67,* 499–501.

Dorr, R. T., & Alberts, D. S. (1985). Vinca alkaloid skin toxicity: Antidote and drug disposition studies in the mouse. *Journal of the National Cancer Institute 74,* 113–120.

Dorr, R. T., Alberts, D. S., & Chen, H. S. (1980). The limited role of corticosteroids in ameliorating experimental doxorubicin skin toxicity in the mouse. *Cancer Chemotherapy and Pharmacology, 5,* 17–20.

Dorr, R. T., Alberts, D., & Stone, A. (1985). Cold protection and heat enhancement of doxorubicin skin toxicity in the mouse. *Cancer Treatment Reports, 69,* 431–437.

Dorr, R. T., & Fritz, W. L. (1980). *Cancer chemotherapy handbook.* New York: Elsevier North-Holland, Inc.

Dorr, R. T., Soble, M. J., & Alberts, D. S. (1988). Efficacy of sodium thiosulfate as a local antidote to mechlorethamine skin toxicity in the mouse. *Cancer Chemotherapy and Pharmacology, 5,* 299–302.

Dorr, R. T., Soble, M. J., Liddie, J. D., & Keller, J. H. (1986). Mitomycin-C skin toxicity studies in mice: Reduced ulceration and altered pharmacokinetics with topical dimethyl sulfoxide. *Journal of Clinical Oncology, 4,* 1399–1404.

Ensminger, W. D. (1984). Management, complications, and evaluation of intra-arterial infusion. In S. B. Howell (Ed.), *Intra-arterial and intra-cavitary cancer chemotherapy* (pp. 33–40). Boston: Martinus Nijhoff, Publishers.

Flowers, R. H., Schwenzer, K. J., Kopel, R. F., Fisch, M. J., Tucker, S. I., & Farr, B. H. (1989). Efficacy as an attachable subcutaneous cuff for the prevention of intravascular catheter-related infection. *Journal of the American Medical Association, 261,* 878–883.

Garnick, M. B., Maxwell, B., Gibbs, R. B., & Richer, T. B. (1984). Intra-vesical doxorubicin for prophylaxis in the management of recurrent superficial bladder carcinoma. An update. In S. B. Howell (Ed.), *Intra-arterial and intra-cavitary cancer chemotherapy* (p. 211). Boston: Martinus Nijhoff, Publishers.

Gaze, N. R. (1978). Tissue necrosis caused by commonly used intravenous infusion. *Lancet, 2,* 417–419.

Goodman, M., & Wickham, R. (1984). Vascular access devices: An overview. *Oncology Nursing Forum, 11,* 16–23.

Gullo, S. M. (1988). Safe handling of antineoplastic drugs: Translating the recommendations into practice. *Oncology Nursing Forum, 15,* 595–601.

Harwood, K., & Bachur, N. (1987). Evaluation of dimethylsulfoxide and local cooling as antidotes for doxorubicin extravasation in a pig model. *Oncology Nursing Forum, 14,* 39–44.

Hirst, M., Tse, S., Mills, D., Levin, L., & White, D. F. (1984). Occupational exposure to cyclophosphamide. *Lancet, 1*(8370), 186–188.

Hubbard, S. M. (1985). Cancer treatment. In B. L. Johnson & J. Gross (Eds.), *Handbook of oncology nursing* (pp. 21–65). New York: A. Wiley Medical Publishers.

Ignoffo, R. T., & Friedman, M. A. (1980). Therapy of local toxicities caused by extravasation of cancer chemotherapeutic drugs. *Cancer Treatment Reviews, 7,* 17–27.

Jackson, I. T., & Robinson, D. W. (1976). Severe tissue damage following accidental subcutaneous infusion of bicarbonate solution. *Scottish Medical Journal, 21,* 200–201.

Jameson, J., & O'Donnell, J. (1983). Guidelines for extravasation of intravenous drugs. *Infusion, 7,* 157–162.

Jenkins, J. (1985). Parenteral chemotherapy. In B. L. Johnson & J. Gross (Eds.), *Handbook of oncology nursing* (p. 557). New York: A. Wiley Medical Publishers.

Johnston-Early, A., & Cohen, M. (1981). Mitomycin-C induced skin ulceration remote from infusion site. *Cancer Treatment Reports, 65,* 529.

Keizer, J. H., & Pinedo, H. M. (1985). Cancer chemotherapy: Alternative routes of drug administration—a review: *Cancer Drug Delivery, 2,* 147–169.

Knobf, M. K., & Fischer, D. S. (1989). *Cancer chemotherapy treatment and care* (3rd ed.). Boston: G. K. Hall Medical Publishers.

Ladik, C. R., Stoehr, G. P., & Maurer, M. A. (1980). Precautionary measures in the preparation of antineoplastics. *American Journal of Hospital Pharmacy, 37,* 1185–1186.

Larson, D. L. (1982). Treatment of tissue extravasation of antitumor agents. *Cancer, 49,* 1796–1799.

Larson, D. L. (1985). What is the appropriate management of tissue extravasation by antitumor agents? *Plastic and Reconstructive Surgery, 75,* 397–401.

Laughlin, R., Landeen, J. M., & Habal, M. (1979). The management of inadvertent subcutaneous adriamycin infiltration. *American Journal of Surgery, 137,* 408–412.

Lawson, M., Bottino, J. C., & McCredie, K. B. (1979). Long term IV therapy: A new approach. *American Journal of Nursing, 79,* 1100–1103.

Legha, S. S., Benjamin, R. S., MacKay, B., Ewer, M., Wallace, S., Valdivieso, M., Rasmussen, S. L., Blumenschein, G. R., & Freireich, E. J. (1982). Reduction of doxorubicin cardiotoxicity by prolonged continuous intravenous infusion. *Annals of Internal Medicine, 96,* 133–139.

Lokich, J., Bothe, A., Fine, N., & Perri, J. (1981). Phase I study of protracted venous infusion of 5-fluorouracil. *Cancer, 48,* 2565–2568.

Lucas, W. E. (1984). Surgical principles of intra-peritoneal access and therapy. In S. B. Howel, (Ed.), *Intra-arterial and intra-cavitary cancer chemotherapy* (pp. 53–71). Boston: Martinus Nijhoff, Publishers.

Luedke, D. W., Kennedy, P., & Rietschel, R. (1979). Histopathogenesis of skin and subcutaneous injury induced by adriamycin. *Plastic and Reconstructive Surgery, 63,* 463–465.

Markman, M. (1984). Medical principles of intra-peritoneal and intra-pleural chemotherapy. In S. B. Howell (Ed.), *Intra-arterial and intra-cavitary cancer chemotherapy* (pp. 61–69). Boston: Martinus Nijhoff, Publishers.

Markman, M., Howell, S. B., & Lucas, W. E. (1984). Combination intra-peritoneal chemotherapy with cis-platin, cytarabine, and doxorubicin for refractory ovarian carcinoma and other malignancies principally confined to the peritoneal cavity. *Journal of Clinical Oncology, 2,* 1321–1326.

Miller, S. A. (1980). Legal implications for the nurse involved in cancer chemotherapy. In R. T. Dorr & W. L. Fritz (Eds.), *Cancer chemotherapy handbook* (pp. 743–754). New York: Elsevier.

Miller, S. A. (1982). Intravenous cancer chemotherapy administration. In A. Plumer (Ed.), *Principles and practices of intravenous therapy* (3rd ed., pp. 277–323). Boston: Little, Brown, & Co.

Miller, S. A. (1988). Safety and the health care worker: Chemotherapy drug handling. *California Nursing Review,* 12–15.

Montrose, P. A. (1987). Extravasation management. *Seminars in Oncology Nursing, 3,* 128–132.

National Study Commission on Cytotoxic Exposure. (1987). Position statement: The handling of cytotoxic agents by women who are pregnant, attempting to conceive or breast feeding. Providence: Rhode Island Hospital.

Neal, A. D., Wadden, R. A., & Chiou, W. L. (1983). Exposure of hospital workers to airborne antineoplastic agents. *American Journal of Hospital Pharmacy, 40,* 597–601.

Niederhuber, D. E., Ensminger, W., & Gyves, J. W. (1982). Totally implanted venous and arterial access system to replace external catheters in cancer treatment. *Surgery, 92,* 706–711.

Nguyen, T., Theiss, J., & Matney, T. (1982). Exposure of pharmacy personnel to mutagenic antineoplastic drugs. *Cancer Research, 42,* 4792–4796.

Okano, T., Ohnuma, T., Efemidis, A., & Holland, J. F. (1983). Doxorubicin induced skin ulcer in the piglet. *Cancer Treatment Reports, 67,* 1075–1078.

Oliver, I., & Schwarz, M. (1983). Use of dimethyl sulfoxide in limiting tissue damage caused by extravasation of doxorubicin. *Cancer Treatment Reports, 67,* 407–408.

Oncology Nursing Society. (1988). *Cancer chemotherapy guidelines, modules I–V.* Pittsburgh: Author.

Oncology Nursing Society. (1989). *Safe handling of cytotoxic drugs. Independent study module.* Pittsburgh: Author.

Owen, O. (1980). Accidental IM injection of mechlorethamine. *Cancer, 45,* 2225–2226.

Penman, D. T., Holland, T. C., Bahna, G. F., Morrow, G., Schmale, A. H., Derogatis, L. R., Carnrike, C. L., Jr., & Cherry, R. (1984). Informed consent for investigational chemotherapy: Patients and physicians perceptions. *Journal of Clinical Oncology, 2,* 849–855.

Pfeifle, C. E., Howell, S. B., & Markman, M. (1984). Totally implanted system for peritoneal access. *Journal of Clinical Oncology, 2,* 1277–1280.

Rieselbach, R. E., Dichior, G. D., & Freireich, E. J. (1962). Subarachnoid distribution of drugs after lumbar injection. *New England Journal of Medicine, 267,* 1273–1278.

Rogers, B., & Emmett, E. A. (1987). Handling antineoplastic agents: Urine mutagenicity in nurses. *Image: Journal of Nursing Scholarship, 19,* 108–113.

Selevan, S. G., Lindbohm, M. L., Hornung, R. W., & Hemminki, K. (1985). A study of occupational exposure to antineoplastic drugs and fetal loss in nurses. *New England Journal of Medicine, 313,* 1173–1178.

Slater, H., Goldfarb, W., & Jacob, H. (1985). Experience with long-term out-patient venous access utilizing percutaneous placed silicone elastomer catheters. *Cancer, 55,* 2074–2077.

Smith, E., Hadidian, Z., & Mason, M. (1967). The single and repeated dose toxicity of dimethylsulfoxide. *Annals of the New York Academy of Science, 14,* 96–109.

Sotaniemi, E. A., Sutinen, S., Arranto, A. J., Sutinen, S., Sotaniemi, K. A., Lehtola, J., & Pelkonen, R. O. (1983). Liver damage in nurses handling cytostatic agents. *Acta Medica Scandinavica, 214,* 181–189.

Speyer, T. L. (1985). The rationale behind intra-peritoneal chemotherapy in gastrointestinal malignancies. *Seminars in Oncology, 12* Suppl. (3), 23–28.

Svingen, B. A., Powis, G., Appel, R., & Scott, M. (1981). Protection against adriamycin induced skin necrosis in the rat by dimethyl-sulfoxide and alpha-tocopherol. *Cancer Research, 41,* 3395–3399.

Swenson, K. K., Eriksson, T. H. (1986). Nursing management of intra-peritoneal chemotherapy. *Oncology Nursing Forum, 13,* 33–39.

Torti, F. M., Bristow, M. R., Howes, A. E., Aston, D., Stockdale, F. E., Carter, S. K., Kohler, M., Brown, B. W., Jr., & Billingham, M. E. (1983). Reduced cardiotoxicity of doxorubicin delivered on a weekly schedule. *Annals of Internal Medicine, 99,* 745–749.

Torti, F. M., & Lum, B. (1984). The biology and treatment of superficial bladder cancer. *Journal of Clinical Oncology, 2,* 505–531.

U.S. Department of Labor, Office of Occupational Medicine, Occupational Safety and Health Administration. (1986). *Work practice guidelines for personnel dealing with cytotoxic (antineoplastic) drugs* (Publication No. 8.1.1). Washington, DC: Author.

Vogelzang, N. (1979). "Adriamycin flare" a skin reaction resembling extravasation. *Cancer Treatment Reports, 63,* 2067–2069.

Von Hoff, D. D., Layard, M. W., Basa, P., Davis, H. L., Von Hoff, A. L., Rozencweig, M., & Muggia, F. M. (1979). Risk factors for doxorubicin induced congestive heart failure. *Annals of Internal Medicine, 91,* 710–717.

Waksvik, H., Klepp, O., & Brogger, A. (1981). Chromosome analyses of nurses handling cytotoxic agents. *Cancer Treatment Reports, 65,* 607–610.

Wallace, S., Carrasco, H., & Charnsangavej, C. (1984). Intra-arterial chemotherapy. In *Current problems in cancer* (pp. 2–55). Chicago: Year Book Medical Publishers.

Wickham, R. (1988). *Techniques for long term venous access.* Fifth National Conference on Cancer Nursing, American Cancer Society, Atlanta.

Wood, H. A., & Ellerhorst-Ryan, J. M. (1984). Delayed adverse skin reactions associated with mitomycin-C administration. *Oncology Nursing Forum, 11,* 14–18.

Wujcik, D. (1983). Meningeal carcinomatosis: Diagnosis, treatment, and nursing care. *Oncology Nursing Forum, 10,* 35–40.

CHAPTER 23

Biologic Response Modifiers

LINDA EDWARDS HOOD
ELIZABETH ABERNATHY

It is hoped that the use of biologic response modifiers (BRMs) or biotherapy in cancer treatment will aid researchers in putting together the missing pieces of the cancer puzzle. In 1981, BRMs were defined by the Subcommittee on BRMs to the Division of Cancer Treatment, National Cancer Institute, as "those agents or approaches that modify the relationship between tumor and host by modifying the host's biological response to tumor cells with resultant therapeutic effects" (Mihich & Fefer, 1983). Biotherapy is based largely on the manipulation of the immune system in an effort to control cancer. Immunologic deficiencies are documented in individuals with cancer. If through the use of BRMs the immune system can be modulated to better destroy malignant cells, then biotherapy will become a prominent treatment for cancer in the future.

MECHANISM OF ACTION

Biologic response modifiers are being researched both clinically and in the laboratory. Even after extensive research, the mechanism of action of many of the agents is not clearly defined. Table 23–1 lists some of the more frequently used agents and their recognized modes of antitumor activity or combinations of activities. Several of the agents have many known antitumor activities; thus for these agents, it is difficult to determine which antitumor capabilities are the most critical. Although the principal mechanism of action of BRMs appears to be immunologic, other systems are also involved. For example, interferon acts both as an

Table 23–1. FUNCTIONS OF BIOLOGIC RESPONSE MODIFIERS

Agent	Mode of Action
Lymphokines (IL 2, interferon-γ)	I
Nonspecific immunomodulating agents (bacille Calmette-Guérin, *Corynebacterium parvum*)	I
Active specific immunizations with tumor cells	I
Interferon or interferon inducers (e.g., alpha, beta, gamma/poly: ICLC, Sendai virus)	I/C
Adoptive immunotherapy (lymphokine-activated killer cells)	C
Tumor necrosis factor	C
Metastasis preventors (laminin fragments and anticoagulation agents)	C
Growth factors (granulocyte colony-stimulating factor, granulocyte-macrophage colony-stimulating factor, erythropoietin)	B

I, immunomodulation; C, direct cytotoxic or cytostatic effect; B, other biologic effects.

immunomodulator and as a cytotoxic agent with direct activity on cancer cells (Trotta, 1986).

Biologic response modifiers can be classified into three major divisions: (1) agents that restore, augment, or modulate the host's immunologic mechanisms; (2) agents that have direct antitumor activity; and (3) agents that have other biologic effects (agents that interfere with tumor cells' ability to metastasize or survive, differentiating agents, or agents that affect cell transformation) (Clark & Longo, 1986).

There are two major groups of BRMs: lymphokines and monokines (Table 23–2). *Cytokine* is a generic term referring to all BRMs released by any body cell.

HISTORICAL BACKGROUND

The overlap between BRM therapy and immunotherapy is considerable. William B. Coley, a surgeon who practiced at New York's Memorial Hospital from 1891 until 1936, is responsible for some of the most interesting early work using the principles of immunotherapy, although the scientific foundations of his research were not clearly defined at the time. At the death of a young woman patient with a malignancy, the disheartened Coley began searching hospital records for clues to explain why after surgically removing a cancerous tumor some patients appeared to be cured and others relapsed very quickly. He found a correlation between patients who developed severe infections and those who remained tumor-free for a prolonged time.

To induce an infectious response in cancer patients, Coley first used live bacteria and later tried filtered toxins, with mixed therapeutic success. What became known as *Coley's toxins* were used clinically until 1975; they provide the background data for tumor necrosis factor (TNF), a BRM that is being clinically researched today. These toxins may have acted as immunotherapy to boost the immune system to recognize, destroy, or clear tumor cells from the body (Goodfield, 1984).

Although the concept of immunotherapy was developed in the 1800s, its application to cancer therapy gained popularity only in the last two decades. In the 1960s, many clinical trials were initiated using injections of bacterial agents, such as bacille Calmette-Guérin, methanol-extruded residue, and *Corynebacterium parvum*. It was hypothesized that exposure to these agents would elicit a nonspecific immune response, thus boosting the body's ability to destroy foreign invaders, such as tumor cells. These experiments produced positive results in selected laboratory animal tumor models (Oldham, 1983).

In 1969, Mathe and Amiel reported successful results of immunotherapy in a small clinical trial of patients with acute lymphoblastic leukemia. Although this success was never replicated, hundreds of clinical trials of nonspecific bacterial agents were conducted. Viruses were used to stimulate tumor cells to produce viral oncolysates, which were injected into the patient in an attempt to stimulate an immune response to the tumor cell. Tumor cells and their products were used to try to stimulate the specific immunity of the patient and to activate either humoral or cell-mediated immunity to slow tumor growth.

Although some results of these clinical trials were positive, the majority were very discouraging, and by the late 1970s, many clinicians had a negative attitude toward immunotherapy (Terry & Rosenberg, 1982). Researchers have suggested that a lack of understanding of immunologic responses and related physiologic and pathophysiologic mechanisms contributed to the failure of these earlier trials (Oldham & Smalley, 1983). The question that now comes to mind is whether we have increased our knowledge sufficiently to develop and utilize immunotherapy.

CLASSIFICATION

Major technologic advances in the last decade have expanded researchers' ability to study BRMs. Through gene cloning, human genes can be placed inside bacteria or yeast cells in culture to produce large quantities of purified human BRMs, including recombinant human interferons, interleukin 2 (IL 2), and TNF (Suppers & McClamrock, 1985) (Fig. 23–1).

Hybridoma technology (Fig. 23–2) has made possible the development of clones of cells that produce specific antibodies against one antigen. *Monoclonal antibodies* (MoAbs), which are antibodies developed to bind with specific types of cancer cells, are used directly in cancer therapy and diagnosis and indirectly in the isolation and purification of other BRMs (Foon, Bernhard, & Oldham, 1982).

Clinically, interferons have been studied more extensively than any other BRM. Approved by the United States Food and Drug Administration in 1986 for therapeutic use in patients with hairy cell leukemia, a chronic B-cell malignancy (Clark & Longo, 1987), interferon-α continues to be studied in many phase II and III trials that have examined various indications, dosages, schedules, and routes of administration. Clinical trials of interferon-γ and interferon-β are also increasing. Research on the use of interferon in combination with radiation therapy, chemotherapy, and other BRMs is also under way (see Chapter 24).

In the last 2 years, considerable attention has been focused on IL 2. This BRM, a lymphokine produced by T lymphocytes, is being examined for direct anti-

Table 23–2. GROUPS OF BIOLOGIC RESPONSE MODIFIERS (BRMs)

BRM Categories	Cell Origin	BRMs
Lymphokines	Lymphocytes	Interleukin 2
		Interferon-γ
		B-cell growth factor
Monokines	Mononuclear phagocytes	Interferon-α
		Colony-stimulating factor
		Tumor necrosis factor
Cytokines	Any stimulated cell	All BRMs

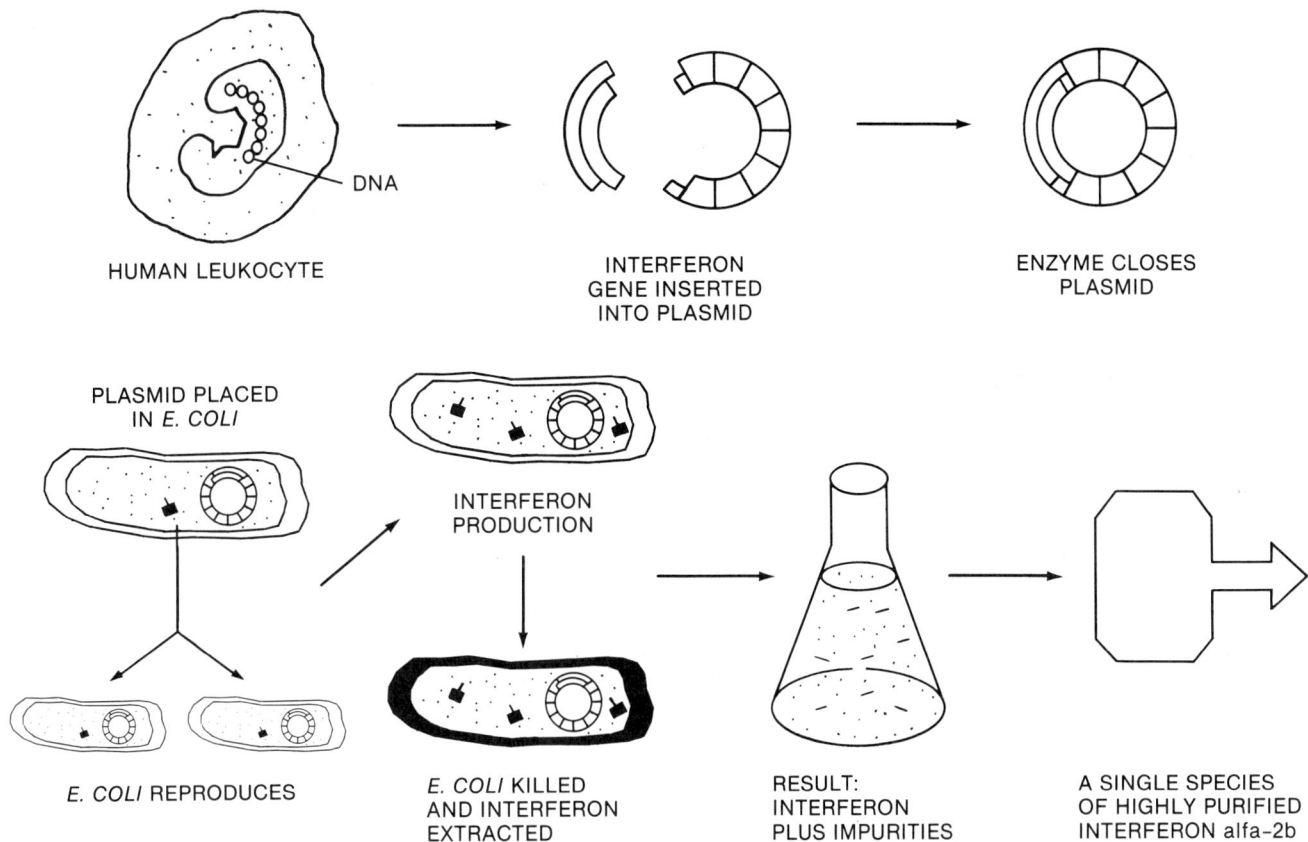

Figure 23–1. Recombinant DNA production of highly purified human interferon-alpha-2b. (Schering Corporation. Reproduced by permission. Copyright © 1986. Schering Corporation. All rights reserved.)

tumor activity as well as for an exciting approach to immunotherapy: adoptive immunotherapy. *Adoptive immunotherapy* has been defined as a "treatment approach in which cells with antitumor reactivity are administered to a tumor-bearing host and mediate either directly or indirectly the regression of established tumor" (Rosenberg, Lotze, Muul, et al., 1985). With this approach, IL 2 mixes with human peripheral blood lymphocytes and generates cells termed *lymphokine-activated killer* (LAK) *cells* that are capable of killing tumor cells.

Currently, a number of medical centers across the United States and abroad are studying IL 2 clinically and in the laboratory to further define its efficacy and delineate methods of reducing the toxicities it produces (West et al., 1987).

Considerable in vitro data but few clinical reports are available on relatively new BRMs, such as colony-stimulating factors (CSFs), antimetastatic agents, and TNF. Multiple clinical trials are under way using CSF, a monokine, in an effort to stimulate production of leukocytes in the stem cells of the bone marrow of cancer patients. For more than a century and particularly since Coley's work, the antitumor effects of bacterial cell products have been recognized (Oettgen & Old, 1987). In 1975, researchers isolated TNF, an agent noted for its ability to induce hemorrhagic necrosis in tumor cells without harming normal tissues. Several phase I trials using escalating doses of TNF are in progress throughout the United States.

TESTING

The approach to testing cytotoxic agents clinically has been to establish the maximum tolerated dose in phase I trials (see Chapter 25). With BRMs, the maximum tolerated dose as well as the optimal immunomodulatory dose must be determined, because lower doses of some BRMs may be more effective in altering various aspects of the immune response than higher doses, or the agent may be effective by different mechanisms at different doses.

NURSING CONSIDERATIONS

Individuals who receive biologic therapy have many of the same needs as individuals who receive investigational or conventional therapy for cancer (Irwin, 1987) (Table 23–3). Although most biotherapy continues to be administered in research settings, agents such as interferon are rapidly becoming more common in therapy in the community setting. Oncology nurses in community agencies and research settings should be well versed in biotherapy.

In the past, nurses caring for individuals receiving immunotherapy were expected to be familiar with basic principles of immunotherapy and to be clinically expert at administering the therapy. Today the role of the nurse caring for these patients has become quite complex and requires the nurse's understanding of the

Immunization

Removal of
antibody secreting
B lymphocytes
from spleen

Isolate myeloma
cell line from
culture

Fusion to make
hybridoma cell
(nuclei also fuse)

Expand hybridoma
in vitro

Concentrate and purify
secreted monoclonal
antibody

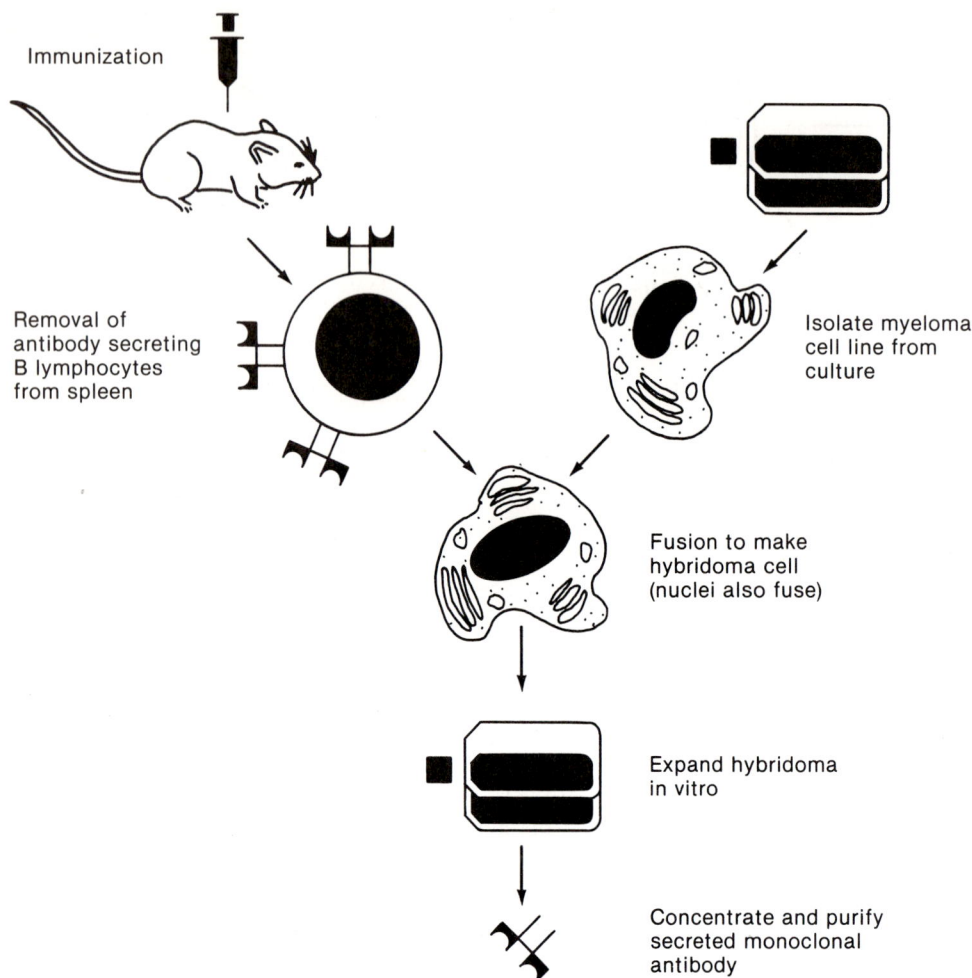

Figure 23–2. The hybridoma technology. (From NeoRx Corporation. K. A. Foon, M.D. Application of monoclonal antibodies in the diagnosis and therapy of cancer, 1988. Reproduced by permission.)

immune system and the different agents that affect it (Abernathy, 1987a).

TUMOR IMMUNOLOGY

Tumor immunology is the study of the relationship between tumor development and growth and the immunologic status of the host. In the late 1800s, Novinsky performed tumor transplantation in dogs and reported that he could successfully carry a tumor through two generations. His work created the basis of transplantation genetics (Gallucci, 1985). During the same era, physicians were observing that some individuals with cancer who developed secondary infections survived for a long time (Gallucci, 1987). Such discoveries led to the theory that the immune system, if properly stimulated, could elicit a response against cancerous cells and control them in the same manner that it controlled infections (Gallucci, 1985). More recently, the discovery of tumor antigens on the surface of cancer cells has fueled curiosity about the interlink between the immune system and tumor control (Bates & Longo, 1985).

An understanding of tumor immunology and biotherapy is built on a basic knowledge of the immune system (Fig. 23–3). It is necessary to understand the

components of the immune system and their function to comprehend this complex new approach to cancer treatment.

Overview of the Immune System

The immune system is a complex network of organs and cells that is responsible for guarding the body against the invasion of harmful elements. When functioning correctly, this system fights off invaders such as viruses, bacteria, fungi, and parasites as well as malignant cells and thus provides a safe habitat for the body. When a breakdown in the system occurs, various diseases proliferate (Abernathy, 1987b).

The defense mechanisms provided by the immune system (immunologic defense mechanisms) can be divided into the first line of host defenses—nonspecific immunity—and the second line of resistance—specific immunity.

Host Defenses

Nonspecific immunity is perhaps the body's most important defense against infection. It is designed to provide immediate protection on the first occasion that

Table 23–3. PATIENTS RECEIVING BIOLOGIC RESPONSE MODIFIERS: RISK FACTORS AND NURSING OBSERVATIONS

Symptoms/Organ-System Side Effects	Potential Risk Factors	Usual Time Frame	Observations
Constitutional Symptoms Headache Fever Chills Myalgias Flu-like symptoms	Age Poor performance status	Acute	• Observe for presence and severity of symptoms (acute symptoms generally abate with repeated dosing)
Fatigue Malaise Weakness	Age Poor performance status Malnutrition Anemia Other medications Inadequate social support system	Chronic	• Monitor use of other medications (e.g., propranolol can contribute to fatigue) • Monitor nutritional status (e.g., weight change) • Monitor hematologic status
Cardiovascular	Cardiac history Unstable hypertension Dehydration Age	Acute and chronic	• Observe orthostatic blood pressure changes with vital signs • Monitor for potential cardiac symptoms
Neurologic	History of seizures History of mood swings, depression Age	Acute and chronic	• Observe for cognitive and mood alterations • Educate family to report subtle changes
Gastrointestinal	History of gastrointestinal disorders	Acute	• Observe for symptoms
Hematologic	History of coagulation disorders Leukemia Multiple myeloma Bone marrow suppression	Chronic	• Routinely monitor complete blood count, differential, platelets, prothrombin time, partial thromboplastin time
Renal/Metabolic	Renal disease	Acute and chronic	• Routinely monitor blood urea nitrogen, creatinine, electrolytes • Monitor for proteinuria in high-risk patients
Hepatic	History of ethyl alcohol use Other hepatotoxic drugs Malnutrition Preexistent liver disease	Chronic	• Obtain baseline liver function tests • Routinely monitor lactose dehydrogenase, alkaline phosphatase, serum glutamic-oxaloacetic transaminase, serum glutamic-pyruvic transaminase, bilirubin • Monitor nutritional status • Monitor ethyl alcohol and other drug intake

(From Irwin, M. M. [1987]. Patients receiving biological response modifiers: Overview of nursing care. *Oncology Nursing Forum, 14* [Suppl. 6], 32–37. Reproduced by permission.)

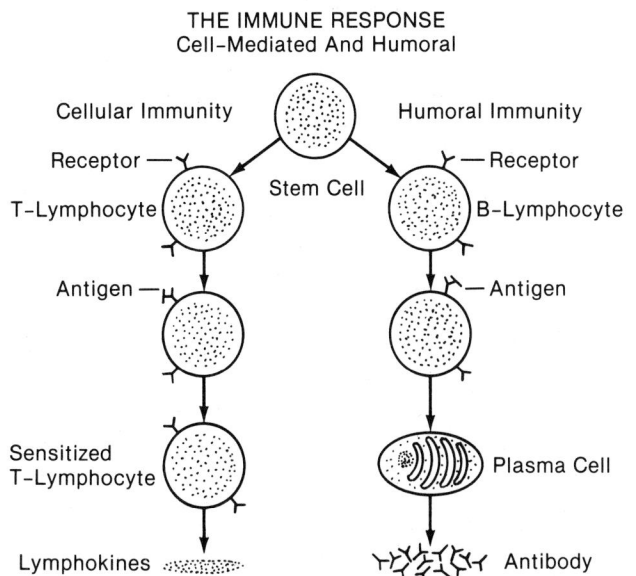

Figure 23–3. Differentiation of the lymphoid stem cell results in two distinct populations of lymphocytes. The B-cell system generates the humoral response, whereas the T-cell system generates the cellular response. (From National Institutes of Health. [1983]. *Understanding the immune system* [USDHHS Publication No. NIH 84-529]. Washington, DC: U.S. Government Printing Office.)

THE IMMUNE RESPONSE
Cell-Mediated And Humoral

the body encounters a foreign invader. Nonspecific immunity is the body's way of protecting itself using the capabilities of its normal anatomy and physiology.

The first line of defense against invaders attempting to enter the body is the physical barrier provided by the intact skin and mucous membranes. However, when the integrity of the skin is broken, for example, from a burn, invasion from foreign cells will occur, thus upsetting the body's homeostasis and allowing disease to flourish. Other examples of nonspecific immunity include the following:

1. The ciliated epithelial lining in the respiratory tract that traps and sweeps away inhaled bacteria.

2. The flushing action and composition of urine that help prevent urinary tract infections.

3. The large quantities of lysozyme, an enzyme in human tears that destroys bacteria.

When these first-line defenses fail to prevent entry of microorganisms into the body, an inflammatory response is activated that attempts to control the infectious growth and systemic invasion. Neutrophils congregate in the area of the invasion and phagocytize the invaders. These are not cells that react specifically with the antigens but are cells that recognize something as foreign and attempt to destroy it (Gallucci, 1987; Gurevich & Tafuro, 1986).

Specific (acquired) immunity is the immune system's response once an invader (antigen) is recognized as potentially harmful and not belonging to the body. An antigen is anything the immune system recognizes as nonself. Once the antigen is recognized as nonself, an army of cells is activated to destroy and dispose of the antigenic material. Antigens are carried on the cell surface of certain tumor cells, viruses, and bacteria. The cells of the immune system are quite sophisticated and develop a memory response. For example, if an individual is exposed to measles, the immune system has been primed for that specific invader. Following reexposure to measles, the immune system immediately identifies and attacks the measles organism to rid the body of the harmful threat. However, it is reactive only for that specific organism and not for any other foreign invader. The immune system must learn about each individual invader to which it is exposed and must develop specific cells (memory lymphocytes and B lymphocytes) that recognize and react to reexposure of the foreign matter; this process is the basis for immunizations (Huffer, Kanapa, & Stevenson, 1986).

The antigen is processed by macrophages before the immune response is generated. Antigen receptors on cell surfaces are responsible for the specificity of the reaction. Each antigen reacts only with one lymphocyte receptor in a manner similar to a lock and key (Hanson & Wigzell, 1985). On binding to the antigen, the lymphocyte is activated. It grows and divides and secretes lymphokines that activate other lymphocytes. The cell's clone has the same specificity as the mother cell and facilitates the specific immune response needed to eliminate that antigen.

Acquired immunity may be divided into two subsystems: (1) humoral immunity and (2) cell-mediated immunity. *Humoral immunity* is made of two serum

proteins derived from stem cells in the bone marrow: antibody molecules (immunoglobulins or Ig) and complement molecules. Immunoglobulins, by their ability to bind to a specific antigen, are capable of neutralizing that invader. Tumor cells express surface antigens that are capable of being recognized as foreign by the immune system. The antibody-antigen reaction is very specific in that an antibody will react only with one particular type of antigen. For example, if the antigen were an *Escherichia coli* bacterium, the body would have to summon an *E. coli* antibody for neutralization. Each immunoglobulin protein consists of two identical heavy chains and two light chains linked by a disulfide bridge (chemical bond). Each of the light chains has a section called the *variable region* that determines to which antigen this particular antibody has the binding capability (Bernier, 1985). Because there are thousands of different antigens from which the body must be protected, the amino acids in the section of the light chains can be sequenced in thousands of different orders.

The heavy chain's amino acid sequences determine the class of the immunoglobulin. The five known classes are IgG, IgA, IgM, IgE, and IgD. The letters that name the heavy chain type of immunoglobulin are from the Greek alphabet (e.g., gamma = IgG). Each of the five classes of immunoglobulins has very specific and independent functions (Table 23-4).

When the body is invaded by a single antigen, a group of white blood cells—B lymphocytes—becomes activated. The B lymphocytes transform into Ig-secreting cells (plasma cells). The first exposure to an antigen is followed by a latent phase during which no antibody levels are detected. This phase is followed by a primary response, during which a rapid rise in serum antibody is detected, then a plateau, and then a decline in antibody level. This reaction time is not immediate and thus allows the spread of the antigen during the body's first exposure.

After the primary response, an immunologic memory is developed whereby on second exposure to the antigen, the latency period is very short, antibody production is much faster, and higher concentrations of antibody are present, again creating the basis for immunization.

This reaction between the antigen and the immunoglobulin signals the activation of complement, the nonspecific component of humoral immunity. The complement system is composed of a series of proteins circulating in an inactive form in the blood stream. These proteins, which are produced by mononuclear

Table 23–4. IMMUNOGLOBULINS

Immuno-globulin (Ig)	Per cent of Ig	Function
IgG	75	Secondary immune responses; activates complement
IgA	15	First-line defense; bacteria
IgM	10	Primary exposure; activates complement
IgE	—	Allergy symptoms
IgD	>1	Function unclear

phagocytes, are mostly regulatory enzymes. However, the last few proteins do not perform regulatory functions but are responsible for the ultimate destruction of the antigen. Complement circulates in a completely inactive form until activated in a "cascading" fashion by the enzyme above it in the cascade.

Complement destroys the antigen by actually "poking" holes in cell membranes, allowing the intracellular fluid to leak out. Complement is nonspecific in its destruction of antigen. Thus normal cells located in the area in which the complement system has been activated will also be destroyed. The destroyed cells are then cleared from the blood stream by mononuclear phagocytes and monocytes (Cooper, 1987).

Cell-mediated immunity is the key line of defense in fighting viral infections, some fungal infections, parasitic disease, and bacteria that are harbored inside cells. Cell-mediated immunity is responsible for delayed hypersensitivity, transplant rejection, and possibly tumor identification and destruction.

A cell-mediated reaction is activated when an antigen binds with an antigen receptor on the surface of a specialized white blood cell, a T lymphocyte. This interaction signals the differentiation of T lymphocytes into five very different subsets: (1) antigen-specific killer T lymphocytes, (2) "suppressor" T lymphocytes, (3) "helper" T lymphocytes, (4) "memory" T lymphocytes, and (5) "lymphokine-producing" T lymphocytes. The functions of the subsets of T lymphocytes are listed in Table 23–5.

The nonspecific component of cell-mediated immunity includes other leukocytes (mononuclear phagocytes and natural killer cells) that destroy and ingest a range of antigens. These cells function under the direction of the T lymphocytes. Mononuclear phagocytes and natural killer cells are nonspecific and are capable of destroying and eliminating a variety of antigens.

It is absolutely essential that all components of the immune system function properly. When a malfunction occurs in any one of the complex components of the system, disease may present itself. These diseases may include allergies, immune deficiency diseases, cancer, immune complex diseases, or autoimmune disease. The diversity of these diseases is tremendous owing to the complex and widespread interfacing of the immune system with the human body.

Immune Surveillance

The hypothesis of immune surveillance is much of the basis for biotherapy. This hypothesis suggests that the immune system is capable of recognizing that cancerous cells are foreign and eliciting an immune response that destroys the cells, thus protecting the host (Herberman, 1983). There are several assumptions from this hypothesis:

1. Cancer cells have surface antigens that are recognizable by the immune system.
2. The immune system through its inherent mechanisms is capable of destroying the cancer cells once they are identified.
3. A failure in the immune system may result in malignancy.

This hypothesis is also expressed while our bodies are creating malignant cells continuously. Not everyone develops a malignancy, however, because the immune system, when functioning correctly, is able to maintain control of the situation by recognizing and destroying the abnormal cells. When the immune system is depressed, the malignant cells are no longer destroyed, and a malignancy develops.

Clinical experience appears to lend support to the hypothesis of immune surveillance (Herberman, 1983; Roth & Foon, 1987). Patients with immunodeficiency states, such as individuals who have acquired immune deficiency syndrome (AIDS) or who have received a transplanted organ and take immunosuppressive agents to avoid rejection, have a higher incidence of cancer. More recent research has linked stress with the suppression of the immune system and the higher risk of developing cancer (Levi, 1987).

The increased incidence of cancer in the elderly also lends support to this theory. As the body ages, the immune system loses its ability to differentiate self from nonself, and autoimmune disorders develop (Groenwald, Fisher, & McCalla, 1987). In addition, the surveillance mechanisms become dulled, and the response to the challenge of antigens is impaired. Abnormal cells may be allowed to proliferate until a malignancy develops.

Histologic evidence of tumor cells being infiltrated with lymphocytes, plasma cells, and macrophages further supports this theory. The evidence suggests that the host's immune system has elicited an immune response to the tumor in an effort to destroy the cells (Berman, 1975).

Tumor Antigens

When a cell becomes malignant, the antigens that appear on the surface of the cell are also transformed

---

Table 23–5. FUNCTIONS OF T LYMPHOCYTES

1. *Killer lymphocytes* are highly antigen specific, capable of killing only cells coated with the specific antigen to which the particular T cell responds and no other. The cell-kill mechanism of these cells is not fully understood. Cytotoxic T cells release granules on their surface membrane (Gallucci, 1987). These granules contain molecules called *perforins* that make holes in the target cell membrane leading to cell destruction.

2. *Memory T lymphocytes* provide "memory" for antigen-specific cell-mediated immune responses. Following immunization with a specific antigen, memory T lymphocytes store the memory of this response so that following reexposure to the antigen, a cell-mediated immune response can occur more rapidly.

3. *Helper T lymphocytes* stimulate enhanced function of other lymphocytes and mononuclear phagocytes.

4. *Suppressor T lymphocytes* reduce the function of other lymphocytes and mononuclear phagocytes. Without the aid of suppressor T lymphocytes, certain autoimmune diseases may occur.

5. *"Lymphokine-producing" T lymphocytes* secrete molecules that allow the T lymphocytes to communicate with one another. Examples of lymphokines include interferon and interleukin 2.

biochemically. The theory is that tumor cells have distinct antigens that are capable of being recognized by the host as foreign and thus provoke an immune response (Bates & Longo, 1985). In humans these antigens are called *tumor-associated antigens* or oncofetal antigens.

Fetal tumor–associated antigens have been isolated on human tumor cells. These antigens appear to be closely associated with tumor growth. Carcinoembryonic antigen and alpha$_1$-fetoprotein are expressed on cells in fetal life and on certain malignant cells (Bates & Longo, 1985).

Tumor Escape Mechanisms

Several theories have been proposed to address the dilemma of how tumors escape mechanisms of immune surveillance. The first is that when the number of tumor cells is low, the cells may be tolerated because antigenic stimulation to the immune system is insufficient. By the time the immune system is properly stimulated, it may be too late because the number of cancer cells is too large for mechanisms of the immune system to destroy them (Gallucci, 1987).

Blocking factors are apparently tumor antigen-antibody complexes that are thought to stimulate suppressor T-cell activity, thus suppressing the immune response. They also may create a barrier that prevents cytotoxic cells from making contact with the tumor cells (Gallucci, 1987).

CLASSIFICATION OF BIOLOGIC RESPONSE MODIFIERS

Monoclonal Antibodies

Monoclonal antibody technology holds great promise for the development of treatments that are specific for the various types of cancer. The immune system's recognition of unfamiliar antigens (molecules of protein and glycoproteins located on tumor cells) and the production of antibodies to recognize these particular antigens provide the potential for targeting treatment specifically to tumor cells, thus sparing normal cells.

Monoclonal antibodies are high molecular weight proteins that are produced by a clone of cells and are meant to attack one specific antigen. The clone of cells originates from a single parent cell and produces only the particular antibody to which the parent cell was sensitive. Monoclonal antibodies therefore will target only one specific antigen and potentially can be used to differentiate cells possessing that antigen from other normal cell antigens.

Historical Background

At the turn of the century, Paul Ehrlich, a pioneer of specific antibacterial agents, applied the phrase "the magic bullet" to the possible targeting of antibodies to tumors (Ehrlich, 1900). Early studies involved administration of sera from recovered cancer patients to patients with active tumors. Occasional short-lived tumor responses in patients with melanoma and renal cell carcinoma were reported. Failure to fully achieve the anticipated success may have been due to two factors. First, the sera contained relatively low amounts of specific antibody, and second, the sera contained many other products and impurities that may have blocked beneficial effects (Moldawer & Murray, 1985). Interest was revived by the purification of the carcinoembryonic antigen and studies by Goldenberg and colleagues on the localization of radio-labeled antibodies in colorectal carcinomas (Pimm, 1987).

The immune system normally scouts the body for any nonself substances or antigens. Ordinarily, when an antigen is recognized and the immune reaction is initiated, various antibody-producing cells are stimulated to secrete different antibodies, which attach to receptors located on the antigen's cell wall. These different antibodies are polyclonal because they are produced by a variety of cells.

In the late 1970s, Kohler and Milstein (1975) developed a method of producing specific MoAbs from cloned cells or hybridomas from mice that had been inoculated with tumor cells. This breakthrough allowed scientists to develop large quantities of identical antibodies specific for a desired antigen.

To make an MoAb by the hybridoma technique (see Fig. 23–2), mice are injected with an antigen that causes their immune systems to react and initiate the production of antibodies. Antibody-producing lymphocytes are harvested from the spleen's reservoir and isolated. Each lymphocyte, which is capable of producing only one antibody, is fused to a mouse myeloma cell. Myelomas are tumors of plasma cells (mature antibody-producing B cells) that live for a very long time. The fused spleen and myeloma cells, called hybridomas, can produce a large quantity of antibody. The antibody that is produced by the hybridoma is isolated and tested to determine whether it possesses the desired specificity. If it does, the hybridoma is grown in culture, in which it produces large quantities of one specific purified antibody; this process explains the reason for the name MoAb (Gallucci, 1985).

With the advances made in the past decade in MoAb technology and the ability to identify antigens on tumor cells with precision, clinical immunology has surpassed the progress of the previous three decades. Now MoAbs can be utilized for a variety of purposes (Table 23–6).

Mechanism of Action

The central issue regarding the future potential of MoAbs is whether tumor-specific antigens exist or whether antigens possessed by tumors are shared with normal tissues. To induce a specific immune response, the tumor cells have to express an antigen specific to or associated with the tumor. But because tumors are derived from normal cells, it cannot be assumed that tumors carry antigens that are different or foreign.

Table 23–6. USES OF MONOCLONAL ANTIBODIES

Diagnostic

1. Early detection of cancer by identifying surface markers of tumor cells and circulating tumor-associated antigens
2. Identification and disabling of activated lymphocytes involved in organ transplant rejection and graft-versus-host disease
3. Identification of lymphocyte antigens and correlation of their functions in the immune response
4. Identification of dysfunction of components of the immune system in cancer and other immune-related diseases
5. Identification of function, isolation, or blockage of growth factors, tumor factors, and other biologic response modifiers, ultimately allowing for manipulation of the immune response
6. Delivery of radioactive isotopes directly to tumor sites, allowing scans to visualize the tumor

Therapeutic

1. Delivery of immunotoxins—target to tumor
   a. toxic agents, such as ricin
   b. chemotherapy, such as doxorubicin and daunomycin
   c. radioactive isotopes for both diagnostic scans and therapeutic delivery of radiation

Some tumor cells do possess certain antigens on their cell membranes that are capable of eliciting an immune response in the host. However, other tumor cells share antigens with the cells of the parent organ from which the tumor arose. Some tumor cells possess antigens that are normally displayed only on fetal tissues, such as carcinoembryonic antigen, which is associated with colon carcinomas and is found on normal fetal gut cells during the first two trimesters of pregnancy, or alpha$_1$-fetoprotein, which is secreted by hepatocellular carcinomas. Other tumor-associated antigens include differentiation antigens, such as the protein antigens on malignant melanoma cells; carbohydrate antigens expressed by carcinomas of the breast and ovary; and glycolipid antigens, which are present in colorectal cancer (Baldwin & Byers, 1987).

The immune response generated against tumor-associated antigens consists of either the formation of antibodies against the antigens or the attachment of various immune cells (stimulated killer lymphocytes and macrophages) to the antibody that is bound to the tumor, which effects tumor cell death. Tumors can escape immunologic attack in a number of ways. Tumor cells can shed their surface antigens or alter their appearance within 2 hours of MoAb exposure, an effect that can last up to 36 hours (Oldham, 1983). Or circulating tumor antigen may bind with the MoAb, blocking its receptor sites and thus preventing it from reaching the tumor cell. Blocking factors may be released by tumor cells to coat the tumor cell surface antigens, preventing recognition and destruction of the tumor (Oldham, 1983). Immune complexes composed of the linked antibody and antigen may be drawn into the cell, where detection of the tumor cell antigen becomes hidden from the immune effector cells. Antigens bound by antibodies create a large complex that is unable to penetrate very deeply into the tumor; therefore, only a small proportion of the tumor cells are attacked. Tumors are heterogenous, with metastases displaying different antigens than the primary one, such that one specific MoAb may not recognize all of the areas of tumor in one individual. Also

neoplastic cells survive with minimal accessibility to blood supply; thus it is difficult for MoAbs to reach many tumor cells.

Clinical Applications

The use of antibodies to mediate specific toxicity for the cancer cell through recruitment of cell-mediated immunity and activation of the complement system is under investigation. Currently, greater anticipated potential is attributed to the ability to link many types of molecules to MoAbs. Each MoAb has its own unique advantages and drawbacks for use in the localization of tumor. Cancer treatment can be enhanced through the use of MoAbs to target the delivery of drugs, toxins, and radioactive substances specifically to the area of tumor (Moldawer & Murray, 1985).

The use of MoAbs to detect early or preinvasive tumor by examining serum samples that may reveal the presence of surface antigens that are different from those of normal tissues also holds great promise in the fight against cancer. For example, distinct surface markers found on testicular carcinoma in situ, melanoma cells, and lymphoma cells possess antigens recognizable by MoAbs that assist pathologists in distinguishing tumor cells from normal cells. Monoclonal antibodies also will be used to define the existence of tumor-associated antigens.

Currently MoAbs are used to purge bone marrow of neoplastic cells before reinfusion for bone marrow transplantation. MoAbs can identify and then disable activated lymphocytes that are responsible for transplant rejection or graft-versus-host disease without causing overall suppression of the immune mechanisms of the host (Baldwin & Byers, 1987). The use of MoAbs to correlate distinct lymphocyte surface antigens with specific functions would allow an understanding of the pathophysiology of immune dysfunction in cancer and other immune-related diseases.

The ability of MoAbs to identify, isolate, or block the function of growth factors, tumor factors, or other BRMs may shed light on the understanding of the development and maintenance of the cell that has undergone neoplastic transformation and the means by which tumor cells may go undetected by the immune system (Thor, Weeks, & Schlom, 1986). Monoclonal antibodies may be used to manipulate the immune system specifically to interfere with the activity of growth factors induced by the tumor and to block other factors secreted by the tumor that induce increased numbers of suppressor lymphocytes to suppress the immune response.

Immunotoxins are created by the linkage of toxins to MoAbs. The toxin bound to the MoAb attaches to the antigenic receptor on the tumor cell membrane and then penetrates into the cytoplasm by endocytosis through smooth invaginations or coated pits of the plasma membrane. Once inside the tumor cell's cytoplasm, protein synthesis is inactivated and cell killing results (Baldwin & Byers, 1987). However, before utilization of such linked immunotoxins, technology must provide methods to be certain that the MoAb will hold on to the toxin until it reaches the tumor cell; otherwise, these toxins could be just as deadly to the host if even one toxic molecule enters the cell cytoplasm.

When MoAbs are linked to radioactive isotopes, scanning for areas of MoAb localization on tumor cells can determine if and where tumor recurrence exists. Such use could guide surgeons regarding the extent of surgery needed to yield total tumor resection based on the presence or absence of antibody in lymph nodes or other tissues surrounding the primary tumor. However, studies with many radiolabeled MoAbs show that only a proportion of the total antibody dose actually localizes in the tumor. A large proportion of the intravenously administered MoAbs remain in the circulation or are distributed in the reticuloendothelial system, for example, in the lungs, liver, and spleen, where the circulation pools blood (Morgan & Foon, 1986). Work continues in an attempt to improve the specificity of the MoAbs in use.

Side Effects

Targeting of drugs conjugated to MoAbs may increase therapeutic efficacy by improving localization and retention of drugs in tumors and by reducing normal tissue toxicity (Baldwin & Byers, 1987). Although great promise exists in the use of MoAbs in the diagnosis and treatment of cancer, a few problems have surfaced. Toxicity to normal cells, although generally mild, must be considered in their use with patients. Side effects related to the administration of MoAbs include fever, chills, flushing, urticaria, rash, nausea, vomiting, headache, and hypotension (Oldham & Smalley, 1983). Allergic types of reactions that may occur are easily treated with corticosteroids, acetaminophen, and antihistamines. However, immune complexes may stagnate within, causing damage to various organ tissues, for example, liver, lungs, or kidneys.

The development of antimouse antibodies has been noted when murine MoAbs are used. Because the murine MoAbs are large molecular weight protein molecules, they can evoke an immune allergic response against themselves. The host may produce antibodies against the injected MoAbs that inactivate their therapeutic effect. The use of human MoAbs may decrease the occurrence of antibodies, but human cell lines are unstable antibody producers (Jakobsen, 1987).

Toxicities associated with MoAbs have not been major and usually are associated with the initial one or two administrations or with rapid intravenous infusions. Clinical toxicities are observed when rapid intravenous infusion rates exceed 5 to 10 mg/hr. Pulmonary symptoms, such as acute dyspnea and mild wheezing, were noted and are felt to be related to lymphocyte clumping or trapping in the lungs. Such clumping in the lungs and in the kidneys was detected by continued monitoring after the administration of MoAbs (Oldham, 1983). These effects were less frequent or were absent with prolonged infusions over 2 to 4 hours.

With some of the human MoAbs, mild erythema at the injection site is the only side effect noted. None of the nausea, fever, or pain associated with murine antibodies was noted with the human antibodies.

Side effects of immunotoxin (MoAbs linked with toxins) administered for 5 days in 22 patients included transient drop in serum albumin level, weight gain, and fluid shifts resulting in mild edema and hypovolemia (Baldwin & Byers, 1987). The linked toxins have shown that they can be administered in large quantities with less toxicity than when they are administered as a single agent. Close observation for severe toxicities may indicate that the toxin has become detached from the MoAb molecule.

Nursing Considerations

Patient Safety. Because MoAbs are high molecular weight proteins, they have the potential to induce the production of host antibodies against themselves. Therefore, the risk of hypersensitivity reactions exists. Resuscitation and intubation equipment should be readily available along with emergency drugs such as parenteral corticosteroids, diphenhydramine, and epinephrine. Patients should be observed closely for at least the first hour after administration of MoAbs, with assessments of vital signs and pulmonary status taken every 15 minutes and additional assessments taken every hour for a period following completion of administration.

Environmental Safety. When radiolabeled MoAbs are utilized, the handling and disposal of radioactive substances and body fluids from the patient are important safety issues. Knowledge of the radioactive element and its half-life should be shared with individuals involved in the clinical care of the patient, although the doses of radioactivity in most cases are not high enough to require isolation. Badges that register the amount of radioactivity to which a health care worker is exposed should be worn. Also, radiation safety teams should monitor the emissions of radioactivity from the patient through body fluids, blood samples drawn, and other procedures. Lead shields and lead-lined specimen containers can be utilized to further minimize individual exposure. The patient's contact with family members and particularly with small children or pregnant women may be limited for a period of time following the administration of the MoAb.

Documentation. Evaluation of the patient's response and communication with the primary physician about any possible allergic reaction, such as hives, wheezing, urticaria, or rash, should be carefully documented. Also the determination about the development of anti-MoAb antibodies should be made before subsequent administrations of the MoAb to avoid anaphylactic shock.

Laboratory tests, frequent blood samples of various sorts, multiple scans, and tumor measurements are necessary in the evaluation of response to a new therapy such as MoAb therapy. Nurses must feel comfortable with the fact that new therapies provide knowledge to the medical community that may evolve into improved treatments in the future, even if the immediate benefit for a specific patient is not readily apparent.

Patient and Family Education and Support. Currently MoAbs are innovative therapy options about which the lay person has very little understanding. Charts, drawings, and printed materials about the immune system and the function of antibodies are useful for the new patient on MoAb therapy. The roles of advocate and interpreter are important for the nurse who cares for patients in the initial studies with new agents when consent forms are presented and initial discussions take place.

Colleague Education. Monoclonal antibodies possess multiple and varied characteristics, including different dosages and administration methods. Health care personnel who will be involved with patients receiving MoAbs need current information to enable them to provide appropriate care.

Interferon

Interferon is a family of cytokines that are glycoproteins produced as part of the cell-mediated immune response by the T lymphocyte after activation by viruses or tumor cells. Interferon is named for its antiviral ability to interfere with the spread of viral infection by affecting the synthesis of viral RNA and protein; it has been found to possess antitumor and immunomodulatory potential as well.

Interferon has potent effects on the immune system as an "immunological hormone" (Gutterman, 1988). It is considered to be the prototype BRM, a natural human protein that can alter the body's immune response to result in detrimental effects to a tumor and, it is hoped, in little toxicity to normal tissues. Interferon has undergone extensive clinical investigation and in 1986 received Food and Drug Administration approval for therapeutic use for hairy cell leukemia; additional approval was granted in 1988 for use in AIDS-related Kaposi's sarcoma and condylomata acuminata (genital warts).

Historical Background

Since the early 1900s, it has been known that viral infection with one agent could prevent simultaneous infection with a second agent. In 1957 Issacs and Lindenmann discovered an agent with antiviral properties and called it *interferon* (Lindenmann, 1982). The production of this agent was an expensive and tedious process that yielded insufficient and impure supplies of interferon. Also, interferon was species specific, which meant that preclinical laboratory research with animals was not useful in predicting toxicity and biologic effects in humans. When antitumor properties were discovered, however, interferon was heralded by the press as a potential miracle cure, and investment capital was provided quickly for its study and production (Gresser & Tovey, 1978).

Technologic advances in the 1970s, such as recombinant DNA gene cloning and increased sophistication of computers and other laboratory equipment, enabled the determination of interferon's molecular structure, the examination of its biologic activity, and, subsequently, the mass production of it in large quantities. DNA is isolated from the human gene responsible for interferon production (see Fig. 23–1). This DNA is then implanted into altered bacteria, which produce mass quantities of interferon. Unlike cultured "human" interferon obtained by the Cantell method (which was a soup-like mixture containing many types of interferons and proteins together within the vat), recombinant interferons consist of only one subtype that was coded on the DNA. This ability to make large quantities of purified human interferon proteins facilitated clinical trials that began in the late 1970s.

Interferon consists of a family of small glycoproteins of three general types that are determined by the type of cell and the substance that stimulates interferon production. Their names are designated by the Greek letters alpha, beta, and gamma. All three are antigenically distinct and possess separate biologic and chemical properties, but all share the ability to prevent viral spread.

Interferon-α possesses more than 16 subtypes. Interferon-$\alpha2_a$ and interferon-$\alpha2_b$ differ in the chemical molecule located on the gene at position 23, with 2_a possessing a lysine group and 2_b possessing an arginine group. Interferon-α is produced by viral, bacterial, or tumor cell stimulation of leukocytes, including T and B lymphocytes, macrophages, natural killer cells, and large granular lymphocytes (Hooks & Detrick, 1985). A single gene exists for the production of interferon-β and interferon-γ; therefore, only one type of each exists. Interferon-β is produced by stimulation of fibroblast or epithelial cells. Interferon-γ is produced by helper and suppressor T lymphocytes as an integral part of the immune response.

Mechanism of Action

The particular biochemical response generated by interferon depends on the type of interferon involved, the responding cell, and the agent against which interferon is reacting—virus, parasite, or tumor.

Antiviral. Interferon was originally identified for its antiviral properties: it is able to induce an antiviral state when a virus attaches to a cell membrane. Interferon stimulates the production of various factors that participate in the events that occur during the immune response to protect cells from a second simultaneous infection. It prevents further viral RNA and protein replication, halting the virus' ability to spread to other body cells (Higgins, 1984).

Interferon is measured in units of antiviral activity based on its ability to inhibit viral multiplication in tissue cultures. One million antiviral units is the common unit for measurement of interferon dosage, also called one megaunit or International Unit (IU). This antiviral activity can vary among lots and types of interferon, which makes comparisons difficult.

Results have been dramatic in interferon treatment of some conditions induced by viral infections, such as the papovavirus, which causes genital and laryngeal warts. Without continued interferon treatment, children with laryngeal papillomatosis would require surgery as often as every 2 to 3 months to remove the warts within their airways (Strander, 1986). Condyloma acuminata is increasing in incidence, surpassing genital herpes. Its response to interferon is good, but the warts tend to recur and thus require retreatment.

Antitumor. Direct antitumor effects have been identified that involve inhibition of tumor growth and cell division. As interferon contacts a tumor cell receptor site, it triggers a number of reactions that arrest or delay the stages of cell division, primarily G_0 to G_1 (Goldstein & Laszlo, 1986; Higgins, 1984).

Interferon also influences the production of other cellular products, enzymes, and lymphokines. These actions can result in differentiating effects on the malignant cell, alterations in malignant cell phenotype and metabolism, or inhibition of important genes, such as oncogenes. Inhibition of oncogene expression can accompany changes in morphology of some cell lines that have undergone neoplastic transformation, such as loss or decrease in tumorigenicity, inhibition of cell proliferation, and return to normal growth of these cells (Clark & Longo, 1987). Variations in the degree of these effects are time and dose related; therefore, the optimal inhibitory dose for various malignancies must be refined as clinical use progresses.

Immunomodulatory. Interferon causes some indirect effects, influencing various immunomodulatory aspects of both cellular and humoral immunity. Some of these effects include the stimulation of cytotoxic T lymphocytes, macrophages, and natural killer cells as well as phagocytic activity.

Interferon also increases the expression of tumor-associated antigens on the tumor cell membrane, which causes the tumor cells to be more recognizable (Goldstein & Laszlo, 1986; Higgins, 1984). B lymphocytes are directed to differentiate into antibody-producing plasma cells. Overall, interferon influences a number of immune activities that enhance the body's ability to recognize and rid itself of tumor growth.

Clinical Applications

Interferon-α. Interferon-α was initially approved by the Food and Drug Administration in June 1986 for use against hairy cell leukemia, a rare, chronic form of B-cell leukemia that is highly sensitive to small amounts of interferon. Hairy cell leukemia is named for the many hair-like projections of cytoplasm that extend from the walls of lymphoid cells. Fewer than 2 per cent of all leukemia cases are hairy cell leukemia. Its symptoms are fatigue, anemia, easy bruising, and frequent infections that are caused by crowding of the bone marrow, which prevents the production of normal blood cells. Before the discovery of interferon's effectiveness, the treatment for about half of these patients was splenectomy. Forty per cent of those undergoing surgery have relapses within 2 years, at which point few interventions effectively control the disease. Patients then die of infections or bleeding (Huang, 1985).

Hairy cell leukemia responds to interferon-α administration in a reported 67 to 90 per cent of patients at low doses of 0.2 to 3.0 IU/m² after 6 to 10 months of daily or three times per week administration (Goldstein & Laszlo, 1986; Oldham, 1985). Responses are evidenced by improvement in hematologic parameters, with increases in platelet counts, production of normal leukocytes, and resolution of anemia. Forty per cent of those responding will have relapses after interferon-α is discontinued, which suggests the need for maintenance therapy or reinduction to maintain remissions. The mechanism of action in hairy cell leukemia is uncertain, but Gutterman (1988) reports that patients who have had complete remissions have demonstrated a restored ability to produce their own endogenous interferon.

Chronic myelogenous leukemia in the benign or chronic phase has also been found to respond to interferon-α. The benign or chronic phase of this disease is characterized by large numbers of leukocytes in the blood, giving the appearance of "purulent blood"; it lasts an average of 3.5 years despite current chemotherapy schedules. The accelerated phase or blastic crisis, or both, follow the chronic phase with their course little affected by chemotherapy. Chronic myelogenous leukemia is associated with increased cytogenetic abnormalities, such as the presence of the Philadelphia chromosome and the activation of various oncogenes and growth factors (Gutterman, 1988).

Complete hematologic responses are achieved at a rate of about 70 per cent in patients treated with interferon-α. However, unlike responses achieved with busulfan or hydroxyurea, continued interferon use induces suppression of the Philadelphia chromosome and reversal of some cytogenetic abnormalities. These response rates with correction of cytogenetic abnormalities have lasted for more than 2 years as the patients in remission continue to be followed (Gutterman, 1988). There is an increased response rate if treatment is started within 6 months of diagnosis.

Interferon-α is also indicated for use against AIDS-related Kaposi's sarcoma. Classic Kaposi's sarcoma is a relatively rare tumor of older men, usually considered to be benign. It appears as flat, macular lesions, primarily in the lower extremities, that are faint pink to reddish-purple. The incidence of this malignancy in young male homosexuals has increased, which observation, in fact, led to the awareness of the AIDS epidemic. It is a multifocal cancer of the skin and connective tissue that does not metastasize to internal organs; however, its spread along the epithelial linings of the visceral mucosa is a poor prognostic indicator.

Response to interferon includes the flattening or disappearance, or both, of the lesions with no evidence of disease on biopsy of prior Kaposi's sarcoma sites. The response is dose related, with 28 to 35 per cent of the responses occurring with high doses. Interferon-α does not correct the immune deficiencies of AIDS, but the incidence of opportunistic infections in responders is reported to decrease.

Other hematologic disorders that show responsiveness to interferon-α include nodular non-Hodgkin's lymphoma, chronic lymphocytic leukemia, and multiple myeloma. Solid tumors have shown less responsiveness to interferon, but some significant responses have been seen in renal cell carcinoma and superficial bladder cancer; in ovarian carcinoma, with intraperitoneal administration of interferon; and in colon cancer, with interferon enhancing the effect of 5-fluorouracil. For more detailed discussions of clinical indications for its use, comprehensive review articles are available (Goldstein, & Laszlo, 1986; Gutterman, 1988; Kirkwood & Ernstoff, 1984).

Interferon-β. Interferon-β is very similar to interferon-α in both its activity and its toxicities, but it is less potent as an antiviral agent. Intramuscularly administered interferon-β becomes bound to local tissues and is destroyed within the muscle. Therefore, higher doses administered by the intravenous route have been necessary to attain adequate serum levels. Investigative clinical trials are not as far along as the trials with interferon-α, but results should be available soon concerning its effectiveness in various malignancies.

Interferon-γ. Interferon-γ has several different biologic effects that differentiate it from either interferon-α or interferon-β. Interferon-γ has more of an activation effect on macrophages and demonstrates a much higher cytotoxic effect in vitro through its role in regulating cytotoxic T cells (Vilcek, Kelke, Jumming, & Yip, 1985). Although early clinical trials of interferon-γ used as a single agent have failed to yield tumor regressions, it does suppress growth and differentiation and interacts with other interferons, TNF, and interleukins to have antiproliferative effects (Gutterman, 1988). It is hoped that continued trials of interferon-γ in combination with other BRMs and chemotherapy will define its role in the future.

Interferon-γ must be administered by intravenous route to achieve detectable serum levels. It is tolerated at much higher doses than those of interferon-α. Its toxicity profile is similar to that of interferon-α with an additional dose-limiting effect involving prolonged systolic hypotension that in some cases lasts 12 to 24 hours after interferon-γ administration.

Side Effects

Toxicity commonly begins to be seen at doses of higher than 1 IU, and severity increases with higher doses (Table 23–7). Tolerance to the acute side effects develops after the first one to three doses of interferon. See the section on "Management of Toxicities" for a more detailed discussion of side effects.

Long-term administration of high doses (greater than 15 IU) may result in cumulative, dose-limiting toxicities. These include unacceptable fatigue, anorexia with weight loss, confusion, and occasionally liver transaminase elevations (Kirkwood & Ernstoff, 1984). Other less frequent toxic effects that are transient and reversible with cessation of therapy include nausea, vomiting, diarrhea, hypotension, central nervous system depression, somnolence, electroencephalogram changes, paresthesias, and proteinuria. Acute cardiac failure with arrhythmias and acute ischemic events are

Table 23–7. INTERFERON SIDE EFFECTS

Frequent	Less Common
Acute	
Fever (to 40°C)	Nausea and vomiting
Chills (and rigors)	Diarrhea
Headaches	Hypotension
Chronic	
Fatigue	Central nervous system changes:
Malaise	Confusion
Anorexia (taste changes)	Depression
Weight loss	Electroencephalogram changes
Mild leukopenia	Mild hepatic dysfunction
Mild thrombocytopenia	Proteinuria
	Cardiac arrhythmias

evidence of a rare life-threatening toxicity, so caution is required in administering high doses of interferon to those with a strong history of cardiovascular disease.

Antibody formation after a median time of 7 months, with the development of high titers of neutralizing antibodies in hairy cell leukemia and chronic myelogenous leukemia patients that resulted in a relapse of the disease, occurred with the administration of interferon-α 2$_a$. Its incidence was not so high with interferon-α 2$_b$, but different testing techniques were used, which caused some controversy over its significance.

Nursing Considerations

The nursing care of individuals undergoing biologic therapies offers a challenge to provide comprehensive care in diverse areas. Other areas of nursing consideration include assessment of the immune response, administration, nursing management of side effects, and patient education and support (Irwin, 1987).

Assessment and Administration. Interferon comes in several subtypes and dilutions. The directions on package inserts for different interferons should be followed carefully in the preparation of the correct dosage and concentration, route of administration, and procedure for reconstitution and maintenance of stability. Advise the patient not to change brands.

Interferon is a nonvesicant, although soreness and redness can occur at sites of subcutaneous or intramuscular injections. Phlebitis may result from prolonged intravenous infusions. Interferon is not known to possess mutagenic properties. A common-sense approach in handling interferon supplies is recommended by the Oncology Nursing Society's *Biological Response Modifiers Guidelines* (1989).

Management of Toxicities. Contrary to original hopes that a natural therapy such as interferon would be nontoxic, interferons can induce significant toxicities. However, the toxicities are dose related and reversible with the cessation of interferon administration. Tolerance to acute toxicities develops with time, but the long-term side effects accumulate (see Table 23–7).

Constitutional. The acute "flu-like syndrome" consisting of fever, chills, malaise, and myalgias occurs in 90 per cent of patients (Quesada, Talpaz, Rios, Kurzrodk, & Gutterman, 1986). Initially chills begin about 2 to 6 hours after administration of the interferon dose and include severe teeth-chattering rigors accompanied by pallor due to peripheral vasoconstriction. The increased muscular activity associated with the shivers causes the body temperature to rise, along with the pulse rate and blood pressure. Blankets and warm beverages may comfort the patient; however, the use of morphine to lessen the severity of muscular contractions may be necessary for the most severe rigors that occur with the highest doses of interferon (Hood, 1988).

Acetaminophen is generally very effective in controlling the fevers, which may peak at 39° to 40° C (102° to 104° F). The use of aspirin, nonsteroidal anti-inflammatory agents, or steroids to block this acute febrile reaction is generally avoided because of fear that the effects of these drugs on the immune system may block the beneficial results of interferon.

This clinical picture of fever and chills resembles the onset of sepsis, and commonly a full infection evaluation is carried out. However, generally this predictable pattern of effects, which is related to the timing of interferon administration and which responds to acetaminophen, allows one to closely observe the otherwise stable patient and await culture results before instituting antibiotic therapy.

The day following interferon administration is usually free of fever, but a "washed-out" feeling with muscular aches and fatigue may persist. Chronic, severe fatigue accumulates over the course of interferon administration, with doses greater than 20 IU/m² needing to be reduced in 50 per cent of patients. Doses of less than 5 IU/m² are more tolerable. Patients may become unable to attend to usual daily activities to the extent that they ignore personal care. Patients should be counseled to take planned rest periods and to anticipate some fatigue so that they will not be overly anxious that these symptoms signal the progression of their malignancy. Administration of interferon in the evening results in less fatigue (Abrams, McClamrock, & Foon, 1985).

Central Nervous System. Up to 70 per cent of patients receiving interferon in initial dose-escalating trials have experienced dose-related central nervous system toxicities (Goldstein & Laszlo, 1986; Quesada, Talpaz, Rios, Kurzrodk, & Gutterman, 1986) (Box 23–1). These include confusion, inability to perform simple calculations or to concentrate, depression, somnolence, electroencephalogram changes with diffuse slowing as with encephalopathies, and paresthesias. At lower doses, patients may note irritability, lack of patience, low motivation, and depression. Patients may forget appointments and become easily disoriented. Headaches can be relieved with acetaminophen.

Many of these neurologic changes are subtle, and patients tend to try to cover up impairments, such that specific testing (e.g., serial sevens, mental status) and questioning of family members should be a routine element in the assessment of patients.

Gastrointestinal. Fewer than one third of patients experience mild nausea, usually during the first week of treatment. This is a constant nausea, seldom accompanied by emesis, which is managed by the use of antiemetics. Mild diarrhea is occasionally reported, also in the initial stages of therapy.

More common gastrointestinal complaints include chronic taste alteration, early satiety, and cumulative anorexia (Mayer, Hetrick, Riggs, & Sherwin, 1984; Quesada et al., 1986). Nutritional counseling is important to help patients maintain their strength and to avoid muscle wasting syndrome. Decreased salivary flow may contribute to the occurrence of stomatitis, caries, and candidiasis, which means that good oral care is important.

Cardiovascular. The acute flu-like syndrome with its associated rigors, tachycardia, cyanosis, and rapid breathing is very stressful for the patient with a history of cardiovascular problems. Sudden cardiac deaths and myocardial infarctions are rare, but precautions are given against the use of high doses of interferon in individuals with a strong history of active cardiac disease and for the careful evaluation of the heart and electrocardiogram before initiating interferon therapy.

Orthostatic hypotension is evident during patient monitoring, although most patients are unaware of it (Laszlo et al., in press). It is managed in most cases by encouraging intake of sufficient fluids and advising patients to avoid sudden changes in position. Hypertensive medications may need to be lowered or discontinued during interferon therapy.

Hematologic, Hepatic, and Renal. These organ toxicities are dose related and disappear when the interferon is discontinued or the dose is lowered. Mild decrease in granulocytes, platelets, and red blood cells is seen during interferon therapy. Transient elevations in serum transaminase levels and mild proteinuria have been reported. Because interferon is cleared via the kidneys, patients with preexisting renal disease should be observed carefully.

Patient Education and Support. Patients need careful explanations, both to educate them regarding their treatment program and to familiarize them with the terminology utilized with BRM therapies. Clarification of misconceptions or preconceptions about the purpose and side effects of interferon is needed to enable the patient to understand how to become an informed participant in the treatment program.

Patients are taught to self-administer the interferon doses; they learn about the preparation of the injection; use of syringes; sterile technique; and proper administration of the injection, including the rotation of subcutaneous injection sites. Patients are also taught to recognize and report toxicities promptly to the health care team to prevent the development of more severe complications.

Supportive counseling has been discussed previously in symptom management. Patients should be monitored closely during the initial doses of interferon, especially elderly patients who are at increased risk of cardiac or neurologic toxicity. Reassurance that acute side effects will lessen as tolerance develops often encourages a patient to stick with the treatment plan for at least 2 weeks rather than drop out. Suggestions of ways to handle the long-term side effects, such as

---

Box 23–1. INTERFERON: NEUROPSYCHIATRIC MANIFESTATIONS

Adams, F., Quesada, J. R., & Gutterman, J. U. (1984). **Neuropsychiatric manifestations of human leukocyte interferon therapy in patients with cancer.** *Journal of the American Medical Association, 252,* 938–941.

This descriptive study was among the first to identify the intense fatigue-asthenia syndrome that accompanies human leukocyte interferon-α therapy as a manifestation of a complex neurotoxicity, with reversible impairment of some higher mental functions.

Ten patients with metastatic renal cell carcinoma (5 men and 5 women), aged 36 to 72 years (median = 54 years), were examined before, 1 week after, and 1 month after continuous, daily intramuscular doses of interferon. The assessment utilized a detailed, structured, clinical mental status examination that was supplemented by tests that were sensitive to neurodynamic and higher mental function alterations. Before interferon treatment, all ten patients were found to be free of psychiatric illnesses or cognitive impairments.

Behavioral changes, manifested as reduced physical activity, were most pronounced in the first week of interferon therapy. Eight patients experienced psychomotor retardation, with slowing of spontaneous movements, speech, and thought. Symptoms of social withdrawal were also displayed. Complaints of decreased energy and disinclination to act or think were severe enough that some activities of eating, grooming, and daily living were ignored. Daily naps were necessary for all patients. Lack of drive and universal loss of libido were noted.

Cognitively fully oriented, all patients appeared duller, inattentive, and disinterested, with five patients complaining of memory and concentration difficulties. Half the patients exhibited speech blockage, with sentences interrupted by periods of silence and staring. Affectively, once interferon therapy started, the pretreatment anxiety of eight patients and the suicidal ideation of four patients ceased. Half of the patients became tearful, emotionally labile, or uncharacteristically irritable.

The sudden appearance and pronouncement of symptoms at the start of interferon therapy, with reversal following discontinuation, implies that they are drug related. Metoclopramide (a dopamine antagonist) was found to reverse some of the neuropsychiatric effects of interferon. It was concluded that these side effects, especially fatigue-asthenia, are manifestations of a complex, diffuse, toxic encephalopathy that interferes primarily with frontal lobe functions, especially those involved with planning, drive, and execution of activities.

---

frequent rest periods, evening injections, use of acetaminophen, and hydration to avoid dehydration, help patients tolerate longer courses of interferon therapy. Quesada and colleagues (1986) summarize the necessary concerns of nurses who care for patients on interferon: "Close observation, attention to diet, careful instruction, and reassurance of the patient will avoid complications from the most severe side effects induced by interferon, thus helping to maintain the patient's performance status and quality of life."

Interleukin 2

Interleukin 2 is a lymphokine that is a BRM (peptide hormone); it is secreted by T lymphocytes, which are capable of directing the function of other cells in the area of an immune response. Interleukin 2 directs the T lymphocytes to multiply into clones capable of performing during an immune response (Morgan, Ruscetti, & Gallo, 1976). Administered alone in high doses as well as in combination with lymphokine-activated killer (LAK) cells in the adoptive immunotherapeutic approach, IL 2 has demonstrated substantial antitumor activity (Lotze et al., 1986).

Historical Background

Interleukin 2 was initially described by Morgan, Ruscetti, and Gallo in 1976 at the National Cancer Institute as "t-cell growth factor." These investigators noted that IL 2 was a small protein that had the ability to sustain the proliferation in vitro of activated T lymphocytes. Although its biology is not fully understood, the protein has been purified, and its gene has been cloned in the past 10 years. The gene for IL 2 has been expressed in bacteria, and recombinant IL 2 is now commercially available for biologic and pharmacologic studies (Morgan et al., 1976).

Mechanism of Action

As a growth factor, IL 2 sustains the proliferation of activated T lymphocytes. T lymphocytes not stimulated by the immune response do not express IL 2 receptors. T lymphocytes activated by antigenic stimulation express IL 2 receptors and will facilitate the multiplication of T lymphocytes under the direction of IL 2. Depending on the subset of activated T lymphocytes that are amplified, IL 2 has several different in vitro immunologic effects. In vivo, the administration of IL 2 has corrected the immune deficit in the athymic nude mouse (Rosenberg et al., 1985) (Box 23–2). In vitro, some of the immunologic abnormalities have been reversed in patients with AIDS. Studies have demonstrated that human lymphocytes incubated with IL 2 develop the ability to lyse human tumor cells in the laboratory. High doses of IL 2 have also been shown to lyse tumor cells in mice (Rosenberg et al., 1985).

Clinical Applications

After evaluating the positive in vivo responses, researchers at the National Cancer Institute's surgery

---

Box 23–2. INTERLEUKIN 2

Rosenberg, S. A., Lotze, M. T., Muul, L. M., Leitman, S., Chang, A. E., Ettinghausen, S. E., Matory, Y. L., Skibber, J. M., Shiloni, E., Vetto, J. T., Seipp, C. A., Simpson, C., & Reichert, C. M. (1985). **Observations on the systemic administration of autologous lymphokine-activated killer cells and recombinant interleukin-2 to patients with metastatic cancer.** *New England Journal of Medicine, 313,* 1485–1492.

This research report was the first to relate the promising effects of administering interleukin 2 (IL 2) and lymphokine-activated killer cells (LAK) to patients with refractory cancer. In this study, 25 patients with metastatic cancer who had failed standard therapy were treated. Patients received both LAK cells, generated from lymphocytes obtained through serial leukapheresis, and up to 90 doses of IL 2.

More than a 50 per cent volume regression was observed in 11 of the 25 patients. One patient with metastatic melanoma obtained a complete remission of 10 months' duration. Partial responses occurred in nine patients with pulmonary or hepatic metastases from melanoma and colon or renal cell cancer and in one patient with a primary unresectable lung adenocarcinoma. Severe toxicities were reported in this study.

More than 50 per cent of all patients gained in excess of 10 per cent of their weight from fluid retention. Pulmonary interstitial edema was seen in 20 patients, and two of these 20 patients required intubation. Fever, chills, and malaise were seen in almost all of the patients. A generalized erythematous rash was seen in 17 of the 25 patients. Adverse effects in all patients disappeared promptly after the IL 2 administration ended.

---

branch began a series of human clinical trials (Rosenberg et al., 1985). Initially in 1984, IL 2 alone was administered to individuals with cancer. The maximum tolerated doses of IL 2 were determined, and side effects were delineated. No antitumor effects were seen in any of the patients. The administration of LAK cells alone to patients with cancer also yielded no positive tumor response.

In 1984, Rosenberg began treating patients with a combination of IL 2 and LAK cells (Rosenberg et al., 1985). Through the studies, it was determined that IL 2 and LAK cells must be combined for antitumor activity to occur. Interleukin 2 and LAK cell therapy is known as *adoptive immunotherapy.* This term implies that there is a transfer of active immunologic cells with the potential to directly or indirectly induce an antitumor response in the patient with a tumor.

The process of treating patients with IL 2 and LAK cells was initially very complex (Fig. 23–4). Patients were admitted and placed on high doses of IL 2, which increases the number of lymphocytes in the body (100,000 U/kg intravenously three times per day for

days 2 through 6 of the first week). The second week involved 5 days of lymphocytopheresis, the purpose of which is to obtain sufficient quantities of lymphocytes to incubate with IL 2 in the laboratory cultures. These lymphocytes then produce LAK cells to be infused back into the patient (in the same manner as other cell transfusions). On the last day of pheresis, the patient receives the IL 2 again in the same doses as the first week, as well as the first round of LAK cell infusions. This complex 2-week process is continued for three doses daily of IL 2 plus LAK cells (Jassak & Sticklin, 1986; Mathe & Amiel, 1969).

The initial results, published in December 1985, reported significant tumor responses in patients with malignant melanoma, colon carcinoma, and metastatic renal cell carcinoma. Researchers became very optimistic that IL 2 given with LAK cells could be a significant breakthrough in cancer treatment (Bylinsky, 1985; Rosenberg et al., 1985). The National Cancer Institute funded six clinical centers across the United States to extend the clinical trials with this agent using this approach. In addition, many other trials were

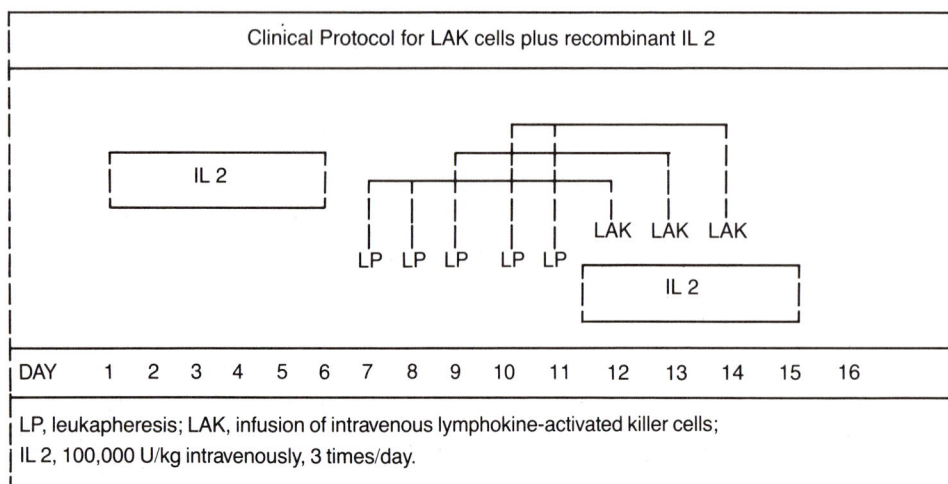

Figure 23–4. Schedule for administration of interleukin 2 (IL 2) and lymphokine-activated killer (LAK) cells. (Adapted from Simpson, C., Seipp, L. A., Rosenberg, S. A. [1988]. The current status and future applications of interleukin-2 and adoptive immunotherapy in cancer treatment. Semin Oncol Nurs *4*[2]:132–141.)

developed that treated hundreds of individuals with cancer in an attempt to refine the process.

Subsequent trials have reported positive effects in using low doses of IL 2 on a continuous basis (West et al., 1987). In these trials, side effects were considerably lessened. Other studies are examining the use of IL 2 plus LAK cells intraperitoneally for diseases such as ovarian and colon carcinomas with no metastasis outside the peritoneal cavity.

Future Applications

Tumor-Infiltrating Lymphocytes. Scientists have reported that lymphocytes that have infiltrated tumors may be extracted and expanded in IL 2 in the laboratory. The tumor-infiltrating lymphocytes can then be infused into the patient, in an effort to mediate tumor regression. Studies have shown these cells to be 50 to 100 times more potent than LAK cells (Simpson, Seipp, & Rosenberg, 1988). Compared with LAK cells, tumor-infiltrating lymphocytes do not require systemic administration of IL 2 to sustain their cytotoxic ability. In the laboratory setting, high-dose cyclophosphamide (Cytoxan 100 mg/kg) appeared to enhance the effect of tumor-infiltrating lymphocytes and IL 2 (Rosenberg, Spiess, & Lafreniere, 1986).

Tumor-infiltrating lymphocytes are prepared by surgically removing a portion of the tumor and dissecting it into pieces that are digested in an enzyme solution. The tumor cell suspension is placed in a culture medium. While in culture, the number of lymphocytes increases as the number of tumor cells decreases. Tumor-infiltrating lymphocytes are administered in the same manner as LAK cells, through a central line catheter. Clinical studies are currently under way (Simpson et al., 1988).

Interleukin 2 and Interferon-β. The combination of IL 2 and interferon-β is being tested in an effort to activate LAK cells and achieve further enhancement of the antitumor response. In preliminary reports of clinical trials with this combination, lower doses of IL 2 may be used, thus lowering toxicities (Rosenberg, 1986).

Cyclophosphamide and Interleukin 2. In laboratory studies, cyclophosphamide (Cytoxan) given concomitantly with IL 2 inhibits the capillary leakage in mice (Rosenstein, Ettinghausen, & Rosenberg, 1986). Cyclophosphamide may also reduce tumor bulk or may remove suppressor cells that interfere with the immune destruction of tumor (North, 1982). Clinical trials are under way to evaluate this treatment approach.

Side Effects

Much controversy exists regarding the pronounced toxicities and expense of adoptive cell therapy with the high doses of IL 2. Patients receiving high doses of IL 2 (33 μg/kg intravenously three times per day for 5 days or longer) have a series of predictable toxicities (Corey & Collins, 1986; Seipp, Simpson, & Rosenberg, 1986; Sticklin, 1987).

Constitutional. Fevers of up to 40.5° C with chills may occur within 2 hours of administering IL 2 and persist until after it has been discontinued. Acetaminophen and nonsteroidal anti-inflammatory drugs control the fever very well.

Headache, malaise, and flu-like symptoms are frequently observed. Nasal congestion, glossitis, and xerostomia have been reported (Jassak & Spiewak, 1987).

Integumentary. The majority of patients develop diffuse erythema that may evolve into a pruritic desquamating rash.

Cardiovascular or Pulmonary. At high doses, systemic vascular resistance drops significantly, producing leaky capillary syndrome with significant hypotension. Intravascular volume depletion occurs, and fluid replacement results in significant amounts of fluid weight gain. Fluid retention is manifested by peripheral edema, ascites, and later by pulmonary interstitial edema that may necessitate intubation. Myocardial infarction has been reported in 1 to 2 per cent of all patients. Arrhythmias have been more frequently reported (Seipp et al., 1986).

Gastrointestinal. Some patients experience severe nausea and vomiting and may have significant diarrhea. Mucositis has developed in many of the patients, along with anorexia.

Neurologic. Confusion is frequently observed in patients after receiving several doses of IL 2. Combativeness, disorientation, increased anxiety, and, rarely, psychosis have been reported. In the presence of brain metastasis, increased cerebral edema has developed (Corey & Collins, 1986).

Renal. Oliguria, proteinuria, and elevations of serum creatinine and blood urea nitrogen are frequently exhibited. Restoration of normal renal function usually occurs within 48 hours of discontinuing IL 2.

Hepatic. Most patients develop hyperbilirubinemia to some degree, with liver enzyme changes suggestive of intrahepatic cholestasis.

Hematologic. Progressive anemia, exacerbated by the leukapheresis procedures, thrombocytopenia, and rise in prothrombin and partial thromboplastin times are frequently reported.

Miscellaneous. An additional complication of cellular therapy has been reported at several study sites. Several cases of hepatitis A were noted in patients treated with IL 2 and LAK cells. This infection was traced back to the human serum added to the tissue culture medium in which LAK cells were generated. All serum has been routinely screened for hepatitis B and human T-lymphotropic virus III.

After completion of the course of therapy, patients generally recover very rapidly and are discharged within 2 to 3 days. There are data to suggest the more IL 2 received the better the potential for tumor cell kill (Rosenberg, 1986). Considering that all of the toxicities are increased with increased doses of IL 2, a fine balance must be attained in optimizing the tumor cell kill and containing the toxicities in a reasonable manner.

Tumor Necrosis Factor

Tumor necrosis factor was named on the basis of its ability to cause necrosis of established tumors in the mouse. It is a monokine produced by activated macrophages and specialized circulating phagocytic monocytes that selectively kills neoplastic cells.

Historical Background

Tumor necrosis factor evolved from the investigations with Coley's toxins in the early 1900s. Coley noted that a recurrent sarcoma, which had continued to regrow after five resections within 3 years, regressed following two episodes of an unusual bacterial infection. Coley began investigations with toxins derived from heat-killed bacteria. Several patients, primarily those with sarcoma, experienced tumor regressions. Side effects included nausea and vomiting, headache, malaise, and fever, which disappeared in 1 to 2 days (Coley, 1893).

One of Coley's toxins was refined by Shear and colleagues (1943), and it was much more potent in inducing hemorrhage and necrosis in mouse tumor implants. This endotoxin was located in the cell wall of gram-negative bacteria. More recent investigations have confirmed that the activity is induced by a byproduct of the host's immune response rather than by the bacteria itself. The name *tumor necrosis factor* was chosen because this toxin appeared to specifically affect tumor without causing undesirable effects in normal tissues (Oettgen & Old, 1987).

Tumor necrosis factor is identical in genetic sequence to cachectin, a macrophage hormone that has been studied for its effects on patients with neoplastic diseases. Chronic infections and cancer have been noted to cause severe wasting with negative calorie and nitrogen balance leading to death, which is felt to result from the effects of cachectin (Beutler & Cerami, 1987).

Mechanism of Action

The production of the monokine TNF by mononuclear phagocytes is induced by most infectious agents, including virus particles and some of the other BRMs. Tumor necrosis factor is the mediator of general inflammation. Its induction of necrosis appears to be related to its ability to diminish tissue perfusion. It alters hemostatic properties of vascular endothelium, inducing a disseminated intravascular coagulation type of effect at a systemic level with local occlusion of tumor vessels. Tumor necrosis factor is directly toxic to vascular endothelial cells, causing the "third spacing" of plasma water and electrolytes into the extravascular spaces. It also induces the release of interleukin 1 by monocytes and endothelial cells, which may elicit the features of endotoxin poisoning: fever, hypotension, neutropenia, and thrombocytopenia (Beutler & Cerami, 1987).

Exposure to TNF activates macrophages to release cytotoxic factors that mediate events leading up to hemorrhagic necrosis. The activated macrophages adhere to endothelial surfaces, enhancing their phagocytic activity. Within a few hours of administration, TNF induces hemorrhagic necrosis. The core of the tumor turns blue-black, owing to the extravasation of blood into the tumor, which may then slough off (Flick & Gifford, 1985). Tumor necrosis factor is effective against established tumors, unlike other bacterial products that must be injected directly into the tumor, such as bacille Calmette-Guérin, a tuberculosis vaccine containing live, attenuated tubercle bacilli, which is used in immunotherapy for melanoma to produce a nonspecific immune reaction against tumor (Beutler & Cerami, 1987).

Tumor necrosis factor, which is comparable to the interferon system, most likely consists of a whole family of cytotoxic factors. However, unlike the interferons, TNF is not species specific. The TNF gene resides on chromosome 6, closely linked to genes that code for lymphotoxin. Gene cloning has allowed the recombinant production of large amounts of highly purified TNF (Oettgen & Old, 1987).

Clinical Applications

Preclinical trials with primates had demonstrated considerable toxicity, including hypotension, acute renal insufficiency, and disseminated intravascular coagulation after administration of recombinant TNF.

The first clinical trials with patients began in the fall of 1985 by defining the effects of subcutaneous and intravenous administration twice weekly for 4 weeks. Doses were escalated each week. Doses ranged from 1 to 250 $\mu g/m^2$ (Chapman et al., 1986). Tumor necrosis factor combined with other BRMs is also beginning to be investigated.

Side Effects

Considerable toxicity is associated with the administration of TNF (Table 23–8). Side effects in 26 human patients studied by Chapman and colleagues (1986) included rigors, fever, and headache. The episodes of rigors lasted 20 to 30 minutes after intravenous administration but were less severe after subcutaneous injection. Fevers higher than 38.5° C were seen in more than 72 per cent of patients after subcutaneous injection and were of longer duration than the fevers in those who had had intravenous injection. More than half of the patients complained of headaches. Mild hypotension with systolic blood pressure lower than 90 mm Hg and responsive to saline infusion occurred in one quarter of the patients. Hypertension during the

Table 23–8. SIDE EFFECTS OF TUMOR NECROSIS FACTOR

Common	Uncommon
Rigors	Hypotension
Fever	Peripheral vasoconstriction
Headache	Hypertension, tachycardia, and
Local inflammation (at	mild chest discomfort during
subcutaneous injection site)	rigors
Nausea and vomiting	Fatigue

severe rigors with systolic blood pressure higher than 200 mm Hg occurred in 37 per cent of patients. Associated tachycardia with mild chest discomfort but no electrocardiogram changes occurred during episodes of rigors in some patients (23 per cent) as well.

Fatigue was more common and more severe after subcutaneous injection, and it continued for several days following administration of the higher doses. No weight loss was observed, and few patients (fewer than 12 per cent) experienced anorexia. Nausea and vomiting occurred only in those patients with prior abdominal disease (Chapman et al., 1986). Central nervous system changes are observed with the high doses being used in trials that are still in the early phase of investigation.

Subcutaneous administration caused an inflammatory reaction, with erythema, induration, and blisters. Local pain was the dose-limiting factor at 200 $\mu g/m^2$. Skin biopsy of injection sites showed congestion and cellular infiltrates of primarily mononuclear cells. Local pain and headaches increased in severity at higher doses, although no increased antitumor effects were observed (Chapman et al., 1986).

Recent reports indicate that tolerance appears to increase with daily administration, allowing greater amounts of TNF to be given than can be well tolerated in a single dose. By this method of administration, two of 28 patients had significant regression of their tumors.

Thymic Hormones

Historical Background

The thymus is located in the chest anterior to the heart and great vessels. It is a rather mysterious lymphoid tissue whose function is still being identified. This organ consists of a dense reticular framework with lymphocytes arranged in the cortex and medulla. The lymphoid tissue receives a rich blood supply. Since the mid 1850s, it had been observed that animals whose thymus gland was removed at birth died of infection. Further discoveries about the immune effects of neonatal thymectomy led to the search for endocrine functions of the thymus (Bach & Carnaud, 1976).

In fewer than 25 years of intensive investigation, the thymus has emerged as the potential master gland of immunity. The thymus secretes an entire family of compounds into the blood stream that influence a patient's immunologic responses. Research further reveals that thymic hormones have an important influence on tissue and organ transplantation, on the development of autoimmune diseases, on immunodeficiency states, and on the immunologic response against tumor development (Goldstein, Schulof, Naylor, & Hall, 1986).

Mechanism of Action

The thymus synthesizes small hormone-like polypeptides that differ in chemical structure and circulate in the blood stream, producing systemic effects similar to those of hormones. Interestingly, some of the thymic hormones induce the stimulation of lymphokines, such as CSF, IL 2, interferon-α, and interferon-γ, which are involved in the molecular events associated with the differentiation and functioning of T lymphocytes (Sztein & Goldstein, 1985).

Thymic hormones can also correct immune function in immune diseases. By increasing numbers and functions of T lymphocytes, by activating other lymphokines with antiviral activity, and by stimulating macrophage populations, thymic hormones help prevent infections in patients with cancer (Chen & Goldstein, 1985). It is well known that cancer treatments result in significant cellular immunodeficiencies and that cancer itself is related to deficits that cause the oncology patient to be prone to viral, bacterial, and fungal diseases.

Clinical Applications

The use of thymic hormones in cancer patients is based on several factors, including their demonstrated activity in several animal systems and their minimal toxicity (Schafer, Goldstein, Gutterman, & Hersh, 1976).

The two best known products—thymosin fraction 5, a partially purified natural compound prepared from the thymus gland, and thymosin-α_1, a potent synthetic component of thymosin fraction 5 that induces helper T cells and lymphokines—are currently in clinical trials with children and adults who have primary and secondary immunodeficiency diseases, including those undergoing cancer therapy, those with pre-AIDS, and those with autoimmune diseases such as rheumatoid arthritis and multiple sclerosis (Goldstein et al., 1986).

The results of the first phase II clinical trial with thymosin-α_1 in patients with small-cell lung cancer who were treated with radiation therapy were encouraging. The disease-free interval and survival rate increased significantly compared with those of patients who received placebo during their radiation therapy. Measurements of immune parameters also showed improvement (Schafer et al., 1976). Therefore, the National Cancer Institute has sponsored two trials to replicate the study and verify the results.

Other trials have employed thymic hormones as adjuncts with chemotherapy and have looked at a variety of cancers, including head and neck cancer and malignant melanoma. Results have shown only minimal effectiveness.

Toxicity

Thymic hormones have thus far been reported to have very mild side effects, only inflammation at the injection site and no organ toxicity. Constanzi and colleagues (1979) reported that patients experienced an increased sense of well-being and ability to function in daily life. Objective improvement included decreased infections and weight gain. Further, other chronic conditions, such as dermatitis, arthritis, and arthralgias, either improved or did not recur.

Nursing Considerations

Administration, route, dosage, and stability of the preparations are the primary concerns of the nurse working with thymic hormones. Education of the patient regarding basic immunology and the purpose of thymic hormones involves the nurse in teaching; representation of the patient who participates in clinical trials with such new agents makes the nurse the patient's advocate.

Growth Factors

Peptide Growth Factors. Normal growth relies on the controlled expression of growth factors. Malignant growth occurs when uncontrolled expression occurs. Platelets, macrophages, and lymphocytes all normally produce peptide growth factors, which in a malignant condition may be stimulated by cancer cell byproducts to increase production of peptide growth factors, which mediate further malignant behavior (Sporn & Roberts, 1988).

The unrestrained growth of cancer cells results from enhanced metabolic activity involving peptide growth factors, their receptors, and intracellular signals they generate by binding to other receptors. Peptide growth factors can influence invasiveness and metastasis of tumors by affecting matrix destruction and synthesis and angiogenesis.

A specific peptide growth factor, transforming growth factor-beta, is produced by cells of the immune system. Transforming growth factor-beta modulates the activity of immune cells, affects matrix syntheses and angiogenesis by cells, and potently inhibits immunoglobulin synthesis by B lymphocytes.

Tumor Growth Factors. Malignant transformation of cancer cells may occur by (1) excessive production, expression, and action of positive autocrine factors; or (2) failure of cells to synthesize, express, or respond to specific negative growth factors. Tumor growth factors are substances secreted by transformed cells; although growth factors secreted by normal cells and tumor growth factors are similar in many ways, normal growth factors do not cause transformation. Growth factors act via a cell surface receptor mechanism, and, in fact, significant similarity has been shown between some growth factor receptors and oncogenic products. Use of MoAbs will help to identify the effects of these growth factors in the etiology and treatment of cancers by demonstrating the effects of blocking these factors and similar manipulations.

Colony-Stimulating Factors. A number of polypeptide growth factors capable of stimulating the proliferation and differentiation of specific hematologic cell lines have been identified and investigated in the past decade.

Granulocyte-macrophage colony-stimulating factor induces colony formation, stimulating a marked response in the total white blood cell count with particular increments in neutrophils and eosinophils and in lymphocytes and reticulocytes as well (Nathan, 1987).

When given by infusion to patients with small-cell lung cancer, granulocyte colony-stimulating factor produced a specific increase in neutrophils. Patients had a significant reduction in the nadir period of neutropenia with a return of neutrophil counts to normal or above by 2 weeks after the initiation of chemotherapy (Bronchud & Dexter, 1989). These two factors are currently being investigated to shorten the period of granulocytopenia during bone marrow transplantation (Nathan, 1987).

Erythropoietin was identified in 1906 as the hormone produced primarily by the kidneys that is responsible for the regulation and control of red blood cell production and maturation. It is fair to say that erythropoietin was the first growth factor described. It has undergone clinical trials for the correction of anemia related to end-stage renal failure and dialysis. Hemoglobin and hematocrit levels returned to normal without the problems associated with repeated blood transfusions, such as iron overload, development of antibodies, or transmission of infectious viral agents. Patients achieve a sense of well-being and levels of energy that enable them to return to normal life styles. Erythropoietin was approved by the Food and Drug Administration in May 1989 for use with end-stage renal disease (Bronchud & Dexter, 1989).

Clinical trials continue to investigate potential uses in oncology. Anemia related to chemotherapy treatment with cisplatin appears to be due to inadequate erythropoietin levels; erythropoietin replacement provided a 35 per cent increase in hematocrit levels without additional blood transfusions (Wood, Nygaard, & Hrushesky, 1989).

Tumor Vaccines

Another type of adoptive immunotherapy involves removal of patients' lymphocytes, sensitization of lymphocytes immunized against tumor cells from the patients' tumors, and return of the sensitized blood cells to the patient.

Before the initiation of biologic therapy with vaccines, the strength of the patient's immune response must be assessed. Skin tests are often used to stimulate a delayed hypersensitivity response, which is measured by the areas of erythema and induration that develop after 48 hours. An anergic response (weak or nonexistent) would be a poor indicator for the ability of therapy to enhance the host's immune response (Cox & Ern, 1980). Various blood samples, including total protein, protein electrophoresis, immunoglobulin assays, complement function, antibody titers, hematologic cell counts with assessment of lymphocyte surface markers, and counts of T and B lymphocytes, are collected and sent for analyses of immune parameters.

Miscellaneous Factors

Cimetidine (commonly used to treat ulcers) has been shown to have a potent modulating effect on the immune system. Histamines lead to activation of suppressor T lymphocytes and release of suppressor factors. Cimetidine blocks this overall suppression, thereby allowing an increased action of the immune system. Antitumor effects have been noted in patients receiving cimetidine alone or in combination with interferon (Osband, 1986).

Antimetastatic Agents

It has been stated that cancer metastasis is the most lethal aspect of neoplastic disease and that a method for eradication of metastasis would be a giant step toward successful therapy (DeVita, 1982). Agents with proposed antimetastatic activity include inhibitors of tumor cell invasion (protease inhibitors and disruptors of microtubule function), antagonists of tumor cell–platelet interactions (prostacyclin thromboxane antagonists, calcium channel blockers), and blockers of tumor cell arrest (laminin fragments) (Allen, Cicone, & Skoff, 1981).

Anticoagulants

Metastatic cells in the blood have been observed to be associated with platelets or fibrin attached to vessel walls. Platelet aggregation interacting with tumor cells assists in the attachment of tumor cells to the vascular endothelium or in the covering of the tumor cell that prevents its recognition and elimination by the natural killer cells. It has been observed that anticoagulant drugs have substantial antimetastatic effects (Gorelik & Herberman, 1986). In mice injected with melanoma, prostacyclin, a very potent antithrombogenic agent, has been shown to reduce pulmonary metastases by 70 per cent and to eliminate liver and spleen metastases entirely.

Angiogenesis Inhibitors

Interest lies in investigating the idea that if tumors recruit new vessels continuously, then inhibition of the angiogenesis factor would lead to tumor atrophy.

Enzymes

Cathepsin B is a lysosomal enzyme that is released primarily by neoplastic tissues. Detection of the activity of this enzyme in serum correlates directly with invasion and metastasis. Attempts to block the activity of this enzyme, such as with an MoAb, may allow interruption of the cascade of biologic events that leads to metastasis (Saito et al., 1980).

SUMMARY

Oldham and Smalley (1983) suggested that biotherapy would become the fourth modality of cancer treatment, with surgery, chemotherapy, and radiation therapy being the standard three. It seems apparent that we are not yet at that point. Further understanding of the immune system and the complex interrelated functions of its components is needed. However, movement toward that goal progresses as research continues to flourish in the field of biotherapy, and new agents or approaches are constantly being examined. Although interferon-α and erythropoietin are the only Food and Drug Administration–approved BRMs today, it is anticipated that by 1991 six additional BRMs will have been approved (Ratafia & Puvinton, 1988).

The potential of biotherapy has been somewhat like a roller coaster ride during the last two decades. When interferon was first investigated in relation to controlling cancer, the media billed it as a cure for cancer. After much research, we have learned that it is very effective—but only with a limited range of malignancies (Kirkwood & Ernstoff, 1988; Roth & Foon, 1987). Interleukin 2 in combination with LAK cells brought another flood of hope for a cancer cure, and again we have had to step back and examine the research for the true role of this therapeutic approach. Expectations have had to be altered, but these trials have given us much information about cancer and the response of the body's immune system to BRMs.

Nurses have and will continue to play an important role in caring for patients receiving BRMs. Now BRMs are being administered not only in research settings but in community hospitals, physicians' offices, and private homes. Suppers and McClamrock (1985) point out that clinical trials with BRMs will demand different nursing approaches than those to which nurses grew accustomed with chemotherapy trials. For example, toxicities may be difficult to determine because they are often subtle, subjective, or cumulative over a period of time. Nurses will need acute observation skills and a systematic approach to patient assessment to detect the effects of BRMs in an individual. Nurses must be familiar with biotherapy and understand the components of the immune system and their function to make these assessments as well as to educate patients about their treatment program. Even if the patient is not receiving biotherapy, the media produce brochures and programs that stimulate many questions from the lay person about biotherapy.

The possibilities for nursing research in this area are vast. Groenwald, Fisher, and McCalla (1987) stressed that oncology nurses are obligated to investigate current methods of caring for individuals receiving BRMs and to make recommendations for improvement in care. With the development of new agents and approaches, nurse researchers should design studies to determine better nursing approaches for caring for individuals receiving biotherapeutic agents. Biotherapy is an exciting field, rich with opportunities and challenges for oncology nurses. Oncology nurses must accept the challenge, educate themselves, and provide quality care for the patient receiving biotherapy.

References

Abernathy, E. (1987a). Biotherapy: An introductory overview. *Oncology Nursing Forum, 14* (Suppl. 6), 13–15.

Abernathy, E. (1987b). How the immune system works. *American Journal of Nursing, 87,* 456–459.

Abrams, P. G., McClamrock, E., & Foon, K. A. (1985). Evening administration of alpha interferon. *New England Journal of Medicine, 312,* 443–444.

Adams, F., Quesada, J. R., & Gutterman, J. U. (1984). Neuropsychiatric manifestations of human leukocyte interferon therapy in patients with cancer. *Journal of the American Medical Association, 252,* 938–941.

Allen, K. V., Cicone, B., & Skoff, A. (1981). Prostacyclin: A potent antimetastatic agent. *Science, 212,* 1270.

Bach, J., & Carnaud, C. (1976). Thymic factors. *Progress in Allergy, 21,* 342–408.

Baldwin, R. W., & Byers, V. S. (1987). Monoclonal antibody targeting of cytotoxic agents for cancer therapy. In V. S. Byers & R. W. Baldwin (Eds.), *Immunology of malignant diseases* (pp. 44–54). Lancaster, England: MTP Press.

Bates, S. E., & Longo, D. L. (1985). Tumor markers: Value and limitations in the management of cancer patients. *Cancer Treatment Reviews, 12,* 163–207.

Berman, L. D. (1975). Immune parameters in the host response to neoplasia: Morphological considerations. In A. E. Reif (Ed.), *Immunity and cancer in man.* New York: Marcel Dekker.

Bernier, G. M. (1985). Antibody and immunoglobulins: Structure and function. In J. A. Bellanti (Ed.), *Immunology III* (pp. 89–105). Philadelphia: W. B. Saunders Co.

Beutler, B., & Cerami, A. (1987). Cachectin: More than a tumor necrosis factor. *New England Journal of Medicine, 316,* 379–385.

Biological response modifiers guidelines: Recommendations for nursing education and practice. (1989). Pittsburgh: Oncology Nursing Society.

Bronchud, M. H., & Dexter, T. M. (1989). Clinical use of haematopoietic growth factors. *Blood, 3,* 66–70.

Bylinsky, G. (1985, November 25). Science scores a cancer breakthrough. *Fortune.*

Chapman, P. B., Lester, T. J., Casper, E. S., Gabrilove, J. L., Kempin, S., Welt, S., Sherwin, S., Old, L. J., & Oettgen, H. G. (1986). Phase I study of recombinant tumor necrosis factor (rTNF). *Proceedings ASCO, 5,* 231.

Chen, J., & Goldstein, A. L. (1985). Thymosins and other thymic hormones. In P. F. Torrence (Ed.), *Biological response modifiers: New approaches to disease intervention* (pp. 121–140). Orlando, FL: Academic Press.

Clark, J., & Longo, D. (1986). Biological response modifiers. *Mediguide to Oncology, 6*(2), 1–10.

Clark, J., & Longo, D. (1987). Interferons in cancer therapy. In V. T. DeVita, S. Hellman, & S. A. Rosenberg (Eds.), *Cancer: Principles and practice of oncology.* Philadelphia: J. B. Lippincott Co.

Coley, W. B. (1893). The treatment of malignant tumors by repeated inoculations of erysipelas: With a report of ten original cases. *American Journal of Medical Science, 105,* 487–511.

Constanzi, J., Daniels, J., Thurman, G., Goldstein, A., & Hokanson, J. (1979). Clinical trials with thymosin. *Annals New York Academy of Sciences, 332,* 148–159.

Cooper, N. R. (1987). The complement system. In P. P. Stobo & J. V. Wells (Eds.), *Basic and clinical immunology (6th ed),* (pp. 114–127). Norwalk, CT: Appleton & Lange.

Corey, B., & Collins, J. (1986). Implementation of an rIL-2/LAK cell clinical trial: A nursing perspective. *Oncology Nursing Forum, 13*(6), 31–34.

Cox, K. O., & Ern, M. (1980). Immunotherapy II. *Cancer Nursing, 3:*307–321.

DeVita, V. T. (1982). Principles of chemotherapy. In V. T. DeVita, S. Hellman, & S. A. Rosenberg (Eds.), *Cancer: Principles and practice of oncology* (pp. 132–155). Philadelphia: J. B. Lippincott Co.

Ehrlich, P. (1900). On immunity with special reference to cell life. *Proceedings of the Royal Society of London, 66,* 424–448.

Flick, D. A., & Gifford, G. E. (1985). Tumor necrosis factor. In P. F. Torrence (Ed.), *Biological response modifiers: New approaches to disease intervention* (pp. 171–218). Orlando, FL: Academic Press.

Foon, K., Bernhard, M., & Oldham, R. (1982). Monoclonal antibody therapy: Assessment by animal tumor models. *Journal of Biological Response Modifiers, 1,* 277–304.

Gallucci, B. B. (1985). Selected concepts of cancer as a disease: From 1900 to oncogenes. *Oncology Nursing Forum, 12*(5), 69–78.

Gallucci, B. B. (1987). The immune system and cancer. *Oncology Nursing Forum, 14*(6), 3–11.

Goldstein, A. L., Schulof, R. S., Naylor, P. H., & Hall, N. R. (1986). Thymosins and anti-thymosins: Properties and clinical applications. *Medical Oncology and Tumor Pharmacotherapeutics, 3,* 211–221.

Goldstein, D., & Laszlo, J. (1986). Interferon therapy in cancer: From imaginon to interferon. *Cancer Research, 46,* 4315–4329.

Goodfield, J. (1984, April). Dr. Coley's toxins. *Science, 84,* 68–73.

Gorelik, E., & Herberman, R. (1986). Role of natural killer cells (NK) cells in the control of tumor growth and metastatic spread. In R. B. Herberman (Ed.), *Cancer immunology: Innovative approaches to therapy* (pp. 151–176). Boston: Martinus Nijhoff Publishers.

Gresser, I., & Tovey, M. B. (1978, October). Antitumor effects of interferon. *Biochimica et Biophysica Acta, 516,* 231–247.

Groenwald, S. L., Fisher, S. G., & McCalla, J. L. (1987). Biological response modifiers. In S. L. Groenwald (Ed.), *Cancer nursing principles and practice* (pp. 387–390). Boston: Jones & Bartlett.

Gurevich, I., & Tafuro, P. (1986). The compromised host. *Cancer Nursing, 9,* 263–275.

Gutterman, J. U. (1988). The role of interferons in the treatment of hematologic malignancies. *Seminars in Hematology, 25,* 3–8.

Hanson, L. A., & Wigzell, H. (1985). *Immunology.* London: Butterworth.

Herberman, R. B. (1983). Lymphoid cells in immune surveillance against malignant transformation. In J. I. Gallin & A. S. Fauci (Eds.), *Advances in host defense mechanisms: Vol. 2: Lymphoid cells* (pp. 241–274). New York: Raven Press.

Higgins, P. G. (1984). Interferons. *Journal of Clinical Pathology, 37,* 109–116.

Hood, L. E. (1988). Interferon: Getting in the way of viruses and tumors. *American Journal of Nursing, 87,* 459–465.

Hooks, J. J., & Detrick, B. (1985). Immunoregulatory functions of interferon. In P. F. Torrence (Ed.), *Biological response modifiers: New approaches to disease intervention* (pp. 57–75). Orlando, FL: Academic Press.

Huang, A. T. (1985, April). *A treatment overview of hairy cell leukemia.* Paper presented at the R. W. Rundles Symposium on Hairy Cell Leukemia and Chronic Lymphocytic Leukemia, Durham, NC.

Huffer, T. J., Kanapa, D. J., & Stevenson, G. W. (1986). *Introduction to human immunology.* Boston: Jones & Barlett.

Irwin, M. M. (1987). Patients receiving biological response modifiers: Overview of nursing care. *Oncology Nursing Forum, 14* (Suppl. 6), 32–37.

Jakobsen, P. H. (1987). Human monoclonal antibodies—still much to learn. *Leukemia, 1,* 521–523.

Jassak, P., & Spiewak, P. (1987). Interleukin-2. *American Journal of Nursing, 87,* 464–465.

Jassak, P., & Sticklin, L. (1986). Interleukin 2: An overview. *Oncology Nursing Forum, 13*(6), 17–22.

Kirkwood, J. M., & Ernstoff, M. S. (1984). Interferons in the treatment of human cancer. *Journal of Clinical Oncology, 2,* 336–352.

Kirkwood, J. M., & Ernstoff, M. S. (1988). A clinical update: The role of interferon in the biotherapy of solid tumors. *Oncology Nursing Forum, 15* (suppl. 6), 3–6.

Kohler, G., & Milstein, C. (1975). Continuous cultures of fused cells secreting antibody of predefined specificity. *Nature, 256,* 495–497.

Laszlo, J., Goldstein, D., Gockerman, J., Hood, L., Huang, A. T., Triozzi, P., Sedwick, W. D., Koren, H., Ellinwood, E. H., & Tso, C. Y. (in press). Phase I studies of recombinant gamma interferon. *Journal of Biological Response Modifiers.*

Levi, S., Herberman, R., Lippman, M., & D'angelo, T. (1987, March 5). Correlation of stress factors with sustained depression of natural killer cell activity and predicted prognosis in patients with breast cancer. *Journal of Clinical Oncology, 3,* 348–353.

Lindenmann, J. (1982). From interference to interferon: A brief historical introduction. In D. A. Tyrrell & D. C. Burke (Eds.), *Interferon: Twenty-five years on* (pp. 3–6). London: The Royal Society of London.

Liotta, L. A. (1986). Molecular biology of metastases: A review of recent approaches. *European Journal of Cancer and Clinical Oncology, 22,* 345–347.

Lotze, M. T., Matory, Y. L., Rayner, A. A., Ettinghausen, S. E., Vetto, J. T., Seipp, C. A., & Rosenberg, S. A. (1986). Clinical effects and toxicity of Interleukin-2 in patients with cancer. *Cancer, 58,* 2764–2772.

Mathe, G., & Amiel, J. (1969). Active immunotherapy for acute lymphoblastic leukemia. *Lancet, 1*(7597), 697–699.

Mayer, D., Hetrick, K., Riggs, C., & Sherwin, S. (1984). Weight loss in patients receiving recombinant leukocyte A interferon (IFLrA): A brief report. *Cancer Nursing, 7,* 53–56.

Mihich, E., & Fefer, A. (1983). *Biological response modifiers: subcommittee report* (Monograph No. 63). Bethesda, MD: National Cancer Institute.

Moldawer, N., & Murray, J. (1985). The clinical uses of monoclonal antibodies in cancer research. *Cancer Nursing, 8,* 207–213.

Morgan, A. C., & Foon, K. A. (1986). Monoclonal antibody therapy of cancer: Preclinical models and investigations in humans. In R. B. Herberman (Ed.), *Cancer immunology: Innovative approaches to therapy* (pp. 177–200). Boston: Martinus Nijhoff Publishers.

Morgan, P. A., Ruscetti, F. W., & Gallo, R. G. (1976). Selective in vitro growth of T-lymphocytes from normal human bone marrows. *Science, 193,* 1007–1008.

Nathan, D. G. (1987). Leukemia and the regulation of hematopoiesis. *Leukemia, 1,* 683–696.

Noble, T. (1987). Muromonab-CD3: Murine monoclonal antibody. *Drug Information Bulletin, 4*(7), 1–4.

North, R. J. (1982). Cyclophosphamide-facilitated adoptive immunotherapy of an established tumor depends on elimination of tumor induced suppressor cells. *Journal of Experimental Medicine, 155,* 1063.

Oettgen, H. F., & Old, L. J. (1987). Tumor necrosis factor. In V. T. DeVita, S. Hellman, & S. A. Rosenberg (Eds.), *Important advances in oncology 1987* (pp. 105–127). Philadelphia: J. B. Lippincott Co.

Oldham, R. K. (1983). Monoclonal antibodies in cancer therapy. *Journal of Clinical Oncology, 1,* 582–590.

Oldham, R. K. (1985). Biologicals for cancer treatment: Interferons. *Hospital Practice, 20,* 71–91.

Oldham, R., & Smalley, R. (1983). Immunotherapy: The old and the new. *Journal of Biological Response Modifiers, 2,* 1–37.

Osband, M. E. (1986). New cancer therapy: Strengthening immune systems. *Oncology News/Update, 1*(6), 1 and 7.

Otter, W. D. (1985). Tumor cells do not arise frequently. *Cancer Immunology Immunotherapy, 19,* 159–162.

Pimm, M. V. (1987). Immunoscintigraphy: Tumor detection with radiolabelled antibody monoclonal antibodies. In V. S. Byers & R. W. Baldwin (Eds.), *Immunology of malignant diseases* (pp. 21–43). Lancaster, England: MTP Press.

Quesada, J. R., Talpaz, M., Rios, A., Kurzrodk, R., & Gutterman, J. U. (1986). Clinical toxicity of interferons in cancer patients: A review. *Journal of Clinical Oncology, 4,* 234–243.

Ratafia, M., & Puvinton, T. (1988, Nov. 17–20). Immunomodulators for cancer. *Cope Magazine.*

Rosenberg, S. A. (1986). Adoptive immunotherapy of cancer using lymphokine-activated killer cells and recombinant interleukin-2. In V. T. DeVita, S. Hellman, & S. A. Rosenberg (Eds.), *Important advances in oncology* (pp. 55–91). Philadelphia: J. B. Lippincott Co.

Rosenberg, S. A., Lotze, M. T., Muul, L. M., Leitman, S., Chang, A. E., Ettinghausen, S. E., Matory, Y. L., Skibber, J. M., Shiloni, E., Vetto, J. T., Seipp, C. A., Simpson, C., & Reichert, C. M. (1985). Observations on the systemic administration of autologous lymphokine-activated killer cells and recombinant interleukin-2 to patients with metastatic cancer. *New England Journal of Medicine, 313,* 1485–1494.

Rosenberg, S. A., Spiess, P., & Lafreniere, R. (1986). A new approach to the adoptive immunotherapy of cancer with tumor-infiltrating lymphocytes. *Science, 233,* 1318–1321.

Rosenstein, M., Ettinghausen, S. E., & Rosenberg, S. A. (1986). Extravasation of intravascular fluid mediated by the systemic administration of recombinant interleukin-2. *Journal of Immunology, 137,* 1735–1742.

Roth, M. S., & Foon, K. A. (1987). Biotherapy with interferon in hematologic malignancies. *Oncology Nursing Forum, 14* (suppl. 6), 16–22.

Saito, O., Sawamura, M., Umezawa, K., Kanai, Y., Furihata, C., Matsushima, T., & Sugimura, T. (1980). Inhibition of experimental blood-borne lung metastases by protease inhibitors. *Cancer Research, 40,* 2539.

Schafer, L. A., Goldstein, A. L., Gutterman, J. U., & Hersh, E. (1976). In vitro and in vivo studies with thymosin in cancer patients. *Annals New York Academy of Sciences, 277,* 609–620.

Seipp, C., Simpson, C., & Rosenberg, S. A. (1986). Clinical trials with IL-2. *Oncology Nursing Forum, 13*(6), 25–29.

Shear, M. J., Turner, F. C., Perrault, A., & Shovelton, T. (1943). Chemical treatment of tumors. V. Isolation of the hemorrhage-producing fraction from Serratia marcescens (Bacillus prodigiosus) culture filtrate. *Journal of the National Cancer Institute, 4,* 81–97.

Simpson, C., Seipp, C. A., & Rosenberg, S. A. (1988). The current status and future applications of interleukin-2 and adoptive immunotherapy in cancer treatment. *Seminars in Oncology Nursing, 4,* 132–141.

Sporn, M. B., & Roberts, A. B. (1988). Peptide growth factors are multifunctional: Review. *Nature, 332*(616), 217–219.

Sticklin, L. (1987). Interleukin-2 and killer T-cells. *American Journal of Nursing, 87,* 468–469.

Strander, H. A. (1986). Interferon in the treatment of human papilloma virus. *Medical Clinics of North America, 70*(Suppl.), 19–23.

Suppers, V., & McClamrock, E. (1985). Biologicals in cancer treatment: Future effects on nursing practice. *Oncology Nursing Forum, 12*(3), 27–32.

Sztein, M. B., & Goldstein, A. L. (1985). Recent advances in thymic hormone research. In P. Chandra (Ed.), *NATO advanced study institute on new experimental modalities in the control of neoplasm* (pp. 137–158). Marates, Italy: NATO.

Terry, W., & Rosenberg, S. (Eds.). (1982). *Immunotherapy of human cancer.* New York: Excerpta Medica.

Thor, A., Weeks, M. O., & Schlom, J. (1986). Monoclonal antibodies and breast cancer. *Seminars in Oncology, 13,* 393–401.

Trotta, P. (1986). Preclinical biology of alpha interferons. *Seminars in Oncology, 13*(3), 3–12.

Vilcek, J., Kelke, H. C., Jumming, L. E., & Yip, Y. K. (1985). Structure and function of human interferon gamma. In R. J. Ford (Ed.), *Mediators of cell growth and differentiation* (pp. 299–313). New York: Raven Press.

West, W. H., Tauer, K. W., Yannelli, J. R., Marshall, G. D., Orr, D. W., Thurman, G. B., & Oldham, R. K. (1987). Constant-infusion recombinant interleukin-2 in adoptive immunotherapy of advanced cancer. *New England Journal of Medicine, 316,* 898–905.

Wood, P., Nygaard, S., & Hrushesky, W. J. M. (1989). Cisplatin-induced anemia is correctable with erythropoietin. *Abstracts on Hematopoietic Growth Factors.* San Antonio, TX: American Society of Hematology.

CHAPTER 24

Multimodal Therapy

ROBERTA P. SCOFIELD
MARCIA C. LIEBMAN
JAMES D. POPKIN

Multimodal therapy is the integration of more than one antineoplastic therapy into a treatment program with the intent of improving therapeutic outcomes, reducing toxicities (when compared with conventional single-modal therapy), or both. Surgery, radiation, and chemotherapy are the modalities that currently form the basic armamentarium of the oncologist considering a multimodal treatment plan. As newer modalities emerge, multimodal therapy might comprise a vast array of differing treatments. Combinations of therapies might include adjuvant chemotherapy, neoadjuvant or induction chemotherapy, bone marrow transplantation, or biologic response modification (see Chapters 23 and 27).

The development of effective anticancer treatment has been a slow and uneven process (Table 24–1). Therapy has evolved through the data derived from early empiric clinical experience and the application of newer hypotheses in successive generations of clinical trials. Current cancer therapy, although far from perfect, has the capability of curing diseases that previously were uniformly fatal. The number of cured cancers continues to increase. Only a few areas in medicine have been able to produce such unequivocal cures. This chapter traces the origins of single treatments, their inherent shortcomings, and the potential exploitation of their combined benefits as multimodal therapy.

EVOLUTION OF SINGLE-AGENT MODALITY THERAPY

Surgery

Surgery was the original cancer treatment. In 1704, Valsalva believed that cancer originated as a local lesion capable of cure by surgery but that it spread by lymphatics to regional lymph nodes and that it tended to recur (Fisher & Gebhardt, 1978). In 1863, Paget wrote that he was "not aware of a single clear instance of recovery . . . that the patient should live for more

Table 24–1. TIME LINE

Year	Event
ca. 500 B.C.	Hippocrates originates the term *carcinoma*.
2nd century A.D.	Galen classifies tumors; calls cancer a systemic disease without a cure.
1700	Hypothesis that cancer starts as a local disease and later spreads.
mid-1800s	Blood-borne tumors detected in the circulation.
	Lymphatic system postulated to be effective barrier to tumor cell dissemination.
1900	Theories of William Halsted.
	Radiation first used for cancer treatment.
1930s	Interstitial radium implanted for treatment of breast cancer.
1940s	Development of chemotherapy.
1955	Presence of tumor cells in venous blood demonstrated.
late 1960s	Effectiveness of combined chemotherapy in Hodgkins's disease demonstrated.
	Adjuvant chemotherapy for breast cancer used.
	Communication between lymphatics and blood-vascular system demonstrated.
late 1970s	Effectiveness of total mastectomy versus radical mastectomy demonstrated.
	Effectiveness of adjuvant chemotherapy demonstrated.
	Effectiveness of conservative surgery and radiation therapy in breast cancer demonstrated.
	Combination chemotherapy in head and neck cancer introduced.
1985	Effectiveness of lumpectomy versus total mastectomy demonstrated.

than ten years free from disease . . . we may . . . dismiss all hope that the operation [mastectomy] will be the final remedy for the disease."

Until the end of the eighteenth century, surgery rarely provided more than palliation with little prospect for cure (Moore, 1867). At the turn of the twentieth century, the name William Halsted became synonymous with the en bloc radical mastectomy. Halsted believed that cancer spread in a contiguous manner from the original growth, moving along surface planes through the vasculature, until it finally penetrated into visceral organs (Halsted, 1907). This concept led to the adoption of even more radical operations in the mid-twentieth century.

Other clinical observations were also used to determine surgical treatment of cancer. In 1869 Ashworth detected the presence of blood-borne tumor cells in the circulation. In 1955, Fisher and Turnbull demonstrated the presence of tumor cells in venous blood of patients undergoing colorectal surgery. Subsequently, this phenomenon became increasingly recognized in patients with both early and advanced cancers. Communication between the lymphatic and the blood-vascular systems was demonstrated in 1966 (Fisher & Fisher, 1966).

No longer was the lymphatic system felt to be the effective barrier to tumor cell dissemination as was originally postulated by Virchow in the mid-1800s. Evidence revealed that the majority of tumor cells entering a lymph node failed to maintain a permanent residence (Fisher & Gebhardt, 1978). The presence of metastases that skip geographically adjacent areas within a lymph node region and the occurrence of disseminated metastases in patients with negative lymph node metastases were further findings contrary to Halstedian theory. These findings form the basis of current concepts of metastasis.

Along with changes in the anatomic concepts of cancer spread, theories of cell kinetics developed, leading to alternative hypotheses regarding cancer cell biology. Mathematic approaches to tumor cell growth were developed. Estimates of the time of neoplastic transformation in solid tumors were calculated by extrapolating backward, using observed tumor doubling times (Table 24–2) (Gullino, 1977). Data indicated that a tumor with a doubling time of 100 days (an average value for breast cancer) grows for years before it becomes clinically apparent. One cancer cell and its progeny must go through about 30 doublings

Table 24–2. TUMOR DOUBLING TIMES

Tumor Type	Mean Doubling Time (in days)
Testicular carcinoma	21
Ewing's sarcoma	22
Osteogenic sarcoma	34
Hodgkin's disease	38
Squamous cell lung cancer	87
Colon carcinoma	96
Breast cancer	129
Adenocarcinoma of the lung	134

(Data from Shackney, McCormick, & Cuchural, 1978.)

(about 10^8 to 10^9 cells) to be detectable by radiograph or palpation. Once a tumor becomes palpable, the cell population must double only three more times to double the tumor diameter again, and in about ten cell doublings the amount of cancerous tissue reaches 1 kg, which would be fatal for most people. The clinical phase of solid tumors (the time when a tumor is large enough to result in morbidity or mortality) occurs during the last one third of the actual duration of untreated disease (Gullino, 1977; Norton & Simon, 1977).

The mathematic model of tumor growth suggests that even when a cancer is detected early, metastatic spread may have already occurred. So-called early detection of cancer generally does not find a chronologically early disease. Experiments on animal models have revealed as many as 3 to 4 million cancer cells entering the blood stream by flowing through only 1 g of tumor tissue (Butler & Gullino, 1975). The great majority of these circulating cancer cells are destroyed, but the higher their number, the higher the frequency of metastases; thus early diagnosis and treatment are essential (Gullino, 1977).

Further clinical trials revealed that in breast cancer, recurrence and survival are independent of the number of axillary nodes removed at surgery (Fisher & Slack, 1970). Patients with the same number of positive nodes had similar prognoses regardless of the number of nodes removed. The National Surgical Adjuvant Breast Project demonstrated in a prospective, randomized fashion that patients who were clinically without axillary node involvement were not significantly different in the incidence of treatment failure, distant metastases, or survival when treated with radical mastectomy versus simple mastectomy and local regional radiation versus simple mastectomy alone (with axillary node dissection if nodes are found to be clinically positive for disease later on) (Fisher et al., 1977). (Box 24–1). The conceptual framework of surgery in cancer was thus undermined by these findings, and alternative hypotheses of tumor biology came into medical practice (Table 24–3). Radiation and antineoplastic chemotherapy were developing treatment modalities for cancer therapy during the beginning and middle of this century, respectively.

Radiation Therapy

Initially, radiation was felt to be merely an adjunct to surgery in early stage disease or a palliative measure in advanced cases (Harris, Levene, & Hellman, 1978; Mitchell, 1988; Tepper, 1989). Subsequently, radiation was shown to have the ability to cure select tumors in their earlier stages (e.g., Hodgkin's disease), but by and large radiation was considered secondary to surgery for most common cancers (e.g., breast, lung, and colorectal). In the last 20 to 30 years, radiation has become a viable alternative to surgery in some cancers (breast cancer [Fisher et al., 1977; Fisher & Wolmark, 1986; Harris et al., 1978], head and neck cancer [Brady & Davis, 1988], sarcomas [Tepper, 1989], and anal

---

Box 24–1. COMPARING SURGICAL INTERVENTIONS FOR BREAST CANCER

Fisher, B., Montague, E., Redmond, C., Barton, B., Borland, D., Fisher, E. R., Deutsch, M., Schwarz, G., Margolese, R., Donegan, W., et al. (1977). **Comparison of radical mastectomy with alternative treatments for primary breast cancer: A first report of results from a prospective randomized clinical trial.** *Cancer, 39,* 2827–2839.

STUDY

Comparison of radical mastectomy with alternative treatments for primary breast cancer.

SAMPLE

1665 women with primary operable breast cancer in 34 institutions in the United States and Canada.

STUDY AIMS

Node-negative women were randomized to groups receiving treatment by radical mastectomy, total mastectomy with regional radiation, or total mastectomy alone. Node-positive women were randomized to treatment groups by radical mastectomy or total mastectomy with regional radiation.

FINDINGS

No statistically significant difference between the three groups of node-negative women in relation to disease-free interval or length of survival. No statistically significant difference between the two groups of node-positive women in relation to disease-free interval or length of survival. (Node-negative women treated with total mastectomy alone who later developed positive nodes were treated with axillary node dissection but were not considered treatment failures; inability to carry out the dissection because of extent of tumor in the axilla was classified as treatment failure.)

DISCUSSION

There was a failure to demonstrate an advantage of treatment of radical mastectomy for either node-negative or node-positive women with primary operable breast cancer.

---

cancer [Salmon, Fenton, & Asselian, 1984]) and a valuable adjunct in others (rectal cancer [Metzger, Ghosh, & Kisner, 1985; O'Connell, Gunderson, & Fleming, 1988] and lung cancer [Klatersky & Sculier, 1986]). This change in focus was directed by the accumulation of clinical evidence that supported a more active role for radiation therapy in primary treatment. The efficacy and toxicity of radiation therapy are critically dependent on dose. The success of radiation therapy depends on multiple factors, including tumor cell type, surrounding normal tissue, time-dose relationships, volume of radiation, and tumor bulk (Harris et al., 1978).

In 1929 and again in 1937, Keynes described primary treatment of localized breast cancer with interstitial radium. His 5-year survival rate for women with either local disease or axillary node involvement was comparable to surgical treatment. Keynes noted that patients with bulky tumors were likely to have local recurrences, which prompted the excisional biopsy of the primary tumor mass. Radiation continued to be used, with improved techniques that allowed better results with decreasing damage to surrounding tissue. Nevertheless, despite advances in radiation therapy, this modality remained a local treatment, similar to

surgery, and could not answer the problem of systemic metastases. Radiation in many instances could provide a cure for a localized tumor mass with the same likelihood as surgery but without the deformity produced by a cancer operation. Limited surgery with radiation has been used with the greatest success in breast cancer (Harris et al., 1978), sarcomas (Tepper, 1989), anal carcinomas (Mitchell, 1988), and, to some degree, head and neck tumors (Brady & Davis, 1988).

Antineoplastic Chemotherapy

Chemotherapy developed after World War II with work on derivatives of mustard gas and antifolates. A narrow therapeutic index resulted in few meaningful improvements in patients who were usually laden with far-advanced disease that had failed to respond to surgery, radiation, or both. Many responses were short lived, and patients' disease sometimes became drug resistant (the tumor no longer responded to the drug); often they later responded to another chemotherapeutic agent. DeVita, Serpick, and Carbone (1970) developed the MOPP (mechlorethamine [Mustargen], vincristine [Oncovin], prednisone, procarbazine) regimen

Table 24–3. TWO DIVERGENT HYPOTHESES OF TUMOR BIOLOGY

Halstedian	Alternative
1. Tumors spread in an orderly defined manner based on mechanical considerations.	1. There is no orderly pattern of tumor cell dissemination.
2. Tumor cells traverse lymphatics to lymph nodes by direct extension, supporting en bloc dissection.	2. Tumor cells traverse lymphatics by embolization, challenging the merit of en bloc dissection.
3. The positive lymph node is an indicator of tumor spread and is the instigator of disease.	3. The positive lymph node is an indicator of a host-tumor relationship that permits development of metastases rather than being the instigator of distant disease.
4. Regional lymph nodes are barriers to the passage of tumor cells.	4. Regional lymph nodes are ineffective as barriers to tumor cell spread.
5. Regional lymph nodes are of anatomic importance.	5. Regional lymph nodes are of biologic importance.
6. The blood stream is of little significance as a route of tumor dissemination.	6. The blood stream is of considerable importance in tumor dissemination.
7. A tumor is autonomous of its host.	7. Complex host-tumor interrelationships affect every facet of the disease.
8. Operable breast cancer is a local-regional disease.	8. Operable breast cancer is a systemic disease.
9. The extent and nuances of operation are the dominant factors influencing patient outcome.	9. Variations in local-regional therapy are unlikely to substantially affect survival.

(Adapted from Fisher, B. [1980]. Laboratory and clinical research in breast cancer: A personal adventure. *Cancer Research, 40,* 3863–3874.)

in the late 1960s, and it quickly became apparent that a major milestone had been reached. Treatment of Hodgkin's disease, which once had had a dismal prognosis in advanced stages, now resulted in frequent clinical and pathologic complete remissions that were durable and tantamount to cure.

Combination chemotherapy—the use of more than one agent in a systematic fashion—became a valuable tool of the oncologist, and the number of curable malignancies increased. Combination chemotherapy permitted different types of drugs to exert toxic effects by different mechanisms, resulting in greater cell kill. The cumulative toxicities on the host were often less than an equipotent single agent that would have to be given in a much larger quantity to exploit the dose-response relationships. Chemotherapy has established its role and now is a potentially curative modality rather than only a palliative one.

MULTIMODAL REGIMENS

Combined modality therapy initially consisted of radiation therapy after potentially curative surgery in breast cancer patients who had a high risk of relapse because of poor prognostic factors (e.g., positive lymph nodes, large primary lesions, multicentric lesions). This approach might have led to improved local control, but because of systemic metastases, patients had little chance of being cured. The use of chemotherapy following surgery for breast cancer first developed in the mid-1960s.

The combination of treatment modalities, based on newer concepts of tumor metastases, actually improved cure rates over surgery alone and therefore became known as *adjuvant therapy. Neoadjuvant* (up-front or induction) *therapy* is treatment that is designed to enhance the primary treatment but is given before rather than after the primary treatment.

Adjuvant Therapy

Nissen-Meyer, Kjellgren, Malmio, Mansson, and Norton (1978) began a collaborative trial in Scandinavia by giving cyclophosphamide immediately after a mastectomy; this therapy demonstrated a significant survival advantage. Numerous studies in breast cancer have established a role for chemotherapy as an adjunct to potentially curative local therapy (Bonadonna & Valagussa, 1987; Fisher & Gebhardt, 1978; Goldie, 1987). Adjuvant chemotherapy may eradicate systemic micrometastases that would elude local therapy, whether it is conservative or radical. Seventy per cent of patients with solid tumors have micrometastatic disease at diagnosis (Ashworth, 1869; Curt & Chabner, 1987; Moore, 1867; Schabel, 1972).

The initial enthusiasm for chemotherapy in breast cancer treatment quickly led to the application of postoperative adjuvant chemotherapy to other cancers with solid tumors, with clinically variable results (Eilber & Eckardt, 1985; Frei & Ervin, 1981). The natural histories of different malignancies are very diverse: two thirds of head and neck cancers recur locally despite surgery, radiation therapy, or both; in breast cancer, less than 5 per cent recur locally. Other diseases are much more chemotherapy resistant than breast cancer (e.g., non-small-cell lung cancer), and adjuvant chemotherapy has not fulfilled the promise expected from breast cancer trials (Klatersky & Sculier, 1986). The anti-Halstedian theories were formulated using a breast cancer model, but in other malignancies, different biologic patterns are apparent.

Neoadjuvant Therapy

The head and neck were among the first cancer sites for the application of neoadjuvant chemotherapy. Despite aggressive local therapy with surgery and radiation, advanced head and neck cancer has a high local relapse rate (Hong & Bromer, 1983). The use of chemotherapy after definitive local therapy was a relatively futile undertaking, with an average of 20 per cent response to drugs administered either as single agents or in combinations (Hong, Schaefer, & Issell, 1982; Jacobs, 1982; Williams, Einhorn, & Velez-Garcia, 1982). Often patients with recurrent disease are malnourished and tolerate aggressive therapy poorly. Theoretically, several advantages and disadvantages in the utilization of neoadjuvant chemotherapy can be postulated (Table 24–4). Indeed, the results with an induction chemotherapy approach were startling: 75 per cent of tumors responded (showing greater than 50 per cent reduction of all measurable disease), and approximately 20 per cent were complete clinical responses (nondetectable disease) (Hong et al., 1979; Randolph et al., 1978). The results of this up-front approach have been encouraging for further evaluations and therapy modifications. Whether cure rates have increased, however, has yet to be demonstrated (Baker, Makuch, & Wolf, 1981; Vogl et al., 1982). Hope still exists that the encouraging results seen with neoadjuvant chemotherapy will be reflected in improved survival rates. The use of more intensive and longer courses of chemotherapy has resulted in higher complete clinical response rates, which may be the key to lengthening survival rates (Hong, Popkin, & Shapshay, 1984).

Current Combination Therapy

Investigations are being conducted to evaluate the results using multimodal therapy, which comprises neoadjuvant chemotherapy, radiation, and limited surgery, compared with the results using radical surgery alone. This is an area of key interest in the treatment of cancers in which standard cancer operations result in major deformities: head and neck cancers (Marcial et al., 1988), limb sarcomas (Eilber, Morton, Eckardt, Grant, & Weisenburger, 1984), and breast cancers (Hortobagyi et al., 1988; Jacquillat et al., 1986).

Table 24–4. ADVANTAGES AND DISADVANTAGES OF NEOADJUVANT CHEMOTHERAPY IN PREVIOUSLY UNTREATED PATIENTS

Disadvantages	Advantages
1. Delay of surgery from complications of chemotherapy.	1. Better performance status and good nutritional status will increase tolerance of chemotherapy in the preoperative patient.
2. Inaccurate knowledge of tumor margins.	2. Intact blood supply of previously untreated tumors has the potential to deliver high concentrations of the drug to the tumor site.
3. Increased immunosuppression.	3. Increased tumor cell kill in rapidly growing tumor cells.
	4. Potential eradication of subclinical microscopic metastatic disease that is not exposed to local treatment.
	5. Enhanced efficacy of planned definitive local treatment by cytoreduction of the primary tumor and nodal metastases.
	6. Continued use of a chemotherapeutic regimen as a maintenance regimen in patients who initially achieved significant response.

(Adapted from Hong, W. K., Shapshay, S. M., Bhutani, R., Craft, M. L., Uemaki, A., Yamaguchi, K. T., Vaughan, C. W., & Strong, M. S. [1979]. Induction chemotherapy in advanced squamous head and neck carcinoma with high dose cisplatinum and bleomycin infusion. *Cancer, 44,* 19–25.)

Table 24–5. CURRENT CHALLENGES FOR MULTIMODAL THERAPY

Colorectal Cancer
Problem: 50% of patients having curative surgery will have local-regional or systemic recurrence
Corrective Action:
1. Early screening
2. Recognition of high-risk patients
3. Adjuvant or combination treatment
   a. Utilization of adjuvant radiotherapy for patients with local rectal carcinoma
   b. Development of newer, more active chemotherapeutic agents
   c. Development of monoclonal antibody studies
   d. Further delineation of the role of radiation therapy in colon cancer (Metzger, Ghosh, & Kisner, 1985; Tepper, 1986)

Breast Cancer
Problem: 80% of patients diagnosed with breast cancer develop systemic disease
Corrective Action:
1. Early recognition with screening mammograms
2. Recognition of high-risk patients
3. Continued development of adjuvant systemic therapy
   a. Determination of optimal duration of chemotherapy for premenopausal patients
   b. Definition of the role of hormonal manipulation with or without chemotherapy for node- or receptor-positive patients
   c. Identification of adjuvant therapy for node-negative patients at risk for recurrence
   d. Further examination of the role of chemotherapy for postmenopausal women

Lung Cancer
Problem: Unless curative surgery can be performed, all patients will develop systemic disease
Corrective Action:
1. Reduction in numbers of persons who smoke
2. Development of effective screening for high-risk patients
3. Improved systemic treatment with newer, more active antineoplastic agents
4. Continued definition of the role of radiation therapy combined with chemotherapy

The poor results that are currently achieved in the treatment of lung cancer may be amenable to improvement with a multimodal approach. In non-small-cell lung cancer, radiation with or without neoadjuvant chemotherapy followed by surgery is being evaluated. Small-cell lung cancer results have reached a plateau in the past 10 years using chemotherapy with or without radiation. The use of alternating chemotherapy drug regimens and the use of surgery in selected cases are current protocols being evaluated by Eastern Cooperative Oncology Group.

Anal carcinoma has been effectively controlled in the majority of cases utilizing chemotherapy concomitantly with radiation, often eliminating sphincter loss from surgery (Mitchell et al., 1988). Current treatment dilemmas exist for the three most common solid tumors that may be resolved as newer combinations and treatment plans become available (Table 24–5).

TOXICITIES AND SIDE EFFECTS

All modalities of antineoplastic therapy have side effects and toxicities. When these therapies are combined, careful consideration must be given to the expected side effects of each modality and to the impact on the patient of the combined side effects. The risk of the combined toxicities should be weighed against the benefit of the expected therapeutic effect of the combined modalities. Ideally, the toxicity from the therapy should be no greater than the sum of the side effects of each modality. Toxicities of multimodal treatment do occur in excess of this ideal because of many factors, including the sequencing of the therapies and the individual component therapies utilized.

Schedule of Therapies

The optimal scheduling of combined therapy regimens has still not been determined. Scheduling options are sequential (each therapy given according to its schedule with no overlap) or concomitant (two or more therapies given at the same time). Sequential administration, although less toxic than combined therapy, may result in inadvertent delays and overall reduced efficacy of the treatment plan. Unexpected side effects may occur when modalities are given sequentially, for example, delayed wound healing or development of anastomotic leaks in the patient who has preoperative radiation therapy.

The most significant problem of concomitant administration is the risk of synergistic toxicity (e.g., radiation and chemotherapy in the treatment of breast cancer). Suggested benefits of concomitant administration include synergism of action with increased treatment efficacy (Klatersky & Sculier, 1986).

Surgery Combinations

When surgery is performed first, the acute and long-term effects of surgery do not appear to influence the side effects of chemotherapy or radiation therapy. Postoperative treatments with chemotherapy or radiation therapy may be delayed to allow for tissue repair necessitated by the surgical approach. Long-term effects of surgery, such as adhesions, fibrosis, abscesses, and fistula formation, may be exaggerated when surgery is combined with radiation therapy, particularly when radiation is given preoperatively. To reduce this problem, intraoperative radiotherapy (radiation directed to a surgically exposed tumor) is being investigated. This combination of modalities offers a greater radiation dose to the tumor site with potential reduction of tissue injury to surrounding normal tissue and reduced potential for altered tissue healing and fistula formation (Goldson, 1981).

Bingham (1986) notes that a larger radiation treatment volume may be required postoperatively for patients with head and neck cancer to achieve a similar degree of local control. The cumulative toxicities from combined surgical and chemotherapy approaches are limited as long as adequate time is allowed for patient recovery after surgery. The most difficult problems are listed in Table 24–6. Problems are usually associated

Table 24–6. TOXICITIES RELATED TO SURGERY AND RADIATION THERAPY COMBINATIONS

Toxicity	Definition	
Delayed wound healing	A longer than normal course of tissue healing that occurs in previously radiated tissue due to radiation-incurred injury to wound.	
	Major:	Requiring operative revision
	Moderate:	Persistent seroma; wound separation greater than 2 cm or hematoma greater than 25 ml
	Minor:	Seroma resolving with aspiration; wound separation less than 2 cm or hematoma less than 25 ml
Fistula or anastomotic leaks	Nonhealing of anastomoses occurs owing to preoperative radiation injury to microvessels in bowel	

(Data from Arbeit, Hilaris, & Brennan, 1987; Stevens, Fletcher, & Allen, 1978.)

with planned preoperative radiation therapy, as well as with surgery that needs to be done on previously irradiated tissue. New surgical techniques are being developed to decrease postradiation complications (Russ, Sonoron, & Gagnon, 1984).

Chemotherapy and Radiation Therapy Combinations

Acute and long-term tissue injury associated with combined radiation and chemotherapy has been identified as more patients are offered this therapy. Injury may accompany both modalities, with acute reactions occurring during or soon after the treatment begins and irreparable damage remaining years after treatment has stopped.

Acute Effects

Acute damage from both radiation and chemotherapy is the result of injury to rapid renewal cell systems, such as those of the bone marrow and gastrointestinal epithelium. In tissue systems with slow renewal time, injury is associated with separate mechanisms in chemotherapy and radiation therapy, thus producing different effects (Rubin, 1984). The primary reason for chemotherapy injury is damage to the parenchymal cellular component. Radiation acts on the stroma, the microcirculation, and the parenchymal cells of tissues. Both mechanisms affect the number of stem cells needed to maintain organ viability. Antineoplastic agents that are cell-cycle specific will interfere with actively dividing cells only during certain portions of the cell cycle. Cells that are in division at the time of exposure to drugs experience acute injury. Irradiated tissue response is also dependent on the mitotic activity of the tissue being radiated, with dividing cells being more sensitive than resting (G_0) cells. The noncycling cells in the G_0 of the cell cycle will express radiation injury as they reenter the cell cycle and divide (Rubin & Casorett, 1968).

Both radiation and chemotherapy may lead to organ damage. The addition of one treatment modality to another can augment expected benefits. Either modality can leave residual injury when large enough doses are used, regardless of which one is used first. Subclinical effects may be uncovered when a second treatment is administered. If injury to tissues or organ systems is present from the initial modality, the immediate addition of a second modality may be fatal. Additional stressors, such as infection or trauma, may produce overt signs of injury due to cumulative subclinical damaging effects of treatment. Age and organ function at the time of initiation of combined treatment can also lower the clinical threshold for injury. Determination of safe doses for both radiation and chemotherapy, when given as combined modalities, is still poorly understood (see Chapter 23). Close patient monitoring must be emphasized when combined chemotherapy and radiation therapy are utilized. Acute toxicities need to be modified by appropriate dose adjustments, careful attention to scheduling of treatment, and observation for early signs of reactions.

Long-Term Effects

Like acute toxicities, utilization of chemotherapy and radiation together raises concerns about long-term effects. Evidence demonstrates that late side effects of combined treatment affect similar organs but via different pathways of injury. Late effects of treatment may be additive and may become evident years after treatment (Table 24–7). As the number of long-term survivors of cancer treatment increases, second malignancies in this group of patients are becoming increasingly evident. In survivors, the incidence of second malignancies can be as high as 15 per cent, which is 20 times the rate in the general population (Byrd, 1983). The risk for leukemia is greatest for patients receiving combined treatment and for those who receive chemotherapy after relapse following radiation-induced remission. Blayney and colleagues (1987) describe the development of secondary leukemia in patients with Hodgkin's disease who had combined modality treatment. Johnson and associates (1986) describe a significantly increased risk in a group of patients who received combined treatment for small-cell lung cancer, in whom the second malignancy was again acute leukemia. The incidence of second malignancies peaks at 11 years and does not appear to rise after that time. Both groups of investigators recommend continued long-term follow-up with observation for secondary malignancies.

TOXICITY MONITORING

Toxicity monitoring is a critical component for nursing in the care of patients receiving combined modality treatment. Smith and Chamorro (1978) proposed a standard care plan for a group of patients receiving combined chemotherapy and radiation treatment for advanced gynecologic cancer. The principle that underscored the monitoring was based on the knowledge of the increased toxicity associated with this combination and the timing of expected side effects.

Monitoring includes early observation for complications related to chemotherapy side effects and radiation therapy side effects. Nursing care should be planned to anticipate the pattern of expected side effects. Initiation of self-care and nursing measures early in the course of treatment can be helpful in reducing the discomfort of the expected side effects (Hassey, 1987). Nursing observations need to be directed at early symptom recognition to attempt to avoid severe reactions to the side effects. Symptoms need to be documented accurately and communicated to members of the team to prevent major complications (Hockenberry & Lane, 1988).

Patient compliance may be a problem with multimodal treatment regimes of long duration. Problems with compliance may be manifested by failure to keep appointments, have necessary laboratory work, or complete all treatments. Although poor compliance has not been described for multimodal programs, Haynes (1976) suggests that therapies of long duration may have lower compliance rates, and Donabedian and Rosenfeld (1964) have found that the cost of therapy is inversely related to compliance. The high number of patient visits observed with multimodal programs has correlated with higher than average medical and out-of-pocket expenses (Lansky, 1979). Nurses monitoring patients on extensive, complicated regimens need to maintain a close consistent relationship with the patient and be alert to early signs of failure to keep appointments as an indicator of future problems with compliance. If compliance becomes a problem, the nurse should explore with the patient the issues that may be leading to the noncompliance and work with the patient to resolve any problems.

PATIENT EDUCATION

Witt, McDonald-Lynch, & Grimmer (1987) discuss the importance of preparatory education for groups of patients receiving adjuvant radiotherapy for cancer of the colon. They stress that education about radiation should begin after surgery, before the patient leaves the hospital. Visiting the radiation suite will introduce the patient to a new team of oncology personnel now involved in the treatment plan. Education should include discussion of potential long-term side effects or complications and symptoms associated with these late effects. Late effect symptoms that occur 6 to 12 months after treatment ends may cause unnecessary concern about disease recurrence. Frequent posttreatment follow-up and a careful symptom history can be helpful in early detection of late effects and can serve as a time for continued patient education.

An integral part of education for patients receiving multimodal therapy is an explanation of how each

Table 24–7. LATE EFFECTS OF CHEMOTHERAPY AND RADIATION THERAPY

Organ System	Agent	Mechanism of Injury	Effect	Threshold Dose	Comments
Heart	Doxorubicin (Adriamycin)	Cytotoxic to cardiomyocytes via direct cell damage to myocyte with resultant loss of contractile component	Congestive heart failure	550 mg/m^2	300–350 mg/m^2 when used with radiation
	Radiation	Myocardial capillary endothelial cell injury that produces myocardial fibrosis with exudate; no damage to myocytes	Myocardial fibrosis (may occur 5–10 years after radiation when doxorubicin given)	45–50 Gy	—
Lungs	Bleomycin	Changes in nucleus in alveolar cells	Alveolitis; parenchymal fibrosis; interstitial changes	400–500 U	When combined with radiation, dose response is increased
	Radiation	Ablation of alveolar cells and release of surfactant; injury to lung vasculature	Arterial hypoxia; decreased blood flow; acute pneumonitis	>6.0 Gy	
Renal	Cisplatin	Acute tubular necrosis and atrophy due to changes in renal tubular cell	Renal failure due to tubular damage	—	Added and enhanced problems occur
	Radiation	Changes in the arteriolar glomerular area	Nephritis due to microvascular damage	5–20 Gy	10 Gy when used with chemotherapy
Liver	Methotrexate 6-Mercaptopurine Doxorubicin (Adriamycin)	Direct effect on hepatocytes	Hepatocellular necrosis and fat replacement	—	—
Skin	Doxorubicin (Adriamycin) Actinomycin D Carmustine	—	Enhancement or "recall" of previous radiation skin reactions when chemotherapy is given	—	—
Central nervous system	Methotrexate (intrathecal and intravenous)	Contacts white matter; damage to vascular choroid plexus; alters drug clearance	Leukoencephalopathy	—	—
	Brain irradiation	Alters capillary permeability of blood-brain barrier	Leukoencephalopathy	—	—
Gastrointestinal (major dose-limiting organ in acute reaction)	5-Fluorouracil	*Acute* mucosal loss	Stomatitis; enteritis; ulceration	—	Late effects occur only with addition of radiation therapy
	Radiation	*Acute* mucosal loss Late progressive endarteritis	Ulceration and infarction necrosis of vessels resulting in fistulae and perforation; slow fibrosis and stricture of bowel	— —	—
Bone marrow (major dose-limiting organ in acute reaction)	Chemotherapy	*Acute* suppression of cycling stem cells	Leukopenia, thrombocytopenia, gradual anemia	—	—
	Radiation	*Acute* suppression of resting cells 10–15% irradiated marrow ablated at doses <30.0 Gy 25–50% irradiated marrow ablated at doses >30.0 Gy 50–75% irradiated marrow ablated but responds quickly due to increased sensitivity to total volume ablated (new islands of hematopoiesis become active; protected marrow compensates with overproduction)	Gradual with time		Recovery of bone marrow suppressed when combined treatment given simultaneously

(Data from Billingham, Bristow, Glatstein, Mason, Masek, & Daniels, 1977; Smith & Chamorro, 1978.)

modality contributes to the overall goals of treatment. Discussion should include concepts of local-regional control versus systemic control. The goal of these discussions should be to help the patient develop a sense of continuity. If the goal of the total treatment plan is unclear or if the relationship among the treatment modalities is unclear, patients may conclude that their situation is dire and the potential for cure is low. Patients receiving more than one treatment form may believe that the first therapy was not successful or that their cancer is especially virulent and requires two or three forms of treatment. The patient must comprehend the cycling of the treatment modalities and the goals of each. The nurse who initiates the treatment teaching plan should be careful to introduce the patient to all members of the treatment team so that the patient knows which caregivers are responsible for each part of the treatment plan. Ideally, when the patient is finished with one modality, the nurse should introduce him or her to the next nurse in the new treatment area.

Patients receiving multimodal therapy should understand not only what symptoms to report but who to contact. The patient and family risk becoming confused about who is responsible if care is not taken to identify for them the primary caregivers and their roles. In addition to recording the name of the nurse or doctor, patients should be encouraged to record the dates and times of treatments or visits to those professionals and what problems were identified and discussed. The division of care between two or more oncology specialties can result in ineffective symptom management. Potential problems include over- or undermedication owing to poor communication by prescribing physicians, duplication of diagnostic studies, and patient or family confusion. Reactivated anxiety over the initial

diagnosis can be a problem as a second therapy is begun. Nurses should be alert for signs of anxiety in a patient beginning radiation after finishing chemotherapy or a patient whose situation is the reverse. Patient histories reveal that beginning a new treatment may raise concerns about the first course of treatment, including fears and anxieties about the initial diagnosis. In summary, the oncology nurse should coordinate the treatment plans for the patient and renew the educational focus of the care plan with the beginning of each new treatment modality.

PATIENT SELECTION

The selection of patients for multimodal treatment is critical to the success of the treatment program. Selection criteria include factors related to the type of cancer and the stage of disease as well as factors inherent in the patient, such as advanced age and presence of other chronic diseases. Side effects may be more pronounced in patients with borderline organ function. Subclinical problems associated with natural aging processes may become apparent as the rigors of intensive combined therapy are undertaken. Careful staging studies need to be done to determine the exact presence of clinical disease so that adequate consideration can be given to ultimate combined local and systemic therapy. Careful assessment must be done to reduce postoperative complications in programs utilizing surgical approaches.

A factor associated with the selection of treatment modality is the presence or absence of the treatment capability in the clinical facility. The lack of radiation treatment facilities will eliminate utilization of combinations including radiation therapy at that clinical facility. Many local community oncology programs do not have radiation therapy capabilities, thus necessitating patient travel to a treatment center. Careful planning and close coordination are necessary to integrate patient travel and to achieve a therapeutic alternative not available locally.

Table 24–8. CURRENT MULTIMODAL COMBINATIONS DEPENDENT ON TUMOR TYPE

Primary Tumor Type	Multimodal Combinations
Breast Cancer	
Stages I, II, III	Adjuvant chemotherapy
	Conservative surgery with radiation with or without chemotherapy
Locally advanced	Neoadjuvant chemotherapy with or without radiation with or without surgery
Head and Neck Cancer	Surgery with or without radiation
	Neoadjuvant chemotherapy with or without radiation with or without surgery
Esophageal Cancer	Surgery with or without radiation
	Chemotherapy with or without radiation with or without surgery
Lung Cancer	
Non-small cell	Chemotherapy with or without radiation with or without surgery
Small cell	Chemotherapy with or without radiation
Anal Cancer	Chemotherapy with radiation
Ovarian Cancer	
Stages I and II	Surgery with adjuvant chemotherapy, radiation, or both
Stages III and IV	Surgery with chemotherapy
Bladder Cancer	Chemotherapy with radiation with or without surgery

FUTURE DIRECTIONS

The results of present and future clinical trials will better define the optimal combination and sequencing of therapies. Currently combinations are being tested clinically in many, if not all, solid tumors (Table 24–8). The continued increase of locally available technologies will make sophisticated combined modalities accessible to patients locally so that they will not need to travel to major cancer centers. Closer cooperation between major centers and cooperative groups or community hospital oncology programs will increase the availability of all therapeutic modalities to patients in their own environment, making more complex care available to more persons with cancer.

Recent oncology nursing literature describes the complex care needed by patients undergoing multimodal therapy. Pretreatment teaching and monitoring of acute side effects and toxicities throughout the course of treatment are critical (Haibeck, 1988; Hassey, 1987; Hockenberry & Lane, 1988; O'Rourke, 1987; Smith & Chamorro, 1978; Witt et al., 1987). Oncology nurses will also be spending more time doing follow-up assessments of persons cured of cancer as nurses monitor for late effects of treatment (Fergusson et al., 1987). Oncology nurses will need a broader area of expertise as interaction and consultation between the surgical, medical, and radiation therapy nurses become more frequent. Case management, in which a health team member coordinates all aspects of care, may become more prevalent to prevent patients from "falling through the cracks" as they go from one treatment modality to another. Patients and families need to be able to identify a member of the treatment team whom they can trust with all aspects of their care.

References

Arbeit, J. M., Hilaris, B. S., & Brennan, M. F. (1987). Wound complications in multimodal treatment of extremity and superficial truncal sarcomas. *Journal of Clinical Oncology, 5*, 480–488.

Ashworth, T. (1869). A case of cancer in which cells similar to those in tumors were seen in the blood after death. *Australian Journal of Medicine, 14*, 146.

Baker, S. R., Makuch, R. W., & Wolf, G. T. (1981). Preoperative cisplatin and bleomycin therapy in head and neck squamous carcinoma. *Archives of Otolaryngology, 107*, 683–689.

Billingham, M. E., Bristow, M. R., Glatstein, E., Mason, J. W., Masek, M. A., & Daniels, J. R. (1977). Adriamycin cardiotoxicity: Endocardial biopsy evidence of enhancement by irradiation. *American Journal of Surgical Pathology, 1*, 17–23.

Bingham, H. G. (1986). Adjuvant chemotherapy. *Surgical Clinics of North America, 66*, 183–188.

Blayney, D., Longo, D. L., Young, R., Greene, M., Hubbard, S., Postal, M., Duffy, P., & DeVita, V. (1987). Decreasing risk of leukemia with prolonged follow-up after chemotherapy and radiotherapy for Hodgkin's disease. *New England Journal of Medicine, 316*, 710–714.

Bonadonna, G., & Valagussa, P. (1987). Current status of adjuvant chemotherapy for breast cancer. *Seminars in Oncology, 14*, 8–22.

Brady, L. W., & Davis, L. W. (1988). Treatment of head and neck cancer by radiation therapy. *Seminars in Oncology, 15*, 29–38.

Butler, T. P., & Gullino, P. M. (1975). Quantitation of cell shedding into efferent blood of mammary adenocarcinoma. *Cancer Research, 35*, 512–516.

Byrd, R. L. (1983). Late effects of treatment of cancer in children. *Pediatric Annals, 12*, 450–460.

Curt, G. A., & Chabner, B. A. (1987). Medical oncology: Decade of discovery. *Internal Medicine, 8*, 47–54.

DeVita, V. T., Serpick, A. A., & Carbone, P. P. (1970). Combination chemotherapy in the treatment of advanced Hodgkin's disease. *Annals of Internal Medicine, 73*, 881–895.

Donabedian, A., & Rosenfeld, L. (1964). Follow-up study of chronically ill patients discharged from hospital. *Journal of Chronic Disease, 17*, 847–862.

Eilber, F. R., & Eckardt, J. (1985). Adjuvant therapy for osteosarcoma: A randomized perspective trial. *Proceedings of the American Society of Clinical Oncology, 4*, 144.

Eilber, F. R., Morton, D. L., Eckardt, J., Grant, T., & Weisenburger, T. (1984). Limb salvage for skeletal and soft tissue sarcomas. *Cancer, 53*, 2579–2584.

Fergusson, J., Ruccione, K., Waskerwitz, M., Perin, G., Diserens, D., Nesbit, M., & Hammond, G. D. (1987). Time required to assess children for the late effects of treatment. *Cancer Nursing, 10*, 300–310.

Fisher, B. (1980). Laboratory and clinical research in breast cancer: A personal adventure. *Cancer Research, 40*, 3863–3874.

Fisher, B., & Fisher, E. R. (1966). The interrelationship of hematogenous and lymphatic tumor cell dessimination. *Surgery, Gynecology and Obstetrics, 122*, 791–798.

Fisher, B., & Gebhardt, M. D. (1978). The evolution of breast cancer surgery: Past, present and future. *Seminars in Oncology, 5*, 385–394.

Fisher, B., Montague, E., Redmond, C., Barton, B., Borland, D., Fisher, E. R., Deutsch, M., Schwarz, G., Margolese, R., Donegan, W., et al. (1977). Comparison of radical mastectomy with alternative treatments for primary breast cancer: A first report of results from a prospective randomized clinical trial. *Cancer, 39*, 2827–2839.

Fisher, B., & Slack, N. H. (1970). Number of lymph nodes examined and the prognosis of breast cancer. *Surgery, Gynecology and Obstetrics, 131*, 79–88.

Fisher, B., & Turnbull, R. B., Jr. (1955). Cytologic demonstration and significance of tumor cells in the mesenteric blood in patients with colorectal carcinoma. *Surgery, Gynecology and Obstetrics, 100*, 102–108.

Fisher, B., & Wolmark, N. (1986). Conservative surgery: The American experience. *Seminars in Oncology, 13*, 425–433.

Frei, E, III, & Ervin, T. J. (1981). Summary and overview. In S. E. Salmon & S. E. Jones (Eds.), *Adjuvant therapy of cancer* (Vol. III, pp. 569–584). New York: Grune & Stratton, Inc.

Goldie, J. H. (1987). Scientific basis for adjuvant and primary (neoadjuvant) chemotherapy. *Seminars in Oncology, 14*, 1–7.

Goldson, A. L. (1981). Past, present, and prospects of intraoperative radiotherapy (IOR). *Seminars in Oncology, 8*, 59–64.

Gullino, P. M. (1977). Natural history of breast cancer. *Cancer, 39*, 2697–2703.

Haibeck, S. V. (1988). Intraoperative radiation therapy. *Oncology Nursing Forum, 15*, 143–147.

Halsted, W. S. (1907). The results of radical operations for the cure of carcinoma of the breast. *Annals of Surgery, 46*, 1–19.

Harris, J. R., Levene, M. B., & Hellman, S. (1978). The role of radiation therapy in the primary treatment of carcinoma of the breast. *Seminars in Oncology, 5*, 403–416.

Hassey, K. M. (1987). Radiation therapy for rectal cancer and the implications for nursing. *Cancer Nursing, 10*, 311–318.

Haynes, R. B. (1976). A critical review of the determinants of patient compliance with therapeutic regimens. In D. L. Sackett & R. B. Haynes (Eds.), *Compliance with therapeutic regimens*. Baltimore: Johns Hopkins University Press.

Hockenberry, M. J., & Lane, B. (1988). Limb salvage procedures in children with osteosarcoma. *Cancer Nursing, 11*, 2–8.

Hong, W. K., & Bromer, R. (1983). Chemotherapy in head and neck cancer. *New England Journal of Medicine, 308*, 75–79.

Hong, W. K., Popkin, J., & Shapshay, S. (1984). Preoperative adjuvant induction chemotherapy in head and neck cancer. In G. Wolff (Ed.), *Head and neck oncology* (pp. 287–300). Boston: Martinus Nijhoff.

Hong, W. K., Schaefer, S., & Issell, B. (1982). A prospective randomized trial of methotrexate versus cisplatinum in the treatment of recurrent squamous cell carcinoma of the head and neck. *Proceedings of the American Society of Clinical Oncology, 1*, 202.

Hong, W. K., Shapshay, S. M., Bhutani, R., Craft, M. L., Uemaki, A., Yamaguchi, K. T., Vaughan, C. W., & Strong, M. S. (1979). Induction chemotherapy in advanced squamous head and neck carcinoma with high dose cisplatinum and bleomycin infusion. *Cancer, 44*, 19–25.

Hortobagyi, G. N., Ames, F. C., Buzdar, A. U., Kau, S. W., McNeese, M. D., Paulus, D., Hug, V., Holmes, F. A., Romsdahl, M. M., Fraschini, G., McBride, C. M., Martin, R. G., & Montague, E. (1988). Management of stage III primary breast cancer with primary chemotherapy, surgery, and radiation therapy. *Cancer, 62*, 2507–2516.

Jacobs, C. (1982). Use of methotrexate and 5FU for recurrent head and neck cancer. *Cancer Treatment Reports, 66*, 1925–1928.

Jacquillat, C. L., Baillet, F., Auder, G., Sellami, M., Facchini, T., Khayat, D., & Weil, M. (1986). Neoadjuvant chemotherapy and conservative treatment in 205 patients with breast cancer. *Proceedings of the American Society of Clinical Oncology, 5*, 69.

Johnson, D., Porter, L., List, A., Hande, K., Hainsworth, J., & Greco, F. (1986). Acute nonlymphacytic leukemia after treatment of small cell lung cancer. *American Journal of Medicine, 81*, 962–968.

Keynes, G. (1929). The treatment of primary carcinoma of the breast with radium. *Acta Radiologica, 10*, 393–402.

Keynes, G. (1937). Conservative treatment of cancer of the breast. *British Medical Journal, 2,* 643–647.

Klatersky, J., & Sculier, J. P. (1986). Nonsurgical combined modality therapy in non-small cell lung cancer. *Chest, 89,* 2895–2935.

Lansky, S. B. (1979). Childhood cancer: Nonmedical costs of illness. *Cancer, 43,* 403–408.

Marcial, V. A., Pajak, T. F., Kramer, S., Davis, L. W., Stetz, J., Laramore, G. E., Jacobs, J. R., Al-Sarraf, M., & Brady, L. W. (1988). Radiation therapy oncology group (RTOG) studies in head and neck cancer. *Seminars in Oncology, 15,* 39–60.

Metzger, U. F., Ghosh, B. C., & Kisner, D. L. (1985). Adjuvant treatment of colorectal cancer. *Cancer Chemotherapy and Pharmacology, 14,* 1–8.

Mitchell, E. P. (1988). Carcinoma of the anal region. *Seminars in Oncology, 15,* 146–153.

Moore, C. H. (1867). On the influence of inadequate operations on the theory of cancer. *Royal Medicine and Society, 1,* 245.

Nissen-Meyer, R., Kjellgren, K., Malmio, K., Mansson, B., & Norton, T. (1978). Surgical adjuvant chemotherapy results with one short course of cyclophosphamide after mastectomy for breast cancer. *Cancer, 41,* 2088–2098.

Norton, L., & Simon, R. (1977). Tumor size, sensitivity to therapy, and design of treatment schedules. *Cancer Treatment Reports, 61,* 1307–1317.

O'Connell, M. J., Gunderson, L. L., & Fleming, T. R. (1988). Surgical adjuvant therapy of rectal cancer. *Seminars in Oncology, 15,* 138–145.

O'Rourke, M. E. (1987). Enhanced cutaneous effects in combined modality therapy. *Oncology Nursing Forum, 14,* 31–35.

Paget, J. (1863). *Lectures on surgical pathology.* London: Green, Longman, Roberts and Green.

Randolph, V., Vallejo, A., Spiro, R. H., Shah, J., Strong, E. W., Huvas, A. G., & Wittes, R. E. (1978). Combination therapy of advanced head and neck cancer: Induction of remissions with diamminedichloroplatinum (II), bleomycin and radiation. *Cancer, 41,* 460–467.

Rubin, P. (1984). Late effects of chemotherapy and radiation: A new hypothesis. *International Journal of Radiation Oncology-Biology-Physics, 10,* 5–34.

Rubin, P., & Casorett, G. W. (1968). *Clinical radiation pathology* (Vols. I–II). Philadelphia: W. B. Saunders Co.

Russ, J. E., Sonoron, G. L., & Gagnon, J. D. (1984). Omental transposition flaps in colorectal carcinoma. *International Journal of Radiation Oncology-Biology-Physics, 10,* 55–62.

Salmon, R. D., Fenton, J., & Asselian, B. (1984). Treatment of epidermoid anal canal cancer. *American Journal of Surgery, 147,* 43–48.

Schabel, F. M., Jr. (1972). Rationale for adjuvant chemotherapy. *Cancer, 39,* 2875–2882.

Shackney, S. E., McCormack, G. W., & Cuchural, G. J. (1978). Growth rate patterns of solid tumors: Their reaction and responsiveness to therapy. An analytic review. *Annals of Internal Medicine, 89,* 107–121.

Smith, D., & Chamorro, T. (1978). Nursing care of patients undergoing combination chemotherapy and radiotherapy. *Cancer Nursing, 1,* 129–134.

Stevens, K. R., Fletcher, W. S., & Allen, C. V. (1978). Anterior resection and primary anastomosis following high dose preoperative irradiation for cancer of the rectosigmoid. *Cancer, 41,* 2065–2071.

Tepper, J. E. (1986). Adjuvant irradiation of gastrointestinal malignancies: Impact on local control and tumor cure. *International Journal of Radiation Oncology-Biology-Physics, 12,* 667–671.

Tepper, J. E. (1989). Role of radiation therapy in the management of patients with bone and soft tissue sarcomas. *Seminars in Oncology, 16,* 281–288.

Vogl, S. E., Lerner, H., Kaplan, B. H., Coughlin, C., McCormick, B., Camacho, F., & Cinberg, J. (1982). Failure of effective initial chemotherapy to modify the course of stage IV (MO) squamous cancer of the head and neck. *Cancer, 50,* 840–844.

Williams, S. D., Einhorn, L. H., & Velez-Garcia, E. (1982). Chemotherapy of head and neck cancer: Comparison of cisplatin and vinblastine and bleomycin (PVB) versus methotrexate (MTX). *Proceedings of the American Society of Clinical Oncology, 1,* 202.

Witt, M., McDonald-Lynch, A., & Grimmer, D. (1987). Adjuvant radiotherapy to the colorectum: Nursing implications. *Oncology Nursing Forum, 14*(3), 17–21.

CHAPTER 25

Implementation of Clinical Trials

JEAN JENKINS
GREGORY CURT

CLINICAL TRIALS DEVELOPMENT

Advances in cancer treatment have occurred largely because of the application of new knowledge gained in basic research in the clinical management of patients with cancer. The term *research* brings to mind the classical laboratory environment with its equipment, white-coated scientists, and experimental animals. This is the environment of basic research in which careful, systematic investigation leads to new ideas for patient treatment. Clinical research, in contrast, is the bridge between the basic research laboratory and the patient's bedside. Clinical trials are carefully controlled experiments aimed at utilizing the smallest number of subjects to determine with statistical confidence the effectiveness of treatments and at the same time maintain patient safety. Information on the various kinds of clinical trials provides the background for defining the important role that nurses play in the scientific development of cancer care.

Whereas some clinical trials test new treatments, others investigate new ways of preventing cancer; screening patients for earlier diagnosis; and detecting the disease in its earliest stages with new imaging modalities, such as magnetic resonance and positron emission (Hender, 1985). Studies are now monitoring the psychological impact of cancer on patients and studying related changes in their quality of life (Ochs, Mulhern, & Kun, 1988). Today's clinical trials are multifaceted, striving not only to improve survival rates of patients with cancer through testing of new therapies but also to determine the safest, most effective treatment available.

Overview

Clinical research is the keystone of modern medicine. In the early 1900s, surgery was the only treatment available to patients with cancer, and few were cured. Local treatments, such as surgical excision, are inadequate for the 70 per cent of patients with solid tumors who have obvious or occult metastatic disease at the time of diagnosis. By the mid 1950s, options for treatment began to increase, with the introduction of both radiotherapy, which improved local disease control, and anticancer chemotherapy. Chemotherapy offered effective treatment for patients with advanced malignancy for the first time.

The progress of cancer therapy has been steady. Although only 20 per cent of patients with cancer survived for 5 years (considered a cure) in the 1930s, improved surgical techniques and the developing field of radiotherapy cured 33 per cent of patients by the 1950s (DeVita et al., 1979). Further improvements in radiotherapy and the development of chemotherapy have improved the cure rate to 50 per cent. Overall, advances have been greatest for patients under the age of 55, for whom the 5-year survival rate reached 59 per cent in 1986 (National Cancer Institute [NCI], 1986a).

Clinical trials have made important contributions through the development of new drugs and through the pioneering of better overall treatments for patients with common cancers. These treatments include limb-sparing procedures for patients with sarcoma; limited surgery for patients with breast cancer; and effective adjuvant chemotherapy for those with lung, colon, and rectal cancers. Development of these treatments occurs through a series of preclinical and clinical investigations. The development of drugs to be administered as chemotherapy is used to discuss this process of investigation.

Preclinical Drug Development

The first step in identifying a new cancer drug is screening or measuring a drug's antitumor activity in a cancer model system. During this phase, the National Cancer Institute's (NCI) computer systems scan the structures of approximately 40,000 new chemicals that are synthesized each year to select novel compounds for testing. Earlier this testing was done against mouse tumors, but for the past 2 years the NCI has begun to screen drugs against a panel of human tumor cell lines that were derived from patients with cancer (Fig. 25–1). This new system, it is hoped, will identify novel structures that will show specific activity against solid tumors of adults. Each year approximately 10,000 compounds are selected for testing, of which ten will pass all the steps needed to reach their first use in patients in what is known as a phase I study (Hubbard, 1981). Although only one in perhaps 50,000 drugs screened will eventually be approved for marketing, all 33 drugs that are commercially available to cancer patients in the United States have undergone such testing (DeVita et al., 1979).

PHASES OF CLINICAL TRIALS

Once preclinical drug development has been completed, clinical trials progress through four phases of testing. These trials are identified as phases I, II, III, and IV. The purpose of the study, the study design, the monitoring required, and the role of the nurse are determined by the phase of the clinical research (Hubbard, 1982).

Phase I

Phase I study is the first testing of new agents in humans. The purpose of phase I clinical trials is to establish the maximum tolerated dose of the agent in various schedules in humans. In addition, pharmacologic tests, or how well the agent is absorbed, what blood levels are achieved, and how the drug is metabolized and eliminated by the body, are important parts of phase I evaluation (Box 25–1).

Although all drugs entering phase I studies are selected carefully for their potential activity against cancer, certain constraints minimize the likelihood that the trials of these drugs will demonstrate a significant antitumor effect during this stage of development. For example, the initial dose must be as safe as possible to avoid possible overdosing. For this reason, the starting dose level of the agent is based on prior animal studies and is usually one tenth of the maximum tolerated dose in mice (Hubbard, 1985). Doses are usually

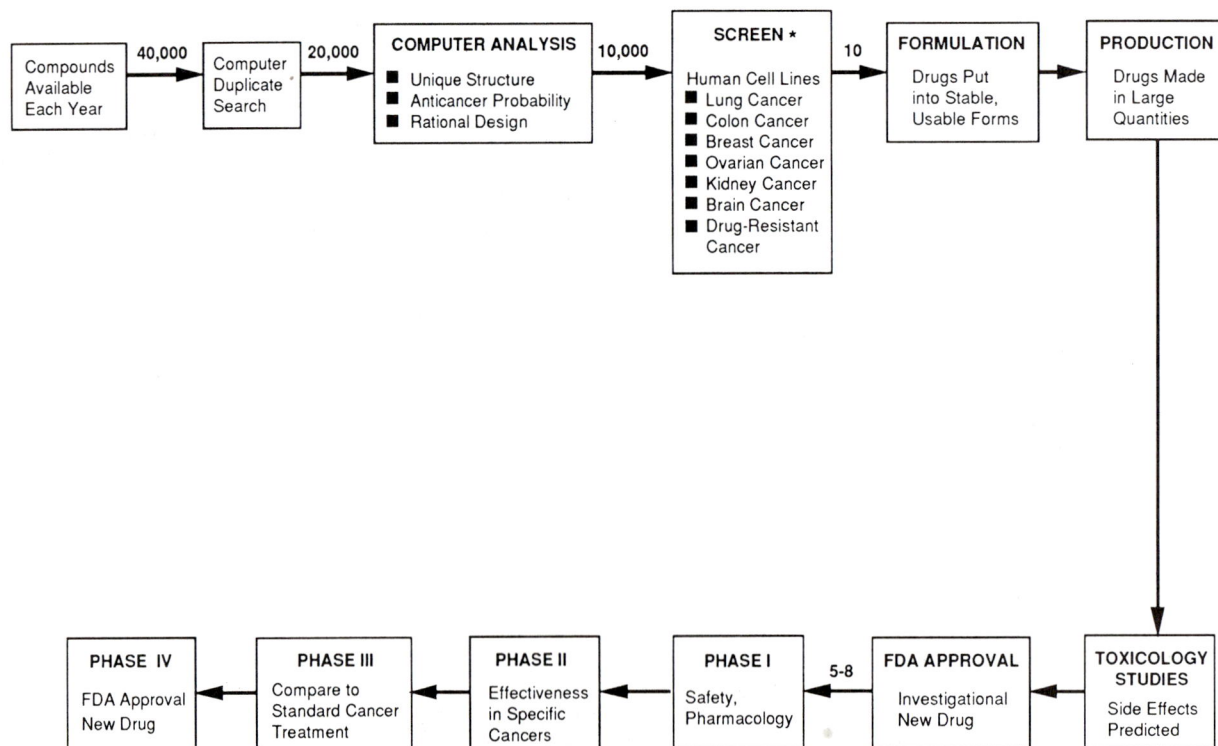

*The new screening system using human cell lines replaces the mouse leukemia screen.

Figure 25–1. How a cancer drug is developed.

Box 25–1. PHASE I STUDY

STUDY

Yarchoan, R., Weinhold, K., Lyerly, H., Gelmann, E., Blum, R., Shearer, G., Mitsuya, H., Collins, J., Myers, C., Klecker, R., Markham, P., Durack, D., Lehrman, S., Barry, D., Fischls, M., Gallo, R., Bolognesi, D., & Broder, S. (1986). **Administration of 3′-azido-3′-deoxythymidine, an inhibitor of HTLV-III/LAV replication, to patients with AIDS or AIDS-related complex.** *Lancet, 1,* 575–580.

SAMPLE

Nineteen patients with AIDS or AIDS-related complex (ARC). All patients received test doses of 3′-azido-3′-deoxythymidine (AZT), after which they received AZT intravenously for 14 days and then oral AZT for 4 weeks according to the following regimens: patients 1–4 received 1.0 mg/kg every 8 hr; patients 5–10 received 2.5 mg/kg every 8 hr; patients 11–15 received 2.5 mg/kg every 4 hr; and patients 16–19 received 5 mg/kg every 4 hr.

MEASURES

In a 6-week clinical trial, four dose regimens of AZT were examined in patients to determine toxicity, tolerable dose, and pharmacokinetics. Patients were monitored for clinical and laboratory changes. Heparinized plasma samples were obtained at various times for measurement of AZT levels.

FINDINGS

AZT was well absorbed from the gut and crossed the blood-brain barrier. Therapeutic levels were maintained with 5 mg intravenously or 10 mg given orally every 4 hr. Side effects were minimal, with headaches and depression of white blood cell counts being the most common. Responses included evidence of clinical improvement (6), and general weight gain of 2.2 kg. Those patients at the higher doses had negative results from viral culture at the end of the 6-week treatment.

LIMITATIONS

The small number of patients provided the answers to the questions of toxicity, appropriate dose, blood, cerebrospinal fluid, and excretion levels of AZT. Although there are some indications of disease response, further larger studies are recommended to determine the effectiveness of AZT in the treatment of AIDS and ARC.

---

escalated via the Fibonacci search scheme (Table 25–1) (Buyser, Staquet, & Sylvester, 1984). This plan requires that three to five patients be treated at each dose level and evaluated for toxicity before advancing to the next level. Dose escalation occurs in smaller increments as the amount is increased because side effects are anticipated at the higher dose levels. Approximately 15 to 20 patients are needed to complete a phase I study.

Table 25–1. FIBONACCI SEARCH SCHEME

Drug Dose	Per Cent Above Preceding Level	Number of Patients Entered
n (mg/m²)	—	3
2 n	100	3
3.3 n	67	3
5.0 n	50	3
7.0 n	40	3
9.0 n	33	3
12.0 n	33	3
16.0 n	33	3

n, beginning dose.
(Modified Buyse, M., Staquet, M., & Sylvester, R. [1984]. *Cancer clinical trials, methods, and practice.* New York: Oxford University Press. Reproduced by permission.)

To minimize the number of phase I patients who receive subtherapeutic doses, new dosing regimens are currently under development (Collins, Zaharko, Dedrick, & Chabner, 1986). One of the most promising is to measure blood levels of the drug in animals that receive the optimal dose. These levels can then be compared with the drug blood levels in the first group of patients being tested. If these levels are far below those observed in the experimental animals, it may be possible to bypass some of the Fibonacci steps to reach the optimal dose in humans more quickly. Already this approach has been used successfully in several phase I studies with the result that fewer patients were needed to complete the trial and more were treated at safe and potentially therapeutic drug doses (Collins, 1988). Different schedules for agent administration may be tested in phase I trials.

Only patients with malignant disease that is unresponsive to standard therapies or for which no standard therapy exists are eligible for phase I studies. Phase I trials are carefully controlled by the drug sponsor (whether the NCI or industry) and must be carried out by approved physicians at centers with expertise in this area. Before participation is allowed, approved physicians must meet certain criteria established by the Cancer Therapy Evaluation Program (CTEP) of the NCI and must be registered. Phase I studies are frequently done by a single institution to maintain the highest level of safety and continuity of data (Cancer Therapy Evaluation Program, 1986).

For phase I studies sponsored by the NCI, principal investigators are required to submit current data biweekly and study summaries every 6 months and at the end of the clinical trial. This requirement is needed to fulfill United States Food and Drug Administration (FDA) regulations. Phase I results are reviewed three times a year at a working group meeting during which all investigators report results and compare pharmacology, toxicities, and treatment responses.

Careful monitoring of phase I studies is essential in providing safety for the patient. A major nursing responsibility is the observation of toxic side effects. To facilitate this observation, a clinical brochure is available for each investigational agent developed by the NCI. This brochure provides information about the rationale for selecting the drug for clinical testing as well as the toxicity levels experienced in the animal studies. Anticipation of similar side effects in humans can allow early recognition of any potentially serious effect of the treatment. The first occurrence of any toxic reaction for phase I trials is reported by telephone to CTEP at 301-496-7957. Such information is used to collate details from diverse settings and to disseminate the information quickly to other investigators working with the drug. Any severe, life-threatening, or fatal event brought about by the new drug must also be reported by phone and later by letter (Cancer Therapy Evaluation Program, 1986).

Nurses frequently collect samples for pharmacokinetic monitoring of a patient on a phase I study. Timed blood samples are drawn to measure rates of drug absorption, metabolism, and excretion. The nurse coordinates or performs the timed studies to ensure both accuracy of the study and comfort of the patient.

The staff nurse contributes to the completeness of a phase I study through early recognition and management of the side effects of treatment. This information is then used to determine whether it is safe to escalate to the next higher drug dosage. Ethical concerns for patients in phase I studies include ensuring that informed consent has been given (discussed later) and emphasizing the patient's contribution to scientific knowledge regardless of the study's results. Patients eligible for phase I trials are often physically and emotionally debilitated and may need special attention to ensure that ethical considerations are addressed. For instance, a patient who is desperately ill may feel there is no other hope and may be easily persuaded to participate in research trials without understanding the total ramifications. Nurses can assist patients to consider the treatment alternatives but should be careful not to overstep a nurse's expertise. A case reported by Gargaro (1978) illustrates the right of the nurse to inform patients of nursing treatments available. The role of the nurse in relation to medical management issues is to be an advocate for the patient and, if

questions still exist regarding treatment options, to be a liaison to the physician to insist that these questions of risks and alternative treatment options be clarified.

Phase II

Phase I studies focus on the evaluation of drug toxicities and the determination of safe drug dosages to be utilized for testing in a phase II trial. Agents entered into phase II study are tested in humans with various types of cancer primarily to determine effectiveness against a given cancer. The most frequently tested tumors include those found in leukemia, lymphoma, and melanoma and in colon, lung, breast, ovarian, and brain cancers (DeVita, 1982). Additional information on toxicity may be determined, and more sophisticated pharmacology studies may also be performed. Many patients eligible for phase II clinical studies have had prior cancer treatment. Their disease may have progressed or become refractory to standard treatment. Patients must also have a tumor that is measurable so that the effectiveness of the agent against cancer can be determined. Responses can then be graded as complete (all tumor regresses), partial (greater than 50 per cent regression), or minimal (less than 50 per cent regression). Pretreatment organ function must be normal, and life expectancy must be a sufficient amount of time for observation. Phase II studies usually require 18 to 30 patients to make a statistical determination about the effectiveness of the drug in specific human tumors (Simon, Wittes, & Ellenberg, 1985). The nurse can best contribute to the completeness of phase II studies by documenting benefits and side effects of the treatment. Patients must be eligible and able to be evaluated to ensure the accuracy of phase II data. The nurse may anticipate and prepare the patient for studies that monitor disease response. Knowledge of the means by which various cancers spread, effects of cancer therapy, and staging procedures required by the protocol will assist the nurse in preparing the patient for participation in phase II study (Box 25–2).

Phase III

The purpose of phase III studies is to compare the effectiveness of an experimental drug or treatment with a standard regimen or treatment. A phase III study applies a more complex design than those of phase I and II studies, which describe a single treatment. Once activity of an agent in a specific tumor has been determined in a phase II study, a comparative phase III study is designed. A phase III study compares established therapy with a new therapy in terms of impact on overall survival, disease-free survival, and quality of life. Patients are stratified by a number of variables that may affect the outcome of the study (age, performance status, tumor grade, stage of disease). These stratifications assist in making the comparative groups equivalent so that valid conclusions

---

Box 25–2. PHASE II STUDY

STUDY

Sessa, C., Gundersen, S., Huinink, W., Renard, J., & Cavalli, F. (1988). **Phase II study of intravenous menogaril in patients with advanced breast cancer.** *Journal of the National Cancer Institute, 80,* 1066–1069.

SAMPLE

Forty patients with advanced breast cancer who had not received anthracycline drugs previously. Patients with recurrent or metastastic breast cancer, or both, who may or may not have had prior treatment, were eligible for this study. Having a measurable level of disease was a prerequisite.

MEASURES

Menogaril was administered every 4 weeks at intravenous doses of 160 mg/m^2 in high-risk patients or 200 mg/m^2 in low-risk patients. The patient's physical examination and history, together with an assessment of lesions, blood tests, and electrocardiogram, were repeated before each cycle. Blood counts were done weekly. Ejection fraction measurements and echocardiograms were done every two cycles. Responses and toxicity were monitored.

FINDINGS

Forty patients entered the study, but 34 were eligible for evaluation for response to therapy and toxicity. The overall response rate was 22 per cent in patients with no prior treatment and 10 per cent in patients with prior therapy. Toxicities included manageable myelosuppression, leukopenia, mild gastrointestinal toxicity, alopecia, phlebitis, erythema at intravenous site, and limited cardiac toxicity.

LIMITATIONS

Extent of disease and number of prior therapies do affect the response of tumor to cytotoxic drugs. Thus the overall response rate of 17 per cent in this study may not predict overall usefulness of menogaril for treatment of breast cancer. The skin toxicity needs to be solved before further evaluation may be possible. Further studies need to be done to determine menogaril's activity and toxic effects.

---

can be drawn from study results. In phase III study, two equally effective treatments may be evaluated to determine whether one is less toxic and therefore preferable (Box 25–3).

Phase III study designs require large numbers of patients to allow comparisons. Unlike phase I and II trials, many Phase III studies are multi-institutional so that adequate numbers can be entered on a study in a timely manner. Patients considered eligible for phase III studies usually have had no prior treatment for cancer. To prevent bias, randomization is made to the standard treatment (control group) versus the new treatment (Ellerberg & Eisenberger, 1985). Because of their size, phase III studies are the most costly and the most difficult to plan and implement. It is in this stage, however, that an improved treatment is discovered and becomes the standard of care. Objective criteria for measuring tumor response and study objectives (survival, disease-free survival) must be clearly defined.

The nursing role in phase III studies includes monitoring patient eligibility and protocol compliance, documenting therapeutic effects and toxicities, and providing continuity of care. Phase III observations may require that the patient make frequent long-term hospital visits to measure the effectiveness of treatment. Delineation of long-term effects of cancer treatment may be a significant factor in determination of the best therapy to offer to future patients.

Phase IV

Phase IV studies are designed to integrate a new agent or treatment into a primary or proven plan. This additional study may elucidate data on the optimum use of the agent. At this stage of study, the drug is known to be effective but is not yet authorized for wide-scale commercial distribution. Long-term follow-up data are needed to show long-term efficacy and any development of other toxicities. Nurses caring for patients receiving phase IV therapy need to provide education and evaluate nursing interventions to decrease the regimen's morbidity.

RESOURCES FOR CLINICAL TRIALS

The NCI sponsors all the major phase I, II, and III cancer clinical trials in the United States. The CTEP

Box 25–3. PHASE III STUDY

STUDY

Pavlosky, S., Maschio, M., Santarelli, T., Muriel, F., Corrado, C., Garcia, I., Schwartz, L., Montero, C., Sanahuja, F., Magnasco, O., Rana, R., & Cavagnaro, F. (1988). **Randomized trial of chemotherapy versus chemotherapy plus radiotherapy for stage I–II Hodgkin's disease.** *Journal of the National Cancer Institute, 80,* 1466–1473.

SAMPLE

A total of 277 patients with untreated Hodgkin's disease, clinical stages I or II, could be evaluated of the 293 patients who were randomized to groups of either six cycles of cyclophosphamide, vinblastine, procarbazine, and prednisone (CVPP) or six cycles of CVPP plus radiation.

MEASURES

A total of 142 patients were treated with CVPP, and 135 were treated with CVPP plus radiation. Extensive documentation of disease was necessary, with clinical examination, bone marrow biopsy, chest radiographs, lymphangiogram, and computed tomographic (CT) scans being done before testing and at the end of the sixth cycle of chemotherapy. Follow-up every 2 months for 2 years and then three times a year indefinitely was necessary. Periodic tests were necessary to follow the disease response. Median time on the study was 43 months for CVPP and 51 months for CVPP plus radiation.

FINDINGS

Complete remissions were obtained in 85 per cent of patients on CVPP and 93 per cent of those receiving CVPP plus radiation. When analysis was done of variables that may have affected overall disease response, two prognostic groups were identified. Both regimens were well tolerated.

LIMITATIONS

The prognostic factors were not defined ahead of this study so stratification for randomization was not done for this phase III trial. Longer follow-up may be necessary to verify the extent of disease response and long-term toxic effects.

---

is responsible for administration and coordination of the majority of the extramural clinical trials. These trials are conducted by the NCI (1) through clinical or comprehensive cancer centers, (2) by cooperative study groups (Table 25–2), or (3) through community clinical

Table 25–2. NATIONAL CANCER INSTITUTE COOPERATIVE CLINICAL TRIALS GROUPS

Multimodality Multidisease Groups
Cancer and Leukemia Group B (CALGB)
Children's Cancer Study Group (CCSG)
Eastern Cooperative Oncology Group (ECOG)
North Central Cancer Treatment Group (NCCTG)
Pediatric Oncology Group (POG)
Southwest Oncology Group (SWOG)

Multimodality Group Devoted to a Major Oncologic Disease or Modality Area
Brain Tumor Study Group (BTSG)
Gynecologic Oncology Group (GOG)
Intergroup Rhabdomyosarcoma Study Group (IRSG)
Lung Cancer Study Group (LCSG)
National Surgical Adjuvant Breast and Bowel Project (NSABP)
National Wilms' Tumor Study Group (NWTSG)
Radiation Therapy Oncology Group (RTOG)

Special Activities Groups
European Organization for Research on Treatment for Cancer (EORTC)—Operations and Statistical Office
Quality Assurance Review Center (QARC)

oncology programs. Collaboration of the NCI and pharmaceutical industry may occur at any step along the drug development process.

The Clinical Oncology Program is the intramural treatment research arm of the NCI (NCI, 1986b). Programs conducted at the Clinical Center, National Institutes of Health, focus on basic and clinical research in surgery, pharmacology, radiobiology, immunology, genetics, and molecular biology. Information about clinical trials in progress is available from Physicians Data Query, which is a clinically oriented database that was developed to make current information on cancer treatment more widely available (Hubbard, Henney, & DeVita, 1987). Physicians Data Query can be accessed directly by computer, by consulting a medical librarian with a connection to Medical Literature Analysis and Retrieval System (MEDLARS), or by telephoning 1-800-4-CANCER (Deininger, Collins, & Hubbard, 1989). This service summarizes information on clinical protocols, state-of-the-art cancer treatment, and physicians who are qualified to treat patients with cancer. Any patient who wishes to and who fits eligibility criteria can take part in a clinical trial. Any well-run clinical trial receives a careful review for scientific validity, humanitarian value, and patient safety to provide protection of human rights.

FEDERAL REGULATIONS OF CLINICAL TRIALS

All clinical trials in the United States must meet criteria established by the Department of Health and Human Services (DHHS) and the FDA (Levine, 1981). Anyone receiving a grant from DHHS must file with the National Institutes of Health a statement of assurance of compliance with the DHHS regulations (Levine, 1986). The five general ethical norms required by these regulations for developing a clinical trial include a good research design, competent investigators, favorable balance of harm versus risk benefit, informed consent, and equitable selection of subjects.

The FDA is given the responsibility and authority by Congress for ensuring the safety of the public (Young, 1981). This governmental agency enforces the laws established by Congress that define the terms under which clinical work with experimental agents may proceed.

All clinical research is required by federal regulations to be reviewed at each participating institution by an institutional review board. Both the DHHS and the FDA have adopted policies designed to ensure the competent function of these boards. Projects must be reviewed by the institution's review board before protocol initiation and at least annually thereafter. The composition of an institutional review board includes physicians, scientists, lawyers, clergy, community members, and nurses. When these boards review pediatric protocols, they should have persons who care for children as members. The institutional review board affords protection for the investigator, the institution, and the patient through protocol review.

PROTOCOL COMPONENTS

A well-designed research trial has a written protocol, which is a clear, well-written plan of action (Cancer Therapy Evaluation Program, 1986). Components of a research protocol are listed in Table 25–3. Clear definitions are essential in communicating the study design to participating investigators. Adherence to the protocol is critical to producing reliable study findings. For multi-institutional protocols, approval from each institution's review board is required. An essential component of a protocol proposal is the provision for informed consent (Tables 25–3 and 25–4). Information in the informed consent form is specific and must be communicated in lay terms to ensure patient understanding. Informed consent results in voluntary study participation or refusal (see "Informed Consent").

APPROACHES TO ALLEVIATING OBSTACLES TO PERFORMING CLINICAL TRIALS

Participation in clinical trials is voluntary. Community physicians should engage in or support activities

Table 25–3. COMPONENTS OF A RESEARCH PROTOCOL

Component	Criteria
Rationale for study	Objectives*
	Scientific data
	Patient selection
Treatment plan	Schedule, dose, route*
	Pharmaceutical information
	Expected toxicities*
Study parameters	Dose modifications
	Criteria for response
	Measurement parameters*
	Off-study criteria
	Records to keep
Statistical criteria	Method of analysis
	Numbers needed for study
	Expected duration of study
Bibliography	Contact persons*
	Informed consent

*To be included in informed consent document.
(Modified from Cancer Therapy Evaluation Program. [1986]. *Investigator's handbook*. Washington, D.C.: National Cancer Institute.)

that will lead to improved patient care (Leviner, 1986), and referrals to clinical trials should begin at the community level. Patients need to be informed of the opportunity for study participation and the advantages of clinical trials. Feelings of hopelessness and fear of abandonment by the primary physician must be addressed so that the patient can hear the options and make an informed decision (Meisel & Roth, 1981).

A major obstacle to conducting clinical trials is the accrual of an adequate sample size to answer the study questions. Some of the reasons reported by Taylor, Maegolese, and Soskolne (1985) for physicians not entering patients on a specific National Surgical Adjuvant Breast Program (NSABP) randomized study include concern that the doctor-patient relationship would be affected by the clinical trial (73 per cent), difficulty with obtaining informed consent (38 per cent), dislike for open discussion involving uncertainty (22 per cent), perceived difficulty in following procedures (9 per cent), and feelings of personal responsibility if the treatments were found to be unequal (8 per cent). The NCI is targeting several of these concerns by physicians in a campaign to publicize clinical trials to physicians and to the general public (Wittes & Friedman, 1988). Several mechanisms for addressing the increased need for information by the patient are being developed, such as video tapes to explain protocols and written materials for the lay person to describe clinical trials.

Table 25–4. INFORMED CONSENT*

Expected benefits from the study
Alternative treatment options
Record confidentiality
Compensation for injury
Participation is voluntary
Withdrawal from the study is possible at any time

*All criteria marked in Table 25–3 with an asterisk (*), expressed in lay terms, are included here as well.
(Modified from Cancer Therapy Evaluation Program. [1986]. *Investigator's handbook*. Washington, D.C.: National Cancer Institute.)

Another obstacle is the attitude of the public toward participation in research. Patients may be reluctant to participate in a clinical trial because such experimentation makes them feel like a "guinea pig." A study by Casselith, Lusk, Miller, and Hurwitz (1982) reported on a population of 295 subjects that included oncology patients, cardiology patients, and members of the general public (Box 25–4). Seventy-one per cent of the respondents felt that it is reasonable for patients to participate in clinical studies. Patients who participate in medical research were perceived to get the best medical care, to benefit others, and to broaden the base on which improved treatments could be developed. The NCI is making an effort to publicize the benefits of clinical trials and is working to make participation in clinical trials socially and medically acceptable for all patients and physicians (Gelber & Goldhirsch, 1989). Nurses can offer information to patients and families or direct them to appropriate resources for information about available treatments. This attention will help the patient and family consider all the benefits and risks and make an informed decision about the best option.

The concern for protection of minors from exploitation is still another obstacle. Treating children in a clinical trial is a special challenge to the research nurse and doctor. Children must be studied to make appropriate treatments available (American Academy of Pediatrics, 1977); indeed, many successful therapies have been pioneered in pediatric oncology. Many of the principles of cancer therapy were established initially in clinical trials involving children (Fletcher, Eyes, & Dorn, 1988). For example, the notion that combinations of drugs could be given in a cyclical fashion to allow for bone marrow nadir and recovery was first tested in childhood leukemias and only later was applied successfully to adults with lymphoma and solid tumors. Clinical trials involving children were the first to establish that teams of surgeons, radiotherapists, and chemotherapists could work together to limit treatment effects without compromising care. These principles, first established in children with soft-tissue sarcomas, were only later applied to adults with breast, bladder, and head and neck cancers. In addition, clinical trials involving children established the principles of supportive care for the febrile, neutropenic patient.

However, emotional response by all involved with the child's care may interfere with the best individual treatment decision. The nurse can play a central role in helping families explore options and evaluate what is best for the child so that the family can make the most informed decision (Cogliano-Shutta, 1986).

Box 25–4. PUBLIC ATTITUDES TOWARD RESEARCH PARTICIPATION

STUDY

Cassileth, B., Lusk, E., Miller, D., & Hurwitz, S. (1982). **Attitudes toward clinical trials among patients and the public.** *Journal of the American Medical Association, 248,* 968–970.

SAMPLE

Total population of 295 subjects, including 104 patients with cancer, 84 cardiology patients, and 107 members of the general public in Philadelphia, Pennsylvania.

MEASURES

Self-report questionnaire of ten multiple-choice questions and one open-ended item regarding opinions on the purpose and ethical status of contemporary clinical research.

FINDINGS

Seventy-one per cent of respondents believed that patients should serve as research subjects to make an important contribution to society. The majority felt that research would increase medical knowledge and help future patients and that any patient could participate. Respondents viewed clinical trials as important, ethical, and a means of attaining superior care.

LIMITATIONS

Participants were being seen at a major university hospital and may view research differently from those in other settings. Additional public participants were selected from nonhealth, nonuniversity jobs but may not be a representative sample because selection for participation was not described. The majority of those responding in the study were white. It would be of interest to repeat a similar study in minority populations in which high incidences of cancer occur.

NURSING RESPONSIBILITIES

Providing information to the patient and family is only one of many responsibilities of the nurse in a research setting as part of the research team. Nurses make significant contributions to the success of clinical investigations by implementing various roles. The first role is that of a staff nurse. The staff nurse is the primary caregiver for the patient. The staff nurse has varied levels of education and experience; administratively, he or she is under the head nurse of a unit or an outpatient area. A nurse who has developed additional skills and has pursued an advanced educational degree may become a clinical nurse specialist in a research setting. The clinical nurse specialist role is that of a consultant, educator, and developer of advanced clinical practice skills. This nurse usually answers to the head nurse or director of the nursing service. The research nurse performs a variation of these roles. This nurse may or may not have an advanced educational degree, may work directly for physicians or nurses, and most often has advanced practice experience. The other role of a nurse in a research setting is that of data manager. Other types of persons can be hired to do the data retrieval and reporting often done by data managers; these positions do not have to be filled by nurses. Data managers often report administratively to the principal investigators of the research study or to the research nurse. As part of the research team, each of these nurses will assume certain responsibilities, depending on the role being implemented (Table 25–5).

Advocacy

Nurses can serve as advocates for patients considering participation in clinical trials. The nurse can be a liaison between the physician and the patient. The nurse identifies concerns, resolves conflicts, or assists as questions develop. Written information such as *What Are Clinical Trials All About?* (Nealon, 1986) is available to patients to assist them in understanding what is involved in participating in clinical trials. This booklet as well as information about disease and treatment alternatives and clarification of unclear information can promote informed patient participation. Printed materials can be obtained by calling the Cancer Information Service at 1–800–4–CANCER.

Informed Consent

Informed consent is a legal and ethical prerequisite for patient participation in clinical trials (see Table 25–4). The nurse is ideally situated to evaluate the patient's understanding of the study and to determine that the decision to participate has indeed been voluntary. The manner in which information is conveyed is important. Consideration of the patient's age, level of education, cultural background, or lack of knowledge may modify the process of obtaining informed consent.

There are always risks associated with experimental treatments (Chabner, Wittes, Hoth, & Hubbard, 1984). It is the responsibility of the principal investigator to develop a complete, clear consent form that states all possible risks known about the agents used in the study. The physician is responsible for seeing that the patient understands the available options, potential risks, and benefits of the treatment alternatives. The consent should be read by the patient, explained by the physician, and clarified by the nurse. Informed consent is a dynamic educative process and is often achieved through oral and written explanations (Varricchio & Jassak, 1989). The informed consent must be signed by the patient and witnessed. The witness can only verify that the signature is that of the patient, not that the patient understands all that is written. Collaboration of the nurse with the rest of the health care team is essential to ensuring that an individual has knowingly consented to medical treatment.

Monitoring

The nurse in a research setting is also responsible for monitoring patients during the study. Depending on the role of the nurse, monitoring may include various kinds of assessment, planning, and documentation. For example, the research nurse and the clinical nurse specialist might review a protocol to monitor the impact of that study on nursing care. A proposed study might include a new method for delivery of drugs, such as intraperitoneal administration which might require in-service demonstrations, changes in policies and procedures, and new equipment for protocol implementation. All nurses should be monitoring patients for how well the patient fits the eligibility criteria of the study. One of the goals of the principal investigator should be to maximize the number of patients who can be evaluated in the study. The nurse's roles may include preparing the patient for studies required to document protocol eligibility and ensuring protocol compliance.

Monitoring responsibilities also include assessing the side effects of treatment on a frequent basis to document the physical and psychological responses of the patient. The staff nurse is often the first to notice unusual or expected symptoms and should report them to the research nurse or the principal investigator. Grading of toxicities such as nausea and vomiting (on a scale of 1 to 4, as in Table 25–6) promotes improved recognition of trends in the study population. Laboratory tests seem to be one of the easiest side effects to quantify and monitor routinely. Monitoring of patients on clinical trials is critical to the accuracy of study results.

Documenting

Side effects of cancer treatment are often noted by the staff nurse. Documentation on the patient's chart

Table 25–5. THE NURSE IN A RESEARCH SETTING

Type	Role	Responsibilities
Staff nurse	Primary caregiver	Knowledge of preclinical information and rationale for basis of study Provision of patient care with optimal safety and comfort Clinical expertise with assessment skills that promote recognition of side effects Patient education Assistance with ensuring informed consent Patient advocacy Documentation of treatment and disease effects Referral to appropriate resources Continuity of care and long-term follow-up Knowledge and application of ethical considerations Awareness of attitudes about research (self) Administration of treatment
Clinical nurse specialist (CNS)	Consultant Educator Advanced practice	Assessment of impact of medical research on nursing responsibilities Planning for implementation of research Preparation and guidance of staff caring for patients Education of staff about theory, rationale, and objectives of research Problem solving Patient and staff advocate Rapid dissemination of information on advances in practice and research Awareness of attitudes about research (self and staff)
Research nurse	Collaborator Liaison	Participate in study design and execution Coordinate smooth implementation of study Assist CNS with education of staff and patients Develop teaching materials specific to protocol Pharmacokinetics Collaboration with all health care resources Liaison between patient and physician, nurse and physician relationships and concerns Awareness of attitudes about research (self and others) Liaison to drug companies and Cancer Therapy Evaluation Program Collection of patient data, review of medical records Monitor trends in side effects for early recognition of response to treatment Assist with data analysis and interpretation Advocate for patient and protocol Assist with summarizing of data for publication
Data manager	Management of research information	Design of data report forms Retrieval of patient information for summary Data entry onto forms or into computer for analysis Analysis of data

is critical to the evaluation of the experimental treatment. Toxicity is generally documented on a scale of 1 to 4, with 4 being the most severe (Vietti, 1980). Standardization of toxicity reporting allows a comparison of toxic effects of various regimens as well as an identification of unacceptable, intolerable, or life-threatening toxicities. Development of standard forms for reporting data promotes computer entry of data and easier analysis. Documentation should include type of toxicity, severity, when the toxicity occurred, and its duration.

Data Management

Nurses in some institutions have assumed the added responsibility of abstracting data from charts. Data collection completed as soon as possible after it is generated ensures data accuracy, protocol compliance, and correction of procedural requirements while the study is in progress. Regular review of data is essential so that unsuspected toxicity or protocol infractions can be noted early. For multi-institutional trials, procedures for ensuring the accuracy and safety of data reporting are implemented. Site visits for training may

be required. Mechanisms for reporting problems and accessing information should be established. Nurses may assist in the collection and analysis of data and the publication of results.

Nursing Research

The nurse in a research setting has opportunities to collaborate as part of the research team, often as a coinvestigator. This role promotes the understanding of the research process and offers opportunities for incorporating nursing issues into medical protocols. Improvement of nursing care to patients may help decrease toxicities of treatment and thus promote greater utilization of medical research results in the community. Examples of research challenges and programs for nurses in the practice setting are provided by Hinshaw (1987). Nursing research may focus on methods of controlling nausea and vomiting, stomatitis, or pain, all of which may decrease treatment morbidity.

Communication

Education, support, administration of therapy, and prevention of toxicity for the patient with cancer re-

Table 25–6. COMMON TOXICITY CRITERIA

Organ/System	Toxicity	Grade				
		0	1	2	3	4
Blood and bone marrow	White blood count	≥4.0	3.0–3.9	2.0–2.9	1.0–1.9	<1.0
	Platelet count	WNL	75.0–normal	50.0–74.9	25.0–49.9	<25.0
	Hemoglobin	WNL	10.0–normal	8.0–10.0	6.5–7.9	<6.5
	Granulocytes/ bands	≥2.0	1.5–1.9	1.0–1.4	0.5–0.9	<0.5
	Lymphocytes	≥2.0	1.5–1.9	1.0–1.4	0.5–0.9	<0.5
	Hemorrhage (clinical)	None	Mild, no transfusion	Gross, 1 to 2 units transfusion per episode	Gross, 3 to 4 units transfusion per episode	Massive, >4 units transfusion per episode
	Infection	None	Mild	Moderate	Severe	Life threatening
Gastrointestinal	Nausea	None	Able to eat Reasonable intake	Intake significantly decreased but can eat	No significant intake	—
	Vomiting	None	1 episode in 24 hr	2 to 5 episodes in 24 hr	6 to 10 episodes in 24 hr	>10 episodes in 24 hr, or requiring parenteral support
	Diarrhea	None	Increase of 2 to 3 stools/day over pretreatment	Increase of 4 to 6 stools/day, or nocturnal stools, or moderate cramping	Increase of 7 to 9 stools/day, or incontinence, or severe cramping	Increase of ≥10 stools/day or grossly bloody diarrhea, or need for parenteral support
	Stomatitis	None	Painless ulcers, erythema, or mild soreness	Painful erythema, edema, or ulcers but can eat	Painful erythema, edema, or ulcers and cannot eat	Requires parenteral or enteral support
Liver	Bilirubin	WNL	—	<1.5 × N	1.5–3.0 × N	>3.0 × N
	Transaminase (SGOT, SGPT)	WNL	≤2.5 × N	2.6–5.0 × N	5.1–20.0 × N	>20.0 × N
	Alkaline phosphatase or 5' nucleotidase	WNL	≤2.5 × N	2.6–5.0 × N	5.1–20.0 × N	>20.0 × N
	Liver—clinical	No change from baseline	—	—	Precoma	Hepatic coma
Kidney, bladder	Creatinine	WNL	<1.5 × N	1.5–3.0 × N	3.1–6.0 × N	>6.0 × N
	Proteinuria	No change	1+ or <3 g/L	2–3+ or 3–10 g/L	4+ or >10 g/L	Nephrotic syndrome
	Hematuria	Negative	Microscopic only	Gross, no clots	Gross, clots	Requires transfusion
	Alopecia	No loss	Mild hair loss	Pronounced or total hair loss	—	—
	Pulmonary	None or no change	Asymptomatic, with abnormality in pulmonary function tests	Dyspnea on significant exertion	Dyspnea at normal level of activity	Dyspnea at rest
Heart	Cardiac dysrhythmias	None	Asymptomatic; transient requiring no therapy	Recurrent or persistent; no therapy required	Requires treatment	Requires monitoring; or hypotension, or ventricular tachycardia, fibrillation
	Cardiac function	None	Asymptomatic; decline of resting ejection fraction by less than 20% of baseline value	Asymptomatic; decline of resting ejection fraction by more than 20% of baseline value	Mild congestive heart failure, responsive to therapy	Severe or refractory congestive heart failure

Table continued on following page

Table 25–6. COMMON TOXICITY CRITERIA *Continued*

Organ/System	Toxicity	Grade 0	1	2	3	4
	Cardiac—ischemia	None	Nonspecific T-wave flattening	Asymptomatic, ST and T wave changes, suggesting ischemia	Angina without evidence for infarction	Acute myocardial infarction
	Cardiac—pericardial	None	Asymptomatic effusion; no intervention required	Pericarditis (rub, chest pain, electrocardiogram changes)	Symptomatic effusion; drainage required	Tamponade; drainage urgently required
Blood pressure	Hypertension	None or no change	Asymptomatic, transient increase of more than 20 mm Hg (D) or to >150/100 if previously WNL. No treatment required	Recurrent or persistent increase of more than 20 mm Hg (D) or to >150/100 if previously WNL. No treatment required	Requires therapy	Hypertensive crisis
	Hypotension	None or no change	Changes requiring no therapy (including transient orthostatic hypotension)	Requires fluid replacement or other therapy but not hospitalization	Requires therapy and hospitalization; resolves within 48 hr of stopping the agent	Requires therapy and hospitalization for >48 hrs after stopping the agent
Neurologic	Neuro—sensory	None or no change	Mild paresthesias; loss of deep tendon reflexes	Mild or moderate objective sensory loss; moderate paresthesias	Severe objective sensory loss or paresthesias that interfere with functioning	—
	Neuro—motor	None or no change	Subjective weakness; no objective findings	Mild objective weakness without significant impairment of function	Objective weakness with impairment of function	Paralysis
	Neuro—cortical	None	Mild somnolence or agitation	Moderate somnolence or agitation	Severe somnolence, agitation, confusion, disorientation, or hallucinations	Coma, seizures, toxic psychosis
	Neuro—cerebellar	None	Slight incoordination, dysdiadokinesis	Intention tremor, dysmetria, slurred speech, nystagmus	Locomotor ataxia	Cerebellar necrosis
	Neuro—mood	No change	Mild anxiety or depression	Moderate anxiety or depression	Severe anxiety or depression	Suicidal ideation
	Neuro—headache	None	Mild	Moderate or severe but transient	Unrelenting and severe	—
	Neuro—constipation	None or no change	Mild	Moderate	Severe	Ileus >96 hr
	Neuro—hearing	None or no change	Asymptomatic; hearing loss on audiometry only	Tinnitus	Hearing loss interfering with functioning but correctable with hearing aid	Deafness not correctable
	Neuro—vision	None or no change	—	—	Symptomatic subtotal loss of vision	Blindness

Table 25–6. COMMON TOXICITY CRITERIA *Continued*

Organ/System	Toxicity	Grade 0	1	2	3	4
	Skin	None or no change	Scattered macular or papular eruption or erythema that is asymptomatic	Scattered macular or papular eruption or erythema with pruritus or other associated symptoms	Generalized symptomatic macular, papular, or vesicular eruption	Exfoliative dermatitis or ulcerating dermatitis
	Allergy	None	Transient rash, drug fever <38° C (100.4° F)	Urticaria, drug fever = 38° C (100.4° F); mild bronchospasm	Serum sickness, bronchospasm requiring parenteral medication	Anaphylaxis
	Fever in absence of infection	None	37.1–38.0° C. (98.7–100.4° F)		>40.0°C >104.0°F less than 24 hr	>40.0° C (104.0° F) for more than 24 hr or fever accompanied by hypotension
	Local	None	Pain	Pain and swelling with inflammation or phlebitis	Ulceration	Plastic surgery indicated
Metabolic	Weight gain or loss	<5.0%	5.0–9.9%	10.0–19.9%	≥20.0%	—
	Hyperglycemia	<116	116–160	161–250	251–500	>500 or ketoacidosis
	Hypoglycemia	>64	55–64	40–54	30–39	<30
	Amylase	WNL	$<1.5 \times N$	$1.5–2.0 \times N$	$2.1–5.0 \times N$	$>5.1 \times N$
	Hypercalcemia	<10.6	10.6–11.5	11.6–12.5	12.6–13.5	≥13.5
	Hypocalcemia	>8.4	8.4–7.8	7.7–7.0	6.9–6.1	≤6.0
	Hypomagnesemia	>1.4	1.4–1.2	1.1–0.9	0.8–0.6	≤0.5
Coagulation	Fibrinogen	WNL	$0.99–0.75 \times N$	$0.74–0.50 \times N$	$0.49–0.25 \times N$	$<0.24 \times N$
	Prothrombin time	WNL	$1.01–1.25 \times N$	$1.26–1.50 \times N$	$1.51–2.00 \times N$	$>2.00 \times N$
	Partial thromboplastin time	WNL	$1.01–1.66 \times N$	$1.67–2.33 \times N$	$2.34–3.00 \times N$	$>3.00 \times N$

WNL, within normal limits; SGOT, serum glutamic-oxaloacetic transaminase; SGPT, serum glutamic-pyruvic transaminase; N, normal or control.
(Unpublished table developed by CTEP. Dr. M. Friedman, personal communication.)

quire special skills and a trusting relationship between patient and nurse. Relationships with physicians involved in research are also based on effective communication, trust, and mutual respect. Collaboration in design, implementation, and follow-up of trials demonstrates recognition that nursing care, education, and research are critical to protocol results. Collaboration is a logical outgrowth when physicians and nurses have shared clinical goals and responsibilities (Hubbard & Donehower, 1980).

Relationships between the research (protocol) nurse and other staff nurses require good communication. Discussion among all health care providers of side effects noted may point out similarities or trends in patients on a specific protocol that should be reported to the investigator. Educational and emotional support for nurses during implementation of protocols that involve high toxicity or require technical skill is essential to maintaining adequate, safe care of patients and in preventing added stress. Stress can result in decreased quality of care as well as significant staff

problems, such as low morale, job dissatisfaction, and high turnover rates (Sarantos, 1988). Aggressive clinical trials may require considerable nursing support of patients, physicians, and one another.

THE IMPORTANCE OF CLINICAL TRIALS

Only a small percentage of cancer patients participate in clinical trials, although such trials often offer the best available cancer treatment (Gross, 1986). Indeed, less than 1 per cent of eligible cancer patients will enter clinical studies. Currently 25,000 patients in the United States are being followed on clinical trials (National Institutes of Health, 1986). Nurses can have an important role in increasing patient awareness of the advantages of clinical trials both for individuals in terms of improved care and for society through the advancement of the understanding of cancer and its treatment. The NCI is planning selected studies designed to enroll larger numbers of patients with the help of community nurses and physicians. These studies will be simple in design and will require minimal statistical support, but they may be able to answer important questions, such as the appropriate duration of hormonal adjuvant therapy for breast cancer patients. Other trials that require more extensive data management and oversight will address the effectiveness of primary adjuvant treatment for patients with lung, head and neck, breast, colon, rectal, and bladder cancers. These trials will have considerable significance for more than 175,000 Americans each year and will be coordinated in national trial efforts through the NCI's cooperative group program.

PRIORITIES IN CANCER CARE

Broader use of clinical trials is one of the many approaches being used to meet the NCI's goal for the year 2000 of reducing cancer mortality by 50 per cent (National Institutes of Health, 1985). Priorities for future clinical trials will focus on immunology, drug resistance, and molecular biology. New drugs will continue to be developed. Transfer of research results to practice offers a continuing challenge to the nurse to be aware of the best treatment alternatives, the newer modes of therapy, and the effects of each on the patient.

SUMMARY

The process of research is a long, expensive, yet exciting road to advancement in the care of patients with cancer. The total time of bringing a treatment from initial screening to commercial availability can last as long as 14 years and can cost between $50 and 70 million (Gross, 1986). The NCI and the FDA are working to accelerate the availability of new drugs through revision of the regulatory process and improvement of participation in clinical trials (Kessler, 1989). As nursing participation in clinical trials increases, the nursing role as principal or coinvestigator in studies dealing with patients' responses to therapy will expand. There are many unknowns in research that challenge and stimulate nurses wanting to become involved in caring for patients in clinical trials. As members of the research team, nurses can utilize assessment, technical, psychosocial, and intellectual skills to advance and contribute to scientific knowledge and thus to overall quality patient care.

References

American Academy of Pediatrics. (1977). Guidelines for the ethical conduct of studies to evaluate drugs in pediatric populations. *Pediatrics, 60,* 10-1–10.11.

Buyse, M., Staquet, M., & Sylvester, R. (1984). *Cancer clinical trial, methods, and practice.* New York: Oxford University Press.

Cancer Therapy Evaluation Program. (1986). *Investigator's handbook.* Washington, DC: National Cancer Institute.

Cassileth, B., Lusk, E., Miller, D., & Hurwitz, S. (1982). Attitudes toward clinical trials among patients and the public. *Journal of the American Medical Association, 248,* 968–970.

Chabner, B., Wittes, R., Hoth, D., & Hubbard, S. (1984). Investigational trials of anticancer drugs: Establishing safeguards for experimentation. *Public Health Reports, 99,* 355–360.

Cogliano-Shutta, N. (1986). Pediatric phase 1 clinical trials: Ethical issues and nursing considerations. *Oncology Nursing Forum, 13*(2), 29–32.

Collins, J. (1988). Pharmacology and drug development. *Journal of the National Cancer Institute, 80,* 790–792.

Collins, J., Zaharko, D., Dedrick, R., & Chabner, B. (1986). Potential roles for preclinical pharmacology in phase 1 clinical trials. *Cancer Treatment Reports, 70,* 73–80.

Deininger, H., Collins, J., & Hubbard, S. (1989). Nurses and PDQ: What's in it for you? *Oncology Nursing Forum, 16,* 547–552.

DeVita, V. (1982). *Cancer treatment* (NIH Publication No. 82-1807). Washington, DC. U.S. Government Printing Office.

DeVita, V., Oliverio, V., Muggia, F., Wiernik, P., Ziegler, J., Goldin, A., Rubin, D., Henney, J., & Shepartz, S. (1979). The drug development and clinical trials programs of the division of cancer treatment, National Cancer Institute. *Cancer Clinical Trials, 2,* 195–216.

Ellerberg, S., & Eisenberger, M. (1985). An efficient design for phase III studies of combination chemotherapies. *Cancer Treatment Reports, 69,* 1147–1152.

Fletcher, J., Eyes, J., & Dorn, L. (1988). Ethical considerations in pediatric oncology. In P. Pizzo and D. Poplack (Eds.), *Principles and practice of pediatric oncology* (pp. 309–320). Philadelphia: J. B. Lippincott Co.

Gargaro, W. (1978). Informed consent. *Cancer Nursing, 1,* 467–468.

Gelber, R., & Goldhirsch, A. (1989). Can a clinical trial be the treatment of choice for patients with cancer. *Journal of the National Cancer Institute, 80,* 886–887.

Gross, J. (1986). Clinical research in cancer chemotherapy. *Oncology Nursing Forum, 13,* 59–65.

Hender, W. (1985). The impact of future technology on oncologic diagnosis. In D. Bragg, P. Rubin, & J. Youker (Eds.), *Oncologic imaging* (pp. 629–644). New York: Pergamon Press.

Hinshaw, A. (1987). Research challenges and programs for practice settings. *Journal of Nursing Administration, 17*(7, 8), 20–26.

Hubbard, S. (1981). Chemotherapy and the cancer nurse. In L. Marino (Ed.), *Cancer nursing* (pp. 287–343). St. Louis: C. V. Mosby Co.

Hubbard S. (1982). Cancer treatment research: The role of the nurse in clinical trials of cancer therapy. *Nursing Clinics of North America, 17,* 763–783.

Hubbard, S. (1985). Principles of clinical research. In B. Johnson & J. Gross (Eds.), *Handbook of oncology nursing* (pp. 67–92). New York: John Wiley & Sons, Inc.

Hubbard, S., & Donehower, M. (1980). The nurse in a cancer research setting. *Seminars in Oncology, 7,* 9–17.

Hubbard, S., Henney, J., & DeVita, V. (1987). A computer data base for information on cancer treatment. *New England Journal of Medicine, 316,* 315–318.

Kessler, D. (1989). The regulation of investigational drugs. *New England Journal of Medicine, 320,* 281–288.

Levine, R. (1981). *Ethics and regulations of clinical research.* Baltimore: Urban & Schwarzenberg.

Levine, R. (1986). Referral of patients with cancer for participation in randomized clinical trials: Ethical considerations. *CA: A Cancer Journal for Clinicians, 36,* 95–99.

Meisel, A., & Roth, L. (1981). What we do and do not know about informed consent. *Journal of the American Medical Association, 246,* 2473–2477.

National Cancer Institute. (1986a). *NCI fact book.* Washington, D.C.: Author.

National Cancer Institute. (1986b). *Report of the division of cancer treatment.* Washington, D.C.: Author.

National Institutes of Health. (1985). *NCI program 1983–84 directors report and annual plan 1986–1990.* (NIH publication #85-2765). Washington, D.C.: U.S. Government Printing Office.

National Institutes of Health. (1986). *DCT program information booklet fiscal year 1986.* Washington, D.C.: National Cancer Institute.

Nealon, E. (1986). *What are clinical trials all about?* (NIH Publication No. 86–2706). Washington, D.C.: U.S. Government Printing Office.

Ochs, J., Mulhern, R., & Kun, L. (1988). Quality of life assessment in cancer patients. *American Journal of Clinical Oncology, 11,* 415–421.

Sarantos, S. (1988). Innovations in psychosocial staff support: A model program for the marrow transplant nurse. *Seminars in Oncology Nursing, 4*(1), 69–73.

Simon, R., Wittes, R., & Ellenberg, S. (1985). Randomized phase II clinical trials. *Cancer Treatment Reports, 69,* 1375–1381.

Taylor, K., Maegolese, R., & Soskolne, C. (1985). Physicians reasons for not entering eligible patients in a randomized trial of surgery for breast cancer. *New England Journal of Medicine, 310,* 1363–1367.

Varricchio, C., & Jassak, P. (1989). Informed consent: An overview. *Seminars in Oncology Nursing, 5*(2), 95–98.

Vietti, T. (1980). Evaluation of toxicity: clinical issues. *Cancer Treatment Reports, 64,* 457–461.

Wittes, R., & Friedman, M. R. (1988). Accrual to clinical trials. *Journal of the National Cancer Institute, 80,* 884–885.

Young, R. (1981). Role of the FDA in cancer therapy research. *Seminars in Oncology, 8,* 447–452.

CHAPTER 26

Blood Component Therapy

PATRICIA F. JASSAK
JOHN GODWIN

The clinical practice of blood transfusion is a development of the latter half of the twentieth century. Practical problems of blood cell typing, cross-matching, development of blood anticoagulants, refrigeration, and storage in plastic were not solved until the 1950s and early 1960s. Twenty-five years later, in 1985, approximately 14,500,000 total blood components were transfused in the United States.

Blood component therapy plays an integral role in the comprehensive care of cancer patients. Advances in the use of blood components have affected the overall survival rate of cancer patients by contributing to the success of new cancer treatments associated with prolonged myelosuppression. One prominent example is the increasing use of bone marrow transplantation since the 1970s (see Chapter 27). Improved responses with combination chemotherapy in chemosensitive tumors have led to the search for even better results, requiring increased dose intensity and supportive transfusion therapy. Intensive transfusion support and the development of new methods to promote blood cell production with cytokines will further the successful development of other new cancer therapies.

The safety of blood products has become a national concern since the recognition in 1982 of the transmission of acquired immune deficiency syndrome (AIDS) by blood transfusion (see Chapter 41). This concern is especially acute in the cancer patient who is frequently exposed to large numbers of blood components. The use of autologous blood (self-donated) in clinical settings has dramatically increased in response to the AIDS crisis. However, the cancer patient is not usually a candidate for autologous donation owing to disease and therapy-related bone marrow depression. In cancer patients, the risk of AIDS transmission by transfusion can be reduced by ensuring donor selectivity, the use of newer screening methods to detect the AIDS virus, and the development of growth factors to promote autologous cell production and decrease transfusion need.

This chapter reviews the principles of blood component therapy with particular attention to the cancer patient. Blood components and the techniques of their administration are described. Practical points are illustrated with clinical examples and reference tables.

BASIC PRINCIPLES OF TRANSFUSION

The most common indication for transfusion in the cancer patient is bone marrow depression (see Chapter 49). *Bone marrow depression* is a general term used to describe a decrease in blood cell production from the marrow. This is in contrast to the various causes of increased cell destruction or sequestration that can occur (e.g., DIC or splenomegaly). Bone marrow depression is manifested as a decrease in one or more blood cell lines (e.g., anemia, thrombocytopenia, or granulocytopenia). The usual cause of bone marrow depression in the cancer patient is the malignancy itself, the therapies the patient is given for cancer, or a nutritional deficiency state. Specific terms for the common types of bone marrow depression are (1) *dysmyelopoiesis*, a primary defect in the bone marrow cells responsible for blood cell formation; (2) *myelophthisis*, a metastatic solid tumor or fibrosis infiltrating the bone marrow; and (3) *myelosuppression*, a chemotherapy- or radiotherapy-induced temporary reduction in the rapidly growing cells in the bone marrow. Nutritional causes of bone marrow depression, such as vitamin B_{12} and iron deficiency, are less commonly seen in the cancer patient. However, nutritional causes should not be overlooked because they are easily reversible.

The need for understanding the basic cause of bone marrow depression in the patient is that some idea of the clinical course and transfusion requirements can be determined from this knowledge. For example, in a patient with myelosuppression, temporary transfusion support is required until the marrow recovers. In myelophthisis, the strategy is to try to reverse the infiltration or fibrosis, if possible, while supporting the patient with transfusions. In dysmyelopoiesis the patient will not recover normal marrow function unless the disorder is cured (e.g., by bone marrow transplant in patients who are eligible). The usual strategy in dysmyelopoiesis is to provide supportive transfusions on an indefinite basis.

Knowledge of the patient's type of cancer will also enable the medical team to anticipate transfusion needs. Different transfusion requirements can be anticipated among malignancies owing to the manifestations of the disease itself or the specific treatment strategies employed. The leukemic patient, for example, requires different blood component support from the patient with a solid tumor. The cardinal feature of leukemia is failure of one or more cell lines in the bone marrow to be produced, whereas solid tumors cause direct bone marrow depression much less frequently. Different treatment strategies for the leukemic patient also result in different transfusion requirements. Leukemic patients are given chemotherapy despite the presence of severe cytopenia. However, when severe cytopenia occurs in patients with solid tumors or other hematologic malignancies, the treatment regimen is usually adjusted by decreasing the dose, extending the length of the recovery period, or doing both. This solution results in less severe marrow depression in solid tumor patients and in a shorter duration of transfusion support for myelosuppression.

SOURCES OF BLOOD COLLECTION

Blood components are available from three different donor sources: homologous, autologous, or directed (designated) donors. Homologous blood is obtained from the general pool of volunteer donors—or, less commonly, paid donors—and is currently the most common source of blood components for patients. Autologous blood is the recipient's own blood that was donated before its anticipated use. Directed or designated donor blood is obtained when the recipient selects or recruits a specific person for blood donation.

When a potential blood donor is seen in a collection center, community blood drive, or hospital, a prescreening interview and tests are conducted to determine donor eligibility. These include an assessment of age, weight, health status, medication use, prior donation history, adequate hemoglobin, and standard blood pressure, pulse, and temperature. Questions are asked to determine past medical history and the presence of risk factors for the development of disease. Persons with a history of certain diseases—e.g., hepatitis—are permanently ineligible candidates for donation. People with known risk factors for transmissible disease (e.g., AIDS or hepatitis) are asked to voluntarily remove themselves from the donor pool. Today most centers allow donors the option of indicating confidentially that their blood should be discarded without specifying a reason.

Directed donor programs have been established in response to the AIDS crisis and are actually mandated by law in some states. Directed donor and homologous units are screened for transmissible diseases and tested for compatibility (Widmann, 1985). When screening tests are positive, the blood units are discarded and the donor informed confidentially. If red blood cell (RBC) incompatibility between the directed donor and the specified recipient is determined, and test results for transmissible disease are negative, the blood is released to the general donor pool.

Autologous donations are recommended to patients undergoing elective surgical procedures. These patients donate a number of units of blood during the month before the anticipated need (Pisciotto, 1989). Autologous transfusions have dramatically increased since the recognition of the transmission of human immunodeficiency virus (HIV) in blood products.

RED BLOOD CELL COMPATIBILITY TESTING

The purpose of red blood cell compatibility testing is to prevent the destruction of the transfused cells. When this destruction occurs, it is called a hemolytic transfusion reaction. To understand compatibility testing it is necessary to briefly review certain concepts of immunology.

An antigen is a molecule that is recognized as foreign ("nonself") by the immune system. *Simply put, an antigen distinguishes self from nonself.* Antigens stimulate B cells of the immune system to produce antibodies and also sensitize monocytes and T cells to react with the antigen. Antibodies are a family of proteins that have in common the ability to bind to antigens. *Antibodies recognize antigens as nonself.* Antigen-antibody binding is one of the major ways that the immune system eliminates foreign substances. Hemolytic transfusion reactions are triggered by antigen-antibody binding. The successful practice of blood transfusion was made possible by the understanding of which red cells were recognized as "foreign" and which were accepted as like "self."

Early in the history of transfusion, it was found that blood from an animal administered to humans was rapidly hemolyzed and the recipient became critically ill. The cells were recognized as foreign by the recipient. However, it was not understood why some attempts at transfusion from one person to another were successful and others failed. In 1900 Landsteiner (1901) found that human red cells will react with the sera of some persons and not others (Box 26-1). He described blood types that were different by virtue of the presence of different red blood cell antigens. He recognized three different blood types, which he called A, B, and O (a fourth group, AB, was later added by Landsteiner's pupils). Red cells contain either an A or B antigen, both, or neither (group O), and serum con-

---

Box 26–1. DISCOVERY OF THE BLOOD GROUPS

Karl Landsteiner is one of twentieth-century medicine's greatest scientists. He is most remembered for his discovery of the blood groups, for which he received the Nobel Prize in Medicine in 1930. In 1900 scientists were beginning to question the phenomena of nature that distinguished one cell from another. Landsteiner was especially interested in differences between cells of the same species. His observations first appeared as a footnote in a paper "Zur Kenntnis der antifermentativen, . . . Blutserums und der Lymphe" (Contribution to the knowledge of the antienzymatic lytic and agglutinating effects of the blood serum and lymph"): "The serum of healthy persons not only has an agglutinating effect on animal corpuscles, but also on human blood corpuscles from different individuals. . . ." The publication of his studies appeared in a later paper: "Über Agglutinationserscheinungen normalen menschlichen Blutes" ("Agglutination phenomena in normal human blood"). In this paper he presented the concept of blood groups in a simple table titled "Concerning the Blood of Six Apparently Healthy Males" (+ denotes agglutination):

Serum from:	Blood cells from:					
	Dr. St.	Dr. Plecn.	Dr. Sturl.	Dr. Erdh.	Zar.	Landst.
Dr. St.	−	+	+	+	+	−
Dr. Plecn.	−	−	+	+	−	−
Dr. Sturl.	−	+	−	−	+	−
Dr. Erdh.	−	+	−	−	+	−
Zar.	−	−	+	+	−	−
Landst.	−	+	+	+	+	−

His interpretation is terse: "In a number of cases (group A), the serum reacts with the cells of another group (group B), but not with those of group A; these A cells are acted upon in the same manner by serum B. In the third group (C), the serum agglutinates the corpuscles of A and B, while the red cells of group C are not acted upon by the sera from A and B."

He was not only reporting the agglutination of one person's red cells by sera from another but also recognizing a pattern, and he concluded that there were two kinds of "agglutinins" (antibodies) in the sera and at least three different kinds of red cells. From the table it can be seen that Dr. Landsteiner was a group "C" or what we now call group O. The pattern of reactions was the key observation, and that fundamental observation has not changed with the passage of time. It was the first opening of one of nature's secrets.

---

tains antibodies to antigens not present on the person's red blood cells (Table 26–1). A great deal is now known about the specific molecular characterization of the ABO blood group antigens and their genetics.

ABO antigens are determined by specific carbohydrates on the developing red blood cell surface, whose synthesis is directed by enzymes from genes on chromosome 9. Initially Landsteiner thought that the O blood type (from the German word *öhne*, meaning "without") had no antigen. However, it is now known that type O has a precursor sugar termed H antigen. The antigens A and B are made by adding additional sugars to the H antigen.

More than 400 different antigens are present on the human red blood cell surface. Families of these antigens with similar antigenic and genetic properties form blood groups. Most of these blood group antigens have been detected serologically (i.e., by noting agglutination of red blood cells by adding serum samples). In

some cases, sera from animals immunized with red blood cells from different animal species are mixed with human red blood cells. The pattern of cross-reactivity of these sera with human cells from large numbers of people are examined to identify groups with common reactions (i.e., blood groups). In other cases, human sera from patients with hemolytic reactions are tested for their pattern of reaction with other human red blood cells. Such investigations were responsible for the discovery of another major blood group, the Rh system (Widmann, 1985). Rh was the name given by Landsteiner and Wiener to the human red blood cell antigen that showed reactivity with sera from animals immunized with red blood cells from the rhesus monkey (*Macaca mulatta*) (Fig. 26–1). Levine and Stetson independently reported an antibody, which later proved to be the same as anti-Rh, in the serum of a mother who had a stillborn infant. Rh antigen is important in hydrops fetalis and hemolytic disease of the newborn. Some blood group antigens are common to many people, and others are extremely rare. Examples of blood groups other than ABO and Rh include Kell, Duffy, Lutheran, and P.

Practical Aspects of Red Blood Cell Compatibility Testing

Each person has a complex red blood cell antigen pattern, and it would be difficult to match blood if all

Table 26–1. ABO BLOOD GROUP AND NATURALLY OCCURRING ANTIBODIES

Red Blood Cell Group	Frequency in Population (%)		Serum Antibody
	Whites	*Blacks*	
A	40	27	Anti-B
B	11	20	Anti-A
AB	4	4	None
O	45	49	Anti-A, anti-B

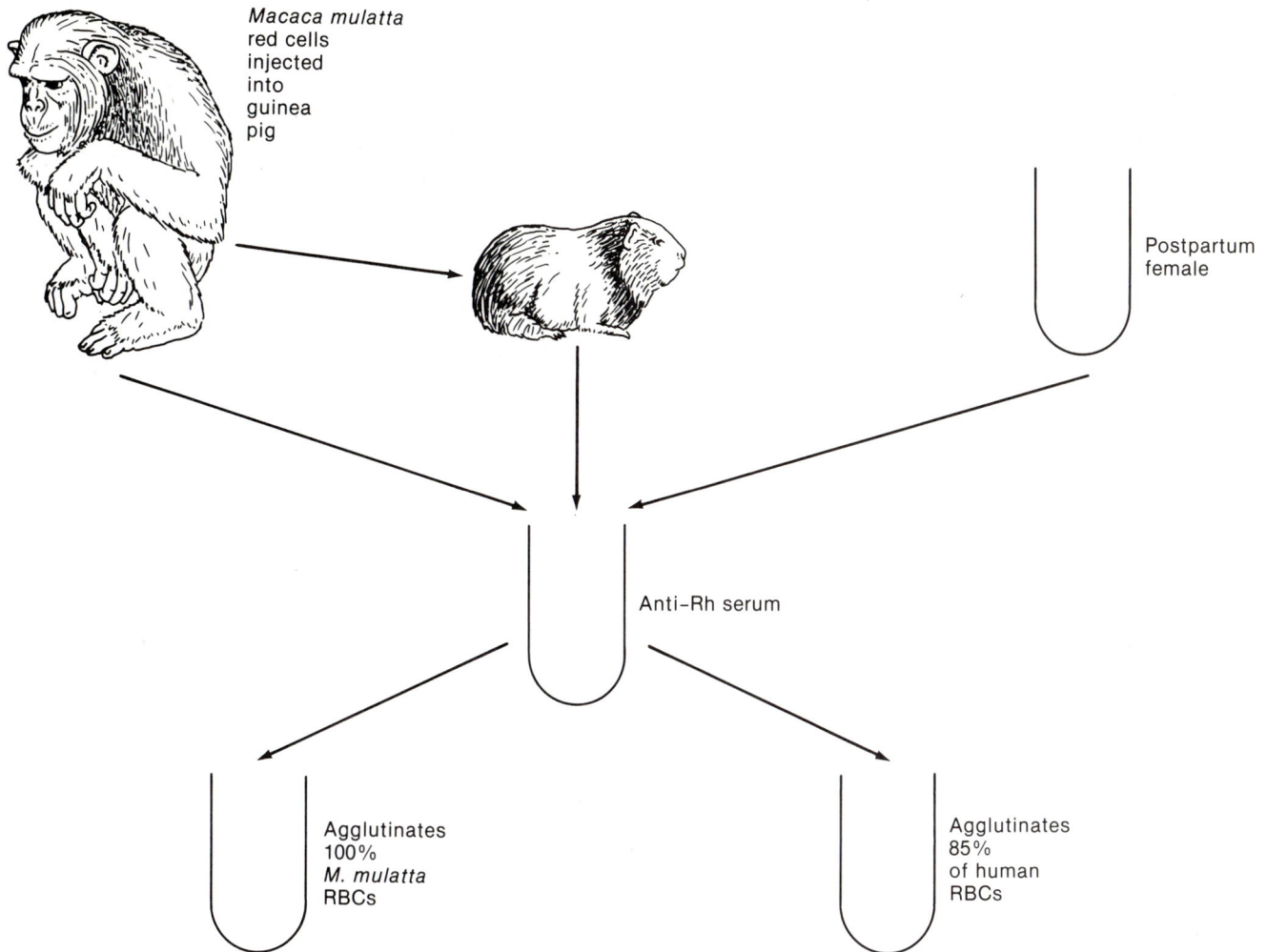

Figure 26–1. Discovery of the Rh blood groups. Landsteiner and Weiner immunized guinea pigs with red blood cells from rhesus monkeys *(Macaca mulatta)*. They found that the serum agglutinated 85 per cent of human red blood cells. They called the determinant on the red blood cells the *Rh factor.* Independently Levin found that the serum from postpartum females with hydrops fetalis agglutinated other human cells in a pattern similar to that of the anti-Rh serum from Landsteiner.

these antigens had to be typed. Although many of these antigens have been associated with hemolytic transfusion reactions, only a few are antigenic enough to commonly give rise to antibodies. Red blood cell compatibility testing involves a series of pretransfusion tests in the blood bank designed to detect antibodies against blood antigens in the recipient's serum and ensure the acceptance of the donor blood by the recipient. The "type and cross-match" order is a request for pretransfusion testing. There are four major parts to a type and cross-match (Table 26–2) (Rutman & Miller, 1985). The first step is to check the records for any previous transfusion.

The second step is to determine the recipient's blood type. In practice only two major blood groups are routinely determined in blood typing: ABO and Rh. ABO-incompatible blood is potentially the most dangerous transfusion, as more than 95 per cent of recipients have naturally occurring anti-A or anti-B antibodies, which can cause an immediate hemolytic reaction. The Rh antigen is highly immunogenic, and antibodies arise after exposure to the Rh antigen in Rh-negative persons. Exposure to the Rh antigen can occur from prior pregnancy or transfusion. Determination of the Rh type is important to prevent immunization in certain Rh negative groups. Rh-negative women of reproductive age should never receive Rh-positive blood, because the immune reaction could result in hemolytic disease of the newborn and death of the fetus in future pregnancies.

The third step is the antibody screen. The recipient's serum is tested for antibodies other than anti-A or anti-B by exposing the serum to a standardized panel of red blood cells, all group O, but with a mixture of the other common blood group antigens. A positive

Table 26–2. PRETRANSFUSION TESTING

Step	Procedure	Rationale
1	Previous records	Compare blood type; determine if prior alloantibody
2	Blood type	ABO, Rh are major groups needed to be determined
3	Antibody screen	Determine if alloantibody present
4	Cross-match	Donor cells and recipient serum

antibody screen means that the patient has antibodies to other blood group antigens, such as Kell or Duffy. These antibodies are termed *alloantibodies* and usually occur when the patient has a history of pregnancy or prior transfusion. Occasionally the presence of such alloantibodies may delay the availability of compatible blood. In some situations the pretransfusion testing is stopped at this point. This is commonly referred to as "type and screen" or "type and hold." Donor units of the same ABO-Rh group are not reserved on the blood bank shelf in response to a type and screen. However, units can be made available rapidly on request.

The fourth step is testing of the donor red cells and recipient serum for direct compatibility. Compatible units are then reserved for a short period of time, usually 24 to 48 hr.

It is always preferable to administer blood of the same type. However, in emergencies or shortages, blood of other ABO groups can be given. Group O recipients can only receive group O. Group A and Group B recipients can receive group O. Group AB can receive either A or B or O red blood cells, although A is more commonly given owing to its availability. Group O is preferrably not given to the AB patient because there is too great a need to use it for Group O persons. A summary of ABO compatible products is found in Table 26–3.

TISSUE COMPATIBILITY ANTIGENS (HLA)

The major histocompatibility antigens among humans are termed HLA (histocompatibility locus antigens). They are found on all cells except red blood cells and serve as tissue recognition sites (Dudjak, 1984). Human chromosome 6 contains several genes (loci) that code for different HLA antigens. The loci have been named HLA-A, HLA-B, and HLA-C. These genes code for the proteins that make up the cell surface antigens referred to as class I antigens. For

example, the HLA-A loci codes for antigens called A1, A2, A3, and so forth; HLA-B codes for BW22 or BW16, and so forth; and HLA-C codes for CW1 or CW2, and so forth. Each person has a pair of HLA genes coding for each of the A, B, and C class I antigens. As with red blood cell antigens, these antigens can be detected serologically by testing different sera using a patient's lymphocytes.

In transfusion therapy, these antigens play an important role when problems with platelet transfusion occur. One of the most common causes of an inadequate platelet increase after transfusion is immune platelet destruction. Multiple red blood cell or platelet transfusions expose the patient to numerous foreign HLA antigens. In some patients, an immune response occurs and alloantibodies (antibodies to other human antigens) to HLA-A, HLA-B, and HLA-C antigens develop (Gmur et al., 1983). These antibodies are responsible for the immune destruction of platelets. This is similar to the problem described earlier under red blood cell compatibilty testing. However, the antibodies that cause the destruction of transfused platelets react not against blood group antigens but instead against tissue antigens (i.e., the HLA) (Churchill & Kurtz, 1988; McLeod, 1980). Platelets contain small amounts of ABO antigens on their surface, but antibodies to red blood cell antigens do not cause increased platelet destruction. Strategies for managing patients with platelet alloantibodies (refractory responders) are identified in Table 26–4 (Menitove, 1983; Sniecinski, O'Donnell, Nowicki, & Hill, 1988).

BLOOD COMPONENTS AND THEIR ADMINSTRATION

Blood component therapy is the transfusion of a specific part of blood rather than whole blood and offers several advantages. First, it conserves precious resources; that is, one unit of donated whole blood provides several components. Dividing blood into components allows the tailoring of treatment for specific problems (e.g., platelets for thrombocytopenia and packed red blood cells for anemia). In addition, it provides an optimal method for patients who require numerous transfusions of a specific blood component. The most frequently used blood components in cancer therapy are packed red blood cells and platelets. Other blood components generally are used for coagulation problems—for example, fresh frozen plasma is administered for clotting factor deficiencies. Table 26–5 lists the most commonly used blood components and their characteristics.

Red Blood Cells

Packed red blood cells (PRBCs) are prepared from a unit of whole blood by removing 200 to 250 ml of plasma. Each unit of PRBCs still contains residual leukocytes, platelets, and plasma proteins, but the granulocytes and platelets become nonfunctional be-

Table 26–3. ABO COMPATIBILITY OF BLOOD COMPONENTS

Blood Component	Recipient Blood Group	Donor Selection
Red blood cells	O	O only
	A	A or O
	B	B or O
	AB	AB, A, B, O
Fresh frozen plasma	O	O, A, B, or AB
	A	A or AB
	B	B or AB
	AB	AB only
Platelet concentrate	O	Any blood group may be used; because a large volume of plasma is given, it is preferable to use ABO compatible component
	A	
	B	
	AB	
Cryoprecipitate	O	All ABO groups acceptable; transfusion of cryoprecipitate may cause positive direct Coombs' test for group A recipients, but rarely hemolysis
	A	
	B	
	AB	

Table 26–4. STRATEGIES FOR TREATING PATIENTS WITH PLATELET ALLOANTIBODIES (REFRACTORY RESPONDERS)

Strategy	Rationale
Single-donor platelet unit, random, by apheresis	Platelets have one HLA type; may raise the platelet count in refractory responders if the recipient does not have antibodies to HLA type transfused
Single-donor platelet unit, family, by apheresis	Sibling of the recipient may have nearly identical HLA type; can raise platelet count in refractory responders (Schiffer & Slichter, 1982); parents and children are not suitable—they are haploidentical (Match only one half the HLA type)
Single-donor platelet unit, HLA-matched, by apheresis (Yankee, Grumet, & Rogentine, 1969)	Determine recipient's HLA-A, B, C type (serologic testing); donors are obtained from a computer registry of known HLA types; availability of service, expense, and rare recipient HLA types are drawbacks; failure to respond suggests poor match or other cause for increased destruction
Autologous platelets	Recipient undergoes apheresis and platelets are stored; this requires special freezing of platelets, which is still experimental; technique is not readily available
Immune interventions	High-dose intravenous gamma globulin (IgG) raises the platelet count in patients with idiopathic thrombocytopenic purpura (Bussel et al., 1983), but does not prevent alloantibody destruction of random-donor platelets (Schiffer et al; 1984); currently there is no effective immune intervention

cause of storage time and conditions (Pisciotto, 1989; Widmann, 1985). PRBCs contain a portion of the anticoagulant-preservative used when obtaining the whole blood. The most commonly used agent is citrate phosphate dextrose with adenine (CPDA-1) (Widmann, 1985). Citrate binds the calcium and is an anticoagulant; phosphate acts as a buffer; dextrose provides energy for red cell metabolism; and adenine serves as a source for adenosine triphosphate synthesis. Packed red blood cells are stored at 4 to 6° C for a shelf life of 35 days. In addition, certain additive solutions are available that extend the shelf life to 42 days, or the unit may be frozen for storage for 7 to 10 years.

Red blood cell transfusion requirements in cancer patients are based on the clinical status as well as the hemoglobin value. Most patients experience symptoms of anemia with a hemoglobin value less than 8.0 g, and this value is frequently used as a guideline for PRBC transfusions (Lichtiger & Huh, 1985).

Patients may become sensitized to the white blood cell and platelet antigens still present in the PRBC unit, which often leads to febrile or allergic transfusion reactions (see discussion on complications later in this chapter). These reactions are more common in patients who have had multiple pregnancies or prior transfusions. Different RBC products containing reduced amounts of unwanted antigens are available for use in these patients (Pisciotto, 1989). Methods to remove unwanted antigens include *filtration*, usually with special in-line white blood cell removal filters; *centrifugation* of the unit in the blood bank with mechanical removal or trapping of white blood cells; *washing* the PRBCs with buffer solutions; and using *frozen* red blood cells (these cells are washed to remove glycerol) (Ciavarella & Snyder, 1988). The use of these products depends on availability, cost, and severity of the patient's reaction.

Platelets

One unit of platelets is obtained from each unit of donated whole blood. Each platelet unit has a volume of approximately 50 ml and contains varying amounts of residual leukocytes and red blood cells (Pisciotto, 1989; Widmann, 1985). Platelet units are stored for 5 days at room temperature (20 to 24° C), with constant gentle agitation. Cold temperatures activate platelets. Multiple units are pooled for each transfusion. For an adult, the average platelet transfusion consists of 6 to 10 units.

In oncology practice, platelets are transfused as needed in cases of bleeding and prophylactically to prevent bleeding. Traditionally, the platelet count used for prophylactic transfusion is 20,000/mm³ (Higby, Cohen, Holland, & Sinks, 1974). Clinical trials in pediatric leukemic patients established that the incidence of hemorrhage increased markedly with platelet counts under 20,000/mm³ (Gaydos, Freireich, & Mantel, 1962). However, recent experience indicates that platelet counts in the range of 10,000 to 20,000/mm³ can be used safely for prophylactic transfusion (National Institutes of Health [NIH], 1989). In these cases, the use of clinical judgment and close observation to detect bleeding is essential (NIH Consensus Conference, 1987a).

Platelets are available in three forms: (1) random-donor, (2) single-donor non-HLA matched, and (3) single-donor HLA matched. A typical random-donor platelet transfusion consists of 4 to 10 single platelet units pooled in a concentrate. Single-donor platelets are obtained by placing the donor on a pheresis machine and collecting approximately 300 ml of platelet-enriched plasma (see Table 26–5). When a donor and recipient are HLA typed and matched, this is referred to as an HLA-matched platelet transfusion. A random-donor platelet transfusion should raise a 70-kg adult's platelet count by 5000 platelets/mm³ per unit trans-

Table 26–5. BLOOD COMPONENT SUMMARY

Component	Available Forms	Indication	Contents	Volume	Infusion Time	Expected Response
Red Blood Cells (RBCs)	RBCs	Signs of anemia (Hgb <8 g)	RBCs; WBCs and platelets are nonfunctional	250–300 ml	2–4 hr	Increase Hgb to 1 gm/dl unit
	Filtered PRBCs	Repeated febrile reactions	RBCs, WBCs (<10⁵), platelets, plasma	200 ml	2–4 hr	Same
Leukocyte-Poor RBCs	Saline-washed PRBCs	Febrile reactions; IgA deficiency with allergic reactions	RBCs, WBCs (<10⁵), platelets, minimal plasma	200 ml	2–4 hr	Same
	Frozen, deglycerolized RBCs	Rare blood type	RBCs, no plasma, minimal WBCs, platelets	180 ml	2–4 hr	Same
Platelets	Random donor (RD)	<20,000 platelet count, bleeding	Multiple units, plasma, WBCs, few RBCs	1 unit = 30–50 ml (8 units pooled ~400 ml)	1 unit over 5–10 min	Increase platelet count to 5000/mm³ per unit in 70-kg adult
	Single donor, non-HLA matched	Severe febrile reactions; or alloantibodies	Single donor, from apheresis; donor may be family or non-related; plasma, WBCs, RBCs	300 ml	30–60 min	Equivalent to 8 units RD platelets (~40,000 increase)
	Single donor, HLA matched	Alloantibodies (refractory responder)	Single donor; HLA-A, B, C matched; plasma, WBCs, RBCs	300 ml	30–60 min	Equivalent to 8 units RD platelets (~40,000 increase)
Granulocytes	Single donor granulocyte concentrate	Documented sepsis with PMN <500; infection worse despite antibiotics	Granulocytes, lymphocytes platelets, some RBCs, plasma	400 ml	45–60 min	Transient (<4 hr) rise in WBC count
Fresh Frozen Plasma (FFP)	From homologous donor pool and frozen within 6 hr	Coagulation factor deficiency	All coagulation factors complement	220 ml	30–60 min	1 unit increases coagulation factors by 5–10%
Cryoprecipitate	From FFP cold-insoluble precipitate after thaw at 4–6°C	Deficiency of factor VIII (coagulant or von Willebrand factor), fibrinogen, or factor XIII	Fibrinogen, factor VIII, factor XIII, minimal immunoglobulins	10–15 ml unit	15–30 min	Increase factor VIII, XIII, and fibrinogen levels

Hgb, Hemoglobin; PMN, polymorphonuclear leukocytes.

fused. A single-donor platelet transfusion raises the platelet count by approximately 40,000 platelets/mm³. In the absence of normal platelet production, platelet transfusions are generally required every 3 days. Severe exogenous losses, including those that occur in the presence of hemorrhage or fever, will increase platelet transfusion requirements.

Monitoring the posttransfusion platelet count is critical in determining the efficacy of a platelet transfusion. In any thrombocytopenic patient, the laboratory result should be verified when first reported. An artificial decrease in platelet count due to "clumping," or aggregation in the test tube, should be ruled out by visual inspection in the laboratory. Often the patient's platelet count is determined on the next morning's blood draw. The result of this blood draw is referred to as a random count. Random counts may be adequate for patients whose conditions are stable, but they are not adequate when there is a question about the patient's

response or when there is active bleeding. Failure of the random count to rise appropriately is an indication of excessive platelet destruction. A 1-hr posttransfusion count should be obtained if the random count does not rise appropriately or if there is active blood loss. Counts 1 hr after transfusion are a good indicator of the efficacy of the transfusion (Daly, Schiffer, Aisner, & Wiernik, 1980). Evidence by O'Connell and colleagues (1988) indicates that 10-min posttransfusion counts are as useful as 1-hr posttransfusion counts for evaluating platelet transfusion efficacy. A series of clinical examples illustrates these points about increased platelet destruction (Table 26–6).

Common causes for the failure of the platelet count to rise appropriately are found in Table 26–7. Immune destruction may be caused by the development of autoantibodies or alloantibodies. Autoantibodies are rarely identified in the cancer patient. When present, the patient usually has a preexisting history of throm-

Table 26–6. CLINICAL EXAMPLES OF PLATELET TRANSFUSIONS

Example	Platelet Counts	Response
70-kg female leukemic patient; day 15 of induction therapy; afebrile; no bleeding; first platelet transfusion, 8 units of random donor (RD) platelets	Pretransfusion: 10,000; random count next morning draw post transfusion: 48,000 (12 hr later)	Appropriate rise in platelet count (5000/unit/kg); no evidence of excessive platelet destruction; next transfusion monitored by random count
70-kg female leukemic patient; day 20 of therapy; temperature 38.5°C, possible pneumonia; 8 units RD platelets	Pretransfusion: 20,000; next morning draw after transfusion: 28,000	Failure of adequate response; this could be no platelet rise or a rapid fall in transfused platelets; need to assess count 1 hr after transfusion to determine cause
70-kg female leukemic patient; day 15; afebrile; heavy menstrual bleeding; 8 units RD platelets given	Pretransfusion: 15,000; post transfusion: 12,000 (6 hr later)	In setting of acute bleed, platelet loss is rapid; need to determine the adequacy of rise with frequent counts at 1 hr post transfusion
70-kg female leukemic patient; day 20; afebrile; no bleeding; 8 units RD platelets given	Pretransfusion: 15,000; the last random count (8 hr after transfusion) was 12,000; 1 hr post transfusion count was 17,000	Refractory response to RD platelets; search for causes listed in Table 26–7; possible alloantibodies; consider HLA typing of patient for HLA matched platelets

bocytopenia—that is, immune thrombocytopenia purpura (ITP). The development of alloantibodies to platelets was discussed earlier under HLA antigens.

Granulocytes

Granulocyte concentrates are prepared by leukapheresis of a single donor. Each concentrate contains white blood cells, platelets, and red blood cells suspended in 200 to 400 ml of plasma (Pisciotto, 1989; Widmann, 1985). Ideally, granulocytes should be transfused immediately after collection. If necessary, they can be stored without agitation at room temperature for up to 24 hr.

The use of granulocytes is controversial (Dutcher, 1986). Abrams and Deisseroth (1985) suggest the use of granulocytes for patients who meet the following criteria: "(1) granulocyte count of less than 500 cells/mm³, (2) early bone marrow recovery not expected, (3) documented gram-negative sepsis, (4) failure to show clinical improvement after the initiation of appropriate broad-spectrum antibiotic coverage, and (5) overall clinical setting and prognosis warranting the use of aggressive clinical supportive measures." Once initiated, granulocyte transfusions are given daily until bone marrow recovery or resolution of the identified clinical indication occurs (Winston, Ho, & Gale, 1982).

Preparing granulocytes is costly and requires expensive technology, close supervision, and 2 to 4 hrs of

Table 26–7. FAILURE OF ADEQUATE PLATELET TRANSFUSION RESPONSE

Mechanism	Clinical Condition
Platelet loss	1. Bleeding
	2. Fever
	3. Infection ± fever
	4. DIC
Sequestration	5. Splenomegaly
Immune destruction	6. Alloantibody
	7. Autoantibody

the donor's time. Although studies have demonstrated the effectiveness of such treatments, the ratio of cost to benefit is high (Wright, 1984). Complications associated with the administration of granulocyte concentrates include pulmonary infiltrates, severe febrile reactions, and transmission of viruses such as cytomegalovirus and hepatitis (Clift & Buckner, 1984; Patterson, 1980). In addition, the concomitant administration of granulocytes and amphotericin B has been reported to produce severe adverse pulmonary reactions (Wright, Robinchaud, Pizzo, & Deisseroth, 1981). However, another study failed to confirm this observation (Dana, Durie, White, & Huestis, 1981). In practice, the administration of amphotericin B and granulocytes should be separated by 4 to 6 hrs because either agent alone may cause a severe allergic reaction. It is unlikely that granulocyte transfusions will alter the clinical course of a neutropenic patient if recovery of bone marrow function is not expected (Higby & Burnett, 1980; Strauss et al., 1981; Winston, Ho, & Gale, 1981).

Plasma Products

Plasma component products routinely available are (1) fresh frozen plasma (FFP) and (2) cryoprecipitate (CRYO). These products are used in cancer patients to treat coagulopathies due to secondary disease states such as disseminated intravascular clotting (DIC) or liver failure (NIH Consensus Conference, 1987b).

Fresh frozen plasma is obtained by centrifugation of whole blood and rapid freezing of the plasma within 6 hr after phlebotomy (Pisciotto, 1989; Widmann, 1985). One unit of FFP has an approximate volume of 200 to 250 ml and may be stored for up to 1 year at −18° C or lower. This blood component should be used to replace coagulation factors and not to expand blood volume or to replace fluid. Fresh frozen plasma is often indicated for replacement of multiple clotting factor deficiencies. All clotting factors are present in FFP at an approximate concentration of 1 unit of factor/ml of FFP. (Pisciotto, 1989; Widmann, 1985). In adults the average or usual replacement is 2 to 4 units of FFP every 6 hr. Transfusion of 2 units of FFP provides a replacement of roughly 10 to 15 per cent of the normal level of each clotting factor. Transfusion of large volumes of FFP is not appropriate for replacing an isolated clotting factor deficiency when an alternative product is available.

Cryoprecipitate is prepared by thawing 1 unit of FFP at 4° C and collecting the precipitate formed (Pisciotto, 1989; Widmann, 1985). It is stable for 1 year at −18° C or lower. Each unit of CRYO has a volume of 10 to 15 ml and contains about 250 mg of fibrinogen, 80 to 120 units of factor VIII:C (procoagulant activity), 40 to 70 per cent of factor VIII:vWf (von Willebrand factor), and 20 to 30 per cent of factor XIII (fibrin-stabilizing factor). Most often CRYO is used to replace deficiencies of fibrinogen and factor VIII. An average dose is 12 to 20 units of CRYO. The frequency of transfusion depends on the half-life of the specific factor replaced.

Costs of Blood Component Therapy

Blood components vary in cost across the country. Current blood component charges reflect five distinct types of fees. These include (1) a processing fee, (2) a product preparation fee, (3) a type and screen fee, (4) a cross-match fee, and (5) an administration fee. The processing fee covers the procurement and handling fee for blood components distributed by the collection facility. The product preparation fee takes into account the special processing that may be required—for example, washing, freezing, or preparing autologous blood. The charge for testing a sample of the recipient's blood for ABO and Rh compatibility is reflected in the type and screen fee. The cross-match fee includes testing a sample of the recipient's blood for serologic incompatibility. Administration fees are basically charges for transfusion equipment, nursing care or the use of an intravenous team, and documentation.

Factors that will influence blood component costs in the future are reduced demand, increased use of autologous blood, reimbursement issues, and new technologies. The availability of artificial blood, colony-stimulating factors that promote normal hematopoiesis, automated collection techniques, and new methods of pretransfusion testing are expected to affect greatly the cost of blood component therapy.

HEMAPHERESIS

Technologic advances have allowed the introduction into clinical medicine of sophisticated cell separators. These machines remove whole blood from the donor, separate it into cellular and plasma components by centrifugation, and return the remaining blood to the donor (Beal & Isbister, 1985). *Hemapheresis* is the general term used for all procedures for which cell separators are used. Hemapheresis is used to provide the cancer patient with selected blood components and, in addition, may function to remove unwanted cellular or plasma elements.

Leukapheresis is the selective collection of leukocytes (usually referring to granulocytes). When therapeutic granulocyte transfusions are indicated, normal donors undergo leukapheresis to provide the granulocyte concentrate. Leukapheresis can be used in leukemic patients with very high white blood cell blast counts. These patients are at risk for leukostasis (white blood cell sludging and obstruction in the microvasculature) of the central nervous system (CNS) and lungs. Leukapheresis is used to acutely lower the white blood cell count. Lymphocytapheresis (the removal of lymphocytes) is used as part of a specific cancer treatment to remove lymphocytes from the cancer patient, which are then incubated in laboratory cultures with interleukin 2 to produce lymphokine-activated killer (LAK) cells (see Chapter 23).

The most common hemapheresis requested is thrombocytapheresis, which is the removal or collection of platelets. Single-donor and HLA-matched platelets are collected from normal donors by this technique (see the earlier section on platelets) (Arrell, 1987).

Plasmapheresis is used to selectively remove plasma components in various disease states. For example, in multiple myeloma, plasmapheresis removes immunoglobulins, reduces the serum viscosity, and thus decreases the patient's acute symptoms related to increased immunoglobulin levels.

COMPLICATIONS OF TRANSFUSION

The adverse effects of transfusion can be characterized by the timing of their occurrence, *immediate (acute)* or *delayed,* and by the mechanism of the reaction, *immunologic* or *nonimmunologic* (Berkman, 1984; Smith, 1984; Walker, 1987). The term *transfusion reaction* generally refers to the immediate immune reactions that can occur from blood component therapy. The most frequent acute nonimmune complication of transfusion is congestive heart failure from volume overload. The most common delayed nonimmune reaction is the transmission of infection. Bacterial contamination of the product is a rare complication. Viral infection, especially non-A, non-B hepatitis, is one of the most common serious risks faced by the blood recipient (Table 26–8). The risk of a hemolytic transfusion reaction is one thousandth and the risk of developing AIDS is one ten-thousandth the risk of developing hepatitis (see Table 26–8). Iron overload is another delayed reaction that is seen after many red blood cell transfusions (usually more than 100). The

Table 26–8. TRANSFUSION RISKS

Complication	Risk per Unit Transfused
Non-A, non-B hepatitis	1:100
Human immunodeficiency virus infection (HIV)	1:40,000 to 1:1,000,000
Fatal hemolytic transfusion reaction	1:100,000

sections that follow discuss the immune and infectious complications of transfusion in greater detail.

Complications Due to Immune Mechanisms

The immediate transfusion reactions due to immunologic causes can be remembered by the acronym: **NOFUN**:aNaphylactic, hemOlytic, Febrile, Urticarial, Noncardiogenic pulmonary edema. These reactions and their mechanisms are summarized in Table 26–9.

Anaphylactic reactions are very rare. They are associated with IgA deficiency and occur in certain patients who develop antibodies to IgA. These reactions can occur after only a few millimeters of blood or plasma have been received. They are characterized by the absence of fever and the presence of acute pulmonary symptoms such as cough and wheezing. Shock commonly accompanies the reaction. Treatment is the same as for any anaphylactic reaction, but prevention should be the goal. Patients with hereditary or acquired immune deficiencies should be considered at risk.

An acute hemolytic reaction is the most dreaded complication of transfusion; fortunately, it occurs rarely. This reaction is usually caused by red blood cell ABO incompatibility (Greenwalt, 1981). Errors in labeling the blood specimen or in identifying the component or patient are the most common causes, which result in the recipient receiving the wrong blood product. The recipient may develop shock, disseminated intravascular coagulation, or acute renal failure, any of which can be fatal. The severity of the reaction is in direct proportion to the amount of transfused incompatible blood and the elapsed time before appropriate intervention. Antibodies to blood group antigens other than the ABO system may cause a hemolytic reaction. Common offenders are antibodies to the blood groups Duffy and Kell. When these antibodies are not detected during initial antibody screening, the transfusion of blood may result in an acute hemolytic reaction.

Febrile reactions (febrile nonhemolytic reaction) are the most common transfusion reactions, and they are usually immune mediated. These reactions are caused by antibodies in the recipient directed against antigens present on granulocytes, platelets, or lymphocytes in the transfused blood components. The fever may occur early in the transfusion or even a few hours after the transfusion is complete. If fever occurs during blood transfusion, a thorough clinical evaluation of the pa-

tient should be undertaken (to isolate the cause of the fever). When fever occurs during transfusion in a leukopenic patient, infection must be considered before the fever can be attributed to a transfusion reaction. Fever can also be a sign of a hemolytic transfusion reaction. The patient should be carefully observed until the cause is determined. Antipyretics and antihistamines are often given before transfusion in *frequently* transfused patients to prevent immune-mediated febrile reactions. Meperidine is extremely effective in relieving the shaking chills that can occur.

Urticarial reactions are thought to be due to antibodies against plasma proteins or soluble factors. These reactions are usually benign, and the transfusion is continued while the reaction is treated with antihistamines. As in the case of fever, urticaria can accompany a more severe reaction such as anaphylaxis or hemolysis. A severe reaction is suspected when the patient does not respond readily to antihistamines as in the benign isolated urticaria reaction.

Noncardiogenic pulmonary edema is also a rare complication of transfusion. The mechanism is not completely understood, but at least two triggers have been described. Antibodies to leukocytes in the donor product may react with recipient white blood cells and cause leukoagglutination in pulmonary capillaries. In other cases, complement is activated by the donor antibodies, which cause recipient cells such as mast cells to release mediators, which then cause leukoagglutination. When noncardiogenic pulmonary edema is suspected, the transfusion should be stopped immediately and supportive measures instituted; some authors recommend steroids. A summary of the types of transfusion reactions, signs and symptoms, and clinical management is found in Table 26–10 (Huestis, Bove, & Case, 1988; Pauley, 1984, 1985; Querin & Stahl, 1983; Rutman & Miller, 1985; Smith, 1984).

Some transfusion reactions occur days after the transfusion and are dramatic reminders of earlier, undetected reactions. Although all are rare, three of the most important problems are (1) delayed hemolytic transfusion reaction, (2) posttransfusion purpura, and (3) graft-versus-host disease.

A *delayed hemolytic transfusion reaction* is characterized by a drop in hemoglobin that may be gradual or sudden and dramatic. The basic mechanism is a rise in antibody titer against the transfused blood. In some patients who are considered to be having a primary immunization, the rise is slow and the hemolysis is gradual over the 2 weeks following the transfusion. In other patients the rise is rapid and is thought to come from an anamnestic response (recall memory immune response). In these cases, when the recipients were tested before transfusion the antibody titers were low so the screening test results (discussed in the section on red blood cell compatibility) were negative. Transfusion of blood then resulted in an anamnestic response, the antibody titer rose after 7 to 10 days, and sudden hemolysis occurred. These patients generally have sudden fever, jaundice, and a marked drop in hemoglobin, but the reaction rarely causes renal problems or shock. The only means of preventing delayed

Table 26–9. IMMEDIATE IMMUNE TRANSFUSION REACTIONS

Reaction	Mechanism
Anaphylaxis	Antibody to IgA (hereditary or acquired IgA deficiency)
Hemolysis, acute	Red blood cell incompatibility
Fever, nonhemolytic	Antibody to donor leukocyte antigens
Urticaria	Antibody to plasma proteins
Noncardiogenic pulmonary edema	Antibody to recipient leukocytes; complement activation

Table 26–10. TRANSFUSION REACTIONS

Type	Signs/Symptoms	Onset	Management
Acute hemolytic	Fever, chills, anaphylaxis, decreased blood pressure, nausea/vomiting, flushing, back pain, hematuria, decreased urine output	Usually during the first 15 min	1. Stop transfusion 2. Resuscitate 3. Notify blood bank 4. Monitor intake and output 5. Medical management: administration of osmotic diuretics and fluids
Febrile nonhemolytic	Fever ± chills, headache, dyspnea, chest pain, decreased blood pressure, nausea/vomiting	Immediately or within 8 hr of transfusion	1. Stop transfusion 2. Notify blood bank 3. Rule out infection 4. Acetaminophen for fever; meperidine for chills; continue transfusion if symptoms not severe
Allergic	Urticaria	During transfusion or within 1–2 hr	1. Decrease transfusion rate 2. Antihistamines 3. Notify blood bank 4. Monitor vital signs
Delayed hemolytic	Decreased hemoglobin level, low-grade fever	7–10 days to weeks	1. Notify blood bank

hemolytic reactions is a thorough and accurate review of the patient's transfusion history.

Another delayed reaction affects platelets. *Posttransfusion purpura* is a rare, immune-mediated thrombocytopenic complication of red blood cell or plasma product transfusion. A patient with a normal platelet count may receive a red blood cell, platelet, or plasma transfusion for a standard indication and 7 to 10 days later suddenly develop severe thrombocytopenia. This phenomenon appears to be produced by an autoantibody directed against a platelet-specific antigen or antigens (Keimowitz, Collins, Davis, & Aster, 1986). The exact mechanism of platelet destruction is not completely understood, but it appears to occur in persons who lack one or more very common platelet-specific antigens. After exposure to the new platelet antigen or antigens during transfusion, the recipient develops antibodies and destroys his or her own platelets as well as those transfused. The paradoxical destruction of the recipient's own platelets may be caused by a coating of the recipient's platelets with antigen-antibody complexes or by a cross-reactivity of the antibody (Barton, 1981). Less than 3 per cent of the population is at risk for this phenomenon, and it does not always occur even when the population at risk is exposed to transfusion.

Graft-versus-host disease (GVHD) is a rare complication of transfusion therapy that has been documented in severely immunocompromised recipients (Leitman, 1985). This complication is a direct result of the transfusion of immunocompetent T lymphocytes, present in whole blood, granulocyte, platelet, and red blood cell fractionated components. The T lymphocytes remain functional for weeks in stored blood, and when the component is administered to an immunocompromised patient with a different set of histocompatible antigens, the T lymphocytes may proliferate, resulting in GVHD. For a detailed explanation of GVHD, see Chapter 27.

Case reports of GVHD in patients with cancer who received blood component therapy have been documented in the literature (Kessinger, et al., 1987; Von Fliedner, Higby, & Kim, 1982). One case report cites the occurrence of GVHD after a transfusion of only 1 unit of PRBCs (Hathaway et al., 1967). Cancer patients at highest risk for developing GVHD from blood component therapy include bone marrow transplant patients and patients with Hodgkin's and non-Hodgkin's lymphoma undergoing combined chemotherapy and radiation.

Irradiating blood components with 15 to 50 Grays (1500 to 5000 rad) abolishes the ability of the T lymphocytes to proliferate without compromising the function of other blood components (Button, DeWolf, Newburger, Jacobson, & Kevy, 1981; McMican, Luban, & Sacher, 1987). The use of irradiated blood components in severely immunocompromised states has been recommended to prevent GVHD (Weiden, 1984). The practice of irradiating blood components is diligently adhered to in the bone marrow transplantation population. In other severely immunocompromised disease states, the cost-benefit ratio of providing irradiated blood products to prevent GVHD has not yet been established (Lind, 1985). However, the prevention of GVHD in populations at high risk warrants the clinical use of irradiated blood components even though the incidence of GVHD is quite rare.

Infectious Complications

The development of non-A, non-B hepatitis is the most frequent serious risk faced by the recipient of a transfusion. Hepatitis A is rarely transmissible by blood transfusion owing to its short period of viremia and the absence of a carrier state. Mandatory testing for hepatitis B surface antigen (HBsAg) in blood products significantly reduced the transmission of hepatitis B. However, testing of blood products for hepatitis B did not produce a decrease in the frequency of posttransfusion hepatitis. Subsequently, it was recognized that another virus, or group of viruses, was or were capable of producing hepatitis after blood transfusion. The term *non-A, non-B hepatitis* refers to the infection caused by this virus(es). Non-A, non-B hepatitis is responsible for approximately 80 to 90 per cent of the hepatitis seen following transfusion, and the remainder represents predominantly hepatitis B. The incubation period of non-A, non-B hepatitis (the time from transfusion to the first rise in serum transaminase) varies from 2 weeks to 4 months. Clinical features of non-A, non-B hepatitis include fever, malaise, loss of appetite, jaundice, and right upper quadrant pain. Jaundice is observed in only 20 per cent of patients and occurs about 1 to 4 weeks after the rise in serum transaminase level. Thus many cases of transfusion hepatitis are "silent." Most patients who develop non-A, non-B hepatitis will have an abrupt increase in their serum transaminase levels followed by a gradual return to normal. Some patients will become chronic carriers of the virus, and some of these will subsequently develop cirrhosis.

Some data indicate that approximately 1 per cent of blood recipients develop posttransfusion hepatitis (Conrad, 1981). The risk of developing hepatitis depends on the number of donors used for each product. Blood products prepared from pools of donors have the greatest risk (e.g., for coagulation factor concentrates). Currently, the most effective means of preventing non-A, non-B hepatitis is the sole use of volunteer blood and the exclusion of donors with a history of risk factors for hepatitis, prior jaundice, or clinical hepatitis. The rejection of blood products with elevated hepatic transaminase enzyme levels (a surrogate marker for hepatitis) is expected to further reduce hepatitis transmission (American Association of Blood Banks, 1988).

The next most important infectious complication of transfusion is cytomegalovirus (CMV) infection. This virus is transmitted by viable leukocytes in the blood product. It is estimated that approximately 6 to 12 per cent of the blood products from the general donor pool are capable of transmitting CMV. The recipients at highest risk for complications of CMV infection are (1) immunocompromised patients, (2) the fetus in utero with primary CMV maternal infection, and (3) premature infants. The complications in these recipients include CMV interstitial pneumonitis, birth defects, and death.

No completely reliable way to prevent CMV infection exists. Because there is no convenient, direct way to detect CMV in the blood, the presence of antibodies to CMV is determined. Blood components that contain anti-CMV antibodies (CMV-positive units) are more likely to transmit the infection. Therefore, in the high-risk populations identified, CMV-negative blood is required for patients who have a low titer of anti-CMV antibodies. These patients have not been exposed to the CMV virus and are considered CMV negative. Most authorities would consider all transplant recipients and leukemic patients who do not have anti-CMV in this high-risk category. Bowden and colleagues (1986) reported that CMV-negative bone marrow transplant patients who received only CMV-negative

blood products had a significantly decreased incidence of CMV infection compared with those patients who received standard blood products without regard to the presence of CMV. Clinical practice has clearly demonstrated that when CMV-positive blood components are given to a CMV-negative bone marrow transplant patient, fatal interstitial pneumonitis or CMV infection of other organs may develop (Meyers, Flournoy, & Thomas, 1986).

NURSING IMPLICATIONS

Oncology nurses play a key role in the administration of blood components to the cancer patient. Nurses must be knowledgeable about transfusion principles, indications for component use, product contents, need for ABO-Rh compatibility, and potential adverse effects. Administration guidelines for nurses to follow to ensure that oncology patients will receive blood components in a safe, efficient manner are identified in Table 26–11 (Blood Component Therapy Committee, 1987; Landier, Barrell, & Styffe, 1987; Mintz et al., 1986).

Standard 170-μm blood filters are required for all blood components and factor concentrates to trap clots. Microaggregate filters have a pore size of 20 to 40 μm. The function of these filters is to remove leukocyte-

Table 26–11. GUIDELINES FOR BLOOD COMPONENT ADMINISTRATION

1. Use universal precautions when handling blood components and contaminated equipment.
2. Identify the patient.
3. Obtain the requested blood specimen.
4. Accurately label the specimen.
5. Administer premedications, such as acetaminophen or diphenhydramine hydrochloride, if ordered.
6. Obtain the ordered blood component from the blood bank.
7. PRIOR TO ADMINISTRATION:
   - Verify physician order
   - Compare donor identification numbers and ABO-Rh compatibility on transfusion record with information on blood component
   - At the bedside, identify patient with full name
   - Request patient to state his or her full name
   - Compare full name and identity of patient with name and identification on blood component and transfusion record
   DO NOT TRANSFUSE COMPONENT IF INFORMATION DOES NOT EXACTLY MATCH
   - Check expiration date and time on blood component
   - Once it is determined that everything is correct, sign the transfusion record
8. Inspect the blood component for color and consistency turning component upside down to gently mix its contents.
9. Prepare filter, tubing, and 0.9 per cent normal saline flush solution.
10. Record patient's baseline vital signs.
11. Start transfusion and record date and time of initiation.
12. Stay with the patient for the first 5 to 15 min to assess for an acute reaction.
13. Record patient's vital signs 15 min after the initiation of the transfusion and as required by policy.
14. Monitor patients frequently during the transfusion.
15. At completion, document patient's condition and complete transfusion record.
16. Place copy of transfusion record in patient's chart and return copy to blood bank.

platelet aggregates that form during blood storage. These filters have been used during massive transfusions and in clinical situations in which an increased risk of noncardiogenic pulmonary edema exists. It is not clear whether the presence of these leukocyte-platelet aggregates produces any direct harm to the patient. Leukocyte-poor filters are now available for red blood cell and platelet component administration. These are used when a leukocyte-poor component is clinically indicated (see earlier sections on red blood cells and platelets).

The physician's order will specify the transfusion rate. All blood components should be infused within 4 hr after initiation. This decreases the risk of bacterial contamination and ensures component stability. The blood bank can divide the unit into two or more parts, dispensing one part at a time when clinically warranted. This allows a longer transfusion period without jeopardizing the blood component or increasing the patient's risk for adverse effects. Once the component is obtained, it must be used (that is, the infusion begun) within 30 min or returned immediately to the blood bank for proper storage.

No medication should be added to blood at any time. Normal saline solution (0.9 per cent) may be added for dilutional purposes, if needed. Other solutions, such as 5 per cent dextrose in water (D_5W), may destroy red blood cells. Lactated Ringer's solution may induce clot formation owing to the presence of calcium. A large-gauge needle (18 gauge) is recommended for peripheral blood administration. However, many oncology patients may have poor access routes, and a 20-gauge needle may be used. In addition, many oncology patients may have some type of venous access device, either an implanted port or a tunneled Silastic central catheter, providing a consistent access route. Blood administration through venous access devices requires adherence to the procedures established by the nurse's institution.

Blood components may be administered via infusion devices. However, the manufacturer or blood bank should be consulted to determine device capabilities, because hemolysis of red blood cells may occur with some models. Blood warmers—devices that warm the blood as it passes through—are used for patients receiving massive amounts of blood over a short time and for patients who have cold agglutinins to prevent adverse reactions.

Thorough and accurate documentation is critical to the transfusion process. Many institutions require frequent monitoring of vital signs (e.g., every 15 min for 1 hr, then every 30 min until the transfusion is complete), although little clinical data exist to support this practice. Taylor, Wagner, and Kraus (1987) undertook a retrospective chart audit to determine when transfusion reactions occurred in relation to vital sign monitoring. They found that fever and chills were the most common reactions reported, with reactions occurring from 30 min to 3 hr 35 min from the onset of the transfusion. Recommendations included staying with the patient for the first 15 min or being readily available and seeing the patient every 5 min for the first 15 min, plus taking of vital signs every 30 min two times and then every hour until the transfusion is completed. A flow sheet identifying assessment criteria to be monitored is helpful in establishing a consistent evaluation of transfusion therapy. Actual symptoms to be assessed, clinical data to be monitored, and the patient's response to therapy can be clearly identified and be useful in planning nursing care.

Blood component therapy is essential in the supportive care of the patient with cancer. Patients and families will request information about the risks of transfusion therapy and participation in a designated donor program. Oncology nurses must have an adequate knowledge base to answer these questions. In addition, nurses must be familiar with their hospital's policies and procedures and be aware of available resources for their own educational needs. No transfusion should be considered routine. Each component administered requires strict adherence to guidelines throughout the transfusion process to provide optimal patient care.

SUMMARY AND FUTURE TRENDS

Knowledge of modern transfusion principles is essential for oncology nursing practice. Nurses are in an optimal position to provide education to the cancer patient and family regarding transfusion practice. The administration of blood products is a treatment directly provided to the patient and monitored almost exclusively by nurses.

New cancer treatments with biologic agents may prove to be effective and less toxic to the bone marrow, thus reducing transfusion support requirements in the future. Recombinant hormonal agents that stimulate hematopoietic cell production are in early clinical trials (Groopman, Mitsuyasu, DeLeo, Oette, & Golde, 1987). These agents may allow cytotoxic therapy to be given with fewer and shorter intervals of bone marrow suppression. However, treatment methods such as high-dose chemotherapy with autologous bone marrow transplant require intensive blood component support. Additionally, the use of such intensive therapies may increase in future clinical practice. An intimate knowledge of the principles of blood transfusion remains essential for the oncology nurse.

References

Abrams, R. A., & Deisseroth, A. (1985). Use of blood and blood products. In V. T. DeVita, S. Hellman, & S. A. Rosenberg (Eds.), *Cancer principles and practice of oncology* (pp. 1920–1940). Philadelphia: J. B. Lippincott Co.

American Association of Blood Banks. (1988, May 13). Hepatitis non-A, non-B virus discovered. *Blood Bank Week*.

Arrell, H. M. (1987). Platelet pheresis. *Nursing, 17,* 92–93.

Barton, J. C. (1981). Nonhemolytic, noninfectious transfusion reactions. *Seminars in Hematology, 18,* 95–121.

Beal, R. W., & Isbister, J. P. (1985). *Blood component therapy in clinical practice.* London: Blackwell Scientific Publications.

Berkman, S. A. (1984). The spectrum of transfusion reaction. *Hospital Practice, 19,* 205–219.

Blood Component Therapy Committee. (1987). *Blood component administration: A guide for nurses.* Arlington, VA: American Association of Blood Banks.

Bowden, R. A., Sayers, M., Flournoy, N., Newton, B., Banaji, M., Thomas, E. D., & Meyers J. D. (1986). Cytomegalovirus immune globulin and seronegative blood products to prevent primary cytomegalovirus infection after marrow transplantation. *New England Journal of Medicine, 314,* 1006–1010.

Bussel, J. B., Kimberly, R. P., Inman, R. D., Schulman, I., Cunningham-Rundles, C., Cheung, N., Smithwick, E. M., O'Malley, J., Barandun, S., & Hilgartner, M. W. (1983). Intravenous gammaglobulin treatment of chronic idiopathic thrombocytopenic purpura. *Blood, 62,* 480–486.

Button, L. N., DeWolf, W. C., Newburger, P. E., Jacobson, M. S., & Kevy, S. V. (1981). The effects of irradiation on blood components. *Transfusion, 21,* 419–426.

Ciavarella, D., & Snyder, E. (1988). Clinical use of blood transfusion devices. *Transfusion Medicine Reviews, 2,* 95–111.

Churchill, W. H., & Kurtz, S. R. (Eds.). (1988). *Transfusion medicine.* London: Blackwell Scientific Publications.

Clift, R. A., & Buckner, C. D. (1984). Granulocyte transfusions. *The American Journal of Medicine, 76,* 631–636.

Conrad, M. E. (1981). Disease transmissible by blood transfusion: Viral hepatitis and other infectious disorders. *Seminars in Hematology, 18,* 122–146.

Daly, P. A., Schiffer, C. A., Aisner, J., & Wiernik, P. H. (1980). Platelet transfusion therapy. One hour posttransfusion increments are valuable in predicting the need for HLA-matched preparations. *Journal of the American Medical Association, 243,* 435–438.

Dana, B. W., Durie, B. G. M., White, R. F., & Huestis, D. W. (1981). Concomitant administration of granulocyte transfusions and amphotericin B in neutropenic patients: Absence of significant pulmonary toxicity. *Blood, 57,* 90–94.

Dudjak, L. A. (1984). HLA typing: Implications for nurses. *Oncology Nursing Forum, 11(5),* 30–36.

Dutcher, J. P. (1986). Platelet and granulocyte transfusions in cancer patients. *Advances in Immunology Cancer Therapy, 2,* 211–249.

Gaydos, L. A. Freireich, E. J., & Mantel, N. (1962). The quantitative relation between platelet count and hemorrhage in patients with acute leukemia. *New England Journal of Medicine, 266,* 905–909.

Gmur, J., von Felton, A., Osterwalder, B., Honegger, H., Hormann, A., Sauter, C., Deubelbeiss, K., Berchfold, W., Metaxas, M., Scali, G., & Frick, P. G. (1983). Delayed alloimmunization using random single donor platelet transfusions: A prospective study in thrombocytopenic patients with acute leukemia. *Blood, 62,* 473–479.

Greenwalt, T. J. (1981). Pathogenesis and management of hemolytic transfusion reactions. *Seminars in Hematology, 18,* 84–94.

Groopman, J. K., Mitsuyasu, R. T., DeLeo, M. J., Oette, D. H., & Golde, D. W. (1987). Effect of recombinant human granulocyte-macrophage colony-stimulating factor on myelopoiesis in the acquired immunodeficiency syndrome. *New England Journal of Medicine, 317,* 593–598.

Hathaway, W. E., Filginiti, V. A., Pierce, C. W., Githens, J. H., Pearlman, D. S., Muschenheim, F., & Kempe, H. (1967). Graft-vs.-host reaction following a single blood transfusion. *Journal of the American Medical Association, 201,* 1015–1020.

Higby, D. J., & Burnett, D. (1980). Granulocyte transfusions: Current status. *Blood, 55,* 2–8.

Higby, D. J., Cohen, E., Holland, J. F., & Sinks, L. (1974). The prophylactic treatment of thrombocytopenic leukemia patients with platelets: A double blind study. *Transfusion, 14,* 440–446.

Huestis, D. W., Bove, J. R., & Case, J. (1988). *Practical blood transfusion* (4th ed.). Boston: Little, Brown & Co.

Keimowitz, R. M., Collins, J., Davis, K., & Aster, R. H. (1986). Post-transfusion purpura associated with alloimmunization against the platelet specific antigen, Bak[A]. *American Journal of Hematology, 21,* 79–88.

Kessinger, A., Armitage, J. O., Klassen, L. W., Landmark, J. D., Hayes, J. M., Larsen, A. E., and Purtilo, D. T. (1987). Graft versus host disease following transfusion of normal blood products to patients with malignancies. *Journal of Surgical Oncology, 36,* 206–209.

Landier, W. C., Barrell, M. L., & Styffe, E. J. (1987). How to administer blood components to children. *Maternal–Child Nursing Journal, 12,* 178–184.

Landsteiner, K. (1901). Über agguluntinationserscheinungen normalen menschlichen Blutes. *Klinische Wochenschrift, 14,* 1132–1145.

Leitman, S. F. (1985). Post transfusion graft-versus-host disease. In D. M. Smith & A. J. Silvergleid (Eds.). *Special considerations in transfusing the immunocompromised patient,* pp. 15–37. Arlington, VA: American Association of Blood Banks.

Levine, P., & Stetson, R. (1939). An unusual case of intra-group agglutination. *Journal of the American Medical Association, 113,* 126–127.

Lichtiger, B., & Huh, Y. O. (1985). Transfusion therapy for patients with cancer. *CA:A Cancer Journal for Clinicians, 35,* 311–316.

Lind, S. E. (1985). Has the case for irradiating blood products been made? *American Journal of Medicine, 78,* 543–544.

McLeod, B. C. (1980). Immunologic factors in reactions to blood transfusions. *Heart and Lung, 9,* 675–681.

McMican, A., Luban, N. L. C., & Sacher, R. A. (1987). Practical aspects of blood irradiation. *Laboratory Medicine, 18,* 299–303.

Menitove, J. E. (1983). Platelet transfusion for alloimmunized patients. *Journal of Clinical Oncology, 2,* 587–609.

Meyers, J. D., Flournoy, N., and Thomas, E. D. (1986). Risk factors for cytomegalovirus infection after human marrow transplantation. *Journal of Infectious Disease, 153,* 478–488.

Mintz, P. D., Grindon, A. J., Tomasulo, P. A., Bergin, J. J., Klein, H. G., Kruskall, M. S., Mercado, S. B., Miller, J. D., & Johnston, M. F. M. (1986). The latest protocols for blood transfusions. *Nursing, 16(10),* 34–41.

National Institutes of Health. (1989, May). Transfusion alert. Indications for the use of red blood cells, platelets, and fresh frozen plasma. Publication No. 89-2974a. Washington, DC: Author.

National Institutes of Health Consensus Conference. (1987a). Platelet transfusion therapy. *Transfusion Medicine Reviews, 1,* 195–200.

National Institutes of Health Consensus Conference (1987b). Fresh frozen plasma: Indications and risks. *Transfusion Medicine Reviews, 1,* 201–204.

O'Connell, B., Lee, E. J., and Schiffer, C. A. (1988). The value of 10 minute post-transfusion platelet counts. *Transfusion, 28,* 66–67.

Patterson, P. (1980). Granulocyte transfusion: Nursing considerations. *Cancer Nursing, 3,* 101–104.

Pauley, S. Y. (1984). Transfusion therapy for nurses. Part 1. *National Intravenous Therapy Association, 7,* 501–511.

Pauley, S. Y. (1985). Transfusion therapy for nurses. Part 2. *National Intravenous Therapy Association, 8,* 51–60.

Pisciotto, P. T. (Ed.). 1989. *Blood transfusion therapy—a physician's handbook* (3rd ed.). Arlington, VA: American Association of Blood Banks.

Querin, J. J., & Stahl, L. D. (1983). 12 simple, sensible steps for successful blood transfusions. *Nursing, 13,* 34–43.

Rutman, R. C., & Miller, W. V. (1985). *Transfusion therapy—principles and procedures* (2nd ed.). Rockville, MD: Aspen Publications.

Schiffer, C. A., Hogge, D. E., Aisner, J., Dutcher, J. P., Lee, E. J., & Papenberg, D. (1984). High dose intravenous gammaglobulin in alloimmunized platelet transfusion recipients. *Blood, 64,* 937–940.

Schiffer, C. A., & Slichter, S. J. (1982). Platelet transfusions from single donors. *New England Journal of Medicine, 307,* 245–247.

Schiffer, C. A., & Wade, J. C. (1987). Supportive care: Issues in the use of blood products and treatment of infection. *Seminars in Oncology, 14,* 454–467.

Smith, L. G. (1984). Reactions to blood transfusions. *American Journal of Nursing, 84,* 1096–1101.

Sniecinski, I., O'Donnell, M. R., Nowicki, B., and Hill, L. R. (1988). Prevention of refractoriness and HLA-alloimmunization using filtered blood products. *Blood, 71,* 1402–1407.

Strauss, R. G., Connett, J. E., Gale, R. P., Bloomfield, C. D., Herzig, G. P., McCullough, J., Maguire, L. C., Winston, D. J., Ho, W., Stump, D. C., Miller, W. V., & Keopke, J. A. (1981). A controlled trial of prophylactic granulocyte transfusions during initial induction chemotherapy for acute myelogenous leukemia. *New England Journal of Medicine, 305,* 597–603.

Taylor, B. N., Wagner, P. L., & Kraus, C. L. (1987). Development of a standard for time-effective patient assessment during blood transfusion. *Journal of Nursing Quality Assurance, 1,* 66–71.

Von Fliedner, V., Higby, D. J., & Kim, U. (1982). Graft-versus-host reaction following blood product transfusion. *American Journal of Medicine, 72,* 951–961.

Walker, R. H. (1987). Special report: Transfusion risks. *American Journal of Clinical Pathology, 88,* 374–378.

Weiden, P. (1984). Graft-versus-host disease following blood transfusions. *Archives of Internal Medicine, 144,* 1557–1558.

Widmann, F. K. (Ed.). (1985). *Technical manual.* Arlington, VA: American Association of Blood Banks.

Winston, D. J., Ho, W. G., & Gale, R. P. (1981). Prophylactic granulocyte transfusions during chemotherapy of acute nonlymphocytic leukemia. *Annals of Internal Medicine, 94,* 616–622.

Winston, D. J., Ho, W. G., & Gale, R. P. (1982). Therapeutic granulocyte transfusions for documented infections. *Annals of Internal Medicine, 97,* 509–515.

Wright, D. (1984), Leukocyte transfusions: Thinking twice. *American Journal of Medicine, 76,* 637–644.

Wright, D. G., Robinchaud, K. J., Pizzo, P. A., & Deisseroth, A. B. (1981). Lethal pulmonary reactions associated with the combined use of amphotericin B and leukocyte transfusions. *New England Journal of Medicine, 304,* 1185–1189.

Yankee, R. A., Grumet, F. C., & Rogentine, G. N. (1969). The selection of compatible platelet donors for refractory patients by lymphocyte HLA typing. *New England Journal of Medicine, 281,* 1212.

CHAPTER 27

Bone Marrow Transplantation

ROSEMARY C. FORD

HISTORICAL PERSPECTIVE

The first bone marrow transplants in humans were conducted in the 1950s in patients with end-stage leukemia. These transplants were unsuccessful in that all the patients relapsed; however, the patients did show hematologic recovery. Extensive laboratory studies based on these early experiments were conducted during the next decade using mice and dogs. By the late 1960s several developments had offered encouragement to again try marrow transplant in humans, including advances in tissue typing, improved techniques for pheresis of blood products, and development of more effective and broad-spectrum antibiotics. Clinical trials resumed in the early 1970s, again with patients considered to be in the end stages of their disease (Box 27–1) (Thomas et al., 1977). Because of the success of these studies, protocols were initiated for patients earlier in their course of treatment, when their physical condition was better (Appelbaum et al., 1988).

Since the early 1970s, the number of long-term transplantation survivors has increased every year. Relapse and long-term survival vary depending on the diagnosis of the patient and the type of transplant (Table 27–1). Along with improved survival rates, the number of centers offering transplantations has also grown, especially in the last decade, with an estimated 160 units currently functioning in the United States (Bortin & Rim, 1986). Cost of care continues to be very high, with hospitalization averaging $100,000 (Kay, Powles, Lawler, & Clink, 1980).

Marrow transplantation remains a highly experimental procedure. Medical research on transplant units continues to focus on finding optimum conditioning therapies, timing of transplantation in the course of the patient's original disease, and preventing or limiting the major complications such as infections and graft-versus-host disease (Gale, 1986).

BONE MARROW TRANSPLANT NURSING AS A SPECIALTY

Bone marrow transplantation (BMT) has become established over the last 20 years as a treatment option for patients with aplastic anemia, hematologic malignancies, selected solid tumors, and some genetic disorders (Appelbaum & Thomas, 1985; Burton, Horowitz, & Gale, 1988; O'Reilly, 1983; Thomas, 1983). As transplantation has become accepted on a wide scale in the medical community, nursing in this area has grown into a specialty. This specialty requires expertise in many established areas of nursing, including oncology, critical care, pediatrics, and psychosocial nursing (Buchsel & Ford, 1988).

There are obvious similarities between oncology nursing and BMT nursing. Most patients who undergo transplantation have a malignant disease, and the types of therapies and nursing approaches used with the patients often are the same as those used routinely with oncology patients. There are, however, some differences between the two specialties. First, although all marrow transplant patients have a life-threatening

---

Box 27–1. THE FIRST LARGE-SCALE MARROW TRANSPLANT STUDY

Thomas, E. D., Buckner, C. D., Banaji, M., Clift, R. A., Fefer, A., Flournoy, N., Goodell, B. W., Hickman, R. O., Lerner, K. G., Neiman, P. E., Sale, G. E., Sanders, J. E., Singer, J., Stevens, M., Storb, R., & Weiden, P. L. (1977). **One hundred patients with acute leukemia treated by chemotherapy, total body irradiation, and allogeneic marrow transplantation.** *Blood, 49,* 511–533.

A milestone in the field was reached with the publication in 1977 of the results of bone marrow transplantation as a treatment for 100 patients with end-stage leukemia. In all 94 patients who lived long enough for engraftment to occur (21 days after transplantation) engraftment did take place. This large-scale study compared various preparation regimens and reported the types and incidence of complications for which marrow transplant patients are at risk. Interstitial pneumonia was the cause of death in 34 patients, 50 patients developed moderate to severe graft-versus-host disease, and 31 patients had relapses.

The most remarkable finding, however, was the 13 patients alive without recurrent leukemia 1 to 4.5 years after transplantation. These patients would not have survived without transplant. This was a major breakthrough in the field of oncology. From these encouraging early results, protocols were implemented for patients earlier in the course of their disease who were in better clinical condition to undergo the rigorous therapy required in marrow transplantation.

---

disease, not all have malignant disease. Second, whereas oncology nurses care for patients of all age groups, transplant patients are a younger population with a median age of 20 years. Many transplant centers use a cut-off age for acceptance into protocol of 50 years. Third, all patients are on elective protocols. Bone marrow transplantation is almost always an experimental procedure and is treatment of choice for only a small number of diseases. Fourth, whereas chemotherapy and irradiation doses are limited in the usual oncology setting because of marrow toxicity, supralethal doses of these therapies provide the basis of treatment in marrow transplant, creating maximum toxicities. Fifth, transplant patients may be treated far from their homes, away from already established support systems. Sixth, the goal of marrow transplantation is always cure. Finally, in addition to requiring the same knowledge base as oncology nurses, BMT nurses need the skills to care for critical-care patients. Dialysis, ventilatory support, and hemodynamic monitoring must all be available to meet the care needs of BMT patients (Kelleher & Jennings, 1988; O'Quin & Moravec, 1988).

TYPES OF MARROW TRANSPLANTS

Transplanted marrow can be obtained from several sources, and the source determines the "type" of transplant the patient receives. To understand how the most appropriate donor is selected, an overview of the tissue typing process is necessary. In searching for a marrow donor, the human leukocyte antigens (HLA) are identified from blood drawn from the patient and all potential donors (Fig. 27–1). These antigens play a role in the immune response (Dudjak, 1984). The HLA-A, HLA-B, and HLA-C loci are identified through a cytotoxic assay using anti-HLA antibodies. The HLA-D locus is identified by a mixed lymphocyte culture of cells from the patient and the potential donors. Reactivity is monitored, and if there is no response, the mixed lymphocyte culture is "negative"

and therefore the HLA-D locus is considered matched (Hansen et al., 1987).

The ABO blood antigens are also identified at this time. A difference in ABO blood groups between patient and donor will not interfere with donor selection; however, it does present unique clinical problems. The marrow infusion may have to be depleted of red blood cells (RBCs) to prevent a hemolytic reaction caused by antibodies still circulating from the patient's original marrow. At times the patient will have to undergo a plasma exchange to eliminate antibodies against the ABO group of the donor. A new method has been utilized in which the patient's plasma is run through a column of synthetic antigens that attract and remove the ABO antibodies (Bensinger, 1984). The patient's own plasma is then returned missing only the ABO antibodies. After transplant, all patients will become the ABO type of their donor.

The most desirable donor in terms of compatibility is an identical twin. Transplants from identical twins are called syngeneic. Transplants from persons other than twins are called allogeneic. Allogeneic donors may or may not be HLA-MLC matched with the patient. These donors are usually siblings; however, other family members can also be used as donors. The odds of a patient matching a sibling are 1 in 4, resulting in only 35 to 40 per cent of patients having a matched sibling (Fig. 27–2) (Appelbaum, 1989; Beatty et al., 1988). Unrelated but HLA-matched donors have been used successfully for patients without related donors (Beatty et al., 1985; McCullough, Hansen, Perkins, Stroncek, & Bartsch, 1989). Mismatched donors have also been used. When the donor and patient differ in only one HLA haplotype, the results are similar to those of patients with matched donors. When differences occur in two or three haplotypes, the incidence of complications is markedly increased (Anasetti, 1989). Figure 27–2 illustrates the chance of finding a suitable donor for patients eligible for transplantation.

Allogeneic transplants are the prototype of transplants for hematologic malignancies. The success rates of allogeneic transplants led to trials of autologous

Table 27–1. RELAPSE AND LONG-TERM SURVIVAL RATES AFTER BONE MARROW TRANSPLANTATION

Disease	Disease Status at Time of Transplantation	Type of Transplant	Relapse (Per Cent)	Long-term Survival* (Per Cent)
Aplastic anemia	No history of blood transfusion	Allogeneic	NA	55–73
	History of blood transfusion	Allogeneic	NA	40–80
Thalassemia	—	Allogeneic	NA	75
Acute lymphocytic leukemia	Remission	Allogeneic	30–50	25–50
	Relapse	Allogeneic	50–70	10–20
	Remission	Autologous	32	43
	Relapse	Autologous	>50	15
Acute nonlymphocytic leukemia	First remission	Allogeneic	10–40	40–70
	Second or subsequent remission	Allogeneic	†	20–50
	First relapse	Allogeneic	†	20–34
	Second or subsequent relapse	Allogeneic	50–70	25–30
	Remission	Autologous	32	40–48
	Relapse	Autologous	>50	30
Chronic myelogenous leukemia	Chronic phase	Allogeneic	12–20	45–70
	Accelerated phase	Allogeneic	40–56	15–28
	Blast crisis	Allogeneic and autologous	50–75	5–15
Lymphoma (Hodgkin's or non-Hodgkin's)	Multiple relapse	Allogeneic and autologous	60	22
		Syngeneic		
	First relapse or second remission	Allogeneic and autologous	41	42
Preleukemia				50
Metastatic neuroblastoma			20	40

NA, not applicable.

*Long-term survival is defined as alive 3 years without evidence of disease.

†No data available.

transplants in patients without a suitable marrow donor. Autologous transplants use the patient's own marrow. When the patient is in remission, marrow is aspirated and frozen. At a later date, usually after the patient has relapsed, the patient then undergoes high-dose conditioning in an attempt to destroy all tumor cells. The marrow is then reinfused back into the patient, sometimes after having been treated in vitro with agents to remove any residual tumor cells (Kemshead et al., 1987; Linch & Burnett, 1986; Yeager et al., 1986).

Each type of transplant has advantages and disadvantages. Autologous transplant recipients experience less regimen-related toxicity than allogeneic transplant recipients (Bearman et al., 1988). Autologous and syngeneic transplants eliminate the complication of graft-versus-host disease (GVHD, to be discussed later in this chapter). Both of these types of transplants, however, have a higher relapse rate than allogeneic

transplants, in which a possible "graft-versus-leukemia" effect has been hypothesized (Butturni, Bortin, & Gale, 1987; Weiden, Flournoy, Sanders, Sullivan, & Thomas, 1981). Analysis of relapse rates suggests that the immunocompetent cells in the allogeneic graft have a role in eliminating residual host leukemia cells beyond the eradication of these cells by the conditioning regimen. It has also been noted that patients who develop GVHD have a lower incidence of recurrent leukemia (Sullivan et al., 1987).

Marrow transplantation is now being tried as a new application in the area of solid tumors. In these patients, who rarely have disease in the marrow, autologous instead of allogeneic transplants have been the prototype. Unfortunately, although substantial response rates have been seen in decreasing the tumors of the patients, the response is usually short-lived (Appelbaum, 1989). Medical research using autologous marrow transplants for solid tumors is still in phase I and II trials, in which optimal patient selection, timing, and dosing of therapy are being studied (Antman & Gale, 1988; Armitage & Gale, 1989; Pinkerton et al., 1987; Williams et al., 1989; Wolff et al., 1989).

THE TRANSPLANTATION PROCESS

Preadmission

The timing of transplantation depends on the patient's diagnosis. Untransfused aplastic anemia patients may be admitted to a transplant unit within a week after diagnosis, whereas patients with chronic leukemia may be admitted 5 years after initial diagnosis. These patients will be at very different stages in terms of

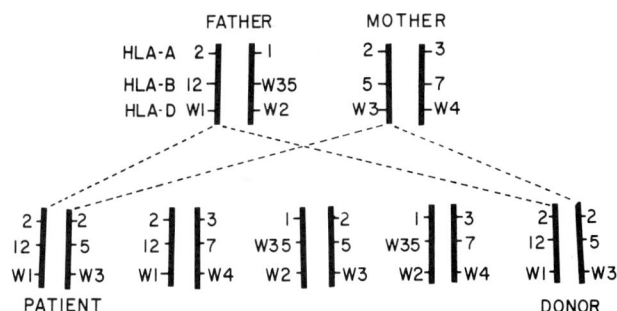

Figure 27–1. Example of the possible combinations of the human leukocyte antigen (HLA) region of chromosome 6 passed to a patient and siblings from the patient's parents. The patient and donor have inherited the same haplotypes and thus are HLA genotypically identical.

CHANCE OF FINDING A DONOR

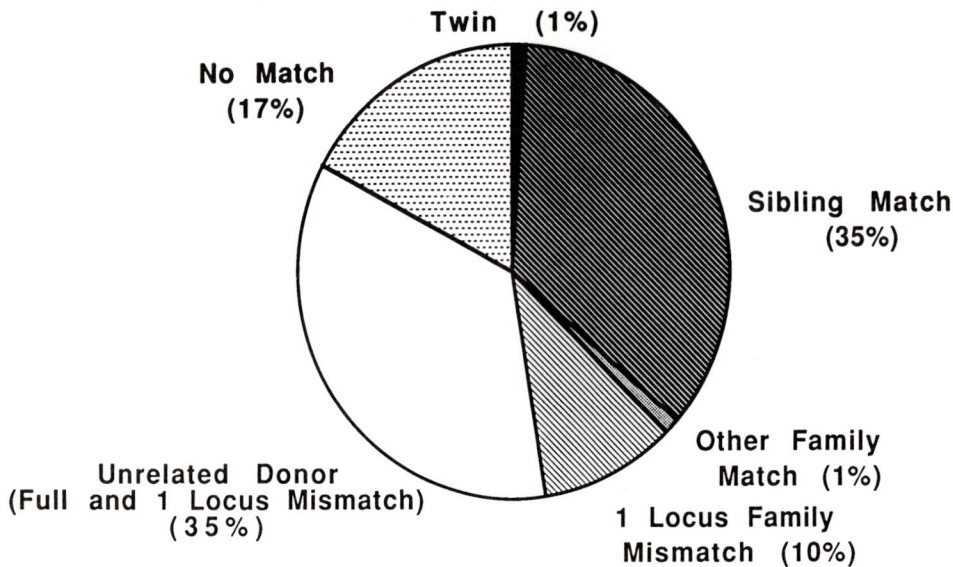

Figure 27–2. Diagram illustrating the probability of finding a marrow donor if current plans for establishing a registry of unrelated bone marrow donors progress as projected. (From Beatty, P. G. et al. [1988]. Probability of finding HLA-matched unrelated marrow donors. *Transplantation, 45,* 714–718. Reproduced by permission.)

their grief in coping with a potentially fatal disease, their knowledge of their disease, and their familiarity with hospital environments. Nurses must individualize patient teaching to match the knowledge base of each patient.

Ideally, at the time of diagnosis, before induction therapy (see Chapter 21) is started, it should be determined whether the patient is a candidate for marrow transplantation. Unfortunately, this is not usually done, and the patient is treated with standard chemotherapy (Appelbaum, 1989). Factors that should be considered are the patient's physical, emotional, and psychological status; the possibility of identifying an acceptable marrow donor; the patient's financial status, including insurance coverage; and the patient's philosophy on entering a research study (Buchsel & Parchem, 1988). Induction therapy could then be coordinated with future conditioning therapy for transplantation should it be necessary. When patients are referred for possible transplantation after usual treatment, conditioning regimens must sometimes be altered in light of previously received toxic regimens (Appelbaum, 1989).

The patient's primary physician usually presents the option of marrow transplantation with a recommendation as to which center to consider; however, it is becoming common for patients to "shop" the various centers to find the one most acceptable. Once a referral is made to a transplant center, the medical staff at the center determines whether the patient is eligible for entry on a current protocol. When the patient is accepted by the center, the patient and the referring physician are notified, and the patient may be placed on a waiting list for an opening at the center. At this time, sperm banking should be discussed with male patients because the irradiation used in conditioning will cause sterility (Buchsel, 1986). The length of the wait is determined by many factors, including the acuteness of the patient's condition, the protocol prior-

ities at the center, and the physical status of the patient. The transplant center should send preliminary information to the referring physician and nurse to aid in patient education. The patient and the donor must both come to the center for about 1 week before admission to confirm the health status of both, the remission status of the patient, and the genetic match of the donor. The health care team should clarify expectations of the patient and family and keep them informed of the results of the preadmission work-up and how these may affect the patient's transplant course. A permanent right atrial dual-lumen, or in some cases triple-lumen, catheter is inserted for venous access if the patient does not already have one in place (Box 27–2).

Admission to the Marrow Transplant Unit

When the patient has completed the preadmission work-up, he or she is admitted to the transplant unit. In a family conference, the inpatient team explains the treatment protocols, responds to concerns, and obtains signatures on research consent forms. The primary nurse should review the teaching begun in the outpatient department and initiate an individualized care plan for this patient.

Conditioning Therapy

The patient begins conditioning therapy to prepare for the marrow transplantation soon after admission. Conditioning consists of high-dose chemotherapy or total body irradiation (TBI), or both, precisely timed (Fig. 27–3). The purpose is to totally eradicate the patient's original marrow and any residual tumor cells.

Box 27–2. COMPARISON OF FLUSH SOLUTIONS FOR HICKMAN CATHETER IRRIGATION

Dr. Robert O. Hickman developed the prototype of the permanent, tunneled right atrial catheter for marrow transplant patients in the mid-1970s. Marrow transplant units continue to conduct research to fine-tune management of these now widely used catheters.

A randomized, double-blind, pilot study was conducted at Fred Hutchinson Cancer Research Center, Seattle, Washington, between February and August 1988, to determine whether there is a difference in thrombotic complications when using normal saline solution and heparinized saline solution, 100 USP u/ml, as a Hickman catheter irrigant in marrow transplant patients. Patients were entered into the study before their catheter placement. They were followed from the day of the catheter insertion until (1) they died or they were first discharged to the outpatient department after marrow transplantation, (2) removal of the catheter, or (3) withdrawal from the study. Those eligible for this protocol had to weigh more than 20 kg and have the catheter inserted at Fred Hutchinson Cancer Research Center.

Data collected included patient demographics, catheter type, catheter insertion and removal dates, antimicrobial therapy (including colonization and cultures), and any catheter-related complications. Catheter complications included inability to infuse through or aspirate from the catheter, line breakage or accidental dislodgment, local and systemic infections, or any event that led to premature removal of the catheter.

A total of 39 patients were entered into the pilot study. Twenty-nine patients were followed from catheter insertion until either their discharge to the outpatient department or their death after transplantation. Six patients withdrew from the study; however, data from their catheters were included in the analysis. Catheters were removed in the remaining four patients. Two catheters were removed for reasons of infection; two catheters were removed because of accidental dislodgment. No catheters were removed because of thrombus formation.

Thrombi occurred in two of 17 catheters in the normal saline solution arm of the project. Right subclavian venous thrombosis occurred in one of 22 patients in the heparinized saline solution arm. On the basis of these findings, the study will proceed, accruing a total of 200 patients, to increase the confidence level of the data.

(Ulz, L. [1988]. *Normal saline solution versus heparinized saline solution for Hickman catheter irrigation.* Unpublished paper.)

Much of the research currently being conducted on transplant units is involved with the dosing, timing, and sequencing of these conditioning therapies. The goal is to find the therapy that provides the best tumor kill with the least toxicity to unaffected major organs (Appelbaum et al., 1989; Bearman et al., 1988). The common chemotherapeutic agent used is cyclophosphamide, given in megadose; however, dimethylbusulfan, cytosine arabinoside, etoposide, melphalan, and carmustine are also used (Appelbaum et al., 1989; Welenglass et al., 1988; Jagganath et al., 1989; Kanfer et al., 1987; Riddall et al., 1988; Schmitz et al., 1988). Total body irradiation can be given from one or two sources at one session or fractionated over several days.

All patients experience side effects during the days of conditioning, including severe nausea, vomiting, and diarrhea. Owing to the severe gastrointestinal response during high-dose chemotherapy infusion, continuous antiemetic coverage is recommended. The antiemetics can cause profound sedation, and nurses must keep the patients arousable while administering optimal antiemetic relief. High-dose cyclophosphamide can cause cardiotoxicity. Electrocardiograms should be taken before each dose to assess for decreased voltage (Hutchison & King, 1983). Hemorrhagic cystitis can also result from high-dose cyclophosphamide. Bladder irrigation and intravenous hydration should be initiated before and continue 24 hr after administration of this medication (Hutchison & King, 1983).

Total body irradiation usually produces less severe nausea and vomiting than high-dose chemotherapy and so requires less antiemetic usage. The patient may become febrile immediately after TBI. Some patients also develop bilateral parotitis (Hutchison & King, 1983).

The Bone Marrow Donor

On or around the last day of conditioning of the patient, the marrow donor is admitted to the hospital to donate marrow. This is a surgical procedure requiring general or spinal anesthesia (Ruggiero, 1988). Multiple aspirations from the anterior and posterior iliac crests of the pelvic bone are performed (Fig. 27–4). The volume of marrow is determined by the size of the donor, with a pediatric donor usually yielding a volume of 300 ml and a male adult donor often yielding a volume of more than 1000 ml. The marrow is filtered

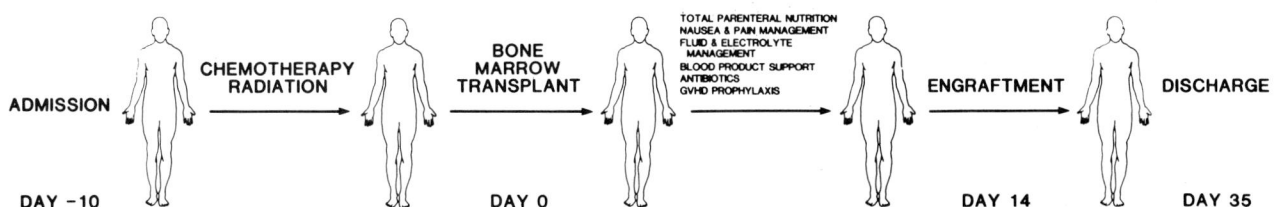

Figure 27–3. Depiction of the process for an allogeneic marrow transplant. In this example, the patient receives conditioning to prepare for the transplant and then receives graft-versus-host-disease (GVHD) prophylaxis per protocol.

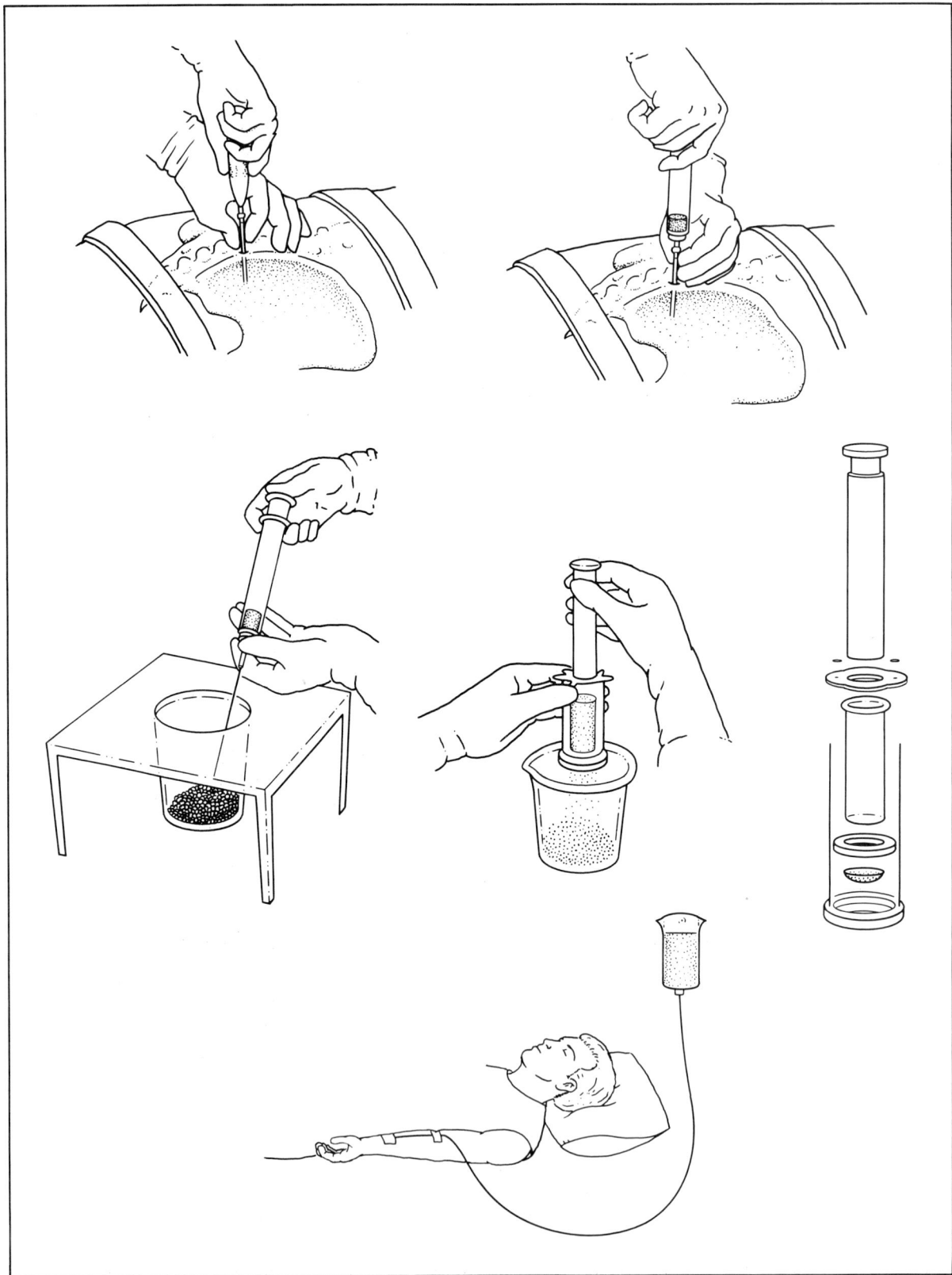

Figure 27–4. Sequence of steps in aspirations of marrow from donor. A large-bore needle is placed in the posterior iliac crest, and multiple aspirations of 3 to 5 ml of marrow are performed. The marrow is placed in a collecting beaker, drawn up in a large syringe, and forced through a coarse metal grid to remove bone and fat particles. The marrow is then placed in a blood administration bag and administered through the patient's central venous catheter.

in the operating room using a large metal mesh to remove bone particles and fat and then is placed in blood administration bags (Holcombe, 1987; Ruggiero, 1988).

The marrow donor may require a RBC transfusion after donation because most of the volume of marrow aspiration is whole blood. Often the marrow donor undergoes pheresis for a unit of blood a week before marrow donation, which is returned during surgery (Ruggiero, 1988). Donors are usually discharged the day after surgery with oral pain medication, prophylactic antibiotics, and ferrous sulfate supplements.

The donors must be included in the planning of care to the patient-family unit. In addition to the discomfort of the actual marrow donation, the donor faces a major inconvenience in time commitment. Some centers require that the donor be in close geographic proximity of the center when the patient begins conditioning therapy to ensure the availability of the donor to donate when the patient is ready to receive the marrow. This requirement could call for a 2- or 3-week time commitment. After donating the marrow, the donor may be needed for platelet or white cell donation. This commitment may spread into months if the patient becomes refractory to platelets from other donors.

The psychological impact of donating marrow must be evaluated for each donor and appropriate interventions planned. Donors at times feel ignored in the larger transplant scheme, in which so much attention is given to the patient. They may not feel satisfactorily thanked for their sacrifice and then may feel guilty for these feelings. If the patient develops complications after transplant, feelings of guilt may again surface for not having good enough marrow, or—in the case of GVHD—of actually causing the problem. A goal should be to help the donor achieve a sense of emotional and intellectual balance before and after the transplant (Ruggiero, 1988).

The Marrow Transplantation

The actual marrow transplantation is a relatively simple procedure. The marrow is infused into the patient's right atrial catheter, similar to a blood transfusion, except that it is not irradiated or filtered. The rate should be as rapid as possible, determined by the patient's fluid status. Care must be taken to prevent fluid overload because of the colloid load being administered. Side effects are rare; however, chills or a rash occasionally occurs. Rarely a patient may develop a pulmonary fat embolus or anaphylaxis. These are dealt with as they would be if they resulted from any other cause.

The First 100 Days after Marrow Transplantation

The focus of care in a transplant unit is on optimum support of the patient after the insult of the chemoirradiation and until the marrow graft begins to function (Fig. 27–5). This support requires expert nursing care. The patient is at tremendous risk of several potentially fatal complications and multiorgan failure (Bearman et al., 1988). These complications are often insidious, with quick but subtle onsets. Routine nursing tasks, such as taking vital signs, weights, and intake and output, often offer the first clues to the development of a complication and must be performed by a professional staff well educated on the implications of their assessment (Ford & Ballard, 1988).

Complications and Side Effects of the Transplantation Process

Acute complications are defined as those occurring during the first 100 days after marrow transplantation (Ford & Ballard, 1988). The major complications seen in patients after transplantation are the result of the conditioning regimen (chemoirradiation) used to prepare for transplantation (Bearman et al., 1988), the lack of a functioning bone marrow, the replacement of the patient's immune system, or iatrogenic (the result of the therapies the patient receives to treat other complications) (Table 27–2). The complications are rarely the result of the patient's original disease. The conditioning is given in supralethal doses, and patients would die if they were not rescued with marrow transplantation.

Figure 27–6 shows a visual representation of the time of onset of the most frequent complications and their peak time of occurrence; it also shows that the complications often occur simultaneously. There are important concepts to keep in mind in understanding the implications of these complications and the nursing care needed to assist patients in the months after transplantation (Ford & Ballard, 1988).

One of these concepts is that the complications are interrelated (Fig. 27–7). One complication can cause or exacerbate another, or the treatment of one can cause or exacerbate another (Storb & Thomas, 1985). Or, the treatment of one complication may have to be modified or terminated because of the development of another complication and so the patient is at risk for the development of the complication originally being treated.

Another concept to keep in mind is that the clinical onset of many of the complications may be subtle, and the clinical manifestations of different complications can be the same. This has major implications for the quality of nursing assessment (Ford & Ballard, 1988). Nurses must be well educated in assessing these patients with complications and in interpreting the results of their assessments. Table 27–3 identifies the complications discussed later in this chapter with the clinical manifestations and nursing implications for each. Further elaboration of nursing care can be found in the appropriate sections in Chapters 47 through 58. The probability of developing these complications and the mortality rate differ for each (Table 27–4).

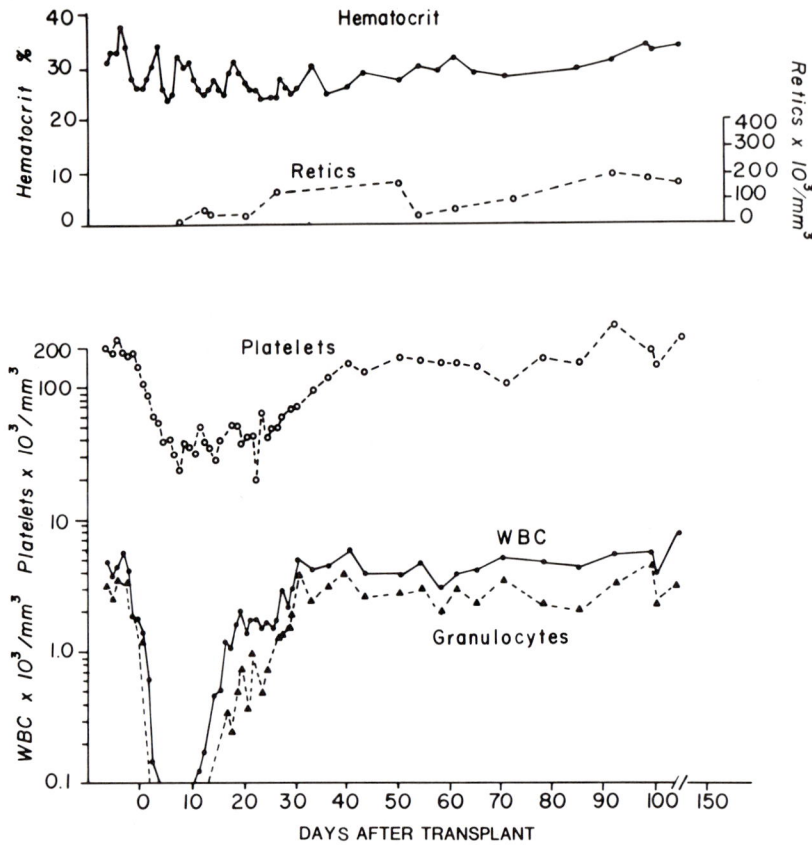

Figure 27–5. Platelet, white blood cell (WBC), and granulocyte counts of a patient from the day before transplant to 100 days after transplant. Day 0 is the day of transplant. Platelet transfusions were administered between days 6 and 27 after transplant. The ordinate is on a log scale to display the very low cell counts.

Table 27–2. CAUSES OF ACUTE AND CHRONIC COMPLICATIONS

Conditioning Regimen (Chemoirradiation Therapies)	Lack of Functioning Marrow	Replacement of Immune System	Iatrogenic Complications
Acute			
Nausea and vomiting	Hemorrhage	Acute GVHD	Renal failure
Diarrhea	Infections		Hypertension
Mucositis	Cytomegalovirus pneumonia		Electrolyte imbalance
Alopecia			
Lethargy			
Veno-occlusive disease			
Interstitial pneumonia			
Chronic			
Cataracts	Late infections	Chronic GVHD	
Sterility			
Delay or lack of puberty			

GVHD, Graft-versus-host disease.

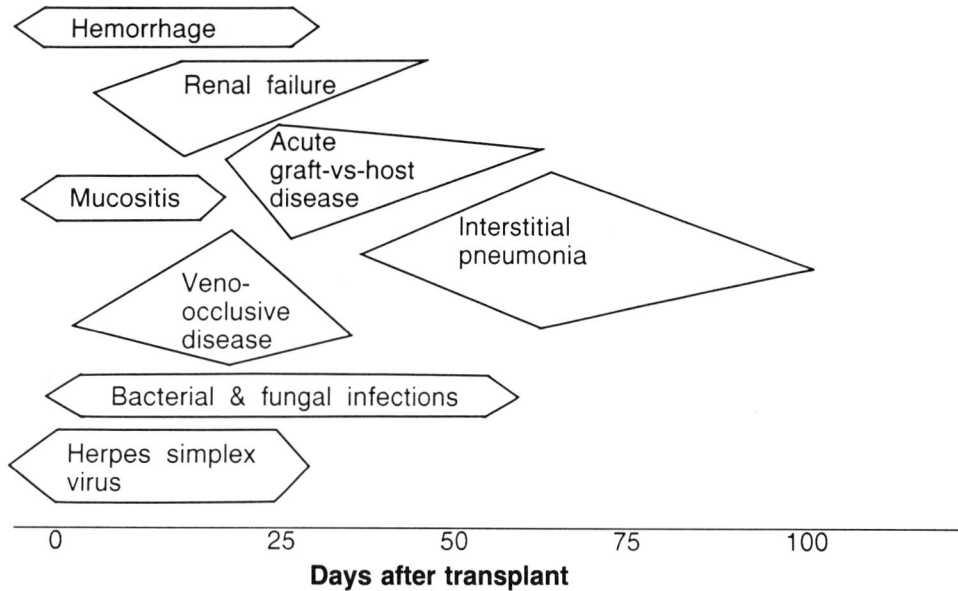

Figure 27–6. The approximate time of onset of the major acute complications after bone marrow transplantation. The peaks in the figures (when present) represent the peak incidence of each complication. (From Ford, R. C., & Ballard, B. [1988]. Acute complications after bone marrow transplantation. *Seminars in Oncology Nursing, 4,* 15–24. Reproduced by permission.)

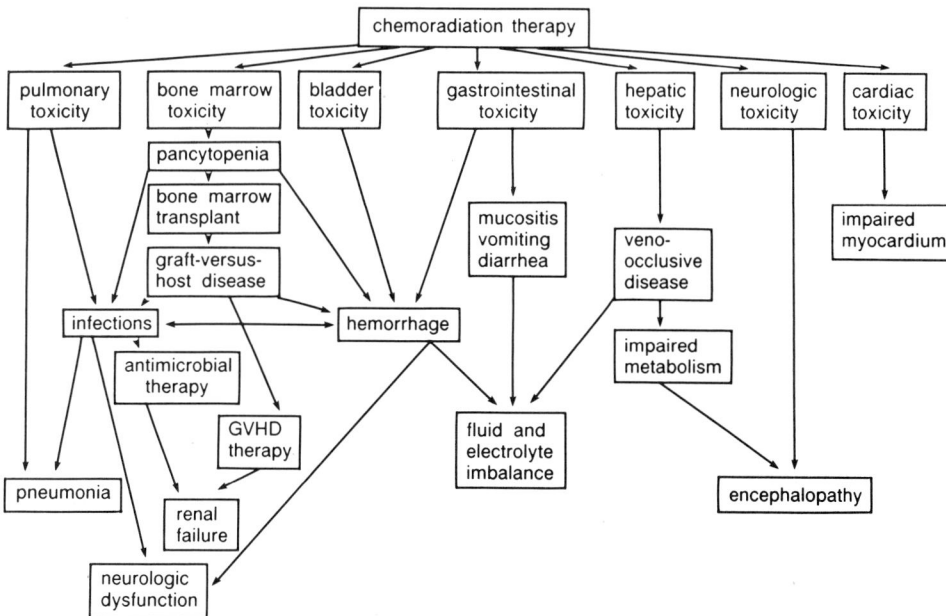

Figure 27–7. The interrelationships among the major acute bone marrow transplantation (BMT) complications, etiologies, and treatments. (From Ford, R. C., & Ballard, B. [1988]. Acute complications after bone marrow transplantation. *Seminars in Oncology Nursing, 4,* 15–24. Reproduced by permission.)

Table 27–3. CLINICAL MANIFESTATIONS AND NURSING IMPLICATIONS OF ACUTE COMPLICATIONS AFTER TRANSPLANTATION

Complication	Clinical Manifestations	Nursing Implications
Mucositis	Initially dry mouth, sore throat, thickening saliva; progressing to copious oral mucus, intense pain, high probability of oral bleeding and infections	• Inspect mouth three times a day, noting color, consistency of mucus, presence of lesions or hemorrhage • Teach patient to perform mouth care with normal saline solution at least every 4 hr • Titrate topical anesthetics and narcotics to patient comfort
Hemorrhage		• Monitor platelet counts • Administer platelets • Avoid invasive procedures when platelet count is less than 50,000 per µl • Avoid medications by intramuscular route
	Epistaxis	• Apply pressure, ice, topicals such as epinephrine, cocaine • In severe cases the nose may need to be packed
	Mouth bleeding often occurs simultaneously with epistaxis	• Assess airway for patency • Keep oral airway at bedside • Apply topicals as for epistaxis • Encourage frequent mouth care with iced saline solution and cautious use of suction
	Central nervous system bleeding	• Frequent neuroassessment • Lumbar puncture only with platelet count >50,000 • Elevate head of bed
	Gastrointestinal bleeding can be frank or occult	• Guaiac test for all vomitus and stools • Avoid nasogastric tubes, enemas, and rectal medications and temperatures
	Genitourinary	• Assess for blood in urine • Irrigate bladder during administration of cyclophosphamide • Prevent trauma during urinary catheter insertion • Administer medroxyprogesterone acetate to stop menstrual bleeding
Nausea and vomiting	Complaints of nausea Emesis Anorexia	• Assess amount, apperance, color, guaiac positivity, consistency of emesis • Titrate routine antiemetics to patient comfort • Administer total parenteral nutrition until symptoms decrease and appetite returns • Encourage compliance with oral medications
Alopecia		• Support patient in coping with body image change • Suggest hats, scarves, wigs
Lethargy		• Encourage patients to ambulate and participate in activities of daily living, schedule times in medication schedule for ambulation, coordinate exercise plan with physical therapists
Veno-occlusive disease	Sudden weight gain, increase in bilirubin, SGOT, and alkaline phosphatase levels Hepatomegaly Ascites Encephalopathy	• Exact assessment of fluid balances and therapy • Check weight twice daily • Measure abdominal girth daily • Postural blood pressure twice daily • Restrict fluids and sodium intake • Monitor narcotic usage in light of changed liver metabolism • Hemodynamic monitoring if indicated
Renal impairment	Doubling of serum creatinine Decreased urine output Decreased quality of urine	• Strict monitoring of intake and output • Check urine specific gravity every 4 hr • Obtain samples for urine electrolyte and sediment determinations • Monitor patient thirst • Postural blood pressure checks • Assess neck veins • Assess for peripheral edema • Monitor patient during dialysis
Graft-versus-host disease	*Initially:* Maculopapular rash Nausea and vomiting Green watery diarrhea Abdominal pain ↑ SGOT *May progress to:* Total body skin sloughing Copious watery guaiac-positive diarrhea Progressive liver failure	• Daily skin assessment • Daily assessment of stools for quantity, consistency, color • Administer fluids to replace gastrointestinal losses • Protect confused patient

Table 27–3. CLINICAL MANIFESTATIONS AND NURSING IMPLICATIONS OF ACUTE COMPLICATIONS
AFTER TRANSPLANTATION *Continued*

Complication	Clinical Manifestations	Nursing Implications
Infections	Fever Increased lethargy Erythema at potential site	• Daily hygiene, including bath, dressing, change bed linen • Oral care every 4 hr • Reverse isolation • Good handwashing techniques • Maintain laminar air flow if available • Obtain cultures (blood, urine, throat, stool, catheter site) routinely and immediately on suspicion of development of infection • Administer antimicrobials • Institute measures to lower temperature
Pneumonia	Tachypnea Diffuse infiltrates on chest radiograph	• Monitor vital signs • Assess breath sounds, quality of respirations, use of accessory respirator, mucositis, skin color, mental status • Support anxious patient and family • Monitor arterial blood gases • Prepare for bronchoalveolar lavage or surgery • Maintain on ventilator

SGOT, serum glutamic-oxaloacetic transaminase.
(Compiled from Cunningham et al., 1986, and Hutchison & King, 1983.)

Mucositis

Mucositis is a side effect that all transplant patients experience. Patients who are irradiated have more severe mucositis than those who only undergo chemotherapy during conditioning (McDonald, Shulman, Sullivan, & Spencer, 1986). Mucositis starts around the day of transplant with dry mouth, sore throat, and thickening saliva (McDonald et al., 1986). It then progresses with increasing secretion of oral mucus and development of pain, often requiring narcotic analgesia. Superimposed infections often complicate the symptoms and bring added risk of hemorrhage. Frequent assessment of the mouth is a routine part of nursing care. Mucositis does not subside until the marrow graft starts to function (see Fig. 27–6) and the new immune system begins to heal the tissue (Mc-

Table 27–4. PROBABILITY OF DEVELOPMENT AND MORTALITY RATE OF ACUTE COMPLICATIONS AFTER TRANSPLANTATION

Complication	Probability of Development (Per Cent)	Mortality Rate* (Per Cent)
Mucositis	100	1
Hemorrhage	†	1
Nausea and vomiting	100	NA
Alopecia	100	NA
Lethargy	100	NA
Veno-occlusive disease	30	15
Renal impairment	25	10
Graft-versus-host disease	50	8
Infections (excluding cytomegalovirus-induced pneumonia)	100	10
Interstitial pneumonia:		
Cytomegalovirus	17	13
Idiopathic	12	8

*Patients may have more than one cause of death.
†Data not available.
NA, not applicable.

Donald et al., 1986). If the oral pain and lesions persist for longer than 3 weeks, oral infection or acute GVHD should be suspected (Kolbinson, Schubert, Flournoy, & Truelove, 1988).

Hemorrhage

Hemorrhage can occur any time after transplantation; however, it is most likely to occur in the first month after transplantation when the patient is not producing megakaryocytes. Epistaxis is the most frequently seen form (Ford & Ballard, 1988). Bleeding can also occur from the mouth, the gastrointestinal tract (Spencer, Shulman, Myerson, Thomas, & McDonald, 1986), and the genitourinary tract (Brugieres et al., 1989); in the head; and at any site of an invasive procedure (see Table 27–3).

Accessibility of blood products is an essential component of the transplantation procedure (Osterwalder, Gratwohl, Reusser, Tichelli, & Speck, 1988; Wulff et al., 1983). Daily blood cell counts must be conducted to determine blood product need. Hematocrit values are generally kept above 30 per cent and platelet levels above 20,000 per µl. All patients require platelet support. Random pooled platelets are administered until the patient becomes refractory, and then family platelets are given (Press, Schaller, & Thomas, 1986). The patient's marrow donor is the best source of platelets. All blood products are irradiated to prevent T lymphocytes from blood donors from initiating a graft-versus-host response (Sullivan & Parkman, 1983; Weiden, Zuckerman, et al., 1981).

Nausea and Vomiting

Nausea and vomiting, which start during the conditioning regimen, can continue for weeks after transplantation. The entire gastrointestinal tract is damaged and takes weeks to repair (Champlin & Gale, 1984a;

Press et al., 1986). Infections of the gastrointestinal tract can prolong nausea and vomiting (Spencer, Hackman, et al., 1986). During this time most patients stop all oral intake (Aker et al., 1982). All patients require total parenteral nutrition to meet their nutritional requirements (Cunningham et al., 1983; Weisdorf et al., 1987). Compliance in taking oral medications is often a major problem. A large amount of nursing effort is focused on creative methods of oral medication administration, timing antiemetics so maximum relief will coincide with medication administration (Hill, Saeger, & Chapman, 1988).

Alopecia

Alopecia occurs about 1 week after transplantation, with the patient's hair regrowing about 2 months after transplantation. Nurses must support patients in dealing with the stress of body image changes.

Lethargy

Lethargy is a usual side effect of conditioning but it is as well related to the antiemetics and analgesics given during this time (Hutchison & King, 1983). Nurses must encourage patients to be as active as possible. Activities of daily living are often major accomplishments for these patients.

Veno-occlusive Disease

Veno-occlusive disease (VOD) is a disease of the liver that is rarely seen in other patient populations. Patients at highest risk are those over the age of 30, those with the most intensive conditioning regimens, and those with a history of liver disease (McDonald et al., 1985, 1986). One third of all transplant patients with malignancy develop VOD (McDonald, 1985). One half of these patients recover, and the other half die, with liver disease being the primary or secondary cause of death (McDonald, 1986).

Veno-occlusive disease occurs during the first 3 weeks after transplantation (McDonald, 1986). The symptoms of VOD are weight gain, ascites, upper right quadrant pain, and elevated bilirubin and serum glutamic-oxaloacetic transamenase (SGOT) levels (McDonald, 1985). This is one of the complications with insidious onset that requires astute nursing assessment. There is no treatment for VOD other than decreasing stress on the liver (McDonald, 1986). This may necessitate cutting back or terminating therapies initiated to prevent other complications, such as infection or GVHD, placing the patient at high risk of developing these.

Renal Impairment or Failure

Renal impairment after transplantation is most often caused by therapy initiated to prevent or treat other complications. Roughly one half of all allogeneic transplant patients develop renal disease, as evidenced by a doubling of their serum creatinine levels (Kennedy et al., 1985; Yee et al., 1985). Risk factors include infection and the subsequent therapies used, having received cyclosporine, or having an intravascular volume deficit, a history of liver disease, or a mismatched transplant (Press et al., 1986; Zager et al., 1989). Combinations of these factors, such as receiving amphotericin and cyclosporine, are especially toxic (Kennedy et al., 1983).

Prevention of renal disease focuses on frequent assessment of renal status through monitoring of serum creatinine levels and the amount and analysis of the patient's urine (Ford & Ballard, 1988). Attention needs to be focused on the daily fluid management of these patients to ensure adequate renal blood flow. Treatment of renal disease entails aggressive frequent assessment of fluid and electrolyte status. At times this can be accomplished only through hemodynamic monitoring (O'Quin & Moravec, 1988).

Nephrotoxic drugs should be decreased and ideally eliminated, although this is rarely possible. Patients may require dialysis support until renal function returns. Mortality associated with dialyzed transplant patients is around 85 per cent; however, cause of death is usually multiorgan system failure (Ford & Ballard, 1988).

Graft-versus-Host Disease

Graft-versus-host disease is unique to marrow transplant patients. In GVHD the immune system of the donor (specifically the T lymphocytes) recognizes the tissue of the patient as foreign and launches an attack (Champlin & Gale, 1984b; Press et al., 1986; Sullivan & Parkman, 1983). Three systems of the body are affected by this disease: the skin (see Color Figure 1), the liver, and the gastrointestinal tract (Champlin & Gale, 1984b; Press et al., 1986). The disease can be manifested in any one or all three systems. Risk factors for developing this disease are age over 30 years, having a donor of the opposite sex, or having a donor who is not a perfect HLA-MLC match (McDonald et al., 1986). Graft-versus-host disease can be fatal in any of the systems. This disease occurs in one half of all allogeneic transplants, with 16 per cent of these patients dying of GVHD or related complications, such as infection, hemorrhage, or liver disease (Press et al., 1986).

The onset of GVHD coincides with engraftment. Diagnosis is difficult because the symptoms are hard to differentiate from lingering side effects of the conditioning regimen or other complications (see Table 27–3 for clinical manifestations). Diagnosis is made on the basis of biopsy of the organ involved, laboratory data, and clinical observation (McDonald et al., 1986; Spencer, Shulman, et al., 1986; Storb & Thomas, 1985).

Much of the medical research conducted on marrow transplant units focuses on protocols to prevent or treat GVHD. All therapies used are toxic, and the optimum therapies, or combination of therapies, that cause the least toxicity are constantly being sought. The goal of preventive therapies is to remove or inactivate the T lymphocytes (McDonald et al., 1986; Storb & Thomas, 1985). Methotrexate has been administered in low doses to slow the growth of new marrow and in so doing slow the production of T lymphocytes. Cyclosporine is an immunosuppressive drug that acts specifically against T lymphocytes and so allows the other cells formed in the bone marrow to grow without interference (Press et al., 1986). Studies have shown that these two medications used in combination are more successful at preventing GVHD than either alone (Storb, Deeg, Farewell, et al., 1986; Storb, Deeg, Whitehead, et al., 1986). Prednisone has also been used for GVHD prophylaxis (Forman et al., 1986). Other therapies used to remove T lymphocytes include monoclonal antibodies made specifically against these cells and soy bean agglutinin, which is added to the marrow component before infusion (Reiser et al., 1981; Storb, Deeg, Whitehead, et al., 1986). Should GVHD occur despite prophylaxis, treatment includes increasing the dosage of cyclosporine and administering monoclonal antibodies, horse antithymocyte globulin, and corticosteroids (Martin et al., 1984; McDonald et al., 1986; Press et al., 1986).

Infections

Infections pose an enormous threat to these patients. There is no population of patients who are more immunosuppressed than marrow transplant patients in the weeks before engraftment of the new marrow. Infections caused by bacterial, fungal, or viral pathogens commonly occur alone or in combination in almost every transplant patient (Meyers & Thomas, 1988; Peterson et al., 1983; Winston et al., 1979). Infections contribute to and often are the major cause of death in transplant patients (Peterson et al., 1983; Young, 1984).

Sites of infection will not resemble those of patients with intact immune systems because there is a lack of white blood cells to make pus and inflammation is usually minimal (van der Meer et al., 1984). Temperature elevation is the main parameter used to detect infection; however, this can also be misleading because other factors, such as irradiation, GVHD, and drug or blood product administration can also elevate temperature (Ford & Ballard, 1988). Pancultures should be obtained daily in patients suspected of being infected, although therapy is often started on a best-guess basis before culture results are known.

Risk factors that increase the chance of developing an infection include prolonged granulocytopenia, GVHD, age over 30 years, being in relapse at time of transplant, and colonization before or early after transplantation (Meyers & Atkinson, 1983; van der Meer et al., 1984). Prevention of infection is a major focus of medical protocols on transplant units. All patients must be on protective isolation in private rooms (Ford & Ballard, 1988).

In many units patients are placed in laminar air flow (LAF) rooms (Peterson et al., 1986). These rooms divide a single room in half with one side sterile (Fig. 27–8). The patient enters the "sterile" side after skin decontamination and remains there until engraftment. All supplies, food, and medications entering the patient's side of the room are "low bacteria" or sterile. The patient continues skin decontamination with antimicrobial soap, powders, and ointments and gut decontamination with oral nonabsorbable antibiotics (Lindgren, 1983). Other prophylactic measures to prevent infections include administration of broad spectrum of intravenous antibiotics, antivirals, and antifungals at the start of the transplant process (Burns & Saral, 1985; Meyers & Atkinson, 1983; Press et al., 1986). It has been found that LAF rooms used with prophylactic systemic antibiotics significantly decrease septicemia (Petersen, et al., 1988). Prophylactic intravenous immune globulins have also proved to be effective in decreasing septicemias (Petersen et al., 1987). Treatment of infection includes administration of appropriate antimicrobials, continued surveillance cultures, and close monitoring of patients for development of further complications, such as septic shock. Antimicrobial treatment is often limited by the patient's renal or hepatic function, which may prevent administration of optimal doses.

A new therapy currently in initial trials in some transplant centers is the use of granulocyte macrophage colony stimulating factor (GMCSF). This biologic response modifier has shortened the period of neutropenia in marrow transplant patients, resulting in fewer days of fever and earlier discharge from the hospital (Nemunaitis et al., 1988). Although this method is very promising, researchers are proceeding carefully because of the unknown ability of this new therapy to stimulate malignant cells or increase the severity of GVHD (Klingemann & Eaves, 1988).

Interstitial Pneumonia: Idiopathic or Cytomegalovirus

Interstitial pneumonia is manifested as adult respiratory distress syndrome (ARDS) with peak onset being around day 60 after transplantation (see Fig. 27–6) (Press et al., 1986). This is perhaps the most insidious of the complications, often occurring after patients have been discharged from the inpatient setting. Patients exhibit a rapid onset of symptoms, including a dry cough, dyspnea, nasal flaring, tachypnea, and rales (Press et al., 1986). Diffuse infiltrates are seen on chest radiographs, and marked hypoxia is demonstrated in arterial blood gas analysis. This is the single greatest cause of death in the first 100 days after transplantation (see Table 27–4) (Buckner et al., 1984).

Medical diagnosis of the cause of the pneumonia is difficult because the process is occurring in the interstices of the lungs and not in the airways. Until recently, a sample of lung tissue was needed to make a definitive diagnosis, and patients underwent open lung biopsy if their platelet counts were high enough to tolerate surgery (Buchner et al., 1984). With the current availability of rapid detection culture technology, it is now possible to obtain accurate results using bronchoalveolar lavage, which eliminates the need for

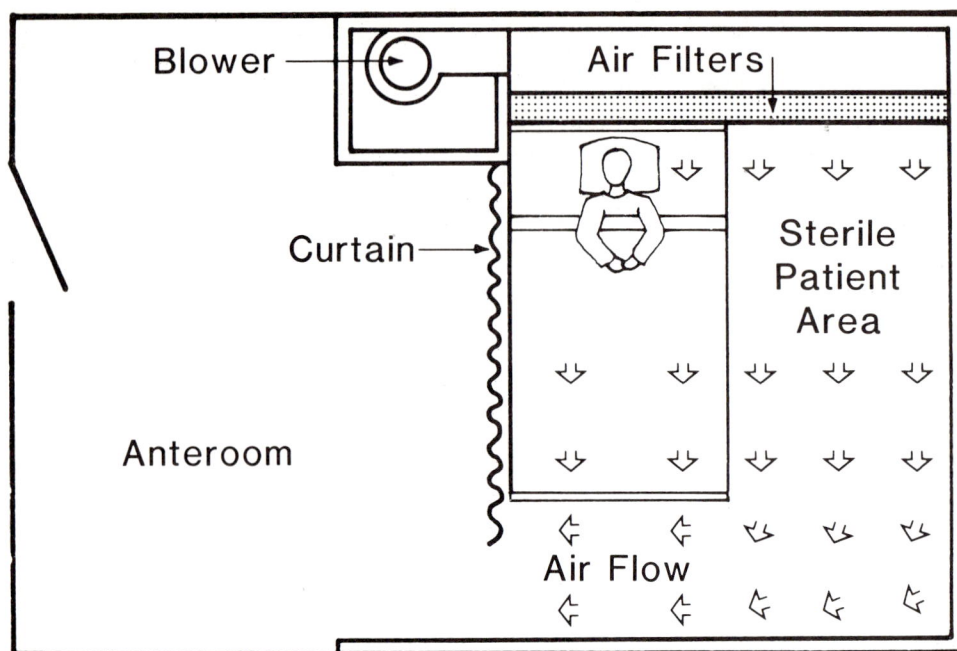

Figure 27–8. Diagram of a laminar air-flow room. The transparent curtain separates the sterile patient zone from the anteroom. Nurses put on sterile attire to enter the room. The patients decontaminate themselves by drinking nonabsorbable antibiotics and applying antibiotic creams and powders to their skin.

surgery, which was so traumatic in the past (Crawford, Hackman, & Clark, 1988; Crawford et al., 1988). Pneumonia is diagnosed as "idiopathic" when no infectious organism can be identified (Springmeyer et al., 1986). These pneumonias are thought to be caused by the irradiation used during conditioning (Press et al., 1986; Springmeyer et al., 1984). Single doses seem to increase the incidence over irradiation doses that are "fractionated" over several days (Buckner et al., 1984; Press et al., 1986). *Idiopathic pneumonia* is responsible for 30 per cent of all pneumonias in these patients (Buckner et al., 1984). If no infectious organism is found after biopsy, the patient is usually treated with ventilatory support and steroids.

Cytomegalovirus (CMV) is the most frequent cause of pneumonia and carries the highest mortality rate (see Table 27–4) (Buckner et al., 1984; Press et al., 1986). Risk factors include previous CMV infection, GVHD, age over 30 years, and exposure to the virus through blood products (Buckner et al., 1984; Meyers, Flournoy, & Thomas, 1986; Press et al., 1986; Springmeyer et al., 1984). In the past, many agents have been tried in the treatment of this pneumonia without success (Krowka, Rosenow, & Hoagland, 1985; Meyers et al., 1983). Ganciclovir and CMV immunoglobulin have shown promise in initial trials (Meyers, 1988). Prevention of this disease is a major focus of medical research, and new agents such as ganciclovir and foscarnet are currently being tried (Meyers, 1988; Sheep et al., 1985). The most promising recent finding is that patients who are seronegative before transplantation and receive marrow from a CMV seronegative donor and blood products that have been screened against CMV do not contract CMV infections (Bowden et al., 1986).

Pneumonia can also be caused by other microorganisms such as other viruses, bacteria, and fungi, which account for approximately 15 per cent of the pneumonias in these patients (Buckner et al., 1984; Press et al., 1986). Many of these can be treated with pharmaceutical agents.

Neurologic Complications

Neurologic complications can occur after marrow transplantation as a result of previous chemotherapy and irradiation, conditioning therapy, or infections, or as a consequence of therapies to control GVHD, such as cyclosporine. Also, organ failure in other systems can lead to central nervous system dysfunction (Davis & Patchell, 1988). Neurotoxicity can be manifested by seizures, cerebellar ataxia, tremor, depression, expressive aphasia, or quadriparesis (Press et al., 1986).

Graft Rejection

Graft rejection, the failure of the new marrow to engraft, has become an increasing problem in recent years. Whereas in early transplant operations the donors were always HLA-matched and the marrow was given to the patient without any manipulation, this is no longer the case. Current studies to increase the available donor pool by using mismatched donors (Beatty et al., 1985), and to decrease the incidence of GVHD by depleting the marrow of T cells before giving it to the patient, have increased the incidence of graft rejection (Anasetti et al., 1989; Martin et al., 1988). Research studies are being formulated to attempt to remove the population of host cells responsible for the rejection or to use growth factors to stimulate the donor's marrow (Appelbaum, 1989).

Psychosocial Responses

The decision to undergo a BMT is a major life crisis for the patient and family. In addition to the very real threat of death, patients experience social isolation, bodily discomfort, major body image changes, and a sense of loss of control (Haberman, 1988; Wiley & House, 1988). These stressors lead to a myriad of emotions, including hope, anger, depression, anxiety, anticipation, guilt, and joy. Pediatric patients often regress, demonstrating behavior of an earlier developmental level (Wiley & House, 1988).

Every aspect of the patient's personal and professional life is disrupted with marrow transplantation. The financial burden is tremendous, including medical expenses for the patient and marrow donor and possibly travel expenses and loss of income for other family members. Patients and their immediate families are often far from usual support systems because of the distance to the transplant center. In some cases, family members who have not been close in the past may be forced by the situation to interact with each other, leading to additional stress.

Nurses have a major role in helping patients cope with the uncertainty and ambiguity of marrow transplantation and in fostering hope (Brack, LaClave, & Blix, 1988). Nurses can plan interventions that give the patient as much control as possible (Haberman, 1988). Fear of the unknown can be decreased through patient education about procedures and potential complications. Nurses can offer strategies such as relaxation, visualization, and distraction for coping with pain and nausea (Haberman, 1988). Pediatric patients should have their developmental levels determined before admission and have activities planned that are appropriate for their age and degree of illness (Kelleher, 1986). Psychosocial assessment and interventions must be a part of every marrow transplant patient's plan of care.

Long-term Complications

The causes of long-term complications after transplantation are the same as those for acute complications. Table 27–5 summarizes chronic complications and the nursing care required (Buchsel, 1986) (Box 27–3).

Chronic Graft-versus-Host Disease

Chronic GVHD occurs in 30 per cent of long-term survivors. As in acute GVHD, it is caused by donor T lymphocytes reacting with the patient's tissue antigens. In addition to the skin, liver, and gut involvement of acute GVHD, the esophagus, eyes, lungs, joints, vaginal mucosa, and other serosal surfaces may be involved (Buchsel, 1986). Chronic GVHD can occur whether patients had acute GVHD or not; however, prognosis is better for those without a history of acute GVHD.

Late Infectious Complications

Late infectious complications are a frequent occurrence in long-term survivors of marrow transplantation. Herpes zoster infections occur in 50 per cent of allogeneic transplant patients in the first year after transplant (Buchsel, 1986). Patients with chronic GVHD are at a higher risk of bacterial pneumonia, septicemia, and sinusitis.

Pulmonary Complications

Pulmonary complications in long-term survivors are thought to be caused by the conditioning regimen and chronic GVHD (Holland, Wingard, Beschorner, Saral, & Santos, 1988). Patients with prior pulmonary problems are at greater risk of chronic pulmonary complications.

Cataracts

Cataracts develop in 20 per cent of patients receiving fractionated irradiation and in 50 per cent of patients receiving single-dose irradiation. The range of time for cataract formation is 1 to 5 years after transplantation. Cataracts can be removed surgically with intraocular lens replacement (Buchsel, 1986).

Retarded Growth and Development in Children

Retarded growth and development in pediatric patients is thought to be caused primarily by irradiation, with chronic GVHD adding to the risk. Bone age seems to be less affected than adrenocortical function, growth hormone levels, and thyroid function. Gonadal dysfunction has been seen in pediatric as well as adult patients after transplantation. Hormonal replacement is being investigated to induce puberty in pediatric patients.

Long-term Survival

The major reason for failure of a marrow transplant is recurrence of the original disease (Appelbaum, 1989; Boyd, Ramberg, & Thomas, 1982). Table 27–1 provides an overview of the major disease categories in which transplantation is offered, with the relapse and long-term survival rates for each.

SUMMARY AND FUTURE TRENDS

As an experimental therapy method, BMT continues to undergo adaptation, incorporating additional therapies and being used in new diagnoses (Osserman et al., 1982; Smith, Shulman, Thomas, Fefer, & Buckner, 1981). Currently, much of the medical research is geared toward decreasing the relapse rate by improving the chemoradiation used in conditioning (Champlin, Jacobs, et al., 1985; Herzig et al., 1985; Shank et al., 1981) or by removing tumor cells with monoclonal antibodies (Badger, Shulman, Peterson, & Bernstein, 1986; Bernstein & Nowinski, 1982; Kemshead et al.,

Table 27–5. CLINICAL MANIFESTATIONS AND NURSING IMPLICATIONS OF CHRONIC COMPLICATIONS AFTER TRANSPLANTATION

Complication	Clinical Manifestations	Nursing Implications
Graft-Versus-Host Disease:		
Skin	Rough, scaly skin Malar erythema Generalized rash Hypo- or hyperpigmentation Dyspigmentation Alopecia Joint contractures Scleroderma Loss of sweating	• Use nonabrasive soaps, lotions, sunscreen • Cosmetic support, makeup, wigs • Range of motion activities • Patient-family education • Monitor compliance with treatment protocols
Liver	Jaundice	• Infection precautions until differential diagnosis is made • Monitor liver function test results • Low fat diet
Oral cavity	Pain, burning, dryness, irritation, soreness, loss of taste Lichenoid changes, atrophy, erythema in oral cavity *Candida* infection Stomatitis Dental caries Xerostomia	• Encourage soft, bland diet • Dental hygiene education, soft toothbrush, flossing • Saline rinses • Dental medicine referral or recommendation • Salivary gland stimulants, sugarless mints, artificial saliva
Ocular	Grittiness, burning of eyes Dry eyes Sicca syndrome	• Artificial tears • Schirmer's tear test: if < 10 mm of wetting, refer to ophthalmologist
Gastrointestinal tract	Anorexia Difficulty eating Painful swallowing Retrosternal pain Weight loss, malabsorption Vomiting	• Serial checking of weight • High calorie food supplements • Recommend nutritional counseling
Vagina	Inflammation Stricture formation causing obstruction of menstrual flow Adhesions Dry vagina Painful intercourse Marital problems	• Water-soluble lubricants • Recommend sexual counseling
Late Infectious Complications		

Bacterial, viral, fungal infections	Fever, wheezing, rales, postnasal drip, signs of infection	• Preventive teaching
		• Mask-wearing until 6 months posttransplantation
		• Obtain cultures
		• Administer antimicrobials
		• Patient teaching should included the following:
		  (a) Avoid infectious persons (measles, chickenpox, mumps)
		  (b) Avoid school or work until 6 months posttransplantation
		  (c) Avoid hot tubs, public swimming pools until 6–9 months posttransplantation
		  (d) Limit number of sexual partners
		  (e) Avoid live virus vaccines

Varicella-zoster virus infection	Lesions, pain, malaise, tenderness, neurologic manifestation	• Relieve pruritus with calamine lotion • Cool compresses • Prevent secondary infection • Obtain cultures • Administer acyclovir
Pulmonary Complications:		
Interstitial pneumonia Cytomegalovirus infection *Pneumocystis carinii* infection	Fever, sepsis, hypotension, lethargy, cough, tachypnea	• Anticipatory preventive teaching • Routine monitoring of vital signs • Chest auscultation and percussion • Monitor pulmonary function test results, arterial blood gases
Restrictive disease	May be asymptomatic or cough	• Anticipatory teaching of pulmonary toilet • Routine monitoring of vital signs • Chest auscultation and percussion

Table 27–5. CLINICAL MANIFESTATIONS AND NURSING IMPLICATIONS OF CHRONIC
COMPLICATIONS AFTER TRANSPLANTATION *Continued*

Complication	Clinical Manifestations	Nursing Implications
Obstructive disease	Decreased ability to perform daily living activities owing to pulmonary insufficiency	• Monitor pulmonary function test results and arterial blood gases
Cataracts	Poor vision	• Anticipatory teaching of BMT risk factors • Ophthalmologist recommendation
Neurologic Complications:		
Leukoencephalopathy	Lethargy Somnolence Dementia Seizures Spastic quadriplegia Coma Personality changes	• Early intervention • Multidisciplinary approach with special education program • Routine neurologic assessments
Psychological Complications	Depression, weight change Altered body image Survival syndrome Sibling rivalry	• Allow patient-family to verbalize feelings • Identify coping mechanisms, personal strengths • Refer to mental health resources
Impaired Growth in Children	Subnormal growth and develpment	• Anticipatory teaching to patients and parents • Annual evaluation of growth pattern • Serial checking of height and weight
Gonadal Dysfunction:		
Female patients	Delayed onset of puberty Premature menopause Sterility	• Careful monitoring of prepubertal girls • Menstrual history • Fertility counseling • Anticipatory teaching and counseling • Sexual counseling
Male patients	Delayed onset of puberty Sterility	• Careful monitoring of prepubertal boys • Fertility counseling • Sperm storage prior to BMT • Anticipatory teaching and counseling • Sexual counseling

(Adapted from Buchsel, P. C. [1956]. Long-term complications of allogeneic bone marrow transplantation: Nursing implications. *Oncology Nursing Forum, 13*[6], 61–70.)

Box 27–3. PSYCHOSOCIAL ADAPTATION AND RECOVERY IN LONG-TERM SURVIVORS OF BONE
MARROW TRANSPLANTATION

Despite improved chances for long-range, disease-free survival, bone marrow transplantation recipients face numerous threats relating to morbidity and mortality. Bone marrow transplantation survivors may be at risk for a host of complications that arise relatively late after transplantation: leukemia relapse, chronic graft-versus-host disease, obstructive pulmonary disease, cataracts, neurologic damage, personality changes, early menopause, and death. Little is known, however, about the explicit effect these medical complications have on survivors' psychosocial well-being and quality of life. We intend to examine the comprehensive impact bone marrow transplantation has on the lives of long-term survivors and their families. An attempt will be made to identify discrete stages of long-term survival and the psychosocial stressors, adaptations, and medical complications that characterize each stage of recovery.

Using a time-series, repeated measures design, we will follow adults who have survived 1 year and beyond at 6-month intervals up to 5 years survival, then yearly thereafter. A large battery of questionnaires will be administered by telephone survey and through the mail. Adaptation and quality of survival will be examined using a wide range of empirical indicators: economic and nutritional status; cognitive impairment; and vocational, physical, psychosocial, and family functioning variables. A better understanding of the problems associated with long-range survival should benefit health care planning for persons at high risk for these problems. Ideally, interventions can be implemented to prevent or minimize the impact of late medical and psychosocial complications of bone marrow transplantation, thereby improving survivors' quality of life.

(Bush, N., & Haberman, M. R. [1990]. *Psychosocial adaptation and recovery in long-term survivors of bone marrow transplantation.* Unpublished paper.)

Example of 24-hr Intravenous Therapy and
Venous Access for a BMT Patient

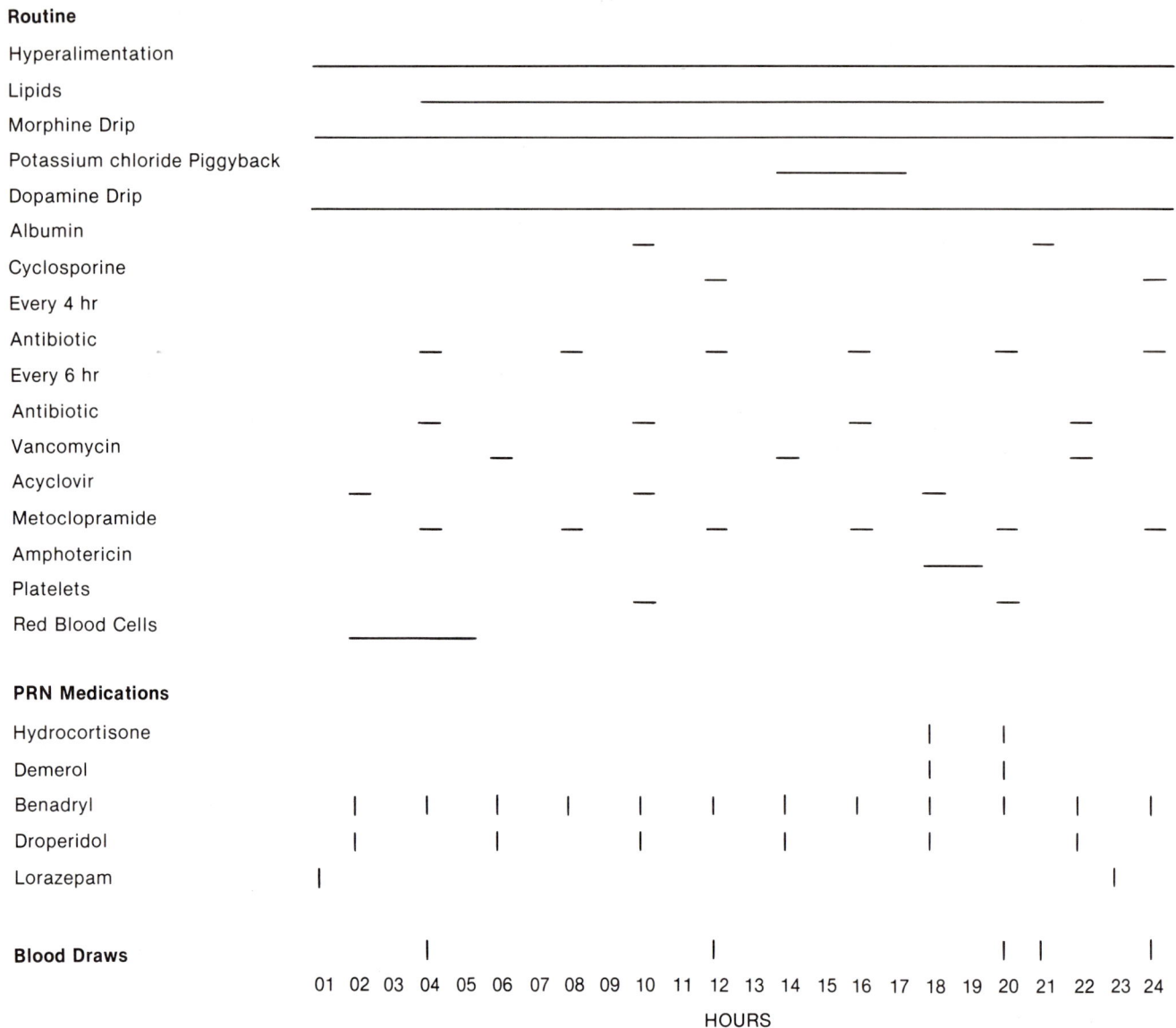

Routine

Hyperalimentation

Lipids

Morphine Drip

Potassium chloride Piggyback

Dopamine Drip

Albumin

Cyclosporine

Every 4 hr

Antibiotic

Every 6 hr

Antibiotic

Vancomycin

Acyclovir

Metoclopramide

Amphotericin

Platelets

Red Blood Cells

PRN Medications

Hydrocortisone

Demerol

Benadryl

Droperidol

Lorazepam

Blood Draws

01 02 03 04 05 06 07 08 09 10 11 12 13 14 15 16 17 18 19 20 21 22 23 24

HOURS

Figure 27-9. Example of the 24-hour intravenous therapy required for a patient in the early weeks after allogeneic transplant, as well as the blood samples required for both research protocols and patient monitoring. The horizontal lines indicate therapies administered by pump over a minimum of 15 minutes; the vertical marks indicate intravenous "push" medications administered by syringe.

1987), using tissue-specific isotopes or antigens (Appelbaum, 1989). Although these regimens offer hope, they increase toxicity (Appelbaum, 1989).

In the future, emphasis will be on increasing the marrow donor pool from unrelated mismatched and cadaveric sources and on improving engraftment with hemopoietic growth factors (Lucas, Quinones, Moses, Nakamura, & Gress, 1988). Major attention will continue to be paid to decreasing the myriad complications following transplantation. The psychological impact of marrow transplantation needs to be examined at the time of the transplant as well as in long-term survivors.

Bone marrow transplantation has offered hope and cure to thousands of patients in the last decades. This success is due in large part to the dedicated professional nurses working in this specialty. Nurses are responsible for orchestrating the coordination of therapies required in clinical research protocols (Fig. 27–9), performing frequent complicated assessments on patients who may develop concurrent multiorgan complications, and supporting patients and families experiencing life crises. The intensity of the care involved, the low patient-to-nurse ratio required, the minimum 30- to 40-day length of hospitalization, and the degree of planned and unplanned change require a staff of dedicated primary care nurses (Kelleher & Jennings, 1988). The professional and personal rewards from making the transplantation experience as optimum for the patient and family as possible, regardless of the eventual outcome, are great for those nurses willing to take on the challenge.

References

Aker, S. N., Cheney, C. L., Sanders, J. E., Lenssen, P. L., Hickman, R. O., & Thomas, E. D. (1982). Nutritional support in marrow graft recipients with single versus double lumen right atrial catheters. *Experimental Hematology, 10*, 732–737.

Anasetti, C., Amos, D., Beatty, P. G., Appelbaum, F. R., Bensinger, W., Buckner, C. D., Clift, R., Doney, K., Martin, P. J., Mickelson, E., Nisperos, B., O'Quigley, J., Ramberg, R., Sanders, J., Stewart, P., Storb, R., Sullivan, K. M., Witherspoon, R. P., Thomas, E. D., & Hansen, J. A. (1989). Effect of HLA compatibility or engraftment of bone marrow on patients with leukemia or lymphoma. *New England Journal of Medicine, 320*, 197–204.

Antman, K., & Gale, R. P. (1988). Advanced breast cancer: High-dose chemotherapy and bone marrow autotransplants. *Annals of Internal Medicine, 108*, 570–574.

Applebaum, F. R. (1989). Allogeneic marrow transplantation for malignancy: Current problems and prospects for improvement. In I. T. Magrath (Ed.), *New directions in cancer treatment* (pp. 143–165). Heidelberg: Springer-Verlag.

Applebaum, F. R., Dahlberg, S., Thomas, E. D., Buckner, C. D., Cheever, M. A., Clift, R. A., Crowley, J., Deeg, H. J., Fefer, A., Greenberg, P. D., Kadin, M., Smith, W., Stewart, P., Sullivan, K., Storb, R., & Weiden, P. (1984). Bone marrow transplantation or chemotherapy after remission induction for adults with acute nonlymphoblastic leukemia—a prospective comparison. *Annals of Internal Medicine, 101*, 581–588.

Applebaum, F. R., Fisher, L. D., Thomas, E. D., & the Seattle Marrow Transplant Team (1988). Chemotherapy versus marrow transplantation for adults with acute nonlymphocytic leukemia: A five-year follow-up. *Blood, 72*, 179–184.

Applebaum, F. R., Petersen, F., Buckner, C. D., Badger, C., Sandmaier, B., Storb, R., & Thomas, E. D. (1989). New preparative regimens prior to marrow transplantation for acute nonlymphoblastic leukemia. In R. P. Gale & R. Champlin (Eds.), *Bone marrow transplantation: Current controversies* (pp. 107–116). UCLA Symposia on Molecular and Cellular Biology, New Series, Vol. 91. New York: Alan R. Liss.

Applebaum, F. R., Storb, R., Buckner, C. D., Ramberg, R. E., Shulman, H. M., Sargur, M., Clift, R. A., Deeg, H. J., Fefer, A., Sanders, J., Singer, J., Stewart, P., Sullivan, K., Witherspoon, R., & Thomas, E. D. (1987). The role of marrow transplantation in the treatment of preleukemia, therapy-related preleukemia, and acute leukemia evolving from preleukemia. In R. P. Gale & R. Champlin (Eds.), *Progress in bone marrow transplantation*. UCLA Symposia on Molecular and Cellular Biology, New Series, Vol. 53. New York: Alan R. Liss.

Applebaum, F. R., Storb, R., Ramberg, R. E., Shulman, H. M., Buckner, C. D., Clift, R. A., Deeg, H. J., Fefer, A., Sanders, J., Self, S., Singer, J., Stewart, P., Sullivan, K., Witherspoon, R., & Thomas, E. D., (1987). Treatment of preleukemic syndromes with marrow transplantation. *Blood, 69*, 92–96.

Applebaum, F. R., Storb, R., Ramberg, R. E., Shulman, H. M., Buckner, C. D., Clift, R. A., Deeg, H. J., Fefer, A., Sanders, J., Stewart, P., Sullivan, K., Witherspoon, R., & Thomas, E. D. (1984). Allogeneic marrow transplantation in the treatment of preleukemia. *Annals of Internal Medicine, 100*, 689–693.

Applebaum, F. R., Sullivan, K. M., Buckner, C. D., Clift, R., Hill, R., Sanders, J. E., Storb, R., & Thomas, E. D. (1987). Treatment of malignant lymphoma at first relapse or second remission with marrow transplantation. In A. Dicke, G. Spitzer, & S. Jagannath (Eds.), *Proceedings of Third International Symposium on Autologous Transplantation* (pp. 275–277). Houston TX, December.

Applebaum, F. R., Sullivan, K., & Thomas, E. D. (1985). Treatment of malignant lymphoma in 100 patients with chemoradiotherapy and marrow transplantation. *Experimental Hematology, 13*, 321 (abstract).

Applebaum, F. R., & Thomas, E. D. (1985). The role of marrow transplantation in the treatment of leukemia. In C. D. Bloomfield (Ed.), *Chronic and acute leukemias in adults*, (pp. 229–262). Boston: Martinus Nijhoff.

Armitage, J. O., & Gale, R. P. (1989). Bone marrow autotransplantation. *American Journal of Medicine, 86*, 203–206.

August, C. S., Serota, F. T., & Koch, P. A. (1984). Treatment of advanced neuroblastoma with supralethal chemotherapy, radiation, and allogeneic or autologous marrow reconstitution. *Journal of Clinical Oncology, 2*, 609–616.

Badger, C. C., Shulman, H., Peterson, A. V., & Bernstein, I. D. (1986). Monoclonal antibody therapy of spontaneous AKR T-cell leukemia. *Cancer Research, 46*, 4058–4063.

Bearman, S. I., Appelbaum, F. R., Buckner, C. D., Peterson, F. B., Fisher, L. D., Clift, R. A., & Thomas, E. D. (1988). Regimen-related toxicity in patients undergoing bone marrow transplant. *Journal of Clinical Oncology, 6*, 1562–1568.

Beatty, P. G., Clift, R. A., Mickelson, E. M., Nisperos, B., Flournoy, N., Martin, P. J., Sanders, J. E., Stewart, P., Buckner, C. D., Storb, R., Thomas, E. D., & Hansen, J. A. (1985). Marrow transplantation from related donors other than HLA-identical siblings. *New England Journal of Medicine, 313*, 765–771.

Beatty, P. G., Dahlberg, S., Mickelson, E. M., Nisperos, B., Opelz, G., Martin, P. J., & Hansen, J. A. (1988). Probability of finding HLA-matched unrelated marrow donors. *Transplantation, 45*, 714–718.

Bensinger, W. I. (1984). Selective removal of A and B isoagglutinins. In A. Pineda (Ed.), *Selective plasma component removal* (pp. 43–70). Mount Kisco, NY: Futura Publishing Co.

Bernstein, I. D., & Nowinski, R. C. (1982). Monoclonal antibody treatment of transplanted and spontaneous murine leukemia. In H. Oettgen & M. Mitchell (Eds.), *Hybridomas in the diagnosis and treatment of cancer* (pp. 97–112). New York: Raven Press.

Bortin, M. M., Horowitz, M. M., & Gale, R. P. (1988). Current status of bone marrow transplantation in humans: Report from the International Bone Marrow Transplant Registry. *Natural Immunity and Cell Growth Regulation, 7*, 334–350.

Bortin, M. M., & Rim, A. A. (1986). Increasing utilization of bone marrow transplantation. *Transplantation, 43*, 229–234.

Bowden, R. A., Sayers, M., Flournoy, N., Newton, B., Banaji, M., Thomas, E. D., & Meyers, J. D. (1986). Cytomegalovirus immune globulin and seronegative blood products to prevent primary cytomegalovirus infection after marrow transplant. *New England Journal of Medicine, 314*, 1006–1010.

Boyd, C. N., Ramberg, R. C., & Thomas, E. D. (1982). The incidence of recurrence of leukemia in donor cells after allogeneic bone marrow transplantation. *Leukemia Research, 6*, 833–837.

Brack, G., LaClave, L., & Blix, S. (1988). The psychological aspects of bone marrow transplant. A staff perspective. *Cancer Nursing, 11*, 221–229.

Brugieres, L., Hartmann, O., Travagli, J. P., Benhammov, E., Pico, J. L., Valteau, D., Kalifa, C., Patte, C., Flamant, F., & Lemerle, J. (1989). Hemorrhagic cystitis following high-dose chemotherapy and bone marrow transplantation in children with malignancies: Incidence, clinical course, and outcome. *Journal of Clinical Oncology, 7*, 194–199.

Buchsel, P. C. (1986). Long-term complications of allogeneic bone marrow transplantation: Nursing implications. *Oncology Nursing Forum, 13*(6), 61–70.

Buchsel, P. C., & Ford, R. C. (1988). Guest editorial. *Seminars in Oncology Nursing, 4*, 1–2.

Buchsel, P. C., & Parchem, C. (1988). Ambulatory care of the bone marrow transplant patient. *Seminars in Oncology Nursing, 4*, 41–46.

Buckner, C. D., Meyers, J. D., Springmeyer, S. C., Sullivan, K. M., Hackman, R. C., Flournoy, N., Clift, R., Storb, R., Witherspoon, R. P., Petersen, F. B., & Thomas, E. D. (1984). Pulmonary complications of marrow transplantation: Review of the Seattle experience. *Experimental Hematology, 12*(Suppl. 15), 1–5.

Burns, W. H., & Saral, R. (1985). Opportunistic viral infections. *British Medical Bulletin, 41*, 46–49.

Butturni, A., Bortin, M. M., & Gale, R. P. (1987). Graft-versus-leukemia following bone marrow transplantation. *Bone Marrow Transplantation, 2*, 233–242.

Champlin, R., & Gale, R. P. (1984a). The early complications of bone marrow transplantation. *Seminars in Hematology, 21*, 101–107.

Champlin, R. E., & Gale, R. P. (1984b). Role of bone marrow transplantation in the treatment of hematologic malignancies and solid tumors. Critical review of syngeneic, autologous and allogeneic transplants. *Cancer Treatment Reports, 68*, 145–161.

Champlin, R., & Gale, R. P. (1987). Acute myelogenous leukemia: Recent advances in therapy. *Blood, 69,* 1551–1562.

Champlin, R. E., Ho, W. G., Winston, G. H., Gale, R. P., Winston, D., Selch, M., Mitsuyasu, R., Lenarsky, C., Elashoff, R., Zighelboim, J., & Feig, S. A. (1985). Treatment of acute myelogenous leukemia: A prospective controlled trial of bone marrow transplantation versus consolidation chemotherapy. *Annals of Internal Medicine, 102,* 285–291.

Champlin, R., Jacobs, A., Gale, R. P., Ho, W., Selch, M., Lenarsky, C., & Feig, S. A. (1985). High-dose cytarabine in consolidation chemotherapy or with bone marrow transplantation for patients with acute leukemia: Preliminary results. *Seminars in Oncology, 12* (Suppl. 3), 190–195.

Clift, R. A., Buckner, C. D., Thomas, E. D., Kopecky, K. J., Appelbaum, F. R., Tallman, M., Storb, R., Sanders, J., Sullivan, K., Banaji, M., Beatty, P. S., Bensinger, W., Cheever, M., Deeg, J., Doney, K., Fefer, A., Greenberg, P., Hansen, J. A., Hackman, R., Hill, R., Martin, P., Meyers, J., McGuffin, R., Neiman, P., Sale, G., Shulman, H., Singer, J., Stewart, P., Weiden, P., & Witherspoon, R. (1987). The treatment of acute nonlymphoblastic leukemia by allogeneic marrow transplantation. *Bone Marrow Transplantation, 2,* 243–258.

Clift, R. A., Buckner, C. D., Thomas, E. D., Sanders, J. E., Stewart, P. S., McGuffin, R., Hersman, J., Sullivan, K. M., Sale, G. E., & Storb, R. (1982). Allogeneic marrow transplantation for acute lymphoblastic leukemia in remission using fractionated total body irradiation. *Leukemia Research, 6,* 409–412.

Clift, R. A., Buckner, C. D., Thomas, E. D., Sanders, J. E., Stewart, P. S., Sullivan, K. M., McGuffin, R., Hersman, J., Sale, G. E., & Storb, R. (1982). Allogeneic marrow transplantation using fractionated total body irradiation in patients with acute lymphoblastic leukemia in relapse. *Leukemia Research, 6,* 401–407.

Crawford, S. W., Bowden, R. A., Hackman, R. C., Gleaves, C. A., Meyers, J. D., & Clark, J. G. (1988). Rapid detection of cytomegalovirus pulmonary infection by bronchoalveolar lavage and centrifugation culture. *Annals of Internal Medicine, 108,* 180–185.

Crawford, S. W., Hackman, R. C., & Clark, J. G. (1988). Open lung biopsy diagnosis of diffuse pulmonary infiltrates after marrow transplantation. *Chest, 94,* 949–953.

Cunningham, B. A., Lenssen, P., Aker, S. N., Gittere, K. M., Cheney, C. L., & Hutchison, M. M. (1983). Nutritional considerations during marrow transplantation. *Nursing Clinics of North America, 18,* 585–596.

Cunningham, B. A., Morris, G., Cheney, C. L., Buergel, N., Aker, S. N., & Lenssen, P. (1986). Effects of resistive exercise on skeletal muscle in marrow transplant recipients receiving total parenteral nutrition. *Journal of Parenteral and Enteral Nutrition, 10,* 558–563.

Davis, D. G., & Patchell, R. A. (1988). Neurologic complications of bone marrow transplantation. *Neurology Clinics, 6,* 377–387.

Dudjak, L. A. (1984). HLA typing: Implications for nurses. *Oncology Nursing Forum, 11*(5), 30–36.

Ford, R. C., & Ballard, B. (1988). Acute complications after bone marrow transplantation. *Seminars in Oncology Nursing, 4,* 15–24.

Forman, S. J., Blume, K. G., Krance, R. A., Miner, P. J., O'Donnell, M. R., Nademanee, A. P., Snyder, D. S., Metter, G. E., & Hill, L. R. (1986). A prospective randomized study on acute graft-versus-host disease (GVHD) in 107 patients with leukemia: Methotrexate/prednisone (CSA/PSE). *Blood, 68* (Suppl. 1), 1004 (abstract).

Gale, R. P. (1986). Analysis of bone marrow transplantation data in man. *Bone Marrow Transplantation, 1,* 3–9.

Goldman, J. M., Apperley, J. F., Jones, L., Marcus, R., Goolden, A. W. G., Batchelor, R., Hale, G., Waldmann, H., Reid, C. D., Hows, J., Gordon-Smith, E., Catovsky, D., & Galton, D. A. G. (1986). Bone marrow transplantation for patients with chronic myeloid leukemia. *New England Journal of Medicine, 314,* 202–208.

Haberman, M. R. (1988). Psychosocial aspects of bone marrow transplantation. *Seminars in Oncology Nursing, 4,* 55–59.

Hansen, J. A., Beatty, P. G., Anasetti, C., Martin, P. J., Mickelson, E., & Thomas, E. D. (1987). Transplantation of hematopoietic stem cells (HSC). *British Medical Bulletin, 43,* 203–216.

Helenglass, G., Powles, R. L., McElwain, T. J., Lakhani, A.,

Milan, S., Gore, M., Nandi, A., Zviable, A., Perren, T., Forgeson, G., Treleavan, J., Hamilton, C., & Millar, J. (1988). Melphalan and total body irradiation (TBI) versus cyclosporine and TBI as conditioning for allogeneic matched sibling bone marrow transplants for acute myeloblastic leukaemia in first remission. *Bone Marrow Transplantation, 3,* 21–29.

Herzig, R. H., Coccia, P. F., Lazarus, H. M., Strandford, S. E., Graham-Pole, J., Cheung, N.-K., Gordon, E. M., Gross, S., Spitzer, T. R., Warkentin, P. I., Fay, J. W., Phillips, G. L., & Herzig, G. P. (1985). Bone marrow transplantation for acute leukemia and lymphoma with high-dose cytosine arabinoside and total body irradiation. *Seminars in Oncology, 12,* (Suppl. 3), 184–186.

Hill, H., Saeger, L., & Chapman, R. (1988). Combination antiemetic therapy in bone marrow transplant patients. Unpublished manuscript.

Holcombe, A. (1987). Bone marrow harvest. *Oncology Nursing Forum, 14*(2), 63–65.

Holland, H. K., Wingard, J. R., Beschorner, W. E., Saral, R., & Santos, G. (1988). Bronchiolitis obliterans in bone marrow transplantation and its relationship to chronic graft-versus-host disease and low serum IgG. *Blood, 72,* 621–627.

Hutchison, M. M., & King, A. H. (1983). A nursing perspective on bone marrow transplantation. *Nursing Clinics of North America, 18,* 511–522.

Jagannath, S., Armitage, J. O., Dicke, K. A., Tucker, S. L., Velasquez, W. S., Smith, K., Vaughan, W. P., Kessinger, A., Horwitz, L. J., Hagemeister, F. B., McLaughlin, P., Cabanill, F., & Spitzer, G. (1989). Prognostic factors for response and survival after high-dose cyclosporine, carmustine, and etoposide with autologous bone marrow transplantation for relapsed Hodgkin's disease. *Journal of Clinical Oncology, 7,* 179–185.

Johnson, F. L., Thomas, E. D., Clark, B. S., Chard, R. L., Hartmann, J. R., & Storb, R. (1981). A comparison of marrow transplantation with chemotherapy for children with acute lymphoblastic leukemia in second or subsequent remission. *New England Journal of Medicine, 305,* 846–851.

Kanfer, E. J., Buckner, C. D., Fefer, A., Storb, R., Appelbaum, F. R., Hill, R. S., Amos, D., Doney, K. C., Clift, R. A., Shulman, H. M., McDonald, G. B., & Thomas, E. D. (1987). Allogeneic and syngeneic marrow transplantation following high dose dimethylbusulfan, cyclophosphamide and total body irradiation. *Bone Marrow Transplantation, 1,* 1–8.

Kay, H. E., Powles, R. L., Lawler, S. D., & Clink, H. M. (1980). Cost of bone marrow transplants in acute myeloid leukemia. *Lancet, 1,* 1067–1069.

Kelleher, J. (1986). Pediatric marrow transplantation. In M. J. Hockenberry & D. K. Coody (Eds.), *Pediatric hematology/oncology: Perspective on care* (pp. 347–363). St. Louis: C. V. Mosby Co.

Kelleher, J., & Jennings, M. (1988). Nursing management of a marrow transplant unit: A framework for practice. *Seminars in Oncology Nursing, 4,* 60–68.

Kemshead, J. T., Treleaven, J., Heath, L., Meara, A. O., Gee, A., & Vogelstad, J. (1987). Monoclonal antibodies and magnetic microspheres for the depletion of leukaemic cells from bone marrow harvested for autologous transplantation. *Bone Marrow Transplantation, 2,* 133–139.

Kennedy, M. S., Deeg, H. J., Siegel, M., Crowley, J. J., Storb, R., & Thomas, E. D. (1983). Acute renal toxicity with combined use of amphotericin B and cyclosporine after marrow transplantation. *Transplantation, 35,* 211–215.

Kennedy, M. S., Yee, G. C., McGuire, T. R., Leonard, T. M., Crowley, J. J., & Deeg, H. J. (1985). Correlation of serum cyclosporine concentration with renal dysfunction in marrow transplant recipients. *Transplantation, 40,* 249–253.

Klingemann, H. G., & Eaves, C. J. (1988). Colony stimulating factors. *Bone Marrow Transplantation, 3,* 177–184.

Kolbinson, D. A., Schubert, M. M., Flournoy, N., & Truelove, E. L. (1988). Early oral changes following bone marrow transplantation. *Oral Surgery, Oral Medicine, Oral Pathology, 66,* 130–138.

Krowka, M. J., Rosenow, E. C., & Hoagland, H. C. (1985). Pulmonary complications of bone marrow transplantation. *Chest, 87,* 237–246.

Linch, D. C., & Burnett, A. K. (1986). Clinical studies of ABMT in acute myeloid leukaemia. *Clinics in Haematology (Autologous Bone Marrow Transplantation), 15,* 167–186.

Lindgren, P. (1983). The laminar air flow room: Nursing practices and procedures. *Nursing Clinics of North America, 18,* 553–561.

Lucas, P. J., Quinones, R. R., Moses, R. D., Nakamura, H., & Gress, R. E. (1988). Alternate donor sources in HLA-mismatched marrow transplantation: T cell depletion of surgically resected cadaveric marrow. *Bone Marrow Transplantation, 3,* 211–220.

Martin, P. J., Hansen, J. A., Torok-Storb, B., Durnam, D., Przepiorka, D., O'Quigley, J., Sanders, J., Sullivan, K. M., Witherspoon, R. P., Deeg, H. J., Appelbaum, F. R., Stewart, P., Weiden, P., Doney, K., Buckner, C. D., Clift, R., Storb, R., & Thomas, E. D. (1988). Graft failure in patients receiving T cell-depleted HLA-identical allogeneic marrow transplants. *Bone Marrow Transplantation, 3,* 445–456.

Martin, P. J., Remlinger, K., Hansen, J. A., Storb, R., Thomas, E. D., & the Seattle Marrow Transplant Team (1984). Murine monoclonal anti-T cell antibodies for treatment of refractory acute graft-versus-host disease (GVHD). *Transplantation Proceedings, 16,* 1494–1495.

McCullough, J., Hansen, J., Perkins, H., Stroncek, D., & Bartsch, G. (1989). The national marrow donor program: How it works, accomplishments to date. *Oncology, 3,* 63–72.

McDonald, G. B., Sharma, P., Matthews, D. E., Shulman, H. M., & Thomas, E. D. (1985). The clinical course of 53 patients with venocclusive disease of the liver after marrow transplantation. *Transplantation, 36,* 603–608.

McDonald, G. B., Shulman, H. M., Sullivan, K. M., & Spencer, G. D. (1986). Intestinal and hepatic complications of human bone marrow transplantation. Parts I & II. *Gastroenterology, 90,* 460–477, 770–784.

Meyers, J. D. (1988). Prevention and treatment of cytomegalovirus infection after marrow transplantation. *Bone Marrow Transplantation, 3,* 95–104.

Meyers, J. D., & Atkinson, K. (1983). Infection in bone marrow transplantation. In D. G. Nathan (Ed.), *Bone marrow transplantation* (pp. 791–811). London: W. B. Saunders Co.

Meyers, J. D., Flournoy, N., & Thomas, E. D. (1986). Risk factors for cytomegalovirus infection after human marrow transplantation. *Journal of Infectious Diseases, 153,* 478–488.

Meyers, J. D., & Thomas, E. D. (1988). Infection complicating bone marrow transplantation. In R. H. Rubin & L. S. Young (Eds.), *Clinical approach to infection in the immunocompromised host* (pp. 525–556). New York: Plenum Press.

Meyers, J. D., Wade, J. C., McGuffin, R. W., Springmeyer, S. C., & Thomas, E. D. (1983). The use of acyclovir for cytomegalovirus infections in the immunocompromised host. *Journal of Antimicrobial Chemotherapy, 12,* 181–193.

Nemunaitis, J., Singer, J., Buckner, C. D., Hill, R., Storb, R., Thomas, E. D., & Appelbaum, F. R. (1988). Use of recombinant human granulocyte macrophage colony-stimulating factor in autologous marrow transplantation for lymphoid malignancies. *Blood, 72,* 834–836.

O'Quin, T., & Moravec, C. (1988). The critically ill bone marrow transplant patient. *Seminars in Oncology Nursing, 4,* 25–30.

O'Reilly, R. J. (1983). Allogeneic bone marrow transplantation: Current status and future directions. *Blood, 62,* 941–964.

Osserman, E. F., Dire, L. B., Dire, J., Sherman, W. H., Hersman, J. A., & Storb, R. (1982). Identical twin marrow transplantation in multiple myeloma. *Acta Haematologica, 68,* 215–223.

Osterwalder, B., Gratwohl, A., Reusser, P., Tichelli, A., & Speck, B. (1988). Hematological support in patients undergoing allogeneic bone marrow transplantation. *Recent Results in Cancer Research, 108,* 44–52.

Petersen, F. B., Bowden, R. A., Thornquist, M., Meyers, J. D., Buckner, C. D., Counts, G. W., Nelson, N., Newton, B. A., Sullivan, K. M., McIver, J., & Thomas, E. D. (1987). The effect of prophylactic intravenous immune globulin on the incidence of septicemia in marrow transplant recipients. *Bone Marrow Transplantation, 2,* 141–148.

Petersen, F. B., Buckner, C. D., Clift, R. A., Lee, S., Nelson, N., Counts, G. W., Meyers, J. D., Sanders, J. E., Stewart, P. S., Bensinger, W. I., Navari, R., & Thomas, E. D. (1986). Laminar air flow isolation and decontamination: A prospective randomized study of the effects of prophylactic systemic antibiotics in bone marrow transplant patients. *Infection, 14,* 115–121.

Peterson, P. K., McGlave, P., Ramsay, N. K. C., Rhame, F., Cohen, E., Perry, G. S., Goldman, A. I., & Kersey, J. (1983). A prospective study of infectious diseases following bone marrow transplantation: Emergence of *Aspergillus* and cytomegalovirus as the major causes of mortality. *Infection Control, 4,* 81–89.

Petersen, F. B., Thornquist, M., Buckner, C. D., Counts, G. W., Nelson, N., Meyers, J. D., Clift, R. A., & Thomas, E. D. (1988). The effects of infection prevention regimens on early infectious complications in marrow transplant patients: A four-arm randomized study. *Infection, 16,* 199–208.

Phillips, G. L., Herzig, R. H., & Lazarus, H. M. (1984). Treatment of resistant malignant lymphoma with cyclophosphamide, total body irradiation, and transplantation of cryopreserved autologous marrow. *New England Journal of Medicine, 310,* 1557–1561.

Pinkerton, C. R., Philip, T., Biron, P., Frapazz, D., Phillipe, N., Zucker, T. M., Bernard, J. L., Philip, I., Kemshead, J., & Favrot, M. (1987). High-dose melphalan, vincristine, and total body irradiation with autologous bone marrow transplantation in children with relapsed neuroblastoma: A phase II study. *Medical and Pediatric Oncology, 15,* 236–240.

Powles, R. L., Morgenstern, G., & Clink, H. M. (1980). The place of bone-marrow transplantation in acute myelogenous leukaemia. *Lancet, 1,* 1047–1050.

Press, O. W., Schaller, R. T., & Thomas, E. D. (1986). Bone marrow transplant complications. In L. H. Toledo-Pereyra (Ed.), *Complications of organ transplantation* (pp. 399–424). New York: Marcel Dekker.

Reisner, Y., Kapoor, N., Kirkpatrick, D., Pollack, M. S., Dupont, B., Good, R. A., & O'Reilly, R. J. (1981). Transplantation for acute leukemia with HLA-A and B nonidentical parenteral marrow cells fractionated with soybean agglutinin and sheep red blood cells. *Lancet, 2,* 327–331.

Riddell, S., Appelbaum, F. R., Buckner, C. D., Stewart, P., Clift, R., Sanders, J. E., Storb, R., Sullivan, K. M., & Thomas, E. D. (1988). High-dose cytarabine and total body irradiation with or without cyclosphosphamide as a preparative regimen for marrow transplantation for acute leukemia. *Journal of Clinical Oncology, 6,* 576–582.

Rivera, G. K., Buchanan, G., Boyett, J. M., Camitta, B., Ochs, J., Kalwinsky, D., Amylon, M., Vietti, T. J., & Crist, W. M. (1986). Intensive retreatment of childhood acute lymphoblastic leukemia in first bone marrow relapse: A pediatric oncology group study. *New England Journal of Medicine, 315,* 273–278.

Ruggiero, M. (1988). The donor in bone marrow transplantation. *Seminars in Oncology Nursing, 4,* 9–14.

Sanders, J. E., Flournoy, N., Thomas, E. D., Buckner, C. D., Lum, L. G., Clift, R. A., Appelbaum, F. R., Sullivan, K. M., Stewart, P., Deeg, H. J., Doney, K., & Storb, R. (1985). Marrow transplant experience in children with acute lymphoblastic leukemia: An analysis of factors associated with survival, relapse and graft-versus-host disease. *Medical and Pediatric Oncology, 13,* 165–172.

Schmitz, N., Gassmann, W., Rister, M., Johannson, W., Suttorp, M., Brix, F., Holthuis, J. J. M., Heit, W., Hertenstein, B., Schaub, J., & Loffler, H. (1988). Fractionated total body irradiation and high-dose VP16-213 followed by allogeneic bone marrow transplantation in advanced leukemias. *Blood, 72,* 1567–1573.

Shank, B., Hopfan, S., Kim, J. H., Chu, F. C. H., Grossbard, E., Kapoor, N., Kirkpatrick, D., Dinsmore, R., Simpson, L., Reid, A., Chui, C., Mohan, R., Finegan, D., & O'Reilly, R. J. (1981). Hyperfractionated total body irradiation for bone marrow transplantation: I. Early results in leukemia patients. *International Journal of Radiation Oncology, Biology, Physics, 7,* 1109–1115.

Sheep, D. H., Dandliker, R. N., de Miranda, P., Burnette, T. C., Cederberg, D. M., Kirk, L. E., & Meyers, J. D. (1985). Activity of 9-[2-hydroxy-1-(hydroxymethyl)ethoxymethyl]guanine in the treatment of cytomegalovirus pneumonia. *Annals of Internal Medicine, 103,* 368–373.

Smith, J. W., Shulman, H. M., Thomas, E. D., Fefer, A., & Buckner, C. D. (1981). Bone marrow transplantation for acute myelosclerosis. *Cancer, 48,* 2198–2203.

Spencer, G. D., Hackman, R. C., McDonald, G. B., Amos, D. E., Cunningham, B. A., Meyers, J. D., & Thomas, E. D. (1986). A prospective study of unexplained nausea and vomiting after marrow transplantation. *Transplantation, 42,* 602–607.

Spencer, G. D., Shulman, H. M., Myerson, D., Thomas, E. D., & McDonald, G. B. (1986). Diffuse intestinal ulceration after marrow transplantation: A clinical-pathological study of 13 patients. *Human Pathology, 17,* 621–633.

Springmeyer, S. C., Hackman, R. C., Holle, R., Greenberg, G. M., Weems, C. E., Myerson, D., Meyers, J. D., & Thomas, E. D. (1986). Use of bronchoalveolar lavage to diagnose acute diffuse pneumonia in the immunocompromised host. *Journal of Infectious Diseases, 154,* 604–610.

Springmeyer, S. C., Silvestri, R. C., Flournoy, N., Kosanke, C. W., Peterson, D. L., Huseby, J. S., Hudson, L. D., Storb, R., & Thomas, E. D. (1984). Pulmonary function of marrow transplant patients: I. Effects of marrow infusion, acute graft-versus-host disease, and interstitial pneumonitis. *Experimental Hematology, 12,* 805–810.

Storb, R. (1987). Critical issues in bone marrow transplantation. *Transplantation Proceedings, 14,* 2774–2781.

Storb, R., Deeg, H. J., Farewell, V., Doney, K., Appelbaum, F., Beatty, P., Bensinger, W., Buckner, C. D., Clift, R., Hansen, J., Hill, R., Longton, G., Lum, L., Martin, P., McGuffin, R., Sanders, J., Singer, J., Stewart, P., Sullivan, K., Witherspoon, R., & Thomas, E. D. (1986). Marrow transplantation for severe aplastic anemia: Methotrexate alone compared to a combination of methotrexate and cyclosporine for prevention of acute graft-versus-host disease. *Blood, 68,* 119–125.

Storb, R., Deeg, H. J., Whitehead, J., Appelbaum, F., Beatty, P., Bensinger, W., Buckner, C. D., Clift, R., Doney, K., Farewell, V., Hansen, J., Hill, R., Lum, L., Martin, P., McGuffin, R., Sanders, J., Stewart, P., Sullivan, K., Witherspoon, R., Yee, G., & Thomas, E. D. (1986). Methotrexate and cyclosporine compared with cyclosporine alone for prophylaxis of acute graft-versus-host disease after marrow transplantation for leukemia. *New England Journal of Medicine, 314,* 729–735.

Storb, R., & Thomas, E. D. (1985). Graft-versus-host disease in dog and man. The Seattle Experience. In G. Moller (Ed.), *Immunological reviews No. 88* (pp. 215–238). Copenhagen: Munksgaard.

Sullivan, K. M., Fefer, A., Witherspoon, R., Storb, R., Buckner, C. D., Weiden, P., Schoch, G., & Thomas, E. D. (1987). Graft-versus-leukemia in man: Relationship of acute and chronic graft-versus-host disease to relapse of acute leukemia following allogeneic bone marrow transplantation In R. L. Truitt, R. P. Gale, & M. M. Bortin (Eds.), *Cellular immunotherapy of cancer* (pp. 391–399). New York: Alan R. Liss.

Sullivan, K. M., & Parkman, R. (1983). The pathophysiology and treatment of graft-versus-host disease. *Clinics in Haematology, 12,* 775–789.

Thomas, E. D. (1983). Marrow transplantation for malignant diseases (Karnofsky Memorial Lecture). *Journal of Clinical Oncology, 1,* 517–531.

Thomas, E. D., Buckner, C. D., Banaji, M., Clift, R. A., Fefer, A., Flournoy, N., Goodell, B. W., Hickman, R. O., Lerner, K. G., Neiman, P. E., Sale, G. E., Sanders, J. E., Singer, J., Stevens, M., Storb, R., & Weiden, P. L. (1977). One hundred patients with acute leukemia treated by chemotherapy, total body irradiation, and allogeneic marrow transplantation. *Blood, 49,* 511–533.

Thomas, E. D., Buckner, C. D., Clift, R. A., Fefer, A., Johnson, F. L., Neiman, P. E., Sale, G. E., Sanders, J. E., Singer, J. W., Shulman, H., Storb, R., & Weiden, P. L. (1979). Marrow transplantation for acute nonlymphoblastic leukemia in first remission. *New England Journal of Medicine, 301,* 597–599.

Thomas, E. D., Clift, R. A., Fefer, A., Appelbaum, F. R., Beatty, P., Bensinger, W. I., Buckner, C. D., Cheever, M. A., Deeg, H. J., Doney, K., Flournoy, N., Greenberg, P., Hansen, J. A., Martin, P., McGuffin, R., Ramberg, R., Sanders, J. E., Singer, J., Stewart, P., Storb, R., Sullivan, K., Weiden, P. L., & Witherspoon, R. (1986). Marrow transplantation for the treatment of chronic myelogenous leukemia. *Annals of Internal Medicine, 104,* 155–163.

Thomas, E. D., Clift, R. A., Hersman, J., Sanders, J. E., Stewart, P., Buckner, C. D., Fefer, A., McGuffin, R., Smith, J. W., & Storb, R. (1982). Marrow transplantation for acute nonlymphoblastic leukemia in first remission. *International Journal of Radiation Oncology, Biology, Physics, 8,* 817–821.

van der Meer, J. W. M., Guiot, H. F. L., van den Brock, P. J., & van Furth, R. (1984). Infections in bone marrow transplant recipients. *Seminars in Hematology, 21,* 123–138.

Weiden, P. L., Flournoy, N., Sanders, J. E., Sullivan, K. M., & Thomas, E. D. (1981). Antileukemic effect of graft-versus-host disease contributes to improved survival after allogeneic marrow transplantation. *Transplantation Proceedings, 13,* 248–251.

Weiden, P. L., Zuckerman, N., Hansen, J. A., Sale, G. E., Remlinger, K., Beck, T. M., & Buckner, C. D. (1981). Fatal graft-versus-host disease in a patient with lymphoblastic leukemia following normal granulocyte transfusions. *Blood, 57,* 328–332.

Weisdorf, S. A., Lysne, J., Wind, D., Haake, R. J., Sharp, H. L., Goldman, A., Schissel, K., McGlave, P. B., Ramsay, N. K., & Kersey, J. H. (1987). Positive effect of prophylactic total parenteral nutrition on long-term outcome of bone marrow transplantation. *Transplantation, 43,* 833–838.

Wiley, F. M., & House, K. U. (1988). Bone marrow transplant in children. *Seminars in Oncology Nursing, 4,* 31–40.

Williams, S. F., Bitran, J. D., Hoffman, P. C., Robin, E., Fullem, L., Beschorner, J., Golick, J., & Golcomb, H. M. (1989). High dose, multiple-alkylator chemotherapy with autologous bone marrow reinfusion in patients with advanced non–small cell lung cancer. *Cancer, 63,* 238–242.

Winston, D. J., Gale, R. P., Meyer, D. V., Young, L. S., & the UCLA Bone Marrow Transplantation Group (1979). Infectious complications of human bone marrow transplantation. *Medicine, 58,* 1–31.

Wolff, S. N., Herzig, R. H., Fay, J. W., LeMaistre, C. F., Frei-Lahr, D., Lowder, J., Bolwell, B., Giannov, C., & Herzig, P. (1989). High-dose thiotepa with autologous bone marrow transplantation for metastatic malignant melanoma: Results of Phase I and II studies of the North American Bone Marrow Transplantation Group. *Journal of Clinical Oncology, 7,* 245–249.

Wulff, J. C., Santner, T. J., Storb, R., Banaji, M., Buckner, C. D., Clift, R., Stewart, P., Sanders, J., Slichter, S., & Thomas, E. D. (1983). Transfusion requirements after HLA-identical marrow transplantation in 82 patients with aplastic anemia. *Vox Sanguinis, 44,* 366–374.

Yeager, A. M., Kaizer, H., Santos, G. W., Saral, R., Colvin, O. M., Stuart, R. K., Brainey, H. G., Burke, P. J., Ambinder, R. F., Burns, W. H., Fuller, D. J., Davis, J. M., Karp, J. E., May, W. S., Rowley, S. D., Sensenbrenner, L. L., Vogelsang, G. B., & Wingard, J. R. (1986). Autologous bone marrow transplantation in patients with acute nonlymphocytic leukemia, using ex vivo marrow treatment with 4-hydroperoxycyclophosphamide. *New England Journal of Medicine, 315,* 141–148.

Yee, G. C., Kennedy, M. S., Deeg, H. J., Leonard, T. M., Thomas, E. D., & Storb, R. (1985). Cyclosporine-associated renal dysfunction in marrow transplant recipients. *Transplantation Proceedings, 17,* 196–201.

Young, L. S. (1984). An overview of infection in bone marrow transplant recipients. *Clinics in Haematology, 13,* 661–667.

Zager, R. A., O'Quigley, J., Zager, B. K., Alpers, C. E., Shulman, H. M., Gamelin, L. M., Stewart, P., & Thomas, E. D. (1989). Acute renal failure following bone marrow transplantation: A retrospective study of 272 patients. *American Journal of Kidney Diseases, 13,* 210–216.

CHAPTER 28

Palliative Support

LESLEY F. DEGNER

A FRAMEWORK FOR HELPING
Palliative Surgery
Palliative Radiotherapy
Palliative Chemotherapy
THE NURSE'S ROLE IN PALLIATIVE SUPPORT

Palliative Care versus Palliative Treatment
Communication and Control
Nursing Interventions
SUMMARY

The shift away from therapy aimed at cure or control of disease marks an important transition for all those involved in a patient's cancer treatment. When therapy fails to produce a response and available treatment options become limited, caregivers may experience discouragement and frustration. Such feelings are intensified if the patient had a high probability of cure at the onset of treatment or if the patient remains disease free but has developed a lethal side effect as a result of aggressive therapy. Caregivers may wonder how to provide help in a context in which cure or control of the disease is not possible and in which death is the inevitable outcome.

Shifts in focus become apparent in patient, family, and staff communication. For the patient and family, progression of the disease can raise questions that previously remained unasked and unanswered: How long do I have? Will I die? Will I suffer? Changes in focus will also be noticeable among caregivers: whereas once they talked about helping the patient "get better," now they talk about helping the patient "feel better." The reduction in number of tests and frequency of blood work is also symbolic of the transition in treatment goals. A frequent concern of the patient and family is that they will be abandoned now that active treatment has failed.

The challenge for nursing is to understand how to provide help within this context. Therapies traditionally viewed as "curative" can be extremely useful even toward the end of life. This chapter focuses on three of these treatments: surgery, radiation, and chemotherapy. Before examining the specific uses of these treatments as forms of palliative support, we need a framework for understanding how to help when cure is no longer possible.

A FRAMEWORK FOR HELPING

The concept of helping is central to most definitions of nursing (Cronenwett, 1983). One model of helping that has proved useful in examining the efficacy of palliative care was described by Brickman and his colleagues (Brickman et al., 1982; Degner, Henteleff, & Ringer, 1987). This model was developed using two dimensions that define responsibility for the origin of problems and responsibility for the resolution of problems. These dimensions permit the distinction of four alternative approaches to helping (Fig. 28–1).

1. Moral Model: people are assigned a large share of responsibility for both creating and solving their problems.

2. Compensatory Model: people are held minimally, if at all, responsible for their problems but are still primarily responsible for finding solutions.

3. Medical Model: people are viewed as being minimally, if at all, responsible for the origin of their problems or for finding solutions to their problems.

4. Enlightenment Model: people are assigned a large share of responsibility for having caused their problems but are believed to be minimally, if at all, responsible for solving them.

The two models that view the person as being responsible for his or her own problems (moral and enlightenment) are not dominant in the care of the dying. Even if the patient has contributed to the occurrence or severity of disease (for example, by smoking or by delay in seeking treatment), health professionals tend to emphasize responsibility for solutions rather than for the origin of the problem at this phase of life. An exception to this generalization may be in caregiver responses to patients dying as a result of acquired immune deficiency syndrome (AIDS), in which the moral model of helping may become dominant. The two models generally used in palliative care

	Attribution of responsibility for the problem	
	High	Low
Attribution of responsibility for finding a solution to the problem — High	Moral Model	Compensatory Model
Attribution of responsibility for finding a solution to the problem — Low	Enlightenment Model	Medical Model

Figure 28–1. Models of helping.

are those in which attribution of responsibility for the problem is low: the medical model and the compensatory model.

The medical model is obviously the dominant model of helping within the acute care hospital. Generally, patients are not held responsible for their illnesses, nor are they held responsible for providing cures for their illnesses. Patients are expected to accept treatment from medical "experts" who have been trained to recognize the problem and to provide whatever treatment is available. As Brickman and colleagues (1982) observed: "Even when the solution is largely one that the person can or must carry out themselves, such as bedrest, the responsibility for prescribing this solution and for judging whether it has been successful rests with the expert." However, the medical model fails when a disease has progressed so far that physicians conclude that recovery is impossible. Patients confronted with this judgment have no resources left unless they have alternatives to the medical model.

The compensatory model is a more appropriate approach to helping within palliative care units and hospices. Patients are not blamed for their problems, but they are seen as having to compensate for the handicaps or obstacles imposed on them with a special kind of effort, ingenuity, or collaboration with others. Helpers see themselves as compensating for resources that the recipients of the help deserve but somehow did not get. The use of family conferences and the active participation of patients in clinical decision making are the clearest indicators of this orientation to helping. Solutions to problems are not prescribed but rather evolve through a process of collaboration among the patient, family, and health professionals. The compensatory model of helping encompasses a joint approach to decision making.

Given this approach to helping, caregivers assist the patient and family in anticipating and preventing complications that could produce *unwanted* suffering. This approach implies that the patient and family are actively involved in defining the degree to which suffering is tolerable and even preferable to accepting additional surgery, radiotherapy, or chemotherapy. After discussing the circumstances in which specific therapies can be useful in palliative care, a series of questions that nurses can use to implement this model of helping are presented and discussed.

Palliative Surgery

There are several circumstances in which surgery can provide palliative benefits (Colapinto, 1985). Although the risk of death from surgery may be high owing to the patient's general debilitated condition, not all patients view this risk in a negative manner. Indeed, some may prefer a death during surgery to one they anticipate will be lingering and potentially painful. Patients and families should understand both the potential risks and benefits of the procedures being offered so that they can make informed choices about accepting or declining further treatment.

Surgery is frequently used to manage malignant obstructions. Obstruction of the small or large bowel is a common problem in patients with a variety of primary and metastatic malignancies (Borass, 1985). Medical therapy that includes explanation, dietary advice, antiemetics, steroids, or antispasmodic agents may be effective for patients with single or even multiple obstructions of the bowel (Twycross & Lack, 1984). In contrast, laparotomy for malignant intestinal obstruction is associated with significant mortality and low median survival (Zollinger, Sternfeld, & Schrelber, 1986).

Patients with colonic obstruction risk progressive bowel distention and resulting perforation and peritonitis. Palliative surgery involves removal of the lesion to prevent distressing symptoms from developing, but when the lesion is technically unresectable, a palliative bypass of the obstruction can relieve or avert symptoms (Borass, 1985). Operative mortality is estimated to be between 10 and 11.7 per cent for resection and 4.9 per cent for bypass (Joffe & Gordon, 1981; Johnson, McDermott, Milne, Price, & Hughes, 1981). Laser photocoagulation has been used as an alternative to surgery to manage malignant obstructions of the gastrointestinal tract, with encouraging results (Brunetaud et al., 1987; Mathus-Vliegen & Tytgat, 1986; Russin, Kaplan, Goldberg, & Barkin, 1986).

The second context in which surgery can be an effective palliative therapy is in the treatment of malignant ascites and pleural effusions. Accumulation of fluid in the peritoneal or pleural cavities can cause the distressing symptoms of abdominal pain and nausea or dyspnea and cough. Although temporary relief through percutaneous drainage of this fluid is frequently beneficial, patients who require multiple paracentesis for recurrent ascites may be candidates for placement of a peritovenous shunt. One study of 40 patients treated with shunts found that 28 experienced effective palliation, with noticeable improvements in strength, appetite, and ambulation (Qazi & Savlov, 1982). Patients with malignant pleural effusions that recur following thoracentesis may be offered closed-tube thoracostomy and pleural stenosis. One randomized trial studied 46 patients with pleural effusions secondary to breast cancer who were treated at first occurrence of the effusion with instillation of either mustine (mechlorethamine) or talc into the pleural cavity. Eighteen of 20 patients in the talc group had no recurrence of pleural fluid, and many experienced long-term benefits (Fentiman, Rubens, & Hayward, 1983). In contrast, pleuradesis by instillation of tetracycline resulted in complete resolution of pleural fluid in only 5 of 32 procedures described in a 10-year retrospective study (Gravelyn, Michelson, Gross, & Sitrin, 1987).

Surgery may also be used to manage extensive local disease, pathologic fractures, and pain. When large, painful, ulcerated, and secondarily infected tumors occur, surgical removal of the entire mass is usually desirable. Complete resection is most applicable to tumors located on an extremity or within the breast (Borass, 1985). Operative stabilization of pathologic fractures can relieve pain, restore function, increase mobilization, and facilitate nursing care (Sim & Pritchard, 1982). Supplementing internal fixation by intramedullary methylmethacrylate has proved particularly successful (Harrington et al., 1976). Surgical insertion of venous access devices has become an approach to managing pain when control cannot be achieved by oral narcotics (Moore, Erikson, Yanes, Franklin, & Gonsalves, 1986).

Palliative Radiotherapy

Nearly half of all radiation therapy treatments are given with a palliative intent. When there is rapid tumor progression or an anticipated short life expectancy, treatment may be given in an accelerated course over 1 or 2 weeks. Radiation tolerance guidelines should be followed even if the patient's life span is expected to be short. The overall goal is to avoid producing debilitating side effects that are worse than the symptoms being treated. Optimally, problems that are amenable to palliative radiotherapy can be anticipated and treated before symptoms escalate (Richter & Cola, 1985).

Spinal cord compression occurs in approximately 5 per cent of all cancer patients, usually owing to metastatic disease. Severe persistent back pain, sensory changes, unexplained constipation, or urinary difficulties may indicate cord compression. Radiotherapy is usually the treatment of choice for these patients, although decompressive laminectomy is sometimes recommended before the onset of radiotherapy. The objective is to reduce or prevent the paralysis that would severely compromise the patient's quality of life by limiting mobility and interfering with bowel and bladder function. Unfortunately, patients with severe dysfunction before treatment have little chance of neurologic improvement (Bruckman & Bloomer, 1978).

Obstruction of the superior vena cava, which is most often experienced by patients with lung cancer, can constitute a radiotherapy emergency (Davenport, Ferree, Blake, & Raben, 1975). Initial high-dose therapy may be required to the thoracic inlet and mediastinum, followed by lower, conventional doses (Lokich & Goodman, 1975). Most patients experience rapid relief of the symptoms of obstruction, which include facial swelling and venous dilation (Schraufnagel, Hill, Leech, & Pare, 1981).

Other problems that are commonly treated with palliative radiotherapy include bone, brain, and skin metastases. A study of alternative radiotherapy treatment approaches for osseous metastases demonstrated that up to 55 per cent of patients treated with protracted schedules experienced long-term and significant pain relief (Blitzer, 1985). Such relief usually occurs within days of the start of radiotherapy and is complete within 1 month after completion of the treatment program. Brain metastases are usually treated with radiation therapy in combination with corticosteroids. Approximately 60 per cent of patients treated with radiation therapy alone experience neurologic im-

provement that lasts 3 to 6 months. Skin metastases, such as those accompanying chest wall recurrence in breast cancer, are also treatable with palliative radiotherapy (Richter & Cola, 1985).

Palliative Chemotherapy

Chemotherapy is most often thought of as curative or as designed to bring about long-term control of the disease. However, systemic or regional chemotherapy may be offered to patients with cancers that have responded poorly to previous therapy or that have metastasized extensively. The objective of palliative chemotherapy is usually to provide time, not for its own sake but for the sake of the patient and family, who must deal with the personal consequences of a fatal disease (Romond, Metcalfe, & Macdonald, 1985). The central issues in designing treatment are the selection of a drug and the adjustment of the drug regimen to achieve tumor control while limiting toxic effects. Patients with various advanced or poor-prognosis diseases may choose to "buy time" by accepting palliative chemotherapy.

Palliative chemotherapy may also be used to ameliorate specific symptoms. Systemic regimens may be used to treat pleural effusions and to reduce recurrent attacks of dyspnea and the need for paracentesis, but the success rate is low (Fentiman et al., 1983). Chemotherapy can also be used as an adjunct to palliative radiotherapy, as in the treatment of superior vena caval obstruction (Schraufnagel et al., 1981). Regional chemotherapy for liver metastases and advanced ovarian carcinoma is being investigated for its usefulness in palliation (Romond et al., 1985). Chemotherapy that is designed to reduce tumor mass and as a result palliate specific symptoms, such as pain secondary to compression of pain-sensitive structures or profound muscle weakness secondary to hypercalcemia (Poe & Radford, 1985), can be effective in selected patients.

THE NURSE'S ROLE IN PALLIATIVE SUPPORT

This review has highlighted the wide range of circumstances in which surgery, radiotherapy, or chemotherapy can be truly "helpful" to patients, even when their life spans are limited. Many nurses believe the implementation of these therapies automatically implies a curative intent, and as a result they become distressed when these treatments are offered to the terminally ill patient (Degner & Beaton, 1987). This misconception must be set aside if the nurse is to assume an effective role in providing palliative support.

The compensatory model of helping implies that caregivers help patients by doing for them what they would do for themselves if they were able. Understanding the potential risks and benefits of palliative surgery, radiotherapy, and chemotherapy provides a sound basis for implementing this model of helping. Most patients want to know that options are available to

---

Box 28–1. PREFERENCES FOR TREATMENT, CASE 1

STUDY

Degner, L. F., & Russell, C. A. (1988). **Preferences for treatment control among adults with cancer.** *Research in Nursing and Health, 11,* 367–374.

SAMPLE

Sixty patients with cancer at various points in their disease trajectories and with a wide variety of cancers. However, more than half had breast cancers, and 73.3 per cent were female.

MEASURE

Card-sort procedure that allowed patients to express their preferences for roles in making decisions about treatment.

FINDINGS

Out of 60 patients, 59 had systematic preferences about keeping, sharing, or giving away control over treatment decision making. Forty-seven of the 59 patients (79.7 per cent) preferred a pattern of joint decision making, which was reflected in the statement: "After my doctor explains the various treatment options, the selection of any therapy is a joint decision between myself and my doctor."

LIMITATIONS

Because patients were at various points in their diagnosis and treatment trajectories, their actual experiences in the health care system may have affected their preferences. The sample was overrepresented in terms of females who had breast cancer and underrepresented in terms of patients who had lung and bowel cancer.

---

reduce their distress, and some will want to play an active role in deciding which of these options is appropriate.

Palliative Care versus Palliative Treatment

If they decline palliative treatment with surgery, radiotherapy, or chemotherapy, patients and families should be informed that the option of palliative care still exists. Described elsewhere in this volume are many approaches to symptom management and psychosocial support that are extremely effective in reducing the distress that usually accompanies the progression of cancer. Nurses should play an active role in communicating the availability of these options to patients and families. The nurse must have knowledge of the resources available within the clinical setting (such as a palliative consultation team) as well as those based in the community. Patients and families may need as much assistance in selecting among alternatives to palliative care as in choosing among alternative palliative treatments.

Communication and Control

An analysis of the literature on communication and cancer (Northouse & Northouse, 1987) reached the

conclusion that loss of control is the single most important problem confronting cancer patients.

Loss of control refers to an individual's perceived inability to make choices which will affect the outcome of events that impinge on his or her life. Specifically for cancer patients, loss of control refers to the feelings of powerlessness and

Table 28–1. TREATMENT DECISION MAKING FOR PALLIATIVE SUPPORT

Nursing Questions	Alternative Answers
1. What is the intent of the treatment being proposed?	Cure, control, or palliation
2. What role does the patient, family, or both want to play in decision making about treatment?	Active collaborative role or passive role that delegates responsibility for making decisions to others
3. What are the potential risks and benefits of the treatment being proposed?	High risk-high benefit Low risk-low benefit High risk-low benefit Low risk-high benefit
4. Have these risks and benefits been clearly communicated to the patient and family?	Yes or no
5. How are the patient and family making their decision about selecting, accepting, or declining further treatment?	Risk-benefit calculation Feeling better-feeling worse calculation
6. What is the time frame for decision making?	Short or prolonged

---

Box 28–2. PREFERENCES FOR TREATMENT, CASE 2

STUDY

Cassileth, B. R., Zupkis, R. V., Sutton-Smith, K., & March, V. (1980). **Information and participation preferences among cancer patients.** *Annals of Internal Medicine, 92,* 832–836.

SAMPLE

Patients (256) who had metastatic cancer, had a median age of 55.5 years, and had been diagnosed for an average of 10 months.

MEASURES

Five-point rating scale of information preferences; two alternative statements about preferred roles in treatment decision making; rating scales about the types and amounts of information preferred; and the Beck Hopelessness Scale.

FINDINGS

Two thirds of patients wanted an active role in decision making, which was reflected in the statement, "I prefer to participate in decisions about my medical care and treatment." Most patients (85 per cent) preferred to receive as much information as possible, good and bad. Age consistently distinguished patients wanting information and active involvement and those preferring a more passive role, with the younger patients preferring a more active role. Patients who preferred active involvement in their care and who wanted as much information as possible were significantly more hopeful than those who did not.

LIMITATIONS

Patients were under treatment in a major urban medical center, and the setting itself may have influenced the patients' information and participation preferences. Patients who seek treatment in large medical centers may differ from those who go elsewhere for cancer treatment.

---

helplessness that result from the inability to predict or have an impact on events surrounding their illness. (p. 18)

Northouse and Northouse (1987) also described three aspects of communication that are of central importance to health professionals: imparting information, communicating hope, and sharing control. The six questions in Table 28–1 provide a clinical guide that nurses can use to communicate information, hopefulness, and a sense of shared decision making within the context of palliative treatment.

Nursing Interventions

Specifying the intent of treatment is the first step in clarifying treatment goals. Medical rounds provide an ideal opportunity for the nurse to ask, What is the intent of this treatment? Alternative answers include cure, control, or palliation. Once the intent has been identified and discussed, it should be clearly communicated to all staff members, both verbally and in writing. Misunderstandings about the goals of treatment can create unnecessary strife between nursing and medical personnel, and the resulting tensions can adversely influence nursing care of the patient.

In the process of providing care, nurses often become aware of the preferences that patients and families have about participating in treatment decision making. Some will want to play an active or collaborative role, and others will simply want to delegate the responsibility for decision making to the physician (Lewis, Haberman, & Wallhagen, 1986). Health care professionals frequently assume that patients or families cannot or should not participate in making decisions about treatment because (1) patients and families do not have the necessary knowledge, and (2) even if they did understand the options, they might suffer irreparable psychological damage from participating, especially if predicted outcomes for the patient were poor (Degner & Beaton, 1987). In contrast to these beliefs, one study found that 78 per cent of a sample of 60 cancer patients preferred a collaborative model of decision making (Box 28–1). Similarly, Dennis (1987) found in a study of 70 medical-surgical patients that those with cancer represented the majority who wanted to be involved in decisions about the diagnosis and treatment of their illness. Patients with cancer who want to play a more active role in decision making have been found to be significantly more hopeful than those who do not (Box 28–2). Eliciting preferences about roles in treatment decision making is one way to facilitate the effectiveness of patients and families in dealing with the health care system. As Dennis

---

Box 28–3. PREFERENCES FOR TREATMENT, CASE 3

STUDY

O'Connor, A. M. (1989). **Effects of framing and level of probability on patients preferences for cancer chemotherapy.** *Journal of Clinical Epidemiology, 42,* 119–126.

SAMPLE

Healthy volunteers (129) and patients with cancer (154). The patients with cancer had a mean age of 54 years, and the sample was 57 per cent female and 44 per cent male. Most of the volunteers (70 per cent) were health professionals.

MEASURE

Treatment choice questionnaire that permitted subjects to choose between two hypothetical treatments: one that produced mild but persistent nausea, diarrhea, and fatigue; and one that had no side effects. The probability of survival for the treatments was systematically varied between 10 per cent and 100 per cent, and subjects were tested in one of three randomly assigned conditions: (1) the probability of survival was given, (2) the probability of death was given, or (3) both the probability of survival, and the probability of death were given.

FINDINGS

Patients had stronger preferences for toxic treatment than did healthy volunteers. Preference for toxic treatment decreased as the probability of survival dropped below 50 per cent. Patients who received probabilities in terms of the chances of dying considered the toxic treatment less desirable than did those in the other two groups.

LIMITATIONS

Patients were presented with a hypothetical rather than an actual treatment decision.

(1987) noted: "Nurses have a central role in identifying patients who want to be involved in making decisions about their care and in providing support for that active involvement."

Although most patients seem to prefer a shared pattern of decision making, many have difficulty achieving this role in their own care (Beisecker, 1988). Patients and families may need explicit invitations to take responsibility for decisions so that they do not automatically assume a passive stance. Robinson and Whitfield (1985) found that patients who were given specific instructions on how to assume a more active role during consultation sessions with their physicians produced more relevant questions and comments than did patients in control groups. Nurses need to communicate their own comfort with the process of sharing control and to provide the means by which patients can participate in this process.

Defining the potential risks and benefits of the proposed treatment is a critical step in deciding among therapies. Perceptions of the severity of risks and the nature of the benefits to be derived from therapy can vary among the patient, family, and caregivers and even among the caregivers. If the consensus is that the proposed treatment has low risks and high potential benefits, the decision to proceed with therapy becomes straightforward. However, when other possible combinations of risks and benefits are defined by partici-

pants (see Table 28–1), decision making can become more complicated and can provoke disagreement about the appropriate course of action. The potential for disagreement is particularly likely when the patient is terminally ill and benefits are defined in terms other than that of survival.

Risk assessment also changes when the chances of survival are low. One study of 154 cancer patients showed that they were willing to sacrifice aspects of their quality of life when chances of survival were high but were less likely to agree to potentially toxic therapy when the chances of survival dropped below 50 per cent. O'Connor (1989) concluded that when the probability of survival drops below 50 per cent, people give up hope of survival and opt for quality of life (Box 28–3). However, it is important to note that a subgroup of patients always preferred treatment even when survival rates were as low as 10 per cent. The challenge for the nurse is to elicit the values that the patient and family attach to the alternative therapies being proposed and to communicate these values effectively within the health care team.

In contrast to these subjective assessments, objective risks and benefits of the proposed therapy can be ascertained by conducting a review of the recent scientific literature. Nurses must be aware that clinical trials of palliative surgery, radiotherapy, and chemotherapy are ongoing and that knowledge about their efficacy is constantly changing. Those patients and families who wish to collaborate in making decisions about treatment deserve to receive the most up-to-date knowledge available.

Various other approaches can be used to judge the advisability of accepting or declining further treatment (Degner & Beaton, 1987). The most common of these, aside from the risk-benefit calculation, is the "feeling better–feeling worse calculation." Patients and families almost always want information about whether the proposed therapy will make the patient feel better or worse, and they use this data as the basis for their decisions. The weight attached to these assessments is often much greater for the recipients of care than for the caregivers, who tend to compartmentalize their thinking into risk-benefit calculations. Communication problems often occur when the patient and family base their decision on whether the patient will feel better or worse as a result of the treatment, but the caregivers base theirs on a risk-benefit calculation. The process of thinking that underlies the decision making of each person needs to be made explicit to avoid such difficulties. The nurse can play a key role in eliciting this information to avoid the escalation of conflicts that will make the patient's care anything but palliative.

The patient's ability to participate in decisions about palliative treatment may become limited if an oncologic emergency occurs. When the time frame for decision making suddenly becomes contracted and the patient is rapidly deteriorating, the family is left in the difficult position of having to decide whether to consent to therapy that is life saving even though it is of palliative intent. Assisting the family to make decisions that are in the patient's best interest is a central role for the nurse. Family members who believe that they did not act appropriately during this critical time may experience considerable difficulty during their bereavement as they consider and reconsider what they "should" have done.

SUMMARY

The more knowledge nurses gain about the efficacy of alternative treatment methods that are useful for palliative support, the more assistance they can provide to patients and families faced with the difficult decision of whether to accept further treatment when the patient's life span is limited. If the nurse adopts the perspective of one who is there to help patients do what they would do for themselves if they were able, the nurse's role in helping the patient becomes clearly defined. The six questions presented in Table 28–1 provide a clinical guide that the nurse can follow to understand what decisions the patient would want to make. The objective is to help the patient and family make an "effective" decision: one that is informed, consistent with their values, and able to be implemented in practice (O'Connor & O'Brien, 1989).

The value of being in the right place to ask the right question at the right time cannot be overestimated. This approach was used by Florence Nightingale to bring about a 60 per cent reduction in hospital mortality for soldiers in the Crimea (Kopf, 1916). Today the same approach can be used by oncology nurses to ensure that palliative support accomplishes the goals that are defined as relevant by terminally ill patients and their families.

References

Beisecker, A. E. (1988). Aging and the desire for information and input in medical decisions: Patient consumerism in medical encounters. *Gerontologist, 28,* 330–335.

Blitzer, P. H. (1985). Reanalysis of the RTOB study of the palliation of symptomatic osseous metastases. *Cancer, 55,* 1468–1472.

Borass, M. C. (1985). Palliative surgery. *Seminars in Oncology, 12,* 368–374.

Brickman, P., Rabinowitz, V. C., Karuza, J., Coates, D., Cohn, E., & Kidder, L. (1982). Models of helping and coping. *American Psychologist, 37,* 368–384.

Bruckman, J. E., & Bloomer, W. D. (1978). Management of spinal cord compression. *Seminars in Oncology, 5,* 135–140.

Brunetaud, J. E., Maunoury, V., Ducrotte, P., Cochelard, D., Cortot, A., & Paris, J. C. (1987). Palliative treatment of rectosigmoid carcinoma by laser endoscopic photoablation. *Gastroenterology, 92,* 663–668.

Cassileth, B. R., Zupkis, R. V., Sutton-Smith, K., & March, V. (1980). Information and participation preferences among cancer patients. *Annals of Internal Medicine, 92,* 832–836.

Colapinto, N. D. (1985). Is age alone a contraindication to major cancer surgery? *Canadian Journal of Surgery, 28,* 323–326.

Cronenwett, L. R. (1983). When and how people help: Theoretical issues and evidence. In P. L. Chinn (Ed.), *Advances in nursing theory development.* Rockville, MD: Aspen.

Davenport, D., Ferree, C., Blake, D., & Raben, M. (1975). Response of superior vena cava syndrome to radiation therapy. *Cancer, 38,* 1577–1580.

Degner, L. F., & Beaton, J. I. (1987). *Life-death decisions in health care.* New York: Hemisphere.

Degner, L. F., Henteleff, P. D., & Ringer, C. (1987). The relationship between theory and measurement in evaluations of palliative care services. *Journal of Palliative Care, 3,* 8–13.

Degner, L. F., & Russell, C. A. (1988). Preferences for treatment control among adults with cancer. *Research in Nursing and Health, 11,* 367–374.

Dennis, K. E. (1987). Dimensions of client control. *Nursing Research, 36,* 151–155.

Fentiman, I. S., Rubens, R. D., & Hayward, J. L. (1983). Control of pleural effusions in patients with breast cancer: A randomized trial. *Cancer, 52,* 737–739.

Gravelyn, T. R., Michelson, M. K., Gross, B. H., & Sitrin, R. G. (1987). Tetracycline pleurodesis for malignant pleural effusions. *Cancer, 59,* 1973–1977.

Harrington, K. D., Sim, F. H., Enis, J. E., Johnston, J. O., Dick, H. M., & Gristina, A. G. (1976). Methylmethacrylate as an adjunct in internal fixation of pathological fracture. *Journal of Bone and Joint Surgery, 58-A,* 1047–1054.

Joffe, J., & Gordon, P. H. (1981). Palliative resection of colorectal carcinoma. *Diseases of the Colon and Rectum, 24,* 355–360.

Johnson, W. R., McDermott, F. T., Milne, B. J., Price, A. B., & Hughes, E. S. R. (1981). Palliative operative management in rectal carcinoma. *Diseases of the Colon and Rectum, 24,* 606–609.

Kopf, E. W. (1916). Florence Nightingale as statistician. *Journal of the American Statistical Association, 15,* 116.

Lewis, F. M., Haberman, M. R., & Wallhagen, M. I. (1986). How adults with late stage cancer experience personal control. *Journal of Psychosocial Oncology, 4,* 26–42.

Lokich, J. J., & Goodman, R. (1975). Superior vena cava syndrome: Clinical management. *Journal of the American Medical Association, 231,* 58–61.

Mathus-Vliegen, E. M. H., & Tytgat, G. N. (1986). Laser ablation and palliation in colorectal malignancy. *Gastrointestinal Endoscopy, 32,* 393–396.

Moore, C. L., Erikson, K. A., Yanes, L. B., Franklin, M., & Gonsalves, L. (1986). Nursing care and management of venous access ports. *Oncology Nursing Forum, 13*(3), 35–39.

Northouse, P. G., & Northouse, L. L. (1987). Communication and cancer: Issues confronting patients, health professionals, and family members. *Journal of Psychosocial Oncology, 5(3)*, 16–46.

O'Connor, A. M. (1989). Effects of framing and level of probability on patient's preferences for cancer chemotherapy. *Journal of Clinical Epidemiology, 42*, 119–126.

O'Connor, A. M., & O'Brien-Pallas, L. L. (1989). Decisional conflict. In G. K. MacFarland & E. A. McFarlane (Eds.), *Nursing diagnosis and intervention* (pp. 573–588). Toronto: C. V. Mosby Co.

Poe, C. M., & Radford, A. I. (1985). The challenge of hypercalcemia in cancer. *Oncology Nursing Forum, 12*(6), 29–34.

Qazi, R., & Savlov, E. D. (1982). Peritoneovenous shunt for palliation of malignant ascites. *Cancer, 49*, 600–602.

Richter, M. P., & Cola, L. R. (1985). Palliative radiation therapy. *Seminars in Oncology, 12*, 375–383.

Robinson, E. J., & Whitfield, M. J. (1985). Improving the efficacy of patients' comprehension monitoring: A way of increasing patients' participation in general practice consultations. *Social Science in Medicine, 21*, 915–919.

Romond, E. H., Metcalfe, M. S., & Macdonald, J. S. (1985). Palliative chemotherapy and hormonal therapy. *Seminars in Oncology, 12*, 384–389.

Russin, D. J., Kaplan, S. R., Goldberg, R. I., & Barkin, J. S. (1986). Neodymium-YAG laser: A new palliative tool in the treatment of colorectal cancer. *Archives of Surgery, 121*, 1399–1403.

Schraufnagel, D. E., Hill, R., Leech, J. A., & Pare, J. A. P. (1981). Superior vena caval obstruction: Is it a medical emergency? *American Journal of Medicine, 70*, 1169–1174.

Sim, F. H., & Pritchard, D. J. (1982). Metastatic disease in the upper extremity. *Clinical Orthopedics and Related Research, 169*, 83–94.

Twycross, R. G., & Lack, S. A. (1984). *Therapeutics in terminal cancer*. London: Pitman.

Zollinger, R. M., Sternfeld, W. C., & Schrelber, H. (1986). Primary neoplasms of the small intestine. *American Journal of Surgery, 151*, 654–658.

CHAPTER 29

Questionable Cancer Therapies

BARRIE R. CASSILETH
JENNIFER M. KLEINBART

FROM HERBAL MEDICINE TO HIGH COLONICS
TODAY'S UNPROVEN CANCER THERAPIES
WHO SEEKS UNORTHODOX THERAPY, WHO
DISPENSES IT, AND WHY

SUGGESTIONS FOR THE NURSE CLINICIAN
SUMMARY

Patients' use of unorthodox or unproven cancer treatments (American Cancer Society, 1964a) represents an important social, economic, and clinical problem. A measure of its magnitude may be gleaned from the fact that the public spends approximately $4 billion on unproven cancer cures per year (U.S. House, 1984). Contrary to stereotypes, patients who seek unproven cancer treatments tend to be well educated, middle to upper class, and not necessarily terminally ill or even beyond hope of cure or remission by conventional treatments (Cassileth, Lusk, Strouse, & Bodenheimer, 1984). Also contrary to stereotypes, today's unorthodox cancer practitioner may very well be a licensed physician: not an oncologist, but a physician who specializes in homeopathic or naturopathic medicine applied to patients with cancer and other major illnesses.

This chapter describes the types of unorthodox cancer practices that have achieved popularity in recent years and the toxic effects often associated with them. It provides research-based suggestions for the health care worker who must deal with a patient who is using or considering an alternative treatment regimen, and it attempts to place the contemporary zeal for unorthodox practices in social and historical perspective. Several terms (unproven, unorthodox, unconventional, alternative) are used here interchangeably, as they are by patients, practitioners, and conventional medical publications, to refer to those treatments and methods deemed by established medicine to be unproven (as in the American Cancer Society's "Unproven Methods" lists), unorthodox or ineffective (as in the American Society of Clinical Oncology's Subcommittee on "Unorthodox" Therapies), fraudulent, questionable, and so on.

FROM HERBAL MEDICINE TO HIGH COLONICS

The most commonly used unorthodox treatment for malignant disease today is metabolic therapy, which is

Supported in part by NIH Grant CA 31147. This chapter is an edited version of an article that appeared in *Cancer Investigation, 4,* 591–598, 1986.

a practitioner-specific combination of diet, megadoses of vitamins and minerals, detoxification by internal cleansing, and spiritual or emotional restoration (Cassileth et al., 1984). Maintenance of these regimens requires a full-time commitment of activity and time by the patient and typically by a family member as well.

Metabolic therapy and other variant treatments are based on a philosophy of health and illness that views disease not as a localized or system-specific disorder but as an expression of systemic pathology. Thus cancer, for example, is perceived as one of many possible expressions of underlying dysfunction. It is the underlying dysfunction, not the symptom (cancer), that is treated.

This philosophy and its implicit self-care components are central to contemporary unorthodox cancer medicine. It is precisely this ideology, rather than the particulars of the treatment regimen per se, that patients acknowledge when they elect the unproven methods route.

Today's unorthodox cures differ importantly from their major twentieth-century predecessors, which were cancer-targeted quasi-medicines in pill or liquid form (Cassileth, 1982). During the early years of this century, liquid cures were introduced, such as Radol, Chamlee's Cancer Specific Purifies-the-Blood Cure, and a host of others (Cramp, 1912). Koch's glyoxilide (distilled water) cure of the 1940s was followed by the Hoxsey treatment in extract and pill form in the 1950s, by injectable krebiozen during the 1960s, and by Laetrile in the 1970s. Each in its own time created a furor at least equal to that aroused in the recent past by Laetrile (Box 29–1).

Contemporary unproven therapies, then, differ in three major ways from the previously popular unorthodox cures of the twentieth century. First, contemporary cures are not pills or potions, but life-style–oriented remedies. (For that reason they cannot be regulated by the United States Food and Drug Administration.) Second, they are not secret formulas known only to their manufacturers but activities of daily living that can be understood and accomplished by patients themselves. Finally, they carry an aura of respectabil-

---

Box 29–1. UNORTHODOX CANCER THERAPY

STUDY

Moertel, C. G., Fleming, T. R., Rubin, J., Kvols, L. K., Sarna, G., Koch, R., Currie, V. E., Young, C. W., Jones, S. E., & Davingnon, J. D. (1982). **A clinical trial of amygdalin (Laetrile) in the treatment of human cancer.** *New England Journal of Medicine, 306,* 201–206.

SAMPLE

Patients with cancer (171) for which no curative or life-extending treatment was known. Only patients who had undergone no surgery, radiation therapy, or chemotherapy for at least 1 month and who were in generally good health were selected.

TREATMENT

Administration of intravenous amygdalin for 21 days followed by an oral low-dose maintenance regimen. "Metabolic therapy," consisting of high doses of vitamins, pancreatic enzymes, and specific diet restrictions, was practiced throughout treatment.

RESULTS

Treatment with amygdalin in combination with metabolic therapy produced no therapeutic benefits: tumor progression was neither arrested nor slowed. Further, significantly toxic effects of amygdalin were demonstrated, as blood cyanide rose to dangerous and potentially fatal levels.

---

ity, even a hint of conventional medicine's blessing, because they are not far removed from orthodox medicine's concerns with diet, life style, environmental carcinogens, and the reciprocal relationship between many emotional and physiologic responses.

Despite these important differences, it is perhaps surprising and reassuring to note that precedents exist for both the scope and the particular emphasis of contemporary unorthodox cures. The nineteenth century, known as the golden age of quackery (Janssen, 1979), produced an abundance of self-cure cults and the following statement from an anonymous physician, published in the *National Quarterly Review* in 1861: "Quackery kills a larger number annually of the citizens of the United States than all the diseases it pretends to cure."

At that time, as now, advocates worked for democratization of medical knowledge, with "every man his own doctor," and for a "holistic" self-care alternative to a disease-oriented, impersonal medical system (Starr, 1982). The nineteenth-century movement arose in response to the development of modern clinical methods with the then new emphasis on disease as stemming from localized pathology.

Today's medical counterculture mirrors the nineteenth-century experience. The contemporary version stems at least in part from an analogous reaction to today's technologic medicine that favors heroic measures to save lives, against which the public attempts to protect itself through living wills, court battles to achieve the "right to die," and demands for "humane" alternatives. Medical specialization offers sophisticated and clinically optimal care, but it also creates dissatisfaction among patients. Written in 1932, the following

comment is equally valid today (Bruhn, 1980). The patient feels: "that there is no one who really sees him or is interested in him as a whole. The cults have capitalized on this failure of modern medicine to view the patient as an entity, and to replace the old family physician with a coordinated specialism" (Reed, 1932).

Alternative cancer medicine today represents a rejection of both conventional medicine and the previous unorthodox emphasis on targeted medications, professional authority, and disease as a localized pathologic response. Instead, investigators note a throwback to nineteenth-century beliefs in disease as a systemic phenomenon, in demystification and simplification of illness, in "natural" cures, and in self-care. Now as then, the counterculture is firmly rooted in a politicized antibureaucracy, antigovernment, and antiregulatory context. Now as then, ambivalence or hostility toward the medical profession is clearly evident.

Table 29–1 illustrates some of the major unorthodox approaches that captured national attention over the decades. The tendency is to view the particular unorthodox fashion of the moment, for example the Laetrile experience of the 1970s, as "unprecedented" (Lerner, 1984). To place recent unorthodox medicine events in perspective, it is important to note the similarities between them and each example in Table 29–1. As was true of Laetrile and as now holds for metabolic regimens, previous unproven methods attracted many thousands of followers; raised a great deal of money for practitioners; and were attacked by the medical establishment, the United States Postal Service, and the Bureau of Chemistry (later the Food and Drug Administration). Reports of worthlessness of most of these cures (and of others not discussed here) were

Table 29–1. EXAMPLES OF MAJOR UNORTHODOX APPROACHES OVER TIME

Era of Popularity in the United States	Unorthodox Approach	Reference
1800–1850	*Thomsonianism* Belief: All disease results from one general cause (cold) and can be cured by one general remedy (heat). Opposed "mineral" drugs and the "tyranny" of doctors. Remedy: Emetics and hot baths.	(Starr, 1982; Thompson, 1825; Thompsonian Record, 1832)
1850–1900	*Homeopathy* Belief: Like cures like ("Law of Similia"); disease results from suppressed itch ("psora"). Remedy: More than 3000 different drugs, each a highly distilled organic or inorganic substance.	(Gardner, 1957; Kaufman, 1971; Starr, 1982)
1890–	*Naturopathy* Belief: Disease results not from external bacteria but from violation of the natural laws of living; drugs are harmful; "natural" products and activities cure. Remedy: Diets, massages, colonic irrigation.	(Gardner, 1957; Kellog, 1923)
1890–	*Early Osteopathy and Chiropracty* Belief: Mechanistic view of the body; disease caused by dislocation of bones in the spine. Rejected drugs and germ theory. Remedy: Spinal manipulation.	(Gardner, 1957; Still, 1897)
1900s	Tablet and ointment cancer cures by B. F. Bye, W. O. Bye, Buchanan, Chamlee, G. M. Curry, L. T. Leach (Cancerol), C. W. Mixer, E. H. Griffith (Radio-sulpho), F. W. Warner, R. Wells (Radol).	(Cramp, 1912)
1920s	"Energy" cancer cures by A. Abrams (radio wave cure), R. B. Brown (radio therapy), A. E. Kay (cosmic energy "vrilium"), D. Ghadiali (spectro-chrome light therapy); E. Cayce's psychic diagnoses and treatments.	(Gardner, 1957)
1940s	W. F. Koch's Glyoxylide.	(American Cancer Society, 1964b; Janssen, 1979; Miller & Howard-Rubin, 1983)
1950s	H. Hoxsey's cancer treatment.	(American Cancer Society, 1964a; Janssen, 1979; Miller & Howard-Rubin, 1983)
1960s	A. C. Ivy's Krebiozen.	(American Cancer Society, 1962; Janssen, 1979; Miller & Howard-Rubin, 1983)
1970s	Laetrile.	(Markle & Petersen, 1980; Moertel, Fleming, Rubin et al., 1982)
1980s	Metabolic therapies: diet, high colonics, vitamins and minerals; Simonton's imagery.	(Cassileth et al., 1984) (Simonton, 1982; Simonton et al., 1981)

published by the American Cancer Society in numerous separate reports, by the *Journal of the American Medical Association* (Cramp, 1912), and in many other publications at the turn of the twentieth century.

Table 29–1 also illustrates the shifting cycles of popular unproven approaches, from the "natural, holistic" alternatives of the nineteenth century (Gardner, 1957) to the quasi-medicines of the early and mid-twentieth century, to today's return to the natural, holistic, diet-oriented regimens. These shifting preferences also may be seen against the prevailing emphases of conventional medicine of the time.

The unorthodox therapies listed in Table 29–1 represent a sampling of the most popular regimens of their era. Olson's list of unproven cancer methods (1977) includes 59 entries for the years 1893 through 1971, and the American Cancer Society's "unproven methods" list is even more extensive.

TODAY'S UNPROVEN CANCER THERAPIES

The covert nature of the most contemporary unorthodox cures and the widespread dissemination of self-care remedies through nonmainstream periodicals and books preclude precise estimates of their popularity. However, new data from a previous study (Cassileth et al., 1984), now based on a national sample of 1000 patients with cancer, reveal the six most common unproven treatments. In descending order of frequency of use, these include metabolic therapy, diet treatments, megavitamin therapy, mental imagery applied for antitumor effect, spiritual or faith healing, and "immune" therapy. The first four are reviewed in this chapter. Spiritual therapy rarely is used independently of other unorthodox or conventional treatments. "Immune" therapy, although popular, is available only at a few sites.

Metabolic therapy, received by 45 per cent of patients who used unorthodox regimens with or without conventional care (Cassileth et al., 1984), rests on the principles that toxins and waste materials in the body interfere with metabolism and healing and that cells lack the nutrients essential to health. Cancer and other chronic illnesses are viewed as the result of degeneration of the liver and pancreas and of the immune and "oxygenation" systems. Treatment is directed at cellular "detoxification and restoration" (Gerson, 1977; Kelly, 1974; Manner, DiSanti, & Michaelsen, 1978).

Although metabolic regimens vary by practitioner, they typically include special diets; detoxification by colonic cleansing; and additional vitamins, minerals, or enzymes (Fig. 29–1).

Metabolic therapies are available from clinics and individual practitioners throughout North America and Europe, with a special concentration of clinics in Mexico. The major medical toxicity associated with metabolic regimens results from colonic irrigation, which is typically given in the form of coffee enemas (to detoxify the liver) or high colonics with coffee, wheatgrass, or other substances.

Deaths from electrolyte imbalance, bowel necrosis and perforation, toxic colitis, amebiasis, hypokalemia, and sepsis caused by colonic irrigation have been reported (Eisele & Reay, 1980; Istre, Kreiss, Hopkins et al., 1982; Markman, 1985). Difficulties associated with the dietary and vitamin components of metabolic therapy are discussed later under regimens involving diet or vitamins exclusively. These components apparently cause fewer problems in the context of metabolic therapy, probably because diets associated with metabolic cures are less restrictive.

Diet treatments consist exclusively of particular, practitioner-specified foods. Dietary cures were tried

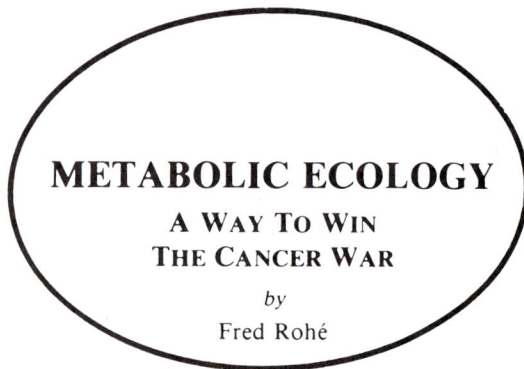

METABOLIC ECOLOGY

A WAY TO WIN
THE CANCER WAR

by
Fred Rohé

— Few people should ever die of cancer.

— There have been over 4,000 Metabolic Ecology victories over cancer.

— Read about the true early warning signs of cancer.

— Read about 23 personal victories over 16 classes of cancer.

— Read about how to be victorious using the most successful strategy against cancer ever devised.

A Note from Dr. Keller
I have read every word of Fred Rohé's *Metabolic Ecology*. It is an exact, up-to-date presentation of my work. This book supersedes my own book, *One Answer to Cancer*, which is now out-of-date, and will not be reprinted.

Figure 29–1. Advertisement for a questionable cancer therapy.

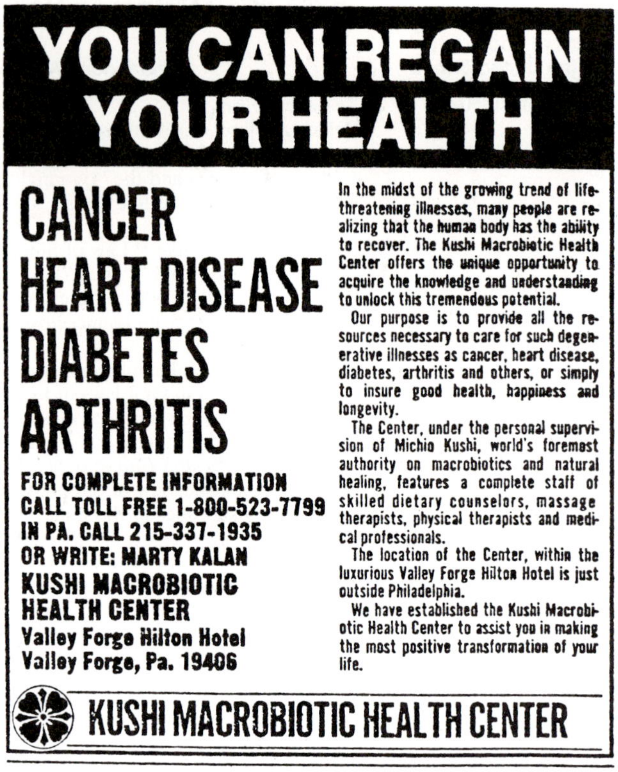

Figure 29–2. Advertisement for a questionable cancer therapy.

by 32 per cent of patients who used unproven methods (Cassileth et al., 1984). A variety of diet therapies exist, from the grape cure to raw foods to wheatgrass extract. Probably the most commonly adopted dietary cure in the United States today is macrobiotic therapy (Fig. 29–2).

The macrobiotic diet, offered by its proponents as both a cancer preventive and a cancer cure, is based on Eastern yin-yang philosophic principles and on a fully formulated alternative concept of human physiology and disease (Esko, 1981; Kohler & Kohler, 1979). A "mother red blood cell" in the intestine is viewed as the sole progenitor of all body cells and organs. Food intake must be carefully balanced to counteract disease. The notion of balance is central to treatment: yin foods are prescribed for yang cancers, and yang foods are prescribed for yin cancers. The macrobiotic diet, expanded after a patient died of malnutrition several years ago, now includes whole grains, some specially cooked vegetables, and miso, a product of soybean fermentation believed to have anticancer properties (Esko, 1981).

Nutritional deficiency, a potential result of dietary cures (Arnold, 1984; Herbert, 1980–1981), is particularly hazardous for patients with cancer. Dietary regimens have a special attraction for the general public today, given conventional medicine's emphasis on dietary restrictions to prevent heart disease and cancer and given the relationship between the consumption of certain foods and the increased incidence of some malignant diseases. Further, patients often make the mistaken but seemingly logical leap from the conventional position that diet may prevent cancer to the unconventional position that diet can cure cancer.

Many unproven cancer therapies come equipped with their own diagnostic techniques. Macrobiotic practitioners use iridology for this purpose. This procedure involves looking at the iris, each pie-shaped segment of which is believed to represent a different organ or body area. A discoloration in the eight-o'clock segment of the right iris, for example, would be diagnostic of liver cancer. An evaluation of iridology, reported in the scientific literature, documented its uselessness (Simon, Worthen, & Mitas, 1979). It may be assumed that reports of at least some macrobiotic cures describe healthy patients who had been diagnosed as having cancer by iridology.

Megavitamins, used by 20 per cent of patients, represents the third most common unorthodox cancer treatment (Cassileth et al., 1984). This therapy involves consumption of large quantities of high-dose vitamins, which are believed to enhance the body's capacity to destroy malignant cells (Berkley, 1978; Newbold, 1979). Excessive vitamin intake can be toxic if not useless (Greenberg, 1975; Herbert & Barrett, 1982; Moertel et al., 1985; Schaumburg et al., 1983). Here again, however, it requires a sophisticated and discerning public to differentiate between unorthodox claims for vitamin cures and conventional medical reports such as this from the *Journal of the American Medical Association*: "Research on Vitamin-Cancer Relationship Getting Big Boost" (Gunby, 1982).

Mental imagery requires the patient to visualize or imagine the destruction of malignant cells (Howard-Ruben & Miller, 1984; Simonton, Matthews-Simonton, & Creighton, 1981). Sixteen per cent of patients used this technique not as a potential emotional benefit but as a means of treating malignant disease (Cassileth et al., 1984). Destruction of cancerous cells is viewed as the result of psychological influence on the immune system, which in turn counteracts the malignant process. Proponents typically describe imagery as part of psychoneuroimmunology (Howard-Ruben & Miller, 1984; Peterson & Markler, 1980; Simonton et al., 1981; Solomon, 1985; Varan, 1989), an emerging field that encompasses scientific investigation (Halvorsen & Vassend, 1987; Locke et al., 1984; Schleifer, Keller, Cammerino, Thornton, & Stein, 1983; Stein, Keller, & Schleifer, 1985), as well as all manner of regimens meant to enhance immune function, such as imagery. Although imagery, stress, and other activities have been shown to alter immune function, the changes are transient. Of greatest significance is the fact that enhanced immune function has never been demonstrated to affect established cancer. According to the American Cancer Society review, imagery's drawbacks include no scientific proof of efficacy, no evidence that personality contributes to the development or cure of cancer, no evidence that stress or imagery affects cancer, possible guilt as a result of inability to cure oneself, and possible abandonment of conventional care (Simonton, 1982).

WHO SEEKS UNORTHODOX THERAPY, WHO DISPENSES IT, AND WHY

Before research was carried out, it was generally believed that patients who sought marginal or unproven medical remedies did so out of ignorance. Such patients were seen as "innocent victims" of quackery (Duffy, 1975) or as "uninformed" (Cobb, 1954) and in need of factual information from the American Cancer Society or the Food and Drug Administration, information likely to dissuade them from adopting unorthodox practices (Olson, 1977). They were assumed to be underprivileged, poor, and uneducated (Bruch, 1974).

The limited number of studies of patients with cancer as well as the more general studies of the use of marginal medicine have taught us that people who use unorthodox therapies are equally or better educated and informed than patients who do not try unorthodox remedies (Avina & Schneiderman, 1978; Bruch, 1974; Cassileth et al., 1984; Kane, Leymaster, Olsen et al., 1974; Lupton, Najman, Payne, Sheehan, & Western, 1978; National Analysts, Inc., 1972; Reed, 1932; Wagenfeld, Vissing, Markle, & Peterson, 1979). Our study indicated that patients who used unorthodox treatments exclusively or in conjunction with conventional therapy tended to be better educated (p<.00001) than patients who used conventional cancer treatment only (Cassileth et al., 1984).

The British royal family uses and supports alternative medicine, and the Prince of Wales made a well-publicized trip to Bristol in 1983 to open a Cancer Help Centre that specializes in "complementary" methods (Baum, 1983). Alternative medicine is said to be one of the few growth industries in contemporary Great Britain (Lister, 1983; Smith, 1983).

In an interesting historical note, Benjamin Franklin wrote in 1731 to his sister: "I know cancer of the breast is often though to be incurable, yet we have here in town a kind of shell made of some wood, cut at a proper time, by some men of great skill which has done wonders in this disease" (Duffy, 1975). The evidence seems "overwhelming" that socioeconomic status is "either independent of use of such therapies or that higher status and better educated individuals are overrepresented among the patients of unorthodox practitioners" (Peterson & Markle, 1981).

If patients fail to conform to an assumed stereotype, so do many unorthodox practitioners. Although some practitioners indeed may be appropriately classified as untrained, unscrupulous quacks and charlatans (Barrett, 1978; Burkhalter, 1977; Glymour & Stalker, 1983; Olson, 1977), others may not. A survey of 100 young physicians in Great Britain, for example, revealed that 86 per cent held favorable views toward alternative medicine and that 43 per cent had referred patients for such treatment (Lister, 1983). Our study showed that of 166 unorthodox practitioners, 51 per cent were M.D.s and 5 per cent were D.O.s. Of these, 18 per cent were board certified in various specialties, not including oncology (Cassileth et al., 1984).

The involvement of educated patients with unproven remedies can be explained in part by the fact that several features of these contemporary cures require time, financial resources, and an educated, questioning approach to illness. One must read the unorthodox literature to learn about alternative remedies, to select among them, and to follow their self-care components.

Patients typically are quite knowledgeable about conventional options as well, having obtained second and third opinions and having read relevant orthodox medical publications. Comparison of conventional and unorthodox options requires a level of involvement and intellect that the passive, poorly educated patient is less likely to display.

Further, unorthodox cancer regimens typically involve travel to often distant alternative clinics; the purchase of equipment, food processing devices, and special foods; and a major commitment of time and energy to the pursuit of such regimens in the patient's home. These are activities that require the financial and human resources consonant with middle and upper socioeconomic status.

But the foregoing is not the whole answer, nor does it explain the tacit approval or active participation of physicians who, one would expect, have been trained to distinguish and deliver rational, scientific therapies, not unproven treatments. A central point, usually not mentioned in the literature, is that *there are no unproven remedies for curable diseases*. In the nineteenth century, quack remedies for tuberculosis abounded, but they vanished when medical science discovered effective treatment for the disease (Lerner, 1984). Some malignant diseases are curable, but the cure rates for the common cancers (such as lung and colon cancer) have remained stable for decades.

Patients see a discrepancy when conventional medical practitioners argue that cancer is a curable disease and their statistics claim a cure rate approaching 50 per cent, but the experience of public figures and their friends and neighbors is that people often die of cancer. The discrepancy and the cure rate data have two important consequences. They shake patients' confidence in the validity and veracity of conventional cancer cure statistics. They encourage patients to seek alternative options because of the potentially erroneous belief that these alternatives cannot offer worse than a 50 per cent chance. Further, unconventional treatments may offer the same opportunity for cure with the added benefit of being "natural" and nontoxic. Conventional cancer medicine, conversely, is dangerous in and of itself. Patients are familiar with the common toxic effects associated with chemotherapy and radiation therapy. And so are physicians.

Thus patients and physicians who turn to unorthodox methods do so in part out of discouragement and despair concerning the realities of orthodox cancer treatment. The medical profession and the media have promised more than can be delivered, and the public has responded by suspending belief and often by seeking alternative therapeutic options.

Yet additional factors contribute to the popularity of today's unproven cancer methods. The social and psychological pressures exerted on the patient with disseminated disease and the hope for cure offered by unorthodox healers (Holland, 1981) play important roles. But many patients use unorthodox methods in lieu of conventional treatment, and others initiate unproven treatments with early-stage or localized disease (Cassileth et al., 1984).

The patient's fear, previous negative experiences with conventional medicine (Barrett, 1978; Burkhalter, 1977), and search for a more supportive therapeutic alliance (Howard-Ruben & Miller, 1984) are cited as reasons for the use of unproven cancer methods. Media overplay of treatments is also cited (Morris, 1975), as is the precept that "you reach people by offering something they want" (Ingelfinger, 1976). That precept, a fundamental law of communications, provides a major clue to the attraction of patients and physicians to unorthodox medicine.

Unorthodox medicine, with its contemporary focus on holistic and self-care, is what many people want. It provides them not only with the particulars of treatments but also with an entire belief system that is consistent with a more general prevailing ideology. Today's unproven methods represent a social movement bound by beliefs in the fundamental importance of nutrition and responsibility for one's own health, by the understanding that conventional medicine cannot cure most cancers, by opposition to technologic therapy and professional bureaucracy, and by repudiation of basic scientific beliefs.

This social movement is called *holistic medicine,* or naturopathy, and it is undergoing a major renaissance today in the United States and abroad. In 1978, the American Holistic Medical Association Conference sponsored a symposium on "Holistic Medicine and Health Care" (Relman, 1979). The holistic or naturopathic movement offers apparently rational, natural alternatives to conventional drugs and surgery plus the appealing emphasis on self-care of the disease and of the total person. It suggests an alternative that has clearly reached people by "offering something they want." It is not typically a rational, safe alternative (Baum, 1983; Glymour & Stalker, 1983; Relman, 1979). Nonetheless, its populist roots and "freedom of choice" theme provide the public with an opportunity to display its dissatisfaction with traditional medicine (Fuks & Modan, 1984; Peterson & Markle, 1980); its preference for nineteenth-century style democratized health care, now wrapped in the banner of patients' rights; and its dislike of bureaucratic, technologic, and specialized care of disease.

SUGGESTIONS FOR THE NURSE CLINICIAN

Nurses generally spend more time with cancer patients than do any other members of the health care team. Accordingly, patients may feel more comfortable expressing concerns to a nurse, including fears and doubts about standard treatments and questions regarding unproven therapies. The nurse, therefore, has the potential to play a crucial role in influencing patients' behavior and decisions concerning treatment options. By establishing open communication with the patient, the opportunity is gained to clarify physician-prescribed treatments and to help the patient sort out information about unorthodox or dubious therapies. Early counseling of patients regarding available treatments can be critical in protecting them from pursuing ineffective, detrimental, or questionable therapies.

Typically, patients inform their caregivers that they are using an unproven therapy; approximately 75 per cent of patients on unorthodox therapies disclose this fact to members of their conventional health care teams (U.S. House, 1984). There may be reason to suspect that even more patients use questionable treatments covertly, perhaps because they fear anger or rejection: 4 per cent of patients said that they were refused continued care because of their use of unorthodox treatments (U.S. House, 1984).

Only a small minority of patients discuss the fact that they are considering the use of unproven methods. The key is for the nurse to initiate a discussion about questionable cancer treatments before the patient starts to use them. A number of health professionals have found the following approach useful. Explain to the patient that he or she is likely to hear about a variety of questionable alternatives to standard cancer treatment. Urge the patient to discuss these at any time. When delivered in a nonjudgmental fashion, this message is likely to result in the patient's initiating a discussion of unproven methods that may be of interest.

If patients sense the possibility of ridicule, disapproval, or rejection, they are unlikely to mention this subject again. In that event, the opportunity to explain the lack of benefit and the toxicities associated with a particular regimen and the resultant ability to dissuade the patient from trying it are lost, as is the opportunity to know what the patient is doing and how that may affect his or her clinical status.

When the patient indicates interest in a particular unorthodox method, it is critical to determine why. What is it about this unproven remedy that the patient finds appealing? What specific aspects of this unorthodox treatment are of interest?

Typically, one can explain why the treatment will not be effective and, at the same time, discuss a possible modification of that component of the treatment of particular interest to the patient. For example, if a special interest in nutrition has drawn the patient to a particular regimen, that patient could be given specific dietary guidelines. A concurrent explanation of how the unorthodox dietary approach could create nutritional deficiencies and other problems should be provided.

It is helpful to request that patients bring copies of materials that they have received from the unorthodox clinic or practitioner. Knowing what information the patient has acquired will enable a more complete assessment to be made, and a broader critique can be given to the patient. Patients who do not read this material critically can be helped to understand where flaws in the logic occur.

Often patients will describe cures that the unorthodox clinic or practitioner claims to have achieved, and these cures are generally cited in the written material from the clinic. Here it is helpful to explain the difference between anecdotal reports and reliable evaluations, for most patients cannot distinguish between the two. It can be pointed out as well that many "miraculous cures" are reported for patients who were not diagnosed by conventional means and who perhaps did not have cancer in the first place. Many practitioners of unproven methods have their own diagnostic techniques, such as forms of iridology, and there are also "self-tests" for cancer diagnosis that can be purchased through the mail. Even many apparently sophisticated patients are not aware that diagnoses can be made only through tissue biopsy analysis or related conventional methods.

Patients frequently turn to questionable methods because they feel that their conventional treatment is not working. This feeling may be their own perception, or it may be the reality. In the former instance, an explanation of how the conventional treatment works, how long it will take to work, possible side effects, and so on will be helpful. In the latter instance, other possibilities may be recommended. These include participation in a conventional clinical trial, a suggestion that should be accompanied by an explanation of what a clinical trial is.

Patients often explain that they are considering an unproven method because it is "less toxic." Toxic reactions are not discussed in brochures from unorthodox clinics, which typically extol the "naturalness" of their regimen compared with the "cutting, burning, and poisoning" of conventional treatments. However, problems associated with the major unproven methods, as described earlier, as well as other toxic reactions associated with these and other questionable remedies should be discussed with the patient.

To deride questionable therapies of interest to patients is to deride the patients themselves and to drive them toward the questionable methods. The patient's interest must be met with the degree of seriousness and thoughtfulness applied by the patient to the unorthodox therapy itself. In addition to the details of conventional therapy and the problems associated with questionable methods, patients contemplating or using unorthodox treatments want a sympathetic ear. They want to be heard as much as they want to obtain information. For the busy nurse, this is perhaps the most difficult need to meet. It is, however, a need that is consistently well met by the unorthodox practitioner, who gives unfailingly of time and concern. Patients who sense inadequate interest and caring on the part of the conventional health care team are more likely than others to seek the ministrations of the questionable therapist.

SUMMARY

Contemporary unorthodox therapies appear unprecedented in their scope and specifics. They are not. We are experiencing a revival of nineteenth-century natural, holistic, self-care medicine. Today this takes the form of metabolic cancer therapy, the most commonly sought alternative of the mid 1980s.

Now, as then, a substantial segment of patients and of the healthy population has rejected what it perceives to be a disease-oriented, technologic, authoritarian health care system. Up to half of cancer patients today consider or use unorthodox treatments. Typically, these treatments are embedded in an ideology that patients find more compelling than what conventional medicine has to offer. This ideology includes an emphasis on self-care, a systemic rather than a localized view of pathology and health, and a belief in the fundamental importance of nutrition and whole-body fitness.

To the extent that patients reject conventional care as they are drawn to unproven alternatives, conventional medicine can and should respond by incorporating those reasonable components of unorthodox therapy that patients find lacking within the traditional health care framework.

References

American Cancer Society. (1962). *Krebiozen and carcalon. Unproven methods of cancer management.* New York: Author.

American Cancer Society. (1964a). *Hoxsey method or Hoxsey chemotherapy. Unproven methods of cancer management.* New York: Author.

American Cancer Society. (1964b). *Koch antitoxins. Unproven methods of cancer management.* New York: Author.

American Cancer Society. (1983). *Macrobiotic diets. Unproven methods of cancer management.* New York: Author.

Arnold, C. (1984). The macrobiotic diet: a question of nutrition. *Oncology Nursing Forum, 11,* 50–53.

Avina, R. & Schneiderman, L. (1978). Why patients choose homeopathy. *Western Journal of Medicine, 128,* 366–369.

Barrett, S. (1978). The health quack: supersalesman of the seventies [Editorial]. *Archives of Internal Medicine 138,* 1065–1066.

Baum, M. (1983). Quack cancer cures or scientific remedies? *Clinical Oncology, 9,* 275–280.

Berkley, G. E. (1978). *Cancer: How to prevent it and how to help your doctor fight it.* Englewood Cliffs, NJ: Prentice-Hall, Inc.

Bowman, B. B., Kushner, R. F., Dawson, S. C. & Levin, B. (1984). Macrobiotic diets for cancer treatment and prevention. *Journal of Clinical Oncology, 2,* 702–711.

Bruch, H. (1974). The allure of food cults and nutrition quackery. *Nutrition Reviews 32,* 63.

Bruhn, J. G. (1980). Specializing in being human. *Southern Medical Journal, 73,* 928–930.

Burkhalter, P. K. (1977, March). Cancer quackery. *American Journal of Nursing, 77,* 451–453.

Cassileth, B. R. (1982). After Laetrile, what? *New England Journal of Medicine, 306,* 1482–1484.

Cassileth, B. R., Lusk, E. J., Strouse, B. A. & Bodenheimer, B. J. (1984). Contemporary unorthodox treatments in cancer medicine: A study of patients, treatments, and practitioners. *Annals of Internal Medicine, 101,* 105–112.

Cobb, B. (1954). Why do people detour to quacks? *Psychiatric Bulletin, 3,* 66–69.

Cramp, A. J. (1912). *Nostrums and quackery and pseudo-medicine.* Chicago: American Medical Association.

Duffy, P. H. (1975). Cancer quackery. *Arizona Medicine, 32,* 724–726.

Eisele, J. W. & Reay, D. T. (1980). Deaths related to coffee enemas. *Journal of the American Medical Association, 244,* 1608–1609.

Esko, E. (1981). *The cancer prevention diet.* Brookline, MA: East-West Foundation.

Fuks, Z., & Modan, B. (1984). The story of "Joseph M."—mass media against "medical bureaucracy." *Public Health Reports, 99,* 338–342.

Gardner, M. (1957). *Fads and fallacies in the name of science.* New York: Dover Publications.

Gerson, M. (1977). *A cancer therapy: Results of fifty cases.* Del Mar, CA: Totality Books.

Glymour, C., & Stalker, D. (1983). Engineers, crank physicians, magicians [Sounding board]. *New England Journal of Medicine, 308,* 960–963.

Greenberg, D. M. (1975). The vitamin fraud in cancer quackery. *Western Journal of Medicine, 122,* 345–348.

Gunby, P. (1982). Research on vitamin-cancer relationship getting big boost. *Journal of the American Medical Association, 247,* 1799–1802.

Halvorsen, R., & Vassend, O. (1987). Effects of examination stress on some cellular immunity functions. *Journal of Psychosomatic Research, 31,* 693–701.

Herbert, V. (1980–1981). *Nutrition cultism: Facts and fictions.* Philadelphia: George F. Stickley Co.

Herbert, V., & Barrett, S. (1982). *Vitamins & "health" foods: The great American hustle.* Philadelphia: George F. Stickley Co.

Holland, J. C. (1981). Patients who seek unproven cancer remedies: A psychological perspective. *Clinical Bulletin, 11,* 102–105.

Howard-Ruben, J., & Miller, N. J. (1984). Unproven methods of cancer management part II: Current trends and implications for patient care. *Oncology Nursing Forum, 11,* 67–73.

Ingelfinger, F. J. (1976). Quenchless quest for questionable cure [Editorial]. *New England Journal of Medicine, 295,* 838–839.

Istre, G. R., Kreiss, K., Hopkins, R. S., Healy, G. R., Benziger, M., Canfield, T. M., Dickinson, P., Englert, T. R., Pompton, R. C., Matthews, H. M., & Simmons, R. A. (1982). An outbreak of amebiasis spread by colonic irrigation at a chiropractic clinic. *New England Journal of Medicine, 307,* 339–342.

Janssen, W. F. (1979). Cancer quackery—the past in the present. *Seminars in Oncology, 6,* 526–536.

Kane, R. L., Leymaster, C., Olsen, D., Woolley, F. R., & Fisher, F. D. (1974). Manipulating the patient: A comparison of the effectiveness of physician and chiropractor care. *Lancet 1,* 1333–1336.

Kaufman, M. (1971). *Homeopathy in America: The rise and fall of a medical heresy.* Baltimore: Johns Hopkins University Press.

Kellog, J. H. (1923). *The natural diet of man.* Battle Creek, MI: Modern Medicine Publishing Co.

Kelley, W. D. (1974). *One answer to cancer.* Beverly Hills International Association of Cancer Victims and Friends, Beverly Hills, CA: The Kelley Foundation.

Kohler, J. C., & Kohler, M. A. (1979). *Healing miracles from macrobiotics.* New York: Parker Publishing Co., Inc.

Lerner, I. J. (1984). The whys of cancer quackery. *Cancer, 53,* 815–819.

Lister, J. (1983). Current controversy on alternative medicine. *New England Journal of Medicine, 309,* 1524–1527.

Locke, S. E., Kraus, L., Leserman, J., Hurst, M. W., Heisel, J. S., & Williams, R. M. (1984). Life change stress, psychiatric symptoms and natural killer cell activity. *Psychosomatic Medicine, 46,* 441–453.

Lupton, G., Najman, J., Payne, S., Sheehan, M., & Western, J. (1978). Demographic characteristics of patients presenting for chiropractic and related forms of treatment. *Community Health Studies, 1,* 51–56.

Manner, H. W., DiSanti, S. J., & Michaelsen, T. L. (1978). *The death of cancer.* Chicago: Advanced Century Publishing Corp.

Markle, G. E., & Peterson, J. C. (1980). *Politics, science, and cancer: The Laetrile phenomenon.* Boulder, Co.: Westview Press, Inc.

Markman, M. (1985). Medical complications of "alternative" cancer therapy [Letter]. *New England Journal of Medicine, 312,,* 1640–1641.

Miller, N. J., & Howard-Rubin, J. (1983). Unproven methods of cancer management, part I: Background and historical perspectives. *Oncology Nursing Forum, 10,* 46–52.

Moertel, C. G., Fleming, T. R., Creagan, E. T., Rugin, J., O'Connell, M. J., & Ames, M. M. (1985). High-dose vitamin C versus placebo in the treatment of patients with advanced cancer who have had no prior chemotherapy: A randomized double-blind comparison. *New England Journal of Medicine, 312,* 137–141.

Moertel, C. G., Fleming, T. R., Rubin, J., Kvols, L. K., Sarna, G., Koch, R., Currie, V. E., Young, C. W., Jones, S. E., & Davignon, J. D. (1982). A clinical trial of amygdalin (Laetrile) in the treatment of human cancer. *New England Journal of Medicine, 306,* 201–206.

Morris, N. (1975). Potential tragedy in public overplay of cancer "cures". *Canadian Medical Association Journal, 113,* 465–470.

National Analysts, Inc. (1972). *A study of health practices and opinions.* Springfield, VA: U.S. Department of Commerce, National Technical Information Service.

Newbold, H. L. (1979). *Vitamin C against cancer.* New York: Stein & Day Publishers.

Olson, K. B. (1977). Drugs, cancer and charlatans. In J. Morton & G. J. Hill (Eds.), *Clinical oncology* (pp. 182–191). Philadelphia: W. B. Saunders Co.

Pelletier, K. R., & Herzing, D. L. (1988). Psychoneuroimmunology: Toward a mindbody model. *Advances, 5,* 27–56.

Peterson, J. C., & Markle, G. E. (1980). Politics, science and cancer: The Laetrile phenomenon. Westview Press, Boulder, CO.

Peterson, J. C., & Markle, G. E. (1981). *Public receptivity to marginal medicine.* Unpublished Manuscript, Department of Sociology, Western Michigan University.

Reed, L. (1932). *The healing cults.* Chicago: University of Chicago Press.

Relman, A. (1979). Holistic medicine [Editorial]. *New England Journal Medicine, 300,* 312–313.

Schaumburg, H., Kaplan, J., Windebank, A., Vick, N., Rasmus, S., Pleasure, D., & Brown, M. J. (1983). Sensory neuropathy from pyridoxine abuse: A new megavitamin syndrome. *New England Journal of Medicine, 309,* 445–448.

Schleifer, S. J., Keller, S. E., Cammerino, M., Thornton, J. C., & Stein, M. (1983). Suppression of lymphocyte stimulation following bereavement. *Journal of the American Medical Association, 250,* 374–377.

Shils, M. E., & Hermann, M. G. (1982). Unproved dietary claims in the treatment of patients with cancer. *Bulletin of the New York Academy of Medicine, 58,* 323–340.

Simon, A., Worthen, D. M., & Mitas, J. A. (1979). An evaluation of iridology. *Journal of the American Medical Association, 242,* 1385–1389.

Simonton, O. C. (1982). (American Cancer Society). Unproven methods of cancer management. *CA: A Cancer Journal for Clinicians, 32,* 58–61.

Simonton, O. C., Matthews-Simonton, S., & Creighton, J. L. (1981). *Getting well again.* New York: Bantam Books.

Smith, T. (1983). Alternative medicine. *British Medical Journal, 287,* 307–308.

Solomon, G. (1985). The emerging field of psychoneuroimmunology. *Advances, 2,* 6–19.

Starr, P. (1982). *The social transformation of American medicine.* New York: Basic Books, Inc.

Stein, M., Keller, S. E., & Schleifer, S. J. (1985). Stress and immunomodulation: The role of depression and neuroendocrine function. *Journal of Immunology, 135,* (Suppl.), 827–832.

Still, A. T. (1897). *The autobiography of A. T. Still.* Kirksville, MO: Author.

Thompson, S. (1825). *Narrative of the life and medical discoveries of Samuel Thompson . . . to which is added an introduction to his new guide to health* (2nd ed). Boston.

Thompsonian Record 1 (1832, December 15).

U.S. House Select Committee on Aging. (1984, May 31). Quackery: A $10 billion scandal. 98th Congress, second session.

Varan, W. J. (1989). Imagery and immunity. *Holistic Living, 6,* 4.

Wagenfeld, M. O., Vissing, Y. M., Markle, G. E., & Peterson, J. C. (1979). Notes from the underground: Health attitudes and practices of participants in the Laetrile movement. *Social Science Medicine, 13A,* 483–485.

EFFECTS OF COMMON ADULT CANCERS

CHAPTER 30

Breast Cancer

M. TISH KNOBF

Carcinoma of the breast is the most common cancer and the leading cause of death among American women between the ages of 35 to 54 years. In 1990 in the United States, an estimated 150,000 women will be diagnosed and 44,000 will die from this malignancy (Silverberg, Boring, & Squires, 1990). Although the incidence of breast cancer is greatest in North America and Europe, it appears to be increasing worldwide at an average rate of 2 per cent per year (Miller, 1987). Death rates due to breast cancer over the last decades are relatively unchanged, despite the increasing incidence. The stability of these mortality figures is most easily explained by improvement in the 5-year survival rates. It is unclear whether the prolonged survival is related to early detection and diagnosis, treatment strategies, or both.

EPIDEMIOLOGY AND ETIOLOGY

The incidence of breast cancer varies around the world. Incidence is highest in North America and the countries of northern Europe and lowest in the Asian and African countries. Incidence rates change substantially for the first- and second-generation descendants of low-risk geographic populations when they migrate to areas in which breast cancer is common. This change strongly suggests that environment and life style are major factors in determining breast cancer risk.

Risk Factors

In the United States, one out of every ten women is expected to be diagnosed with breast cancer in the course of her lifetime. History of a previous breast cancer, age older than 40 years, late menopause, no children or first pregnancy after age 30, and family history of breast cancer are recognized risk factors; diet, obesity, benign breast disease, oral contraceptive use, radiation exposure, and replacement estrogen use are potential risk factors that continue to be studied (Table 30–1). Although risk factors have been identified, the exact etiology for the development of breast

Table 30–1. RISK FACTORS ASSOCIATED WITH BREAST CANCER

Factor	Degree of Risk	Comments
Female gender	Increased	99% of all breast cancers occur in women and 1% in men.
History of a previous breast cancer	Increased	The risk of developing a cancer in the opposite breast is five times greater than for the average population at risk.
Age > 40	Increased	Incidence increases with age and peaks in the fifth decade.
Menstrual history: Early menarche or late menopause or both	Increased	The risk of breast cancer rises as the interval between menarche and menopause increases; shortening the interval by castration reduces the risk, especially if performed in women younger than 35 years of age (Brinton, Williams, & Hoover, 1979; Trichopoulos, MacMahon, & Cole, 1968).
Reproductive history: Nulliparity First child born after 30 years of age	Increased	Childless women have an increased risk as do women who bear their first child near or after the age of 30 years.
Family history: Mother or sister or both	Increased	Risk increases two to three times if a mother or sister has had breast cancer and is further increased if the relative was diagnosed during the premenopausal state and if the cancer was bilateral (Anderson, 1974; Anderson & Bodzich, 1985).
Diet	Controversial	Animal data and descriptive epidemiology of breast cancer incidence strongly suggest an association of dietary factors, specifically a high fat diet, with an increased risk of breast cancer. The National Academy of Science recommends decreasing total fat intake to 30% of available calories.
Alcohol	Unknown	A suggested small increase in risk with moderate alcohol consumption has been reported, although limitations in methodology have been cited, and results require confirmation.
Obesity	Controversial	Weight, height, obesity, and increased body mass have been reported to be associated with an increased risk of breast cancer.
Ionizing radiation	Increased	Three groups of women who received low-level radiation exposure demonstrated an increased breast cancer risk, which was particularly notable if the exposure occurred in the early years (<30 years) (Land, Boice, Shore, Norman, & Tokwnaga, 1980).
Benign breast disease	None	Fibrocystic breast disease is not associated with breast cancer. However, biopsy-proven atypical hyperplasia is associated with an increased risk (Dupont & Page, 1985).
Oral contraceptives	None	There is no evidence yet to suggest a causal relationship between oral contraceptives and incidence of and survival from breast cancer (Rosner, Lane, & Brett, 1985).
Exogenous hormones	Controversial	Several studies report no link with replacement hormones and breast cancer, and those that do appear to identify only subsets of patients at risk: those who have taken replacement estrogens for very long periods of time and those who have taken large cumulative doses (Brinton, Hoover, Szelko, & Fraumeni, 1981; Ross et al., 1980).

cancer is unknown. Epidemiologic data and clinical observations have led some to the hypothesis that a multistep process is responsible. A four-step process consisting of an initiation event, a promotional event, a transformation, and an early-to-late progression is suggested, which is consistent with current beliefs in cancer biology as described in Chapter 13.

Screening and Early Detection

Age is the only risk factor identified for the majority of women diagnosed with breast cancer. The risk predictably rises for women nearing the age of 40 years and persists at a significant level for the following 20 years. Education about the disease, the signs and symptoms, and the benefits of early detection is essential (see Chapter 17).

The goal of screening in breast cancer is to detect cancers at the earliest stage possible, because the extent of tumor at diagnosis is correlated with survival. Women who have small tumors and no spread to the axillary lymph nodes have a very good long-term prognosis compared with those who have large tumors and axillary lymph nodes that test positive.

Physical examination, breast self-examination (BSE), and mammography are three methods of screening proposed by the American Cancer Society (Table 30–2). Educational reinforcement is necessary particularly for mammography because concern persists among women about radiation exposure from annual examinations. The benefit of identifying tumors that are too small or that cannot be detected by physical examination must be communicated and stressed to the public on an ongoing basis. Ultimately, the benefit

Table 30–2. SCREENING FOR BREAST CANCER

Method	Age	Frequency
Physical examination by health care professional	20–40	Every 3 years
	>40	Annually
Breast self-examination	≥20	Monthly
Mammography	35–40	Baseline
	40–50	Every 1–2 years
	>50	Annually

is translated into long-term survival for the woman diagnosed with early-stage breast cancer.

BIOLOGIC CHARACTERISTICS

Anatomy

The breast is a glandular organ, consisting of lobes, ducts, connective tissue, fat, a nipple, and an areola (Fig. 30–1). The entire organ is enclosed by fascia that separates the breast tissue and skin anteriorly and posteriorly by the chest wall muscles. The pectoralis major and minor muscles lie between the breast and rib cage. The axillary lymph nodes are the primary drainage site for the breast, followed by the internal mammary and supraclavicular nodes. The composition of the breast changes with age, primarily because of hormonal influences. Following maturation of the ducts and lobules after menarche, the breast is exposed to hormonal alterations (estrogen and progesterone) with

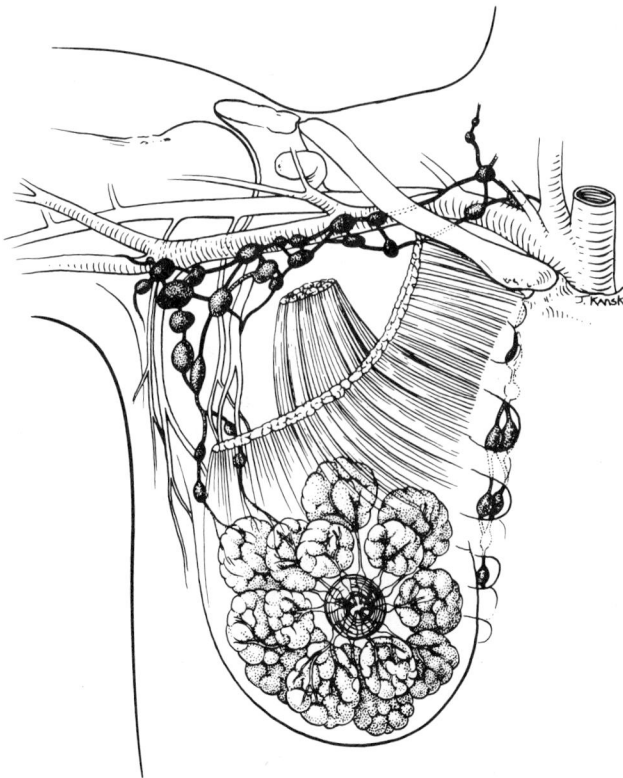

Figure 30–1. Anatomic figure at the breast. This schematic representation of the breast substance shows the lobules in the periphery of the ductal system with the major ducts draining each portion of the periphery. The axillary drainage is primarily in a lateral fashion, first to the low axilla, then to the mid axilla at the lateral aspect of the axillary vein, and then to the apex of the axilla at the point where the axillary vein passes beneath the clavicle and becomes the subclavian vein. The apical axillary nodes then drain to the supraclavicular region. The medial and central aspect of the breast drains to the internal mammary lymph nodes through the pectoral musculature. (From Wilson, R. E. [1984]. Evaluation of a woman with a breast mass. In C. H. Pfeiffer & J. B. Mulliken [Eds.], *Caring for the patient with breast cancer* [p. 24]. Reston, VA: Reston Publishing Company. Reproduced by permission.)

each menstrual cycle. These changes affect the ducts, lobules, and breast tissue, which over time results in an increase in the percentage of fatty tissue.

Pathology

Breast carcinomas arise primarily from epithelial cells, with the origin being either ductal or lobular. These carcinomas are invasive or noninvasive. The term *infiltrating* is synonomous with invasive and the term *in situ* with noninvasive. Invasive ductal carcinoma accounts for 70 to 80 per cent of all breast cancers. Some have specific histologic features, but others do not and are described as not otherwise specified (NOS) (American Joint Committee, 1987). Histologically, there are variants, but the clinical course and treatment approaches are essentially uniform. Lobular carcinomas account for 2 to 3 per cent of all invasive tumors and behave similarly to those of ductal origin.

Historically, the noninvasive carcinomas have represented less than 5 per cent of breast cancer that is diagnosed. However, the incidence of the detection of ductal carcinoma in situ has risen dramatically to 15 to 20 per cent with the widespread use of screening mammography (Schmitt, Silen, Sadowsky, Connolly, & Harris, 1988).

Prognostic Factors

Axillary lymph node status is the single most important prognostic determinant. The pathologic status of the axillary nodes is the most valuable predictor of recurrence and survival. Women with negative-nodes have a 70 to 75 per cent chance of being disease free at 10 years compared with only 20 to 25 per cent of node-positive patients, if no adjuvant therapy is received. The prognosis for node-positive patients worsens as the number of nodes involved increases (Fisher, Slack, Katrych, & Wolmark, 1975; Valagussa, Bonadonna, & Veronessi, 1978).

Hormone receptor content is an important prognostic factor as well and is becoming a more critical element in planning treatment. Hormone receptors are cytoplasmic proteins, which in breast cancer act as receptors for estrogen and progesterone. These receptors are located on either the surface or the interior of the cell. Although the precise mechanism is unknown, once estrogen is bound to the receptor, a series of biologic steps occur that allow a hormonal influence to alter the cell's activity. Patients are considered to be estrogen-receptor (ER) or progesterone-receptor (PR) positive or negative based on the binding capacity. Values are expressed as femtomoles (fmol) of 3H-estradiol bound per milligram of cytosol protein, generally with less than 10 considered negative and more than 10 considered positive. Some values differ slightly, however, and the guidelines from specific laboratories and the method used to determine the ER and PR receptor value must be consulted for reference. Tumors

---

Box 30–1. FACTORS AFFECTING SURVIVAL IN BREAST CANCER

STUDY

Freeman, H., & Wasfie, T. J. (1989). **Cancer of the breast in poor black women.** *Cancer, 63,* 2562–2569.

SAMPLE

708 patients with breast cancer who were diagnosed and treated or followed, or both, at Harlem Hospital Center in New York between 1964 and 1986.

METHOD

Retrospective analysis using the patients' charts, outpatient follow-up records, and tumor registry records.

FINDINGS

The majority of patients were black and of low economic status, and nearly half had no medical coverage. Treatment consisted of surgery for 512 patients (72 per cent) and radiation or chemotherapy or both for 94 patients (13 per cent). One hundred two patients (14 per cent) refused treatment or died before it was initiated. Overall 5- and 10-year survival rates for the surgical patients were 39 per cent and 27 per cent, respectively. These survival figures are low compared with black women nationally and very low compared with white women. The low rates are thought to be associated with the fact that 49 per cent of the patients in this study presented with stages III and IV disease. The investigators conclude that multiple factors associated with a low socioeconomic status may explain the survival disparities between poor Americans and those who are middle class and affluent.

---

that are ER positive are generally hormonally responsive, tend to be more well differentiated, have low proliferative activity, are uncommonly associated with visceral metastases, and indicate a better chance of survival as compared with ER-negative tumors (Clark, Osbourne, & McGuire, 1984; Fisher et al., 1975; Osbourne, 1987).

Progesterone receptor content is a recognized prognostic factor alone, and it adds significantly to the predictive value of ER (Clark et al., 1984; Fisher et al., 1975; Osbourne, 1987). Tumors with high ER content are likely to have high PR content, and that combination constitutes a favorable subset of patients. The quantitative values are directly related to response and length of predicted disease-free survival. Progesterone receptor may be a better marker for hormone reponsiveness. In patients who had sequential biopsies for PR, those who converted from PR positive to PR negative following endocrine therapy had a significantly shorter survival time (Gross, Clark, Chamness, & Maguire, 1984). It is hypothesized that this loss of PR may be related to the emergence of resistant cells lacking PR with the gradual elimination of the hormone-sensitive population (Osbourne, 1987).

Other factors that may influence the prognosis of breast cancer patients include histologic features of the tumor, tumor size, age, weight, race, socioeconomic status, and newer discoveries such as growth factors, cell kinetics, and oncogenes. A major histologic feature correlated with survival has been tumor grade, a simple grading system that estimates tumor differentiation. The majority of studies have shown that poorly differentiated tumors are associated with a shorter disease-free and overall survival period (Dawson, Ferguson, & Karrison, 1982; Freedman, Edwards, McConnell, & Downham, 1979).

Cell kinetics and the DNA content of cells have been the focus of many investigators. Thymidine-labeling index and DNA flow cytometry are methods that determine the proliferative activity, the percentage of cells in S phase, and the DNA content (ploidy status) of the tumor. Patients who have a high thymidine-labeling index and aneuploid tumors (those with altered DNA content) have a higher risk for recurrence, early relapse, and shorter survival time when compared with patients who have low S-phase activity and diploid tumors (Clark & McGuire, 1989; Silvestrini et al., 1986). An important consideration is the number of unfavorable factors for any given patient. The greater the number of poor prognostic features, the worse the prognosis (Box 30–1) (Fisher, Redmond, & Brown, 1986; Rosen, Kinne, Lesser, & Hellman, 1986).

STAGING

Staging classifies patients clinically and pathologically according to the extent of disease. A clinical staging system has been adopted by the American Joint Commission on Cancer Staging and End Results Reporting (Tables 30–3 and 30–4). This TNM system evaluates clinically the extent of cancer according to tumor size (T), axillary lymph node involvement (N), and presence or absence of metastases (M). The staging work-up includes a complete history and physical ex-

Table 30–3. TNM CLASSIFICATION OF BREAST CANCER

T (tumor)	T_0 No evidence of tumor
	T_{1s} In situ carcinoma
	T_1 Tumor is 2 cm or less at greatest dimension
	T_2 Tumor is less than 2 cm but not greater than 5 cm at greatest dimension
	T_3 Tumor is greater than 5 cm at greatest dimension
	T_4 Any size tumor with extension to chest wall or skin
N (nodes)	N_0 No palpable homolateral axillary nodes
	N_1 Movable homolateral axillary nodes
	N_2 Homolateral axillary nodes that are considered to contain cancer and are fixed
	N_3 Homolateral supraclavicular or infraclavicular nodes
M (metastasis)	M_0 No evidence of distant metastases
	M_1 Distant metastases

Table 30–5. INFLUENCE OF NODAL SUBGROUPS ON THE FIVE-YEAR RELAPSE-FREE SURVIVAL

Nodal Group	CTR* %	CMF 12* (1st Study) %	CMF 12* (2nd Study) %	CMF 6* %	CMFP → AV† %
1	57	74	73	71	82
1–3	51	66	70	75	76
>3	32	34	36	51	28
4–10	36	40	40	51	41
>10	11	18	17	50	11

*Premenopause and postmenopause.
†Postmenopause aged 65 years or younger.
CTR, control; CMF, cyclophosphamide, methotrexate, and fluorouracil; CMFP, cyclophosphamide, methotrexate, fluorouracil, and prednisone; AV, doxorubicin (Adriamycin), vincristine.
(From Bonadonna, G., & Valagussa, P. [1985]. Adjuvant systemic therapy for resectable breast cancer. *Journal of Clinical Oncology, 3,* 259–276. Reproduced by permission.)

amination; a hematologic and chemical blood profile; and a chest radiograph, mammogram, and baseline bone scan. Because of the exceedingly small yield and economic factors, liver and spleen scans generally are not recommended.

Clinical staging guides the individual patient and physician in evaluating treatment options and provides data for comparison of therapies and outcomes in various stages of breast cancer. The major limitation of the clinical staging system is the high false-positive and false-negative rates of the clinical examination of the axilla. Because axillary lymph node status is the strongest prognostic factor, pathologic staging, particularly for the patient with locally resectable breast cancer, is required. Pathologic staging is a simple two-stage classification: stage I indicates no axillary lymph node involvement, and stage II indicates nodal involvement. Because the extent of axillary nodal involvement is related to prognosis, stage II may be divided into categories of one to three, four to nine, and more than ten positive nodes, the last category being associated with a poor prognosis, even if adjuvant therapy is administered (Table 30–5).

CLINICAL FEATURES AND DIAGNOSIS

Signs and Symptoms

The most common presenting symptom is a lump or thickening in the breast. More than 90 per cent of lumps are discovered by the woman herself, and only 20 to 25 per cent are malignant in nature. Nipple discharge, nipple retraction, scaly skin around the

Table 30–4. CLINICAL STAGING FOR BREAST CANCER*

Stage	Tumor	Node	Metastasis
I	T_1	N_0	M_0
II	T_2	N_{0-1}	M_0
IIIA	T_3	N_{0-1}	M_0
IIIB	T_{1-3}	N_2	M_0
IV	T_4	any N	M_0
	any T	any N	M_1

*See Table 30–3 for descriptions of T, N, and M values.

nipple, and skin changes (dimpling, "peau d'orange," or inflammation) are less frequently observed and are symptoms that are often associated with a more advanced stage of cancer.

Diagnosis

Once a lump has been detected, a physical examination by a physician is recommended. A cyst, a benign tumor, and a malignant tumor are the possiblities for a palpable breast mass. If a cyst is suspected, needle aspiration may be attempted. If aspiration is successful, the lump will decrease in size significantly or will disappear, and the patient should have a follow-up visit. Ultrasonography, a noninvasive diagnostic test without any radiation exposure, can distinguish between a fluid-filled cystic lump and a solid one. Ultrasonography is a valuable clinical tool that can aid in avoiding an invasive procedure such as a biopsy. In women in the high-risk age group, mammography should also be performed. If a tumor is suspected, a mammogram and a biopsy should be scheduled. Mammography is the superior breast imaging tool; yet false-negative results have been reported as high as 30 per cent. Thus negative findings on a mammogram do not preclude a decision to perform a biopsy on a clinically suspicious mass (Mann et al., 1983).

The incidence of suspicious findings on mammography in asymptomatic women appears to be increasing, perhaps because of numbers of women obtaining mammograms, increasing low-cost mammography, mobile mammography vans that travel to communities, third-party reimbursement practices, and advances in technologic equipment. Mammographic findings that may indicate malignancy include asymmetry, clusters of microcalcifications, spicular masses, and masses with a sunburst appearance (Kopans, Meyer, & Sadowsky, 1984; Martin, 1983; Paulus, 1987).

With a nonpalpable mass and a suspicious mammogram, a needle localization biopsy is indicated. Because this is a collaborative procedure with a radiologist and surgeon, often taking place in two separate environments, patients require information on the specific procedures, duration, time, and predicted outcome (Habegger & Ellerhorst-Ryan, 1988). Approaches to diagnosing a palpable breast mass include fine-needle aspiration, core-needle biopsy, and incisional or excisional biopsies. Fine-needle aspiration of solid breast masses to determine malignancy is a recognized diagnostic procedure in a setting in which physicians have extensive experience and in which pathologic expertise is also available (Bell, Hajdu, Urban, & Gaston, 1983). Cytologic diagnosis cannot distinguish noninvasive from invasive carcinoma; thus if a positive cytologic result is reported, a tissue biopsy is required (Wilson, 1984a). A TruCut needle allows the surgeon to obtain a core of tissue (similiar to a bone marrow biopsy) that is ample for diagnostic examination but may not be sufficient for hormone receptor assays, depending on the method used. This approach, however, is not recommended for small resectable tumors and is generally reserved for patients with large breast masses, for whom treatment options would be limited. Excisional biopsy is recommended whenever possible, particularly for early-stage breast cancer, in which options for treatment are defined. The goal is to remove the entire tumor mass with an area of surrounding normal tissue.

Nursing Practice

Recognizing that only two out of every ten lumps discovered are malignant does not alleviate a woman's fear. Emotional support and education regarding the pending procedures are major nursing concerns. For many women, this may represent a first experience with mammography. A thorough explanation of the test should be given and supplemented by written materials. For invasive procedures, patients must know where to report, which health care professional will be involved, how the procedure will be performed, and how long it will take. They also should be informed about the need for anesthesia, predictable side effects, follow-up care, and when the results will be available. Nurses in ambulatory health care settings as well as hospitals are challenged with meeting patients' educational needs. The contribution of the nurse specialist in providing information and support to this patient population is recognized (Bloom, Ross, & Burnell, 1978; Thompson, 1983). Approaches include providing educational materials, coordinating the various health care team and department members toward a unified approach in delivery, and evaluating the type of care.

Predictable side effects and follow-up care are specific to the type of biopsy performed, the surgeon's technique, and the complexity of the surgical procedure. General guidelines following a breast biopsy include the following: (1) expect mild to moderate discomfort, for which pain relief measures will be prescribed; (2) wear a supportive bra for 24 hours to enhance comfort; (3) avoid strenuous arm activity for the first few days; (4) expect sutures, if present, to be removed in 5 to 7 days and anticipate that the area will be ecchymotic and tender with gradual dissolution (Wiley, 1981). Indentation at the biopsy site will fill in with fat in a month or two, and significant alterations

are rare if incisions follow recommended guidelines according to location of the mass (Fig. 30–2A and B).

Following diagnosis, the nurse continues to provide information and support, expanding the focus to help the patient, spouse, and family process the information to optimize their coping strategies and facilitate decision making (Brody, 1980; McHugh, Christman, & Johnson, 1982; Messerli, Garamedi, & Romano, 1980; Wellisch, Jamison, & Pasnaw, 1978). The decision-making process is a complex phenomenon that is influenced by many variables (Fig. 30–3), and health care providers must give patients and families adequate time to process information, review options, and seek a second opinion, if desired. Nursing assessment and interventions at this stage provide a foundation for rehabilitation that can be communicated to colleagues involved in the patient's care.

PRIMARY TREATMENT

Stages I and II, Early-Stage Breast Cancer

Local Regional Control

The goal of surgery for stages I and II breast cancer is to control local regional disease. Surgical approaches have been modified as new theories of breast cancer have evolved and as radical surgery has failed to alter mortality rates. The theory in the 1900s on which radical surgery was based proposed that breast cancer metastasized in an orderly sequence from the breast to lymph nodes to distant sites. In the last decade, major advances in the understanding of the biology of cancer have occurred. Heterogeneity, genetic instability of cancer cells, tumor burden, and intrinsic drug resistance all support the observation that breast cancer is a systemic disease, which means that micrometastases could be present at the initial presentation with or without nodal involvement (Bonadonna & Valagussa, 1985; Fisher & Gebhart, 1978; Goldie, 1983; Spremulli & Dexter, 1983). Consequently, current efforts focus on achieving optimal local regional control and identifying prognostic factors that discriminate patients likely to harbor micrometastases.

The modified radical mastectomy has been the standard of care since the 1970s. Radical surgery offers no survival advantage over modified approaches, yet it carries a significant psychological morbidity and alterations in body image and function. The modified radical mastectomy is synonymous with total mastectomy and axillary lymph node dissection; it includes removing the breast and lymph nodes and preserving the pectoralis major muscle with or without preservation of the pectoralis minor muscle (Maier, Leber, Rosemond, Goldman, & Tyson, 1977).

Breast-preserving surgery combined with radiotherapy is an alternative approach for women who have small tumors (≤4 cm). This approach involves removing the tumor along with some adjacent normal tissue (referred to as lumpectomy, tylectomy, local excision,

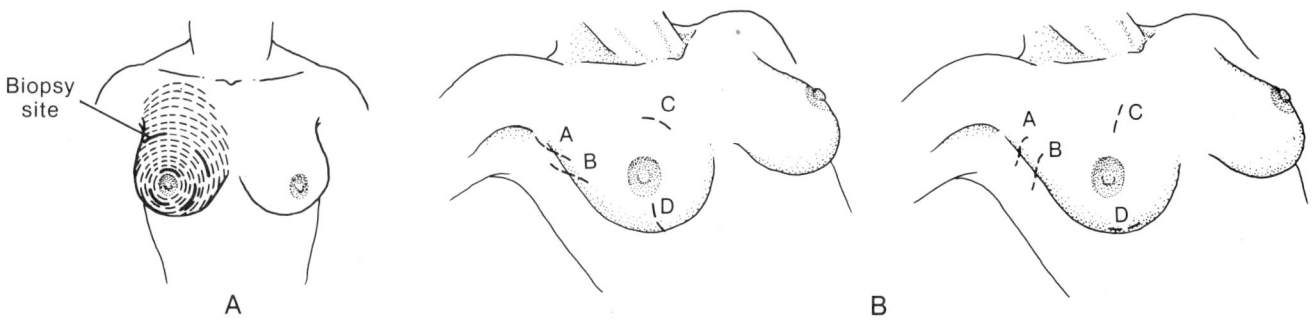

Figure 30–2. Recommended biopsy sites of the breast. *A,* Curvilinear (Langer's) lines, showing ideal incision placement for optimal cosmetic result. *B,* Examples of incision for peripheral malignant lesions. *(Left)* Recommended. *(Right)* Poor. (From Kinne, D. W., & Kopans, D. B. [1987]. Physical examination and mammography in the diagnosis of breast disease. In J. R. Harris, S. Hellman, I. C. Henderson, & D. W. Kinne [Eds.], *Breast diseases,* [pp. 54–85]. Philadelphia: J. B. Lippincott Co. Reproduced by permission.)

partial mastectomy, wide excision, segmental mastectomy, or tumorectomy), axillary node dissection, and radiotherapy for about 6 weeks (Box 30–2). Radiotherapy is delivered to the entire breast and the tumor bed area with external electron beam boost. Iridium implants as a method to provide a boost to the tumor site have declined dramatically in favor of the electron beam (see Chapter 20).

Conservative surgery and irradiation for women with small tumors are equivalent to mastectomy for local control and survival and they preserve the breast (Clark, Wilkinson, Mahoney, Reid, & MacDonald,

1982; Fisher et al., 1985; Veronesi et al., 1981). Considerations for conservative breast surgery and irradiation include the size of the tumor, the existence of more than one foci of tumor, and the extent of microcalcifications on mammographic findings (Recht et al., 1986). For example, a centrally located tumor in a small breast may require removal of a relatively large volume of the total breast tissue and the nipple-areola complex, which would compromise the cosmetic outcome significantly.

The extent of the axillary lymph node dissection is an important issue. These lymph nodes are divided

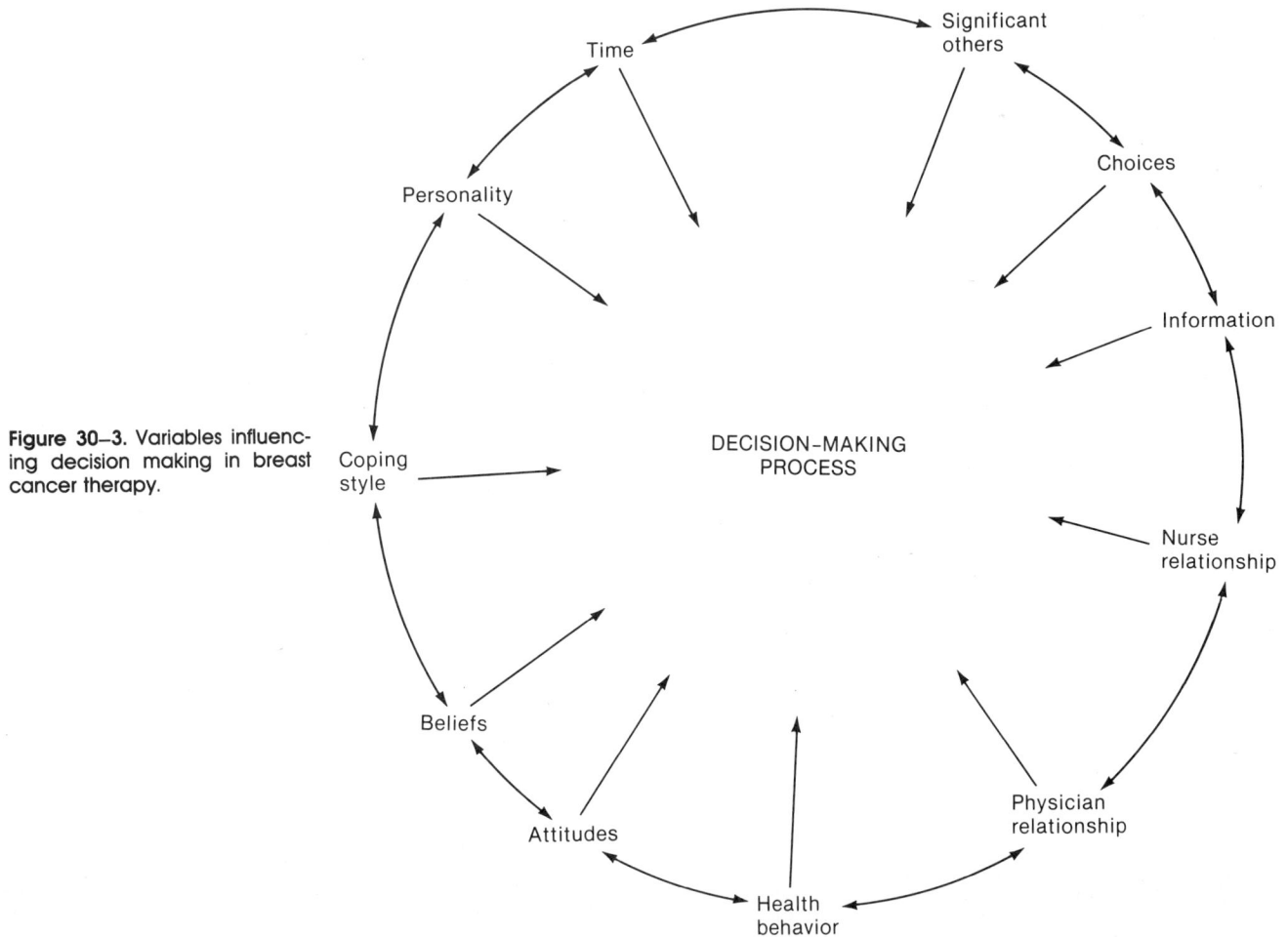

Figure 30–3. Variables influencing decision making in breast cancer therapy.

Box 30–2. PRIMARY THERAPY FOR BREAST CANCER

STUDY

Fisher, B., Redmond, C., Poisson, R., Margolese, R., Wolmark, N., Wickerham, L., Fisher, E., Deutsch, M., Caplan, R., Pilch, Y., Glass, A., Shibata, H., Lerner, H., Terz, S., & Sidorovich, L. (1989). **Eight-year results of a randomized clinical trial comparing total mastectomy and lumpectomy with or without irradiation in the treatment of breast cancer.** *New England Journal of Medicine, 320,* 822–828.

SAMPLE

1855 women with stage I or II breast cancer randomized to groups of total mastectomy (n = 590), lumpectomy (n = 636), or lumpectomy and irradiation (n = 629).

FINDINGS

No significant differences were found in the rates of disease-free, distant-disease-free, and overall survival among the three treatment groups. However, there was a significantly greater increase in the incidence of ipsilateral breast recurrences for women who underwent only lumpectomy when compared with those who had lumpectomy followed by irradiation. The investigators conclude that these data continue to support breast conservation approaches in the treatment of stages I and II breast cancer but note that irradiation reduces the local tumor recurrence risk in patients treated with lumpectomy.

---

into three levels (Fig. 30–4). Level I is tissue between the latissimus dorsi muscle and the lateral border of the pectoralis minor muscle; level II is tissue from the lateral border of the latissimus dorsi to the lateral and medial borders of the pectoralis minor muscle, with clearing of the axillary vein; and level III is tissue between the medial border of the pectoralis minor and Halsted's ligament (Danforth et al., 1986; Kinne, 1987b).

Excision of the axillary contents from levels I and II is recommended to achieve adequate nodal dissection for prognostic information and local disease control (Danforth et al., 1986; Fisher & Wolmark, 1986). Several researchers recommend a full axillary dissec-

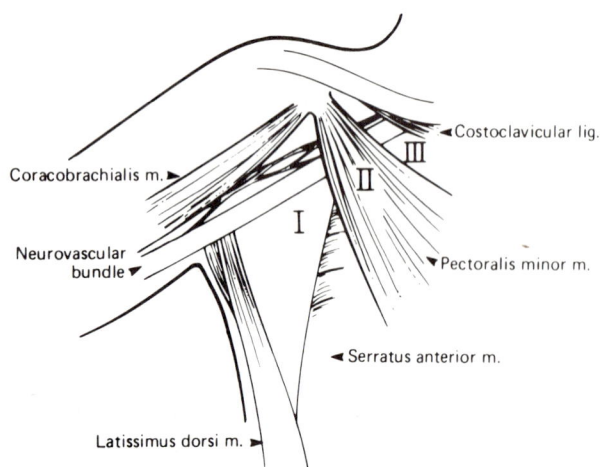

Figure 30–4. Levels of axillary lymph nodes. (From deMoss, E. et al. [1983]. Complete axillary lymph node dissection before radiotherapy for primary breast cancer. In J. R. Harris, S. Hellman, & W. Silen [Eds.], *Conservative management of breast cancer* [p. 166]. New York: J. B. Lippincott Co. Reproduced by permission.)

tion (levels I to III) to check patients with clinically suspicious nodes and to investigate the possibility of "skipped" metastases, that is, level I nodes testing negative but level II or III nodes testing positive for tumor. The incidence of level III nodes testing positive when lower level nodes test negative is very small. Axillary sampling is a vague, imprecise term that does not define boundaries and should not be used (Fisher & Wolmark, 1986; Kinne, 1987b).

Nursing Practice

The goal of nursing care is to promote physical and psychological recovery. It is important to note that physical and psychological responses are similar in all women regardless of choice of mastectomy or conservative surgery with radiotherapy. Ganz and colleagues (1987) investigated 50 women with breast cancer during the first month after primary treatment and confirmed these clinical observations (Figs. 30–5 and 30–6).

The postoperative period should focus on meeting basic needs (Table 30–6), and because hospital stays today rarely exceed 5 days, and more often average 2 to 4 days, written information to supplement verbal teaching is strongly recommended. Discharge instructions can facilitate self-care at home and have the potential to decrease anxiety levels (Table 30–7). Communication among the surgeon, inpatient nurses, ambulatory care nurses, and other involved health care providers is essential to the patient's rehabilitation. The nurse in the ambulatory care setting has the unique opportunity to coordinate and evaluate the patient's rehabilitation from diagnosis through long-term follow-up.

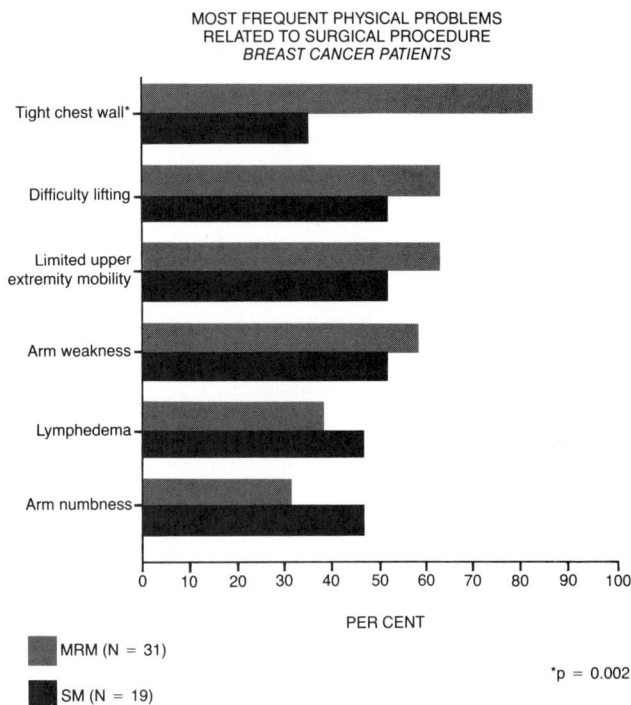

MOST FREQUENT PHYSICAL PROBLEMS
RELATED TO SURGICAL PROCEDURE
BREAST CANCER PATIENTS

MRM (N = 31)

SM (N = 19)

*p = 0.002

Figure 30–5. Frequent physical problems related to surgical procedure in women with breast cancer who have had mastectomy or segmental mastectomy with axillary node dissection. MRM = modified radical mastectomy; SM = segmental mastectomy. (From Ganz, P. A., Schag, C. C., Polinsky, M. L., Heinric, R. L., and Flack, V. [1987]. Rehabilitation needs and breast cancer: The first month after primary therapy. *Breast Cancer Research and Treatment, 10,* 243–253. Reproduced by permission.)

Complications of Breast Surgery

The majority of complications associated with a modified radical mastectomy are related to the axillary lymph node dissection, which is the longest and technically the most difficult part of the surgical procedure. Problems specific to breast removal are integrated into the discussion of sequelae following axillary lymph node dissection. Seroma, hematoma, infection, nerve injury, muscle atrophy, arm swelling, and impaired shoulder function are potential complications of dissecting the axillary nodes. Seroma is a fluid accumulation in the operative site with an observed incidence of 4.2 to 32 per cent (Aitken & Minton, 1983; Lotze, Duncan, Gerber, Woltering, & Rosenberg, 1981; Martinez & Clarke, 1984; Say & Donegan, 1974). Major preventive strategies are the placement of continuous closed suction drains and the suturing of skin flaps to deep structures (Aitken & Minton, 1983). Initiation of early range of motion exercises (postoperative day 1) has been shown to increase the amount and duration of drainage. Delay of 7 to 10 days for initiation of physical rehabilitative exercises did not alter range of motion function when evaluated at 3 and 6 months, and therefore it is recommended that active motion exercises be delayed for at least 1 week (Lotze et al., 1981).

The guideline for removal of closed continuous suction drains is based on amount of drainage, generally 25 to 30 ml per 24 hours (Aitken & Minton, 1983; Lotze et al., 1981). Drainage from the chest wall tubes

subsides rather soon, but axillary drainage may persist for 7 to 14 days. In a clinical analysis of 88 patients with breast cancer who had axillary dissection with or without breast removal, drains remained in place for an average of 10.7 days (McKhann & Knobf, 1986). Seromas occurred in 15 per cent of patients regardless of the average number of days the drain had been in place, the preceding 24-hour drainage, the number of nodes removed at surgery, and the surgical techniques. Treatment of seroma is aspiration, and if fluid accumulation persists after several taps, placement of a Penrose drain and prescription of a course of antibiotics is recommended.

Sensory changes secondary to trauma to the nerves or transection of the nerves occur in patients with axillary dissection and mastectomy. Although surgeons attempt to keep as many nerves intact as possible, trauma may result in muscular atrophy and sensory changes (Table 30–8). The subjective complaints include numbness, weakness, increased skin sensitivity, itching, heaviness, "pins and needles," and phantom breast sensations, all of which may change in character and persist for up to 1 year (Lierman, 1988; Nail, Jones, Guiffre, & Johnson, 1984). Once initial recovery is achieved from surgery, sensory changes are the most frequent chronic complaint of patients for the first year and sometimes longer. Patients need continual reassurance and confirmation that the recovery process is gradual, although for some, full sensation to the area may not return.

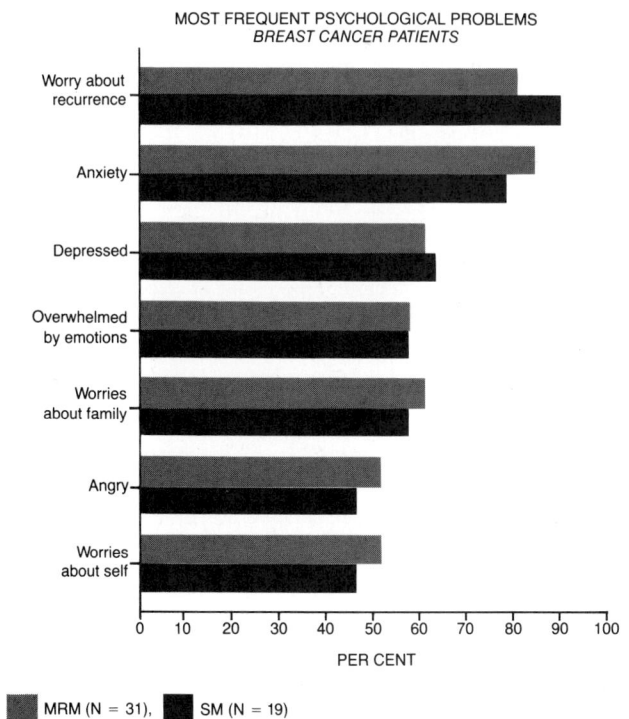

MOST FREQUENT PSYCHOLOGICAL PROBLEMS
BREAST CANCER PATIENTS

MRM (N = 31), SM (N = 19)

Figure 30–6. Frequent psychological problems in women with breast cancer who have had mastectomy or segmental mastectomy and axillary dissection. MRM = modified radical mastectomy; SM = segmental mastectomy. (From Ganz, P. A., Schag, C. C., Polinsky, M. L., Heinric, R. L., and Flack, V. [1987]. Rehabilitation needs and breast cancer: The first month after primary therapy. *Breast Cancer Research and Treatment, 10,* 243–253. Reproduced by permission.)

Table 30–6. NURSING CARE FOR THE WOMAN WITH BREAST CANCER

Patient with Axillary Node Dissection

Physical

Begin exercises 24 hr after surgery. Demonstrate limited exercises involving the hand, wrist, and elbow such as squeezing a ball, flexing fingers, touching hand to shoulder, and circular wrist motions.

Communicate with the surgeon about further exercise, considering factors of wound healing, status of suture line, and drainage. Identify the time to begin further exercise, usually about 1 week later or after the drains and sutures are removed.

Demonstrate range of motion exercises for upper extremity and shoulder. Encourage normal (preoperative) use of arm following drain removal.

Stress the importance of continuing range of motion exercises of arm and shoulder on a daily basis for at least the first 6 months. Suggest arm elevation for at least 30 min at a time if inactivity is prolonged.

Discuss the potential complications of infection and edema.

Review with the patient methods of preventing infection:

Avoid breaks in the skin (wear gloves when gardening, thimble when sewing, electric razor for shaving axilla; avoid trauma to cuticles and injections in that arm).

If a break in the skin occurs, wash with soap and water and cover. Call the physician for any signs of warmth, swelling, or redness in the area.

Avoid constriction of circulation in that arm such as tight sleeves, snug fitting wrist jewelry, or carrying very heavy objects for prolonged periods of time. Strenuous exercise or use of the arm should be interrupted at 20-min intervals.

Avoid burns. Suggest tanning gradually in the sun and use of sun screens; use of oven mitts to prevent stove burns.

Discuss initial care of the axilla such as avoiding depilatory creams, strong deodorants, and shaving under the arm. Advise the patient to check with the nurse and physician at follow-up visits for guidelines on when it is safe to resume shaving the axilla and using deodorants.

Identify when the sutures will be removed.

Discuss with the patient that numbness around the incision and arm is common. Describe changes in sensation in arm and axilla over time and explain why this happens.

Early Detection

Discuss with the patient the importance of breast self-examination. Identify the pamphlet in the volunteer visitation packet or provide a similar brochure.

Psychosocial

Diagnosis of cancer/extent of disease

Allow the patient to verbalize her feelings about the diagnosis, fears, and concerns.

Incorporate the spouse or significant other in care and communication as much as possible.

Discuss with the physician the pathology of the axillary nodes.

Identify when the patient may be expected to learn the results.

Identify the patient's perception and significance of the pathology of the axillary nodes.

If axillary lymph nodes are involved with cancer, identify the physician's plan for additional therapy. Assess the patient's response and need for support and information.

Suggest readings for the patient from the popular lay press on cancer and breast cancer.

For patients who will receive irradiation, provide information on therapy.

Volunteer visitation programs

Identify what types of volunteer visitation programs are available through your institution or local American Cancer Society for women with breast cancer.

Discuss the opportunity to have a volunteer visit with the patient. If desired, make the referral as soon as possible since hospital stays are relatively short today. (Acquire a physician's order if required in your institution.)

Discuss the volunteer visit with the patient later. Review the exercises, hand/arm care, and information in the kit. Clarify any misconceptions.

Sexual Relationship

Identify that sexual relationship, specifically intercourse, may be resumed at any time, as desired.

Postmastectomy Patient

Physical

Discuss with the patient that slight redness around the surgical site sutures and some tightness and swelling in the area are normal.

If dressings over the incision are still required, discuss how often they should be changed, the procedure, and what supplies are to be used.

Describe the healing process over time.

If discomfort remains, identify where it exists and the degree. Describe relief measures such as pain medication and relaxation techniques.

Cosmesis

Demonstrate the use of the temporary prosthesis and bra extender (if the patient has received a kit from a Reach to Recovery volunteer). Explain the "lightness" of the temporary prosthesis and need to secure well in her bra. Assure the patient that this will not be a problem with the heavier permanent form.

Discuss with the patient that it is best to wait a few weeks to be fitted for a permanent breast form. This will allow resolution of any postoperative swelling and incisional healing.

Assure the patient that very few to no changes will be needed in her present wardrobe.

Assess the patient's need for any further information about reconstructive breast surgery.

Psychosocial

Discuss the mastectomy with the patient. Encourage the patient to express her feelings and concerns about the loss of the breast, the incision, and relationship with spouse or significant other.

Identify with the patient sources of support for her over the next few months, such as spouse, family, friends, clergy.

Sexual Relationships

Discuss with the patient that initially a soft pillow or the temporary prosthesis in a comfortable bra may provide padding to alleviate any fear of discomfort during sexual relations and to avoid confrontation of the surgical area.

(From Knobf, M. T. [1985]. Primary breast cancer: Physical consequences and rehabilitation. *Seminars in Oncology Nursing 1,* 214–224. Reproduced by permission.)

Table 30–7. PATIENT DISCHARGE INSTRUCTIONS
FOLLOWING BREAST CANCER SURGERY

Dressings

Incision

There will be a dry gauze dressing over the incision when you
leave the hospital. It is not necessary to change this dressing
until you return to see the doctor.

Drain site

A small dry dressing will be around the site where the drain is
placed. Often there is some leakage of fluid around the drain.
Check the gauze dressing for drainage and change if soiled.
Some leakage is normal, but if the dressing becomes soaked
more than once a day, call your doctor.

Drains

Your nurse has shown you how to empty the reservoir from your
drain and how to measure the volume of drainage. You should
empty the drain twice a day and record the measurements.

Drains are generally removed when drainage is about 30 ml in 24
hr.

Drains are often removed at the same time as the stitches,
generally 7 to 10 days after surgery.

Bathing

Sponge baths or tub baths, making certain that the area of the
drain and incision stay dry, are permitted. You may shower after
the stitches and drains are removed.

Hand and Arm Care

You can begin using your arm for normal activities such as eating
or combing your hair. Exercises involving the wrist, hand, and
elbow such as flexing your fingers, circular wrist motions, and
touching hand to shoulder are very good. More strenuous
exercises can usually be resumed after the drains have been
removed.

Comfort

Some discomfort or mild pain is expected following surgery, but
within 4 to 5 days, most women have no need for medication or
require something only at bedtime.

Numbness in the area of the surgery and along the inner side of
the arm from the armpit to the elbow occurs in virtually all
patients. It is a result of injury to the nerves that provide
sensation to the skin in those areas. Women have described
sensations such as heaviness, pain, tingling, burning, and "pins
and needles." These sensations change over the months and
usually resolve by 1 year.

Support and Information

Pamphlets on exercises, hand and arm care, and general facts
about breast cancer are available from your nurse or volunteer
visitor. The American Cancer Society has volunteers who have
had surgery similar to yours and are available to visit you.

Lymphedema has been reported in 6.7 to 70 per
cent of patients, occurring as early as 2 months after
surgery and up to 15 to 20 years later (Aitken &
Minton, 1983; Markowski, Wilcox, & Helm, 1981;
Stillwell, 1969; Treves, 1957). The major risk factor is
removal of the axillary lymph nodes. If no further
aggravating factors are present, such as infection,
trauma, or radiation, and if sufficient collateral pathways develop, adequate lymphatic drainage will be
maintained. But the patient *always* remains at risk
because of the surgical interruption of the lymph
vessels.

To determine if any statsis is present, the arm is
measured 5 to 10 cm above and below the olecranon
process and compared with the opposite side (Aitken
& Minton, 1983; Markowski et al., 1981). Lymphedema is defined as the difference between one extremity and its opposite of 1.0 to 1.5 cm; it is categorized

as mild if the difference is 3 cm, moderate if it is 3.0
to 5.0 cm, and severe if it is greater than 5 cm. Mild
lymphedema may not be observed clinically, yet it is a
warning sign for increased risk. Patients should be
asked if they notice a difference between the two
extremities (fit of clothes, heaviness), and measurements should be taken periodically and documented in
the record. Once lymphedema occurs, management is
aimed at prevention of further lymph accumulation.
Elevation, mild exercise, massage, salt restriction,
avoidance of local heat and trauma, and elastic support
are basic interventions. A patient should be measured
for an elastic support sleeve when the swelling is at a
minimal level and should be reevaluated every 2 to 3
months for a replacement (Zeissler, Rose, & Nelson,
1972). For moderate to severe lymphedema, an intermittent compression sleeve may be indicated. One of
the newer products (Lympha Press) is designed with
overlapping cells and shorter cycle times (Zelikowski,
Manoach, Giler, & Urca, 1980). Patients must have
realistic expectations of the amount of benefit from
such an intervention, and they may require ongoing
support to cope with this chronic problem.

Complications of Radiotherapy

Fatigue, breast edema, skin reactions, and breast
tenderness are symptoms that are frequently associated
with breast irradiation, whereas hyperpigmentation,
fibrosis, rib fractures, pneumonitis, arm edema, and
myositis are uncommonly observed (Clark et al., 1982;
Clarke, Martinez, & Cox, 1983; Harris & Hellman,
1983; Montague, 1984). Two sets of investigators attempted to refine this database through the initiation
of patient questionnaires. Patients were queried retrospectively about their symptoms, and they reported
breast soreness (65 to 82 per cent), breast tenderness
(50 per cent), arm swelling (53 per cent), pain (75 per
cent), fatigue (82 per cent), and ipsilateral arm numbness (41 per cent) (Schain et al., 1983; Shannon-Bodner
& Flynn, 1987). Trying to discriminate accurately
which symptoms are secondary to irradiation and which

Table 30–8. NERVES INVOLVED IN BREAST
CANCER SURGERY

Nerve	Innervation	Potential Injury
Intercostobrachial	Axilla/upper arm	Numbness in axilla and upper arm and diminished sweat production
Anterior thoracic—medial	Lower half of pectoralis major Pectoralis minor	Muscle atrophy
Anterior thoracic—lateral	Upper half of pectoralis major	Muscle atrophy
Posterior thoracic	Serratus anterior	Increased prominence of scapula tip ("winged scapula deformity")
Thoracodorsal	Lattissimus dorsi	Weakness in adduction and internal rotation

(From Knobf, M. T. [1985]. Primary breast cancer: Physical
consequences and rehabilitation. *Seminars in Oncology Nursing, 1,*
214–224. Reproduced by permission.)

to surgery is challenging and often impossible; to the patient, it is irrelevant. Teeple (1987) conducted the first prospective study that attempted to determine the onset, duration, frequency, and severity of symptoms during treatment using the Symptom Profile Tool, adapted from King and colleagues (1985).

Skin changes, fatigue, sleep disturbance, sore throat, eructation, changes in breast sensations, and alterations in daily activity were reported. Descriptions of skin changes included increased itching, tenderness, swelling, redness, dryness, and temperature that was uncomfortably hot. These changes were experienced universally by the end of the third week of treatment. Eructation was a newly identified symptom occurring in virtually all patients at the onset of treatment, but it persisted in only 38 per cent by the fifth and sixth weeks. Changes in breast sensations were experienced by 75 per cent of subjects and were described as "electric shock-like sensations" that lasted only moments but occurred throughout the day and night. The major limitation of this study is its small sample size of 8 subjects, yet it suggests that our current database of preparatory information (Table 30–9) may require

further study and incorporation of patient subjective responses over time.

Breast Reconstruction

Removal of the breast is a significant loss, and the impact on body image and adjustment is well documented. The cosmetic benefit for women who receive breast-preserving surgery and irradiation is a more intact body image. Compared with mastectomy patients, irradiated patients have fewer negative feelings about themselves nude, resume sexual relations earlier, and experience less change in body satisfaction (Beckman, Johansen, Richardt, & Blichert-Toft, 1983; Sanger & Reznikoff, 1981; Schain et al., 1983).

Having a choice of therapy appears to have a positive influence on satisfaction, coping, and outcome (Leinster, Ashcroft, Slade, & Dewey, 1989; Morris & Ingham, 1988). Two variables of age and concern about appearance, however, may be important to consider before surgery is done. When patients were offered a choice, younger age and greater concern for physical

---

Table 30–9. PATIENT GUIDELINES FOR BREAST IRRADIATION

General Information
- There will be several persons involved in your care: physician, nurse, technologist, physicist, and receptionist. You will see your doctor and nurse once a week. If you have questions or a problem arises, notify them sooner.
- The schedule is daily visits Monday through Friday for about 6 weeks. Appointments can be made to accommodate your work schedule or other activities.

Treatments
- The first visit will include special x-rays (called simulation) of the chest area. Your skin will be marked to outline the treatment area. A common way to mark is with Castaderm, a purple indelible ink. It is important that these marks are not removed during the treatment course.
- The treatments are invisible, silent, painless, and have no odor. Machines may make a whirring or clicking sound, which is normal.
- You will be alone in the room during the actual treatment, which may vary from 1 to 3 min. The entire procedure may take longer if positioning is required by the staff. You will be monitored constantly even while you are alone in the room.
- There are three to five areas that may receive treatment. These areas, also called fields include different sides of the breast, around the collarbone, center of the chest, and under the arm.
- The usual position is with your hand behind your head. This may cause slight discomfort during your first few treatments due to your surgery. To ease the discomfort, continue your arm exercises, and if necessary take medication 1 hr before treatment.

Possible Reactions and Care Measures
- Side effects are usually minimal and do not appear until the second or third week of treatment. The most common are feeling tired and skin changes. Report any changes to your nurse and doctor.
- If you feel tired, you may find it helpful to plan an afternoon nap or an early bedtime.
- You may be more comfortable during treatment if you wear a loose-fitting bra.
- It is best to avoid perfumes, soaps, or any other such substances on the area being treated.
- You may shower, but use warm water. Be careful not to remove the markings if Castaderm was used (wash but do not use soap and scrub the area; rinse and gently pat dry).
- Your breast may become swollen, and the area around your incision may become firm. These are expected reactions and will subside over time.
- Wearing soft, light clothing may help reduce irritation of your skin. A cotton T-shirt may be more comfortable than a bra and very helpful to protect your clothing from the Castaderm markings.
- Your skin may become pink, swollen, dry, or itchy during the second or third week of treatment. Report these changes to your nurse. A cream or light sprinkling of cornstarch on the area may help the itching. Lotions that are gentle and soothing include Nivea, Eucerin, Aquaphor, and Lubriderm.
- Occasionally, the skin may blister. Report this to your nurse or physician so that he or she can monitor you and suggest the best treatment. Skin changes will generally go away within 1 to 3 weeks.
- If the area under your arm is treated, the hair and sweat glands will likely be affected. This means that hair may not regrow there, and you may not perspire. This may be for a short time or may last for long periods of time.
- To avoid further skin irritation, cover the treated area when you go into the sun. Also, avoid heating pads, hot water bottles, or ice packs to the area.
- Your skin may appear tan after the treatment is completed and remain that way for some time. Your skin may also be somewhat more sensitive for a short time. Remember, we are only talking about the skin in the areas being treated. Care for the rest of your body and skin in your usual way.

(Data from Heery, M. [1984]. Unpublished patient teaching pamphlet, (Yale University School of Nursing.)

appearance correlated with choosing radiation over mastectomy when mastectomy was offered as the only viable option; and immediate reconstruction was chosen over no reconstruction or a delayed procedure.

The nurse should explore with the patient her feelings about the loss, her relationship with her partner, when appropriate, and her adaptation to the prosthesis or reconstructed breast. For women who do not choose immediate reconstruction, a temporary prosthesis should be provided. The American Cancer Society's Reach to Recovery volunteer visitor program can provide a temporary breast form and suggest sources for purchase of a permanent form. A variety of permanent breast forms are available (Table 30–10). Evaluation, usage, and satisfaction with the breast form must be integrated into follow-up care.

Breast reconstruction is the alternative to achieve symmetry and preserve body image. Reconstructive surgery creates a breast mound. The most common procedures are implantation of a silicone prosthesis or placement of a tissue expander under the pectoralis muscle. Generally, a 1- to 3-day hospital admission is required for either implant procedure.

Historically, tissue expanders were an option for women with an inadequate amount of skin and soft tissue. Today physician preference, experience, and ability to evaluate symmetry as the process takes place may be additional factors influencing this choice. Like the permanent implant, the tissue expander can be placed at the time of mastectomy or any time thereafter. The tissue expander is initially filled with 75 to 200 ml of normal saline; in 2 to 6 weeks after surgery, it is injected with varying amounts of normal saline (30 to 200 ml) every 1 to 3 weeks (D'Angelo & Gorrell, 1989). Expansion continues until it slightly exceeds cosmetic symmetry to optimize tissue stretch and to prepare for placement of a permanent prosthesis.

Other reconstructive procedures include the latissimus dorsi flap or the transverse rectus abdominis flap, which use autologous tissue and skin (Dinner & Dowden, 1984; Hutcheson, 1986; Snyderman, 1983). These procedures require more extensive surgery and longer hospitalization and recovery time yet can achieve a more natural symmetry and can provide an option to the patient who is not a candidate for implant reconstruction.

The goal of breast reconstruction to achieve symmetry and replicate the normal contour of a breast has not yet been perfected, particularly for women who are 40 to 60 years of age. To optimize symmetry, surgery on the opposite breast is often considered, such as mastopexy for a sagging breast, reduction

Table 30–10. TYPES OF PERMANENT BREAST PROSTHESES AVAILABLE

Brands and Types of Prostheses	Main Characteristics	Major Advantages and Disadvantages
Amoena brands	Silicone gel with a smooth, shiny covering and side wings.	Made for left and right breasts; secures to chest wall and bra forms; has air vents that ensure ventilation; has a concave back that decreases skin friction; must be warmed before placement.
Comfort 2000	Similar to the Amoena brand but has a flat back; worn in a bra with a specially designed pocket.	May cause scar irritation.
Cameo natural breast prosthesis	Made of organic material called Kunsleakahout, which is also used for creating artificial veins and skin; is worn directly on the skin; has 3 small air holes for ventilation; has nipple on form.	Not filled with liquid or silicone so there is no danger of leaking or shrinking; hygienic and odorless; chlorine- and salt-waterproof; made in left and right breast forms; warms quickly and remains at room temperature.
Nearlyme	Has side tapers that fill in the hollow under the arm and top tapers too that help fit the form closer to the chest wall (especially important for those who have undergone a radical mastectomy); must be worn in bra and may need to use a breast form cover for comfort; made of nonstick polyurethane filled with silicone; no nipple on form.	Designs for both radical and modified radical mastectomies are available; has left and right breast forms; may be worn in chlorinated or salt water or in sauna.
Cherish II	Soft, mobile silicone gel encased in a smooth silicone elastomer skin; has a base seam to ensure dimensional stability; no need for a breast form cover in most cases; has nipple on breast form.	One breast form only; has graduated weights.
Trulife	Has foam and liquid breast forms; has nipple on form; must be worn with cotton covers for comfort; oil-filled prosthesis has sponge back.	No seams to irritate skin; has only one breast form; oil-filled form is the least expensive, but it does not last as long as the form model.
Carefree	Silicone gel prosthesis with a Silastic rubber skin; available in pink or brown.	Does not breathe well; less preformed; one breast form available.
Custom breast prosthetics	Customized prosthesis using a preoperative impression; made with silicone.	Costs $600.

(From Keohan, S. M. [1987]. Patient rehabilitation nursing. In J. R. Harris, S. Hellman, I. C. Henderson, & D. W. Kinne [Eds.], *Breast diseases* [pp. 656–668]. Philadelphia: J. B. Lippincott Co. Reproduced by permission.)

mammoplasty for a very large breast, or augmentation mammoplasty for a small contralateral breast. Nipple and areola reconstructions are options that often can be performed in 1-day surgery centers.

Although reconstruction is technically feasible today for almost any patient, the patient's expectations and stage of disease and the timing and type of procedure are factors that are weighed carefully before a decision is made. Consideration for reconstructive surgery begins with a physical and psychosocial assessment, a description of the procedure and potential complications, and a discussion about the expectations of cosmetic improvement. Controversy persists about stage of disease and timing of the procedure (immediate versus delayed), although opinions appear to be based largely on clinical judgement and personal preference rather than on hard data (Frazier & Noone, 1985). Complications of breast reconstruction include hematoma, infection, delayed wound healing, and capsular contractions (if an implant was used).

Teaching should begin before the operation and should be reinforced with written guidelines when the patient is discharged. Implant reconstruction is the most common practice, and general guidelines for care at home include restrictions on bathing and daily activities, comfort measures, drainage, incisional care, and massage exercises (Table 30–11).

Stage III, Locally Advanced Breast Cancer

Ten to 30 per cent of breast cancer patients present with locally advanced stage III disease, which includes tumors that can be defined as operable ($T_3 N_{0-1} M_0$) or inoperable ($T_4 N_{2-3} M_0$). Stage III disease is associated with a high incidence of local and distant recurrence and a poor 5-year survival rate. Surgery, radiation therapy, and chemotherapy have been used alone and in combination, but the most appropriate therapy or combination of therapies remains controversial. For operable stage III disease, surgery with or without radiation or high-dose radiation alone may be recommended.

Although local control rates have improved with this approach, prognosis is poor because of the incidence of distant metastases. Combination chemotherapy or chemohormonal therapy followed by mastectomy with or without radiation appears to improve the local control rate and may influence disease-free and overall survival rates (Cardenas et al., 1987; Lippman et al., 1986; Sheldon, Parker, & Cady, 1987; Wilson, 1984b). Clinical trials with autologous bone marrow transplantation are in progress and may have a role in breast cancer therapy in advanced stages of disease and for patients at high risk for recurrence (Antman & Gale, 1988) (see Chapter 27).

Noninvasive Breast Cancer

Intraductal or ductal carcinoma in situ (DCIS) previously was observed in 0.8 to 5.0 per cent of all breast cancers, typically as palpable lesions. Its incidence has risen to 15 to 20 per cent of all women who undergo screening mammography. The lesions in DCIS are usually small and nonpalpable. Intraductal carcinoma in situ is characterized by multicentricity but is restricted primarily to the ipsilateral breast (Betskill, Rosen, & Lieberman, 1978; Carter & Smith, 1977). In one study evaluating mastectomy specimens of women who had a positive biopsy result for DCIS, the incidence of multicentricity in the remaining breast was 66 per cent (Carter & Smith, 1977); occult invasive cancers have been observed in 6 to 21 per cent of specimens (Carter & Smith, 1977; Lagios, Westdahl, Margolini, & Rose, 1982). It is estimated that up to 40 per cent of patients treated with excision alone for DCIS will develop an invasive carcinoma over a latent 10-year period (Betskill et al., 1978; Page, Dupont, Rogers, & Landenberger, 1982). These data and those from pathologic studies of mastectomy specimens suggest that excision alone is insufficient for most patients. One exception may be the patient who has a very small tumor (≤ 2 mm) that was detected by mammography, has breasts that are easily examined clinically, is informed of the risk, and has no other risk factors (Lagios et al., 1982).

Mammographic findings of clusters of microcalcifications or soft tissue densities have been reported in approximately 40 per cent of patients, often in asymptomatic patients who had negative results in clinical examinations. This finding confirms that less than half of the lesions are detectable on radiographs. Mastectomy was promoted for decades as the treatment of choice, but wide excision and radiation is an alternative for some patients (Findlay & Goodman, 1983; Montague, 1984; Recht et al., 1986). Axillary lymph node metastases are uncommon, and therefore axillary dissection is generally not indicated. One exception may be women with extensive DCIS, in whom the likelihood of positive nodes may be increased.

Lobular carcinoma in situ (LCIS) occurs in younger women and is characterized by multicentricity and a generally less aggressive natural history and better survival rates (Carter & Smith, 1977; Fryberg, Santiago, Betskill, & O'Brien, 1987; Rosen, 1987). The risk of developing an invasive cancer occurs in a minority of patients but not until 15 or more years have passed. Lobular carcinoma in situ is almost always an incidental finding on a pathology report and is often undetected by mammography (Senofsky et al., 1986). Pathologic interpretation and clinical applicability are controversial. Fryberg and colleagues (1987) present an excellent review. Treatment is equally controversial. With bilateral mastectomy, the cure rate is 100 per cent, but this solution is perceived as overtreatment by many. Other options include ipsilateral mastectomy with contralateral mirror image biopsy or wide local excision with or without contralateral biopsy and close follow-up. More recently, support has increased for the conservative approach because of the natural history and the good prognosis if subsequent disease develops and is detected early.

The incidence of in situ carcinomas restricts the

Table 30–11. DISCHARGE GUIDELINES FOR PATIENTS WITH IMPLANT BREAST RECONSTRUCTION

Incision

A small gauze dressing over the incision should be changed once a day. Small amounts of clear odorless fluid or slightly blood-tinged drainage is common. Sutures, if present, will be removed 1 to 2 weeks after surgery by your physician.

Drains

Drainage tubes may be present if your reconstruction was performed at the same time as your mastectomy.

Bathing

Sponge baths or tub baths are permitted, keeping the incision dry. Once the sutures are removed, showers are permitted, and the incisional area should be washed gently. Once the incision begins healing, application of vitamin E oil or cream, cocoa butter, or aloe-based cream will moisturize the area and may enhance the healing process.

Comfort

Because the surgery involves operating on muscle, there will be some pain and discomfort. You will be given a pain medication to take at home that will keep you comfortable.

Daily Activities

General household activities and mild exercise, such as walking, are permitted. Strenuous exercise, heavy lifting, and extreme stretching should be avoided for 4 to 6 weeks to allow time for the muscle over the implant to heal. Driving a car may be resumed in 1 to 2 weeks. When in a car, the seat belt should always be worn to protect the reconstructed breast in case of an abrupt stop. Sexual relations can be resumed after you leave the hospital. However, avoid heavy pressure on the reconstructed breast for 4 to 6 weeks, which includes not sleeping on your stomach.

Return to Work

The type of job you have dictates when you can return to work. If no strenuous activity is required, you may return as early as 1 week after surgery. But as with the exercise restriction, it is recommended to wait 4 to 6 weeks if your job involves heavy physical activity.

Care of the Reconstructed Breast

Bra

Immediate reconstruction: Delay wearing a bra for several weeks to optimize blood supply to the muscle and skin. A very soft, stretchy bra with no wires could be worn if needed for a special occasion.

Delayed reconstruction: Begin wearing a bra immediately and for 24 hours a day for 2 weeks. The bra should be slightly supportive without seams.

Sun

Use a number 15 sunscreen if you are exposed to the sun. The blood supply of the skin over the implant has been interrupted by surgery and may be more vulnerable to sun exposure and burning.

Massage Exercises

Massage of the reconstructed breast helps the breast become softer, more natural looking, and aids in preventing the development of scar tissue around the implant. Exercises should be done *at least* two to three times; the more the better. To do the exercises, firmly press the breast on both sides, the top, and the bottom with the palm of your hand. Do this for a full minute. Then press the breast together with one or both hands for 15 to 20 seconds. Repeat this exercise five times. Your doctor and nurse will demonstrate the exercises for you and tell you when you should begin.

(Data from Pfeiffer, C. H., & Mullikne, J. B. [1984]. *Caring for the patient with breast cancer* [pp. 202–204]. Reston, VA: Reston Publishing Co.; and Knobf, T., & Stahl, R. [1987]. *Breast reconstruction: What to do after an implant*. Patient education pamphlet, Yale Comprehensive Cancer Center, New Haven, CT.)

average physician's experience, perhaps with the exception of those at large university or cancer centers. Therefore, treatment decisions will likely be controversial and subject to discussions and case presentations, and patients should be encouraged to enter clinical trials, if available. The patient's role in decision making for the treatment of in situ carcinomas is stressful because many women have difficulty understanding that the treatment options are the same as those for truly invasive cancer. Nurses in the ambulatory care setting are a resource for information, questions, clarification of issues, reassurance, and support.

SYSTEMIC TREATMENT OF BREAST CANCER

The purpose of systemic treatment of breast cancer is to prevent distant recurrence, as used in the adjuvant setting, to improve the response and durability of response in locally advanced cancer, and to treat patients who have relapsed with distant metastases. Mortality has been relatively unaffected by surgery or radiation because patients die of disseminated, not local, disease. One approach to changing the mortality statistics is systemic treatment administered at the time

of diagnosis and surgery when the tumor burden is small and the number of resistant cells is low or nonexistent. Several years of experience with adjuvant therapy have demonstrated improvement in survival rates while highlighting the heterogeneity of breast cancer and the fact that survival benefits accrue to subsets of patients only.

Adjuvant Therapy

Henderson (1987) provides a concise historical review, beginning with the practice of oophorectomy following mastectomy in premenopausal women some 40 years ago. The ovaries were either removed or irradiated, and a definite survival advantage could not be determined from these early adjuvant hormonal studies. The next generation of studies conducted between 1958 and 1970 involved short courses of chemotherapy administered in the immediate postoperative period, referred to as perioperative. Although one such perioperative study, now with a 20-year follow-up, reports a survival advantage for the treated versus the control group (Nissen-Meyer, Host, Ljellgren, Mansoon, & Nonn, 1986), short-term single-agent therapy was replaced by combination drug therapy as the kinetic theory of chemotherapy evolved. Beginning in the 1970s and up to the present time, trials focus on particular subsets of patients and factors that influence the efficacy of therapy, such as specific antineoplastic agents, hormones, timing, duration, dose, regimen of choice, long-term effects, cell kinetics, and tumor biology. The following discussion of these controversial issues intends to provide convincing evidence to support the concept of clinical trials in breast cancer to more accurately identify subsets of patients at risk and to determine optimal therapy. Nurses in both surgical and medical oncology specialty areas are critical to the success of clinical research. They can encourage patient participation, provide information to the patient and family, and monitor patient side effects, and they are invaluable in determining the quality of data collected on the tolerance and toxicity of systemic adjuvant therapy.

Duration of Therapy

Clinical trials from the 1970s consisting of 12 to 24 months of adjuvant chemotherapy, demonstrated a survival advantage to certain subsets of patients. In an attempt to decrease both long- and short-term toxicity, shorter courses of 4 to 6 months were compared with the previous 1- to 2-year course of therapy. A review of five major trials from cancer centers and cooperative groups failed to demonstrate any advantage to prolonged therapy (Henderson, Gelman, Harris, & Canellos, 1986), and some data suggest that the shorter courses may be more beneficial (Bonadonna et al., 1985). Thus in the absence of a definite survival advantage, short-term therapy offers several potential advantages to the patient, such as decreased severity of long- and short-term toxicity and less total drug

exposure, which may be important in the development of acquired drug resistance.

Regimen of Choice

The choice of drugs and regimens is influenced by the knowledge gained from clinical trials over the last 20 years and the degree of risk for subsets of patients. Combination chemotherapy was shown to be superior to single alkylating agent treatment (Fisher et al., 1975), and the combination of cyclophosphamide, methotrexate, and fluorouracil (CMF) represents a standard for multidrug adjuvant breast therapy in practice and a reference in the design of many clinical trials. For example, in the premenopausal subgroup of women who have one to three positive axillary nodes, it is unlikely that adding drugs to the basic CMF regimen improves results, yet an increase in toxicity can be appreciated (Tormey et al., 1984). In contrast, the addition of vincristine and prednisone to CMF may be worthwhile for postmenopausal patients at high risk, that is, those who have more than four positive nodes (Wood et al., 1985). Nodal involvement as a measure of tumor burden is a critical prognostic factor. Premenopausal patients with one to three positive nodes who are treated with adjuvant chemotherapy have a survival advantage, but as the number of positive axillary nodes increases, prognosis is greatly altered despite therapy (Fig. 30–7). Such data have prompted investigators to develop innovative and more aggressive approaches for higher risk patients, such as the addition of doxorubicin. Some investigators have substituted doxorubicin for methotrexate in the CMF regimen, whereas others have compared CMF-based regimens with a subsequent or alternating doxorubicin regimen. At the present time, the role of doxorubicin

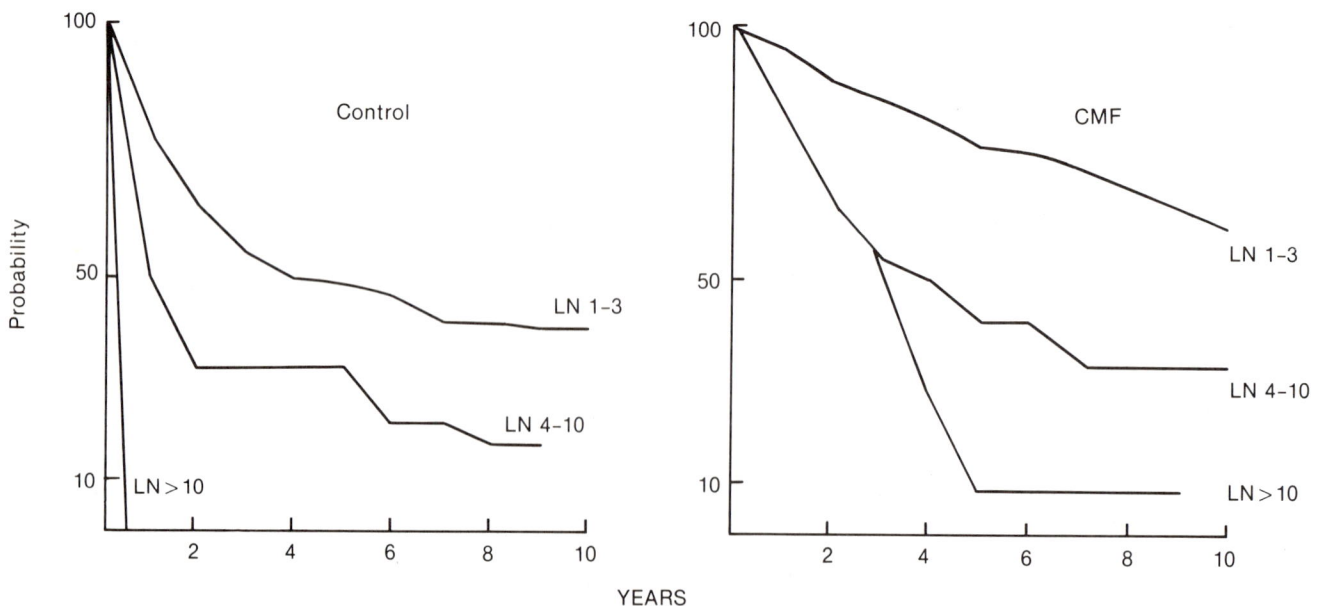

Figure 30–7. First cyclophosphamide, methotrexate, and fluorouracil (CMF) program (CMF = 12 cycles versus control = no treatment): comparative relapse-free survival time in premenopausal women related to lymph node (LN) subsets. (From Bonadonna, G., Valagussa, P., Rossi, A., Tancini, G., Brambilla, C., Zambetti, M., & Veronesi, U. [1985]. Ten year experience with CMF-based adjuvant chemotherapy in resectable breast cancer. *Breast Cancer Research and Treatment, 5,* 95–115. Reproduced by permission.)

in routine practice, that is, outside of a clinical trial, remains controversial, although recently doxorubicin appears to be more commonly prescribed.

Timing

In routine clinical practice, adjuvant therapy is initiated within 4 to 6 weeks after surgery. The optimal time to begin chemotherapy is unknown. Some investigators promote the neoadjuvant or perioperative approach in which drugs are administered after biopsy specimens are taken, at the time of surgery, or both, with or without subsequent courses of treatment (Ragaz, 1986). This rationale is based on concepts of tumor biology, including genetic mutations, development of resistant cells, and tumor cell burden. Another unresolved issue is optimal timing of chemotherapy with definitive radiotherapy. It is generally agreed that chemotherapy should be administered early on, but whether it is given before, concurrently, or in a sandwich technique with radiation has yet to be defined. Concurrent administration with CMF regimens is feasible with an accepted incidence of increased skin reactions (O'Rourke, 1987). Concomitant administration of doxorubicin and radiotherapy is not recommended, but doxorubicin-based combinations given before or after primary radiation are safe (Lippman et al., 1986). Dose reductions should be based on absolute granulocyte counts because of the lymphopenia that can occur secondary to irradiation.

Hormone Therapy

Adjuvant endocrine therapy regained status when the relatively nontoxic antiestrogen tamoxifen became available. A review of nine published studies of tamoxifen versus no treatment or placebo concluded that relapse-free survival is significantly prolonged, as is probably overall survival for postmenopausal women with positive nodes (Pritchard, 1987). Response appears proportional to the quantity of the receptor levels (Fisher et al., 1983; Rose et al., 1985); prescribing for more than 2 years is safe and may provide a continued

benefit to patients (Senofsky et al., 1986). Tamoxifen combined with cytotoxic therapy remains controversial. Although a disease-free survival advantage has been demonstrated for postmenopausal patients, the benefit of chemo-hormonal therapy over tamoxifen alone on overall survival is yet to be determined (Fisher et al., 1990; Tormey & Jordan, 1984).

Node-Negative Patients

Although node-negative patients are in the better prognostic group, 25 to 30 per cent will eventually relapse by 10 years and die of their disease. Efforts have focused on identifying subsets of higher risk patients within the node-negative group who may benefit from adjuvant therapy. Negative estrogen receptors, large tumors, a high thymidine labeling index, and a high percentage of S-phase cells as measured by DNA flow cytometry are all reported to have prognostic value (Clark & McGuire, 1989; Meyer & Province, 1988; Silvestrini et al., 1986).

Many patients with negative axillary nodes were included in earlier clinical trials with large numbers of node-positive patients. However, the numbers are small, and patients were not stratified for high-risk factors. Four major study groups have conducted randomized clinical trials of patients with node-negative breast cancer and estrogen receptor-negative tumors; some patients were given adjuvant chemotherapy and some no therapy (Fisher, Redmond, et al., 1989; Ludwig Breast Cancer Study Group, 1989; Mansour et al., 1989; Valagussa, 1989). With a median follow-up of 3 to 5 years, all of these trials report a disease-free survival advantage for treated patients (Table 30–12). An overall survival advantage has been reported only by the Milan group (Valagussa et al., 1989), but the follow-up time is much too short to make definitive conclusions on the effect of treatment on overall survival.

Adjuvant tamoxifen has been reported to be beneficial to women with breast cancer regardless of menopausal, nodal, or hormone receptor status (Baum, 1985; Scottish Cancer Trial, 1987). However, conclu-

Table 30–12. RELAPSE-FREE SURVIVAL IN ADJUVANT CHEMOTHERAPY TRIALS WITH NODE-NEGATIVE, ESTROGEN RECEPTOR-NEGATIVE PATIENTS

Study Group	Number of Patients	ER− (n)	RFS (%) Rx	RFS (%) Control	Average Follow-up	P Value
Intergroup (Mansour et al., 1989) 6 cycles CMF	406	310	83	71	3 years	0.005
NSABP (Fisher, Redmond, et al., 1989) Sequential MTX-5-FU-LCV	679	679	80	71	4 years	0.003
Ludwig (Ludwig Breast Cancer Study Group, 1989) Single-course CMF (perioperative)	1275	402	77	68	4 years	0.02
Milan (Valagussa, Brambilla, & DiFronzo, 1989) CMF × 12 cycles	90	90	88	47	5 years	0.001

CMF, cyclophosphamide, methotrexate, and fluorouracil; MTX, methotrexate; 5-FU, 5-fluorouracil; LCV, leucovorin.

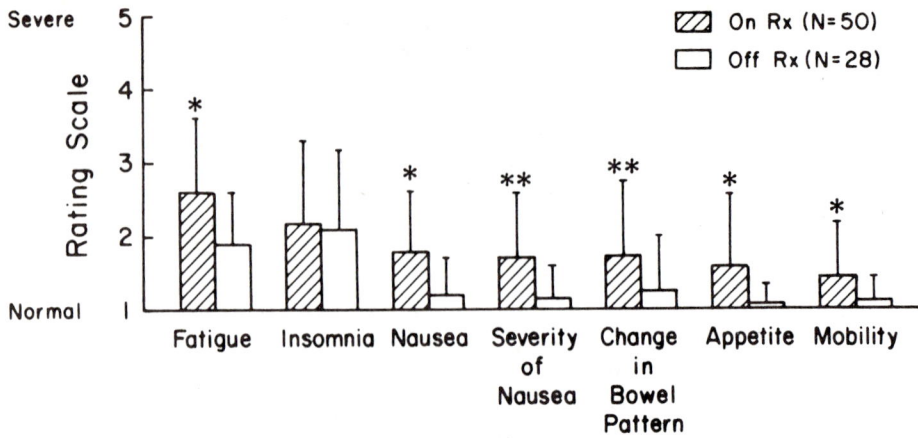

Figure 30–8. Physical distress rated by subjects who received adjuvant chemotherapy. *P ≤ 0.01; **P ≤ 0.05. (From Knobf, M. T. [1986]. Physical and psychologic distress associated with adjuvant chemotherapy in women with breast cancer. *Journal of Clinical Oncology, 4*, 678–684. Reproduced by permission.)

sions about the efficacy of tamoxifen in premenopausal patients with negative nodes cannot be made from those studies because the numbers were small and the data on hormone receptor status were not adequate. The National Surgical Adjuvant Breast and Bowel Project conducted randomized clinical trials of 2644 women with node-negative breast cancer and estrogen receptor-positive tumors, some of whom were given tamoxifen and some placebo for 5 years (Fisher, Costantino, et al., 1989). With a 4-year median follow-up, a significant disease-free survival benefit is noted for the treated group (83 per cent) versus the placebo group (77 per cent). An advantage was observed for both the younger (less than 49 years) and older (more than 50 years) women who received treatment. As with the adjuvant chemotherapy trials, follow-up is still too limited to evaluate the effect on overall survival.

Toxicity

The incidence, frequency, and severity of side effects associated with adjuvant therapy are influenced by the specific drugs, multidrug regimens, combination therapy, hormonal therapy, and duration of treatment. Although a wide variety of side effects have been observed, the most common include nausea, vomiting,

hair loss, fatigue, weight gain, and symptoms associated with menopause. Knowledge of the incidence of symptoms is important but may not be sufficient to determine the degree of severity or distress associated with side effects. Therefore, the nurse's ability to prepare the patient and focus the interventions may be circumscribed.

Knobf (1986) attempted to assess the degree of physical and psychological distress in 78 patients who received adjuvant chemotherapy with CMF with or without vincristine and prednisone (50 patients on therapy, 28 patients completed therapy) (Knobf, 1986). Mild physical distress (Fig. 30–8), mild to moderate psychological distress (Fig. 30–9), minimal life-style changes, some alterations in sexual relationships secondary to menopausal symptoms, and significant weight gain were reported by subjects. The low ratings of physical distress were unexpected; yet using the same symptom distress assessment tool, Ehlke (1988) confirmed these data. Fatigue, insomnia, and nausea were perceived as most distressful and received similar ratings in both studies.

Nausea, vomiting, and hair loss are three side effects feared by patients for whom chemotherapy is recommended. They are, however, not specific for women with breast cancer on adjuvant chemotherapy, and Chapter 22 provides guidelines for predicting and man-

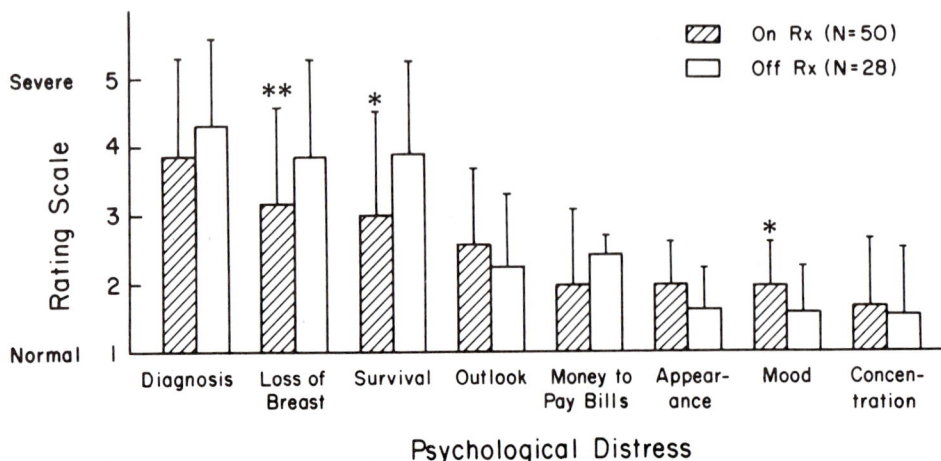

Figure 30–9. Psychological distress rated by women who received adjuvant chemotherapy. *P ≤ 0.01; **P ≤ 0.05. (From Knobf, M. T. [1986]. Physical and psychologic distress associated with adjuvant chemotherapy in women with breast cancer. *Journal of Clinical Oncology, 4*, 678–684. Reproduced by permission.)

aging these side effects. Fatigue, weight gain, and symptoms of menopause are reviewed here because of their documented incidence in this patient population.

Fatigue

Fatigue is common as part of the disease process, is associated with various cancer therapies, and is correlated with physical and psychological symptoms. Average ratings of distress for fatigue on a 1 to 5 scale for women on adjuvant chemotherapy were in the range of 2.3 to 2.6 (Ehlke, 1988; Knobf, 1986). In a prospective study of 37 women during their first two courses of adjuvant chemotherapy, more than half of the subjects reported fatigue; they described symptoms of whole-body tiredness, anxiety, tired legs, wanting to lie down, forgetfulness, and eye strain (Piper, Friedman, Hartigan, Post, & Smith, 1989). It is hoped that nursing research will continue in this area and guide our patient teaching and development of interventions for the future.

Weight Change

An average weight gain of 4 kg has been observed in patients receiving systemic adjuvant chemotherapy regardless of menopausal status, receptor content, pretreatment weight, duration of therapy, or ingestion of steroids (Bonadonna et al., 1985; Heasman, Sutherland, Campbell, Elhakim, & Boyd, 1985; Knobf, 1986; Knobf, Mullen, Xistris, & Moritz, 1983; Subramanian, Raich, & Walker, 1981). The total amount of weight gained appears to be slightly greater for women on steroids, for premenopausal patients, and for those on chemotherapy for longer periods of time (Foltz, 1985; Heasman et al., 1985; Knobf, 1986). Increased appetite, decreased activity, increased caloric intake, mild nausea, mood changes, and decreased serum estradiol levels have been associated with weight gain (Foltz, 1985; Grindel, Cahill, & Walker, 1989; Heasman et al., 1985; Knobf, 1986; Mukhopadhyay & Larkin, 1986). The incidence of drug-induced ovarian failure as defined by the presence or absence of amenorrhea secondary to chemotherapy does not appear to influence weight gain (Table 30–13). The causes of weight gain remain elusive, and patient distress is well recognized. Counseling and nutritional interventions are indicated, but clinical experience with patients has not proved that these interventions are successful, particularly during treatment. Aerobic exercise appears to be the first intervention to modulate the mild nausea associated with treatment and to promote weight control in this patient population (Box 30–3) (Winningham

Table 30–13. INCIDENCE OF WEIGHT GAIN (KG) IN PREMENOPAUSAL WOMEN ON CMF ADJUVANT CHEMOTHERAPY

	CMF 12	CMF 6
Without amenorrhea	5 ± 4.6	4.1 ± 4.7
With amenorrhea	5.2 ± 4.7	3.7 ± 3.5

(Data from Bonadonna, G., & Valagussa, P., Milan Cancer Institute, unpublished.)

& MacVicar, 1988; Winningham, MacVicar, Bondoc, Anderson, & Minton, 1989).

Menopausal Symptoms

The majority of women 40 years or older on adjuvant chemotherapy can be expected to develop some degree of drug-induced ovarian failure that is progressive with drug cycles (Fisher, Sherman, & Rockette, 1979; Rose & Davis, 1980; Samaan, deAsis, Buzdar, & Blumenstein, 1978). Associated menopausal symptoms of hot flashes, sweats, headaches, decreased vaginal lubrication, and dyspareunia have been reported (Rose & Davis, 1980; Tarpy & Rothwell, 1983). Information and counseling are critical. Adjuvant endocrine therapy with tamoxifen is associated with hot flashes, vaginal discharge, and irregular menses, particularly in younger women (Fisher, Costantino, et al., 1989). Menopausal symptoms disrupt routine activities and interfere significantly with sleep. Drug therapy may be indicated to control or minimize symptoms (Chapman, 1982). Diphenhydramine (Benadryl) at bedtime may be useful to minimize sleep deprivation, and low-dose clonidine has been reported to reduce the incidence of hot flashes (Clayden, Bell, & Pollard, 1974; Laufer, Erlik, Meldrum, & Judd, 1982; Yanes, Ross, Yanes, et al., 1987).

Treatment of Metastatic Disease

The greatest risk of relapse in breast cancer occurs within the first 2 to 3 years after diagnosis. Although 90 per cent of those who relapse do so by the fifth year, recurrences have been observed as long as 20 to 25 years later. Bone is the most common site of relapse (40 to 60 per cent), followed by lung (15 to 20 per cent), pleura (10 to 14 per cent), soft tissue (7 to 15 per cent), and liver (5 to 15 per cent) (Canellos, 1987). The mainstay of treatment for metastatic disease is hormone and cytotoxic therapy. Indications for surgery and radiotherapy are limited, with the most common being palliative radiotherapy for symptomatic bone metastases (Petrek, 1987). Selection of treatment is influenced by menopausal status, receptor content, specific metastatic site or sites, and aggressiveness of the tumor (Figs. 30–10 and 30–11).

Endocrine Therapy

Hormonal manipulation has been used for decades in the treatment of breast cancer, but not until the discovery of hormone receptors could the selection of patients be refined. Estrogen receptor-negative patients rarely respond; an overall response rate in the range of 30 per cent has been observed, but a higher response rate of 50 to 60 per cent may be achieved with ER-positive patients. Average responses last 12 to 18 months, and response rates are related to the quantity of receptor protein. Clinical experience indicates that postmenopausal patients respond more often than premenopausal patients; bone and soft tissue are

---

Box 30–3. EFFECT OF AEROBIC EXERCISE ON PATIENTS WITH BREAST CANCER

STUDY

Winningham, M. L., MacVicar, M. G., Bondoc, M., Anderson, J. I., & Minton, J. (1989). **Effect of aerobic exercise on body weight and composition in patients with breast cancer on adjuvant chemotherapy.** *Oncology Nursing Forum, 16,* 683–689.

SAMPLE

24 women with breast cancer who had completed at least one cycle but not more than 6 cycles of CMF (cyclophosphamide, methotrexate, and fluorouracil) or CMFVP (cyclophosphamide, methotrexate, fluorouracil, vincristine, and prednisone) adjuvant chemotherapy.

INTERVENTION

An experimental group (n = 12) participated in an aerobic exercise program, and a control group (n = 12) continued normal daily activities.

MEASURES

Body composition using multiple-site skin fold measurements to determine the relationship among weight, per cent body fat, and patterns of fat distribution.

FINDINGS

Aerobic exercise had a moderating effect on gain in body fat. Although both groups gained weight (the control group gained a mean of 1.99 kg; the experimental group gained 0.82 kg), there were significant differences between the groups for skin fold measurements and per cent body fat. Body fat increased in the control group, whereas body fat was reduced in the experimental group, and lean body tissue increased.

LIMITATIONS

Small sample size, inability to control for chemotherapy protocols, and lack of dietary intake data.

---

the most responsive metastatic sites; and patients who respond to one hormonal therapy will likely respond to another. There are many endocrine correlations with breast cancer, and approaches to inhibit growth are either ablative or additive (Fig. 30–12). The surgical ablative therapies are gradually being replaced by systemic therapy with tamoxifen, aminoglutethimide, and megestrol acetate (Megace) (Buchanon et al., 1986; Henderson, 1987; Legha, 1988). Although side effects are tolerated reasonably well, patients may experience a flare that is defined as transient increased bone pain or hypercalcemia.

Progestins such as megestrol acetate have similar response rates in the 30 per cent range and are associated with few side effects except that of weight gain. Increased appetite and fluid retention are implicated in weight gain, which is observed in as many as 50 per cent of treated patients.

Aminoglutethimide is a drug that blocks adrenal steroid synthesis. The adrenal gland is a major source of estrogen in the postmenopausal woman, aminoglutethimide therapy and, in essence produces a medical adrenalectomy. Because of the complex feedback mechanisms in the endocrine system, a steroid replacement is recommended with aminoglutethimide therapy, usually hydrocortisone 40 mg per day in physiologically divided doses. Side effects of lethargy, visual blurring, maculopapular rash, and dizziness occur in 25 to 50 per cent of the patients during the first 6 weeks of treatment but usually disappear thereafter (Henderson, 1987).

Although the exact sequence of endocrine therapies is unknown, response to endocrine therapy is associated with a prolonged survival. Whether this prolonged survival is due to multiple therapeutic responses to endocrine therapy or to the presence of less aggressive disease is also unknown.

Chemotherapy of Recurrent Disease

Only a few clinical predictors exist for response to chemotherapy. A good performance status, a long disease-free survival, and an absence of liver metastases are favorable factors, whereas pretreatment weight loss, extensive disease, anemia, and prior chemotherapy or radiotherapy are associated with a poorer

Diagnosis of Metastatic Disease

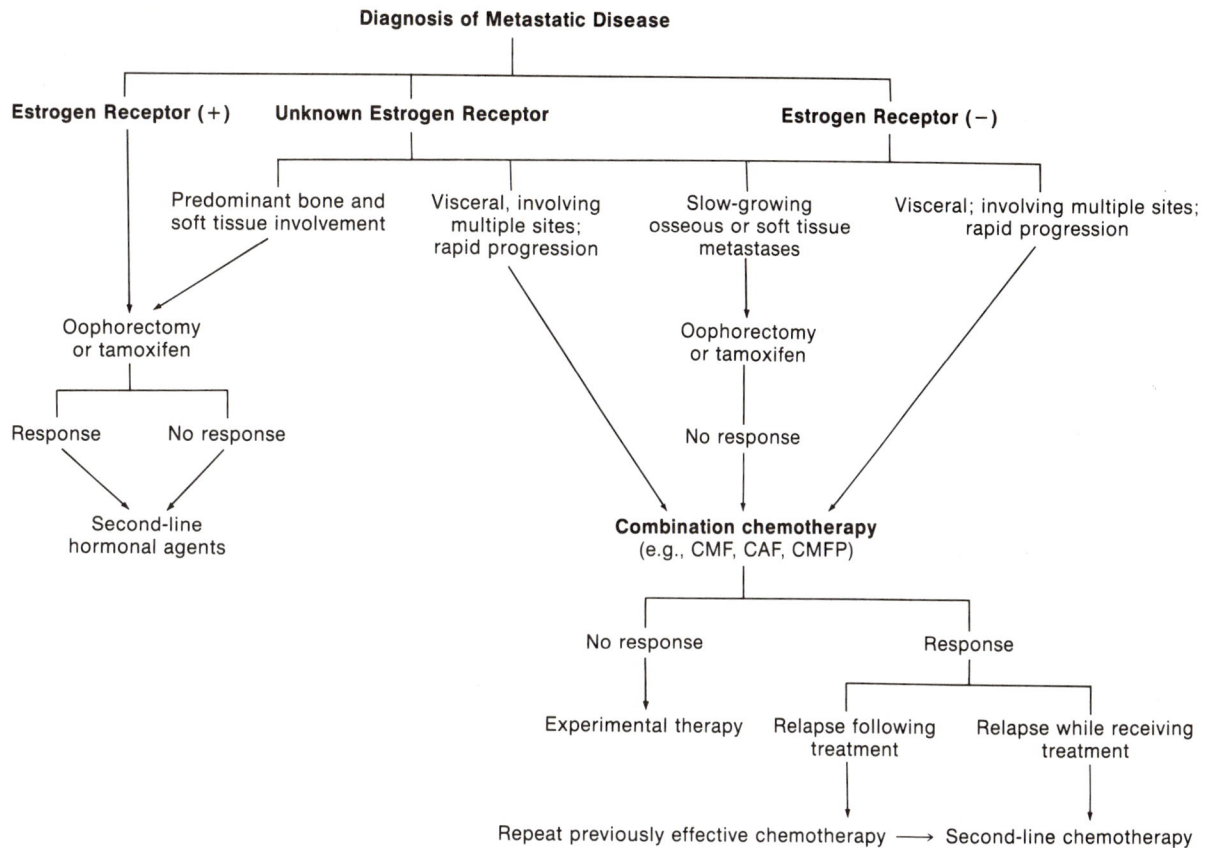

Figure 30–10. Selection of therapy for premenopausal patients with metastatic breast cancer. CMF, cyclophosphamide, methotrexate, and fluorouracil; CAF, cyclophosphamide, doxorubicin (Adriamycin), and fluorouracil; CMFP, cyclophosphamide, methotrexate, fluorouracil, and prednisone. (From Canellos, G. P. [1987]. Selection of therapy. In J. R. Harris, S. Hellman, I. C. Henderson, & D. W. Kinne [Eds.], *Breast diseases* [pp. 385–394]. Philadelphia: J. B. Lippincott Co. Reproduced by permission.)

response rate and prognosis (George & Hoogstraten, 1978; Swenerton, 1979). Hundreds of studies of chemotherapy in advanced breast cancer have been done, and several conclusions can be drawn (Harris, Hellman, Canellos, & Fisher, 1985). Combination chemotherapy is superior to single-agent therapy, producing an average response rate of 50 per cent, with a median duration of response ranging from 6 to 12 months. Complete responders are very uncommon and are not associated with a significantly prolonged survival. The average survival time following metastatic disease is 18 to 36 months. The combination of chemotherapy and hormone therapy may increase the response rate, but thus far it has not increased the duration of response or survival. Sequential non-cross-resistant regimens have not yet demonstrated any advantage to response rates or survival.

Many chemotherapeutic drugs have been studied in breast cancer; cyclophosphamide, methotrexate, 5-fluorouracil, doxorubicin, vincristine, and vinblastine are used routinely in clinical practice. Frequently used combination regimens are presented in Table 30–14. Side effects and interventions are reviewed in Units V and VIII. Predictable side effects are related primarily to single-agent therapy and must be weighed carefully according to dose, duration, and scheduling when combining one drug with another. Increasing the database for predictable toxicity of combination chemo-

therapy regimens is needed to improve patient preparation and to plan interventions.

Innovative strategies to improve the response rate have included using established drugs in new ways, such as administering moderate doses of methotrexate and 5-fluorouracil sequentially and giving continuous vinblastine infusions. In general, these new strategies have not changed the status of chemotherapy in breast cancer. New drugs with potential for advanced breast cancer therapy include bisantrene, 4'-demethoxydaunorubicin, 4'-deoxydoxorubicin, elliptinium acetate, 4'-epidoxorubicin, mitolactol, mitomycin, mitoxantrone, prednimustine, and vindesine (Henderson, Hayes, Come, Harris, & Canellos, 1987). A major advantage to some of these drugs is decreased toxicity; the new anthracycline derivatives, for example, are less cardiotoxic than doxorubicin. Clinical trials are ongoing for evaluation of these newer agents, and accurate documentation of subjective responses and nonhematologic toxicity is a critical task for the nurse caring for patients participating in clinical trials.

Many problems are associated with advanced disease and sites of metastases in breast cancer. Hypercalcemia, spinal cord compression, and development of brain metastases are complications of the disease. The nurse must know the symptoms of these complications, must provide careful assessment of their severity, and must identify the individual's degree of risk for them.

Diagnosis of Metastatic Disease

```
Estrogen Receptor (+)        Unknown Estrogen Receptor        Estrogen Receptor (−)
```

Visceral involving multiple sites; rapid progression

Predominant bone and soft tissue involvement; slow progression or affecting patients aged 65 years or older

Visceral; involving multiple sites; rapid progression

Tamoxifen

Response   No response

Aminoglutethimide or megestrol acetate

No response

Tamoxifen

Response   No response

Second-line hormonal therapy

No response ⟶ **Combination Chemotherapy**
(e.g., CMF, CAF, CMFP)

Response   No response

Experimental treatment

Relapse following treatment   Relapse while receiving treatment

Repeat previously effective chemotherapy   Second-line chemotherapy

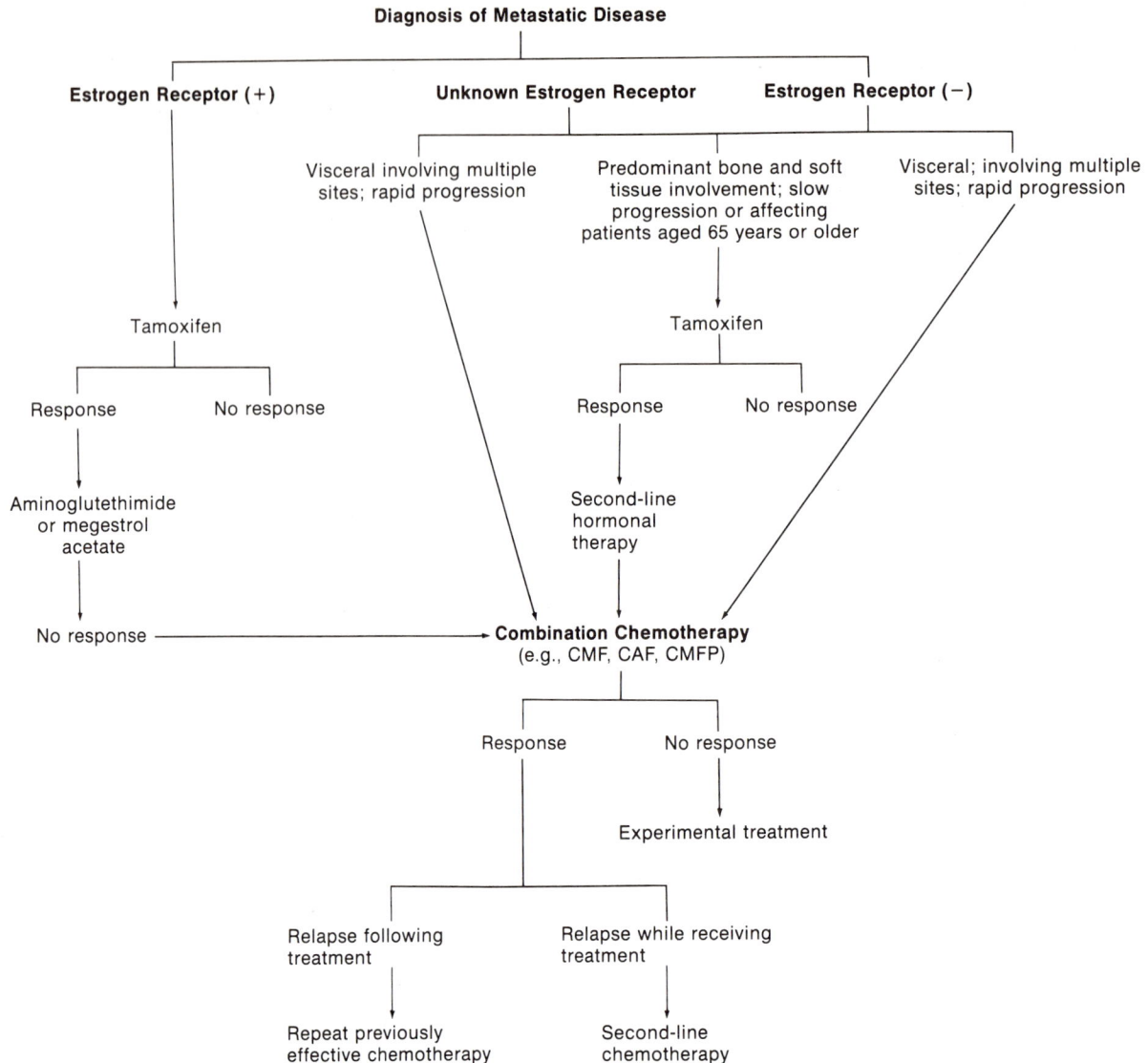

Figure 30–11. Selection of therapy for perimenopausal and postmenopausal women with metastatic breast cancer. CMF, cyclophosphamide, methotrexate, and fluorouracil; CAF, cyclophosphamide, doxorubicin (Adriamycin), and fluorouracil; CMFP, cyclophosphamide, methotrexate, fluorouracil, and prednisone. (From Canellos, G. P. [1987]. Selection of therapy. In J. R. Harris, S. Hellman, I. C. Henderson, & D. W. Kinne [Eds.], *Breast diseases* [pp. 385–394]. Philadelphia: J. B. Lippincott Co. Reproduced by permission.)

Other disease-related problems include pathologic fractures, liver metastases, carcinomatous meningitis, anemia, pleural effusions, lymphedema, and local chest wall recurrences. All of these represent major nursing challenges for care delivery and are detailed in Units V, VII, and VIII.

MALE BREAST CANCER

Breast cancer in men is uncommon, representing less than 1 per cent of all cancer in males. Its natural history is very similar to that of breast cancer in women (Erlichman, Murphy, & Elhakin, 1984; Kinne, 1987a; Ouriel, Lotze, & Hinshaw, 1984), with the major exception being age at onset. The average age of onset for men is 60 to 65 years. Other differences include presentation with a slightly more advanced stage of

disease and greater percentage of hormone receptor-positive tumors (Kinne, 1987a). The majority of patients present with a firm, painless subareolar mass and a histologic diagnosis of infiltrating ductal carcinoma. Patterns of recurrence and survival as influenced by pathologic stage of axillary lymph nodes are similiar to those for women.

Primary treatment is usually modified radical mastectomy, and adjuvant therapy is recommended for pathologic stage II disease. Postoperative radiotherapy may be recommended for improved local disease control. Treatment of recurrent disease is based on hormone receptor status. Orchiectomy or administration of tamoxifen are the first-line treatment choices; additive second-line endocrine therapy is somewhat more controversial. Data on chemotherapy responsiveness are sparse, and therefore it is difficult to make any specific recommendations.

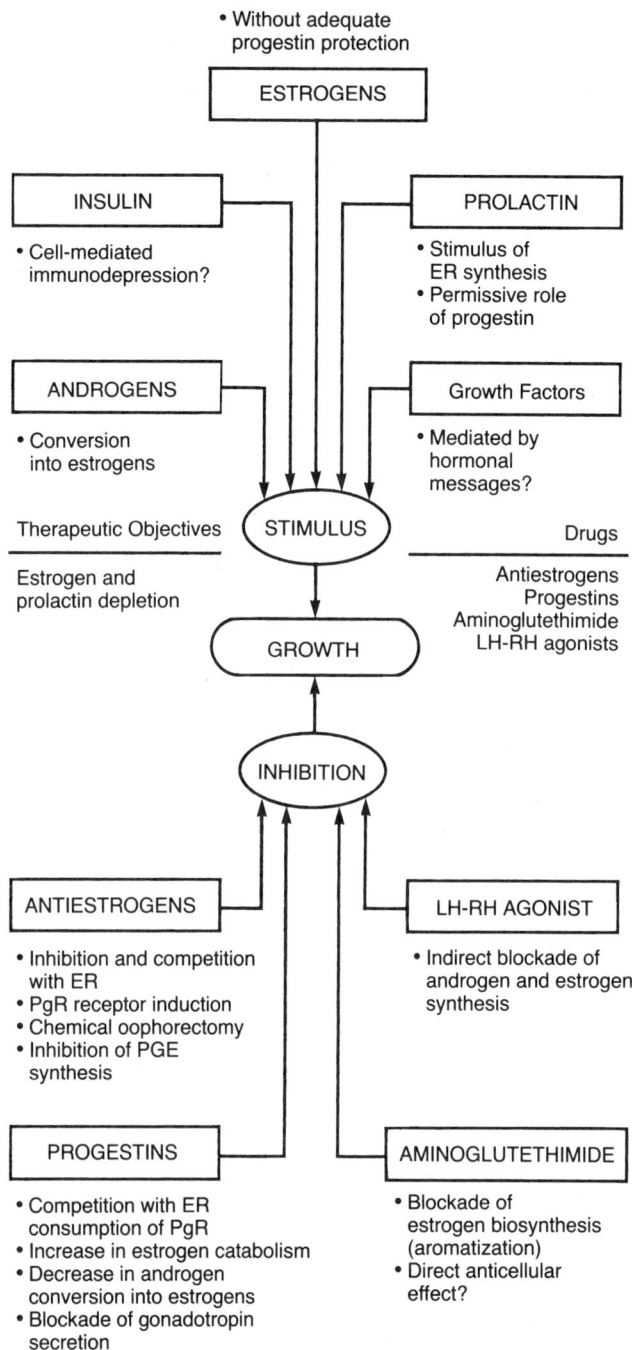

Figure 30–12. Endocrine correlations in breast cancer. ER, estrogen receptor; LH-RH, luteinizing hormone-releasing hormone; PgR, progesterone receptor; PGE, prostaglandin E. (From Robustelli della Cuna, G. [1988]. Principles of endocrine therapy. In G. Bonadonna & G. Robustelli della Cuna [Eds.], *Handbook of medical oncology,* [3rd ed. pp. 255–271]. Milan: Masson Publishers. Reproduced by permission.)

Table 30–14. COMMON CHEMOTHERAPY REGIMENS FOR BREAST CANCER

Drug	Dosage
CMF (Bonadonna et al., 1976)	**Every 28 days:**
Cyclophosphamide	$100/m^2$ days 1–14 po
Methotrexate	$40\ mg/m^2$ days 1 and 8 IV
5-Fluorouracil	$400\ mg/m^2$/days 1 and 8 IV
CMF (Bonadonna et al., 1986)	**Every 21 days:**
Cyclophosphamide	$600\ mg/m^2$ day 1 IV
Methotrexate	$40\ mg/m^2$ day 1 IV
5-Fluorouracil	$600\ mg/m^2$ day 1 IV
FAC (Blumenschein, Cardenas, Freirich, & Gottleib, 1974)	**Every 21 days:**
5-Fluorouracil	$500\ mg/m^2$ days 1 and 8 IV
Doxorubicin (Adriamycin)	$50\ mg/m^2$ day 1 IV
Cyclosphosphamide	$500\ mg/m^2$ day 1 IV
CAF (Smalley, Bartolucci, Vogel, & Krauss, 1977)	**Every 21 days:**
Cyclophosphamide	$500\ mg/m^2$ day 1 IV
Doxorubicin (Adriamycin)	$50\ mg/m^2$ day 1 IV
5-Fluorouracil	$500\ mg/m^2$ day 1 IV
CMFVP (Smalley et al., 1977)	**Every 28 days:**
Cyclophosphamide	$400\ mg/m^2$ day 1 IV
Methotrexate	$30\ mg/m^2$ days 1 and 8 IV
5-Fluorouracil	$400\ mg/m^2$ days 1 and 8 IV
Vincristine	1 mg days 1 and 8 IV
Prednisone	20 mg po qid days 1–7
Cooper Regimen (Cooper, Holland, & Gidewell, 1979)	
Cyclophosphamide	2 mg/kg/day po × 9 months
Methotrexate	0.7 kg/week for 8 weeks, then every other week for 7 months
5-Fluorouracil	12 mg/kg/week for 8 weeks, then every other week for 7 months
Vincristine	0.035 mg/kg/week IV × 5 weeks, then once a month
Prednisone	0.75 mg/kg/day po × 10 days, then ½ the dose for 10 days, ¼ dose for 10 days, 5 mg/day × 20 days, then discontinue.

IV, intravenously; po, orally; qid, four times a day.

References

Aitken, D. R., & Minton, J. P. (1983). Complications associated with mastectomy. *Surgical Clinics of North America, 63,* 1331–1362.

American Joint Committee on Cancer. (1987). *Manual for staging cancer* (3rd Ed.). Chicago: Author.

Anderson, D. E. (1974). Genetic study of breast cancer: Identification of a high risk group. *Cancer, 34,* 1090–1097.

Anderson, D. E., & Bodzich, M. D. (1985). Bilaterality in familiar breast cancer patients. *Cancer, 56,* 2092–2098.

Antman, K., & Gale, R. B. (1988). Advanced breast cancer: High dose chemotherapy and bone marrow auto transplants. *Annals of Internal Medicine, 108,* 570–574.

Baum, M. (1985). Controlled trial of tamoxifen as single adjuvant agent in management of early breast cancer: Analysis at six years of Nolvadex Adjuvant Trial Organization. *Lancet, 1,* 836–839.

Beckman, J., Johansen, L., Richardt, C., & Blichert-Toft, M. (1983). Psychological reactions in younger women operated on for breast cancer. *Danish Medical Bulletin, 30,* 10–13.

Bell, D. A., Hajdu, S. I., Urban, J. A., & Gaston, J. P. (1983). Role of aspiration cytology in the diagnosis and management of mammary lesions in office practice. *Cancer, 51,* 1182–1189.

Betskill, W. L., Rosen, P. P., & Lieberman, P. H. (1978). Intraductal carcinoma. *Journal of the American Medical Association, 239,* 1863–1867.

Bloom, J. R., Ross, R. D., & Burnell, E. (1978). The effect of social support inpatient adjustment after breast surgery. *Patient Counseling Health Education, 1,* 1–19.

Blumenschein, G., Cardenas, J. O., Freirich, J., & Gottleib, J. (1974). FAC chemotherapy for breast cancer. *Proceedings of the American Society for Clinical Oncology, 15,* 193 (Abstract).

Bonadonna, G., Brusamolino, E., Valagussa, P., Rossi, A., Brugnatelli, L., Brambilla, C., DeLena, M., Tancini, G., Bajetta, E., Musumeci, R., & Veronessi, U. (1976). Combination chemotherapy as an adjuvant treatment in operable breast cancer. *New England Journal of Medicine, 294,* 405–410.

Bonadonna, G., & Valagussa, P. (1985). Adjuvant systemic therapy for resectable breast cancer. *Journal of Clinical Oncology, 3,* 259–275.

Bonadonna, G., & Valagussa, P. (1986). Adjuvant chemoendocrine therapy in breast cancer. *Journal of Clinical Oncology, 4,* 451–454.

Bonadonna, G., Valagussa, P., Rossi, A., Tancini, G., Brambilla, C., Zambetti, M., & Veronessi, U. (1985). Ten year experience with CMF-based adjuvant chemotherapy in resectable breast cancer. *Breast Cancer Research and Treatment, 5,* 95–115.

Bonadonna, G., Zambetti, M., Valagussa, P., Bignami, P., Di-Fronzo, G., & Silvestrini, R. (1986). Adjuvant CMF in node negative breast cancer. *Proceedings of the American Society for Clinical Oncology, 5,* 74 (Abstract No. 290).

Brinton, L. A., Hoover, R. N., Szelko, M., & Fraumeni, J. F. (1981). Menopausal estrogen use and the risk of breast cancer. *Cancer, 47,* 2519–2522.

Brinton, L. A., Williams, R. R., & Hoover, R. N. (1979). Breast cancer risk factors among screening program participants. *Journal of the National Cancer Institute, 62,* 37–44.

Brody, D. S. (1980). The patient's role in clinical decision making. *Annals of Internal Medicine, 93,* 718–722.

Buchanon, R. B., Blamyey, R. W., Durrant, K. R., Howell, A., Paterson, A. G., Preece, P. E., Smith, D. C., Williams, C. J., & Wilson, R. G. (1986). A randomized comparison of tamoxifen with surgical oophorectomy in premenopausal patients with advanced breast cancer. *Journal of Clinical Oncology, 4,* 1326–1330.

Canellos, G. P. (1987). Selection of therapy. In J. R. Harris, S. Hellman, I. C. Henderson, & D. W. Kinne (Eds.), *Breast diseases* (pp. 385–391). Philadelphia: J. B. Lippincott Co.

Cardenas, J., Ramirez, T., Noriega, J., DeLaGarze, J., Gonzalez, F., & Labastida, M. (1987). Multidisciplinary therapy for locally advanced breast cancer. An update. *Proceedings of the American Society for Clinical Oncology, 6,* 67 (Abstract No. 261).

Carroll, K. K., & Braden, L. M. (1985). Dietary fat and mammary carcinogenesis. *Nutrition and Cancer, 6,* 254–259.

Carroll, R. M. (1981). The impact of mastectomy on body image. *Oncology Nursing Forum, 8,* 29–32.

Carter, D., & Smith, R. I. (1977). Carcinoma in situ of the breast. *Cancer, 40,* 1189–1193.

Chapman, R. M. (1982). Effect of cytotoxic therapy on sexuality and gonadal function. *Seminars in Oncology, 9,* 84–94.

Clark, G. M., & McGuire, W. L. (1989). New biologic prognostic factors in breast cancer. *Oncology, 3,* 49–54.

Clark, G. M., Osbourne, C. K., & McGuire, W. L. (1984). Correlations between estrogen receptor, progesterone receptor and patient characteristics in human breast cancer. *Journal of Clinical Oncology, 2,* 1102–1109.

Clark, R. M., Wilkinson, R. H., Mahoney, L. J., Reid, J. G., & MacDonald, W. D. (1982). Breast cancer: A 21-year experience with conservative surgery and radiation. *International Journal of Radiation Oncology, Biology, and Physics, 8,* 967–975.

Clarke, D., Martinez, A., & Cox, R. S. (1983). Analysis of cosmetic results and complications in patients with stage I and II breast cancer treated by biopsy and radiation. *International Journal of Radiation Oncology, Biology, and Physics, 9,* 1807–1813.

Clayden, J. R., Bell, J. W., & Pollard, P. (1974). Menopausal flushing: Double-blind trial of a non-hormonal medication. *British Medical Journal, 1,* 409–412.

Cooper, R. G., Holland, J. F., & Gidewell, O. (1979). Adjuvant chemotherapy of breast cancer. *Cancer, 44,* 793–798.

Danforth, D. N., Findlay, P. A., McDonald, H. D., Lippman, M. E., Reichart, C. M., D'Angelo, T., et al. (1986). Complete axillary node dissection for Stage I & II carcinoma of the breast. *Journal of Clinical Oncology, 4,* 655–662.

D'Angelo, T. M., & Gorrell, C. R. (1989). Breast reconstruction using tissue expanders. *Oncology Nursing Forum, 16,* 23–27.

Dawson, P. J., Ferguson, D. J., & Karrison, T. (1982). The pathologic findings of breast cancer in patients surviving 25 years after radical mastectomy. *Cancer, 50,* 2131–2138.

Dinner, M. I., & Dowden, R. V. (1984). Breast reconstruction: State of the art. *Cancer, 53,* 809–814.

Dupont, W. D., & Page, D. L. (1985). Risk factors for breast cancer in women with proliferative breast disease. *New England Journal of Medicine, 312,* 145–151.

Ehlke, G. A. (1988). Symptom distress in breast cancer patients receiving chemotherapy in the out-patient setting. *Oncology Nursing Forum, 15,* 343–346.

Erlichman, C., Murphy, K. C., Elhakin, T. (1984). Male breast cancer: A 13-year review of 89 patients. *Journal of Clinical Oncology, 2,* 903–909.

Findlay, P., & Goodman, R. (1983). Radiation therapy for the treatment of intraductal carcinoma of the breast. *American Journal of Clinical Oncology, 6,* 281–285.

Fisher, B. (1983). Relation of estrogen and/or progesterone receptor content of breast cancer to patient outcome following adjuvant chemotherapy. *Breast Cancer Research and Treatment, 3,* 355–364.

Fisher, B., Bauer, M., Margolese, R., Poisson, R., Pilch, Y., Redmond, C., Fisher, E., Wolmark, N., Deutsch, M., Montague, E., Saffer, E., Wickerman, L., Lerner, H., Gloss, A., Shibata, H., Deckers, P., Ketchem, A., Oishi, R., & Russell, I. (1985). Five year results of a randomized clinical trial comparing total mastectomy and segmental mastectomy with or without radiation in the treatment of breast cancer. *New England Journal of Medicine, 312,* 665–673.

Fisher, B., Costantino, J., Redmond, C., Poisson, R., Bowman, D., Couture, J., Dimitrov, N., Wolmark, N., Wickerham, D. L., Fisher, E., Margolese, R., Robidoux, A., Shibata, H., Terz, J., Paterson, A. H. G., Feldman, M. I., Farrar, W., Evans, J., Lickley, H. L., & Ketner, M. (1989). A randomized clinical trial evaluating tamoxifen in the treatment of patients with node-negative breast cancer who have estrogen-receptor-positive tumors. *New England Journal of Medicine, 320,* 479–484.

Fisher, B., Fisher, E. R., Redmond, C., & Brown, A. (1986). Tumor nuclear grade, estrogen receptor and progesterone receptor: Their value alone or in combination as indicators of outcome following adjuvant therapy for breast cancer. *Breast Cancer Research and Treatment, 7,* 117–160.

Fisher, B., & Gebhart, M. C. (1978). The evolution of breast cancer surgery: Past, present and future. *Seminars in Oncology, 5,* 385–395.

Fisher, B., Redmond, C., Brown, A., Wickerham, L., Wolmark, N., Allegra, J., Escher, G., Lippman, M., Savlov, E., Wittliff, J., & Fisher, E. R. (1983). Influence of tumor estrogen and progesterone levels on the response to tamoxifen and chemotherapy in primary breast cancer. *Journal of Clinical Oncology, 1,* 227–241.

Fisher, B., Redmond, C., Dimitrov, N. V., Bowman, D., Legault-Poisson, S., Wickerham, L., Wolmark, N., Fisher, E., Margolese, R., Sutherland, C., Glass, A., Foster, R., Caplan, R., et al. (1989). A randomized clinical trial evaluating sequential methotrexate and flourouracil in the treatment of patients with node-negative breast cancer who have estrogen-receptor-negative tumors. *New England Journal of Medicine, 320,* 473–478.

Fisher, B., Redmond, C., Poisson, S., Dimitrov, N., Margolese, R., Bowman, D., Glass, A., Robidoux, A., Wickerham, D., Wolmark, N., & Jochimsen, P. (1990). Increased benefit from addition of Adriamycin and cyclophosphamide (AC) to tamoxifen (TAM, T) for positive node TAM-response postmenopausal breast cancer patients: Results from NSABP B-16. *Proceedings of the American Society of Clinical Oncology, 9:*20.

Fisher, B., Sherman, B., & Rockette, H. (1979). L-Phenylalanine-mustard (L-PAM) in the management of premenopausal patients with primary breast cancer. *Cancer, 44,* 847–857.

Fisher, B., Slack, N., Katrych, D., & Wolmark, N. (1975). Ten year follow up results of patients with carcinoma of the breast in a cooperative clinical trial evaluating surgical adjuvant chemotherapy. *Surgery, Gynecology and Obstetrics, 140,* 528–531.

Fisher, B., & Wolmark, N. (1986). Conservative surgery: The American experience. *Seminars in Oncology, 13,* 425–433.

Foltz, A. (1985). Weight gain among stage II breast cancer patients: A study of five factors. *Oncology Nursing Forum, 12,* 21–26.

Frazier, T. G., & Noone, R. B. (1985). An objective analysis of immediate simultaneous reconstruction in the treatment of primary carcinoma of the breast. *Cancer, 55,* 1202–1205.

Freedman, L. S., Edwards, D. W., McConnell, E. M., & Downham, D. Y. (1979). Histological grade and other prognostic factors in relation to survival of patients with breast cancer. *British Journal of Cancer, 40,* 44–55.

Fryberg, E. R., Santiago, F., Betskill, W. L., & O'Brien, P. H.

(1987). Lobular carcinoma in situ of the breast. *Surgery, Gynecology and Obstetrics, 164,* 285–301.

Ganz, P. A., Schag, C. C., Polinsky, M. L., Heinrich, R. L., & Flack, V. (1987). Rehabilitation needs and breast cancer: The first month after primary therapy. *Breast Cancer Research and Treatment, 10,* 243–253.

George, S. L., & Hoogstraten, B. (1978). Prognostic factors in the initial response to therapy by patients with advanced breast cancer. *Journal of the National Cancer Institute, 60,* 731–736.

Goldie, J. H. (1983). Drug resistance and cancer chemotherapy strategy in breast cancer. *Breast Cancer Research and Treatment, 3,* 129–136.

Graham, S. (1987). Alcohol and breast cancer. *New England Journal of Medicine, 316,* 1211–1213.

Grindel, C. G., Cahill, C. A., & Walker, M. (1989). Food intake of women with breast cancer during the first six months of chemotherapy. *Oncology Nursing Forum, 16,* 401–407.

Gross, G. E., Clark, G. M., Chamness, G. C., & Maguire, W. (1984). Multiple progesterone receptor assays in human breast cancer. *Cancer Research, 44,* 836–840.

Habegger, D., & Ellerhorst-Ryan, J. M. (1988). Needle localization for non-palpable breast lesions. *Oncology Nursing Forum, 15,* 192–194.

Harris, J. R., & Hellman, S. (1983). Primary radiation therapy for early breast cancer. *Cancer, 51,* 2547–2552.

Harris, J. R., Hellman, S., Canellos, G. P., & Fisher, B. (1985). Cancer of the breast. In V. T. DeVita, S. Hellman, S. A. Rosenberg (Eds.), *Cancer: Principles and practices of oncology* (pp. 1119–1177). Philadelphia: J. B. Lippincott Co.

Heasman, K. Z., Sutherland, H. J., Campbell, J. A., Elhakim, T., & Boyd, N. F. (1985). Weight gain during adjuvant chemotherapy for breast cancer. *Breast Cancer Research and Treatment, 5,* 195–200.

Henderson, I. C. (1987). Adjuvant systemic therapy of early breast cancer. In J. R. Harris, S. Hellman, I. C. Henderson, & D. W. Kinne (Eds.), *Breast diseases* (pp. 398–428). Philadelphia: J. B. Lippincott Co.

Henderson, I. C., Gelman, R. S., Harris, J. R., & Canellos, G. P. (1986). Duration of therapy in adjuvant chemotherapy. *NCI Monographs, 1,* 95–98.

Henderson, I. C., Hayes, D. F., Come, S., Harris, J. R., & Canellos, G. (1987). New agents and new medical treatments for advanced breast cancer. *Seminars in Oncology, 14,* 34–64.

Howe, G. R., Sherman, G. J., Seminciew, R. M., & Miller, A. B. (1981). Estimated benefits and risks of screening for breast cancer. *Canadian Medical Association Journal, 124,* 399–403.

Hutcheson, H. A. (1986). TAIF: New option for breast reconstruction. *Nursing '86, 2,* 52–53.

King, K., Nail, L., Kreamer, K., Strohl, R., & Johnson, J. E. (1985). Patients descriptions of the experience of receiving radiation therapy. *Oncology Nursing Forum, 12,* 55–61.

Kinne, D. W. (1987a). Male breast cancer. In J. R. Harris, S. Hellman, I. C. Henderson, & D. W. Kinne (Eds.), *Breast diseases* (pp. 557–583). Philadelphia: J. B. Lippincott Co.

Kinne, D. W. (1987b). Primary treatment of breast cancer surgery. In J. R. Harris, S. Hellman, I. C. Henderson, & D. W. Kinne (Eds.), *Breast diseases* (pp. 259–284). Philadelphia: J. B. Lippincott Co.

Knobf, M. K. (1986). Physical and psychological distress associated with adjuvant chemotherapy in women with breast cancer. *Journal of Clinical Oncology, 4,* 678–684.

Knobf, M. K., Mullen, J., Xistris, D., & Moritz, D. A. (1983). Weight gain in women with breast cancer on adjuvant chemotherapy. *Oncology Nursing Forum, 10,* 28–33.

Kopans, D., Meyer, J. E., & Sadowsky, N. (1984). Breast imaging. *New England Journal of Medicine, 310,* 960–967.

Lagios, M. D., Westdahl, P. R., Margolini, F. R., & Rose, M. R. (1982). Duct carcinoma in situ. *Cancer, 53,* 700–704.

Land, C. E., Boice, J. D., Shore, R. E., Norman, J. E., & Tokwnaga, M. (1980). Breast cancer risk from low dose exposure to ionizing radiation. Results of parallel analysis of three exposed populations of women. *Journal of the National Cancer Institute, 65,* 353–376.

Laufer, L. R., Erlik, Y., Meldrum, D. R., & Judd, H. L. (1982). Effect of clonidine on hot flashes in postmenopausal women. *Obstetrics and Gynecology, 60,* 583–586.

Legha, S. S. (1988). Tamoxifen in the treatment of breast cancer. *Annals of Internal Medicine, 109,* 219–228.

Leinster, S. L., Ashcroft, J. J., Slade, P. D., & Dewey, M. E. (1989). Mastectomy versus conservative surgery: Psychosocial effects of the patients choice of treatment. *Journal of Psychosocial Oncology, 7,* 179–192.

Lierman, L. M. (1988). Phantom breast experiences after mastectomy. *Oncology Nursing Forum, 15,* 41–44.

Lippman, M. E. (1983). Efforts to combine endocrine and chemotherapy in the management of breast cancer: Do two and two equal three? *Breast Cancer Research and Treatment, 3,* 117–127.

Lippman, M. E., Sorace, R. A., Bagly, C., Danforth, D. W., Lichter, A., & Wesley, M. (1986). Treatment of locally advanced breast cancer using primary induction chemotherapy with hormonal synchronization followed by radiation with or without debulking surgery. *NCI Monograph, 1,* 153–159.

Lotze, M. T., Duncan, M. A., Gerber, L. H., Woltering, E. A., & Rosenberg, S. A. (1981). Early vs. delayed shoulder motion following axillary dissection. *Annals of Surgery, 193,* 288–295.

The Ludwig Breast Cancer Study Group. (1989). Prolonged disease free survival after one course of perioperative adjuvant chemotherapy for node-negative breast cancer. *New England Journal of Medicine, 320,* 491–496.

Maier, W., Leber, D., Rosemond, G. P., Goldman, L. I., & Tyson, R. R. (1977). The technique of modified radical mastectomy. *Surgery, Gynecology and Obstetrics, 145,* 69–74.

Mann, B. D., Giuliano, E., Bassett, L. W., Barber, M., Hallouer, W., & Morton, D. (1983). Delayed diagnosis of breast cancer as a result of normal mammograms. *Archives of Surgery, 118,* 23–24.

Mansour, E. G., Gay, R., Shatila, A. H., Osborne, C. K., Tormey, D. C., Gilchrist, K. W., Cooper, M. R., & Falkson, G. (1989). Efficacy of adjuvant chemotherapy in high risk node-negative breast cancer. *New England Journal of Medicine, 320,* 485–490.

Markowski, J., Wilcox, J. P., & Helm, P. A. (1981). Lymphedema incidence after postmastectomy therapy. *Archives of Physical Medicine and Rehabilitation, 62,* 449–452.

Martin, J. E. (1983). Breast imaging techniques. *Radiologic Clinics of North America, 21,* 149–153.

Martinez, A. A., & Clarke, D. (1984). Treatment results, cosmesis and complications in stage I and II breast cancer patients treated by excisional biopsy and irradiation. In F. C. Ames, G. R. Blumenschein, & E. D. Montague (Eds.), *Current controversies in breast cancer* (pp. 369–381). Austin: University of Texas Press.

McHugh, N. G., Christman, N. J., & Johnson, J. (1982). Preparatory information: What helps and why. *American Journal of Nursing, 82,* 78–82.

McKann, C. F., & Knobf, M. K. Unpublished data. (1985). Department of Surgery, Yale University School of Nursing.

Messerli, M. L., Garamedi, C., & Romano, J. (1980). Breast cancer: Information as a technique of crisis intervention. *American Journal of Orthopsychiatry, 50,* 728–731.

Meyer, J. S., & Province, M. (1988). Proliferative index of breast carcinoma by thymidine labeling: Prognostic power independent of state, estrogen and progesterone receptors. *Breast Cancer Research and Treatment, 12,* 191–204.

Miller, A. B. (1987). Breast cancer epidemiology and prevention. In J. R. Harris, S. Hellman, I. C. Henderson, & D. W. Kinne (Eds.), *Breast diseases* (pp. 87–102). Philadelphia: J. B. Lippincott Co.

Miller, A. B., Kelly, A., Choi, N. W., Matthews, V., Morgan, R. W., Munan, L., Burch, J. D., Feather, J., Howe, G. R., & Jain, M. (1978). A study of diet and breast cancer. *American Journal of Epidemiology, 107,* 499–509.

Montague, E. D. (1984). Conservative surgery and radiation therapy in the treatment of operable breast cancer. *Cancer, 53,* 700–704.

Morris, J., & Ingham, R. (1988). Choice of surgery for early breast cancer: Psychosocial considerations. *Social Science and Medicine, 27,* 1257–1262.

Mukhopadhyay, M. G., & Larkin, S. (1986). Weight gain in cancer patients on chemotherapy. *Proceedings of the American Society for Clinical Oncology, 5,* 254 (Abstract No. 992).

Nail, L., Jones, L. S., Giuffre, M., & Johnson, J. E. (1984). Sensations after mastectomy. *American Journal of Nursing '84, 9,* 1121–1124.

Nissen-Meyer, R., Host, H., Ljellgren, K., Mansoon, B., & Nonn,

T. (1986). Treatment of node negative breast cancer patients with short course chemotherapy immediately after surgery. *NCI Monographs, 1,* 125–128.

O'Rourke, M. E. (1987). Enhanced cutaneous effects in combined modality therapy. *Oncology Nursing Forum, 14,* 31–35.

Osbourne, C. K. (1987). Receptors. In J. R. Harris, S. Hellman, I. C. Henderson, & D. W. Kinne (Eds.), *Breast diseases* (pp. 210–232). Philadelphia: J. B. Lippincott Co.

Ouriel, K., Lotze, M. T., & Hinshaw, J. R. (1984). Prognostic factors of carcinoma of the male breast. *Surgery, Gynecology and Obstetrics, 159,* 373–376.

Page, D. L., Dupont, W. D., Rogers, L. W., & Landenberger, M. (1982). Intraductal carcinoma of the breast: Follow up after biopsy only. *Cancer, 49,* 751–758.

Partsch, H., Mostbeck, A., & Leitner, G. (1980). Experimental investigations on the effect of a pressure wave massage apparatus (Lympha-press) in lymphedema. *Phlebologie Proktologie, 2,* 124–128.

Paulus, D. D. (1987). Imaging in breast cancer. *CA: A Cancer Journal for Clinicians, 37,* 133–150.

Petrck, J. A. (1987). Surgery for metastatic disease. In J. R. Harris, S. Hellman, I. C. Henderson, & D. W. Kinne (Eds.), *Breast diseases* (pp. 391–394). Philadelphia: J. B. Lippincott Co.

Piper, B., Friedman, L., Hartigan, K., Post, B., & Smith, J. (1989). Fatigue patterns over time in women receiving CMF chemotherapy for breast cancer. *Oncology Nursing Society, 16* (Suppl.), 217 (Abstract No. 355).

Pritchard, K. I. (1987). Current status of adjuvant endocrine therapy for resectable breast cancer. *Seminars in Oncology, 14,* 23–33.

Ragaz, J. (1986). Emerging modalities for adjuvant therapy of breast cancer: Neoadjuvant chemotherapy. *NCI Monographs, 1,* 145–152.

Recht, A., Connolly, J. L., Schnitt, S. J., Cady, B., Love, S., Osteen, R. T., Patterson, W. B., Shirley, R., Silen, W., Come, S., Henderson, I. C., Silver, B., & Hams, J. (1986). Conservative surgery and radiation therapy for early breast cancer: Results, controversies, and unsolved problems. *Seminars in Oncology, 13,* 434–449.

Rose, C., Mouridsen, H. T., Thorpe, S. M., Anderson, J., Bilchert-Toft, M., & Anderson, K. W. (1985). Anti-estrogen treatment of postmenopausal breast cancer patients with high risk of recurrence: 72 months of life table analysis and steroid hormone receptor status. *World Journal of Surgery, 9,* 765–774.

Rose, D. P., & Davis, T. E. (1980). Effects of adjuvant chemohormonal therapy on the ovarian and adrenal function of breast cancer patients. *Cancer Research, 40,* 4043–4047.

Rosen, P. P. (1987). The pathology of breast carcinoma. In J. R. Harris, S. Hellman, I. C. Henderson, & D. W. Kinne (Eds.), *Breast diseases* (pp. 147–209). Philadelphia: J. B. Lippincott Co.

Rosen, P. P., Kinne, D. W., Lesser, M., & Hellman, S. (1986). Are prognostic factors for local control of breast cancer treated by primary radiotherapy significant for patients treated by mastectomy? *Cancer, 57,* 1415–1420.

Rosner, D., Lane, W. W., & Brett, R. P. (1985). Influence of oral contraceptives on the prognosis of breast cancer in young women. *Cancer, 55,* 1556–1562.

Ross, R. K., Paganini-Hill, A., Gerkins, V. A., Mack, T. M., Pfeffer, R., Athur, M., & Hendersen, B. E. (1980). A case control study of menopausal estrogen therapy and breast cancer. *Journal of the American Medical Association, 243,* 1635–1639.

Samaan, N. A., deAsis, D. W., Buzdar, A. U., & Blumenstein, G. R. (1978). Pituitary-ovarian function in breast cancer patients on adjuvant chemoimmunotherapy. *Cancer, 41,* 2084–2087.

Sanger, C. K., & Reznikoff, M. (1981). A comparison of the psychological effects of breast saving procedures with modified radical mastectomy. *Cancer, 48,* 2341–2346.

Say, C. C., & Donegan, W. (1974). A biostatistical evaluation of complications from mastectomy. *Surgery, Gynecology and Obstetrics, 138,* 370–376.

Schain, W., Edwards, B. K., Gorrell, C., Moss, E. V., Lippman, M. E., Gerber, L., et al. (1983). Psychosocial and physical outcomes of primary breast cancer therapy: Mastectomy vs. excisional biopsy and irradiation. *Breast Cancer Research and Treatment, 3,* 377–382.

Schatzkin, A., Jones, Y., Hoover, R. N., Taylor, P. R., Brinton, L. A., Zeigler, R., Hariby, E. B., Carter, C. L., Licitra, L. M.,

Dufour, M. C., & Larson, D. B. (1987). Alcohol consumption and breast cancer in the epidemiologic follow up study of the first national health and nutrition examination survey. *New England Journal of Medicine, 316,* 1169–1180.

Schnitt, S. J., Silen, W., Sadowsky, N., Connolly, J. L., & Harris, J. R. (1988). Ductal carcinoma in situ (intraductal carcinoma) of the breast. *New England Journal of Medicine, 318,* 898–903.

Scottish Cancer Trial. (1987). Adjuvant tamoxifen in the management of operable breast cancer: The Scottish trial—report from the Breast Cancer Trials Committee. *Lancet, 2,* 171–175.

Senofsky, G. M., Wanebo, H. J., Wilhelm, M. L., Pope, T. L., Fechner, R. E., & Kaiser, D. L. (1986). Has monitoring the contralateral breast improved the prognosis in patients treated for primary breast cancer? *Cancer, 57,* 597–602.

Shannon-Bodner, R. M., & Flynn, K. T. (1987). Symptom distress of women treated with conservative surgery and primary radiation therapy for carcinoma of the breast. *Oncology Nursing Forum, 14* (Suppl.), Abstract No. 234.

Sheldon, T. A., Parker, L. M., & Cady, B. (1987). Management of locally advanced breast cancer. In J. R. Harris, S. Hellman, I. C. Henderson, & D. W. Kinne (Eds.), *Breast diseases* (pp. 563–570). Philadelphia: J. B. Lippincott Co.

Silverberg, E., Boring, C. C., & Squire, T. S. (1990). Cancer statistics, 1990. *CA: A Cancer Journal for Clinicians, 40,* 9–26.

Silvestrini, R., Daidone, M. G., DiFronzo, G., Morabito, A., Valagussa, P., & Bonadonna, G. (1986). Prognostic implication of labeling index versus estrogen receptors and tumor size in node negative breast cancer. *Breast Cancer Research and Treatment, 7,* 161–169.

Smalley, R. V., Bartolucci, A., Vogel, C., & Krauss, S. (1977). A comparison of cyclophosphamide, adriamycin, 5-flourouracil (CAF) and cyclophosphamide, methotrexate, 5-flourouracil, vincristine and prednisone (CMFVP) in patients with metastatic breast cancer. *Cancer, 40,* 625–632.

Snyderman, R. K. (1983). Breast reconstruction today. *Breast Cancer Research and Treatment, 3,* 5–13.

Spremulli, E. N., & Dexter, D. L. (1983). Human tumor cell heterogeneity and metastasis. *Journal of Clinical Oncology, 1,* 496–509.

Stillwell, G. K. (1969). Treatment of postmastectomy lymphedema. *Modern Treatment, 6,* 396–412.

Subramanian, V. P., Raich, P. C., & Walker, B. K. (1981). Weight gain in breast cancer patients undergoing chemotherapy. *Breast Cancer Research and Treatment, 1,* Abstract No. 170.

Swenerton, K. D., Legha, S. S., Smith, T., Hortobagyi, G. N., Gehan, E. A., Yap, H., Guttermne, J. U., & Blumenschein, G. R. (1979). Prognostic factors in metastatic breast cancer treated with combination chemotherapy. *Cancer Research, 39,* 1552–1562.

Tarpy, C., & Rothwell, S. (1983). Menses and related menopausal symptomatology of the breast cancer patient on chemotherapy. *Proceedings of the Oncology Nursing Society,* Abstract No. 15, p. 50.

Teeple, C. (1987). *Symptoms associated with primary radiation therapy for breast cancer: The six week experience.* Unpublished master's thesis, Yale University School of Nursing, New Haven, CT.

Thompson, L. (1983). The specialist nurse as a resource person and practitioner. Improving care for patients with breast cancer. *Proceedings of the Second European Conference on Clinical Oncology,* 22–41 (Abstract).

Tormey, D. C., & Jordan, V. G. (1984). Long term tamoxifen adjuvant therapy in node positive breast cancer: A metabolic and pilot clinical study. *Breast Cancer Research and Treatment, 4,* 297–302.

Tormey, D. C., Taylor, S. G., Kalish, L. A., Olsen, J. E., Grage, T., & Gray, R. (1984). Adjuvant systemic therapy in premenopausal (CMF, CMFP, CMFPT) and postmenopausal (observation, CMFP, CMFPT) women with node positive breast cancer. In S. E. Jones & S. E. Salmon (Eds.), *Adjuvant chemotherapy of cancer, IV* (pp. 359–368). Orlando, FL: Grune & Stratton, Inc.

Treves, N. (1957). Lymphedema after radical mastectomy. *Cancer, 10,* 444–459.

Trichopoulos, D., MacMahon, B., & Cole, P. (1968). Menopause and breast cancer risk. *Journal of the National Cancer Institute, 41,* 315–329.

Valagussa, P., Bonadonna, G., & Veronesi, U. (1978). Patterns of relapse and survival following radical mastectomy. *Cancer, 41,* 1170–1178.

Valagussa, P., Brambilla, C., & DiFronzo, G. (1989). Adjuvant CMF in node-negative (N−) and estrogen receptor negative (ER−) breast cancer: Updated results. *Proceedings of the American Society for Clinical Oncology,* No. 75, Abstract 8, p. 21.

Veronesi, U., Saccozzi, R., DelVecchio, M., Banfi, A., Clemente, C., & Delena, M. (1981). Comparing radical mastectomy and quantrantectomy, axillary dissection and radiotherapy in patients with small cancers of the breast. *New England Journal of Medicine, 305,* 6–11.

Wellisch, D. K., Jamison, K. R., & Pasnau, R. O. (1978). Psychosocial aspects of mastectomy II. The man's perspective. *American Journal of Psychiatry, 135,* 543–546.

Wiley, R. R. (1981). Postbiopsy care. *American Journal of Nursing '81,* 1660–1662.

Wilson, R. E. (1984a). Evaluation of the woman with a breast mass. In C. H. Pfeiffer & J. B. Mulliken (Eds.), *Caring for the patient with breast cancer* (pp. 21–35). Reston, VA: Reston Publishing.

Wilson, R. E. (1984b). Surgical management of locally advanced and recurrent breast cancer. *Cancer, 53,* 752–757.

Winningham, M. L., & MacVicar, M. G. (1988). The effect of aerobic exercise on patient reports of nausea. *Oncology Nursing Forum, 15,* 447–450.

Winningham, M. L., MacVicar, M. G., Bondoc, M., Anderson, J. I., & Minton, J. P. (1989). Effect of aerobic exercise on body weight and composition in patients with breast cancer on adjuvant chemotherapy. *Oncology Nursing Forum, 16,* 683–689.

Wood, W. C., Weiss, R. B., Tormey, D. C., Holland, J. F., Henry, P. H., Leone, L. A., Rafla, S., Silver, R. T., Carey, R. W., Lesnick, G. J., Weinberg, V. E., & Korzun, A. (1985). A randomized trial of CMFVP as adjuvant chemotherapy in women with node positive stage II breast cancer: A CALGB study. *World Journal of Surgery, 9,* 714–718.

Wynder, E. L., & Rose, D. P. (1984). Diet and breast cancer. *Hospital Practice, 19,* 73–88.

Yanes, B., Ross, S., Yanes, B. S., et al. (1987). Treatment of hot flashes in patients with breast carcinoma. *Proceedings of the American Society for Clinical Oncology, 6,* 269 (Abstract).

Zeissler, R. H., Rose, G. B., & Nelson, P. A. (1972). Postmastectomy lymphedema: Late results of treatment in 385 patients. *Archives of Physical Medicine and Rehabilitation, 53,* 159–166.

Zelikowski, A., Manoach, M., Giler, S., & Urca, I. (1980). Lymphapress, a new pneumatic device for treatment of lymphedema of the limbs. *Lymphology, 13,* 68–73.

Lung Cancer

ADA M. LINDSEY

The incidence of lung cancer is continuing to increase at a rapid rate; approximately 149,000 new cases are diagnosed and 130,000 deaths are reported per year. Lung cancer remains the most common cause of cancer mortality for men, and in the United States, it has now surpassed breast cancer as a cause of death for women (Choi, Grillo, & Huberman, 1986; Silverberg, 1985). The prognosis for lung cancer patients remains poor. Most people have metastatic disease at the time of diagnosis; thus the 5-year survival rate is very low, less than 10 per cent (Choi et al., 1986; Olsen, Block, & Tobias, 1984).

There are two major classifications of bronchogenic carcinoma; small-cell lung cancer (SCLC) and non-small-cell lung cancer (non-SCLC). The non-SCLCs are further classified as squamous cell or epidermoid lung cancer, adenocarcinoma, and large-cell carcinoma. The ratio of incidence of non-SCLC to SCLC is 3 to 1. In the United States, the incidence of adenocarcinoma has increased, and that of squamous cell carcinoma has decreased (Reyes, Chua, & Aranha, 1987; Valaitis, Warren, & Gamble, 1981). The increase is occurring in both men and women, but women have a propensity for developing adenocarcinoma. Thus the increased incidence of lung cancer in women partially accounts for the change in relative frequency of adenocarcinoma.

RISK FACTORS AND INCIDENCE

The primary risk factor in the development of bronchogenic carcinoma is longer total exposure to cigarette smoking (including number of cigarettes smoked, age when smoking began, duration of smoking, and tar and nicotine content of cigarettes smoked) (Table 31–1) (Loeb, Ernster, Warner, et al., 1984; Stayner & Wegman, 1983). The population at greatest risk for developing lung cancer are male smokers older than

45 years of age. Although the majority of lung cancer incidence occurs in those older than 50 years of age, the greatest prevalence of lung cancer is observed in those 65 years of age or older (Flehinger, Melamed, Zaman, et al., 1984; Fontana, Sanderson, Taylor, et al., 1984; Frost, Ball, Levin, et al., 1984; Loeb et al., 1984).

Data available suggest that in addition to cigarette smoking, industrial and environmental pollutants are risk factors for lung cancer development. Other carcinogenic substances associated with increased risk include asbestos, ionizing radiation, hydrocarbons, chromium, and nickel (Filderman, Shaw, & Matthay, 1986; Frank, 1982). Asbestos exposure in cigarette smokers increases the risk of lung cancer 80 to 90 times (Craighead & Mossman, 1982). Older men and women who have been smoking at least a pack of cigarettes a day for most of their lives and men and women who have been exposed to cigarette smoking and occupational or environmental carcinogens are at risk for developing lung cancer. These individuals remain at risk even after the exposure is removed because the development of lung cancer is a long-term process.

A smoker's risk of developing lung cancer decreases from a sixteenfold to about a fivefold increase approximately 5 years after cessation of smoking and in 15 years approaches the risk of developing lung cancer for those who have never smoked (Doll & Hill, 1964). Thus following cessation of smoking, the risk of de-

Table 31–1. RISK FACTORS IN DEVELOPMENT OF LUNG CANCER

Cigarette smoking
Industrial and environmental pollutants
  Asbestos
  Ionizing radiation
  Hydrocarbons
  Metals (e.g., nickel, silver, chromium)
  Chloromethyl ethers

veloping lung cancer progressively decreases for 10 to 15 years. The role of passive smoking in the development of lung cancer in nonsmokers was studied by pooling data from three large investigations. The risk was greater for older women whose husbands were heavy smokers; the histologic types of cancer that occurred were squamous and small-cell carcinomas (Dalager et al., 1986).

The rates of lung cancer are higher among those who consume alcohol and those in the lower socioeconomic groups. Because cigarette smoking and alcohol consumption are associated with greater risk for development of (lung) cancer, Marino and Levy (1986) proposed health promotion as a requisite for primary cancer prevention in pediatric practice.

Considerable interest has been shown in the role of diet in the prevention of cancer and the inhibition of tumor growth. Although some specific dietary constituents have been associated with some cancers, very little evidence supports any dietary constituent as having a preventive role in lung cancer development (Colditz, Stampfer, & Willett, 1987). However, there may be some protective effect from daily dietary intake of green and yellow vegetables (Palgi, 1984). Refer to Chapter 12 for more detail on the causes of cancer.

Trends in lung cancer incidence and mortality show a continual increase. The incidence is almost double that of two decades ago. The current annual lung cancer incidence rate is 90 men and 31 women per 100,000 (Choi et al., 1986). In 1985, lung cancer resulted in approximately 125,000 deaths (Silverberg, 1985). In the year 2000, projections indicate the diagnosis of 300,000 new cases. Partial explanations for this increase include an increase in the number of women who smoke, increased exposure to carcinogens in natural and occupational environments, more sophisticated diagnostic techniques, and more accurate classification. Reviews of current information about lung cancer have been published (Choi et al., 1986; Ershler, Socinski, & Greene, 1982; Filderman & Matthay, 1985; Filderman et al., 1986; Geddes, 1979; Hande & Des Prez, 1984).

Nurses can assist in the identification of individuals at risk for lung cancer and can encourage them to engage in disease prevention behaviors, for example, to stop smoking, or to change jobs or minimize occupational environmental risks. The nurse also can educate these individuals and their families about risk factors for development of lung cancer and can provide follow-up consultation and surveillance to ensure that these individuals take advantage of early detection and screening programs.

HISTOLOGIC TYPES

Small-Cell Lung Cancer

Approximately 20 to 25 per cent of lung cancers are histologically classified as small-cell carcinoma. This type of cancer and squamous cell cancer are most frequently linked with cigarette smoking. Approxi-

mately 80 per cent of these tumors are located centrally and submucosally. Small-cell cancer is the most aggressive type of lung cancer; it spreads rapidly to submucosal vessels and regional lymph nodes (Yesner & Carter, 1982). Small-cell cancer has a cell doubling time of approximately 30 days (Table 31–2) (Bone & Balk, 1982). Thus at the time of diagnosis, 70 to 90 per cent of the patients have extensive metastatic disease (Yesner & Carter, 1982). Owing to the frequent occurrence of micrometastases, SCLC is considered to be a systemic disease at diagnosis (Hande & Des Prez, 1982). A survival rate of more than 1 year is more likely for those with limited disease. Prognosis and survival remain poor even in the few patients with SCLC who present with limited disease and have had surgical resection. The failure of curative resection results from the presence of undetectable, subclinical metastases. Although SCLC cells are quite sensitive to irradiation, failure with radiation therapy also occurs due to the presence of occult metastases. Thus considering that SCLC is usually disseminated at the time of diagnosis, chemotherapy is usually the first treatment of choice. Although the response to treatment with multiple agents is high initially, the duration of the response is short (6 to 8 months). Because of the frequent central location of the tumor, compression of the bronchial lumen may occur. The occurrence of paraneoplastic syndromes is more frequent with this tumor type (Carr, 1981; Hansen & Pedersen, 1986; Lindsey, Piper, & Carrieri, 1981). Examples of paraneoplastic syndromes that occur with SCLC include Cushing's syndrome (ectopic production of adrenocorticotropin hormone by malignant lung tissue that stimulates excess production of adrenal gland glucocorticoids) and syndrome of inappropriate antidiuretic hormone secretion (ectopic production of antidiuretic hormone by malignant lung tissue) (see "Clinical Manifestations").

Squamous Cell Carcinoma

Squamous cell carcinoma currently represents about 30 to 35 per cent of all lung cancers. The majority of these tumors also occur centrally but are seen anywhere in the lung. Because of the central location and the tendency for local invasion, bronchial obstruction does occur. There is also a tendency for ulceration and bleeding with squamous cell carcinoma. This type of cancer is much more frequent in males; approximately 90 per cent of the cases are seen in men. The cell doubling time is approximately 100 days, and early

Table 31–2. HISTOLOGIC TYPES OF LUNG CANCER

Histologic Cell Type	Percentage of Lung Cancers	Cell Doubling Time (days)
Small cell	20–25	30
Non-small cell		
Squamous cell	30–35	100
Adenocarcinoma	33	180
Large-cell carcinoma	10–15	100

metastases are less common than is invasion of local structures (see Table 31–2) (Bone & Balk, 1982). This histologic type is more prone to cavitation. Squamous cell carcinoma occurs in areas in which the bronchial epithelium has been chronically damaged (Gazdar, Carney, & Minna, 1983; Yesner & Carter, 1982).

Patients may present with obstructive atelectasis, pneumonitis, and/or hemoptysis (Filderman & Matthay, 1985). The tumor may also impinge on other thoracic structures such as the mediastinum, chest wall, ribs, or diaphragm. An inflammatory response and an early positive sputum cytologic evaluation are common findings; these sometimes are observed before changes appear in the chest radiograph (Woolner, Fontana, & Cortese, 1984; Yesner & Carter, 1982).

Adenocarcinoma

Adenocarcinoma is now the most common type of lung cancer in some geographic areas. This increase in incidence is attributable in part to the increased incidence of lung cancer in women and in part to changes in histologic criteria for diagnosis. Adenocarcinoma represents about 33 per cent of all bronchogenic cancers (Valaitis et al., 1981). These tumors frequently are small and occur peripherally. Adenocarcinoma is seen in areas of previous pulmonary damage with fibrosis, or it may arise from bronchial glands or peripheral mucosa. As a result of its origin, mucin production is frequent (Mathews, McKay, & Lukeman, 1983). The cell doubling time is approximately 180 days (see Table 31–2) (Bone & Balk, 1982). Adenocarcinoma is most often detected by a routine chest radiograph; at the time of diagnosis, patients frequently are asymptomatic (Mathews et al., 1983). However, adenocarcinoma has a tendency toward early metastasis, and approximately 40 per cent of patients are considered to have unresectable tumor at the time of diagnosis. Due to the more common peripheral location of this tumor type, an early positive sputum cytologic finding is rare.

Large-Cell Carcinoma

Large-cell carcinomas are extremely undifferentiated forms of other types of lung cancer. About 10 to 15 per cent of lung tumors are categorized as large-cell carcinoma. Because tumors with unclear differentiation may be classified as large-cell carcinoma, this percentage may be an overestimate of the actual incidence. Usually they are large, bulky, peripheral tumors, and they can occur in any part of the lung. They are known to mimic other types of lung cancer. The cell doubling time is approximately 100 days (see Table 31–2) (Bone & Balk, 1982). Early invasion of the mediastinum and central nervous system occurs.

Non-Small-Cell Lung Cancers

Non-small-cell lung cancers represent three (squamous cell, adenocarcinoma, large-cell carcinoma) of the four histologic groups of lung cancer; 70 to 80 per cent of the lung cancers can be classified into these three subgroups. If these tumors are localized, surgery is the treatment of choice; however, in only a small percentage of the cases (10 to 15 per cent) are the tumors considered to be surgically resectable at the time of diagnosis. The 5-year survival rate for those few judged to have operable tumors is approximately 30 to 40 per cent. Because most patients with lung cancer have disseminated disease at the time of diagnosis, chemotherapy is used as the major treatment modality.

The remaining lung cancers, about 5 per cent, are classified as relatively uncommon types, such as carcinoid tumors and mucoepidermoid lung cancer. Mixed histologic types of lung cancer have been found on examination of tumor specimens. Recent evidence supports the idea that all types of lung tumors may have a common stem cell origin. Mixed cell tumors are thought to be the result of the secondary development of different cell types (Yesner & Carter, 1982). Some tumors may undergo differentiation, for example, small cell to adenocarcinoma or squamous cell lung cancer (Carney, 1986).

In addition to histologic classification, tumors may be characterized as endocrine or non-endocrine producing and by the biologic marker or markers expressed. The histologic cell type, degree of differentiation, and paraneoplastic expression are related to prognosis.

CLINICAL MANIFESTATIONS

The presenting clinical manifestations for lung cancer diagnosis are diverse because they may be due to one or more of the following: the primary tumor; metastatic involvement, either local or distant; or systemic, paraneoplastic expression. Some patients who are asymptomatic are diagnosed with lung cancer following a routine chest radiograph. Approximately 15 per cent of those with lung cancer are asymptomatic at diagnosis (Filderman & Matthay, 1985).

Clinical manifestations caused by local involvement of proximal airways include coughing, hemoptysis, dyspnea, and vague chest pain. Coughing occurs as a symptom of lung cancer in about 40 per cent of cases; however, it may also be due to the chronic bronchitis frequently seen in those with a history of cigarette smoking. A change in an existing cough should be determined. Infection may occur if clearance of mucous secretions from airways is impaired. In lung cancer, a developing cough or a change in cough may be the result of a central airway obstruction or a bronchial mucosal ulceration.

In more than half the cases, hemoptysis is the initial symptom of lung cancer. Dyspnea also commonly occurs and is associated with increased coughing and sputum production. Dyspnea may be the result of atelectasis distal to the tumor. Dyspnea is a subjective symptom defined as difficult, uncomfortable breathing. Dyspnea may occur at any point along the disease continuum; it may be present at diagnosis or may begin later with advancing disease. Obstructive tumors, pleural effusions, pneumonitis, and cachexia are among the factors contributing to dyspnea. In a study of 30 lung cancer patients experiencing dyspnea, Brown and colleagues (1986) reported that these patients had significant dyspnea and felt extreme fatigue. Over an 8-week period, their activity decreased significantly due to progressive weakness associated with disease progression (Box 31–1 presents a summary of this study). Foote and colleagues (1986) described nursing therapies that may be useful in ameliorating the discomforts of dyspnea. These include relaxation, planning for activity, body positioning, and instruction in breathing techniques.

Lung cancer can occlude airways and invade or compress blood vessels. Wheezing, usually localized unilaterally, is due to airway obstruction from the tumor, but wheezing is an infrequent complaint. Most commonly, lung cancer involves the central airways; only about 20 per cent occurs in the periphery. Frequently patients present with atelectasis.

Weight loss is a clinical feature characteristic of lung cancer. At the time of diagnosis, weight loss for the preceding 6 months is an important factor in determining prognosis. The survival time of patients who have sustained a 5 per cent weight loss is significantly shorter than that of patients who have not experienced a weight loss (Chlebowski, Heber, & Block, 1983; Costa et al., 1981; DeWys, Begg, Lavin, et al., 1980). In one large study, 57 per cent of the SCLC patients and 61 per cent of the non-SCLC patients had experienced weight loss in the preceding 6 months; the median survival time of those who presented with weight loss was approximately 2 months less than that of those who presented without weight loss (DeWys et al., 1980). Decreased dietary intake was shown to account for weight loss during chemotherapy for SCLC patients (Lindsey & Piper, 1985). A case study of a patient with SCLC who showed progressive weight loss is reported by Lindsey and colleagues (1982). Weight loss as one component of cancer cachexia is described elsewhere (Lindsey, 1986a, 1986b; Lindsey, Piper, & Stotts, 1982).

As many as 40 per cent of patients present with chest pain described as being a nonspecific, dull intermittent ache that is on the same side as the tumor. (Spiro, 1984). Chest pain associated with a rib or pleuritic pain is indicative of metastatic disease. Pancoast's tumor, which grows in the apex of the lung, may cause shoulder pain (described later).

Extension of the tumor to the pleural surface of the

Box 31–1. PERCEPTIONS OF DYSPNEA

STUDY

Brown, M. L., Carrieri, V. L., Janson-Bjerklie, S., & Dodd, M. J. (1986). **Lung cancer and dyspnea: The patient's perception.** *Oncology Nursing Forum, 13*(5), 19–24.

PURPOSES

To determine and describe patterns of dyspnea sensation; to identify coping and adaptive strategies used by lung cancer patients; to determine the relationship between activity and dyspnea.

SAMPLE

Thirty adults (17 males, 13 females) experiencing dyspnea with lung cancer. The mean age was 63 years; the mean smoking history was 60 pack years.

PROCEDURES

The patients were interviewed twice over a 2-month interval. They completed the following questionnaires: American Thoracic Society Respiratory Disease Questionnaire, Grade of Breathlessness Scale, Dyspnea Visual Analog Scale, and Karnofsky Performance Scale. Data from the patients' medical records included type and stage of lung cancer and treatment.

MAJOR FINDINGS

- Patients experienced significant dyspnea and extreme fatigue.
- Patients experienced loss of concentration and memory when short of breath.
- Patients experienced loss of appetite when short of breath.
- Degree of breathlessness did not change over the 2-month interval.
- Activity decreased significantly with progressive weakness and advancing malignancy.
- Patients were able to describe both short- and long-term strategies for managing dyspnea.

lung results in a pleural effusion. Usually the amount of the effusion is large; unless treatment yields significant tumor regression, the fluid rapidly reaccumulates following removal of the fluid.

At the time of diagnosis, the majority of lung cancer patients have either regional or distant metastases and will seek health care for symptoms occurring as a result of the metastases. An example is hoarseness. It occurs secondary to involvement of the left recurrent laryngeal nerve at the left hilum.

A potentially life-threatening syndrome occurs with superior vena cava obstruction, and it requires treatment. Patients present with upper hemibody edema, appearance of collateral venous circulation on upper body, and increased jugular venous pressure (Sculier et al., 1986). The syndrome occurs secondary to peritracheal lymphadenopathy and results in compression of the great veins that drain the head and upper trunk. It is seen more often in patients with SCLC; it occurs in approximately 7 to 12 per cent of the cases. Because of the anatomic location of the superior vena cava, the preponderance is in those with tumors in the right lung. The symptoms include severe headache occurring with cough, blackouts after bending or on rising, dyspnea, and dysphagia. General facial puffiness and periorbital edema may occur. Emergency treatment directed at relieving the edema is required. Diuretics and dexamethasone have been used, but treatment of the tumor by radiation, chemotherapy, or both may be the most useful.

Cancer occurring in the lung apex (superior sulcus) may invade the brachial nerve roots; this extension is associated with brachial neuritis. Pancoast described the syndrome associated with tumors involving the superior (apical) sulcus. Patients present with pain, wasting of muscles of the hand, and Horner's syndrome. If the eighth cervical and first thoracic segments of the sympathetic nerve trunk are involved, symptoms indicating Horner's syndrome are observed (Cohen, 1982). These include a small pupil, partial ptosis of the eyelid, enophthalmos, and ipsilateral absence of thermal sweating on the face.

Tumor extension through the pericardium results in pericarditis and abnormalities in cardiac rhythm. Cardiac output may be diminished if the tumor causes a pericardial effusion.

Local spread of lung cancer occurs initially in the hilar glands and usually is present at diagnosis. Metastatic involvement of peritrachael and subcarinal nodes is evident at diagnosis in a third or more of the patients, and spread to supraclavicular lymph nodes and deep cervical chain nodes is observed in about 20 per cent of the patients. Metastatic involvement results in symptomatic disease. Older patients at diagnosis have less incidence of metastatic disease, and a significant decrease in frequency of metastatic disease has been reported in studies of elderly lung cancer patients. (Ershler et al., 1982; Suen, Lau, & Yermakov, 1974).

Evidence of systemic disease or the distant effects of lung cancer include lymph node, bone, liver, and central nervous system metastases and paraneoplastic phenomena. Neurologic involvement from intracere-

bral metastases may be the presenting pathology for lung cancer; complaints include headache and unsteadiness or difficulty in walking.

Some patients present with bone pain; the ribs, vertebrae, humerus, and femoral bones are those with the most frequent occurrence of metastases. Pathologic fractures may be the presenting symptom. Bone marrow involvement occurs in 25 to 50 per cent of cases of SCLC (Carney & Minna, 1982; Muss, Jackson, Richard, et al., 1984) (see also Chapter 14.)

Symptoms of hepatic metastases occur later; only a few patients newly diagnosed with lung cancer have indications of liver involvement. The usual changes include an increasingly firm, irregular, enlarged liver. If the metastases are small and isolated, liver function tests will remain in the normal range. Jaundice and anorexia may occur. Early liver involvement may be observed more commonly in those with SCLC of the bronchus.

Ectopic hormone secretion has been associated with lung cancer. Some patients present with endocrine-related pathologies such as Cushing's syndrome that result from increased ectopic secretion of adrenocorticotropic hormone from the lung tumor. This syndrome occurs in about 5 per cent of the cases of SCLC. A case study of an SCLC patient presenting with Cushing's syndrome as a result of ectopic production of adrenocorticotropic hormone has been reported by Lindsey and colleagues (1981). Another endocrine-related syndrome seen particularly in patients with SCLC that results from ectopic hormone production by the tumor is the syndrome of inappropriate antidiuretic hormone secretion (SIADH). It occurs in 5 to 10 per cent of the cases of SCLC. These patients present with high urine osmolality, low serum sodium, and plasma osmolality reflecting a retention of fluid; they may show confusion, lethargy, or other mental disturbances. The presence of SIADH is associated with a poor prognosis. Hypercalcemia may occur as a result of ectopic secretion of parathyroid hormone from squamous cell lung cancer. Hypercalcemia usually occurs in association with a large tumor mass. These paraneoplastic syndromes are most commonly seen with SCLC but do occur with other lung cancers (Carr, 1981; Neal, Kosinski, Cohen, & Orenstein, 1986).

Clubbing of the fingers occurs in up to a third of the cases of lung cancer; it is observed more frequently in patients with squamous cell tumors.

An osteitis may occur during the course of lung cancer. The distal parts of the radius, ulna, tibia, and fibula are the most frequently involved bones. Swelling, erythema, and tenderness occur with the symmetric proliferation of subperiosteal tissue of the wrists and ankle joints. This condition is referred to as hypertrophic pulmonary osteoarthropathy. It is seen more frequently with squamous cell carcinoma.

Benedict (1989) reported on her study designed to determine the incidence of suffering associated with lung cancer (Box 31–2 presents a summary of this study). Only 10 per cent of her sample of 30 adults with primary pulmonary malignancies reported no suffering, whereas 50 per cent indicated "very much"

Box 31–2. LUNG CANCER AND SUFFERING

STUDY

Benedict, S. (1989). **The suffering associated with lung cancer.** *Cancer Nursing, 12,* 34–40.

PURPOSE

To determine the incidence of suffering associated with lung cancer.

SAMPLE

Thirty adults (26 males, 4 females) with primary pulmonary malignancy. The mean age was 60 years (range 43 to 74); the mean smoking history was 50 pack years.

PROCEDURES

The patients participated in a structured interview that included questions about physical, psychological, and interactional aspects of cancer. Suffering was rated on a 5-point Likert-type scale for each of the aspects under study.

MAJOR FINDINGS

- Ten per cent of the patients experienced no suffering.
- Fifty per cent of the patients experienced very much suffering.
- Suffering was statistically greater in those patients with known metastatic disease versus those with no known metastatic disease.
- The sources of greatest suffering were disability, pain, anxiety, changed daily activities, weakness, and fatigue.

---

suffering. There was a statistically significant difference in the amount of suffering associated with psychological aspects between those with known metastatic disease and those with no known metastatic disease. Disability, pain, anxiety, changed daily activities, and weakness and fatigue were reported as the sources of greatest suffering (see Box 31–2). The suffering associated with physical aspects was found to be greater than that reported for psychological and for interactional aspects of the lung cancer experience.

These findings have implications for nursing care. First, it is important to recognize the high incidence of suffering experienced by lung cancer patients and the fact that more suffering is associated with the physical aspects of the disease. If the sources of greatest suffering are made explicit, such as from disability, pain, or weakness and fatigue, the nurse can provide suggestions or nursing actions for the patient and family that may alleviate or ameliorate the sources of suffering. For example, the nurse can discuss and arrange for analgesic administration that allows the patient to be functional but also relieves the pain.

In addition to detection of symptoms of lung cancer and assessment and surveillance of the progression or regression of these symptoms, the nurse has a major responsibility for assisting the patient with symptom management. Examples include suggesting that the patient limit activity; assisting the patient with essential activity when pain and dyspnea are most severe; providing for nutritional intake when the patient is most comfortable; and providing small amounts of high-calorie, high-protein food frequently when anorexia is present. Provision of oxygen and instruction in breathing techniques may be required. Nursing care is based on the specific clinical manifestations that the patient experiences, and these include a range from local to systemic manifestations.

SCREENING

Early detection through large screening programs has shown only very limited success in reducing mortality. In the Mayo Lung Project, 9211 male smokers who were older than 45 years of age were followed from 1972 to 1982 (Woolner, Fontana, Sanderson et al., 1981). The control group had an annual chest radiograph, and a sputum specimen was collected for cytologic study; the close surveillance group had the same screening every 4 months. At the time of the report (1982), 78 in the control group and 109 in the close surveillance group were diagnosed with lung cancer. The great majority were diagnosed by chest radiograph. Despite the screening effort, only about half were determined to have operable disease at the time of diagnosis. The conclusion from this long-term screening project is that the detection of new cases of lung cancer is low compared with the expense involved.

Results of a large cooperative screening project (National Cancer Institute Cooperative Early Lung

Cancer Detection Programs) indicated that chest radiographs and sputum cytologic evaluations were both useful (Melamed et al., 1984). The central squamous cell cancers were detected by cytologic studies, whereas the peripheral large-cell carcinomas and adenocarcinomas were detected by chest radiographs. Less than 10 per cent of the cancers were detected simultaneously by both screening procedures.

For detection of lung cancer on radiograph, the tumor must be in the range of 1 cm in diameter. This size requires 30 doublings, by which time metastases have occurred (Geddes, 1979). Thus early detection of lung cancer by chest radiographic screening is unlikely. At 40 doublings, the tumor burden usually results in death (Bone & Balk, 1982).

TUMOR MARKERS

The production of ectopic hormones by some lung cancers has been reported for years; however, no marker has yet been identified that can be used for screening for lung cancer (Hansen & Pedersen, 1986; Lindsey et al., 1981). Although it is not yet possible to use tumor markers to diagnose or specify the tumor burden of lung cancer in individual patients, the measurement levels in groups of patients have been correlated with stage of disease. With tumor regression from treatment, the levels of tumor markers are observed to decrease. A number of tumor markers have been measured in serum specimens from SCLC patients; these include adrenocorticotropic hormone, antidiuretic hormone, oxytocin, carcinoembryonic antigen, and calcitonin. Patients with SCLC have higher levels of ectopic hormone and other peptides than do patients with other histologic types of lung cancer. Levels of two enzymes, neuron-specific enolase and creatine kinase BB, have been found to be elevated in patients with untreated SCLC (Akoun, Scarna, Milleron, Benichoun, & Herman, 1985; Carney, Zweig, Ihde, et al., 1984; Johnson et al., 1984). Studies reporting incidence of ectopic hormone and other peptide production in SCLC patients are reviewed elsewhere (Hansen & Pedersen, 1986). Measurement of tumor markers in the cerebral spinal fluid of lung cancer patients with the derivation of a ratio of cerebral spinal fluid and plasma concentrations has been suggested as a potential means for determining the presence of brain metastases.

DIAGNOSIS

Diagnostic techniques include the use of chest radiographs, sputum cytologic evaluations, fiberoptic bronchoscopy and transthoracic needle aspiration biopsy to obtain tissue specimens, and computed tomographic (CT) scans (Loke, Matthay, & Ieda, 1982). The diagnosis of lung cancer must be histologically or cytologically confirmed from tissue or sputum specimens, respectively. Centrally located tumors have a higher percentage of positive sputum cytologic evaluations than do peripherally located tumors. For the most accurate diagnostic results, a series of three or four sputum specimens should be collected and subjected to cytologic examination. Bronchoscopy is also useful in diagnosing centrally located tumors. Bronchoscopy done with a fiberoptic instrument passed through a nostril is a common diagnostic procedure. It is used for visualization of the tracheobronchial tree, including access to upper lobes, and for obtaining bronchial biopsy specimens and brushings. Tumor tissue can also be obtained through the use of bronchial needle aspiration technique. Transthoracic needle biopsies are most useful for diagnosing the more peripherally located tumors and for obtaining pleural and mediastinal tissue (Wang & Terry, 1983). Because pneumothorax is a complication of transthoracic needle biopsies, observation for this problem is critical.

Computed tomography is an important adjunct to chest radiographs in the diagnosis of lung cancer; it is particularly useful in evaluating the mediastinal lymph node involvement and the extent of disease (Heitzman, 1986). It is most helpful in the staging of bronchogenic carcinoma, for example, in the identification of metastases in the central nervous system or other extrapulmonary sites. Computed tomography and radiographs are also used in evaluating the response to therapy. The use of CT in lung cancer diagnosis and management is reviewed elsewhere (Heitzman, 1986). The most sensitive imaging technique for detecting bone metastases is the radionuclide bone scan (Waxman, 1986). Bone metastases are seen at diagnosis for approximately 40 per cent of the patients with SCLC but only 10 per cent of those with non-SCLC.

The nurse should describe the specifically ordered diagnostic procedures to the patient and family; this description should include what will occur and what the patient is to do. Again, assessment and surveillance for recovery or complications following the specific procedures are the nurse's responsibility.

STAGING

Staging follows the diagnosis and histologic classification of lung cancer. Extensive efforts have been directed to accurate staging of lung cancer because selection of treatment and subsequent survival are predicated on accurate assessment of the extent of tumor involvement. There is a high correlation between tumor metastases and prognostic survival.

For non-SCLCs, the TNM (tumor, node, metastasis) classification is used for staging (Table 31–3). The T subscript reflects the extent of the primary tumor, the N subscript reflects the absence or presence of lymph node (hilar or mediastinal) involvement, and the M subscript reflects the existence of distant metastases. For stage III, T_3, N_2, and M_1 are the most important criteria (Choi et al., 1986).

For SCLC, the limited or extensive classifications are used more frequently for staging than the TNM system. Limited classification refers to tumors that are confined to the ipsilateral hemithorax; extensive clas-

Table 31–3. TNM CLASSIFICATION FOR STAGING NON-SMALL-CELL LUNG CANCERS

Stage	Tumor	Node	Metastasis
I	T_1	N_0	M_0
	T_1	N_1	M_0
	T_2	N_0	M_0
II	T_2	N_1	M_0
III	T_3	N_{0-2}	M_{0-1}
	T_{1-3}	N_2	M_{0-1}
	T_{1-3}	N_{0-2}	M_1

Key: T_1 = 3.0 cm or less in diameter without evidence of invasion

T_2 = more than 3.0 cm in diameter or any size with invasion of visceral pleura or associated atelectasis or pneumonitis extending to hilar region

T_3 = any size tumor with direct extension to adjacent structure

N_0 = no demonstrable metastasis

N_1 = metastasis to peribronchial or ipsilateral hilar lymph nodes

N_2 = metastasis to mediastinal lymph nodes

M_0 = no known distant metastasis

M_1 = distant metastasis

sification refers to tumors that have spread beyond the ipsilateral hemithorax and adjacent lymph nodes. The limited or extensive categories are more useful for SCLC because with the rapid extrathoracic spread of small-cell lung tumors, most would be classified as stage III at diagnosis. The prognosis for those classified as stage I or II is also poor due to the undetected micrometastases (Filderman et al., 1986). In staging for SCLC, bone marrow aspiration and biopsy may be performed because bone marrow involvement has been observed to occur in as many as 50 per cent of the cases (Muss et al., 1984).

For more accurate staging of lung cancer, CT scans are used. Direct tumor extension into mediastinal, pleural, or other structures is better identified with CT scans; for example, metastatic disease in the adrenal gland can be detected. If operability is a question, mediastinoscopy may be used for those with a positive CT scan of the mediastinum to confirm metastatic disease. A tissue sample is obtained to determine if mediastinal involvement is inflammatory or malignant. Using a mediastinoscopy, the presence or absence of mediastinal (paratrachael and subaortic) lymph node involvement is used to determine operability for lung cancer. Generally, a poor prognosis is associated with positive mediastinal nodes (Spiro, 1984). More extensive information about staging procedures is reviewed elsewhere (Bone & Balk, 1982; Feinstein & Wells, 1982; Filderman et al., 1986; Mountain, 1986; Tisi, Friedman, Peters, et al., 1983).

Another staging system has been proposed to better account for specific differences, such as extent and distance of lymph node involvement and histology (Tisi et al., 1983). The proposed new staging system for lung cancer has been described in detail (Mountain, 1986). This change has been proposed because differences in effectiveness of treatment and survival were observed in patients classified according to the original TNM staging. Variations in the extent and location of involvement showed differences in survival patterns within the original staging schema. These changes are important because of the implications for prognosis and choice of therapy. Those included in the new stage I have T_1 or T_2 tumors with no metastasis, and they have the best prognosis; the new stage II includes those with T_1 or T_2 tumors with intrapulmonary lymph node metastasis. Stage III has been divided into IIIA and IIIB groups, designating those considered to have operable disease (IIIA) and those considered to have inoperable disease (IIIB) because of more extensive extrapulmonary involvement, such as spread to the contralateral lymph nodes (mediastinal, hilar, supraclavicular, or scalene) or pleural effusion. Those with distant metastases are classified as stage IV.

The specific histologic cell type and the degree of differentiation are related to prognosis. Generally, those diagnosed with squamous cell carcinoma have a better prognosis than those with other types of lung cancer. Prognosis is associated not only with type of lung tumor but also with location and size of tumor, extent of spread, and absence of complications such as pleural effusion or paraneoplastic syndrome.

The prognosis for those with a small (<3.0 cm) peripheral tumor is better than for those with larger or more centrally located tumors (Mountain, 1983). The 5-year survival rate for those with metastatic disease in mediastinal lymph nodes or contralateral hilar or cervical nodes is 3 per cent, whereas it is about 30 per cent for those with no evidence of metastatic disease at the time of surgery. Performance status and weight also have been shown to be predictors of survival (DeWys et al., 1980; Feinstein & Wells, 1982).

TREATMENT

The management of lung cancer depends on the histologic cell type and the extent and pattern of invasion and spread. Generally, the treatment of lung cancer is not terribly effective. There is no really effective therapy for lung cancer patients with disseminated disease.

Surgery

If the mediastinal nodes are determined to be disease free, then surgery is usually the initial procedure. Functional or performance status is also considered in determining treatment. Surgery may be the choice of treatment when there is no evidence of metastatic spread beyond the ipsilateral hemithorax and when other patient characteristics, such as respiratory, cardiac, and cerebral status, are determined to be satisfactory for a favorable surgical outcome.

Surgery is the choice of treatment for patients with stage I or II non-SCLC. For tumor removal, segmental or wedge resections can be used to preserve lung tissue, but lobectomy or pneumonectomy is the more usual approach. The choice of procedure depends on location, size, and extent of tumor spread. Those being considered for surgical resection should have a forced expiratory volume in 1 second (FEV_1) greater than 2 liters and a predicted postpulmonary resection FEV_1 of 800 ml or greater (Olsen et al., 1984). This value is necessary to ensure adequate respiratory function following surgery, that is, to prevent respiratory insufficiency.

Before surgery, the nurse may have to assist the patient with airway clearance measures to improve ventilatory capacity. Examples of these measures are to teach the patient coughing and deep breathing techniques, to assist with postural drainage, or to provide for inhalation of aerosol solutions. Smoking cessation may be advised before surgery. If infection is present, antibiotic administration will be prescribed. Nursing actions include explanations about the surgical procedure and about what is expected after surgery. Postoperatively, the patient is likely to have mechanical ventilatory assistance for a short time, but positive pressure ventilation is discontinued to prevent or minimize stress to sutured tissues. Following extubation, coughing and deep breathing exercises are necessary; splinting the incision will help decrease the pain as will timing the exercises with analgesic administration. Position the individual to facilitate lung expansion.

Nursing care depends on the surgical procedure used. For example, with a lobectomy, chest tubes with a closed drainage system may be used, whereas following a pneumonectomy, chest tubes will be clamped to allow filling of the thoracic cavity to prevent mediastinal shift. Thus it is critical that the nurse knows what procedure has been done and understands the underlying physiologic alterations to determine the appropriate specific nursing actions.

Survival rate decreases as size of tumor increases. Thus for those with more extensive disease, the evidence of increased survival rate with surgery is more controversial. Those with stage I disease have an 80 per cent 1-year survival rate and a 50 per cent 5-year survival rate following surgical resection (Choi et al., 1986). Those with stage II disease have a 20 to 35 per cent 5-year survival rate; the success rate is associated with histologic type. The median survival of those with stage III disease is approximately 1 year following surgery. Because at the time of diagnosis, those with SCLC frequently have extensive intrathoracic disease and evidence of extrathoracic disease, surgical resection is not generally a choice (Baker, Ettinger, Ruckdeschel, Eggleston, & McKneally, 1987).

Surgical resection may be done for other than curative purposes; for example, tumor excision can prevent invasion of the chest wall or involvement of ribs and intercostal spaces, which can result in severe pain. Surgery may be used in conjunction with adjuvant radiation therapy or in combination with chemotherapy or with chemotherapy alone.

Pulmonary resection may not be possible for those who have coexisting chronic lung disease or compromised pulmonary function. For example, the elderly may have diminished pulmonary function. Wedge resection or sleeve resection may be used as an alternative to lobectomy in poor-risk patients.

From a review of prognostic factors for patients with inoperable lung cancer, the initial Karnofsky performance score, the extent of disease, and the weight loss in the preceding 6 months were the most important prognostic factors (Stanley, 1980).

Radiation Therapy

Radiation therapy is rarely curative for lung cancer, although a small percentage of patients survive 5 years following therapy. Initially, complete regression is seen in about half of those undergoing radiation therapy; however, there is a high incidence of local recurrence. The failure of radiation may be due to the presence of radio-resistant hypoxic tumor cells. Neutron therapy may be more effective against hypoxic cells; thus the combination of conventional cobalt-60 radiation and neutrons may improve control of local lung cancer. In the best circumstances, the 5-year cure rate using radiation therapy is only 10 to 15 per cent (Choi et al., 1986). Despite the local effectiveness of the radiation, the survival rate remains low because of distant metastatic involvement.

Radiation is more successful for those with small, peripheral, non-SCLC tumors with no evidence of metastases (Hande & Des Prez, 1982; Hoffman, Albain, Bitran, et al., 1984; Perez, Pajak, Rubin, Simpson, Mohiuddin, et al., 1987). Patients with limited squamous cell carcinoma are those for whom radiation therapy has been the most effective. Although SCLC is quite sensitive to radiation, chemotherapy is the first treatment of choice because of the high frequency of extrathoracic metastatic disease with this type of lung cancer. Primarily radiation is used for patients with unresectable tumors, for those with regional lymph node involvement, and for those with direct invasion of other thoracic structures. For increased effectiveness of the therapy, the patient should be able to tolerate a 6- to 7-week course of therapy.

Radiation therapy has also been used preoperatively and postoperatively, but the benefit at those times remains controversial (Filderman & Matthay, 1985). Following tumor resection, radiation therapy may be prescribed for patients who have tumor cells at tissue margins (Hande & Des Prez, 1982). Radiation may be preferable for those who have resectable tumors but who may not be able to tolerate surgery.

Radiotherapy may be used for palliation of symptoms that result from compression or infiltration of intrathoracic structures by the tumor. For example, it has been shown to improve atelectasis resulting from lung cancer. It is also employed for palliation in chest wall invasion and for relief of bone pain, intractable cough, dyspnea, and hemoptysis. Radiation is used to treat complications such as bronchial obstruction, superior vena cava syndrome, and rib invasion; it is also used prophylactically for possible central nervous system involvement (Cox, 1981).

Prophylactic brain irradiation has been used for those with adenocarcinoma of the lung, but there is no evidence of increased duration of survival (Filderman & Matthay, 1985). Evidence supports the use of prophylactic cranial irradiation for those SCLC patients who show complete remission. This prophylaxis is important because cerebral metastases can occur with relapse of SCLC. Radiation is also employed in the treatment of metastatic central nervous system involvement (Carney & Minna, 1982; Greco & Oldham, 1979). Prophylactic cranial irradiation has been shown to decrease incidence of cerebral metastases and to improve survival, but this improvement has not been statistically significant (Blechen, 1984).

Contraindications for the use of curative irradiation include inadequate respiratory reserve, pleural effusion, distant metastases, large tumor, weight loss greater than 4.5 kg, and a Karnofsky performance status of less than 70. These contraindications are similar to those that also exclude surgery as the choice of treatment.

Complications from radiation therapy increase as the dose increases and as the extent of normal tissue included in the field increases. For example, the incidence of fibrosis has been shown to increase with increased dose (Van Houtte, Piron, Lustman-Marechal, Osteaux, & Henry, 1980). Pulmonary fibrosis can result from permanent damage to the alveolar endothelium, and the extent of fibrosis is related to the amount of tissue irradiated. Some patients will experience dyspnea as a later consequence of this radiation-induced pulmonary fibrosis. Most patients usually have pulmonary fibrosis following chest radiation therapy but are asymptomatic. One complication that occurs 1 to 3 months after chest irradiation is pneumonitis; the patient experiences dyspnea and a nonproductive cough. Corticosteroids may be used for symptomatic relief, although the efficacy of this treatment is debatable; recovery usually occurs within a few weeks. Because of their effect on respiratory function, pneumonitis and fibrosis can influence the patient's quality of life (Wickham, 1986). If they are severe, respiratory complications may result in death.

Other complications are radiation-induced myelitis that occurs when protection of the spinal cord has been inadequate and pericarditis that results from inclusion of the heart in the irradiated field. Following postradiation dysphagia, long-term effects may be observed in the esophagus. Toxicities resulting from therapy have been described in detail elsewhere (Wickham, 1986).

Nurses have a role in explaining the use of radiation therapy and in helping the patient minimize the side effects, such as anorexia, nausea, and fatigue. Because the therapy requires long-term, almost daily treatment, it is important for the nurse to help the patient adhere to the scheduled therapy. The nurse also needs to be alert for clinical manifestations of the complications associated with radiation and to participate in the therapeutic management of the specific complication. It is important to understand that these complications may occur some time after radiation therapy has been completed.

Chemotherapy

Reviews of the effectiveness of chemotherapy in the treatment of SCLC and non-SCLC are reported else-where (Greco, Johnson, Hainsworth, & Wolff, 1985; Klastersky & Sculier, 1985; Livingston, 1986; Zinreich, Baker, Ettinger & Arder, 1984). The drugs most commonly used alone or in some combination for treatment of non-SCLC are doxorubicin, methotrexate, cyclophosphamide, cisplatin, etoposide (VP-16-213), and vindesine. An increase in survival time after using these agents is not yet well demonstrated. Most of the drugs in the chemotherapeutic regimen are associated with considerable side effects (morbidity).

Chemotherapy is the main treatment for SCLC. Chemotherapy is less effective for non-SCLCs, except that survival time has been observed to lengthen with the use of cisplatin. Small-cell lung cancer is more sensitive to chemotherapy than are non-SCLCs; however, the response occurs for only a short time, and relapse is frequent. The most effective agents include cyclophosphamide in combination with vincristine and doxorubicin, methotrexate, etoposide or (VePesid). Procarbazine, cisplatin, and lomustine (CCNU) are also used. Generally there is an initial response rate in 80 to 95 per cent of the patients, but prolonged survival occurs only in 2 to 12 per cent of the SCLC patients. For patients with limited disease, the median survival time is approximately 10 to 12 months (Carney & Minna, 1982); for those with extensive disease, it is even less—approximately 8 to 9 months (Hoffman et al., 1984).

Tumor resistance to the drugs occurs; in new trials, attempts are being made to include non-cross-reactive agents to delay tumor resistance. Sequencing different drug combinations is another strategy to delay drug resistance; however, failure occurs with the emergence of drug-resistant cells. Little evidence suggests that a truly non-cross-resistant drug regimen has been identified for successful therapy for SCLC (Livingston, 1986).

Autologous bone marrow infusion has been used to reestablish hematopoiesis when severe myelosuppression is a result of therapy. Monoclonal antibodies to SCLC can be used for in vitro removal of tumor cells from bone marrow when autologous transplantation is required for high-dose chemotherapy (Okabe, Kaizu, Fujisawa, Watanabe, & Takaku, 1985).

Trials have included the use of warfarin as an anticoagulant, based on the concept that further growth of metastases may be prohibited. The evidence to date shows no real survival benefit.

The major nursing care associated with chemotherapy frequently includes administration of the prescribed agents, assisting the patient in managing the side effects experienced, assessing for signs and symptoms of toxicities specific to the agents used, and monitoring patient responses. Again, as is true for radiation therapy, the nurse can play a role in helping the patient understand the principles of the therapy and the necessity for completing the prescribed treatment protocol.

Combination Therapy

Some investigators have shown improved complete response rates and survival using combination radiation therapy of the primary limited small-cell tumor along with chemotherapy (Choi, Carey, Kaufman, Grillo, Younger, & Wilkins, 1987; Perry, Eaton, Propert, Ware, Zimmer, et al., 1987). Response rates in the elderly being treated for SCLC are similar to the responses of others (Clamon, Audeh, & Pinnick, 1982).

The success of surgical adjuvant therapies for non-SCLC patients has been reviewed (Holmes, 1986). For those non-SCLC patients whose disease is considered inoperable, combined radiation therapy for control of locoregional involvement and chemotherapy for control of distant metastases are used. However, survival rates have not improved greatly; systemic recurrence remains a problem. Response rates to chemotherapy for those with advanced non-SCLC range from 25 to 40 per cent; for those whose disease is limited to the thorax, the response rates are 50 to 70 per cent. New active non-cross-resistant drugs need to be developed.

The most common first site of recurrence in patients treated for adenocarcinoma and large-cell undifferentiated carcinoma is extrapulmonary, usually the brain (Holmes, 1986). The most common first site of recurrence for squamous cell carcinoma is local; postoperative radiation therapy results in decreased incidence of local recurrence in patients with squamous cell cancer but has not been shown to prolong survival significantly (Holmes, 1986).

Immunotherapy

Lung cancer is an immunosuppressive disease; that is, some lung cancer patients have a depressed immune response, and lymphocytes that have infiltrated the tumor have depressed activity (Holmes, 1986). These immune system defects may contribute to the rapid disease progression. In a study of anorexia and immune response in patients with SCLC, the only patient who was alive 1 year after diagnosis remained responsive to two out of three skin test antigens (Lindsey & Piper, 1986). Despite attempts of treatment with immunotherapy, evidence remains controversial. Improvement in duration of survival after treatment with nonspecific immunoadjuvants has not been shown to occur (see Chapter 23 on biologic response modifiers for more detail).

Although monoclonal antibodies (MoAbs) have been made in response to lung cancer antigens, the antigenic and biologic heterogeneity of SCLC in particular results in the lack of antibody specificity and thus limits the utility of this approach for treatment (Carney, 1986). Monoclonal antibodies were used to demonstrate the presence of SCLC cells in bone marrow specimens that had been considered to be tumor free and to demonstrate bone marrow metastases in patients who had been determined clinically to have limited disease (Bernal & Speak, 1984). These antibodies have potential value in the preparation of bone marrow for autologous transplantation, because specific MoAbs lyse the SCLC cells that are present in the ex vivo bone marrow. The concept is that the creation of specific MoAbs or other biologic response modifiers has the potential to eliminate any residual microscopic drug-resistant cells; until these cells are eradicated, therapy remains ineffective in improving survival rates. Over the past two decades, little change has occurred in the survival rates for new lung cancer patients.

PSYCHOSOCIAL ASPECTS

Germino and McCorkle (1985) described the awareness of diagnosis, prognosis, and treatment in patients with a recent diagnosis of lung cancer compared with that of a group of patients with first-time myocardial infarction. The lung cancer patients were receiving radiation therapy. Those with cancer expressed higher, although not statistically significant, acknowledged awareness and symptom distress scores at 1 and 2 months after diagnosis. Lung cancer patients with higher symptom distress also expressed significantly higher acknowledged awareness.

Driever and McCorkle (1984) followed these same two groups of patients at 3 and 6 months after diagnosis to compare the concerns expressed at those times. They classified their concerns into four categories: patient status, patient activities, patient symptoms, and patient attitude. The concerns were then rated in a range from "doing well" to "doing poorly." Fifteen lung cancer patients responded at both 3 and 6 months. Lung cancer patients expressed greater severity (poorer) for patient status and symptoms, but both groups expressed a positive attitude overall. Box 31–3 presents a summary of this study.

Cooper studied 15 lung cancer patients and their spouses to determine the effects of the diagnosis on family relationships (Cooper, 1984). The spouses indicated that they did not share their fears and that they talked less often than they were perceived to by the patients. The majority of couples also showed a discrepancy in their perceptions of closeness in the marital relationships. The spouses expressed more signs of stress than did the patients. Although the sample size was small, Cooper provided some implications for practice, such as including the family as a focus for intervention; providing time to interact with family members for support, information, and opportunity to express concerns; and providing for further contact following hospital discharge (see also Chapter 5).

SUMMARY

In those who have no metastatic spread, non-SCLCs are potentially curable by surgery but are relatively resistant to chemotherapy and radiation. For those with SCLC, surgery is relatively ineffective due to the frequent existence of metastatic disease, but the tumor cells are responsive to radiation and chemotherapy. At the time of diagnosis, only about 20 per cent of lung cancer patients have localized tumor.

Box 31–3. PATIENT CONCERNS POSTDIAGNOSIS

STUDY

Driever, M. J., & McCorkle, R. (1984, June). **Patient concerns at 3 and 6 months postdiagnosis.** *Cancer Nursing, 7,* 235–241.

PURPOSE

To determine and compare the concerns expressed by patients with lung cancer or myocardial infarction at 3 and 6 months after diagnosis.

SAMPLE

Fifteen lung cancer patients; 29 myocardial infarction patients. There were 15 males and 29 females in the sample, and the age range extended from 31 to 83 years.

PROCEDURES

Two open-ended questions were asked during a telephone interview at 3 and 6 months after diagnosis: "How are things going?" and "How are you managing?" The concerns expressed by patients were classified into four categories: (1) patient status, (2) activities, (3) symptoms, and (4) attitude. The responses were judged on a four-point scale from doing well to doing poorly.

MAJOR FINDINGS

- Myocardial infarction patients reported doing better than did lung cancer patients.
- For the lung cancer patients, there was more variation in the reports on how they felt they were doing, the level and quality of their activities, the symptoms they experienced, and their outlook.
- The concerns expressed at 3 months after diagnosis were not significantly different at 6 months after diagnosis.

For those whose tumors do not respond to treatment, therapy is changed, and if the tumor remains unresponsive after different therapeutic regimens have been used, therapy may be withheld. (See Chapter 45 for more detailed descriptions of care.)

For some lung cancer patients with extensive disease, supportive care with antibiotics, analgesics, and bronchodilators may be the treatment of choice. For some, quality of life may be increased with symptom management rather than with aggressive anticancer therapy. For more information, see Chapter 28 on palliative support.

References

Akoun, G. M., Scarna, H. M., Milleron, B. H., Benichoun, M. R., & Herman, D. P. (1985). Serum neuron-specific enolase: A marker for disease extent and response to therapy for small cell lung cancer. *Chest, 87,* 39.

Baker, R. R., Ettinger, D. S., Ruckdeschel, J. D., Eggleston, J. C., McKneally, M. F., Abeloff, M. D., Woll, J., & Adelstein, D. J. (1987). The role of surgery in the management of selected patients with small-cell carcinoma of the lung. *Journal of Clinical Oncol, 5,* 697–702.

Benedict, S. (1989). The suffering associated with lung cancer. *Cancer Nursing, 12,* 34–40.

Bernal, S., & Speak, J. A. (1984). Membrane antigen in small cell carcinoma of the lung defined by monoclonal antibody SMI. *Cancer Research, 44,* 266–270.

Blechen, N. M. (1984). Management of small cell cancer: Radio therapy. In W. Duncan (Ed.), *Recent results in cancer research: Lung cancer* (pp. 65–78). New York: Springer-Verlag.

Bone, R. C., & Balk, R. (1982). Staging of bronchogenic carcinoma. *Chest, 82,* 473–480.

Brown, M. L., Carrieri, V. L., Janson-Bjerklie, S., & Dodd, M. J. (1986). Lung cancer and dyspnea: The patient's perception. *Oncology Nursing Forum, 13*(5), 19–24.

Carney, D. N. (1986). Recent advances in the biology of small cell lung cancer. *Chest, 89*(4 Suppl.), 253S–257S.

Carney, D. N., & Minna, J. D. (1982). Small cell cancer of the lung. *Clinics in Chest Medicine, 3,* 389–398.

Carney, D. N., Zweig, M. H., Ihde, D. C., Cohen, M. H., Makuch, R. W., & Gazdor, A. F. (1984). Elevated serum creatine kinase BB levels in patients with small cell lung cancer. *Cancer Research, 44,* 5399–5403.

Carr, D. T. (1981). Malignant lung disease. *Hospital Practice, 17,* 97–115.

Chlebowski, R. T., Heber, D., & Block, J. B. (1983). Lung cancer cachexia. In F. A. Greco (Ed.), *Biology and management of lung cancer* (pp. 125–142). Boston: Martinus Nijhoff Publishers.

Choi, N. C., Carey, R. W., Kaufman, S. D., Grillo, H. C., Younger, J., & Wilkins, E. W. (1987). Small cell carcinoma of the lung. *Cancer, 59,* 6–14.

Choi, N. C., Grillo, H. C., & Huberman, M. S. (1986). Cancer of the lung. In B. Cody (Ed.), *Cancer manual* (pp. 166–177). Boston: American Cancer Society Massachusetts Division, Inc.

Clamon, G. C., Audeh, M. W., & Pinnick, S. (1982). Small cell lung carcinoma in the elderly. *Journal of American Geriatric Society, 30,* 299–302.

Cohen, M. H. (1982). Natural history of lung cancer. *Clinics in Chest Medicine, 3,* 229–241.

Colditz, G. A., Stampfer, M. J., & Willett, W. C. (1987). Diet and lung cancer: A review of the epidemiologic evidence in humans. *Archives of Internal Medicine, 147,* 157–160.

Cooper, E. T. (1984, August). A pilot study on the effects of the diagnosis of lung cancer on family relationships. *Cancer Nursing, 7,* 301–308.

Costa, G., Lane, W. W., Vincent, R. G., Siebold, J. A., Aragon, M., & Bewley, P. T. (1981). Weight loss and cachexia in lung cancer. *Nutrition and Cancer, 2,* 98–103.

Cox, J. D. (1981). The role of radiation therapy for carcinoma of the lung. *Yale Journal of Biology and Medicine, 54,* 195–200.

Craighead, J. E., & Mossman, B. T. (1982). The pathogenesis of asbestos-related diseases. *New England Journal of Medicine, 306,* 1446–1455.

Dalager, N. A., Pickle, L. W., Mason, T. J., Correa, P., Fontham, E., Stemhagan, A., Buffler, P. A., Ziegler, R. G., & Fraumeni, J. F. (1986). The relation of passive smoking to lung cancer. *Cancer Research, 46,* 4808–4811.

DeWys, W. D., Begg, C., Lavin, P. T., Band, R. P., Bennett, M. J., Bertino, R. J., Cohen, H. M., Douglas, Jr., O. H., Engstrom, F. P., Ezdinli, Z. E., Horton, J., Johnson, J. G., Moertel, G. C., Oken, M. M., Perlia, C., Rosenbaum, C., Silverstein, N. M., Skeel, T. R., Sponzo, W. R., & Tormey, C. D. (1980). Prognostic effect of weight loss prior to chemotherapy in cancer patients. *American Journal of Medicine, 69,* 491–497.

Doll, R., & Hill, A. B. (1964). Mortality in relation to smoking: Ten year observations of British doctors. *British Medical Journal, 1,* 1399–1410.

Driever, M. J., & McCorkle, R. (1984, June). Patient concerns at 3 and 6 months postdiagnosis. *Cancer Nursing, 7,* 235–241.

Ershler, W. B., Socinski, M. A., & Greene, C. J. (1982). Bronchogenic cancer, metastases, and aging. *Journal of the American Geriatric Society, 31,* 673–676.

Feinstein, A. R., & Wells, C. K. (1982). Lung cancer staging: A critical evaluation. *Clinics in Chest Medicine, 3,* 291–305.

Filderman, A. E., & Matthay, R. A. (1985, November/December). Update on lung cancer. *Respiratory Therapy, 15*(6), 21–31.

Filderman, A. E., Shaw, C., & Matthay, R. A. (1986). Lung cancer in the elderly. *Clinics in Geriatric Medicine, 2,* 363–383.

Flehinger, B. J., Melamed, M. R., Zaman, M. B., Heelan, T., Perchick, B. W., & Martini, N. (1984). Early lung cancer detection: Results of the initial (prevalence) radiologic and cytologic screening in the Memorial Sloan Kettering study. *American Review of Respiratory Disease, 130,* 555–560.

Fontana, R. S., Sanderson, D. R., Taylor, W. F., Woolner, B. L., Miller, E. W., Muhm, R. J., & Uhlenhopp, A. M. (1984). Early lung cancer detection: Results of the initial (prevalence) radiologic and cytologic screening in the Mayo Clinic Study. *American Review of Respiratory Disease, 130,* 561–564.

Foote, M., Sexton, D. L., & Pawlik, L. (1986). Dyspnea: A distressing sensation in lung cancer. *Oncology Nursing Forum, 13*(5), 25–31.

Frank, A. L. (1982). The epidemiology and etiology of lung cancer. *Clinics in Chest Medicine, 3,* 219–228.

Frost, J. K., Ball, W. C., Levin, M. L., Tockman, S. M., Baker, R. R., Carter, D., Eggleston, C. J., Erazan, Y., Gupta, K. P., Khouri, F. N., Marsh, R. B., & Stitik, P. F. (1984). Early lung cancer detection: Results of the initial (prevalence) radiologic and cytologic screening in the Johns Hopkins Study. *American Review of Respiratory Disease, 130,* 549–554.

Gazdar, A. F., Carney, D. N., & Minna, J. D. (1983). The biology of non-small cell lung cancer. *Seminars in Oncology, 10,* 3–19.

Geddes, D. M. (1979). The natural history of lung cancer: A review based on rates of tumour growth. *British Journal of Diseases of the Chest, 73,* 1–17.

Germino, B., & McCorkle, R. (1985). Acknowledged awareness of life-threatening illness. *International Journal of Nursing Studies, 22,* 33–44.

Greco, F. A., Johnson, D. H., Hainsworth, J. D., & Wolff, S. N. (1985). Chemotherapy of small cell lung cancer. *Seminars in Oncology, 12*(4, Suppl. 6), 31–37.

Greco, F. A., & Oldham, R. K. (1979). Small-cell lung cancer. *New England Journal of Medicine, 301,* 355–358.

Hande, K. R., & Des Prez, R. M. (1982). Chemotherapy and radiation therapy for non-small cell lung carcinoma. *Clinics in Chest Medicine, 3,* 399–414.

Hande, K. R., & Des Prez, R. M. (1984). Current perspectives in small cell lung cancer. *Chest, 85,* 669–677.

Hansen, M., & Pedersen, A. G. (1986). Tumor markers in patients with lung cancer. *Chest, 89*(4 Suppl.), 219S–224S.

Heitzman, E. R. (1986). The role of computed tomography in the diagnosis and management of lung cancer. *Chest, 89*(4 Suppl.), 237S–241S.

Hoffman, P. C., Albain, K. S., Bitran, J. D., & Golomb, M. H. (1984). Current concepts in small cell carcinoma of the lung. *CA: A Cancer Journal for Clinicians, 34,* 269–281.

Holmes, E. C. (1986). Surgical adjuvant therapy of non-small cell lung cancer. *Chest, 89*(4 Suppl.), 295S–300S.

Johnson, D. H., Marangos, P. J., Forbes, J. T., Hainsworth, J. D., Welch, V. R., Hande, K. R., & Greco, A. F. (1984). Potential utility of serum neuron-specific enolase levels in small cell carcinoma of the lung. *Cancer Research, 44,* 5409.

Klastersky, J., & Sculier, J. P. (1985). Chemotherapy of non-small cell lung cancer. *Seminars in Oncology, 12*(4, Suppl. 6), 38–48.

Lindsey, A. M. (1986a). Cachexia. In V. Carrieri, A. M. Lindsey, & C. West (Eds.), *Pathophysiological phenomena in nursing: Human responses to illness* (pp. 122–136). Philadelphia: W. B. Saunders Co.

Lindsey, A. M. (1986b). Cancer cachexia: Effects of the disease and its treatment. *Seminars in Oncology Nursing, 2,* 19–29.

Lindsey, A. M., & Piper, B. F. (1985). Anorexia and weight loss: Indicators of cachexia in small cell lung cancer. *Nutrition and Cancer, 7*(1 & 2), 65–76.

Lindsey, A. M., & Piper, B. F. (1986). Anorexia, serum zinc, and immunologic response in small cell lung cancer patients receiving chemotherapy and prophylactic cranial radiation. *Nutrition and Cancer, 8,* 231–238.

Lindsey, A. M., Piper, B. F., & Carrieri, V. L. (1981). Malignant cells and ectopic hormone production. *Oncology Nursing Forum, 8,* 13–15.

Lindsey, A. M., Piper, B. F., & Stotts, N. (1982). The phenomenon of cancer cachexia: A review. *Oncology Nursing Forum, 9*(2), 38–42.

Livingston, R. B. (1986). Current chemotherapy of small cell lung cancer. *Chest, 89*(4 Suppl.), 258S–263S.

Loeb, L. A., Ernster, V. L., Warner, K. E., Abbotts, J., & Laszio, J. (1984). Smoking and lung cancer: An overview. *Cancer Research, 44,* 5940–5958.

Loke, J., Matthay, R. A., & Ieda, S. (1982). Techniques for diagnosing lung cancer. *Clinics in Chest Medicine, 3,* 321–329.

Marino, L. B., & Levy, S. M. (1986). Primary and secondary prevention of cancer in children and adolescents: Current status and issues. *Pediatric Clinics of North America, 33,* 975–993.

Mathews, M. J., McKay, B., & Lukeman, J. (1983). The pathology of non-small cell carcinoma of the lung. *Seminars in Oncology, 10,* 34–55.

Melamed, M. R., Flehinger, B. J., Zaman, M. B., Heelan, R. T., Perchick, W. A., & Martini, N. (1984). Screening for early cancer. *Chest, 86,* 44–53.

Mountain, C. F. (1983). Therapy of stage I and stage II non-small cell lung cancer. *Seminars in Oncology, 10,* 71–80.

Mountain, C. F. (1986). New international staging system for lung cancer. *Chest, 89*(4 Suppl.), 225S–233S.

Muss, H. B., Jackson, D. V., Jr., Richards, F., White, D. R., & Cooper, M. R. (1984). Bone marrow evaluation in small cell lung cancer. *American Journal of Clinical Oncology, 6,* 59–63.

Neal, M. H., Kosinski, R., Cohen, P., & Orenstein, J. M. (1986). Atypical endocrine tumors of the lung. *Human Pathology, 17,* 1264–1277.

Okabe, T., Kaizu, T., Fujisawa, M., Watanabe, J., & Takaku, F. (1985). Clinical application of monoclonal antibodies to small cell lung cancer. *Japanese Journal of Medicine, 24,* 250–256.

Olsen, G. N., Block, A. J., & Tobias, J. A. (1984). Prediction of postpneumonectomy pulmonary function using quantitative macroaggregate lung scanning. *Chest, 66,* 13–16.

Palgi, A. (1984). Vitamin A and lung cancer: A perspective. *Nutrition and Cancer, 6,* 105–120.

Perez, C. A., Pajak, T. F., Rubin, P., Simpson, J. R., Mohiuddin, M., Brady, L. W., Perez-Tamayo, R., & Rotman, M. (1987). Long-term observations of the patterns of failure in patients with unresectable non-oat cell carcinoma of the lung treated with definitive radiotherapy. *Cancer, 59,* 1874–1881.

Perry, M. C., Eaton, W. L., Propert, K. J., Ware, J. H., Zimmer, B., Chahinian, A. P., Skarin, A., Carey, R. W., Kreisman, H.,

Faulkner, C., Comis, R., & Green, M. R. (1987). Chemotherapy with or without radiation therapy in limited small-cell carcinoma of the lung. *New England Journal of Medicine, 316,* 912–918.

Reyes, C. V., Chua, D., & Aranha, G. V. (1987). Changing incidence of adenocarcinoma of the lung: A brief review. *Journal of Surgical Oncology, 35,* 50–51.

Sculier, J. P., Evans, W. K., Feld, R., De Boer, G., Payne, D. G., Shepherd, F. A., Pringle, J. F., Yeoh, J. L., Quirt, I. C., Curtis, J. E., & Herman, J. G. (1986). Superior venal caval obstruction syndrome in small cell lung cancer. *Cancer, 57,* 847–851.

Silverberg, E. (1985). Cancer statistics; 1985. *Cancer, 35,* 19–35.

Spiro, S. G. (1984). Diagnosis and staging. In W. Duncan (Ed.), *Recent results in cancer research: Lung cancer* (pp. 16–29). New York: Springer-Verlag.

Stanley, K. E. (1980). Prognostic factors for survival in patients with inoperable lung cancer. *Journal of the National Cancer Institute, 65,* 2532.

Stayner, L. T., & Wegman, D. H. (1983). Smoking, occupation, and histopathology of lung cancer: A case control study with the use of the Third National Cancer Survey. *Journal of the National Cancer Institute, 70,* 421–426.

Suen, K. C., Lau, L. L., & Yermakov, V. (1974). Cancer and old age: An autopsy study of 3535 patients over 65 years old. *Cancer, 33,* 1164–1168.

Tisi, G. M., Friedman, P. J., Peters, R. M., Pearson, G., Carr, D., Lee, R. E., & Selaury, O. (1983). Clinical staging of primary lung cancer. *American Review of Respiratory Disease, 127,* 659–664.

Valaitis, J., Warren, S., & Gamble, D. (1981). Increasing incidence of adenocarcinoma of the lung. *Cancer, 47,* 1042–1046.

Van Houtte, P., Piron, A., Lustman-Marechal, J., Osteaux, M., & Henry, J. (1980). Computed axial tomography (CAT) contribution for dosimetry and treatment evaluation in lung cancer. *International Journal of Radiation Oncology, Biology, Physics, 6,* 995–1000.

Wang, K. P., & Terry, P. B. (1983). Transbronchial needle aspiration in the diagnosis and staging of bronchogenic carcinoma. *American Review of Respiratory Disease, 127,* 344–347.

Waxman, A. D. (1986). The role of nuclear medicine in pulmonary neoplastic processes. *Seminars in Nuclear Medicine, 41,* 285–295.

Wickham, R. (1986). Pulmonary toxicity secondary to cancer treatment. *Oncology Nursing Forum, 13*(5), 69–76.

Woolner, L. B., Fontana, R. S., & Cortese, D. A. (1984). Roentgenographically occult lung cancer: Pathologic findings and frequency of multicentricity during a 10-year period. *Mayo Clinic Proceedings, 59,* 453–466.

Woolner, L. B., Fontana, R. S., Sanderson, D. R., Miller, E. W., Muhm, R. J., Taylor, F. W., & Uhlenhopp, A. M. (1981). Mayo lung project. *Mayo Clinic Proceedings, 56,* 544–547.

Yesner, R., & Carter, D. (1982). Pathology of carcinoma of the lung. *Clinics in Chest Medicine, 3,* 257–289.

Zinreich, E. S., Baker, R. R., Ettinger, D. S., & Arder, S. E. (1984). New frontiers in the treatment of lung cancer. *CRC Critical Reviews in Oncology/Hematology, 3,* 279–308.

CHAPTER 32

Genitourinary Cancers

JULENA LIND
ROBERT J. IRWIN, JR.

Cancers of the prostate, kidney, and bladder are common in adults. Testicular cancer, although uncommon, is important to discuss because it is the most common cancer in young men between 25 and 30 years of age. Figure 32–1 shows the tumor sites and routes of metastases in men.

PROSTATIC CANCER

Definition and Incidence

The prostate is a small, firm organ made up of glands and musculature enclosed in a fibrous capsule through which the urethra passes as it exits the bladder. It is a secondary sex organ whose only known function is its contribution to seminal fluid. Figure 32–2 illustrates the anatomic relationships of the prostate.

Prostate cancer accounts for approximately 20 per cent of all cancers in men and 10 per cent of all cancer deaths (Silverberg & Lubera, 1989).

Epidemiology and Etiology

The peak incidence of prostatic cancer is in men between 60 and 70 years of age. In fact, it is found incidentally on routine autopsy examination in most men older than 70 years. The highest rate of prostatic cancer in the world is among black Americans; the lowest incidence is found among Japanese men. There is a fortyfold difference between the incidence of prostatic cancer in black Americans and Japanese men (Doll, 1978).

Three major factors are hypothesized to contribute to the causation of prostatic cancer: age, infectious agents, and endocrine factors. Age is the most important variable yet described. Prostatic cancer in men under 40 years old is rare. Black men in Los Angeles, for example, have a one in four risk of developing clinically significant prostatic cancer by 85 years of age (Ross, Paganini-Hill, & Henderson, 1988b).

Although they are not completely understood, hormonal interactions seem to play a role in the development of prostate cancer. For example, prostatic cancer does not develop in eunuchs, and many cases of metastatic disease respond to hormonal manipulation (Perez, Ihde, Fair, & Labrie, 1985). Furthermore, although prostatic cancer is difficult to induce in animal models, subcutaneous testosterone alone can produce this cancer in rats (Noble, 1980).

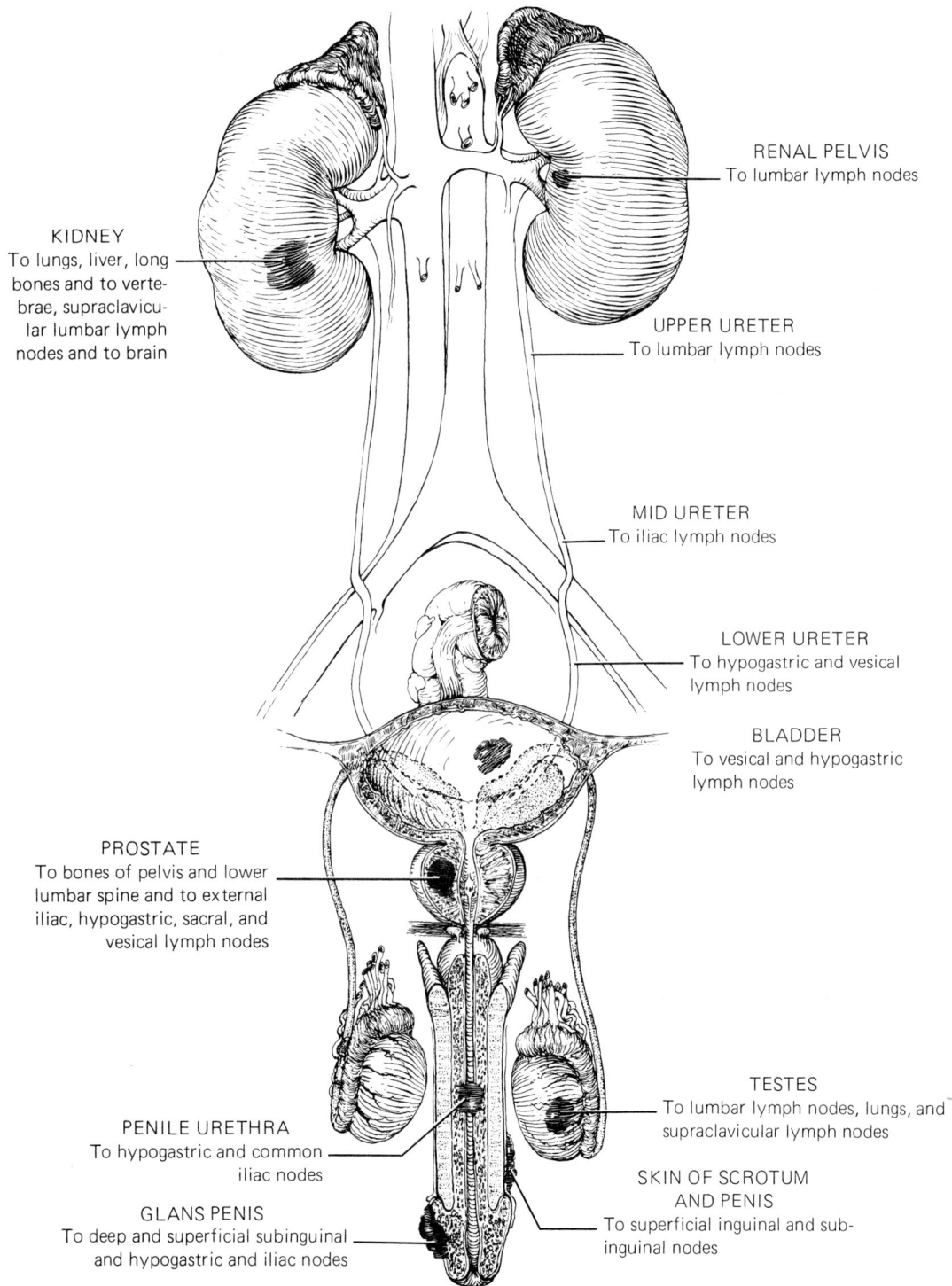

RENAL PELVIS
To lumbar lymph nodes

KIDNEY
To lungs, liver, long
bones and to verte-
brae, supraclavicu-
lar lumbar lymph
nodes and to brain

UPPER URETER
To lumbar lymph nodes

MID URETER
To iliac lymph nodes

LOWER URETER
To hypogastric and vesical
lymph nodes

BLADDER
To vesical and hypogastric
lymph nodes

PROSTATE
To bones of pelvis and lower
lumbar spine and to external
iliac, hypogastric, sacral, and
vesical lymph nodes

TESTES
To lumbar lymph nodes, lungs, and
supraclavicular lymph nodes

PENILE URETHRA
To hypogastric and common
iliac nodes

SKIN OF SCROTUM
AND PENIS
To superficial inguinal and sub-
inguinal nodes

GLANS PENIS
To deep and superficial subinguinal
and hypogastric and iliac nodes

Figure 32–1. Sites of tumor origin and metastases in the male. (From Smith, D. R. [1981]. Tumors of the genitourinary tract. In D. R. Smith [Ed.], *General urology* [10th ed., p. 272]. Los Altos, CA: Lange. Reproduced by permission.)

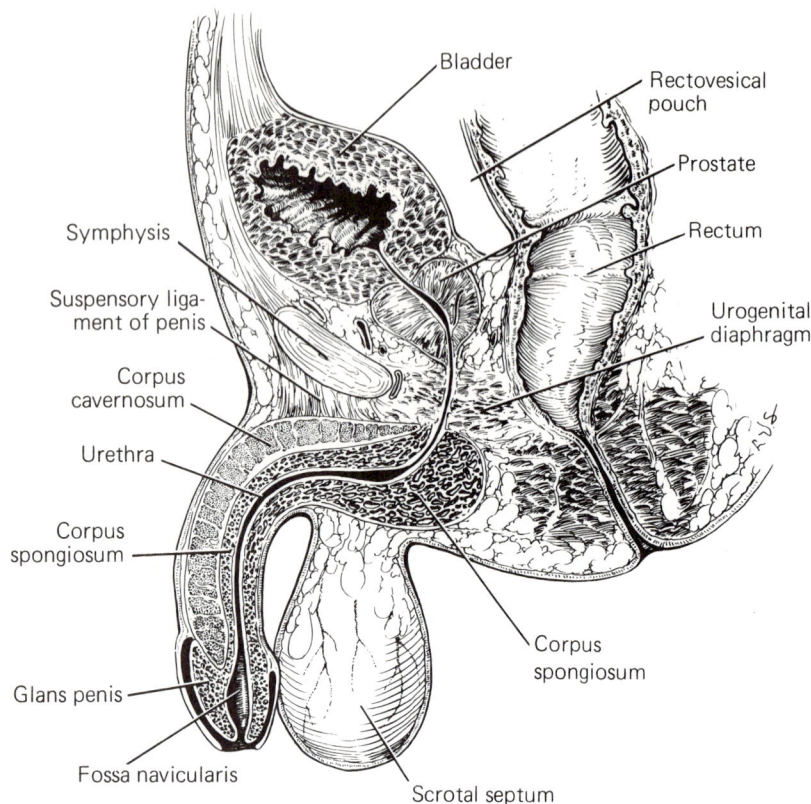

Figure 32–2. Relations of the bladder, prostate, seminal vesicles, penis, urethra, and scrotal contents. (From Smith, D. R. [1981]. Tumors of the genitourinary tract. In D. R. Smith [Ed.], *General urology* [10th ed., p. 9]. Los Altos, CA: Lange. Reproduced by permission.)

Biology and Natural History

Prostatic cancers are almost always adenocarcinomas, which vary in differentiation and appearance. They are generally staged according to an A, B, C, D system (Fig. 32–3); however, the tumor-nodes-metastasis (TNM) system is also used (Table 32–1).

Also used more frequently today is the Gleason classification. This is a system of histopathologic grading based on the glandular pattern of the tumor at relatively low magnification. Combining clinical staging and histopathologic grading helps predict the biologic potential of prostate cancer (Gleason et al., 1974; Kramer, Spahr, Brendler, Glenn, & Paulson, 1980; Layfield et al., 1984).

Local spread to the seminal vesicles and the bladder is common. Prostatic cancer also disseminates hematogenously to the bones and rarely to the lungs and liver. The disease spreads via the lymphatics to the pelvic lymph nodes, then to the periaortic nodes, and occasionally to the supraclavicular nodes. In fact, as many as one third of the men with early disease (stage B and low volume stage C) have evidence of metastases to the pelvic lymph nodes (Waisman & Mott, 1978).

In the last two decades, the survival rates for prostatic cancer have increased significantly (Silverberg & Lubera, 1989). Five-year survival after prostatectomy for stage A is 88 to 91 per cent, and for stage B, 73 to 81 per cent (Middleton, Smith, Melzer, & Hamilton, 1986). Survival rates for advanced cancer are much less encouraging (Kramer et al., 1980) (Table 32–2).

Presenting Signs and Symptoms

On rectal examination the gland normally feels rubbery. In early cancer it will feel like a nonraised, firm nodule that may have a sharp edge. However, less than 10 per cent of prostate cancers detected on routine examinations are discovered early enough for potential cure. Unfortunately, there are no real symptoms in early-stage disease, and small tumors are easily missed. Later tumors might be detected as a hard lump on rectal examination or as an unexpected finding during histologic examination of transurethral resection specimens.

Urinary disorders such as frequency, dysuria, and obstruction are common presenting symptoms. A frequent symptom of late disease is bone pain related to metastasis.

Differential Diagnosis

The urinary tract symptoms of benign prostatic hypertrophy closely resemble cancer. Because only 50 per cent of prostatic nodules are malignant tumors, it is imperative to establish a tissue diagnosis. This is most commonly done by needle aspiration or biopsy (Layfield et al., 1984). A hardened area felt on rectal examination could also be the result of prostatitis, tuberculosis, fibrous benign prostatic hypertrophy (BPH), or prostatic calculi.

Determination of serum prostatic acid phosphatase by either biochemical or radioimmunologic assay should be included in the prostatic cancer work-up.

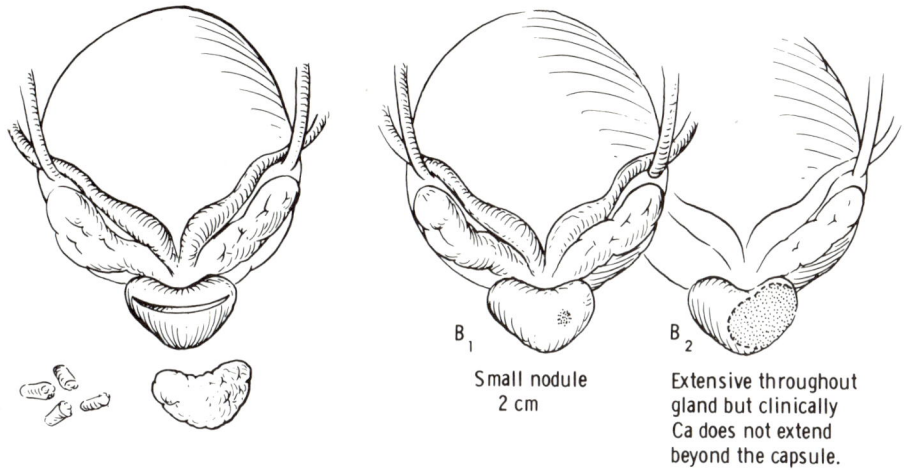

STAGE A (I)

Unsuspected clinically.
Incidental pathologic finding following TURP or open enucleation. Isolated microscopic finding, grade I.

STAGE B (II)

B₁ Small nodule 2 cm

B₂ Extensive throughout gland but clinically Ca does not extend beyond the capsule.

Clinically completely confined prostate. Normal acid phosphatase. No significant urinary symptoms present.

(5-15% Incidence)

Figure 32–3. Prostate cancer staging according to clinical and radiologic estimates of tumor involvement. TURP, transurethral resection of the prostate; Ca, carcinoma. (From Skinner, D. G. [1973]. Current concepts concerning carcinoma of the prostate. In L. Nyhus [Ed.], *Surgery annual* [p. 393]. New York: Appleton-Century-Crofts. Reproduced by permission.)

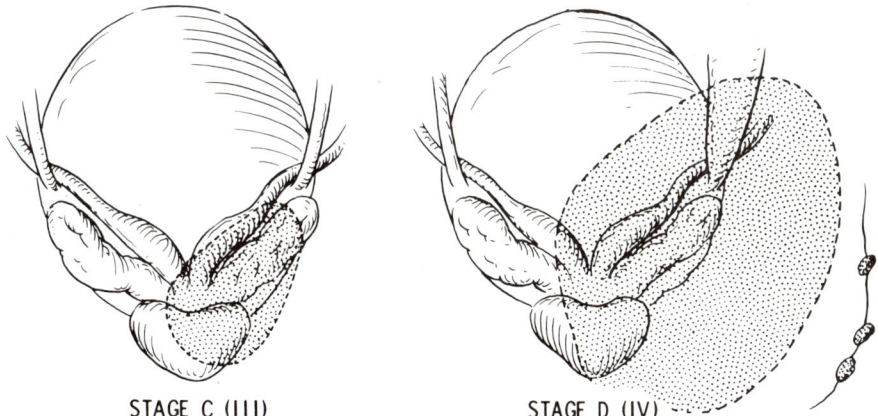

STAGE C (III)

Ca extends beyond the capsule, involving the seminal vesicles, bladder neck or lateral pelvic wall. Urinary symptoms prostatism.

(15-30% Incidence)

STAGE D (IV)

Ca extends beyond the pelvis with soft tissue, bony or pelvic lymph node metastases, or hydronephrosis from ureteral obstruction. Acid phosphatase elevated 76%.

(60-80% Incidence)

Table 32-1. TNM STAGING OF PROSTATIC CANCER

Primary Tumor (T)

TX	Minimum requirements to assess the primary tumor cannot be met
T_0	No tumor present
T_{1A}	No palpable tumor; on histologic sections no more than three high-power fields of carcinoma found.
T_{1B}	No palpable tumor; histologic sections reveal more than three high-power fields of prostatic carcinoma
T_{2A}	Palpable nodule less than 1.5 cm in diameter with compressible, normal-feeling tissue on at least three sides
T_{2B}	Palpable nodule more than 1.5 cm in diameter or nodule or induration in both lobes
T_3	Palpable tumor extending into or beyond the prostatic capsule
T_{3A}	Palpable tumor extending into the periprostatic tissues or involving one seminal vesicle
T_{3B}	Palpable tumor extending into the periprostatic tissues, involving one or both seminal vesicles; tumor size more than 6 cm in diameter
T_4	Tumor fixed or involving neighboring structures

Nodal Involvement (N)

The regional nodes are those within the true pelvis; all others are distant nodes. Histologic examination is required for stages N_0 through N_3.

NX	Minimum requirements to assess the regional nodes cannot be met
N_0	No involvement of regional lymph nodes
N_1	Involvement of a single homolateral regional lymph node
N_2	Involvement of contralateral, bilateral, or multiple regional lymph nodes
N_3	A fixed mass present on the pelvic wall with a free space between this and the tumor

Distant Metastasis (M)

MX	Minimum requirements to assess the presence of distant metastasis cannot be met
M_0	No (known) distant metastasis
M_1	Distant metastasis present

(From Beahrs, O. H., & Myers, M. H. [eds.]. [1983]. *Manual for staging of cancer* [2nd ed., pp. 106–161]. Philadelphia: J. B. Lippincott Co. Reproduced by permission.)

More than 80 per cent of men with stage D disease have an increased serum acid phosphatase level (McCullough, 1988). A bone scan and an excretory urogram (intravenous pyelogram, or IVP) are also usually performed.

Because the sudden discovery of prostatic cancer may take the asymptomatic patient and his family by complete surprise, nursing interventions should focus on education and emotional support. Helping the patient and family to understand the implications of his treatment options—for example, possible impotence or incontinence—is a significant challenge.

Treatment

Surgery

Radical prostatectomy is the surgical removal of the entire prostate, including the true prostatic capsule,

Table 32-2. 5-YEAR SURVIVAL, PROSTATIC CANCER

	Whites (per cent)	Blacks (per cent)
All stages	72	60
Localized	85	79
Spread	48	32

(Data from Silverberg, E., & Lubera, J., 1989.)

the seminal vesicles, and a portion of the bladder neck. It can be done with or without pelvic lymph node dissection (Fig. 32–4). Radical prostatectomy is indicated for stage A and stage B disease, particularly in situations in which the patient is younger, has no metastases, and has a normal acid phosphatase level (Paulson, Stone, Walther, Tucker, & Cox, 1986). The perineal and retropubic approaches are commonly used (Fig. 32–5).

Transurethral resection of the prostate (TURP) also plays a role in treatment. Although it is not used as a curative method, TURP is used to treat obstructive disease in advanced cancer. It may also reveal an unsuspected cancer when used as a treatment for BPH.

Complications after radical prostatectomy include impotence, infection, and urinary incontinence. It is thought that post–radical prostatectomy impotence is a result of damage to autonomic nerves posterolateral to the prostate, which are required for physiologic erections. The Walsh and Mostwin (1984) retropubic prostatectomy (which carefully avoids injury to the pelvic nerves) has shown fewer problems with impotence and incontinence.

Nursing implications involve initially exploring preoperative concerns regarding sexual competence. People in general may hold certain prejudices concerning sexuality in the older adult, which the nurse should avoid. Teaching should be geared to the role of the prostate in sexual activity and alleviating misconceptions that all sexual activity is over (Heinrich-Rynning (1987). The reader is referred to Chapter 53, for an in-depth discussion of sexuality.

Immediate postoperative nursing responsibilities include maintaining catheter presence and patency, preventing urinary tract infection, and administering antispasmodics to decrease the discomfort caused by bladder spasms (Lind, 1987). Interestingly, clot retention after radical prostatectomy is less of a problem than it is after simple prostatectomy.

Radiotherapy

Radiotherapy has been used for curative, adjunctive, and palliative treatment of prostate cancer. A 1986 study reported comparable results in patients treated with definitive external beam radiotherapy as compared with those who had undergone surgery (Pilepich, Bagshaw, Asbell et al., 1986). The patient selection criteria in this study included those with clinical stages A2 and B disease, negative staging lymphadenectomy, negative bone scan, and normal acid phosphatase levels. However, an earlier Veterans Administration study reported a higher relapse rate in the patients treated with radiotherapy (Paulson et al., 1982).

Radiotherapy has also been attempted as an adjunct to surgery. Postoperative irradiation for patients with localized disease does not offer any apparent advantage (Paulson, Stone, Walther, Tucker, & Cox, 1986). When clinical stage B disease is found to be pathologic stage C disease after radical prostatectomy, preoperative adjuvant therapy can decrease the incidence of local recurrence (Gibbons et al., 1986).

Prophylactic radiotherapy of the regional lymphatics

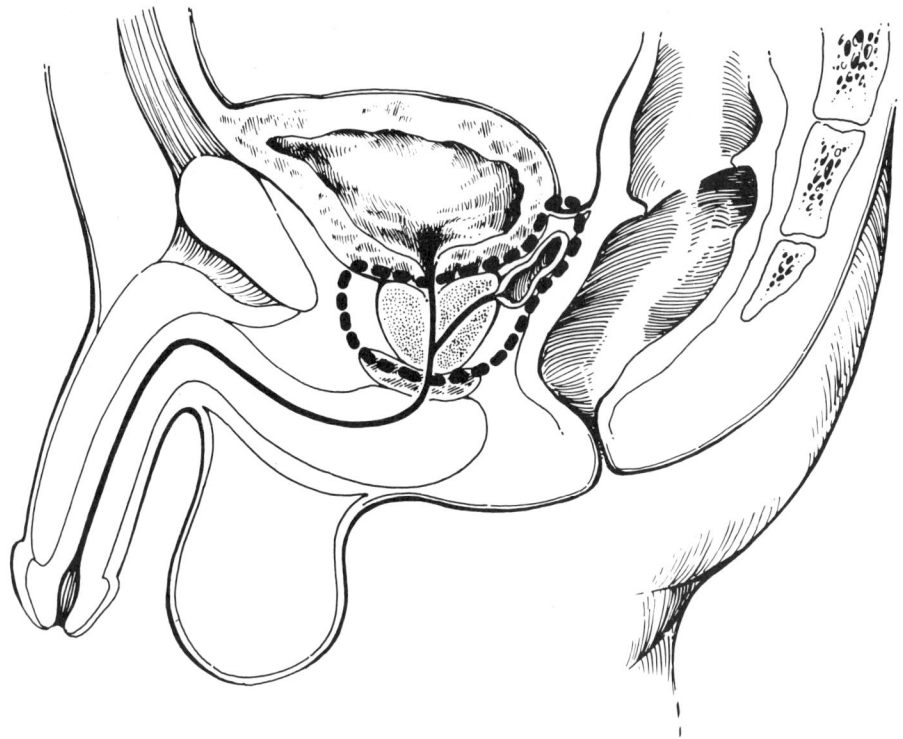

Figure 32–4. Surgical boundaries of a radical prostatectomy. (From Swanson, D. [1981]. Cancer of the bladder and prostate: The impact of therapy on sexual function. In A. von Eschenbach & D. Rodriguez [Eds.], *Sexual rehabilitation of the urologic cancer patient* [p. 93]. Boston: G. K. Hall. Reproduced by permission.)

is often used in patients who are at significant risk of harboring tumor deposits in the regional lymph nodes. Data reported in 1986 revealed no apparent benefit of elective periaortic irradiation in patients with detectable disease confined to the pelvis (Pilepich, Krall, Johnson et al., 1986).

Common side effects of radiotherapy to the prostate are proctitis, diarrhea, and urinary frequency. Potency rates of 60 per cent are possible, although this finding probably applies to younger patients (Bagshaw, 1988).

Internal radiotherapy via direct implantation has also been used to treat prostate cancer. When the disease

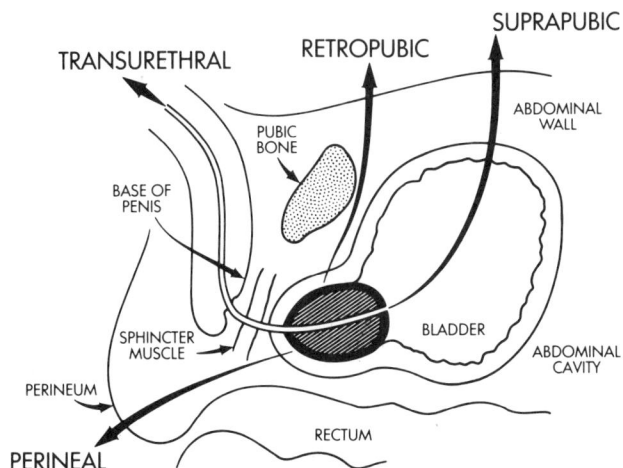

Figure 32–5. Surgical approaches to prostatectomy. (From Henrich-Rynning, T. [1987]. Prostatic cancer treatments and their effects on sexual functioning. *Oncology Nursing Forum, 14*[6], 39. Reproduced by permission.)

is localized to the pelvis, internal radiation can increase the dose directly to the prostate and decrease the exposure to the surrounding tissue. Radioactive iodine (^{125}I) is commonly used (Carlton, 1988). Wound infection, proctitis, and fistula formation are occasional complications described in up to 25 per cent of the patients treated with ^{125}I. However, potency was preserved in 70 to 90 per cent of the patients who were previously potent (Carlton, 1988).

A newer afterloading technique using iridium (^{192}Ir) has been described, with equivocal results (Bosch et al., 1986). Although early morbidity is low, there is significant later morbidity, including proctitis, ulceration, progressive obstructive symptoms, incontinence, and impotence (Bosch et al., 1986).

Radiation-induced cystitis usually occurs during the first 2 to 3 weeks of therapy. Education by the nurse would include encouraging the patient to drink at least 2 liters of fluid per day and explaining the benefits of antispasmodics and analgesics in decreasing the discomfort. See Chapter 20 for detailed information on the nursing care of patients experiencing radiation-induced proctitis and dermatitis.

Nursing care of the patient with afterloading interstitial implants (^{192}Ir) should be done quickly to reduce radiation exposure to the nursing personnel; however, seed implants pose minimal risk. Provided that the patient's urine is promptly disposed of, there is no risk to others from ^{125}I radiation because this isotope's decay is by beta emission. Patients are understandably concerned about radiation exposure, and every attempt should be made to provide reassurance for them and their families.

Chemotherapy

Chemotherapy plays a limited role in the treatment of advanced, hormonally unresponsive prostatic cancer. Both single-agent and combination protocols have been attempted. Agents tested include cyclophosphamide, methotrexate, doxorubicin, 5-fluorouracil, cisplatin, vincristine, prednisone, and melphalan (Einhorn, 1988; Graham et al., 1986).

Hormonal Manipulation

Hormonal treatment of adenocarcinoma of the prostate is based on the assumption that prostatic cancer cells are androgen dependent (Paulson, 1988). This treatment is indicated for patients with advanced cancer, but it plays no role in the therapy of patients with localized disease. Dihydrotestosterone is the principal intracelluar androgen. Blocking androgen formation or utilization will theoretically arrest tumor growth.

Hormonal manipulation can take the following forms:

- administration of estrogen
- administration of drugs that interfere with androgens
- orchiectomy
- adrenalectomy (surgical and medical)
- hypophysectomy

Diethylstilbestrol (DES), 1 to 3 mg orally, is the estrogen usually given. Side effects of DES include thromboembolic disease, congestive heart failure, decreased libido, impotence, and gynecomastia. In some settings, breast irradiation is routinely performed to prevent gynecomastia (Fass, Steinfeld, Brown, & Tessler, 1986). Drugs that interfere with androgen metabolism, such as cyproterone acetate, and medroxyprogesterone acetate (Depo-Provera) were compared as a treatment for advanced cancer, patients treated with medroxyprogesterone acetate had a less favorable course with shorter duration of survival. There were no significant differences between DES and cyproterone acetate (Pavone-Macaluso et al., 1986). A new drug, buserelin, which is given either subcutaneously or via nasal spray, is a luteinizing hormone–releasing hormone (LH-RH) agonist that causes sustained suppression of circulating testosterone. This is achieved by depleting the pituitary of luteinizing hormone–releasing factor (LHRF), which is necessary for the testicular production of testosterone (Rajfer et al., 1986; Waxman et al., 1986). Initial results show promise but are not superior to those with DES.

Bilateral orchiectomy decreases plasma testosterone levels, but to virtually unmeasurable levels. Adrenalectomy (either surgical or chemical with aminoglutethamide) blocks adrenal androgens and is used for those persons who originally responded to hormonal therapy but who have relapsed (de Kernion, 1985). Hypophysectomy (surgical removal of the pituitary) ablates both the adrenal and testicular production of androgens, but it is rarely used because of profound endocrine complications.

The most significant nursing implications related to hormonal manipulation include patient teaching regarding the side effects of DES, particularly sodium retention, the potential for cardiac complications, and feminization effects (Lind & Nakao, 1987).

Recurrence and Palliative Treatment

Most prostatic cancers are advanced at the time of diagnosis, and treatment reflects this. Bone metastases to the vertebrae, pelvis, femur, and ribs are very common. Subsequently, pain management is often an issue.

Endocrine manipulation is the usual palliative treatment, although it may be coupled with radiotherapy. Chemotherapy has also been attempted but with only limited success (Huben & Murphy, 1988).

Nursing management for patients with recurrent disease focuses on providing for pain relief, teaching the patient how to manage the side effects of hormonal therapy, and offering emotional support.

BLADDER CANCER

Definition and Incidence

Bladder cancer accounts for about 4 to 5 per cent of all cancers in the United States. In 1987, there were approximately 45,400 new cases of bladder cancer and 10,600 deaths (Silverberg & Lubera, 1989). The greatest number appear on the mucosal lining of the bladder. The incidence of bladder cancer in men is three times greater than that in women, and the age-adjusted bladder cancer rate in white men is almost twice that in blacks (Ross, Paganini-Hill, & Henderson, 1988a).

Epidemiology and Etiology

Bladder cancer is typically seen in industrialized rather than in underdeveloped countries. The exception to this generalization is countries such as Egypt, where exposure to the parasite *Schistosoma haematobium* is common.

Hypothesized etiologic factors include cigarette smoking, exposure to the industrial chemicals called arylamines (used in textile and rubber industries), and exposure to *Schistosoma haemotobium* (squamous cell cancer of the bladder [Ross et al., 1988a]).

Biology and Natural History

Most bladder cancers in the United States are transitional cell carcinomas arising from the transitional epithelium of the mucosal lining. Within the classification of transitional cell carcinoma are the subdivisions of carcinoma in situ and papillary or solid tumors. Although 90 per cent of the cases are localized at the time of diagnosis, as many as 30 to 90 per cent of patients will develop recurrent cancers (Herr, 1987).

Table 32–3. BLADDER CANCER STAGING SYSTEMS

1946 Jewett-Strong	1952 Jewett	1952 Marshall		1974, TNM Clinical	1974, TNM Pathological
		0	No tumor in definitive specimen	T_0	P_0
			Carcinoma in situ	T_{IS}	P_{IS}
A	A		Papillary tumor without invasion	T_1	P_1
		A	Invasion of lamina propria		
B	B_1	B_1	Superficial } Muscle invasion	T_2	P_2
	B_2	B_2	Deep	T_{3A}	P_3
C	C	C	Invasion of perivesical fat	T_{3B}	
		D_1	Invasion of contiguous viscera / Pelvic nodes	T_{4A-B}	P_4 / N_{1-3}
		D_2	Distant metastases / Nodes above aortic bifurcation		M_1 / N_4

(From deKernion, J. B. [1985]. Cancer of the bladder. In C. Haskell, *Cancer treatment* [2nd ed., p. 371]. Philadelphia: W. B. Saunders Co. Reproduced by permission.)

The most common staging systems used in the United States are the Jewett-Strong system (modified by Marshall) and the tumor, nodes, and metastases (TNM) system. See Table 32–3 for a compilation of these systems.

The overall 5-year survival for whites is 76 per cent; for blacks, it is 55 per cent (Silverberg & Lubera, 1989) (Table 32–4).

Presenting Signs and Symptoms

Gross hematuria is the most common presenting symptom. Other symptoms include irritability of the bladder (dysuria, frequency, or urgency). Symptoms associated with large tumor growth may also be present. For example, tumor pushing on the internal urethral orifice can cause urinary hesitancy and decreased force and caliber of the stream. Obstruction of the ureters can cause flank pain and result in hydronephrosis.

Differential Diagnosis

In the evaluation of any patient with gross hematuria, an intravenous pyelogram (IVP) can help evaluate a suspected bladder tumor by possibly showing the tumor itself or by showing evidence of ureteral obstruction. Cystoscopy provides not only tumor visualization but also an opportunity to perform a biopsy and palpate the tumor. Urine cytology can help in the evaluation of those patients who have hematuria and are suspected

Table 32–4. 5-YEAR SURVIVAL BLADDER CANCER

	Whites (Per cent)	Blacks (Per cent)
All stages	77	56
Localized	88	80
Spread	41	25

(Data from Silverberg, E., & Lubera, J., 1989.)

of having a malignancy (Lieskovsky, Ahlering, & Skinner, 1988).

Nursing implications at the time of diagnosis include patient and family teaching about what to expect from the diagnostic tests. For example, patients may be anesthetized for cystoscopy. Following the procedure, patients are advised to drink plenty of fluids and to expect some hematuria. As another example, it is useful to know that urine cytology specimens are more reliable if they are not obtained as the first voided specimen of the day. If the specimens are not sent immediately for analysis, the urine should be refrigerated. A further nursing role involves clarifying for the patient and family the test results. If cancer is found, they will need assistance in understanding their treatment options. It must be emphasized here that if cystectomy is indicated, choosing a setting for treatment with access to an enterostomal therapist is extremely important. The patient's future adjustment to treatment and his or her quality of life very well might depend on interactions with an enterostomal therapist.

Treatment

Surgery

Surgical therapy depends on the pathologic stage of the tumor. Provided that the lesion penetrates no more deeply than the mucosa, every attempt is made to preserve the bladder. Therapy for disease of lower stages (0 to A) is generally intravesical chemotherapy and transurethral resection of recurrent disease. More advanced disease (stages B to C) can only be managed by radical cystectomy and urinary diversion. The rare exception to this is when the lesion is solitary, is in the dome of the bladder, and specimens from random mucosal biopsies remote from the tumor are normal. In this case, a partial cystectomy can be performed. Frequently, pelvic lymph node dissection is included

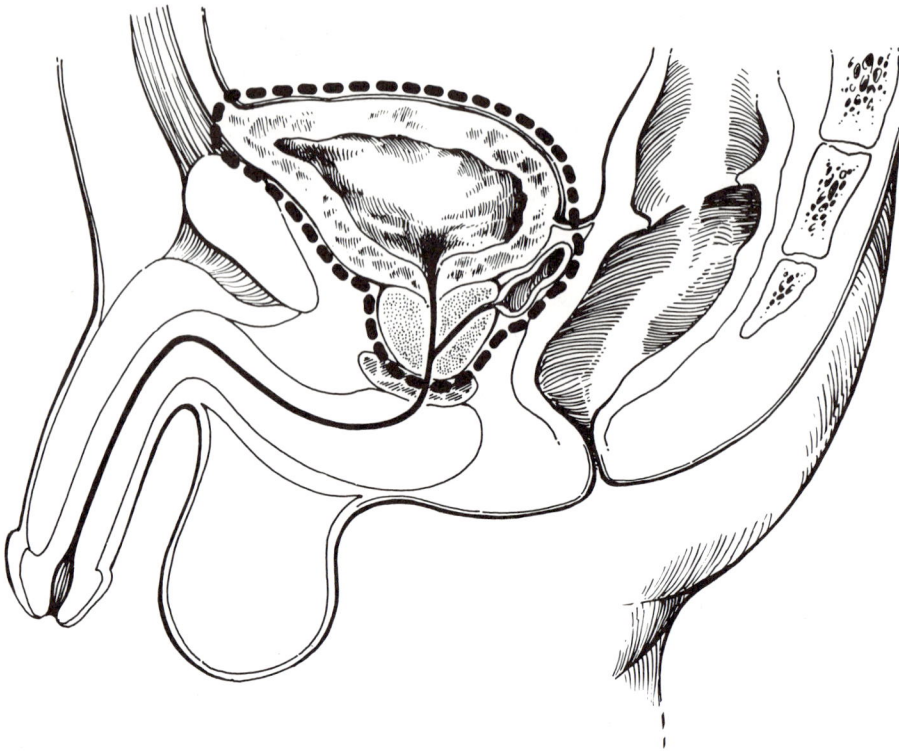

Figure 32–6. Surgical boundaries of a radical cystectomy in a man. (From Swanson, D. [1981]. Cancer of the bladder and prostate: The impact of therapy on sexual function. In A. von Eschenbach & D. Rodriguez [Eds.], *Sexual rehabilitation of the urologic cancer patient* [p. 102]. Boston: G. K. Hall. Reproduced by permission.)

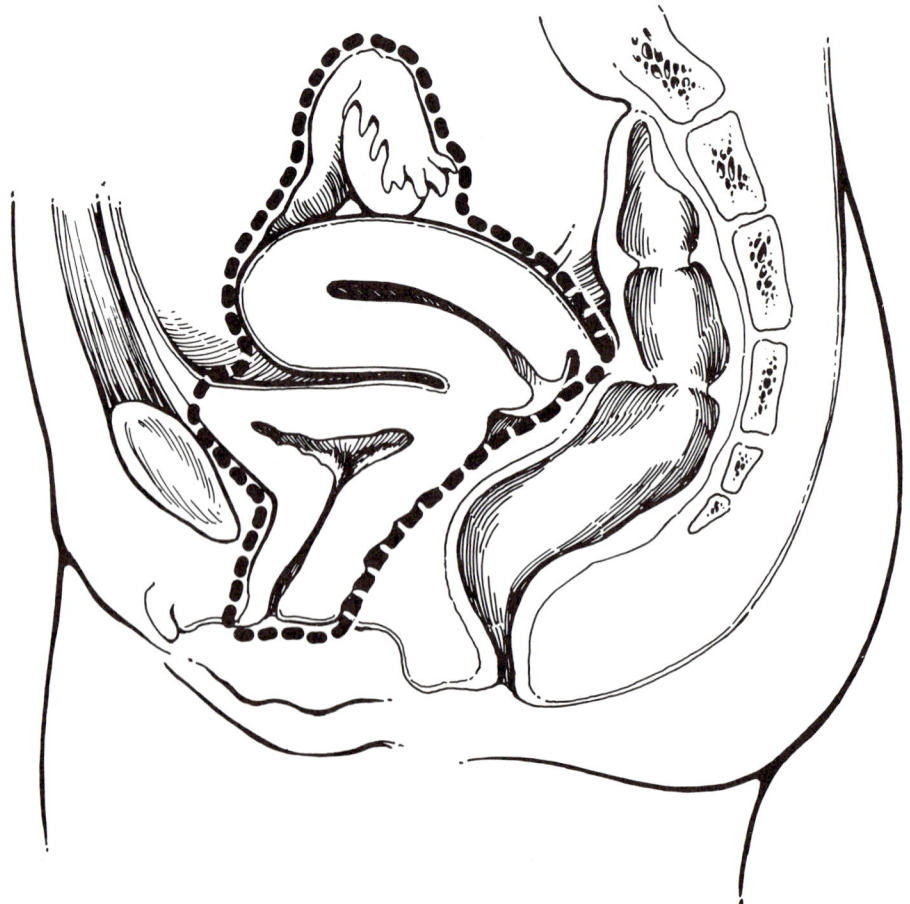

Figure 32–7. Surgical boundaries of a radical cystectomy in a woman. (From Swanson, D. [1981]. Cancer of the bladder and prostate: The impact of therapy on sexual function. In A. von Eschenbach & D. Rodriguez [Eds.], *Sexual rehabilitation of the urologic cancer patient* [p. 103]. Boston: G. K. Hall. Reproduced by permission.)

at the time of cystectomy in an effort to prevent local pelvic recurrence. Figure 32–6 shows radical cystectomy boundaries in men, and Figure 32–7 shows the boundaries for women.

The urinary diversion associated with radical cystectomy may be an intestinal conduit (such as an ileal conduit) or a continent urinary reservoir. Figure 32–8 shows an ileal conduit, and Figure 32–9 pictures one type of continent urinary reservoir, which is constructed with a piece of ileum. This technique was first described by Kock and colleagues (1982) and was introduced into the United States by Gerber (1983). Most of the reported experience with this procedure is limited to southern California (Gerber, 1983; Montie, MacGregor, Fazeo, & Lavery, 1986; Skinner, Boyd, & Lieskovsky, 1984).

Ureterosigmoidostomy, a procedure in which the ureters are implanted into the sigmoid colon and urine is then excreted through the rectum, is rarely done today.

Nursing Implications. Potential problems occurring in the first month after creation of an ileal conduit include wound infections, enteric fistulas, urine leaks, ureteral obstruction, bowel obstruction, and pelvic abscesses (Boyd, Lieskovsky, & Skinner, 1988). Late complications include stomal stenosis, peristomal hernias, chronic pyelonephritis, ureteroileal obstruction, intestinal obstruction, calculi, and metabolic problems with hyperchloremic acidosis.

Unlike a fecal diversion, the urinary diversion should produce urine from the time of surgery, and a urinary appliance is needed. Ideally, a urinary stoma should protrude 1.25 to 2 cm (0.5 to 0.75 inch) above the skin to allow the urine to drain into the aperture of an appliance (Lind & Nakao, 1987).

The color of the stoma should be checked frequently in the early postoperative period. Normal color is deep pink to dark red. A dusky appearance could indicate stoma necrosis.

Because the intestine normally produces mucus, mucus will be present in all urinary diversions that use bowel segments. Excessive mucus can, on occasion, clog the urinary appliance. Increasing fluid intake to 3 liters per day will help.

Skin care and the pouching of the stoma are important nursing considerations. Several excellent sources describe these techniques (Broadwell & Jackson, 1982; Lind & Nakao, 1987; Watt, 1986).

Patient teaching is vital for the person with a new urinary diversion. Concepts that should be emphasized include leakage prevention to protect peristomal skin, comfort and ease in handling the various pieces of equipment, early identification of kidney infections, and resources to call on when at home. Body image issues should also be addressed. Teaching should not begin until the patient's physical discomfort has subsided and the physiologic state has returned more or less to normal. Enterostomal therapists are skilled

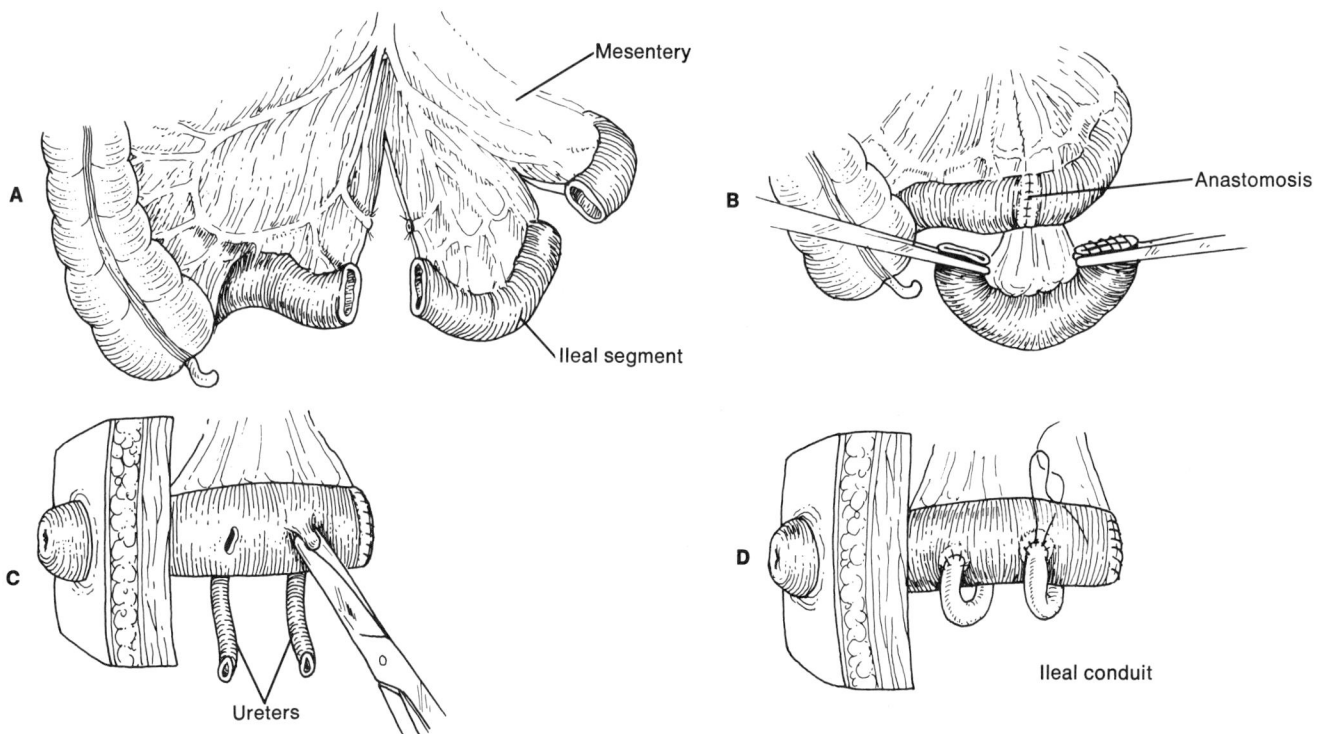

Figure 32–8. Ileal conduit. A, A segment of ileum is isolated from the gastrointestinal tract with its mesenteric blood flow. B, The gastrointestinal tract is reanastomosed. One end is sutured closed, and the other end will be used to form an abdominal stoma. C, The ureters, which are located retroperitoneally, are brought into the abdominal cavity. Incisions are made in the conduit for ureteral implantation. D, The abdominal stoma is matured, and the ureters are anastomosed to the ileum segment in an end-to-side fashion. (From Broadwell, D. C., & Jackson, B. S. [1982]. A primer: Definitions and surgical techniques. In D. C. Broadwell & B. S. Jackson [Eds.], *Principles of ostomy care* [p. 93]. St. Louis: C. V. Mosby Co. Reproduced by permission.)

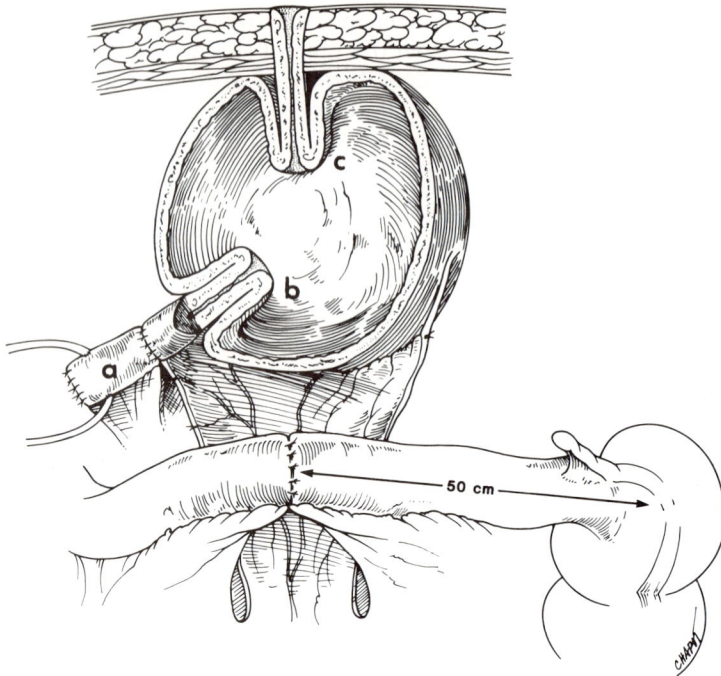

Figure 32–9. The continent ileal reservoir. *(a)* The original ileal conduit with implanted ureters. *(b)* The reflux-preventing nipple valve. *(c)* The continence-maintaining nipple valve. (From Gerber, A. [1983]. The Kock continent ileal reservoir for supravesical urinary diversion. *American Journal of Surgery, 146,* 16. Reproduced by permission.)

specialists in technical matters and help the patient and family learn that a normal life is possible with an ileal conduit.

Complications after radical cystectomy with placement of a continent ileal reservoir, such a Kock pouch, include incontinence, difficult catheterization, urinary reflux, obstruction, bacteriuria, electrolyte imbalances, or absorptive deficits (Montie et al., 1986).

Immediate postoperative nursing concerns for the patient who has had a Kock pouch include checking the stoma for ischemia and irrigating the Medena tube with normal saline solution to wash out both clots and mucus, which might plug the pouch (Lind & Nakao, 1987; Montie et al., 1986). Three to 4 weeks after the operation, when the Medena tube is removed, the nurse will teach the patient to perform self-catheterizations, first every 2 to 3 hr and then every 4 to 6 hr during the day and once at night (Lind & Nakao, 1987; Skinner et al., 1984). Figure 32–10 shows the method of emptying the pouch. With a continent ileal reservoir, there is no need for an external appliance, and intubation of the pouch can duplicate normal bladder function.

A radical cystectomy with urinary diversion affects many aspects of sexual function. The cause of erectile dysfunction after radical cystectomy is similar to that associated with radical prostatectomy for prostatic cancer. However, patients can still achieve orgasm (Schover, von Eschenbach, Smith & Gonzalez, 1984). Because the prostate and seminal vesicles are removed, men experience dry orgasms without emission of semen but still have normal muscle contractions (Schover, Evans, & von Eschenbach, 1986). Women may experience some physiologic problems during intercourse as a result of a shortened vagina. The reader is referred to Chapter 53 for specific information on sexual counseling.

Radiation Therapy

Definitive radiotherapy in bladder cancer is generally reserved for patients who are not candidates for surgery (Skinner & Lieskovsky, 1988). However, outside the United States, invasive bladder cancer frequently is

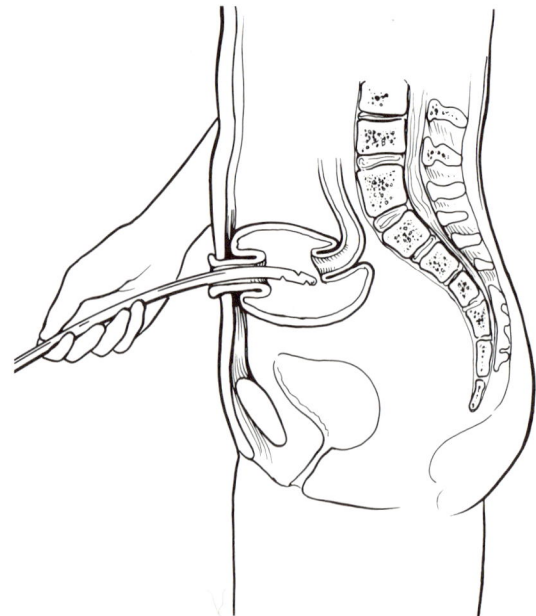

Figure 32–10. Emptying the continent ileal reservoir. (From Montie, J. E., MacGregor, P. S., Fazio, V. W., & Lavery, I. [1986]. Continent ileal reservoir [Kock pouch]. *Urology Clinics of North America, 13,* 254. Reproduced by permission.)

treated primarily by radiotherapy (Duncan & Quilty, 1986).

Preoperative radiotherapy has been advocated in an effort to reduce pelvic recurrence and decrease the possibility of tumor spread during surgery. A typical protocol utilizing high-dose, short-course radiotherapy is 1600 to 2000 Gy (rad) delivered in fractionated doses over 4 days. A more conventional course would include 4000 to 4500 Gy delivered in 4 to 6 weeks (Skinner & Lieskovsky, 1988). Although preoperative radiotherapy can now be safely combined with surgery, most studies have shown no significant improvement in cure in those patients who received radiation (Skinner & Lieskovsky, 1988).

Laser surgery to treat invasive bladder cancer has also been attempted. One clinical trial demonstrated that neodymium YAG laser treatment in patients with clinical stage B1 and some stage B2 disease appears to be capable of eradicating the local lesion within the bladder wall (Smith, 1986).

Complications of radiotherapy include radiation enteritis or colitis and skin reactions. See Chapter 20 for a discussion of nursing care of radiation complications.

Chemotherapy

For superficial, low-grade disease, intravesical chemotherapy (direct instillation of drug into the bladder) has been used to increase the concentration of drug in the area where the tumor cells are located. It may aid in decreasing recurrence by eliminating the residual tumor and stem cells (Herr, 1987).

Thio-TEPA is the drug most commonly used. However, mitomycin C, bacillus Calmette-Guérin (BCG), and doxorubicin (Adriamycin) have also been used (Herr, 1987; Smith, Chisholm, Newsom, & Hargreave, 1986).

Nursing implications include assessment of myelosuppression and handling precautions while the drug(s) are being instilled. See Chapters 21 and 22 for a discussion of myelosuppression and handling precautions.

Recurrence and Palliative Treatment

Superficial recurrences are managed by repeated transurethral resection and intravesical chemotherapy. Provided that they do not develop invasive disease, patients have a 95 per cent 5-year survival. Invasive bladder tumors spread rapidly to the regional lymph nodes and by direct extension into the adjacent structures. About 50 per cent of patients with high-stage, high-grade tumor will have relapses after cystectomy (Daniels, Skinner, & Lieskovsky, 1988). Surgical treatment is seldom used to palliate symptoms in these patients.

Chemotherapy as a treatment for advanced bladder cancer has been investigated and may achieve a complete response in 40 to 50 per cent of the patients (Daniels et al., 1988), but relapse is inevitable. Single-agent therapy using cisplatin, methotrexate, or vinblastine has been attempted with partial responses of short duration. Cisplatin has produced the longest responses (Fass et al., 1986).

Various combination protocols have been tested. Cisplatin, doxorubicin, and cyclophosphamide is one combination protocol that has demonstrated both complete and partial responses in patients with advanced bladder cancer (Daniels et al., 1988). Methotrexate and vinblastine combinations have also demonstrated responses (Ahmed et al., 1985).

The combination programs with higher doses seem to result in higher complete response rates. Unfortunately, they also result in more significant side effects. Nursing management of the side effects of high doses of cisplatin and doxorubicin is challenging. Nausea and vomiting, renal toxicity, ototoxicity, myelosuppression, and the potential for extravasation all must be considered. See Chapter 21 for a more in-depth discussion of these side effects and their nursing implications.

TESTICULAR CANCER

Definition and Incidence

Testicular cancer is a rare tumor that arises in embryonal tissue. Although rare, it is the most common solid tumor in men between 25 and 35 years of age. Dramatic improvement in the management of this disease has been one of cancer's real success stories. The key to this success was the simultaneous development of effective combination chemotherapy and reliable, noninvasive techniques to assess the extent of disease and its response to treatment (Ellis & Sikora, 1986).

Epidemiology and Etiology

Although testicular tumors are uncommon, their incidence is increasing among young white men (Henderson, Ross, & Pike, 1988; Netherell, Drake, & Sikora, 1984).

Cryptorchidism is one of the hypothesized etiologic factors in testicular cancer. Relative risk of testicular cancer in men with an undescended testicle is 3 to 14 times that of normal men (Henderson et al., 1988).

Exogenous estrogens have also been implicated in the causation of testicular cancer. There is an increased risk in the male offspring of women exposed to DES in the first trimester of pregnancy and in women exposed to the estrogen-progestin combinations that have been used frequently as diagnostic tests to confirm pregnancy (Henderson et al., 1988).

Biology and Natural History

Most testicular tumors (97 per cent) arise from germ tissue and are called *germinal tumors*. The following is a list of the various types of germinal testicular tumors.

Seminoma (germinoma) (up to 40 per cent of all testes tumors)

Typical (most common)
Anaplastic
Spermocytic
Nonseminomatous germ cell testicular tumors
(NSGCTT)
Embryonal
Teratocarcinoma
Teratoma
Choriocarcinoma

Many tumors, however, are mixed and contain several distinct elements. There are several staging systems used for cancer of the testis. Two of the most common (Richie, 1988) are described in Table 32–5. A TNM system is also used (Table 32–6).

Survival from testicular cancer has improved dramatically in the last decade. The overall 5-year survival is 89 per cent in whites and 78 per cent in blacks (Silverberg & Lubera, 1989). Patients with early-stage seminomas treated by radiotherapy experience a 5-year survival of more than 90 per cent (Graham & Bagshaw, 1983). The cumulative survival rate for stage II disease is 69 per cent (Smith, 1988). In later stages the prognosis is not as favorable.

Stage I nonseminomatous tumors have a reported 5-year survival of 99 per cent; stage II has a survival of 95 per cent (Fraley, Narayan, Vogelzang, Kennedy, & Lange, 1985). Those patients with disseminated nonseminomatous tumors have an extraordinary long-term survival of approximately 70 per cent (Einhorn, 1988).

Table 32–5. STAGING OF TESTICULAR TUMORS

Walter Reed General Hospital*	Skinner†
I$_A$: Confined to testis; no clinical or radiographic evidence of spread	A: Same, but includes no positive nodes on node dissection
I$_B$: Same as IA, but at lymph node dissection metastases to iliac or para-aortic lymph nodes are found	B: Disease below diaphragm, normal mediastinum, normal chest radiograph
II: Disease below diaphragm, with no spread to visceral organs; clinical or radiographic evidence of metastases to para-aortic, femoral, inguinal, and iliac lymph nodes	B$_1$: <6 positive nodes that are well encapsulated and show no extension into retroperitoneal fat
II+: Palpable abdominal mass (≥ 5 cm)	B$_2$: >6 positive nodes that are encapsulated and may or may not show extension into retroperitoneal fat; any node >2 cm
III: Disease above diaphragm or spread to body organs (clinical radiograph)	B$_3$: Bulky, palpable abdominal mass (>5 cm)
	C: Metastases above diaphragm or liver involvement

*From Maier, J. E., & Sulak, M. H. (1973). Proceedings: Radiation therapy in malignant testis tumors. II. Carcinoma. *Cancer, 32,* 1212–1216.

†From Skinner, D. G. (1969). Non-seminomatous testis tumors: A plan of management based on 96 patients to improve survival in all stages by combined therapeutic modalities. *Journal of Urology,* 115, 65–69.

(From Richie, J. [1988]. Diagnosis and staging of testicular cancer. In D. G. Skinner & G. Lieskovsky [eds.], *Diagnosis and management of genitourinary cancer* [p. 501]. Philadelphia: W. B. Saunders Co. Reproduced by permission.)

Table 32–6. TNM STAGING OF TESTICULAR TUMORS

Primary Tumor (T)

TX	Minimal requirements cannot be met (in the absence of orchiectomy, TX must be used)
T$_0$	No evidence of primary tumor
T$_1$	Tumor limited to body of the testis
T$_2$	Tumor extends beyond the tunica albuginea
T$_3$	Involvement of the rete testis or epididymis
T$_{4A}$	Invasion of the spermatic cord
T$_{4B}$	Invasion of the scrotal wall

Nodal Involvement (N)

NX	Minimum requirements cannot be met
N$_0$	No evidence of involvement of regional lymph nodes
N$_1$	Involvement of a single homolateral regional lymph node, which, if inguinal, is mobile
N$_2$	Involvement of contralateral or bilateral or multiple regional lymph nodes, which, if inguinal, are mobile
N$_3$	Palpable abdominal mass present or fixed inguinal lymph nodes
N$_4$	Involvement of juxtaregional nodes

Distant Metastasis (M)

MX	Not assessed
M$_0$	No (known) distant metastasis
M$_1$	Distant metastasis present

(From Beahrs, O. H., & Myers, M. H. [eds.] (1983). *Manual for staging of cancer* [2nd ed, pp. 166–167]. Philadelphia: J. B. Lippincott Co. Reproduced by permission.)

Presenting Signs and Symptoms

Two thirds of patients have a history of painless enlargement of the testes. Other symptoms include a dragging sensation in the scrotum and rarely a painful mass owing to intratesticular bleeding. Symptoms related to spread of the disease include lumbar pain and abdominal or supraclavicular pain caused by enlarged lymph nodes.

Differential Diagnosis

Epididymitis and hydrocele both occasionally mimic the symptoms of testis cancer.

Diagnostic procedures commonly used in testicular cancer include the following:

- Manual palpation of testes and surrounding structures
- Radical inguinal orchiectomy (as biopsy)
- Radiologic techniques
  Chest radiograph (for lung metastases)
  Computed tomographic (CT) scan of chest (detects lung metastases)
  Abdominal and pelvic CT scan (detects retroperitoneal nodes)
  Excretory urogram
- Laboratory studies
  Serum α-fetaprotein (AFP)
  Serum human chorionic gonadotropin–β subunit (hCG–β)

The laboratory studies determining AFP and hCG–β are used as preoperative tumor markers, and because they reflect the clinical course of the disease, they are very important in the staging of testicular cancer (Horwich & Peckham, 1986).

Elevated serum AFP levels are never seen in men

with *pure* seminomas and therefore help to indicate the presence of a nonseminomatous testicular tumor. Because liver damage can also produce elevated AFP levels, hepatotoxicity from chemotherapy or radiotherapy should be ruled out.

About 50 to 60 per cent of patients with nonseminomatous testicular tumors will have an elevated hCG–β level, and occasionally patients with pure seminomas will also have elevated levels of hCG (Richie, 1988). HCG is normally produced only in pregnant women.

Nursing implications regarding detection of testicular cancer should include educating the public about testicular self-examination (TSE). A 1986 report stated that a moderate percentage of professional men had knowledge of TSE but that very few practiced it. Of those who knew about TSE, none had learned about it from a nurse (Blesch, 1986).

Patient and family education is the other important nursing function at this time. Young, otherwise healthy young men with testicular cancer need help in understanding their treatment and its sequelae. They especially need help with their sexuality and body image concerns. The psychosocial dynamics may also be complex. Independent young adults are often forced to be dependent again on their parents. Nurses can help both the young men and their parents to adjust to the situation.

Treatment for Seminomatous Tumors

Surgery

High radical inguinal orchiectomy, in which the testis, the epididymis, a portion of the vas deferens, and portions of the gonadal lymphatics and blood supply are removed, is routinely done as a diagnostic step.

The remaining testicle will produce enough testosterone to maintain sexual capacity (Bracken, 1981); the orchiectomy has no defined adverse effect on sexual potency or fertility in the otherwise normal patient (Brenner, Vugrin, & Whitmore, 1985). However, studies have shown that a large percentage of men with testicular cancer have a lower sperm count even before treatment (Brenner et al., 1985).

Radiotherapy

Because seminomas are extremely radiosensitive, external beam radiotherapy, directed to the perineum, is used to treat stages A, B1, and B2 disease (stages I, IIA, IIB) (Smith, 1988). If there is retroperitoneal involvement, the mediastinal and supraclavicular nodes will also be irradiated.

Complications associated with pelvic irradiation include fatigue, diarrhea, and azoospermia. Radiotherapy, although it does not affect libido or potency, causes infertility in many men. Moderate oligospermia to azoospermia has been reported after a single testicular dose of 8 to 50 cGy (Levison, 1986; Rowley et al., 1974).

Nursing implications include teaching the patient and family to manage the side effects of radiotherapy and providing information on sexuality issues.

Chemotherapy

Patients with advanced seminoma (stages B3 and C [IIC, III, and IV]) are candidates for chemotherapy, with or without radiotherapy to the pelvis (Smith, 1988). Most protocols use a combination of cisplatin, vinblastine, and bleomycin, with or without doxorubicin (Mendenhall, Williams, Einhorn, & Donohue, 1981). Because this protocol is very similar to the one used for nonseminomatous testicular tumors, the reader is referred to that section for complications and nursing implications.

Treatment for Nonseminomatous Tumors

Surgery

Although orchiectomy is a standard part of surgical "diagnosis," the role of bilateral retroperitoneal lymph node dissection after orchiectomy in treating nonseminomatous germ cell tumors (NSGCTT) remains controversial. Several years ago, the principal NSGCTT treatments were surgery versus radiotherapy, neither of which provided much hope for cure of advanced or bulky disease. Today with chemotherapy, most patients with advanced disease at presentation can be cured, and the debate has shifted to ways in which to reduce treatment morbidity (Fraley et al., 1985).

Advocates of retroperitoneal lymph node dissection (RPLND) believe that it facilitates staging and that it decreases the number of patients who would otherwise need chemotherapy because the tissue that is most likely to contain metastases is removed. Therefore, it has a role as a curative procedure, which, if successful, means the avoidance of chemotherapy (Fraley et al., 1985). Others find that the benefit would be only to a few patients and that many would be subjected to the risks of major surgery unnecessarily (Ellis & Sikora, 1986).

Because many autonomic nerves necessary for ejaculation are located in the retroperitoneal area, infertility may result from this surgery (Bracken, 1981). However, one series reported spontaneous return of normal ejaculatory ability after 3 years in 50 per cent of patients (Fraley et al., 1985).

Nursing implications after RPLND include observation for infection and bleeding immediately after the operation and later patient education regarding sexuality.

Radiotherapy

Because nonseminomatous germ cell tumors are relatively radioresistant, radiotherapy is not routinely used in the United States to treat these tumors.

Chemotherapy

The major role of chemotherapy in NSGCTT is in disseminated disease. In August 1974, early studies were begun at Indiana University using a combination of cisplatin, vinblastine, and bleomycin (PVB) (Einhorn & Donohue, 1977). The results of this chemotherapy combination on NSGCTT has been remarkable and has revolutionized the treatment of testicular cancer. Einhorn (1988) reported a regularly achieved 80 per cent 5-year disease-free survival for patients with disseminated disease.

However, the PVB regimen is highly toxic. Leukopenia, sepsis, nausea and vomiting, and cisplatin-induced nephrotoxicity are common. Raynaud's phenomenon is also a long-term side effect associated with vinblastine therapy.

Another combination using etoposide instead of vinblastine may avoid the long-term morbidity of Raynaud's phenomenon and decrease the added effects of vinblastine and cisplatin (Ellis & Sikora, 1986; Muggia, 1985).

During the same time that the PVB regimen was being tested in Indiana, various combinations of vinblastine, actinomycin D, cyclophosphamide, and cisplatin (VAB programs) were being evaluated at Memorial Sloan-Kettering Hospital (Vugrin, Whitmore, & Sogani, 1981). The results of most of the early VAB programs were inferior to those for PVB, probably because of the intermittent use of cisplatin (Einhorn, 1988).

Because the majority of patients with NSGCTT are living longer than 5 years, the focus has turned to evaluation of long-term side effects and survival. One such long-term effect is indicated in the reports over the last 10 years of cases of acute leukemia in men treated for testicular cancer (Hoekman, Huinink, Egbers-Bogaards, McVie, & Somers, 1984; Johnson, Luedke, Sapiente, & Naidu, 1980; van Imhoff et al., 1986).

Nursing implications for those men treated with chemotherapy are related to the significant side effects of the PVB and the VAB regimens. See Chapter 21 for nursing management of the side effects of cisplatin, bleomycin, vinblastine, actinomycin D, and cyclophosphamide.

Sexuality is also an important nursing concern. In one study of men treated for metastatic NSGCTT with a bilateral RPLND and VAB, only 11 per cent retained ejaculatory ability. The results are better if only unilateral node dissection is done. However, the majority of the patients in the study denied any change in libido (Brenner et al., 1985).

Recurrence and Palliative Treatment

Testicular cancer spreads to the retroperitoneal lymph nodes, to the lungs, and rarely to the brain and liver.

As mentioned previously, chemotherapy is used for advanced disease, both seminomatous and nonseminomatous tumors. In tumors that have been refractory to the PVB regimen, combinations of etoposide, cisplatin, or bleomycin or ifosfamide are being evaluated (Einhorn, 1983).

Nursing implications for late-stage disease are directed primarily toward relieving the side effects associated with chemotherapy. Emotional support for the patients and families is also very important. This disease affects primarily young men, and the family might include wife, small children, and siblings as well as parents. Concern for all of the members of the family will be an important nursing consideration.

CANCER OF THE KIDNEY

Definition and Incidence

There are two major types of kidney cancer: renal cell and transitional cell cancer of the renal pelvis. It is not a common cancer and accounts for only about 2 per cent of all cancers. Renal cell cancer, which occurs in the parenchyma of the kidney, is also known as renal adenocarcinoma, renal cell carcinoma, cancer of the kidney, and hypernephroma. Renal cell cancer accounts for 85 per cent of all kidney tumors and is the only type of kidney cancer discussed in this chapter.

Epidemiology and Etiology

There is a 2 to 1 male predominance in kidney cancer. This disease is rare in people under 35 years of age (Paganini-Hill, Ross, & Henderson, 1988).

The rate of renal cell cancer is high in Scandinavia and low in Japan. The North Central part of the United States, especially Minnesota, has the highest kidney cancer incidence in the United States (Newsom & Vugrin, 1987).

Cigarette smoking has been linked to the incidence of renal cell cancer. One study estimated that 43 per cent of renal cell cancer in Los Angeles is attributable to cigarette smoking (Yu, Mack, & Hanisch, 1986). The highest risk appears to be in the heaviest smokers (Paganini-Hill et al., 1988).

A hormonal association also appears likely. Diethylstilbestrol and estradiol both have induced kidney tumors in rats (Kirkman, 1952). There is little doubt that human renal cell tumors are under some sort of hormonal influence, but the nature of that influence remains controversial (Newsom & Vugrin, 1987).

Coffee consumption has been implicated as causing renal cell cancer, but the results have been conflicting and need further clarification (Newsom & Vugrin, 1987; Paganini-Hill et al., 1988; Yu et al., 1986).

The data also suggest an increased risk of malignancy in patients on chronic hemodialysis (Matas, Simmons, & Kjellstrand, 1975; Sutherland, Glass, & Gabriel, 1977).

Biology and Natural History

Renal cell cancer is divided into two major groups: clear cell tumors and granular cell tumors. Figure 32–

11 describes the staging system for cancer of the kidney.

Presenting Signs and Symptoms

Gross hematuria is present in more than 40 per cent of patients with renal cell cancer (Pritchett, Lieskovsky, & Skinner, 1988). Pain, described as a dull, aching flank pain, also is a common presenting symptom. Finally, a palpable abdominal mass has also been noted on presentation. However, it is rare for these three classic symptoms to appear simultaneously (Pritchett et al., 1988). A wide variety of other vague symptoms also are seen, including fever, weight loss, anemia, and hypercalcemia, which occur infrequently.

Differential Diagnosis

The differential diagnosis is that of a renal mass, most commonly renal cysts and renal tumors. Diagnosis is usually made radiographically because of the variety of presenting symptoms and nonspecific laboratory findings. The advent of renal ultrasound and CT scanning has greatly simplified making the distinction between simple cysts and renal cancer. In many cases, renal angiography is no longer necessary. Tests used in the diagnosis and staging of renal cell cancer include the following: kidneys, ureters, bladder radiograph (KUB), excretory urogram (IVP), nephrotomogram, renal sonogram, renal CT scan, and renal angiogram.

The role of magnetic resonance imaging (MRI) is not yet determined. It does not appear to be better than CT in identifying regional or metastatic disease (Paulson, 1987).

Nursing implications involve education about the nature of the diagnostic tests. Allaying misunderstandings about the implications of losing a kidney might also be important.

Treatment

Surgery

Radical nephrectomy is the removal of the kidney and associated tumor, the adrenal gland, the surrounding perinephric fat within Gerota's fascia, and Gerota's fascia itself. This is the treatment of choice for localized renal cell cancer, which also includes tumor extension into the renal vein and vena cava. There is no role for nephrectomy in patients with disseminated disease.

Regional retroperitoneal lymph node dissection is often routinely performed in association with radical nephrectomy even though there are no solid data supporting its use in improving survival (Skinner & Lieskovsky, 1988).

Nursing implications during the immediate postoperative period include pain management and prevention of postoperative complications. Pain can be quite severe after nephrectomy. As a result of the position on the operating table, the patient experiences not only incisional pain but also muscular strain. Use of moist heat, massage, and pillows to support the back while the patient is lying on his or her side can provide relief.

Postoperative nursing interventions include prevention of atelectasis and pneumonia, monitoring renal function of the remaining kidney, anticipating paralytic ileus, monitoring for bleeding, and preventing infection at the incision site.

Radiotherapy

Most renal cell tumors are radioresistant. However, radiotherapy has been used both preoperatively and postoperatively as an adjunct to nephrectomy. Although this treatment is somewhat controversial, in a review of accumulated data regarding radiotherapy investigators concluded that neither preoperative nor

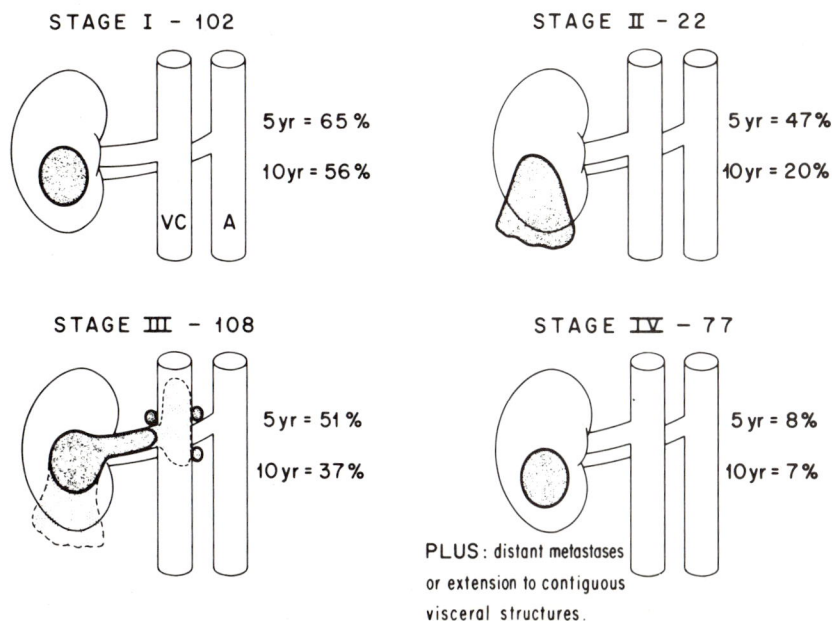

Figure 32–11. Five- and 10-year survival after nephrectomy in 309 patients with renal cell cancer according to the pathologic stage of the lesion. (From Skinner, D. G. [1972]. The surgical management of renal cell carcinoma. *Journal of Urology, 107,* 707. © by Williams & Wilkins, 1972. Reproduced by permission.)

postoperative radiotherapy has been beneficial (deKernion, 1986; Paulson, 1987).

Chemotherapy

There is no effective adjunctive chemotherapy for renal cell carcinoma (deKernion, 1986).

Immunotherapy

Although renal cell cancer has been highly resistant to both chemotherapy and hormonal therapy, preliminary studies suggest that it is particularly susceptible to adoptive immunotherapy with lymphokine-activated killer (LAK) cells plus recombinant interleukin 2 (IL 2) (Belldegrun, Uppenkamp, & Rosenberg, 1988). The use of IL 2 alone has been clinically examined in patients with advanced disseminated disease (Rosenberg, Lotze, & Muul, 1987; West, Tauer, & Yanelli, 1987). However, complete and partial responses have been much higher when combined with LAK cells (Rosenberg, Lotze, & Muul, 1987).

This treatment, however, is complicated, toxic, and expensive (Fowler, 1988). One regimen requires five leukaphereses on consecutive days for a single treatment course. After that, the lymphocytes are incubated with IL 2 for 3 to 4 days. Patients are often monitored in the intensive care unit because, although LAK cell infusions alone are well tolerated, high-dose IL 2 has caused many complications, including malaise, fever, hepatic dysfunction, thrombocytopenia, somnolence, disorientation, and pulmonary edema. Respiratory distress, coma, and even myocardial infarctions have occurred in a few cases (Fowler, 1988).

Other investigators have examined the use of interferon-α in the treatment of patients with advanced renal cell cancer and have shown that it has modest activity, with overall response rates between 15 and 20 per cent. The side effects reported have been tolerable (Sarna, Figlin, & deKernion, 1987).

Recurrence and Palliative Treatment

Renal cell cancer spreads to the medullary portion of the kidney, to the renal vein (sometimes into the vena cava), and to the lungs, bones, brain, and liver. About 30 per cent of patients have metastases at the time of diagnosis.

Palliative nephrectomies are rarely done today. The principal local complications of bleeding, pain, and fever can usually be controlled better by angiographic infarction using a wide variety of materials. The nursing implications for angiographic infarction include watching for hemorrhage.

Chemotherapy has no great impact on metastatic renal cell cancer (Pritchett et al., 1988).

Hormonal therapy in the form of progestational agents or therapy has shown responses in rats (Bloom, 1971). Medroxyprogesterone acetate (Depo-Provera) and megestrol acetate (Megace) have been used with modest rates of response (Bloom, 1971). Although the mild toxicity of hormonal therapy makes it use appealing, responses do not significantly improve survival, and this method has largely been abandoned (Pritch et al., 1988).

As mentioned earlier, therapy employing LAK and IL 2 has been tested in patients with advanced or recurrent disease. Responses thus far have been encouraging. Nursing implications associated with this experimental therapy include extensive patient education and support and intensive monitoring of the severe side effects, such as hypotension, fever, hepatic dysfunction, thrombocytopenia, and disorientation or somnolence.

References

Ahmed, T., Yagoda, A., & Needles, B. (1985). Vinblastine and methotrexate for advanced bladder cancer. *Journal of Urology, 133*, 602–604.

Bagshaw, M. A. (1988). Radiation therapy for cancer of the prostate. In D. G. Skinner & G. Lieskovsky (Eds.), *Diagnosis and management of genitourinary cancer* (pp. 325–445). Philadelphia: W. B. Saunders Co.

Belldegrun, A., Uppenkamp, I., & Rosenberg, S. A. (1988). Antitumor reactivity of human lymphokine activated killer (LAK) cells against fresh and cultured preparations of renal cell cancer. *Journal of Urology, 139*, 150–155.

Blesch, K. S. (1986). Health beliefs about testicular cancer and self-examination among professional men. *Oncology Nursing Forum, 13*(1), 29–33.

Bloom, H. J. (1971). Medroxyprogesterone acetate (Provera) in the treatment of metastatic renal cancer. *British Journal of Cancer, 25*, 250–252.

Bosch, P. C., Forbes, K. A., Prassinichai, S., Miller, J. B., Golji, H., & Martin, D. C. (1986). Preliminary observations on the results of combined temporary 192-iridium implantation and external beam irradiation for carcinoma of the prostate. *Journal of Urology, 135*, 722–725.

Boyd, S. D., Lieskovsky, G., & Skinner, D. G. (1988). Cutaneous urinary diversion in the cancer patient. In D. G. Skinner & G. Leiskovsky (Eds.), *Diagnosis and management of genitourinary cancer* (pp. 634–648). Philadelphia: W. B. Saunders Co.

Bracken, R. B. (1981). Cancer of the testis, penis and urethra: The impact of therapy on sexual function. In A. von Eschenbach & D. Rodriguez (Eds.), *Sexual rehabilitation of the urologic cancer patient* (pp. 108–127). Boston: G. K. Hall.

Brenner, J., Vugrin, D., & Whitmore, W. (1985). Effect of treatment on fertility and sexual function in males with metastatic nonseminomatous germ cell tumors of testis. *American Journal of Clinical Oncology (Cancer Clinical Trials), 8*, 178–182.

Broadwell, D. C., & Jackson, B. S. (Eds.). (1982). *Principles of ostomy care.* St. Louis: C. V. Mosby Co.

Carlton, C. E. (1988). Radioactive isotope implantation for cancer of the prostate. In D. G. Skinner & G. Lieskovsky (Eds.), *Diagnosis and management of genitourinary cancer* (pp. 446–453). Philadelphia: W. B. Saunders Co.

Daniels, J. R., Skinner, D. G., & Lieskovsky, G. (1988). Chemotherapy of carcinoma of bladder. In D. G. Skinner & G. Lieskovsky (Eds.), *Diagnosis and management of genitourinary tumors* (pp. 313–322.) Philadelphia: W. B. Saunders Co.

deKernion, J. B. (1985). Cancer of the bladder. In C. Haskell (Ed.), *Cancer treatment* (2nd ed., pp. 367–381). Philadelphia: W. B. Saunders Co.

deKernion, J. B. (1986). Renal cell carcinoma. *Journal of Urology, 136*, 882.

Doll, R. (1978). Geographic variation in cancer incidence: A clue to causation. *World Journal of Surgery, 2*, 595–602.

Duncan, W., & Quilty, P. M. (1986). The results of a series of 963 patients with transitional cell carcinoma of the urinary bladder primarily treated by radical megavoltage x-ray therapy. *Radiotherapy and Oncology, 7*, 299–310.

Einhorn, L. H. (1983). An overview of chemotherapeutic trials in advanced cancer of the prostate. In D. G. Skinner (Ed.), *Urological cancer* (pp. 89–100). New York: Grune & Stratton, Inc.

Einhorn, L. H. (1988). Chemotherapy of disseminated testicular cancer. In D. G. Skinner & G. Lieskovsky (Eds.), *Diagnosis and management of gentourinary cancer* (pp. 526–531). Philadelphia: W. B. Saunders Co.

Einhorn, L. H., & Donohue, J. P. (1977). Cis-diamminedichloroplatinum, vinblastine and bleomycin combination chemotherapy in disseminated testicular cancer. *Annals of Internal Medicine, 87,* 293–298.

Ellis, M., & Sikora, K. (1986). The current management of testicular cancer. *British Journal of Urology, 59,* 2–9.

Fass, D., Steinfeld, A., Brown, J., & Tessler, A. (1986). Radiotherapeutic prophylaxis of estrogen-induced gynecomastia: A study of late sequel. *International Journal of Radiation Oncology, Biology, Physics, 12,* 407–408.

Fowler, J. E. (1988). Adoptive immunotherapy using lymphokine-activated killer cells. *Journal of Urology, 139,* 148–149.

Fraley, E. E., Narayan, P., Vogelzang, N. J., Kennedy, B. J., & Lange, P. (1985). Surgical treatment of patients with stages I and II nonseminomatous testicular cancer. *Journal of Urology, 134,* 70–73.

Gerber, A. (1983). The Kock continent ileal reservoir for supravesical urinary diversion. *American Journal of Surgery, 146,* 15–21.

Gibbons, R. P., Cole, B. S., Richardson, R. G., Correa, R. J., Brannen, G. E., Mason, J. T., Taylor, W. J., & Hafermann, M. D. (1986). Adjuvant radiotherapy following radical prostatectomy: Results and complications. *Journal of Urology, 135,* 65–68.

Gleason, D. F., Mellinger, G. T., & the Veteran's Administration Cooperative Urological Research Group. (1974). Prediction of prognosis for prostatic adenocarcinoma by combined histological grading and staging. *Journal of Urology, 111,* 58–64.

Graham, L. D., & Bagshaw, M. (1983). Treatment of testicular germinomas. In D. G. Skinner (Ed.), *Urological cancer* (pp. 281–300). New York: Grune & Stratton, Inc.

Graham, S. D., Laszlo, J., Walker, A., Berry, W. R., Cox, E. B., & Paulson, D. F. (1986). Value of cyclophosphamide or melphalan as combined chemotherapy in hormonally unresponsive prostatic carcinoma. *Urology, 28,* 404–408.

Heinrich-Rynning, T. (1987). Prostatic cancer treatments and their effects on sexual functioning. *Oncology Nursing Forum, 14*(6), 37–41.

Henderson, B. E., Ross, R. K., & Pike, M. C. (1988). Epidemiology of testicular cancer. In D. G. Skinner & G. Lieskovsky (Eds.), *Diagnosis and management of genitourinary cancer* (pp. 46–52). Philadelphia: W. B. Saunders Co.

Herr, H. (1987). Intravesical therapy—a critical review. *Urology Clinics of North America, 14,* 399–404.

Hoekman, K., Huinink, W. W. T. B., Egbers-Bogaards, M., McVie, J. G., & Somers, R. (1984). Acute leukemia following therapy for teratoma. *European Journal of Cancer and Clinical Oncology, 20,* 501–502.

Horwich, A., & Peckham, M. J. (1986). Transient tumor marker elevation following chemotherapy for germ cell tumors of the testis. *Cancer Treatment Reports, 70,* 1329–1331.

Huben, R. P., & Murphy, G. P. (1988). Management of advanced cancer of the prostate. In D. G. Skinner & G. Lieskovsky (Eds.), *Diagnosis and management of genitourinary cancer* (pp. 473–482). Philadelphia: W. B. Saunders Co.

Johnson, D. C., Luedke, D. W., Sapiente, R. A., & Naidu, R. G., (1980). Acute lymphocytic leukemia developing in a male with germ cell carcinoma: A case report. *Medical and Pediatric Oncology, 8,* 361–365.

Kirkman, H. (1952). Estrogen-induced tumors of the kidney. II. Effect of dose, administration, type of estrogen, and age on the induction of renal tumors in intact male golden hamsters. *Journal of the National Cancer Institute, 13,* 757–771.

Kock, N. G., Nilson, A. E., Nilsson, L. O., Horlen, L. J., Philipson, B. M., (1982). Urinary diversion via a continent ileal reservoir: Clinical results in 12 patients. *Journal of Urology, 128,* 469–475.

Kramer, S. A., Cline, W. A., Farnharm, R., Carson, C. C., Cox, E. B., Hinshaw, W., & Paulson, D. F. (1981). Prognosis of patients with stage D1 prostatic carcinoma. *Journal of Urology, 125,* 817–819.

Kramer, S. A., Spahr, J., Brendler, C., Glenn, J., & Paulson, D. F. (1980). Experience with Gleason's histopathologic grading in prostatic cancer. *Journal of Urology, 124,* 223–225.

Layfield, L. J., Mukamel, E., Hilborne, L. H., Hannah, J. B., Glasgow, B. J., Ljung, B., & deKernion, J. B. (1984). Cytological grading of prostatic aspiration biopsy: A comparison with the Gleason grading system. *Journal of Urology, 138,* 798–800.

Levison, V. (1986). The effect on fertility, libido, and sexual function of post-operative radiotherapy and chemotherapy for cancer of the testicle. *Clinical Radiology, 37,* 161–164.

Lieskovsky, G., Ahlering, T., & Skinner, D. G. (1988). Diagnosis and staging of bladder cancer. In D. G. Skinner & G. Lieskovsky (Eds.), *Diagnosis and management of genitourinary cancer* (pp. 264–280). Philadelphia: W. B. Saunders Co.

Lind, J. (1987). Prostate cancer. In C. R. Ziegfeld (Ed.), *Core curriculum for oncology nursing* (pp. 129–136). Philadelphia: W. B. Saunders Co.

Lind, J., & Nakao, S. L. (1987). Urologic and male genital malignancies. In S. Groenwald (Ed.), *Cancer nursing principles and practice* (pp. 700–745). Boston: Jones & Bartlett.

Matas, A. J., Simmons, R. L., & Kjellstrand, C. M. (1975). Increased incidence of malignancy during chronic renal failure. *Lancet, 1,* 883–886.

McCullogh, D. L. (1988). Diagnosis and staging of prostatic cancer. In D. G. Skinner & G. Lieskovsky (Eds.), *Diagnosis and management of genitourinary cancer* (pp. 405–416). Philadelphia: W. B. Saunders Co.

Mendenhall, W. L., Williams, S. D., Einhorn, L. H., & Donohue, J. P. (1981). Disseminated seminoma: Re-evaluation of treatment protocols. *Journal of Urology, 126,* 493–496.

Middleton, R. G., Smith, J. A., Melzer, R. B., & Hamilton, P. E. (1986). Patient survival and local recurrence rate following radical prostatectomy for prostatic carcinoma. *Journal of Urology, 136,* 422–424.

Montie, J. E., MacGregor, P. S., Fazio, V. W., & Lavery, I. (1986). Continent ileal reservoir (Kock pouch). *Urology Clinics of North America, 13,* 251–260.

Muggia, F. M. (1985). Testicular cancer and the legacy of chemotherapy. *Cancer Chemotherapy and Pharmacology, 15,* 1–5.

Nethersell, A. B. W., Drake, L. K., & Sikora, K. (1984). The increasing incidence of testicular cancer in East Anglia. *British Journal of Cancer, 50,* 377–380.

Newsom, G. D., & Vugrin, D. (1987). Etiologic factors in renal cell adenocarcinoma. *Seminars in Nephrology, 7,* 109–116.

Noble, R. (1980). Production of Nb rat carcinoma of the dorsal prostate and response of estrogen-dependent transplant to sex hormones and tamoxifen. *Cancer Research, 40,* 3547–3550.

Paganini-Hill, A., Ross, R. K., & Henderson, B. E. (1988). Epidemiology of renal cell cancer. In D. G. Skinner & G. Lieskovsky (Eds.), *Diagnosis and management of genitourinary cancer* (pp. 32–39). Philadelphia: W. B. Saunders Co.

Paulson, D. F. (1987). Treatment strategies in renal carcinoma. *Seminars in Nephrology, 7,* 140–151.

Paulson, D. F. (1988). Role of endocrine therapy in the management of prostatic cancer. In D. G. Skinner & G. Lieskovsky (Eds.), *Diagnosis and management of genitourinary cancer* (pp. 464–472). Philadelphia: W. B. Saunders Co.

Paulson, D. F., Lin, G. H., Hinshaw, W., Stephani, S., & the Uro-Oncology Research Group. (1982). Radical surgery vs. radiotherapy for adenocarcinoma of the prostate. *Journal of Urology, 128,* 502–504.

Paulson, D. F., Stone, A. R., Walther, P. J., Tucker, J. A., & Cox, E. B. (1986). Radical prostatectomy: Anatomical predictors of success or failure. *Journal of Urology, 136,* 1041–1043.

Pavone-Macaluso, M., deVoogt, H. J., Viggiano, G., Barasolo, E., Lardennois, B., dePauw, M., & Sylvester, R. (1986). Comparison of diethylstilbestrol, cyproterone acetate and medroxyprogesterone acetate in the treatment of advanced prostatic cancer: Final analysis of a randomized phase III trial of the European Organization on Treatment of Cancer Urological Group. *Journal of Urology, 136,* 624–631.

Perez, C. A., Ihde, D. C., Fair, W. R., & Labrie, F. (1985). Cancer of the prostate. In V. T. DeVita, Jr., S. Hellman, & S. A. Rosenberg (Eds.), *Cancer: Principles and practice of oncology* (2nd ed. pp. 929–960). Philadelphia: J. B. Lippincott Co.

Pilepich, M. V., Basgshaw, M. A., Asbell, S. O., Hanks, G. E., Krall, J. M., Emami, B. N., & Bard, R. H. (1986). Definitive radiotherapy on resectable (stage A2 and B) carcinoma of the prostate—results of a nationwide overview. *International Journal of Radiation Oncology, Biology, Physics, 13,* 659–663.

Pilepich, M. V., Krall, J. M., Johnson, R. J., Sause, W. T., Perez, C. A., Zinninger, M., & Martz, K. (1986). Extended field (peri-aortic) irradiation in carcinoma of the prostate—analysis of RTOG 75–06. *International Journal of Radiation Oncology, Biology, Physics, 12*, 345–351.

Pritchett, T. R., Lieskovsky, G., & Skinner, D. G. (1988). Manifestations and treatment of renal parenchymal tumors. In D. G. Skinner & G. Lieskovsky (Eds.), *Diagnosis and management of genitourinary cancer* (pp. 337–361). Philadelphia: W. B. Saunders Co.

Rajfer, J., Handelsman, D. J., Crum, A., Steiner, B., Peterson, M., & Swerdloff, R. S. (1986). Comparison of the efficacy of subcutaneous and nasal spray buserelin treatment in the suppression of testicular steroidogenesis in men with prostatic cancer. *Fertility and Sterility, 46*, 104–110.

Richie, J. (1988). Diagnosis and staging of testicular cancer. In D. G. Skinner, & G. Lieskovsky (Eds.), *Diagnosis and management of genitourinary cancer* (pp. 498–507). Philadelphia: W. B. Saunders Co.

Rosenberg, S. A., Lotze, M. T., & Muul, L. M. (1987). A progress report on the treatment of 157 patients with advanced cancer using lymphokine-activated killer cells and interleukin-2 or high-dose interleukin-2 alone. *New England Journal of Medicine, 316*, 889–891.

Ross, R. K., Paganini-Hill, A., & Henderson, B. E. (1988a). Epidemiology of bladder cancer. In D. G. Skinner & G. Lieskovsky (Eds.), *Diagnosis and management of genitourinary cancer* (pp. 23–31). Philadelphia: W. B. Saunders Co.

Ross, R. K., Paganini-Hill, A., & Henderson, B. E. (1988b). Epidemiology of prostate cancer. In D. G. Skinner & G. Lieskovsky (Eds.), *Diagnosis and management of genitourinary cancer* (pp. 40–45). Philadelphia: W. B. Saunders Co.

Rowley, M. J., Leach, D. R., Warner, G. A., & Heller, C. G. (1974). Effect of graded doses of ionizing radiation in the human testes. *Radiation Research, 59*, 665–678.

Sarna, G., Figlin, R., & deKernion, J. B. (1987). Interferon in renal cell carcinoma. *Cancer, 59*, 610–612.

Schover, L. R., Evans, R., & von Eschenbach, A. C. (1986). Sexual rehabilitation and male radical cystectomy. *Journal of Urology, 136*, 1015–1017.

Schover, L. R., von Eschenbach, A. C., Smith, D. B., & Gonzalez, J. (1984). Sexual rehabilitation of urologic cancer patients: A practical approach. *Cancer, 34*, 66–68.

Silverberg, E., & Lubera, J. (1989). Cancer statistics, 1989. *CA: A Cancer Journal for Clinicians, 39*, 3–20.

Skinner, D. G., Boyd, S. D., & Lieskovsky, G. (1984). Clinical experience with the Kock continent ileal reservoir for urinary diversion. *Journal of Urology, 132*, 1101–1107.

Skinner, D. G., & Lieskovsky, G. (1988). Management of invasive and high grade bladder cancer. In D. G. Skinner & G. Lieskovsky (Eds.), *Diagnosis and management of genitourinary cancer* (pp. 684–703). Philadelphia: W. B. Saunders Co.

Smith, J. A. (1986). Treatment of invasive bladder cancer with a neodymium:YAG laser. *Journal of Urology, 135*, 55–57.

Smith, R. A. E., Chisholm, G. D., Newsom, J. E., & Hargreave, T. B. (1986). Superficial bladder cancer: Intravesical chemotherapy and tumor progression to muscle invasion or metastases. *British Journal of Urology, 58*, 659–663.

Smith, R. B. (1988). Testicular seminoma. In D. G. Skinner & G. Lieskovsky (Eds.), *Diagnosis and management of genitourinary cancer* (pp. 508–515). Philadelphia: W. B. Saunders Co.

Sutherland, G. A., Glass, J., & Gabriel, R. (1977). Increased incidence of malignancy in chronic renal failure. *Nephron, 18*, 182–184.

van Imhoff, G. W., Sleijfer, D. T., Breuning, M. H., Anders, G., Mulder, N. H., & Halie, M. R. (1986). Acute nonlymphocytic leukemia 5 years after treatment with cisplatin, vinblastine, and bleomycin for disseminated testicular cancer. *Cancer, 57*, 984–987.

Vugrin, D., Whitmore, W., & Sogani, P. C. (1981). Combined chemotherapy and surgery in treatment of advanced germ cell tumors. *Cancer, 47*, 2228–2231.

Waisman, J., Mott, L. J. (1978). Pathology of neoplasms of the prostate gland. In D. G. Skinner & J. B. deKernion (Eds.), *Genitourinary cancer* (pp. 310–343). Philadelphia: W. B. Saunders Co.

Walsh, P. C., & Mostwin, J. C. (1984). Radical prostatectomy and cystoprostatectomy with preservation of potency. Results using a new nerve-sparing technique. *British Journal of Urology, 56*, 694–699.

Watt, R. C. (1986). Nursing management of a patient with a urinary diversion. *Seminars in Oncology Nursing, 2*, 265–269.

Waxman, J. H., Sandow, J., Man, A., Barnett, M. J., Hendry, W. F., Besser, G. M., Oliver, R. T. D., & Magill, P. J. (1986). The first clinical use of depot buserelin for advanced prostatic carcinoma. *Cancer Chemotherapy and Pharmacology, 18*, 174–175.

West, W. H., Tauer, K. W., & Yanelli, J. R. (1987). Constant-infusion recombinant interleukin-2 in adoptive immunotherapy of advanced cancer. *New England Journal of Medicine, 316*, 898–900.

Yu, M. C., Mack, T., & Hanisch, R. (1986). Cigarette smoking, obesity, diuretic use and coffee consumption as risk factors for renal cell carcinoma. *Journal of the National Cancer Institute, 77*, 351–356.

CHAPTER 33

Gastrointestinal Cancers

GRACEANN EHLKE

Cancers of the gastrointestinal system account for the largest number of cancers in any one body system. Because of the location of many of the gastrointestinal organs, the prognosis of many of these cancers has been poor. Better screening techniques and new treatment protocols show promise of a decrease in mortality rates. For example, with esophageal cancer, several new treatments have become available that have caused optimism for "cure" with some types of the disease. The most common sites for gastrointestinal cancer for adults are identified in Figure 33–1.

CANCER OF THE ESOPHAGUS

Definition and Incidence

The incidence of esophageal cancer in the United States is increasing slightly. The estimated incidence for 1985 was 9400 and for 1989 was 10,100 (Silverberg, 1985; Silverberg & Lubera, 1989). Esophageal cancer is more common in men than in women and is most frequently seen in those older than 60 years.

In the United States, the mean survival for patients with esophageal carcinoma is presently between 3 and 20 months. Five-year survival rate is less than 5 per cent.

Epidemiology and Etiology

Esophageal cancer is common in Japan, the southern shore of the Caspian Sea (Iran), and northern China.

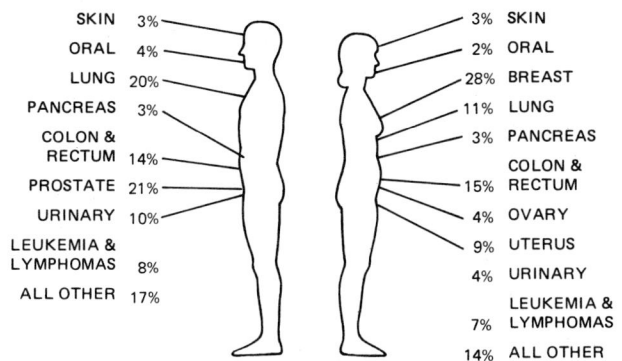

† Excluding nonmelanoma skin cancer and carcinoma in situ.

Figure 33–1. Estimated cancer incidence by site and sex, 1989. (From Silverberg, E., & Lubera, J. A. [1989]. Cancer statistics, 1989. *CA: A Cancer Journal for Clinicians, 39,* 3–32. Reproduced by permission.)

485

In the United States, esophageal cancer is common in North Carolina and Washington, DC.

Conditions that increase the risk of development of esophageal cancer include Barrett's esophagus, Plummer-Vinson syndrome, a history of head and neck squamous carcinoma, untreated achalasia or lye stricture of long duration, hereditary tylosis, nontropical sprue, and diverticulum of the pharynx or esophagus.

Additional risk factors include alcohol consumption and smoking. Dietary factors include deficiencies in iron or zinc, hot (temperature) beverages, and silica dust (Iranian bread).

Biology and Natural History

Table 33–1 lists the different histologic types of esophageal cancer. The tumor, nodes, and metastases (TNM) staging of esophageal cancer is listed in Table 33–2.

The mean survival in esophageal cancer is extremely low, frequently because it is diagnosed in an advanced stage. With esophageal cancer, prognosis may depend on location of the tumor: 20 per cent of the tumors are in the upper one third of the esophagus, 37 per cent are in the middle of the esophagus, and 43 per cent are in the lower third. Tumors in the upper esophagus are very difficult to treat with current therapies and have a poorer prognosis than lower third tumors.

Presenting Signs and Symptoms

A major indication of cancer of the esophagus is dysphagia for solids and eventually liquids, which is associated with weight loss. When dysphagia occurs, the lumen of the esophagus may be reduced by 75 per

Table 33–1. MALIGNANT ESOPHAGEAL TUMORS

Epithelial Tumors
  Squamous cell carcinoma
    Well differentiated
    Moderately differentiated
    Poorly differentiated
  Variants of squamous cell carcinoma
    Spindle cell carcinoma
    Pseudosarcoma and carcinosarcoma
    Verrucous carcinoma
    In situ carcinoma
  Adenocarcinoma
    Adenoacanthoma
  Adenoid cystic carcinoma (cylindroma)
  Mucoepidermoid carcinoma
  Adenosquamous carcinoma
  Carcinoid
  Undifferentiated carcinoma
    Oat cell carcinoma
Nonepithelial Tumors
  Leiomyosarcomas
  Malignant melanoma
  Myoblastoma
  Choriocarcinoma
  Rhabdomyosarcoma

(Data from Rosenberg, Schwade, & Vaitkevicius, 1982, p. 505.)

cent. Odynophagia is present in approximately 50 per cent of the cases and is an indication of poor prognosis; this may reflect compression of spinal nerves and mediastinal involvement. Hoarseness is usually a symptom when the laryngeal nerve is affected. A chronic cough may be noted in patients with an esophageal-tracheal (ET) fistula, or it may be seen as a result of aspiration. Autopsy results reveal that nearly 50 per cent of the patients have bronchopneumonia.

The most serious symptoms are hoarseness and chronic cough. In addition, hemoptysis usually implies that the aorta is involved.

Differential Diagnosis

Diagnosis of some types of esophageal cancer can be made via chest radiograph. In these cases, a posterior tracheal stripe has been described as an indication of esophageal cancer of the upper and middle portions of the esophagus (Putnam, Curtis, Westfried, & McLoud, 1978). In approximately 50 per cent of the patients, this stripe could be seen on radiographs 6 months before the patient developed symptoms of esophageal cancer.

For those patients with dysphagia, a barium swallow is usually ordered. This is a procedure for diagnosis of many esophageal tumors.

Esophagoscopy allows a tissue diagnosis. It is accurate 96 per cent of the time (Bruni & Nelson, 1975). Gallium or cobalt-bleomycin tracers are taken up by squamous cell cancers and have been reliable indicators of tumor in some cases.

In studies by Moss and co-workers (1981) and Quint and associates (1985a and 1985b) the investigators found that computed tomography (CT) is effective and more reliable than magnetic resonance imaging (MRI) in the identification of esophageal cancer; however, it is not accurate in detecting extent of disease. On the other hand, endoscopic ultrasound (EUS) is a promising development in the diagnosis of esophageal cancer. In this procedure, endoscopy is merged with ultrasound technology. This technique is effective in measuring depth of penetration of the tumor.

Additional diagnostic procedures include exfoliative cytology by esophageal lavage and balloon-mesh cytology. With the balloon-mesh cytology, a catheter with a balloon on the end is inserted through the mouth. The balloon is covered with a nylon mesh covering. Before withdrawing the catheter, the balloon is inflated. As the catheter is removed, the nylon mesh covering of the balloon collects cells that adhere to it.

Treatment

Because esophageal cancer is frequently diagnosed in an advanced stage, treatment for cure of the disease is usually not possible. However, if the tumor is diagnosed in an early stage, both radiation and surgery can be used to cure the disease.

Most of the treatment methods currently in use are

Table 33–2. TNM STAGING FOR ESOPHAGEAL CANCER

Primary Tumor (T)

T_0 No demonstrable tumor

T_{IS} Carcinoma in situ

T_1 Tumor involves 5 cm or less of esophageal length with no obstruction or complete circumferential involvement or extraesophageal spread

T_2 Tumor involves more than 5 cm of esophagus and produces obstruction with circumferential involvement of the esophagus but no extraesophageal spread

T_3 Tumor with extension outside the esophagus involving mediastinal structures

Regional Lymph Nodes (N)

Cervical esophagus (cervical and supraclavicular lymph nodes)

N_0 No nodal involvement

N_1 Unilateral involvement (moveable)

N_2 Bilateral involvement (moveable)

N_3 Fixed nodes

Thoracic esophagus (nodes in the thorax, not those of the cervical supraclavicular or abdominal areas)

N_0 No nodal involvement

N_1 Nodal involvement

Distant Metastases

M_0 No metastases

M_1 Distant metastases. Cancer of thoracic esophagus with cervical, supraclavicular, or abdominal lymph node involvement is classified as M^1

(Data from Rosenberg, Schwade, & Vaitkevicius, 1982, p. 509.)

for palliation of the disease. There are four main purposes of palliative treatment. The first is to open the esophageal lumen. This may be done by surgery, radiation therapy, dilation, prosthesis, laser, or tumor probe.

The second goal is to slow the growth of the tumor. These treatments include surgery, radiation therapy, or chemotherapy.

The third purpose of palliative treatment—to seal a fistula—is done with a prosthesis.

The final purpose of palliative treatment is to provide nutrition. Usually this is done via a gastrostomy or jejunostomy.

One chemotherapy protocol that has been shown to have an effect on esophageal cancer is a combination using a continuous infusion of 5-fluorouracil (5-FU) for 21 days in addition to cisplatin.

Another popular treatment for esophageal carcinoma is endoscopic laser therapy (ELT). Laser therapy works by vaporizing neoplastic tissue. Other thermal devices are also used to treat esophageal cancer, most notably bipolar electrocoagulation. This treatment uses heat at the cancer site, and its popularity is attributable to a decrease in problems usually associated with laser treatment. For example, laser treatment is not usually effective in tumors in the upper portion of the esophagus because the laser cannot be positioned adequately for such tumors. A second problem with laser treatment is that smoke may develop in the treatment area, which decreases visibility. The bipolar probe does not present these problems.

Nursing Care

The major problems for patients with esophageal cancer are nutritional ones. Therefore, the primary nursing diagnosis for a patient with esophageal cancer is *alteration in nutrition*.

Patients with esophageal cancer will have an alteration in nutrition owing to an inability to take in food.

This causes difficulty in swallowing, which results from constriction of the esophagus by the tumor. The alteration in nutrition leads to a decrease in weight and cachexia. For additional problems related to alteration in nutrition, see Chapter 47.

This nursing diagnosis is also a major problem for patients with gastric cancer. Trying to maintain a nutritional state that will enable the individual to undergo treatment for the disease is a major challenge for the nurse.

GASTRIC CARCINOMA

Definition and Incidence

The incidence of gastric cancer has steadily decreased in the last 55 years. Evidence of this decline is noted in the decline in cancer death rates per 100,000 population from more than 30 in 1930 to less than 10 in 1985 (American Cancer Society, 1989). The peak age for gastric cancer is 55 to 65 years (Burn & Welbourn, 1975), and the male-to-female ratio is 3:2 in favor of men (Burn & Welbourn, 1975); however, mortality rates for women are one half those for men (Waterhouse, 1984).

Epidemiology and Etiology

The highest incidence of gastric cancer occurs in Japan (see Box 33–1) followed by Chile (Waterhouse, 1984). The mortality rate of this cancer is high, with the 1988 mortality rate at 14,400 (Silverberg & Lubera, 1989). Considering all stages of disease, approximately 16 per cent of persons with gastric cancer live 5 years. However, of those with localized disease, 75 per cent live 5 years (Silverberg, 1987).

Gastric cancer has been linked etiologically to heredity, diet, socioeconomic status, and other carcinogens, such as exposure to dust in coal mines and

---

Box 33–1. CANCER MORTALITY AMONG JAPANESE-AMERICANS

Haenszel, W., & Kurihara, M. (1968). **Studies of Japanese migrants: 1. Mortality from cancer and other diseases among Japanese in the United States.** *Journal of the National Cancer Institute,* 40(1), 43–68.

Cancer mortality among Japanese-Americans for 1959–1962, emphasizing contrasts of Issei-Nisei experience, is reviewed and compared with earlier findings. Japanese migrant experience concerning changes in cancer risk appears generally consistent with those of other groups migrating to the United States. Stomach cancer mortality rates among Issei and Nisei are more closely aligned to the high rates in Japan than to the low rates in the United States. On the other hand, mortality rates for cancer of the colon among Japanese (particularly men) have risen to almost equal the higher risks prevailing for United States whites. An atypical feature of Japanese migrant experience was the persistence among Issei and Nisei women of the low breast cancer risks characteristic of Japan, with no apparent tendency to rise to the host population level.

---

potteries. One of the main hypotheses on causation relates to preservation of foods through refrigeration as a major factor in the decrease of gastric cancer (Waterhouse, 1984). This hypothesis is controversial, however, because other investigators hypothesize that the decrease relates to a decrease in gastric atrophy in adults (Hill, 1984).

Biology and Natural History

Of the several classification systems used for gastric cancer, the one used most frequently is that of Lauren (1965). In this classification, gastric cancer is defined as intestinal-type or diffuse gastric cancer. The characteristics of these two types of cancers are given in Table 33–3. The staging of gastric cancer is illustrated in Figure 33–2 and described in Table 33–4.

The prognosis of gastric cancer depends on the stage of disease. Early gastric carcinoma, if treated surgically, carries 5-year survival rates of 85 to 90 per cent (Biasco et al., 1987; Kidokoro, 1971). Early gastric cancers that remain untreated become advanced gastric cancers in 3 to 8 years (Okabe, 1971). The 5-year survival rate for advanced gastric cancer is 16 per cent.

Table 33–3. THE CHARACTERISTICS OF DIFFUSE VERSUS INTESTINAL-TYPE GASTRIC CANCERS

	Diffuse	Intestinal
Relative age at onset	Slightly younger	Slightly older
Male-to-female ratio	Approximately 1	>1
Location	Often in the cardia	Mainly antral
Blood group association	Group A	None
Associated diseases	Pernicious anemia Hypogammaglobulinemia	Atrophic gastritis Intestinal metaplasia
Gross morphology	Ulcerous	Polypoid
Prognosis	Poor	Better
Familial association	Strong	Weak
Environmental association	Weak	Strong

(With permission from Hill, M. J. [1984]. Aetiology of gastric cancer. *Clinics in Oncology, 3,* 237–249.)

Presenting Signs and Symptoms

With early gastric cancer, abdominal pain is a frequent symptom. In a study by Biasco and colleagues (1987), all patients with depressed lesions or ulcerated lesions had abdominal pain (48 of 80 patients). Other symptoms of early gastric cancer frequently noted by Biasco and co-workers were anorexia, nausea, vomiting, and weight loss. In most other studies, however, (Macdonald, Gunderson, & Adson, 1982; Morton, Poulter, & Pandya, 1983), the patients' presenting complaints were vague abdominal symptoms that are usually thought to be related to ulcer disease. According to Morton and colleagues (1983), other early signs of gastric cancer include fullness, belching, regurgitation, and pain after meals and (dyspepsia).

Differential Diagnosis

At the present time, the best diagnostic tool for gastric carcinoma is endoscopy. In the study by Biasco and co-workers (1987), 82.5 per cent of the early gastric cancers were correctly diagnosed with endoscopy versus 43.5 per cent with barium studies. Other diagnostic tools that may be used include indirect radiology, gastric juice factors (fetal sialoglycoprotein and lactic dehydrogenase), serum tests (tetracycline test), urine test (Diagnex Blue test), gastric juice (pH, alpha-acid glycoprotein, and carcinoembryonic antigen [CEA]) and serologic tests (alpha$_1$-fetoprotein, CEA, and pepsinogen I).

Treatment

Surgery

The major curative treatment of gastric cancer is surgery. Most often a subtotal gastrectomy is done with removal of only that portion of the stomach that is diseased. In addition, the omentum and associated lymph nodes are removed. Other organs that may be removed include the spleen and the distal portion of the pancreas. In addition, splenic or pancreatic lymph nodes, or both groups of nodes, may be removed. The best survival rates are found in the Japanese studies,

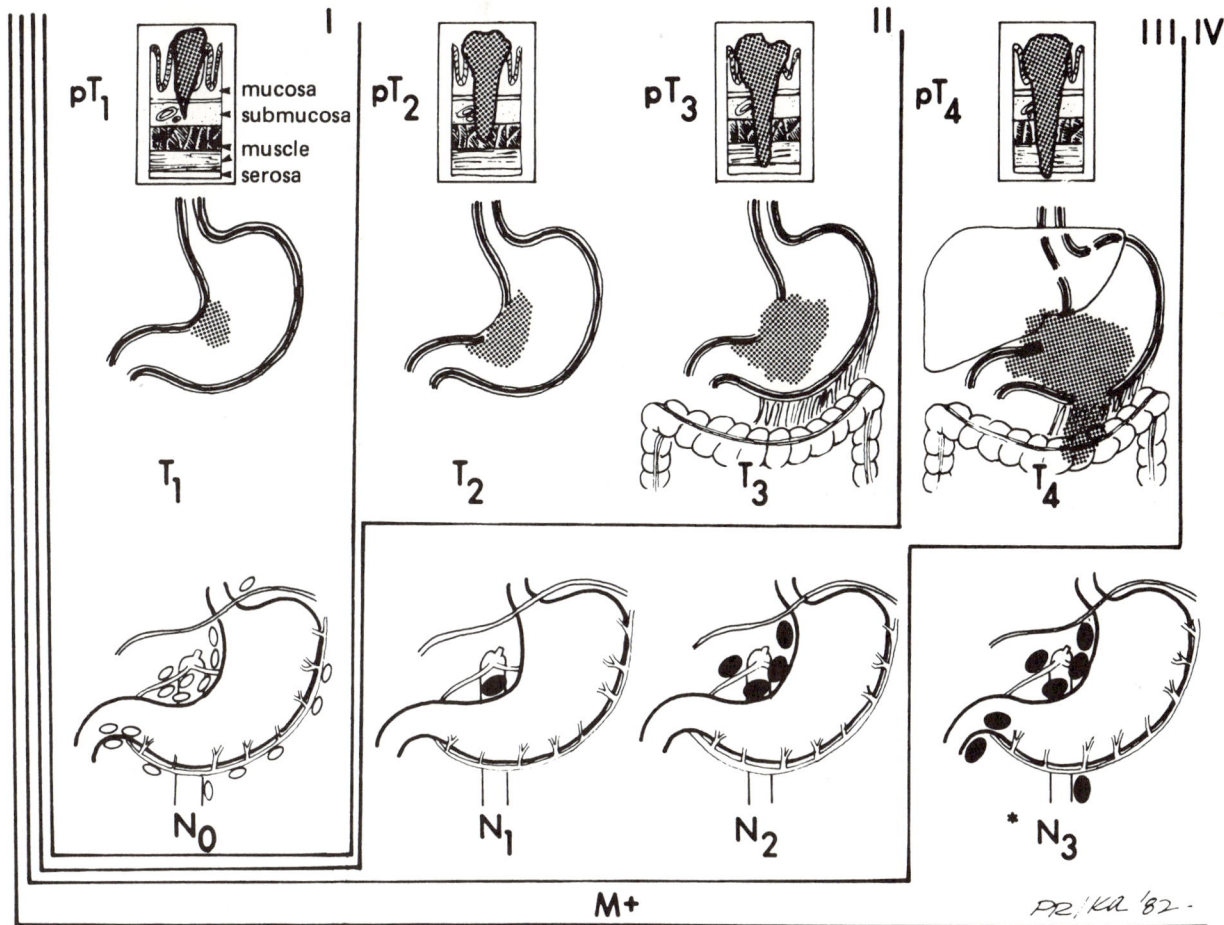

Figure 33–2. Stage of disease according to degree of involvement of stomach tissue. Tumor *(T)* categories: Tumor categorization is essentially a postsurgical classification, although with new tumor imaging techniques, it may be possible to determine depth of penetration. Progression is through layers of viscera, mucosa, and submucosa, muscle, seros, and contiguous structures. Node *(N)* categories: The distance of nodes from a primary site is used: less than 3 cm or greater than 3 cm (N_1 versus N_2) in regional nodal areas of lesser and greater curvature; juxtaregional nodes are N_3. Stage grouping: T category determines stage. Positive nodes are stage III as long as they are resectable (N_1–N_3). Stage IV applies to metastases and unresectable lymph nodes (N_3). American Joint Committee for Cancer Staging and End-Results Reporting (AJC) versus Union International contra le Cancrum (UICC) classification: Differences relate to clinical T categories only. T_1 is similar, but the UICC's T_2 and T_3 refer to occupying more than half of one region or an entire region with deep infiltration that is not defined. T_4 involves more than one region and invasion to a contiguous structure. The UICC-pTNM system is identical to that of AJC, and both are postsurgical classifications. N categories and stage grouping systems are similar. (From Morton, J. M., Poulter, C. A., & Pandya, K. J. [1983]. Alimentary tract cancer. In P. Rubin, R. F. Bakemeier, & S. K. Krackov [Eds.], *Clinical oncology—a multidisciplinary approach* [pp. 154–176]. New York: American Cancer Society. Reproduced by permission.)

most likely because of the high percentage of early gastric cancers that are resected and to the wide resections that are done. Outside Japan, there are no systematic guidelines regarding standardized surgical treatment. In the West, extensive surgery has had high postoperative morbidity and mortality rates.

Radiation

Radiation is frequently used to treat gastric cancer in combination with surgery. The types of radiation employed include preoperative, intraoperative, and postoperative. Intraoperative radiation has been used mainly in Japan. Preoperative radiation, although helpful in shrinking some types of gastric cancers, requires irradiating large areas to effect tumor shrinkage. Postoperative radiation can usually be confined to a more specific, definitive location.

Radiation is also utilized in combination with che-

motherapy. The most frequently chosen chemotherapy protocols are 5-FU; 5-FU and CCNU; and 5-FU, doxorubicin (Adriamycin), and mitomycin C (FAM). The combination of chemotherapy and radiation therapy carries a better prognosis than does radiation alone.

Chemotherapy

Advanced gastric cancer has also been treated with chemotherapy alone. The most frequently used single agent has been 5-FU. Mitomycin C has been used with a 21 per cent response rate for a period of 1 to 3 months (Earl, Coombes, & Schein, 1984). BCNU and methyl-CCNU have also been used as single agents in the treatment of advanced gastric cancer. Both of these nitrosoureas are less effective than either 5-FU or mitomycin C when used as single agents. Additional single agents that have been tried in the treatment of

Table 33–4. STAGE GROUPING OF STOMACH CANCER AND TNM CLASSIFICATION

Stage	Tumor	Node	Metastasis
I	T_1	N_0	M_0
II	T_2	N_0	M_0
	T_3	N_0	M_0
III	T_1, T_2, T_3	N_1, N_2	M_1
	T_1, T_2, T_3 (Resectable for cure)		
	T_4 (Resectable for cure)	Any N	M_0
IV	T_1, T_2, T_3 (Not resectable for cure)	N_3	M_0
	T_4 (Not resectable for cure)	Any N	M_0
	Any T	Any N	M_1

(Data from Morton, Poulter, & Pandya, 1983, p. 160.)

advanced gastric cancer are doxorubicin, cis-dichloro-diammineplatinum, methotrexate, hydroxyurea, chlorambucil, dacarbazine, triazinate, 4-epiadriamycin, razoxane, 4-methanesulfon-m-anisididi, and dihydroxyanthracenedione (Earl et al., 1984).

A number of combination chemotherapy regimens have been used in the treatment of advanced gastric cancer (Table 33–5). The best response rate has been generated with the FAM protocol. Currently it is thought that sequencing the usual FAM protocol so that the regimen begins with doxorubicin followed by 5-FU and mitomycin C, produces even better results than does the standard protocol (Panettiere & Heilbrun, 1979). Another protocol that has generated exciting results (63 per cent response rate) consists of high-dose methotrexate, high-dose 5-FU, and doxorubicin.

Chemotherapy has also been used as adjuvant therapy, but results have been mixed. The most positive findings were produced with the 5-FU and methyl-CCNU protocol (Gastrointestinal Tumor Study Group, 1982) and with a mitomycin protocol used in Japan (Imanaga & Nakazato, 1977).

In summary, the treatment of gastric cancer consists of multiple therapy combinations. The prognosis for gastric cancer remains poor because of the high number of patients who present initially with advanced disease. Early diagnosis and continued research on treatment protocols for this disease offer the best future hope for improved prognosis.

Nursing Care

As with esophageal cancer, nutrition is a major problem for the person with gastric cancer. In addition,

Table 33–5. EXAMPLES OF COMBINATION CHEMOTHERAPY REGIMENS FOR ADVANCED GASTRIC CANCER

5-FU and BCNU
5-FU and methyl-CCNU
5-FU and mitomycin C
5-FU, cyclophosphamide, and methyl-CCNU
5-FU, mitomycin C, and cytosine arabinoside
5-FU, doxorubicin (Adriamycin), and mitomycin C (FAM)

Table 33–6. HISTOLOGIC CLASSIFICATION OF MALIGNANT INTESTINAL TUMORS

Adenocarcinoma	Adenosquamous carcinoma
Mucinous adenocarcinoma	Undifferentiated carcinoma
Signet ring carcinoma	Unclassified carcinoma
Squamous cell carcinoma	

(Data from World Health Organization, 1978.)

these patients frequently have problems with abdominal pain, which in many cases is due to damage to the gastric mucosa caused by the cancer. Therefore, it is not uncommon for gastric cancer patients to have an *alteration in comfort*.

This type of pain is not seen as frequently in other types of gastrointestinal cancer. Pain experienced by colorectal cancer patients is most often related to perforation of the bowel or obstruction. Unfortunately, in many cases, this is the problem that initially brings the client to the health care system.

Irritation and ulceration of the gastric mucosa cause the stomach cancer patient to have abdominal pain that is sometimes severe. Sometimes the pain results in the patient who is unable to eat experiencing anorexia. Other patients complain of pain after meals. Other gastrointestinal symptoms that may accompany the pain are nausea or vomiting (or both), abdominal fullness, belching, regurgitation, or dyspepsia. Because of these symptoms associated with the abdominal pain, weight loss frequently occurs. If unchecked, this weight loss may lead to a cachexic state, which frequently is irreversible.

For further information on *alteration in comfort,* see Chapter 50. Because of the nutritional problems associated with an alteration in comfort, the gastric cancer patient will also have an alteration in nutrition. Information on this nursing diagnosis can be found in Chapter 47.

COLORECTAL CANCER

Definition and Incidence

Colorectal cancer is a common malignancy. In 1989, it was estimated to rank third in men and second in women (Silverberg & Lubera, 1989). For 1989, the anticipated incidence of colorectal cancer was 151,000 (73,000 men, 78,000 women) (Silverberg & Lubera, 1989). This figure represents an increased incidence from the 1985 statistics of 150,200 (67,100 men, 73,100 women) (Silverberg, 1985). The majority of cases of colorectal cancer are seen in persons older than 50 years. When colorectal cancer occurs before the age of 50, there usually is a history of familial polyposis or ulcerative colitis.

Epidemiology and Etiology

In the United States the mortality rate of colorectal cancer is second only to that of lung cancer. Geographically, the incidence of colorectal cancer is higher in

Table 33–7. TUMOR (T) AND NODE (N) CLASSIFICATION OF COLON CANCER

UICC		AJC
T_1/pT_1	Mucosa or submucosa only	T_1
T_2/pT_2	Muscle or serosa	T_2
T_{3A}/pT_{3A}	Extension to contiguous structures No fistula	T_3
T_{3B}/pT_{3B}	Extension to contiguous structures with fistula	T_4
T_4/pT_4	Extension beyond contiguous structures	T_5
N	No regional node involvement	N_0
N_1	Regional nodes	N_1
N_4	Juxtaregional nodes	

UICC, Union International Contra le Cancrum: AJC, American Joint Committee for Cancer Staging and End-Results Reporting: pathologic (postsurgical) stage.
(Data from Morton, J. M., Poulter, C. A., & Pandya, K. J., 1983, p. 170.)

the Western world, owing primarily to the diet high in refined carbohydrates. A classic study compared Japanese people in Japan, Hawaii, and the mainland United States (Haenszel & Kurihara, 1968) and found that people in Japan had the highest incidence of gastric cancer, those in Hawaii were second, and those on the mainland United States had the lowest incidence of gastric cancer. On the other hand, mainland residents had the highest incidence of colorectal cancer, those in Hawaii were second, and people in Japan had the lowest incidence of colorectal cancer (Haenszel & Kurihara, 1968).

In addition to familial polyposis and ulcerative colitis, diverticulosis, hemorrhoids, adenomatous polyps, villous adenoma, and diet are main contributors to the development of colorectal cancer. Because the Western diet is high in refined carbohydrates, transit through the colon is slow, and as a result, the extended presence of bile acids may result in carcinogenic effects on the bowel tissue (Hill, 1979).

Persons with a family history of colon cancer are at greater risk for the development of the disease. Also at risk are those with a previous history of breast or female genital tract cancer (Doughty, 1986).

Biology and Natural History

The histologic classification of intestinal tumors is given in Table 33–6. Adenocarcinomas constitute approximately 95 per cent of all colorectal cancers (Boarini, 1987).

Table 33–8. TUMOR (T) AND NODE (N) CLASSIFICATION OF RECTAL CANCER

T_1/pT_1	Mucosa or submucosa only
T_2/pT_2	Muscle or serosa
T_{3A}/pT_{3A}	Extension to contiguous structures No fistula
T_{3B}/pT_{3B}	With fistula
T_4/pT_4	Extension beyond contiguous structures
N_0	No regional node involvement
N_1	Regional
N_4	Juxtaregional

p, pathologic (postsurgical) stage. (Data from Morton, J. M., Poulter, C. A., & Pandya, K. J., 1983, p. 170.)

Table 33–9. STAGE GROUPING OF COLON CANCER AND TNM CLASSIFICATION

Stage	Tumor	Node	Metastasis
I	T_1	N_0	M_0
IB	T_2	N_0	M_0
II	T_3, T_4	N_0	M_0
III	Any T	N_1	M_0
IV	Any T	N_4	M_0
	Any T	Any N	M_1

(Data from Morton, J. M., Poulter, C. A., & Pandya, K. J., 1983, p. 170.)

Staging for colorectal cancer include the Broder Dukes, and TNM methods of classification. Broder's classification system focuses on anaplasticity and degree of differentiation of cells (Broder, 1925; Morton et al., 1983). The Dukes classification depends on depth of spread of the tumor and whether or not nodal metastases are present, according to the following system

- Invasion into submucosa, muscle. No nodal or distant metastasis.
- Invasion through serosa. No nodal or distant metastasis.
- Invasion through serosa. Involvement of regional nodes.
- Distant metastasis (Morton et al., 1983).

The TNM classification for both colon cancer and rectal cancer is given in Tables 33–7 and 33–8.

The staging of colorectal cancer is frequently based on the tumor and node classification. The staging of both colon and rectal cancer may be seen in Tables 33–9 and 33–10 and Figure 33–3.

Although the Dukes system of classification is frequently used, it does not always separate patients into appropriate prognostic groups. There are many ways in which prognosis is evaluated in colorectal cancer patients. Asymptomatic patients have the best prognosis. Duration of symptoms is also indicative of prognosis, with patients who have an acute episode of symptoms having the poorest prognosis. Analysis of the relationship of age to prognosis reveals that persons under 30 years old have a very poor prognosis (5-year survival rate of 19.5 per cent) (Sugarbaker et al., 1982) and those 70 years old and older have the best 5-year survival rate (67.2 per cent) (Block & Enker, 1971). Prognosis has been linked to CEA levels in the peripheral blood.

Table 33–10. STAGE GROUPING OF RECTUM CANCER AND TNM CLASSIFICATION

Stage	Tumor	Node	Metastasis
IA	T_1	N_0	M_0
IB	T_2	N_0	M_0
II	T_3, T_4	N_0	M_0
III	Any T	N_1	M_0
IV	Any T	N_4	M_0
	Any T	Any N	M_1

(Data from Morton, J. M., Poulter, C. A., & Pandya, K. J., 1983, p. 170.)

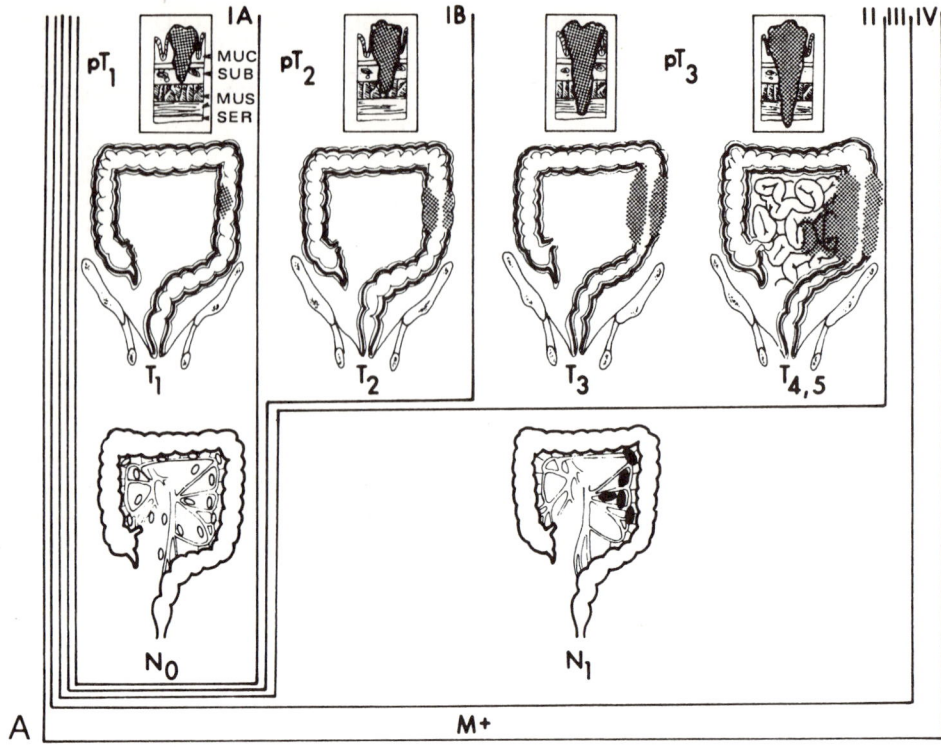

Key:

MUC = Mucosa.

SUB = Submucosa.

MUS = Muscle.

SER = Serosa.

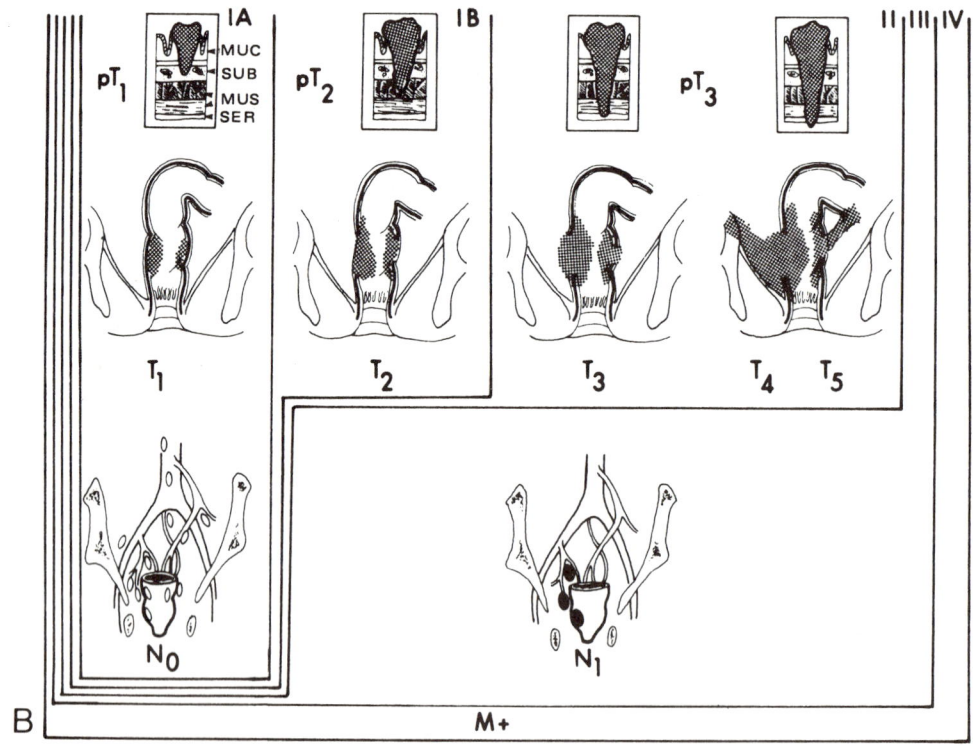

Figure 33–3. Staging of colon *(A)* and rectal *(B)* cancer. Tumor *(T)* categories: The depth of penetration is the most important criterion but for some unknown reason is carried to five categories. The order of progression for hollow viscera is a stage for each layer: mucosal, muscle, serosa (T_1 to T_3). Extension to extramural structures also characterizes T_3, fistula in T_4, and adjacent organs T_5, which are superfluous. Node *(N)* categories: The regional nodes are either negative or positive and are confined to the course of the inferior mesenteric artery and vein. Stage grouping: This is awkward but essential. It groups favorable T lesions (T_1 and T_2) as stage I because of ease of resection. Unfavorable T_3 to T_5 lesions are grouped as stage II. Positive nodes are stage III, and metastases that include nodes beyond the inferior mesenteric are stage IV. American Joint Committee for Cancer Staging and End-Results Reporting (AJC) versus Union International contra le Cancrum (UICC) classification: The UICC has approximately four categories but confuses the standard categories of visceral organs by lumping muscle and serosal invasion into T_2. The UICC T_3 (A and B) is equivalent to the AJC's T_4 and T_5. The UICC's T_4 category is quite absurd. It has primary tumor extending to the immediately adjacent organs, which for the AJC, would be a T_6. There is an additional UICC N_4 category for juxtaregional nodes, whereas N_2 and N_3 are noted as not being applicable. (From Morton, J. M., Poulter, C. A., & Pandya, K. J. [1983]. Alimentary tract cancer. In P. Rubin, R. F. Bakemeier, & S. K. Krackov [Eds.], *Clinical oncology—a multidisciplinary approach* [pp. 154–176]. Reproduced by permission.)

Patients with high CEA levels have been found to have a poor prognosis because invasion of the veins has already taken place (Sugarbaker et al., 1982).

Clinical Features and Diagnosis

Although CEA levels mentioned earlier are important in the diagnosis of colorectal cancer, by far the most important tests are the digital rectal examination, the Hemoccult test, and sigmoidoscopy. Half of all rectal cancers can be detected by rectal examination alone.

The signs and symptoms of colorectal cancer depend on the location of the tumor. However, the most common signs of colorectal cancer include rectal bleeding, anemia, and a change in stool. Other possible indications of colorectal cancer include melena, tenesmus, abdominal pain, constipation, or diarrhea. Two major problems that bring the client to the health care system are obstruction or perforation of the bowel. Unfortunately, these two problems are indications of a poor prognosis.

Treatment

Surgery

In the last 30 years, survival rates have not changed for colon cancer treated with surgery (Bouwman & Weaver, 1988). However, surgery is the primary treatment of colorectal cancer, with the focus of surgery being the removal of the primary tumor as well as any regional spread. Surgery must be a part of the treatment plan if cure is the goal.

Surgical approaches include a segmental resection, a radical resection, or a supraradical resection. Patients undergoing radical or supraradical resections do no better than those with segmental resections (Sugarbaker et al., 1982). Reports indicate also that patients with more than five positive lymph nodes have a poor prognosis regardless of how radical the surgery is.

The number of bowel colostomy surgery cases has decreased over the years. Reasons for the reduction in the number of colostomies done include the following: early diagnosis of some colorectal tumors, a new procedure dealing with electrical coagulation of involved

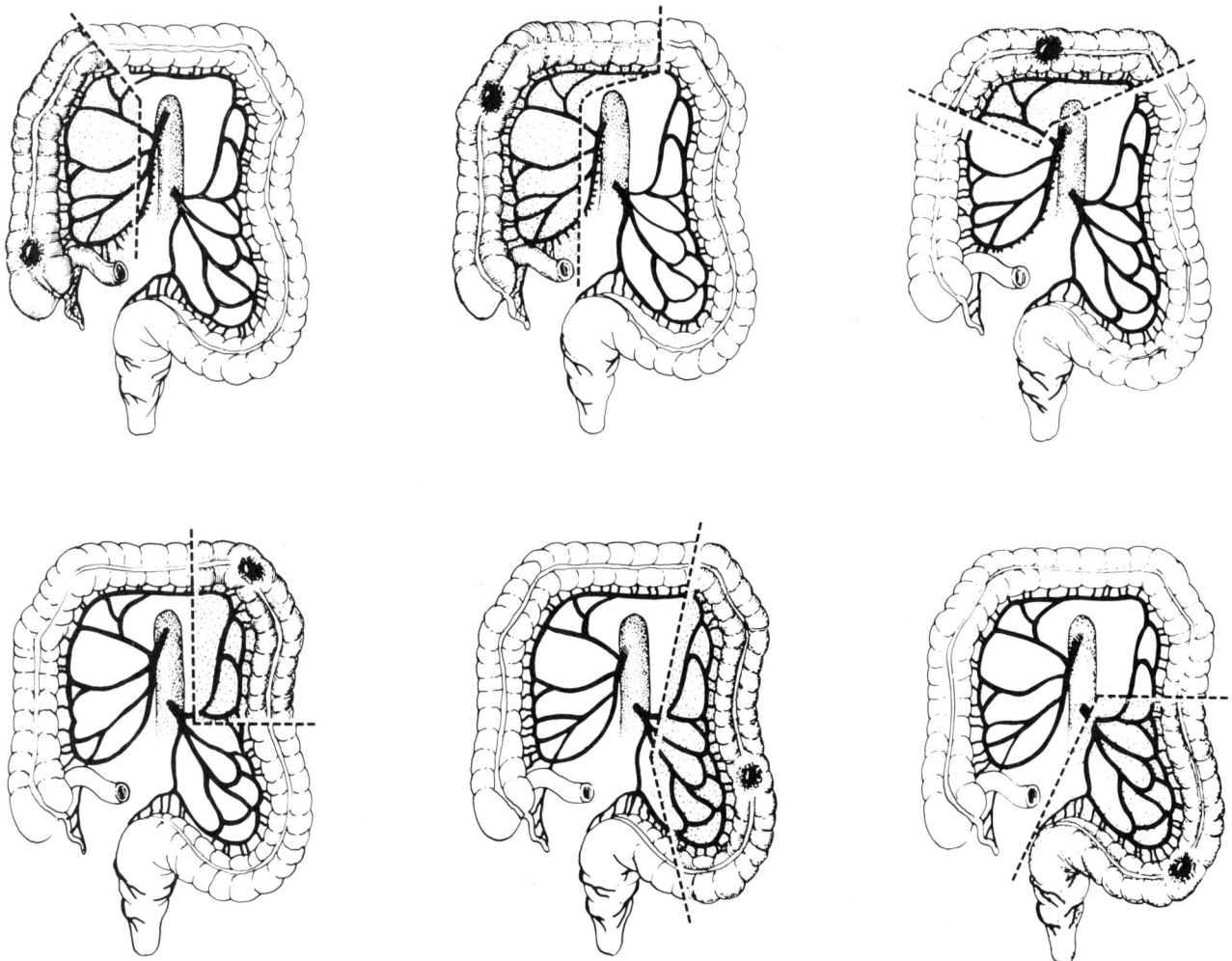

Figure 33–4. Colon cancer operative sites. The boundaries of the resection are dictated by lymphatic drainage patterns that parallel the blood supply. (From Evans, J. T., & Dayton, T. [1988]. Colon, rectum and anus. *In*: Lawrence, P. F. [Ed.]: Essentials of General Surgery [pp. 207–230]. © 1988, the Williams & Wilkins Co., Baltimore.)

tissue, and the availability of "end-to-end mechanical anastomosers (EEA staplers) ..." (Bouwman & Weaver, 1988). These staplers allow for more anastomoses to be done with shorter segments of the rectal stump.

Two groups of patients constitute the majority of candidates for colostomy surgery: patients who have had surgery with removal of the rectum, and patients who are at high risk for infection. The infection usually results from bowel obstructions or perforations. Various operative sites for colon cancer are shown in Figure 33–4.

Radiation Therapy

Radiation therapy is also used in the treatment of colorectal cancer, either to increase cure rates or to aid in the palliation of the disease. Currently radiation is used preoperatively, postoperatively, or both pre- and postoperatively with surgery being performed between the two periods. In addition, radiation may be used in combination with both surgery and chemotherapy or with just chemotherapy.

Colorectal tumors respond as well to radiation as other tumors (Herskovic & Han, 1988). The major problem related to irradiation of the bowel is the sensitivity of normal tissues. In many cases, these normal tissues are unable to tolerate the dose of radiation being delivered to the colorectal cancer.

It is easier to radiate the fixed portion of the bowel (ascending colon, descending colon, rectum, and hepatic and splenic flexures) than the mobile portion of the bowel (transverse colon and sigmoid colon). With the mobile portions of the bowel there is a tendency for peritoneal seeding, which would necessitate that a larger portion of the abdomen be radiated. With the fixed portion of the bowel, the metastases tend to be local (Herskovic & Han, 1988).

Chemotherapy

Chemotherapy used in the treatment of colorectal cancer has not been as effective as in other types of cancer. Single agents used in the treatment of the disease are 5-FU, the nitrosoureas, or mitomycin C. By far the most common agent used is 5-FU. (See Box 33–2.) The response rate to this chemotherapy agent ranges between 8 and 85 percent (Moertel, 1978). Usually a response rate of less than 20 per cent is the recognized figure for 5-FU in the treatment of colorectal cancer (Poplin & Baker, 1988). The optimal dose, frequency, and mode of administration of 5-FU have yet to be determined.

Combination chemotherapy has also been used in the treatment of advanced disease. Although it is believed that combination chemotherapy should improve response rates, to date this evidence has been lacking. Various studies have been done with 5-FU in combination with leucovorin, methotrexate, lavamasol, methyl-CCNU, vincristine, streptozocin, cisplatin, interleukin 2 (IL 2), and lymphokine-activated killer (LAK) cells.

Many studies have been carried out using chemotherapy as adjuvant therapy for colorectal cancer. The benefit of this treatment for colon cancer remains unclear (Wicks, 1986).

For rectal cancer at the present time, surgery with adjuvant chemotherapy and local radiation should be used (Poplin & Baker, 1988).

Nursing Care

As with the esophageal and gastric cancer patients, the colorectal patients have nutritional problems. In addition, at one time or another, they are prone to develop an *alteration in bowel elimination* (Dobkin & Broadwell, 1986). The various treatments used for colorectal cancer may also cause fluid and electrolyte imbalances as well as malabsorption problems owing to changes in levels of enzymes frequently associated with the gastrointestinal system (Table 33–11). These enzyme changes also occur frequently in patients who have cancer of the pancreas.

CANCER OF THE PANCREAS

Definition and Incidence

Cancer of the pancreas is on the rise in the United States, with an estimated number of cases for 1989 of 27,000 (Silverberg & Lubera, 1989). The estimated incidence for 1985 was 25,200 (Silverberg, 1985). This form ranks fifth as a cancer-related death, after lung, breast, colorectal, and prostate cancers, in decreasing order. Fewer than 1 per cent of persons with cancer of the pancreas live longer than 5 years (del Regato & Spjut, 1977). Cancer of the pancreas consists of 2 to 3 per cent of all cancers. At the present time, cancer of the pancreas is more common in blacks (Moosa, 1980), and the peak incidence is around age 60 years (Silverberg & Lubera, 1989).

Epidemiology and Etiology

Pancreatic cancer has no known cause, although chronic pancreatitis has been associated with the disease (Adams, Poulter, & Pandya, 1983). Other etiologic factors include cigarette smoking (Kahn, 1966) and possibily chemicals or alcohol. Coffee may be an inducer. In addition, there is a sixfold increase of pancreatic cancer in diabetic women.

Biology and Natural History

The most common histologic classification of pancreatic carcinomas is that found in Table 33–12. In addition to pancreatic carcinoma, there are islet cell tumors, some of which secrete insulin. Staging of pancreatic cancer is done according to the TNM classification (Table 33–13).

Box 33–2. COMPARISON OF TREATMENT SCHEDULES FOR COLORECTAL CANCER

Budd, G. T., Fleming, T. R., Bukowski, R. M., McCracken, J. D., Rivkin, S. E., O'Bryan, R. M., Balcerzak, S. P., & Macdonald, J. S. (1987). **5-Fluorouracil and folinic acid in the treatment of metastatic colorectal cancer: A randomized comparison. A Southwest Oncology Group Study.** *Journal of Clinical Oncology, 5, 272–277.*

To determine the clinical applicability of the observation of enhanced cytotoxicity of 5-fluorouracil (5-FU) in vitro in the presence of excess reduced folates, the Southwest Oncology Group (SWOG) performed a randomized trial evaluating two dose schedules of 5-FU and folinic acid (FA) in 128 patients with metastatic colorectal cancer. Of 125 eligible patients, 62 were randomized to groups to receive bolus FA (200 mg/m² days 1 through 4) by continuous 4-day infusion (infusion arm), whereas 63 were randomized to groups to receive bolus FA (200 mg/m² days 1 through 5) in addition to 5-FU (325 mg/m² days 1 through 5) by bolus injection (bolus arm). The toxicities of the two schedules differed, with stomatitis being more severe in the infusion arm and leukopenia being more severe in the bolus arm. The response rates and survival data for the two arms are nearly identical. The median survival of patients on the infusion arm is 11.0 months and of patients on the bolus arm, 10.3 months. The infusion arm produced one complete response (CR) and 12 partial responses (PRs), for a major response rate of 21 per cent of eligible patients. The bolus arm produced three CRs and 11 PRs, for a major response rate of 22 per cent of eligible patients. The response rate is minimally superior to recent cooperative group studies of colorectal cancer, but the response rate and survival experience are within the range of experience for treatment with 5-FU alone.

The prognosis for pancreatic cancer remains grim, with less than 1 per cent of the patients surviving 5 years (del Regato & Spjut, 1977). There are a number of reasons for these statistics. First, in a study by Cubilla and Fitzgerald (1979), only 14 per cent of the patients had disease confined to the pancreas. Second, metastatic spread throughout the abdomen occurs easily owing to the location of the pancreas. Third, the pancreas has a rich blood and lymphatic system (Macdonald, Gunderson, & Adson, 1982).

Some signs and symptoms of pancreatic cancer occur in all forms, whereas others are related to either the type of pancreatic cancer or the location of the pancreatic cancer. With the exception of jaundice, many of the signs and symptoms—weight loss, weakness, anorexia, nausea, vomiting, depression, asthenia, and gaseousness (Adams et al., 1983;) (Macdonald, Gunderson, & Adson, 1982)—are not specific for pancreatic symptoms but could be related to any number of other problems that occur with other syndromes or diseases.

Jaundice is frequently seen in patients with cancer of the head of the pancreas. Although it is not an early sign, jaundice is usually accompanied by pain, a frequent symptom in pancreatic cancer patients.

When the body of the pancreas is involved, the patient experiences back pain. With pancreatic carcinoma of the tail of the pancreas, many of the symptoms are related to metastases; consequently, the patient exhibits an abdominal mass, weight loss, and weakness (Adams et al., 1983).

If the tumor is one in which insulin is produced and excreted, the patient may complain of all of the symptoms related to an insulin reaction, which include fatigue, hypoglycemia, diaphoresis, pallor, and malaise. If the condition continues uncorrected, the patient's mental status will deteriorate and coma will result (Adams et al, 1983).

Because of the location of the pancreas, the patient may have other signs or symptoms related to metastatic disease or obstruction. Therefore, the nurse should be alert for indications of liver or gastrointestinal involvement.

Differential Diagnosis

Diagnosis has most frequently been done with radiographic tests, such as upper gastrointestinal tests. Computed tomography and ultrasonography are also frequently used. Arteriography, transhepatic thin-needle cholangiography, and endoscopic retrograde choledochopancreatography (ERCP) have in recent years been found to be valuable in diagnosing some types of gastrointestinal system tumors. Several tumor markers are elevated with pancreatic cancer. These include CEA, pancreatic oncofetal antigen (POA), and alpha-fetoglobulin. Serum immunoreactive elastastase I also has been found to be a sensitive marker for pancreatic cancer (Hamano, Hayakawa, & Kondo, 1987). Additional items that may be helpful in the diagnosis of pancreatic cancer are gastrin, insulin, glucagon, human chorionic gonadotropin, C-peptide, ribonuclease, and calcitonin (Macdonald, Gunderson, & Cohn, 1982).

Treatment

Surgery

A major treatment for pancreatic cancer is surgery. Surgery usually consists of either the Whipple procedure or a total pancreatectomy. If a total pancreatectomy is done, there may be major problems with the management of both the endocrine and the exocrine functions of the pancreas. In a limited number of cases the patients have had more radical surgery (Fortner, 1973, 1980). This operation is referred to as a regional pancreatectomy and involves "not only a total pancreatectomy and extensive lymph node dissection, but also includes removal of the portal vein, transverse mesocolon, and the adjacent soft tissue" (Macdonald, Gunderson, & Cohn, 1982). In addition to these op-

Table 33–11. NURSING CARE PLAN FOR A PATIENT WITH A COLOSTOMY

Assessment	Interventions	Expected Outcomes
Nursing Diagnosis: Alteration in comfort—pain		
Intensity of pain will be influenced by activity of disease process, surgery, or psychological factors; fear of injuring stoma may cause patient to restrict movements that intensify pain	Report and document nature and site of pain Medicate for pain as needed Reposition and use proper support measures as needed; assure patient that position change will not injure stoma Encourage patient to verbalize Actively listen and provide support Document relief from pain	Verbalizes or displays relief from pain and demonstrates ability to assist in care through use of general comfort measures
Nursing Diagnosis: Potential alteration in nutrition—less than body requirements		
May be undernourished from disease process or illness; some foods are gas- and odor-forming in the digestive process and individual sensitivities to some foods may result in diarrhea or constipation; bulk and residue may need to be restricted depending on bowel activity	Do thorough nutritional assessment; confer with physician and dietitian to correct deficiencies Provide nutrition high in protein and calories to repair tissue and prevent weight loss Identify offensive foods and temporarily restrict them from diet; gradually reintroduce one food at a time Document those foods that are a source of flatus (e.g., carbonated drinks, beer, beans, cabbage family, onions, fish, and highly seasoned foods) or odor (e.g., onions, cabbage family, eggs, fish, and beans) Increase use of yogurt, buttermilk, and cranberry juice Discuss the mechanics of swallowed air as a factor in the formation of flatus and some ways patient can exercise control Avoid cellulose products (e.g., peanuts) Exercise caution in the dietary intake of prunes, dates, stewed apricots, strawberries, grapes, bananas, cabbage family, beans, and nuts Discuss with the physician the patient's nutritional needs and have the dietitian discuss meal planning with the patient and significant others before discharge	Patient is able to plan a diet that meets nutritional needs and limits gastrointestinal disturbances
Nursing Diagnosis: Potential fluid volume deficit		
Preoperatively, patient may have been dehydrated from emesis, diarrhea, diaphoresis, and nothing by mouth order	Monitor intake and output carefully, including liquid stool Monitor blood pressure, pulse, and weight Monitor hematocrit and electrolyte levels Intravenous fluid and electrolyte replacement Instruct patient about need for increased fluid intake during warm weather months May need to decrease salt intake	Adequate hydration maintained
Nursing Diagnosis: Injury; potential for infection		
Myelosuppression may be present owing to disease process; potential fecal contamination at time of surgery; debilitated state may also influence state of myelosuppression	Review signs and symptoms of possible infection Monitor complete blood counts and platelet counts as indicated Avoid medications that may mask signs of infection (e.g., Tylenol) Provide adequate nutrition, including fluids Monitor any temperature elevations Emphasize good hygiene Promote adequate rest and exercise periods Protect from sources of infection	No evidence of infection
Nursing Diagnosis: Fear—disease with poor control or cure history		
Fear and anxiety may be common problems because life may be threatened and normal coping mechanisms may fail	Review with patient and significant others his or her previous experience with cancer Assist patient and significant others in recognizing and clarifying fears and to begin developing coping strategies for those fears; may be helpful to coach person by use of examples of coping skills used by others	Patient and significant others verbalize fears and begin to deal with them effectively; coping mechanisms are identified and the level of anxiety is reduced

Table 33–11. NURSING CARE PLAN FOR A PATIENT WITH A COLOSTOMY *Continued*

Assessment	Interventions	Expected Outcomes
Nursing Diagnosis: Potential impairment of skin integrity		
No sphincter control of stoma, stool, and flatus flow from ostomy; peristomal skin is susceptible to breakdown from bacteria or enzymes in the effluent; consistency of effluent will be affected by the disease process, location of the ostomy, and medications	Measure stoma and order the correct size and make of an odor-proof drainable pouch Use effective skin barriers, such as Stomahesive (Squibb), karaya gum, Reliaseal (Davol), and similar products Opening on adhesive backing of pouch should only be ⅛ inch larger than the base of the stoma with adequate adhesiveness left to apply pouch Provide proper equipment to empty and cleanse ostomy pouch when necessary	

This care plan identifies some of the major nursing diagnoses that a patient with a colostomy might *initially* have.
(Data from Doenges, M. E., Jeffries, M. F., & Moorhouse, M. F., 1984, pp. 285–292, 677–688.)

erations aimed at cure, surgery may be done for palliative reasons. If the patient is jaundiced, however, there is an increased risk of operative morbidity.

Radiation Therapy

Radiation therapy may be used as adjuvant therapy after surgery or for palliative reasons. In a Massachusetts General Hospital study, 50 per cent of the patients treated with adjuvant radiation after surgery had no recurrence (Macdonald, Gunderson, & Cohn, 1982). Palliative radiation has also been successful for this disease. Radiation combined with chemotherapy produces even better survival rates than radiation alone.

Both single-agent chemotherapy and combination chemotherapy have been used to treat pancreatic carcinoma. The single agents most commonly used are 5-fluorouracil, mitomycin C, and streptozocin. Response rates vary, with the best data indicating an approximately 20 per cent partial response rate for 5-FU (Carter & Comis, 1975; Macdonald, Gunderson, & Cohn, 1982; Smith & Schein, 1979). Combination chemotherapy most often involves 5-FU plus another agent, most frequently a nitrosourea or antitumor antibiotic. In some of studies reported (Lokich & Skarin, 1973; Waddell, 1973; Moertel & Lavin, 1977), the combination chemotherapy is more effective than the single-agent chemotherapy.

HEPATOCELLULAR CARCINOMA
Definition and Incidence

Primary liver cancer (hepatocellular carcinoma) is among the ten most common cancers in the world

Table 33–12. HISTOLOGIC CLASSIFICATION OF PANCREATIC CARCINOMA

Type	Percentage of Patients
Duct cell adenocarcinoma	75
Giant cell carcinoma	4
Adenosquamous carcinoma	4
Mucinous cystadenocarcinoma	1
Acinar cell adenocarcinoma	1
Others	15

(Data from Macdonald, Gunderson, & Cohn, 1982, p. 564.)

(Zhou, De Tolla, Custer, & London, 1987). It is estimated that there will be 250,000 new cases of hepatocellular carcinoma each year (World Health Organization, 1983). The American Cancer Society estimates that the 1989 incidence of primary liver cancers and cancers of the biliary passages will be 14,500 with a slightly greater incidence in men (7500) than in women (7000) (Silverberg & Lubera 1989). Worldwide, hepatocellular carcinoma constitutes 2 per cent of all cancers, and it is most common in persons 60 to 70 years old (Adams et al., 1983). These malignancies of the liver, gallbladder, and biliary tract will result in 11,400 deaths (Silverberg & Lubera, 1989).

Epidemiology and Etiology

Approximately 80 per cent of hepatocellular carcinomas have been attributed to hepatitis B virus. In the United States, 50 per cent of hepatocellular cancer patients have cirrhosis (Macdonald, Gunderson, & Adson, 1982). Other etiological factors related to hepatocellular cancer include intestinal parasites, hemochromatosis, and aflatoxin from moldy peanuts (Adams, Poulter, & Pandya, 1983). Geographically a high association of liver cancer occurs in countries where hepatitis B virus infections are high, such as the

Table 33–13. TUMOR (T) AND NODE (N) CLASSIFICATION OF PANCREATIC CANCER

T_1	Limited to pancreas; <2 cm
T_2	Limited to pancreas; 2–6 cm
T_3	>6 cm
T_4	Extrapancreatic direct extension to contiguous structures
N_0	No metastatic nodes
N_1	One regional group found to be involved at laparotomy
N_2	≥2 regional groups involved
N_3	Clinical evidence of regional lymph node involvement
N_4	Involvement of juxtaregional nodes

(Reprinted with permission from Adams, J. T., Poulter, C. A., & Pandya, K. J. [1983]. Cancer of the major digestive glands: Pancreas, liver, bile ducts, gallbladder. In P. Rubin, R. F. Bakemaier, & S. K. Krackov [Eds.], *Clinical oncology—a multidisciplinary approach* [p. 180]. New York: American Cancer Society.)

Table 33–14. HISTOLOGIC CLASSIFICATION OF MALIGNANT TUMORS OF THE LIVER

Hepatocellular carcinoma (liver cell carcinoma)
Cholangiocarcinoma (intrahepatic bile duct carcinoma)
Bile duct cystadenocarcinoma
Combined hepatocellular and cholangiocarcinoma
Hepatoblastoma
Undifferentiated carcinoma

(Reprinted with permission from Adams, J. T., Poulter, C. A., & Pandya, K. J. [1983]. Cancer of the major digestive glands: Pancreas, liver, bile ducts, gallbladder. In P. Rubin, R. F. Bakemaier, & S. K. Krackov [Eds.], *Clinical oncology—a multidisciplinary approach* [p. 185]. New York: American Cancer Society.)

People's Republic of China, where cancer ranks third in men and fourth in women. Also, in China this is the most common malignancy in persons 15 to 34 years old (Zhou, et al., 1987). It has also been found that steroids may be a cause of primary liver cancer, particularly oral contraceptives and the androgens (Levine et al., 1976).

Biology and Natural History

The histologic classification of malignant liver tumors can be seen in Table 33–14. There are two major types of malignant tumors—those involving liver cells (hepatomas) and those involving bile duct cells (cholangiomas). The usual metastatic spread of liver tumors is to the regional lymph nodes, brain, and lungs.

No particular staging system is used for liver tumors. The prognosis for hepatocellular cancer is poor. For patients with resectable disease, the 5-year survival rate is 33 per cent (Foster & Berman, 1977). For those patients whose disease is associated with cirrhosis, the 5-year survival rate is zero.

Signs and Symptoms

The presenting signs and symptoms of hepatocellular carcinoma depend on whether or not cirrhosis is present. When cirrhosis is present, the patient's condition deteriorates rapidly, liver failure develops, and death occurs. From diagnosis to death is approximately 2 months (Moertel, 1975).

For patients without cirrhosis, the initial symptoms may be vague complaints of pain, anorexia, weakness, bloating, and a feeling of abdominal fullness (Mosby, 1967). As the disease progresses, the pain becomes more intense, and approximately 70 per cent of the patients have pain and weight loss (Adams et al., 1983). Other signs of liver damage that may be present include an enlarged liver, ascites, and portal hypertension. Jaundice, if present, is mild (Adams et al. 1983).

Differential Diagnosis

In diagnosing hepatocellular carcinoma, it is important to differentiate it from other liver conditions, such as metastatic liver disease. Metastatic liver disease is the most common type of liver tumor. After the history and physical examination, liver function tests should be done. These may indicate elevated levels of bilirubin and alkaline phosphatase. Elevated levels of $alpha_1$-fetoprotein are most frequently associated with hepatocellular carcinoma. In addition, a needle biopsy should be done. Radioisotope scans, CT, and ultrasonography are other diagnostic tools frequently used in the diagnosis of hepatocellular carcinoma.

Treatment

Cure of hepatocellular carcinoma can only be done with surgery. The recommended operation is total hepatic lobectomy (Adams et al., 1983; Brasfield, Bowden, & McPeak, 1972), which has a mortality rate of 20 per cent (Foster & Berman, 1977).

Radiation therapy has not been effective against primary liver tumors in most cases. However, in a study by Phillips and Murikami (1960), regression of the tumor was seen. When radiation is used in combination with chemotherapy, positive results have been obtained.

Chemotherapy used alone has not had a good response rate. In an Eastern Cooperative Oncology Group study using oral 5-FU, the agent was found to be totally ineffective (Falkson, Moertel, Lavin, Pretorius, & Carbone, 1978). It appears that chemotherapy administered systemically or by direct infusion provides better results than chemotherapy administered orally. In addition to 5-FU, other single agents used in the treatment of hepatocellular carcinoma include doxorubicin and neocarzinostatin. Combination chemotherapies identified by Macdonald, Gunderson, & Adson (1982) are listed in Table 33–15.

The following chemotherapy protocols have been used in conjunction with radiation:

1. 5-FU, cyclophosphamide, methotrexate, and vincristine (Cochrane, Murray-Lyon, Brinkley, & Williams, 1977). In this study, some of the patients were treated with this chemotherapy protocol. The other patients received this protocol in conjunction with radiation. Those who received only the chemotherapy had a better response than those who received both treatments.

2. Intrahepatic arterial doxorubicin with 5-FU in combination with radiation was effective against the disease.

GALLBLADDER AND BILIARY SYSTEM
Definition and Incidence

The biliary duct system consists of the gallbladder, common bile duct, cystic duct, common hepatic duct,

Table 33–15. COMBINATION CHEMOTHERAPY USED IN THE TREATMENT OF HEPATOCELLULAR CARCINOMA

5-FU and BCNU
5-FU and doxorubicin (Adriamycin)
5-FU and mitomycin C
5-FU and streptozocin
5-FU and methyl-CCNU
Adriamycin and bleomycin

and right and left hepatic ducts. Cancers of the gallbladder and biliary duct system are rare; at the present time, they are estimated to affect men slightly more frequently than women (Silverberg & Lubera, 1989), most commonly between the ages of 60 and 70 years.

The incidence of cancer of the gallbladder and biliary system is increasing slightly, from an estimated incidence of 13,400 in 1985 to 14,500 for 1989. These incidence rates also include cancers of the liver, and when they are combined, these cancers have a greater incidence in men (7500) than in women (7000) (Silverberg, 1985; Silverberg & Lubera, 1989). However, cancer of the gallbladder is found more frequently in women.

Epidemiology and Etiology

The cause of the biliary system tumors is related primarily to cholelithiasis (Adams et al., 1983). Liver fluke infestation and presence of other parasites are directly related to the development of bile duct cancer. In some cases, this type of cancer has been associated with ulcerative colitis (Levin, et al., 1976).

Biology and Natural History

The most common type of gallbladder cancer is adenocarcinoma, which is found in approximately 85 per cent of all the patients. Other forms of gallbladder cancer include anaplastic and squamous cell carcinomas and adenoacanthomas.

There is no anatomic staging done for either cancer of the gallbladder or cancer of the biliary system. Most of the cancers are advanced when found.

Prognosis

The mortality rate for this cancer, as for other cancers of the hepatobiliary system, is poor. It is estimated that 11,400 persons in the United States with biliary system cancer will die of this disease in 1989 (Silverberg & Lubera, 1989).

Presenting Signs and Symptoms

The most common symptom of cancer of the gallbladder is pain and that of the biliary system is jaundice. Other symptoms of cancer of the gallbladder are anorexia, nausea and vomiting, and weight loss. These symptoms are found in approximately 60 per cent of the patients (Macdonald, Gunderson, & Adson, 1982). When seen with cancer of the gallbladder, jaundice is usually indicative of advanced disease. Other symptoms of biliary system cancers may include pruritus and hepatomegaly.

In assessing the patient for gallbladder or biliary system disease, the clinician needs to realize that the symptoms are similar to those for benign disease. It is always important to assess the client for jaundice, which is usually first noted in the sclera or gums. In addition, complaints of pruritus should be discussed with the health team. Dark urine may also be an indication of disease.

Differential Diagnosis

Diagnostic tests usually done in cancer of the gallbladder include radiography of the gallbladder and liver chemistry tests. An elevated alkaline phosphatase level is indicative of liver involvement (Adams et al., 1983).

Common diagnostic tests done for the biliary system cancers include ERCP and liver chemistry tests. In addition to elevations in alkaline phosphatase, bilirubin level is usually elevated as well.

The 5-year survival rate of patients with cancers of the biliary system is approximately 33 per cent. The 5-year survival rate for gallbladder cancers ranges between 2.6 and 6 per cent, depending on the extensiveness of the surgical treatment (Dowdy, 1969).

Treatment

Surgery

Cancers of the gallbladder and biliary system are usually treated surgically. According to Adams and co-workers (1983), complete removal of the gallbladder is the only way to cure gallbladder cancers. This is also the case with the biliary ducts. In some cases, portions of the liver also may need to be resected along with affected lymph nodes. Although Macdonald, Gunderson, & Adson (1982) indicate that wedge resections may be done with early tumors of the gallbladder, in most cases the disease is advanced when found.

Radiation Therapy

Radiation therapy has been found to have a good palliative role in the treatment of this disease. Because the failure rate with surgical treatment alone is high, it is believed that radiation therapy may be useful as adjuvant treatment (Kopelson, Chu, Douchette, & Gunderson, 1980). The amount of radiation delivered to these patients varies from low doses to a radical dose used as the primary treatment. When radiation is the primary treatment, there is evidence that patients remain disease free for from 6 to 26 months (Pilepich & Lambert, 1978). External beam radiation has also been used preoperatively with good results (Vaittinen, 1970).

Chemotherapy

Adjuvant chemotherapy has not been used frequently in the treatment of cancer of the gallbladder or the biliary duct system. In the few cases in which it has been used, 5-FU is the drug of choice. The other two protocols that have been tried include (1) 5-FU, mitomycin C, and BCNU, and (2) 5-FU with either methyl–1-(2-chloroethyl)–3-cyclohexyl–1-nitrosourea (methyl-CCNU) or streptozocin (Adams et al., 1983). In all cases, the results have been favorable.

SUMMARY

Of all the body systems, the gastrointestinal system continues to have the highest incidence of cancer. Because of the difficulty in early diagnosis of most of the cancers of this system, the prognosis remains poor. However, with early diagnosis, the 5-year survival rates of gastrointestinal cancers do increase dramatically. Although great strides are being made in medical management, nursing assessments of patients with gastrointestinal complaints could play a major role in decreasing the morbidity and mortality associated with this disease.

References

Adams, J. T., Poulter, C. A., & Pandya, K. J. (1983). Cancer of the major digestive glands: Pancreas, liver, bile ducts, gallbladder. In P. Rubin, R. F. Bakemeier, & S. K. Krackov (Eds.), *Clinical oncology—a multidisciplinary approach* (pp. 178–189). New York: American Cancer Society.

American Cancer Society. (1989). *Cancer facts and figures.* Atlanta, GA: Author.

Biasco, G., Paganelli, G. M., Azzaroni, D., Grigioni, W. F., Merighi, S. M., Stoja, R., Villanacci, V., Rusticali, A. G., Cuoco, D. L., Caporale, V., & Barbara, L. (1987). Early gastric cancer in Italy. *Digestive Diseases and Science, 12,* 113–120.

Block, G. E., & Enker, W. E. (1971). Survival after operations for rectal carcinoma in patients over 70 years of age. *Annals of Surgery, 174,* 521–527.

Boarini, J. (1987). Gastrointestinal malignancies: Colon and rectum. In S. L. Groenwald (Ed.), *Cancer nursing: principles and practices* (pp. 544–557). Boston: Jones & Bartlett Publishers, Inc.

Bouwman, D. L., & Weaver, D. W. (1988). Colon cancer: Surgical therapy. *Gastroenterology Clinics of North America, 17,* 859–872.

Brasfield, R. D., Bowden, L., McPeak, C. J. (1972). Major hepatic resection for malignant neoplasm of the liver. *Annals of Surgery, 176,* 171–177.

Broder, A. C. (1925). The grading of carcinoma. *Minnesota Medicine, 8,* 726–730.

Bruni, H., & Nelson, R. (1975). Carcinoma of the esophagus and cardia: Diagnostic evaluation in 113 cases. *Journal of Thoracic and Cardiovascular Surgery, 70,* 367–370.

Budd, G. T., Fleming, R. M., Bukowski, R. M., McCracken, J. D., Rivkin, S. E., O'Bryan, R. M., Balcerzak, S. P., & Macdonald, J. S. (1987). 5-Fluorouracil and folinic acid in the treatment of metastatic colorectal cancer: A randomized comparison. A Southwest Oncology Group Study. *Journal of Clinical Oncology, 5,* 272–277.

Burn, I. A., & Welbourn, R. B. (1975). Cancer of the stomach. In Sir Rodney Smith (Ed.), *Gastric surgery: Surgical forum* (pp. 121–148). Boston: Butterworth's.

Carter, S. K., Comis, R. L. (1975). Adenocarcinoma of the pancreas, prognostic variables, and criteria of response. In M. J. Staquet (Ed.), *Cancer therapy: Prognostic factors and criteria of response* (p. 237). New York: Raven Press.

Cochrane, A. M., Murray-Lyon, I. M., Brinkley, D. M., & Williams, R. (1977). Quadruple chemotherapy versus radiotherapy in treatment of primary hepatocellular carcinoma. *Cancer, 40,* 609–614.

Cubilla, A. L., & Fitzgerald, P. J. (1979). Cancer of the pancreas (non-endocrine): A suggested morphologic classification. *Seminars in Oncology, 6,* 285.

del Regato, J. A., & Spjut, H. J. (1977). Cancer of the digestive tract. In J. A. del Regato & H. J. Spjut (Eds.), *Ackerman and del Regato's cancer: Diagnosis, treatment and prognosis* (5th ed., pp. 572–611). St. Louis: C. V. Mosby Co.

Dobkin, K. A., & Broadwell, B. C. (1986). Nursing considerations for the patient undergoing colostomy surgery. *Seminars in Oncology Nursing, 2,* 249–256.

Doenges, M. E., Jeffries, M. F., & Moorhouse, M. F. (1984). *Nursing care plans—nursing diagnoses in planning patient care.* Philadelphia: F. A. Davis Co.

Doughty, D. B (1986). Colorectal cancer: Etiology and pathophysiology. *Seminars in Oncology Nursing, 2,* 235–241.

Dowdy, G. S., Jr. (1969). *The biliary tract.* Philadelphia: Lea & Febiger. (1969).

Earl, H. M., Coombes, R. C., & Schein, P. S. (1984). Cytotoxic chemotherapy for cancer of the stomach. *Clinics in Oncology, 3,* 351–369.

Falkson, G., Moertel, C. G., Lavin, P., Pretorius, F. J., & Carbone, P. P. (1978). Chemotherapy studies in primary liver cancer: A prospective randomized trial. *Cancer, 42,* 2149–2156.

Fortner, J. G. (1973). Regional resection of cancer of the pancreas: A new surgical approach. *Surgery, 73,* 307.

Fortner, J. G. (1980, March). Regional pancreatectomy and other radical approaches to pancreatic cancer. International Meeting on Pancreatic Cancer, New Orleans.

Foster, J., & Berman, M. (1977). *Solid liver tumors.* Philadelphia: W. B. Saunders Co.

Gastrointestinal Tumor Study Group. (1982). Controlled trial of adjuvant chemotherapy following curative resection for gastric cancer. *Cancer, 49,* 1116–1122.

Haenszel, W., & Kurihara, M. (1968). Studies of Japanese migrants: 1. Mortality from cancer and other diseases among Japanese in the United States. *Journal of the National Cancer Institute, 40,* 43–68.

Hamano, H., Hayakawa, T., & Kondo, T. (1987). Serum immunoreactive elastase in diagnosis of pancreatic diseases. *Digestive Diseases and Sciences, 33,* 50–56.

Herskovic, A., & Han, I. (1988). The role of radiation in the distal bowel. *Gastroenterology Clinics of North America, 17,* 887–903.

Hill, M. J. (1979). Bacterial metabolism and colon cancer. *Nutrition and Cancer, 1,* 46–50.

Hill, M. J. (1984). Aetiology of gastric cancer. *Clinics in Oncology, 3,* 237–249.

Imanaga, H., & Nakazato, H. (1977). Results of surgery for gastric cancer and effect of adjuvant mitomycin C on cancer recurrence. *World Journal of Surgery, 1,* 213–221.

Kahn, H. A. (1966). The Dorn study of smoking and mortality among U.S. veterans: Report on 8 and one half years of observation. *National Cancer Institute Monograph, 19,* 1–125.

Kidokoro, T. (1971). Frequency of resection, metastasis and five years survival rate of early gastric carcinoma in a surgical clinic. *Gann Monograph Cancer Research, 11,* 45–49.

Kopelson, G., Chu, A. M., Douchette, J. A., & Gunderson, U. (1980). Extra-hepatic biliary tract metastases from breast cancer. *International Journal of Radiation Oncology, Biology, Physics, 6,* 497–504.

Lauren, P. (1965). The two histological main types of gastric carcinoma: Diffuse and so-called intestinal type carcinoma. An attempt at a histoclinical classification. *Acta Pathologica et Microbiologia Scandinavica, 64,* 31–49.

Levin, B., Riddell, R. H., & Kirsner, J. B. (1976). Management of precancerous lesions of the gastrointestinal tract. *Clinical Gastroenterology, 5,* 827.

Lokich, J. J., Skarin, A. T. (1973). Combination therapy with 5-fluorouracil (5-FU) and 1,3 Bis(2 Chlorethyl)–1-nitrosourea (BCNU) for disseminated gastrointestinal carcinoma. *Cancer, Chemotherapy Reports, 56,* 653.

Macdonald, J. S., Gunderson, L. L., & Adson, M. A. (1982). Cancer of the hepatobiliary system. In V. T. Devita, Jr., S. Hellman, & S. A. Rosenberg (Eds.), *Cancer: Principles and practice of oncology* (pp. 590–615). Philadelphia: J. B. Lippincott Co.

Macdonald, J., Gunderson, L., & Cohn, I., Jr. (1982). Cancer of the pancreas. In V. T. DeVita, Jr., S. Hellman, & S. A. Rosenberg (Eds), *Cancer: Principles and practice of oncology* (pp. 563–589). Philadelphia: J. B. Lippincott Co.

Moertel, C. G. (1975). Clinical management of advanced gastrointestinal cancer. *Cancer, 36,* 675.

Moertel, C. G. (1978). Chemotherapy of gastrointestinal cancer. *New England Journal of Medicine, 299,* 1049–1059.

Moertel, C. G., & Lavin, P. T. (1977). An evaluation of 5-FU, nitrosourea, and lactone combinations in the therapy of upper gastrointestinal cancer. *Proceedings of the American Society of Clinical Oncology, 18,* 344.

Moosa, A. R. (Ed.). (1980). *Tumors of the pancreas.* Baltimore: Williams & Wilkins.

Morton, J. M., Poulter, C. A., & Pandya, K. J. (1983). Alimentary tract cancer. In P. Rubin, R. F. Bakemeier, & S. K. Krackov (Eds.), *Clinical oncology—a multidisciplinary approach* (pp. 154–176). New York: American Cancer Society.

Mosby, R. V. (1967). Primary malignant tumors of the liver. A review of the clinical and pathologic characteristics of 47 cases and a discussion of current diagnostic techniques and surgical management. *Surgery, 61,* 674–686.

Moss, A. A., Schnyder, P., Theoni, R. F., & Margulis, A. R. (1981). Esophageal carcinoma pre-therapy staging by computed tomography. *American Journal of Radiology, 136,* 1051–1056.

Okabe, H. (1971). Growth of early gastric cancer. In T. Murakami (Ed.) *Gann monograph on cancer research* (pp. 67–69). Tokyo: University of Tokyo Press.

Panettiere, F. J., & Heilbrun, L. (1979). Comparison of two different combinations of Adriamycin, mitomycin C, and 5-FU in the management of gastric carcinoma. A SWOG study. *Proceedings of the American Society of Clinical Oncology* (Abstract No. C-102, p. 315).

Pilepich, M. U., & Lambert, P. M. (1978). Radiotherapy of carcinomas of the extrahepatic biliary system. *Radiology, 127,* 767.

Poplin, E., & Baker, L. (1988). Colon cancer: Medical therapy. *Gastroenterology Clinics of North America, 17,* 873–886.

Putman, C., Curtis, A., Westfried, M., & McLoud, T. (1978). Thickening of the posterior tracheal stripe. A sign of squamous cell carcinoma of the esophagus. *Radiology, 126,* 597–601.

Quint, L. E., Glazer, G. M., & Orringer, M. B. (1985). Esophageal imaging by MR and CT: Study of normal anatomy and neoplasms. *Radiology, 156,* 727–731.

Quint, L. E., Glazer, G. M., Orringer, M. B., & Gross, B. H. (1985). Esophageal carcinoma: CT findings. *Radiology, 155,* 171–175.

Rosenberg, J. C., Schwade, J. G., & Vaitkevicius, V. (1982). Cancer of the esophagus. In V. T. Devita, Jr., S. Hellman, & S. A. Rosenberg (Eds.), *Cancer: principles and practice of oncology* (pp. 499–533). Philadelphia: J. B. Lippincott Co.

Silverberg, E. (1985). Cancer statistics, 1985. *CA: A Cancer Journal for Clinicians, 35,* 19–35.

Silverberg, E. (1987). Cancer statistics, 1987. *CA: A Cancer Journal for Clinicians, 37,* 2–19.

Silverberg, E., & Lubera, J. A. (1989). Cancer statistics, 1989. *CA: A Cancer Journal for Clinicians, 39,* 3–32.

Smith, F. P., Schein, P. S. (1979). Chemotherapy of pancreatic cancer. *Seminars in Oncology, 6,* 368.

Sugarbaker, P. H., Macdonald, J. S., & Gunderson, L. L. (1982). Colorectal cancer. In V. T. DeVita, Jr., S. Hellman, & S. A. Rosenberg (Eds.), *Cancer: principles and practice of oncology* (pp. 643–723). Philadelphia: J. B. Lippincott Co.

Vaittinen, E. (1970). Carcinoma of the gallbladder: A study of 390 cases diagnosed in Finland, 1953–1967. *Annales Chirurgiae et Gynaecologiae Fenniae, 29* (Suppl.), 7.

Waddell, W. R. (1973). Chemotherapy for carcinoma of the pancreas. *Surgery, 74,* 420.

Waterhouse, J. A. H. (1984). Epidemiology of stomach cancer. *Clinics in Oncology, 3,* 221–236.

Wicks, L. J. (1986). Treatment modalities for colo-rectal cancer. *Seminars in Oncology Nursing, 2,* 242–247.

World Health Organization. (1978). *International histologic classification of tumors,* Nos. 1–20. Geneva: Author.

World Health Organization Scientific Group on Prevention and Control of Hepatocellular Carcinoma. (1983). Prevention of primary liver cancer: Report on a meeting of a WHO scientific group. *Lancet, 1,* 463–465.

Zhou, X., DeTolla, L., Custer, R. P., & London, W. T. (1987). Iron, ferritin, hepatitis B surface and core antigens in the livers of Chinese patients with hepatocellular carcinoma. *Cancer, 59,* 1430–1437.

CHAPTER 34

Gynecologic Cancers

LUCY K. MARTIN
PATRICIA S. BRALY

The recent emergence of gynecologic oncology as a recognized subspecialty of obstetrics and gynecology is appropriate not only because of the frequency of diagnosis of these cancers but also because of the rapid advances being made in this field. It was estimated that in 1988 more than 70,000 women would be diagnosed as having a new gynecologic cancer and during that year, more than 23,000 women would die of their cancers. Marked reduction in the mortality rate has been achieved for those gynecologic cancers for which an effective screening mechanism or means of early diagnosis exists (such as the Papanicolaou smear for premalignant and early cervical cancer) and for those in which a sensitive tumor marker and effective chemotherapy have been identified (such as gestational trophoblastic neoplasia and ovarian germ cell cancers). However, for other cancers, such as epithelial ovarian cancer, in which the majority of cases are diagnosed in advanced stages, much more needs to be done before a positive impact on survival can be expected. The goals of improving not only survival but also quality of life for women with gynecologic cancers can only be accomplished with a true team approach, which is the subject of this chapter.

CARCINOMA OF THE UTERINE CERVIX

Incidence

Cancer of the cervix has dropped from second to sixth place in cancers afflicting women in the United States (Smith, 1976). The number of new cases expected to be diagnosed in 1988 was 12,900, with an expected 7000 deaths. This decrease is due primarily to the availability and use of the Papanicolaou-Traut smear as a screening device.

Epidemiology

The median age for the occurrence of cancer of the cervix is 51 years. Preinvasive conditions—dysplasia or carcinoma in situ—may be found 10 to 15 years earlier than invasive carcinoma. Those populations at risk include women with a history of early sexual activity, women with a large number of sex partners before the age of 20 years, those who have had multiple deliveries, cigarette smokers, and those in the lower socioeconomic strata (Table 34–1).

Etiology

A strong relationship between infection with the human papillomavirus (HPV) types 16 and 18 and cervical intraepithelial neoplasia (CIN) has been demonstrated (Campion, Singer, Clarkson, & McCance, 1985) (Box 34–1). HPV infections are increasing rapidly in the United States in the female population under 30 years of age (Lovejoy, 1987). The increasing incidence of CIN progressing to carcinoma in situ (CIS) and invasive cervical cancer in younger women appears to be more common than was previously the case. In addition, cervical cancer is known to develop in many women despite previous screening; the possibility of false-negative readings can be decreased with multiple screenings. This information has led the American College of Obstetricians and Gynecologists (ACOG) to advocate yearly Papanicolaou smears for essentially

Table 34–1. RISK FACTORS ASSOCIATED WITH CANCER OF THE UTERINE CERVIX

Personal Factors
Infection: Human papillomavirus (HPV), herpes simplex 2
Addiction to cigarettes
Multiple sexual partners
Abnormal squamocolumnar junction
Possible Factors
Oral contraceptives
Wine
Poor personal hygiene with respect to intercourse
Intercourse during menses
Douching frequently
Low socioeconomic status
Male Partner Factors
Addiction to cigarettes
Multiple sex partners
Intercourse with prostitutes
Carcinogenic work environment
Penile warts (caused by HPV)
Former spouses with history of cervical cancer

all women. Nursing practice implications, according to Lovejoy (1987), are to urge women to obtain annual Papanicolaou smears and to avoid known risks.

Biology and Natural History

Cervical cancer is divided into premalignant and invasive forms. The premalignant lesions may sometimes spontaneously regress (Table 34–2 and Fig. 34–1). The International Federation of Gynecology and Obstetrics (FIGO) staging system is used to describe the original distribution of invasive cancer of the cervix (Table 34–3). Eighty-five to 90 per cent of all cervical cancers arise from the squamous epithelium, approximately 10 per cent are adenocarcinomatous in origin, and 1 to 5 per cent are other, rare types. The junction between the squamous epithelial lining of the ectocervix and the columnar epithelial lining of the endocervix is referred to as the transformation, squamocolumnar junction, or transitional zone. This zone undergoes a process of migration from being located laterally on the ectocervix during adolescence to finally lying high up in the endocervical canal in postmenopausal women

Table 34–2. CLASSIFICATION OF PREMALIGNANT LESIONS OF THE CERVIX

Classification	Description
Low Grade	
CIN I	Mild dysplasia
	Cellular changes associated with human papillomavirus (HPV)
High Grade	
CIN II	Moderate cellular dysplasia
CIN III	Severe cellular dysplasia
Carcinoma in situ	

CIN, cervical intraepithelial neoplasia. (Adapted with permission from Lundberg, G. D. [1988]. The 1988 Bethesda system for reporting cervical/vaginal cytological diagnoses, National Cancer Institute Workshop. *Journal of the American Medical Association, 262*, 931–934.)

Box 34–1. VENEREAL TRANSMISSION OF HPV INFECTION

STUDY

Campion, M. J., Singer, A., Clarkson, P. K., & McCance, D. J. (1985). **Increased risk of cervical neoplasia in consorts of men with penile condylomata acuminata.** *Lancet, 2,* 943–946.

SAMPLE

The study group consisted of 25 women with no evidence of cervical intraepithelial neoplasia who had been the sole partners of men with long-standing penile condylomata acuminata (HPV infection) for at least 1 year. The control group consisted of 20 women who had been regular sexual partners of men with nonspecific urethritis but not with HPV infection for at least 1 year. None of the women of either group used barrier contraception.

MEASURES

Microbiology and serology: urethral, high vaginal, and endocervical swabs and smears taken for culture to exclude *Candida, Trichomonas, Haemophilus vaginalis, Chlamydia trachomatis,* and *Neisseria gonorrhoeae,* and blood was taken to test for syphilis. Cytology and colposcopy: Papanicolaou smear and colposcopic examination were obtained to look for cellular changes as evidence of genital wart virus infection and changes signaling intraepithelial neoplasia. Cervical washings: done with 5 per cent acetic acid; cervix was reexamined for whitish epithelium within the squamocolumnar junction that suggests HPV or cervical intraepithelial neoplasia (CIN). Biopsies: specimens taken from suspicious areas; one examined by pathologists for CIN and one sent for DNA-DNA hybridization for identification of type of HPV.

FINDINGS

Nine of 25 women (36 per cent) were diagnosed as having HPV or CIN infection (or both), compared with none of the control group. Nineteen of 25 (76 per cent) had a recent history or currently had condylomata acuminata. None of the control group had clinical evidence of HPV infection. Forty per cent of the control group had other venereal diseases. Nine of 25 (36 per cent) had abnormal Papanicolaou smears. Five of the nine (56 per cent) had clinical HPV infection in genital tract. None of the control group had abnormal Papanicolaou smears or abnormal findings on colposcopy. Eight of the nine had CIN I–III. One of the nine had HPV infection only, and one of the nine had CIN III only. Seven of the nine had both CIN and HPV infection. Seven of the nine had HPV type 16 DNA.

DISCUSSION

This study confirms the venereal transmission of HPV infection. It also confirms that the male partner with penile HPV infection constitutes a route of infection to his partner, who may subsequently develop CIN. Premalignant cervical infections with HPV type 16 may be the ones most likely to progress to CIN. Clinical infection with HPV type 16 and incidence of CIN are increasing in young women especially. Women with abnormal Papanicolaou smears should be questioned as to whether the partner has penile condylomata acuminata, and an effort should be made to treat men and women with wart virus infections to decrease the virus reservoir. The use of barrier contraception should be encouraged.

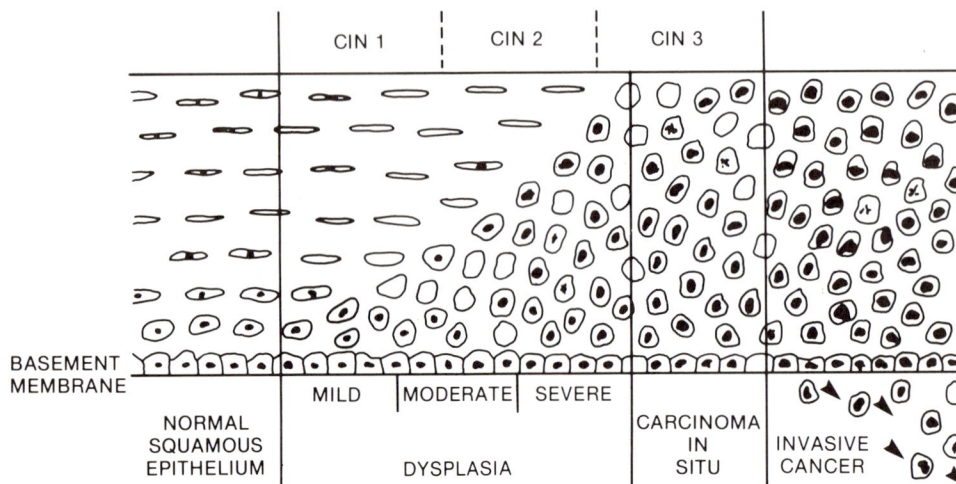

Figure 34–1. Diagram of phases of premalignant lesions of the cervix. (From Jones, H. W., Wentz, A. C., & Burnett, L.S. [1988]. *Novak's textbook of gynecology* [11th ed.]. © 1988. The Williams & Wilkins Co., Baltimore. Reproduced by permission.)

Table 34–3. FIGO STAGING SYSTEM FOR CANCER OF THE CERVIX UTERI

Preinvasive Carcinoma

Stage 0	Carcinoma in situ, intraepithelial carcinoma.
	(Cases of stage 0 should not be included in any therapeutic statistics.)

Invasive Carcinoma

Stage I	The carcinoma is strictly confined to the cervix (extension to the corpus should be disregarded).
Stage IA	Preclinical carcinomas of the cervix, that is, those diagnosed only by microscopy.
Stage IA1	Minimal microscopically evident stromal invasion.
Stage IA2	Lesions detected microscopically that can be measured. The upper limit of the measurement should not show a depth of invasion of more than 5 mm taken from the base of the epithelium, either surface or glandular, from which it originates, and a second dimension, the horizontal spread, must not exceed 7 mm. Larger lesions should be staged as Ib.
Stage IB	Lesions of greater dimensions than stage Ia2 whether seen clinically or not. Preformed space involvement should not alter the staging but should be specifically recorded so as to determine whether it should affect treatment decisions in the future.
Stage II	The carcinoma extends beyond the cervix but has not extended onto the pelvic wall. The carcinoma involves the vagina, but not the lower third.
Stage IIA:	No obvious parametrial involvement.
Stage IIB:	Obvious parametrial involvement.
Stage III	The carcinoma has extended on to the pelvic wall. On rectal examination, there is no cancer-free space between the tumor and the pelvic wall. The tumor involves the lower third of the vagina. All cases with hydronephrosis or nonfunctioning kidney.
Stage IIIA:	No extension onto the pelvic wall.
Stage IIIB:	Extension onto the pelvic wall or hydronephrosis (or both) or nonfunctioning kidney.
Stage IV	The carcinoma has extended beyond the true pelvis or has clinically involved the mucosa of the bladder or rectum. A bullous edema as such does not permit a case to be allotted to stage IV.
Stage IVA:	Spread of the growth to adjacent organs.
Stage IVB:	Spread to distant organs.

(Data from *Gynecology Oncology Group pathology manual* [unpublished]).

(DiSaia & Creasman, 1989). Squamous metaplasia is defined as the encroachment of the squamous epithelium on the area normally occupied by the columnar epithelium (Rivlin et al., 1986). This is a common finding in adolescent and pregnant women, and it may increase the vulnerability of immature cervical cells to a carcinogen. Squamous cell carcinoma of the cervix is manifested as four typical lesion types. An exophytic lesion, the most common type, is located on the external cervix; this type is friable, polyp-like, fungating and bleeds easily. This lesion arises in the endocervix or ectocervix. A cervix that is rock-hard to palpation usually is a sign of an infiltrating invasive

type of lesion in which tumor infiltrates deeply into the cervical stroma. The third type is an ulcerating lesion that appears to have eroded a portion of the cervix. A fourth type spreads superficially along the surface of the cervix. Lesions associated with adenocarcinoma of the cervix arise from the mucus-secreting glands of the endocervix and may not become visible for some time. They continue to grow within the cervix, causing it to bulge and become characteristically barrel shaped. These lesions have a high incidence of nodal metastasis and high failure rate for cure, regardless of treatment.

Prognosis

Although it is difficult to estimate prognosis for invasive cervical cancer accurately, 5-year survival results from treatment with surgery or radiation alone range from 60 to 90 per cent. Poor prognostic factors that have been identified are increased primary tumor size, tumor extension outside of the cervix, and the presence of adenocarcinoma or other aggressive histologic cell types. Because of the problem of potential systemic metastasis of the disease, one current practice option is to give postoperative radiation to patients with positive pelvic nodes in an attempt to prevent this spread and to increase survival. However, no statistically significant increase in survival has been shown with this treatment plan (DiSaia & Creasman, 1989).

The Papanicolaou Smear

Although the Papanicolaou smear is used only as a screening device, it is essential that it be performed correctly. Papanicolaou smears are frequently performed by nurse practitioners. The results obtained often form the basis for the decision to proceed in a diagnostic work-up. For a Papanicolaou smear to be representative, cells must be obtained from the cervical transformation zone. For accuracy, a sample should be scraped with a spatula from the external portio of the cervix and a second sample obtained by swirling a moist cotton swab or brush within the cervical canal. Nursing implications include taking care that the specimen is promptly placed in saline or sprayed with a fixative and not allowed to air dry. Contamination with lubricating jelly may render the specimen useless (White, 1986). The woman should be instructed to avoid douching and intercourse and not to use any vaginal medications before the smear, which should be postponed if menstrual flow is heavy (Lovejoy, 1987) (Fig. 34–2).

As a result of new findings implicating HPV in cervical cancer, a new test has been developed that permits examination of the DNA structure of the specimen for the presence of HPV. This new test, called ViraPap, is still under investigation, but it may in the future be performed routinely along with the Papanicolaou smear (ViraPap, 1987). A new system of reporting Papanicolaou smear results has also recently been advocated by experts in the field. The Bethesda System for Reporting Cervical-Vaginal Cytological Di-

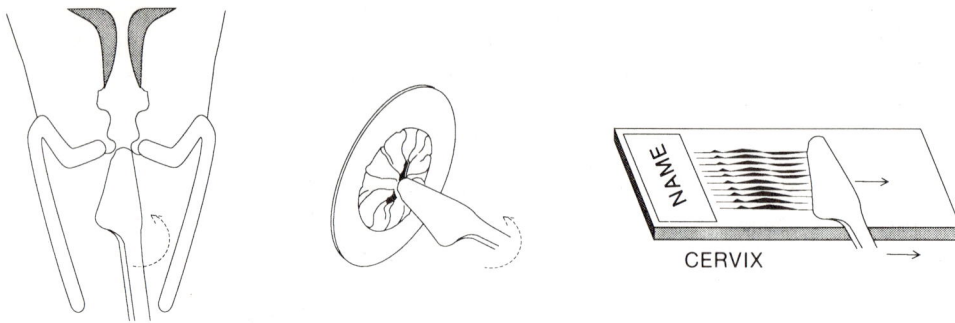

Sample the squamocolumnar junction using the heart-shaped end of a cervical spatula, rotating it 360 degrees. Apply a thin smear to the slide and immerse in fixative.

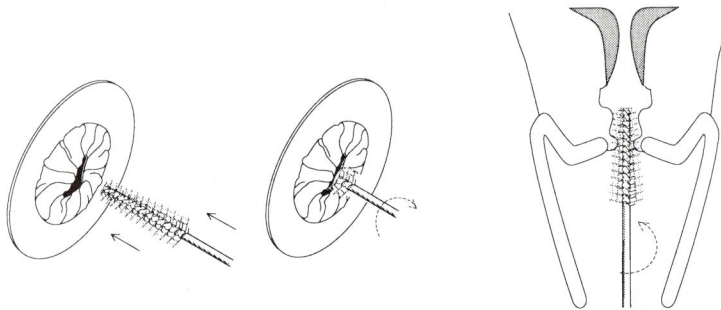

Figure 34–2. The Papanicolaou procedure. (Courtesy of P. Townsend, graphic artist.)

Sample the endocervix by gently inserting a Cytobrush (Hollywood, FL) dipped in saline, until only the bristles closest to the handle are exposed. Rotate one-quarter to one-half turn. Remove.

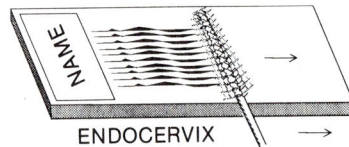

Prepare the slide by rolling and twisting the brush with moderate pressure across the slide.

agnoses has less ambiguity than the current Papanicolaou system, is congruent with current histopathologic terminology, and has been adopted by major cancer centers as the reporting system of choice (Lundberg, 1988).

Cervical Intraepithelial Neoplasia

Diagnosis

A definitive diagnosis of either premalignant or invasive cervical lesions always requires a histologic tissue examination under the microscope.

Colposcopy. Colposcopy is the technique of choice for determining the source of abnormal cells seen on the Papanicolaou smear. After application of 3 per cent acetic acid to the transformation zone of the cervix, the examiner visually inspects the entire zone through a colposcope (a low-power microscope). A moistened swab or endocervical speculum is often used to manipulate the exocervical os to increase visualization of the transformation zone in the endocervical

canal. The increased ratio of nucleus to cytoplasm in abnormal cells causes the suspected areas to look whiter than the surrounding area, and a biopsy may then be performed (Wilbanks, 1984). Whitened epithelium, mosaic structure, punctation, and atypical vessels are all examples of abnormal patterns that may be seen, for which a biopsy is indicated. Atypical vessels may indicate the presence of invasive cancer, whereas the other patterns are more typical of CIN.

An endocervical curettage (ECC) should be performed as part of every colposcopic evaluation unless the patient is pregnant. A curette is inserted into the endocervix without cervical dilation. The entire upper half of the endocervical canal is scraped first, followed by the lower half. Patients should be informed that the procedure is moderately painful but not lengthy. Some patients may choose to premedicate themselves with a nonnarcotic analgesic such as acetaminophen, ibuprofen, or aspirin. The same preexamination instructions as those given for the Papanicolaou smear apply to preparing the patient for the ECC. The specimen should be placed on a 2 × 2 piece of paper towel, folded, and placed in a fixative immediately. During colposcopy, punch biopsies of the external cervix are also taken under direct visualization. A cotton pledget should be held firmly against the cervix and Monsel's solution or silver nitrate applied to the area to stop any bleeding. Postbiopsy instructions include avoidance of douching, intercourse, and tampons for 2 weeks (Wilbanks, 1984). The Papanicolaou smear cytology, ECC, and biopsies constitute the recommended current outpatient diagnostic evaluation as long as all the tests reveal the same degree of CIN or invasive cancer. Figure 34–3 depicts a schema for further evaluation and management of the patient with an abnormal Papanicolaou smear.

Cone Biopsy. Cold knife conization or a cone biopsy is necessary if the ECC is positive, if invasive cancer has not been ruled out, or if there is a major discrepancy between the Papanicolaou smear and the biopsy results. If the patient wishes to preserve fertility, this technique may be employed as a treatment of CIN as well as a diagnostic technique. During the procedure, a cone of cervical tissue is excised. The apex of the cone contains part of the external os. It is sometimes performed through a colposcope or the surgeon may be guided by the previous colposcopy diagram. Iodine is helpful to stain the area for increased visualization (Fig. 34–4).

Conization usually requires general anesthesia, but most patients do not need to be admitted to the hospital unless there is heavy bleeding or other complications. For those patients requiring inpatient observation, routine postoperative monitoring of vital signs and vaginal bleeding from hemorrhage or perforation of the operative site should be carried out. Cervical stenosis, incompetence, and mechanical infertility are rare complications and are related to the amount of endocervix removed (DiSaia and Creasman, 1989).

Management

After satisfactorily establishing the diagnosis of preinvasive disease, several outpatient treatments may be employed. The goal of treatment is to completely obliterate the transformation zone.

Cryosurgery. At present, cryosurgery appears to be the most innocuous and effective treatment option. It is relatively painless, is low cost, can be done on an outpatient basis, and has demonstrated efficacy in eradicating the disease. The gas refrigerant is usually carbon dioxide or nitrous oxide. Larger tanks provide more consistent pressure required for a rapid freezing of the tissue. DiSaia and Creasman (1989) describe a double-freeze technique. The correct size of probe (selected to encompass the entire abnormality) is coated with lubricating jelly and applied to the cervix until an ice ball 4 to 5 mm in diameter is formed. The cervix is allowed to thaw for 2 to 3 min and the probe is reapplied to form another 4 to 5 mm ice ball. The ice ball should take no more than 2 to 3 min to form. Patients should be instructed by the nurse that a watery discharge will be present for approximately 2 weeks, to use peri-pads, and to refrain from intercourse and the use of tampons until the watery discharge has resolved.

Laser Surgery. The newest of the current treatments, laser surgery, is another treatment option. Laser stands for *light amplification by stimulated emission of radiation.* The laser is mounted on a colposcope. The beam vaporizes tissue and must reach a depth of 5 to 7 mm to be effective (Butts, 1977). Physicians and nurses should take precautions to protect the eyes, use nonreflective surfaces, and eliminate inflammatory agents. Smoke and steam that may contain HPV are created with the tissue vaporization; therefore, masks should be worn and a suction tube must be attached to the

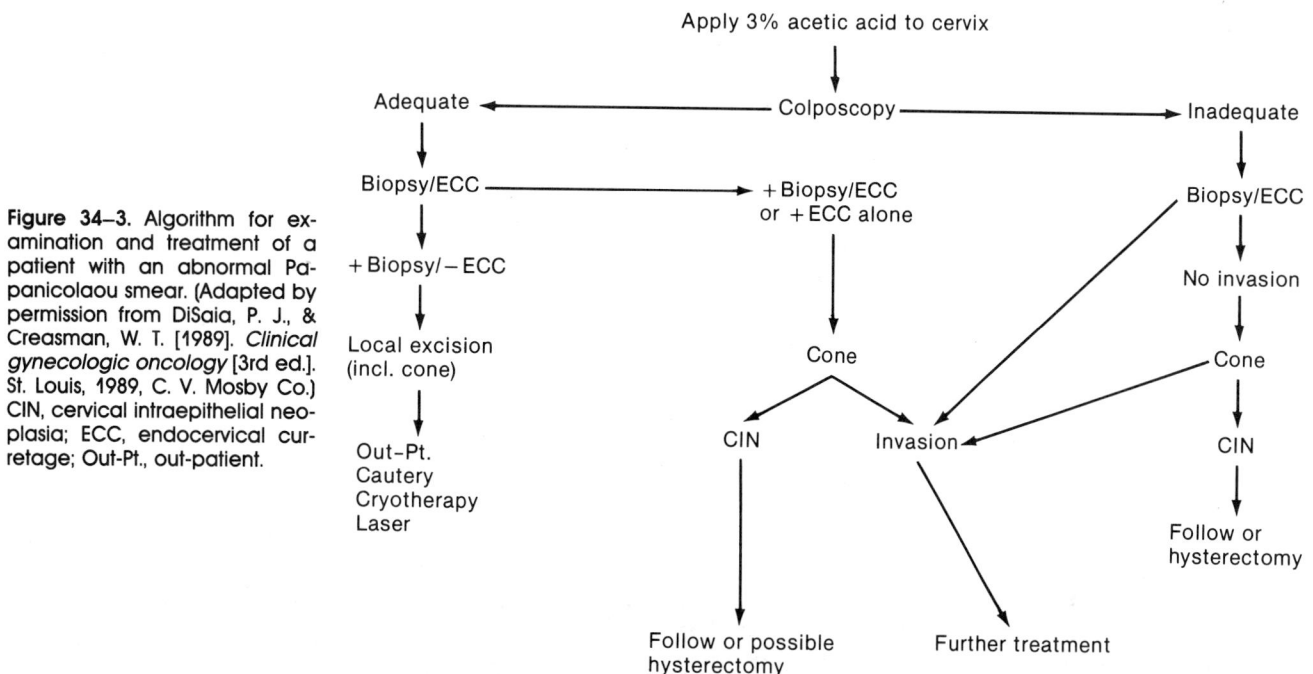

Figure 34–3. Algorithm for examination and treatment of a patient with an abnormal Papanicolaou smear. (Adapted by permission from DiSaia, P. J., & Creasman, W. T. [1989]. *Clinical gynecologic oncology* [3rd ed.]. St. Louis, 1989, C. V. Mosby Co.) CIN, cervical intraepithelial neoplasia; ECC, endocervical curretage; Out-Pt., out-patient.

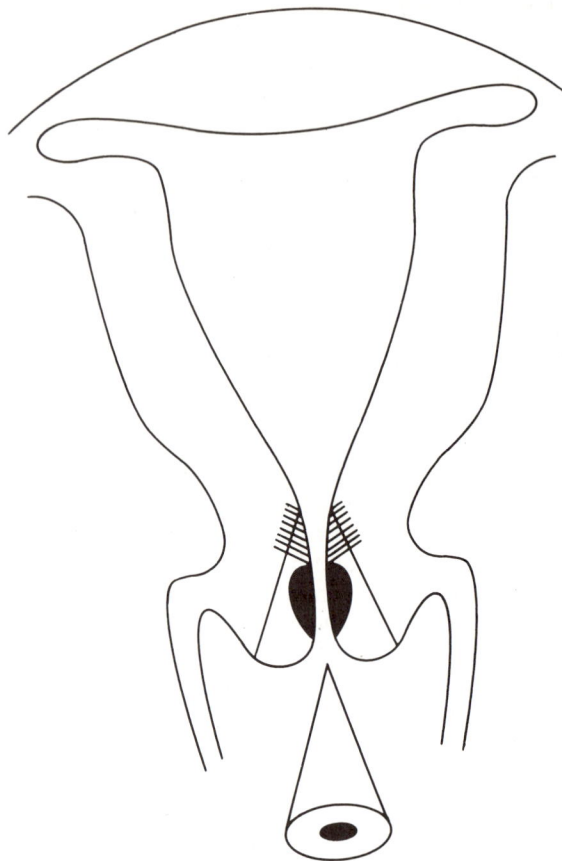

Figure 34–4. Endocervical cone biopsy. (Reproduced by permission from DiSaia, P. J., & Creasman, W. T. [1989]. *Clinical gynecologic oncology* [3rd ed.]. St. Louis, 1989, C. V. Mosby Co.)

speculum. Patients should be informed that some pain occurs during the procedure, that it will take longer than cryosurgery, and that there may be some bleeding afterward. Pads should be worn and intercourse avoided until spotting and any discharge subsides.

Hysterectomy. The patient with CIN who desires no more children and permanent sterilization may choose hysterectomy after examining the other options.

Regardless of the method of treatment for CIN, all patients must be followed up for evidence of recurrence. A Papanicolaou smear is usually taken at 3-month intervals for 2 years, and thereafter every 6 months for an additional 3 years. Abnormal Papanicolaou smears always require reevaluation.

Microinvasive Carcinoma of the Cervix

Confusion has surrounded this disease entity owing to the multiplicity of terms used to define it and the lack of agreement in anatomic description. The Society of Gynecologic Oncology, in 1974, agreed to accept the following definition of a microinvasive lesion or *early stromal invasion.* A microinvasive carcinoma occurs when the tumor penetration into the stroma from the basement membrane is less than 3 mm deep and

there is no evidence of lymphatic or vascular involvement.

Management

Simple hysterectomy is the treatment of choice only for cases in which there is solely microinvasion, but as the volume increases and becomes confluent, the condition is treated the same as microcarcinoma or occult cancer (stage IB) because the risk of lymphatic and vascular involvement (and therefore lymph node metastasis) increases.

Carcinoma of the Cervix

Diagnosis and Staging

No single symptom occurs that heralds cervical cancer. Contact bleeding, which results from mere touching such as occurs during coitus or a pelvic examination, is the symptom most frequently associated with cervical cancer. The blood is characteristically bright red (Barber, 1980). The bleeding can vary from a thin, watery, pink discharge to a continuous bloody discharge or frank hemorrhage. Late symptoms include development of pain referred to the leg or flank, which is most often secondary to invasion of the sciatic nerve or pelvic sidewall. Hematuria and renal failure relate to bladder involvement and ureteral obstruction. Rectal bleeding or obstruction attributable to invasion of the rectum are also symptoms of advanced disease. Unilateral or bilateral lower extremity lymphedema indicates lymphatic or venous blockage by tumor extending to the pelvic sidewall. A preterminal condition is often accompanied by uremia, massive hemorrhage, and profound cachexia with inanition (DiSaia & Creasman, 1989). After thorough history, physical, and pelvic examinations under anesthesia (EUA), bimanual and rectal included, biopsy specimens are obtained and further tests are done to clinically stage the patient's cancer. Radiologic studies include a chest radiograph, intravenous pyelogram (IVP), and barium enema. Rectosigmoidoscopy and cystoscopy are often performed at the time of the EUA. Nursing interventions include providing the patient with the information necessary to understand the work-up process and to assist with the physical examination and ensuring that the patient's privacy and comfort needs are met. Simple explanations of the scheduled tests increase the knowledge and decrease the anxiety of the patient during this pretreatment period.

Management

After definitive diagnosis and staging are completed, treatment is begun. In most cases, stages IIB and above are treated with radiation therapy. A long-standing controversy has existed as to the optimal treatment for stages I and IIA cervical cancer. Statistics reveal that there is no significant difference in survival rates among patients undergoing surgery alone, surgery plus adjuvant postoperative radiation therapy, and radiation therapy alone for stages I and IIA disease (DiSaia & Creasman, 1989). Advantages of surgery are that ovarian function and vaginal elasticity are preserved; mortality rate and the occurrence of postoperative ureterovaginal fistula are much less than 1 per cent. Surgical therapy can proceed in the presence of pregnancy, moderate obesity, inflammatory disease of the bowel and pelvis, preexistant radiotherapy, and a concurrent pelvic neoplasm such as an ovarian tumor. However, surgical treatment can be done only if the patient can withstand the rigors of general anesthesia and radical surgery. Radiation therapy, on the other hand, can be used for most patients, and it avoids the immediate risks of radical surgery. It cannot, however, be instituted in the presence of any of the conditions mentioned earlier for choosing surgery (pregnancy, and so forth). In addition, vaginal tissue integrity is sacrificed, permanent injury to normal organs can occur, and there is a real possibility of the occurrence of a second neoplasm as a late effect of the radiation therapy. The tenacious barrel-shaped lesion associated with adenocarcinoma of the cervix is often treated with combined multimodality treatment of surgery and radiation (DiSaia & Creasman, 1989).

Surgery. Simple, total, or extrafascial hysterectomy (type I) ensures the removal of all cervical tissue but does not require dissection of adjacent structures. It is employed for carcinoma in situ, early stromal invasion, and microinvasive carcinoma of the cervix. This procedure may also be used after preoperative radiation of adenocarcinoma of the cervix and for the similarly barrel-shaped squamous cell carcinomas of the endophytic type that arise in the endocervix. The modified radical hysterectomy (type II) is preferred to the more extended versions because of decreased postoperative complications of bladder atony and obstipation. Less paracervical tissue is dissected, and only the upper one third of the vagina is removed. Vital nerve tracts are spared (DiSaia & Creasman, 1989). A pelvic lymphadenectomy is also performed. More deeply invasive (> 5 mm) carcinomas and recurrent cervical cancer after previous irradiation are most often treated with this procedure as long as the cervix is not grossly expanded with tumor. The more commonly seen procedure is the Meigs or Wertheim radical hysterectomy (type III) and pelvic lymphadenectomy. This procedure involves wide excision of parametrial tissue along with the uterosacral ligaments and the upper half of the vagina. Bladder atony and obstipation are more frequent after this procedure (Robertson, 1986). There is a trend toward less radical resections for early lesions and occult microscopic disease.

Complications. Bladder dysfunction appears to be directly related to the extent of the surgery. The patient may lose the awareness of the need to void and often must perform the Credé maneuver (bending forward while seated) to completely empty the bladder (Lamb, 1985). This appears to be related to damage to the nerve supplying the detrusor muscle to the bladder and in most cases resolves over time. Formation of lymphocysts or seromas may occur after lymphadenectomy when there is inadequate internal drainage of the retroperitoneal space. If the lymphocyst is large enough to obstruct the ureteral urine flow or becomes infected, a reoperation may be necessary to drain the sequestered fluid. Percutaneous drainage is sometimes accompanied by infection. Pulmonary embolism, secondary to deep pelvic or leg vein thrombosis, is sometimes seen postoperatively. Prophylactic perioperative minidose heparinization is sometimes instituted in high-risk patients such as those with a history of thromboembolic disease, varicositis, or excessive obesity. Postoperative radiation therapy is used in situations in which the findings at surgery included positive lymph nodes, unclear surgical margins, or a tumor that is large and deeply invasive into the cervix. A delay of no more than 4 to 6 weeks is usually recommended for wound healing to occur.

Radiation Therapy. In practice radical surgery has often been reserved for younger, healthy stage I and stage IIA patients; radiation therapy is employed for treatment of the remainder of the population. The postoperative therapy is administered by either external beam or internal brachytherapy or a combination of both (DiSaia & Creasman, 1989). Whole pelvis irradiation is administered optimally on a linear accelerator megavoltage machine, which will deliver rays to the deeper internal structures with little injury to the skin. Usually 40 or 50 grays (Gy) are delivered in a 4- to 6-week period in fractionated doses.

Brachytherapy. Internal radiation therapy, or brachytherapy, is usually accomplished by application of a sealed intracavitary radiation source. In internal radiotherapy a very concentrated dose is administered in and around the tumor site, and the dosage falls off rapidly so that adjacent structures are not greatly affected (Hassey, 1985) (Fig. 34–5).

Radioisotopes such as cesium-137 or radium-226 are administered by means of a Fletcher-Suit system consisting of a tandem and colpostats (ovoids) (Fig. 34–6).

An alternative method used for carcinoma of the cervical stump and more advanced or asymmetrical

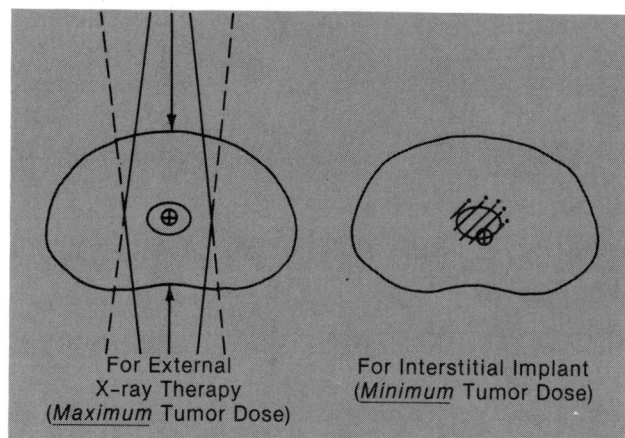

Figure 34–5. Comparison of tumor dose for internal and external radiation. (From Hilaris, B. S. [1975]. *Handbook of interstitial brachytherapy.* Acton, Massachusetts: Publishing Sciences Group, Inc. Reproduced by permission.)

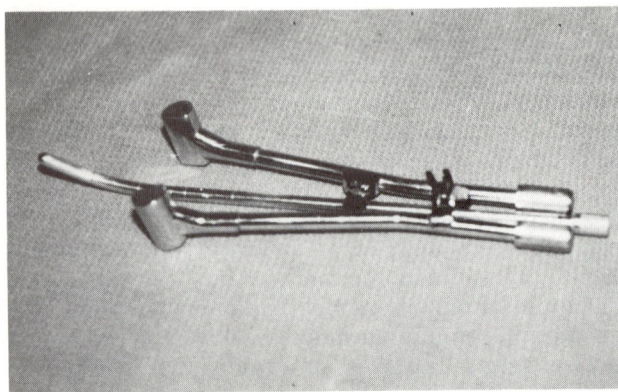

Figure 34–6. Fletcher-Suit system with tandem and colpostats.

disease is application of an interstitial source such as iridium-192 via needle implants attached to a vaginal template and obturator (Fig. 34–7).

Usually two applications 2 weeks apart, each lasting 36 to 50 hrs, are administered after completion of the course of external radiotherapy. The patient is considered radioactive during the time when the internal sources are in place. In an effort to minimize staff exposure to radiation, the sources are usually "afterloaded" when the applicators or implants have been properly placed into the patient during general anesthesia and the patient is back in her room. Remote afterloading machines have been developed that withdraw the radioactive sources from the patient and reinsert them when bedside care is completed. Bedside care should be limited to 30 min each shift, or less if possible (Hassey, 1985). See Chapter 20 for additional implications for nursing care.

Complications of Radiation Therapy. Complications are seen both acutely during treatment and with delayed onset and are usually confined to the irradiated area when the patient is managed appropriately. Table

Table 34–4. EARLY AND LATE INTERNAL AND EXTERNAL RADIATION SIDE EFFECTS AND COMPLICATIONS

Internal	External
Early	
Rectal tenesmus	Diarrhea
Passage of mucus and blood	Abdominal cramping
Dysuria	Dysuria
Urinary frequency	Urinary frequency
Erythema: 1 week	Fatigability
Exudation: 2 weeks	Leukopenia
Slough: 6 to 8 weeks	
Scar: 6 months	
Contracture	
Late	
Proctitis—thickened mucosa, thin, atrophic, mucosal ulceration	
Radiation enteritis	
Bowel obstruction	
Hematuria	
Urinary fistula ($<1\%$)	
Small bowel fistula	
Rectovaginal fistula	
Ureteral obstruction	
Vaginal stenosis	
Fibrotic uterus	

(Data from DiSaia, P. J., & Creasman, W. T. [1989]. *Clinical gynecologic oncology* [3rd ed.]. St. Louis: C. V. Mosby Co.)

34–4 lists the common complications associated with radiation therapy. Both early and late complications can occur and the late sequelae are directly proportional to the occurrence and severity of the early complications. Vaginal dilators are prescribed to prevent vaginal stricture after irradiation. Figure 34–8 depicts vaginal dilators in graduated sizes. Table 34–5 identifies appropriate vaginal care instructions for patients. Refer to Chapter 20 for discussion of interventions for specific problems and side effects.

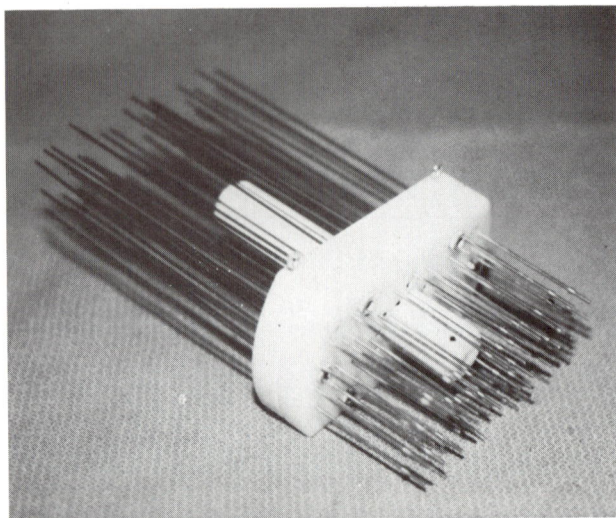

Figure 34–7. Vaginal template with needles (17 G) and obturator in place for interstitial implant.

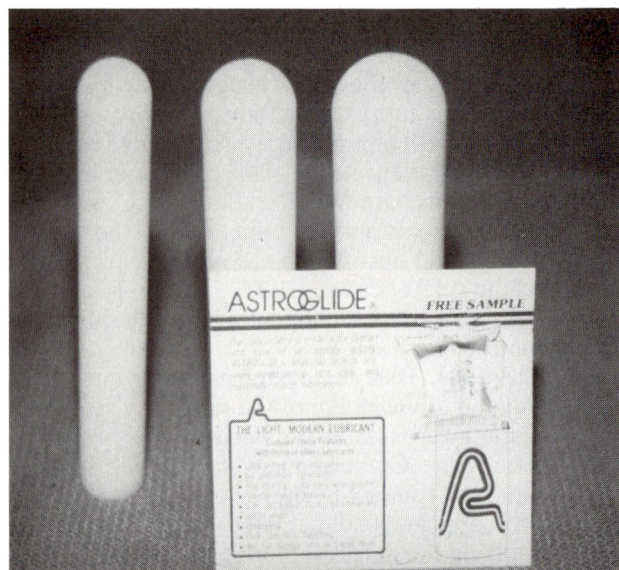

Figure 34–8. Vaginal dilators. *Left to right:* small (2.1 cm), medium (2.8 cm), large (3.4 cm).

Table 34–5. VAGINAL CARE DURING AND AFTER PELVIC IRRADIATION

For the first 2 weeks, have partner use condom to decrease irritation to the mucosa from sperm.

Discomfort with intercourse begins at approximately the third week.

Refrain from intercourse when discomfort and mucositis begin.

Begin using vaginal dilator 2 weeks after therapy is finished, daily for 10 min.

Use dilator every other day thereafter for the rest of patient's life.

Dilation may be omitted on the day patient has intercourse.

Vaginal Dilation

  Make sure dilator is clean.

  Start with the small size dilator.

  Apply water-soluble lubricant or prescribed cream to the dilator.

  Insert dilator between the labia gently and firmly.

  Remove and reinsert three to four times over a period of 10 min. Clean well with soap and water.

  Dilation may be done at the same time as a bath, using water as the lubricant if patient is not using a cream that is prescribed.

  Douching is not necessary.

(Data from Richards & Hiratzka, 1986; Strohl, 1986.)

Recurrent Carcinoma of the Cervix

Regardless of primary treatment, follow-up is essential for early diagnosis of recurrence. Examinations, including a Papanicolaou smear, should be done every 3 to 4 months. Thirty-five per cent of all patients with invasive cervical cancer will experience recurrence or have residual disease even after therapy (Dericks, 1974). Recurrence will most likely appear within 2 years after completion of treatment. Metastasis is rare. The suspicious site should be biopsied and examined for histologic confirmation. Central recurrences carry a more favorable prognosis (Mattingly & Thompson, 1985).

Management

The goal of most treatment for recurrence is palliation only. Radiation outside the original field may be given for relief of symptoms and comfort for the uncommon occurrence of bone metastasis. Chemotherapy has not proved to be effective for definitive treatment of recurrence. The tumor often recurs within a hard shell of previously irradiated tissue and is not accessible via the blood stream. Historically, squamous cell cancers have not proved to be vulnerable to chemotherapeutic agents, and the majority of all cervical cancers are of this type. Finally, many cytotoxic agents are also nephrotoxic and could not be excreted in a timely manner owing to the prevalence of ureteral obstruction in this patient population. The occurrence of ureteral obstruction is a difficult management problem. Patients who have had no previous irradiation are best treated with a urinary diversion (ileal conduit) procedure within radiation after the operation. When irradiation has been administered previously, many physicians opt to treat the patient with palliative comfort measures only, after consultation with the patient and family. The patient usually dies from the progression of irreversible uremia (DiSaia & Creasman, 1989). Alternatively, nephrostomy tube diversion is usually successful in reversing the uremia and prolonging life, but the quality of life may be poor.

Table 34–6. EVALUATION FOR PELVIC EXENTERATION PROCEDURE FOR RECURRENCE

Pelvic examination

Chest radiograph, computer tomographic scan of abdomen and pelvis

Creatinine clearance, liver function tests, prothrombin time, partial thromboplastin time

Lymphangiogram*

Bone scan,* Liver scan*

Scalene node biopsy*

Exploratory laparatomy

Psychological evaluation

*Done as necessary. (Data from DiSaia, P. J., & Creasman, W. T. [1989]. *Clinical gynecologic oncology* [3rd ed.]. St. Louis: C. V. Mosby Co.)

Pelvic Exenteration

A few patients exhibiting central recurrence may be suitable for a pelvic exenteration. Anterior, posterior, or total pelvic exenteration may be performed (see Fig. 34–9). A stringent work-up of the patient is performed to rule out extrapelvic disease, tumor fixed to the pelvic wall, or cancer with ureteral obstruction in the posterior part of the pelvis (Table 34–6) (Barber, 1980).

Unilateral leg edema, sciatica, and ureteral obstruction accompany unresectable, recurrent pelvic disease. All three must be present to justify halting efforts toward salvage with an exenteration. If the patient fails in any of the parameters of the evaluation, exenteration may not be performed. Construction of a neovagina using a segment of bowel or myocutaneous grafts may be done at the time of the exenterative procedure, if possible (DiSaia & Creasman, 1989). The angle, dimensions, and tissue flexibility are close to anatomically correct (circumference, 12 to 14 cm; depth 13 to 15 cm) for patients to engage in satisfying sexual intercourse (Hampton, 1986). With newer operative stapling techniques, rectal anatomy and function can be preserved in some cases by utilizing a very low descending colon-to-anus, end-to-end anastamosis (Trelford & Williams, 1984). Complications are numerous and occur at predictable times during the postoperative period (Table 34–7).

Table 34–7. POSTOPERATIVE COMPLICATIONS ASSOCIATED WITH PELVIC EXENTERATION

Early

  Pulmonary embolism, pulmonary edema, MI, CVA, hemorrhage

Later (second week)

  Sepsis because of pelvic abscess or diffuse pelvic cellulitis

Later

  SBO because of adherence to denuded surface of pelvic floor or previous irradiation; small bowel fistula related to SBO or irradiation

Long-term

  Urinary obstruction of ileal conduit; pyelonephritis because of hydronephrosis

MI, Myocardial infarction; CVA, cerebrovascular accident; SBO, small bowel obstruction.

(Data from DiSaia, P. J., & Creasman, W. T. [1989]. *Clinical gynecologic oncology* [3rd ed.]. St. Louis: C. V. Mosby Co.)

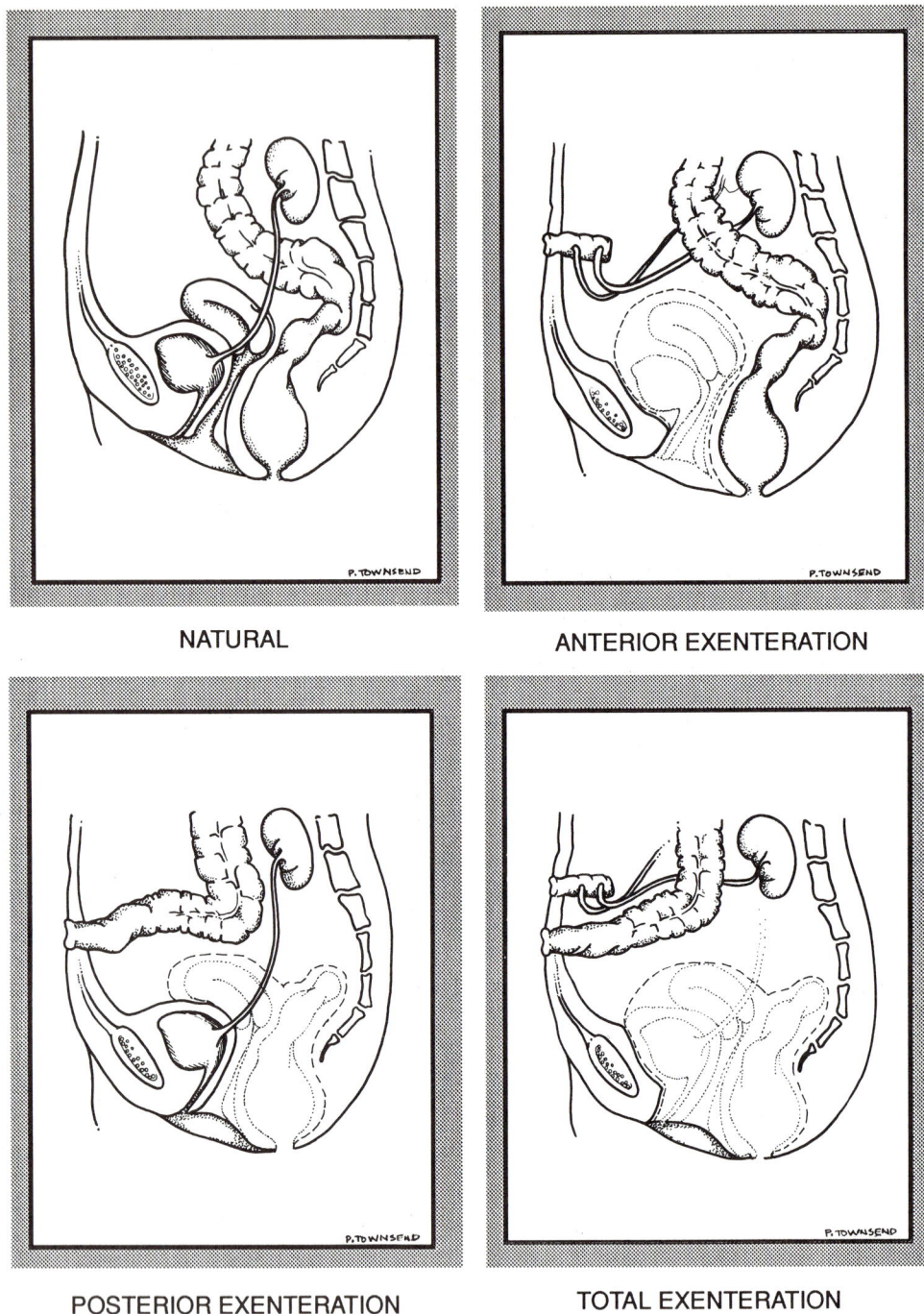

NATURAL

ANTERIOR EXENTERATION

POSTERIOR EXENTERATION

TOTAL EXENTERATION

Figure 34–9. Pelvic exenteration procedures. (Courtesy of P. Townsend, graphic artist.)

Nursing care after pelvic exenteration is complex and involves careful observation and coordination of caretakers (Tables 34–8 and 34–9).

Survival

Survival statistics vary according to patient selection criteria. Symptom-free patients with a favorable work-up preoperatively survive longer than those who had symptoms or abnormalities on work-up. Survival for this group can be more than 50 per cent at 2 years after surgery (DiSaia & Creasman, 1989).

Fistulas

Fistulas are abnormal tracts occurring between two areas of the body not normally in direct communication with each other. They are named for the two connected structures. Of all fistulas formed, 10 per cent occur in gynecologic cancer patients (Boarini, Bryant, & Irgang, 1986). Table 34–10 lists situations that increase the likelihood of fistula development.

The three most commonly occurring fistulas are of the rectovaginal, enterocutaneous, and vesicovaginal types. Rectovaginal or vesicovaginal fistulas may occur

Table 34–8. NURSING CARE PLAN FOR THE PATIENT UNDERGOING PELVIC EXENTERATION

Assessment	Interventions	Expected Outcomes
Nursing Diagnosis: Potential for impaired physical mobility related to presence of lymphedema arising from absence of lymph nodes		
Assess lower extremities (LE) for presence of edema	No intravenous (IV) lines or needlesticks to LE's Prohibit use of knee gatch, pillows under knees Elevate LE in stockinette sling on IV pole or on pillows Consult Rehabilitation personnel for pneumatic intermittent compression stocking therapy; obtain order for measurement and construction of Jobst type pressure garment for permanent control; discharge instructions concerning protection of extremity	Patient's LE is free of edema Patient demonstrates no increase in edema
Nursing Diagnosis: Impaired physical mobility related to healing myocutaneous graft donor sites		
Assess LE for full range of motion (ROM)	ROM every shift, passive and active; consult Rehabilitation personnel	Patient demonstrates full ROM in bilateral LE
Nursing Diagnosis: Potential for sexual dysfunction related to neovaginal stricture		
Assess size of neovagina Assess healing status of neovagina	Obtain compatible size set of vaginal dilators or use syringe covers in gradually increasing sizes; instruct patient in dilation regimen (see Chapter 31); discuss alternatives to coitus with patient: masturbation, mutual masturbation, oral-genital maneuvers, erotic films; stimulation of erogenous body areas (buttocks, breasts, neck, inner thighs), nudity, and snuggling are other nondemand pleasuring activities	Neovagina will maintain normal anatomic circumference
Nursing Diagnosis: Potential for infection related to pelvic abscess, cellulitis, or wound dehiscence		
Assess for presence of fever (Palpate abdomen for warmth or presence of exudate from suture line, drains, vagina, rectal area, and for pain and tenderness; examine dressings for color and odor)	Wound care as specified: wet to wet, wet to dry dressings every 4 hr; take vital signs every 4 hr	Patient vital signs within normal limits; abdominal area clean and dry

(Data from Grunberg, K. J. [1986]. Sexual rehabilitation of the cancer patient undergoing ostomy surgery. *Journal of Enterostomal Therapy, 13,* 148–152; Grunberg, K. J. [1986]. Spotlight: Sex counselling called crucial for patients with pelvic or genital surgery. *Oncology Nurse Bulletin, 3,* 12; Grunberg, K. J. [1986]. Practice corner: Sexuality and the person with cancer. *Oncology Nursing Forum, 13* [2], 87; Dericks, V. C. [1974]. *Nursing care of patients with extensive surgery: Pelvic exenteration.* American Cancer Society Professional Education Publication, Publ. No. 3363-PE; and Herberth, L., & Gosnell, D. [1987]. Nursing diagnosis for oncology nursing practice. *Cancer Nursing, 10,* 41–51.)

Table 34–9. NURSING DIAGNOSES ASSOCIATED WITH PELVIC EXENTERATION

Altered urinary elimination related to construction of diversional conduit (Chapter 32)

Altered bowel elimination related to construction of colostomy (Chapter 33)

Sexual dysfunction related to presence of ostomies and neovagina (Chapter 53)

Body image disturbance related to loss of anatomic and functional bladder or anus, or both (Chapter 52)

Self-esteem disturbance related to change in physical abilities and normal roles (Chapter 53)

Self-toileting deficit related to uncontrolled new ostomies (Chapter 33)

Knowledge deficit related to presence of new colostomy and conduit (Chapter 33)

Activity intolerance related to muscle weakness (Chapter 54)

Potential for impaired skin integrity related to fistula formation in previously irradiated skin in conjunction with repair of bowel obstruction (Chapter 34)

Impaired home maintenance management related to prolonged hospitalization (Chapter 70)

Alteration in nutrition—less than body requirements, related to increased metabolic needs for healing (Chapter 47)

(Data from Herberth, L., & Gosnell, D. [1984]. Nursing diagnosis for oncology nursing practice. *Cancer Nursing, 10,* 41–51.)

after irradiation therapy in the presence of persistent or recurrent tumor. Because of this, all patients should have a careful pelvic or rectal examination and undergo biopsy to document the presence or absence of tumor

Table 34–10. PREDISPOSING FACTORS LEADING TO FISTULA FORMATION

Recurrent tumor

Incidental enterotomy at the time of surgery

Anastomotic dehiscence after surgical bypass for intestinal obstruction

Intraoperative disruption of blood flow to pelvic structures

Previous irradiation

(Data from Boarini, Bryant, & Irrgang, 1980.)

before attempted repair of the fistula or diversion. Fistulas are classified as high output (> 500 ml/24 hr), low output (< 500 ml/24 hr), or minimal output (< 100 ml/24 hr). Principles of fistula management include physiologic stabilization of the patient, assessment of the fistula, and implementation of treatment for the fistula (Boarini et al., 1986). Refer to Tables 34–11 and 34–12 for the nursing care plan for patients with fistulas related to gynecologic malignancies and for other nursing diagnoses associated with the presence of a fistula.

ADENOCARCINOMA OF THE UTERINE CORPUS

Incidence

Cancer of the endometrium is the most common of the gynecologic cancers and its incidence is rising.

Table 34–11. NURSING CARE PLAN FOR PATIENTS EXPERIENCING FISTULA(S) RELATED TO GYNECOLOGIC CANCERS

Assessment	Intervention	Expected Outcome
Nursing Diagnosis: Impaired skin integrity, related to abnormal communication between colon, small intestine, bladder, ureter, or vagina and skin		
Determine output status (high or low)	*Low Output:* Apply transparent dressing as prophylactic protection	Patient's skin remains dry
Evaluate characteristics of effluent, skin condition, number of fistulas, and location of orifices	Apply ointments with each dressing change (useful with suction catheter in fistula if unable to use pouch)	Patient reports increased comfort
	Apply skin sealant to perifistular skin to decrease excoriation when frequent tape removal occurs; apply under barriers with adhesives to prevent inadvertent denuding of epidermis	Macerated skin, if present, shows evidence of reepithelialization
	High Output: Apply skin barriers in presence of caustic drainage	
Nursing Diagnosis: Alteration in bowel elimination, related to incontinence through the enterovaginal fistula		
Evaluate for fecal drainage from vagina	*Low Output:* Frequent pad changes and perineal care	Patient reports control of fecal drainage
	Apply ointment or skin barrier to perineum	Vaginal mucosa remains intact
	High Output: Insert vaginal diaphragm–type device connected to over-side drainage bag; Remove and clean every shift	Patient reports no odor
		Patient expresses increased comfort
Nursing Diagnosis: Fluid volume deficit: electrolyte imbalance, related to increased drainage through the fistula		
Determine 24-hr volume loss	Record daily weight and intake and output	Patient maintains normal electrolyte status
Observe for symptoms of dehydration and and electrolyte balance	Monitor ongoing electrolyte levels	Patient maintains normal fluid balance
Evaluate electrolyte studies	*Minimal Output:* Apply absorbent dressings, secure with stockinette, rolled gauze, or Montgomery straps every 1–4 hr	Patient expresses feelings of increased control over drainage
Evaluate fluid intake and output	Apply charcoal-impregnated dressing over fistulas	Patient reports increased comfort
Observe for odor	*Low or High Output:* Apply pouch over skin barrier	Patient reports no odor
	Empty pouch when ⅓ full or connect to over-side drainage while in bed	Patient demonstrates increased mobility
	Change pouch every 24 hr	
	Consult E. T. nurse for assistance with difficult anatomic fistulas	

(Data from Irrgang & Bryant, 1984; Fitzgerald, 1982; Herberth & Gosnell, 1987.)

Table 34–12. NURSING DIAGNOSES ASSOCIATED WITH THE PRESENCE OF FISTULA(S)

Alteration in nutrition, related to increased metabolic requirements from the presence of a fistula (Chapter 47)
Potential for infection, related to abscess formation or presence of necrotic tissue (Chapter 19)
Powerlessness, related to loss of control of normal body functions (Chapter 52)
Body image disturbance, related to impaired bowel or bladder function (Chapter 52)
Sexual dysfunction, related to altered bowel or bladder function and altered role (Chapter 53)
Impaired mobility, related to the presence of drainage control devices or the frequency of dressing changes (Chapter 54)
Impairment of urinary elimination: incontinence, related to presence of a vesicovaginal fistula (Chapter 32)
Social isolation: rejection, related to foul odors from the presence of fistula drainage or necrotic tissue (Chapter 51)
Alteration in comfort, related to impaired skin integrity owing to fistulas (Chapter 50)
Sleep pattern disturbance, related to frequency of dressing changes owing to presence of fistula (Chapter 58)

(Data from Herberth & Gosnell, 1987.)

Increased availability of medical care, increased numbers of women alive at the susceptible age, incorporation of the dysplastic conditions into the diagnostic criteria, and unknown environmental factors are among the probable explanations for this rise. Cancer of the endometrium represents 7 per cent of all cancers in women. It was anticipated that in 1988 34,000 new cases would occur and that 3000 women would die (Silverberg & Lubera, 1988). Although cancer of the endometrium is increasing in younger women, it is primarily a disease affecting women in the peri- and postmenopausal years and appears a decade later than cervical cancer. Five per cent of cases are diagnosed before the age of 40 years, 20 per cent between the ages of 40 and 50 years, and 70 per cent after 50 years of age (DiSaia & Creasman, 1989).

Epidemiology and Etiology

Hormonal imbalance is the single most important causative factor (Smith, 1986). Aberrant pituitary function may be the common factor that links the predisposing conditions. Obesity, nulliparity, late onset of menopause, diabetes mellitus, and hypertension are frequently correlated with endometrial cancer (DiSaia & Creasman, 1989). The presence of the hormone estrogen normally decreases with age. It is thought that the lower concentrations of estrogen may stimulate an increased production of postmenopausal estrogen precursors, primarily androstenedione, in a negative feedback fashion. This prehormone is also produced in increased amounts in the presence of obesity or hepatic disease and when the endometrium has continuous stimulation by unopposed estrogen, creating a state of hyperestrogenism, such as is seen in Stein-Leventhal syndrome. Table 34–13 lists the symptoms of unopposed estrogen stimulation.

Androstenedione is converted to estrone, the most prevalent postmenopausal estrogen. Estrone is consid-

Table 34–13. SYMPTOMS OF UNOPPOSED ESTROGEN STIMULATION

Early menarche
Delayed onset of ovulation
Premature cessation of ovulation
Extremely heavy menses
Menses continuing beyond 50 years of age
Idiopathic sterility
Endometrial polyps and hyperplasia
History of more than one spontaneous abortion
Severe cystic disease of the breasts

(Data from Barber, 1980.)

ered a carcinogen and may lead to the development of endometrial hyperplasia in postmenopausal women (Barber, 1980). Exogenous estrogens may also play a role in the development of endometrial cancer. Conjugated estrogens taken to prevent or control the symptoms of menopause, vaginal estrogen creams, or estrogen ingested as additives to meats have been correlated to the development of hyperplasia and cancer (Horwitz & Feinstein, 1978).

Biology and Natural History

Endometrial Hyperplasia

Endometrial cancer is often discussed in conjunction with a condition known as endometrial hyperplasia much in the same way that cervical cancer is discussed along with cervical intraepithelial neoplasia. Endometrial hyperplasia is generally considered a precursor of endometrial carcinoma, and the relative risk is increased in the presence of the same risk factors discussed for endometrial carcinoma. Table 34–14 describes the three types of hyperplasia and their relative risks for progressing to adenocarcinoma of the endometrium (DiSaia & Creasman, 1989).

Adenocarcinoma of the Endometrium

Three main cell types are seen in endometrial tumors. Columnar glandular epithelium is the normal cell type. Adenocarcinoma can be a well-differentiated noninvasive tumor. Twenty per cent of adenocarcinomas are adenoacanthomas, a mixed form of adenocarcinoma with benign squamous metaplastic encroachment. The third type is adenosquamous carcinoma, in which both cell types represented are malignant. Ad-

Table 34–14. TYPES OF HYPERPLASIA IN ENDOMETRIAL CANCER

Cystic hyperplasia ("swiss cheese hyperplasia")
  No malignant potential
Adenomatous hyperplasia
  Considered a precancerous condition of endometrial carcinoma
Atypical adenomatous hyperplasia
  Further divided into mild, moderate, and severe stages (the last is considered carcinoma in situ); this type is often treated as if it were cancer.

(Data from DiSaia & Creasman, 1989.)

enosquamous and clear cell carcinoma, a rare subvariant type, carry the poorest prognoses. Unlike cervical cancer, cancer of the endometrium is more likely to metastasize (Fig. 34–10). Patients with high-grade tumors, lesions involving the lower uterus or cervix, and deep invasion into the myometrium are most at risk for metastasis (Barber, 1980). Regardless of cell type, the advanced disease takes the form of a fungating mass, has areas of hemorrhage and necrosis, and bleeds easily.

Prognosis

Prognosis appears to be related to the presence or absence of certain factors before primary treatment and possibly the type of pathogenic disease the patient exhibits. Bokhman (1983) hypothesizes that the patient who does not fit into the typical pattern (obesity, hyperlipidemia, and signs of hyperestrogenism) may have a poorer prognosis. This group tends to have deeply invasive, high-grade tumors in advanced stage and lymph node involvement and have the poorest 5-year survival rate (58 per cent). Table 34–15 lists other prognostic factors.

Diagnosis and Staging

Young Patients

The profile of the young patient who develops endometrial cancer is one of obesity with a history of anovulation. Spotting and protracted heavy menstrual periods are an indication for further work-up for cancer.

Older Patients

The normal pattern for cessation of menstruation during menopause is periods that become scantier and farther apart over time. Other patterns of bleeding that occur after menopause are cause for concern. This sometimes is ignored and assumed to be irregularity accompanying the "change of life." Any bleeding that occurs 12 months after menses have stopped is considered abnormal (Haskell, 1985). Symptoms of advanced disease include generalized abdominal carcinomatosis caused by tumor studding of the entire peritoneal cavity, pain, intestinal obstruction, ascites, and possibly

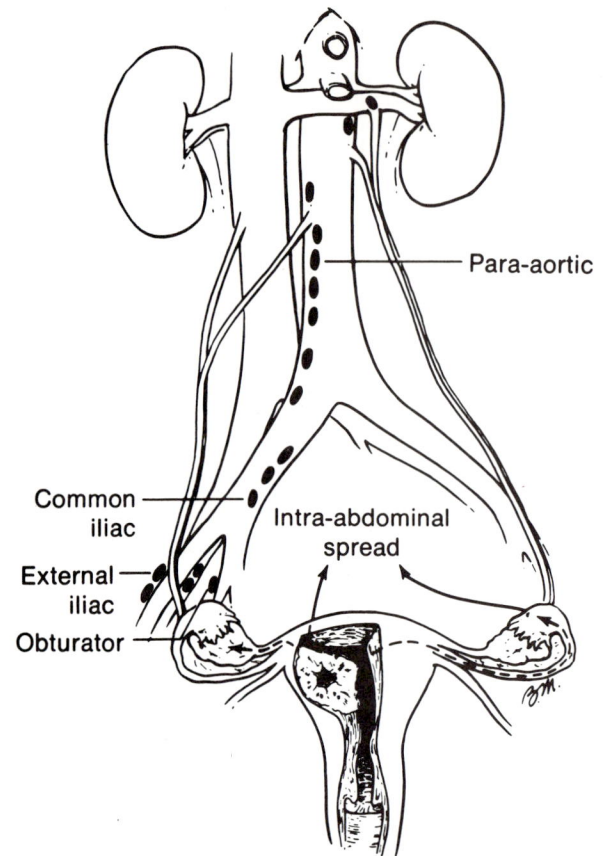

Figure 34–10. Metastatic spread pattern for endometrial carcinoma. (Reproduced by permission from DiSaia, P. J., & Creasman, W. T. [1989]. *Clinical gynecologic oncology* [3rd ed.]. St. Louis: C. V. Mosby Co.)

hemorrhage (Haskell, 1985). Histologic confirmation is necessary for diagnosis. Endometrial biopsy or aspiration and endocervical curettage, although uncomfortable, can be performed on an outpatient basis and are associated with little morbidity. Nursing responsibilities include an explanation of the procedure, including the fact that there is some discomfort. The patient should be advised to take a nonnarcotic analgesic such as acetaminophen, ibuprofen, or aspirin (if not contraindicated) before the procedure. Peri-pads may be required for the first 24 to 48 hr after the biopsy. The presence of a preinvasive abnormality in any of the specimens mandates proceeding with a formal fractional dilation and curettage and possible cone biopsy. Often a measurement of the uterus is taken and an EUA is included. Although general anesthesia is required, the trend is to perform this procedure on an outpatient basis in a day surgery setting. Nursing implications include appropriate preoperative teaching, including taking nothing by mouth and instruction on control of postoperative vaginal bleeding, drainage, cramping, and pain control. With confirmation of endometrial carcinoma, a diagnostic work-up and clinical staging should be done. Table 34–16 lists the evaluation studies necessary before initiation of therapy. The FIGO classification system is used to describe the stages of endometrial carcinoma (Table 34–17).

Table 34–15. PROGNOSTIC FACTORS AFFECTING SURVIVAL OF ENDOMETRIAL CARCINOMA

Cell type
Degree of differentiation
Size of the uterus
Stage of the disease at diagnosis
Depth of uterine muscle invasion
Presence of cancer cells in the peritoneum at time of surgery
Lymph node involvement
Ovarian and cervical invasion

(Adapted from DiSaia, P. J., & Creasman, W. T. [1989]. *Clinical gynecologic oncology* [3rd ed.]. St. Louis: C. V. Mosby Co.)

Table 34–16. PRETREATMENT EVALUATION OF THE ENDOMETRIAL CANCER PATIENT

Outpatient
Thorough history and physical examination, which includes pelvic, rectal, and rectovaginal examination, dilatation and curettage, endocervical curettage
Preoperative
Routine blood studies, clotting values
Chest radiograph
Intravenous pyelogram
Sigmoidoscopy,* barium enema*
Brain, liver, bone scans*

*Done when metastasis is suspected.
(Data from Barber, 1980; DiSaia & Creasman, 1989.)

The grade of the tumor plays a major role in the pathologic aspect of the staging process. The cell type is always classified according to degree of differentiation: grade I, well-differentiated; grade II, moderately differentiated; and grade III, poorly differentiated.

Treatment

The stage and grade of the tumor are taken into consideration when treatment is planned. Figure 34–11 diagrams the current management of stage I endometrial cancer.

Radiation is usually given postoperatively for patients with poor prognostic indicators, such as high-grade tumor, deep myometrial invasion, cervical involvement, and disease in the pelvic and para-aortic lymph nodes. For stage II disease, two forms of treatment appear to be effective—surgery (radical hysterectomy and pelvic lymphadenectomy followed by radiation for positive nodes) and external radiation with 40 to 50 Gy with one application of brachytherapy

Table 34–17. FIGO CLASSIFICATION SYSTEM FOR STAGING ENDOMETRIAL CARCINOMA

Stage 0 Carcinoma in situ. Histologic findings suspicious of malignancy.
(Cases of stage 0 should not be included in any therapeutic statistics.)
Stage I The carcinoma is confined to the corpus.
Stage IA: The length of the uterine cavity is 8 cm or less.
Stage IB: The length of the uterine cavity is more than 8 cm.
The stage I cases should be subgrouped with regard to the histologic type of the adenocarcinoma as follows:
G1: highly differentiated adenomatous carcinoma.
G2: differentiated adenomatous carcinoma with partly solid areas.
G3: predominantly solid or entirely undifferentiated carcinoma.
Stage II The carcinoma has involved the corpus and the cervix.
Stage III The carcinoma has extended outside the uterus but not outside the true pelvis.
Stage IV The carcinoma has extended outside the true pelvis or has obviously involved the mucosa of the bladder or rectum. A bullous edema, as such, does not permit a case to be allotted to stage IV.

(Data from *Gynecology Oncology Group pathology manual* [unpublished].)

followed by hysterectomy and bilateral salpingo-oophorectomy 6 weeks later. A third alternative is the treatment described for stage I, grade 2 and grade 3 in Figure 34–11 if no disease is visible on the cervix and suspicion of parametrial disease is absent. Occult stage II disease (i.e., stage II with endocervical disease found in the operative specimen) is also managed as stage I, grade 2 and grade 3 disease (DiSaia & Creasman, 1989). In most cases stages III and IV are treated with surgery, radiation, hormones, and chemotherapy (Fig. 34–12).

Recurrence

Endometrial carcinoma often recurs locally either inside the vaginal vault or above the upper vagina. Some local recurrences can be treated with surgery or radiation or a combination of the two with an overall good result and long-term survival. The recurrences that occur beyond the vagina are difficult to treat successfully with either surgery or radiation. Often, hormonal therapy or chemotherapy becomes the treatment of choice in this situation.

Hormonal Therapy

Progestins, in use for more than 20 years, do produce a response in approximately one third of all patients with recurrent carcinoma of the endometrium. Tumors that are well-differentiated respond better than moderately or poorly differentiated lesions. Recently, malignant uterine tissue has been examined in studies to determine the presence or absence of estrogen and progesterone receptors (Creasman et al., 1980). Well-differentiated tumors contain more estrogen and progesterone receptors than those that are poorly differentiated. Because of this discovery, it is likely that estrogen and progesterone receptor analyses will be done on all biopsied uterine tissue and, depending on the results, progestin therapy will be initiated or the patient will be placed on cytotoxic agents. Progestin therapy is continued unless progression of disease is noted. Patients should be instructed regarding the side effects of progestins, such as nausea, depression, rash, mild fluid retention, and mild liver function abnormalities, including jaundice (Skeel, 1982). Table 34–18 lists commonly prescribed progestins (DiSaia & Creasman, 1989).

Chemotherapy

One study noted that patients with few estrogen or progesterone receptor sites had a significantly greater response rate to a combined chemotherapy regimen of doxorubicin (Adriamycin), cyclophosphamide (Cy-

Table 34–18. PROGESTINS

Medroxyprogesterone (Depo-Provera), 400 mg IM daily
Medroxyprogesterone (Provera), 150 mg PO daily
Megestrol acetate (Megace), 160 mg PO daily

IM, Intramuscularly; PO, orally.

Stage I, Grade 1

↓

Total abdominal hysterectomy; → Positive peritoneal ← Stage I, Grade 2 and Grade 3
bilateral salpingo-oophorectomy; cytology
peritoneal cytology

↓

Phosphorus-32
(32 p)

Total abdominal hysterectomy; bilateral salpingo-oophorectomy, selective pelvic and para-aortic lymphadenectomy, peritoneal cytology

↓

Grade 2

Grade 2, more than superficial muscle involvement

Disease in uterus only

↓

Grade 3, with superficial muscle involvement

Grade 3, more than superficial muscle involvement

↓

No further therapy necessary

45-50 Gy whole-pelvis radiation

Disease extends beyond uterus

↓

Disease extends beyond uterus → Consider 45-50 Gy whole-pelvis or 20-30 Gy whole-abdomen radiation; consider chemotherapy or progestins

↓

Extend field to include para-aortic nodes if metastasis present

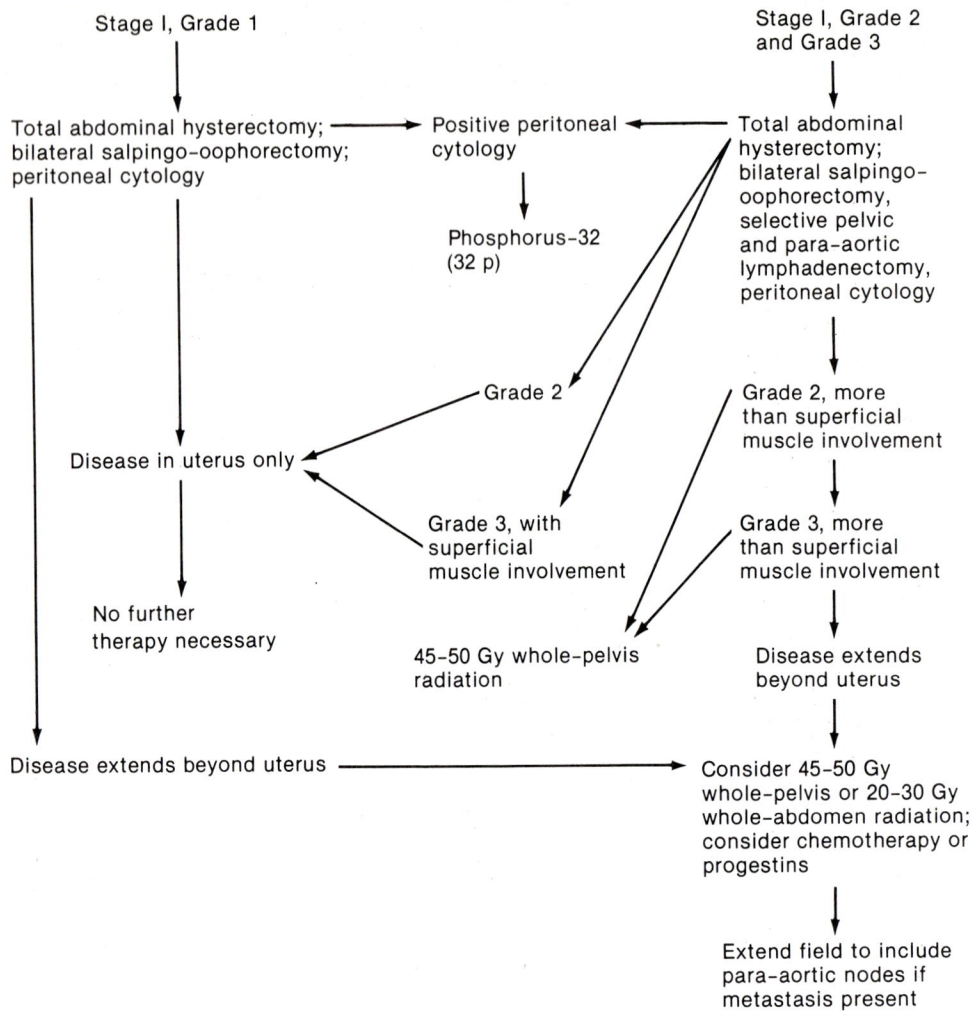

Figure 34-11. Schema for management of stage I endometrial carcinoma. (Adapted by permission from DiSaia, P. J., & Creasman, W. T. [1989]. *Clinical gynecologic oncology* [3rd ed.]. St. Louis: C. V. Mosby Co.)

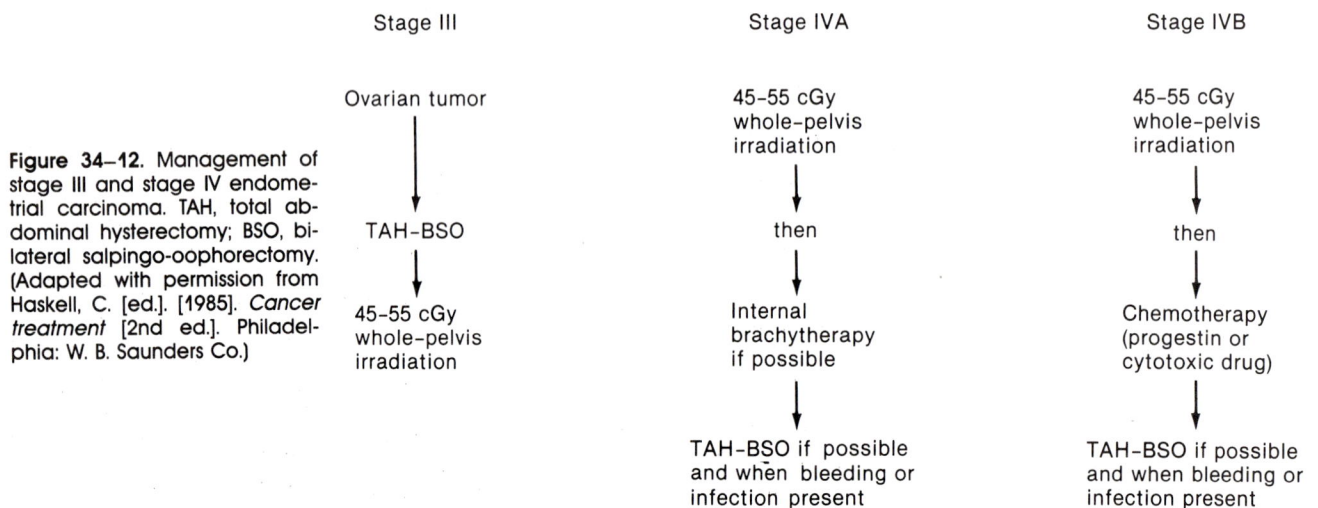

Figure 34-12. Management of stage III and stage IV endometrial carcinoma. TAH, total abdominal hysterectomy; BSO, bilateral salpingo-oophorectomy. (Adapted with permission from Haskell, C. [ed.]. [1985]. *Cancer treatment* [2nd ed.]. Philadelphia: W. B. Saunders Co.)

Stage III

Ovarian tumor

↓

TAH-BSO

↓

45-55 cGy whole-pelvis irradiation

Stage IVA

45-55 cGy whole-pelvis irradiation

↓

then

↓

Internal brachytherapy if possible

↓

TAH-BSO if possible and when bleeding or infection present

Stage IVB

45-55 cGy whole-pelvis irradiation

↓

then

↓

Chemotherapy (progestin or cytotoxic drug)

↓

TAH-BSO if possible and when bleeding or infection present

Table 34–19. NURSING DIAGNOSES ASSOCIATED WITH
ADVANCED ENDOMETRIAL CARCINOMA

Potential for infection related to presence of necrotic parametrial
tumor (Chapter 34)

Alteration in nutrition—less than body requirements, related to
increased metabolic rate owing to presence of tumor
(Chapter 47)

Potential fluid volume deficit—intracellular, intravascular, related
to the presence of ascites (Chapter 34)

Alteration in fluid volume (excess)—extracellular, interstitial,
related to presence of ascites (Chapter 34)

Potential activity intolerance related to fatigue owing to poor
nutritional status (Chapters 47 and 58)

Total self-care deficit (Chapter 55)

Impaired home maintenance management related to prolonged
hospitalization (Chapter 70)

Ineffective breathing pattern related to presence of ascites
(Chapter 34)

Alteration in comfort related to pelvic pain (Chapter 50)

Fear related to hemorrhage episodes (Chapter 57)

Body image disturbance related to gynecological surgery
(Chapter 52)

Sexual dysfunction related to presence of tumor in vagina
(Chapter 53)

Spiritual distress related to grieving and dying process (Chapter 56)

(Data from Herberth & Gosnell, 1987.)

toxan), 5-fluorouracil, and vincristine (Oncovin) than
those with greater numbers of receptor sites (Kauppila,
1980). Overall, neither single agent nor combination
chemotherapy has increased survival. With increased
use of receptor analysis in the determination of individual patient therapy, response rates may increase.

Table 34–19 lists other nursing diagnoses associated
with endometrial cancer.

SARCOMA OF THE UTERUS

Sarcoma of the uterus constitutes approximately 3
to 5 per cent of uterine cancers. Refer to DiSaia and
Creasman's book (1989) for a complete discussion of
this subject.

OVARIAN CANCER

Incidence

Cancer of the ovary ranks fourth in fatalities among
cancers of women in the United States. It represents
23 per cent of all gynecologic cancers but is responsible
for nearly 47 per cent of all deaths of women afflicted
by cancer of the genital tract. Silverberg and Lubera
(1988) estimated that 19,000 new cases would occur
and 12,000 women would die from ovarian cancer in
1988. Of great concern is the lack of progress in
identifying a cause for this deadly disease.

Epidemiology and Etiology

Most ovarian cancers occur in women between 50
and 59 years of age. There may be genetic components
to the pathogenesis, and this is currently being studied.

Environmental factors play a role in that the highest
frequency is found in highly industrialized countries
with the exception of Japan. Life-style behaviors such
as ingestion of a diet high in saturated fat may also be
implicated. Other, as yet unproven hypotheses include
the use of chemicals and carcinogens in the genital
area, with upward migration and absorption of the
toxins into the ovaries and fallopian tubes, and the
presence of the mumps virus because of its known
gonadotropic potential. Nursing implications include
taking as accurate a history as possible when interviewing patients, including exposure to environmental carcinogens or viruses and pertinent life-style patterns.
Runowicz (1987) has described the profile of the high-
risk patient as white, nulliparous, and infertile, having
a positive family history of ovarian cancer, and living
an upper socioeconomic life style.

Biology and Natural History

Ovarian neoplasms arise from cells that were present
during the four stages of early embryologic ovarian
development. Table 34–20 depicts the four stages, the
types of cancers that are derived from cells present
during these stages, and the ages when they are most
likely to occur.

The ovary is also a vulnerable site for metastasis
from other primary cancer sites, such as the breast,
gastrointestinal tract, and endometrium, and from lymphomas. Typically, all forms of ovarian cancer spread

Table 34–20. DERIVATION OF OVARIAN NEOPLASMS AND
AGE GROUP AFFECTED

First developmental stage: coelomic epithelium cells. Most
  prevalent over 50 years of age; 80% of tumors
  Serous tumor
  Mucinous tumor
  Endometrioid tumor
  Mesonephroid (clear cell) tumor
  Brenner tumor
  Undifferentiated carcinoma
  Carcinosarcoma and mixed mesodermal tumor

Second developmental stage: arrival of germ cells and proliferation
  of coelomic epithelium and mesenchyme. Most prevalent
  before 20 years of age.
  Teratoma
    Mature teratoma (dermoid cyst)
    Immature teratoma
  Dysgerminoma
  Embryonal carcinoma
  Endodermal sinus tumor
  Choriocarcinoma
  Gonadoblastoma

Third developmental stage: ovary divided into cortex and medulla
  Granulosa-theca cell tumors
  Sertoli-Leydig tumors
  Gynandroblastoma
  Lipid cell tumors

Fourth developmental stage: development of cortex and involution
  of medulla
  Fibroma
  Lymphoma
  Sarcoma

(Adapted from DiSaia, P. J., & Creasman, W. T. [1989]. *Clinical
gynecologic oncology* [3rd ed.]. St. Louis: C. V. Mosby Co.)

insidiously along the peritoneum and the surfaces of abdominal organs, encompassing all of the structures of the upper abdomen. The tumor may be of varying consistencies, ranging from a rocky hardness to a rubbery or even a cyst-like quality. This phenomenon is caused by a rapid growth of the tumor away from the main sources of blood supply (Barber, 1980). Ovarian size diminishes with age until the ovary is not palpable in a postmenopausal woman. The normal premenopausal ovary is approximately $3.5 \times 2 \times 1.5$ cm. During early menopause (the first 2 years), it decreases in size to $2 \times 1.5 \times 0.5$ cm and ultimately shrinks to $1.5 \times 0.75 \times 0.5$ cm during the next 2 to 5 years (DiSaia & Creasman, 1989). This is important to keep in mind because a woman who is more than 2 years beyond the menopause but has an ovary of premenopausal size in reality may have an ovarian tumor (palpable postmenopausal syndrome).

Borderline Malignant Epithelial Neoplasms

Borderline malignant epithelial neoplasms account for 15 per cent of all ovarian cancers, are composed of low-grade serous cystadenocarcinomas and mucinous tumors, and have characteristic histologic features. Although the great majority of these are cured with surgery only, if left untreated they may recur, seed the peritoneum, and eventually cause death.

Prognosis

Long-term survival for ovarian cancer is related to certain prognostic factors. Well-differentiated epithelial tumors of a low grade, small residual tumor volume after surgery (< 2 cm in any one focus), and additional adjuvant treatment after the initial surgery influence survival significantly. Overall survival is 31 per cent after 5 years. The survival rate for the borderline cystadenocarcinomas is as high as 95 per cent after 10 years (DiSaia and Creasman, 1989). Five-year figures are given in Table 34–21.

Diagnosis

Ovarian cancer is rarely diagnosed early. Seventy per cent of all patients already have metastasis outside

Table 34–21. FIVE-YEAR SURVIVAL RATES FOR EPITHELIAL OVARIAN CANCER

Stage	Per Cent
IA	70
IB	64
IC	50
IIA	52
IIB or IIC	42
III	13
IV	4

(Adapted from DiSaia, P. J., & Creasman, W. T. [1989]. *Clinical gynecologic oncology* [3rd ed.]. St. Louis: C. V. Mosby Co.)

Table 34–22. NONMALIGNANT OVARIAN MASSES

Cysts
  Germinal inclusion cyst
  Follicular cyst
  Corpus luteum cyst
  Pregnancy luteoma
  Theca lutein cyst
  Sclerocystic ovaries
Cystic tumors from epithelium
  Serous cystoma
  Endometrioma
  Mucinous cystoma
  Mixed forms
Tumors from stroma of epithelium
  Fibroma, adenofibroma
  Brenner tumor
Tumors from germ cells
  Dermoid (benign cystic teratoma)

(Adapted from DiSaia, P. J., & Creasman, W. T. [1989]. *Clinical gynecologic oncology* [3rd ed.]. St. Louis: C. V. Mosby Co.)

the pelvis at diagnosis. These neoplasms grow rapidly and without pain. However, it is a nursing responsibility to encourage any woman older than 40 years of age who complains of persistent low-grade or vague abdominal symptoms of mild indigestion, abdominal discomfort, or urinary abnormalities to seek further evaluation (Sargis, 1983). These symptoms are frequently minimized either by the patient or physician and may persist for months before the tumor itself becomes clinically detectable as it grows within the pelvis (15 cm in size). Compression of the surrounding organs occurs, causing urinary frequency, indigestion, and a feeling of "pressure." Unfortunately, the most frequent presentation is that of a grossly enlarged abdomen accompanied by ascites. Late symptoms may include hemorrhage from the necrotizing tumor, sepsis, and profound cachexia. Patients appear gaunt and alert. Often they are hungry but cannot eat without immediately experiencing nausea and vomiting. Gastrointestinal obstruction often occurs and death usually ensues within 6 months of its onset.

Exploratory laparotomy is the only accurate method for diagnosing ovarian cancer. There are a multitude of causes for ovarian and abdominal enlargement, and some of these are benign. Table 34–22 lists nonmalignant causes for ovarian masses and their cells of origin.

Table 34–23 compares characteristics of benign and malignant tumors found at pelvic bimanual examination. Even though early diagnosis is important, a careful diagnostic preoperative work-up should be completed (Table 34–24). Paracentesis is not per-

Table 34–23. CHARACTERISTICS OF BENIGN AND MALIGNANT TUMORS

Benign	Malignant
Cystic	Solid, semisolid
Smooth walled	Irregular
Mobile	Fixed
Unilateral	Bilateral
<8 cm	Associated with nodules in cul de sac
	Ascites

(Adapted from DiSaia, P. J., & Creasman, W. T. [1989]. *Clinical gynecologic oncology* [3rd ed.]. St. Louis: C. V. Mosby Co.)

Table 34–24. DIAGNOSTIC EVALUATION FOR
OVARIAN CANCER

Thorough history
Multisystem physical examination
Pelvic, bimanual examination, and Papanicolaou smear
Proctosigmoidoscopy*
Hematologic studies, urinalysis
Blood chemistry tests
Chest radiograph
Intravenous pyelogram, barium enema
Gastrointestinal series*

*Where indicated.
(Adapted from DiSaia, P. J., & Creasman, W. T. [1989]. *Clinical gynecologic oncology* [3rd. ed.]. St. Louis: C. V. Mosby Co.)

formed to avoid inadvertent rupture of the tumor and resultant spillage.

Staging

Ovarian cancer is staged surgically. Care is taken not to rupture the tumor. Optimally, the operative note will document if rupture occurs or if it had occurred before the operation spontaneously and will record the source of the specimens (peritoneal washings or ascitic fluid). All suspicious areas are removed for pathologic study if possible. An attempt is made to remove all foci of tumor larger than 2 cm. Residual disease is the most important predictor of response to chemotherapy, greater even than the stage of disease. Tables 34–25 and 34–26 list the components of the initial extirpative surgery and the FIGO staging for primary carcinoma of the ovary.

Treatment

Surgery

Borderline Malignant Epithelial Neoplasms. In most cases, conservative therapy is chosen. If the lesion is unilateral, a unilateral salpingo-oophorectomy with or without contralateral biopsy is acceptable. Some controversy exists regarding biopsy of the remaining ovary owing to the high incidence of scarring and resulting

Table 34–25. COMPONENTS OF THE INITIAL
EXTIRPATIVE SURGERY

Midline abdominal incision
Cytologic examination of ascites
Systematic examination of all of abdominal contents: pelvis, peritoneum, diaphragm, omental apron, lymph nodes
Cytologic washing of peritoneum, pelvis, side gutters, and diaphragm
Total abdominal hysterectomy; bilateral salpengo-oophorectomy
Partial omentectomy
Appendectomy
Lymphadenectomy
Tumor debulking to leave no lesion greater than 2 cm behind

(Adapted from DiSaia, P. J., & Creasman, W. T. [1989]. *Clinical gynecologic oncology* [3rd ed.]. St. Louis: C. V. Mosby Co.; and Runowicz, C. D. [1987]. Ovarian cancer. *Mediguide to Oncology, 7* [2], 1–5.)

Table 34–26. FIGO STAGING SYSTEM FOR CANCER
OF THE OVARY

Based on findings at clinical examination or surgical exploration, or both. The histology is to be considered in the staging, as is cytology as far as effusions are concerned. It is desirable that a biopsy be taken from suspicious areas outside the pelvis.

Stage I	Growth limited to the ovaries.
Stage IA	Growth limited to one ovary; no ascites. No tumor on the external surface; capsule intact.
Stage IB	Growth limited to both ovaries; no ascites. No tumor on the external surfaces; capsules intact.
Stage IC*	Tumor either stage IA or IB but with tumor on surface of one or both ovaries; or with capsule ruptured; or with ascites present containing malignant cells or with positive peritoneal washings.
Stage II	Growth involving one or both ovaries with pelvic extension.
Stage IIA	Extension or metastases, or both, to the uterus or tubes (or both).
Stage IIB	Extension to other pelvic tissues.
Stage IIC*	Tumor either stage IIA or IIB, but with tumor on surface of one or both ovaries; or with capsule(s) ruptured; or with ascites present containing malignant cells or with positive peritoneal washings.
Stage III	Tumor involving one or both ovaries with peritoneal implants outside the pelvis or positive retroperitoneal or inguinal nodes. Superficial liver metastasis equals stage III. Tumor is limited to the true pelvis but with histologically proved malignant extension to small bowel or omentum.
Stage IIIA	Tumor grossly limited to the true pelvis with negative nodes but with histologically confirmed microscopic seeding of abdominal peritoneal surfaces.
Stage IIIB	Tumor of one or both ovaries with histologically confirmed implants of abdominal peritoneal surfaces none exceeding 2 cm in diameter. Nodes are negative.
Stage IIIC	Abdominal implants greater than 2 cm in diameter or positive retroperitoneal or inguinal nodes, or both.
Stage IV	Growth involving one or both ovaries with distant metastases. If pleural effusion is present, there must be positive cytology to allot a case to stage IV. Parenchymal liver metastasis equals stage IV.

*To evaluate the impact on prognosis of the different criteria for allotting cases to stage IC or IIC, it would be of value to know (1) if rupture of the capsule was (a) spontaneous or (b) caused by the surgeon, or (2) if the source of malignant cells detected was (a) peritoneal washings or (b) ascites.
(Data from *Gynecology Oncology Group pathology manual* [unpublished]).

infertility. A comprehensive staging laparotomy should be done, which includes inspection and biopsy of multiple peritoneal sites, sampling of pelvic and para-aortic lymph nodes, biopsy of the omentum, and possibly endometrial curettage. Nursing management includes instructing the patient of the increased risk of recurrence. The incidence of occult metastasis ranges from 12 to 43 per cent for epithelial neoplasms (Kaempfer & Major, 1986). Childbearing should occur within the space of a few years, followed by reexploration and removal of the remaining ovary. When bilateral involvement is present, more radical treatment is necessary; in such cases total abdominal hysterectomy and bilateral salpingo-oophorectomy with careful inspection of the entire abdominal cavity as described previously is performed. Germ cell tumors, common in young women, are treated with unilateral salpingo-oophorectomy and vigorous chemotherapy, which allows preservation of the remaining gonad and permits possible childbearing at a later date (Kaempfer & Major, 1986). Management is controversial owing to the previously mentioned risks associated with conservative management. Further studies will assist in clarification of these issues.

Serous, Mucinous, Endometrial, and Clear Cell Types. These cell types are the most common epithelial cancers of the ovary and act similarly in both stage and grade. They also resemble each other in response to treatment, prognosis, and survival. Table 34–27 describes therapy for stages I to IV epithelial cell types.

The Concept of Cytoreductive Surgery

The aim of cytoreductive surgery is to debulk the poorly vascularized larger portions of the tumor. It is hypothesized that the residual tumor volume responds aggressively by stimulating growth and cell kinetics. This may result in increasing the efficacy and cell kill of the postoperative chemotherapy. The goal of current therapy is to leave no single focus of cancer larger than 2 cm, or less if possible, anywhere in the abdomen.

Radiation Therapy

In certain circumstances radiotherapy is employed as an adjuvant treatment after laparatomy when there is minimal residual disease volume. Techniques used are external irradiation of the total abdomen and pelvis and instillation of intraperitoneal phosphorus-32 (^{32}P). Use of radiation therapy has decreased as the effectiveness of chemotherapy has increased. Significant difficulties exist related to the tumor and its abdominal location when attempting to administer therapeutic doses of radiation.

Further studies are needed to determine the role of radiation as compared with chemotherapy for earlier stage II disease.

Intraperitoneal Instillation of ^{32}P. This technique has been used in stage II patients with microscopic residual disease and is advocated by some practitioners for use in stage III patients when second-look procedures reveal persistent microscopic intra-abdominal lesions as well (Stehman, 1987). A Tenckoff catheter is inserted and proper placement and free flow are determined by instillation of fluid and a radiopaque substance. Table 34–28 outlines a procedure for instillation of ^{32}P. Nursing implications include ensuring that the patient turns frequently to distribute the isotope throughout the peritoneal cavity and initiating comfort measures as required.

Chemotherapy

Chemotherapy has proved to be effective as an adjunctive treatment after the initial primary surgery. Ideally, 80 to 90 per cent of the tumor volume has been removed with the cytoreductive surgical effort. Theoretically, most of the residual tumor cells are left in a state in which they are vulnerable to the effects of chemotherapy. Residual cells will be in varying phases of the cell cycle. The cell cycle nonspecific, alkylating agents have proved to work most effectively against sluggish tumors. In gynecologic oncology, the following alkylating agents have been used for early stage disease:

Cyclophosphamide (Cytoxan)
Chlorambucil (Leukeran)
Melphalan (Alkeran)
Triethylenethiophosphoramide (thio-TEPA)

However, those cells recovering from treatment with alkylating agents have demonstrated increased susceptibility to cycle-specific agents. This information has spurred a search for effective single-agent and multiagent chemotherapies for treatment of ovarian cancer. Other single-agent, cycle-specific, nonalkylating agents that have been variably effective for early stage disease are

Doxorubicin (Adriamycin)
Hexamethylmelamine (HMM)
Methotrexate
Cis-diamminedichloroplatinum (cisplatin)
5-Fluorouracil (5-FU)

Cisplatin has emerged as the most beneficial drug when used as a single agent or in combination with other drugs. DiSaia and Creasman (1989) recommend aggressive removal of the tumor and combination multiagent chemotherapy as the optimal approach for improving patient survival in advanced ovarian cancer.

Table 34–27. PRIMARY SURGICAL TREATMENT OF STAGES I TO IV EPITHELIAL CELL TYPES

Stage IA, IB, IC	*Staging* TAH-BSO, omentectomy, pelvic and para-aortic lymphadenectomy *Treatment:* P intraperitoneally; plus alkylating agents* except for grade 1 histologic type
Stage I, grade 3	Add multiagent chemotherapy
Stage IIA, IIB	*Staging:* TAH-BSO, omentectomy, pelvic and para-aortic lymphadenectomy *Treatment:* P intraperitoneally; abdominal* and pelvic external irradiation; systemic chemotherapy* (single- or multiagent) if grade 2 or 3 plus pelvic irradiation; 12 months of single or multiagent chemotherapy* and second-look operation
Stages III and IV	*Staging:* TAH-BSO, omentectomy, pelvic and para-aortic lymphadenectomy *Treatment:* Tumor debulking and multiagent chemotherapy

*Options of treatment. TAH-BSO, total abdominal hysterectomy with bilateral salpengo-oophorectomy.
(Data from DiSaia, P. J., & Creasman, W. T. [1989]. *Clinical gynecologic oncology* [3rd ed.]. St. Louis: C. V. Mosby Co.)

Table 34–28. PROCEDURE FOR INSTILLATION OF [32]P

Perforated (Tenckoff) catheter placed into peritoneal cavity
Instillation of 500 ml normal saline solution
Instillation of Hypaque or technetium
Fluoroscopy used to confirm adequate distribution
15 mCi of ^{32}P in 500 ml normal saline solution instilled quickly
Patient turned: Trendelenburg, 15 min; right side, 15 min; left
  side, 15 min; feet down, 15 min

(Data from DiSaia, P. J., & Creasman, W. T. [1989] *Clinical gynecologic oncology* [3rd ed.]. St. Louis: C. V. Mosby Co.)

Runowicz (1987) cites four of the most effective combinations in Table 34–29.

Chapters 21 and 22 contain specific nursing diagnoses and intervention strategies for patients undergoing combination chemotherapy regimens. The accepted minimum number of chemotherapy treatment cycles has not been determined. In actuality, owing to the short-term toxicities of doxorubicin and cisplatin, patients may tolerate as few as four cycles. Second-look operations assist in determining the need for further treatment (Runowicz, 1987).

Recurrence

Second-Look Laparotomy. In the 1940s Wangenstein performed an exploratory laparotomy in some of his patients in hopes of detecting early recurrences (DiSaia, 1989). Ovarian cancer implants itself in and behind niches in the abdominal cavity, and these foci can go undetected until they are many centimeters in diameter, even with sophisticated noninvasive surveillance techniques such as computed tomography (CT) and magnetic resonance imaging (MRI). With the knowledge of these limitations, gynecologic surgeons have employed the second-look operation to assess the control or extent of disease after a course of treatment in selected patients. Second-look operations allow the surgeon (1) to restage a cancer previously staged improperly or that had not been staged at all, (2) to evaluate effectiveness of standard and investigational chemotherapy regimens, and (3) to assess the possibilities of discontinuing further treatment in patients who have received an adequate course of chemotherapy and who appear disease-free clinically (DiSaia &

Table 34–29. MULTIAGENT CISPLATIN CHEMOTHERAPY REGIMENS

CAP	Cyclophosphamide (Cytoxan) Doxorubicin (Adriamycin) Cis-diamminedichloroplatinum (cisplatin)
AP	Adriamycin Cisplatin
CP	Cytoxan Cisplatin
CHAP	Cytoxan Hexamethylmelamine (HMM) Adriamycin Cisplatin

(Adapted from Runowicz, C. D. [1987]. Ovarian cancer. *Mediguide to Oncology*, 7[2], 1–5. Copyright 1987, Lawrence Della Corte Publications, Inc.)

Table 34–30. COMPONENTS OF THE SECOND-LOOK PROCEDURE

Review original operative note
Exploratory laparotomy:
  Cephalocaudal incision
  Serial cytologic washings: peritoneum, pelvis, side gutters, and
    subdiaphragm
  Biopsy of scraping of underside of diaphragm
  Inspection of all peritoneal surfaces, pelvic peritoneum, pelvic
    organs
  Excision of omentum, appendix
  Biopsies of previous tumor site and all adhesions
  Random biopsies
  Lymph node sampling

(Adapted from DiSaia, P. J., & Creasman, W. T. [1989]. *Clinical gynecologic oncology* [3rd ed.]. St. Louis: C. V. Mosby Co.; and Runowicz, C. D. [1987]. Ovarian cancer. *Mediguide to Oncology*, 7[2], 11–12.)

Creasman, 1989). There is some controversy because abdominal surgery in this patient population is not without risk. Smith (1976) found that the only patients for whom a second-look procedure was appropriate were those with clinical remission of their disease. Stehman (1987) postulates that second-look operations should be done outside the investigational setting very cautiously. Patients previously treated with cisplatin have probably had the best chance at control of their disease, because no other agent has proved to be as effective and no changes would be made in the management of the patient regardless of the outcome of the surgery (Stehman, 1987). The procedure, if undertaken, must proceed as meticulously as the original cytoreductive procedure to be of any evaluative or therapeutic benefit. Table 34–30 lists components of a second-look procedure.

When recurrence is documented, previously untried second-line chemotherapy combinations are the treatment of choice. The goal is a partial response and control of symptoms, such as malignant effusions. Surgery is reserved occasionally for those patients who had localized disease at the second-look operation, but generally it is not advised.

Investigational Approaches. Research is under way that may soon make it possible to alter the patient's immune response mechanisms by using monoclonal antibodies as transporters of new therapies. Work is also being conducted to develop antigens that will alter and intensify the patient's innate antigenic response to ovarian cancer cells. Exploration of the efficacy of diagnostic tumor markers, such as CA125, continues; these would permit earlier diagnosis and determination of recurrence, thus increasing survival (Rutledge, 1986). One of the more promising approaches is intraperitoneal chemotherapy.

Intraperitoneal Chemotherapy

Administration of chemotherapy via direct instillation into the peritoneum is currently being investigated at a number of institutions. Pharmacologically, drugs suitable for intraperitoneal instillation must have certain properties (Table 34–31).

Table 34–31. PROPERTIES OF DRUGS SUITABLE FOR INTRAPERITONEAL USE

Pharmacologic advantage: slow peritoneal and rapid total body clearance
Steep dose-response relationship: increased concentrations mean increased cytotoxicity
Cytotoxic levels present in systemic circulation as well as in peritoneal cavity
Tolerable peritoneal toxicity level

(Adapted from Ozols, R. F. [1986]. Intraperitoneal chemotherapy. *Mediguide to Oncology*, 5[4], 1–5. Copyright 1986, Lawrence Della Corte Publications, Inc.)

In most cases, ovarian cancer is limited to the serosal surfaces of the peritoneal cavity and its contents. This pattern of tumor spread makes it ideal for local instillation of a cytotoxic agent. Sensitivity to combination chemotherapy has yielded 60 to 80 per cent partial response rates but low complete remissions. Complete response rates are correlated with prolonged survival, and therefore these efforts are justified if technical difficulties can be overcome (Ozols, 1986). Patients with slight residual disease confined to the abdominal cavity who have had an extirpative surgery are considered appropriate candidates. Fluid must be able to be distributed throughout the abdomen for optimal efficacy of this local therapy. Two types of catheter placements are used to achieve this result. A percutaneously inserted Tenckoff catheter, frequently used for home peritoneal dialysis patients, was the first catheter utilized and still is used in selected circumstances, such as obesity. Implanted ports, such as the Port-a-Cath (Pharmacia Nu-Tech, Piscataway, NJ) have gained favor because no external site care is required between treatments. In both types of catheters a tip with multiple exit perforations is placed in the peritoneal cavity. Contrast material can be injected to assess fluid distribution, ascitic fluid specimens can be withdrawn for cytologic study, and fluids and chemotherapeutic agents can be instilled, allowed to remain for a time and drained. Hoff (1987) states that the Port-a-Cath requires increased infusion time owing to the small lumen size of the Huber needle, which is required to access the port. When multiple consecutive instillations are anticipated, the percutaneous Tenckoff catheter is more appropriate because of its increased flow rate (Hoff, 1987) (Fig. 34–13).

Drugs that have proved to be effective systemically for ovarian cancer have been used in intraperitoneal trials as well. Table 34–32 lists drugs and toxicities associated with their use.

In these trials, cisplatin displayed the most cytotoxic activity and is considered the drug of choice. Combination chemotherapy trials with cisplatin are currently under way. Doxorubicin (Adriamycin), cyclophosphamide (Cytoxan), 5-FU, and analogues of cisplatin such as carboplatin are being evaluated in varying combinations. To date, unfortunately, improvement in progression-free intervals or survival has not been documented (Stehman, 1987). Significant problems associated with the Tenckoff catheter have been noted, including loss of the capacity to drain owing to the

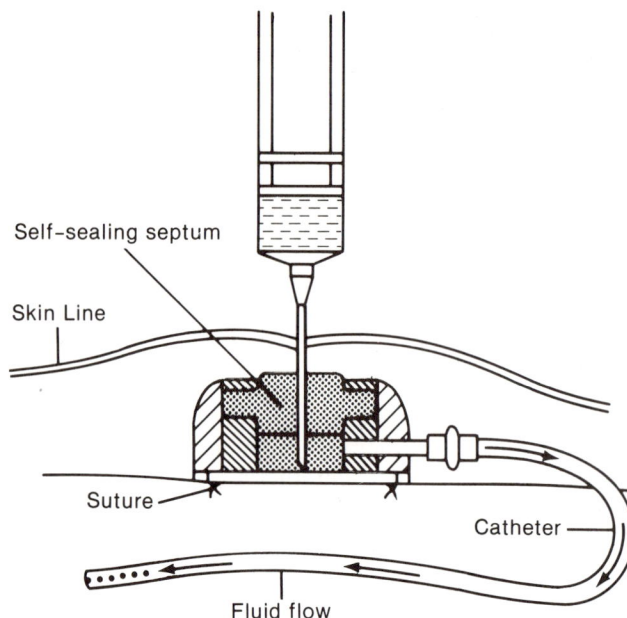

Figure 34–13. Port-A-Cath implanted peritoneal access device. (Courtesy of Port-A-Cath, Piscataway, NJ.)

adherence of a fibrin sheath at the catheter tip, adhesion of the catheter to the abdominal structures, kinking, pain associated with the presence of the catheter, and infection, which is a greater problem with the externalized Tenckoff than with the implanted port. Nursing implications include skill in accessing the implanted port, close observations of the patient during intraperitoneal chemotherapy, and patient education (Hoff, 1987) (Table 34–33).

Terminal Management

The goal of end-stage management of this group of patients is maintenance of quality of life. Despite statistics, patients with cancers considered "unresectable" have responded to cytoreduction favorably. In addition, others have outlived their odds after multiple surgical procedures and chemotherapeutic regimens. It is always justified to offer hope for relief of symptoms and comfort if not cure. Table 34–34 lists frequent problems associated with very advanced ovarian carcinoma and appropriate medical interventions.

Table 34–32. CYTOTOXIC DRUGS EVALUATED FOR INTRAPERITONEAL USE

Drug	Toxic Effect
Methotrexate	Peritoneal irritation
5-Fluorouracil	Myelosuppression, mucositis, severe abdominal pain
Doxorubicin (Adriamycin)	Sterile peritonitis
Cisplatin	No local irritation, neuropathy, myelosuppression, and nephropathy

(Data from DiSaia, P. J., & Creasman, W. T. [1989]. *Clinical gynecologic oncology* [3rd ed.]. St. Louis: C. V. Mosby Co.)

Table 34–33. NURSING CARE PLAN FOR THE PATIENT UNDERGOING INTRAPERITONEAL CHEMOTHERAPY

Assessment	Interventions	Expected Outcomes
Nursing Diagnosis: Health management deficit: related to intraperitoneal chemotherapy		
Assess current knowledge of patient regarding intraperitoneal chemotherapy	Describe anatomic placement of catheter, show patient a catheter Discuss postoperative care and radiologic studies, short- and long-term side effects of chemotherapy; discuss complications: fever, chills, nausea and vomiting, diarrhea, abdominal pain or expansion, shortness of breath	Patient and significant others will accurately verbalize expectations of this treatment
Nursing Diagnosis: Alteration in fluid volume: excess fluid volume related to retained IP fluid		
Inspect "dialysis" tubing for kinks Check for clamped tubing in outflow system Check height of tubing Consider if fibrin sheath has formed intraperitoneally	Separate intake and output lines for IP instillations Total intake and output every 4 hr Flush catheter with 10 ml of normal saline solution to lift away fibrin sheath Straighten tubing if kinked and keep tubing lower than insertion site	Intake will not exceed output by >500 ml
Nursing Diagnosis: Alteration in comfort: pain, related to IP fluid infusion		
Assess all pain parameters	Infuse IP fluids at a slower rate Reposition to attempt to distribute fluid evenly Analgesics per orders as necessary	Patient verbalizes comfort; fewer requests for analgesics; able to sleep for longer periods at a time
Nursing Diagnosis: Potential for infection: peritonitis, related to irritation of cytotoxic drugs		
Assess for abdominal rigidity, distention, rebound tenderness Auscultate abdomen for decreased bowel sounds Check IP fluid cultures Check if febrile	Vital signs 4 hr; antibiotics as ordered; culture of peritoneal fluids; aseptic technique	Patient shows no signs of infection

(Data from Eriksson & Swenson, 1986; Herberth & Gosnell, 1987; Hoff, 1987; Swenson & Eriksson, 1986.)

Malignant Effusions

Patients with late-stage ovarian cancer often have ascites and pleural effusion, or both. Meigs' syndrome is a common manifestation in which the patient has ascites, hydrothorax, and grossly enlarged tumor in the abdomen. It is supposed that lymphatics transversing the diaphragm drain into the pleura. This syndrome resolves after tumor removal. Table 34–35 lists probable causes of malignant effusions.

Management should be limited to paracentesis or thoracentesis to relieve symptoms such as respiratory compromise or pain. Patients often receive short-term relief of gastrointestinal problems and of nausea and vomiting as well. Nursing implications during these procedures include assisting the patient to attain a comfortable position, using comfort measures such as pillows, and proper preparation of the aspirated specimen for laboratory or cytologic analysis. Table 34–36 is a nursing care plan for the patient with advanced ovarian cancer.

Table 34–34. PROBLEMS AND MEDICAL INTERVENTIONS IN ADVANCED OVARIAN CANCER

Problems	Medical Interventions
Fluid and electrolyte imbalance owing to paracentesis or thoracentesis	Replacement of fluids, orally and intravenously via vascular access device
Malnutrition, hunger, nausea, vomiting from displacement of intestines by ascites or obstruction	Intravenous alimentation
Intermittent episodes of small and large bowel obstruction owing to carcinomatosis	Surgical bypass, gastrostomy, jejunostomy
Recurrent malignant effusions	Peritoneovenous shunt insertion; paracentesis, thoracentesis, chest tube placement; pleurodesis with tetracycline

(Data from DiSaia & Creasman, 1989.)

Table 34–35. PROBABLE CAUSES OF MALIGNANT EFFUSIONS

Obstruction of lymphatic vessels
Obstruction of venous circulation
Serous membrane inflamed by tumor
Elevated portal pressure
Disseminated studding on right diaphragmatic peritoneal surfaces
Increased production of fluid by nonimplanted peritoneal surfaces

(Data from DiSaia, P. J., & Creasman, W. T. [1989]. *Clinical gynecologic oncology* [3rd ed.]. St. Louis: C. V. Mosby Co.)

Table 34–36. NURSING CARE PLAN FOR THE PATIENT WITH ADVANCED OVARIAN CANCER

Assessment	Interventions	Expected Outcomes
Nursing Diagnosis: Alteration in nutrition, related to extrinsic pressure on gastrointestinal tract or obstruction of gastrointestinal tract by tumor		
Calorie count for 24 hr; assess for weight loss; assess previous food habits	*Intact gastrointestinal tract:* Small frequent meals of patient's choice Position from 30 to 90 degrees for maximal stomach expansion *Obstructed gastrointestinal tract* Obtain interim order for nasogastric tube; discuss with attending physician the option of gastrostomy or jejunostomy placement; explore options with patient; analgesics as necessary	Patient's weight will remain stable Patient will express increased ability to eat; intestines will be decompressed Patient able to ingest food via tube: nasogastric, gastrostomy, or jejunostomy Decreased requests for narcotic analgesic
Nursing Diagnosis: Alteration in fluid volume—excess, related to malignant effusions of ascites or pleural fluid		
Palpate abdomen for fluid wave or percuss for dullness Auscultate bowel sounds Observe skin turgor Assess vein filling Check for edema Assess for weight gain Measure abdominal girth	Position patient at most comfortable angle between 30 and 90 degrees Prepare patient for paracentesis; assist with paracentesis Dress and observe paracentesis site for leakage Apply urostomy pouch with drainage bag for continued leakage Accurate intake and output determinations Encourage intake of fluids	Volume of ascites will diminish or stabilize
Nursing Diagnosis: Impaired gas exchange: related to extrinsic pressure of pleural fluid on lungs		
Auscultate breath sounds; listen for a pleural friction rub; observe for respiratory distress	Prepare patient for thoracentesis Assist with thoracentesis; dress thoracentesis site and observe for leakage *Recurrent effusion:* Prepare patient for chest tube insertion Set up chest drainage collection system Assist with insertion Dress insertion site with occlusive dressing Monitor chest drainage output Prepare patient for pleurodesis (instillation of tetracycline into the pleural space) Premedicate patient with analgesic Assist with pleurodesis; rotate patient every 5 min to distribute the sclerosing agent	Pleural effusion will diminish in volume or stabilize Patient will demonstrate adequate respirations

(Data from Herberth & Gosnell, 1987; Rosetti, 1985.)

CANCER OF THE VAGINA

Incidence

Cancer of the vagina is the rarest type of gynecologic cancer. One per cent of all genital cancers are of this type. Approximately 300 deaths occur per year from vaginal cancer. Cancer of the vagina occurs most frequently in women older than 70 years of age (Barber, 1980). Another rare type of vaginal cancer, clear cell adenocarcinoma, suddenly appeared in a cluster during the 1960s and continues to appear in diminishing numbers. The population most affected by this type is between the ages of 7 and 29 years, with the most common age at diagnosis being 19 years. Thus far, 500 cases have been reported.

Epidemiology and Etiology

Primary Cancer of the Vagina

It has been hypothesized that irritation of the vagina such as from trauma, chronic pessary usage for a prolapsed uterus, intercourse, or use of chemical carcinogens, as in sprays and douches, plays a role in the development of squamous cell carcinoma of the vagina, but a relationship has never been established. Current theory now considers that cancer in this location may be an extension of a previous cancer of the cervix, vulva, or endometrium. This is referred to as a wide field of origin of a multicentric disease (Marcus, 1961). A previous positive history of any of these and an advanced age appear to be the most likely risk factors (White, 1986).

DES-related Cancer of the Vagina

Clear cell adenocarcinoma of the vagina is linked to the treatment of women with diethylstilbestrol (DES) during pregnancy, which was done in the 1940s and 1950s to prevent spontaneous abortions. This resulted in the exposure of as many as 6 million female fetuses to DES (Orr & Shingleton, 1986).

Biology and Natural History

Squamous Cell Carcinoma

The premalignant forms of disease seen in cervical cancer are also seen in this type of vaginal cancer.

Table 34–37. PREMALIGNANT CLASSIFICATIONS OF VAGINAL DYSPLASIA

Vaginal intraepithelial neoplasia (VAIN)	
VAIN I	Mild dysplasia
VAIN II	Moderate dysplasia
VAIN III	Severe dysplasia
Carcinoma in situ	

(Data from DiSaia, P. J., & Creasman, W. T. [1989]. *Clinical gynecologic oncology* [3rd ed.]. St. Louis: C. V. Mosby Co.)

Nomenclature for the premalignant lesions is given in Table 34–37.

Premalignant lesions may develop as primary lesions, after radiation therapy, or as a multifocal abnormality. Vaginal intraepithelial neoplasia may occur many years after treatment for cervical or vulvar cancer. The lesion most often occurs in the upper one third of the vagina. When an invasive lesion is present, it may appear as a round or oblong ulcer with elevated smooth edges, with an excavated crater in the center. Unchecked, it will spread upward to the rectovaginal septum and the cervix, and it will invade the vaginal tissue. If located low in the vagina, the tumor metastasizes to the inguinal and deep pelvic nodes (DiSaia & Creasman, 1989).

Clear Cell Adenocarcinoma

In contrast to squamous cell carcinoma, this type usually appears on the upper part of the vagina, but on the anterior wall. In all cases, adenosis, a condition in which glandular epithelium is present in the vagina, accompanies clear cell adenocarcinoma. The lesion is frequently raised and soft, and it bleeds easily. It is known to invade the nearby tissue early and metastasize through the lymphatics (Barber, 1980)

A very few vaginal cancers are sarcomas of the spindle cell or botryoides type; the latter mainly affects children. Also seen are endodermal sinus tumors which have a very poor prognosis of less than 2 years. Malignant melanoma is a very rare type of vaginal malignancy. It is treated aggressively with surgery but still has a survival of less than 5 per cent at 5 years.

Diagnosis and Staging

Squamous Cell Carcinoma

The patient usually seeks medical treatment because of a bloody vaginal discharge, which is the most frequent presenting symptom. If it is invasive, the lesion is usually visible on examination and the patient has irregular or postmenopausal bleeding. Urinary frequency or retention is sometimes seen owing to the proximity of the lesion to the neck of the bladder. Diagnosis is often delayed, most probably because of the patient's age, infrequency of pelvic examinations in this age group, and lack of sexual activity. Implications for patient education include informing the elderly patient to report any discharge or episodes of bleeding and encouraging the patient to have an annual

Table 34–38. DIAGNOSTIC EXAMINATION FOR DES-EXPOSED WOMEN

Thorough history (teratogens, fertility problems, spontaneous abortions)
Physical examination:
   Speculum examination
   Lugol's staining of entire area
   Cervical and vaginal Papanicolaou smears
   Colposcopy
   Careful bimanual examination with palpation of entire vagina and cervix
   Biopsy of suspicious nodules

(Data from Orr, J. W., & Shingleton, H. M. [1986, Fall]. Effects of in-utero exposure to DES: An update. *Your Patient and Cancer*, pp. 9–15.)

pelvic examination. Once diagnosed, a staging work-up similar to that for invasive cervical cancer should proceed. A barium enema should also be included to rule out rectal invasion. Staging is done clinically (see Table 34–38 for FIGO staging).

Clear Cell Adenocarcinoma

Twenty per cent of patients with clear cell adenocarcinoma of the vagina are usually asymptomatic, and the rest have abnormal bleeding. The cervix can have a hood-like appearance, surrounded by a collar or with a pseudopolyp protruding from it. The uterus is often hypoplastic and may be the anatomic basis for the infertility problems often experienced by this patient population. Staging is also performed clinically for clear cell vaginal cancer. Table 34–39 lists components of a diagnostic physical examination (Orr & Shingleton, 1986).

Prognosis

Squamous Cell Carcinoma

Survival is affected by several factors. The increased volume of tumor in the body, the fact that squamous cell cancers are not very radiosensitive, the high grade of this tumor type, and finally the fact that the vagina is relatively thin and is adjacent to both the rectum and bladder all contribute to the overall poor long-term survival of this group of patients. The 5-year survival rate is between 30 and 35 per cent (DiSaia & Creasman, 1989).

Table 34–39. CLINICAL STAGING OF INVASIVE CANCER OF THE VAGINA: FIGO SYSTEM

Stage 0	Carcinoma in situ, intraepithelial carcinoma.
Stage I	The carcinoma is limited to the vaginal wall.
Stage II	The carcinoma has involved the subvaginal tissue but has not extended on to the pelvic wall.
Stage III	The carcinoma has extended on to the pelvic wall.
Stage IV	The carcinoma has extended beyond the true pelvis or has involved the mucosa of the bladder or rectum. A bullous edema as such does not permit allotment of a case to stage IV.

(Data from *Gynecology Oncology Group pathology manual* [unpublished]).

Clear Cell Adenocarcinoma

The stage at which the cancer is discovered, the prevalent histologic pattern, and the age of the patient are all important prognostic factors that influence survival. It has not yet been possible to determine long-term follow-up, but currently the overall 5-year survival rate approaches 80 per cent.

Management

Squamous Cell Carcinoma

Therapy for carcinoma in situ of the vagina should be individualized according to age, degree of sexual activity, and patient preference. Radiation therapy is the preferred treatment for all stages of vaginal cancer. Although it does involve complications, radiotherapy is tolerated better in this population of older patients. One exception is when the tumor is located in the lower one third of the vagina; in such cases it is preferable to perform a radical inguinal node dissection to prevent early lymph node invasion and then follow this with radiation therapy. Three methods of administering radiation are utilized: external beam to the pelvis, vaginal intracavitary radiation using a tandem and colpostats (see Fig. 34–6), or interstitial vaginal implant using an obturator and vaginal template (see Fig. 34–7). The depth of invasion is an important consideration in determining which treatment method to use. Most often a course of radiation is given with or without a boost to the local area, followed by a course of intracavitary brachytherapy in one of the two methods described earlier. Table 34–40 lists the different combinations of methods used for the various stages of vaginal cancers (DiSaia & Creasman, 1989).

Clear Cell Adenocarcinoma

In contrast to most cancers, follow-up has been for less than 10 years in these patients. Clear guidelines for the best therapy are nonexistent. This disease tends to metastasize early, although the tumor is not a deeply invasive one. With this information available, appropriate treatment seems to be aggressive, radical surgery, including lymphadenectomy followed by radiotherapy for patients with positive lymph nodes for early stages and radiation therapy alone for tumors of later stages (Table 34–41) (DiSaia & Creasman, 1989).

Recurrence

Squamous Cell Carcinoma

Nearly 50 per cent of these cancers recur locally within 2 years. Distant metastasis is rare. Chemotherapy is not effective. Resection of inguinal lymph nodes and a combination of internal and external radiotherapy appears to be promising and without the severe morbidity associated with ultraradical surgery in this primarily elderly population (DiSaia & Creasman, 1989).

Clear Cell Adenocarcinoma

Distant metastasis is more common with this type of vaginal cancer, which tends to make it more difficult to control. Surgery and radiation have sometimes been effective, and efforts to find an effective chemotherapy regimen continue but so far have been without success. Neither single-agent nor combination chemotherapy seems to work. Patients have not responded objectively to treatment with progestational agents (DiSaia & Creasman, 1989).

CANCER OF THE VULVA

Incidence

Vulvar cancer constitutes 3 to 5 per cent of all gynecologic malignancies. The incidence of this cancer

Table 34–40. RADIATION THERAPY OF SQUAMOUS CELL VAGINAL CARCINOMA

Stage	Type of Therapy					
	External		Intracavitary		Interstitial	
In situ surgery	AND		60 Gy/72 hr	OR	Implant—if less than 0.5 cm, use a single-plane implant	
I and II Large tumors	40–50 Gy and over 5–6 wk	AND	60 Gy/72 hr or 40 Gy/48 hr × 2, 2 wk apart	OR	Implant 60 Gy/72 hr or 40 Gy/48 hr × 2, 2 weeks apart	
Small tumors					Implant 60–70 Gy/72 hr	
Absent uterus	40–50 Gy	AND	Ovoids and transvaginal cone	OR	Implant 60–70 Gy/72 hr	
III and IV	50 Gy over 5–6 wk; 10–20 Gy boost	AND			Large volume multiplane implant	

(Adapted from DiSaia, P. J., & Creasman, W. T. [1989]. *Clinical gynecologic oncology* [3rd ed.]. St. Louis: C. V. Mosby Co.)

Table 34–41. MANAGEMENT OF CLEAR CELL ADENOCARCINOMA OF THE VAGINA

Stage	Surgery	Radiotherapy
I (upper ⅓ of vagina)	Radical hysterectomy; bilateral pelvic lymphadenectomy; upper vaginectomy	Positive lymph nodes: 50 Gy to whole pelvis
I (lower ⅔ of vagina)	Radical hysterectomy; bilateral pelvic lymphadenectomy; total vaginectomy with reconstruction	Positive lymph nodes: 50 Gy to whole pelvis
II	? Pelvic exenteration if irradiation fails	50 Gy to whole pelvis; transvaginal cone; or interstitial implant
III and IV	? Pelvic exenteration if irradiation fails	60 Gy to whole pelvis; interstitial implant

(Adapted from DiSaia, P. J., & Creasman, W. T. [1989]. *Clinical gynecologic oncology* [3rd ed.]. St. Louis: C. V. Mosby Co.)

in younger women is rising, and it is the fourth most common gynecologic cancer.

Epidemiology and Etiology

Women in their mid-60s and older are most affected with cancer of the vulva, although 15 per cent of all vulvar cancers occur in women younger than 40 years old. Historically, obesity, diabetes, hypertension, and arteriosclerosis are correlated with vulvar cancer. However, this correlation may be because these conditions are frequently present in the older female population. Hygiene and age have also been linked with this cancer, because it is more common in the poor and the elderly. There is a strong association between the development of vulvar cancer and the presence of condylomata acuminata (genital warts), caused by Virus HPV as well as herpes simplex II virus (HSV), but no evidence has appeared to confirm either HPV or HSV as a cause for vulvar cancer (Barber, 1980; DiSaia & Creasman, 1989).

Biology and Natural History

The vulva is a structure consisting primarily of skin, and nearly 90 per cent of all cancers of the vulva are of the epidermoid type. Other types of cancers arising in the vulva are melanoma (4.8 per cent), sarcoma, basal cell carcinoma, adenocarcinoma (this often oc-

curs in the Bartholin's gland), and undifferentiated types. Vulvar disease occurs in premalignant forms similar to cervical and vaginal disease, and there is a probability that a cancer originating in one area manifests itself at different locations in a skip-lesion fashion (Marcus, 1961).

Vulvar Dystrophies and Intraepithelial Neoplasias

A variety of conditions may produce visible changes in the vulva but are not necessarily premalignant conditions (Table 34–42). Dystrophies have minimal potential for transforming to malignant lesions, but vulvar intraepithelial neoplasias (VIN) may progress to invasive carcinoma over many years. Table 34–43 contains a description of the appearance of the various dystrophies.

Invasive Vulvar Carcinoma

Seventy per cent of the lesions of invasive vulvar carcinoma appear on the labia and 13 per cent on the clitoris (Rivlin et al., 1986). A small, hard nodule, which usually arises from a previous area of VIN,

Table 34–42. VULVAR PREMALIGNANT CONDITIONS

Hyperplastic dystrophy	Without atypia
	With atypia
Lichen sclerosus	
Mixed dystrophy (lichen sclerosus with foci of epithelial hyperplasia)	
Paget's disease	
Vulvar intraepithelial neoplasia	
VIN I	Mild dysplasia
	Atypical hyperplasia
VIN II	Moderate dysplasia
VIN III	Severe dysplasia
Carcinoma in situ	

(Adapted from DiSaia, P. J., & Creasman, W. T. [1989]. *Clinical gynecologic oncology* [3rd ed.]. St. Louis: C. V. Mosby Co.)

Table 34–43. EXTERNAL APPEARANCE OF PREMALIGNANT VULVAR DISEASES

Disease	Description
Hyperplastic dystrophies	Small or extensive lesions, with white patches, redness, fissures, scars from scratching
Lichen sclerosus	Parchment-like, rough skin surface, or diffuse, macular, pale, or wet. Fissures, cracks, ecchymoses; labia minora retracted into labia majora, clitoris buried in adhesions, shrunken introitus
Mixed dystrophy	Discrete circumscribed areas of hyperplastic dystrophy and lichen sclerosus
Paget's disease	Moist, reddish lesions
Cellular atypia	No gross external changes; sometimes white, red, or pigmented areas present

(Adapted from Rivlin, M. E., Morrison, J. C., & Bates, G. W. [1986]. *Manual of clinical problems in obstetrics and gynecology* [2nd ed.]. Boston: Little, Brown & Co.)

begins to ulcerate. Another common presentation is a wart-like, cauliflower-type growth that does not break down. All cell types of invasive vulvar carcinoma spread in the same pattern via the lymphatics (DiSaia & Creasman, 1989) (Fig. 34–14).

Invasive vulvar carcinoma grows slowly and spreads to the adjacent structures, perineum, anus, vagina, and pubic bone.

Diagnosis and Staging

Fifty per cent of all patients have had symptoms for 2 to 16 months before seeking treatment or receive medical treatment only. Pruritus is the most common symptom for those with VIN. When it is located on the mucosa, VIN appears red, pink, or macular; if located on the skin it is pale or whitened. In invasive vulvar cancer, long-standing pruritus, a mass, or lump is often present. For appropriate evaluation, the perineum and vulva must be inspected with a bright light. All suspicious-appearing areas, including pigmented regions, are biopsied using a punch technique to obtain 4- to 6-mm cones of tissue. Gelfoam is punched out and plugged into the biopsy sites to prevent bleeding, and the area is covered with a dressing. Patients should be instructed to watch for any bleeding and to leave the dressings in place for 24 hr (DiSaia & Creasman, 1989). Instructions should also include avoidance of irritating laundry detergent, hygienic sprays, tight

Table 34–44. CLINICAL STAGING FOR INVASIVE VULVAR CARCINOMA: FIGO SYSTEM

Stage I	All lesions confined to the vulva with a maximum diameter of 2 cm or less and no suspicious groin nodes.
Stage II	All lesions confined to the vulva with a diameter greater than 2 cm and no suspicious groin nodes.
Stage III	Lesions extending beyond the vulva without grossly positive groin nodes or lesions confined to the vulva with suspicious or grossly positive groin nodes.
Stage IV	Lesions extending beyond the vulva with grossly positive nodes or involvement of mucosa of rectum, bladder, or urethra, or involvement of bone. Patients with distant or palpable deep pelvic masses are included with stage IV.

(Data from *Gynecology Oncology Group pathology manual* [unpublished]).

clothing, and synthetic underwear, which permit heat and moisture to be trapped in the perineal area. The patient's bathing practices should be reviewed, with education as necessary.

Staging is best done by a combination of surgical and histologic data rather than from a clinical basis owing to the multiplicity of presentations of this disease. Table 34–44 presents the FIGO system for staging invasive vulvar carcinoma.

Prognosis

Prognostic parameters identified for vulva cancer are the size of the lesion and the grade of the tumor. Invasion of less than 5 mm without lymph or blood vessel involvement is a favorable prognostic factor. The 5-year survival rate approaches 90 per cent for all patients, regardless of stage, when lymph node invasion is negative. The rate drops quite rapidly to 50 to 60 per cent if any lymph nodes are positive at the time of surgery (DiSaia & Creasman, 1989).

Treatment

Premalignant Intraepithelial Neoplasias and Dystrophies

Removal of the involved area of the vulva will arrest the disease at this stage. This is accomplished in various ways, and the decision should be based on the extent and location of the lesions and the patient's preference. Surgically, the procedure of choice for extensive or multifocal disease is a skinning vulvectomy and split-thickness skin graft with preservation of the clitoris. The skin graft is usually taken from the buttocks. Bed rest for 6 to 7 days is usually required. Nursing measures to promote adherence of the skin graft to the vulvar area would include inspection of the area for suppuration under the graft and maintaining a clean, dry perineum. A transparent dressing may be in place, or application of a heat lamp to the donor site three times a day for 20 min may be ordered instead if the site is covered with Xeroform gauze. The donor site is

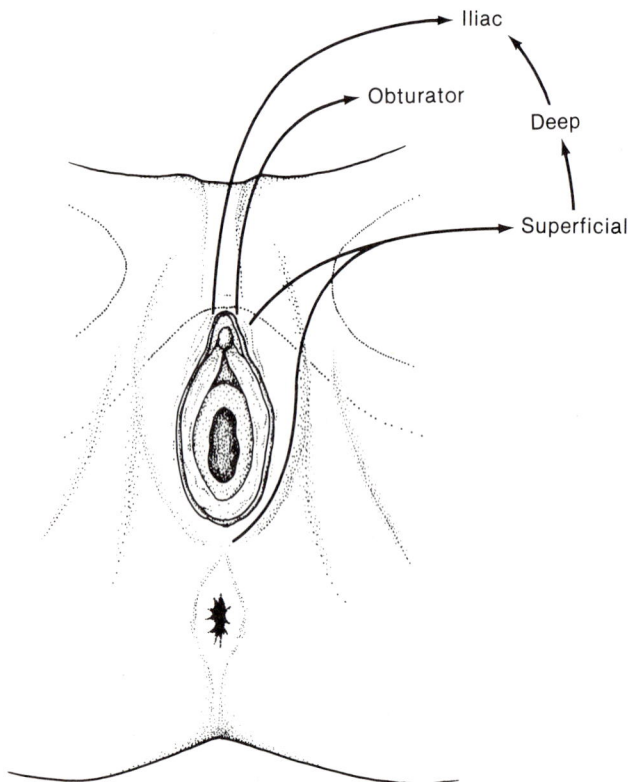

Figure 34–14. Lymph node spread pattern for vulvar carcinoma. (Reproduced by permission from DiSaia, P. J., & Creasman, W. T. [1989]. *Clinical gynecologic oncology* [3rd ed.]. St. Louis: C. V. Mosby Co.)

Table 34–45. ALTERNATIVE TREATMENT METHODS FOR PREMALIGNANT VULVAR LESIONS

Therapy	Advantages	Disadvantages
Destructive cautery	Excellent cosmetic result	Necrotic ulcer may develop
Laser		2–5 treatments required General anesthesia required because of pain Bleeding and infection
Cryosurgery		Pain
Topical 5-fluorouracil		Pain with denudation Lengthy healing period Poor patient compliance Must be applied three times per day for 1 month

(Data from DiSaia, P. J., & Creasman, W. T. [1989]. *Clinical gynecologic oncology* [3rd ed.]. St. Louis: C. V. Mosby Co.)

painful when exposed to the air, and coverage with a transparent dressing or Xeroform gauze that remains in place will minimize the discomfort. Patients report the cosmetic result and ability to achieve orgasm to be satisfactory (DiSaia & Creasman, 1989). Table 34–45 discusses other treatment methods and their advantages and disadvantages.

Early Invasive Vulvar Carcinoma

An investigational approach has been developed based on the concept of the known lymph node spread pattern of vulvar cancer (DiSaia & Creasman, 1989). The goal is to preserve as much sexual function and to provide the best possible cosmetic result while ensuring cure of the disease. When the primary lesion is less than 1 cm and the depth of invasion is less than 5 mm, the patient is prepared preoperatively for the normally accepted procedural approach of a classic radical vulvectomy and bilateral groin dissection, in the event that positive lymph nodes are encountered (Fig. 34–15). The investigational procedure involves a bilateral exploration of the groin and removal of the *sentinel* lymph nodes—those that would be invaded first by the vulvar cancer. These nodes are examined immediately and analyzed as frozen section specimens. If these nodes are positive, the classic procedure is carried out. If the nodes are negative, the incisions are closed, wound drains are placed, and a wide local excision of the involved vulvar area is performed. Subcutaneous tissue is removed, and margins of 3 cm on all sides of the specimen are established. The defect is either approximated and closed primarily or a split-thickness skin graft, usually from the thigh, is sutured into the defect. A pressure stent is applied to the grafted site to promote adhesion. Nursing care would be as described for the skinning vulvectomy procedure. Midlabial, unilateral lesions less than 2 cm are being treated in some cases with a bilateral groin dissection and hemivulvectomy. This minimizes disfigurement even further for patients for whom this type of treatment is appropriate (DiSaia & Creasman, 1989).

Invasive Carcinoma of the Vulva

The ultraradical procedure—radical vulvectomy and bilateral groin dissection—is the most effective treatment for the advanced stages of vulvar cancer (see Fig. 34–15).

Bilateral groin dissections and vulvectomy are made through separate incisions. The perivulvar skin with a 2- to 3-cm margin, labia majora, labia minora, and glans clitoris are all removed. Pelvic exenteration, bilateral groin dissection, and radical vulvectomy are performed in selected advanced cases when the disease is central and not adherent to the pelvic sidewall. The morbidity associated with this type of surgery, especially in the elderly population, is high, and the 5-year survival is only 16 per cent. Boronow (1973) has encouraged the use of preoperative pelvic and groin irradiation. Six weeks after irradiation, the patient undergoes a radical vulvectomy with or without a groin dissection. The cure rate is similar, and the patient is spared the assault of a massive surgery (Mattingly & Thompson, 1985). Table 34–46 lists the complications associated with radical vulvectomy and groin dissection.

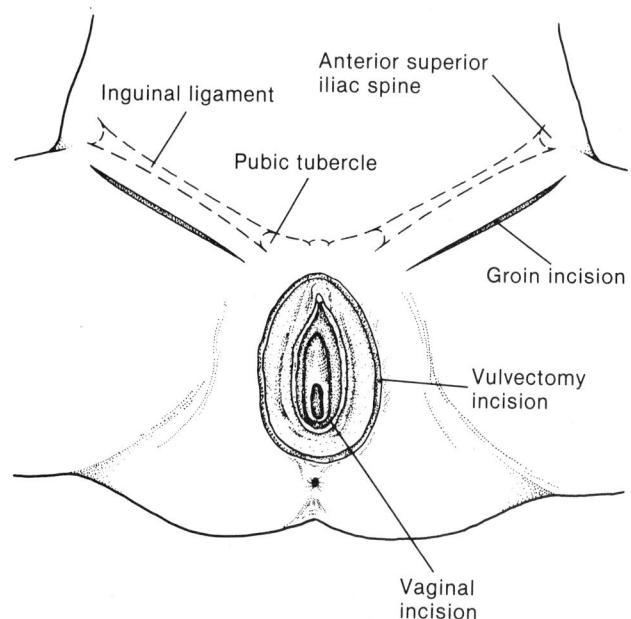

Figure 34–15. Radical vulvectomy and bilateral groin dissection are made through three separate incisions. The labia majora, labia minora, glans clitoris, and perivulvar skin to a 2- to 3-cm margin are removed. (From Mattingly, R. F., & Thompson, J. D. [1985]. *Operative gynecology* [6th ed.]. Philadelphia: J. B. Lippincott Co. Reproduced by permission.)

Table 34–46. COMPLICATIONS OF RADICAL VULVECTOMY AND MEASURES UTILIZED TO CORRECT THEM

Complication	Corrective Measure
Infection of skin flaps (15%)	Suction drainage; three-incision
Necrosis of skin flaps	technique, rapid debridement, split-thickness skin grafts if necessary
Serous drainage (200–300 ml per day)	Large drainage catheters
Lymphedema (25–30%)	Custom fitted Jobst pressure stocking
Cystocele, rectocele	Reconstruction of perineum with muscle grafts
Venous thrombosis	Mini-dose heparin, mechanical compression stockings postoperatively
Retroperitoneal hematoma	Drain insertion, percutaneous vaginal evacuation
Hernia	Long-lasting suture materials
Vaginal stenosis	Exteriorization of the more elastic vaginal mucosa to minimize circular scarring
Negative body image	Perineal reconstruction, using gracilis muscle grafts or split-thickness skin grafts

(Derived from Mattingly, R. F., & Thompson, J. D. [1986]. *Operative gynecology* [6th ed.]. Philadelphia: J. B. Lippincott Co.)

Recurrence

Patients with pelvic recurrent disease are best treated with wide local excision of the lesion and irradiation to the groin. Within 2 years, 80 per cent of recurrences will appear. More than half of the recurrences are near the site of the original lesion.

GESTATIONAL TROPHOBLASTIC NEOPLASMS

Incidence

The term *hydatidiform* comes from the Greek *hydatis*, meaning a droplet. Hydatidiform mole has been recognized as a disease entity since it was described by Hippocrates in AD 400. One in every 1200 women in the United States, and 1 in 120 in the Orient, will have a molar pregnancy. Malnutrition with protein deficiency and closely spaced, multiple pregnancies are thought to be etiologic factors (Barber, 1980). *Gestational trophoblastic neoplasia* (GTN) is the term given to the spectrum of trophoblastic diseases (hydatidiform mole, invasive mole, and choriocarcinoma). It is considered the most curable of all gynecologic malignancies.

Table 34–47. RISK FACTORS FOR DEVELOPING MORE EXTENSIVE GTN AFTER HYDATIDIFORM MOLE

Normal or large-sized uterus at diagnosis
Enlarged ovaries
Enlarged ovaries and uterus
Evacuation done between 11 and 15 weeks' gestation
?Oral contraceptive ingestion
Complete mole type
Associated thecal luteal cyst

(Derived from DiSaia, P. J., & Creasman, W. T. [1989]. *Clinical gynecologic oncology* [3rd ed.]. St. Louis: C. V. Mosby Co.)

Epidemiology and Etiology

Older women have hydatidiform moles more frequently than younger women. Risk factors for developing invasive moles or choriocarcinoma after having a mole are listed in Table 34–47.

Biology and Natural History

An understanding of the embryology of fertilization is required before discussing the specific pathophysiology of gestational trophoblastic neoplasias. Figure 34–16 describes the embryologic development and implantation of a trophoblast.

Hydatidiform Mole

An abnormal proliferation occurs in the villi of the placenta within the uterus. The most notable features are hydropic (droplet-like) changes in the stromal layer and absence of blood vessels. The ovary may develop

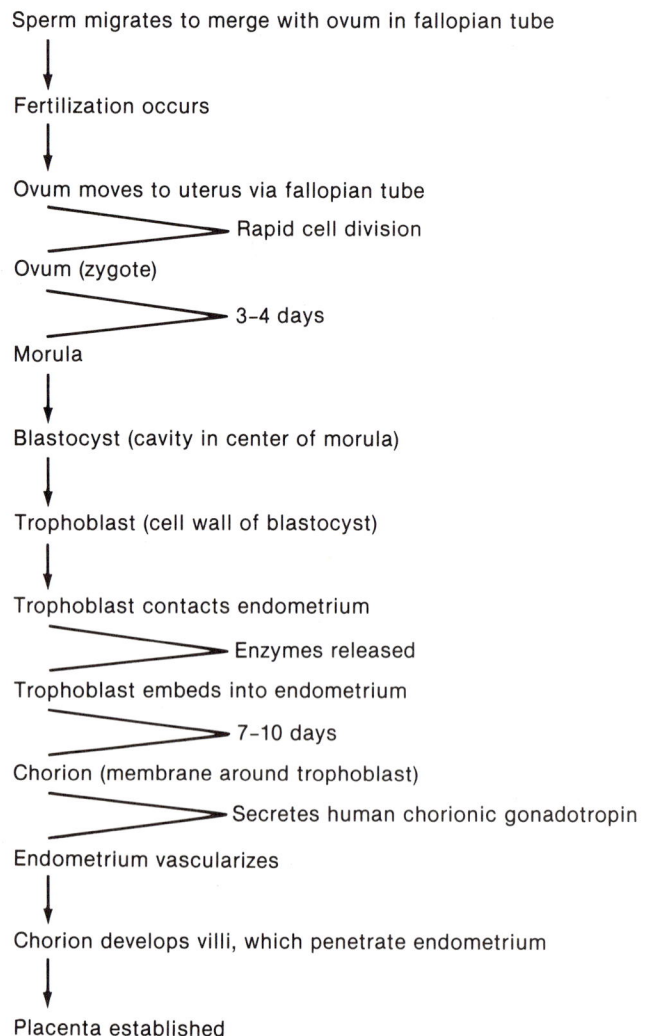

Sperm migrates to merge with ovum in fallopian tube

↓

Fertilization occurs

↓

Ovum moves to uterus via fallopian tube
⟶ Rapid cell division

Ovum (zygote)
⟶ 3–4 days

Morula

↓

Blastocyst (cavity in center of morula)

↓

Trophoblast (cell wall of blastocyst)

↓

Trophoblast contacts endometrium
⟶ Enzymes released

Trophoblast embeds into endometrium
⟶ 7–10 days

Chorion (membrane around trophoblast)
⟶ Secretes human chorionic gonadotropin

Endometrium vascularizes

↓

Chorion develops villi, which penetrate endometrium

↓

Placenta established

Figure 34–16. Embryologic development and implantation of the trophoblast. (Adapted from Dickinson, C. L. [1984]. Choriocarcinoma: A multifaceted challenge. *Oncology Nursing Forum, 11*[1], 32–36.)

Table 34–48. CLASSIFICATION OF GESTATIONAL TROPHOBLASTIC NEOPLASIAS

Nonmetastatic gestational trophoblastic disease
(present only in uterus)
Metastatic gestational trophoblastic neoplasias
   Good prognosis metastatic gestational trophoblastic
     neoplasia (GPMGTN)
   Poor prognosis metastatic gestational trophoblastic
     neoplasia (PPMGTN)

(Modified from DiSaia, P. J., & Creasman, W. T. [1989]. *Clinical gynecologic oncology* [3rd ed.]. St. Louis: C. V. Mosby Co.)

Table 34–50. EVALUATION FOR GTN

Thorough detailed history and physical examination
Chest radiograph
Liver scan
Intravenous pyelogram
Blood and serum chemistry tests
hCG level
CT scan of abdomen, pelvis, and head
Ultrasound of pelvis

(Modified from DiSaia, P. J., & Creasman, W. T. [1989]. *Clinical gynecologic oncology* [3rd ed.]. St. Louis: C. V. Mosby Co.)

very large thecal luteal cysts. A complete mole will only contain these structures. In contrast, a partial mole will have swollen villi and a less hydropic appearance and may contain an umbilical cord, amniotic membranes, or even a fetus. Both types secrete excessive amounts of human chorionic gonadotropin (hCG).

Gestational Trophoblastic Neoplasia

Table 34–48 lists the classification of GTN. The tissue in any of the three classifications may be molar tissue or choriocarcinoma cells. Choriocarcinoma invades the muscles and blood vessels of the uterus, destroys tissue, and causes necrosis and hemorrhage.

Diagnosis and Staging

Hydatidiform Mole

Cardinal symptoms of the hydatidiform mole are missed periods and vaginal bleeding that ranges from rusty brown spotting to bright red hemorrhage. Often a patient may pass tissue that is grape-like in appearance. One third of the patients have nausea and vomiting. Unusual, first-trimester preeclampsia is considered almost singularly diagnostic for hydatidiform mole. A few patients will manifest hyperthyroidism. The uterus is usually larger than its expected size in half of the patients. Fifteen per cent of the patients have large thecal luteal cysts. Table 34–49 lists methods and clues for diagnosis.

Gestational Trophoblastic Neoplasia

Most patients have abnormal uterine bleeding. If the patient was pregnant recently and GTN appears, it is easier to confirm a diagnosis. In some cases, only

metastatic disease is present and the primary lesion may be unknown. Diagnosis is possible if a high index of suspicion is maintained by the physician (Barber, 1980). A thorough evaluation is required to establish a diagnosis (Table 34–50).

Prognosis

With the discovery of the benefit of chemotherapy in 1956, the mortality rates reversed from 90 per cent to a remission rate of 80 to 90 per cent (Barber, 1980).

Management of Gestational Trophoblastic Neoplasms

Hydatidiform Mole

Evacuation of the uterus is the most effective method of treatment. Suction dilation and curettage is usually performed, and moderate blood loss is not uncommon. Intravenous oxytocin (Pitocin) is begun partway through the procedure to initiate involution of the uterus. As involution occurs, an instrumental curettage is done, and the specimens are sent for pathologic examination. This procedure is often performed on an outpatient basis. Nursing considerations would include very specific instruction to the patient regarding the danger of hemorrhage and the importance of returning for follow-up, avoidance of intercourse until drainage ceases, and contraception information for when intercourse resumes. Simple hysterectomy may also be done if the patient does not wish future pregnancies. Further treatment with chemotherapy is necessary when there is a rise in the hCG level, when the hCG level reaches a plateau and stabilizes, or when metastases are discovered. Regular follow-up is essential (DiSaia & Creasman, 1989). Table 34–51 lists a typical follow-up plan.

Table 34–49. METHODS FOR DIAGNOSIS OF HYDATIDIFORM MOLE

Analysis of specimen of passed tissue
Pregnancy test hCG > 1,000,000 IU/L, in addition to the
   following:
   Enlarged uterus and vaginal bleeding
   Amniography if uterus is the size of a 14 weeks' gestation
   X-ray film reveals honeycomb pattern
   Ultrasound reveals snowflake pattern

(Derived from Barber, H. R. K. [1980]. *Manual of gynecologic oncology*. Philadelphia: J. B. Lippincott Co.)

Table 34–51. FOLLOW-UP FOR HYDATIDIFORM MOLE

hCG levels every week until negative 3 times
hCG levels every other month for 1 year
Chest radiograph after evacuation
Physical examination with pelvic examination every 2 weeks until
   hCG test is negative
Physical examination every 3 months for 1 year
Contraception for 1 year

(Adapted from DiSaia, P. J., & Creasman, W. T. [1989]. *Clinical gynecologic oncology* [3rd ed.]. St. Louis: C. V. Mosby Co.)

Gestational Trophoblastic Neoplasia

Nonmetastatic Trophoblastic Disease. Treatment of nonmetastatic trophoblastic disease is 100 per cent successful. Single-agent chemotherapy using high-dose methotrexate with citrovorum rescue is the most effective therapy. If preservation of fertility is not an issue for the patient, early hysterectomy hastens the achievement of remission. Hysterectomy is performed as secondary therapy if remission is not achieved with chemotherapy alone.

Metastatic Trophoblastic Disease. Two other categories of GTN exist and are differentiated by criteria other than histologic differences. Table 34–52 is a comparison between the criteria for good prognosis metastatic gestational trophoblastic neoplasia (GPMGTN) and poor prognosis metastatic gestational trophoblastic neoplasia (PPMGTN).

Good Prognosis Metastatic Gestational Trophoblastic Neoplasia (GPMGTN). Therapy is also 100 per cent successful for this category of patients and consists of the same regimen as that for NMTD. Methotrexate, however, is not given in a high-dose regimen. If methotrexate therapy fails, dactinomycin is administered. Multiagent protocols are then attempted for resistant disease (DiSaia & Creasman, 1989).

Poor Prognosis Metastatic Gestational Trophoblastic Neoplasia (PPMGT). A less favorable but improving outcome occurs with this group of patients. Statistics also have improved along with gains in the ability to support the patients effectively during aggressive courses of multiagent chemotherapy regimens. Current therapy consists of methotrexate, dactinomycin, and chlorambucil chemotherapy and concurrent brain or liver irradiation if metastatic disease is documented in these sites. An overall remission rate of 92 per cent has been achieved. All patients who failed to go into remission had a diagnosis of choriocarcinoma rather than invasive mole (Lurain, 1982).

Recurrence

Recurrence develops most often in patients who had advanced initial disease. Remission can be achieved again in 100 per cent of patients in both the nonmeta-

Table 34–52. COMPARISON OF CRITERIA FOR GOOD PROGNOSIS METASTATIC GTN (GPMGTN) AND POOR PROGNOSIS METASTATIC GTN (PPMGTN)

Criteria	GPMGTN	PPMGTN
Brain or liver metastases	None	Present
Urine hCG level	<100,000 IU in 24 hr	>100,000 IU in 24 hr
Serum hCG level	<40,000 IU/ml	>40,000 IU/ml
Previous chemotherapy	None	Failed
Previous pregnancy	<4 months ago	>4 months ago
Previous term pregnancy	No	Yes

(Derived from DiSaia, P. J., & Creasman, W. T. [1989]. *Clinical gynecologic oncology* [3rd ed.]. St. Louis: C. V. Mosby Co.)

Table 34–53. FOLLOW-UP FOR GESTATIONAL TROPHOBLASTIC NEOPLASIA

Chemotherapy as indicated until three normal weekly hCG levels have been obtained
Give 1 to 3 courses of chemotherapy after hCG levels reach normal as back-up
Pelvic examination every 2 months for 1 year
hCG levels every 2 weeks for 3 months
hCG levels monthly for 3 months
hCG levels bimonthly for 6 months
hCG levels semiannually
Contraception for 1 year

(Adapted from DiSaia, P. J., & Creasman, W. T. [1989]. *Clinical gynecologic oncology* [3rd ed.]. St. Louis: C. V. Mosby Co.)

static and good prognosis categories. Nearly 90 per cent of the patients in the poor prognosis category can achieve remission. Use of aggressive multiagent chemotherapy, switching to different combinations if resistance develops, and very close follow-up are the keys to achieving increasingly favorable results (Table 34–53).

SUMMARY

In summary, the field of gynecologic oncology is making rapid advancements. The almost daily achievements in this specialty are a reflection of advances in multiple areas: epidemiology, diagnostic techniques, radiation therapeutics, surgical expertise, chemotherapeutics, and investigative approaches. The continued dedication of many health care providers is needed to synthesize these advances into practical methods for improving the quality of life and survival for these patients.

References

Barber, H. R. J. K. (1980). *Manual of gynecologic oncology.* Philadelphia: J. B. Lippincott Co.

Boarini, J. H., Bryant, R. A., & Irrgang, S. J. (1986). Fistula management. *Seminars in Oncology Nursing, 2,* 287–292.

Bokhman, J. V. (1983). Two pathogenic types of endometrial carcinoma. *Gynecologic Oncology, 15,* 10.

Boronow, R. C. (1973). Therapeutic alternative to primary exenteration for advanced vulvovaginal cancer. *Gynecologic Oncology, 1,* 233.

Butts, P. (1977). Female reproductive organs: Postop safeguards. In Nursing77 books. Horsham, PA: Intermed Communications.

Campion, M. J., Singer, A., Clarkson, P. K., & McCance, D. J. (1985). Increased risk of cervical neoplasia in consorts of men with penile condylomata acuminata. *Lancet, 2,* 943–946.

Creasman, W. T., McCarty, K. S., Sr., & McCarty, K. S., Jr. (1980). Clinical correlation of estrogen, progesterone binding proteins in human endometrial adenocarcinoma. *Obstetrics and Gynecology, 55,* 63.

Dallenbach-Hellweg, G. (Ed.). (1981). *Cervical cancer.* New York: Springer-Verlag.

Dericks, V. C. (1974). *Nursing care of patients with extensive surgery: Pelvic exenteration.* American Cancer Society Professional Education Publication Pub. No. 3363-PE. New York: American Cancer Society.

Dickinson, C. L. (1984). Choriocarcinoma: A multifaceted challenge. *Oncology Nursing Forum, 11*(1), 32–36.

DiSaia, P. J., and Creasman, W. T. (1989). *Clinical gynecologic oncology* (3rd ed.). St. Louis: C. V. Mosby Co.

Eriksson, J. H., & Swenson, K. K. (1986). Your guide to intraperitoneal chemotherapy. *Oncology Nursing Forum, 13*(5), 77–81.

Fitzgerald, J. (1982). Vaginal fistulas: One management method. *Journal of Enterostomal Therapy, 9*, 25–26.

Gosnell, D. (1987). Nursing diagnosis for oncology nursing practice. *Cancer Nursing, 10*, 41–51.

Grunberg, K. J. (1986). Sexual rehabilitation of the cancer patient undergoing ostomy surgery. *Journal of Enterostomal Therapy, 13*, 148–152.

Grunberg, K. J. (1986). Spotlight: Sex counselling called crucial for patients with pelvic or genital surgery. *Oncology Nurse Bulletin, 3*, 12.

Grunberg, K. J. (1986). Practice corner: Sexuality and the person with cancer. *Oncology Nursing Forum, 13*(2), 87.

Gynecology Oncology Group Pathology Committee. (1987). *Gynecology Oncology Group pathology manual* (unpublished).

Hampton, B. G. (1986). Nursing management of a patient following pelvic exenteration. *Seminars in Oncology Nursing, 2*, 281–286.

Haskell, C. (Ed.). (1985). *Cancer treatment* (2nd ed.). Philadelphia: W. B. Saunders Co.

Hassey, K. (1985). Demystifying care of patients with radioactive implants. *American Journal of Nursing, 85*, 788–792.

Herberth, L., & Gosnell, D. (1987). Nursing diagnosis for oncology nursing practice. *Cancer Nursing, 10*, 41–51.

Hoff, S. T. (1987). Concepts in intraperitoneal chemotherapy. *Seminars in Oncology Nursing, 3*, 112–117.

Horwitz, R. I., & Feinstein, A. F. (1978). Alternative analytic methods for case-control studies of estrogens and endometrial cancer. *New England Journal of Medicine, 299*, 1090.

Irrgang, S., & Bryant, R. (1984). Management of the enterocutaneous fistula. *Journal of Enterostomal Therapy, 11*, 211–225.

Kaempfer, S. H., & Major, P. (1986). Fertility considerations in the gynecologic oncology patient. *Oncology Nursing Forum, 13*, 23–27.

Kauppila, A. (1980). Treatment of advanced endometrial adenocarcinoma with combined cytotoxic therapy. *Cancer, 246*, 2162.

Lamb, M. A. (1985). Sexual dysfunction in the gynecologic oncology patient. *Seminars in Oncology Nursing, 1*, 9–17.

Lovejoy, N. C. (1987). Precancerous lesions of the cervix. Personal risk factors. *Cancer Nursing, 10*, 2–14.

Lundberg, G. D. (1988). The 1988 Bethesda system for reporting cervical/vaginal cytological diagnoses (National Cancer Institute Workshop). *Journal of the American Medical Association, 262*, 931–934.

Lurain, J. R. (1982). Fatal gestational trophoblastic disease: An analysis of treatment failures. *American Journal of Obstetrics and Gynecology, 144*, 391.

Marcus, S. L. (1961). Multiple squamous cell carcinomas involving the cervix, vagina, and vulva: The theory of multicentric origin. *American Journal of Obstetrics and Gynecology, 80*, 802.

Mattingly, R. F., & Thompson, J. D. (1985). Te *Linde's operative gynecology*. Philadelphia: J. B. Lippincott Co.

Orr, J. W., & Shingleton, H. M. (1986). Effects of in-utero exposure to DES: An update. *Your Patient & Cancer*, pp. 9–15.

Ozols, R. F. (1986). Intraperitoneal chemotherapy. *Mediguide to Oncology, 5*(4), 1–5.

Richards, S., & Hiratzka, S. (1986). Vaginal dilatation post pelvic irradiation: A patient education tool. *Oncology Nursing Forum, 13*(4), 89–91.

Rivlin, M. E., Morrison, J. C., & Bates, G. W. (1986). *Manual of clinical problems in obstetrics and gynecology* (2nd ed.). Boston: Little, Brown.

Robertson, C. (1986). Treatment modalities for gynecological cancers. *Seminars in Oncology Nursing, 2*, 275–280.

Rossetti, A. C. (1985). Nursing care of patients treated with intrapleural tetracycline for control of malignant pleural effusion. *Cancer Nursing, 8*, 103–109.

Runowicz, C. D. (1987). Ovarian cancer. *Mediguide to Oncology, 7*, 1–5.

Rutledge, F. (1986). Ovarian cancer today. *Innovations in Oncology*, pp. 11–12.

Sargis, N. M. (1983). Detecting ovarian cancer: A challenge for nursing assessment, *Oncology Nursing Forum, 10*(2), 48–52.

Silverberg, E., & Lubera, J. A. (1988). Cancer statistics, 1988. *Ca-A Cancer Journal for Clinicians, 38*, 5–220.

Skeel, R. T. (Ed.) (1982). *Manual of cancer chemotherapy*. Boston: Little, Brown.

Smith, D. B. (1986). Gynecological cancers: Etiology and pathophysiology. *Seminars in Oncology Nursing, 2*, 270–274.

Smith, J. P. (1976). Second-look operation in ovarian carcinoma. *Cancer, 38*, 1438.

Stehman, F. B. (1987). The value of second-look laparotomy in ovarian cancer. *Oncology, 1*(8), 50–51.

Strohl, R. (1986). Practice corner: Advising women receiving pelvic irradiation. *Oncology Nursing Forum, 13*(2), 86.

Swenson, K. K., & Eriksson, J. H. (1986). Nursing management of intraperitoneal chemotherapy. *Oncology Nursing Forum, 13*(5), 33–39.

Trelford, J. D., & Williams, C. F. (1984). Pelvic exenterations. *Journal of Enterostomal Therapy, 11*(2), 55–58.

ViraPap: Human papillomavirus DNA detection kit (Product release document). (1987). Life Technologies, Inc./Molecular Diagnostics. Gaithersburg, MD: Bethesda Research Laboratories.

White, L. N. (1986). Cancer risk assessment. *Seminars in oncology nursing, 2*, 184–190.

Wilbanks, G. D. (1984). Cervical intraepithelial neoplasia. In J Sciarra (Ed.) *Gynecology and obstetrics* (rev. ed., Vol. 4). Philadelphia: Harper and Row.

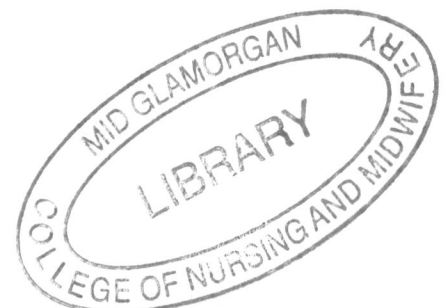

CHAPTER 35

Hematopoietic and Immunologic Cancers

COLETTE CARSON
MARY E. CALLAGHAN

The hematopoietic and immunologic malignancies are diseases in which there is a proliferation of malignant cells that derive originally from the bone marrow, thymus, and lymphatic tissue. Blood cells that originate in the bone marrow are called hematopoietic cells; those that originate in the thymus and lymphatic tissue are called lymphoid cells. In general, when the bone marrow and peripheral blood are major sites of involvement, the neoplasm is classified as a leukemia. Neoplasms that originate in the lymphatic tissue are collectively referred to as malignant lymphomas. Lymphoid cells differ from hematopoietic cells in both anatomic distribution and function; therefore, their neoplastic proliferation is usually distinguishable. Oc-casionally, differentiating between a leukemia and a lymphoma may be difficult. The distinction between non-Hodgkin's lymphoma and lymphocytic leukemia becomes blurred when a lymphoma infiltrates the bone marrow or results in large numbers of malignant lymphocytes entering the peripheral blood from tissues other than the bone marrow.

Hematologic malignancies meet immunologic criteria that describe their development as a malignant process. Malignant proliferation of hematopoietic and lymphoid cells is usually marked by monoclonality, that is, cells arising as a single clone, whereas normal tissues are composed of a mixture of cells. Wherever the malignant clone proliferates—lymphoid tissues, bone marrow, extranodal organs, or all of these—it has the advantage of replacing normal cell lines (Rapaport, 1987). In both leukemia and non-Hodgkin's lymphomas, the proliferating cell often takes the characteristics of a normal cell in a specific phase of maturation. Instead of progressing to the next stage of development, the cell becomes fixed and continues to proliferate in its immature phase. The names of specific leukemia and lymphoma subtypes (e.g., acute myeloid leukemia, small cleaved cell lymphomas) often represent the description of the normal cellular counterpart in a particular maturational phase.

The clinical manifestations of specific hematologic malignancies present an array of symptoms that require nursing intervention. It is the purpose of this chapter to describe the disease process and treatment, identify nursing issues, and refer the reader to specific chapters for a more in-depth review of nursing measures.

LEUKEMIAS

The leukemias are classified along with lymphomas, multiple myeloma, and Waldenström's macroglobulinemia as hematologic malignancies. The common characteristic of all the leukemias is an "unregulated proliferation in the bone marrow of a cell of hematopoietic origin" (Rapaport, 1987). The malignant cell has a growth advantage over normal cells and replaces the normal elements in all areas of hematopoietic bone marrow.

The leukemias are described by the particular cell type of origin. Most originate in the white blood cell lines, but occasionally they can begin in the megakaryocyte line or the erythroid line.

The leukemias are classified on the basis of their cellular differentiation. The acute leukemias describe disease in which differentiation is very minimal, with early forms of cells or blasts being the cell type. The chronic leukemias describe diseases in which the malignant cells have some degree of differentiation. The following discussion describes the major leukemias and their treatment in the adult population.

Acute Lymphoblastic Leukemia

Overview

Acute lymphoblastic leukemia (ALL) is a hematologic malignancy of uncontrolled proliferation and accumulation of immature lymphocytes and their progenitors (Henderson, 1983). Although ALL is the most common childhood malignancy, it accounts for only 20 per cent of adult leukemias (Henderson & Han, 1986). This discussion reviews current ideas about adult ALL.

Etiology

The exact etiology of ALL is unknown, but several factors have been implicated. These factors include radiation, chemicals and drugs, viruses, and genetic abnormalities.

Certain genetic disorders, for example, Down's syndrome, ataxia, and telangiectasia, are associated with an increased risk of developing ALL in children (Berenson, Zigelboim, & Gale, 1985). In adults, the evidence for this etiologic factor is less clear-cut. In one study, chromosomal abnormalities were identified in approximately 66 per cent of patients with ALL (Bloomfield et al., 1983). The data in this study suggest that chromosomal abnormalities influence prognosis in adults with ALL, but no evidence regarding a causal factor has been documented.

The survivors of the atomic bomb have shown an increased incidence of both ALL and acute myelogenous leukemia (AML), probably due to the effects of ionizing radiation. The increased incidence of leukemia with exposure to high levels of ionizing radiation is well established, but studies attempting to link low-level radiation to the development of adult leukemia have not shown such an association (Berenson et al., 1985).

The documentation linking the exposure to chemicals to the increased incidence of developing leukemia is stronger for AML than for ALL. Benzene exposure has been reported as increasing the incidence of ALL, as well as that of AML (Berenson et al., 1985). After treatment with chemotherapy, the development of leukemia has been reported as a result of the therapy; the leukemia that develops is usually AML, although ALL has been reported.

Exogenous retroviruses (RNA tumor viruses) are known to cause leukemia and lymphoma in chickens, cats, cows, and primates (Jacobs & Gale, 1986). In humans the identification of human T-cell leukemia/ lymphoma virus (HTLV) has been demonstrated in patients with T-cell lymphoproliferative malignancies (Blayney et al., 1983; Bloomfield et al., 1983). Although viruses have been identified in some patients with ALL, the cause of most cases is undetermined.

Despite the research and technologic advances, the cause of ALL in most patients will be unknown. Evidence supports a multifactorial approach to its development, yet most patients may never have a factor that is associated with the development of ALL.

Nurses can help dispel false information and educate patients and their families regarding what is currently known about etiologic factors when the patient begins to ask "Why me?"

Classification

Two classification systems have been developed that describe the types of ALL. The first is based on the morphologic description of the disease and is called the French-American-British classification system (FAB). The FAB classification recognizes three types of lymphoblasts: L_1, L_2, and L_3 (Bennett et al., 1976). In childhood ALL, 85 per cent of patients have L_1 morphology with relatively few having L_2 or L_3. In adult ALL, L_1 and L_2 are common, with a preponderance of L_2. L_3 morphology represents a small percentage of patients with ALL (Hoelzer & Gale, 1987).

There has been controversy surrounding the use of the FAB classification and its ability to thoroughly describe the heterogeneous ALL population as well as to determine prognostic variables. Another classification has been developed that is being utilized with some success.

This approach to the classification of ALL is based on immune properties of the leukemia cells (Bennett et al., 1976). The subtypes include the common T-, B-, or null-cell ALL. The subtypes are based on the detection on the cell surface of one of the following: the common ALL antigen (CALLA), T-cell antigens, or immunoglobulin molecules or B-cell markers (Bennett et al., 1976). The null-cell type has none of the cell surface features.

Prognostic variables in adult ALL have been studied, although less frequently than those in childhood ALL, to identify patients in high-risk groups. Investigations correlating the FAB classification with prognosis have produced contradictory results (Hoelzer & Gale, 1987).

Data from studies evaluating prognosis in the immunologic classification seem to indicate that adults with T-cell ALL have the best prognosis, those with common ALL have an intermediate prognosis, and those with null-cell ALL have a slightly inferior prognosis. Patients with B-cell ALL have the least favorable prognosis (Hoelzer & Gale, 1987).

Other factors are reported to influence negatively the remission rates. These include male sex, initial presentation with central nervous system leukemia, high white blood count on presentation, older age, and presence of a mediastinal mass (Jacquillat et al., 1978). These factors have been reported to influence a poorer prognosis but do not always confirm a poor prognosis. A 1980 study reported that the only significant prognostic finding in its group was that patients presenting with a white blood count greater than 35×10^9/L had a lower probability of surviving 3 years (Amadori et al., 1983).

Studies investigating prognostic variables originate in various centers, and conclusions drawn must not be taken as definitive predictors of outcomes in individual patients. Patients are individuals with unique diseases that may respond very differently to similar treatment regimens.

Clinical Features

The clinical features of acute leukemia are outlined in Table 35–1 (Henderson, 1983). The classic clinical features of fatigue, fever, bruising, and pallor are manifestations of failure of normal bone marrow. Most patients have these symptoms less than 3 months (Henderson, 1983). Common laboratory findings include leukocytosis with immature blasts or cells, anemia, thrombocytopenia, and bone marrow packed with poorly differentiated lymphoid blast cells. The peripheral leukocyte count can range from 1000 to 400,000/mm³. Although more commonly seen in patients with chronic myelogenous leukemia (CML) blast crisis and AML, intravascular clumping of leukemia cells may occur in patients with blast counts in excess of 100,000/mm³ (Berenson et al., 1985).

Other clinical features associated with ALL are lymph node enlargement, hepatic or splenic enlargement, meningeal leukemia, bone or joint pain, genitourinary manifestations including hematuria, cystitis, pyelonephritis, priapism, renal failure, hyperuricemia, uric acid nephropathy, and testicular involvement (Henderson, 1983). These symptoms are related to leukemic infiltration of extramedullary lymphatic tissue.

Infections are common in patients presenting with disease and as a cause of death. Acute lymphoblastic leukemia causes marked impairment in the host defense system (Berenson et al., 1985). There is a marked reduction in the number of phagocytic leukocytes and an impairment in ability to mobilize against infection. Patients with ALL show a decreased response to mutagen, have reduced delayed hypersensitivity reactions, and often have low levels of immunoglobulins at diagnosis (Berenson, 1985). Diagnosis is based on morphologic and cytochemical analysis of bone marrow.

Treatment

The treatment of ALL is generally divided into two phases termed *induction therapy* and *postremission therapy*. The purpose of induction chemotherapy is to eradicate all detectable leukemic cells, induce a remission, and restore normal bone marrow function. Postremission therapy usually consists of central nervous system prophylaxis, consolidation-intensification chemotherapy, and maintenance chemotherapy. The goal of postremission therapy is to eradicate undetectable leukemic cells and thereby prevent a relapse.

The terminology utilized in describing postremission therapy can be confusing. Consolidation-intensification chemotherapy usually refers to therapy given after remission has been achieved and restoration of normal bone marrow has occurred. This therapy can involve high-dose chemotherapy, use of new agents to help prevent drug resistance, or, less often, readministration of the induction regimen (Hoelzer & Gale, 1987). Maintenance follows consolidation and involves less intensive therapy.

Specific drugs utilized in the treatment of adult ALL have been reviewed elsewhere (Hoelzer & Gale, 1987). At present, most induction regimens include vincristine, prednisone, daunorubicin, and L-asparaginase (Hoelzer & Gale, 1987). Consolidation-intensification chemotherapy is considered useful, but specific drugs and duration of therapy have not been determined. As in maintenance therapy, which is important in the treatment of childhood ALL, the drugs and duration of therapy are yet to be determined in adult ALL.

In general, current chemotherapy regimens utilizing an anthracycline, usually daunomycin, can achieve 70 to 80 per cent remission rates. With optimal postremission therapy, 3- to 5-year actuarial leukemia-free survival has been achieved in 20 to 35 per cent of unselected patients (Champlin & Gale, 1987). Survival is difficult to predict because of the varying prognostic variables.

Table 35–1. CLINICAL FEATURES OF ACUTE LEUKEMIA RELATED TO PATHOPHYSIOLOGY

Symptoms	Signs	Laboratory Abnormalities	Cause
Fatigue, weakness	Pallor, lethargy, weakness	Anemia, hypocalcemia, hypercalcemia, hypomagnesemia	Marrow failure, release of cellular ions and metabolites
Weight loss	Weight loss		Reduced food intake, anemia, hepatosplenomegaly, increased catabolism
Bleeding in skin, mucous membranes, gums, or gastrointestinal or genitourinary tracts	Purpura, gum oozing or hypertrophy, hematuria, melena	Thrombocytopenia, hypofibrinogenemia, reduced factors V or VIII, increased fibrin split products	Marrow failure, DIC
Infection of skin, throat, gums, or respiratory or urinary tracts	Fever, chills, tissue infiltrates, pyoderma gangrenosum	Granulocytopenia; radiographic evidence of pneumonia, sinusitis, and the like; positive cultures	Marrow failure, granulocytopenia, immunodeficiency
Headache, nausea, vomiting, blurred vision, cranial nerve dysfunction	Papilledema, cranial nerve palsy, meningeal irritation	Spinal fluid pleocytosis, reduced CSF sugar, increased CSF protein	Meningeal, CNS, or nerve infiltration, compression, or both
Bone pain and tenderness	Increased bone tenderness	Periosteal elevation, bone destruction by x-rays, abnormal bone marrow, pressure fibrosis	Local leukemic infiltration
Abdominal fullness, anorexia	Hepatosplenomegaly, abdominal tenderness	Hyperfibrinogenemia, elevated SGOT or SGPT, alkaline phosphatase	Infiltration of abdominal viscera
Enlarged lymph nodes or tumor masses	Enlarged lymph nodes or masses in node areas, skin, breast, or testes	Abnormal liver or spleen biopsy results, abnormal bone scan results	Local tumor growth or infiltration
Oliguria	Oliguria	Concentrated urine, elevated BUN, elevated uric acid	Dehydration, uric acid nephropathy, DIC
Obstipation	Abdominal fullness, tenderness	Abnormal results for scans or radiographic contrast studies	Local infiltration or obstruction, calcium/magnesium imbalance

DIC, disseminated intravascular coagulation; CSF, cerebrospinal fluid; SGOT, serum glutamic-oxaloacetic transaminase; SGPT, serum glutamic-pyruvic transaminase; BUN, blood urea nitrogen; CNS, central nervous system.
(Data from Henderson, 1983.)

Central Nervous System Prophylaxis

In childhood ALL, the role of central nervous system prophylaxis in prolonging survival is well documented (Berenson et al., 1985). In adult ALL, the usefulness of central nervous system prophylaxis in prolonging survival has been difficult to document. In general, most treatment regimens in adult ALL include intrathecal methotrexate with or without central nervous system irradiation (Hoelzer & Gale, 1987).

Relapsed and Resistant Leukemia

Hoelzer and Gale (1987) have reviewed the experimental drugs utilized in patients who have relapsed and resistant ALL. The most active regimens appear to be moderate- to high-dose methotrexate with L-asparaginase or folinic acid rescue, the combination of teniposide and cytarabine, and high-dose cytarabine in combination with amsacrine or an anthracycline.

Limited studies utilizing immunotherapy have not shown convincing benefit to patients. Studies utilizing monoclonal antibodies are in progress, but no complete responses have been reported (Hoelzer & Gale, 1987).

Bone Marrow Transplantation

Champlin and Gale (1987) have reviewed the data evaluating bone marrow transplantation (BMT) in adult ALL. In patients with advanced disease, the 2- to 4-year survival rate is 10 to 20 per cent. Patients in first or second remission have a 2- to 4-year survival rate of 30 to 50 per cent. These statistics are utilizing allogeneic transplants and vary in different studies.

Autologous bone marrow transplantation in adult ALL has been performed. Disease-free survival of approximately 20 per cent in 2 years is reported in individuals with ALL in second or third remission (Champlin & Gale, 1987). The value of autologous transplantation in ALL remains an area for further critical investigation.

Nursing Care

The mainstay in the treatment of ALL is effective elimination of leukemic cells in the bone marrow by chemotherapeutic agents. The resultant pancytopenia is a nursing challenge. Nursing care of patients receiving treatment for ALL requires an integrated knowledge of blood component therapy; of management of infection in immunosuppressed patients; of management of patients experiencing alteration in elimination, alteration in skin integrity, alteration in protective mechanisms, alteration in comfort, and alteration in nutritional status; and of the psychosocial problems of facing a life-threatening illness. Refer to Unit VIII for elaboration of these specific nursing interventions.

Acute Myelogenous Leukemia

Overview

Acute myelogenous leukemia (AML) or acute non-lymphocytic leukemia (ANLL) is a group of diseases in which an abnormal hematologic stem cell gives rise to a monoclonal population of myeloid cells whose ability to differentiate beyond early forms is impaired (Rai & Montserrat, 1987). These abnormal cells have a growth advantage, and therefore blasts and other early forms eventually replace the normal hematopoietic marrow cells. This disease is characterized by a proliferation and accumulation of malignant myeloblasts or other immature myeloid cells. The cell lines that can be affected by the malignancy are the granulocytic, monocytic, erythroid, and megakaryocyte.

Etiology

The exact etiology of AML is unknown. Like ALL, several factors have been implicated. These factors include radiation, chemicals and drugs, viruses, and genetic abnormalities.

Acute myelogenous leukemia occurs with increased frequency in several congenital disorders including Down syndrome, Klinefelter's syndrome, Fanconi's anemia, osteogenesis imperfecta, and Wiskott-Aldrich syndrome (Bloomfield et al., 1983).

The effects of ionizing radiation on the survivors of the atomic bomb are well documented with the increased incidence of leukemia, especially AML (Cronkite, Maloney, & Bond, 1960; Graham, 1960; Heysel et al., 1960). Exposure to chemicals has been associated with an increased incidence of AML. The association of benzene exposure and AML has been noted (Vigliani & Sart, 1964). Chloramphenicol, phenylbutazone, alkylating agents, procarbazine, and the nitrosoureas are the drugs most commonly associated with the development of AML, although the association is identified in few patients (Vigliani & Sart, 1964).

A relationship between RNA viruses and myeloid leukemias in animals has been found, but viral cancer in humans has not been identified (Blayney et al., 1983). An interest in cellular oncogenes has been evident. Cellular oncogenes are closely related to RNA tumor viruses called viral oncogenes (Blaney et al., 1983). The cellular oncogenes have been found near sites of chromosomal rearrangements common in AML, but there is no evidence yet that the oncogenes are directly involved in the development of AML.

Classification

The FAB classification is a widely accepted classification system for AML. This system is based on the morphologic description of the malignant cell line involved. Table 35–2 describes this classification (Rapaport, 1987). Acute myelogenous leukemia with granulocyte differentiation includes acute undifferentiated leukemia (M_1), acute myelogenous leukemia (M_2) with maturation to or beyond promyelocyte stage, and acute

Table 35–2. FRENCH-AMERICAN-BRITISH CLASSIFICATION OF ACUTE MYELOGENOUS LEUKEMIA

	Designation	Predominant Cell Type
M_1	(undifferentiated myelocytic)	Myeloblasts
M_2	(myelocytic)	Myeloblasts, promyelocytes, myelocytes
M_3	(promyelocytic)	Hypergranular promyelocytes
M_4	(myelomonocytic)	Promyelocytes, myelocytes, promonocytes, monocytes
M_{5A}	(monoblastic)	Monoblasts
M_{5B}	(differentiated monocytic)	Monoblasts, promonocytes, monocytes
M_6	(erythroleukemic)	Erythroblasts
M_7	(megakaryocytic)	Megakaryocytes

(Data from Rapaport, 1987.)

progranulocytic leukemia (M_3). The M_4, M_5, and M_6 types of AML show varying cell types as indicated in the table and are less common than the previously described types. Cytogenic studies are being utilized to further classify different types of AML, and surface marker analysis is being used to characterize cell types of very early blast forms (Rapaport, 1987).

Clinical Features

The clinical presentation of patients with AML usually reflects the degree of replacement of normal bone marrow by leukemic cells. Table 35–1 summarizes the various symptoms associated with acute leukemia. Zigelboim, Foon, and Gale (1985) estimate that 20 per cent of patients present with symptoms of anemia, pallor, weakness, and fatigue.

Bleeding is another important manifestation of this disease. Twenty to 50 per cent of patients with AML will have moderately severe thrombocytopenia at the time of diagnosis. The severe thrombocytopenia is usually related to decreased platelet production or increased consumption of cells from infection, hypersplenism, and, rarely, disseminated intravascular coagulation. Patients with acute promyelocytic leukemia (M_3) can have additional coagulation abnormalities (Gale & Foon, 1986). These coagulation abnormalities include hypofibrinogenemia, abnormal Factors V and VII, increased fibrin degradation products, and circulating anticoagulants. These abnormalities present unique challenges in the induction phase of a patient with acute promyelocytic leukemia.

Patients with AML commonly present with infection (Gale & Foon, 1986). Because of myeloid leukemic involvement, the neutrophils are decreased and can function abnormally. Bacterial infections are most common, but fungal, viral, and protozoal infections can occur.

Patients will also present with physical complaints that reflect the infiltration of normal tissues with leukemic cells. Bone or joint pain can reflect infiltration of the bone marrow. Hepatomegaly, splenomegaly, and lymph node enlargement have been reported in 10 to 60 per cent of patients. Renal abnormalities may occur as a result of direct infiltration; gout from increased uric acid and gastrointestinal symptoms, including distention, satiety, and obstipation as a result of organ infiltration, are reported (Zigelboim et al., 1985).

Skin lesions can occur. The most common skin lesions are petechiae related to thrombocytopenia. Leukemic skin infiltrates are uncommon but can be found in patients with monocytic and myelomonocytic leukemia, relapsed or resistant leukemia, and high white blood cell counts (Rapaport, 1987). In addition to skin infiltrates, patients with monocytic leukemia can have hypertrophied gums, oral ulcers, palpable spleen, anorectal ulcerations, and central nervous system involvement (Rapaport, 1987).

Central nervous system involvement in AML is uncommon but is primarily seen in patients with monocytic (M_2) and myelomonocytic leukemia (Zigelboim et al., 1985). When patients experience headaches, diplopia, changes in mental status, cranial nerve palsies, and papilledema, central nervous system involvement is suspected.

Acute myelogenous leukemia is diagnosed by bone marrow aspiration and evidence from biopsy specimens. One classic feature of AML is the presence of Auer rods on the leukemic blast (Graham, 1960). The other method of distinguishing myeloblasts from lymphoblasts is to use a histochemical stain that demonstrates peroxidase activity (Henderson, 1983). More recently, monoclonal antibodies have been used to identify some types of AML, but these need further development (Griffin et al., 1986).

Prognostic variables have been investigated in an attempt to identify patients who will respond favorably to therapy. Gale and Foon (1987) have summarized the pretreatment variables that may influence treatment outcomes. In general, older age, previous cancer, previous therapy, and chromosomal abnormalities are variables that are associated with unfavorable prognosis. A favorable prognosis is associated with patients in the younger age group, with the presence of Auer rods, and with a shorter time between treatment and complete remission.

Treatment

The goal of induction therapy in AML is to achieve hematologic remission. Hematologic remission is generally defined as the reduction of leukemia cells to undetectable levels; restoration of bone marrow function, including normalization of hemoglobin, granulocytes, and platelets; resolution of hepatosplenomegaly; and return to a normal performance status (Gale & Foon, 1987).

Various drug regimens have been utilized in the treatment of AML. Table 35–3 lists the various multi-chemotherapy drug regimens (Gale & Foon, 1986). In general, most centers use cytarabine (200 mg/m²/day) for 7 days by continuous infusion and 3 days of daunorubicin (Griffin et al., 1986). In patients younger than 60 years, daunorubicin doses range from 45 to 75 mg/m²/day. In patients older than 60 years, lower doses of daunorubicin are sometimes given because of the toxicity at higher doses. Addition of other drugs to

Table 35–3. COMBINATION INDUCTION CHEMOTHERAPY FOR ACUTE MYELOGENOUS LEUKEMIA

Cytarabine + 6-thioguanine or mercaptopurine
Cytarabine + vincristine + prednisone + cyclophosphamide
Cytarabine + daunorubicin + 6-thioguanine (5 days)
Cytarabine + doxorubicin or daunorubicin (7 days)
Cytarabine + daunorubicin + 6-thioguanine (7 days)

(Data from Gale & Foon, 1986.)

this regimen have not improved the results sufficiently to be statistically significant.

It is not unusual for patients to undergo two induction courses to obtain a remission. The drugs used at the second induction may be the same ones used during the first induction, or the regimen may be different. Once remission has been achieved, the goal becomes one of preventing relapse. If no further therapy is given, recurrence of leukemia occurs in a majority of patients. It is believed that recurrence is related to the presence of residual leukemic cells that are undetectable by current methods. The approach to preventing relapse is to administer chemotherapy to the patient in remission (Gale & Foon, 1987).

Various protocols have been employed in the chemotherapy of postremission AML. Gale and Foon (1987) reviewed these protocols, stating that most contained two to six additional cycles of cytosine arabinoside (ara-C) and 6-thioguanine with or without daunomycin. They found that occasionally other drugs were used alone or in combination. These drugs included 5-azacytidine, amsacrine, methotrexate, prednisone, vincristine, cyclophosphamide (Cytoxan), doxorubicin (Adriamycin), and carmustine.

More recently, high-dose cytosine arabinoside (HDARAC) has been utilized in postremission therapy. The doses range from 1 to 3 g/m² IV q 12 hours for 12 doses on days 1 through 6 of the regimen. The results indicate complete remissions approaching 80 per cent. More investigations with this regimen are being carried out in induction regimens.

Another chemotherapy regimen currently being investigated is high-dose cytoxan (50 mg/kg) and VP-16 (3600 mg/m²) without bone marrow transplant for high-risk and relapse leukemias. This regimen has produced about 30 per cent remission rates in patients who have relapsed after initial therapy (Brown et al., 1990). Studies are continuing to determine the role of this therapy for leukemia.

The efficacy of the individual protocols is difficult to evaluate because most of them have been utilized in nonrandomized studies. Most studies indicate median remission of 9 to 16 months, regardless of the protocol used (Gale & Foon, 1987).

Because of the various reports, results, and uncontrolled data, most centers administer one to three cycles of chemotherapy to patients in remission. These chemotherapy regimens usually consist of the same drugs used to obtain remission or new drugs to prevent cross resistance. Once sustained remission has been accomplished, the question of continued chemotherapy in the form of maintenance therapy can be addressed.

The efficacy of maintenance therapy has been reviewed by Gale and Foon (1987). In general, studies have shown little or no benefit in continuing therapy 1 to 3 years after remission. Most centers currently do not utilize maintenance therapy in the treatment of AML.

Most patients relapse within 1 to 2 years. Remission can be achieved in 25 to 50 per cent of patients with resistant or recurrent leukemia. The drugs that have been utilized are summarized in Table 35–4 (Gale & Foon, 1987).

Although remission in resistant or relapsed leukemia may occur, the duration of remission is short. Remission of more than 1 year occurs in less than 10 per cent of responding patients (Gale & Foon, 1987). Given these small numbers, the use of BMT is often considered (see Chapter 27).

Before the advent of chemotherapy, the median survival for patients with AML was 3 months (Tivey, 1954). Within current drug regimens, remission occurs in 60 to 80 per cent of patients (Berenson et al., 1985). The median duration of remission has been reported to be 9 to 16 months, with some reports of 20 to 40 per cent of patients in remission for 2 years or more (Gale & Foon, 1987). Despite these advances, AML remains a fatal disease for the majority of patients.

Bone Marrow Transplantation

Bone marrow transplantation has been utilized in the treatment of AML. Several centers utilizing allogeneic transplants report continuous disease-free survival of 45 to 57 per cent at 2 to 5 years after transplantation (Santos, 1989). These figures have led some investigators to recommend that allogeneic BMT be the treatment of choice for patients under the age of 50 who have a suitable donor. This issue remains controversial, however. Studies continue to ascertain the role of BMT in patients in first remission.

Autologous BMT is currently being investigated at various centers. Results are preliminary, and further studies need to be carried out (see also Chapter 27).

Nursing Care

Nursing care of patients with AML can be very challenging. The goal of therapy is to achieve remis-

Table 35–4. USEFUL DRUGS IN RESISTANT ACUTE MYELOGENOUS LEUKEMIA*

Cytarabine + daunorubicin†
High-dose cytarabine + L-asparaginase
High-dose cytarabine + daunorubicin
High-dose cytarabine + amsacrine
Amsacrine ± other drugs
Mitoxantrone
Aclarubicin
Cytarabine analogues
Harringtonine
High-dose methotrexate + L-asparaginase
Epipodophyllotoxins
2,5-Piperazinedione
Zinostatin

*Drugs are ranked in estimated order of efficacy.
†In patients who are receiving limited therapy or who are off therapy for prolonged periods (Gale & Foon, 1987.)

sion. To accomplish this means that bone marrow hypoplasia and pancytopenia will occur. Nursing care is critical during the recovery period of bone marrow after chemotherapy.

The newer regimens utilizing high dose chemotherapy offer newer challenges for oncology nurses. With total white blood cell counts below 500 and platelet counts below 20,000, life-threatening infection and bleeding are common problems. Nursing assessment and intervention are critical components in the care of patients with these problems. Knowledge of the administration and side effects of chemotherapy agents, as well as the administration of blood components is important for nursing intervention. Chapters 21, 22, 26, 27, 47, 48, and 50 will help prepare nurses to care for a patient with AML.

Chronic Lymphocytic Leukemia

Overview

Chronic lymphocytic leukemia (CLL) is a hematologic malignancy characterized by proliferation and accumulation of relatively mature-looking but immunologically ineffective lymphocytes. It is the most common leukemia in Western countries, accounting for about 30 per cent of all leukemia cases (Foon & Gale, 1986). It is extremely rare in the Orient.

Chronic lymphocytic leukemia generally occurs in older individuals (median age is 60), although occasionally it can develop in young adults and even children. It occurs twice as often in males as in females.

Etiology

The exact etiology of CLL is unknown, but various factors seem to be important. Chronic lymphocytic leukemia has been the most common type of leukemia associated with familial leukemia (Rundles, 1982a). Although CLL has a propensity to occur in closely related individuals, there is no definite pattern of inheritance. Although extra chromosomes have been found in some CLL patients (most notably trisomy 12 in 30 per cent of CLL patients), no chromosome abnormality has yet been identified as specific for CLL. Other specific chromosomal abnormalities that would be characteristic of CLL have *not* been found (Whang-Peng & Knutsen, 1980).

In CLL, the malignant transformation occurs most frequently in the B lymphocyte, with a small proportion occurring in T lymphocytes (Foon & Gale, 1987). The malignant cells have a long life and a low proliferative capability and tend to be immunologically dysfunctional.

In general, patients' first symptoms of the disease are fatigue and reduced exercise tolerance, enlargement of superficial lymph nodes, or splenomegaly (Rundles, 1982a). In many patients, the signs and symptoms have occurred gradually so that a specific date of onset is unknown. In about a quarter of the patients, the diagnosis is discovered by accident, in a

Table 35–5. RAI CLINICAL STAGING SYSTEM FOR CHRONIC LYMPHOCYTIC LEUKEMIA

Stage	Findings at Diagnosis
0	Lymphocytes in blood 15,000 × 100⁹/L or higher, and 40% or more lymphocytes in marrow
I	Above plus enlarged lymph nodes
II	Above plus splenomegaly, hepatomegaly, or both
III	Above plus anemia (Hb <11 g/dL)
IV	Above plus thrombocytopenia (platelets <100,000/μl)

(Data from Rai et al., 1975.)

routine examination, during which enlarged lymph nodes, splenomegaly, or abnormal blood counts are found (Rundles, 1982a).

Classification

Two types of staging systems have been utilized to describe CLL. The Rai system categorizes patients into 5 stages on the basis of the lymphocyte count and the presence or absence of lymphadenopathy, splenomegaly, hepatomegaly, anemia, and thrombocytopenia (Rai et al., 1975). Table 35–5 summarizes the Rai system. Stage 0 represents patients at low risk, stages I to II patients are at intermediate risk, and stages III and IV patients are considered to be at high risk.

The Binet system categorizes patients into 3 groups. Table 35–6 describes this schema (Binet et al., 1981). The prognosis for patients with stage A disease equals that of the general population; for patients with stage B disease, median survival is approximately 7 years; and for patients with stage C disease, median survival is less than 2 years.

Other staging systems have been introduced in the literature, but most clinicians utilize either the Rai or the Binet system. The limitation of these staging systems is that they cannot predict for some patients in the low and intermediate risk groups (Binet's A and B and Rai's 0, I, and II) who will have an indolent course and good prognosis and those patients in the group whose disease is aggressive and progresses rapidly (Rai & Montserrat, 1987).

Natural History

During the early phase of CLL, no treatment is given. Patients are usually asymptomatic, but as time

Table 35–6. BINET STAGING SYSTEM OF CHRONIC LYMPHOCYTIC LEUKEMIA

Stage	Findings at Diagnosis
A	Lymphocytosis in blood 15,000 × 1⁹/L or higher, and 40% or more lymphocytes. No anemia or thrombocytopenia and less than three areas of nodal involvement.
B	Above with three or more areas of lymphoid involvement and enlarged lymph nodes, spleen, or liver. No anemia or thrombocytopenia.
C	Above with anemia (Hb <11 g/dL in men or <10 g/dL in women) or thrombocytopenia (<100,000 × 10⁹/L) regardless of the number of areas of lymphoid involvement.

(Data from Binet et al., 1981.)

goes on, fatigue and reduced exercise tolerance may worsen. Lymph nodes gradually increase in size with new lymph nodes becoming involved. The spleen enlarges, and hepatomegaly may develop. Lymph tissue may grow in unusual areas, such as the scalp, orbit, subconjunctiva, pharynx, pleura, lung parenchyma, walls of the gastrointestinal tract, liver, prostate, and gonads. Obstructive jaundice can occur from periportal infiltration, and, very rarely, congestive heart failure can occur as a result of myocardial infiltration (Rundles, 1982a).

As the CLL becomes more aggressive and advanced, patients may experience severe fatigue; recurrent or persistent infection with fevers, pallor, edema, or thrombophlebitis from nodal obstruction; and increasing back tenderness and pain (Rundles, 1982a).

The absolute lymphocytic count in CLL ranges from 10 to 150 × 10³/μl, but counts up to 1000 × 10³/μl can occur in patients who are untreated. The abnormal lymphocytes in CLL are smaller than the lymphoblasts and myeloblasts of acute leukemia. Therefore, the incidence of thrombotic and embolic complications is small (Rundles, 1982a).

As the tumor burden of lymphoid tissue increases, the proportion of normal marrow precursors decreases until eventually only lymphocytes remain in the marrow (Rundles, 1982a). It is not unusual for the differential white blood cell count of these patients to contain 90 to 100 per cent lymphocytes with only a few of the other types of white blood cells in the peripheral blood. As replacement of the marrow with lymphocytes occurs, granulocytopenia, thrombocytopenia, and anemia occur and can be mild to severe. Most patients will die from the complications related to pancytopenia.

Treatment

The treatment of CLL varies, depending on the stage of disease. In general, no data suggest that treatment of patients with elevated leukocyte counts and lymphadenopathy prolongs survival. In one study, patients with stages I and II, or A, were given chlorambucil alone, chlorambucil with prednisone, or no treatment (Shapiro et al., 1984). No advantage in survival was shown in any group. In general, when patients experience organomegaly or cytopenias, treatment is then initiated. Several treatment modalities have been utilized in the treatment of CLL.

Chemotherapy. The chemotherapy used in the treatment of CLL is either a single-agent or a multiagent regimen. The initial treatment for patients who require intervention is usually chlorambucil or cyclophosphamide with or without prednisone.

Chlorambucil is the most common drug. The usual dose is 0.1 to 0.2 mg/kg/day until the disease is controlled or toxicity is experienced; then the dose is reduced. Pulse therapy is given in a dose of 0.4 to 0.6 mg/kg once every 2 to 4 weeks. A response rate of 60 per cent is common using chlorambucil, with 10 to 20 per cent complete remission reported (Foon & Gale, 1987). Pulse therapy is utilized because it is reported to cause less hematologic toxicity (Knospe, Lolb, & Huguley, 1974).

Cyclophosphamide is reported to be as effective as chlorambucil (Huguley, 1977). It is often administered to patients who are unresponsive to chlorambucil. The usual dose is 2 to 3 mg/kg/day or 20 mg/kg every 2 to 3 weeks.

Corticosteroids are utilized to control the increase in leukocytic count and to treat the immune-mediated hemolytic anemia and thrombocytopenia (Prednisone and prednisolone, 1970). Prednisone is given as 20 to 60 mg/m² body surface area. Corticosteroids are not prescribed alone in the treatment of CLL.

In patients with advanced disease, combination chemotherapy with cyclophosphamide (Cytoxan), vincristine, and prednisone (CVP) has been used as has cyclophosphamide, hydroxydaunorubicin (Adriamycin), vincristine (Oncovin), and prednisone (CHOP) (Huguley, 1977; Prednisone and prednisolone, 1970). The advantages of both have been reported in the literature.

New drug therapies are being investigated in the treatment of CLL. Pentostatin (2'-deoxycoformycin) has shown activity in controlling lymphoid malignancies, including CLL. Initial studies utilizing this drug identified considerable toxicities, although current studies testing pentostatin at low-dose levels indicate toxicities have been reduced (Grever et al., 1985).

Another drug that has shown antilymphocytic activity is 2-chlorodeoxyadenosine (2-CDA). In one study, 78 per cent of patients had a reduction of circulating lymphocytes, with 55 per cent of patients demonstrating objective clinical responses (Piro, Carrera, Beutler, & Carson, 1988). Investigations with this drug continue.

Fludarabine is another drug under investigation (Keating et al., 1989). Complete responses have occurred in 13 per cent of patients in this study. Further investigations are continuing to establish the schedule for dosing and the length of response to treatment.

In summary, patients who develop organomegaly or cytopenia are initially treated with single-agent chemotherapy. As the disease progresses, multiagent chemotherapy is utilized to control the disease. Investigations continue to find drugs that are more effective in the treatment of CLL.

Biologic Response Modifiers. The role of monoclonal antibodies is being investigated in the treatment of CLL. Treatment with T-101 monoclonal antibody, or a similar antibody, has shown some activity or response in patients with CLL, but these studies are in the early phases of investigation (Foon et al., 1983).

Another approach utilizing monoclonal antibodies is the development of anti-idiotype monoclonal antibodies. These antibodies are "tailor-made" specifically for an individual patient's tumor cells (Foon & Gale, 1986). This approach is in the early stages of investigation and has limited applicability to individual patients.

Interferon, another biologic response modifier, has been studied in patients with CLL (Figlin, 1989; Foon et al., 1985). Although reported responses from the initial trials have been low in numbers, interferon's activity in combination with alkylating agents and as maintenance therapy continues to be investigated in patients with CLL (Figlin, 1989).

Splenectomy. The benefits of splenectomy in patients with CLL have been debated over the years. Today splenectomy is used in selected patients with hemolytic anemia, thrombocytopenia, pancytopenia, and painful splenomegaly (Foon & Gale, 1986). Only in these unusual cases is splenectomy recommended.

Radiotherapy. The primary role of radiation therapy in CLL is one of palliation and symptom control. Radiation therapy is generally used to treat enlarged lymph nodes, painful bony lesions, or massive splenomegaly that is resistant to chemotherapy (Rundles, 1982a). Splenic radiation has also been utilized to treat painful splenomegaly, progressive lymphocytosis, anemia, and thrombocytopenia (Byhardt, Brace, & Wiernic, 1975).

Leukapheresis. When the number of circulating white blood cells is great enough to produce vascular thrombosis or embolism in patients who are unresponsive to chemotherapy, removal of the lymphocytes by pheresis has been utilized (Curtis, Hersh, & Freirich, 1972). Leukapheresis does not treat the disease, and therefore, when discontinued, the problem of increasing white blood cells continues. Routine use of leukapheresis is probably not justified but in selected patients may be beneficial for a period of time.

Systemic Complications of CLL. Table 35–7 identifies the complications experienced by patients who have CLL (Henderson & Han, 1986). These complications usually occur as the disease advances and becomes refractory to therapy.

Nursing Care

Nursing care of patients with CLL begins with the initial diagnosis. Patient and family education about the disease and its treatment is an important area in which nurses can intervene. Questions and issues related to treatment versus no treatment will have to be

Table 35–7. SYSTEMIC COMPLICATIONS IN CHRONIC LYMPHOCYTIC LEUKEMIA AND THEIR MANAGEMENT

Condition	Management
Hypogammaglobulinemia and recurrent infections	Gammaglobulin (intramuscularly) Gammaglobulin (intravenously) Appropriate antibiotics
Immune-mediated anemia; thrombocytopenia and neutropenia	Prednisone Immunosuppressive agents Splenectomy Gammaglobulin (intravenously)
Hyperviscosity syndrome (rare)	Plasmapheresis Prednisone Chemotherapy
Hyperuricemia (rare)	Hydration Allopurinol
Hypercalcemia (very rare)	Hydration Diuretics Prednisone Calcitonin

(Data from Henderson & Han, 1986.)

clarified for patients. Nurses can assist the medical team in identifying and clarifying questions.

As the disease progresses, education related to the treatment and the side effects of treatment must be undertaken with patients and families (see Chapters 20 and 21). As patients experience the symptoms of the disease and the complications associated with CLL, nursing care becomes an integral part of the treatment.

Bone marrow replacement with ineffective lymphocytes results in neutropenia, thrombocytopenia, and anemia. Chapter 49 provides nursing interventions for these problems.

Infiltration of bone and other organs with lymphocytes will cause the patient pain. Chapter 50 discusses comfort measures nurses can provide.

Hemolytic anemia associated with CLL requires the nurse to have expertise in blood component therapy. Patient education and support are important because some patients may require weekly transfusions. Other complications associated with CLL—hyperviscosity syndrome, hyperuricemia, and hypercalcemia—although uncommon, are challenging to the nursing and medical team.

Patients with CLL can live long lives. As the disease progresses, quality of life issues become important. Toward the end of their lives, many patients spend increasing time in hospitals with recurrent infections and bleeding and are dependent on blood transfusions. Emotional support of patients and families during times of crisis are important in nursing care.

Chronic Myelogenous Leukemia

Overview

Chronic myelogenous leukemia accounts for approximately 20 to 30 per cent of the adult leukemias. It is a relatively rare disease in children. The peak incidence of CML has been in the fourth decade of life but has been found to be shifting to a later age. This leukemia occurs more frequently in men than in women (Rundles, 1982b).

Etiology

Exposure to radiation has been implicated in the development of CML. The exposure of the Japanese in Hiroshima and Nagasaki during the atomic bomb explosions demonstrated the leukogenic effects of single-dose radiation (Cronkite et al., 1960). After a 3-year latency period, the yearly incidence of leukemia in survivors gradually increased to its maximum by 7 years and then began to fall. Yet at 14 years, the rate still exceeded the national average for incidence of CML in the general population. The most common leukemias among the survivors were CML and AML (Heysel et al., 1960).

Other evidence associating radiation exposures with development of CML was demonstrated in patients with ankylosing spondylitis, who were treated with radiotherapy in Great Britain (Graham, 1960). After

a 6-year latency period, the incidence of leukemia increased to 12 times that of the normal population. Chronic myelogenous leukemia was the most common leukemia in these cases.

Although radiation exposure can be an etiologic factor, very few patients with CML are exposed to unusual amounts of radiation. Approximately one person in 15 or 20 who develops the disease has had unusual exposure to any form of radiation or chemical (Rundles, 1982b). Any chemical capable of damaging hematopoietic stem cells is potentially leukogenic, although identification of causative agents can be difficult. The chemical that has clearly been identified as one that increased the incidence of myelogenous leukemia in humans is benzene associated with heavy occupational exposure (Vigliani & Sart, 1964).

In most cases, the etiology of CML is unknown. Nurses can educate as well as allay the fears of patients who look for something that they may have done to cause this disease.

Biologic Manifestations

Chronic myelogenous leukemia is a hematologic malignancy that results from the development of an abnormal hematopoietic stem cell that gives rise to offspring that have the Philadelphia chromosome (Rundles, 1982b). With the development of cytogenetic studies and the enzyme marker G-6-PD (glucose-6-phosphate dehydrogenase), it has been established that CML is a clonal disorder resulting from the malignant transformation of a pluripotent hematopoietic stem cell (Rapaport, 1987).

The chromosome abnormality, found in 90 to 95 per cent of patients, is thought to be a key element in the steps of the malignant transformation. These chromosomal rearrangements are associated with translocation and activation of cellular oncogenes (Champlin, 1986).

The transformed malignant stem cell in CML shows a marked increase in proliferation of marrow granulocytic and occasionally megakaryocytic progenitor and precursor cells (Rundles, 1982b). The marrow cells with increased proliferation seem to have a growth advantage and to overproduce in the marrow itself, replacing normal myeloid cells and expanding into the peripheral blood. Thus large numbers of immature and mature granulocytic cells accumulate in the blood. With further expansion into the peripheral blood, the malignant cells proliferate in the spleen, replacing the normal lymphoid elements of that organ, and accumulate in the sinusoids of the liver (Rapaport, 1987). This extramedullary proliferation results in enlargement of both the spleen and the liver. It is believed that the increase in myeloid production is not due to an accelerated proliferation of cells but to a massive expansion in the cells that are committed to myeloid production.

Diagnosis

The diagnosis of CML is based on sustained granulocytosis, which is usually associated with splenomegaly; a low leukocyte alkaline phosphatase (LAP score); and the presence of the Ph^1 chromosome. Myeloid cells at all stages of differentiation are found in the peripheral blood, and they appear to be normal in morphology. Platelet counts are usually normal or slightly depressed. A bone marrow aspiration is obtained for cytogenic studies to confirm the presence of the Ph^1 chromosome (Champlin, 1986). Chemical abnormalities associated with CML include hyperuricemia, low LAP score, increase in vitamin B_{12} levels, increase in lactate dehydrogenase, and increase in K^+ (Rundles, 1982b).

Clinical Phases

Chronic myelogenous leukemia is characterized by three phases: chronic, accelerated, and acute. During the chronic phase, there is an overproduction of relatively normal granulocytes that respond to treatment. At diagnosis, patients will experience malaise, fatigue, lack of exercise tolerance, and weight loss (Rundles, 1982b). As the disease progresses, aching in the bones that contain red blood cell marrow, tenderness in the lower half of the sternum, and discomfort and fullness in the upper abdomen that indicate hepatosplenomegaly, are present.

The symptoms usually subside with treatment, and patients may be asymptomatic during these periods from 1 to 4 years. After this period, the signs and symptoms gradually become worse and less responsive to treatment.

The accelerated phase is characterized by progressive symptoms and resistance to chemotherapy. Systemic symptoms (fever, night sweats, weight loss), increasing hepatosplenomegaly, lymphadenopathy, and extramedullary leukemia are common manifestations (Champlin, 1986). The blood counts that were so responsive to therapy during the chronic phase now become unresponsive.

The acute phase is highlighted by a significant increase in the blast count and further progression of anemia, thrombocytopenia, or myelofibrosis (Champlin, 1986). Extramedullary leukemia with tumors or diffuse infiltration involving skin, mucous membranes, lymph nodes, orbit, pleurisy, synovia, extradural tissues, peripheral nerves, and meninges occurs in approximately 40 per cent of patients. Most patients will develop the acute or blast crisis phase in which the disease now resembles acute leukemia (Keating et al., 1989). Approximately 5 to 10 per cent of patients move from a chronic phase, in which the disease seems to be controlled, to a sudden acute or blast crisis phase (Rundles, 1982b).

During this phase, the manifestations of CML resemble those of acute leukemia. The cells no longer differentiate to mature granulocytes, and maturation arrest occurs at the blast or promyelocyte stage of maturation. The blast crisis generally occurs in one of two forms: myeloid and lymphoid (Boggs, 1974). Approximately 70 per cent of patients will develop a myeloblastic acute leukemia, and the remaining 30 per cent will develop a lymphoblastic leukemia (Rosenthal,

Canellos, DeVita, & Gralnick, 1977). To determine the appropriate treatment, it is important to determine whether the blast crisis is of lymphoid or myeloid origin.

Treatment

The purpose of treating CML is to control the white blood cell count and to relieve symptoms. The growth of malignant cells is controlled by chemotherapeutic agents, the two most common being busulfan and hydroxyurea. Busulfan is given in pulses for several weeks and then is discontinued after white blood cell counts return to normal. The usual dosage is 1 to 4 mg/day until normal results are achieved. During the busulfan treatment, peripheral blood counts must be monitored to prevent life-threatening pancytopenia. After prolonged use of busulfan, pulmonary fibrosis, skin pigmentation, hypogonadism, or a muscle-wasting syndrome with features of Addison's disease may develop (Haut, Abbott, Wintrobe, & Cartwright, 1961).

Hydroxyurea, which must be given daily, is another commonly used drug that effectively suppresses myelopoiesis. It provides more erratic control of the leukemia and requires monitoring of blood counts every week. The most common dosage is 500 mg to 2 g/day (Kennedy, 1972).

The chemotherapy drugs control the growth of the malignant cells but do not eradicate the disease. Patients who achieve normal white blood cell counts continue to have Ph^1 chromosome–positive cells in their bone marrow (Champlin, 1986). Chemotherapy relieves the symptoms of the disease, but no single agent has been shown to delay the development of a blast crisis or to prolong survival.

Splenectomy has been suggested as a potential treatment of CML. In general, splenectomy has not proved to be beneficial in prolonging the chronic phase or the patient's survival (Italian Cooperative Group, 1984). In patients with painful splenomegaly, anemia produced by hypersplenism, or severe thrombocytopenia, splenectomy may be considered. The decision to do a splenectomy in a patient with CML is difficult to make because of the complications from the operation and the propensity of these patients to develop extreme thrombocytosis after the operation (Champlin, 1986).

Combination chemotherapy has been attempted in patients with CML. It has resulted in significant toxicity and has provided no convincing evidence that the duration of the chronic phase is prolonged or that the probability of survival is improved (Cunningham et al., 1979).

Interferon is beginning to be evaluated for the treatment of CML. In initial studies, interferon has been effective in controlling granulocytosis and thrombocytosis in CML (Talpaz et al., 1987). The effectiveness of interferon will need further study to determine its role in the treatment of CML.

The prognosis for patients in the acute phase is poor. Once patients have entered the acute phase, survival without treatment may be limited to 2 to 6 months.

Patients who present with the acute lymphocytic

leukemia–type crisis are treated with ALL standard therapy: vincristine and prednisone. At least one half of these patients will respond to this therapy with complete remission that can last from 2 to 18 months, utilizing aggressive induction or cyclical reinduction therapy (Janossy et al., 1979).

Patients who present with the acute myelogenous leukemia–type crisis do not respond to vincristine and prednisone, nor do they respond to the type of therapy utilized for acute myelogenous leukemia. Only 20 to 30 per cent achieve a remission with this intensive chemotherapy, and their remissions are brief (Cunningham et al., 1979).

Bone Marrow Transplantation

In the past several years, BMT has been utilized to treat CML. Approximately 65 per cent of patients in the chronic phase who received syngeneic transplants and 20 per cent who were treated in blast crisis have achieved complete remission (Champlin, 1986). Allogeneic transplantation has yielded a complete remission rate of 63 per cent in the chronic phase and 12 per cent in the acute phase (Champlin, 1986). Younger patients tolerate this procedure better than do older patients. Most centers do not perform transplant operations on patients older than 50 years. Investigation into the role of BMT as a treatment measure in CML continues.

Nursing Care

Nursing care of patients with CML revolves around the education and treatment of patients and family members. During the chronic phase, educating the patient and family about the disease and the initial chemotherapy is important. As the disease progresses and as patients develop more symptoms, nursing care will address alteration in protective mechanisms, nutritional status, and comfort and other areas, depending on the manifestations of disease progression (see Chapters 47 through 58).

Hairy Cell Leukemia

Overview

Hairy cell leukemia is described as a lymphoproliferative disease similar to CLL (Golde & Koeffler, 1985). It is usually seen in patients older than 30 years of age; the ratio of males to females is 5:1. It represents 2 per cent of all leukemias (Cawley, Burns, & Hayhoe, 1980).

Etiology

The etiology of hairy cell leukemia is unknown. Little information is available on environmental factors associated with this disease (Jacobs, 1986).

Clinical Features

Hairy cell leukemia is considered primarily a B-lymphocyte disorder. The term *hairy* describes the projections on the abnormal lymphocyte that are characteristic of the disease (Golde & Koeffler, 1985).

Patients may be asymptomatic, but they usually present with symptoms caused by splenomegaly, pancytopenia, or infection (Golomb et al., 1978). Splenomegaly is present in 80 to 90 per cent of patients, whereas the presence of lymphadenopathy is unusual (Golde & Koeffler, 1985; Golomb et al., 1978). Patients may experience moderate to severe pancytopenia (Golde & Koeffler, 1985).

Splenectomy Treatment

When patients become symptomatic, treatment for hairy cell leukemia is initiated. Splenectomy is usually the first treatment. The cytopenias related to the splenic sequestration are improved by splenectomy, although not completely in most cases. Splenectomy is usually beneficial to all patients, but approximately half will require further therapy at a later date (Golomb et al., 1978).

Chemotherapy

Hairy cell leukemia progresses in two different forms. One, in which the bone marrow is replaced by hair cells, causes pancytopenia. In the other, the disease appears with an increasing white blood cell count and resembles a leukemia (Golomb et al., 1978). Usually chemotherapy is required for both forms of disease.

Various drug regimens have been utilized with varying effects: chlorambucil as a single agent, and multi-agent regimens that contained rubidazone, ara-C, cyclophosphamide, and high-dose methotrexate and leucovorin rescue have been used (Golomb et al., 1978). Studies of 2′-deoxycoformycin have shown complete bone marrow remission can be achieved and may be long-lasting (Urba et al., 1989). This drug needs further investigation before it is approved by the Food and Drug Administration.

2-Chlorodeoxyadenosine (2-CDA) is a new lymphocyte-selective, antineoplastic drug under clinical investigation. A study by Piro and colleagues (1990) indicates that 2-CDA has become an effective therapy for hairy cell leukemia. In 12 patients treated with 2-CDA, 11 patients obtained complete remission, the longest remission being 3.8 years. Trials are continuing with this drug to evaluate long-term complete remissions.

The treatment of choice at present is the interferons, although 2-CDA may become the most effective therapy. Interferon has shown high response rates in large numbers of patients (Golomb et al., 1978). The length of response to the interferons is now being investigated. Approximately 80 per cent of patients treated with interferon-α achieve beneficial clinical responses, but there are few complete responders (<10 per cent) (Figlin, 1989).

Radiation Therapy

Radiation therapy provides symptomatic relief of bone pain. In hairy cell leukemia, bone involvement can occur that causes lytic bone lesions (Jacobs, 1986). Bilateral hip joint involvement with pain and necrosis of the joint is the most common symptom (Jacobs, 1986). Radiation therapy to local areas of involvement can provide symptomatic relief of pain and radiographic changes of lytic bone lesions.

Nursing Care

Some patients with hairy cell leukemia have a very indolent course with little nursing intervention required. Others require nursing care similar to that performed for CLL, depending on presenting symptoms. Infection is a major cause of death; therefore, alteration in protective mechanisms is an important problem. Alteration in comfort because of splenomegaly or bone lesions will be another area for nursing interventions. As pancytopenia develops, nursing skills related to blood component therapy and administration of chemotherapeutic agents will be necessary. As with the other leukemias, nursing care will be an integral part of the team approach.

LYMPHOMAS

The lymphomas consist of two major subtypes: Hodgkin's disease and non-Hodgkin's lymphomas. In 1932 Thomas Hodgkin first described a disease that was characterized by progressive enlargement of the lymph nodes. Many years later, Hodgkin's disease became distinct from other lymphomas when the giant Reed-Sternberg cell was recognized in some lymphomas and not in others. This differentiation resulted in the classification of Hodgkin's disease, which is characterized by the presence of Reed-Sternberg cells, and non-Hodgkin's lymphomas, which are characterized by an absence of Reed-Sternberg cells. Although both diseases have some similarities, they are distinctly different in cellular origin, pattern of spread, and response to treatment. They are addressed separately with references to similarities and differences throughout the text.

Hodgkin's Disease

Overview

The treatment for Hodgkin's disease and the survival rate have improved dramatically in the past two decades. Once a fatal disease, the current 5-year survival rate is estimated to be between 80 and 90 per cent; the 10-year survival rate is an estimated 60 to 70 per cent. Much of this success is attributable to understanding the disease process and to technicologic advances in radiotherapy and complex chemotherapeutic methods.

According to the American Cancer Society (1989), an estimated 7400 new cases of Hodgkin's disease will occur in 1989. This number represents approximately 1 per cent of all cancers, which means that Hodgkin's disease is not common. Hodgkin's disease may develop at any age, from early childhood to advanced old age. A bimodal curve of age incidence is found, with a peak in the United States in the mid to late twenties and a second peak after the age of 50 years. The young adult group is composed equally of men and women, and the predominant disease is the nodular sclerosis subtype. Among older patients, men exceed women. Survival and disease-free survival decrease as age increases (American Cancer Society, 1989; DeVita, Hellman, & Rosenberg, 1985).

Etiology

The etiology of Hodgkin's disease is unknown, although many theories have been explored. Several peculiar characteristics of Hodgkin's disease have implicated viral, possibly genetic, and environmental factors.

Findings suggest that an infectious process, possibly viral, may be involved. Long-standing observations have indicated a defective T-cell functioning and a persistent immune system deficiency in patients with Hodgkin's disease. Similarities have also been noted between Hodgkin's disease and graft-versus-host disease. The autoimmune response could be indicative of a virus and lack of T-cell response. Other studies have indicated an increased risk of Hodgkin's disease with a prior history of infectious mononucleosis; however, an etiologic association of Hodgkin's disease with Epstein-Barr virus has not been confirmed. Other nonconclusive observations include a higher than expected incidence in the disease in siblings of the same sex and an increased risk of Hodgkin's disease with higher economic and educational status (DeVita et al., 1985; Haskell & Parker, 1985).

Studies presenting results that contradict the viral contagious bias have indicated that although siblings have demonstrated a higher risk for contracting Hodgkin's disease, it is very rare to observe this pattern with marital partners. In addition, health professionals caring for patients with Hodgkin's disease have not shown an increased incidence (Haskell & Parker, 1985). Despite interesting findings, it is not known what causes the disease or what is required to prevent it.

Origin and Spread

Although information is inconclusive regarding the cause of Hodgkin's disease, there has been greater understanding of the tumor's clinical behavior, including its pattern of spread and prognostic indications, such as histologic type and extent of disease.

In the 1960s and 1970s a large number of patients at clinical research centers underwent very careful clinical evaluations and laporatomies, which precisely identified the extent of abdominal disease. Important information regarding the origin and spread of disease resulted from these studies.

It appears that Hodgkin's disease arises as a single focal area, beginning in lymph nodes in more than 90 per cent of patients. In the early stages, the disease remains confined to lymph nodes for a variable period, making diagnosis sometimes difficult until multiple nodes are involved. Kaplan (1981) and Rosenberg (1986) have documented that in the majority of cases, Hodgkin's disease spreads in predictable patterns from the original site to lymph nodes in other areas. Disease usually spreads to adjacent lymph nodes. This orderly pattern of contiguous spread is most evident in nodular sclerosing Hodgkin's disease. For example, a lesion that originates in the mediastinum will first spread to nodes in the lower neck and then to nodes in the upper retroperitoneal area. Figure 35–1 represents the orderly pattern of contiguous lymphoid spread characteristic of Hodgkin's disease (Rosenberg, 1986).

There are exceptions. Other histologic types may also spread contiguously, but some lesions first noted in the cervical region skip the mediastinum and spread to retroperitoneal nodes without causing intrathoracic disease. It is suggested that spread occurs by retrograde flow in the thoracic duct. It is also possible that disease begins in the retroperitoneum but does not become evident until it spreads to the cervical nodes.

Disease spreads to extranodal areas by direct extension; for example, it spreads from hilar lymph nodes to lungs—a vascular invasion—which then results in hematogenous dissemination. When the spleen becomes involved, it is usually evidence of hematogenous dissemination and raises the possibility of liver and bone marrow involvement. Conversely, no evidence of splenic disease would suggest an absence of hematogenous dissemination to other organs. By this predictable pattern of spread, the spleen represents the final lymph node area of involvement before hematogenous dissemination occurs. Therefore, the most important fact influencing both staging and treatment is that Hodgkin's disease is a unifocal disease that usually spreads in a contiguous manner (DeVita, 1982; Haskell & Parker, 1985; Lacher, 1985; Rapaport, 1987).

Histopathologic Classification

Hodgkin's disease differs histologically from other lymphomas. In Hodgkin's disease, the diagnostic cell—the Reed-Sternberg cell—rarely predominates on a biopsy section and sometimes is difficult to find. Most of the tumor mass is usually composed of lacunar cells and numerous inflammatory cells that are presumed not to be neoplastic. The Reed-Sternberg cell is multinucleated, and each nucleus contains a giant nucleolus. Mononuclear cells with neoplastic features are also evident and are sometimes referred to as Hodgkin's cells or pre-Sternberg cells. These cells alone may not be distinctive enough to diagnose Hodgkin's disease without the presence of Reed-Sternberg cells (Rapaport, 1987).

According to the Rye classification, which was developed in the 1960s and is widely used, Hodgkin's disease is divided into four categories. The histopathologic identification reflects the host's resistance and subsequently the prognosis, which proceeds from favorable to less favorable. The four categories are listed in Table 35–8: lymphocyte predominance, nodular sclerosis, mixed cellularity, and lymphocyte depletion.

The first and last subgroups are the least common. The lymphocyte predominance subgroup has a good prognosis and is most commonly found in young males with localized cervical node involvement; the lymphocyte depletion subgroup has the least favorable prognosis; biopsy specimens indicate an increased number of Reed-Sternberg cells and a breakdown of normal cellular components. Lymphocyte depletion is indicative of a breakdown in host resistance. The two more common subtypes, nodular sclerosis and mixed cellularity, fall between lymphocyte predominance and lymphocyte depletion in degree of neoplastic cells and prognosis.

The nodular sclerosis subtype is most often seen in younger patients and twice as frequently in women as in men. Because these large so-called lacunar cells are predominant, it is sometimes impossible to find Reed-Sternberg cells. All subtypes except nodular sclerosis may develop into a less favorable subtype (Haskell & Parker, 1985; Rapaport, 1987).

As prognostic indicators, the histologic subtypes are dependent on other important variables, which include volume and site of disease, extent of disease spread, and presence of systemic symptoms (known as staging); age; and sex.

Clinical Presentation

One characteristic symptom of Hodgkin's disease generally is progressive, painless, "rubbery" lymph node enlargement, usually localized in the neck region in 60 to 80 per cent of cases (DeVita et al., 1985). Most patients are asymptomatic, but 40 per cent of patients may have associated B symptoms (systemic symptoms) of fever, night sweats, and unexplained weight loss. Occasionally a patient is diagnosed after a mediastinal mass is discovered on a routine chest radiograph or after a persistant cough provokes a visit to a physician. When disease originates in the retroperitoneal area, it may be accompanied by prolonged fever. Rarely, a patient may present with complaints indicative of an extranodal lesion, for example, gastrointestinal bleeding or pain due to obstruction.

Other disorders with similar characteristics are infectious mononucleosis, acquired immune deficiency syndrome (AIDS), or other infectious inflammations.

Diagnosis and Staging

The initial evaluation of Hodgkin's disease requires an adequate surgical specimen for the histologic diagnosis. A detailed clinical history is required that establishes the presence or absence of systemic symptoms, including fever, night sweats, and weight loss. A complete physical examination includes an examination of all lymph node chains, including Waldeyer's ring, and

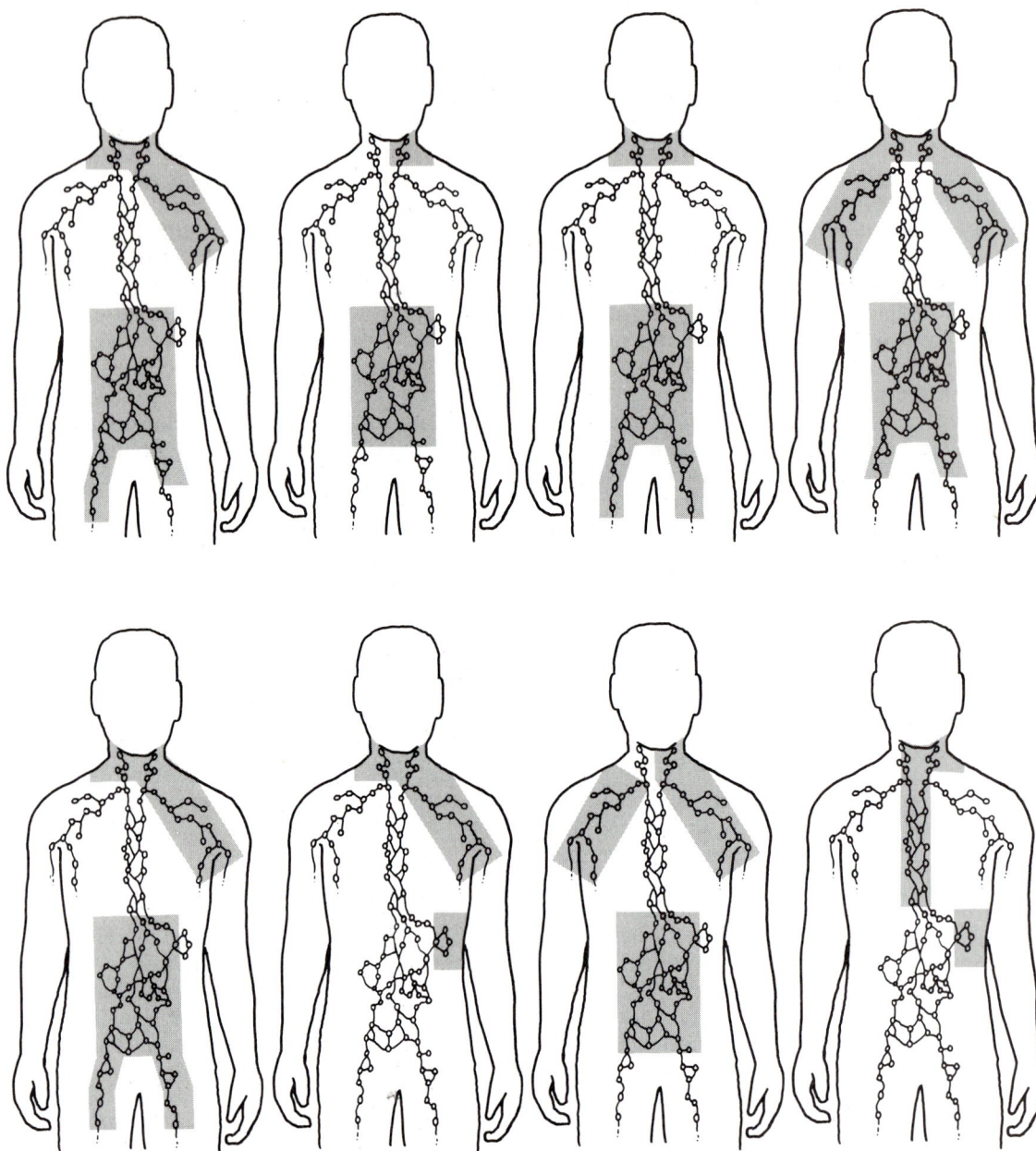

Figure 35–1. Orderly pattern of contiguous lymphoid spread in Hodgkin's disease. (From Rosenberg, S. A. [1986]. Hodgkin's disease: No stage beyond cure. *Hospital Practice, 21* [8], 91–98, 101–108. Reproduced by permission.)

a determination of abdominal involvement, such as that of the liver and spleen. Specific laboratory and radiologic procedures are listed in Table 35–9.

Extent of Disease. The extent or stage of disease strongly influences the choice of treatment and must be carefully determined in each patient. This process is referred to as staging. *Clinical staging* usually refers to all procedures except a staging laparotomy. *Pathologic staging* refers to findings indicated from a staging laparotomy.

After the initial staging work-up is completed, the extent of the disease is staged by a widely used system called the Ann Arbor Staging Classification of Hodgkin's disease (Table 35–10). The Ann Arbor system divides Hodgkin's disease into four stages based on the extent of disease involvement. Stages range from a

single node or region of involvement (stage I) to a diffuse disseminated involvement (stage IV). In the first three stages, extranodal involvement is delineated using the subscript E, meaning direct extension rather than that of hematologic dissemination, as in stage IV. Additionally, all stages are given the letter A to indicate the absence of systemic symptoms or the letter B to indicate the presence of systemic symptoms. Patients with B symptoms have unexplained fever, night sweats, or weight loss of more than 10 per cent of body weight in the preceding 6 months. The presence of B symptoms indicates a less favorable prognosis.

Laparotomy. A number of investigators are now questioning the routine application of staging laparotomies in Hodgkin's disease. The procedure includes a splenectomy, liver biopsy, and excisional biopsies of the retroperitoneal nodes. Laparotomies increase the accuracy of staging patients with Hodgkin's disease beyond that achieved by clinical methods. There is no question that the use of laparotomies in research treatment centers has provided important information on the origin and spread of Hodgkin's disease. The controversy rests on the issues of whether—and if so, when—to perform surgical staging laparotomies.

Studies at Stanford University Medical Center, where laparotomies are performed routinely, indicated that the disease was more extensive in 22 per cent of patients clinically staged and less extensive in 9.6 per cent of patients (Rosenberg, 1986). Changes in a patient's stage after laparotomy occur in about one third of patients, and appropriate treatment is given. The procedure should be performed only if the information obtained will potentially change the course of treatment and not just change the stage of the disease (Bonadonna, Valagussa, & Santoro, 1986).

Staging laparotomies are usually restricted to patients in whom radiotherapy alone will be used for treatment. Patients with a clinical stage of IIIB or IV Hodgkin's disease require chemotherapy and therefore would not be candidates for a staging laparotomy. Similarly, patients with a clinical stage of IB, IIB, or IIA with mediastinal involvement generally require chemotherapy and radiotherapy (combined modality) and would not be candidates for laparotomy. Therefore, candidates eligible for staging laparotomy given no medical contraindications are patients with clinical stages of IA, IIA without mediastinal involvement, and IIIA Hodgkin's disease (Ultmann & Bitran, 1989). Because the clinical staging process is not always absolute, some claim advantages to doing staging laparotomies on all patients who are not clearly in stage IV. Nevertheless, the routine use of staging laparotomies should only be considered at institutions that conduct clinical trials in which the results of therapy can be related to sites and volume of disease (DeVita, 1982).

Table 35–8. RYE CLASSIFICATION OF HODGKIN'S DISEASE

Subgroup	Major Histologic Features	Approximate Frequency (%)
Lymphocyte predominance	Abundant normal-appearing lymphocytes with or without benign histiocytes; occasionally nodular, rare Reed-Sternberg cells	2–10
Nodular sclerosis	Nodules of lymphoid tissue separated by bands of collagen; numerous variants of Reed-Sternberg cells	40–80
Mixed cellularity	Pleomorphic infiltrate of eosinophils, plasma cells, histiocytes, and lymphocytes, with numerous Reed-Sternberg cells	20–40
Lymphocyte depletion	Paucity of lymphocytes with numerous Reed-Sternberg cells, diffuse fibrosis and necrosis	2–15

(Adapted from Rosenberg, S. A. [1986]. Hodgkin's disease: No stage beyond cure. *Hospital Practice, 21*[8], 91–98, 101–108.)

Table 35–9. LABORATORY AND RADIOLOGIC PROCEDURES USED IN DETERMINING THE EXTENT OF DISEASE IN HODGKIN'S DISEASE

Study or Procedure	Function
Laboratory Studies	
CBC, platelet count, ESR	Evidence of peripheral blood involvement
Liver function tests, particularly serum alkaline phosphatase	Hepatic involvement
Urinalysis and renal function tests	Proteinuria
Radiographic Studies	
For thoracic disease: Chest radiographs, posteroanterior and lateral; whole lung tomograms (if abnormal chest radiograph)	Visualizes mediastinal masses, hilar and paratracheal lymphadenopathy
For abdominal disease: CT scan of the abdomen	Can visualize lymph node enlargement in areas not seen on lymphangiogram; visualizes tumor nodules in spleen and liver
Bilateral lower lymphangiogram (dye injected into lymphatic channels in both feet)	Internal structural changes in a node from Hodgkin's disease may be evident on lymphangiogram but not on a CT scan because the node may not be large enough
Intravenous pyelogram	
Bilateral bone marrow biopsy	To obtain histologic report of marrow. Sometimes omitted in young patients with early disease I and II with favorable histologic results on lymph node biopsy

CBC, complete blood count; ESR, erythrocyte sedimentation rate; CT, computed tomography.

Disadvantages of doing a staging laparotomy include the risk of significant morbidity (0.7 per cent) and mortality (0.7 per cent) that is associated with the surgical procedure. Infection is always a possibility and is confounded by the immunosuppressive effects of radiation therapy, chemotherapy, and anergy from the disease itself. To decrease the risk of pneumococcal pneumonia, a prophylactic pneumococcal vaccine is sometimes given before a planned splenectomy (Ultmann & Bitran, 1989).

Prognosis

Many factors influence the prognosis of Hodgkin's disease in an individual patient. Although current treatment has resulted in a dramatic increase in survival, some patients still respond poorly. Many factors contribute to a favorable or a less favorable prognosis (Table 35–11).

The prognosis of Hodgkin's disease is dependent on several variables, including the histologic classification

Table 35-10. ANN ARBOR STAGING SYSTEM FOR HODGKIN'S DISEASE AND NON-HODGKIN'S LYMPHOMA

Stage	Definition
I	Involvement of a single lymph node region (I) or of a single extralymphatic organ or site (I_E).
II	Involvement of two or more lymph node regions on the same side of the diaphragm (II) or involvement of an extralymphatic organ or site and one or more lymph node regions on the same side of the diaphragm (II_E).
III	Involvement of lymph nodes on both sides of the diaphragm (III), which may also be accompanied by localized involvement of extralymphatic organs or sites (III_E) or involvement of the spleen (III_S), or both (III_{SE}).
IV	Diffuse or disseminated involvement of one or more extralymphatic* organs or tissues, with or without associated lymph node involvement.

Each stage is subclassified by the presence (B) or absence (A) of one or more of the following unexplained symptoms:
Weight loss >10% over 6 months
Fever >38° C
Night sweats

*Extralymphatic may include the following sites: lung, bone, bone marrow, liver, or brain.

as it reflects host resistance and therefore the prognosis. The extent and volume of disease at diagnosis—less being better—are equally important influential prognostic variables. Other factors include age, older age being associated with decreased host resistance and decreased tolerance to aggressive therapy; and gender, women having a better prognosis than men, which is associated with the proclivity for young women to have nodular sclerosing Hodgkin's disease. The nodular sclerosis subtype inherently has less dissemination to extranodal sites. The presence of systemic B symptoms is associated with a less favorable prognosis (Rapaport, 1987).

Treatment

The goal of management of Hodgkin's disease is cure. The success of the treatment for Hodgkin's disease has improved dramatically over the past 20 years. Several factors have contributed to this success. They include:

- The orderly process by which the disease spreads and the ability to stage the disease clinically and pathologically.

Table 35-11. VARIABLES IN THE PROGNOSIS OF HODGKIN'S DISEASE

Favorable	Less Favorable
Clinical Factors	
Young age	Older age (over 60)
Stages IA, IIA, III1A	Bulky mediastinal disease
	Stage III2B or IVA or B
	B symptoms
	Male sex
Histologic Factors	
Lymphocyte predominance	Lymphocyte depletion
Few Reed-Sternberg cells	Many Reed-Sternberg cells

(Data from Rapaport, 1987.)

- Modern megavoltage techniques in radiation therapy, which allow beam direction to specific sites but shield normal tissue to prevent unnecessary damage. Consequently, tumoricidal doses of radiation can be administered, thus eradicating disease.
- Combination chemotherapy (e.g., mechlorethamine [Mustargen], vincristine [Oncovin], procarbazine, and prednisone [MOPP], doxorubicin [Adriamycin], bleomycin, vinblastine, and dacarbazine, [ABVD]), which is curative in many patients with disseminated disease.

Treatment of Hodgkin's disease is based, for the most part, on the stage of disease rather than on the histologic type. Various forms of treatment include radiation therapy, combination chemotherapy, and combined methods, which include both radiation therapy and chemotherapy prescribed at different intervals.

The basic goal of radiation therapy is the eradication of all tumor in a specific tissue volume or in all sites of disease. Radiation fields used in treating Hodgkin's disease are shown in Figure 35-2. Hodgkin's disease is very radiosensitive, and it has been documented that eradication of tumor is proportional to the dose of radiation administered. Thus the therapeutic objective is to give the maximum dose possible to eradicate disease without compromising normal tissue (Kaplan, 1981).

Patients with stage IA or IIA disease can obtain a complete response following either involved field or subtotal nodal irradiation. It has not been determined whether radiation limited to involved fields results in a decrease in long-term survival as compared with "extended field" or "total nodal" irradiation. The last two techniques eradicate suspected disease as well as known disease. Ten-year survival ranges from 90 per cent to 76 per cent, respectively.

Patients with stage IB or IIB disease have a higher rate of relapse after radiation therapy than patients with stage IA or IIA disease. Therefore, treatment of early-stage disease with B symptoms is often combination chemotherapy.

Patients with stage IIIA disease present a more controversial therapeutic group. There are several approaches to treatment for these patients. Some institutions recommend radiation therapy, followed by salvage treatment with chemotherapy on relapse. Total nodal irradiation as a primary treatment has been associated with a 5-year relapse-free survival. Because of the efficacy of salvage chemotherapy, rates of 10-year freedom from second relapse are similar to those of combined methods (radiation and chemotherapy) in one study (82 per cent versus 86 per cent) (Willett et al., 1987b). Other institutions, such as Stanford and Yale, recommend combined modality for patients with stage IIIA disease. Studies have indicated an improvement in 10-year survival in patients treated with radiation therapy and chemotherapy compared with those treated with total nodal irradiation alone (79 per cent versus 57 per cent) (Hoppe, Cox, Rosenberg, & Kaplan, 1982).

In patients with advanced disease, defined as stage

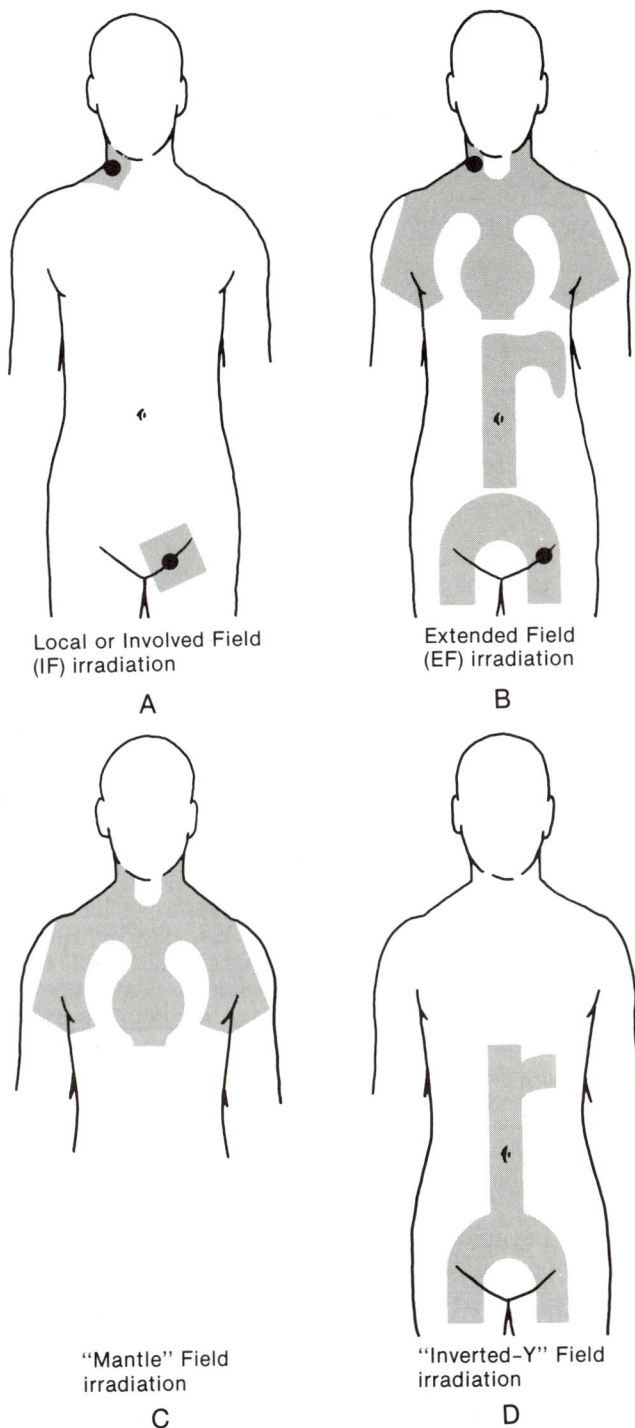

Figure 35–2. Radiation fields in the treatment of Hodgkin's disease. (From Haskell, C. M., & Parker, R. G. [1985]. Hodgkin's disease. In C. Haskell, *Cancer treatment* [2nd ed., pp. 758–788]. Philadelphia: W. B. Saunders Co. Reproduced by permission.)

IIIA with five or more nodules in the spleen, stage IIIB, or stage IVA or IVB, combination chemotherapy is clearly the treatment of choice. Various regimens have been evaluated over the years, with cures using chemotherapy alone ranging from 25 to 60 per cent in advanced disease (Rosenberg, 1986). The first successful combination of drugs—the well-known and widely used MOPP regimen—was developed by DeVita and

colleagues in 1964 at the National Cancer Institute (NCI). The combination mechlorethamine, vincristine (Oncovin), procarbazine, and prednisone regimen is given in 28-day cycles, with 2 weeks of treatment and 2 weeks of recovery period. This combination of drugs is administered for at least six courses, or two courses beyond evidence of disease for consolidation. The results of the NCI experience after a 20-year study demonstrated that 84 per cent of patients treated with MOPP had a complete remission, 66 per cent remained disease free for 10 years, and overall disease-free survival was 54 per cent at 15 years (DeVita, 1982). The Stanford group recommends chemotherapy plus total lymphoid irradiation for patients who have stage IIIA disease with splenic involvement and for stages IVA and IVB. A staging laparotomy is done to confirm splenic involvement in stage IIIA patients.

Over the years, several other chemotherapy or combined modality programs have been compared with the success of MOPP. The approach is to use a different non-cross-resistant regimen. These combinations support the Goldie-Goldman hypothesis that the earlier the tumor is exposed to all potential therapeutic methods, the better the chance of avoiding refractoriness to treatment, which is the greatest obstacle to cure (Goldie, Goldman, & Guaduskus, 1982).

The best and most studied is the ABVD combination of drugs doxorubicin (Adriamycin), bleomycin, vinblastine, and dacarbazine, developed by Bonadonna and colleagues in Milan. ABVD has the advantage of efficacy without showing evidence of the sterility and secondary malignancies found in patients receiving MOPP (Bonadonna et al., 1988). Many clinical trials are still ongoing, comparing ABVD and MOPP as primary treatments or alternating the two drug regimens and thus providing a non-cross-resistant regimen. The Bonadonna group after an 8-year comparative study, has found that alternating cycles of ABVD and MOPP is superior to using either one alone (84 per cent versus 64 per cent) (Binet et al., 1981). Other combinations are being studied with the intent of reducing the toxicities of the current regimens. Table 35–12 lists the various chemotherapeutic agents used in the treatment of Hodgkin's disease.

The success of chemotherapy, like that of radiation therapy, is dependent on the dosage and timing of the drug. Reduction of the dose or dose rate by as little as 20 per cent in animal models can totally abolish the curative effect of combination chemotherapy (DeVita, 1982). Because of some of the severe side effects from the most successful regimens (MOPP, ABVD), patients may request dose and schedule changes to avoid disruption in their life styles. It is extremely important for the oncology nurse to explain to the patient that such alterations will decrease the effectiveness of treatment and ultimately may lead to the loss of life. The importance of side-effect management is critical to help patients accept and tolerate life-saving therapy.

Side Effects

The most commonly used chemotherapy regimens, MOPP and ABVD, cause nausea and vomiting. Antic-

Table 35–12. CHEMOTHERAPY REGIMENS FOR HODGKIN'S DISEASE

Regimen	Dosage
MOPP	
Mechlorethamine	6 mg/m², IV, days 1 and 8
Vincristine	1.4 mg/m², IV, days 1 and 8 (maximum 2.0 mg)
Procarbazine	100 mg/m², PO, days 1 to 14
Prednisone	40 mg/m², PO, days 1 to 14 (cycles 1 and 4 only)
Cycles repeated every 4 weeks.	
COPP	
Cyclophosphamide	600 mg/m², IV, days 1 and 8
Vincristine	1.4 mg/m², IV, days 1 and 8 (maximum 2.0 mg)
Procarbazine	100 mg/m², PO, days 1 to 14
Prednisone	40 mg/m², PO, days 1 to 14 (cycles 1 and 4 only)
Cycles repeated every 4 weeks, as described for MOPP.	
MVPP	
Mechlorethamine	6 mg/m², IV, days 1 and 8
Vinblastine	6 mg/m², IV, days 1 and 8
Procarbazine	100 mg/m², PO, days 1 to 14
Prednisone	40 mg/m², PO, days 1 to 14
Drug administration during a 42-day cycle with 4 weeks of rest.	
ABVD	
Doxorubicin	25 mg/m², IV, every 2 weeks
Bleomycin	10 units/m², IV, every 2 weeks
Vinblastine	6 mg/m², IV, every 2 weeks
Dacarbazine	375 mg/m², IV, every 2 weeks
Maximum total cumulative dose of doxorubicin 450 mg/m² and 450 units bleomycin.	
Dosage of drugs reduced for bone marrow suppression.	
B-CAVe	
Bleomycin	5.0 units/m², IV, days 1, 28, 35
CCNU	100 mg/m², PO, day 1
Doxorubicin	60 mg/m², IV, day 1
Vinblastine	5 mg/m², IV, day 1
Cycles repeated every 6 weeks (if blood counts permit) to a total of 9 cycles.	

IV, intravenously; PO, orally.

ipatory nausea and vomiting are not unusual and should be prevented. In one study of patients with Hodgkin's disease, conditioned responses were usually firmly developed by the fourth or fifth course of treatment (Devlin, Maguire, Phillips, & Crowther, 1987; Devlin, Maguire, Phillips, Crowther, & Chambers, 1987). Early recognition and avoidance of anticipatory nausea and vomiting are the most effective nursing interventions. Regular nausea and vomiting require skilled nursing prevention and intervention and are discussed in Chapter 47. Other side effects such as hair loss are related to administration of individual drugs and are discussed in Chapter 22. It is extremely important to assist the patient in controlling these difficult side effects to maintain optimal curative doses.

Fatigue and lack of energy during treatment and at 1 year after treatment had been reported in several studies of patients with Hodgkin's disease. Preparing the patient for this reaction may help to reduce anxiety should it occur (Fobair, 1986).

Patients receiving radiation to the chest experience sore throats, difficulty swallowing, nausea, and vomiting. The nutritional status of the patient may be compromised owing to difficulties in eating and lack of appetite. Radiation to the abdominal and pelvic areas can cause the patient discomfort from diarrhea, which then leads to fluid and electrolyte loss. Good skin care is essential, because a common side effect in radiation therapy is skin desquamation. Measures for nursing intervention are addressed in Chapter 20.

Complications of Treatment

Years ago, many of the following complications were not evident. In fact, they are truly an indication of success in the treatment of Hodgkin's disease. The acute toxicity and long-term complications of treatment are proportional to the ability to cure and keep the patient free of disease.

Hypothyroidism. Late complications of high-dose irradiation include chronic hypothyroidism. Hypothyroidism is most common in patients receiving radiation to the cervical nodes and can be expected to occur in 60 to 70 per cent of patients (Golde & Koeffler, 1985). A thyroid-stimulating hormone (TSH) level should be followed periodically after treatment to evaluate for thyroid hormone replacement.

Sterility. MOPP chemotherapy is known to cause sterility. Several studies have indicated that fertility may still be possible for some young patients treated for Hodgkin's disease (teens to early twenties). Little suppression of fertility occurs in young women; suppression is greater in men receiving MOPP (DeVita, 1982; Horning, Hoppe, & Kaplan, 1981). Men receiving MOPP and mechlorethamine, vinblastine, procarbazine, and prednisone (MVPP) chemotherapy show evidence of permanent azoospermia, testicular atrophy, and elevated follicle-stimulating hormone after one or two cycles of treatment. Before treatment, men should be given the opportunity to store sperm.

Women receiving MOPP chemotherapy have associated ovarian failure after six cycles of MOPP. Alternating MOPP and ABVD reduces the number of MOPP cycles and therefore the risk of sterility. Horning and colleagues (1981) found that even after intensive treatment with combination chemotherapy for Hodgkin's disease, women became pregnant and delivered normal children. A woman undergoing a staging laparotomy should have an oophoropexy in case subsequent radiation affects the abdomen or pelvic area. Radiation therapy can result in the loss of ovarian function even with these precautions in 30 to 70 per cent of patients receiving pelvic irradiation (Cooley & Cobb, 1986; Horning et al., 1981).

Second Malignancy. Among chemotherapy drugs commonly used for Hodgkin's disease, nitrogen mustard, chlorambucil, procarbazine, and lomustine (CCNU) are the ones most associated with therapy-related leukemias. In addition, patients treated with chemotherapy and radiation therapy (combined modality) are at greater risk for late-onset acute leukemia and non-Hodgkin's lymphoma. These risks mandate making a careful assessment by the physician before recommending combined modality therapy for stage IIIA disease and limiting treatment to one therapy or the other in early disease. All patients receiving combined modality therapy need long-term follow-up.

Non-Hodgkin's Lymphomas

Overview

Non-Hodgkin's lymphomas are a heterogeneous group of malignant neoplasms that originate in the lymphoid compartment of the immune system. It has long been recognized that they possess a wide and often bewildering spectrum of clinical and biologic behavior from indolent to very aggressive. As previously mentioned, the boundaries that separate non-Hodgkin's lymphomas from other diseases, for example, lymphocytic leukemia and lymphocyte-predominant Hodgkin's disease, are often difficult to determine. Non-Hodgkin's lymphomas can be defined as malignancies of the lymphatic tissue, with the exception of Hodgkin's disease, acute and chronic lymphoid leukemias, multiple myeloma, Waldenström's macroglobulinemia, and hairy cell leukemia (Haskell & Parker, 1985).

In the United States, non-Hodgkin's lymphomas occur three times as often as Hodgkin's disease. The American Cancer Society (1989) estimates that approximately 32,000 new cases and 17,300 deaths will occur in 1989. For reasons that are not understood, the incidence of lymphoma is increasing yearly, especially in patients with autoimmune deficiencies (e.g., AIDS). The peak age incidence is higher than that for Hodgkin's disease, with about 25 per cent of cases occurring between the ages of 50 and 59 years and the greatest risk occurring between the ages of 60 and 69 years, with males predominating.

Etiology

The cause of non-Hodgkin's lymphoma remains unknown, although several theories have been postulated. A number of lymphomas have been associated with chromosome translocations and rearrangement of proto-oncogenes (e.g., bcl-2, c-myc). These changes may be important to the etiology and progression of the disease. In addition, certain viruses and the competence of the immune system play a role in some lymphomas.

Current data suggest an etiologic role for the HTLV 1 in some adult T-cell lymphomas. This virus has been strongly associated with adult T-cell malignancies in the Caribbean, parts of South Africa, and southwestern Japan. The HTLV 1 infection has also been found in patients with AIDS and subsequent lymphomas.

Burkitt's lymphoma, which is confined almost exclusively to Africa, is associated with the presence of the Epstein-Barr virus, a lymphotropic herpes virus. The precise role of this virus is unknown.

Compared with the general population, individuals with congenital and acquired immunodeficiencies (e.g., AIDS) and those receiving immunosuppressive treatment are at increased risk for developing non-Hodgkin's lymphoma. Inheritable immunodeficient states include Wiskott-Aldrich syndrome and Bloom's syndrome. Non-Hodgkin's lymphoma is 45 to 100 times more common among organ transplant patients (particularly renal), with lymphomas accounting for 29 per cent of cancers in these patients receiving immunosuppressive therapy (Sarna & Kagan, 1985a; Ultmann & Jacobs, 1985). Other patients predisposed to non-Hodgkin's lymphoma are those with autoimmune diseases, such as rheumatoid arthritis and systemic lupus erythematosus.

As mentioned, chromosomal abnormalities have also been linked with both immunodeficiency and lymphoma. Genetic abnormalities of chromosome 14 are recognized in many follicular lymphomas and in Burkitt's lymphoma.

Pathophysiology

To understand the different lymphomas and to appreciate the lymphoma classification systems, it is helpful to review the process of lymphocyte maturation. Lymphomas, for the most part, are the malignant counterpart of the maturing lymphocyte. Therefore, different lymphomas are related to different maturational phases of the lymphocyte. In the process of lymphocytic maturation, the early lymphocyte continues to mature in a predictable manner into an immunocompetent lymphocyte. In non-Hodgkin's lymphoma, an abnormal proliferation of neoplastic cells occurs that resembles a phase or site of maturation. Instead of progressing to the next phase, the cells remain fixed at one phase of development and continue to proliferate. These neoplastic cells may also take on functional characteristics and activities of their normal counterparts. It is possible to predict some of the clinical manifestations of non-Hodgkin's lymphoma based on characteristics of the predominant cell (or normal cell counterpart). The neoplastic cells often retain the surface of their cell of origin. Therefore, it is also possible to group these cells according to surface markers or phenotypic properties (Foon, Schroff, & Gale, 1982).

Lymphocytes consist of two functional classes of cells in the immune system: the T lymphocyte, which is involved in regulation of antibody synthesis and cellular immune processes, and the B lymphocyte, which contributes to the humoral immune response that requires antigen sensitization for maturation to occur. A third class of lymphocytes, the natural killer cells, occurs early in the T-cell lineage and does not require prior sensitization by antigen. In considering the nature of each lymphoma, it is helpful to visualize the specific site of lymphocytic maturation that is related to each neoplastic entity. Figure 35–3 illustrates lymphoid maturation and theoretic sites for development of non-Hodgkin's lymphomas. The lymphoid stem cell is programmed via the bone marrow to become a T-cell or B-cell precursor, respectively. B-

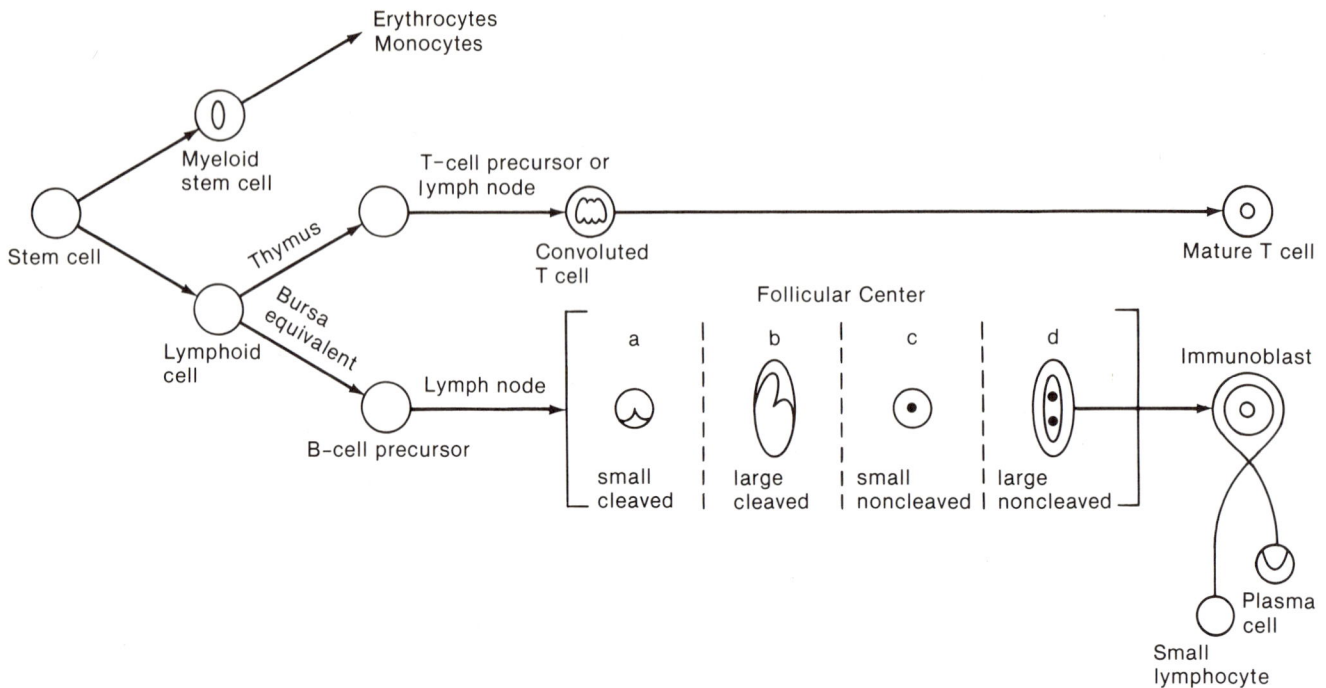

Figure 35–3. Maturation of the lymphocyte.

cell maturation occurs in the follicles of the lymph node after exposure to an antigen. B cells can be divided into four cytologic types that represent different stages of maturation and that contribute to the new classification system: (1) small cleaved, (2) large cleaved, (3) small noncleaved, and (4) large noncleaved. In some lymphoma classification systems, lymphomas are given names that are based on characteristics of their location in the activation process, for example, small cleaved cell lymphoma. The majority of lymphomas, approximately 70 per cent, are B-cell lymphomas. Lymphoid malignancies of T-cell origin are less common, consisting of approximately 20 to 30 per cent of lymphomas (Jaffe, 1986).

Cellular Origin. The cells of the immune system have different locations in the peripheral lymph nodes. Because lymphoma cells often retain certain characteristics of their cell of origin, it is often possible to relate tumors to their function and anatomic properties. Figure 35–4 depicts the normal lymph node architecture and areas in which malignancies may arise. Normal lymph nodes include B cells, T cells, and histiocytes. Approximately 10 per cent of lymphomas are of unknown origin, and less than 1 per cent are from true histiocytes.

Clinical correlations have been established that recognize the more indolent nature of nodular architecture and small cleaved lymphocytic cytologic characteristics and the more aggressive nature of diffuse architecture and large-cell characteristics.

Classification of Non-Hodgkin's Lymphomas

The many different categorization systems for non-Hodgkin's lymphomas have led to controversy and confusion and have made interpretation of treatment difficult for many practitioners. The Working Formulation of non-Hodgkin's Lymphoma for Clinical Usage was developed from a National Cancer Institute international cooperative study (1982). Table 35–13 lists the working formulation, which supersedes other classification systems. In the working formulation, tumors are divided into low-, intermediate-, and high-grade lymphomas, depending on the activity of the specific lymphoma. Lymphomas listed under each category are defined by histologic, anatomic, and immunomorphic characteristics (National Cancer Institute, 1982). Because many readers may be most familiar with the Rappaport or Lukes classification systems, they are compared in Table 35–13.

Most clinical protocols divide lymphomas into two broad categories: (1) indolent, or low grade, and (2) aggressive, or intermediate and high grade. Patients with low-grade non-Hodgkin's lymphoma usually have a relatively long survival, with or without aggressive treatment. Tumors can be controlled with chemotherapy, but they are rarely cured. High-grade tumors may result in death for the patient within 1 or 2 years, but paradoxically, with aggressive treatment, certain subsets of patients can be cured. Manifestations of specific lymphomas are addressed in a following section.

Clinical Presentation

The clinical presentation of patients with non-Hodgkin's lymphoma is similar to that of Hodgkin's disease and various other disorders involving the lymph system. Because palpable nodes are often found on normal individuals, differential diagnosis is dependent on size, shape, feel, and location of lymph nodes. Differences in clinical features of Hodgkin's disease and non-

Sinuses
Malignant Histiocytosis

Perifollicular
Lymphocytic Lymphoma
Intermediate Differentiation

Follicles
Nodular (Follicular) Lymphoma
Burkitt's Lymphoma

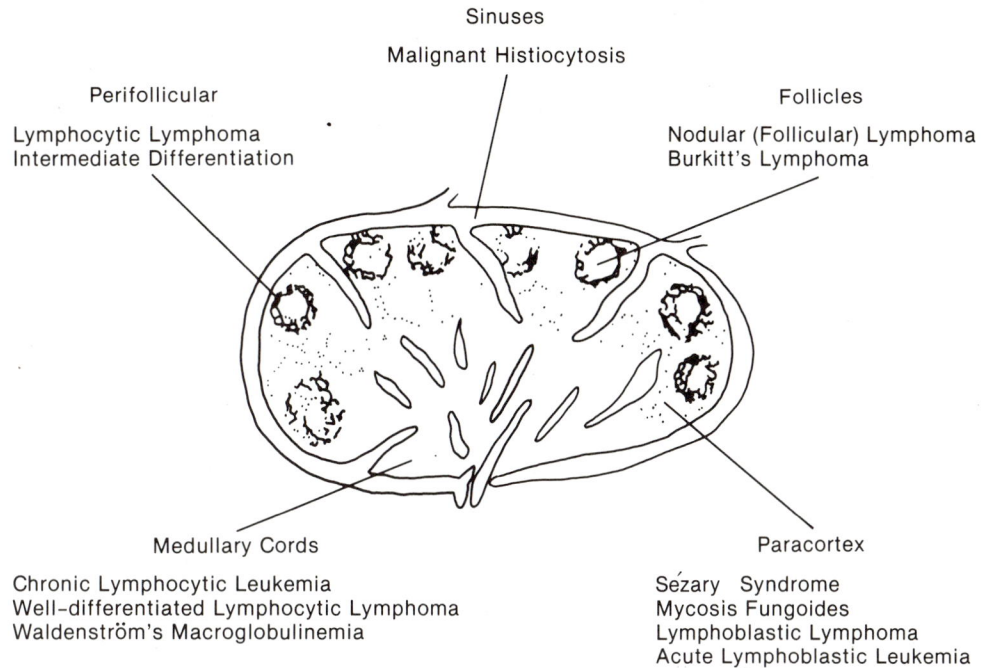

Figure 35–4. Lymph node. Non-Hodgkin's lymphomas according to functional anatomy. (From Mann, R. B., Jaffe, E. S., & Bernard, C. W. [1972]. Malignant lymphomas—a conceptual understanding of morphological diversity. *American Journal of Pathology, 94*, 103–191. Reproduced by permission.)

Medullary Cords
Chronic Lymphocytic Leukemia
Well-differentiated Lymphocytic Lymphoma
Waldenström's Macroglobulinemia

Paracortex
Sezary Syndrome
Mycosis Fungoides
Lymphoblastic Lymphoma
Acute Lymphoblastic Leukemia

Hodgkin's lymphoma are noted in Table 35–14. The most frequent clinical presentation in Hodgkin's disease and non-Hodgkin's lymphoma is painless superficial lymphadenopathy. A history of waxing and waning lymphadenopathy over a period of months is not unusual. Except for an awareness of lymph node enlargement, patients with lymphadenopathy are generally asymptomatic.

Systemic symptoms (fever, weight loss, night sweats) may be present but are more frequently seen in Hodgkin's disease and do not have as strong an association with poor prognosis as they do in Hodgkin's disease. Nodal involvement in Hodgkin's disease is typically axial (cervical, mediastinal, and para-aortic), whereas primary involvement of mesenteric nodes or extranodal sites, such as bone, gastrointestinal track, and brain, is rare. In contrast, non-Hodgkin's lymphoma is commonly more extensive, most often stage III or stage IV disease at diagnosis (DeVita et al., 1985). Non-Hodgkin's lymphoma frequently involves lymphoid sites such as epitrochlear nodes and Waldeyer's tonsillar ring. Localized disease is uncommon; extranodal disease, bone marrow infiltration, and bulky disease are often characteristic features. Truly localized disease is rare, appearing in approximately 10 per cent of patients who present with non-Hodgkin's lymphoma (DeVita et al., 1985).

Manifestations of Specific Lymphomas

Low-Grade Lymphoma. Lymphomas that exhibit a nodular type of histologic pattern display a more indolent behavior pattern than those possessing a diffuse histologic and therefore more aggressive nature. Low-grade lymphomas, according to the working formulation, consist of small lymphocytic lymphomas and follicular lymphomas, both small cleaved cell and mixed small cleaved cell. The corresponding Rappa-

port equivalents are listed in Table 35–13. Nearly all low-grade lymphomas are neoplasms of mature B-cell origin. The terms *good risk, indolent, favorable,* and *low-grade* as categorizing lymphomas are often used synonymously, although even in these subgroups there is a degree of clinical heterogeneity. These lymphomas are characterized by considerably longer survival, but various treatment approaches have failed to yield permanent cures.

Most often, patients with low-grade lymphomas present with widespread disease. Because of the indolent nature of the disease, patients remain asymptomatic, and therefore the disease remains unnoticed. By the time the patient is diagnosed, the low-grade lymphomas show wide dissemination of disease to lymph nodes, bone marrow, and occasionally the liver. Mediastinal lymph node involvement is less common than in Hodgkin's disease, but abdominal lymphadenopathy may be evident and is far more common in non-Hodgkin's lymphoma than in Hodgkin's disease.

Spontaneous regression of disease has been observed in various subtypes of lymphoma (Horning & Rosenberg, 1984). It has occurred in approximately 5 to 15 per cent of low-grade lymphomas and may occur in previously untreated patients or in patients who have relapsed after treatment. Duration can last longer than a year or can be indefinite. Though exciting when it occurs, the cause of spontaneous regression is unknown.

Histologic conversion over time from a low grade to a higher, more aggressive grade is also evident in low-grade lymphomas. Progression is from nodular to diffuse and from small to large cell (Acker et al., 1987). In one study, progression was evident 6 months later in 30 per cent of patients with an original diagnosis of low-grade lymphoma at biopsy (Hubbard et al., 1982). The most common progression is from nodular, poorly differentiated lymphoma (NPDL, Rappaport) or follic-

Table 35–13. CLASSIFICATION OF MALIGNANT NON-HODGKIN'S LYMPHOMAS

Working Formulation for Classification of Non-Hodgkin's Lymphomas for Clinical Usage	Rappaport Classification Equivalent	Lukes Classification
Low Grade		
Small lymphocytic	Diffuse well-differentiated lymphocytic (DWDL)	Small lymphocytic and plasmacytoid lymphocytic
Follicular, small cleaved cell	Nodular poorly differentiated lymphocytic (NPDL)	Small cleaved FCC,* follicular only or follicular and diffuse
Follicular, mixed small cleaved cell	Nodular mixed lymphoma (NML)	Small cleaved FCC, follicular; large cleaved FCC, follicular
Intermediate Grade		
Follicular, predominantly large cell	Nodular histiocytic lymphoma (NHL)	Large cleaved or noncleaved FCC, or both, follicular
Diffuse, small cleaved cell	Diffuse poorly differentiated lymphoma (DPDL)	Small cleaved FCC, diffuse
Diffuse, mixed small and large cell	Diffuse mixed lymphocytic-histiocytic (DML)	Small cleaved, large cleaved, or large noncleaved FCC, diffuse
Diffuse large cell	Diffuse histiocytic lymphoma (DHL)	Large cleaved or noncleaved FCC, diffuse
High Grade		
Large cell, immunoblastic	Diffuse histiocytic lymphoma (DHL)	Immunoblastic sarcoma, T-cell or B-cell type
Large cell, lymphoblastic	Lymphoblastic, convoluted or nonconvoluted	Convoluted T cell
Small noncleaved cell	Undifferentiated, Burkitt's and non-Burkitt's diffuse undifferentiated lymphoma (DUL)	Small noncleaved FCC
Miscellaneous		
Composite		
Mycosis fungoides		
Histiocytic		
Extramedullary plasmacytoma		
Unclassifiable		

*Follicular center cell.
(Modified from the National Cancer Institute-sponsored study of the classifications of non-Hodgkin's lymphomas. [1982]. *Cancer, 49,* 2112–2135.)

ular small cleaved cell lymphomas (working formulation) to more aggressive lymphoma. In a Stanford study, the risk of conversion has been estimated to be approximately 60 per cent. Histologic conversion has occurred in patients who have had prior treatment as well as in patients who have had no prior treatment

(Horning & Rosenberg, 1984). Therefore, additional biopsy specimens are often examined if the disease progresses, the disease progression changes rate, or the disease resists treatment so that the treatment can be directed at the new histologic pattern. Patients may also present with divergent histologic patterns at the initial staging evaluation. In a study conducted at the NCI, of a total of 101 patients who had multiple tissue sites biopsied, 18 patients had a nodular pattern in one site and a diffuse pattern in another (Hubbard et al., 1982). In addition, diffuse involvement as well as areas of nodularity may occasionally be evident in a single biopsy specimen.

Although the picture regarding low-grade lymphomas initially appears optimistic, the disease is usually fatal. Clinical morbidity and life-threatening problems are related to increasing tumor bulk. Eventually symptoms include fever, night sweats, weight loss, and infection. Bone marrow involvement and renal and hepatic dysfunction are manifested in widespread disease.

Aggressive Non-Hodgkin's Lymphomas. Patients with aggressive lymphomas exhibit a large-cell or mixed histologic pattern. Before the improvement of combination chemotherapy, complete remissions for patients with intermediate and high-grade lymphomas were rare, with median survival for those with diffuse histologic findings being rarely more than a year. These findings were attributed to the fact that most patients presented with advanced-stage disease and a rapidly growing tumor. Typically, aggressive lymphomas exhibit high-fraction tumor growth with rapid doubling times. Paradoxically, these aggressive lymphomas respond better to chemotherapy, and therefore have a greater potential for cure, than do most low-grade, indolent lymphomas. Salvage therapy after relapse results in few and short-term remissions, although many combinations of drugs, radiation therapy, and biologic response modifiers have allowed a greater potential for cure.

Table 35–14. CLINICAL DIFFERENCES IN HODGKIN'S DISEASE AND NON-HODGKIN'S LYMPHOMA

Characteristic	Hodgkin's Disease	Non-Hodgkin's Lymphoma
Nodes	Contiguous spread	Noncontiguous
Extranodal disease	Uncommon	More common involvement of gastrointestinal tract, testes, bone marrow
Site of disease	Mediastinal involvement common in 50% of patients	Mediastinal involvement less common (20%)
	Bone marrow involvement uncommon	Bone marrow involvement common
	Liver involvement uncommon	Liver involvement common
Extent of disease	Often localized	Rarely localized (10%)
B symptoms	Common (40%)	Uncommon (20%)

(Adapted from DeVita, V. T., Jr., Hellman, S., & Rosenberg, S. A. [1985]. *Cancer: Principles and practice of oncology* [2nd ed.]. Philadelphia: J. B. Lippincott Co.)

Diagnosis and Staging

Once a histopathologic diagnosis is established by lymph node biopsy, further clinical evaluation is needed to determine the sites and extent of disease involvement. This process, referred to as *staging*, is necessary to plan effective treatment methods and to establish parameters to follow the patient's response to therapy. It is also helpful in predicting the clinical course and prognosis of the specific lymphoma.

Studies useful for the clinical evaluation of non-Hodgkin's lymphoma are listed in Table 35–15. The extent of clinical examination is based on the histologic findings and the type of treatment expected for a specific lymphoma. For example, if a patient has a positive bone marrow biopsy result and therefore has stage IV disease, other invasive tests are not necessary. Patients are required at a minimum to have a history and physical examination, a complete blood count, a chest radiograph, screening chemistries, a urinalysis, an abdominal computed tomographic (CT) scan, and a bone marrow examination.

Several factors indicate the need for a bone marrow aspirate early in the evaluation process. In patients with low-grade lymphomas, 50 to 95 per cent have bone marrow involvement at presentation, which establishes the presence of stage IV disease (Ultmann & Jacobs, 1985). Patients with intermediate or high-grade lymphomas are less likely to have bone marrow involvement, with the exception of those who have lymphoblastic lymphomas. Because of the importance of a thorough bone marrow examination, it is recommended that core biopsies be obtained from each posterior iliac crest.

Computed tomography is very useful in patients with non-Hodgkin's lymphoma for assessing any abnormalities observed after baseline studies. A chest CT scan is required for patients with evident abnormalities on chest radiographs. The abdominal CT scan is valuable because it visualizes nodal and extranodal disease, picking up enlarged nodes greater than 2 cm. The CT scan can visualize the size but not the architecture of the node. It is used to evaluate the upper abdominal, mesenteric, splenic, and hepatic lymph nodes, all of which are commonly involved in non-Hodgkin's lymphoma. In addition, the abdominal CT scan demonstrates hepatic and splenic enlargement and a potential emergency—hydronephrosis. The CT scans are useful in stages III and IV disease to provide a baseline for later evaluation of complete response from therapy (Clouse et al., 1985).

In contrast, the lymphangiogram provides a very accurate evaluation of lower abdominal involvement, such as the lower aortic, iliac, and retroperitoneal lymph nodes. This test is used in clinical stages I and II disease, after all other noninvasive evaluations have been negative, to verify early-stage disease. The importance of verifying early-stage disease is because cure can be achieved with treatment of local radiation therapy. A lymphangiogram is not recommended for patients with large mediastinal involvement, pulmonary disease, or extensive retroperitoneal involvement.

These restrictions limit the use of this test in non-Hodgkin's lymphoma, which typically affects the older patient with bulky disease.

For the majority of patients, accurate assessment of extent of disease and subsequent treatment can be made based on the results of the previously mentioned tests. A staging laparotomy is not utilized in non-Hodgkin's lymphoma because, in contrast to Hodgkin's disease, the majority of non-Hodgkin's lymphoma patients present with disease below the diaphragm and do not require further staging work-up. Therefore, laparotomy, if used, is reserved for the few patients with clinical stage I_E and II_E disease in whom evidence of abdominal involvement would change the course of treatment from radiation therapy to combination chemotherapy.

The Ann Arbor staging classification for Hodgkin's disease (see Table 35–10) is also used for staging non-Hodgkin's lymphoma but has some deficiencies when applied in non-Hodgkin's lymphomas. This staging system does not account for facts such as histologic findings, bulk of disease, and site of disease such as extranodal involvement, all of which are important prognostic indicators in non-Hodgkin's lymphoma.

Treatment

The treatment of malignant non-Hodgkin's lymphoma is a rapidly evolving area with the continuous introduction of new drugs, drug regimens, and other therapeutic methods such as autologous bone marrow transplantation, monoclonal antibodies, and biologic response modifiers. Radiation alone is a limited option that is used for early-stage disease. Chemotherapy or combined modality therapy represents the most common treatment, because most patients present with late-stage disease. Chemotherapy regimens have evolved over the past several years with different combinations of non-cross-resistant drugs now being utilized for optimum benefit. Because the goal is cure, especially with the aggressive lymphomas, regimens are often vigorous and cause side effects such as nausea, vomiting, hair loss, and infection. Nursing support is crucial throughout the treatment phase to assist the patient in preventing and managing side effects.

Indolent Lymphomas—Low Grade. Various treatment approaches have failed to demonstrate durable remissions in low-grade lymphomas, although these lymphomas are characterized by a relatively long survival. Indolent lymphomas have demonstrated a high sensitivity to a wide range of chemotherapeutic agents (with complete remissions ranging from 60 to 70 per cent), but the duration of remissions is short (between 17 and 24 months). Unfortunately, at 4 years, 80 per cent of patients initially treated have relapsed. At 5 years, the survival rate is greater than 70 per cent, but at 10 years it is less than 30 per cent (Young, 1987).

Treatment of patients with low-grade lymphomas is controversial. Owing to the failure of current therapeutic approaches of chemotherapy or radiation therapy to "cure" indolent lymphomas, many physicians

Table 35–15. STUDIES USEFUL IN THE CLINICAL EVALUATION OF LYMPHOMA

Study	Indication	Usefulness
Complete blood count (including differential and platelet count)	All patients	Direct evidence for peripheral blood involvement Indirect evidence for bone marrow involvement or immune hemolytic anemia
Erythrocyte sedimentation rate (ESR)	All patients	Nonspecific; baseline data for subsequent follow-up
Urinalysis	All patients	Screen for proteinuria
Routine chemistries (including calcium and uric acid)	All patients	Hypercalcemia, hyperuricemia, elevated lactate dehydrogenase, electrolyte abnormalities, and acidosis may reflect complications of lymphoma
Liver function tests	All patients	If abnormal, may suggest hepatic involvement
Kidney function tests	All patients	If abnormal, may suggest direct renal parenchymal involvement, hydronephrosis due to retroperitoneal lymphadenopathy; may be secondary to hypercalcemia, hyperuricemia, or paraproteinemia
Serum protein electrophoresis (SPEP)	All patients	Detection of paraprotein
Serum immunoelectrophoresis with quantitation	All patients with an abnormal SPEP	Identification and quantitation of the paraprotein
Chest x-ray (CXR)	All patients	Screen for mediastinal, hilar, and paratracheal lymphadenopathy, and parenchymal involvement
Bone marrow aspirate and four bone core biopsies	All patients	Documents bone marrow involvement (pathologic stage IV disease)
Lumbar puncture with cytology	Diffuse histiocytic lymphoma with a positive result on a bone marrow scan Lymphoblastic lymphoma Undifferentiated lymphoma Any histology with an unexplained alteration in mental status	Documents central nervous system involvement
Abdominal/pelvic computed tomographic (CT) scan	All patients	Evaluates lymph node enlargement in the porta hepatis, splenic hilum, para-aortic region, mesentery, and retroperitoneum; liver and splenic involvement, presence or absence of hydronephrosis
Chest CT scan	All patients with an abnormal CXR	Further evaluation of suspected lymphadenopathy, mediastinal masses, or parenchymal disease
Intravenous pyelogram	All patients with a renal abnormality on CT scan	Further evaluation of renal abnormalities; however, this procedure may be contraindicated in the presence of paraproteinemia or renal failure due to hypercalcemia or hyperuricemia
Gallium scan	Patients with intermediate and high-grade lymphomas	Sensitivity varies with histology and location of disease. It is most sensitive for diffuse histiocytic lymphoma above the diaphragm*
Bone scan	All patients	Baseline data; all abnormal areas must be evaluated by a radiologic examination*
Liver-spleen scan	All patients	Baseline data; may suggest hepatic or splenic involvement*
Lymphangiogram	Patients with clinical stage I and II disease above the diaphragm with a negative abdominal/pelvic CT scan in whom the discovery of abdominal disease would alter treatment	Detects abnormalities in lymph node architecture in the lower para-aortic, retroperitoneal, and iliac lymph nodes. Provides a guide for the surgeon if a staging laparotomy is performed; any abnormal lymph node must be removed if the laparotomy is to be considered adequate*

*If any abnormalities are found, they require biopsy confirmation before changing the treatment based on these studies. When abnormal, these are useful parameters for following a patient's response to therapy.
(From Ultmann, J. E., & Jacobs, R. H. [1965]. The non-Hodgkin's lymphomas. *CA: A Cancer Journal for Clinicians, 35,* 36.)

advocate observing the patient and initiating therapy when symptoms require intervention. Following this policy of watchful waiting, 50 per cent of patients will avoid treatment for more than 1 to 3 years, 10 per cent will avoid treatment for longer than 5 years, and approximately 30 per cent will have partial spontaneous regression of disease that may be prolonged but not permanent (Connors, Fisher, & Armitage, 1989). Stanford, NCI, and other institutions have conducted randomized trials comparing observation with combination chemotherapy followed by total nodal irradiation. Although early treatment has demonstrated longer remissions, long-term survival appears to be equal. At present, there is no convincing data to suggest that early, more aggressive treatments have any survival benefit, although clinical trials are ongoing.

The most common chemotherapeutic agents used to treat low-grade lymphomas are listed in Table 35–16. The main chemotherapeutic agents employed are alkalating agents, usually chlorambucil and cyclophosphamide, and corticosteroids, usually prednisone. For the less than 10 per cent of patients with stage I or II disease, involved field radiation therapy is the treatment of choice. Prognosis is good for these patients, with an expected 50 to 80 per cent chance of disease-free survival exceeding 10 to 20 years, with some variation by site and age (Connors et al., 1989).

Aggressive Lymphomas. The aggressive lymphomas are all considered to be intermediate or high-grade lymphomas as defined by the working formulation, except for lymphoblastic lymphoma and Burkitt's lymphoma. The probability of remaining free of disease after 10 years is currently better for patients with diffuse aggressive lymphomas than for those with indolent lymphomas. In the last decade, a major change in the prognosis of aggressive lymphomas has evolved with the advancement of chemotherapeutic regimens. Chemotherapy regimens are listed in Table 35–17.

Early lymphoma studies in the 1970s introduced the first combination chemotherapy regimen: cyclophosphamide, vincristine, and prednisone (CVP or COP). This combination regimen was reported by DeVita and colleagues after successfully employing the MOPP regimen in Hodgkin's disease. If complete remission was not obtained after three cycles of these drugs, cure was not considered likely. Such partial response is considered to represent resistance, and therefore further chemotherapy would not be effective. Survival plateaus were achieved in approximately 30 per cent of patients (Connors et al., 1989).

Subsequently, several institutions developed second- and third-generation treatment programs that utilized a combination of six to eight chemotherapy drugs. Owing to the aggressive nature of the non-Hodgkin's lymphomas, the goal was to give more drugs in less time through marrow-sparing non-cross-resistant drugs (see Table 35–17) (Goldie et al., 1982; Skarin, 1986). The best-known regimens include COP-BLAM-III, MACOP-B, and Pro-MACE-CytaBOM. Some regimens add mid-cycle chemotherapy: chemotherapy is interspersed between the main cycle because disease regresses quickly, but often it regrows before the next

Table 35–16. THERAPY IN ADVANCED LOW-GRADE LYMPHOMAS

Regimen	Dosage*
Defer therapy/careful observation	—
Single-Agent Chemotherapy	
Cyclophosphamide or	1.5–2.5 mg/kg/day (orally)
chlorambucil	0.1–0.2 mg/kg/day (orally)
(continue therapy until CR is achieved and for 2 years as maintenance therapy)	
Prednisone	30–50 mg/kg/day (orally) × 4 weeks
(optional: may be started with a single drug)	
Combination Chemotherapy	
CVP	
Cyclophosphamide	400 mg/m² (orally) days 1–5
Vincristine	1.4 mg/m² (maximum 2.0 mg) day 1
Prednisone	100 mg/m² (orally) days 1–5
(repeat every 21 to 28 days until CR; CVP × four cycles as consolidation followed by CVP every 3 months as maintenance for a total of 2 years)	
COPP	
Cyclophosphamide	600 mg/m² days 1 and 8
Vincristine	1.4 mg/m² (maximum 2.0 mg) days 1 and 8
Procarbazine	100 mg/m² (orally) days 1–14
Prednisone	40 mg/m² (orally) days 1–14
(repeat every 21 days)	
CHOP	
Cyclophosphamide	750 mg/m² day 1
Doxorubicin	50 mg/m² day 1
Vincristine	1.4 mg/m² (maximum 2.0 mg) day 1
Prednisone	100 mg (orally) days 1 to 5
(repeat every 21–28 days)	

Whole-Body Irradiation
30 rad per week for a total of 150 rad
Boost irradiation to all initial sites of involvement, mantle or minimantle, Waldeyer region, whole abdomen, and pelvis; 2000 rad in 2–3 weeks in each field

Combined Modality
CVP + total lymphoid irradiation (TLI)
CVP, as above, for three cycles followed by TLI including 4400 rad to Waldeyer's ring, mantle, and inverted-Y; 3000 rad to whole abdomen
CVP is given again for three or more cycles until CR is achieved; the dose of cyclophosphamide is reduced to 300 mg/m² (orally) days 1 to 5
CHOP + irradiation
Phase I: CHOP is given every 28 days as above for four cycles, except prednisone is given for 8 days
Phase II: 150 rad total body irradiation for extensive disease, or 3500 rad local irradiation for local disease
Phase III: CHOP for four cycles every 8 weeks

*Drug is given intravenously unless otherwise stated. CR, complete remission.
(Adapted from Ultmann, J. E., & Jacobs, R. H. [1985]. The non-Hodgkin's lymphomas. *CA: A Cancer Journal for Clinicians, 35,* 66–87.)

cycle of chemotherapy begins. These regimens have produced complete remission in approximately 80 per cent of patients with aggressive large-cell lymphomas (Coleman et al., 1987). These results are especially

Table 35–17. CHEMOTHERAPY REGIMENS FOR NON-HODGKIN'S LYMPHOMA—AGGRESSIVE

Regimen	Drugs	Dosage (mg/m²)	Days of Treatment	Frequency
1. C-MOPP:	Cyclophosphamide	650 IV	1 and 8	q 28 days
	Vincristine (Oncovin*)	1.4 IV	1 and 8	
	Procarbazine	100 PO	1 to 14	
	Prednisone	40 PO	1 to 14	
2. CHOP	Cyclophosphamide	750 IV	1	q 21 days
	Doxorubicin (Adriamycin†)	50 IV	1	
	Vincristine (Oncovin*)	1.4 IV	1 and 5	
	Prednisone	100 PO	1 to 5	
3. CHOP-LEO	Cyclophosphamide	750 IV	1	q 21 days
	Doxorubicin (Adriamycin†)	50 IV	1	
	Vincristine (Oncovin*)	1.4 IV	1 and 5	
	Prednisone	100 PO	1 to 5	
	Bleomycin	4 IV	1 and 5	
4. BCVP	Carmustine (BCNU)	60 IV	1	q 21 days
	Cyclophosphamide	1000 IV	1	
	Vincristine (Oncovin*)	1.4 IV	1	
	Prednisone	100 PO	1 to 15	
5. BACOP	Cyclophosphamide	650 IV	1 and 8	q 28 days
	Doxorubicin (Adriamycin†)	25 IV	1 and 8	
	Vincristine (Oncovin*)	1.4 IV	1 and 8	
	Bleomycin	5 IV	15 and 21	
	Prednisone	60 PO	15 to 28	
6. COMLA	Cyclophosphamide	1500 IV	1	q 21 days
	Vincristine (Oncovin*)	1.5 IV	1, 8, and 15	
	Methotrexate	120 IV	22, then weekly × 7	
	Leucovorin	25 PO	q 6 hr × 4, 24 hr after MTX	
	Cytosine arabinoside	300 IV	22, then weekly × 7	
7. m-BACOD	Methotrexate	200 IV	8 and 15; LV 10 mg/m² po q6h × 8; 9 and 16	q 21 days
	Bleomycin	4 IV	1	
	Doxorubicin (Adriamycin†)	45 IV	1	
	Cyclophosphamide	600 IV	1	
	Vincristine (Oncovin*)	1.0 IV	1	
	Dexamethasone	6 PO	1 to 5	
8. PROMACE-MOPP (flexitherapy)	Cyclophosphamide	650 IV	1 and 8	q 28 days
	Doxorubicin (Adriamycin†)	25 IV	1 and 8	
	Epipodophyllotoxin (VP-16-213)	120 IV	1 and 8	
	Prednisone	60 PO	1 to 14	
	Methotrexate	1500 IV	14 (LV 50 mg/m² q6h × 5 day 15)	
	Standard MOPP		after remission	q 28 days
9. COP-BLAM-I	Cyclophosphamide	400 IV	1	
	Vincristine (Oncovin*)	1 IV	1	
	Prednisone	40 PO	1 to 10	q 21 days
	Bleomycin	15 IV (total)	14	
	Doxorubicin (Adriamycin†)	40 IV	1	
	Procarbazine (Matulane)	100 PO	1 to 10	
10. ACOMLA	Doxorubicin (Adriamycin†)	40 IV	1	
	Cyclophosphamide	1000 IV	1	
	Vincristine (Oncovin*)	2 IV total	1, 8, 15	q 3 months
	Methotrexate	120 IV	22, 29, 35, 43, 50, 57, 64, 71	
	Leucovorin	25 PO total	24 hrs after MTX, q6h × 6	
	Ara-C	300 IV	1 hr after MTX on same days	
11. Pro-MACE (day 1) Cytaboma (day 8)	ProMace	see above	1 (no MTX)	
	Cytarabine	300 IV	8	q 21 days
	Bleomycin	5 IV	8	
	Methotrexate	120 IV	8	
	Leucovorin	25 PO	9 q6h × 4, 24 hrs after MTX	
12. COP-BLAM-III	Cyclophosphamide	350 IV (Escalate to 500)	1 and 22	
	Vincristine (Oncovin*)	1 IV	1 to 2; 22 to 23 (cont. IV infusion)	q 6 weeks
	Prednisone	40 IV	1 to 5; 22 to 27	
	Bleomycin	7.5 IV	1 (IV push) 1 to 5; 22 to 23 (cont. IV infusion)	
	Doxorubicin (Adriamycin†)	35 IV (Escalate to 50)	1 and 22	
	Procarbazine (Matulane)	100 PO	1 to 5; 22 to 27	
13. MACOP-B	Methotrexate	400 IV	Weeks 2, 6, 10	
	Doxorubicin (Adriamycin†)	50 IV	Weeks 1, 3, 5, 7, 9, 11	
	Cyclophosphamide	350 IV	Weeks 1, 3, 5, 7, 9, 11	
	Vincristine (Oncovin*)	1.4 IV	Weeks 2, 4, 6, 8, 10, 12	
	Bleomycin	10U IV	Weeks 4, 8, 12	
	Prednisone	75 PO	Daily, dose tapered over the last 15 days	
	Co-trimoxazole	2 tablets PO	Twice daily throughout	

*Manufactured by Eli Lilly and Company, Indianapolis, IN.
†Manufactured by Adria Laboratories, Columbus, OH.
IV, intravenously; LV, leucovorin; MTX, methotrexate; PO, orally.
(From Skarin, A. T. [1986]. Diffuse aggressive lymphomas: A curable subset of non-Hodgkin's lymphomas. *Seminars in Oncology, 13*[4], 10–25.)

significant because the response rate includes patients with previously described poor prognostic factors such as bulky abdominal disease. It is important to treat the patient with as full a dose as possible, because the most important factor affecting outcome is dose intensity (Coleman et al., 1987; DeVita, Hubbard, Young, & Longo, 1988; Goldie et al., 1982; Skarin, 1986). Patients are treated to a documented complete response as determined by prior staging. Those patients in subsets requiring prophylactic central nervous treatment or who have bulky disease may also require consolidated radiotherapy.

Patient selection for these regimens is important for disease characteristics and patient tolerance. Age appears to be a limiting factor, with drug toxicity being more formidable in patients older than 50 years of age.

Side Effects

Studies have suggested a strong relationship between the side effects of disease and treatment and the patient's psychological morbidity (Devlin, Maguire, Phillips, & Crowther, 1987; Devlin, Maguire, Phillips, Crowther, & Chambers, 1987). The strain of coping with side effects as well as the fear that cancer is spreading results in varying degrees of anxiety and depression. The oncology nurse can provide support by educating the patient about potential physical and psychological side effects of treatment (Fobair et al., 1986).

The intensity of treatment regimens for aggressive lymphomas results in potential side effects and toxicities. Side effects have included substantial hematologic and mucosal difficulty, such as infection and mucositis (Coleman et al., 1987). Nursing observation for signs and symptoms of infection is critical. Mucositis remains a continual problem because many patients remain neutropenic throughout treatment. Nursing interventions regarding good and safe oral hygiene and preventive measures are discussed in Chapter 48. Hair loss should be anticipated with the treatment of regimens including doxorubicin and cyclophosphamide. Patient preparation involving wig selection and potential body image concerns requires nursing intervention (see Chapter 52).

Major toxicities resulting from chemotherapy include pulmonary, related to bleomycin, and severe neuropathy, either gastrointestinal or peripheral, as a result of vincristine therapy.

Oncologic Emergencies

Patients with progressive lymphoma are at risk for several oncologic emergencies such as superior vena cava syndrome in patients with mediastinal masses, spinal cord compression from tumor growth, and tumor lysis syndrome as a result of the rapid breakdown of cells from aggressive chemotherapy. Patients with central nervous system involvement are at risk for intracranial pressure. Oncologic emergencies are discussed extensively in Chapter 57.

Patients with gastric lymphomas have a high incidence of perforation with treatment, particularly with bulky disease. Often these patients will undergo a debulking procedure before receiving chemotherapy, such as a subtotal gastrectomy, and in some cases a total gastrectomy. When treating a patient with known gastric involvement, it is important to educate the patient about the signs and symptoms of perforation and the urgency of reporting this emergency (Jacobs, 1988).

Cutaneous T-Cell Lymphoma—Mycosis Fungoides

Mycosis fungoides is a rare cutaneous lymphoma of the T lymphocyte. In the United States, this malignant skin disease affects only 400 to 600 patients per year, who range from 45 to 69 years of age at diagnosis. First described by French physician Alibert in 1806, the name *mycosis fungoides* resulted from the mushroom-like appearance of the tumors. Although indolent in nature, with a median survival of 8 to 10 years, systemic spread to peripheral blood, lymph nodes, and other organs is common. The prognosis is highly dependent on the stage of disease, which is determined by the type of skin lesions and peripheral blood, lymph node, and visceral involvement (Sarna & Kagan, 1985b; Winkler & Bunn, 1983).

The cause of mycosis fungoides is not known but has been correlated with factors such as exposure to chemicals, family history of Hodgkin's disease and lymphoma, and defects in host immune surveillance. The disease often appears superficially with a variety of skin lesions.

Three clinical stages have been identified: (1) premyotic or erythematous, (2) plaque, and (3) tumor. The first stage is characterized by a general itching and superficial skin eruptions of varying sizes (Stabb, 1980). At this early stage, the disease can be confused easily with other skin disorders, such as psoriasis and dermatitis. The lesions may wax and wane and spontaneously disappear and reappear. These lesions usually appear approximately 6 years before most patients are diagnosed. Usually the relentless itching and fear of contagion lead the patient to seek diagnosis (Winkler & Bunn, 1983). The premyotic stage may last from several months to 10 years.

The plaque stage of mycosis fungoides is an aggravated symptom and causes great discomfort. This stage is characterized by an irregular thickening of the skin, with raised and irregularly shaped plaques, which may be accompanied by palpable lymph nodes. Lesions are no longer transitory and may lead to painful fissures of the palms and soles. Scalp involvement may result in alopecia. Itching may become an annoying symptom, especially if it was present in the premyotic phase (Hallowach, McFadden, & Supik, 1984; Sarna & Kagan, 1985b; Stabb, 1980).

The tumor stage is characterized by mass lesions, which can appear in previously normal skin, in plaques, or in previous mycotic lesions. They may appear anywhere but are most often found in the face and body folds such as the axillae, groin, cubital folds, neck, and breasts (Winkler & Bunn, 1983). The most frequent cause of death with cutaneous T-cell lymphoma is infection followed by progressive dissemination.

Treatment for mycosis fungoides includes topical as well as systemic chemotherapy, radiation therapy, biologic response modifiers, and supportive care. Patients respond better with early treatment, but at present there is no cure.

Innovative nursing care is required for the patient with mycosis fungoides, which includes skin care, infection control, and nutritional support. Comfort measures are necessary for pruritus and pain relief (see Chapters 3 and 4). The psychosocial impact of this disease, including the insult to body image and self-esteem, presents multifaceted challenges for nursing intervention.

Problems Associated with Survivorship

The successful treatment of the lymphomas has resulted in cure for many patients and progressively longer lives for others. Studies of patients with Hodgkin's disease and non-Hodgkin's lymphoma have identified several physiologic and psychological difficulties of long-term survival.

Lack of energy or tiredness is a common complaint often accompanied by depression. In a study of patients with Hodgkin's disease, 37 per cent of patients complained that their energy had not adequately returned. For others, it took 12 to 18 months following treatment for energy to return (Fobair et al., 1986). Loss of libido and problems with infertility have been documented in patients with Hodgkin's disease. Impairment or disturbance of short-term memory may be a short- or long-term effect. Anxiety and fear of relapse and further treatment are also problems but appear to decrease as the patient lives longer free of disease (Devlin, Maguire, Phillips, & Crowther, 1987; Devlin, Maguire, Phillips, Crowther, & Chambers, 1987; Fobair et al., 1986).

The failure of some patients to return to work or to resume normal activities years after treatment is cause for early intervention. Those returning to work often experience job discrimination or difficulties at work and problems obtaining insurance. Marital difficulties and an increase in divorce among survivors of Hodgkin's disease has been attributed to role changes, stress of treatment, and anger at the well spouse. Educating the patient about potential psychosocial difficulties during treatment and recovery is a suggested intervention to decrease the impact of these difficulties once they occur (Fobair et al., 1986). As patients continue to live longer, the problems associated with survivorship and the role of the nurse in preventing some of these problems need further study.

Future Treatments

Current studies are using various and new types of biologic response modifiers in the treatment of low-grade lymphomas. Biologicals are used alone or in combination with other biologicals, chemotherapy, radioactive molecules, or toxins (see Chapter 23). Other areas of research include the consequences of higher doses of chemotherapy, with or without whole body irradiation, followed by autologous bone marrow transplantation. Encouraging preliminary results of this research as a salvage program for patients who have had relapses after treatment have been identified (Applebaum & Thomas, 1983; Takvorian, 1987).

References

Acker, B., Hoppe, R. T., Cooby, T. V., Cox, R. S., Kaplan, H. S., & Rosenberg, S. A. (1987). Histologic conversion in the non-Hodgkin's lymphomas. *Journal of Clinical Oncology, 1,* 11–16.

Amadori, S., Meloni, G., Baccarini, M., Haanen, C., Willemze, R., Corbelli, G., Drenthe-Schonk, A., Lopes Cardozo, P., Tura, S., & Mandelli, F. (1983). Long term survival in adolescent and adult lymphoblastic leukemia. *Cancer, 52,* 30–34.

American Cancer Society. (1989). Cancer statistics 1989. *CA: A Cancer Journal for Clinicians, 39*(1).

Applebaum, F. R., & Thomas, E. D. (1983). Review of the use of marrow transplantation in the treatment of non-Hodgkin's lymphoma. *Journal of Clinical Oncology, 1,* 440–447.

Bennett, J. M., Catovsky, D., Daniel, M. T., Flandrin, G., Galton, D. A. G., Gralnick, H. R., & Sultan, C. (1976). Proposals for the classification of the acute leukemias. *British Journal of Hematology, 33,* 451–458.

Berenson, J., Zigelboim, J., & Gale, R. (1985). Acute lymphoblastic leukemia. In C. Haskell, *Cancer treatment* (2nd ed., pp. 706–721). Philadelphia: W. B. Saunders Co.

Bergsagel, D. E., Alison, R. E., Bean, H. A., Brown, T. C., Bush, R. S., Clark, M. N., Chua, T., Dalley, D., DeBoer, G., Gospodarowicz, M., Hasselback, R., Perrault, D., & Rideout, D. F. (1982). Results of treating Hodgkin's disease without a policy of laparotomy staging. *Cancer Treatment Reports, 66,* 717–732.

Binet, J. L., Auquier, A., Dighiero, G., Chastang, C., Piguet, H., Goasguen, J., Vaugier, G., Potron, G., Colona, P., Oberling, F., Thomas, M., Tchernia, G., Jacquillat, C., Boivin, P., Lesty, C., Duault, M. T., Monconduit, M., Belabbes, S., & Gremy, F. (1981). A new prognostic classification of chronic lymphocytic leukemia derived from multivariable survival analyses. *Cancer, 48,* 198–206.

Blayney, D. W., Jaffe, E. S., Blattner, W. A., Cossman, J., Robert-Guroff, M., Longo, D. L., Bunn, P. A. Jr., & Gallo, R. C. (1983). The human T-cell leukemia/lymphoma virus associated with American adult T-cell leukemia/lymphoma. *Blood, 62*[2], 401–405.

Bloomfield, C. D., Rowley, J. D., Goldman, A. I., Lawler, S. D., Walker, L. M., & Mitelman, F. (1983). For the Third International Workshop on chromosomal abnormalities and their clinical significance in acute lymphoblastic leukemia. *Cancer Research, 43,* 868–873.

Boggs, D. R. (1974). Hematopoietic stem cell theory in relation to possible lymphoblastic conversion of chronic myeloid leukemia. *Blood, 44,* 449–453.

Bonadonna, G., Santoro, A., Simonetta, V., & Valagussa, P. (1988). Treatment strategies for Hodgkin's disease. *Seminars in Hematology, 25*(2), 51–57.

Bonadonna, G., Valagussa, P., & Santoro, A. (1986). Alternating non-cross-resistant combination chemotherapy or MOPP in stage IV Hodgkin's disease: A report of 8 year results. *Annals of Internal Medicine, 104,* 739–748.

Brown, R. A., Herzig, S. N., Wolff, D., Frei-Lalr, L., Piniero, L., Bolwell, B. S., Lowder, J. N., Harden, E. A., Hande, K. R., & Herzig, G. P. (1990). High dose etoposide and cyclophosphamide without bone marrow transplantation for resistant hematologic malignancy. *Blood, 76*(3), 473–479.

Byhardt, R. W., Brace, W. C., & Wiernic, P. H. (1975). The role of splenic irradiation in chronic lymphocytic leukemia. *Cancer, 35,* 1621–1625.

Cawley, J. C., Burns, G. F., & Hayhoe, F. G. J. (1980). *Hairy cell leukemia*. Berlin: Springer-Verlag.

Champlin, R. E. (1986). Chronic myelogenous leukemia in leukemia therapy. In R. P. Gale (Ed.), *Leukemia therapy* (p. 148). Boston: Blackwell Scientific Publications.

Champlin, R. E., & Gale, R. P. (1987). Bone marrow transplantation for acute leukemia: Recent advances and comparison with alternative therapies. *Seminars in Hematology, 24*, 55–67.

Clouse, M., Harrison, D., Grassi, C. J., Costello, P., Edwards, S. S., & Wheeler, H. (1985). Lymphangiography, ultrasonography, and computed tomography in Hodgkin's disease and non-Hodgkin's lymphoma. *Journal of Computed Tomography, 9*, 1–7.

Coleman, M., Gerstein, G., Topilow, A., Lebowicz, J., Berhardt, B., Chiarieri, D., Silver, R., Pasmantier, M. W. (1987). Advances in chemotherapy for large cell lymphoma. *Seminars in Hematology, 24*, 8–20.

Connors, J. M., Fisher, R. I., & Armitage, J. O. (1989, December). *Decision making in the treatment of malignant lymphoma*. American Society of Hematology Educational Session, Atlanta, GA.

Cooley, M., & Cobb, S. C. (1986). Sexual and reproductive issues for women with Hodgkin's disease I. Overview of issues. *Cancer Nursing, 9*, 188–193.

Cronkite, E. P., Maloney, W. C., & Bond, V. P. (1960). Radiation leukogenesis: An analysis of the problem. *American Journal of Medicine, 28*, 673.

Cunningham, I., Gee, T., Dowling, M., et al. (1979). Results of treatment of Ph^1 + chronic myelogenous leukemia with an intensive treatment regimen (L-5 protocol). *Blood, 53*, 375–393.

Curtis, J. E., Hersh, E. M., & Freirich, E. M. (1972). Leukapheresis therapy of chronic lymphocytic leukemia. *Blood, 39*, 163.

DeVita, V. T. (1982). Hodgkin's disease: Conference summary and future directions. *Cancer Treatment Reports, 66*, 1045–1055.

DeVita, V. T., Jr., Hellman, S., & Rosenberg, S. A. (1985). *Cancer: Principles and practice of oncology* (2nd ed.). Philadelphia: J. B. Lippincott Co.

DeVita, V. T., Jr., Hubbard, S., Young, R., & Longo, D. (1988). The role of chemotherapy in diffuse aggressive lymphoma. *Seminars in Hematology, 25*, 2–10.

Devlin, J., Maguire, P., Phillips, P., & Crowther, D. (1987). Psychological problems associated with diagnosis and treatment of lymphomas II: Prospective study. *British Medical Journal, 295*, 955–957.

Devlin, J., Maguire, P., Phillips, P., Crowther, D., & Chambers, H. (1987). Psychological problems associated with diagnosis and treatment of lymphomas I: Retrospective study. *British Medical Journal, 295*, 953–954.

Elison, R. R., Holland, J. F., Weil, M., Jacquillat, C., Boiron, M., Bernard, J., Sawitsky, A., Rosner, F., Gussoff, B., Silver, R., Karanas, A., Cuttner, J., Spurr, C., Hayes, D., Blom, J., Leone, L. A., Haurani, F., Kyle, R., Hutchison, J. L., Forcier, R. J., & Moon, J. H. (1968). Arabinoside cytosine: A useful agent in the treatment of acute leukemia in adults. *Blood, 32*, 507–523.

Figlin, R. A. (1989). Biotherapy in clinical practice. *Seminars in Hematology, 26*(No. 3, Suppl. 3), 15–24.

Fobair, P., Hoppe, R. T., Bloom, J., Cox, R., Varghese, A., & Spiegel, D. (1986). Psychosocial problems among survivors of Hodgkin's disease. *Journal of Clinical Oncology, 4*, 805–813.

Foon, K. A., Bottina, G. D., Abrams, P. G., Fer, M. F., Longo, D. L., Schoenberger, C. S., & Oldham, R. K. (1985). A phase II trial of recombinant leukocyte A interferon for patients with advanced chronic lymphocytic leukemia. *American Journal of Medicine, 78*, 216–220.

Foon, K. A., & Gale, R. P. (1986). Chronic lymphocytic leukemia. In R. P. Gale (Ed.), *Leukemia therapy* (p. 165). Boston: Blackwell Scientific Publications.

Foon, K. A., & Gale, R. P. (1987). Staging and therapy of chronic lymphocytic leukemia. *Seminars in Hematology, 24*, 264–274.

Foon, K. A., Schroff, R. W., & Gale, R. P. (1982). Surface markers on leukemia and lymphoma cells: Recent advances. *Blood, 60*, 1–19.

Foon, K. A., Schroff, R. W., Mayer, D., Sherwin, S. A., Oldham, R. K., Bunn, P. A., & Hsu, S. (1983). Monoclonal antibody therapy of chronic lymphocytic leukemia and cutaneous T-cell lymphoma: Preliminary observations. In B. E. Boss, R. E. Langman, I. S. Trowbridge, & R. Dulbecco (Eds.), *Monoclonal antibodies and cancer* (pp. 38–53). New York: Academic Press.

Gale, R. P., & Foon, K. A. (1986). Acute myelogenous leukemia. In R. P. Gale (Ed.), *Leukemia therapy*. Boston: Blackwell Scientific Publications.

Gale, R. P., & Foon, K. A. (1987). Therapy of acute myelogenous leukemia. *Seminars in Hematology, 24*, 40–54.

Gattiker, H. H., Wiltshaw, E., & Galton, A. G. (1981). Spontaneous regression in non-Hodgkin's lymphoma. *Cancer, 45*, 2627–2632.

Golde, D. W., & Koeffler, H. P. (1985). Hairy cell leukemia. In C. Haskell, *Cancer treatment* (2nd ed.). Philadelphia: W. B. Saunders Co.

Goldie, J. H., Goldman, A. J., & Guaduskus, G. A. (1982). Rationale for the use of alternating non-cross resistant chemotherapy. *Cancer Treatment Reports, 66*, 39.

Golomb, H. M., Catovsky, D., & Golde, D. W. (1983). Hairy cell leukemia. A clinical review based on 71 cases. *Annals of Internal Medicine, 99*, 485–486.

Gomez, G. A., Reese, P. A., Nava, H., Panahon, A. M., Barcos, M., Stutzman, L., Han, T., & Henerson, E. S. (1984). Staging laparotomy and splenectomy in early Hodgkin's disease. *American Journal of Medicine, 77*, 205–210.

Graham, D. C. (1960). Leukemia following x-ray therapy for ankylosing spondylitis. *Archives of Internal Medicine, 105*, 51.

Greenberger, J., Mauch, P., Canellow, G., & Larson, R. (1989, December). *Controversies in Hodgkin's disease*. American Society of Hematology Educational Session, Atlanta, GA.

Grever, M. R., Leiby, J. M., Krant, E. H., Wilson, H. W., Niedhart, J. A., Wall, R. L., & Bacerzak, S. P. (1985). Low dose deoxycoformycin in lymphoid malignancy. *Journal of Clinical Oncology, 3*, 1196.

Griffin, J. D., Davis, R., Nelson, D. A., Davey, F. R., Mayer, R. J., Schiffer, C., McIntyre, O. R., & Bloomfield, C. D. (1986). Use of surface marker analysis to predict outcome of adult acute myeloblastic leukemia. *Blood, 68*, 1232–1241.

Hallowach, S., McFadden, M. E., & Supik, K. (1984). Mycosis fungoides: A nursing perspective. *Oncology Nursing Forum, 11*(1), 20–34.

Haskell, C. M., & Parker, R. G. (1985). Hodgkin's disease. In C. Haskell, *Cancer treatment* (2nd ed., pp. 758–788). Philadelphia: W. B. Saunders Co.

Haut, A., Abbott, W. S., Wintrobe, M. M., & Cartwright, G. E. (1961). Busulfan in the treatment of chronic myelocytic leukemia: The effect of long term intermittent therapy. *Blood, 117*, 1–19.

Henderson, E. S. (1983). Acute leukemias—general considerations in hematology. In W. J. Williams, E. Beutler, A. J. Erslev, & M. A. Lichtman, *Hematology* (p. 221). New York: McGraw-Hill Book Co.

Henderson, E. S., & Han, T. (1986, Nov./Dec.). Current therapy of acute and chronic leukemia in adults. *CA: A Cancer Journal for Clinicians, 36*, 322–350.

Heysel, R., Britt, A. M., Woodbury, L. A., Nishimura, E. T., Ghase, T., Hoshino, T., & Yamasaki, M. (1960). Leukemia in Hiroshima atomic bomb survivors. *Blood, 15*, 313.

Hoelzer, D., & Gale, R. O. (1987). Acute lymphoblastic leukemia in adults. Recent progress, future direction. *Seminars in Hematology, 24*, 27–34.

Hoelzer, D., Thiel, E., Loffler, H., Buchner, T., Boaenstein, D., Engelhardt, R., Ruhl, N., Ganser, A., & Messerer, D. (1985). Treatment of adult T-ALL with intensive chemotherapy. *Blood, 66*(Suppl. 1), 201A.

Hoppe, R. T., Cox, R. S., Rosenberg, S. A., & Kaplan, H. S. (1982). Prognostic factors in pathologic stage III Hodgkin's disease. *Cancer Treatment Reports, 66*, 743–749.

Horning, S. J., Hoppe, R. T., & Kaplan, H. S. (1981). Female reproductive potential after treatment for Hodgkin's disease. *New England Journal of Medicine, 304*, 1377–1382.

Horning, S. J., & Rosenberg, S. A. (1984). The natural history of initially untreated low-grade non-Hodgkin's lymphoma. *New England Journal of Medicine, 311*, 1471–1475.

Hubbard, S. M., Chabner, B. A., DeVita, V. T., Simon, R., Bernard, C. W., Jones, R. B., Garvin, A. J., Canellos, G. P., Osborne, C. K., & Young, R. C. (1982). Histologic progression in non-Hodgkin's lymphoma. *Blood, 59*, 258–264.

Huguley, C. M., Jr. (1977). Treatment of chronic lymphocytic leukemia. *Cancer Treatment Review, 4*, 261–273.

Italian Cooperative Group on Chronic Myeloid Leukemia. (1984). Results of a prospective study of early splenectomy in chronic myeloid leukemia. *Cancer, 54*, 333–338.

Jacobs, A. (1986). Hairy cell leukemia. In R. P. Gale (Ed.), *Leukemia therapy*. Boston: Blackwell Scientific Publications.

Jacobs, A. D., & Gale, R. P. (1986). Acute lymphoblastic leukemia in adults. In R. P. Gale (Ed.), *Leukemia therapy* (pp. 71–98). Boston: Blackwell Scientific Publications.

Jacobs, C. (1988, September). Lymphomas: *Diagnosis, staging and principles of treatment.* Oncology Nursing: A National Conference on Today's Clinical Issues, San Francisco.

Jacquillat, C., Weil, M., Auclerc, M. F., Chastang, C., Flandrin, G., Israel, V., Schaison, G., Degos, L., Boiron, M., & Bernard, J. (1978). Prognosis and treatment of acute lymphoblastic leukemia. *Cancer Chemotherapy and Pharmacology, 1*, 113–122.

Jaffe, E. S. (1986). Relationship of classification to biologic behavior of non-Hodgkin's lymphomas. *Seminars in Oncology, 13*(4):3–9.

Janossy, G., Woodruff, R. K., Pippard, M. J., Prentice, G., Hoffbrand, A. V., Paxton, A., Lister, T. A., Bunch, C., & Greaves, M. F. (1979). Relation of *"lymphoid"* phenotype and response to chemotherapy incorporating vincristine, prednisone in the acute phase of Ph[1] positive leukemia. *Cancer, 43*, 426–434.

Kaplan, H. S. (1981). Hodgkin's disease: Biology, treatment, prognosis. *Blood, 57*, 813–822.

Keating, M. J., Kantarjian, H., Talpaz, M., Radman, J., Koller, C., Barlogie, B., Velasquez, W., Plunkett, H., Freirich, E. J., & McCredie, K. B. (1989). Fludarabine: A new agent with major activity against chronic lymphocytic leukemia. *Blood, 74*, 19–25.

Kennedy, B. J. (1972). Hydroxyurea therapy in chronic myelogenous leukemia. *Cancer, 29*, 1052–1056.

Knospe, W. H., Lolb, V., Jr., & Huguley, C. M., Jr. (1974). Biweekly chlorambucil treatment of chronic lymphocytic leukemia. *Cancer, 33*, 555–562.

Lacher, M. J. (1985). Hodgkin's disease: Historical perspective, current status, and future directions. *CA: A Cancer Journal for Clinicians, 35*, 88–94.

Lukes, R. J. (1979). The immunologic approach to the pathology of malignant lymphomas. *American Journal of Clinical Pathology, 72*, 657.

Mann, R. B., Jaffe, E. S., & Bernard, C. W. (1972). Malignant lymphomas—a conceptual understanding of morphological diversity. *American Journal of Pathology, 94*, 103–192.

National Cancer Institute sponsored study of classifications of non-Hodgkin's lymphomas. Summary and description of a working formulation for clinical usage. The non-Hodgkin's lymphoma classification project. (1982). *Cancer, 49*, 2112–2135.

Paryane, S., Hoppe, R. T., Burke, J. S., Sneed, P., Dawley, D., Cos, R. S., Rosenberg, S. A., & Kaplan, H. S. (1983). Extralymphatic involvement in diffuse non-Hodgkin's lymphoma. *Journal of Clinical Oncology, 1*, 682–687.

Piro, L., Carrera, C., Beutler, E., & Carson, D. (1988). 2-Chlorodeoxyadenosine: An effective new agent for the treatment of chronic lymphocytic leukemia. *Blood, 72*, 1069–1073.

Piro, L. D., Carrera, C. J., Carson, D. J., & Beutler, E. (1990). Lasting remissions in hairy cell leukemia induced by a single infusion of 2-chlorodeoxyadenosine. *New England Journal of Medicine, 322*, 1117–1121.

Prednisone and prednisolone. (1970). In R. B. Livingston & S. K. Carter (Eds.), *Single agents in cancer chemotherapy* (pp. 337–358). New York: IFF/Preview Data.

Rai, K. R., & Montserrat, E. (1987). Prognostic factors in chronic lymphatic leukemia. *Seminars in Hematology, 24*, 252–256.

Rai, K. R., Sawitsky, A., Cronkite, E. P., Chanana, A., Levy, R. N., & Pasternak, B. S. (1975). Clinical staging of chronic lymphocytic leukemia. *Blood, 46*, 219–234.

Rapaport, S. I. (1987). *Introduction to hematology*. Philadelphia: J. B. Lippincott Co.

Rosenberg, S. A. (1986). Hodgkin's disease: No stage beyond cure. *Hospital Practice, 21*(8), 91–98, 101–108.

Rosenthal, S., Canellos, G. O., DeVita, V. T., & Gralnick, H. R. (1977). Characteristics of blast crisis in chronic granulocytic leukemia. *Blood, 49*, 705.

Rundles, R. W. (1982a). Chronic lymphocytic leukemia. In W. J. Williams, E. Beutler, A. J. Erslev, & M. A. Licheman (Eds.), *Hematology* (p. 983). New York: McGraw-Hill Book Co.

Rundles, R. W. (1982b). Chronic myelogneous leukemia. In W. J. Williams, E. Beutler, A. J. Erslev, & M. A. Licheman (Eds.), *Hematology* (pp. 196–214). New York: McGraw-Hill Book Co.

Santos, G. (1989). Marrow transplantation in acute nonlymphocytic leukemia. *Blood, 75*, 901–908.

Sarna, G. P., & Kagan, R. A. (1985a). Non-Hodgkin's lymphomas. In C. Haskell, *Cancer treatment* (2nd ed., pp. 789–828). Philadelphia: W. B. Saunders Co.

Sarna, G. P., & Kagan, R. A. (1985b). Mycosis Fungoides. In C. Haskell, *Cancer treatment* (2nd ed., pp. 829–845). Philadelphia: W. B. Saunders Co.

Shapiro, L., Shustic, C., Anderson, K., & Sawitsky, A. (1984). Intermittent chlorambucil in chronic lymphocytic leukemia: A randomized trial of treatment versus observation in early stage of disease. *Proceedings of the American Society of Clinical Oncology, 3*, 191 (Abstract).

Skarin, A. T. (1986). Diffuse aggressive lymphomas: A curable subset of non-Hodgkin's lymphomas. *Seminars in Oncology, 13*(4):10–25.

Stabb, M. A. (1980, February). Mycosis fungoides: A rare cutaneous malignant lymphoma with multifaceted nursing challenges. *Cancer Nursing*, pp. 17–25.

Straus, D. J. (1986). Strategies in treatment of Hodgkin's disease. *Seminars in Oncology, 13*(4):26–33.

Takvorian, T. (1987). Autologous bone marrow transplantation for non-Hodgkin's lymphoma. *Advances in Oncology, 3*(2):27–30.

Talpaz, M., McCredie, K. B., Trujillo, J., Kantarjian, H. M., Keating, M. J., & Guttermen, J. (1987). Clinical investigation of human alpha interferon in chronic myelogenous leukemia. *Blood, 69*, 1280–1288.

Tivey, H. (1954). The natural history of untreated acute leukemia. *Annals of the New York Academy of Science, 60*, 322.

Ultmann, J. E., & Bitran, J. D. (1989). Current recommendations for the staging and restaging of lymphoma. *Current Opinion in Oncology, 1*, 17–22.

Ultmann, J. E., & Jacobs, R. H. (1985). The non-Hodgkin's lymphomas. *CA: A Cancer Journal for Clinicians, 35*, 66–87.

Urba, W., Baseler, M., Kopp, W., Steis, R., Clark, J., Smith, I. J., Coggin, D., & Longo, D. (1989). Deoxycoformin-induced immunosuppression in patients with hairy cell leukemia. *Blood, 73*, 38–46.

Vigliani, E. C., & Sart, G. (1964). Benzene and leukemia. *New England Journal of Medicine, 271*, 872.

Whang-Peng, J., & Knutsen, T. (1980). Lymphocytic leukemias, acute and chronic. *Clinical Hematology, 9*, 87.

Willett, C. G., Linggood, R. M., Meyer, J., Orlow, E., Lindfors, K., Doppke, M. S., & Aisenberg, A. C. (1987a). Results of treatment of stage IA and IIA Hodgkin's disease. *Cancer, 59*, 1107–1111.

Willett, C. G., Linggood, R. M., Meyer, J., Orlow, E., Lindfors, K., Doppke, M. S., & Aisenberg, A. C. (1987b). Results of treatment of stage 3A Hodgkin's disease. *Cancer, 59*, 27–30.

Winkler, C. F., & Bunn, P. A. (1983). Cutaneous T-cell lymphoma: A review. *CRC Critical Reviews in Oncology/Hematology, 1*, 49–92.

Young, R. C. (1987). Combination chemotherapy in advanced non-Hodgkin's lymphoma. *Advances in Oncology, 3*(2), 20–26.

Zigelboim, J., Foon, K., & Gale, R. (1985). Acute myelogenous leukemia. In C. Haskell, *Cancer treatment* (2nd ed., pp. 694–706). Philadelphia: W. B. Saunders Co.

Head and Neck Cancers

JEAN L. REESE

Although cancers of the head and neck region constitute only 5 per cent of all cancers, their effects can produce multiple and severe challenges to physical and psychosocial well-being. Cancerous processes in the paranasal sinuses, nasal and oral cavities, salivary glands, pharynx, and larynx can affect speech, appearance, eating, and breathing. Any one or a combination of these altered functions makes psychosocial adjustment difficult. In addition, the person with head and neck cancer often bears concomitant health problems associated with aging, malnutrition, smoking, and alcohol abuse.

Environmental factors and personal habits are often closely associated with the development of cancer in the head and neck region. Although squamous cell carcinomas constitute the majority of tumors in this region, the biologic behavior of this cell type varies considerably from site to site. A difference of even a few centimeters within the same site of the same tumor type can result in a different natural history (Harnsburger & Dillon, 1987). Location, stage of development on discovery, and treatment alternatives all influence survival rates.

TRENDS

Head and neck cancer is increasing among women, the elderly, and blacks. Social habits changed considerably after World War II, and women are now smoking cigarettes and drinking alcoholic beverages to greater extents. Head and neck cancer among women, like lung cancer, is likely to continue increasing.

For three decades starting with the 1940s, the male-to-female ratio for patients with newly diagnosed cancers of the mouth and pharynx was 4:1. In the 11 years spanning 1964 to 1975, this ratio decreased to 3:1 in a series of 788 patients (McGuirt, 1979). From 1975 through 1980 the male-to-female ratio in 533 new cases was 2:1 (McGuirt, 1983). This last series of patients, obtained from the tobacco states, probably forecasts the changes that are yet to occur nationwide. The combined usage of snuff and alcohol by women in this population contributed to the predominance of lesions in the mouth and pharynx.

More than 50 per cent of all cancers occur in persons over 65 years old. This percentage holds, with slight variation in different sites, for the elderly who have cancers of the head and neck (Baranovsky & Myers, 1986). The numbers of these cancers will more than likely increase because of the larger numbers of people who will be aging in the next decades. Of 758 patients observed in a London clinic between the years 1975 and 1981, 57 per cent were 61 years of age and older (Lampe, Lampe, & Skillings, 1986). Carcinomas in this group most frequently developed in the buccal mucosa, hard palate, soft palate, and tongue. In addition, the 56 per cent 5-year survival rate for the over–61 age group compared unfavorably with the 79 per cent survival rate among patients aged 40 years or less.

Both incidence and death rates have been increasing more rapidly among blacks than among whites. This increase is particularly evident among young blacks. A review of 1066 tumor registry cases in New Jersey revealed that the proportion of patients aged 45 years or younger was 14 per cent blacks and only 2.9 per cent whites. Two- and 5-year survival rates were 23 and 5 per cent, respectively, for blacks, compared with 40 and 13 per cent for whites. Unfortunately, 61 per cent of these 70 patients had stage III or IV tumors on diagnosis regardless of race. Factors thought to be related were poor nutrition, earlier tobacco and alcohol consumption, and other environmental or personal factors (Slotman, Swaminathan, & Rush, 1983). Another concern is the use of smokeless tobacco by teenagers, in whom oral mucosal changes are evident (Poulson, Lindenmuth, & Greer, 1984).

ORAL CAVITY AND PHARYNX

Definition

Oral cavity cancer occurs in the lips, oral tongue, floor of the mouth, buccal mucosa, upper and lower gingiva, retromolar trigone, and hard palate (Fig. 36–1).

The pharynx, composed of the nasopharynx, oropharynx, and hypopharynx, extends from the base of the skull superiorly to the level of the esophagus inferiorly. The soft palate forms the floor and anterior wall of the nasopharynx. The eustachian tube orifice and the adenoids are located in the nasopharynx. The extensive submucosal capillary lymphatic plexus present in the nasopharynx leads to frequent metastasis from this region to the neck. The oropharynx includes the base of the tongue, the tonsillar area, the soft palate, and the posterior pharyngeal wall. The base of the tongue is bounded by the circumvallate papillae anteriorly, by the epiglottis posteriorly, and by the glossopharyngeal sulcus laterally. The hypopharynx extends from the level of the hyoid bone to the lower border of the cricoid cartilage, where the esophagus begins. The pharyngeal walls, pyriform sinus, and postcricoid area make up the hypopharynx (Kornblut, 1987; Mahboubi & Sayed, 1982).

Incidence, Mortality, and Survival Rates

Cancer of the Mouth and Pharynx

Cancers in regions other than the larynx and salivary glands ("other mouth and pharynx" cancers) occur in the United States at an annual incidence rate of 13.5 for men and 5.3 for women (Table 36–1); mortality rates with these cancers are 4.3 and 1.6 per 100,000,

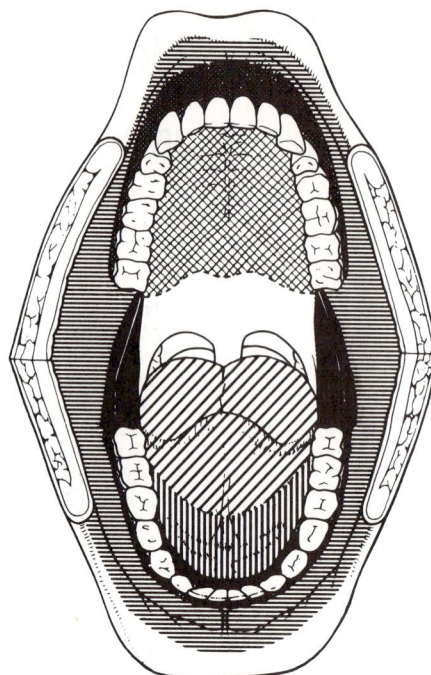

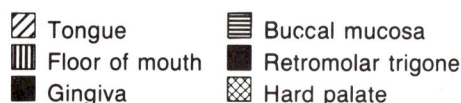

Legend:
- ▨ Tongue
- ▥ Floor of mouth
- ■ Gingiva
- ▤ Buccal mucosa
- ■ Retromolar trigone
- ▩ Hard palate

Figure 36–1. Anatomic sites within the oral cavity. (From Shah, J. P., Shemen, L. J., & Strong, E. W. [1987]. Buccal mucosa, alveolus, retromolar trigone, floor of mouth, hard palate, and tongue tumors. In S. E. Thawley & W. R. Panje [Eds.], *Comprehensive management of head and neck tumors, vol. 1* [p. 552]. Philadelphia: W. B. Saunders Co. Reproduced by permission.)

respectively (Devesa et al., 1987) (Table 36–2). For 1989, 30,600 new cases were expected to occur in the buccal cavity and oral pharynx; estimated deaths from cancer in this region were 8650 (Silverberg & Lubera, 1989) (Table 36–3). This estimate accounts for approximately 3 per cent of the new cancer cases and nearly 2 per cent of new cancer deaths.

The incidence rates of mouth and pharyngeal cancers (excluding salivary glands and lip) have remained fairly stable since the late 1940s for white men, but the rate has increased more than 50 per cent for white women (Devesa et al., 1987). White men, however, have more than double the incidence rate of women.

More than 90 per cent of all oral and pharyngeal cancers occur in people over 45 years old (Mahboubi & Sayed, 1982). An exception arises with nasopharyngeal carcinomas, of which 15 to 20 per cent appear in persons under 30 years old (Cassisi, 1987). In the late 1940s, incidence rates for mouth and pharynx cancers increased with each decade of age. Most recently, however, these rates show a different pattern, with the peak incidence occurring in the 65 to 69 year age group (see Table 36–1). Mortality rates increased from the early 1950s to mid-1980s for white women with a decrease for white men in the same time period (Devesa et al., 1987).

The incidence of oral cancers varies widely internationally. Oral cancer accounts for no more than 5 per

Table 36–1. SELECTED AGE-SPECIFIC AVERAGE ANNUAL INCIDENCE RATES FOR HEAD AND NECK CANCERS PER 100,000 WHITE MEN (M) AND WOMEN (F) IN FIVE GEOGRAPHIC AREAS IN THE UNITED STATES

Cancer Type			Age Ranges						
			35–39	45–49	55–59	65–69	75–79	85+	AA
Mouth and pharynx	F	(1947–1950)	0.7	4.5	10.4	16.0	12.8	27.3	3.4
tumors (other	F	(1983–1984)	1.0	4.8	17.4	28.1	19.9	18.9	5.3
than larynx or	M	(1947–1950)	2.5	6.2	25.8	51.5	77.3	113.0	12.5
salivary glands)	M	(1983–1984)	2.6	14.7	45.5	66.1	56.3	50.6	13.5
Larynx	F	(1947–1950)	—	1.2	1.9	1.8	2.2	—	0.5
	F	(1983–1984)	0.6	2.3	4.9	7.3	5.4	2.1	1.5
	M	(1947–1950)	0.9	4.6	20.6	21.3	26.5	14.6	5.6
	M	(1983–1984)	0.9	6.5	28.5	46.8	44.3	30.2	9.0
Salivary glands	F	(1947–1950)	0.7	2.9	5.2	7.1	6.2	4.8	1.9
	F	(1983–1984)	0.8	1.0	1.7	1.9	2.4	3.7	0.8
	M	(1947–1950)	2.0	0.9	4.1	5.5	18.4	18.2	1.8
	M	(1983–1984)	0.4	0.8	1.7	3.7	6.5	12.9	1.0

AA, average annual age-adjusted (1970 standard) incidence rates per 100,000 population.
(Data from Devesa et al., 1987, pp. 748, 752.)

cent of all cancers in Western countries but represents almost 50 per cent of all cancers in some parts of India (Mahboubi & Sayed, 1982). The age-adjusted death rate for men is above 10 per 100,000 in Hong Kong, France, Singapore, the Bahamas, Puerto Rico, and Hungary. Hong Kong has the highest death rate for women at 6.6 per 100,000, followed by Singapore, Kuwait, Panama, and Puerto Rico. The United States ranked thirteenth (men) and eleventh (women) in death rate from oral cancers in 1980–1981 (Silverberg, 1983).

Untreated oral cavity cancers have resulted in mortality rates of 50 per cent at 13 months and 75 per cent at 20 months (Shimkin, 1951). Survival rates vary depending on the site of cancer in the mouth, with the malignant gradient increasing as the site of the cancer moves posteriorly in the oral cavity. Thus cancer of the lip has the best survival rate when compared with other oral structures (Mahboubi & Sayed, 1982). Shah, Shemen, & Strong (1987) compared data from four surveys of patients who had cancer of the oral cavity. A greater percentage of oral tongue and floor of the mouth cancers were diagnosed at stage I than either cancers of the buccal mucosa or palate. Five-year survival rates for all four sites treated at stage I were well above 70 per cent, with floor of the mouth cancers registering nearly 90 per cent survival. When diagnosed at stage IV, floor of the mouth cancers had, after 5 years, a survival rate of 32 per cent, compared with

less than 20 per cent for the other three sites. Although cancers of the oral cavity of stage T_1 hold an optimistic outlook when treated, early diagnosis is not commonplace (Sisson, 1985). One half of the oral cancers, when diagnosed, are associated with lymphadenopathy (Mashberg & Samit, 1989). See Table 36–4 for tumor (T) categories of the oral cavity.

Cancer of the Tongue

An estimated 6000 new cancer cases in the United States arise annually from the tongue; estimated deaths from cancer of the tongue number 1950 annually (Silverberg & Lubera, 1986). The lateral border of the middle third of the tongue is the most common site for cancers; the dorsum, tip, and ventral surfaces are the least common sites (Batsakis, 1987). About 75 per cent of the cancers occur in the mobile portion of the tongue, and the remainder originate in the posterior third of the tongue.

Floor of the Mouth Carcinomas

Floor of the mouth carcinomas are nearly as common as those occurring in the tongue. Originating in the midline or next to the frenulum, lesions can extend into the tongue via the ventral surface and to the anterior mandible before detection. Metastasis to the cervical lymph nodes occurs in 35 to 70 per cent of the cases but develops later in the disease process than does metastasis from cancer of the tongue (Batsakis, 1987).

Table 36–2. AGE-ADJUSTED (1970 STANDARD) MORTALITY RATES PER 100,000 POPULATION FOR WHITE MEN AND WOMEN IN THE UNITED STATES FOR SELECTED TIME PERIODS

Years	Mouth and Pharynx (Other than Larynx or Salivary Glands)		Larynx		Salivary Glands	
	M	F	M	F	M	F
1950–54	5.2	1.2	2.6	0.3	0.5	0.5
1960–64	5.3	1.4	2.7	0.3	0.5	0.5
1970–74	5.1	1.6	2.8	0.3	0.4	0.4
1983–84	4.3	1.6	2.5	0.4	0.3	0.4

(Data from Devesa, et al., 1987, pp. 764, 766.)

Carcinoma of the Palate

Carcinoma of the palate frequently occurs in men in their sixties. The tumors are usually ulcerated, are surrounded by leukoplakia, and have indistinct borders. The size of the tumor has more bearing on outcome than does location on the hard palate (Batsakis, 1987).

Table 36–3. ESTIMATED NEW CANCER CASES AND CANCER DEATHS BY SEX (SELECTED SITES)

Site	Total	Male	Female
All Sites	1,010,000 (502,000)*	505,000 (266,000)	505,000 (236,000)
Buccal Cavity and Pharynx (oral)	30,600 (8,650)	20,600 (5775)	10,000 (2875)
Lip	4200 (100)	3700 (75)	500 (25)
Tongue	6000 (1950)	3900 (1300)	2100 (650)
Mouth	11,700 (2600)	7000 (1600)	4700 (1000)
Pharynx	8700 (4000)	6000 (2800)	2700 (1200)
Larynx	12,300 (3700)	10,000 (3000)	2300 (700)

*Figures in parentheses represent estimated cancer deaths.

(From Silverberg, E., & Lubera, J. [1989]. Cancer statistics, 1989. *CA: A Cancer Journal for Clinicians, 39,* 12–13. Reproduced by permission.)

Signs and Symptoms

Oral Cavity Carcinomas

A painless mass present for varying periods of time, persistent ulceration, difficulty wearing dentures, local or referred pain to the jaw or ear, and blood-tinged sputum are common complaints with oral cavity carcinomas. Later complaints include dysphagia, difficulty chewing, or changes in articulation. Some lesions may be discovered during a dental examination. In other cases, patients first note a mass in the neck (Kornblut, 1987).

Mashberg and Samit (1989) emphasize that mucosal erythroplasia rather than leukoplakia is the earliest visual sign of oral and pharyngeal carcinomas. In addition, if mucosal redness or inflammation persists for more than 14 days in the high-risk areas (floor of the mouth, ventrolateral tongue, and soft palate) without obvious cause, the area should be biopsied (Mashberg & Samit, 1989).

Nasopharyngeal Cancers

Malignant tumors in the nasopharyngeal area overwhelmingly arise in epithelial tissue (Weiland, 1987). Presenting symptoms are vague and variable. A painless enlarged neck node is a common first indicator of tumor presence. Nasal discharge (sometimes bloody), nasal stuffiness, and hypernasal speech are other indicators. Spread of the tumor can produce unilateral conductive hearing loss, atypical facial pain, and paresthesias, diplopia, trismus, nasal regurgitation, tongue paralysis, and shoulder weakness (Panje, 1987).

Table 36–4. DEFINITION OF TUMOR (T) CATEGORIES OF THE ORAL CAVITY

T_1	Greatest diameter of primary tumor 2 cm or less
T_2	Greatest diameter of primary tumor more than 2 cm but not more than 4 cm
T_3	Greatest diameter of primary tumor more than 4 cm
T_4	Massive tumor more than 4 cm in diameter, with deep invasion involving antrum, pterygoid muscles, base of tongue, or skin of neck

(From Baker, H. W. [1983]. Staging of cancer of the head and neck: Oral cavity, pharynx, larynx, and paranasal sinuses. *CA: A Cancer Journal for Clinicians, 33,* 131. Reproduced by permission.)

Oropharyngeal Cancers

Cancers of the oropharynx tend to be highly metastatic, aggressive, and undifferentiated. The majority of these cancers are beyond the T_1 designation when first seen (Batsakis, 1987). Tumors of the base of the tongue frequently occur without ulceration. Weiland (1987) postulated that tumor spread relates to the mobile nature of the tongue, which "milks" tumor cells into the lymphatic channels. Cancer of the tongue metastasizes more frequently to the cervical lymph nodes than does any other primary intraoral site (Batsakis, 1987). Kornblut (1987) cautioned that almost all tongue lesions are much more extensive than what is usually apparent. This extensiveness is confirmed by the 40 per cent cervical node involvement on initial presentation. Up to 20 per cent of the nodal involvement may be bilateral, reflecting the pattern of lymphatic drainage in the region. Tumors often are visually apparent or palpable at presentation; other manifestations include local pain and dysphagia (Kornblut, 1987).

Hypopharyngeal Cancers

Hypopharyngeal cancers occur most frequently in men in their sixth and seventh decades of life. The pyriform sinus is most commonly involved, with moderately to poorly differentiated squamous cell carcinoma accounting for most of the cancers (Weber & Manzione, 1986). The common presenting symptoms include a sore throat and neck mass. Localized pain with swallowing and referred pain to the ear are also typical (Marks, 1987). Weight loss and dysphagia occur with enlargement of the tumor (Thawley & Sessions, 1987). See Table 36–5 for staging of pharyngeal tumors.

Risk Factors

Persons in the lower socioeconomic groups have a higher incidence of oral and pharyngeal cancers. Unskilled workers have a higher risk rate than professionals, perhaps reflecting exposure to more irritating substances in the environment (Wynder & Stellman, 1977).

Tobacco is strongly associated with oral and pharyn-

Table 36–5. DEFINITION OF TUMOR (T) CATEGORIES OF THE PHARYNX

Tumor	Nasopharynx (Includes Posterosuperior and Lateral Walls)	Oropharynx (Includes Faucial Arch, Tonsil, Base of Tongue, Pharyngeal Wall)	Hypopharynx (Includes Pyriform Sinus, Postcricoid Area, Posterior Hypopharyngeal Wall)
T_1	Tumor confined to one site of nasopharynx or no tumor visible (biopsy only)	Tumor 2 cm or less in greatest diameter	Tumor confined to site of origin
T_2	Tumor involving two sites (both posterosuperior and lateral walls)	Tumor more than 2 cm but not more than 4 cm in greatest diameter	Extension of tumor to adjacent region or site without fixation of hemilarynx
T_3	Extension of tumor into nasal cavity or oropharynx	Tumor more than 4 cm in greatest diameter	Extension to adjacent region or site with fixation of hemilarynx
T_4	Tumor involvement of skull or cranial nerve or both	Massive tumor more than 4 cm in diameter, with invasion of bone, soft tissues of neck, or root (deep musculature) of tongue	Massive tumor involving bone or soft tissues of neck

(From Baker, H. W. [1983]. Staging of cancer of the head and neck: Oral cavity, pharynx, larynx, and paranasal sinuses. *CA: A Cancer Journal for Clinicians, 33,* 130–133. Reproduced by permission.)

geal cancers. Chewing "pan," a mixture of betel leaf (a climbing pepper), areca (or betel) nut, lime (calcium hydroxide), and catechu, is common in India where oral carcinomas abound (Muir, 1967). The effect of tobacco is multiplied by the ingestion of alcohol (Flanders & Rothman, 1982). Also, data from the study by Mashberg, Garfinkel, and Harris (1981) suggest alcohol has an independent role in the development of oral cancer.

Other identified risk factors include poor nutrition and poor oral hygiene (Silverberg & Lubera, 1989). Previously, physical irritation was believed to be associated with oral carcinoma development. Currently, the evidence suggests that chronic oral irritation has little influence on the development of squamous cancers. The oral sites receiving the most trauma (tip of tongue, gingiva, cheeks, and hard palate) are those with the lowest incidence of squamous cell cancers. As mentioned earlier, the three intraoral areas that most frequently show squamous cell carcinoma are the floor of the mouth, the ventrolateral tongue, and the soft palate complex (Mashberg & Samit, 1989).

Boot and shoe manufacturers and repairers have exhibited an increased incidence of buccal cavity cancer owing to exposure to noxious substances in their work. In addition, cotton, wool, and asphalt workers have had a higher than expected incidence for mouth and pharyngeal cancers (Saracci, 1985). Sun exposure has long been associated with the development of lower lip cancer in outdoor workers.

Leukoplakia, a relatively common mucosal disorder, becomes malignant in about 5 to 6 per cent of the cases. Although leukoplakia appears most commonly on commissures, progression of leukoplakia to a malignant lesion occurs most frequently on the tongue (Banoczy, 1977).

Asian Chinese have a high rate of nasopharyngeal carcinomas. The Chinese eat salted fish high in ni-

trosamine but have low vitamin C intake. Vitamin C blocks the nitrosification of amines and is thought to help prevent the disease (Ho, 1978). The relationship of the Epstein-Barr virus (EBV) to nasopharyngeal carcinoma is well established, with antibodies being produced in response to the virus (Ho, 1976). Genetic predisposition, environmental factors, and exposure to EBV are variables associated with increased risk of nasopharyngeal carcinomas.

Diagnosis

Locating the site of the tumor is of great importance for exact staging. The site determines the pattern of lymphatic drainage, which, in turn, affects surgical and radiation treatments and prognosis.

Needle and simple open biopsies are common methods of determining tissue histology. The use of toluidine blue to differentiate the margins of squamous cell carcinoma is helpful with leukoplakia or erythroplasia (Peterson, Overholser, Bergman, & Beckerman, 1986). Routine radiographs of the area serve initially to localize a suspected lesion, whereas chest radiographs rule out lung metastasis. Computed tomography (CT) shows soft tissue densities as well as bony structures, muscles, fascial planes, opacification, and enlarged lymph nodes (Peterson et al., 1986; Weber & Manzione, 1986).

Medical Treatment

Surgery and Radiation

The choice between radiation or surgery as the initial treatment hinges on many factors. Tumor location and volume, patterns of spread, and the impact of treatment on function, rehabilitation, and cosmesis are a few of the considerations (Parsons & Million, 1987). With lip lesions, irradiation or local excision is used. Neck dissection is performed for metastatic disease, not for prophylaxis. Cancers of the lower gingiva that are less than 3 cm require wide local excision with radiation. Initial surgical treatment produces better results than does radiation (Parsons & Million, 1987). Tumors over 3 cm are treated with radical excision, radical neck dissection, and postoperative radiation (Elias, 1986).

Survival rates for T_1 and early T_2 lesions of the mouth floor are similar whether treated with irradiation or surgical excision (Parsons & Million, 1987). Invasive tumors, regardless of size, require wide excision with reconstruction using tongue or nasolabial skin flaps. Deltopectoral or pectoralis major myocutaneous flaps are used for more extensive surgical removal of a tumor, and ipsilateral radical neck dissection is highly recommended. If the tumor is close to the midline, the suprahyoid lymph nodes are removed. If positive nodes are present contralaterally, a modified neck dissection is in order (Elias, 1986).

If surgical removal is chosen for small lesions of the buccal mucosa, a 2-cm margin and the underlying muscle are excised (Elias, 1986). Also, a larger irradiation treatment volume is indicated for tumors of the buccal mucosa (Parsons & Million, 1987). Cheek reconstruction with skin flaps, radical neck dissection, and postoperative irradiation is required after removal of large, invasive tumors.

Tumors of the hard palate require wide resection involving partial or total maxillectomy. Plans for use of an obturator with an upper denture are completed before surgery. Radical neck dissection is not performed unless lymph nodes are involved. High-grade malignant salivary tumors, epidermoid carcinoma, and cylindroma require radiation (Elias, 1986).

Nasopharyngeal tumors are treated by irradiation because surgical removal is nearly impossible and bilateral metastases develop early. However, some extensive surgical procedures are being initiated with an infratemporal fossa or transparotid approach (Panje, 1987). Five-year survival rates after radiotherapy have ranged from 37 to 57 per cent. Five-year survival rates for persons with T_4 stage disease have ranged from 0 to 29 per cent, whereas rates for persons with T_1 stage cancers have ranged from 60 to 76 per cent (Fu, 1987).

Tumors of the anterior two thirds of the tongue that are 2 cm or less can be treated equally well with radiation or partial glossectomy. Although combined external beam and interstitial irradiation have been successful, partial glossectomy demands less treatment time and causes minimal speech and swallowing problems (Parsons & Million, 1987). Larger lesions necessitate total or subtotal glossectomy, regional lymphadenectomy, and irradiation (Elias, 1986).

Base of the tongue lesions have access to a rich lymphatic bed that penetrates the pharyngeal wall. Poor prognosis is associated with squamous cell carcinomas in this area. Surgical management includes glossectomy, partial or total laryngectomy about 23

per cent of the time, and radical neck dissection followed by irradiation (Elias, 1986). Trials using combined methods such as bleomycin and radiation have been initiated with these lesions. Because soft palate tumors do not metastasize early, surgical resection or radiation is recommended at stage I. If metastasis does develop, radical neck dissection is performed. Small tonsillar tumors can be resected through an intraoral approach followed by irradiation (Elias, 1986). Again, large tumors warrant wide resection, including the pharyngeal wall, radical neck dissection, and irradiation.

Tumors of the hypopharynx, because of their late discovery, usually require a laryngopharyngectomy with a radical neck dissection. The overall 5-year survival rate of about 30 per cent has predisposed physicians to use radiation therapy initially and to reserve surgery for recurrence of residual disease (Elias, 1986).

Chemotherapy

Chemotherapy has been used skeptically in the treatment of head and neck cancers. Drug trials have been largely unimpressive, failing to control such variables as dose schedules, response criteria, and eligibility criteria (Eisenberger, Posada, Soper, & Wittes, 1985). Chemotherapy is not effective for those in whom local therapy has already failed, because positive responses usually are short-lived. Somewhat better results have occurred when chemotherapy is used in the initial treatment phase, usually before surgery or radiation. Combining multidrug chemotherapy with radiotherapy also has been shown to increase local tumor response. However, this combined method has not been successful in decreasing the incidence of distant metatases, and tissue reactions have often necessitated interruption of treatment (Fu, 1985). Because the optimal timing for administration of drugs and radiotherapy has not been established, specific schedules that maximize tumor response might still be identified.

The emergence of significant drug resistance, manifested in the lack of distant control, continues to frustrate treatment efforts. It remains unclear whether such high resistance results from specific characteristics of the tumor cells involved or because of widespread compromises in physiologic status associated with tobacco and alcohol use and malnutrition.

NASAL CAVITY AND PARANASAL SINUSES

Definition

The nasal cavity connects laterally with the maxillary sinuses and superiorly with the frontal, ethmoid, and sphenoid sinuses. The nasal epithelium is interspersed with mucus-secreting glands and islands of squamous epithelium (Batsakis, 1979; Redmond, Sass, & Roush, 1982). The nasal passageway acts as a sieve, warmer, and humidifier for the inhaled air. The paranasal sinuses supply additional mucus to the nasal cavity (Rice & Stanley, 1987).

Incidence, Mortality, and Survival Rates

The annual adjusted incidence rates of sinonasal cancers (SNC) is 0.8 for men and 0.5 for women per 100,000 in the United States. According to the Third National Cancer Survey Incident Cases, the cancers occur most frequently in the internal nose and maxillary sinus, followed by the ethmoid sinus. Women have more cancers of the internal nose, whereas men have a greater proportion of maxillary sinus cancers (Redmond et al., 1982). Several studies have found up to 80 per cent of sinus cancers originating in the maxilla (Batsakis, 1979). Squamous cell carcinoma is the most frequent neoplasm (80 to 90 per cent) in both the nose and sinus. Adenocarcinoma (7 to 15 per cent), transitional cell carcinoma, and sarcoma follow in decreasing order (Batsakis, 1979). Adenocarcinomas of the ethmoid sinus have a low frequency of metastatic spread and occur more commonly before age 65 years. Squamous cell carcinomas develop more frequently in people over 65 years old (Klintenberg, Olofsson, Hellquist, & Sokjer, 1984).

Five-year relative survival rates for localized lesions are about double those of regional spread. Local recurrence is the most common cause of failure, with 30 to 40 per cent of recurrences developing in the nasal cavity and ethmoidal-sphenoid complex. The maxillary sinus has about a 60 per cent local recurrence rate, with metastasis taking place 20 to 25 per cent of the time (Moss, 1987). Because advanced lesions resist current treatment modalities, 60 to 75 per cent of the patients with sinonasal carcinomas die slowly within 5 years (Batsakis, 1979). Treatment with radiation alone for unresectable lesions results in a 12 to 19 per cent 5-year survival rate. Malignant tumors of the paranasal sinuses involve the orbit and sinus wall in 60 per cent of the cases, of which 45 per cent will require exenteration (Conley & Baker, 1979).

Risk Factors

Data abstracted from the Registrar General in 1958, 1961, and 1971 for male workers in England and Wales consistently showed that the unskilled possessed a higher standardized mortality rate for sinonasal cancer than other classes of workers, particularly in the most recent twenty years (Fraumini, 1978; Redmond et al., 1982). Numerous environmental substances have been implicated, including nickel, chromium, wood dust, boot and shoe dust, wool dust, mustard gas, isopropyl oil, nitrosamines, aromatic hydrocarbons, and radium. Because of the low incidence rate of sinonasal cancers in the general population, even a small increase in a group exposed to these substances is sufficient to constitute increased risk (Redmond et al., 1982).

Signs and Symptoms

Tumors arising from the paranasal sinuses are usually asymptomatic, and diagnosis occurs late in the disease progression. Moreover, symptoms may be present for several months before a definitive diagnosis is made, and bone destruction is likely to have occurred (Wang, 1983). Symptoms are often mistaken for upper respiratory infections or inflammation of the sinuses (Rice & Stanley, 1987). Stuffy noses, headaches, and facial pains appear months before other symptoms create suspicion. Facial deformation, orbital and dental displacement, cranial nerve involvement, and bone destruction herald advanced disease (Pearson, 1987). Unilateral nasal obstruction raises concern about sinus tumor (Chaudry, Gorlin, & Mosser, 1960). The staging for carcinoma of the sinuses is not as well established as that for other head and neck tumors. Definitions of tumor categories of maxillary sinus involvement are given in Table 36–6.

Diagnosis

Knowing the extent of the tumor is paramount for determining treatment. This determination is based on a history and on direct and indirect examination of nasal cavity and nasopharynx. Computed tomographic scans and tomograms aid detection of bony and soft tissue changes.

Medical Treatment

Surgery and Radiation

Radiation or surgical removal or both is employed, depending on the extent of the tumor (Wang, 1983). Surgical intervention with irradiation has produced better results than irradiation alone. Survival rates have ranged from 29 to 48 per cent for combined therapies, compared with 10 to 34 per cent for irradiation alone (Tong, 1986).

Table 36–6. DEFINITION OF TUMOR (T) CATEGORIES OF THE MAXILLARY SINUS

Ohngren's line, a theoretical plane joining the medial canthus of the eye with the angle of the mandible, divides the maxillary antrum into an anteroinferior portion (the infrastructure) and a posterosuperior portion (the suprastructure)

T_1	Tumor confined to the antral mucosa of the infrastructure with no bone erosion or destruction
T_2	Tumor confined to the suprastructure mucosa without bone destruction, or to the infrastructure with destruction of medial or inferior walls only
T_3	More extensive tumor invading skin of cheek, orbit, anterior ethmoid sinuses, or pterygoid muscles
T_4	Massive tumor with invasion of cribiform plate, posterior ethmoids or sphenoid sinuses, nasopharynx, pterygoid plates, or base of skull

(From Baker, H. W. [1983]. Staging of cancer of the head and neck: Oral cavity, pharynx, larynx, and paranasal sinuses. *CA: A Cancer Journal for Clinicians, 33,* 130–133. Reproduced by permission.)

Surgical procedures may leave the patient with a severe facial deformity requiring specially made prosthetic devices to cover cavities and aid swallowing and articulation. These devices need to be skillfully made to minimize detection without hindering removal and reinsertion.

Craniofacial surgery has increased as an option to remove tumors involving the base of the skull. The team approach, incorporating head and neck surgeons, neurosurgeons, microvascular surgeons, radiologists, anesthesiologists, and prosthodontists, has helped to advance this therapy (Schramm, 1987). The patient and family must understand the potential dangers, expected functional ability, and possible complications. The sequelae, depending on the surgical approach and anatomic position of the tumor, may include loss of smell, loss of vision, numbness of the face, temporary facial paralysis, and facial deformities.

SALIVARY GLANDS

Definition

The salivary glands are divided into the major glands, comprising the parotid, submandibular, and sublingual glands, and the minor salivary glands, found in the mucous membrane throughout the upper aerodigestive tract.

The triangularly shaped parotid gland extends from the zygomatic arch to below the mandible and from the sternocleidomastoid to the midportion of the masseter muscle. This gland lies deeply behind the ascending ramus of the mandible, anterior to the external auditory canal and mastoid process. The lobes of the parotid are distinguished on the basis of their location vis à vis the facial nerve. The portion of the gland overlying the facial nerve (80 per cent) is considered superficial and that portion lying under the facial nerve (20 per cent) is called deep. The parotid or Stensen's duct penetrates the buccinator muscle from the anterior portion of the parotid and exits at the level of the second maxillary molar. The transverse facial artery (from the external carotid) and vein often run parallel to the duct (Johns & Kaplan, 1987).

The auriculotemporal nerve, arising from the mandibular branch of the trigeminal, supplies parasympathetic secretomotor innervation to the parotid. After parotidectomy, redness and sweating may occur over the distribution of this nerve after eating. This phenomenon, known as Frey's syndrome, results from faulty regeneration of the secretory nerve fibers to the sweat glands in the skin (Johns, 1980).

The submandibular gland lies within the space formed by the digastric muscle bellies, the inferior border of the mandible, the mylohyoid muscle, the hypoglossus muscle, and the genioglossus muscle. The marginal mandibular, lingual, and hypoglossal nerves traverse this area. The sublingual glands lie within the anterior floor of the mouth above the mylohyoid muscle and are in close proximity to the lingual and hypoglossal nerves. The minor salivary glands are scattered throughout the oral cavity and pharynx.

Incidence, Mortality, and Survival Rates

Malignant tumors of the major salivary glands are rare, the incidence rate being 0.8 to 1.0 per 100,000 for the years 1983 and 1984. Higher incidence rates occur in the older age groups in both sexes (Devesa et al., 1987) (see Table 36–1). Mortality during this same time frame was less than 1.0 per 200,000, slightly less than that during the three previous decades (see Table 36–2). The parotid gland is involved in approximately 90 per cent of salivary gland neoplasms; about 80 per cent of these are benign and 20 per cent are malignant. Tumors of the submandibular gland are rare, representing about 10 per cent of all salivary gland neoplasms; however, up to 50 per cent of submandibular tumors are malignant. Sublingual neoplasms are very rare, but close to 80 per cent are malignant. Tumors of the minor salivary glands also develop rarely, but about 60 per cent are malignant (Fried, 1986; Shidnia, Hornback, Hamaker, & Lingeman, 1980; Spiro, 1986).

As with other cancers of the head and neck, the type of tumor, location, and extent of disease have a major effect on the outcome. Five-year survival rates differ widely between low-grade (96 per cent) and high-grade (51 per cent) tumors, as well as between staging levels (Spiro, 1985). Undifferentiated tumors record the worst survival rates for the parotid gland—30 to 44 per cent at 5 years and 22 to 25 per cent at 10 years (Johns, 1980).

Risk Factors

Occurrence of salivary gland tumors is associated with prior radiation exposure in the head and neck region. Persons living in or near Hiroshima have shown a 2.6 times higher incidence of salivary gland tumors than those not exposed to radiation from the atomic bomb (Takeichi, Hirose, & Yamamoto, 1976).

Signs and Symptoms

Malignant salivary neoplasms often appear as well-demarcated, localized, firm masses. A painful, large, firm preauricular mass with complete facial nerve paralysis is the classic picture of advanced malignant parotid tumor. Most submandibular and minor salivary gland malignancies are manifested clinically as enlarging masses that may be tender or painful. If the tumor invades the lingual or hypoglossal nerves in the submandibular triangle, clumsiness of the tongue and loss of sensation may ensue (Boles, 1985).

Diagnosis

Parotid tumors present a diagnostic problem because of their notorious heterogeneity. More than 20 categories of epithelial tumors exist with variations within some categories (Fechner, 1985).

Needle aspiration biopsy is viewed favorably as a diagnostic method. Johns and Kaplan (1987) state that the routine sialograms, radionuclide images, and ultrasonograms are not helpful in determining diagnosis and rarely alter therapeutic approaches. Open biopsy is used to make a diagnosis when other methods have failed and to plan palliative radiation or chemotherapy (Johns & Kaplan, 1987).

Medical Treatment

Surgery and Radiation

A parotid tumor less than 4 cm in size can be removed by a subtotal parotidectomy that preserves the facial nerve (Spiro, 1985). Conversely, large stage III tumors require a radical parotidectomy with facial nerve sacrifice. Facial nerve repair with an autogenous nerve graft is accomplished at the time of surgery, and regional flaps are used to cover extensive resection. Large high-grade tumors are associated with limited survival, regardless of how radical a surgical procedure is performed (Spiro, 1985). Postoperative external radiation reduces the otherwise high rate of local and neck recurrence for patients with stage II and stage III tumors (Conley, 1987). Radiation treatment may be primary or adjunctive, depending on the tumor characteristics, the skill of the medical personnel, and the patient's wishes (Conley, 1987).

LARYNX

Definition

The larynx extends from the superior tip of the epiglottis (anterior surface included) to the inferior margin of the cricoid cartilage. The larynx is divided into three regions—supraglottic, glottic, and subglottic (Fig. 36–2). Embryologically, the glottis develops from paired structures that fuse at the anterior commissure; this line of fusion serves to retard the spread of tumors. The absence of midline divisions in the supraglottis and subglottis allows tumors in these areas to spread circumferentially. In addition, anatomic structures that separate the supraglottis from the glottis and the subglottis from the glottis prevent extraglottic tumors from immediate extension into the glottis. Consequently, hoarseness develops later in the course of the disease, making early detection less frequent (van Nostrand, 1987).

Incidence, Mortality, and Survival Rates

The 1987 annual adjusted incidence rate for cancer of the larynx among whites in the United States is 9.0 for men and 1.5 for women per 100,000 (Devesa et al., 1987). Cancer of the larynx occurs in every country, with men consistently having a higher incidence rate than women. However, the estimated number of laryngeal cancer deaths among women in the United States has more than doubled, from 300 in 1969 to 700 in 1987. Estimated laryngeal cancer deaths for men in the United States rose from 2500 to 3100 in the same time period but have remained stable since 1983 (Grant & Silverberg, 1969; Silverberg, 1983; Silverberg & Lubera, 1987). The supraglottic, glottic, and subglottic regions of the larynx have a ratio of tumor occurrence of 40:59:1, respectively, in the United States (Austen, 1982). Five-year survival rates for whites in the United States increased 14 per cent from 1960 to 1983. Blacks, however, had a 1 per cent reduction in survival rates from 1974 to 1983 (Silverberg & Lubera, 1987). Without treatment, 90 per cent of persons afflicted with cancer of the larynx die within 3 years (Shimkin, 1951).

The most frequent abnormalities (90 per cent) arise from the squamous cell. Other cell types are verrucous carcinoma, carcinosarcoma, adenocarcinoma, lymphoma, and sarcoma. The squamous cell abnormality that will most likely become cancerous is keratosis with atypia (Romm, 1986).

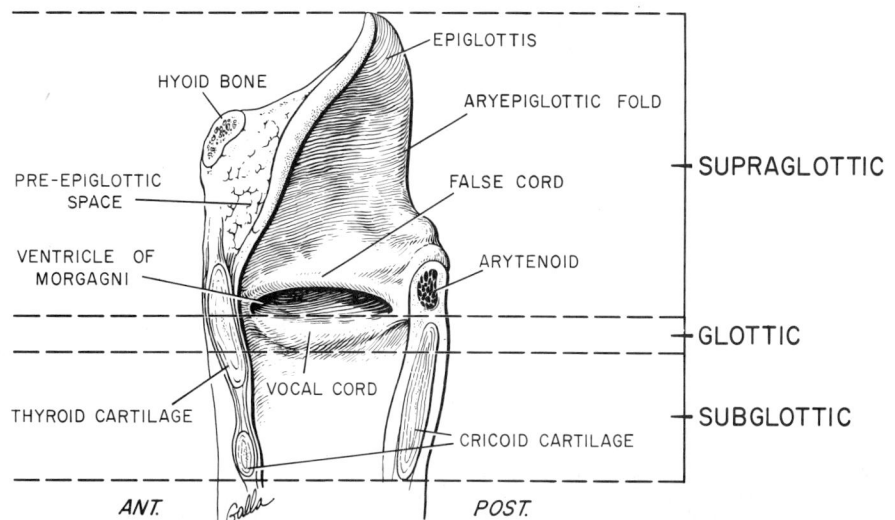

Figure 36–2. Diagram showing anatomic subdivision of the larynx into supraglottic, glottic, and subglottic. (From Wang, C. C. [1987]. Radiation therapy of laryngeal tumors: Curative radiation therapy. In S. E. Thawley & W. R. Panje [Eds.], *Comprehensive management of head and neck tumors, vol. 1* [p. 906]. Philadelphia: W. B. Saunders Co. Reproduced by permission.)

EPIGLOTTIS
HYOID BONE
ARYEPIGLOTTIC FOLD
PRE-EPIGLOTTIC SPACE
FALSE CORD
SUPRAGLOTTIC
VENTRICLE OF MORGAGNI
ARYTENOID
VOCAL CORD
GLOTTIC
THYROID CARTILAGE
CRICOID CARTILAGE
SUBGLOTTIC
ANT.
POST.

Risk Factors

Laryngeal cancer, as with most other head and neck cancers, is closely associated with smoking and alcohol consumption. Using data from the Third National Cancer survey, Flanders and Rothman (1982) found a moderate synergy between alcohol and tobacco, with the resulting risk being approximately 50 per cent greater than if the effects of the two were simply additive. Smoking is associated with the development of squamous cell carcinoma in all portions of the larynx. In addition, the type of cigarette smoked has a bearing on the incidence (Wynder & Hoffman, 1982; Wynder & Stellman, 1977). Increased incidence of laryngeal cancer also occurs among persons who work with asbestos and wood. Communities in which paper, chemicals, or petroleum are manufactured show a higher incidence of laryngeal cancer (Austen, 1982; Cowles, 1983). Templar (1987) concluded that there is not enough evidence to link therapeutic radiation with increased occurrence of laryngeal tumors. Decreased amounts of vitamins A and C in the diet have been associated with increased risks of laryngeal cancer (Graham, Mettlin, & Marshall, 1981).

Signs and Symptoms

Persons who become hoarse see, on the average, three physicians in an attempt to identify the cause, and as many as 8 months can elapse before a diagnosis of laryngeal cancer is made. Any hoarseness that persists longer than 2 weeks should be evaluated by a physician skilled in throat examination techniques (Griffith et al., 1979).

Symptoms depend on location, size, and degree of invasion (Table 36–7). If the tumor develops on a vocal fold, intermittent hoarseness appears early in the course of the disease, and the tumor can be diagnosed at stage I. Conversely, a tumor arising subglottically may progress to stage III before definitive symptoms

appear. Supra- and subglottic tumors may be asymptomatic until the vocal folds are involved or a suspicious node arises in the neck. A mild persistent sore throat may be the only indication of a stage II supraglottic tumor. At stage IV, symptoms become very similar regardless of the original tumor site: pain radiating to the ear, dysphagia, dyspnea, neck mass, and odynophagia (Templar, 1987). Palpation of all the outer surfaces of the laryngeal skeleton is important to detect masses. Table 36–8 contains the definition of T categories for laryngeal tumors.

Diagnosis

The diagnostic work-up includes viewing the larynx with a mirror (indirect laryngoscopy), a flexible fiberoptic endoscope, or a laryngoscope—or all three. Radiographic studies, xerography, and CT add other dimensions to the diagnostic process.

Medical Treatment

Surgery and Radiation

As with many types of cancers, early diagnosis increases the chance of cure. Stage T_1 vocal fold lesions are treated equally well by radiation or by local excision. The T_2 glottic lesion may be treated with either a hemilaryngectomy or radiation, although the surgical approach tends to have better survival rates (Johns, 1980; Wang, 1987). Total laryngectomy is recommended for most stage T_3 glottic lesions. Neck dissections are also advocated with stages T_3, N_0, or N_1. Positive nodes indicate adjuvant irradiation therapy. Stage T_4 lesions require total laryngectomy with radical neck dissection and postoperative irradiation (Kirchner, 1985). The majority of supraglottic lesions can be treated adequately with a horizontal supraglottic partial laryngectomy. Although early stage T_1 supraglottic

---

Table 36–7. SIGNS AND SYMPTOMS OF CANCER OF THE LARYNX

Stage	Supraglottic	Glottic	Subglottic
I	Sensation of local irritation or no symptoms	Hoarseness if on mobile vocal fold	No symptoms
II	Sore throat, mild, persistent Hoarseness if vocal fold involved	Hoarseness Irritation of throat	Mild sensation of irritation or no symptoms
III	Sore throat, localized Hoarseness is probable Odynophagia Single neck mass, 3 cm on same side as other symptoms	Voice reduced to stage whisper Neck mass (possible)	Hoarseness if vocal folds are invaded Dyspnea if tumor is bulky
IV	Pain radiating to ear Hoarseness Odynophagia Neck mass Dysphagia Dyspnea	Pain radiating to ear Severe hoarseness Odynophagia Unilateral or bilateral nodes (probable) Dyspnea Cough	Pain referred to ear Neck mass Odynophagia Dysphagia Dyspnea

(From Templer, J. [1987]. *Clinical evaluation of the larynx.* In S. E. Thawley & W. R. Panje [Eds.], *Comprehensive management of head and neck tumors* [vol. 1, p. 876]. Philadelphia: W. B. Saunders Co. Reproduced by permission.)

Table 36–8. DEFINITION OF TUMOR (T) CATEGORIES OF THE LARYNX

Tumor	Supraglottis (Includes False Vocal Folds, Arytenoids, Epiglottis)	Glottis (Includes True Vocal Folds Including Anterior and Posterior Commissures)	Subglottis
T_1	Tumor confined to site of origin with normal mobility	Tumor confined to glottis with normal mobility	Tumor confined to the subglottic region
T_2	Tumor involves adjacent supraglottic site or glottis without fixation	Supraglottic or subglottic extension of tumor with normal or impaired cord mobility	Tumor extension to vocal folds with normal or impaired cord mobility
T_3	Tumor limited to larynx with fixation or extension to involve postcricoid area, medial wall of pyriform sinus or pre-epiglottic space	Tumor confined to larynx with cord fixation	Tumor confined to larynx with vocal fold fixation
T_4	Massive tumor extending beyond the larynx to involve oropharynx, soft tissues of neck, or destruction of thyroid cartilage	Massive tumor with thyroid cartilage destruction or extension beyond the confines of the larynx	Massive tumor with cartilage destruction or extension beyond the confines of the larynx

(From Baker, H. W. [1983]. Staging of cancer of the head and neck: Oral cavity, pharynx, larynx, and paranasal sinuses. *CA: A Cancer Journal for Clinicians, 33,* 132. Reproduced by permission.)

lesions can be treated with irradiation, if radiotherapy fails a total laryngectomy must be performed (Kirchner & Owen, 1977). Postoperative complications include fistula formation and wound infections (Sheman & Spiro, 1986).

A supraglottic laryngectomy, while preserving the voice, invites aspiration. A total laryngectomy, on the other hand, avoids the problem of aspiration but requires a major adjustment in communication. Persons can learn to communicate by means of esophageal speech, artificial larynges, or voice buttons placed in a primary tracheoesophageal fistula.

NURSING MANAGEMENT

Prevention

The high correlation of smoking and alcohol consumption with head and neck cancer demands unrelenting education of the public and individual discouragement of usage by health professionals—who themselves do not smoke or abuse alcohol. In my opinion, the most potent deterrent to smoking and alcohol abuse for young people is a significant adult who does not smoke or abuse alcohol.

The nurse can operate in the prevention arena at several levels: contacting government representatives to condemn the political and economic advantages that the tobacco industry enjoys, supporting local or national groups that are trying to invoke laws curbing usage of addictive substances, and presenting educational programs in elementary and secondary schools as well as in the community at large. The opportunities to inform patients of the risks and to give information on where help can be obtained abound in the clinical setting. Of particular value is the nurse who has experienced withdrawal and can interact with a patient

on a level unavailable to nurses who have not endured that process.

The newly diagnosed patients tend to be more receptive to changing their personal habits because of perceived vulnerability and knowing the results of that habit (Schleper, 1989). Teaching patients oral self-examination skills empowers them to improve their health status. Knowledge of the symptoms arising from cancerous lesions alerts patients to changes that otherwise may be discounted.

Detection

The higher incidence of cancer in older adults than in middle-aged adults requires the nurse who works with the elderly to be aware of the signs and symptoms of head and neck cancer. Institution of regular assessments for residents of extended care facilities may be successful in spotting early lesions during the quiet progression of head and neck tumors. Inspection of the oral cavity is of particular significance because asymptomatic cancerous lesions remain undetected. Mashberg and Samit (1989) describe these lesions as characterized by "innocuous-appearing red inflammatory or erythroplastic mucosal changes, ... [the] lesions are less than 2 cm in diameter; are predominantly red, with or without a white component; and are smooth, granular, or minimally elevated." Schleper (1989) compiled a list of signs and symptoms related to specific structures of the head and neck (Table 36–9).

Patient Preparation for Treatment

Treatment methods include surgery, radiation, and chemotherapy (see Chapter 20 for nursing care related to irradiation). Surgical intervention for head and neck tumors ranges from minor to extremely complex. Prep-

Table 36–9. SITE-SPECIFIC HEAD AND NECK ASSESSMENT AND SYMPTOMS

Direct and Indirect Assessment	Signs and Symptoms

Larynx (Indirect assessment)
Supraglottis
  Epiglottis
  Aryepiglottic folds
  Arytenoid cartilages
  False vocal folds
Glottis
  True vocal folds
  Commissures
Subglottis
  Area below true vocal folds to inferior border of cricoid
    cartilage
  Rare site of tumor occurrence
	Inquire about:
	Supraglottis
	  Voice change—absence of higher pitched voice tones
	  Throat pain
	  Dysphagia, odynophagia
	  Referred otalgia
	  Stridor or dyspnea
	  Cervical adenopathy
	    Upper jugular
	    Midjugular
	Glottis
	  Persistent hoarseness (hallmark symptom)
	  Sore throat
	  Stridor or dyspnea
	Subglottis
	  Same as glottis

Hypopharynx (Indirect assessment)
Absent thyroid cartilage crepitus when moving laryngeal
  framework over the cervical spine
	Inquire about:
	Throat pain
	Referred ear pain
	Dysphagia
	Cervical adenopathy
	  Upper jugular
	  Midjugular

Cervical esophagus (Indirect assessment) "Silent area"	**Inquire about:** Dysphagia Recent unexplained weight loss of 10 lb or more Hemoptysis Regurgitation

Cervical lymphatics
Superior horizontal group
  Facing patient, palpate this U-shaped group of nodes:
    Preauricular and parotid
    Submandibular and submaxillary
    Submental
    Postauricular and mastoid
    Occipital
Vertical nodes
  Jugular chain (anterior to sternocleidomastoid muscle;
    palpate standing behind patient)
    Subdigastric and jugulodigastric
    Midjugular
    Low jugular
  Posterior cervical or spinal accessory chain (anterior to
    trapezius; posterior to sternocleidomastoid)
  Check motor function of cranial nerve XI
Inferior horizontal nodes
  Supraclavicular (often indicative of distant metastasis)
	Palpate for:
	Nodes >1 cm
	Firm to hard consistency
	Limited mobility or fixed
	Spherical, matted, or poorly defined
	Nontender
	Subdigastric nodes: most common site for metastasis

Major salivary glands
Parotid
Submandibular
Sublingual
	Observe for:
	Mass over gland
	  With pain
	  Without pain
	Facial palsy
	Note swelling of duct openings in oral cavity

Assess symmetry of: Face Neck	**Inspect for:** Asymmetry or masses Deficits of cranial nerve VII Jugular distention

Inspect skin surfaces of:
Face
  Scalp
  Skinfolds
Neck
	Inspect for:
	Persistent ulcerations
	Pink, red, or white elevated lesions with a waxy appearance,
	  telangiectasias, and central umbilication or ulceration
	Inspect pigmented lesions for changes in color, size, shape,
	  surface, or elevation

Table 36–9. SITE-SPECIFIC HEAD AND NECK ASSESSMENT AND SYMPTOMS *Continued*

Direct and Indirect Assessment	Signs and Symptoms

Nasal cavity, paranasal sinuses (indirect assessment of sinuses)—these tumors are often misdiagnosed
Frontal sinus
  Palpate under supraorbital margin
Ethmoid, maxillary
  Palpate infraorbital margin
  Palpate under the inferior border of the maxilla and zygoma
Assess motor functions of cranial nerves:
  III, IV, VI
  Sensory function of cranial nerve V
Inspect nasal cavity for:
  Symmetry
  Discharge or odor
  Lesions or color changes
  Patency
  Optional: cranial nerve I
	Inquire and observe for:
	Asymmetry, pain or numbness over involved sinus, cheeks, upper alveolar ridge
	Proptosis, diplopia, epiphora, headaches
	Unilateral nasal obstruction, bleeding, discharge, anosmia
	In oral cavity: unexplained loosening of upper molars, upper denture, or upper partial plate

Nasopharynx (Indirect assessment): "Silent" area. Symptoms are noted later than for other head and neck sites
Inspect tympanic membranes for:
  Bulging
  Retraction
  Fluid
  Intactness
  Color changes or lesions
Inspect nasal cavity (as above)
Inspect soft palate for:
  Symmetry
	Inquire and observe for:
	Unilateral nasal obstruction
	Epistaxis or blood in postnasal drip
	Ear symptoms or the stopped-up ear
	Nasal voice quality
	Cervical adenopathy:
	  Posterior cervical
	  Jugular chain

Oral cavity, oropharynx
Inspect and palpate:
  Lips, buccal and labial mucosa
  Gums, teeth (if present), or alveolar ridges
  Retromolar trigones
  Hard and soft palates
  Dorsal, ventral, lateral surfaces of oral tongue
  (Check motor function of cranial nerves V, XII)
  Floor of mouth
  Tonsillar fossae and pillars
  Base of tongue (mirror examination)
  Oropharyngeal wall: check motor functions of cranial nerves IX, X
	Observe especially in the U-shaped area previously described for the following:
	Painless color changes
	  Erythroplasia
	  Leukoplakia
	  Pigment changes
	Persistent ulcerations
	Mass or thickening
	Unilateral or specific sore throat
	Referred otalgia
	Dysphagia, odynophagia
	Pain, numbness, or tingling
	Trismus, deficits of cranial nerves IX, X, or XII
	Cervical adenopathy
	  Subdigastric
	  Submandibular

(From Schleper, J. R. [1989]. Prevention, detection, and diagnosis of head and neck cancers. *Seminars in Oncology Nursing, 5,* 144–145. Reproduced by permission.)

aration and continuing support of the patient to meet this challenge on a day-to-day basis falls to the nurse.

Preoperative Care

Sigler (1988) puts the nurse's preoperative assessment into perspective when she advises gaining some insight into the basic life style of the patient. Areas to probe are usual daily activities, eating habits, living arrangements, and availability of the support of significant others. From this information, likely problems can be addressed. Explanations about incisions, tubes, alterations in airway, swallowing, or speech and changes in appearance must be given in terms and in ways the patient can understand.

Postoperative Care

Airway Management. Airway management for patients with surgery of the oral cavity or pharynx entails

keeping the temporary tracheostomy patent. Instillation of sterile saline solution in small amounts (2 to 5 ml) stimulates coughing and allows easier expulsion of thick mucus. Suctioning with sterile equipment may be done as often as every hour depending on the amount of mucus produced. As the patient becomes more ambulatory, the ability to cough up secretions increases and the need for suctioning decreases. Humidification, by ultrasonic nebulization or oxygen mist, provides an essential element in liquefying secretions in the early postoperative period.

Usually plastic disposable cuffed tracheostomy tubes are used to prevent aspiration of oral secretions until the patient gains control of swallowing. I agree with Sigler's preference (1989) to release the cuff around the tracheostomy tube every shift to remove secretions that have collected above the cuff. The amount of tension the cuff exerts on the tracheal wall can be controlled by checking the amount of pressure in the cuff's bladder using a sphygmomanometer, 10 ml syringe, and stopcock.

The inner cannula holds the key to maintenance of a patent airway. It can be removed, without risking the loss of the airway, if it suddenly becomes plugged. Disposable versus reusable inner cannulas have been shown to save time in the cleansing procedure with no difference in the infection rate (Wagner & Sigler, 1988). After the need for a cuffed tracheostomy tube passes, it is replaced by a metal tracheostomy tube.

Corking of the tracheostomy tube allows evaluation of the patient's ability to breathe through the upper aerodigestive tract before removing the tube. If the patient has an adequate airway through the aerodigestive tract and can clear secretions through the mouth, the tracheostomy tube is removed. The tracheostomy incision closes without suturing by applying an airtight pressure dressing over it. The patient is instructed to press fingers over the dressing when coughing to prevent air flow from separating the incision.

If a total laryngectomy is performed, the sequence of events varies slightly with respect to the type of airway device used after the cuffed disposable plastic tube is removed. A plastic stent may be placed in the tracheal stoma to reduce contraction of the stomal opening.

Complications, such as fistula formation, may require reinsertion of a cuffed plastic tracheostomy tube. The cuffed tracheostomy tube prevents secretions from draining into the lungs and also provides a seal for mechanical hyperinflation of the lungs.

Regional Flap Management. The success of reconstructive surgery of the head and neck using a flap rests on the viability of that flap. The use of myocutaneous and free flaps revolutionized the surgical treatment of head and neck cancers. After surgery, the nurse's responsibility centers on maintaining flap viability. Because the myocutaneous flap crosses the neck to its destination, all constricting items around the neck are avoided, such as gown ties, humidification mask cords, and tracheostomy ties. Plastic cuffed tracheostomy tubes may be held in place with sutures rather than ties the first few days after the operation. Humidification delivery by T-piece rather than mask obviates the use of an elastic band encircling the neck. Changes in the temperature and color of a flap need to be reported immediately to the surgeon. The blood flow in free flaps may be monitored with Doppler ultrasound. Loss of the Doppler signal indicates the need for immediate wound evaluation and possible exploration (Sigler, 1988).

Neck dissection includes dermal lifting to expose the underlying structures and requires either pressure dressing or drain placement. The dermis must adhere to the underlying structures to reestablish its blood supply. Functioning drains help prevent the occurrence of hematomas or seromas. Drains are attached to collecting devices and are removed when the daily output becomes scant. In addition to measuring the drain output, the nurse observes the color of the drainage. If it becomes milky rather than reddish, chyle is leaking owing to accidental severance of a lymphatic duct during surgery.

Neck dissection incisions often leak serous fluid, which is removed with hydrogen peroxide followed by normal saline solution and sometimes ointment application. Draining material and its crusting around the tracheostomy stoma require gentle cleansing and application of a tracheostomy bib to absorb secretions. Zinc oxide ointment may be applied on the skin below the tracheostomy stoma for protection from secretions; however, the value of this action has not been established under controlled circumstances.

Communication. The patient with a tracheostomy is without a voice. The patient's call light or some other communication device must always be within reach. Labeling the public address apparatus with the room numbers of patients who cannot speak reminds nurses to tell the patient by public address that they will respond immediately when a call comes in. Paper and pen, flash cards, and pictorial boards are examples of ways in which the patient can let the nursing staff know what is needed. After removal of the tracheostomy tube, the patient may have difficulty with articulation as a result of the oral cavity or pharyngeal surgery. Listening and verifying the communication are essential nurse behaviors to gain the confidence of the patient.

For the patient who has had a total laryngectomy, the loss of voice is permanent. For those persons who have had hemilaryngectomies or supraglottic laryngectomies, the removal of the tracheostomy tube allows return of the voice, albeit somewhat altered from its original timbre. Loss of the voice results in an inability to sing, whistle, make quick verbal retorts, laugh, or change voice inflections. The voice conveys much more than words; it holds emotions—joy, pain, anger, fear, delight. This revelation of self to the world is gone for the laryngectomee. Replacements, such as with esophageal speech, the voice button, or the artificial larynges, give the laryngectomee a means to communicate, but they lack the expressiveness of the "normal" voice. Yet it is not unusual for an individual with a laryngectomy to overcome this handicap and continue a life style with style.

Camouflaging the stoma may be important to some laryngectomees. Bibs, ascots, lace collars, or shirts with a tie provide cover for appearance in public and prevent inhalation of small particles. The laryngectomee must unlearn some reflexes: covering the mouth when coughing, blowing on liquids to cool them, and blowing the nose. Other restrictions include prohibition of swimming or fishing from a boat. As the integration of this change occurs within the self, the patient may develop depression, especially if alternative forms of communication are difficult and if talking was a major way of meeting emotional needs.

Nutrition. Nutrition can be a problem preoperatively as well as postoperatively for the head and neck cancer patient. Preoperatively, patients often suffer from deficient intake owing to alcoholism or dysphagia. Postoperatively, a patient may have insufficient intake because of swallowing difficulties and aspiration (Box

---

Box 36–1. ALTERED SWALLOWING PROCESSES

Logemann, J. A. (1985). **Aspiration in head and neck surgical patients.** *Annals of Otology, Rhinology, Laryngology, 94,* 373–376.

One of the major problems occurring after surgical removal of aerodigestive tract cancer is aspiration with swallowing. This study identified what sequence of the swallowing process is altered with several types of surgical treatments for cancer of the aerodigestive tract that result in aspiration.

A total of 30 patients were studied, of whom 16 had partial laryngectomies, 13 had surgically treated oral cancer, and one had a resection of the posterior pharyngeal wall. Of the 16 patients with partial laryngectomy, 5 had hemilaryngectomies and 11 had supraglottic laryngectomies.

A videofluorographic examination using three consistencies of barium and two views yielded information to appraise the swallowing sequence. The patients with hemilaryngectomies had normal oral control of the bolus during the oral stages of the swallow and a normal swallowing reflex. The problems occurred in the laryngeal adduction and reduced pharyngeal peristalsis phases. The patients with supraglottic laryngectomies showed aspiration before, during, and after the swallow. Most prevalent problems were reduced vocal fold adduction and reduced laryngeal elevation. For the oral cancer patient groups, different deglutition problems occurred depending on the site of the resection. Those patients with anterior composite resection showed only oral disorders. All of them aspirated before the swallow because of reduced tongue control and because part of the bolus entered the pharynx before swallowing was begun. The lateral composite patients showed either a delayed swallowing reflex, reduced tongue control, or reduced pharyngeal peristalsis. Eight patients showed a combination of problems.

The information about the effect of food consistency showed that there is no single best food consistency that aids swallowing for dysphagic patients. The food consistency should be matched with the physiology of each patient's swallow.

The author strongly recommends that a modified barium swallow be the method used to attain the correct information about the physiology of a patient's swallowing, because this uses a small amount of food and keeps the radiographic tube focused on the oral cavity and pharynx for 10 to 30 seconds after the swallow. Identifying the cause of aspiration in the head and neck cancer patient results in application of the correct management technique for improved swallowing.

36–1). This is particularly true of patients who have had surgery that interferes with the changing positions of the upper areodigestive tract structures that control swallowing (Logemann, 1989).

The process of swallowing encompasses four phases: oral preparation and the oral, pharyngeal, and esophageal phases. The functions of any one of these phases or combinations thereof can be altered with surgery. Drooling, pocketing of food in the lateral sulcus, and losing food into the pharynx while chewing are examples of swallowing problems (Logemann, 1989). Procedures that are used to help with swallowing include postural changes and alterations in food consistencies, exercises to strengthen muscles and increase jaw range of motion, and exercises with specific instructions to change the coordination of the swallow (Logemann, 1979). (See Chapter 47 for nutritional needs of the cancer patient).

Psychosocial Aspects. Persons who have cancer of the head and neck often have a history of alcoholism and, with it, lack of close personal relationships, unstable work histories, and dysfunctional family interactions. Characteristics of dependence, inability to change habits, and poor adaptive coping skills make adjustment to the disfigurement and dysfunction from the treatment methods especially difficult (Dropkin, 1989). Other factors that impede adjustment are isolation, fear of rejection, negative changes in family interaction, and the patient's dependence on physical appearance for self-concept.

The alterations in appearance and function of speech, swallowing, or breathing require self-image adjustments and learning of self-care tasks. Dropkin (1989) postulates that the increase in performance of

tasks occurs between postoperative days 4 and 5 because of the interaction between staff and the teaching of new tasks, which decrease the patient's initial anxiety about interaction with others. Task performance by the patient was interpreted as acceptance of the physical change and usually preceded social affiliative behaviors (see Chapter 52 for discussion of alterations in body image).

If the family interaction is dysfunctional, a spouse or significant other can hinder the progress of the patient in accepting physical changes and taking care of physical needs. Trying to alter long-standing interaction patterns during the short hospitalization period is unrealistic. Giving information about what to expect, both physically and psychologically; listening to concerns and giving direction; and including significant others in home care planning will—it is hoped—provide some stability for the patient and family.

Not all patients who have major head and neck surgery are alcoholics or have dependency needs. Many travel through the grieving process without unusual aberrations and retain their self-esteem despite physical changes. The team approach, with nurses coordinating the work of social workers, pastors, dietitians, speech therapists, physical therapists, and surgeons for physical and pyschosocial support of the patient, increases the probability of a better life adjustment to the treatment outcomes.

References

Austen, D. F. (1982). Larynx. In D. Schottenfeld & J. F. Fraumeni (Eds.), *Cancer epidemiology and prevention* (pp. 554–563). Philadelphia: W. B. Saunders Co.

Baker, H. W. (1983). Staging of cancer of the head and neck: Oral cavity, pharynx, larynx, and paranasal sinuses. *CA: A Cancer Journal for Clinicians, 33*, 130–133.

Banoczy, J. (1977). Follow-up studies in oral leukoplakia. *Journal of Maxillofacial Surgery, 5*, 69–75.

Baranovsky, A., & Myers, M. H. (1986). Cancer incidence and survival in patients 65 years of age and older. *CA: A Cancer Journal for Clinicians, 36*, 26–41.

Batsakis, J. G. (1979). Cancer of the nasal cavity and the paranasal sinuses. In *Tumors of the head and neck* (2nd ed., pp. 177–178). Baltimore: Williams & Wilkins.

Batsakis, J. G. (1987). Pathology of tumors of the oral cavity. In S. E. Thawley & W. R. Panje (Eds.), *Comprehensive management of head and neck tumors* (vol. 1, pp. 480–515). Philadelphia: W. B. Saunders Co.

Boles, R. (1985). Carcinoma of the submandibular minor salivary glands. In P. B Chretien, M. E. Johns, D. P. Shedd, E. W. Strong, & P. H. Ward (Eds.), *Head and neck cancer* (vol. 1, pp. 225–227). Proceedings of the International Conference, Baltimore, 1984. St. Louis: C. V. Mosby Co.

Cassisi, N. J. (1987). Clinical evaluation of pharyngeal tumors. In S. E. Thawley & W. R. Panje (Eds.), *Comprehensive management of head and neck tumors* (pp. 614–629). Philadelphia, W. B. Saunders Co.

Chaudry, A. P., Gorlin, R. J., & Mosser, D. G. (1960). Carcinoma of the antrum: A clinical and histopathologic study. *Oral Surgery, 13*, 269–281.

Conley, J. (1987). Controversies regarding therapy of tumors of the salivary glands. In S. E. Thawley, & W. R. Panje (Eds.), *Comprehensive management of head and neck tumors* (pp. 1151–1156). Philadelphia, W. B. Saunders Co.

Conley, J., & Baker, D. L. (1979). Management of the eye socket in cancer of the paranasal sinuses. *Archives of Otolaryngology, 105*, 702–705.

Cowles, S. R. (1983). Cancer of the larynx: Occupational and environmental associations. *Southern Medical Journal, 76*, 894–898.

Devesa, S. S., Silverman, D. T., Young, J. L., Jr., Pollack, E. S., Brown, C. C., Horm, J. W., Percy, C. L., Myers, M. H., McKay, F. W., & Fraumeni, J. F., Jr. (1987). Cancer incidence and mortality trends among whites in the United States, 1947–84. *Journal of the National Cancer Institute, 79*, 701–770.

Dropkin, M. J. (1989). Coping with disfigurement and dysfunction after head and neck cancer surgery: A conceptual framework. *Seminars in Oncology Nursing, 5*, 213–219.

Eisenberger, M., Posada, J., Soper, W., & Wittes, R. (1985). The current status of chemotherapy. In R. E. Wittes (Ed.), *Head and neck cancer* (vol. 2, pp. 181–220). New York: John Wiley & Sons.

Elias, E. G. (1986). Surgical management of head and neck neoplasia. In D. E. Peterson, E. G. Elias, & S. T. Sonis (Eds.), *Head and neck management of the cancer patient* (pp. 255–274). Boston: Martinus Nijhoff.

Fechner, R. E. (1985). Diagnosis of salivary gland neoplasms. In P. B. Chretien, M. E. Johns, D. P. Shedd, E. W. Strong, & P. H. Ward (Eds.), *Head and neck cancer* (vol. 1, pp. 219–222). Proceedings of the International Conference, Baltimore, 1984. St. Louis: C. V. Mosby Co.

Flanders, W. D., & Rothman K. J. (1982). Interaction of alcohol and tobacco in laryngeal cancer. *American Journal of Epidemiology, 115*, 371–379.

Fraumeni, J. F., Jr. (1978). Geographic distribution of head and neck cancers in the United States. *Laryngoscope* (Suppl. No. 8) *88*, 40–43.

Fried, M. P. (1986). Neoplasms of the salivary glands. In D. E. Peterson, E. G. Elias, & S. T. Sonis (Eds.), *Head and neck management of the cancer patient* (pp. 201–229). Boston: Martinus Nijhoff.

Fu, K. K. (1985). Concurrent radiotherapy and chemotherapy. In R. E. Wittes (Ed.), *Head and neck cancer* (vol. 2, pp. 221–248). New York: John Wiley & Sons.

Fu, K. K. (1987). Treatment of tumors of the nasopharynx: Radiation therapy. In S. E. Thawley & W. R. Panje (Eds.), *Comprehensive management of head and neck* tumors (vol. 1, pp. 649–662). Philadelphia: W. B. Saunders Co.

Graham, S., Mettlin C., & Marshall, J. (1981). Dietary factors in

the epidemiology of cancer of the larynx. *American Journal of Epidemiology, 113*, 675–680.

Grant, R. N., & Silverberg, E. (1969). *Cancer statistics—1969* (p. 7). New York: American Cancer Society.

Griffith, G. L., Meeker, W. R., & McMahan, A. (1979). Management of carcinoma of the larynx. *Journal of the Kentucky Medical Association, 77*, 169.

Harnsburger, H. C., & W. P. Dillon (1987). Imaging tumors of the central nervous system and extracranial head and neck. *CA: A Cancer Journal for Clinicians, 37*, 225–245.

Ho, H. C. (1976). Epstein-Barr virus and specific IgA and the IgC serum antibodies in nasopharyngeal carcinoma. *British Journal of Cancer, 34*, 655–660.

Ho, H. C. (1978). An epidemiologic and clinical study of nasopharyngeal carcinoma. *International Journal of Radiation Oncology, Biology, Physics, 4*, 181–198.

Johns, M. E. (1980). Parotid cancer: A rational basis for treatment. *Head and Neck Surgery, 3*, 132–141.

Johns, M. E., & Kaplan, M. J. (1987). Surgical therapy of tumors of the salivary glands. In S. E. Thawley & W. R. Panje (Eds.), *Comprehensive management of head and neck tumors* (pp. 1104–1138). Philadelphia, W. B. Saunders Co.

Kirchner, J. A. (1985). Treatment of laryngeal cancer. In P. B. Chretien, M. E. Johns, D. P. Shedd, E. W. Strong, & P. H. Ward (Eds.), *Head and Neck Cancer* (vol. 1, pp. 199–201). Proceedings of the International Conference, Baltimore, 1984. St. Louis: C. V. Mosby Co.

Kirchner, J. A., & Owen, J. R. (1977). Five hundred cancers of the larynx and pyriform sinus. *Laryngoscope, 87*, 1288–1303.

Klintenberg, C., Olofsson, J., Hellquist, H., & Sokjer, H. (1984). Adenocarcinoma of the ethmoid sinuses. *Cancer, 54*, 482–488.

Kornblut, A. D. (1987). Clinical evaluation of tumors of the oral cavity. In S. E. Thawley & W. R. Panje (Eds.), *Comprehensive management of head and neck tumors* (pp. 460–479). Philadelphia, W. B. Saunders Co.

Lampe, H. B., Lampe, K. M., & Skillings, J. (1986). Head and neck cancer in the elderly. *Journal of Otolaryngology, 15*, 235–238.

Logemann, J. A. (1989). Swallowing and communication rehabilitation. *Seminars in Oncology Nursing, 5*, 205–212.

Mahboubi, E., & Sayed, G. B. (1982). Oral cavity and pharynx. In D. Schottenfeld & J. F. Fraumeni, Jr. (Eds.), *Cancer epidemiology and prevention* (pp. 583–595). Philadelphia: W. B. Saunders Co.

Marks, J. E. (1987). Treatment of tumors of the hypopharynx: Radiation therapy. In S. E. Thawley & W. R. Panje (Eds.), *Comprehensive management of head and neck tumors* (pp. 756–774). Philadelphia: W. B. Saunders Co.

Mashberg, A., Garfinkel, L., & Harris, S. (1981). Alcohol as a primary risk factor in oral squamous carcinoma. *CA: A Cancer Journal for Clinicians, 31*: 146–155.

Mashberg, A., & Samit, A. M. (1989). Early detection, diagnosis, and management of oral and oropharyngeal cancer. *CA:A Cancer Journal for Clinicians, 39*, 67–88.

McGuirt, W. F. (1979). Complications of radical neck dissection: A survey of 788 patients. *Head and Neck Surgery, 1*, 481–487.

McGuirt, W. F. (1983). Head and neck cancer in women—a changing profile. *Laryngoscope, 93*, 106–107.

Moss, W. T. (1987). Radiation therapy for tumors of the nasal cavity. In S. E. Thawley & W. R. Panje (eds.), *Comprehensive management of head and neck tumors* (pp. 344–352). Philadelphia: W. B. Saunders Co.

Muir, C. S. (1967). The oral cavity. In R. W. Raven & F. J. C. Roe (Eds.), *The prevention of cancer* (pp. 71–77). London: Butterworths.

Panje, W. R. (1987). Treatment of tumors of the nasopharynx: Surgical therapy. In S. E. Thawley & W. R. Panje (eds.), *Comprehensive management of head and neck tumors* (vol. 1, pp. 662–683). Philadelphia: W. B. Saunders Co.

Parsons, J. T., & Million, R. R. (1987). Radiation therapy of tumors of the oral cavity. In S. E. Thawley & W. R. Panje (Eds.), *Comprehensive management of head and neck tumors* (vol. 1, pp. 516–535). Philadelphia: W. B. Saunders Co.

Pearson, B. W. (1987). Surgical therapy of the nasal cavity and paranasal sinuses. In S. E. Thawley & W. R. Panje (Eds.), *Comprehensive management of head and neck tumors* (vol. 1, pp. 353–367). Philadelphia: W. B. Saunders Co.

Peterson, D. E., Overholser, C. D., Jr., Bergman, S. A., & Beckerman, T. (1986). Initial detection and evaluation: Intraoral neoplasms. In D. E. Peterson, E. G. Elias, & S. T. Sonis (Eds.), *Head and neck management of the cancer patient* (pp. 163–177). Boston: Martinus Nijhoff.

Poulson, T. C., Lindenmuth, J. E., & Greer, R. O. (1984). A comparison of the use of smokeless tobacco in rural and urban teenagers. *CA: A Cancer Journal for Clinicians, 34,* 248–261.

Redmond, C. K., Sass, R. E., & Roush, G. C. (1982). Nasal cavity and paranasal sinuses. In D. Schottenfeld & J. F. Fraumeni, Jr. (Eds.), *Cancer epidemiology and prevention* (pp. 519–535). Philadelphia: W. B. Saunders Co.

Rice, D. H., & Stanley, R. B., Jr. (1987). Surgical therapy of nasal cavity, ethmoid sinus, and maxillary sinus tumors. In S. E. Thawley & W. R. Panje (Eds.), *Comprehensive management of head and neck tumors* (pp. 368–389). Philadelphia, W. B. Saunders Co.

Romm, S. (1986). Cancer of the larynx: Current concepts of diagnosis and treatment. *Surgical Clinics of North America, 66,* 109–118.

Saracci, R. (1985). Occupation. In M. P. Vessey & M. Gray (Eds.), *Cancer risks and prevention* (pp. 99–118). Oxford: Oxford University Press.

Schleper, J. R. (1989). Prevention, detection, and diagnosis of head and neck cancers. *Seminars in Oncology Nursing, 5,* 139–149.

Schramm, V. L., Jr. (1987). Craniofacial surgery for sinus tumors. In S. E. Thawley & W. R. Panje (Eds.), *Comprehensive management of head and neck tumors* (Vol. 1, pp. 390–407). Philadelphia: W. B. Saunders Co.

Shah, J. P., Shemen, L. J., & Strong, E. W. (1987). Buccal mucosa, alveolus, retromolar trigone, floor of mouth, hard palate, and tongue tumors. In S. E. Thawley & W. R. Panje (Eds.), *Comprehensive management of head and neck tumors* (vol. 1, pp. 551–563). Philadelphia: W. B. Saunders Co.

Sheman, L. J., & Spiro, R. H. (1986). Complications following laryngectomy. *Head and Neck Surgery, 8,* 185–191.

Shidnia, H., Hornback, N. B., Hamaker, R., & Lingeman, R. (1980). Carcinoma of major salivary glands. *Cancer, 45,* 693–697.

Shimkin, M. B. (1951). Duration of life in untreated cancer. *Cancer, 4,* 1–8.

Sigler, B. A. (1988). Nursing care of the head and neck cancer patient. *Oncology, 2*(12), 49–53.

Sigler, B. A. (1989). Nursing care of patients with laryngeal cancer. *Seminars in Oncology Nursing, 5,* 160–165.

Silverberg, E. (1983). Cancer statistics, 1983. *CA: A Cancer Journal for Clinicians, 33,* 17.

Silverberg, E., & Lubera, J. (1986). Cancer Statistics, 1986. *CA: A Cancer Journal for Clinicians, 36,* 20.

Silverberg, E., & Lubera, J. (1987). Cancer Statistics, 1987. *CA: A Cancer Journal for Clinicians, 37,* 3–19.

Silverberg, E., & Lubera, J. (1989). Cancer statistics, 1989. *CA: A Cancer Journal for Clinicians, 39,* 3–20.

Sisson, G. A. (1985). Cancer of the oral cavity. In P. B. Chretien, M. E. Johns, D. P. Shedd, E. W. Strong, & P. H. Ward (Eds.), *Head and neck cancer* (vol. 1, pp. 168–169). Proceedings of the International Conference, Baltimore, 1984. St. Louis: C. V. Mosby Co.

Slotman, G. J., Swaminathan, A. P., & Rush, B. F., Jr. (1983). Head and neck cancer in a young age group: High incidence in black patients. *Head and Neck Surgery, 5,* 293–298.

Spiro, R. H. (1985). Tumors of the parotid gland. In P. B. Chretien, M. E. Johns, D. P. Shedd, E. W. Strong, & P. H. Ward (Eds.), *Head and neck cancer* (vol. 1, p. 223). Proceedings of the International Conference, Baltimore, 1984. St. Louis: C. V. Mosby Co.

Spiro, R. H. (1986). Salivary neoplasms: Overview of a 35-year experience with 2,807 patients. *Head and Neck Surgery, 8,* 177–184.

Takeichi, N., Hirose, F., & Yamamoto, H. (1976). Salivary gland tumors in atomic bomb survivors, Hiroshima, Japan. I. Epidemiologic observations. *Cancer, 38,* 2462–2468.

Templer, J. (1987). Clinical evaluation of the larynx. In S. E. Thawley & W. R. Panje (eds.), *Comprehensive management of head and neck tumors* (vol. 1, pp. 868–886). Philadelphia, W. B. Saunders Co.

Thawley, S. E., & Sessions, D. G. (1987). Surgical therapy of hypopharyngeal tumors. In S. E. Thawley & W. R. Panje (Eds.), *Comprehensive management of head and neck tumors* (vol. 1, pp. 774–812). Philadelphia: W. B. Saunders Co.

Tong, D. Y. (1986). Radiotherapeutic management of head and neck neoplasia. In D. E. Peterson, E. G. Elias, & S. T. Sonis (Eds.), *Head and neck management of the cancer patient* (pp. 275–297). Boston: Martinus Nijhoff.

van Nostrand, A. W. P. (1987). Pathology of laryngeal tumors. In S. E. Thawley & W. R. Panje (Eds.), *Comprehensive management of head and neck tumors* (vol. 1, pp. 887–905). Philadelphia: W. B. Saunders Co.

Wagner, R. L., & Sigler, B. (1988). The efficacy of a disposable inner cannula in tracheostomy associated with head and neck surgery. *Society of Otorhinolaryngology Head Neck Nursing, 6*(2), 13–17.

Wang, C. C. (1983). *Radiation therapy for head and neck neoplasms: Indications, techniques and results* (pp. 213–221). Boston: John Wright, PSG Inc.

Wang, C. C. (1987). Radiation therapy of laryngeal tumors: Curative radiation therapy. In S. E. Thawley & W. R. Panje (Eds.), *Comprehensive management of head and neck tumors* (vol. 1, pp. 906–925). Philadelphia: W. B. Saunders Co.

Weber, A. L., & Manzione, J. V. (1986). Diagnostic radiology for head and neck neoplasms with emphasis on computerized tomography. In D. E. Peterson, E. G. Elias, & S. T. Sonis (Eds.), *Head and neck management of the cancer patient* (pp. 191–199). Boston: Martinus Nijhoff.

Weiland, L. H. (1987). Pathology of pharyngeal tumors. In S. E. Thawley & W. R. Panje (Eds.), *Comprehensive management of head and neck tumors* (vol. 1, pp. 630–648). Philadelphia: W. B. Saunders Co.

Wynder, E. L., & Hoffmann, D. (1982). Tobacco. In D. Schottenfeld & J. F. Fraumeni (Eds.), *Cancer epidemiology and prevention* (pp. 277–292). Philadelphia: W. B. Saunders Co.

Wynder, E. L., & Stellman, S. D. (1977). Comparative epidemiology of tobacco related cancer. *Cancer Research, 37,* 4608–4622.

Endocrine Cancers

MICHELE GIRARD DONEHOWER

Endocrine tumors as a group are relatively rare, and although many oncology nurses may not see large numbers of patients with endocrine cancers, nursing care of these patients is challenging. The clinical spectrum of the endocrine tumors ranges from the most indolent to the most virulent of neoplasms. The clinical presentation is complex and frequently combines tumor symptoms with unusual endocrine syndromes. Knowledge of the pathophysiologic processes involved aids in astute observation and assessment and provides a scientific basis for educating patients about their disease and its management.

Advances in the treatment of endocrine tumors have generally been slow. Randomized clinical trials to evaluate new treatment approaches and studies to identify characteristics of the diseases and prognostic variables are difficult to conduct because of the rarity of these tumors and the resultant problems with adequate patient accrual.

THYROID CANCERS

Incidence

Although they are the most common of the endocrine cancers, thyroid neoplasms account for just over 1 per cent of the total number of cancers and approximately 0.2 per cent of cancer deaths (Silverberg & Lubera, 1989). Incidence is higher in women than in men, and the majority of cases occur in people between the ages of 25 and 65 years (Third National Cancer Survey, 1975).

Risk Factors

Radiation exposure to the head and neck area, especially in infancy and childhood, is the only well-documented etiologic factor for thyroid cancers (Favus et al., 1976; Refetoff et al., 1975). Before the 1950s, there was a widespread practice of treating benign diseases, such as tonsillitis, with radiation. In 1950, the first reports of postirradiation thyroid carcinoma in children raised the possibility of irradiation as an etiologic factor (Duffy & Fitzgerald, 1950) (Box 37–1). This theory was subsequently supported by numerous other studies (Favus et al., 1976; Refetoff et al., 1975; Wilson, Platz, & Block, 1970). Generally a latency period of 5 to 10 years elapses after exposure before thyroid tumors develop, but an increased risk for development of these cancers persists for at least

---

Box 37–1. CANCER OF THE THYROID IN CHILDREN

STUDY

Duffy, B. J., & Fitzgerald, P. J. (1950). **Cancer of the thyroid in children: A report of 28 cases.** *Journal of Clinical Endocrinology, 10,* 1296–1308.

SAMPLE

28 children between the ages of 4 and 18 years with carcinoma of the thyroid.

PURPOSE OF STUDY

These authors analyzed the records of all patients in the above sample for the purposes of (1) examining the tumor characteristics and biologic behavior of cancer of the thyroid in children, (2) identifying possible etiologic factors, and (3) emphasizing the importance of including thyroid cancer in the differential diagnosis of tumors of the neck in children.

RESULTS

The most significant finding of this study was that 9 of 28 patients who developed thyroid cancer had been treated with external radiation for "enlargement of the thymus." Twenty-six of 28 patients had cervical lymph node involvement at diagnosis; 23 of 28 patients had well-differentiated thyroid cancers; and the age of onset correlated with puberty in 25 cases.

DISCUSSION

In addition to providing descriptive information pertaining to histology, progression of disease and treatment of thyroid cancer in this sample, Duffy and Fitzgerald were the first investigators to examine the relationship between external irradiation of the head and neck and the development of thyroid cancer. Although the authors were reluctant, at that time, to propose a cause-and-effect relationship between these irradiation practices and the development of cancer, their studies raised questions prompting further analysis of cases of childhood thyroid cancer and, ultimately, identified head and neck irradiation during childhood as a definitive etiologic factor.

---

35 years in exposed subjects (Favus et al., 1976). In contrast, no relationship has been established between iodine–131 (^{131}I) therapy for hyperthyroidism and the development of thyroid cancer (Holm, Dahlquist, Israelsson, & Lundell, 1980).

An association may exist between prolonged stimulation of secretion of thyroid-stimulating hormone (TSH) secondary to severe iodide restriction or partial thyroid gland resection and the development of thyroid tumors, but this hypothesis has been consistently supported only in animal studies (Williams, 1979).

Approximately 25 per cent of medullary thyroid cancers occur as part of genetically transmitted multiple endocrine neoplasia (MEN) syndromes (Saad et al., 1984).

Prognostic Factors

Important prognostic factors include histologic type, age, and extent of disease at the time of diagnosis, with histologic features being the greatest determinant of overall survival (Kerr et al., 1986). Patients with papillary carcinomas, those under 50 years of age, and

Table 37–1. HISTOLOGIC CLASSIFICATION OF THYROID CARCINOMAS

Tumor Type	Tissue of Origin	Incidence of All Thyroid Cancers* (Per Cent)	Survival (Per Cent) (Reference)
Papillary	Follicular cells	33–73	93 (20 yr) (McConahey et al., 1986)
			92 (10 yr) (Mazzaferri et al., 1977)
Follicular	Follicular cells	14–33	94 (10 yr) (Lang et al., 1986)
			73 (5 yr) (Crile et al., 1985)
			43 (10 yr) (Crile et al., 1985)
Medullary	Parafollicular cells (C cells)	5–10	78.2 (5 yr) (Saad et al., 1984)
			57.5 (10 yr) (Saad et al., 1984)
Anaplastic	Follicular cells	10	0 (5 yr) (Nel et al., 1985)

*Greenfield (1987).

those with limited disease have the most favorable prognosis. A symptom cluster of dysphonia, dysphagia, and dyspnea appears to confer a worse prognosis and probably reflects locally invasive disease (Kerr et al., 1986). In medullary thyroid carcinoma, gender has also been identified as a prognostic factor, with women having a significantly better prognosis (Schroder et al., 1988).

Classification and Staging

Malignant thyroid neoplasms have been divided into four major types, although other rarer forms of primary thyroid cancer (e.g., sarcoma, lymphoma) make up approximately 5 per cent of thyroid cancers. The histologic classification of the major types of thyroid carcinomas is given in Table 37–1. The American Joint Committee on Cancer has incorporated histologic type and age in its most recent staging system of thyroid cancer because of the prognostic significance of these factors (Table 37–2) (Beahrs, Henson, Hutter, & Myers, 1988).

Biology and Natural History

Papillary and follicular carcinomas are well-differentiated cancers that closely resemble their tissue of origin within the thyroid gland (Table 37–1). These tumors generally follow an indolent clinical course even in the presence of nodal involvement or distant metastases, whereas the anaplastic (undifferentiated) types behave more aggressively and are associated with severe morbidity secondary to rapid invasion of contiguous structures (Leeper, 1985). With anaplastic carcinomas, death frequently occurs within months of diagnosis. A histologic progression from well to poorly differentiated carcinoma has been suspected in cases in which there is a sudden change in the rate of growth in a known papillary adenocarcinoma (Mazzaferri et al., 1977). This may reflect end-stage behavior in the natural history of that tumor.

Medullary carcinoma of the thyroid (MCT) varies in its clinical behavior. The majority of patients show an indolent course, but those patients with MEN type IIB (Table 37–3) have a particularly aggressive form of MCT (Saad et al., 1984).

Clinical Manifestations

Frequently, an asymptomatic mass discovered incidentally by the patient or on routine physical examination is the first indication of disease. Anaplastic masses are more likely to have symptoms indicative of local invasion or compression: hoarseness, dysphagia, stridor, and referred ear pain (Leeper, 1985). Symptoms of hormonal imbalance may be present if tumor growth has resulted in actual destruction of the thyroid gland or if the tumor itself is producing excess thyroid hormone. A severe, watery diarrhea syndrome is seen in approximately 25 per cent of cases of MCT with an increased incidence in advanced disease (Saad et al., 1984).

Diagnostic Evaluation

Although the incidence of thyroid nodules is common, the development of cancer within a nodule is

---

Table 37–2. STAGING CLASSIFICATION OF THYROID CARCINOMAS

DEFINITION OF TNM

Primary Tumor (T)

TX	Primary tumor cannot be assessed
T_0	No evidence of primary tumor
T_1	Tumor 1 cm or less in greatest dimension limited to the thyroid
T_2	Tumor more than 1 cm but not more than 4 cm in greatest dimension limited to the thyroid
T_3	Tumor more than 4 cm in greatest dimension limited to the thyroid
T_4	Tumor of any size extending beyond the thyroid capsule

Regional Lymph Nodes (N)

Regional lymph nodes are the cervical and upper mediastinal lymph nodes.

NX	Regional lymph nodes cannot be assessed
N_0	No regional lymph node metastasis
N_1	Regional lymph node metastasis
N_{1A}	Metastasis in ipsilateral cervical lymph node(s)
N_{1B}	Metastasis in bilateral, midline, or contralateral cervical or mediastinal lymph node(s)

Distant Metastasis (M)

MX	Presence of distant metastasis cannot be assessed
M_0	No distant metastasis
M_1	Distant metastasis

STAGE GROUPING

Separate stage groupings are recommended for papillary or follicular, medullary, and undifferentiated.

Papillary or Follicular

	UNDER 45 YEARS	45 YEARS AND OLDER
Stage I	Any T, Any N, M_0	T_1, N_0, M_0
Stage II	Any T, Any N, M_1	T_2, N_0, M_0
		T_3, N_0, M_0
Stage III		T_4, N_0, M_0
		Any T, N_1, M_0
Stage IV		Any T, any N, M_1

Medullary

Stage I	T_1	N_0	M_0
Stage II	T_2	N_0	M_0
	T_3	N_0	M_0
	T_4	N_0	M_0
Stage III	Any T	N_1	M_0
Stage IV	Any T	Any N	M_1

Undifferentiated

All cases are stage IV

Stage IV	Any T	Any N	Any M

Note: All categories may be subdivided into (A) solitary tumor and (B) multifocal tumor (the largest determines the classification).
(From Beahrs, O. H., Henson, D. E., Hutter, R. V. P. & Myers, M. H. [Eds]. [1988]. *Manual for staging of cancer* [3rd ed., p. 58]. Philadelphia: J. B. Lippincott Co. Reproduced by permission.)

relatively uncommon. Diagnosis remains difficult owing to the nonspecific nature of the tests used to evaluate nodules.

With the refinement of fine-needle aspiration biopsy, this technique has become a first-line diagnostic tool in the evaluation of thyroid nodules (Friedman, Toriumi, & Mafee, 1988). It is the only method that can differentiate benign from malignant nodules with a high degree of accuracy. Fine-needle aspiration is performed by introducing a 22-gauge needle into the nodule and aspirating tissue for cytologic examination. Fine-needle aspiration has a reported false-negative rate of 0.3 to 10 per cent and a false-positive rate of 0 to 2.5 per cent (Frable, 1986).

Radionuclide scanning is indicated when fine-needle aspiration is inadequate, the findings reveal benign changes, or the thyroid is diffusely enlarged (Friedman et al., 1988). Scans provide useful clinical information regarding the functional status of a nodule but lack specificity in differentiating malignant from benign tissue. Functional nodules are those that produce and secrete thyroid hormones. They are called "hot" nodules because the radioactive isotope is concentrated in the nodule and appears as an area of increased uptake on the scan. Because most malignant nodules produce lower amounts of thyroid hormones than normal thyroid tissue, they appear "cold" on scan. Technetium–99m is the preferred agent for initial thyroid scanning. A follow-up scan with radioactive iodine may be performed to confirm a true functional or "hot" nodule noted on a technetium–99m scan (Friedman et al., 1988).

Ultrasonography has limited applications in the evaluation of thyroid malignancies (Freitas, Gross, Ripley, & Shapiro, 1985). These include evaluating changes in the size of thyroid nodules after thyroxine suppressive therapy, guiding fine-needle aspiration, and detecting recurrent disease. Both magnetic resonance imaging (MRI) and computed tomography (CT) scans provide information for treatment planning by delineating the extent of disease within the thyroid and surrounding structures (Friedman et al., 1988).

Thyroid function studies are nondiagnostic for cancer. Only the measurement of serum calcitonin may be helpful in confirming a diagnosis of MCT. This test is used as a tumor marker for the detection and postoperative management of patients with MCT (Baylin & Wells, 1981).

Table 37–3. CLINICAL FEATURES OF MULTIPLE ENDOCRINE NEOPLASIA (MEN) SYNDROMES

MEN-I	MEN-IIA	MEN-IIB
Hyperparathyroidism	*Medullary carcinoma of the thyroid (generally indolent course)	*Medullary carcinoma of the thyroid (frequently virulent course)
Pancreatic islet cell tumors		
Pituitary tumors		
Adrenal cortex tumors	Pheochromocytoma	Pheochromocytoma
Thyroid tumors	Hyperparathyroidism (frequent)	Mucosal neuromas
		Bony abnormalities
		Puffy eyes
		Prominent jaw
		Hyperparathyroidism (rare)

*Affects 100 per cent of patients with this syndrome.

Treatment

Surgery

Surgery is recommended as initial therapy for all thyroid cancers, but the extent of the surgery and the postoperative treatment management vary and continue to be areas of controversy among clinicians (Leeper, 1985; McConahey, Hay, Woolner, vanHeerden, & Taylor, 1986). Rational selection of a therapeutic approach should take into consideration age, histologic type, and extent of disease as they relate to prognosis.

Although total lobectomy may be an acceptable procedure in papillary carcinoma when the lesion is less than 2 cm and confined to one lobe, microscopic foci in the contralateral lobe have been detected in up to 87 per cent of cases (Tollefsen, Shah, & Huvos, 1972). Therefore, many clinicians suggest at least a near-total or a total thyroidectomy in all well-differentiated and medullary cancers of the thyroid because of the much higher incidence of recurrence in patients treated with less radical surgery (Clark et al., 1988). In contrast, the extent of cervical lymph node dissection for patients with metastatic cervical lymphadenopathy did not affect recurrence or survival in patients with papillary carcinoma or MCT (Mazzaferri et al., 1977; Saad et al., 1984).

Nursing management requires an awareness of the potential complications that can occur. Postoperatively, patients should be observed for signs of tetany, because hypoparathyroidism is the most frequent complication, occurring in 6 to 8 per cent of patients (Mazzaferri et al., 1977; McConahey et al., 1986). The likelihood of permanent hypoparathyroidism is significantly higher in patients undergoing total thyroidectomy. These patients may require lifelong administration of calcium and vitamin D replacement. If some parathyroid tissue has been preserved, normal function will gradually return.

Bilateral damage to the recurrent laryngeal nerves during surgery results in permanent vocal cord paralysis in less than 2 per cent of cases (Mazzaferri et al., 1977; McConahey et al., 1986). With near-total thyroidectomy, the nerve on one side can be salvaged and only temporary hoarseness will result.

Unless a patient has experienced respiratory distress owing to extensive local disease, airway complications generally are a transient intra- and early postoperative management problem. Nevertheless, nurses should be alert to the possibility of respiratory obstruction, which can result from (1) recurrent laryngeal nerve damage, which can cause vocal cord spasms, (2) tracheal compression from hemorrhage, (3) local edema, or (4) tetany (Cassmeyer, 1987).

Patients should be monitored for 12 to 24 hr after surgery for hemorrhage. Excessive bleeding can be assessed by checking the back of the surgical dressing under the neck and shoulders. Respiratory distress, a sensation of choking, or dysphagia may indicate bleeding into and compression of adjacent structures. If symptoms are not relieved by loosening the wound dressing, the nurse may be instructed to remove surgical clips or sutures (Cassmeyer, 1987). An emergency tracheostomy may be necessary.

Because of the loss of endocrine function after all or part of the thyroid gland is removed, most patients are given thyroid replacement to prevent myxedema (Hubert, 1986). Levothyroxine (Synthroid) is the most commonly used preparation.

Radiation Therapy

^{131}I therapy is used for the ablation of thyroid remnants after surgery and for the treatment of known residual or metastatic disease outside the confines of the thyroid (Greenfield, 1987). Ablation and treatment with ^{131}I is not indicated in medullary or undifferentiated thyroid cancers, which are unable to concentrate and retain this radioisotope (Table 37–1).

About 4 to 6 weeks after surgery for differentiated thyroid cancers, ablation of any remaining normal thyroid tissue is done with ^{131}I. The purpose of pretreatment ablation is to destroy any remaining ^{131}I-concentrating tissues in the thyroid bed and create a hypothyroid state that stimulates increased secretion of TSH (Freitas, Gross, Ripley, & Shapiro, 1985). This prepares the patient for ^{131}I therapy by promoting uptake of ^{131}I in remaining tumor deposits and metastatic foci. Exogenous administration of bovine TSH may be required if residual tumor is secreting enough thyroid hormone to suppress endogenous TSH (Blahd, 1985). It should be used cautiously because of the high incidence of hypersensitivity reactions with repeated doses.

In contrast to ^{131}I ablation, in which a relatively fixed dose of radioactive iodine is given, optimal ^{131}I therapy requires dosimetry calculations to deliver the maximally tolerated dose with minimal toxicity (Freitas et al., 1985). Systemic effects include nausea and vomiting, inflammation of the salivary glands, bone marrow suppression, and, rarely, pulmonary radiation fibrosis and leukemia (Freitas et al., 1985). Treatment doses are given at 4- to 6-month intervals until there is no

---

Table 37–4. GUIDELINES FOR PATIENTS RECEIVING IODINE–131 (^{131}I)

Planning
Order ^{131}I at least 48 hr in advance. Schedule patient for hospital admission.

Room Preparation
Charcoal filters in room air system and exhaust vent in hallway.
Must cover with plastic bags: telephone, food table, basin faucet handles, nurse call set.
Disposable mats next to bed, commode, and shower.
Seat liners for commode.
Two radiation waste containers in room (laundry and foods or paper).

Patient Preparation
Instruct patient on how to replace and dispose of covers and mats.
Instruct patient to keep outside door closed and bathroom door open at all times.
Obtain vital signs and blood and urine samples before ^{131}I administration.

Administration
Patient must wear hospital gown with a "chuck" around neck and in lap.
Personnel administering ^{131}I should wear gown, gloves, and mask.
Vial containing ^{131}I should be vented in nuclear medicine hood to allow any volatile ^{131}I to escape just before administration.
Patient is to sit on side of bed in front of ^{131}I in lead vial on covered table.
Instruct patient to open vial with T-bar, insert drinking straw, put small amount of water in vial (running it down the straw so it does not splash).
Swish and then swallow several cups of water to rinse ^{131}I from oral cavity.
Do not remove straw from vial; bend it over and carefully place lead cap on.

Initial Survey
Within 15 min, measure the radiation exposure rate at 1 m from the midline of patient's abdomen in both anteroposterior and lateral directions. Calculate the average. Patient may be released when same readings show less than 30 mCi of ^{131}I—usually about 48 to 72 hr after 100 mCi was given, but highly variable.
Posted on room door must be room diagram showing safety shields position, inventory-survey form with initial activity and exposure rate, nursing instructions, and decontaminating form.
Do not collect urine unless lead container is available and there is specific reason.

Safety
Nursing recommendations: No pregnant nurses should care for patients receiving ^{131}I. Nurses should not be assigned to care for more than one radioactive patient a month. At 30 mCi ^{131}I discharge, exposure rate is 100 cGy/hr at 25 cm.
Visiting is discouraged: limit to ½ hr/day/visitor; no children under 18 years or pregnant women. Visitors should wear gown, gloves, and mask and sit in a designated chair across the room. If they come close to patient, they should sit behind a lead shield.
Patients should wear hospital gown, not personal clothing (^{131}I is found in breath, sweat), and should leave bed only to go to bathroom or to a designated chair.
Patient should drink copious amounts of water to speed release of unused radioactive agent, shower frequently, and flush toilet several times after each use. Men should urinate seated.
No personal items should be used except those to be disposed of at discharge.
After discharge: sleep alone for 3 days. Do not hold children closely for 3 days.

(From Greenfield, L. D. [1987]. Thyroid tumors. In C. A. Perez & L. W. Brady [Eds.], *Principles and practice of radiation oncology* [pp. 1150–1151]. Philadelphia: J. B. Lippincott Co. Reproduced by permission.)

evidence of functioning tumor on whole body imaging studies (Leeper, 1985). Thyroid hormone replacement is restarted immediately after therapy to permanently suppress TSH, which may act as a growth stimulus for thyroid follicular cells (Greenfield, 1987).

Patients generally require inpatient admission for administration of ^{131}I owing to the higher doses given for therapy. Radiation precaution procedures are instituted and may vary among hospitals, but sample guidelines are listed in Table 37–4 (Greenfield, 1987). Refer to Chapter 20 for other considerations relating to brachytherapy.

External irradiation can be used in conjunction with ^{131}I in patients with inoperable, residual, or metastatic differentiated thyroid cancers (Lindberg, 1980). With this approach, long-term local control of residual disease has been reported in tumors with poor ^{131}I uptake (Simpson & Carruthers, 1978). Treatment of anaplastic carcinomas with ^{131}I and external irradiation has not been effective owing to the radioresistance of this type of thyroid neoplasm, but a study combining a hyperfractionated radiation therapy schedule with low-dose doxorubicin as a radiosensitizer for hypoxic, radioresistant tumor cells has yielded excellent results with local control (Kim & Leeper, 1983).

Chemotherapy

To date, the role of chemotherapy in the treatment of thyroid cancer has been limited to palliation in patients with locally uncontrolled or widely metastatic disease (Greenfield, 1987). Only doxorubicin has demonstrated any significant antitumor activity, with response rates of around 20 per cent (Poster et al., 1981).

ADRENAL CANCER: ADRENOCORTICAL CARCINOMA

Adrenal neoplasms can arise from tissue within the cortex or medulla of the gland. Because of the physiologic diversity of these two areas, adrenocortical and adrenal medullary tumors are discussed separately.

Incidence

The estimated incidence of malignant tumors of the adrenal cortex is approximately 2 cases per million per year (Ferber, Hardy, Gerhardt, & Solomon, 1962). The average age at presentation is 40 to 50 years, but tumors are found in all age groups (Javadpour, Waltering, & Brennan, 1980). Sex distribution is equal, but women have a slightly higher incidence of functional tumors (Cohn, Gottesman, & Brennan, 1986). Bilateral involvement is uncommon (Hutter & Kayhoe, 1966). There are no definitive etiologic factors for adrenocortical cancers.

Biology and Natural History

Adrenocortical carcinomas are aggressive tumors, usually large and frequently metastatic at the time of diagnosis (Cohn et al., 1986; Didolkar, Bescher, Elias, & Moore, 1981). This is due, in part, to the anatomic protection afforded the adrenal glands within the abdominal cavity, which prevents early detection. Overall, the 5-year survival rates range from 16 to 30 per cent despite surgery, chemotherapy, or radiation therapy (Didolkar et al., 1981; Haq et al., 1980). Histologic grade appears to be the most significant determinant of survival, with poorly differentiated adrenocortical carcinomas carrying the poorest prognosis (Karakovsis, Rao, & Moore, 1985).

Classification and Staging

Clinically, adrenocortical carcinomas can be classified as functional (hormone-producing) or nonfunctional, with the vast majority being functional and producing excess androgen, estrogen, or cortisol. Brennan (1985) proposed a simple staging classification (Table 37–5), which discriminates between disease confined to the adrenal and locally invasive or metastatic disease.

Clinical Presentation

Because the adrenal cortex produces glucocorticoids and mineralocorticoids, patients with functional tumors will have symptoms and clinical findings related to hypersecretion of these hormones. Characteristic symptoms of adrenal endocrine syndromes are listed in Table 37–6.

In nonfunctional lesions, presenting symptoms are related to local pressure, necrosis, or hemorrhage secondary to an enlarging intra-abdominal mass (Cohn et al., 1986; Didolkar et al., 1981).

Diagnostic Evaluation

Although clinical presentation alone may be suggestive of an adrenal neoplasm, studies of adrenocortical function are important to confirm the presence of excess hormone production. Patients with adrenocor-

Table 37–5. STAGING OF ADRENOCORTICAL CARCINOMA

Stage	Extent of Tumor
I	Tumor <5 cm Negative nodes No local invasion No metastases
II	Tumor >5 cm Negative nodes No local invasion No metastases
III	Positive nodes or local invasion
IV	Positive nodes and local invasion or distant metastases

(Adapted with permission from Brennan, M. F. [with MacDonald, J. S.] [1985]. Cancer of the endocrine system. In V. T. DeVita, Jr., S. Hellman, & S. A. Rosenberg (Eds.), *Cancer: Principles and practice of oncology* [2nd ed., p. 1199]. Philadelphia: J. B. Lippincott Co.)

Table 37–6. CLINICAL MANIFESTATIONS OF ADRENOCORTICAL HORMONE EXCESS

Hormone	Syndrome	Clinical Manifestations
Aldosterone	Conn's syndrome (aldosteronism)	Hypernatremia, hypokalemia, hypertension, neuromuscular weakness and paresthesias, electrocardiographic and renal function abnormalities
Cortisol (ACTH)	Cushing's syndrome	Acid-base imbalance, hypertension, obesity, osteoporosis, hyperglycemia, psychoses, excessive bruising, renal calculi
Sex hormones (testosterone, estrogen, and progesterone)	Virilization (in women)	Male pattern baldness, hirsutism, deepening voice, breast atrophy, decreased libido, oligomenorrhea
	Feminization (in men)	Gynecomastia, breast tenderness, testicular atrophy, decreased libido

tical carcinoma commonly excrete large amounts of 17-ketosteroids if excessive glucocorticoid or sex steroid production is occurring (Samaan & Hickey, 1987). After laboratory confirmation of a hormone-producing adrenal tumor, CT scan is invaluable in localizing the tumor and further delineating nodal involvement or metastatic disease (Thompson & Cheung, 1987). Reports regarding the ability of MRI to discriminate benign adenomas from adrenocortical carcinomas and pheochromocytomas will increase the use of this diagnostic tool and may ultimately improve the early detection of asymptomatic adrenal masses (Chang et al., 1987; Doppman et al., 1987).

Treatment

Surgery

Surgery is the primary and only potentially curative treatment for all adrenal tumors. Complete resection of tumor may not always be possible because of invasion into adjacent vital structures, but maximal debulking should be undertaken to alleviate symptoms and optimize the effectiveness of postoperative systemic therapy (Didolkar et al., 1981). Surgical treatment can be curative for stage I tumors.

Corticosteroids are administered in high doses preoperatively to prevent acute adrenal insufficiency during surgery and are continued for at least 24 hr after the operation. Patients undergoing bilateral adrenalectomy will require lifelong replacement therapy. A suggested outline for patient teaching is listed in Table 37–7. In patients who have had only unilateral adrenalectomy, replacement doses of steroids will be rapidly tapered and discontinued as function of the contralateral adrenal gland returns (Brennan, 1987).

After adrenalectomy, patients require intensive monitoring because of the potential for addisonian crisis, serious fluid and electrolyte disturbances, and hypoglycemia (Cassmeyer, 1987). Poor wound healing and infection can be a major postoperative complication because of the immunosuppressive effects of corticosteroid therapy. Strict aseptic technique should be maintained for wound care.

Chemotherapy

Although prolonged tumor regression has been reported in isolated patients treated with mitotane (o,p'-DDD) (Jarabak & Rice, 1981), responses are generally of short duration (Haq et al., 1980) and do not significantly affect length of survival (Cohn et al., 1986). The drug is poorly tolerated at higher doses, causing significant lethargy, muscle weakness, and gastrointestinal toxicity. Patient tolerance has been improved with reduced doses (Jarabak & Rice, 1981). Because of its postulated mechanism of action in necrosing segments of the adrenal cortex, corticosteroid replacement is necessary during therapy (Thompson & Cheung, 1987).

Radiation Therapy

The role of irradiation in the management of adrenocortical carcinoma is limited to the palliation of bone pain, and this method has not been effective in controlling bulky residual disease (Brennan, 1987).

ADRENAL CANCER: PHEOCHROMOCYTOMA

Incidence

Pheochromocytoma is a rare catecholamine-secreting tumor that occurs predominantly in adults and does not appear to have a gender predilection. Approxi-

Table 37–7. TOPIC OUTLINE FOR PATIENTS NEEDING REPLACEMENT DOSES OF CORTICOSTEROIDS

A. Function of adrenal glands
  1. Secretion of corticosteroids
  2. Action of glucocorticoids and mineralocorticoids in body
B. Medication regimen
  1. Ingestion with meals or snacks
  2. Glucocorticoids
    a. ⅔ of dose at 8 A.M.
    b. ⅓ of dose at 4 P.M.
  3. Mineralocorticoids: Full dose at 8 A.M.
  4. Technique for parenteral administration if unable to retain oral form of drugs
  5. Rationale for carrying drugs on person at all times
C. Complications
  1. Signs and symptoms of adrenal insufficiency: Anorexia, nausea and vomiting, fatigue, weakness, dehydration, mental status changes, increased pulse and respiratory rate, dizziness
  2. Signs and symptoms of excessive drug therapy: Rapid weight gain, round face, edema, hypertension
  3. Effects of stressors on daily corticosteroid requirements
  4. Ability of corticosteroids to mask infection
  5. Purpose and method of obtaining a Medic Alert bracelet or necklace
  6. Indications for contacting a physician

mately 5 to 10 per cent of pheochromocytomas are malignant, and they differ from benign cases only in their invasive and metastatic behavior (Samaan, Hickey, & Shutts, 1988). Bilateral occurrence is rare. Ninety per cent of cases arise from adrenal medullary tissue, with the remaining cases detected in ectopic sites of catecholamine-secreting tissues (Samaan et al., 1988). Pheochromocytoma occurs sporadically in the population or is inherited as part of a MEN syndrome.

Clinical Presentation

Symptoms result from excess secretion of epinephrine and norepinephrine and include hypertension (either episodic or sustained), excessive perspiration, headache, nervousness, palpitations, nausea, vomiting, abdominal or chest pain, blurred vision, and syncope.

Diagnostic Evaluation

Elevated levels of catecholamines can be documented with measurement of 24-hr urine samples for catecholamines (vanillylmandelic acid, metanephrines) and can aid in confirming the diagnosis (Bravo, Taranzi, Gifford, & Stewart, 1979). Pharmacologic tests using drugs that trigger release of catecholamines by the tumor are no longer used because of the risks of hypertensive crisis.

Once abnormal urinary test results have been documented, localization of the adrenal tumor and ectopic or metastatic disease is done with noninvasive radiologic procedures such as CT or ^{131}I-metaiodobenzylguanidine (MIBG) scan (Bravo & Gifford, 1984). The last mentioned technique uses an agent that mimics norepinephrine and is taken up by catecholamine-producing cells, thereby localizing extra-adrenal pheochromocytomas anywhere in the body (Sisson et al., 1981).

Treatment

Surgery

Aggressive surgical resection of all accessible disease and metastases is indicated for malignant pheochromocytoma, although it may not be possible to remove all active (functional) tissue (Brennan, 1985; Hull, 1986). Patients are routinely given alpha-adrenergic blocking agents after a definitive diagnosis is made to minimize the potential for uncontrolled release of catecholamines during localization procedures and surgery (Hull, 1986). Myocardial damage may be present at the time of surgery as a result of prolonged exposure to epinephrine and norepinephrine, thereby placing the patient at a higher intraoperative risk for cardiovascular complications (Hull, 1986). After removal of the tumor, rigorous monitoring is required because profound shock can develop owing to the dramatic decrease in circulating catecholamine levels (Bravo &

Gifford, 1984). Adequate volume replacement is of paramount importance.

After surgery, patients with malignant pheochromocytoma are maintained on alpha- and beta-adrenergic blocking agents and alpha-methyl-paratyrosine, which reduces the production of catecholamines indefinitely, to prevent recurrence of symptoms (Hull, 1986).

Chemotherapy

Because of the rarity of this tumor, the role of cytotoxic chemotherapy has not been evaluated in any large series of patients, but Averbuch and colleagues (1988) reported an overall response rate of 57 per cent in 14 patients with unresectable malignant pheochromocytoma treated with combined cyclophosphamide, vincristine, and dacarbazine.

Radiation Therapy

Radiation is not used in the treatment of pheochromocytoma.

PITUITARY TUMORS

Incidence

Pituitary tumors account for approximately 10 per cent of symptomatic intracranial neoplasms (Post & Muraszko, 1986). They are found in all age groups but most commonly in middle-aged and older patients, with both sexes being affected equally (Kovacs & Horvath, 1987).

Biology

The majority of pituitary tumors are slow-growing, benign neoplasms confined to the sella turcica, although some exhibit more aggressive, invasive behavior (Kovacs & Horvath, 1987).

Classification

Adenomas arise from cells in the anterior lobe of the pituitary gland, and early classification schemes were based on the chemical staining properties of tumor cells. This classification was of little value because of the lack of correlation between staining characteristics, level of cellular differentiation, and hormone content (Scheithauer et al., 1986). More sophisticated laboratory techniques have permitted a more functional categorization of pituitary adenomas, which are now classified primarily according to their morphology and endocrinologic activity (Scheithauer et al., 1986). The major hormones secreted by pituitary adenomas are prolactin, growth hormone (GH), adrenocorticotropic hormone (ACTH), TSH, follicle-stimulating hormone (FSH), and luteinizing hormone

(LH). Tumors are frequently named according to the hormone secreted (e.g., prolactinomas, GH-secreting adenomas). Pituitary adenomas are also classified according to size. Microadenomas are tumors smaller than 10 mm in diameter and macroadenomas are larger (Ciric, 1985). Microadenomas are associated with a better overall prognosis because generally they are confined to the sella turcica and are easily resectable (Scheithauer et al., 1986).

Clinical Presentation

Headache occurs in approximately 20 per cent of patients with pituitary tumors (Levin, Sheline, & Gutin, 1989). Other symptoms that may be observed are related to either excess secretion of pituitary hormones, hypopituitarism, or mass effect of the tumor (Ciric, 1985).

Prolactin-secreting tumors are the most common pituitary tumors (Levin et al., 1989; Scheithauer et al., 1986). These tumors cause clinical symptoms of amenorrhea and galactorrhea, which are detected most easily in premenopausal women. Early detection is not as likely in nonmenstruating women, and presenting symptoms in this group are generally from the compressive effect of the expanding tumor (Dollar & Blackwell, 1986).

Overproduction of GH results in acromegaly (pituitary gigantism), and initial clinical manifestations are nonspecific: lethargy, headache, and paresthesias. Late effects include weight gain, hypertension, cardiomegaly, and abnormal growth in bone width or length (Bullock & Rosendahl, 1988).

Cushing's disease is caused by hypersecretion of ACTH. Common clinical findings include obesity, hirsutism, muscle weakness, glucose intolerance, and hypertension. LH-, FSH-, and TSH-secreting adenomas are unusual (Ciric, 1985).

Widespread endocrine abnormalities result from loss of pituitary hormonal action on target organs throughout the body. The clinical effects of hypopituitarism attributable to destruction of normal anterior pituitary tissue or impairment of the hypothalamic-pituitary axis are listed in Table 37–8.

Table 37–8. CLINICAL EFFECTS OF HYPOPITUITARISM

Hormone	Target Tissue	Clinical Effects
ACTH	Adrenal cortex	Postural hypotension; impaired tolerance of stress (trauma, surgery); can lead to shock
Prolactin FSH LH	Gonads	Gonadal atrophy; loss of reproductive function; decreased gonadal hormones
TSH	Thyroid	Hypothyroidism (fatigue, slow or slurred speech, bradycardia, decreased reflexes, cold intolerance)
GH	Bones, muscles, organs	Decreased bone growth, lethargy, hypoglycemia

ACTH, Adrenocorticotropic hormone; FSH, follicle-stimulating hormone; LH, luteinizing hormone; TSH, thyroid-stimulating hormone; GH, growth hormone.

Because of its strategic location within the skull, the mass effect of a growing pituitary neoplasm can cause compression of surrounding critical structures, including the optic chiasm, hypothalamus, and cranial nerves (Levin, Sheline, & Gutin, 1989). Patients with involvement of the optic nerves or chiasm may experience loss of visual acuity or visual field defects (Ciric, 1985).

Diagnostic Evaluation

The first step in evaluating a patient with a suspected pituitary tumor includes endocrinologic testing to determine whether hypersecretion of any of the pituitary hormones is present. Laboratory documentation of elevated hormone levels aids in confirming the diagnosis of a functional pituitary adenoma and provides baseline information for assessing response to subsequent therapy (Ciric, 1985).

Radiologic diagnostic tests provide additional information on the structure of both functional and nonfunctional tumors. The most useful techniques in delineating tumor size and extension outside the confines of the gland are CT and MRI. In patients with macroadenomas, carotid angiography may also be indicated to further delineate the surrounding vasculature (Kaufman et al., 1987).

Treatment

Surgery

Selection of a treatment method is contingent on the size and extent of the tumor. Surgery is the single most effective treatment for pituitary microadenomas and results in long-term local control for approximately 85 per cent of patients (Chun, Masko, & Hetelekidis, 1988). With few exceptions, the trans-sphenoidal approach (access through the mouth into the sphenoid sinus and up into the sella turcica) has largely replaced the transfrontal technique (craniotomy), which provided better visualization of the area, but was associated with higher morbidity and mortality (Laws, 1987). Whenever possible, salvage of normal pituitary tissue is desirable to avoid panhypopituitarism.

The most common complications of surgery are diabetes insipidus (DI), cerebrospinal fluid (CSF) leak, and meningitis. Diabetes insipidus is observed in 30 to 50 per cent of patients (Laws, 1982), but even in completely hypophysectomized patients, it is usually temporary because the hypothalamus assumes the secretory function of the pituitary in releasing antidiuretic hormone (ADH). In the immediate postoperative period, patients will have extremely dilute urine, and adequate fluid replacement is essential to prevent hypovolemia.

Because the dura is disrupted during entry into the sella turcica, CSF can drain from the wound site. Activities that increase intracranial pressure, such as coughing, sneezing, and bending over, are to be avoided to minimize the possibility of CSF leakage

(Cassmeyer, 1987). Patients should be assessed for persistent postnasal drip and constant swallowing. Any drainage noted should be tested for glucose, because CSF differs from normal nasal drainage in that CSF contains glucose.

Aseptic technique is essential during wound care because of the increased risk of meningitis in patients after intracranial surgery. The suture line is located within the oral cavity if the trans-sphenoidal approach has been used. The mouth can be rinsed with normal saline solution and cleansed with a Toothette or cotton swab. Regular toothbrushing is contraindicated until healing occurs because of the possibility of disrupting the suture line (Cassmeyer, 1987).

Radiation Therapy

External irradiation is frequently used in conjunction with surgery to decrease the incidence of local recurrences (Chun et al., 1988). It can be given immediately after surgery or as salvage therapy after recurrence. By employing a combined approach, local control can be achieved in almost 95 per cent of patients (Chun et al., 1988; Levin et al., 1989).

Radiation therapy is rarely used as the sole treatment modality because maximal response to therapy may be delayed for months to years, which renders this approach impractical for hypersecreting tumors (Halberg & Sheline, 1987).

Chemotherapy

Traditional cytotoxic chemotherapy has been of limited usefulness because of difficulties in administering concentrations of drug high enough to cross the blood-brain barrier without causing prohibitive toxicity (Kornblith, Walker, & Cassady, 1985). Instead, the focus has been on pharmacologic manipulation of pituitary hormone secretion.

Bromocriptine, a dopamine agonist, has been effective in most prolactin-secreting tumors not only by reducing levels of this hormone but also by reducing tumor size (Molitch et al., 1985). Bromocriptine is not considered curative when used alone, and the drug must be continued indefinitely, because discontinuation can result in rapid regrowth of the tumor (Dollar & Blackwell, 1986). Considerable controversy surrounds the use of this agent, but several studies now support the short-term (4 to 6 weeks) preoperative treatment of prolactinomas with bromocriptine to reduce tumor size and increase resectability (Bevan et al., 1987; Hubbard et al., 1987; Molitch et al., 1985). Long-term treatment may hinder surgical resection because of the development of tumor necrosis and fibrosis.

A long-acting somatostatin analogue, SMS 201–995 (Sandoz, Hanover, NJ), shows promise in the preoperative treatment of GH-producing macroadenomas by suppressing GH hypersecretion (Barkan et al., 1988). Maximal tumor reduction occurs after 8 to 12 weeks of therapy, and GH levels remained within the normal range in 80 per cent of patients postoperatively (Barkan et al., 1988).

PARATHYROID TUMORS

Incidence

Parathyroid carcinoma is extremely rare, causing only 1 per cent of all cases of primary hyperparathyroidism (Shane & Bilezidian, 1982). It affects men and women with equal frequency and can occur as part of a MEN syndrome.

Biology and Natural History

This tumor is slow growing but can metastasize late in the course of disease to regional nodes, liver, and lung (Schantz & Castleman, 1973). Death generally occurs as a result of the renal and cardiac effects of prolonged hypercalcemia (McCance et al., 1987). First-year survival appears to be less than 50 per cent; less than 35 per cent of patients survive 10 years (Schantz & Castleman, 1973; Shane & Bilezidian, 1982).

Clinical Presentation

Clinical manifestations result from the effect of parathyroid hormone (PTH) on the kidneys, bone, gastrointestinal tract, and neuromuscular system. Hypersecretion of PTH results in hypercalcemia and leads to the development of renal calculi, demineralization of bone, gastrointestinal disturbances, pancreatitis, muscle weakness, and lethargy. A neck mass can be palpated in 30 to 50 per cent of patients (Schantz & Castleman, 1973; Shane & Bilezidian, 1982).

Treatment

Surgery

Surgical removal of the carcinoma is indicated in all cases, although 30 to 65 per cent of patients will have recurrent disease even after apparent complete resection of the tumor (Schantz & Castleman, 1973). Because of the indolent nature of this tumor, patients with recurrent tumor who have symptoms of hypercalcemia can obtain long-term palliation with additional surgery (Flye & Brennan, 1981).

Chemotherapy or Radiation Therapy

Experience with chemotherapy and radiation therapy in the management of metastatic disease is limited but these treatment methods do not appear to affect survival (Bukowski et al., 1984; Shane & Bilezidian, 1982).

Symptom management is the focus of treatment for patients with bone pain and hypercalcemia. Pharmacologic agents that block PTH or lower serum calcium level are employed for palliation of symptoms. Calcitonin, diphosphonates, and mithramycin have been used with limited success for short-term management of hypercalcemia. The role of a parathyroid hormone antagonist is currently being explored (Rosenblatt, 1986).

MULTIPLE ENDOCRINE NEOPLASIAS

Hyperplasia or neoplasia of endocrine cells can occur in a single site or involve several different endocrine glands or tissues. The term *multiple endocrine neoplasia* has been used to describe constellations of endocrine abnormalities (Norton, Doppman, & Jensen, 1989). Three distinct MEN syndromes have been described (see Table 37–3).

Patients who have any tumor identified as a component of one of the MEN syndromes should be evaluated for the presence of other tumors. The MEN syndromes are transmitted genetically in an autosomal dominant fashion. Consequently, it has been recommended that screening of all family members in an affected kindred be done in an effort to increase the early detection of lesions in asymptomatic persons (Norton et al., 1989).

Although each component of MEN syndromes is treated independently, patients with more than one tumor at the time of diagnosis will need to have decisions made regarding which tumor to treat first.

APUDOMAS

Overview

Tumors arising from cells that share the common biochemical characteristics for *a*mine *p*recursor *u*ptake and *d*ecarboxylation (APUD) were first described by Pearse (1977) and unified into the APUD concept, which provides a framework for relating a variety of hormonally active tumors arising in diverse sites. These cells have been detected in the thyroid, adrenal medulla, sympathetic nervous system, and gastroenteropancreatic organs. The incidence of APUD-derived gastrointestinal and pancreatic endocrine tumors is extremely rare, but a brief discussion is warranted because increased detection of these tumors has been made possible with advances in radioimmunoassay techniques.

Carcinoid Tumors

Carcinoid tumors are examples of APUD neoplasms and occur most frequently within the gastrointestinal tract, especially the appendix and small intestine (Moertel, 1987). They are slow-growing tumors that may be discovered incidentally because patients are frequently asymptomatic until the disease is well advanced (Thompson et al., 1985). The most common presenting signs with symptomatic tumors are obstructive symptoms, pain, and malignant carcinoid syndrome (MCS). This syndrome is manifested by diarrhea, facial flushing, and heart disease and is usually indicative of metastatic disease in the liver (Moertel, 1987). Symptoms are thought to be related to excess production of serotonin.

Treatment

Surgical resection is indicated for most carcinoid tumors, but the extent of the surgical procedure required varies according to location and size of the primary tumor. Tumors larger than 2 cm require more radical surgery, because they routinely metastasize (Moertel, 1987).

Several approaches have been employed for palliation of MCS symptoms in patients with unresectable disease. Somatostatin analogues that inhibit the release of a variety of hormones, including serotonin, have been used with some success (Kvols et al., 1986). Also, cyproheptadine (Periactin) has been effective in controlling diarrhea related to MCS (Moertel, 1987).

In general, cytotoxic chemotherapy is not recommended with metastatic carcinoid tumors. Multiple agents have been investigated, but response rates have been low and of short duration and therefore do not appear to justify the significant toxicity associated with their administration (Moertel, 1987). Hepatic artery occlusion (via ligation or embolization), which is aimed at decreasing oxygenation of tumor in the liver, thereby causing cell death, has been somewhat successful in transiently relieving symptoms (Moertel, 1987; Odurney & Birch, 1985).

Five-year survival depends on the site of the primary tumor and varies from 52 to 99 per cent for all stages of disease (Godwin, 1975).

SUMMARY

Technologic advances as well as epidemiologic studies have provided new information regarding specific characteristics of many of the endocrine neoplasms. This knowledge is translating into new approaches for (1) modifying the hormonal effects of these tumors within the body, (2) identifying persons at risk for the development of endocrine tumors, and (3) improving early detection with laboratory and radiologic techniques. Nurses caring for patients with endocrine cancers must keep abreast of the advances in this field to educate patients and provide knowledgeable care.

References

Averbuch, S., Steakley, C. S., Young, R. C., Gelmann, E. P., Goldstein, D. S., Stull, R., & Keiser, H. R. (1988). Malignant pheochromocytoma: Effective treatment with a combination of cyclophosphamide, vincristine, and dacarbazine. *Annals of Internal Medicine, 109,* 267–273.

Barkan, A. M., Lloyd, R. V., Chandler, W. F., Hatfield, M. K., Gebarshi, S. S., Kelch, R. P. & Beitins, I. Z. (1988). Preoperative treatment of acromegaly with long-acting somatostatin analog SMS 201–995: Shrinkage of invasive pituitary macroadenomas and improved surgical remission rate. *Journal of Clinical Endocrinology and Metabolism, 67,* 1040–1048.

Baylin, S. B., & Wells, S. A. (1981). Management of hereditary medullary thyroid cancer. *Clinics in Endocrinology and Metabolism, 10,* 367–377.

Beahrs, O. H., Henson, D. E., Hutter, R. V. P., & Myers, M. H. (Eds.) (1988). *Manual for staging of cancer* (3rd ed., pp. 57–59). Philadelphia: J. B. Lippincott Co.

Bevan, J. S., Adams, C. B. T., Burke, C. W., Morton, K. E., Molyneux, A. J., Moore, R. A., & Esiri, M. M. (1987) Factors in the outcome of transsphenoidal surgery for prolactinoma and non-functioning pituitary tumors, including pre-operative bromocriptine therapy. *Clinical Endocrinology, 26,* 541–556.

Blahd, W. H. (1985). Treatment of thyroid cancer. *Comprehensive Therapy, 11*(9), 26–32.

Bravo, E. L., & Gifford, R. W. (1984). Pheochromocytoma: Diagnosis, localization and management. *New England Journal of Medicine, 311,* 1298–1303.

Bravo, E. L., Taranzi, R. C., Gifford, R. W., & Stewart, B. H. (1979). Circulating and urinary catecholamines in pheochromocytoma: Diagnostic and pathophysiologic implications. *New England Journal of Medicine, 301,* 682–686.

Brennan, M. F. (1987). Adrenocortical carcinoma. *CA: A Cancer Journal for Clinicians, 37,* 348–365.

Brennan, M. F. (with MacDonald, J. S.) (1985). Cancer of the endocrine system. In V. T. DeVita, S. Hellman, & S. A. Rosenberg (Eds.), *Cancer: Principles and practice of oncology* (2nd ed., pp. 1179–1241). Philadelphia: J. B. Lippincott Co.

Bukowski, R. M., Sheelar, L., Cunningham, J., & Esselstyn, C. (1984). Successful combination chemotherapy for metastatic parathyroid carcinoma. *Archives of Internal Medicine, 144,* 399–402.

Bullock, B. L., & Rosendahl, P. P. (1988). *Pathophysiology: Adaptations and alterations in function* (2nd ed., pp. 498–500). Glenview, IL: Scott, Foresman & Co.

Cassmeyer, V. L. (1987). Interventions for persons with problems of the endocrine system: Pituitary, thyroid, parathyroid, and adrenal glands. In W. J. Phipps, B. C. Long, & N. F. Woods (Eds.), *Medical-surgical nursing: Concepts and clinical practice* (3rd ed., pp. 549–600). St. Louis: C. V. Mosby Co.

Chang, A., Glazer, H. S., Lee, J. K. T., Ling, D, & Heiken, J. P. (1987). Adrenal gland: MR imaging. *Radiology, 163,* 123–128.

Chun, M., Masko, G. B., & Hetelekidis, S. (1988). Radiotherapy in the treatment of pituitary adenomas. *International Journal of Radiation Oncology, Biology, Physics, 15,* 305–309.

Ciric, I. (1985). Pituitary tumors. *Neurology Clinics, 3,* 751–766.

Clark, O. H., Levin, K., Zeng, Q., Greenspan, F. S., & Siperstein, A. (1988). Thyroid cancer: The case for total thyroidectomy. *European Journal of Cancer and Clinical Oncology, 24,* 305–313.

Cohn, K., Gottesman, L., & Brennan, M. (1986). Adrenocortical carcinoma. *Surgery 100,* 1170–1177.

Crile, G., Pontius, K. I., & Hawk, W. A. (1985). Factors influencing the survival of patients with follicular carcinoma of the thyroid gland. *Surgery, Gynecology, and Obstetrics, 160,* 409–416.

Didolkar, M. S., Bescher, R. S., Elias, E. G., & Moore, R. H. (1981). Natural history of adrenocortical carcinoma: A clinicopathologic study of 42 patients. *Cancer, 47,* 2153–2161.

Dollar, J. R., & Blackwell, R. E. (1986). Diagnosis and management of prolactinomas. *Cancer and Metastases Review, 5,* 125–138.

Doppman, J. L., Reinig, J. W., Dwyer, A. J., Frank, J. P., Norton, J., Loriaux, E., & Keiser, H. (1987). Differentiation of adrenal masses by magnetic resonance imaging. *Surgery, 102,* 1018–1025.

Duffy, B. J., & Fitzgerald, P. J. (1950). Cancer of the thyroid in children: A report of 28 cases. *Journal of Clinical Endocrinology, 10,* 1296–1308.

Favus, M. J., Schneider, A. B., Stachura, M. E., Arnold, J. E., Ryo, V. Y., Pinsky, S. M., Colman, M., Arnold, M. J., & Frohman, L. A. (1976). Thyroid cancer occurring as a late consequence of head and neck irradiation: Evaluation of 1056 patients. *New England Journal of Medicine, 294,* 1019–1025.

Ferber, B., Hardy, V. H., Gerhardt, P. R., & Solomon, M. (1962). Cancer in New York State, exclusive of New York City, 1941–1960. Albany, New York Bureau of Cancer Control, New York State Department of Health.

Flye, M. W., & Brennan, M. F. (1981). Surgical resection of metastatic parathyroid carcinoma. *Annals of Surgery, 193,* 425–435.

Frable, W. J. (1986). The treatment of thyroid cancer. The role of fine needle aspiration. *Archives of Otolaryngology—Head and Neck Surgery, 112,* 1200–1203.

Freitas, J. E., Gross, M. D., Ripley, S., & Shapiro, B. (1985). Radionuclide diagnosis and therapy of thyroid cancer: Current status report. *Seminars in Nuclear Medicine, 15,* 106–131.

Friedman, M., Toriumi, D. M., & Mafee, M. F. (1988). Diagnostic imaging techniques in thyroid cancer. *American Journal of Surgery, 155,* 215–223.

Godwin, D. J. (1975). Carcinoid tumors: An analysis of 2837 cases. *Cancer, 36,* 560–569.

Greenfield, L. D. (1987). Thyroid tumors. In C. A. Perez & L. W. Brady (Eds.), *Principles and practice of radiation oncology* (pp. 1126–1156). Philadelphia: J. B. Lippincott Co.

Halberg, F. J., & Sheline, G. E. (1987). Radiotherapy of pituitary tumors. *Endocrinology and Metabolism Clinics, 16,* 667–683.

Haq, M. M., Legha, S. S., Samaan, N. A., Bodey, G. P., & Burgess, M. A. (1980). Cytotoxic chemotherapy in adrenal cortical carcinoma. *Cancer Treatment Reports, 64,* 909–913.

Holm, L. E., Dahlquist, I., Israelsson, A., & Lundell, G. (1980). Malignant thyroid tumors after iodine–131 therapy. *New England Journal of Medicine, 303,* 188–191.

Hubbard, J. L., Scheithauer, B. W., Abboud, C. F., & Laws, E. L., Jr. (1987). Prolactin secreting adenomas: The preoperative response to bromocriptine treatment and surgical outcome. *Journal of Neurosurgery, 67,* 816–821.

Hubert, J. P. (1986). Papillary carcinoma of the thyroid. *Comprehensive Therapy, 12*(8), 20–26.

Hull, C. J. (1986). Phaeochromocytoma: Diagnosis, preoperative preparation and anesthetic management. *British Journal of Anaesthesiology, 58,* 1453–1468.

Hutter, A. M., & Kayhoe, D. E. (1966). Adrenal cortical carcinoma: Clinical features of 138 patients. *American Journal of Medicine, 41,* 572–580.

Jarabak, J., & Rice, K. (1981). Metastatic adrenal cortical carcinoma: Prolonged regression with mitotane therapy. *Journal of the American Medical Association, 246,* 1706–1707.

Javadpour, N., Waltering, E., & Brennan, M. F. (1980). Adrenal neoplasms. *Current Problems in Surgery, 17,* 1–52.

Karakousis, C. P., Rao, U., & Moore, R. (1985). Adrenal adenocarcinomas: Histologic grading and survival. *Journal of Surgical Oncology, 29*(2), 105–111.

Kaufman, B., Kaufman, B. A., Arafah, B. M., Roessmann, V., & Selman, W. R. (1987). Large pituitary gland adenomas evaluated with magnetic resonance imaging. *Neurosurgery, 21,* 540–546.

Kerr, D. J., Burt, A. D., Boyle, P., MacFarlane, G. J., Storer, A. M., & Brewin, T. B. (1986). Prognostic factors in thyroid tumors. *British Journal of Cancer, 54,* 475–482.

Kim, J. H., & Leeper, R. D. (1983). Treatment of anaplastic giant and spindle cell carcinoma of the thyroid gland with combination Adriamycin and radiation therapy: A new approach. *Cancer, 52,* 954–957.

Kornblith, P. L., Walker, M. D., & Cassady, J. R. (1985). Neoplasms of the central nervous system. In V. T. DeVita, Jr., S. Hellman, & S. A. Rosenberg (Eds.), *Cancer: Principles and practice of oncology* (2nd ed., pp. 1437–1510). Philadelphia: J. B. Lippincott Co.

Kovacs, K., & Horvath, E. (1987). Pathology of pituitaty tumors. *Endocrinology and Metabolism Clinics, 16,* 667–683.

Kvols, L. K., Moertel, C. G., O'Connell, M. J., Schutt, A. J., Rubin, J., & Hahn, R. G. (1986). Treatment of the malignant carcinoid syndrome: Evaluation of a long-acting somatostatin analog. *New England Journal of Medicine, 315,* 663–666.

Lang, W., Choritz, H., & Hundeshagen, H. (1986). Risk factors in follicular thyroid carcinomas. *American Journal of Surgical Pathology, 10,* 246–252.

Laws, E. R., Jr. (1982). Complications of transsphenoidal microsurgery for pituitary adenomas. In M. Brock (Ed.), *Modern neurosurgery* (Vol. 1, pp. 181–191). New York: Springer-Verlag.

Laws, E. R., Jr. (1987). Pituitary surgery. *Endocrinology and Metabolism Clinics, 16,* 647–665.

Leeper, R. D. (1985). Thyroid cancer. *Medical Clinics of North America, 69,* 1079–1096.

Levin, V. A., Sheline, G. E., & Gutin, P. H. (1989). Neoplasms of the central nervous system. In V. T. DeVita, Jr., S. Hellman, & S. A. Rosenberg (Eds.), *Cancer: Principles and practice of oncology* (3rd ed., pp. 1557–1611). Philadelphia: J. B. Lippincott Co.

Lindberg, R. D. (1980). External beam radiation in thyroid cancers. In G. H. Fletcher (Ed.), *Textbook of radiotherapy* (3rd ed., pp. 384–388). Philadelphia: Lea & Febiger.

Mazzaferri, E. L., Young, R. L., Oertel, J. E., Kemmerer, W. T., & Page, C. P., (1977). Papillary thyroid carcinoma: The impact of therapy in 576 patients. *Medicine, 56*, 171–196.

McCance, D. R., Kenny, B. D., Sloan, J. M., Russell, C. F. J., & Hadden, D. R. (1987). Parathyroid carcinoma: A review. *Journal of the Royal Society of Medicine, 80*, 505–509.

McConahey, W. M., Hay, I. D., Woolner, L. B., vanHeerden, J. A., & Taylor, W. F. (1986). Papillary thyroid cancer treated at the Mayo Clinic, 1946 through 1970: Initial manifestations, pathologic findings, therapy, and outcome. *Mayo Clinic Proceedings, 61*, 978–996.

Moertel, C. G. (1987). An odyssey in the land of small tumors. *Journal of Clinical Oncology, 5*, 1503–1522.

Molitch, M. E., Elton, R. L., Blackwell, R. E., Caldwell, B., Chang, R. J., Jaffe, R., Joplin, G., Robbins, R. J., Tyson, J., Thorner, M. O., & The Bromocriptine Study Group. (1985). Bromocriptine as primary therapy for prolactin-secreting macroadenomas: Results of a prospective multicenter study. *Journal of Clinical Endocrinology and Metabolism, 60*, 698–705.

Nel, C. J. C., van Heerden, J. A., Goellner, J. R., Gharib, H., McConahey, W. M., Taylor, W. F., & Grant, C. S. (1985). Anaplastic carcinoma of the thyroid: A clinicopathologic study of 82 cases. *Mayo Clinic Proceedings, 60*, 51–63.

Norton, J. A., Doppman, J. L., & Jensen, R. T. (1989). Cancer of the endocrine system. In V. T. Devita, Jr., S. Hellman, & S. A. Rosenberg (Eds.), *Cancer, Principles and practice of oncology* (3rd ed., pp. 1269–1344). Philadelphia: J. B. Lippincott Co.

Odurney, A., & Birch, S. J. (1985). Hepatic arterial embolization in patients with metastatic carcinoid tumors. *Clinical Radiology, 36*, 597–602.

Pearse, A. G. E. (1977). The diffuse neuroendocrine system and the APUD concept: Related endocrine peptides in brain, intestine, pituitary, placenta, and anuran cutaneous glands. *Medical Biology, 55*, 115–125.

Post, K. D., & Muraszko, K. (1986). Management of pituitary tumors. *Neurology Clinics, 4*, 801–820.

Poster, D. S., Bruno, S., Penta, J. Pina, K., & Catane R. (1981). Current status of chemotherapy in the treatment of advanced carcinoma of the thyroid gland. *Cancer Clinical Trials, 4*, 301–305.

Refetoff, S., Harrison, J., Karanfilski, B. T., Kaplan, E. L., De-Groot, L. J., & Bekerman, C. (1975). Continuing occurrence of thyroid carcinoma after irradiation to the neck in infancy and childhood. *New England Journal of Medicine, 292*, 171–175.

Rosenblatt, M. (1986). Peptide hormone antagonists that are effective in vivo. Lessons from parathyroid hormone. *New England Journal of Medicine, 315*, 1004–1011.

Saad, M. F., Ordinez, N. E., Rashid, R. K., Guido, J. J., Hill, C. S., Hickey, R. C., & Samaan, N. A. (1984). Medullary carcinoma

of the thyroid. A study of the clinical features and prognostic factors in 161 patients. *Medicine, 63*, 319–342.

Samaan, N. A., & Hickey, R. C. (1987). Adrenocortical carcinoma. *Seminars in Oncology, 14*, 292–296.

Samaan, N. A., Hickey, R. C., & Shutts, P. E. (1988). Diagnosis, localization, and management of pheochromocytoma: Pitfalls and follow-up in 41 patients. *Cancer, 62*, 2451–2460.

Schantz, A., & Castleman, B. (1973). Parathyroid carcinoma: A study of 70 cases. *Cancer, 31*, 600–605.

Scheithauer, B. W., Kovacs, K., Laws, E. R., Jr., & Randall R V. (1986). Pathology of invasive pituitary tumors with special reference to functional classification. *Journal of Neurosurgery, 65*, 733–744.

Schroder, S., Bocker, W., Baisch, H., Burk, C. G., Arps, H., Meiners, I., Kastendieck, H., Heitz, P. V., & Kloppel, G. (1988). Prognostic factors in medullary thyroid carcinomas: Survival in relation to age, sex, stage, histology, immunocytochemistry, and DNA content. *Cancer, 61*, 806–816.

Shane, E., & Bilezidian, J. P. (1982). Parathyroid carcinoma: A review of 62 patients. *Endocrine Reviews, 3*, 218–226.

Silverberg, E., & Lubera, J. (1989). Cancer statistics, 1989. *CA: A Cancer Journal for Clinicians, 39*, 3–20.

Simpson, W. J., & Carruthers, J. S. (1978). The role of external radiation in the management of papillary and follicular thyroid cancer. *American Journal of Surgery, 136*, 457–460.

Sisson, J. C., Frager, M. S., Valk, T. W., Gross, M. D., Swanson, D. P., Wieland, D. M., Tobes, M. C., Bierwaltes, W. H., & Thompson, N. W. (1981). Scintigraphic localization of pheochromocytoma. *New England Journal of Medicine, 305*, 12–17.

Third National Cancer Survey: Incidence data. (1975). National Cancer Institute Monograph 41. Bethesda, MD: U.S. Dept of Health, Education, & Welfare, Public Health Service, National Institutes of Health.

Thompson, G. B., vanHeerden, J. A., Martin, J. K., Schutt, A. J., Ilstrup, D. M., & Carney, J. A. (1985). Carcinoid tumors of the gastrointestinal tract: Presentation, management, and prognosis. *Surgery, 98*, 1054–1063.

Thompson, N. W., & Cheung, P. S. (1987). Diagnosis and treatment of functioning and nonfunctioning adrenocortical neoplasms including incidentalomas. *Surgical Clinics of North America, 67*, 423–436.

Tollefsen, H., Shah, J. P., & Huvos, A. G. (1972). Papillary carcinoma of the thyroid: Recurrence in the thyroid gland after initial surgical treatment. *American Journal of Surgery, 124*, 468–472.

Williams, E. D. (1979). The aetiology of thyroid tumors. *Clinics in Endocrinology and Metabolism, 8*, 193–207.

Wilson, S. M., Platz, C., & Block, G. M. (1970). Thyroid carcinoma after irradiation: Characteristics and treatment. *Archives of Surgery, 100*, 330–337.

38

Soft Tissue and Bone Sarcomas

AMY SMITH-BRASSARD

SOFT TISSUE SARCOMAS	BONE SARCOMAS
Definition and Incidence	Definition and Incidence
Epidemiology	Etiology
Biology of Sarcomas	Biology of Bone Sarcomas
Diagnosis of Soft Tissue Sarcomas	Diagnosis
Specific Histologic Types	Specific Histologic Types
Treatment	Treatment

SOFT TISSUE SARCOMAS

Definition and Incidence

By definition soft tissue is the extraskeletal supportive structures arising from the mesoderm. These connective tissues include muscles, tendons, fat, and synovial and fibrous tissues. This heterogeneous group of tissues constitutes approximately 50 per cent of the body weight.

Soft tissue sarcomas are tumors arising from these connective tissue structures. Although there are numerous classifications of sarcomas, they are grouped together owing to similarities in pathologic appearance, presentation, and natural history of the disease. Sarcomas can occur most anywhere in the body but are most commonly found in the extremities. Because of the many types of soft tissue sarcomas and their low incidence, an accepted means to treat these tumors has not been established.

According to the 1990 Cancer Facts and Figures (American Cancer Society, 1990), an estimated 5700 new cases of soft tissue sarcomas would have been diagnosed in 1990, with approximately 3100 deaths. The incidence of soft tissue sarcomas is higher in children under 15 years, ranking behind leukemias, lymphomas, and tumors of the central and sympathetic nervous systems (Pizzo, Miser, Cassady, & Filler, 1985).

Epidemiology

No definable causes or trends have been noted in the incidence of soft tissue sarcomas. A genetic predisposition has not been found, although isolated cases of soft tissue sarcomas among siblings have been documented (Howard & Casten, 1963). Cases of genetic disorders have been linked to the development of sarcomas, but these are rare. An example is a neuro-fibrosarcoma in patients with von Recklinghausen's

disease (Heard, 1963). An erroneous belief is that a causal relationship exists between trauma and the development of a soft tissue sarcoma. There is no scientific evidence that this occurs; instead, it is most likely the trauma that brings attention to the preexisting tumor. Viral agents likewise have not been linked directly to the development of sarcomas. However, within the past decade medical researchers have reported a much higher incidence of Kaposi's sarcoma in association with the acquired immune deficiency syndrome (AIDS). Previously Kaposi's syndrome was seen mainly in elderly men of Jewish or Mediterranean origin. The disease in AIDS patients is a more aggressive form involving the viscera and lymphatic system.

Reports have linked soft tissue sarcomas and environmental exposure to phenoxyacetic acids and chlorophenols (Hardell & Sandstrom, 1979). There have been case reports of patients developing soft tissue sarcomas years after radiation therapy for a malignant tumor such as breast cancer or Hodgkin's disease (Halpern, Greenberg, & Suit, 1984; O'Neill, Cocke, Mason, & Hurley, 1982).

Other conditions and environmental factors associated with soft tissue sarcomas are listed in Table 38–1.

Biology of Sarcomas

In the embryo, three germ layers are found: endoderm, ectoderm, and mesoderm. The primitive mesoderm develops into such organs as the heart, kidneys, and gonads; the hematopoietic, lymphatic, reticuloendothelial tissues; and bone, muscle, and soft connective tissues. Tumors arising from these tissues are termed sarcomas. Although tumors that arise from epithelial tissue are usually called carcinomas, epithelial cells that line blood vessels or organs actually arise from the mesoderm. For this reason, tumors that arise from the endothelium are also termed sarcomas.

Because connective tissue is found throughout the

Table 38–1. CONDITIONS AND ENVIRONMENTAL FACTORS ASSOCIATED WITH SOFT TISSUE SARCOMAS

Previous scars
Long-standing lymphedema
Irradiation for
    Tuberculosis of the skin
    Thyroid disease
Exposure to
    Asbestos
    Thorium dioxide (Thorotrast)
    Arsenic
    Polyvinyl chloride
Genetically linked disease
    Neurofibromatosis
    Tuberous sclerosis
    Gardner's syndrome
    Basal cell nevus syndrome
AIDS (Kaposi's sarcoma)

(From Goodman, T. L. [1987]. Sarcomas of soft tissue and bone. In M. S. Rosenthal, J. Carignan, & B. Smith [Eds.], *Medical care of the cancer patient.* Philadelphia, W. B. Saunders Co. Reproduced by permission.)

body, soft tissue sarcomas can occur nearly anywhere. In a review by Potter and co-workers (1985) of 307 cases of soft tissue sarcoma, nearly 50 per cent were in the lower extremity, 37.4 per cent at above the knee, 19.2 per cent in an upper extremity, and 27.4 per cent in the trunk region.

Owing to the variety of types and the low rate of occurrence, soft tissue sarcomas often represent a difficult diagnostic decision for the pathologist. Table 38–2 lists the histologic types of soft tissue sarcomas. These tumors vary in histologic features and behavior, making treatment decisions challenging and difficult.

Soft tissue sarcomas usually first appear as asymptomatic soft tissue masses. These tumors often grow insidiously, so that early detection is difficult. Soft tissue sarcomas take the path of least resistance in their growth, pushing surrounding tissues before them. They compress surrounding tissue, and so the tumors can grow quite large before clinical symptoms develop. This tumor forms a pseudocapsule yet contains invasive extensions of malignant tissue (Rosenberg, Suit, & Bakes, 1985). Local signs of tumor besides the presence of a mass include peripheral neuralgia, paralysis, or ischemia if the tumor is impinging on nerve or vascular supply. The tumors may also obstruct bowel, ureters, or mediastinal structures (Pories, Murinson, & Rubin, 1983).

Disagreement exists among pathologists on grading systems for soft tissue sarcomas. Necrosis and mitotic rate are important factors in determining the grade of the tumor.

One of the most important factors in the outcome of patients with soft tissue sarcomas is believed to be the histologic grade (G) of the primary tumor, rather than the histopathologic type. G_1 tumors are well differentiated, G_2 are moderately differentiated, and G_3 are poorly differentiated. Anatomic staging uses the TNM classification plus an A or B to denote tumors that are less than or greater than 5 cm. Table 38–3 lists the anatomic staging and stage grouping for soft tissue sarcomas. It is important to note the rare occurrence of nodal involvement. With the exception of

rhabdomyosarcomas and synoviosarcomas, soft tissue sarcomas rarely infiltrate surrounding lymph nodes but instead tend to metastasize via the hematogenous route (Pories et al., 1983).

It is this hematogenous dissemination and local invasion into surrounding tissues that generally dictate a poor prognosis. Another prognostic factor is location—for example, trunk versus extremity. The primary site influences resectability and ability to cure the tumor. In the extremity, proximal lesions are believed to be less curable than distal lesions (Rosenberg et al., 1985). Age and sex seem to have little influence on prognosis with the exception of fibrosarcomas, which tend to do better in children (Enterline, 1981). An estimated 80 per cent of all lesions recur in about 2 years after surgical resection (Lindberg, Martin, & Romsdahl, 1975; Shiu, Castro, & Hajdu, 1975). More than 50 per cent of cases recur as pulmonary lesions. Local recurrence is the next most common site. Aggressive pulmonary resection for isolated lesions is

Table 38–2. HISTOLOGIC TYPES OF SOFT TISSUE SARCOMAS

Tumors of fibrous tissue
    (Fibromatosis)
    Fibrosarcoma
Tumors of adipose tissue
    Liposarcoma
        Well differentiated
        Myxoid
        Round cell
        Pleomorphic
Tumors of smooth muscle
    Leiomyosarcoma
    Leiomyosarcoma, epithelioid variant
Tumors of striated muscle
    Rhabdomyosarcoma
        Pleomorphic
        Alveolar
        Embryonal
        Mixed
Tumors of vascular origin
    Angiosarcoma
    Lymphangiosarcoma
    Hemangiopericytoma (malignant)
Tumors of synovial tissue
    Synovial sarcoma
Tumors of mesothelium
    Malignant mesothelioma
Tumors of neurogenic origin
    Neurogenic sarcoma (malignant schwannoma)
        Neurogenic sarcoma—uncomplicated
        Neurogenic sarcoma with melanocytic, osseous, chondroid, or glandular metaplasia
Tumors of "histiocytic" origin
    Malignant fibrous histiocytoma
    Giant cell tumor of soft parts
Tumors of cartilaginous origin
    Extraskeletal myxoid chondrosarcoma (chordoid sarcoma)
Tumors of debatable origin
    Kaposi's sarcoma
    Dermatofibrosarcoma protuberans
    Clear cell sarcoma
    Epithelioid sarcoma
    Alveolar soft part sarcoma
    Small round cell sarcoma
        Extraskeletal Ewing's sarcoma
        Other

(From Enterline, H. T. [1981]. Histopathology of sarcomas. *Seminars in Oncology, 8,* 133–135. Reproduced by permission.)

Table 38–3. STAGING OF SOFT TISSUE SARCOMAS

Anatomic Staging	Stage Grouping				
Primary Tumors (T)	Stage I				
T_1 Tumor less than 5 cm	IA	G_1	T_1	N_0	M_0
T_2 Tumor 5 cm or greater	IB	G_1	T_2	N_0	M_0
T_3 Tumor that grossly invades bone, major vessel, or major nerves	Stage II				
	IIA	G_2	T_1	N_0	M_0
Node Involvement (N)	IIB	G_2	T_2	N_0	M_0
N_0 No histologically verified metastases to lymph nodes	Stage III				
N_1 Histologically verified regional lymph node	IIIA	G_3	T_1	N_0	M_0
metastases	IIIB	G_3	T_2	N_0	M_0
	IIIC	Any G	$T_{1,2}$	N_1	M_0
Histopathology Grade (G)					
G_1 Low grade	Stage IV				
G_2 Moderate grade	IVA	Any G	T_3	Any N	M_0
G_3 High grade	IVB	Any G	Any T	Any N	M_{1-4}

(From Pories, W., Murinson, D., & Rubin, P. [1983]. Soft tissue sarcomas. In P. Rubin [Ed.], *Clinical oncology: A multidisciplinary approach* [pp. 308–324]. New York: American Cancer Society. Reproduced by permission.)

recommended. Without resection, the median survival after pulmonary mestastases have developed is 6 to 12 months (Rosenberg et al., 1985).

Diagnosis of Soft Tissue Sarcomas

As with any suspected malignancy, the medical work-up should include history, physical examination, soft tissue radiograph of the affected part, computed tomographic (CT) scan or magnetic resonance imaging (MRI) of the region, plus radiographs and CT scans of the lung. The nurse during this early period can provide explanations and offer support to the patient. The diagnostic period is filled with fears and anxieties.

The histologic grade of the tumor is the most important factor in prognosis and in treatment decisions. Usually a needle biopsy does not provide adequate tissue samples necessary to determine the correct histologic grade and pathologic type of the tumor. For this reason, an incisional biopsy is usually done to diagnose a soft tissue mass. The site of the biopsy should be carefully placed so as not to compromise an excisional biopsy later. Incisional biopsies on an extremity should be placed longitudinally so to not interfere with muscle group excisions during a major curative surgical procedure.

Occasionally an arteriogram may be obtained to visualize the vascular supply of the tumor. A bone scan may delineate bone invasion or more likely periosteal reaction to nearby tumor growth and increased blood supply. During any surgical biopsy, extra caution is necessary to prevent development of hematomas. These can result in further spread of the tumor.

Because soft tissue sarcomas rarely invade lymph nodes, a lymphangiogram has little diagnostic value.

In summary, CT scans are invaluable in the diagnosis of soft tissue sarcomas. An incisional biopsy is recommended for adequate tissue sampling. For pathologists, accuracy in diagnosis is difficult owing to the low number of cases seen and the variety of tumor types classified as soft tissue sarcomas.

Specific Histologic Types

A summary of diagnostic facts and histologic presentations is given in Table 38–4.

Fibrosarcomas most often develop in an extremity, usually the thigh. Although they can be locally aggressive, fibrosarcomas may have delayed metastases. Fibrosarcomas in early childhood are associated with lower rates of metastases and tend to have a more positive prognosis (Fraumeni, Vogel, & Easton, 1968).

Liposarcomas occur most commonly in the adult population. They have a strong predilection to appear in proximal lower extremities, such as the buttock, thigh, groin, and retroperitoneal area (Enterline, 1981). Liposarcomas rarely develop from previous lipomas. In fact, most atypical fatty lesions occurring in the skin are benign. Liposarcomas similar to other soft tissue sarcomas tend to have pseudoencapsulation, making local excisions difficult.

Rhabdomyosarcomas are muscle tumors that can be separated into three types. The first, *pleomorphic* rhabdomyosarcoma, is the least common. It occurs in late middle age and has a predilection for such muscle groups as the quadriceps, adductors, biceps, and brachialis (Pories et al., 1983). It has a high tendency for local recurrence. *Alveolar* rhabdomyosarcoma occurs most commonly in children and young adults. It is considered a very aggressive tumor with a poor prognosis. The third type, *embryonal* rhabdomyosarcoma, is the most common form. It also occurs most often in young children with a high percentage involving the head and neck area. Startling success has been achieved with combination chemotherapy after surgical excision.

Leiomyosarcomas are rare tumors of smooth muscle arising in visceral sites, such as the uterus, gastrointestinal tract, and retroperitoneum. They tend to metas-

Table 38–4. DETECTION AND DIAGNOSIS OF SOFT TISSUE SARCOMA

	Average Age	Sex Prevalence	Most Common Site	Most Common Presentation	Average Size (cm)	Histologic Pattern of Growth	Histologic Grade	Most Common Stage	Average 5-year Survival (%)
Malignant tumors of fibrous tissue									
Malignant fibroblastic fibrous histiocytoma	45	Male	Trunk	Superficial	10	Arranged	Low	I	85
Malignant histiocytic fibrous histiocytoma	50	Male	Knee	Deep	15	Epithelioid	—*	II	55
Malignant pleomorphic fibrous histiocytoma	50	Male	Buttock and Arm	Deep	5	Disarranged	—	III	50
Desmoid tumor	25	Male	Arm and Thigh	Deep	5	Spreading	Low	I	95
Fibroblastic fibrosarcoma	45	Male	Thigh	Deep	10	Arranged	High	III	40
Pleomorphic fibrosarcoma	50	Male	Thigh	Deep	15	Disarranged	High	III	35
Malignant tumors of tenosynovial tissue									
Biphasic tenosynovial sarcoma	35	Male	Knee	Deep	10	Alveolar	—	II	55
Monophasic tenosynovial sarcoma	24	Male	Thigh	Deep	15	Spreading	High	III	30
Epithelioid sarcoma	25	Male	Forearm	Superficial	2	Epithelioid	—	II	65
Clear cell sarcoma	30	Male	Leg	Deep	5	Epithelioid	High	II	55
Chordoid sarcoma	40	Male	Hand	Superficial	2	Lacy	Low	0	75
Malignant tumors of adipose tissue									
Well-differentiated liposarcoma	55	Male	Trunk	—	5	Lacy	Low	I	95
Myxoid liposarcoma	40	Male	Thigh	Deep	10	Lacy	Low	II	95
Lipoblastic liposarcoma	45	Male	Thigh	Deep	10	Epithelioid	High	III	50
Fibroblastic liposarcoma	45	Male	Thigh	Deep	10	Arranged	High	III	60
Pleomorphic liposarcoma	55	Male	Thigh	Deep	20	Disarranged	High	III	45
Malignant tumors of muscle									
Leiomyosarcoma	55	Female	Leg	—	5	Spreading	—	II	60
Leiomyoblastoma	50	Female	—	Deep	5	Epithelioid	—	II	60
Embryonal rhabdomyosarcoma	10	Male	Thigh	Deep	15	Epithelioid	High	III	65
Rhabdomyoblastoma	20	Male	—	Deep	5	Epithelioid	High	II	40
Pleomorphic rhabdomyosarcoma	50	Male	Thigh	Deep	20	Disarranged	High	III	25
Malignant tumors of vessels									
Hemangiosarcoma	45	Male	Trunk	—	5	Alveolar	High	III	30
Hemangiopericytoma	40	Male	—	Deep	10	Alveolar	—	II	60
Kaposi's sarcoma	55	Male	Leg	Superficial	2	Alveolar	Low	0	90
Lymphangiosarcoma	50	Female	Arm	—	5	Alveolar	High	III	10
Malignant tumors of peripheral nerves									
Malignant peripheral nerve tumor	40	Female	Thigh	Deep	15	Spreading	—	II	60
Primitive neuroectodermal tumor	25	Male	Trunk	Deep	5	Epithelioid	High	III	30
Extraskeletal malignant bone tumors									
Osteogenic sarcoma	50	Male	—	Deep	15	Disarranged	High	III	15
Chondrosarcoma	45	Male	Thigh	Deep	15	Lacy	—	II	60
Ewing's sarcoma	20	Male	Thigh	Deep	5	Epithelioid	High	III	—
Miscellaneous malignant soft tissue tumors									
Malignant granular cell tumor	45	Female	—	Superficial	5	Epithelioid	—	II	75
Alveolar soft part sarcoma	35	Female	Thigh	Deep	15	Epithelioid	—	III	50
Malignant lymphoma	—	—	Thigh	Deep	10	—	—	—	—
Granulocytic sarcoma	20	Male	—	Deep	5	Epithelioid	High	III	5
Plasmacytoma	50	—	—	Deep	10	—	High	III	45
Malignant mesenchymoma	45	—	—	Deep	10	—	—	—	—
Postirradiation sarcoma	—	—	—	Deep	10	—	High	III	75
Undifferentiated soft tissue sarcoma	—	—	—	Deep	—	—	High	—	—

*All dashes mean that no data are available.

(From Pories, W., Murinson, D., & Rubin, P. [1983]. Soft tissue sarcomas. In P. Rubin [ed.], *Clinical oncology: A multidisciplinary approach* [pp. 308–324]. New York: American Cancer Society. Reproduced by permission.)

tasize widely, and long-term prognosis is generally poor.

Synovial sarcomas or malignant synoviomas arise from mesenchymal cells in the vicinity of tendons, bursae, or joints. Despite their name, they rarely involve the joint itself. Pain and swelling herald a palpable mass, sometimes by many months. As with most soft tissue sarcomas, the synovial variety has a predilection for the extremities and occurs most often in young adults. A longitudinal study of 784 patients from Memorial Hospital (Cadman, Soule, & Kelly, 1965) showed a 40 per cent 5-year survival, with smaller tumors (less than 5 cm) having a much better prognosis. Wide excision with radiation therapy or amputation is usually the treatment of choice.

Malignant mesothelioma, although rare, is well known owing to its correlation with asbestos exposure. This cancer arises in both the pleura and peritoneum and tends to be seen in the older male population. The prognosis is poor, with more than 50 per cent of patients succumbing to the disease within the first year.

Neurogenic sarcoma, malignant schwannoma, and neurofibrosarcoma are spindle cell tumors arising from nerves. Often these tumors are associated with von Recklinghausen's disease or neurofibromatosis. The average age of onset is 40 years, with the nerves involved most commonly being the sciatic, medial, or spinal nerves and the brachial plexus (Enterline, 1981). These tumors tend to have a high mitotic rate and aggressive behavior.

Malignant fibrous histiocytomas vary in histologic presentation, making a confirmed pathologic diagnosis difficult. These tumors arise from histiocytes and are found almost anywhere in the body but most commonly in the thigh. Histiocytomas are usually present in the deep musculature, which contributes to its late detection and high metastatic rate. These tumors are radiosensitive, which helps in tumor control. As with most soft tissue sarcomas, they have a higher rate of occurrence in men between the ages of 40 and 60 years.

Sarcomas of vascular endothelial origin include the angiosarcomas, lymphangiosarcomas, and hemangiopericytoma. Angiosarcomas occur most commonly in the skin, breast, and liver. They are usually poorly defined lesions manifested by a bruise-like appearance. The tumor forms a mass of anastomosing channels, which typically extends farther and deeper than it appears. This "iceberg effect" must be taken into consideration in planning treatments (Enterline, 1981). Lymphangiosarcomas most commonly arise in chronically edematous extremities, such as in the arm of a postmastectomy patient. Although their incidence is low, the rate increases in those patients who received radiation after a radical mastectomy. Hemangiopericytomas are rare soft tissue sarcomas, difficult to diagnose, which can appear most anywhere in the body and at any age. Survival patterns vary (Shiu et al., 1975; Simon & Enneking, 1976), but the tumor's behavior depends on mitotic growth, size, and necrosis.

The incidence of Kaposi's sarcoma has risen dramatically since AIDS has gained prominence. Before this, Kaposi's sarcoma was known as a blood vessel sarcoma that had occurred in the United States in mostly Jewish or Italian men over 65 years old. The lesions appear as bluish-black nodules or plaques, usually on the lower distal extremities. In elderly men the disease pursues a relatively indolent course and responds well to local irradiation. Kaposi's sarcoma in association with AIDS is a much more aggressive disease with visceral involvement, requiring systemic therapy. Etoposide (VP–16–123), vinblastine, and interferon have shown to be effective agents in treating this epidemic form of Kaposi's sarcoma. The combination of doxorubicin, bleomycin, and vinblastine has had success (Odajnyk & Muggia, 1985). There is also a higher incidence of Kaposi's sarcoma among blacks from Africa. If the disease is not treated early, the nodules can become locally aggressive, resulting in large, ulcerative masses. If the sarcoma is allowed to progress, an infiltrative form develops with woody fibrosis, brawny edema, and bone destruction (Ziegler, Templeton, & Vogel, 1984). A comparison of the different forms of Kaposi's sarcoma is given in Table 38–5.

Treatment

The management of the patient with a soft tissue sarcoma usually involves a multidisciplinary effort. The oncology nurse plays a pivotal role in the support and teaching of patients as the treatment plan evolves. The major goal is to eradicate the tumor with minimal loss of function.

The first step in optimal control of the disease is surgical excision with a microscopic tumor-free margin. Because sarcomas spread along tissue planes, a "shelling out" procedure is inadequate. If a pseudocapsule is removed, it is highly likely that the tumor will recur locally (Shieber & Graham, 1962). For this reason, a simple excision is usually inadequate treatment.

The excision of a soft tissue sarcoma should be done by a wide en bloc resection. This should include previous biopsy sites and a wide expanse of muscles, tendons, fascia, neurovascular structures, and lymph nodes. The entire specimen should be removed at one time without violating any tumor (Shiu & Hajdu, 1981). Preferably a margin of 2 to 3 cm is left (Pories et al., 1983).

En bloc resections of truncal sarcomas depend on the skill and ingenuity of the surgeon. In an extremity, however, if a wide resection is not possible, the alternative is amputation in selected cases. Indications for amputation include the following (Pories et al., 1983).

- The mass cannot be encompassed by wide excision.
- An operation would leave a useless extremity with compromised vascular or neurologic supply.
- The mass is a recurrence from a previously excised tumor.
- The tumor is difficult to palliate owing to pain, odor, and so forth.

In a large retrospective study at Memorial Hospital from 1949 to 1968, investigators found that amputations did lower recurrence rates at the stump site; however, 5- and 10-year survival rates were also lower than those for patients receiving en bloc resections (Shiu et al., 1975). This may be attributable to the fact that the original tumors were more involved. Nonetheless, this finding points to the need to combine adjuvant or additional therapy with surgery.

Both preoperative and postoperative radiation therapy has been used for many years as an adjunct in the treatment of soft tissue sarcomas. Radiation is used to treat the microscopic extensions of tumor. This can spare the patient extensive surgery. Using radiation in an adjunctive and more limited fashion avoids the late sequelae of high-dose radiotherapy (Tepper, 1989). With improved equipment and higher dosing, clinical responses are being seen, although clinical trials to prove efficacy are lacking.

Before surgery, 5000 to 6000 cGy are given in the hope that reduction in tumor bulk will occur. An advantage of preoperative radiation therapy is that it reduces the risk of intraoperative contamination of vascular space by viable tumor cells (Goodman, 1987). Another advantage is that patients who would have needed an amputation if surgery had been done initially may now be eligible for limb preservation procedures (Tepper, 1989). Surgery should take place 2 to 3 weeks after radiation. Postoperative radiation is used to sterilize an area that has known residual microscopic tumor or is at risk for developing recurrent disease. Lindberg

Table 38–5. KAPOSI'S SARCOMA

	Classic (Sporadic)	African (Endemic)	AIDS (Epidemic)
Skin lesions	Legs, feet	Extremities*	Widely dispersed
Mucosal involvement	Rare	Rare	Common (oral, anal)
Lymph node involvement	Rare	Uncommon*	Frequent
Response to treatment	Excellent	Excellent	Poor
Indolent course	Common	Common*	Unusual

*The lymphadenopathic form, predominant in children, is the exception.
(From Ziegler, J. L., Templeton, A. C., & Vogel, C. L. [1984]. Kaposi's sarcoma: A comparison of classical, endemic and epidemic forms. *Seminars in Oncology, 11,* 50. Reproduced by permission.)

and colleagues reviewed 100 patients who received adjunct radiation therapy after surgical excision. They found that 20 per cent of the patients had a local recurrence, compared with an estimated 50 per cent of patients expected to develop recurrences after surgery alone. An important unresolved issue is whether resection plus radiation is better therapy when trying to preserve the limb than radical surgery or amputations. To answer this question, a randomized study was done evaluating amputation plus chemotherapy versus excision, radiation therapy, and chemotherapy (Rosenberg & Glatstein, 1981). Results revealed that the 5-year survival rates of the two groups were similar (83 per cent for excision plus radiation and chemotherapy and 88 per cent for amputation) (Rosenberg et al., 1982). Because most soft tissue sarcomas occur in an extremity, the desire to salvage the limb is paramount for the patient. The nurse is instrumental in helping patients explore their options. According to Rosenberg and co-workers (1985), probably the best treatment is radical excision, which usually involves amputation. There is a higher risk of local recurrence otherwise. Refer to Chapter 20 for nursing care of the patient receiving radiation therapy.

Despite the success of achieving local control with surgery and radiation therapy, the 5-year survival rate of patients with soft tissue sarcoma is only 40 to 60 per cent overall (Goodman, 1987). The multimodality approach has improved 5-year survivals in patients with high-grade soft tissue sarcomas of an extremity to 70 to 80 per cent (Yang & Rosenberg, 1989). The main cause of death is disseminated disease. The role of adjuvant chemotherapy is being scrutinized. In the 1970s, trials with doxorubicin alone and with doxorubicin in combination with cyclophosphamide, dacarbazine (DTIC), and vincristine showed an increase in survival (Yap et al., 1980). As mentioned, the study by Rosenberg and colleagues (1982) demonstrated an increased survival in those patients receiving chemotherapy as opposed to the group not receiving systemic therapy (57 per cent versus 83 per cent). This is one of a few randomized trials to date that has shown a statistically significant difference in overall survival for patients receiving adjuvant therapy (Goodman, 1987). This increase in survival, however, has been seen only in patients with soft tissue sarcoma of an extremity. In a randomized trial of patients with head, neck, and trunk sarcomas, the 3-year disease-free survival was 77 per cent with chemotherapy, compared with 49 per cent without chemotherapy. However, there was no difference in overall survival (Glenn et al., 1985).

It appears that adjuvant chemotherapy with a combination of drugs including doxorubicin increases disease-free and overall survival in patients with high-grade sarcomas of an extremity (Rosenberg et al., 1985). The role of adjuvant chemotherapy in sarcomas elsewhere in the body is doubtful at the present time.

Multiple drug combinations, usually involving doxorubicin, cyclophosphamide, DTIC, vincristine, and methotrexate, have been tried in disseminated soft tissue sarcomas. Doxorubicin is considered the drug of choice whether used alone or in combination. The Southwest Oncology Group has randomized patients to one of three study arms: doxorubicin plus DTIC; doxorubicin, DTIC, and cyclophosphamide; or doxorubicin, DTIC, and actinomycin D. The median survivals in each group were 37, 45, and 50 weeks, respectively (Consensus Conference, 1985). Chemotherapy in advanced soft tissue sarcoma offers hope for partial response and a prolongation of survival, but this result is short lived. Until new agents are developed, the long-term survival in soft tissue sarcoma will remain poor.

BONE SARCOMAS

Definition and Incidence

Primary malignant tumors of bone are rare, constituting about 0.5 per cent of all cancers (Dahlin & Unni, 1986). The incidence of bone tumors is highest during adolescence, when it reaches a rate of 3 per 100,000. Osteogenic sarcoma is considered the most common primary malignant bone tumor. However, multiple myeloma, a nonosseous cancer of the bone marrow, is actually the most prevalent type of bone tumor. Chondrosarcoma is the most common malignant cartilage tumor. Most bone cancers are actually metastases from a separate primary carcinoma (Rubin, Evarts, & Boros, 1983).

An "osteogenic" tumor is one that arises from tissues such as bone, cartilage, fibrous tissue, or bone marrow. Therefore, the term *osteogenic* is a general classification and not specific for the various histologic subtypes. Malignant bone tumors do not necessarily arise from their benign counterparts. A list of bone tumors classified according to cell type is given in Table 38–6.

Most bone tumors involve the appendicular skeleton, usually the knee joint.

Table 38–6. PERCENTAGE OF PRIMARY TUMORS OF BONE ACCORDING TO MAYO CLINIC RECORDS

Histologic Type	Per Cent	Benign	Malignant
Hematopoietic	39.8		Myeloma
			Malignant lymphoma
Chondrogenic	21.3	Osteochondroma	Primary chondrosarcoma
		Chondroma	Secondary chondrosarcoma
		Chondroblastoma	Dedifferentiated chondrosarcoma
		Chondromyxoid fibroma	Mesenchymal chondrosarcoma
Osteogenic	19.2	Osteoid osteoma	Osteosarcoma
		Osteoblastoma	Parosteal osteosarcoma
Unknown origin	10.3	Giant cell tumor	Ewing's tumor
			Malignant giant cell tumor
			Adamantinoma
Histiocytic	0.7	Fibrous histiocytoma	Malignant (fibrous) histiocytoma
Fibrogenic	3.7	Metaphyseal fibrous defect (fibroma)	Desmoplastic fibroma
			Fibrosarcoma
Notochordal	3.1		Chordoma
Vascular	1.7	Hemangioma	Hemangioendothelioma
			Hemangiopericytoma
Lipogenic	0.1	Lipoma	Liposarcoma
Neurogenic	0.1	Neurilemoma	
Total	100		

(From Dahlin, D., & Unni, K. K. [1986]. *Bone tumors.* Courtesy of Charles C Thomas, Publisher, Springfield, Illinois.)

Etiology

Because primary bone tumors are relatively rare, etiologic information is often taken from studies on osteogenic sarcomas. This disease occurs 1.5 to 2 times more often in males. Owing to the high incidence in children and adolescents, it is speculated that areas of rapid growth may be more susceptible to developing a neoplasm (Dahlin & Unni, 1986). Metabolic stimulation from Paget's disease has been linked to the development of osteosarcomas (Goodman, 1987). Radiation has also been a culprit in the development of osteogenic sarcomas, chondrosarcomas, and fibrosarcomas (Miller & Miller, 1981). Research on laboratory animals has shown a relationship between a virus-induced osteosarcoma and the human variant (Storm, Morton, Eilber, & Saxton, 1981).

Biology of Bone Sarcomas

Bone sarcomas have their own specific characteristics, which aid the physician in diagnosis and treatment. The tumors are composed of spindle cells that grow centrifugally and form a pseudocapsule. Around the tumor is a zone of reactive tissue, which usually contains inflammatory cells. Tumors often interdigitate with surrounding tissue through this reactive zone. An important yet ominous characteristic of bone sarcomas is the ability to break through the pseudocapsule and form satellite lesions. High-grade sarcomas have the ability to develop "skip metastases," which are tumor nodules within the same bone but not in continuity. These are believed to be caused by embolization of tumor cells within the marrow sinusoids (Malawer, Abelson, & Suit, 1965). Skip metastases are usually indicators of poor prognosis.

Bone sarcomas, like soft tissue sarcomas, spread along the path of least resistance. Their growth is characterized by compression of normal tissue, resorption of bone by reactive osteoclasts, and direct destruction of tissue (Malawer et al., 1965).

Low-grade malignant tumors remain relatively localized with occasional nodules being found within the reactive zone. These lesions can be treated successfully by surgery alone if a margin of normal bone is allowed. Malignant, high-grade bone sarcomas have a normal history of rapid growth and metastasis. Bone tumors disseminate through the blood, usually to the pulmonary bed. High-grade tumors warrant the use of systemic therapy.

The staging of bone tumors is given in Table 38–7. A surgical staging system (SSS) describes the staging of bone sarcomas based on grade, location, and node or metastasis (GTM) (Enneking, Spanier, & Goodman, 1980). Grade designations include low (G_1) or high (G_2). Site of tumor may be intracompartmental (T_1) or extracompartmental (T_2). High-grade sarcomas tend to be T_2 lesions. Lymph nodes and metastasis (M) are represented by either M_0 or M_1.

Diagnosis

Radiographic evaluation, patient history of pain, and tissue biopsy are integral to the diagnosis of a bone sarcoma. Patient history often includes complaints of pain and sometimes of swelling. Occasionally a mass

Table 38–7. STAGING OF BONE SARCOMAS

Stage	Grade	Site
IA	Low (G_1)	Intracompartmental T_1
IB	Low (G_1)	Extracompartmental T_2
IIA	High (G_2)	Intracompartmental T_1
IIB	High (G_2)	Extracompartmental T_2
III	Any G, regional or distant metastasis	Any T

(From Enneking, W. F., Spanier, S. S., & Goodman, M. A. [1980]. A system for the surgical staging of musculoskeletal sarcoma. *Clinical Orthopedics, 153,* 106–120. Reproduced by permission.)

is felt as an extension of the primary tumor. Routine radiographs are the most informative method of depicting the type of bone destruction and the margin between tumor and normal bone (Cooper, McLeod, & Beabout, 1983). Three types of destructive bone patterns are seen on radiographs (Lodwick, 1966). The first is the geographic pattern, which has a slow rate of growth; the edge of tumor presumably indicates the edge of destroyed bone. The second pattern is the so-called moth-eaten pattern, which represents an intermediate growth rate and usually tumor extension beyond the radiographic lesion. The third pattern is a permeated pattern, which indicates rapid growth extending longitudinally within the bone. Radiographic findings will include periosteal reaction and both lytic and blastic features.

Tomography is helpful in delineating tumor margins, internal mineralization, and pathologic fractures (Cooper et al., 1983). The major contribution of CT scans in the diagnostic phase is to determine the extent of the tumor process. Computed tomography is more helpful in assessing lesions of the central skeleton than those of the extremities. In the preoperative staging, CT scans of the chest are very important in depicting metastatic lesions of the lung.

The isotope bone scan is helpful in detecting additional lesions, but owing to its nonspecificity, this technique is not particularly helpful in defining characteristics of the lesions.

Angiography plays a very minor role in the diagnosis of bone tumors, especially since the advent of CT scans, which can delineate vascular involvement.

A high alkaline phosphatase level is indicative of bone destruction and can be of diagnostic value. Aggressive bone tumors may also cause an increase in serum calcium level and urinary calcium excretion (Rubin et al., 1983).

An accurate diagnosis requires an open biopsy to obtain sufficient tissue. As with soft tissue sarcomas, the biopsy site should be chosen that will not interfere with a definitive surgical procedure. For example, the incision should not be placed where an amputation flap may be needed. Likewise a biopsy site needs to be planned so that the region can be removed en bloc with the tumor resection. Previously, a tourniquet was used to prevent hematogenous dissemination of tumor cells during surgery. However, this method did not improve long-term survival, and it is no longer advocated (Sim, Ivins, & Pritchard, 1978). Often a biopsy and definitive resection will be done at the same time. This requires a frozen section and a pathologist who is experienced in diagnosing malignant bone tumors.

If extensive surgery is expected at the time of the biopsy, the patient needs teaching before the operation so that he or she will know what to expect. If an amputation is being considered as the treatment of choice, the health team needs to explain this to the patient and allow the patient adequate time to explore how he or she feels about the loss of a limb. This topic is covered in more detail later in this chapter.

Specific Histologic Types

Owing to the rarity of these tumors, only chondrosarcomas and osteogenic sarcomas are discussed here. Ewing's sarcoma is predominantly a pediatric tumor and is not described in this chapter.

Chondrosarcoma is a malignant tumor composed of cells that produce hyaline cartilage. The tumor has a long, slow evolution, and some variants are so similar to their benign counterparts that diagnosis is difficult; thus mismanagement can occur (Shives, Wold, Dahlin, & Beabout, 1983). Ordinary chondrosarcoma occurs most often in middle-aged or older adults. The diaphysis of the femur is the most common site. Patients with a low-grade tumor have a longer disease-free and overall survival than those with higher grade lesions. Five-year survival is approximately 50 per cent (Pritchard, Lunke, Taylor, Dahlin, & Medley, 1980).

Osteosarcoma accounts for about 20 per cent of all bone sarcomas. Although osteogenic sarcoma tends to occur in adolescents and young adults, Paget's disease is a known precursor of osteosarcoma, accounting for a secondary peak incidence in the fifth and sixth decades of life. It affects men more often than women, and about 50 per cent of tumors occur in the distal part of the femur. Most patients with osteosarcomas have a long history of pain and swelling, occasionally revealing a palpable mass. Osteosarcoma is usually a destructive lesion with indistinct borders. It generally extends into the cortex and even into adjacent soft tissue. Osteosarcomas metastasize to the periphery of the lung, as opposed to deep within lung tissue. Metastasis tends to occur within the first 2 years after diagnosis.

Treatment

A multimodality approach of surgery, radiotherapy, and chemotherapy is most often used in the treatment of bone sarcomas. Most research studies have been done on osteogenic sarcomas as the prototype.

For many years, the standard treatment of bone tumors was amputation of the limb. In more recent years, limb-sparing procedures have become common when it is believed that local control can be achieved. Limb-sparing surgery is a procedure that removes a soft tissue or bone sarcoma while preserving the extremity's function and cosmetic appearance. Treatment is dictated by the grade and staging of the tumor (see Table 38–7). Low-grade lesions can be treated more conservatively, whereas a high-grade tumor requires more aggressive therapy. Simple excision or curettage is used in benign or low-grade tumors as long as adequate excision of the tumor is achieved. If the tumor is not thoroughly removed, recurrence is likely. An en bloc resection is possible if wide enough margins can be achieved yet still leave useful function of the limb. According to Sim (1983), the criterion for conservative surgery is that the tumor be largely interosseous and involve a short segment of bone. Any extraosseous extension should be small.

If at the time of surgery it is known that the margin is not clear or the wound is contaminated with tumor cells, it is best to carry out amputation. In young patients who are still growing, the expected limb-length discrepancy makes limb-sparing techniques difficult (Shiu & Hajdu, 1981). However, a new expandable internal prosthesis has been developed that equalizes the limb length as the child grows (Lewis, Bloom, Esquieres, Kenan, & Ryniker, 1987). An amputation should leave a margin of 8 to 10 cm of healthy tissue. In large, extensive lesions, an adequate margin may mean disarticulation to include possible skip metastases.

Despite radical surgery, either by excision or amputation, only 25 to 30 per cent of patients survived 2 years. Similarly, despite local control, 80 per cent of patients died from pulmonary metastases (Jaffe, Frei, Traggis, & Bishop, 1974). Micrometastases were believed to have been present, probably at diagnosis, and needed to be treated systemically. In the 1970s both doxorubicin and high-dose methotrexate were found to be effective agents in extending survivals after amputation (Jaffe, 1972). Technologic advances at this time enhanced limb-sparing procedures because bone replacement could be done with cadaver allografts or internally fixed metallic prostheses. Metal endoprostheses, usually of titanium, are currently used most often.

Arterial infusion combines local and systemic therapy because some drug escapes the local area to produce systemic effects. In a study by Storm and co-workers (1981), preoperative intra-arterial doxorubicin was given (30 mg/24 hr for three days), followed by radiation therapy and radical excision with reconstruction. These patients then received postoperative adjuvant therapy with doxorubicin and high-dose methotrexate. This group's response was compared with that of patients who underwent an amputation and received the same adjuvant chemotherapy; a slightly longer disease-free interval was found in the former group. This study shows that it is possible to maintain an intact extremity, a prolonged survival, and improved quality of life. Benjamin (1989) has successfully used intra-arterial cisplatin and intravenous doxorubicin in patients undergoing limb salvage surgery. High-dose methotrexate is added after surgery in poor responders. Disease-free survival is 70 per cent at 3 years using the intra-arterial cisplatin at the NIH Consensus Conference on Limb-Sparing Treatment of Adult Soft Tissue and Osteosarcomas (1985), the conclusion was reached that disease-free survival and overall survival were comparable for selected patients treated with limb-sparing versus amputation. Limb-sparing surgery is the treatment of choice when local tumor can be completely resected. Other methods are included, depending on the protocol at a particular institution. Examples of these methods are preoperative radiation, preoperative chemotherapy, postoperative radiation, postoperative chemotherapy, or combinations thereof.

Limb-sparing procedures are not warranted for lesions in which it is impossible to achieve adequate margins or lesions that involve major vessels or nerves.

Some evidence suggests that adjuvant chemotherapy is beneficial in long-term survival in osteosarcoma (Consensus Conference, 1985).

Chemotherapy is advocated for advanced disease. Jaffe and colleagues (1974) achieved disease-free survival in 50 per cent of the patients using a vincristine and high-dose methotrexate regimen.

Cortes and associates (1972) reported using doxorubicin (30 mg/m^2 for 3 days every 4 to 6 weeks), with resulting long-term survivals of up to 5 years. Ettinger and co-workers (1986) have obtained results by alternating doxorubicin (30 mg/m^2 for 3 days) with cisplatin (110 mg/m^2 every 3 weeks).

Rosen and colleagues (1979) have obtained excellent long-term survivals with "neoadjuvant" chemotherapy of high-dose methotrexate, doxorubicin, bleomycin, cyclophosphamide, and dactinomycin given 4 to 16 weeks before surgery. Neoadjuvant therapy avoids delay in treatment by causing necrosis and usually makes less aggressive surgical procedures possible.

Surgical resection of accessible pulmonary metastases is recommended when warranted by the patient's condition (Consensus Conference, 1985).

Bone sarcomas vary in their sensitivity or resistance to radiotherapy. Osteogenic sarcomas and chondrosarcomas are considered radioresistant, and how they respond to radiation depends on the degree of cell differentiation. The role of radiation in osteosarcomas is not clearly defined except to enhance tumor necrosis either before or after surgery. In a few research settings, hyperthermia has been tried in the treatment of locally advanced and bulky sarcomas that have been unresponsive to other treatment methods (Storm et al., 1981). Research continues at major cancer centers throughout the world to try to find the treatment that is the least debilitating yet still ensures long-term survival in patients with bone sarcomas.

Because osteosarcoma is most common in adolescents, patients have body image and peer group identification as major developmental tasks (Nirenberg, 1985). It goes without saying that a cancer diagnosis is a shock to the patient and family. The adolescent must be included in treatment plans and decisions. The nurse plays a major role in helping the patient understand the treatments. The numerous body changes, such as alopecia, nausea, vomiting, mucositis, and change in mobility, must be dealt with in an open and caring manner. The potential or actual loss of a limb can be devastating. Initiating early contact with physical therapists facilitates rehabilitation and adjustment to using a limb prosthesis. The patient experiences a range of emotions, including anger, fear, resentment, guilt, shock, depression, and denial. Patients need an atmosphere of acceptance and understanding so they can freely express feelings and behaviors without fear of being rejected (Fedora, 1985). An oncology nurse should act as an advocate, explaining procedures and protocols, answering questions, and showing genuine concern about a patient's welfare. Peer support groups are available at numerous centers, which are invaluable to young cancer patients who need to share their experiences.

Although sarcomas are rare tumors, the aggressive treatments to achieve cures demand united and supportive approach by the health team.

References

American Cancer Society. (1990). *Cancer facts and figures, 1988.* New York: Author.

Benjamin, R. S. (1989). Regional chemotherapy for osteosarcoma. *Seminars in Oncology, 16,* 323–327.

Cadman, N. L., Soule, E. H., & Kelly, P. J. (1965). Synovial sarcoma—an analysis of 14 tumors. *Cancer, 18,* 613–627.

Consensus Conference. (1985). Limb-sparing treatment of adult soft tissue sarcomas and osteosarcomas. *Journal of the American Medical Association, 254,* 1791–1794.

Cooper, K. L., Mcleod, R. A., & Beabout, J. W. (1983). Radiologic evaluation. In F. H. Sim (Ed.), *Diagnosis and treatment of bone tumors: A team approach* (pp. 9–14). Thorafare, NJ: Slack.

Cortes, E. P., Holland, J. F., Wang, J. J., & Sinks, L. F. (1972). Doxorubicin in disseminated osteosarcoma. *Journal of the American Medical Association, 22,* 1132–1138.

Dahlin, D., & Unni, K. K. (1986). *Bone tumors.* Springfield, IL: Charles C. Thomas.

Enneking, W. F., Spanier, S. S., & Goodman, M. A. (1980). A system for the surgical staging of musculoskeletal sarcoma. *Clinical Orthopedics, 153,* 106–120.

Enterline, H. (1981). Histopathology of sarcomas. *Seminars in Oncology, 8,* 133–135.

Ettinger, L. J., Douglass, H. O., Mindell, E. R., Sinks, L. F., Tebbi, C. K., Risseuw, D., & Freeman, A. I. (1986). Adjuvant Adriamycin and cisplatin in newly diagnosed nonmetastatic osteosarcoma of the extremity. *Journal of Clinical Oncology, 4,* 353–362.

Fedora, N. L. (1985). Fighting for my leg . . . fighting for my life. *Orthopaedic Nursing, 4*(5), 39–42.

Finkel, M. P., Biskis, B. O., & Reilly, C. A. (1971). Interaction of FBJ osteosarcoma virus and with Sr–90 and with Sr–90 osteosarcomas. In R. L. Clark, R. W. Cumley, & J. E. McCoy (Eds.), *Oncology* (vol. 1). Chicago: Year Book Medical Publishers.

Fraumeni, J. F., Vogel, C. L., & Easton, J. M. (1968). Sarcomas and multiple polyposis in a kindred. A genetic variety of hereditary polyposis? *Archives of Internal Medicine, 12,* 57–61.

Glenn, J., Kinsella, T., Glatstein, E., Tepper, J., Baker, A., Sugarbaker, P., Sindelar, W., Roth, J., Brennan, M., Costa, J., Seipp, C., Wesley, R., Young, R. C., & Rosenberg, S. A. (1985). A randomized prospective trial of adjuvant chemotherapy in adults with soft tissue sarcomas of the head and neck, breast, and trunk. *Cancer, 55,* 1206–1214.

Goodman, T. L. (1987). Sarcomas of soft tissue and bone. In S. Rosenthal, J. Carignan, & B. Smith (Eds.), *Medical care of the cancer patient.* Philadelphia: W. B. Saunders Co.

Halpern, E. C., Greenberg, M. S. & Suit, H. D. (1984). Sarcoma of bone and soft tissue following treatment of Hodgkin's disease. *Cancer, 53,* 232–236.

Hardell, L., & Sandstrom, A. (1979). Case control study: Soft tissue sarcomas and exposure to phenoxyacetic acids or chlorophenols. *British Journal of Cancer, 39,* 711–717.

Heard, G. (1963). Malignant disease in von Recklinghausen's neurofibromatosis. *Proceedings of the Royal Society of Medicine, 56,* 502–503.

Howard, G. M & Casten, V. G. (1963). Rhabdomyosarcoma of the orbit in brothers. *Archives of Ophthalmology, 70,* 319–322.

Jaffe, N. (1972). Recent advances in the chemotherapy of metastatic osteosarcoma. *Cancer, 30,* 1627–1638.

Jaffe, N., Frei, E., Traggis, D., Bishop, Y. (1974). Adjuvant methotrexate and citrovorum factor treatment of osteogenic sarcoma. *New England Journal of Medicine, 291,* 994–997.

Lewis, M. M., Bloom, N., Esquieres, E., Kenan, S., & Ryniker, D. M. (1987). The expandable prosthesis. *AORN Journal, 46,* 457–470.

Lindberg, R. D., Martin, R. G., & Romsdahl, M. M. (1975). Surgery and postoperative radiotherapy in the treatment of soft tissue sarcomas in adults. *American Journal of Roentgenology, Radium Therapy, and Nuclear Medicine, 123,* 123–129.

Lodwick, G. S. (1966). Solitary malignant tumors of bone. *Seminars in Roentgenology, 1,* 293–313.

Malawer, M., Abelson, H., & Suit, H. (1985). Sarcomas of bone. In V. T. DeVita, S. Hellman, & S. A. Rosenberg (Eds.), *Cancer: principles and practice* (pp. 1293–1342). Philadelphia: J. B. Lippincott Co.

Miller, E. C., & Miller, J. A. (1981). Mechanisms of chemical carcinogenesis. *Cancer, 47,* 1055–1064.

Nirenberg, A. (1985). The adolescent with osteogenic sarcoma. *Orthopaedic Nursing, 4,* 11–15.

Odajnyk, M. A., & Muggia, F. M. (1985). Treatment of Kaposi's sarcoma: Overview and analysis by clinical setting. *Journal of Clinical Oncology, 3,* 1277–1285.

O'Neill, N. B., Cocke, W., Mason, D., & Hurley, E. J. (1982). Radiation induced soft tissue fibrosarcoma: Surgical therapy and salvage. *Annals of Thoracic Surgery, 33,* 624–628.

Pizzo, P. A., Miser, J. S., Cassady, J. R., & Filler, R. M. (1985). Solid tumors of childhood. In V. T. DeVita, S. Hellman, & S. A. Rosenberg (Eds.), *Cancer: principles and practice* (pp. 1511–1589). Philadelphia: J. B. Lippincott Co.

Pories, W., Murinson, D., & Rubin, P. (1983). Soft tissue sarcomas. In P. Rubin (Ed.), *Clinical oncology: A multidisciplinary approach* (pp. 308–324). New York: American Cancer Society.

Potter, D. A., Glenn, J., Kinsella, T., Glatstein, E., Lack, E. E., Restrepo, C., White, D. E., Seip, C. A., Wesley, R., & Rosenberg, S. A. (1985). Patterns of recurrence in patients with high grade soft tissue sarcomas in adults. *Journal of Clinical Oncology, 3,* 353–366.

Pritchard, D. J., Lunke, R. J., Taylor, W. F., Dahlin. D. C., & Medley, B. E. (1980). Chondrosarcoma: A clinicopathologic and statistical analysis. *Cancer, 45,* 149–157.

Rosen, G., Marcove, R. C., Caparros, B., Nirenberg, A., Kosloff, C., & Huvos, A. G., (1979). Primary osteogenic sarcoma. The rationale for preoperative chemotherapy and delayed surgery. *Cancer, 43,* 2163–2177.

Rosenberg, S. A., & Glatstein, E. J. (1981). Perspectives on the role of surgery and radiation therapy in the treatment of soft tissue sarcomas of the extremities. *Seminars in Oncology, 8,* 190–200.

Rosenberg, S. A., Suit, H., & Baker, L. (1985). Sarcomas of soft tissues. In V. T. DeVita, S. Hellman, & S. A. Rosenberg (Eds.), *Cancer: principles and practice* (pp. 1247–1291). Philadelphia: J. B. Lippincott Co.

Rosenberg, S. A., Tepper, J., Glatstein, E., Costa, J., Baker, A., Brennan, M., deMoss, E., Seipp, C., Sindelar, W., Sugarbaker, P., & Wesley, R. (1982). The treatment of soft tissue sarcomas of the extremities. Prospective randomized evaluations of (1) limb-sparing surgery plus radiation therapy compared with amputation and (2) the role of adjuvant chemotherapy. *Annals of Surgery, 196,* 305–315.

Rubin, P., Evarts, C. M., & Boros, L. (1983). Bone tumors. In P. Rubin (Ed.), *Clinical oncology, a multidisciplinary approach* (pp. 296–306). New York: American Cancer Society.

Shieber, W., & Graham, P. (1962). An experience with sarcomas of soft tissue in adults. *Surgery, 52,* 295–313.

Shiu, M. H., Castro, E. B., & Hajdu, S. I. (1975). Surgical treatment of 297 soft tissue sarcomas of the lower extremity. *Annals of Surgery, 182,* 597–602.

Shiu, M. H., & Hajdu, S. I. (1981). Management of soft tissue sarcoma of the extremity. *Seminars in Oncology, 8,* 172–179.

Shives, T. C., Wold, L. E., Dahlin, D. C., & Beabout, J. W. (1983). Chondrosarcoma and its variants. In F. H. Sim (Ed.), *Diagnosis and treatment of bone tumors: A team approach* (pp. 211–225). Thorafare, NJ: Slack.

Sim, F. H. (1983). Principles of surgical treatment. In F. H. Sim (Ed.), *Diagnosis and treatment of bone tumors: A team approach* (pp. 25–35). Thorafare, NJ: Slack.

Sim, F. H., Ivins, J. C., & Pritchard, D. J. (1978). Surgical treatment of osteogenic sarcoma at the Mayo Clinic. *Cancer Treatment Reports, 62,* 205–211.

Simon, M. A., & Enneking, W. F. (1976). The management of soft tissue sarcomas of the extremities. *Journal of Bone and Joint Surgery, 58-A,* 317.

Storm, F. K., Morton, D. L., Eilber, F. R., & Saxton, R. E. (1981). Sarcoma: Etiology and advances in therapy with immunotherapy, limb salvage surgery and hyperthermia. *Seminars in Oncology, 8,* 229–236.

Tepper, J. E. (1989). Radiation therapy in treatment of sarcomas. *Seminars in Oncology, 16,* 281–288.

Yang, J. C., & Rosenberg, S. A. (1989). Surgery for adult patients with soft tissue sarcomas. *Seminars in Oncology, 16,* 289–296.

Yap, B. S., Baker, L. H., Sinkovic, J. G., Rivkin, S. E., Bottomley, R., Thigpen, T., Burgess, M., Benjamin, R., & Bodey, G. (1980). Cyclophosphamide, vincristine, Adriamycin, and DTIC (CY-VADIC) combination chemotherapy for the treatment of advanced sarcomas. *Cancer, 64,* 90–98.

Ziegler, J. L., Templeton, A. C., & Vogel, O. L. (1984). Kaposi's sarcoma: A comparison of classical, endemic and epidemic forms. *Seminars in Oncology, 11,* 47–52.

CHAPTER 39

Central Nervous System Tumors

CONNIE R. ROBINSON
SR. CALLISTA ROY
MARGARET L. SEAGER

BRAIN

Introduction

The central nervous system (CNS) is composed of several major cell types that are important in understanding the function of the brain and spinal cord and the field of neuro-oncology nursing. Before beginning a discussion of the tumors of the CNS, it may be useful for the reader to refer to Figure 39–1 for a brief orientation to the anatomy of the CNS. A review of basic neuroanatomy would be helpful as well. In Figure 39–2 the types of CNS glial cells are shown. Not shown is the glial cell of the peripheral nervous system, the Schwann cell. Figure 39–3 illustrates the various shapes of neurons. In addition, because the terminology of neuro-oncology is complex, definitions of terms are given in Box 39–1.

Definition and Incidence

Definition

Tumors that arise within the intracranial cavity have many unusual features. A discrepancy exists between their histologic nature and their biologic behavior. In addition, their location can be crucial because many vital structures may be involved. Also, the presence of the blood-brain barrier partially shields the tumor from the systemic circulation (Salcman & Kaplan, 1986). All tumors of the CNS can pursue a "malignant" course to death because they grow within a unique environment, that is, a confined space. Even histologically benign and well-differentiated tumors require prompt diagnosis and management to ensure an optimal outcome for the patient. Intracranial and intraspinal tumors produce signs and symptoms primarily through expanding, compressing, and displacing vital neural tissue (Levin & Wilson, 1978).

Unlike extracranial tumors, tumors of the CNS, even malignant ones (dedifferentiated or anaplastic tumors), rarely metastasize outside of the CNS. Brain tumors arise primarily from adult glial cells that constitute the glioma-astrocytoma series and from connective tissue that constitutes the sarcomas. Some believe tumors arise from developmental cells. Both points of view are discussed later. Tumors range from nonmalignant to highly malignant. Benign gliomas may recur as

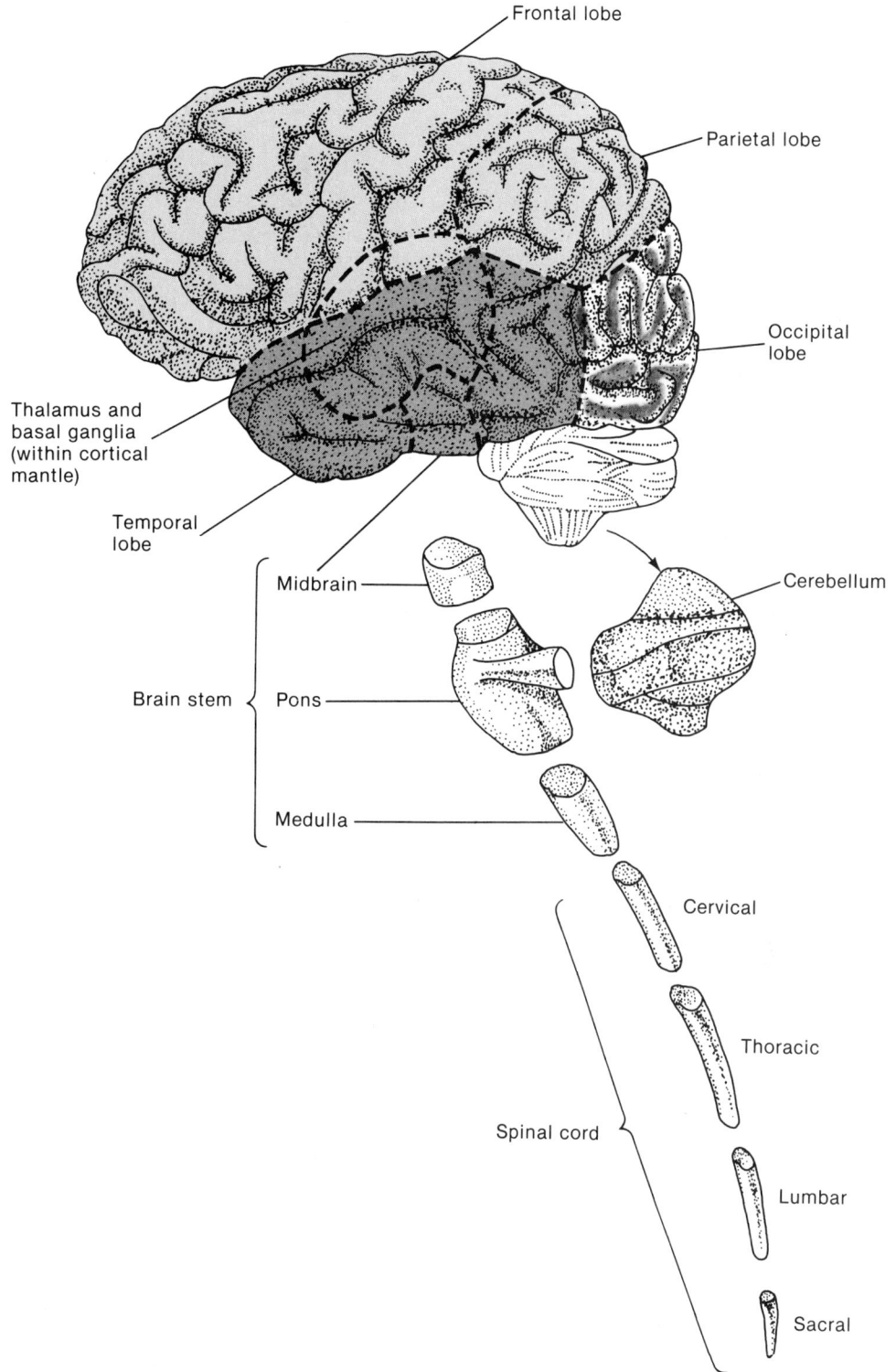

Figure 39-1. Exploded view showing the major components of the central nervous system. Also shown are the four major divisions of the cerebral cortex: the occipital lobe *(darker color)*, parietal lobe *(lighter color)*, frontal lobe *(hatching)*, and temporal lobe *(stippling)*. (From Cohen, D. H., & Sherman, S. M. [1988]. The nervous system. In R. M. Berne & M. N. Levy (Eds.), *Physiology* [p. 74]. St. Louis: C. V. Mosby Co. Redrawn from Kandel, E. R., & Schwartz, J. H. [1981]. *Principles of neuroscience.* New York: Elsevier Science Publishing Co. Used with permission.)

malignant ones. Outcomes depend not only on the nature of the tumor but also on its size and location at the time of diagnosis.

Incidence and Epidemiology

Tumors of the CNS account for close to 10 per cent of the neurologic problems encountered in a general hospital population (Wilson, 1977). Overall, the inci-

dence of primary brain tumors is approximately 10,000 cases per year (other sources report 15,000 to 17,000 cases per year), and the incidence of spinal cord tumors is approximately 4000 cases per year (Kornblith, Walker, & Cassady, 1987). Tumors of the CNS are found in excess of 16.1 per 100,000 population. The majority of these tumors are malignant and astroglial in origin (Levin & Wilson, 1978). Brain tumors of all types represent the second leading cause of cancer

OLIGODENDROCYTE
IN WHITE MATTER

FIBROUS
ASTROCYTE

End
foot

Blood
vessel

PERINEURONAL
OLIGODENDROCYTE

PROTOPLASMIC
ASTROCYTE

Neuron

Blood
vessel

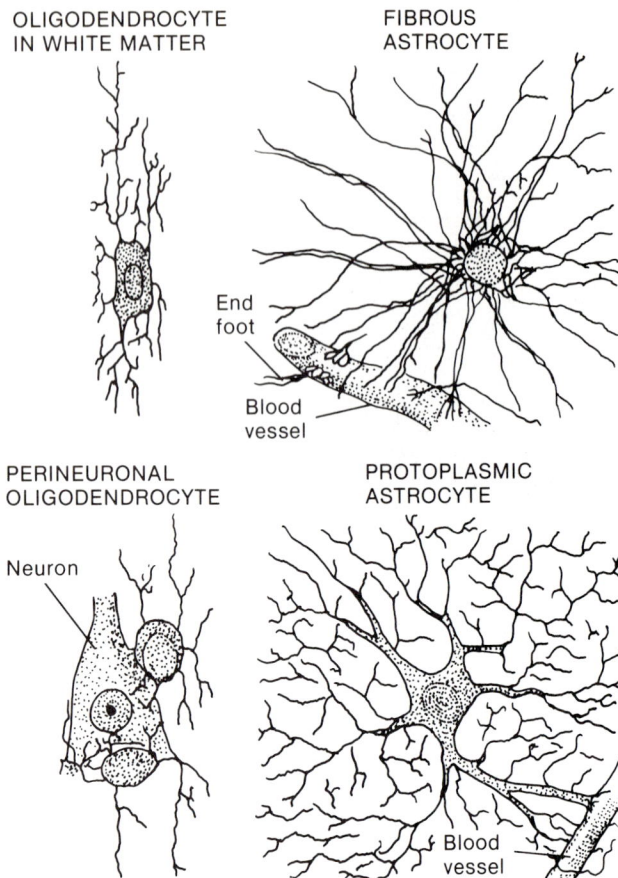

Figure 39-2. Neuroglial cells in the mammalian brain. Neuroglial cells stained with silver impregnation. Oligodendrocytes and astrocytes represent the principal neuroglial cell groups in the vertebrate brain. They are closely associated with neurons and form end feet on blood vessels. (From Kuffler, S. W., & Nicholls, J. G. [1976]. *From neuron to brain* [p. 258]. Sunderland, MA: Sinauer Associates, Inc. After Penfield, 1932. Used with permission.)

deaths in children and the fourth leading cause of cancer deaths in middle-aged adult males (Salcman & Kaplan, 1986). The incidence of metastatic tumors in the CNS has increased two times over the past several decades possibly owing to better diagnostic techniques and better systemic control of the primary tumor, which has resulted in longer life expectancy (Levin & Wilson, 1978), and perhaps owing to the increasing incidence of lung cancer.

Tumors occur in two major peaks across the life span: one in childhood between the ages of 3 and 12 years and the second in later life between the ages of 50 and 70 years (Kornblith et al., 1987). In children younger than 15 years, tumors of the CNS are the second most frequent type of cancer, exceeded only by leukemia (Humphreys, 1982; Morley, 1973). The tumors that occur in children differ histologically and physiologically from those that occur in adults. Nearly two thirds of the pediatric tumors arise in the cerebellum, brain stem, or midbrain-thalamus region and are therefore infratentorial. Approximately three fourths are gliomas. Most adult tumors are supratentorial cortical or within the cerebral hemisphere. The most common tumor type is glioblastoma (Cobb & You-

mans, 1982; Morley, 1973). The incidence of all types of brain tumor is shown in Figure 39-4.

Primary tumors of the CNS arise predominantly from the glia cells. Neurons give rise to tumors much more rarely. Males and females are affected equally, although some tumor types are more common in one sex than in the other (astrocytomas are more common in males, and meningiomas are more common in females). See Figure 39-5 for the incidence of brain tumors according to age.

Etiology

Convincing evidence is lacking for any particular factor (chemical, viral, or traumatic) as the cause of brain tumors in humans. However, some interesting research regarding causes is important to mention.

Genetic

Evidence of genetic factors is weak but cannot be ignored. Some tumors have a hereditary component in three developmental disorders, of which von Recklinghausen's neurofibromatosis is an example. Inheritance is through an autosomal dominant gene (Butler, Brooks, & Netsky, 1982). Also, neurofibromatosis is an inherited genetic condition with an autosomal dominant pattern. Certain tumor types show some evidence of chromosomal abnormalities. For example, in persons with meningiomas, chromosome 22 frequently has been found to contain abnormalities (Kornblith et al., 1987). The significance of these chromosomal abnormalities is not known.

Environmental Factors

There is also little evidence that CNS tumors in humans are linked to environmental carcinogens (Kornblith et al., 1987), although many chemicals have carcinogenic activity in animals and produce CNS tumors in these animal models.

Viruses

Likewise, no evidence exists for viral causes of tumors in humans, although evidence for this in animals is of interest. A type of slow virus has produced astrocytomas in animals, and it is postulated that this type of slow virus may account for some of the difficulties of isolating the organism in humans (Kornblith et al., 1987). Patients with primary CNS lymphomas have a high incidence of infection with the Epstein-Barr virus, and tissue from the tumors contains the Epstein-Barr virus genome.

In lymphoma and Epstein-Barr infection, immunosuppression may play a role. Transplant recipients have a markedly increased risk of primary lymphoma of the brain, as do patients with AIDS.

Trauma

Trauma has been considered a cause of meningeal or glial tumors. A traumatic cause probably can be

BIPOLAR CELL
FROM RETINA

MITRAL CELL FROM
OLFACTORY BULB

PYRAMIDAL CELL
FROM CORTEX

Dendrite

Dendrite

Dendrite

Cell
body

Cell
body

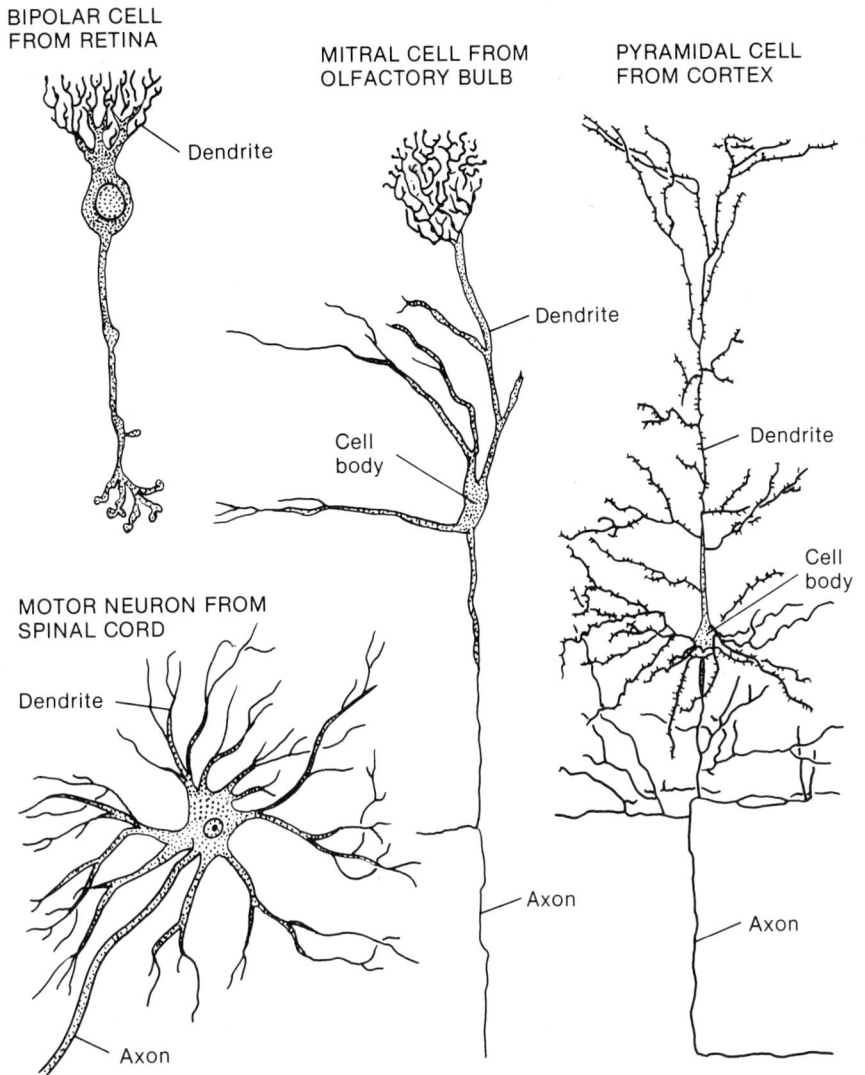

Figure 39–3. Shapes and sizes of neurons. The cells have processes, the dendrites, on which other neurons form synapses. Each cell in turn makes connections with other neurons. (From Kuffler, S. W., & Nicholls, J. G. [1976]. *From neuron to brain* [p. 9]. Sunderland, M. A.: Sinauer Associates, Inc. Used with permission.)

MOTOR NEURON FROM
SPINAL CORD

Dendrite

Axon

Axon

Axon

accepted for a small number of meningiomas. However, in most cases trauma probably initiates or aggravates clinical symptoms of a tumor already in existence (Butler et al., 1982).

Radiation

Sarcomas are reported to occur frequently after radiation therapy; carcinomas are rare; and gliomas are as yet unreported following radiation. The interval between radiation and symptoms of tumor ranges from 5 to 20 years. The mechanisms of radiation-induced tumors are uncertain (Butler et al., 1982).

Chemicals

Anthracene compounds when applied topically have produced CNS tumors in animals. Nitroso compounds can convert glial cells to neoplasms in animals (Butler et al., 1982).

Biology and Natural History

Biology of Central Nervous System Tumors

Tumors grow by expansion, infiltration, or both. Growth by expansion is by proliferation of cells, fluid accumulation related to hemorrhage, increased permeability of blood vessels, and swelling and edema. Benign tumors such as meningiomas seldom infiltrate but expand, surrounded by capsules of connective tissue. Malignant tumors both expand and infiltrate especially around blood vessels in the brain (Butler et al., 1982). Generally, although not always, benign tumors tend to be more localized and malignant tumors more invasive.

The patterns of spread of tumors in the CNS differ from those of other tumors. There is no lymphatic system within the CNS. Spreading through the vascular system does occur but only rarely and mostly with operative intervention. Whether this phenomenon is due to the immunologically privileged status of the CNS or whether the short life expectancy of most

Box 39–1. GLOSSARY OF TERMS IN NEURO-ONCOLOGY

Anaplasia: an assessment of cytologic malignancy as opposed to biologic malignancy. Consists of an assessment of cell and nucleus size and staining characteristics, necrosis, mitoses, and invasiveness.

Apraxia: a disturbance in the execution of learned movements of lips, tongue, or hand, for example, in the absence of paralysis or paresis.

Association fibers: long bundles of fibers that connect the association areas (not receiving primary sensory input) of the brain; the corpus callosum is one such bundle that connects association areas of all four lobes of one hemisphere of the brain with the other.

Astrocytes: one of the five broad types of glial cells, so named because of their star shape.

Astroglial: glial cells of the astrocyte type.

Ataxia: failure or irregularity of muscular coordination.

Atlas: the first cervical vertebra of the spinal column.

Autosomal dominant: gene located on a chromosome other than the sex chromosome; affected individual has a 50 per cent chance of passing it on to an offspring.

Axis: the second vertebra of the spinal column.

Bitemporal hemianopia: the loss of vision in both temporal fields.

Cauda equina: nerve roots in the lumbosacral region that descend almost vertically and because of their length and appearance are called the "horse's tail."

Cerebellopontine angle: the angle formed by the approximation of the cerebellum and pons, the area in which the auditory nerve from the cochlea of the inner ear enters the brain stem.

Cingulate gyrus: located on the medial portion of the brain above the corpus callosum, a part of the limbic lobe on the medial portion of the hemispheres.

Contrecoup: an injury that occurs opposite the site of a sudden strike or blow to the head.

Conus medullaris: the tapered portion of the spinal cord below the twelfth thoracic vertebra.

Corpus callosum: the bundle of association fibers that links the left and right hemispheres.

Cranial nerves: a set of 12 nerves that conveys sensory and motor information primarily from and to the head.

Dedifferentiation: the loss of normal differentiation, cell organization, and specific function; it is a measure of the loss of resemblance of tumor cells or tissue to the cells or tissue of origin.

Dermatome: the area of skin innervated by sensory nerve fibers from a single spinal dorsal (toward back) root nerve.

Developmental cells: immature cells that will develop further and mature into the adult cells, the types of which are differentiated or distinct from one another.

Differentiated: maintains normal cell organization and specific function; groups of like cells but different from other groups of cells.

Drift: a gradual and aimless shift in position of one of the patient's arms when both are extended in front by the patient, whose eyes are closed.

Dura mater: a double layer of fibrous tissue that encloses the brain and spinal cord. The outer layer attaches to the cranial bones, and the inner layer encloses venous sinuses and forms partitions within the brain, e.g., the tentorium. Outermost to the pia mater and arachnoid.

Dysnomia: errors in naming or inability to recall names. Patient may describe objects by function rather than name.

Embryonal cells: cells of the embryo that will develop into the central nervous system (or cells that determine any specific structure).

Encephalopathy: headaches, confusion, drowsiness, dizziness, vomiting, blurring of vision, seizures, and focal signs as a result of varied conditions such as hypertension, liver failure, drugs, and others.

Ependymal cells: cells that line the inner surface of the brain, ventricles, and fluid spaces.

Evoked potential: the change in ongoing electrical activity of neurons as a result of stimulation of any part of the sensory pathways; recorded by surface electrodes on the scalp.

Extradural: outside the dura; extradural tumors are invasive tumors from adjacent vertebrae or metastatic ones from a distant source.

Extramedullary: intradural or within sheaths of spinal nerves.

Falx cerebri: a crescent-shaped extension of dura mater; projects into the longitudinal cerebral fissure separating the right and left hemispheres.

Foramen magnum: an opening in the skull that transmits the medulla, eleventh cranial nerves, arteries, and ligaments.

Gamma radiation: a stream of photons or waves of electromagnetic radiation emitted when an atomic nucleus undergoes transition from one energy level to another.

Ganglion cell: a type of neuron; also, nerve cell bodies that collect and form a swelling in a specific location for a particular function; also found in the retina and elsewhere.

Germ cells: cells arising from the neural tube of the developing embryo.

Glial cells: of 5 types: astrocytes, oligodendrocytes, ependymal cells, microglia, and neuroglial precursors; provide support and possibly some metabolic and nutritional roles for the neurons.

Hemianopia: the loss of half of both right and left visual fields; of various types, e.g., bitemporal hemianopia.

Hemiparesis: muscle weakness that affects one side of the body.

Hemiplegia: muscle paralysis that affects one side of the body.

Hypothalamic-chiasmal derangement: a malfunction of the hypothalamus and of vision as a result of midline tumor, e.g., craniopharyngioma pressing on these structures; signs and symptoms may include fluid and temperature imbalance and hormonal imbalances as well as visual disturbances.

Hypothalamus: a bilateral structure consisting of a collection of neuronal cell bodies (nuclei) located below the thalamus and forming the floor and inferior lateral walls of the third ventricle; involved in many basic functions such as feeding, sexual behavior, sleep, temperature and endocrine regulation, emotional expression, and daily rhythms.

Immunologically privileged: the brain is virtually isolated from and unaffected by the immune system owing to the blood-brain barrier; therefore, transplanted tissue potentially has a better "take" in the brain.

Infratentorial: refers to structures lying below the tentorium cerebelli that is the dura separating the occipital lobes from the cerebellum; the brain stem is largely an infratentorial structure; forms the posterior fossa.

Intramedullary: within the substance of the spinal cord; neuronal and glial tissue.

Leptomeninges: the arachnoid and the pia mater together are known as the leptomeninges.

Lesser wings of sphenoid bones: forming part of the interior structure of the orbit.

Meninges: the dura mater, pia mater, and arachnoid membrane.

Microglia: small glial cells located in perivascular spaces that give rise to primary lymphomas (formerly called reticulum cell sarcoma or microglioma) of the brain.

Midbrain: short portion of the brain between the pons and the cerebral hemispheres.

Morphologic features: characteristics of the cell and subcellular structures, size, shape, and organization; (e.g., orderliness of growth, inhibition of growth when in contact with adjacent cell); cell structures can be identified by these features.

Nerve roots: consist of bundles of fibers that enter and exit the cord in an orderly fashion at each segmental level; motor nerves exit the anterior or front side of the cord, and sensory fibers enter the posterior or back of the cord.

Neuroaxis: (neuraxis) an imaginary line drawn the length of the central nervous system that divides it into symmetric parts.

Neuroglial precursors: developmental cells that give rise to adult neuronal and glial cells.

Nonfluent dysphasia: a type of impairment of speech caused by damage to the part of the central nervous system that controls speech (Broca's area); patients may comprehend speech and language but be unable to express themselves; primarily a motor disorder; tendency to use only meaningful content words.

Obstructive hydrocephalus: an enlargement in the ventricles and cerebrospinal fluid spaces with an abnormal collection of cerebrospinal fluid due to mechanical blockage of the spaces and thus the flow of cerebrospinal fluid.

Olfactory grooves: located in the ethmoid bone of the skull, supporting the olfactory bulb.

Oligodendroglia: a type of glia cell that is responsible for myelinization (insulation) of axons in the central nervous system; Schwann cells myelinate the peripheral nerves.

Optic chiasm: the structure formed by the crossing of some of the left and right optic nerves as they course their way to the occipital lobe; above the pituitary body and adjacent to the hypothalamus, midline tumors press on this structure and cause visual deficits.

Parenchyma: glial, neuronal, and other structures of the central nervous system.

Pia mater (pia): the thin connective tissue that lies close to the brain and carries the blood vessels that supply the nervous tissue.

Pineal area: a knob-like, midline structure close to the third ventricle; regulates gonad function.

Pons: a midbrain structure in front of the cerebellum and above the medulla; contains tracts to and from the periphery as well as several cranial nerve nuclei; various clinical syndromes result from tumors in this area.

Primitive cells: toward the undifferentiated cell.

Proton beam radiation: the use of a radioactive nuclide that emits alpha rays; the shortest penetration of tissue of the three kinds of rays: alpha (positively charged particle), beta (electron), and gamma (photon).

Purkinje cell: a major neuron cell type of the cerebellum.

Radicular pain: results from disturbance of the spinal nerve or spinal root that carries sensory or motor information to and from certain segments of the cord.

Spinal nerve roots: each level of the spinal cord gives rise to spinal roots (front-motor and back-sensory), which exit the cord separately and then join to form the spinal nerve.

Subarachnoid: the space between the arachnoid membrane and the pia mater in which cerebrospinal fluid circulates.

Superior parasagittal surface of sphenoid bones: sphenoid bone extends from temporal surface internally to form portions of the orbit: top surface along sagittal suture.

Supratentorial: all structures above the tentorium: includes the four major lobes (left and right) comprising the two hemispheres.

Sylvian region: regions of the temporal, frontal, and parietal lobes that lie close to the sylvian fissure; the fissure dividing the temporal lobe from the frontal and parietal lobes.

Tentorium: a section of the dura that separates the occipital lobes from the cellebellum and is the border between the anterior and posterior fossae or vaults.

Thalamus: a large, oval, gray mass (cell bodies of neurons) located on each side of the third ventricle that contains several major nuclear groups with specific functions; all sensory information travels through the thalamus, from which it is relayed to the cortex.

Transsphenoidal microsurgery: surgery that uses stereotaxic coordinates and the microscope in which the operation is performed through the sphenoid bone (behind the nose), making a craniotomy (opening of the skull) unnecessary.

Tuberculum sellae: a smooth fossa in the medial portion of sphenoid bone adjacent to the pituitary.

Ventricles: a communicating system of four cavities within the brain, containing cerebrospinal fluid, two lateral ventricles, and the third and fourth ventricles.

Ventricular drainage: shunting of cerebrospinal fluid from the ventricles to the peritoneal cavity or to the cisterna magna (space in the arachnoid between the medulla and the cerebellar hemispheres) to bypass obstruction to the circulation of fluid in the spaces.

von Recklinghausen's disease: a disorder characterized by the development of multiple tumors of the spinal or cranial nerves, tumors of the skin, and cutaneous pigmentation; meningiomas and gliomas may be associated.

Wernicke-like aphasia: dysphasia is more appropriate because the loss of the function of speech is rarely total (aphasia); Wernicke-like refers to a greater loss of the sensory component than of the motor component of speech; patient speaks easily, engages in conversational exchange, and appears to be making an effort to communicate, but little meaning is conveyed in the partial phrases, disjointed clauses, and incomplete sentences.

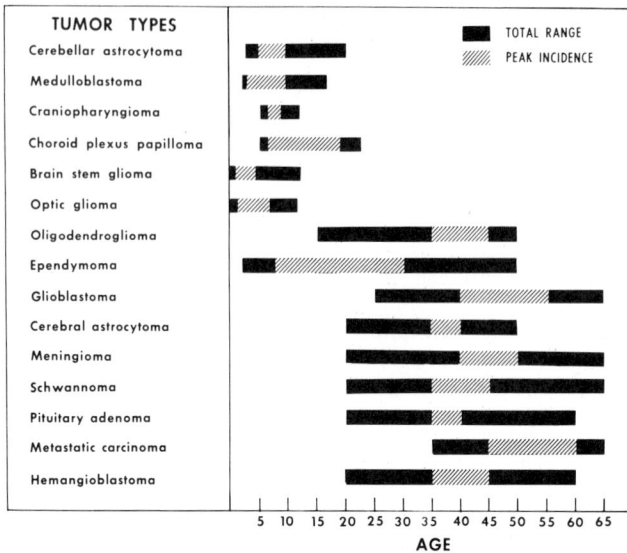

Figure 39–4. Chart showing approximate age distribution and peak incidence of major types of brain tumors. (From Butler, A. B., Brooks, W. H., & Netsky, M. G. [1982]. Classification and biology of brain tumors. In J. R. Youmans [Ed.]. *Neurological surgery* [Vol. 5, 2nd ed., p. 2683]. Philadelphia: W. B. Saunders Co. Reproduced by permission.)

patients does not allow time for metastases to become evident or whether some other factor is operative is unclear (Kornblith et al., 1987).

Tumors of the CNS spread locally and through cerebrospinal fluid (CSF) seeding. The intracranial astrocytomas are capable of invading normal tissue to a remarkable degree and can be found at sites distant from the primary focus. This phenomenon has led some to wonder whether these lesions have multifocal origins. Some tumors seed through the CSF much more than others. Seeding occurs along the surface of the brain to local sites and by "drop metastases," in which cells or groups of cells fall by way of the CSF to the spinal subarachnoid space and form secondary tumors. As a result nerve roots and coverings of the cord may become involved. All sites in the spinal cord are vulnerable to this type of spread, but the lumbosacral area is most frequently involved.

Gliomas rarely metastasize at a distant location; they do invade locally to an extreme degree, grow relatively slowly, and have a varied cell population (heterogeneity). Gliomas produce a variety of growth factors related to the oncogenes. Malignant gliomas have a cell population that divides rather slowly and may even vary from week to week. Gliomas have a marked hypervascularity, probably as a result of other factors (tumor angiogenesis factor) produced by the tumor. This hypervascularity may account for the peritumoral edema associated with gliomas (Kornblith et al., 1987).

Classification

The general principles that govern the statistical classification of tumors were established by a subcommittee of the World Health Organization (WHO) Expert Committee on Health Statistics (Zulch, 1979). For flexibility and ease of coding, three separate clas-

sifications were needed. These are by (1) anatomic site, (2) histologic type, and (3) degree of malignancy. The WHO has used primarily histologic type and degree of malignancy in classifying central nervous system tumors (Zulch, 1979). It is the most comprehensive classification of all systems used and of all types of tumors. Tumors of the CNS are classified by histologic type into 12 major categories with many subdivisions (Batzdorf & Selch, 1985; Zulch, 1979). (For the reader who needs the fully expanded histologic WHO classification of tumors of the nervous system, see Table 39–1 from Cobb & Youmans [1982]. Also, see Zulch [1979, pp. 43–62] for definitions and explanatory notes.) Anatomic classification can be found in the International Classification of Diseases (World Health Organization, 1977).

In an attempt to simplify and clarify, variations of a classification scheme have been developed by several well-known and respected researchers and clinicians; much more experience is needed, however, and confusion reigns in the literature. The most confusion lies in the effort to sort out gliomas and neurogliomas. Therefore, examples of simplified classification schemes are presented later. Finally, a classification scheme for the purposes of this text is presented.

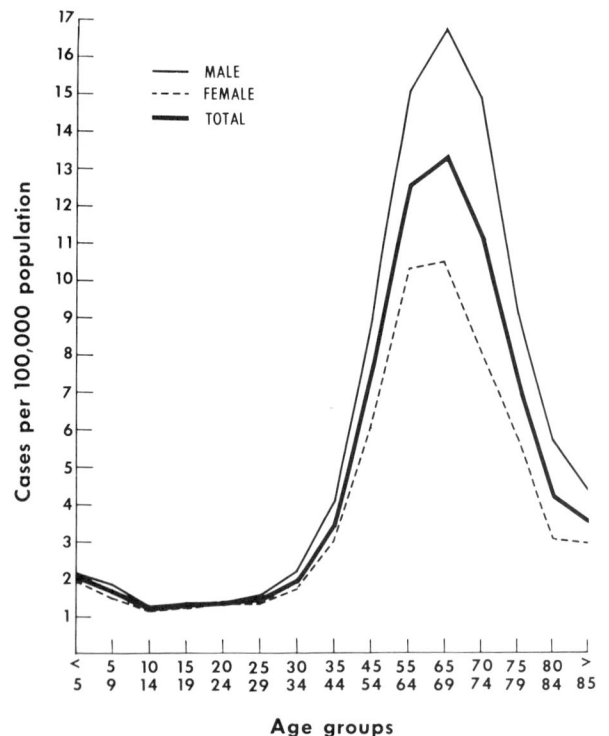

Figure 39–5. The incidence of all types of brain tumors in the United States in 1966 is shown according to 5-year age groups. (Data from U.S. Department of Health, Education and Welfare, Public Health Service [1968]. *Vital statistics rates in the United States 1940–1960.* Washington, DC: U.S. Government Printing Office; from Butler, A. B., Brooks, W. H., & Netsky, M. G. [1982]. Classification and biology of brain tumors. In J. R. Youmans [Ed.], *Neurological surgery* [Vol. 5, 2nd ed., p. 2682]. Philadelphia: W. B. Saunders Co. Reproduced by permission.)

Table 39-1. WORLD HEALTH ORGANIZATION BRAIN TUMOR CLASSIFICATION

Tumors of Neuroepithelial Tissue

Astrocytic tumors
  Astrocytoma
    Fibrillary
    Protoplasmic
    Gemistocytic
  Pilocytic astrocytoma
  Subependymal giant cell astrocytoma (ventricular tumor
    of tuberous sclerosis)
  Astroblastoma
  Anaplastic astrocytoma
Oligodendroglial tumors
  Oligodendroglioma
  Mixed oligoastrocytoma
  Anaplastic oligodendroglioma
Ependymal and choroid plexus tumors
  Ependymoma
    Variants
    Myxopapillary ependymoma
    Papillary ependymoma
    Subependymoma
  Anaplastic ependymoma
  Choroid plexus papilloma
  Anaplastic choroid plexus papilloma
Pineal cell tumors
  Pineocytoma
  Pineoblastoma
Neuronal tumors
  Gangliocytoma
  Ganglioglioma
  Ganglioneuroblastoma
  Anaplastic gangliocytoma and ganglioglioma
  Neuroblastoma
Poorly differentiated and embryonal tumors
  Glioblastoma
    Variants
    Glioblastoma with sarcomatous component
    Giant cell glioblastoma
  Medulloblastoma
    Variants
    Desmoplastic
    Medullomyoblastoma
  Medulloepithelioma
  Primitive polar spongioblastoma
  Gliomatosis cerebri

Tumor of Nerve Sheath Cells

Neurilemoma
Anaplastic neurilemoma
Neurofibroma
Anaplastic neurofibroma

Tumors of Meningeal and Related Tissues

Meningioma
Meningeal sarcoma
Xanthomatous tumors
Primary melanotic tumors
Others

Primary Malignant Lymphomas

Tumors of Blood Vessel Origin

Hemangioblastoma
Monstrocellular sarcoma

Germ Cell Tumors

Germinoma
Embryonal carcinoma
Choriocarcinoma
Teratoma

Other Malformative Tumors and Tumor-Like Lesions

Craniopharyngioma
Rathke's cleft cyst
Epidermoid cyst
Dermoid cyst
Colloid cyst of the third ventricle
Enterogenous cyst
Other cysts
Lipoma
Choristoma
Hypothalamic neuronal hamartoma
Nasal glial heterotopia

Vascular Malformations

Capillary telangiectasia
Cavernous angioma
Arterio-venous malformation
Venous malformation
Sturge-Weber disease

Tumors of the Anterior Pituitary

Pituitary adenomas
Pituitary adenocarcinoma

Local Extension from Regional Tumors

Glomus jugulare tumors
Chordoma
Chondroma
Chondrosarcoma
Olfactory neuroblastoma
Adenoid cystic carcinoma
Other

Metastatic Tumors

Unclassified Tumors

(From Cobb, C. A., & Youmans, J. R. [1982]. Glial and neuronal tumors of the brain in adults. In J. R. Youmans [Ed.], *Neurological surgery* [Vol. 5, 2nd ed., p. 2685]. Philadelphia: W. B. Saunders Co. Reproduced by permission.)

One of the most commonly used and earliest developed classification systems for intracranial tumors is that of Bailey and Cushing, which was revised by them in 1920 (Table 39–2) (Butler et al., 1982). Glial and neural tumors are classified and graded as well as intracranial tumors that arise from other types of cells found in the brain, for example, lymphomas, sarcomas, pineal tumors, and metastatic tumors.

Some investigators believe that CNS tumors derive from developmental cells. Twenty cell types have been identified in the development of the nervous system, and 14 types of glial tumors are presumably derived from these cells. Figúre 39–6 (Butler et al., 1982) is a diagram of the 20 types of cells identified in the development of the nervous system. From these the 14 types of glial and neurologlial tumors presumably derived from the 20 normal cells are shown.

However, it is commonly accepted by others (e.g.,

Table 39–2. MODIFIED BAILEY-CUSHING CLASSIFICATION

Astrocytoma
Oligodendroglioma
Ependymoma
Medulloblastoma
Glioblastoma multiforme
Pinealoma (teratoma)
Ganglioneuroma (ganglioglioma)
Neuroblastoma (sympathicoblastoma)
Papilloma of choroid plexus
Mixed
Unclassified

(From Butler, A. B., Brooks, W. H., & Netsky, M. G. [1982]. Classification and biology of brain tumors. In J. R. Youmans [Ed.], *Neurological surgery* [Vol. 5, 2nd ed., p. 2664]. Philadelphia: W. B. Saunders Co. Reproduced by permission.)

neuropathologists, neurosurgeons) that brain and spinal cord tumors develop from dedifferentiation of adult cells as opposed to developmental cells. These adult cells are stimulated by known and unknown factors to give rise to tumors (Butler et al., 1982).

Kernohan and Sayre (1952) developed a continual series of gradations of tumors in which they used primarily histologic and biologic characteristics (Table 39–3).

For simplicity, Salcman and Kaplan (1986) classify tumors by location rather than by histology. In this system, all CNS tumors are classified into three broad groups: intrinsic, extrinsic, and congenital. Intrinsic tumors include those arising from adult glial cells or capillary cells. Examples are astrocytoma, oligoden-

droglioma, and ependymoma. In their most malignant form, each of these tumors converges toward a more primitive and highly malignant lesion known as glioblastoma multiforme. Those arising from capillary cells include lymphoma and hemangioblastoma. Extrinsic tumors include those arising from the coverings of the brain and cranial nerve roots and from the pituitary gland. These are usually benign and compress the neural parenchyma from without. Included in this category are meningioma, acoustic schwannoma, and the pituitary adenomas. Congenital tumors arise from primitive cells and are almost always located in the midline. They are relatively more frequent in the younger age groups. These include craniopharyngiomas, dermoids, epidermoids, pineal tumors, and medulloblastomas.

Butler and colleagues (1982) suggest an even simpler and more reasonable compromise of the classifications of brain tumors. This classification contains three major categories: (1) glial tumors, (2) neural tumors, and (3) connective tissue tumors. They further suggest that readers who desire an even simpler approach may group the first three types of glial tumors (astrocytoma, oligodendroglioma, and ependymoma) into one group in which the life span of patients usually is measured in years rather than months, as with medulloblastoma or glioblastoma, the last two of the five types of glial tumors in this system. Ganglioneuroma and neuroblastoma are two types of tumors that contain neural tissue rather than the more commonly found gliomas. A third

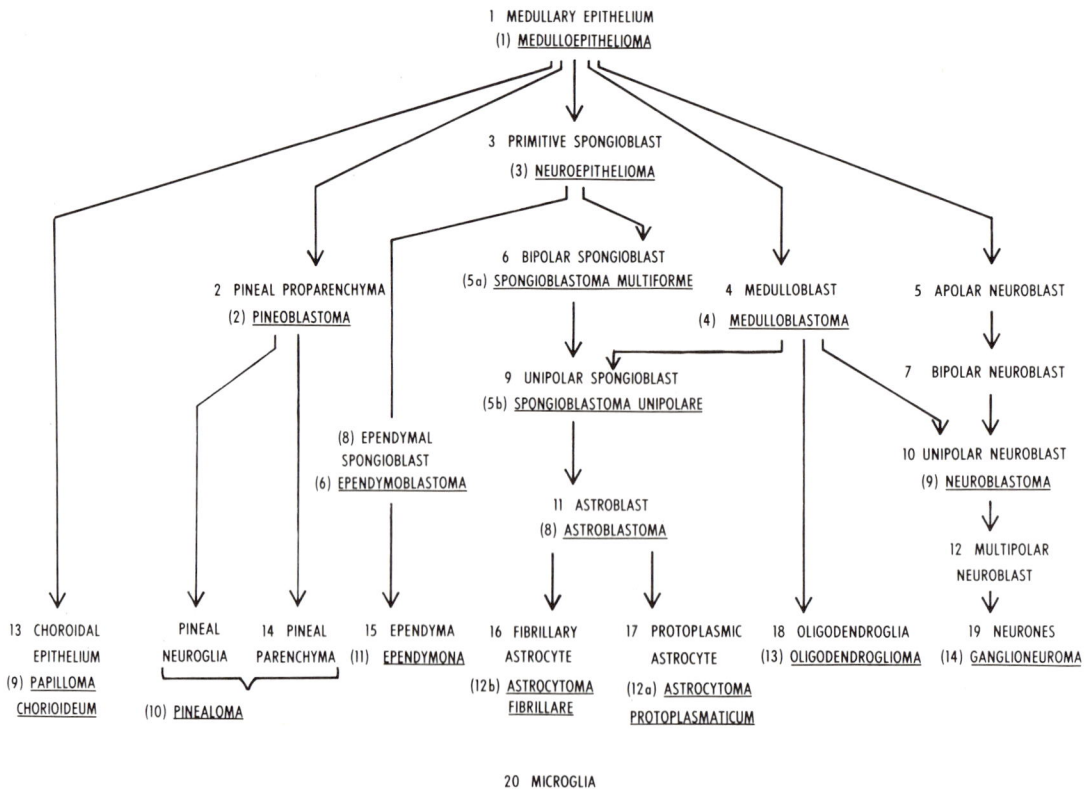

Figure 39–6. Twenty types of cells identified in the development of the nervous system (numbered) with the 14 types of glial tumors presumably derived from these cells (numbered in parentheses). (From Butler, A. B., Brooks, W. H., & Netsky, M. G. [1982]. Classification and biology of brain tumors. In J. R. Youmans [Ed.], *Neurological surgery* [Vol. 5, 2nd ed., p. 2661]. Philadelphia: W. B. Saunders Co. Reproduced by permission.)

Table 39–3. KERNOHAN AND SAYRE CLASSIFICATION OF CENTRAL NERVOUS SYSTEM TUMORS

New Names	Old Names (with new names in parentheses)
Astrocytoma grades 1–4	Astrocytoma (astrocytoma grade I) Astroblastoma (astrocytoma grade II) Spongioblastoma polare (left out) Glioblastoma multiforme (astrocytoma grades III and IV)
Ependymoma grades 1–4	Ependymoma (ependymoma grade I) Ependymoblastoma (ependymoma grades II–IV) Neuroepithelioma (left out) Medulloepithelioma (ependymoma grade IV)
Oligodendroglioma grades 1–4	Oligodendroglioma (oligodendroglioma grades I–IV) Oligodendroblastoma (oligodendroglioma grades II–IV)
Neuroastrocytoma	Neurocytoma Ganglioneuroma (neuroastrocytoma grade I) Gangliocytoma Ganglioglioma Neuroblastoma Spongioneuroblastoma (neuroastrocytoma grades II–IV) Glioneuroblastoma
Medulloblastoma	Medulloblastoma

(From Zulch, K. J. [1986]. *Brain tumors.* [p. 15]. New York: Springer-Verlag. Reproduced by permission.)

overall tumor type is sarcoma, which arises from connective tissue in the brain. In this simplified scheme, only the most commonly encountered tumors are grouped. No attempt is made to list all tumors or categories.

When a cell begins the process of becoming a tumor of any type, it is said to undergo dedifferentiation (see Box 39–1). Generally, tumors are divided into two categories: benign or malignant. Tumors of the same cellular type are then divided into 4 grades, I through IV, based on the degree of cellular anaplasia (malignancy). In grade I tumor cells, differentiation ranges from almost 100 per cent to 75 per cent; in Grade IV tumor cells, only 0 to 25 per cent of the cells are differentiated (Butler et al., 1982). A single cell of astrocytoma can become a glioblastoma multiforme, as can oligodendrogliomas and ependymomas when they recur. However, the biology of the tumor—its invasiveness—rather than the histology is more important in determining the outcome for the patient. Usually a patient with a better differentiated tumor will live longer than a patient with a poorly differentiated one. Parenthetically, one must consider anatomic site as well.

In summary, CNS tumors may be classified as benign or malignant, as gliomas, neuromas, or sarcomas. Some may be graded I through IV, by Kernohan (Butler et al., 1982), according to the degree of dedifferentiation or anaplasia. Malignancy in the cranium is not, however, solely determined by cell of origin, and some tumors that are classified as benign may in fact produce malignant responses (Butler et al., 1982);

therefore, clinical classification and consideration is also important. Further, the behavior of tumors of the same type varies in different patients. See Table 39–4 for a summary of classifications and grades of human intracranial tumors.

The following discussion of major, commonly encountered tumors is from the WHO classification. For purposes of this chapter the categories are collapsed, and a reasonable compromise of all classifications is used. In addition, for each tumor type, discussion includes characteristics (classification and natural history), signs and symptoms, treatment, and survival (Table 39–5 presents a summary). The percentages of occurrence of tumor types are summarized by age and location in Table 39–6.

Gliomas. Approximately 60 per cent of all primary CNS tumors are gliomas, which arise from glial cells. There are five distinct types of glial cells: astrocytes, oligodendroglia, ependymal cells, microglia, and neuroglial precursors. Each gives rise to tumors with different biologic and anatomic characteristics (Kornblith et al., 1987).

Astrocytomas, as a group, arise from astrocytes, which are the majority of the intraparenchymal cells of the brain. Astrocytomas range from benign to highly malignant. The benign ones include cerebellar astrocytomas, juvenile pilocytic astrocytomas, and optic nerve gliomas. Malignant forms include the graded series of astrocytomas, with the last being the highly malignant glioblastoma multiforme. Grade I astrocytomas are primarily hypercellular. In grade II and above there is a gradual progression of vascular proliferation and nuclear changes. Grade III astrocytomas have malignant cytologic features, and in grade IV there is a significant amount of necrosis and hemorrhage and marked variation in cell size and detail (Kornblith et al., 1987). Progression from benign to malignant processes include more rapid growth, tumor doubling, and loss of morphologic features (Box 39–2).

Astrocytomas constitutes about 25 per cent of cerebral gliomas and is the most frequent primary tumor of adults (Levin & Wilson, 1978; Salcman & Kaplan, 1986). It may occur anywhere in the brain or spinal cord but is most often found in the cerebrum, cerebellum, hypothalamus, optic nerve and chiasm, and pons. It grows slowly and infiltrates and has a tendency to form large cavities or pseudocysts. Calcium deposits in the tumor may be seen on a computed tomography (CT) scan. Many astrocytomas undergo malignant degeneration and become mixed astrocytomas and glioblastomas. In about half the patients, the initial symptom is focal or generalized seizure. Up to two thirds have recurrent seizures during the course of their illness. Headaches and other signs of increased intracranial pressure are relatively late phenomena. Temporal lobe lesions give rise to slight character and personality changes, moodiness, pseudoneurotic symptoms, and episodes suggestive of schizophrenia. Hemiparesis may be a symptom of frontal lobe glioma and may appear as only a slight drift of an outstretched arm, a mild limp, and enhanced tendon reflexes; it may remain slight for a long time. Language difficulties

STUDY

Piepmier, J. M. (1987). **Observations on the current treatment of low-grade astrocytic tumors of the cerebral hemispheres.** *Journal of Neurosurgery, 67,* 177–181.

SIGNIFICANCE

Low-grade astrocytic tumors of the cerebral hemispheres make up 15 per cent of treated brain neoplasms, and 50 per cent of these may evolve into anaplastic astrocytomas or glioblastomas. With no reliable method of predicting changes in the tumor's biologic activity, there is a need for studies to evaluate current treatment. Prior reports predate computed tomography (CT) scans and standardized radiation treatment, and thus it is difficult to rely on them for assessments of recent experience in tumor management. Prior reports also had wide variations in management techniques; therefore, this 10-year review of patients from one institution, all with comparable treatment and data, can help better understand the outcome of current treatment.

DESIGN

This is a correlational design using a retrospective review of hospital records, pathology reports, operative notes, radiation therapy reports, CT scans, and autopsy reports. Direct communications with treating physicians and hospital tumor registry records were also used.

SAMPLE

Each patient had to have a histologically confirmed low-grade astrocytic tumor of the cerebral hemispheres without evidence of anaplasia, nuclear pleomorphism, or coagulation necrosis. These patients were treated at a single hospital, including their preoperative evaluation, surgery, radiation therapy, and follow-up care; all irradiated patients were treated in the same manner; CT had been used to improve the ability to localize the lesion, to define the tumor boundary, and to document regrowth; complete and detailed records were available, sixty patients treated between 1975 and 1985 were entered. Ages varied from 0 to 80 years, and sex division was 60 per cent male and 40 per cent female.

VARIABLES

A summary table lists 30 categories of recorded clinical data for the study population. Some are continuous variables such as age and duration of symptoms; others are dichotomous or discrete variables, such as radiation therapy—yes or no—and extent of surgery—total, subtotal, or biopsy. The first 29 variables were evaluated for their potential influence on survival; thus they may be considered the independent variables. The dependent variable, survival data, was recorded as the length of time from diagnosis to death or latest follow-up evaluation. Operative deaths were defined as death within 30 days or during the same hospitalization. Deaths were otherwise noted to result from the tumor or from other causes. Surviving patients were characterized as having no tumor, stable tumor, or tumor status unknown.

DATA ANALYSIS

Survival curves were obtained by the Kaplan-Meier method. Parameters with $p < 0.05$ were further evaluated by a Cox regression analysis while adjusting for covariates.

FINDINGS

For the entire population, age, presence of tumor cyst, and tumor enhancement on CT were associated with survival. Age was the most significant factor in predicting survival when age was dichotomized as under 40 years and 40 and over. Regression analysis adjusting for age revealed that the presence of cystic tumors was no longer significant. Tumors that enhanced on CT scanning with intravenous administration of contrast material carried a poor prognosis when compared with nonenhancing tumors ($p < 0.008$). This significance was also present when adjusting for age ($p < 0.05$).

COMMENTS

This study shows the difficulty in defining optimal treatment and in providing prognostic information for even one type of central nervous system tumor. The strong suggestion of age-dependent variation in biologic activity of low-grade astrocytic tumors is important, as is noting CT enhancement as another indicator of biologic activity of the lesions. Pursuing an understanding of these characteristics of the biologic processes may be a productive line of research. In the meantime, this report shows some of the controls that can be used to do prospective studies with randomized treatment groups to begin to answer basic questions about low-grade tumors and to improve the management of these lesions and the survival of persons with these tumors.

Table 39–4. CLASSIFICATION AND GRADES OF HUMAN INTRACRANIAL TUMORS

Tumor	Grade I Benign	Grade II Semi-	Grade III Semi-	Grade IV Malignant
Angioblastoma	+ + +			
Choroid plexus papilloma	+ + +		+	
Craniopharyngioma	+ + +			
Chordoma	+ + +	+ +	+	
Epidermoid	+ + +			
Gangliocytoma (-glioma)	+ + +	+ +	+	
Meningioma	+ + +		+	
Neurilemoma	+ + +		+	
Paraganglioma	+ + +			
Pineocytoma	+ + +	+ +		
Pituitary adenoma	+ + +	+		
Subependymoma	+ + +			
Pilocytic astrocytoma	+ + +			
Astrocytoma		+ +	+	
Oligodendroglioma		+ +	+	
Ependymoma	+ +	+ + +	+	+
Germinoma				+ + +
Glioblastoma				+ + +
Lymphomas			+	+ + +
Medulloblastoma + PNET				+ + +
Pinealoblastoma				+ + +
Sarcoma				+ + +
Metastases				+ + +

+ + +, usual; + +, less frequent; +, rare; PNET, primitive neuroectodermal tumor.

(From Jellinger, K. [1987]. Pathology of human intracranial neoplasia. In K. Jellinger [Ed.], *Therapy of malignant brain tumors* [p. 12]. New York: Springer-Verlag. Reproduced by permission.)

and sensory changes are also frequently slight. Symptoms may be present for 10 years or longer before the diagnosis is made. In cerebral astrocytoma, the average survival after the first symptom is 67 months; in cerebellar astrocytoma, the average survival is 89 months (Adams & Victor, 1985).

Optic nerve glioma of childhood is another example of a subgroup of astrocytoma and is characterized by slow growth over a period of years, with an evolution from benign to malignant (Kornblith et al., 1987). Eighty-five per cent occur before the age of 15 years and are twice as frequent in girls as in boys. Initial symptoms include visual problems. Treatment includes surgical excision and radiation. Survival is lengthy unless the tumor becomes dedifferentiated and invasive (Adams & Victor, 1985).

Glioblastoma multiforme (grade IV, astrocytoma) is a highly malignant, highly vascular tumor that infiltrates extensively. Necrosis, hemorrhage, and thrombosis are often present in varying degrees. It accounts for 20 per cent of all intracranial tumors, for about 55 per cent of all tumors of the glioma group, and for more than 90 per cent of gliomas of the cerebral hemispheres in adults (Adams & Victor, 1985). Peak incidence is in midlife, and it occurs twice as often in men as in women. Approximately half of these tumors are bilateral, and a small percentage have several foci. They are thought to arise through anaplasia of mature astrocytes.

Symptoms are diffuse, and seizures occur in 30 to 40 per cent. In most cases, symptoms have been present for 3 to 6 months before diagnosis is established. The tumor may become large and diffuse before deranging cerebral functioning. Less than one fifth of all patients survive for 1 year after the onset of symptoms. Approximately 10 per cent survive more than 2 years. Surgery plus radiation extends median survival from only 14 weeks with surgery alone to beyond a year. Chemotherapy prolongs the median survival only slightly. The immediate cause of death is cerebral edema, increased intracranial pressure, and temporal lobe–tentorial herniation. Glioblastoma and malignant astrocytoma have the worst prognosis of any common solid tumor (Salcman & Kaplan, 1986).

Oligodendrogliomas are most often found in the 40- to 50-year age group and constitute approximately 5 to 7 per cent of all intracranial gliomas. They arise from oligodendroglia, which are satellite cells that are involved in the process of myelination. Often oligodendrogliomas are indistinguishable from other gliomas and are in fact frequently mixed (oligodendroglioma-astrocytoma). Oligodendrogliomas are usually benign but occasionally may be malignant. The presence of a significant portion of oligodendroglia in an astrocytoma is a favorable sign (Kornblith et al., 1987). Calcification is often associated with oligodendrogliomas.

This tumor frequently (80 per cent) occurs in the cerebrum, primarily in the frontal lobes, deep in the white matter with little or no surrounding edema. Sometimes it occurs as an intraventricular tumor (15 per cent), and it rarely occurs in other parts of the brain and spinal cord. There may be meningeal dissemination of the tumor (but this occurs less frequently than with medulloblastoma and glioblastoma). Malignant degeneration occurs in approximately one third of the cases.

Oligodendrogliomas grow slowly. Symptoms may appear from 28 to 70 months before surgical intervention. The first symptom in one half the patients is focal

Table 39–5. SUMMARY OF CHARACTERISTICS OF COMMON TUMOR TYPES

	Classification	Natural History	Symptoms	Treatment	Survival
Astrocytomas	Benign to highly malignant; histology varies by grade; in grade IV, variation in cell size and detail is marked	Grows slowly and infiltrates; tends to form large cavities or pseudocysts; progress from benign to malignant	Seizures, personality changes, slight hemiparesis, language difficulties, and sensory changes, depending on location; later headaches and other signs of increased intracranial pressure	Surgery with as complete an excision as possible; sometimes irradiation; chemotherapy for recurrence or for malignant degeneration	Average for cerebral tumors is less than 5 years; for cerebellar tumors, less than 7 years
Optic nerve glioma	Subgroup of astrocytoma occurring mainly in young males	Slow growth over years with evolution from benign to malignant	Visual problems	Surgical excision; irradiation	Lengthy unless tumor becomes dedifferentiated and invasive
Glioblastoma multiforme	Grade IV astrocytoma; malignant, highly vascular; half are bilateral, and some have multifoci	Symptoms appear 3 to 6 months before diagnosis; necrosis hemorrhage and thrombosis are present in varying degrees; infiltrates extensively; immediate cause of death is cerebral edema, IICP and temporal lobe–tentorial herniation	Diffuse symptoms, then more focal seizures	Surgery followed by irradiation; chemotherapy only slightly effective	Less than 20% survive 1 year after onset of symptoms; approximately 10% survive longer than 2 years
Oligodendrogliomas	Frequently mixed oligodendroglioma-astrocytoma; usually benign, occasionally malignant; relatively avascular with tendency to encapsulate	Associated calcification; little surrounding edema; may be meningeal dissemination; grows slowly	Focal or generalized seizures in 70%; some have early signs of IICP; one third have focal signs, e.g., hemiparesis	Surgery and irradiation; chemotherapy especially with anaplasia	Ten-year survival after treatment as high as 50% Mean survival time is 5 years
Ependymoma	Some are densely cellular and anaplastic; others are better differentiated; more complex and variable than other gliomas	Time from onset of symptoms varies from 4 weeks in most malignant types to 7 to 8 years; grows into the ventricles, adjacent brain, or spinal cord tissue	Depends on location; in fourth ventricle, like medulloblastoma	Surgery with as complete resectiona as possible; irradiation; chemotherapy sometimes used with malignant types and at recurrence	Varies; in some studies, 47% died within 1 year, but 13% were alive after 10 years; in more benign cases, 10-year survival about 55 to 60%
Meningioma	Benign (some malignant)	More common in persons who have had prior radiation to the scalp or cranium; involves the dura and often erodes the cranial bones; may have neurologic signs 10 to 15 years before diagnosis	Sometimes none; general neurologic changes; eventual IICP, but less frequent than gliomas	Surgery of tumor if operable; irradiation for incomplete removal or for inoperable cases	Permanent cure with 24 to 76% recurrence in complete removal; for malignant meningoma, survival less than 5 years
Medulloblastomas	Origin PNET; aggressive and always malignant; invasive and not encapsulated; found primarily in children; more prevalent in males	Symptoms 1 to 5 months before diagnosis; originates in cerebellum and spreads by way of cerebrospinal fluid Can fill and infiltrate floor of fourth ventricle Seeding may occur on meningeal surfaces and around spinal cord	Listlessness, vomiting, morning headaches; later, stumbling gait, frequent falls, squinting; papilledema, dizziness, nystagmus	Complete surgical excision; highly radiosensitive; chemotherapy at recurrence; shunt may be necessary	Extent of disease at time of diagnosis defines risk; poor; less than 75% resection, under age 4, positive cerebrospinal fluid cytologies, metastasis to cord, leptomeninges, cerebrum, or seeding of cerebellum—25 to 30% chance of remaining disease free for 5 years; good: 65 to 70% remain disease free for 5 years
Neural tumors	Ganglion cell tumors; benign to malignant; occur in young patients in frontotemporal or parietal cortex	Extremely rare; clearly demarcated but not encapsulated	Related function of frontotemporal and parietal cortex	Surgery	Data unavailable; one patient reportely survived 23 years after surgery
Lymphomas	Arise probably from lymphocytes; affect persons in immunodeficient states, e.g., patients with AIDS and those having transplants	Time from first symptoms to surgery: 3 months; clinical course same as glioblastoma	Focal signs more common than IICP; personality change; dementia; seizures	Surgical biopsy; irradiation and steroids; shunting for diffuse spread to meninges	Improvement with radiotherapy sometimes short

Table 39–5. SUMMARY OF CHARACTERISTICS OF COMMON TUMOR TYPES *Continued*

	Classification	Natural History	Symptoms	Treatment	Survival
Sarcomas	Derived from connective tissue; unique in tending to metastasize to nonneuronal tissues in brain	Rare; slow to fast growing; some have developed 5 to 10 years after gamma radiation for other tumors	Depend on site and rapidity of growth; seizures occur in 25%, headache, papilledema, spontaneous hemorrhage	Surgery	Twelve months to 5 years; longer than 2 years if nonanaplastic
Metastases	Occure primarily in frontal lobes; most common primary source is bronchogenic carcinoma, followed by breast, kidney, stomach, and bowel carcinoma; usually circumscribed and solid	Course similar to glioblastoma multiforme; may be more than one lesion with regional vasogenic edema; with leukemia, one third have diffuse infiltration of the meninges and cranial and spinal nerve roots	Depend on site. Commonly headache, mental and behavioral abnormalities, seizures, focal weakness, ataxia, aphasia, and IICP	Systemic chemotherapy ineffective, as is surgical treatment; irradiation and steroids for multiple tumors; radiation, vincristine, and intrathecal methotrexate for children with lymphoblastic leukemia	Approximately 6 months; longer with bone versus brain metastases; prolonged survival of treated children; some complications of necrotizing leukoencephalopathy
Acoustic neuromas	Benign and do not undergo malignant transformations; oval and encapsulated	Initially within the auditory canal, then grow out into areas of cerebellopontile angle and can damage brain stem and cranial nerves	Hearing loss, vertigo, tinnitus, balance disturbance; later headache, facial pain, unsteady gait, facial weakness, and sensory loss	Surgical removal	Usually facial nerve is preserved and sometimes the acoustic nerve
Pineal tumors	Often low- or intermediate-grade malignancy; discrete firm mass; also highly malignant embryonal tumors, locally invasive	May reproduce the normal structure of the gland, extend into the third ventricle and seed along the neuroaxis; obstructive hydrocephalus, ocular pathway compression	Headache, nausea, vomiting, lethargy, ataxias, and inability to look upward	Microscopic surgery; shunting; some are radioresistant, others very radiosensitive	Survival rates vary with histology and extent of disease; malignant types initially responsive but recur rapidly; are 5-year survivors
Craniopharyngiomas	Because of strategic location, behaves as malignant	May be congenital with subtle and long-standing symptoms; may press on or adhere to hypothalamic structures	Pituitary hypothalamic-chiasmal derangement; IICP	Surgical excision; management of temperature and water balance	Mortality ranges from 5 to 8%
Pituitary tumors	Nonfunctional: act by pressure; functional: hormonal changes	May compress the optic chiasm and other surrounding structures	Endocrine abnormalities. Visual problems.	Proton beam radiation; transsphenoidal microsurgery; hormone treatment and bromocriptine	Excellent; 99 to 100% success with surgery

IICP, increased intracranial pressure.
PNET, primitive neuroectodermal tissue.

Table 39–6. SUBDIVISIONS OF MAJOR CEREBRAL TUMORS BY AGE OF OCCURRENCE AND LOCATION IN THE BRAIN

Location	Infancy and Adolescence (0–20 Yr) Tumor Type	Percentage of All Tumors	Middle Age (20–60 Yr) Tumor Type	Percentage of All Tumors	Old Age (>60 yr) Tumor Type	Percentage of All Tumors
Supratentorial	Cerebral hemispheral glioma	10–14	Glioblastoma multiforme	25	Glioblastoma multiforme	35
			Meningioma	14	Meningioma	20
	Craniopharyngioma	5–13	Astrocytoma	13	Metastases	10
	Ependymoma	3–5	Metastases	10		
	Choroid plexus papilloma	2–3	Pituitary tumors	5		
	Pinealoma	1.5–3				
	Optic glioma	1–3.5				
	Total	16–25				
Infratentorial	Cerebellar		Metastases	5	Acoustic neuroma	20
	Astrocytoma	15–20	Acoustic neuroma	3	Metastases	5
	Medulloblastoma	14–18	Meningioma	1	Meningioma	5
	Brain stem glioma	9–12	Sarcoma	?		
	Ependymoma	4–8				
	Total	41–58				

(From Butler, A. B., Brooks, W. H., & Netsky, M. G. [1982]. Classification and biology of brain tumors. In J. R. Youmans [Ed.], *Neurological surgery* [Vol. 5, 2nd ed., p. 2664]. Philadelphia: W. B. Saunders Co. Reproduced by permission.)

or generalized seizures. Seventy per cent of the patients eventually develop seizures. Fifteen per cent may have early signs of increased intracranial pressure (IICP). However, at the time of surgery only about one half have signs of IICP, and one third have focal signs—primarily those of hemiparesis. Mean survival time after surgery is 5 years. Half of the patients have recurrences within a few months following surgery (Adams & Victor, 1985).

Ependymoma is more complex and variable than the other gliomas. Some, termed epithelial ependymomas, are densely cellular and anaplastic. Others are better differentiated. These tumors arise from differentiated ependymal cells that line the ventricles of the brain and central canal of the spinal cord and have cilia that assist in CSF movement. These tumors grow into the ventricles or adjacent brain tissues. In the brain, the most common site is the fourth ventricle; in the spinal cord, it is the lumbosacral region.

Approximately 5 per cent of all intracranial gliomas are ependymomas (slightly higher in children, 8 per cent). Forty per cent of the infratentorial ependymomas occur in the first decade of life. Supratentorial ependymomas occur evenly throughout life.

Symptoms depend on location. For example, ependymoma of the fourth ventricle produces symptoms much like those of medulloblastoma. Cerebral lesions produce seizures in approximately one third of cases. Length of time from onset of symptoms to surgery varies from 4 weeks in the most malignant types to 7 to 8 years. Prognosis and survival depend on degree of anaplasia. In some studies 47 per cent died within a year, but 13 per cent were alive after 10 years. In the more benign group of ependymomas, 10-year survival can be as high as 55 to 60 per cent (Adams & Victor, 1985).

Meningioma is a benign tumor and accounts for approximately 15 per cent of all primary intracranial tumors. It is more common in women, with the highest incidence in the seventh decade. Persons who have had radiation to the scalp or cranium are particularly vulnerable to this tumor and develop it at an earlier age than those who have not had prior radiation. The cell of origin is not precisely known. It usually occurs in the sylvian region, superior parasagittal surface of the frontal and parietal lobes, olfactory grooves, lesser wings of the sphenoid bones, tuberculum sellae, superior surface of the cerebellum (throughout the surface of the brain), cerebellopontine angles, and spinal canal. Meningiomas involve the dura and often erode cranial bones.

The surface tumors often are found at autopsy in middle-aged and elderly adults and have caused no symptoms. Other patients may have neurologic signs 10 to 15 years before the diagnosis is made. Increased intracranial pressure eventually occurs but less frequently than with gliomas. Surgery may afford permanent cure if the tumor's location allows complete removal. For incomplete removal and inoperable cases, radiation is beneficial. Various series of studies report a 24 to 76 per cent recurrence when removal is incomplete. If the meningioma becomes malignant, survival is less than 5 years (Adams & Victor, 1985).

Medulloblastomas are found primarily in children and are more prevalent in males than in females. The cell of origin was thought to be neuroglial. Recent evidence suggests that it originates from primitive neuroectodermal tissue; therefore, it is a primitive neuroectodermal tumor (PNET). The tumor is aggressive and is always malignant. It is invasive and not encapsulated. It originates in the cerebellum and can spread by way of the CSF pathways to meningeal surfaces and around the spinal cord. Some fill the fourth ventricle and infiltrate the floor of that ventricle (Adams & Victor, 1985).

Symptoms may have been present between 1 and 5 months before diagnosis. Typically, the child becomes listless, vomits repeatedly, and has a morning headache. Later, stumbling gait, frequent falls, and squinting may occur. Papilledema, dizziness, and nystagmus are frequent. With surgery, radiation, and chemotherapy, two thirds of the patients survive 5 years. Extent of disease at diagnosis determines survival. Children considered at poor risk for survival are under 4 years of age; have less than 75 per cent surgical resection; have positive cerebrospinal fluid (CSF) cytology; and have metastasis to the spinal cord, leptomeninges, or cerebrum or seeding of the cerebellum. These children have only a 25 to 30 per cent chance of remaining symptom free for 5 years. However, patients who are good risks have a 65 to 70 per cent chance of remaining disease free for 5 years. Shunting of the CSF may be necessary. Surgical excision should be as complete as possible. The tumor is highly radiosensitive. The entire neuroaxis is irradiated. Chemotherapy has been shown to be beneficial at recurrence (Adams & Victor, 1985).

Neural Tumors. The ganglion cell tumors—ganglioglioma and ganglioneuroma—are examples of neural tumors. In ganglioglioma, astrocytic components predominate; in the ganglioneuroma, abnormal neurons predominate. Ganglion cell tumors usually occur in the frontotemporal or parietal cortex. They occur in young patients and range from benign to malignant. These tumors are extremely rare and are clearly demarcated but not encapsulated. Symptoms are related to the anatomic site (Kornblith et al., 1987). Surgery may be indicated. Survival statistics are unavailable, but Cobb and Youmans (1982) report one patient survived 23 years after surgery.

Lymphoma. Lymphomas arise probably from B lymphocytes and occur primarily in any part of the cerebrum, cerebellum, or brain stem. The lesions may occur singly or in multiple locations and are ill-defined and infiltrative. The same clinical course is seen in lymphoma as is seen in glioblastoma. The average length of time from first symptoms to diagnosis and surgery has been approximately 3 months. Focal signs are more common than are signs of IICP. These are personality change, dementia, seizures, and other focal neurologic symptoms.

Patients with immunodeficiency states are particularly likely to develop this type of tumor. Therefore, it is often seen in patients with acquired immune deficiency syndrome (AIDS) and patients who receive immunosuppressive drugs for long periods of time, such as after renal or other organ transplants. Before the AIDS era, CNS lymphomas accounted for 1 per cent of all lymphomas. Now some estimate that it will become the most common primary CNS tumor by the 1990s. Lymphoma has always been more common in males; it still is, although this may change. Also, the peak incidence has been in the fourth, fifth, and sixth decades, but AIDS likely will lower the age of incidence. Some patients with lymphoma have been shown to have the Epstein-Barr virus.

Craniotomy, for removal of single tumors, may be done. A single biopsy specimen is taken for diagnosis when multiple tumors exist. Radiation and steroids are highly effective, although improvement is short-lived. Chemotherapy has produced variable results (Adams & Victor, 1985).

Sarcomas. Sarcomas of the brain are derived from connective tissue elements. These tumors are rare and account for 1 to 2 per cent of all primary intracranial tumors. A few sarcomas have developed 5 to 10 years after gamma radiation for other tumors. These tumors are unique in their tendency to metastasize to nonneuronal tissue in the brain. They are slow to fast growing (Adams & Victor, 1985). Seizures occur in 25 per cent of the patients. Headache, papilledema, and spontaneous hemorrhage also are symptoms. Surgery may be indicated. Survival has been reported to vary from 12 months to 5 years and is longer than 2 years if the tumor is nonanaplastic (Cobb & Youmans, 1982).

Metastatic Tumors. Metastatic tumors constitute approximately 10 per cent of all intracranial tumors. The most common primary tumor is bronchogenic carcinoma, followed by carcinoma of the breast, kidney, stomach, and bowel. Metastatic malignant melanoma is also a common tumor of the cerebral hemisphere. Metastatic tumors occur primarily in the frontal lobes and less frequently in other areas of the brain; apparently, this is a function of the regional volume in proportion to total brain mass. Smaller structures have fewer metastatic lesions (Wilson, 1977).

The appearance of the tumor is that of any carcinomatous lesion. Usually the tumor is circumscribed and solid; there may be more than one lesion with regional vasogenic edema. Presenting symptoms are those of cerebral lesions that are described later. Patients with metastatic carcinoma of the brain have a course similar to those with glioblastoma multiforme.

Systemic chemotherapy is ineffective against most cerebral metastases. The average period of survival is about 6 months, including patients who have had surgically treated single metastases. Patients with metastases to the bony structures live longer (Adams & Victor, 1985). For single lesions, surgery can be done and followed by radiation therapy. For multiple tumors, irradiation and steroids are the treatment of choice.

Infiltration of the CNS occurs in patients with nonsolid tumors as well. There is a high incidence (about one third) of diffuse infiltration of the meninges, the cranial nerves, and the spinal nerve roots in patients with leukemia. The incidence is greater with lympho-

cytic than with myelocytic leukemia and is higher in children with acute lymphocytic (lymphoblastic) leukemia. The use of radiation therapy, vincristine, and intrathecal methotrexate has been associated with prolonged survival of children with acute leukemia. Unfortunately, there has been also a significant number of patients with necrotizing leukoencephalopathy (discussed later). This complication may appear within several days or months after completion of therapy. In most cases, death occurs, and most who die are under the age of 5 years.

Other Tumors. *Acoustic schwannomas* are the largest group of tumors at the cerebellopontine angle, accounting for 70 per cent of these tumors (Salcman & Kaplan, 1986). Schwannomas (often referred to in the literature as neuromas) grow in association with several cranial nerves. The acoustic nerve is involved most frequently. The tumors actually arise from the superior vestibular branch of the eighth cranial nerve but are called acoustic schwannomas by force of tradition and common usage.

These tumors are benign and do not undergo malignant transformation. They are usually 2 to 3.5 cm, oval, and encapsulated. Acoustic schwannomas grow in relation to both the auditory and vestibular portions of the eighth cranial nerve. Initially they are entirely in the auditory canal, but gradually they grow out into the area of the cerebellopontine angle, where they come into contact with vital brain stem centers. They also damage other cranial nerves, such as the facial nerve.

Progressive hearing loss is an early signal, although in a few cases only vestibular symptoms occur (Kornblith et al., 1987). Other expected symptoms include vertigo, tinnitus, and disturbed sense of balance. Because these tumors can compress other cranial nerves and grow into the posterior fossa, headache, facial pain, unsteady gait, facial weakness, and sensory loss are common symptoms (Adams & Victor, 1985). Acoustic schwannomas occur occasionally as part of von Recklinghausen's neurofibromatosis, and this is likely to occur at a young age (under 21) and to be bilateral.

Bilateral tumors after age 26 usually are classified as central neurofibromatosis. The usual tumor in adults appears as a single tumor. The highest incidence is in the fifth and sixth decades and affects both sexes equally. By the time of diagnosis, the clinical picture is quite complex. Other cranial nerves may be affected owing to proximity to the eighth nerve. A CT scan can detect larger tumors; x-ray tomography is used for smaller ones. Treatment is surgical. In most cases the facial nerve can be preserved and in some cases the acoustic nerve as well (Adams & Victor, 1985).

Pineal tumors are unified by their location and include pineal area astrocytoma. Often they are of low- or intermediate-grade malignancy. Two distinctive tumors (dysgerminoma and pineloblastoma) of this region are of germ cell origin (Kornblith et al., 1987). These tumors reproduce the structure of the pineal gland, enlarge the gland, become locally invasive, extend into the third ventricle, and seed along the neuroaxis. They resemble astrocytomas and may have varying degrees of malignancy. Obstructive hydrocephalus, headache, nausea and vomiting, lethargy, ataxia, and inability to look upward are the major symptoms. Survival rates vary with histology. Because of their location, pineal tumors are among the most difficult brain tumors to remove. However, surgery is important because some of these masses are radioresistant.

Teratomas—benign and arising from misplaced embryonic tissue from other parts of the body—occur here also and are treated with radiotherapy (Adams & Victor, 1985). Highly malignant embryonal tumors develop in the pineal location as well. The tumors are initially responsive to treatment but recur rapidly (Kornblith et al., 1987). Children, adolescents, and young adults are affected primarily. Males are affected more than females. Signs of IICP are present. Technical advances in surgery (use of the operating microscope) now make this tumor operable, although at a high risk. Shunting and radiation may also be used. Several patients have survived 5 years after the removal of the tumor.

Craniopharyngiomas are located in the suprasellar region and because of the strategic location can behave as malignant tumors. They may press on or adhere to the hypothalamic structures. They are found primarily in children but may occur at a later age and are thought to be congenital tumors. Symptoms commonly include pituitary-hypothalamic-chiasmal derangement. Often IICP is present. Symptoms are often subtle and long-standing. The tumor can be excised successfully in a majority of cases. After surgery, careful management of temperature and water balance is needed. Mortality ranges from 5 to 8 per cent (Adams & Victor, 1985).

Pituitary tumors include both nonfunctional (producing their effect by pressure on surrounding structures) and functional hormonal tumors. They are age linked, becoming increasingly numerous with each decade. By the eightieth year, small adenomas are found in more than 20 per cent of pituitary glands. Only a few enlarge the sella. Usually they arise in the anterior pituitary. They may compress the optic chiasm and other surrounding structures. Usually they are recognized because of endocrine abnormalities and visual problems. In both men and women, 60 to 79 per cent secrete prolactin, 10 to 15 per cent secrete growth hormone, and a few secrete adrenocorticotropic hormone. Proton beam radiation or transphenoidal microsurgery are used. Hormone imbalance must be treated. In many cases a dopamine agonist, bromocriptine, is the only treatment needed or is used in conjunction with others (Adams & Victor, 1985).

The prognosis and outcome of the occurrence of any tumor is made by the informed opinion of the pathologist and clinician as a result of previous collaborative experience and joint correlative studies in neuro-oncology. Again, in this field it must be noted that two tumors of similar cellularity, mitotic rate, and other characteristics in fact usually do not exhibit the same biologic behavior (Zulch, 1979).

Clinical Features

Pathophysiology

The cranial cavity has a restricted volume and contains three elements: brain, CSF, and blood. Because all are relatively incompressible, any increase in bulk in one means that one or both of the others must decrease in volume. The converse is also true: a decrease in volume of one results in an increase in volume of one or both of the other components. The pressures must remain constant at all times. When the bulk of one component increases beyond the compensatory capacity of the other components, IICP occurs with some significant consequences for the patient.

Tumors first displace CSF from the ventricles and subarachnoid space into the spinal subarachnoid space and the perioptic subarachnoid space. Pressures are transmitted undiminished throughout the brain and spinal cord spaces. Lumbar pressure rises, and pressure in the optic nerve increases owing to diminished venous drainage, which results in papilledema (Adams & Victor, 1985).

Pressure in the microvasculature surrounding the tumor rises, and this increase along with the release of tumor factors damages the blood-brain barrier. Fluid accumulates around the tumor site in the brain (vasogenic edema). An increase in venous pressure and in CSF pressure results in diminished resorption of CSF and further edema. With an increase in venous pressure, arterial pressure also increases and is accompanied by bradycardia. Carbon dioxide accumulates in the vasomotor centers of the medulla and carotid bodies, resulting in cardiovascular changes and in respiratory changes (irregularity and arrest) (Adams & Victor, 1985). The preceding changes occur in the sequence described—early to late.

Brain Edema. A prominent feature of cerebral tumors is brain edema. Malignant intracerebral tumors (specifically glioblastomas and metastatic tumors) cause the greatest degree of cerebral edema (Wilson, 1977). Vasogenic edema occurs as a result of the processes discussed earlier; that is, tumor growth and release of tumor factors. It is seen almost exclusively in the white matter of the brain. Cytotoxic edema or cellular edema occurs as a result of hypoxic injury to the cells. Hypoxia results in a failure of the adenosine triphosphate–sodium (ATP–Na) pump; sodium accumulates within the cells, and water follows. A third type of edema commonly identified is interstitial edema. Fluid seeps into the periventricular tissues and occupies space between cells. It occurs when pressure (specifically from CSF) is high (Adams & Victor, 1985).

Most patients with brain tumors have regional swelling of tissue (vasogenic edema). Regional pressure changes lead to displacement of structures, impairment of function, and possibly to herniation. Simultaneously, cardiovascular and respiratory changes occur.

Herniation. Herniation is important when considering brain tumor effects. The cranial cavity is divided into several compartments by sheets of relatively rigid dura. The falx cerebri divides the brain into right and left hemispheres, and the tentorium separates the cerebellum from the occipital lobes. Pressure from tumors shifts the brain tissue from an area where pressure is high to another where pressure is lower.

This shifting may result in three well-known types of herniation. Brain tissue (the cingulate gyrus) may be shifted from one hemisphere to another under the falx cerebri, which is known as subfalcial herniation. Or the medial portion of the temporal lobe may herniate through the tentorium where the midbrain passes. Great pressure is exerted on the midbrain and subthalamus and the blood vessels supplying those structures. This is known as tentorial herniation. The third type of commonly known herniation is that which occurs through the foramen magnum: cerebellar–foramen magnum herniation. It may be caused by unilateral, bilateral, cerebellar, or frontal lesions. The lethal effects are the result of medullary compression (Adams & Victor, 1985).

Clinical manifestations of brain tumors are of three kinds: nonspecific effects of IICP, such as headache; secondary effects related to displacement of structures within the intracranial cavity; and focal effects related to direct involvement of the brain and cranial nerves (Wilson, 1977).

Presenting Signs and Symptoms. According to Adams and Victor (1985), these signs and symptoms may be classified into 4 categories: (1) hardly any symptoms and slight bewilderment, slowness in comprehension, or loss of capacity to sustain continuous mental activity; (2) early indication of cerebral disease in the form of a seizure or other dramatic symptom, yet evidence not clear enough for a diagnosis of brain tumor; (3) signs of IICP with or without localizing signs; and (4) symptoms so definite that an intracranial lesion is undoubtedly present.

Changes in Mental Function. These changes are often diffuse and vague and must be elicited from someone who knows the patient well. Signs and symptoms include a lack of persistence in tasks, undue irritability, emotional lability, inertia, faulty insight, forgetfulness, reduced range of mental activity, indifference to common social practices, and lack of initiative and spontaneity. The fact that all these complaints may be attributed falsely to worry, anxiety, and depression sometimes leads to a longer time between their onset and diagnosis. Adams and Victor (1985) call this behavior *psychomotor asthenia* to distinguish it from depression or other similar symptoms. Patients usually accept these changes and complain only of being weak, tired, or dizzy. In fact they may display inordinate drowsiness, apathy, equanimity, or stoicism. Within a few weeks or months these symptoms become more prominent. The dullness and drowsiness may increase gradually and can progress to stupor or coma.

Tumors most likely to cause these symptoms are ones that involve long association fibers (frontal, temporal, and corpus callosum gliomas). Many of these symptoms are related to IICP and are unrelated to the site and nature of the lesion. In subjects older than 60 years of age, an even more skillful evaluation of symptoms must be done again, in collaboration with someone who knows the patient well.

Headaches. Headaches are an early symptom in about one third of patients with tumors. The symptoms vary, but what they may have in common is that they occur during the night or are present on awakening in the morning and have a deep, nonpulsitile quality. Sometimes CSF pressure is normal during the initial time that headaches are present. Tumors above the tentorium produce headaches on the same side and in the vicinity of the tumor—in the orbital-frontal, temporal, or parietal region. Posterior fossa or subtentorial tumors cause headaches on the same side behind the ear or in the occipital region. With IICP, bifrontal or bioccipital headache occurs regardless of tumor location (Adams & Victor, 1985).

Seizures. Twenty to 50 per cent of all patients with brain tumors have either focal or generalized seizures. They may occur singly or in a series and may follow other symptoms or precede them by weeks or months (Adams & Victor, 1985).

Increased Intracranial Pressure. Classic signs and symptoms of IICP are seen initially in some patients with tumors. These signs include periodic bifrontal and bioccipital headaches that awaken the patient during the night or are present on awakening, projectile vomiting, mental torpor, unsteady gait, bowel and bladder incontinence, and papilledema. These signs and symptoms need immediate attention because they can result at any time in coma and death (Adams & Victor, 1985).

In summary, the most frequent combination of complaints in adults includes headache, weakness, personality change, and seizures (Salcman & Kaplan, 1986).

Specific or Localized Signs and Symptoms. Such specific signs and symptoms of intracranial tumors may occur in addition to the more diffuse ones discussed earlier. With a knowledge of neuroanatomy and neurophysiology, the location of the lesion may be determined by neurologic findings. *Unilateral lesions of the right frontal lobe* can cause left hemiplegia, slight elevation in mood, difficulty in adapting to new situations, loss of initiative, and occasional primitive grasping and sucking reflexes. *Left frontal lobe lesions* can cause right hemiplegia and nonfluent dysphasia, with or without some apraxia of lips, tongue, or hand movements. *Bifrontal lesions* can cause variable degrees of bilateral hemiplegia; spastic bulbar palsy; severe impairment of intellect; lability of mood; dementia; and prominent primitive grasp, suck, and snout reflexes.

The effects of *temporal lobe syndromes* can range from impairment of perception and spatial judgment to severe impairment of recent memory. Auditory hallucinations and aggressive behavior can occur. Lesions of the *nondominant temporal lobe* can produce minor perceptual problems and spatial disorientation. Involvement of the *dominant temporal lobe* can produce dysnomia, impaired perception of verbal commands, and Wernicke-like aphasia. Bilateral disease of the temporal lobes is rare in comparison with that found in frontal lobes. *Parietal lobe syndromes* affect sensory more than motor modalities (Levin & Wilson, 1978).

The *optic chiasm syndromes* are often produced by pituitary adenomas and less commonly by craniopharyngiomas and meningiomas (Levin & Wilson, 1978). Sixty per cent of patients with these syndromes have defects in the visual field when they seek medical care. The defect is usually partial or complete bitemporal hemianopia. The tumor presses upward on the optic chiasm and affects the upper temporal quadrants first.

Some *remote effects of neoplasia* on the nervous system have been identified. These are called *paraneoplastic disorders* and are linked with cancer more frequently than could be accounted for by chance. The nervous system has not been directly invaded or compressed by the tumor, yet symptoms occur. One example of this disorder is carcinomatous cerebellar degeneration. Carcinoma of the lung; ovarian carcinoma; and lymphoma, particularly Hodgkin's disease; and carcinoma of the breast, uterus, bowel, and other viscera have been implicated in the syndrome. Cerebellar symptoms have an insidious onset and progress over weeks to months. In about one half the cases cerebellar symptoms are recognized before those of the associated neoplasm. The presence of antibodies to Purkinje cells of the cerebellum have been documented in patients with ovarian carcinoma. Little can be done to modify symptoms, although partial or complete remission has occurred with removal of the primary tumor (Adams & Victor, 1985).

Diagnosis

Diagnosis begins with a detailed review of the patient's history and observations by family members. A thorough neurologic examination follows. Then CT scans and radiographs of the skull are taken. Magnetic resonance imaging (MRI) and positron-emission tomography (PET) are recently developed imaging procedures that have revolutionized diagnosis and treatment. Other procedures that may be employed are audiograms, radionuclide scans, evoked potential studies, electroencephalograms, vestibular tests, psychometric tests, and others. Arteriograms are done if the CT scan has not clarified the problem sufficiently (Adams & Victor, 1985).

Chest Radiographs

Chest radiographs are routinely done because bronchogenic carcinomas account for more cerebral metastases than any other primary malignant tumor (Morley, 1973).

Skull Radiographs

Radiographs of the skull may be done and are abnormal in 50 per cent of patients with astrocytomas of the cerebral hemispheres (Cobb & Youmans, 1982).

Brain Scanning

Brain scanning (radionuclide scanning or gamma encephalography) has been used for more than 20 years. The type of tumor affects the amount of radioactive nucleotide uptake. The timing of the scan is also important (Morley, 1973). Technetium 99m is currently the tracer most often used. Although computed tomography has superceded brain scanning, the latter is useful in following patients who harbor primary or metastatic tumors and those who develop subarachnoid spread of tumor.

Computed Tomography Scan

The CT scan is one of the first tests done after the potential patient has been identified. This test is extraordinarily useful, and more than 95 per cent of all lesions are detected in the initial study (Salcman & Kaplan, 1986). The location, appearance, and extent of peritumoral edema can be determined. In many cases, CT scans have allowed the designation of tumors as benign or malignant (Levin & Wilson, 1978). Computed tomography scanning is based on the principle that x rays when transmitted through a given body (e.g., tumor) from 360-degree polar space can define that body. The x-ray transmissions are reconstructed by a computer for visual imaging. Usually, the initial CT scans are done without a contrast agent. If contrast is used and the tumor is enhanced, a break in the blood-brain barrier and a more active tumor are indicated.

Magnetic Resonance Imaging

Nuclear magnetic resonance imaging combines the anatomic precision of CT scans with some information about metabolic parameters of the brain. Grey and white matter can be differentiated with MRI, and thus greater anatomical detail is provided. It is particularly useful in posterior fossa imaging because bone artifact is absent in MRI (Beaney, 1986). This technique is a rapidly evolving one. Magnetic resonance imaging sees through bone and is done with the patient in a large magnet, which provides a uniform static magnetic field. Hydrogen nuclei are magnetized, and the recovery or relaxation to their original state induces an electric signal in a receiver coil surrounding the patient. This signal is measured, and the image of the brain is reconstructed (Beaney, 1986).

Magnetic resonance imaging is also useful in imaging cysts, other fluid collections, hematomas, and vascular abnormalities. Acoustic neuromas can be well defined because the temporal bone essentially produces no signal. Magnetic resonance imaging is most applicable in imaging the CNS (Paushter, Modic, Borkowski, Weinstein, & Zeman, 1984). Briefly, CT scans demonstrate calcification, and MRI shows water content of tumors. In 1988 a new contrast substance, gadolinium, was released for use in the United States for CNS enhancement only. Its use has resulted in a remarkable improvement in the resolution of the images produced.

Positron-Emission Tomography

Positron-emission tomography is not routinely available for diagnosis but has provided new insights in brain tumors. It does not compete with CT scanning or with MRI for anatomic localization of the tumor. Rather, PET scanning complements the other techniques by giving information on regional cerebral blood flow; in addition, some determinations of metabolic factors and oxygen utilization can be made with PET scanning. It is a noninvasive technique in which biologic tracers labeled with short-lived positron-emitting radionuclides are administered. A detector system or imaging device then shows the fate of the nucleotide in the brain (Beaney, 1986).

Cerebrospinal Fluid Withdrawal

Cerebrospinal fluid withdrawal (lumbar puncture) is dangerous and could produce herniation. Under the appropriate circumstances, it is done, and pressure determinations are useful (Morley, 1973).

Electroencephalogram

An electroencephalogram may be of considerable value, especially when the tumor is within the brain rather than extrinsic to it, as in meningioma, for example. There may be a localized dysrhythmia corresponding to the region of the tumor. A normal record does not necessarily exclude tumor, however (Morley, 1973).

Echoencephalography

Echoencephalography is done by applying a transducer first to one side of the head and then to the other. The transducer both emits and receives pulsed ultrasound waves. These are reflected from the side of the third ventricle and can demonstrate a shift from the midline by space-occupying lesions (Morley, 1973). This test is easily performed and requires relatively simple equipment. Often it is done at the bedside when signs of deterioration are evident. However, CT would then be used for a more definitive assessment of progressive pathology.

Cerebral Angiography

Cerebral angiography is often done when signs and symptoms of brain tumor are present. It can be helpful in localizing the tumor and determining its type (Levin & Wilson, 1978).

Pneumoencephalography

Pneumoencephalography is done when air contrast studies are needed to visualize the fourth ventricle or the aqueduct, for example. A water-soluble iodinated contrast agent, *metrizamide,* is largely replacing air in most cases (Levin & Wilson, 1978). These contrast studies are especially useful in the diagnosis of spinal cord tumors. Extradural tumors can be distinguished from intradural tumors, and often intradural extramedullary spinal cord tumors can be distinguished from intramedullary ones.

Chemical Markers

Chemical markers in the blood and in the CSF have a role in some tumors. Patients suspected of having pituitary tumors, for example, may have serum prolactin and other serum hormones studied (Salcman & Kaplan, 1986).

Stereotaxic Biopsy

Stereotaxic biopsy may be done for diagnostic purposes so that the appropriate treatment can be matched to the tumor type.

Treatment

Treatment of brain tumors depends on the biologic behavior of the tumor. Benign tumors grow slowly, are noninvasive, and are therefore amenable to total surgical removal in most cases (Kornblith et al., 1987). Rarely, do they recur because of incomplete removal or conversion to a malignant tumor.

Malignant tumors are invasive but rarely metastasize outside the CNS. Often these tumors grow slowly but can rapidly become fatal because they exist in a confined space and produce pressure changes inside the intracranial vault.

Malignant gliomas rarely metastasize distantly but do invade local tissue to an extreme degree, grow relatively slowly, and have a marked variation in cell population or heterogeneity (Kornblith et al., 1987). There is clear gradation of malignancy, from low-grade glioma with a relatively favorable prognosis to glioblastoma with a grim outlook. Heterogeneity of the tumors makes them difficult to treat.

Tumor growth factors suggest that the tumors may become autonomous and self-stimulating (Kornblith et al., 1987). At this time, no means of limiting these growth factors exists. In addition, the fact that the cells are dividing slowly makes treatment difficult because therapy is aimed at the rapidly cycling cell population.

Unfortunately, treatment of malignant gliomas is mostly palliative. With regard to the host-tumor interaction, the tumor and its defenses are more effective than the host and its response to the tumor (Kornblith et al., 1987). Survival rates from time of diagnosis for common brain tumors are shown in Table 39–7.

Surgery

Surgical removal is the treatment of choice for many tumors. Sometimes, however, surgery cannot be done because the tumor is located in vital tissue. Also, complete removal is often difficult owing to the invasiveness of the lesion. However, survival of the patient with medulloblastoma, for example, is correlated with the extent of the surgical resection (Salcman & Kaplan, 1986). Often surgery is followed by radiation, as in the case of medulloblastoma, in which whole-axis radiation of the brain and spinal cord has been used.

Table 39–7. SURVIVAL RATES FROM TIME OF DIAGNOSIS FOR COMMON BRAIN TUMORS

Tumor	Percentage Surviving		
	1 yr	**2 yr**	**5 yr**
I. Intrinsic (glial) tumors*			
Astrocytoma grade 1	90	87	76
Astrocytoma grade 2	85	75	58
Astrocytoma grade 3	39	18	6
Glioblastoma multiforme	32	11	0
Ependymoma	50	47	25
II. Extrinsic (benign) tumors			
Meningioma†	100	95	90
III. Congenital tumors*			
Craniopharyngioma		81‡	76
Medulloblastoma		70	56

*All patients received surgery and radiation
†Excludes postoperative deaths
‡Three-year survival
(From Salcman, M., & Kaplan, R. S. (1986). Intracranial tumors in adults. In A. R. Moosa, M. C. Robson, & S. C. Schimpff [Eds.], *Comprehensive textbook of oncology* [p. 627]. Baltimore: Williams & Wilkins. Adapted with permission.)

Radiation

Differences in radiosensitivity of tumors do exist. It is seen clinically that medulloblastoma is often rapidly responsive, whereas astrocytomas are not (Kornblith et al., 1987).

Whole-Axis Radiation. Frequently, the brain and spinal cord of patients with some types of tumors are irradiated after surgical removal of the tumor to prevent subsequent seeding and because the entire tumor cannot be removed. An example is in medulloblastoma in children, noted previously. To achieve 50 to 75 per cent 5-year survival for malignant astrocytoma in adults, a combination of surgery and irradiation is required (Salcman & Kaplan, 1986). The survival of patients with malignant astrocytoma can be correlated with the total dose of radiation received. In a typical treatment plan, for example, daily fractions of 180 rads are given until the whole brain has been irradiated to a total of 4500 rads and until an additional 1800 rads are delivered to the operative site (Salcman & Kaplan, 1986).

The biology of some tumors (hypoxic and poorly vascularized, metabolically quiescent and noncycling, and relatively circumscribed) has led to more aggressive focal irradiation and to interstitial irradiators instead of whole-head teletherapy.

Interstitial Brachytherapy. The implantation of ribbons of seeds containing two frequently used isotopes is common. Iodine-125 and iridium-192 are often used. After the tumor type is identified, commonly by biopsy, and candidacy for brachytherapy is established, an extensive plan using CT scanning is developed by the neuro-oncology team. Maps for implantation of catheters into the tumor are drawn up. Using stereotactic surgery the procedure is usually done in the operating room under local anesthesia. After the patient is stabilized, a repeat CT scan is done for verification of catheter placement and for potential intraoperative complications such as bleeding or pneumocephalus. Finally, the radiation sources are brought to the intensive care unit, and under sterile technique the dummy ribbons are replaced with the radioactive sources (Randall, Drake, & Sewchand, 1987).

Chemical Sensitizers. Given along with radiation or chemotherapy, chemical sensitizers and *hyperthermia* of the tumor site are procedures that are being used to some extent and may enhance therapeutic outcomes in the future treatment of CNS tumors.

Radiation necrosis is a complication of this type of treatment and is not unique to patients with brain tumors. It also occurs in children who have leukemia and have been treated prophylactically by cranial irradiation. From 1 to 12 weeks (most often 6 to 12 weeks) after radiation, a transient encephalopathy can appear, with signs and symptoms of IICP, drowsiness, nausea, and exacerbation of preexisting neurologic deficit. Although uncommon with proper dosing, radiation necrosis can occur from 4 months to 9 years (most often from 1 to 2 years) after radiation therapy.

Chemotherapy

Systemic chemotherapy for CNS tumors does present problems because the tumors are at least partially shielded by the blood-brain barrier and because of other factors. The blood-brain barrier is an anatomic barrier that prevents large molecules from diffusing into the brain. The barrier consists of two components: tight junctions between endothelial cells of CNS capillaries and "feet" or processes of astrocytes that encase the cerebral capillaries (Garroutte, 1981). Modification of the blood-brain barrier has been attempted by use of internal carotid artery infusions of 25 per cent mannitol, which produced transient, reversible, osmotic disruption of the blood-brain barrier and resulted in a several-fold increase of methotrexate (Kornblith, et al., 1987). Modification of the microenvironment of the brain may be of greater interest in the future. Chemotherapy is often polychemotherapy and is used in combination with other types of treatment.

BCNU, a nitrosourea, has been in use for more than 10 years and has been employed widely in the treatment of malignant astrocytomas (Salcman & Kaplan, 1986). It does cross the blood-brain barrier, as do most nitrosoureas. BCNU has been shown to have a membrane-specific effect. In some treatment centers, it is usually initiated at the conclusion of radiation for this tumor type. At other centers, BCNU may be reserved for use when the tumor recurs. A typical protocol includes an initial dose of 100mg/m²/day for 3 days. This is administered intravenously every 8 weeks until a total dose of 1500 to 2000 mg/m² is achieved or until hematologic complications require a reduction of the doses. The drug treatment may be discontinued if the patient becomes worse from the tumor growth. Patients may be monitored for interstitial pulmonary fibrosis, a complication of this treatment.

Other chemotherapeutic agents are used. These include CCNU, a nitrosourea that can be given in a single oral dose of 120 to 130 mg/m² body surface area at 6 to 8 week intervals (Wilson, Levin, & Hoshino, 1982). Procarbazine (a cell cycle nonspecific agent) does cross the blood-brain barrier. Vincristine does not cross it and is of limited use (Wilson et al., 1982). Diaziquone (Aziridinylbenzoquinone, AZQ) has been found to have a specific effect on tumor cell mitochondria. Cisplatin appears to affect the cytoskeleton of the cell.

Clinical worsening may occur in some patients early in their treatment with chemotherapy. This occurs as a result of effective therapy when tumor cells die and lysed cells produce adjacent edema. The brain is inefficient in disposing of these dead cells (Levin & Wilson, 1978).

Immunotherapy

The need for a specialized class of lymphocytes that can kill glial tumor cells has led to the discovery of autologous lymphocytes activated by interleukin 2 (IL 2) that are capable of destroying autologous tumor cells (Kornblith, et al., 1987). Autologous cells are used in an attempt to boost the inadequate biologic defenses of patients with gliomas. Interferon has been used with patients who have gliomas. Some positive results were seen. Further evaluation is needed.

Corticosteroid Therapy

Corticosteroids are used in patients who have CNS tumors and are effective in reducing the peritumoral edema (Jellinger, 1987). Recurrent malignant astrocytoma, for example, is often very sensitive to high-dose corticosteroid therapy (up to 100 mg of dexamethasone or 500 mg of methylprednisolone per day). There appears to be no direct oncolytic effect on the tumor per se (Salcman & Kaplan, 1986).

Palliative Therapy

Palliative treatment includes ventricular drainage—ventriculoperitoneal, ventriculocisternal, for example.

An Ommaya reservoir can be implanted in a tumor resection cavity or ventricle and can be used for intrathecal administration of cytostatic drugs (Voth, 1987). See Chapter 22 for a more in-depth discussion of the Ommaya reservoir.

Factors Affecting the Outcome of Treatment

The prognosis for a person with a malignant brain tumor is not a good one in most instances. However, there are certain variables that affect the eventual outcome. The first is the histology of the tumor. The more aggressive tumors have a poorer prognosis. Glioblastoma multiforme grow rapidly, and long-term survival is virtually nonexistent. Low-grade astrocytomas, however, often have a survival of considerably more than 5 years.

The second factor is the age of the patient at diagnosis. In adults, the younger patients are better able to withstand surgery and follow-up treatment. Their bodies may even utilize therapy more advantageously. The very young, under 3 or 4 years of age, are sometimes at a disadvantage because they may not be given as high a dose of radiation therapy.

Third, the higher the patient's performance or Karnofsky rating, the better the chance of doing well and surviving longer. Individuals who are debilitated and have severe neurologic deficits tolerate treatments with more difficulty. They are more susceptible to medical complications that may limit therapy.

Finally, the extent of surgical resection may influence the time to tumor progression. An extensive tumor resection decreases tumor burden, which may improve or limit the patient's neurologic deficits and thereby improve the patient's performance rating. It also allows for more effective radiation and chemotherapy. Although there is no way to predict how any given individual will respond to therapy or how long that person will survive, the previously mentioned factors can play a role in determining the answers.

SPINAL CORD TUMORS

Definition and Incidence

Primary tumors of the spinal cord have almost the same cell composition as intracranial tumors. However, the incidence of spinal cord tumors is vastly different. Both primary and metastatic cord tumors are less common than cerebral tumors, with an occurrence of 1:7 to 1:10, depending on the population studied (Batzdorf & Selch, 1985). The percentage of each tumor type also is different. Furthermore, the primary cord tumors tend to grow more slowly than their intracranial counterparts, thus providing the possibility for excellent survival with extensive and vigorous microsurgery.

One similarity among CNS tumors relates to their location within bony structures. The spinal cord is contained within the bony vertebral column, just as the brain is contained within the skull, with little room for displacement. A small mass (1 to 10 g) may result in extensive dysfunction. Tumor growth creates a neuro-oncologic emergency with impending cord compression. Inattention invariably results in progressive paralysis, whereas prompt action may prevent or lessen such drastic effects.

Anatomically, tumors of the spinal cord are classified in relation to the dura. Extradural tumors are usually secondary, or metastatic, in nature, but sarcoma, lymphoma, myeloma, and choloroma occur as well. Intradural tumors may be of the cord itself, that is, intramedullary, or they may develop on the nerve roots or coverings of the cord, in which case they are called extramedullary. Tumors located in the substance of the cord are usually gliomas, including both astrocytomas and ependymomas. These present difficult problems in surgical removal. However, the extramedullary lesions are often removable when situated on the nerve roots (e.g., neurofibroma) or associated with the coverings (e.g., meningiomas). Walker (1982) provides a summary of spinal neoplasms by location and origin based on three reported series (Table 39–8).

Looking specifically at the incidence of primary spinal cord tumors by type, Wilson (1977) notes that meningiomas occupy first place, accounting for approximately 30 per cent of all tumors. Nerve sheath tumors follow closely with an incidence of 25 per cent. Gliomas account for 15 to 20 per cent of spinal cord tumors, and the remainder, such as congenital and vascular tumors, are comparatively uncommon. Incidence by site shows that the thoracic region accounts for approximately half of spinal cord tumors because the thoracic canal is long; there is a predilection of meningiomas for the thoracic spine; and finally, the thoracic spine lies in close proximity to the mediastinum, thus providing for direct extension of tumors from mediastinal lymph nodes that are involved in metastatic carcinomas of the breast and lung as well as lymphomas. The cervical and lumbar regions contain about equal proportions of the remaining occurrences, with the sacrum being involved only rarely.

Etiology and Epidemiology

For the most part, as noted by Batzdorf and Selch (1985), nothing is known about the etiology of spinal

Table 39–8. LOCATION AND ORIGIN OF SPINAL NEOPLASM

Location and Origin	Percentage of All Cases
I. Extradural (45%)	
A. Metastatic (solid tumors)	25
B. Sarcoma	7
C. Lymphoma	4
D. Myeloma, chloroma	5
E. Other	4
II. Intradural (55%)	
A. Extramedullary (33%)	
1. Neurofibroma	12
2. Meningioma	15
3. Congenital tumors (epidermoid 3.6%)	5
4. Other	1
B. Intramedullary (22%)	
1. Glioma (ependymoma 5.3%, astrocytoma 4.7%)	14
2. Vascular tumors	6
3. Other	2

(From Walker, M. [1982]. Brain and peripheral nervous system tumors. In J. F. Holland & E. Frei, III [Eds.], *Cancer medicine* [p. 1625]. Philadelphia: Lea & Febiger. Reproduced by permission.)

cord tumors, and the considerations related to ongoing research as discussed with respect to cerebral tumors apply. Primary spinal tumors have been associated with central von Recklinghausen's disease, and thus genetic influences are recognized for this tumor type.

The epidemiology of spinal cord tumors has not been studied separately from that of other CNS tumors. However, Levin and Wilson (1978) point out that meningiomas exhibit a striking dominance in females, arising at both the foramen magnum and the thoracic spine. Reports on the original primary site of metastatic tumors have been varied and tend to reflect the hospital population studied and the relative aggressiveness of palliative treatment of systemic cancer. One report from a large brain tumor service (Levin & Wilson 1978) noted that almost 10 per cent of spinal tumors originated from an intracranial primary CNS tumor. The majority were related to spinal subarachnoid seeding from medulloblastoma, with ependymoma, malignant astrocytoma, and germinoma following in that order.

Natural History, Pathology, and Diagnosis

A tumor produces its effects on the cord or nerve roots in several ways that affect the clinical features of disease. Pathologically, the tumor may act by direct pressure on the neural elements; by interference with circulation; by pressure on veins or arteries of the pia; and, less commonly, by numerous extradural venous occlusions, that is, by metastatic infiltration or extradural encirclement. The *Manual for Staging Cancer* does not provide a staging guide for spinal tumors (Batzdorf & Selch, 1985).

The spinal canal itself is rigid and confining. Furthermore, there may be as little as 1 to 2 mm of space surrounding the normal cord. Nonetheless, the cord can adjust to a mass that grows slowly. It is common for cord tumors to grow slowly over several years, compressing the cord into a thin ribbon with minimal neurologic signs. In addition to speed of growth, softness of the tumor is an important factor in the type of damage to the spinal cord. A soft meningioma or neurinoma may have a consistency little different from that of the spinal cord. Slow growing, soft tumors allow for adjusting the circulation of the cord. With hard tumors, motion of the spine causes contusion and possible glial changes. Similarly, rapidly developing pressure, as in the case of malignant and metastatic tumors, is very poorly handled by the cord. According to Greenwood (1973), the cord apparently responds by swelling and choking itself off so that paralysis may be complete within a few hours.

Symptoms of spinal cord tumors relate to two effects: those that are local, indicating the tumor's location along the spinal axis, and those that are distal, indicating the remote effects of involvement of motor and sensory long tracts within the spinal cord. Local spinal pain can be an important clue in making an early diagnosis, especially in metastatic tumors. Pain usually precedes progressive neurologic deficit. Such pain may be relatively diffuse over the involved area of the spine, but it often has a radicular component if one or more nerve roots are compressed, stretched, or infiltrated by the tumor. Radicular pain is encountered in the extremities or may be perceived as a band-like pain across the dermatomes of the trunk. Distention of the dura from intradural or intramedullary tumors causes pain, but this pain is rarely as severe as that with extradural and extramedullary tumors.

Neurologic manifestations include motor and sensory deficits as well as loss of sphincter control. Sensory abnormalities usually are due to pressure on long tracts, but occasionally they may be due to involvement of the posterior horns or substantia gelantinosa. This difference is reflected in symptoms of, and eventual recovery from, loss of position sense. Motor weakness commonly begins unilaterally and develops asymmetrically, although with severe cord compression, the deficit tends to become symmetric. More generally, a characteristic motor weakness is noted, which is spastic if the tumor lies above the conus medullaris or flaccid if it is at or below the conus. Motor weakness is accompanied by sensory impairment that begins in the feet.

Greenwood (1973) points out that cerebellar involvement is too often ignored in tumors of the spinal cord. Ataxia and hypotonia may be marked, or the patient's gait may be only slightly unstable, but he or she is unable to jump, hop, or stand on one foot. Deep tendon reflexes are usually hyperactive, plantar responses become extensor responses, and superficial abdominal reflexes disappear. However, patients with diffuse meningeal involvement of the cauda equina or individual nerve roots often show loss of deep tendon reflexes that are associated with pain and weakness. Batzdorf and Selch (1985) note that sphincter problems are more common as an early sign of an intramedullary tumor. The clinician is alert to suspect spinal cord or cauda equina compression in a patient known to have cancer who develops an acute urinary retention.

The evolution of motor and sensory loss can follow a common pattern that has two elements: (1) a distinct segmental loss at the level of involvement, and (2) a dysfunction below the level of the lesion. In determining the level of deficit, it is noted that the cord level, below the atlas and axis in the cervical and thoracic areas, will be approximately two levels above the vertebral level. This is because the skeleton grows more rapidly than the spinal cord elongates. Furthermore, the spinal cord ends at L1–2, and, therefore, the lumbar spinal segments are found between T11–12 and the sacral segments at L1–2. Below this point is the cauda equina.

In addition to the common pattern, as is the case with any spinal cord dysfunction, many variations are possible. For example, occasionally the major pressure effect is exerted by contrecoup with a very soft tumor on one side of the cord compressing the spinal cord against the harder bone on the opposite side, thus producing symptoms contralateral to the lesion (Greenwood, 1973). Lateral compression of the cord may cause a partial Brown-Séquard syndrome, with loss of motor function, vibration perception, and position sense below and on the side of the lesion, as well as contralateral loss of pain and temperature sensation (Walker, 1982).

Diagnosis can usually be made with a high degree of accuracy on the basis of a detailed history and neurologic examination. Currently the use of CT scan and MRI complements the diagnostic value of plain radiographs and myelography. Spinal column films can demonstrate bony destruction or vertebral collapse, and vertebral lytic or blastic lesions are evident in 80 per cent of metastatic spinal tumors. In the majority of spinal tumors, myelography indicates not only the tumor's location within the spinal axis but also its relationship to the dura and spinal cord. Computed tomographic scanning in conjunction with metrizamide myelography is a particularly useful diagnostic tool. Magnetic resonance imaging has rapidly become a definitive test for delineating the extent of spinal lesions and their anatomic categories because of its ability to image through bone and to provide detailed views of soft tissue changes.

Treatment

Treatment is determined by tumor type and location in relationship to the spinal cord and dura. If a lesion is likely to be of a primary type, then surgical resection or at least biopsy is usually indicated (Kornblith, et al., 1987). Microsurgery is used, and laser and ultrasonic suction has proved to be of value as well. Preservation of sensory and motor functions can be aided by the intraoperative use of spinal cord–evoked potentials. Incomplete removal of primary tumors is often followed by postoperative radiotherapy. Chemotherapy has not yet shown consistent results.

Medical management of secondary tumors is largely determined by the origin of the tumor, the presence of other metastatic sites, and the general condition of the patient. In general, external-beam irradiation is the treatment of choice (Kornblith, et al., 1987). In a patient known to harbor a tumor highly responsive to radiotherapy, chemotherapy, or both, the spinal metastasis should be treated by one or both of these measures on an emergency basis. Surgical intervention for rapid decompression is employed for a patient evidencing acute spinal cord compression with quickly evolving dysfunction. Surgery may also be indicated for a patient with a radioresistant tumor.

In discussing the prognosis of spinal cord tumors, two major factors must be considered: (1) preservation and restoration of neural function and (2) local tumor control and survival. Prognosis for recovery of neural function is inversely proportional to the severity of the deficit at the time of therapy and the duration of neurologic symptoms. A slow-growing tumor generally has a better prognosis. Total tumor removal is possible in most spinal neurofibromas and meningiomas. However, residual tumor foci may result in recurrences. Metastatic spinal tumors are not amenable to total resection, and other types of tumor vary considerably in this regard.

Batzdorf and Selch (1985) comment as follows about these variations: primary intraparenchymatous tumors may or may not lend themselves to total removal. Intraspinal ependymomas often can be totally removed surgically, but total removal is rarely accomplished with astrocytomas; ependymomas may recur, although usually after a long period of time. Finally, these same authors note that primary malignant gliomas of the spinal cord have a poor prognosis for survival. Most patients live less than 2 years after combined surgery and radiation therapy.

With metastatic tumors of the spinal cord, death likely results from the primary condition. Primary spinal cord tumors usually cause death by one of two mechanisms. High cervical cord tumors, that is, those at or above C4 level, may produce respiratory embarrassment, whereas tumors growing lower in the cord more often lead to chronic urinary tract disease.

NURSING CARE FOR PATIENTS WITH CENTRAL NERVOUS SYSTEM TUMORS

Caring for persons with tumors of the brain and spinal cord involves the full range of nursing knowledge and skill in neuroscience nursing, acute and long-term cancer care, rehabilitation, and care of the dying. Nursing has a long heritage of scientific and philosophic beliefs about the holism of the human being (Roy, 1988). The person is viewed as a perceiving, knowing, and feeling being who acts and relates with purposeful choice and values (Roy, 1982). The central nervous system is the key to these functions. Therefore, CNS tumors are seen as striking at the core of humanness and as having the most drastic effects on the person. Each unique human characteristic listed can be altered during the course of the diagnosis and treatment of the tumors. Accordingly, the challenges for nursing care are exceedingly complex.

This complexity can be approached by discussing the effects of central nervous system cancers and their treatment on the person and the family. The effects will differ and the types of nursing care required will change as human functions of the person change. The effects can be seen within what Roy (1984) refers to as modes of adaptation. For these patients, effects in the physiologic mode often require acute nursing care. The patient with a central nervous system tumor is dealing particularly with role changes during the rehabilitation and long-term care stages of illness. Effects on self and relationships are a prime concern in care of the dying patient.

Physiologic Effects: Acute Care

Tumors of the CNS have widespread physiologic effects that range from headaches and seizures to pain and incontinence. The implications of the physiologic effects for planning nursing care vary with the nature and course of the disease. Generally the phases of diagnosis and initial treatment of these tumors are times of significant physiologic change, and thus the demand for acute care nursing is high. This care involves symptom monitoring and control as well as family support and patient advocacy activities.

These tumors may be slow growing. For persons with glioblastoma multiforme, there is generally an average of 3 to 6 months of symptoms before diagnosis; for those with meningioma or acoustic neuroma, there may be as many as 15 years of symptoms. In these cases, patients and families bring a long history of vague complaints, such as headache or sensory changes, that have not been definitively diagnosed and treated. The suggestion of the diagnosis of a CNS tumor brings some relief that an answer at last may be found, together with the horror of what this diagnosis might mean. Few persons, whether lay persons or health care professionals, can perceive initially the full impact that such a diagnosis holds.

The importance of a primary care nurse in oncology for persons with tumors of the CNS is noted frequently. A nurse with good rapport can help the patient and family sort out the sequence of symptom development that is the key to an accurate history, which affects the choice of diagnostic tests as well as treatment. As treatment choices are made and carried out, the constant contact with a knowledgeable nurse can facilitate such decision making and can do much to restore "the morale of the patient's family unnerved by the shock of serious illness" (Greenwood, 1973).

For other patients, the onset of illness may be rapid. Seizures are not an uncommon presenting symptom of brain tumors, occurring in 30 to 40 per cent of patients with glioblastoma multiforme and in more than 66 per cent of patients with recurrent tumors. As brain tumors displace vital neural tissue, symptoms of increased intracranial pressure may occur with or without localization. Patients with frontal tumors may experience decreased levels of consciousness or sudden loss of affect. Occipital tumors will alter vision, and cerebellar tumors may cause ataxia. Patients with central hemisphere tumors and spinal cord tumors may present with a variety of motor and sensory changes. All of these symptoms are shocking and distressing to patients and to those around them. Again, the nurse can help determine the symptom pattern and sequence of development. From the beginning of the diagnostic studies, the nurse helps the patient and family plan for the future in a confident and realistic manner.

When a diagnosis of brain tumor or spinal cord tumor—even a potentially benign lesion—is made, the patient and family are justified in seeking a second opinion, especially when the course of treatment outlined by the surgeon seems too aggressive or not aggressive enough. There is little doubt that surgery is the treatment of choice; however, the surgical procedures recommended vary from a biopsy to an aggressive resection. Also to be considered are the postoperative treatments of irradiation and possibly chemotherapy.

Each individual, with the help and support of family

members, must make an informed decision, which, of course, is true regarding all forms of cancer treatment. Patients with brain tumors may not be competent or may have a limited capacity to make these decisions, however. Such symptoms as decreased levels of consciousness, dementia, aphasia, and behavioral or personality changes may make it difficult or impossible for the patient to have input. When a second opinion is obtained, those involved may receive a broader view of all that is involved. In an enlightened situation, a surgeon may have a team, including a nurse and social worker, who can help explain and counsel the patient and family. With the nurse's guidance and support, the final decision lies with the patient, family, and physicians.

Once a decision has been made to proceed with treatment, an informed consent or a series of consents must be obtained. It is an awesome responsibility to sign a consent for surgery on the brain or spinal cord and for subsequent irradiation and possibly chemotherapy. It becomes even more difficult for the patient, those responsible for the patient, and the health professional when the patient's judgment is questionable. Because of their location in the brain, some tumors may cause euphoria, decreased memory, or lack of ability to make well thought out decisions.

Often patients do not realize that their capacity is diminished and will insist on making decisions. The professionals working with these patients want them to take an active role in all aspects of treatment that will affect their life and health. Nurses particularly are prepared to value these goals. However, sometimes that is not possible, and others must assist both the patient and the doctor. In these cases, it is more crucial than ever that all treatments, side effects, and potential outcomes be explained carefully. The consent then can be signed by the patient and those responsible for the patient. When the nurse knows the patient and family over time, changes in mentation can be noted, and the patient's wishes at a time of higher level cognitive functioning may be represented effectively at a later time by the nurse. In extreme situations, it may be necessary to apply for medical power of attorney or to obtain a court order for permission to proceed with potentially life-saving surgery and therapy.

Nursing care of patients undergoing surgical treatment for CNS tumors and radiation procedures such as interstitial brachytherapy requires the practice of advanced neuro-oncology nursing. Some key features of this practice can be highlighted here. In preoperative teaching, the nurse discusses intravenous fluids, anesthesia, catheters, pain, medications, and the intensive care setting. In addition, unique details are added, such as instruction regarding head shaving. When health care workers spend many hours of the day on a neurosurgical unit, it is easy to forget how shocking a shaved head will look to the person and the family.

As in any preoperative situation, the nurse recognizes that learning is compromised by fear. In CNS surgery in particular, instruction requires careful assessment of the person's cognitive and emotional states as well as the crucial need for information. When

tumors of the CNS are secondary to a primary cancer, the patient also may need help in the maintenance of altered body function due to prior surgical treatment, for example, tracheostomy care, ileostomy-colostomy care, and the like.

Following surgery, there are three broad fields of nursing responsibility: daily needs, recognition of neurologic deterioration, and rehabilitation. The nurse provides for food, fluids, cleanliness, comfort, bladder and bowel care, and drug administration with an awareness of the neurologic disability attendant to the disease and its treatment and the consequent limitations and expectations of function. Early recognition of signs of progressive cerebral or spinal cord compression caused by postoperative hematoma is crucial. Neurologic checks that must be done at regular intervals include level of consciousness, blood pressure, pulse, respiration, and sensory and motor function. Complications of craniotomy that the neuro-oncology nurse is prepared to recognize and assist in managing include IICP from hemorrhage, edema, and obstruction of CSF flow; respiratory complications of atelectasis, pneumonia, and pulmonary embolism; wound infection and meningitis; dural fistulas; imbalances of fluids, electrolytes, and hormones; steroid insufficiency; seizures; and common surgical risks such as venous phlebitis, thrombophlebitis, abdominal distention, gastrointestinal ulceration, and urinary tract infection.

Neuro-oncology nurses at times will be responsible for radiation control and safety as patients undergo specialized procedures. Randall and colleagues (1987) describe the basic principles of exposure reduction—time, distance, and shielding—as they apply to brachytherapy applications. Special attention is given by the nurse to the comfort and relaxation to be provided to these patients, who must remain essentially alone in one room for more than 2 days. In addition, nurses working in these situations are vigilant in providing the information necessary to make a decision to remove the radiation source prematurely, for example, rapid deterioration in neurologic, cardiac, or respiratory status that warrants constant assessment, intervention, or both, or procedures that require contact with the patient for longer than 15 minutes in close proximity to the source, such as intubation or central line placement.

Effects on Roles: Rehabilitation and Long-Term Care

The drastic physiologic effects of CNS tumors cause great changes in what a person is able to do in life, that is the roles he or she can play. As neurologic symptoms appear, whether rapidly or slowly, and as treatment proceeds, the person shifts from being wife and mother, husband and father, sibling, son or daughter, person in the work force, or retiree to being a person in rehabilitation and long-term care.

These role changes are particularly dramatic in situations in which the patient is no longer able to make responsible decisions. A spouse or son or daughter may have to take on a more dominant role. This may mean a whole gamet of changes from doing all the driving to caring for the patient the way a parent cares for a child. The ability to drive an automobile seems to be considered a basic right in the United States. To take away that right, especially as it is symbolized by the possession of a state license, can generate open hostility and feelings of worthlessness for some people. However, seizure activity, visual field loss, lack of judgment, or motor paresis may mean the loss of ability to drive safely. In a highly mobile society, the majority of adult roles are restricted by an inability to drive or to manage alone on public transportation. Often at this time, the patient has even greater transportation needs that are related to chemotherapy schedules, follow-up medical evaluations, and so forth.

Children in the family are particularly vulnerable to the parent's role changes. It is difficult for a 2 or 3 year old to understand why the parent is not able to talk or is more intolerant of noise than usual. After that age, an explanation and a repeated reinforcement of that explanation may be helpful. When the patient is a child, family role problems may be magnified. The siblings may feel neglected because the mother or father is spending so much time with the sick child. Talking to a family therapist or a knowledgeable and caring professional can help.

For patients with CNS tumors, ongoing treatment involves rehabilitation that aims to restore and maintain function in regard to certain reasonable goals and to promote the maximum health possible. Rehabilitation nurses have expertise in providing care to individuals and groups with actual or potential disability that interrupts or alters function and life satisfaction. According to the Association of Rehabilitation Nurses, their specialized knowledge and clinical skills reflect the profound impact of disability on individuals and recognize its impact in the magnitude of disruption to physical, social, emotional, economic, and vocational status. Greenwood (1973) notes that after surgery for a CNS tumor, body and mental mobilization should be as rapid as the patient's limbs and mind will allow. The specialized skills of the physical and occupational therapists are of great importance, but the nurse provides both the coordination of the therapists' activities and often the challenge, motivation, and support that the patient needs.

After the drama of recovery from CNS surgery, it takes some refocusing to begin the long task of rehabilitation. Early return to familiar surroundings is encouraged to build the patient's ambition and determination necessary to regain maximum function and health. Although the resumption of as normal as possible a level of physical and intellectual activities is encouraged, return to work may be delayed lest minor temporary shortcomings damage the worker's reputation in the eyes of the employer. The nurse works with the patient, family members, and other associates to plan and implement the specific goals of rehabilitation.

Effects on Self and Relationships: Care of the Dying

All that has been written and said about the threat of malignant disease on the integrity of the person can certainly apply to persons with CNS tumors. In addition, these people suffer some unique threats to self and their relationships to others. Initially, patients fear that they are going to "lose their minds" or become "vegetables." Dementia and coma are very real aspects of many of these tumors.

It is probably those who fall between normality and coma who suffer most. These people and their families often become isolated from other family members and friends. It is hard for a friend to carry on a conversation with someone who cannot remember, may be acting slightly silly, or just cannot follow what is being said. Some friends will make the extra effort, but as time passes and the patient slowly deteriorates, even visits from these people might drop off. Often the patient does not realize what is happening, but the caregiver understands and may feel bitter. Familiar faces and routines can be important, and maintaining as normal an environment as possible can help to avoid the confusion and harm that can occur when the patient is isolated from others.

Throughout the course of CNS tumor disease, the nurse and the family assess when to initiate more support systems as patients move from an independent to a more dependent status, that is, as patients become less able to feed themselves, walk to the bathroom alone, get out of bed unaided, bathe, read, see, or swallow. The Karnofsky Rating Scale (Table 39–9) often is used to mark major changes in independent functioning.

It is not always easy for a spouse, an adult child, or a friend to relate to someone who is harboring a brain tumor. Children will have particular difficulty because of their limited understanding. Adults may resent the new duties that they have taken on because of the patient's illness at the same time that they grieve for the person whom they once knew but who has changed. All of those relating to the patient need much help and support. Generally, many cancer support groups are available in major population areas. However, most of these groups do not deal with the specific problems generated by CNS tumors. Sometimes families obtain more help from groups that deal with brain damage as opposed to cancer or from individual ther-

Table 39–9. KARNOFSKY RATING SCALE

100	Normal
90	Able to carry on normal activity; minor symptoms
80	Normal activity with effort; some symptoms
70	Cares for self; unable to carry on normal activity
60	Requires occasional assistance; cares for most needs
50	Requires considerable assistance and frequent care
40	Disabled; requires special care and assistance
30	Severely disabled; hospitalized
20	Very sick; active supportive treatment needed
10	Moribund

apists. Ideally, support groups would exist that focused on the problems faced by patients with malignant CNS tumors and their families.

Eventually most patients with malignant brain tumors will succumb to their disease, as will many patients with spinal cord tumors. With increasing frequency, patients at the terminal stage are being cared for at home. As a tumor increases in size, the amount of cerebral edema also increases. Treatment with steroids may delay this process and enhance the person's feeling of well-being for a time. Given the structure of the brain within the skull, edema eventually causes IICP and shift of vital structures. The terminal course is one of slowly decreasing level of consciousness and increasing neurologic deficits. As hemiparesis progresses to hemiplegia or dementia progresses to coma, the need is for more constant care. The caregiver's need for support and assistance also increases. Again, if there has been a neuro-oncology primary care nurse involved with the family, the nurse can provide much help and guidance, often by telephone.

In addition, providing information about home care services is important. An increasing number of agencies are offering services from full-time nurses or aides to respite time help. Hospices are also available with direct care services as well as support and advice. The person caring for a comatose patient may need to learn how to turn, suction, tube feed, and safely medicate the person. However, just as important is ensuring that caregivers receive support and respite so that they can be as effective as possible in providing that care. The family will benefit from these services throughout the acute and long-term or rehabilitative as well as terminal stages of the person's disease.

SUMMARY

In this chapter we have discussed tumors of the brain and spinal cord: their natural history, clinical features, diagnosis, and treatment. These particular disease processes have been noted to be complex and far-reaching in their effects on the person physiologically and in role functioning, self-concept changes, and relationships. Some key factors of nursing management at acute, long-term and rehabilitative, and dying stages have been highlighted, along with some notion of the range of advanced practice knowledge and skill that this care requires.

References

Adams, R. D., & Victor, M. (1985). Intracranial neoplasms. In R. D. Adams & M. Victor, *Principles of neurology* (pp. 474–509). New York: McGraw-Hill Book Co.

Batzdorf, U., & Selch, M. (1985). Brain tumors. In C. M. Haskell, *Cancer treatment* (2nd ed., pp. 653–687). Philadelphia: W. B. Saunders Co.

Beaney, R. P. (1986). Functional aspects of human brain tumors as studied by positron emission tomography. In N. M. Bleehen (Ed.), *Tumors of the brain* (pp. 63–82). New York: Springer-Verlag.

Butler, A. B., Brooks, W. H., & Netsky, M. G. (1982). Classification and biology of brain tumors. In J. R. Youmans (Ed.), *Neurological surgery* (Vol. 5, 2nd ed., pp. 2659–2701). Philadelphia: W. B. Saunders Co.

Butler, A. B., & Netsky, M. G. (1982). Classification and biology of brain tumors. In J. R. Youmans (Ed.), *Neurological surgery* (Vol. 3, 2nd ed., pp. 1297–1339). Philadelphia: W. B. Saunders Co. (Originally published 1973)

Cobb, C. A., & Youmans, J. R. (1982). Glial and neuronal tumors of the brain in adults. In J. R. Youmans (Ed.), *Neurological Surgery* (Vol. 5, 2nd ed., pp. 2759–2835). Philadelphia: W. B. Saunders Co.

Cohen, D. H., & Sherman, S. M. (1988). The nervous system and its components. In R. M. Berne & M. N. Levy (Eds.), *Physiology* (p. 74). St. Louis: C. V. Mosby Co.

Garroutte, B. (1981). *Survey of functional neuroanatomy* (p. 25). Greenbrae, CA: Jones Medical Publishers.

Greenwood, J., Jr. (1973). Spinal cord tumors. In J. R. Youmans (Ed.), *Neurological Surgery* (Vol. 3, 2nd ed., pp. 1514–1534). Philadelphia: W. B. Saunders Co.

Humphreys, R. P. (1982). Posterior cranial fossa brain tumors in children. In J. R. Youmans (Ed.), *Neurological Surgery* (Vol. 5, 2nd ed., pp. 2733–2785). Philadelphia: W. B. Saunders Co.

Jellinger, K. (1987). Pathology of human intracranial neoplasia. In K. Jellinger (Ed.), *Therapy of malignant brain tumors* (pp. 1–90). New York: Springer-Verlag.

Karnofsky, D. A., & Buchenal, J. H. (1949). The clinical evaluation of chemotherapeutic agents in cancer. In C. M. MacLeod (Ed.), *Evaluation of chemotherapeutic agents* (pp. 191–205). New York: Columbia University Press.

Kernohan, J. W., & Sayre, G. P. (1952). Tumors of the central nervous system. *Atlas of Pathology* (Section X, Fascicles 35 and 37). Washington, DC: Armed Forces Institute of Pathology.

Kornblith, P. L., Walker, M. D., & Cassady, J. R. (1987). *Neurologic oncology*. New York: J. B. Lippincott Co.

Kuffler, S. W., & Nicholls, J. G. (1976). *From neuron to brain* (pp. 9 & 258). Sunderland, MA: Sinauer Associates, Inc.

Levin, V. A., & Wilson, C. B. (1978). Clinical characteristics of cancer in the brain and spinal cord. In S. T. Crooke (Ed.), *Cancer for medical students* (Vol. 2, pp. 3–53). New York: Academic Press.

Morley, T. P. (1973). Intrinsic tumors of the cerebral hemispheres. In J. R. Youmans (Ed.), *Neurological Surgery* (Vol. 3, 2nd ed., pp. 1340–1387). Philadelphia: W. B. Saunders Co.

Paushter, D. M., Modic, M. T., Borkowski, G. P., Weinstein, M. A., & Zeman, R. K., (1984). Magnetic resonance: Principles and applications. *Medical Clinics of North America, 68,* 1393–1421.

Piepmeier, J. M. (1987). Observations on the current treatment of low-grade astrocytic tumors of the cerebral hemispheres. *Journal of Neurosurgery, 67,* 177–181.

Randall, T. M., Drake, D. K., & Sewchand, W. (1987). Neurooncology update: Radiation safety and nursing care during interstitial brachytherapy. *Journal of Neuroscience Nursing, 19,* 315–320.

Roy, C. (1982). Historical perspective of the theoretical framework for the classification of nursing diagnosis. In M. J. Kim & D. A. Moritz (Eds.), *Classification of nursing diagnoses.* New York: McGraw-Hill Book Co.

Roy, C. (1984). *Introduction to nursing: An adaptation model.* Englewood Cliffs, NJ: Prentice-Hall, Inc.

Roy, C. (1988). An explication of the philosophical assumptions of the Roy adaptation model. *Nursing Science Quarterly, 1,* 26–34.

Salcman, M., & Kaplan, R. S. (1986). Intracranial tumors in adults. In A. R. Moosa, M. C., Robson, & S. C. Schimpff (Eds.), *Comprehensive textbook of oncology* (pp. 617–629). Baltimore: Williams & Wilkins.

Voth, D. (1987). Neurosurgery of malignant brain tumors. In K. Jellinger (Ed.), *Therapy of malignant brain tumors* (pp. 91–129). New York: Springer-Verlag.

Walker, M. (1982). Brain and peripheral nervous system tumors. In J. F. Holland & E. Frei III (Eds.), *Cancer medicine* (pp. 1603–1629). Philadelphia: Lea & Febiger.

Wilson, C. B. (1977). Tumors of the central nervous system. In J. H. Horton & G. J. Hill (Eds.), *Clinical oncology* (pp. 588–617). Philadelphia: W. B. Saunders Co.

Wilson, C. B., Levin, V., & Hoshino, T. (1982). Chemotherapy of brain tumors. In J. R. Youmans (Ed.), *Neurological surgery* (Vol. 5, 2nd ed., pp. 2733–2758). Philadelphia: W. B. Saunders Co.

World Health Organization (1977). *Manual of the international statistical classification of diseases, injuries, and causes of death, 1975 revision*. Geneva: Author.

Zulch, K. J. (1979). *Histological typing of tumors of the central nervous system* (pp. 11–24, 43–62). Geneva: World Health Organization.

Zulch, K. J. (1986). *Brain tumors* (p. 15). New York: Springer-Verlag.

Skin Cancers

ALICE J. LONGMAN

Skin cancers are estimated to develop in more than 500,000 people annually, and they lead all other cancers in the rate of increase (American Cancer Society, 1988). Directly visible and easily accessible, skin cancers offer a unique opportunity for early detection, early diagnosis, early treatment, and cure (Gumport, Harris, Roses, & Kopf, 1981).

DEFINITION AND INCIDENCE

The vast majority of skin cancers are highly curable basal cell carcinomas and squamous cell carcinomas. The most serious skin cancer is malignant melanoma, which affects approximately 26,000 men and women each year. In the last 50 years, the incidence of malignant melanoma has increased 1000 per cent. At present, the incidence of malignant melanoma is increasing at the rate of 3.4 per cent each year. Skin cancers account for an estimated 7800 deaths per year—5800 from malignant melanoma and 2000 from other skin cancers (American Cancer Society, 1988). Skin cancer is not only a public health problem: it is also a rapidly worsening one.

SKIN STRUCTURE AND CARCINOGENESIS

The sun or, more precisely, ultraviolet radiation from the sun is the major etiologic factor in the development of skin cancer. Exposure to the sun and ultraviolet radiation has a cumulative effect; thus the signs of skin cancer appear years after the exposure (Berkman, 1985; Schleper, 1984; Stewart, 1987).

The epidermis is the outer layer of the skin, and the entire epidermis is replaced every 15 to 30 days (Stewart, 1987). Fibrous protein keratin, the end product of the maturing epidermal cells that make up the stratum

corneum, is found in the epidermis. Keratin's thickness in the stratum corneum varies, offering the greatest protection in areas such as the palms of the hands and the soles of the feet. Keratinocytes undergo changes in shape, structure, and composition as they are gradually pushed toward the surface in a continuing process (Berkman, 1985).

The inner layer of the epidermis, the stratum basalis, has basal keratinocytes. Interspersed within the basal cells are melanocytes, which synthesize the pigment melanin. Melanin, a brownish-black pigment, protects the epidermis and the superficial dermal vasculature. It does this by simultaneously activating previously synthesized melanin to produce tanning and activating the melanin production cycle to create delayed tanning. Pigment is nature's sunscreen, and the more a person has, the greater the protection (Fig. 40–1).

Basal cell carcinoma and squamous cell carcinoma are named for the cells from which they develop. Basal cells lie in the lowest part of the epidermis, which is the outermost layer of skin (see Color Figure 2). Most of the epidermis is composed of squamous cells. Ker-

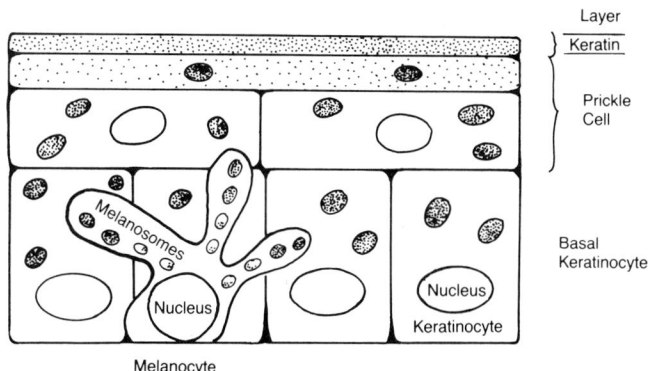

Figure 40–1. Schematic drawing of the epidermis. (Courtesy of James J. Nardlund, M.D. and the Skin Cancer Foundation. Berkman, J. [1985]. The skin remembers. *Cancer News, 39,* 2–4.)

Table 40–1. INCIDENCE, CLINICAL CHARACTERISTICS, AND COMMON SITES OF PRINCIPAL CUTANEOUS CANCERS

Incidence	Clinical Characteristics	Common Sites
Basal Cell Carcinoma Most common form of skin cancer; occurs primarily in persons exposed to prolonged or intense sunlight, especially Caucasians with light eyes, light hair, and fair complexions.	*Nodulo-ulcerative basal cell cancer:* Elevated lesions with umbilicated, ulcerated centers; raised waxy or "pearly" borders; moderately firm. *Superficial basal cell cancer:* Barely elevated plaques, usually with crusted and erythematous centers and raised, thread-like pearly borders; often multiple.	Nose, eyelids, cheeks, and trunks. Uncommon on palms and soles. Metastases are extremely rare.
Squamous Cell Carcinoma Less common than basal cell carcinoma; occurs primarily on areas exposed to actinic radiation and on vermilion border on lips.	Appearance varies from an elevated nodular mass to a punched-out ulcerated lesion to a fungating mass. Unlike basal cell carcinomas, squamous cell carcinomas are opaque.	75% occur on head, 15% on hands, and 10% elsewhere. Can metastasize to regional lymph nodes; in more advanced lesions, visceral (especially pulmonary) metastasis can occur.
Malignant Melanoma Far less common than basal or squamous cell carcinoma. Currently about 14,000 new cases per year in the United States.	Usually irregularly pigmented (black, gray, white, blue, brown, red); often less than 2.5 cm in diameter. May be flat or elevated, eroded or ulcerated; outline usually irregular, often with notch; frequently mildly symptomatic (e.g., pruritic).	Backs of men and women, legs of women, less common in areas unexposed to sun; metastasize via lymphatics and blood vessels, often first to regional lymph nodes.

(From Gumport, S. L., Harris, M. N., Roses, D. F., & Kopf, A. W. [1981]. The diagnosis and management of common skin cancers. *CA: A Cancer Journal for Clinicians, 31,* 79–90. Reproduced by permission.)

atinocytes reach the stratum spinosum or "prickle cell" layer and become elongated and flat. Within these cells, squamous cell carcinoma begins (see Color Figure 3). Malignant melanoma arises from pigment cells (see Color Figure 4).

Several age-related changes occur in the skin. The outer layer of the stratum corneum flattens and thins with age (Berliner, 1986a). Chemicals are able to pass through more easily. As subcutaneous fat decreases, skin elasticity, shape, and support are lost. The collagen fibers stiffen, and glutamic acid and lysine that are needed for elastin formation decrease. Wrinkles and sagging skin result. Changes in melanin production that occur account for changes in skin and hair color (Berliner, 1986b).

A spectrum of radiant electromagnetic energy is produced by the sun. Ultraviolet light is of the greatest photobiologic importance and is divided into wavelengths known as A, B, and C (Schleper, 1984; Stewart, 1987). The wavelengths emanating from the sun range from 200 nanometers (nm) to more than 18,000 nm (Stewart, 1987). The skin is damaged by ultraviolet radiation in the 200 to 400 nm range. Longer waves (320 to 400 nm) are known as ultraviolet A or UV-A; rays falling in a shorter range (290 to 320 nm) are ultraviolet B, or UV-B; and the shortest waves 200 to 290 nm) are ultraviolet C, or UV-C (Stewart, 1987). The worst damage to the skin in the form of short-term erythema and carcinogenesis following long-term exposure is attributed to UV-B. Ultraviolet C rays are largely filtered by the ozone layer in the stratosphere (Lawler & Schreiber, 1989; Stewart, 1987).

The skin responds to ultraviolet light by becoming reddened. The UV-A rays stimulate the cells to produce melanin. Other nearby cells begin dividing and making their way to the surface, carrying the melanin with them. Ultraviolet B rays dilate the blood vessels lying near the skin's surface. The reddening phase of sunburn is caused by the increased circulation of the blood to these injured vessels. Ultraviolet light continues to thicken and break down the network of supportive collagen and elastic fibers in the dermis (Berkman, 1985).

NONMELANOMA SKIN CANCERS

Basal cell carcinoma is the most common form of skin cancer (Gumport et al., 1981; Schleper, 1984). The actual incidence of basal cell carcinoma may be higher than reported because it may be treated as a problem of little consequence. Areas of the body that receive the greatest exposure to sunlight are the most common sites for basal cell carcinoma (Table 40–1).

The two major types of basal cell carcinoma are nodulo-ulcerative and superficial. Nodulo-ulcerative basal cell carcinoma is characterized by (1) an elevated lesion, (2) an umbilicated, ulcerated center with raised margins, and (3) a moderate firmness to the touch (Gumport et al., 1981; Longman, 1987; Schleper, 1984). The lesion has a pearly or waxy gleam (Fig. 40–2). Superficial basal cell carcinoma appears as a superficial, sharply marginated plaque with a raised, pearly, thread-like border. The center is usually crusted, scaly, and erythematous. There are often multiple lesions, and they frequently appear on the trunk of the body. Irregular local extension is the principal problem of management. Other less common types of basal cell carcinoma include the cystic and pigmented varieties (Gumport et al., 1981).

Squamous cell carcinoma is the predominant skin cancer in skin that has been exposed to ionizing radia-

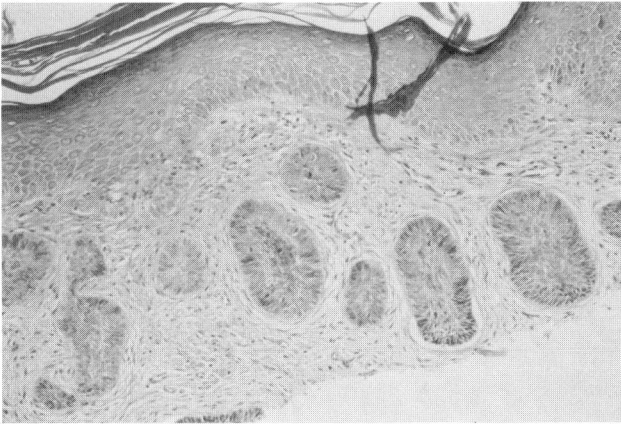

Figure 40–2. Basal cell carcinoma. (Courtesy of Libby Edwards, M.D.)

tion, carcinogenic chemicals, or trauma (see Table 40–1). Actinic keratosis is implicated in the development of squamous cell carcinoma and is considered a premalignant state. Bowen's disease is also considered an in situ squamous cell carcinoma.

The appearance of squamous cell carcinoma varies from an elevated, erythematous, nodular mass with varying amounts of scaling or crusting to an ulcerative lesion or fungating mass (Gumport et al., 1981; Longman, 1987; Schleper, 1984). In contrast to basal cell carcinomas, squamous cell carcinomas are opaque (Fig. 40–3). Squamous cell carcinomas may metastasize to the regional lymph nodes.

MALIGNANT MELANOMA

Malignant melanoma is potentially the most lethal of the skin cancers (see Table 40–1). Melanomas originate from melanocytes and more often than not from a nevus or mole (see Color Figure 5). Nevi or moles are aggregates of melanocytes that are present at birth (Friedman, Riegel, & Kopf, 1985; Goldsmith, 1979; Green et al., 1986; Lawler & Schreiber, 1989).

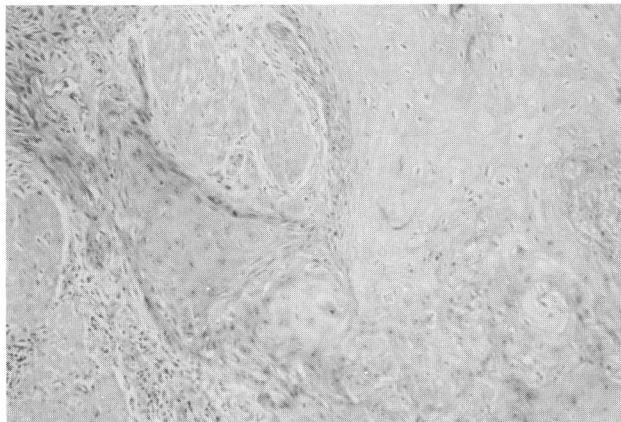

Figure 40–3. Squamous cell carcinoma. (Courtesy of Libby Edwards, M.D.)

Epidemiology

Several epidemiologic factors are important in the prevention and early diagnosis of malignant melanoma. The incidence and mortality rates of melanoma have risen dramatically in the last several decades. Evidence suggests that malignant melanoma is related to exposure to ultraviolet radiation. Precursor lesions such as dysplastic nevi and certain congenital melanocytic nevi give rise to malignant melanoma (Fraser & McGuire, 1984; Friedman et al., 1985; Houghton, 1987).

Ninety per cent of melanomas arise in the skin, and the rest develop in the eye and the mucous membranes of the mouth and anus (Fig. 40–4). The prognosis is good if the lesion is localized and thin. Prognosis depends on several features of the primary tumor: (1) depth of invasion, (2) anatomic site, (3) thickness, (4) presence or absence of ulceration, and (5) growth pattern. Another factor is the sex of the person with melanoma (Houghton, 1987), because steroid hormones may affect the etiology and behavior of the lesion.

CLASSIFICATION OF CUTANEOUS MELANOMAS

Cutaneous melanomas are classified as follows:

1. Lentigo maligna melanoma. This type of melanoma is the slowest growing and least aggressive. It most often occurs in a premalignant lesion.

2. Nodular melanoma. This type of melanoma is extremely aggressive and metastasizes rapidly unless treated early. It may occur on any part of the body.

3. Superficial spreading melanoma. This is the most common type of melanoma. It develops as a slower growing, pigmented, macular lesion and often has red, blue, or white areas.

4. Acral-lentiginous melanoma. This variety develops as a growing pigmented lesion on the palms of the hand, on the soles of the feet, and under the nails. It is commonly seen in blacks, Hispanics, and Orientals (Friedman et al., 1985; Houghton, 1987; Schleper, 1984).

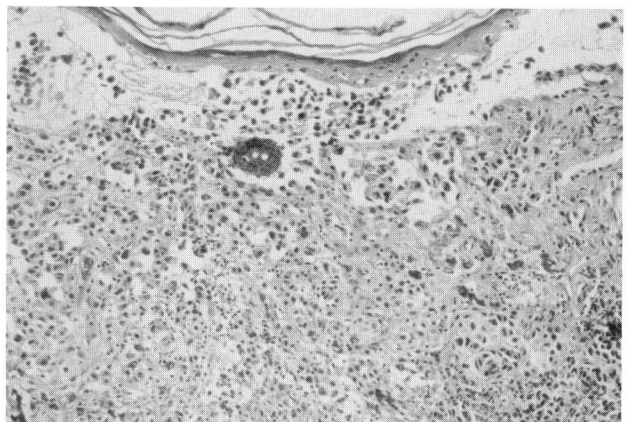

Figure 40–4. Malignant melanoma. (Courtesy of Libby Edwards, M.D.)

The characteristic features of early malignant melanoma are similar. They can be remembered by thinking of A B C D: *A* for asymmetry, *B* for border irregularity, *C* for color variegation, and *D* for diameter (Friedman et al., 1985). Early lesions tend to grow asymmetrically. As the melanocytes in early melanoma extend horizontally within the epidermis in an uncontrolled fashion, the borderline of early lesions is irregular and exhibits characteristic notching or scalloping. Early lesions appear as flat and pigmented with various tones of brown. Layering of melanin is uneven, which results in color variegation. The diameter is usually greater than 6 mm. The earlier the diagnosis of malignant melanoma, the higher the survival rate (Gumport et al., 1981; Houghton, 1987).

RISK FACTORS ASSOCIATED WITH NONMELANOMA SKIN CANCERS

Ultraviolet radiation from sunlight (UV-B spectral range, 290 to 320 nm) is the major risk factor in the development of skin cancers. The increase in the incidence of skin cancers among Caucasians can be attributed in part to changes in life style with subsequent changes in clothing styles, ideas about sunbathing and tanning, and alterations in the ozone layer of the atmosphere (Frank-Stromborg, 1985, 1986; Lawler & Schreiber, 1989; Schleper, 1984; Stair, 1985). Thus prolonged exposure to ultraviolet radiation from the sun is the major exogenous factor in the development of nonmelanoma skin cancers and melanoma.

Other exogenous factors related to the development of squamous cell carcinoma in particular are exposure to ionizing radiation; chemical carcinogens; and petroleum, including coal, tar, pitch, and creosote preparations. Radiologists and uranium miners are at occupational risk for skin cancer, as are individuals who received small repeated doses of radiation for the treatment of acne. Chemical carcinogens include arsenicals in agriculture sprays, psoralens for the treatment of psoriasis, and chemical fumes and burns from molten metals. A history of repeated trauma or chronic infection such as topical ulcers or burns resulting in scarification also predisposes an individual to skin cancer (Fraser & McGuire, 1984; Longman, 1987; Stair, 1985).

Endogenous factors in the development of skin cancer include fair or freckled complexion; red, blond, or light brown hair; light-colored eyes, xeroderma pigmentosum or albinism; and immunodeficiency or suppression. Those at risk because of immunodeficiency or suppression include individuals who have received renal or heart transplants and patients with lymphoproliferative carcinomas (White, 1986b).

Premalignant states or lesions have been described as placing persons at risk for squamous cell carcinoma and are as follows:

1. Actinic and senile keratosis. These lesions are usually found on sun-exposed skin such as the head, neck, hands, and arms. The lesions are slightly elevated, well circumscribed, and reddened with a rough or scaly surface. Malignant transformation is slow and rare.

2. Seborrheic keratosis. The lesion is benign, brownish, sharp in delineation, and flat and can arise from indolent warts. Malignant transformation is rare.

3. Arsenic keratosis. The lesions appear as hard, corn-like areas on the palms of the hands or the soles of the feet and appear to be surrounded by warts. Associated skin surfaces may be diffusely pigmented. Malignant transformation is rare.

4. Bowen's disease. The lesion may appear on any part of the body as a single, slightly raised papule that gradually increases in size. It is superficial and red and eventually crusts but does not heal completely. This lesion is referred to as squamous cell carcinoma in situ (Caldwell, McCormack, Goldsmith, & Rubin, 1983; Schleper, 1984; White, 1986b).

RISK FACTORS FOR MALIGNANT MELANOMA

Exposure to ultraviolet radiation is thought to be the major risk factor for malignant melanoma (Fraser & McGuire, 1984; Friedman et al., 1985; Lawler & Schreiber, 1989). Evidence indicates that the incidence of melanoma is highest in areas receiving the greatest sunlight exposure, such as the "sunbelt" states. There is also speculation that malignant melanoma may be due to intense, intermittent exposure to ultraviolet radiation rather than prolonged exposure. Other factors increasing the risk of developing malignant melanoma are family history of the disease, presence of melanocytic nevi, light complexion, history of sunburns, and susceptible age (Friedman et al., 1985; Lawler & Schreiber, 1989).

Two types of acquired nevi are also implicated in the development of malignant melanoma: commonly acquired nevi, which rarely become malignant, and dysplastic nevi, which sometimes become malignant (Fraser & McGuire, 1984; McGuire, 1984, 1985). Commonly acquired nevi are aggregates of melanocytes, which become most noticeable during the middle years. Caucasian adults have approximately 25 to 40 commonly acquired nevi located mainly on skin above the waist. These moles are small (less than 5 mm), round, and uniformly tan or brown. Dysplastic nevi are often larger than 5 mm; irregular in shape; and mixtures of tan, brown, black, and red or pink. They occur most commonly on the back but do appear on the scalp, breasts, and buttocks. Dysplastic nevi occur as a result of atypical cell development in the melanocytes. A newly recognized precancerous mole pattern, dysplastic nevus syndrome, is confirmed when irregular, variably pigmented moles appear and dysplasia is verified by biopsy specimens (Fraser & McGuire, 1984). Two subtypes of dysplastic nevus syndrome have been described: the familial variant and the sporadic variant. The familial variant affects persons who may or may not have melanoma but have a family history for dysplastic nevi, malignant melanoma, or both (Box 40–1). Those individuals who may or may not have

---

Box 40–1. GENE MAPPING

Bale, S. J., Dracopoli, N. C., Tucker, M. A., Clark, W. H., Jr., Fraser, M. C., Stanger, B. Z., Green, P., Donis-Keller, H., Housman, D. E., & Greene, M. H. (1989). **Mapping the gene for hereditary cutaneous malignant melanoma-dysplastic nevus to chromosome 1p.** *New England Journal of Medicine, 320,* 1367–1372.

Researchers from the National Cancer Institute, Massachusetts Institute of Technology, and the University of Pennsylvania School of Medicine have identified the location of the gene responsible for familial malignant melanoma with the use of molecular genetic techniques and multipoint linkage analysis. Six melanoma-prone families, 99 relatives, and 26 spouses underwent full-skin examinations for the presence of dysplastic nevi and melanoma. Biopsy specimens obtained before and during the study were reviewed as were blood specimens for Rh typing, lymphocyte separation, and direct DNA extraction.

To isolate the gene location, the DNA from the participants was evaluated to analyze the area of chromosome 1 thought to contain the melanoma gene. The researchers then measured how often a crossover event of DNA occurred between an individual's two copies of chromosome 1 during meiosis.

Little recombination between the gene for malignant melanoma was found. On further evaluation, it was determined that the most likely location for the malignant melanoma gene was between these two points. A starting point has been established for investigators to use molecular techniques to identify the melanoma gene and characterize its function. The information should assist in the understanding of the causes of familial melanoma.

---

melanoma and have no family history of dysplastic nevi, melanoma, or both are included in the sporadic subtype (Greene et al., 1986).

NURSING IMPLICATIONS

Oncology nurses have unique opportunities to expand public awareness of the long-term effects of sun exposure on the skin. Formal and informal activities have been described in the literature (Nevidjon, 1986; Ramstack, White, Hazelkorn, & Meyskens, 1986). Knowledge about exposure of the skin to sunlight, different types of skin, and systematic and periodic skin assessment is important if nurses are to make an impact on the prevention and early detection of skin cancers.

ASSESSMENT OF SKIN EXPOSURE

Several factors are important in assessing the impact of exposure to sunlight on skin. These include time of day during exposure, geographic area, altitude and weather conditions, time of year, and length of exposure (Lawler & Schreiber, 1989; Schleper, 1984). Ultraviolet rays are more direct from 10:00 A.M. to 2:00 P.M., and caution should be exercised during this time of day. On a cloudy day, roughly 70 to 80 per cent of the UV-B rays penetrate the clouds and reach the earth. Various surfaces such as snow, water, and sand reflect the sun's rays. Additionally, there are more direct rays from May to October. Certain areas of the world receive sun all year long; in the United States, areas roughly south of a horizontal line from North Carolina to southern California are affected. Those who live or vacation in higher altitudes should be alerted to the fact that there is less atmosphere to filter out the UV-B rays. In tropical areas, more UV-B rays reach the earth. Thus caution should be exercised in relation to sun exposure in these areas.

SKIN TYPES AND SUN PROTECTION

A person's skin type is determined by genetic history and pigmentation and erythema histories (Anders & Leach, 1983; Berkman, 1985). Six sun reaction types have been described (Table 40–2). Knowledge of an individual's skin type determines both natural protection and response to the sun. The minimal erythema dose, or the amount of time unprotected skin can be exposed to sunlight before reddening occurs, is useful in determining sun protection factor needs. The development of sunscreens and sunblocks has made it possible to decrease solar damage to the skin (Table 40–3). Recommendations for the use of sunscreens include the use of commercial sunscreens with a sun protection factor of greater than 10, for example, PreSun and Pabanol; the use of commercial sunblocks that have the active ingredients of titanium dioxide, zinc oxide, talc, iron oxide, and kaolin; and the reapplication of sunscreen every 2 to 3 hours during long sun exposure. For those taking thiazides, sulfonamides, or other photosensitizing drugs, sunscreens containing benzophenones are recommended.

EXAMINATION OF THE SKIN

Complete and thorough examination of the skin is important and to be encouraged if early detection is to become a reality (Friedman et al., 1985). The examination should be systematic and done annually by physicians or nurses. Self-examination of the skin should be performed monthly in a well-lighted area. The following procedure is recommended:

1. Inspect and palpate all accessible skin surfaces including smooth skin, skin folds, mucosal surfaces, and epidermal appendages.

2. Assess preexisting lesions of the skin, such as moles, freckles, warts, birthmarks, and scars.

3. Inspect the scalp and entire hairline and palpate the scalp.

Table 40–2. HOW TO DETERMINE SKIN TYPE AND PHOTOPROTECTION NEEDS

Skin Type	UV-B/MED mJ/cm	Pigmentation/Erythema History	Genetic History
I	10–20	Has a very poor ability to tan; burns easily and severely, then peels	Very fair skin, freckling evident Blue, green, grey eye color Blond, red, or brown hair Unexposed skin is white
II	20–30	Tans minimally or lightly following exposure, usually burns easily, resulting in a painful burn	Fair skin, unexposed skin is white Blue, green, grey, or brown eye color Blond, red, or brown hair
III	30–40	Tans gradually following exposure, burns moderately	"Average" Unexposed skin is white Hair and eye color usually brown
IV	40–50	Burns minimally, tans well with initial exposure	White or light brown skin Unexposed skin is white or light brown Dark hair and eye color (Mediterraneans, Orientals, Hispanics)
V	50–60	Tans easily and profusely, rarely burns	Brown skin, unexposed skin is brown (American Indian, East Indian, Hispanic)
VI	50–60	Deeply pigmented, never burns	Black skin, unexposed skin is black (African and American blacks, Australian and South Indian Aborigines)

A skin type is determined by assessing the person's history of reaction to noonday sun in June following a period of minimal solar exposure. Exposure to 20 to 30 min of natural sunlight in June at sea level equals 15 to 25 ml/cm^2 of UV-B. MED, minimal erythema dose.
(From Anders, J. E., & Leach, E. E. Sun versus skin. © 1983, *American Journal of Nursing, 83,* 1015–1020. Reprinted by permission.)

4. Inspect the face, lips, and neck, including the posterior neck and postauricular areas.

5. Inspect and palpate all surfaces of the upper extremities.

6. Inspect and palpate the skin of the back, buttocks, and back of legs.

7. Inspect the external genitalia. In women, the skin folds of the labia and perineum should be separated to adequately view the surfaces. Men should inspect all sides of the penis and scrotal sac.

8. Inspect and palpate the anterior surfaces of the legs and feet.

9. Inspect and palpate all hairy surfaces, including those beneath axillary, thoracic, and pubic hair.

10. Note the characteristics of normal moles.

With practice, skin self-examination can be accomplished quickly and easily. Guidelines are available from the American Cancer Society, the National Cancer Institute, and the Skin Cancer Foundation.

CLINICAL FEATURES, DIAGNOSIS, AND PROGNOSIS

Because most skin cancers are highly visible on the exposed surfaces of the body, early signs can be

Table 40–3. GUIDE TO SUN PROTECTION

Degree of Protection	Sun Protection Factor	Examples of Sunscreens
Minimal sun protection	2 to 4	Coppertone Dark Tanning
Moderate sun protection	4 to 6	Sea & Ski Golden Tan
Extra sun protection	6 to 8	Maxafil
Maximal sun protection	8 to 15	PreSun 8
Ultra sun protection	15 or more	Sundown 15 Ultra Protection

detected readily. Early signs of nonmelanoma skin cancer are (1) a sore that does not heal, (2) a persistent lump or swelling, and (3) changes in skin markings (Caldwell et al., 1983; Gumport et al., 1981). These changes in skin markings are related to size, color, surface, shape, surrounding skin, sensation, and elevation (see Table 40–1). Late signs include a roughened area of skin that scabs over, rescabs, and fails to heal and a persistent ulcer. A confirmed tissue diagnosis is essential to definitive treatment. With adequate treatment, basal cell carcinoma is highly curable (90 to 95 per cent). Squamous cell carcinoma is also highly curable (75 to 80 per cent), but the recurrence of lesions is the major complication. The tumor may metastasize to the lymph nodes.

The characteristic clinical features of malignant melanoma are related to changes in skin markings. These include changes in color, size, shape, elevation, surface, surrounding skin, sensation, and consistency (Table 40–4). Although there is variegation in color change, red or black, or both, are the most significant. Enlargement of a mole with concurrent changes in surface and shape is noteworthy. If the mole is already black, there may be a new raised area, which creates a high index of suspicion for malignant melanoma (Friedman et al., 1985; Meyskens, 1984). The appearance of new moles is also of critical importance. The association between thickness of the lesion and survival is strong. Persons who have thin (less than 0.76 mm) melanoma lesions have a high cure rate (95 to 100 per cent) following removal of the melanoma (Friedman et al., 1985; Meyskens, 1984). Thus the most important prognostic feature of malignant melanoma is the size of the lesion at the time of its removal. Special considerations associated with maligant melanoma are primary melanoma of the eye, primary mucosal mela-

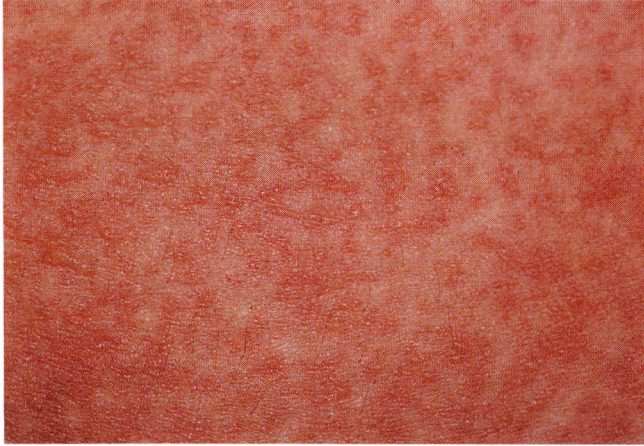 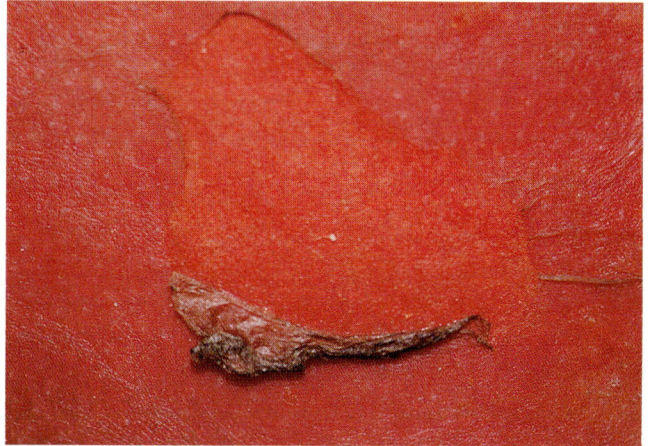

A

B

Color Figure 1. Typical raised maculopapular rash on a patient with severe skin graft-versus-host disease on day 34 after bone marrow transplantation *(A)*, which progressed to skin sloughing by day 46 *(B)*.

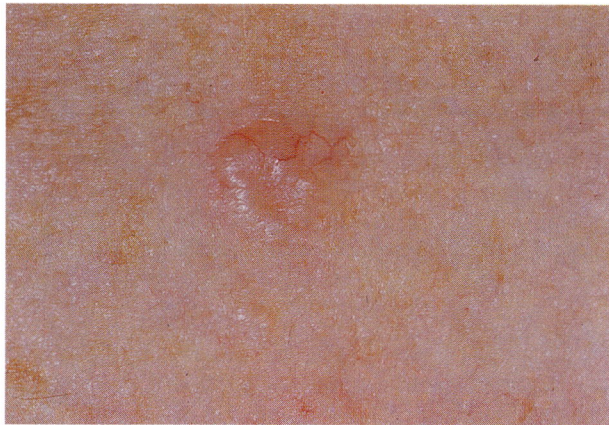

Color Figure 2. Basal cell carcinoma. (Courtesy of Anna Graham, M.D.)

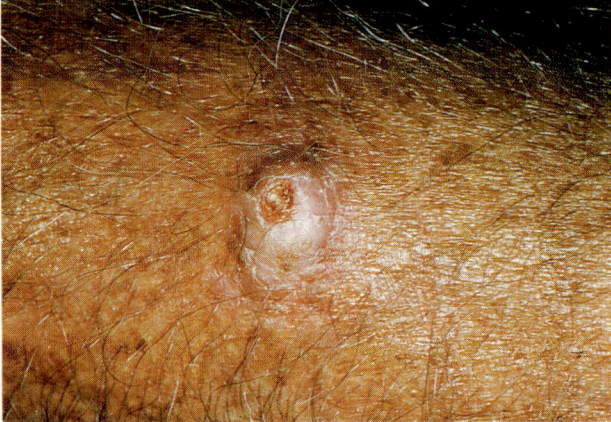

Color Figure 3. Squamous cell carcinoma. (Courtesy of Anna Graham, M.D.)

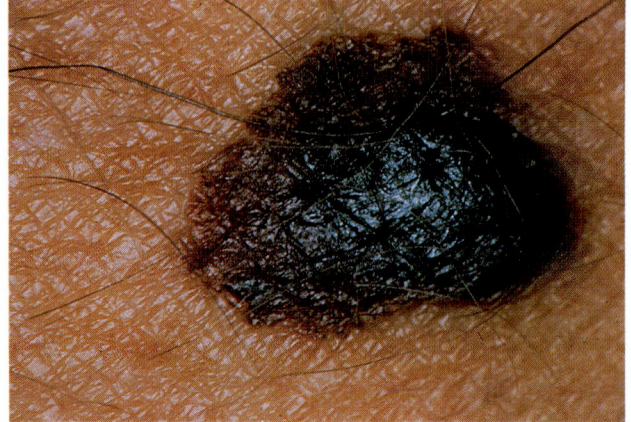

Color Figure 4. Malignant melanoma. (Courtesy of Anna Graham, M.D.)

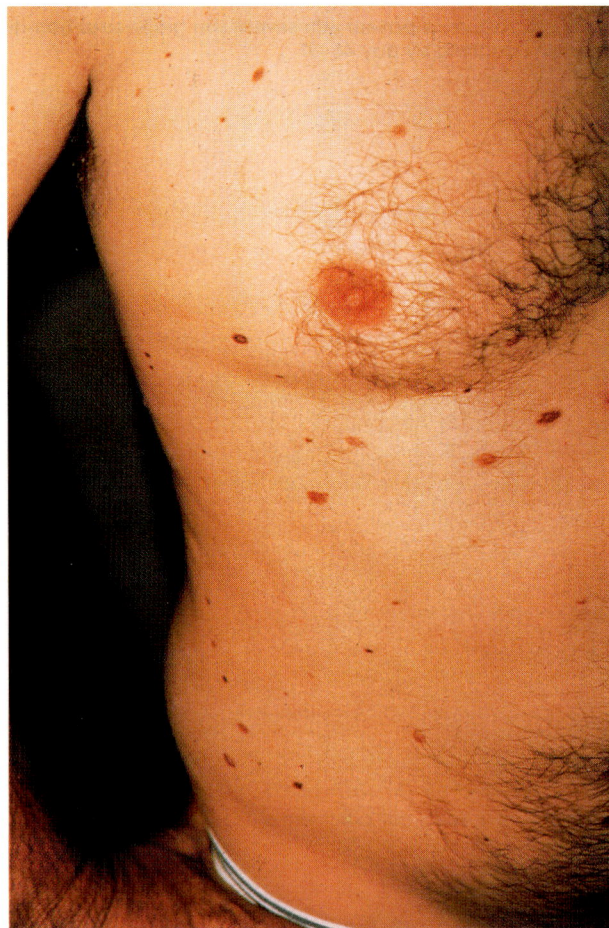

Color Figure 5. Dysplastic nevi. (Courtesy of Libby Edwards, M.D.)

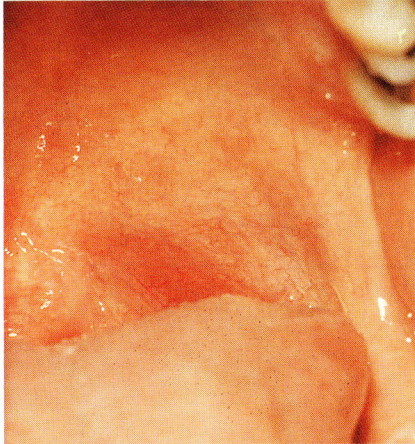

A

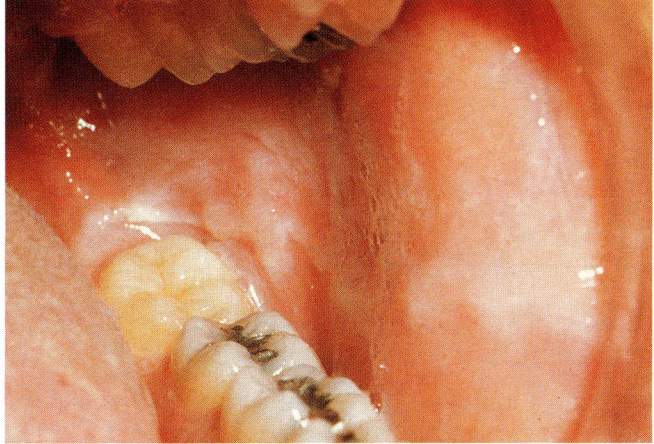

B

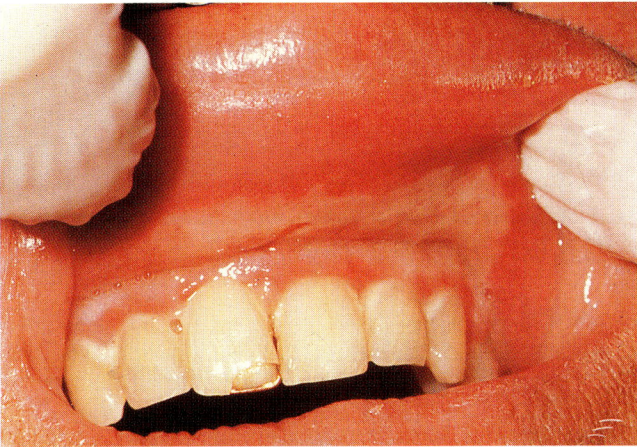

C

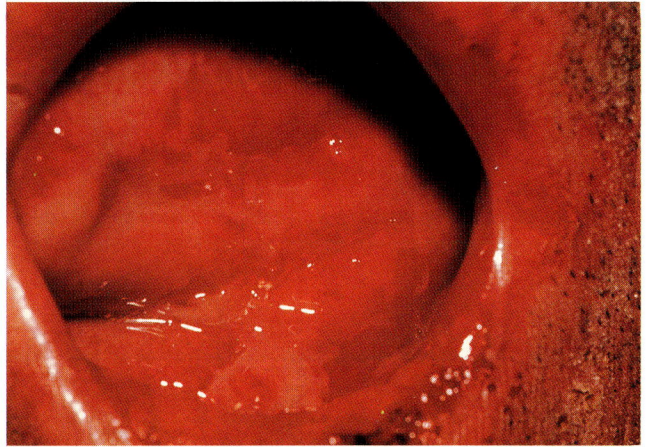

D

Color Figure 6. Examples of stomatitis. *A,* grade 0; *B,* grade I; *C,* grade II; *D,* grade III. (Courtesy of Mark M. Schubert, D.D.S., M.S.D., Oral Medicine Oncology Support Services, School of Dentistry, University of Washington, Seattle.)

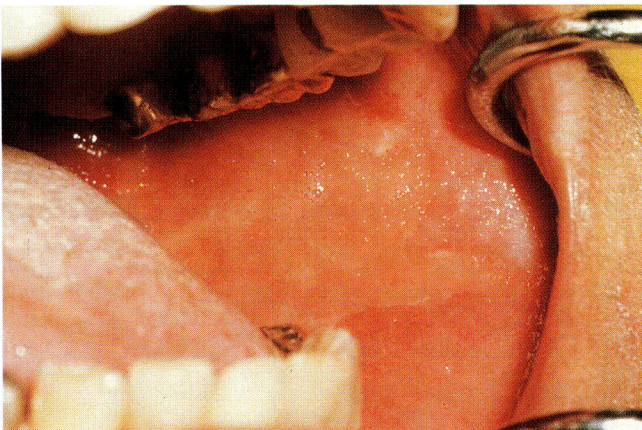

Color Figure 7. Pseudomembrane formation on buccal mucosa as a result of radiation therapy. (Courtesy of Mark M. Schubert, D.D.S., M.S.D., Oral Medicine Oncology Support Services, School of Dentistry, University of Washington, Seattle.)

Category	Voice	Swallow	Lips	Tongue	Saliva	Mucous membranes	Gingiva	Teeth, Dentures, or denture bearing area
Tools for Assessment	Auditory assessment	Observation	Visual/palpatory	Visual/palpatory	Tongue blade	Visual assessment	Tongue blade and visual assessment	Visual assessment
Methods of Measurement	Converse with patient	Ask patient to swallow. To test gag reflex, gently place blade on back of tongue and depress	Observe and feel tissue appearance of tissue	Feel and observe appearance of tissue	Insert blade into mouth, touching the center of the tongue and the floor of the mouth	Observe appearance of tissue	Gently press tissue with tip of blade	Observe appearance of teeth or denture bearing area
1 *Numerical and descriptive rating*	Normal	Normal swallow	Smooth and pink and moist	Pink and moist and papillae present	Watery	Pink and moist	Pink and stippled and firm	Clean and no debris
2 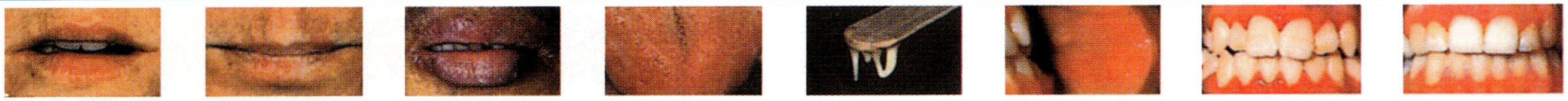	Deeper or raspy	Some pain on swallow	Dry or cracked	Coated or loss of papillae with or without redness	Thick or ropy	Reddened or coated (increased whiteness) without ulcerations	Edematous with or without redness	Plaque or debris in localized areas (between teeth if present)
3 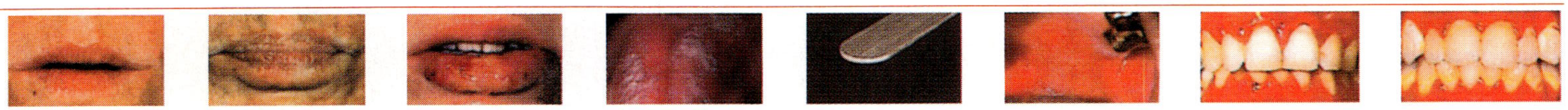	Difficulty talking or painful	Unable to swallow	Ulcerated or bleeding	Blistered or cracked	Absent	Ulcerations with or without bleeding	Spontaneous bleeding or bleeding with pressure	Plaque or debris generalized along gum line or denture bearing area

Color Figure 8. The oral assessment guide. (From June Eilers, R.N., M.S.N., et al., University of Nebraska Medical Center, Omaha, 2-84, rev. 5-84, 4-85, 11-85, and Halbrand, Inc., Willoughby, OH. Reproduced by permission.)

Table 40–4. DANGER SIGNS OF MALIGNANT MELANOMA

Change in Color
Especially multiple shades of dark brown or black; red, white, and blue; spread of color from the edge of the lesion into surrounding skin
Change in Size
Especially sudden or continuous enlargement
Change in Shape
Especially development of irregular margins
Change in Elevation
Especially sudden elevation of a previously macular pigmented lesion
Change in Surface
Especially scaliness, erosion, oozing, crusting, ulceration, bleeding
Change in Surrounding Skin
Especially redness, swelling, satellite pigmentations
Change in Sensation
Especially itching, tenderness, pain
Change in Consistency
Especially softening or friability

(From Friedman, R. J., Rigel, D. S., & Kopf, A. W. [1985]. Early detection of malignant melanoma: The role of physician examination and self-examination of the skin. *CA: A Cancer Journal for Clinicians, 35,* 130–151. Reproduced by permission.)

noma, local advanced disease, and metastasis to the brain (Meyskens, 1984).

TREATMENT OF NONMELANOMA SKIN CANCERS

The goal of treatment for nonmelanoma skin cancers is to eradicate the tumor and yet attain an acceptable cosmetic result. Definitive treatment depends on the location and size of the lesion, exact histologic type, possible extension into nearby structures, previous treatment, and age and general condition of the patient (Caldwell et al., 1983; Gumport et al., 1981).

An accurate histologic diagnosis is achieved by (1) excisional biopsy with 0.5 to 1.0 cm margins if the lesion is small and (2) incisional biopsy, including a 1.0 cm margin for larger lesions. These procedures give adequate specimens with margins in all directions. Often an excisional biopsy is considered definitive therapy.

Surgery for nonmelanoma skin cancer is indicated if the lesion invades bone or cartilage. Planning must be done for acceptable cosmetic results, which can include local rotation flaps or full-thickness skin grafts. Additionally, curettage and electrodesiccation for small lesions are done. Mohs's microscopically controlled surgery removes the cancer in multiple progressive layers and is useful if the tumor margins are difficult to determine or the lesion has reappeared. Cryosurgery using thermocouples is another method of surgical treatment (Caldwell et al., 1983; Gumport et al., 1981).

Radiation therapy is also used in the treatment of nonmelanoma skin cancers when inadequate tumor margins are shown. In a location such as the eyelids, radiation therapy might be the treatment of choice because surgical excision could involve extensive reconstructive surgery. A high fractionated schedule (4500 rad/3 weeks in 200 rad daily fractions) with attention to shielding offers excellent results. If bone and cartilage are involved, a combined approach of radiation, surgery, radiation is often successful (Caldwell et al., 1983; Gumport et al., 1981).

Treatment of premalignant actinic keratosis is topical 5-fluorouracil (5-FU). Shielding exposed areas from repeated sun is a first step. Topical applications of 5-FU are also used in the treatment of multiple keratotic lesions. Therapy usually lasts for at least 2.5 months, and healing usually occurs within 2 weeks of cessation of treatment. For unusual recurrent skin cancers that are no longer manageable by surgery or radiation, or both, various agents have been used through arterial infusion, local injection, and topical application. Although these agents are not curative, difficult lesions may be controllable for periods of time. Two immunotherapeutic agents, dinitrochlorobenzene and triethyleneimmunibenzoquinone, have also been used in the treatment of skin cancers. Vitamin A or retinoic acid has been suggested as a chemopreventive agent (Gumport et al., 1981).

Table 40–5. CLINICAL AND MICROSTAGING CLASSIFICATION METHODS FOR MALIGNANT MELANOMA

Clinical Staging	Clark's Five Levels of Cutaneous Invasion
Stage I Localized melanoma without metastasis to distant or regional lymph nodes 1. Primary melanoma untreated or removed by excisional biopsy 2. Locally recurrent melanoma within 4 cm of primary site 3. Multiple primary melanomas	*Level I* Melanoma located above the basement membrane (basal lamina) of the epidermis. These legions are essentially in situ, are extremely rare, and present no danger. *Level II* Melanoma invades through the basement membrane down to the papillary dermis.
Stage II Metastasis limited to regional lymph nodes 1. Primary melanoma present or removed with simultaneous metastasis 2. Primary melanoma controlled with subsequent metastasis 3. Locally recurrent melanoma with metastasis 4. In-transit metastasis beyond 4 cm from primary site 5. Unknown primary melanoma with metastasis	*Level III* Melanoma at this level is characterized by filling and widening by melanoma cells of the papillary dermis at its interface with the reticular dermis. Characteristically, there is no invasion of the underlying reticular layer. *Level IV* These lesions show melanoma penetration into the reticular dermis.
Stage III Disseminated melanoma 1. Visceral or multiple lymphatic metastases, or both 2. Multiple cutaneous or subcutaneous metastases, or both	*Level V* Melanoma at this level is evident by its presence in the subcutaneous tissue.

(From Goldsmith, H. S. [1979]. Melanoma: An overview. *CA: A Cancer Journal for Clinicians, 29,* 194–215. Reproduced by permission.)

Box 40–2. ARIZONA SUN AWARENESS PROJECT

Southern Arizona receives one of the highest intensities of ultraviolet radiation in the United States. The sun is a mixed blessing, and people in southern Arizona are at risk for developing skin cancer because of the high sun intensity, latitude (32°N), altitude (2410 feet), and skies that are clear for more than 190 days.

The high intensity of ultraviolet radiation in southern Arizona has been confirmed with the use of a Robertson-Berger sunburn meter (one of 21 in the United States) under the auspices of the National Oceanic and Atmospheric Administration, which is studying ozone concentration. The meter detects solar ultraviolet radiation below 330 nm (UV-B), the response varying with decreasing wavelength. The data produced by the meter have been termed the *sunburn unit* (SBU). The SBU is equal to a minimal erythema dose or the amount of UV-B radiation that will produce redness within 24 hr after exposure.

The Robertson-Berger sunburn meter at the Arizona Health Sciences Center prints the sun intensity data on paper tape every 30 min. The sun intensity index is reported to the local newspapers and to the television stations for the weather news reports.

A sample report follows.

Sun Intensity Prediction (predictions are for untanned Caucasians, assuming no clouds)

Minutes in sun today to redden skin

Time	Minutes
9 A.M.	60
10 A.M.	39
11 A.M.	26
Noon	21
1 P.M.	19
2 P.M.	23
3 P.M.	31
4 P.M.	60

(Data from Arizona Sun Awareness Project, University of Arizona Cancer Center.)

TREATMENT OF MALIGNANT MELANOMA

Most malignant melanomas are thought to have two growth phases, radial and vertical. Early melanocytic hyperplasia occurs at the epidermal-dermal junction and is characterized by horizontal growth. As the tumor becomes aggressive, it grows vertically, and it is this vertical growth that is thought to define the prognosis.

The major staging system for malignant melanoma is (1) local disease (stage I), (2) regional nodal disease (stage II), and (3) disseminated disease (stage III) (Table 40–5). Increasingly, a four-stage system that divides stage I into two stages—local primary lesion and local recurrence—is being described (Johnson, 1987; Meyskens, 1984). Clark's five levels of cutaneous invasion are a simple and useful classification that divides the skin into five levels and recognizes the vertical invasion of melanoma (see Table 40–5).

Diagnosis of malignant melanoma is usually made by an excisional biopsy because it yields a specimen with a border several millimeters in diameter. Step sections of the biopsy at 3 mm or closer intervals throughout the specimen should be ordered. Subsequent metastatic work-up procedures, such as chest radiographs and liver-spleen scans, are important to rule out dissemination.

Surgery is the mainstay of treatment for malignant melanoma. Wide, local excision that leaves a 3- to 5-cm margin, if anatomically possible, is required. Large borders frequently require split-thickness skin grafting. Nodal dissection is advocated but remains controversial. Therefore, lymph node dissection may be performed for the purpose of a biopsy (Johnson, 1987; Meyskens, 1984). Symptoms caused by intestinal obstruction, neurologic deficits, pain, or chronic ulceration of skin nodules may be relieved by surgical resection.

The prognosis for disseminated disease is generally poor. The usefulness of adjuvant chemotherapy remains questionable. The most consistently active drugs have been dacarbazine and carmustine. Response rates have been 20 per cent and 10 to 15 per cent, respectively, and have occurred largely in subcutaneous, skin, and pulmonary sites. Additional drugs included in treatment protocols are cyclophosphamide, procarbazine, hydoxyurea, methotrexate, and interferon. Certain chemotherapeutic agents have been perfused by arterial infusions to an involved extremity. Intra-arterial isolation perfusions are done following surgical removal of the tumor mass to prevent local recurrences or metastases. The drugs used are L-phenylalanine mustard (L-PAM) and dacarbazine; systemic toxicity is rare and mild (Johnson, 1987; Meyskens, 1984).

The most common agent to stimulate an immunologic response in those with malignant melanoma is bacille Calmette-Guérin (BCG). Given intradermally by multipuncture technique, BCG is a nonspecific stimulator of immune response (Johnson, 1987; Meyskens, 1984). The precise role of BCG is still uncertain, but it has had some success in the prevention of recurrence and increased duration of survival. A local inflammatory response with ulceration, pain, or both is a result of BCG injections but is temporary. Other investigational treatment includes the use of vitamin A or retinoids and hyperthermia.

Radiation therapy may be used for symptomatic

Box 40–3. WELL-BEING IN SURVIVORS OF MALIGNANT MELANOMA

STUDY

Dirksen, S. R. (1989). **Perceived well-being in malignant melanoma survivors.** *Oncology Nursing Forum, 16,* 352–358.

PURPOSE

This study examined well-being in survivors of malignant melanoma. Based on a review of the literature, a conceptual framework was developed that identified locus of control, social support, and self-esteem as having an effect on well-being.

SAMPLE

Thirty-one survivors of malignant melanoma participated in the study. A cancer survivor was defined as someone who was diagnosed with cancer 5 years ago and has been disease free since treatment was completed. The participants, 12 men and 19 women, had a mean age of 55.2 years. Melanoma sites were most frequently the back, shoulder, leg, or arm.

MEASURES

The Cancer Health Locus of Control (CHLC) scale was used to index internal, powerful others, and chance locus of control. Norbeck's Social Support Questionnaire (NSSQ) was used to assess the multiple dimensions of social support. Self-esteem was assessed by the Coopersmith Self-Esteem Inventory (SEI), and well-being was measured by the Index of Well-Being. To examine the demographic and situational characteristics of the sample, descriptive statistics were used. To test the strength of the predicted relationships in the conceptual framework, multiple regression was used.

FINDINGS

Greater understanding of the factors that influence perceived well-being in these survivors was confirmed. Those individuals with internal locus of control had a greater sense of well-being. With a higher level of self-esteem, an increased perception of well-being ensued, and the greater the perception of support, the higher the level of self-esteem. Exogenous variables, number of chronic illnesses, and treatment with immunotherapy and vitamin A were found to have an effect on well-being. Internal locus of control and self-esteem had a direct positive effect on well-being.

NURSING IMPLICATIONS

Survivors engaged in a variety of activities to exercise control over their cancer. Specific actions were mentioned by these survivors. Nursing interventions proposed are a beginning attempt to identify the long-term rehabilitation aspects of nursing care for cancer survivors.

---

metastases. To reduce pain and prevent pathologic fractures subsequent to bone lesions, radiation is most effective.

PROGNOSIS

Skin cancers offer a unique opportunity for early detection, early diagnosis, early treatment, and cure. For basal cell carcinoma, the cure rates are equally high for surgery and irradiation. Although its metastatic ability is poor, basal cell carcinoma can create extensive local spread. Acceptable cosmetic results are achieved with full-thickness skin grafts.

For squamous cell carcinoma, recurrence of the lesion is the major complication. Surgery and irradia-

tion have equally high cure rates. Follow-up visits two to four times a year are recommended.

Malignant melanoma is the most serious skin cancer, and the most important prognostic feature is the size of the lesion at the time of diagnosis and treatment. The survival rate is correlated with the depth of invasion and location of the lesion. However, the difficult and unpredictable problem of hematogenous dissemination has not been solved.

SUMMARY

Perhaps the greatest contributions nurses can make are those related to the prevention and early detection of skin cancers. By encouraging individuals to become "sun aware," skin cancers can be recognized early

(Box 40–2). Young adults in particular should be educated about the cumulative effects of prolonged sun exposure (Frank-Stromborg; 1986; Lawler & Schreiber, 1989; White; 1986a). The avoidance of tanning salons and sun lamps cannot be overemphasized. For older persons, the risks of skin cancers should be carefully explained. Individuals who are identified as being at high risk for malignant melanoma can reduce their chances of developing the disease with appropriate teaching and support. Skin self-examination should be taught and the procedure verified on contacts with clients in whatever setting they are seen.

The nonmetastatic behavior of basal cell carcinoma can be carefully explained, particularly to older patients. The need for follow-up, however, must be reinforced. For individuals with squamous cell carcinoma, periodic examinations must be conducted to evaluate the sites for potential recurrence.

For individuals with malignant melanoma, follow-up is crucial. Early and prompt treatment of recurrence is of the utmost importance. There should be an open and optimistic approach in discussing feelings and attitudes about the impact of a life-threatening illness (Box 40–3). The nursing profession is in a unique position to deal with the public health problem of skin cancer.

References

American Cancer Society. (1988). *Cancer facts and figures, 1988.* New York: Author.

Anders, J. E., & Leach, E. E. (1983). Sun versus skin. *American Journal of Nursing, 83,* 1015–1020.

Berkman, S. (1985). The skin remembers. *Cancer News, 39*(2):2–4.

Berliner, H. (1986a). Aging skin. *American Journal of Nursing, 86,* 1138–1141.

Berliner, H. (1986b). Aging skin: Part two. *American Journal of Nursing, 86,* 1259–1261.

Caldwell, E. H., McCormack, R. M., Goldsmith, L. A., & Rubin, P. (1983). Skin cancer. In P. Rubin (Ed.), *Clinical oncology for medical students and physicians* (6th ed., pp. 222–229). New York: American Cancer Society.

Frank-Stromborg, M. (1985). The role of the nurse in early detection of cancer: Population sixty-six years of age and older. *Oncology Nursing Forum, 13*(3), 66–74.

Frank-Stromborg, M. (1986). The role of the nurse in cancer detection and screening. *Seminars in Oncology Nursing, 11,* 191–199.

Fraser, M. C., & McGuire, D. B. (1984). Skin cancer's early warning system. *American Journal of Nursing, 84,* 1232–1236.

Friedman, R. J., Riegel, D. S., & Kopf, A. W. (1985). Early detection of malignant melanoma: The role of physician examination and self-examination of the skin. *CA: A Cancer Journal for Clinicians, 35,* 130–151.

Goldsmith, H. S. (1979). Melanoma: An overview. *CA: A Cancer Journal for Clinicians, 29,* 194–215.

Greene, M. H., Clark, W. H., Tucker, M. A., Elder, D. E., Kramer, K. H., Guerry, D., Witmer, W. K., Thompson, J., Matazzo, I., & Fraser, M. C. (1986). Acquired precursors of cutaneous malignant melanoma. *New England Journal of Medicine, 213,* 91–97.

Gumport, S. L., Harris, M. N., Roses, D. F., & Kopf, A. W. (1981). The diagnosis and management of common skin cancers. *CA: A Cancer Journal for Clinicians, 31,* 79–89.

Houghton, A. N. (1987, Winter). A refresher on melanoma: Suggestions toward prevention: Clues to early detection. *Your Patient and Cancer,* pp. 13–18.

Johnson, B. L. (1987). Malignant melanoma. In S. L. Groenwald (Ed.), and *Cancer nursing principles and practice* (pp. 684–692). Monterey, CA: Jones Bartlett Publishers, Inc.

Lawler, P. E., & Schreiber, S. (1989). Cutaneous malignant melanoma: Nursing's role in prevention and early detection. *Oncology Nursing Forum, 16,* 345–352.

Longman, A. (1987). Skin cancer. In C. R. Ziegfeld (Ed.), *Core curriculum for oncology nursing* (pp. 117–127). Philadelphia: W. B. Saunders Co.

McGuire, D. B. (1984). Impact of hereditary melanoma on families. *Cancer Nursing, 7,* 451–459.

McGuire, D. B. (1985). Preventive health practices and educational needs in families with hereditary melanoma. *Cancer Nursing, 8,* 29–36.

Meyskens, F. L. (1984). Malignant melanoma clinical diagnosis quiz, Bristol Laboratories, 8(3), 2–21. St. Louis: C. V. Mosby Company.

Nevidjon, B. (1986). Cancer prevention and early detection: Reported activities of nurses. *Oncology Nursing Forum, 13,* 46–80.

Ramstack, J. L., White, S. E., Hazelkorn, K. S., & Meyskens, F. L. (1986). Sunshine and skin cancer: A school-based skin cancer prevention project. *Journal of Cancer Education, 1*(2):1–8.

Schleper, J. R. (1984). Cancer prevention and detection: Skin cancer. *Cancer Nursing, 7,* 67–84.

Stair, J. C. (1985). Knowledge deficit related to prevention and early detection of nonmelanoma skin cancers (basal cell and squamous cell carcinoma, including Bowen's disease). In J. C. McNally, J. C. Stair, & E. T. Somerville (Eds.), *Guidelines for cancer nursing practice* (pp. 27–31). Orlando, FL: Grune & Stratton, Inc.

Stewart, D. S. (1987). Indoor tanning: The nurse's role in preventing skin damage. *Cancer Nursing, 10,* 93–99.

White, L. N. (1986a). Cancer prevention and detection: From twenty to sixty-five years of age. *Oncology Nursing Forum, 13*(2), 59–64.

White, L. N. (1986b). Cancer risk assessment. *Seminars in Oncology Nursing, 11,* 184–190.

CHAPTER 41

AIDS and the Spectrum of HIV Disease*

ANNE M. HUGHES
JEROME SCHOFFERMAN

The phenomenon known as acquired immune deficiency syndrome (AIDS) was unrecognized before 1981. At that time, the first case reports of *Pneumocystis carinii* pneumonia and Kaposi's sarcoma in previously healthy gay men were described. These unusual illnesses were associated with profound cell-mediated immune deficiency and became the harbingers of the AIDS epidemic (Centers for Disease Control [CDC], 1981).

Since those first cases were reported to the Centers for Disease Control (CDC), 121,645 persons have been diagnosed with AIDS as of January 1990. Of that number 72,578 (60 per cent) have died. During the single year between February 1989 and January 1990, 36,682 cases of AIDS (30 per cent of the total) were reported to the CDC (CDC, 1990).

By the end of 1992, an estimated 365,000 persons will be diagnosed with AIDS in the United States (Heyward & Curran, 1989). Furthermore, it is estimated that between 1 and 1.5 million persons currently are infected with human immunodeficiency virus (HIV), the retroviral etiologic agent that causes AIDS (Coolfont Report, 1986). Evidence suggests that 50 per cent of persons already infected with HIV will develop AIDS within 10 years (Cohn, 1989).

This chapter presents an overview of the epidemiology, pathophysiology, and medical and nursing management of AIDS and the spectrum of HIV disease. In addition, references are cited that provide more detailed information (Broder, 1987; DeVita, Hellman, and Rosenberg, 1988; Flaskerud, 1989; Gee & Moran, 1988; Lewis, 1988; Sande & Volberding, 1988).

---

*Adapted from Hughes, A. M., Martin, J. P., & Frank, P. (1990). *AIDS home care and hospice manual* (2nd ed.). San Francisco: Visiting Nurses and Hospice of San Francisco.

EPIDEMIOLOGY

Transmission of HIV

There are three established routes of transmission of the HIV virus. Ninety per cent of the reported cases of AIDS have been transmitted by only *one* of these three routes: (1) contact with secretions (semen, vaginal secretions) during intimate sexual activities (64 per cent); (2) contact with blood while sharing needles during intravenous drug use (21 per cent) and during blood or blood product transfusion (4 per cent); and (3) contact via placental exchange or intrapartum or breast milk, in maternal-fetal/infant transmission (1 per cent). Seven per cent of the reported AIDS cases have *more than one* route; e.g., male homosexual contact and intravenous drug use. In the remaining 3 per cent of cases, the route of transmission has not been established (CDC, 1990).

Although HIV has been recovered in tears, urine, saliva, cerebrospinal fluid, and alveolar fluid, no evidence indicates that these body fluids can transmit the virus from an infected person to another individual. Moreover, there is no evidence to suggest that HIV can be transmitted through casual contact (Friedland & Klein, 1987).

Despite what appears to be a growing spectrum of disease associated with HIV infection, the groups most at risk for AIDS in the United States have remained largely unchanged. These risk groups include (1) homosexual and bisexual men, (2) intravenous drug users, (3) male or female heterosexuals who have sexual contact with persons infected with HIV, (4) hemophiliacs, and (5) persons who received blood or blood product transfusions before 1985 when widespread testing became available (CDC, 1987a). Table 41–1

647

Table 41–1. CUMULATIVE NUMBER AND PERCENTAGE OF REPORTED AIDS CASES IN THE UNITED STATES BY RISK GROUP AMONG ADULTS AND ADOLESCENTS THROUGH JANUARY 1990

Risk Group	Number	Percentage
Homosexual or bisexual male	72,153	60
Intravenous (IV) drug user	25,200	21
Homosexual male and IV drug user	8326	7
Hemophilia or coagulation disorder	1099	1
Heterosexual contact	5853	5
Transfusion, blood or components	2923	2
Other	4036	3
TOTAL	119,590	100

(From CDC. [1990, February]. HIV/AIDS surveillance report—United States AIDS program through January, 1990.)

shows the number and percentage of reported AIDS cases by risk group among adults and adolescents (CDC, 1990). It *must* be noted, however, that risk group membership does not in and of itself place an individual at risk for AIDS. Rather, it is the practice of high-risk behavior that defines relative risk.

Demographic Profile of Persons with AIDS

Most persons receiving their index or AIDS-qualifying diagnosis are young and middle-aged adults. Nearly 87 per cent of all reported cases of AIDS have been in men and women from 20 to 49 years of age (CDC, 1989c).

Females represent 10 per cent of all AIDS cases and 50 per cent of all pediatric AIDS cases (CDC, 1989c). Women most at risk for AIDS are those who use intravenous drugs or who are sexual partners of infected men. More than 50 per cent of all reported cases of AIDS in women are in women who are intravenous drug users. Women and sexually active adolescent females who are infected with HIV and become pregnant have a 50 per cent chance of giving birth to children who will develop AIDS (Grossman, 1988).

Blacks (27 per cent) and Hispanics (15 per cent) account for 42 per cent of all reported AIDS cases among adults and adolescents. Blacks (52 per cent) and Hispanics (20 per cent) account for 72 per cent of AIDS cases in adult and adolescent females. Among children reported to have AIDS, 77 per cent are black or Hispanic. Black infants and children represent 53 per cent of all AIDS cases in children under the age of 13 (CDC, 1989c).

Children and AIDS

The diagnosis of AIDS in an infant is complicated by both the need to rule out a congenital immune deficiency and the presence of passively acquired maternal antibodies, which may be detected for as long as 18 months after birth (Armann, 1985; Grossman, 1988). In addition, the clinical presentation of AIDS

in children may vary from that seen in adults. Children may present with more bacterial infections, chronic swelling of the parotid gland, and lymphoid interstitial pneumonia, which are uncommon clinical presentations in adults or adolescents. Developmental delays are common (Armann, 1985).

From a health services utilization standpoint, it has been noted that children with AIDS tend to have longer lengths of stay in hospitals as compared with adults with AIDS, often because of an ill parent or caregiver and an inadequate number of foster care homes (Arno & Hughes, 1987). Geographically, almost one third of all pediatric AIDS cases in the United States are concentrated in the metropolitan New York City area (CDC, 1989c). Table 41–2 shows the breakdown of pediatric AIDS cases by risk or exposure category.

Of the 2055 pediatric AIDS cases reported to the CDC as of January 31, 1990, 58 per cent (99 cases) were related to intravenous drug use, that is, the mother of the child was an intravenous drug user (857, 42 per cent) or had sexual relations with an intravenous drug user (342, 17 per cent) (CDC, 1990). These data suggest that prevention efforts that target women, in particular intravenous drug users or women who have partners who are intravenous drug users, would decrease the perinatal spread of HIV.

HIV Prevention Strategies

At the present time, no vaccine is available to prevent HIV infection. Given the three well-documented modes of HIV transmission, prevention strat-

Table 41–2. CUMULATIVE NUMBER AND PERCENTAGE OF REPORTED PEDIATRIC AIDS CASES IN THE UNITED STATES (INCLUDING CHILDREN UNDER 13 YEARS OF AGE) BY EXPOSURE CATEGORY AS OF JANUARY 31, 1990

Exposure Category	Number	Percentage
Hemophiliac or coagulation disorder	108	5
Mother with or at risk for AIDS or HIV infection	1675	82
Intravenous (IV) drug use	857	
Sex with IV drug user	342	
Sex with bisexual male	39	
Sex with persons with hemophilia	7	
Born in Pattern 2 country (includes Caribbean islands and parts of Africa)	178	
Sex with person born in Pattern 2 country	7	
Sex with transfusion recipient with HIV infection	10	
Sex with person with HIV infection, risk not specified	65	
Recipient of blood transfusion or tissue	35	
Has HIV infection, risk not specified	135	
Recipient of transfusion of blood, blood components, or tissue	217	11
Undetermined	55	3
TOTAL	2055	100

(From CDC. [1990, February]. HIV/AIDS surveillance report—United States AIDS program through January, 1990.)

egies rest on these principles: (1) preventing sexual transmission of HIV infection, (2) preventing HIV infection through sharing needles and syringes, (3) preventing HIV infection from donated blood and blood products, (4) preventing HIV infection from mother to infant, and (5) preventing HIV infection through occupational exposure (Fauci, Macher, Longo, et al., 1984).

All sexually active individuals are at risk for infection with HIV. Sexual transmission of HIV can best be prevented by avoiding anal or vaginal intercourse with persons infected with HIV or persons believed to be at risk for HIV infection. Using effective barrier techniques during intercourse (i.e., condoms) along with spermicides (which kill the virus) and dental dams during oral sex may decrease transmission of HIV. In September 1989, the CDC published guidelines regarding HIV risk assessment that are based on sexual health history and counseling recommendations regarding safer sex techniques, especially condom use (Box 41–1) (CDC, 1989e).

Intravenous drug users are at particular risk for acquiring and transmitting HIV infection. Brickner and colleagues (1989) identified four strategies to prevent the spread of HIV in this population: (1) voluntary, confidential HIV testing; (2) free, but carefully controlled, distribution of sterile needles and syringes; (3) accessible drug detoxification and methadone mainte-

nance programs; and (4) health education regarding safer sex techniques, perinatal transmission of HIV, and sterilization techniques for needles and syringes if sterile "works" are not available and continued drug use is likely. These investigators also pointed out that contrary to some commonly held beliefs and attitudes of health care professionals, many intravenous drug users have changed their behavior to reduce their risk of HIV infection.

Efforts by the CDC and blood banks to date have significantly reduced the risk of HIV infection from contaminated blood or blood products to between 1 in 100,000 to 1 in 1,000,000. As early as 1983, individuals at high risk for HIV infection were asked to refrain from donating blood. Beginning in 1985, all donated blood was tested for antibodies to HIV. Heat treatment of clotting factor VIII concentrates has further reduced the danger of HIV transmission to hemophiliacs. Despite the relative safety of the blood supply in the United States today, the CDC recommends that individuals who received blood or blood product transfusions between 1978 and 1985 be counseled regarding their possible exposure to HIV (Friedland & Klein, 1987).

Mother-to-infant transmission can best be prevented if women infected with HIV or women whose male sexual partners are infected do not become pregnant. Programs to identify, screen, and counsel women in

---

Box 41–1. INFORMATION ON SAFE SEX

STUDY

Moran, T. A., Lovejoy, N., Viele, C., Dodd, M. J., & Abrams, D. I. (1988). **Information needs of homosexual men diagnosed with AIDS or AIDS-related complex.** *Oncology Nursing Forum, 15,* 311–314.

METHODS

Descriptive stratified survey design using convenience sample. Data collection instrument included six open-ended questions. Sample accrued in fall 1985.

SAMPLE

Sixty-five self-identified homosexual or bisexual men with confirmed AIDS or ARC diagnosis: 92 per cent were Caucasian, mean age was 34 years, and average education was 15.3 years.

FINDINGS

Most subjects (52 per cent) wanted additional information regarding safe sex. Forty-nine per cent reported their health care provider offered no help in addressing their sexual needs. Half of the subjects obtained safe sex information from community organizations. In general, subjects credited themselves for changing their sexual behavior.

IMPLICATIONS FOR PRACTICE

This study suggests that, in 1985 at least, health care providers were not seen as effective health educators for persons with AIDS or ARC with respect to sexual information and the prevention of HIV transmission. Nurses can play a pivotal role in providing education and counseling regarding safe sex practices and in exploring how intimacy needs can be met by persons infected with HIV.

high-risk groups (e.g., intravenous drug users, women with histories of multiple sexually transmitted diseases or multiple partners) are ways to reduce the vertical transmission of HIV infection from mother to fetus or infant. As discussed earlier, perinatal transmission of HIV accounts for 80 per cent of all pediatric AIDS cases, so its prevention would significantly decrease the problem of HIV disease in children (Armann, 1985; Grossman, 1988).

Finally, reducing the risk of occupational exposure to HIV rests primarily in acknowledging the real risk (albeit low, < 0.5 per cent prevalence rate) and its attendant fear (CDC, 1989a; Gerbert, 1988). In 1987, the CDC recommended the adoption of universal blood and body substance precautions to reduce the risk of HIV transmission in health care settings. Basically, these precautions stress that *all* patients should be assumed to be infected with HIV and other blood-borne pathogens. Appropriate barrier protection (gloves, gowns, mask, goggles) should be worn based on the health care worker's judgment regarding the likelihood of contact with a body substance (CDC, 1987b).

Given that HIV is blood borne, nurses drawing blood, whether from a peripheral vein or a central line, and nurses starting peripheral intravenous lines are advised to wear gloves while performing these tasks and to wash their hands after removing their gloves. However, *needlestick injuries* while recapping or breaking needles *pose the greatest risk of accidental HIV exposure* for nurses and other health care workers. The CDC urges all health care workers not to recap or break a needle from the syringe hub or manually manipulate a used needle or syringe and to dispose of all used needles in puncture-resistant containers located as close to the area of use as possible (CDC, 1989a).

PATHOPHYSIOLOGY

Human Immunodeficiency Virus

The virus that causes AIDS was described simultaneously by three different researchers and was known by three names: AIDS-related virus (ARV), lymphadenopathy-associated virus (LAV), and human T cell lymphotrophic virus type III (HTLV-III). In June 1986, an agreement was reached among AIDS researchers to use a common name for the virus—human immunodeficiency virus (HIV). This is now the accepted term (Gallo, 1988).

Human immunodeficiency virus belongs to a subgroup or classification of viruses known as retroviruses. The term *retrovirus* means that the virus carries its genetic code in RNA. Retroviruses have an enzyme called *reverse transcriptase* that transcribes RNA to DNA, which is incorporated into the genetic material of the host cell. The virus lives within the host cell, replicating itself and integrating with the host cell. As the cell divides, all progeny cells are infected also (Ho, Pomerantz, & Kaplan, 1987). Retroviruses character-

istically are pathogenic for a long time. In the case of HIV, lifelong infection may be expected (Curran, 1985; Lovejoy, 1988).

Human immunodeficiency virus has an affinity for a subclass of T lymphocytes called helper T cells or T4 cells. After being infected, the helper T cell can produce more virus and can release HIV "buds" into the general circulation to infect more lymphocytes. Many HIV-infected T4 cells are dormant. When activated, however, the helper T cells can act like "a virus factory." An invasion of HIV into a helper T cell eventually results in the death of that T cell. As the body produces more helper T cells to combat the invading virus, the virus infects more lymphocytes, and the viral burden, or viral load, is increased. It is the immune system's eventual depletion of helper T cells and its inability to produce more lymphocytes, or functional lymphocytes, that results in the development of diseases diagnostic of AIDS. Evidence suggests that HIV affects other components of the immune system, specifically B cells and macrophages. Macrophages serve as a reservoir of HIV. Some asymptomatic persons who are seropositive for HIV antibody show some

Table 41–3. SUMMARY OF CLASSIFICATION SYSTEM FOR HUMAN IMMUNODEFICIENCY VIRUS (HIV) INFECTION

Group	Description
1	*Acute HIV infection* Transient signs and symptoms at the time of, or shortly after, initial infection with HIV; a mononucleosis-like syndrome, with or without aseptic meningitis.
2	*Asymptomatic HIV infection* No signs or symptoms of HIV infection; may include those persons with abnormal hematologic or immunologic, or both, laboratory findings consistent with HIV infection.
3	*Persistent generalized lymphadenopathy* Palpable lymph nodes at two or more extrainguinal sites persisting for more than 3 months in the absence of a concurrent illness or condition that might explain these findings.
4	*Other HIV disease* A. *Constitutional disease* is defined as one or more of the following: fever > 1 month, involuntary weight loss of greater than 10% baseline, or diarrhea persisting > 1 month: e.g., HIV wasting syndrome; B. *Neurologic disease* is defined as one or more of the following: dementia, myelopathy, or peripheral neuropathy in the absence of a concurrent illness or condition that might explain these findings; C. *Secondary infectious diseases* are defined as the diagnosis of infectious disease associated with HIV infection and/or at least moderately indicative of a defect in cell-mediated immunity (e.g., opportunistic infections such as *Pneumocystis carinii* pneumonia); D. *Secondary cancers* are defined as the diagnosis of one or more kinds of cancer associated with HIV infection and/or at least moderately indicative of a defect in cell-mediated immunity (e.g., Kaposi's sarcoma, primary lymphoma of the brain, non-Hodgkin's lymphoma); E. *Other conditions in HIV infection* are defined as the presence of other clinical findings or diseases, not classifiable above, that may be attributed to HIV infection or at least moderately indicative of a defect in cell-mediated immunity.

(From CDC. [1986]. Classification system for HTLV-III/LAV infections. *MMWR, 35,* 334–338.)

immunologic and hematologic impairment (Bowen, Lane, & Fauci, 1985a, 1985b).

Human immunodeficiency virus also infects cells in the central and peripheral nervous systems (Gallo, 1988). This characteristic of the virus accounts for the increasing number of neurologic and psychiatric complications seen in persons with AIDS (Dilley & Boccellari, 1988; Price et al., 1988). Researchers have recovered HIV from intestinal lining and have speculated that it also directly infects bone marrow (Haseltine & Wong-Staal, 1988; Kaplan, 1988).

Spectrum of HIV Infection

Investigators now believe that HIV may cause other diseases and pathologic changes that are not part of the CDC case definition of AIDS. The clinically evident damage caused by HIV infection is seen in reported AIDS cases; the clinically silent damage caused by HIV and its progression is still being identified. Furthermore, AIDS may not occur in every person infected by the virus, although data suggest that 50 per cent will eventually develop AIDS within 10 years (Cohn, 1989). Some persons who are asymptomatic and feel well may be carriers of the virus and may unknowingly infect others who will subsequently be diagnosed with AIDS. Table 41–3 shows pathophysiologic changes associated with HIV. These changes represent a clinical spectrum of HIV infection, from the initial acute infection with the virus to the diagnosis of opportunistic diseases. This classification system of HIV infection was developed by the CDC (1986).

Acute HIV Infection (CDC Group 1)

The initial manifestation of HIV infection may be a mononucleosis-like syndrome of sudden onset, lasting 2 to 3 weeks during the first few weeks following infection with HIV. This acute, self-limiting viral illness noted in various prevalence studies in 53 to 93 per cent of subjects is associated with the individual's HIV infection seroconversion (Tindall et al., 1988). Acute seroconversion illness is often characterized by neurologic and dermatologic findings (e.g., meningitis, neuropathies, affective or cognitive impairments, and rash or urticaria) in addition to the mononucleosis-like signs and symptoms: fever, pharyngitis, lymphadenopathy, arthralgia, myalgia, headache, lethargy, malaise, anorexia, nausea, and diarrhea (Tindall et al., 1988). The availability of serologic HIV testing has made it possible to identify many symptomatic and asymptomatic persons who have been exposed to the virus and are assumed to be potential transmitters of HIV. Screening tests to determine seropositivity to HIV are discussed in the following section.

Screening Methods for HIV

Infection with HIV is confirmed by one of four methods: (1) detection of HIV antigen, (2) detection of HIV-specific antibodies, (3) viral culture of HIV, and (4) detection of HIV viral genome (Chaisson, 1988). Viral culture and viral genome testing (polymerase chain reaction or PCR) are expensive and are used primarily for research purposes. Therefore, the most frequently employed screening methods are antibody testing and antigen testing.

Screening for HIV infection has been and still is extremely controversial because of the complex ethical and psychosocial ramifications. Countless incidents of discrimination and stigmatization of persons infected with HIV have occurred following the disclosure, often unauthorized, of test results. The public welfare and the public's right to know have been used to justify mandatory testing and abdication of individual autonomy and right to privacy. Given the serious psychosocial implications of HIV testing, informed consent must be obtained and pre- and posttest counseling must be made available (Bennett & Gee, 1988). To date, most states do not require that a confirmed positive HIV test be reported (the diagnosis of AIDS, on the other hand, must be reported). As a result, epidemiologists have been at a disadvantage in obtaining valid incidence and prevalence rates of HIV infection. Recently, confidential testing for HIV has gained more support from the medical community and from many community groups with the finding that antiviral therapy with zidovudine (azidothymidine, AZT) in asymptomatic patients who are seropositive for HIV and who have CD4 (T4) cell counts can significantly delay the progression of AIDS (Volberding et al, 1990; National Institute, 1989).

The two most commonly used HIV antibody tests are enzyme-linked immunosorbent assay (ELISA) and western blot (CDC, 1989d). Other antibody tests include the indirect immunofluorescent antibody (IFA), which is used to test for IgM and IgG. Because the ELISA is more apt to give false-positive test results, especially in populations with a low prevalence of HIV, the western blot is routinely done on all HIV-positive sera to confirm the positive test results. Because antibody tests require the presence of HIV-specific antibodies to confirm infection, there is a window of time— up to 3 to 6 months following infection—when these tests may give false-negative test results in a person who is indeed infected with HIV (Project Inform, 1988; Tindall et al., 1988).

Viral antigen can be detected at the time of HIV seroconversion illness. The HIV p24 antigen is the most commonly used test not only to diagnose acute HIV infection but also to monitor viral activity during the course of infection. In most individuals, HIV antigen disappears with the detection of HIV antibodies. Persistent or recurrent antigenemia is often associated with disease progression (Tindall et al., 1988). Table 41–4 diagrams the progression of HIV infection with the available HIV testing methods and the CDC classification system of HIV disease.

Asymptomatic HIV Infection (CDC Group 2)

The incubation period from infection with HIV to emergence of symptomatic disease has been estimated

Table 41–4. PROGRESSION OF HIV INFECTION USING AVAILABLE HIV SCREENING METHODS AND THE CDC CLASSIFICATION SYSTEM

	HIV Infection	Acute HIV Seroconversion Illness	Asymptomatic/ Development/Detection of HIV Antibodies	Persistent Generalized Lymphadenopathy	Progression of HIV Disease to AIDS
Time	0	2–4 weeks	4 weeks–6 months*	4 weeks–10 years + ?	?2–10 years +
HIV Screening Tests	HIV p24 antigen(?) Polymerase chain reaction	HIV p24 antigen Viral culture Polymerase chain reaction (PCR); IFA test for IgM	IFA for IgM IFA for IgG ELISA WB	HIV antibody tests (ELISA, WB, IFA for IgG)	HIV antibody tests plus HIV p24 antigen Beta-2 microglobulin
HIV in CDC Classification System		Group 1	Group 2	Group 3	Group 4

*There are some isolated reports of individuals with repeated negative HIV antibody tests and detectable HIV antigen 6–14 months before seroconversion by ELISA (Tindall et al., 1988). HIV, human immunodeficiency virus; CDC, Centers for Disease Control; IFA, indirect fluorescent antibody; ELISA, enzyme-linked immunosorbent assay; WB, western blot; AIDS, acquired immune deficiency syndrome.

to be as long as 10 years (Cohn, 1989). However, not all persons infected with the virus develop AIDS. The San Francisco city clinic cohort study, which has monitored men 8.5 years since seroconversion, reported the following: 52 per cent developed AIDS, 22 per cent developed advanced HIV symptoms, 11 per cent had persistent generalized lymphadenopathy, and 15 per cent continued to be asymptomatic (Lifson et al., 1989). It has been suggested that the route of transmission and amount and frequency of viral inoculum may also influence the natural history of HIV infection (Friedland & Klein, 1987). The role of co-factors (e.g., concurrent infections, life-style factors such as substance abuse) in enabling HIV to cause disruptive pathophysiologic changes is being investigated by several researchers (Bowen et al., 1985b; Castro, Hardy, & Curran, 1986; Francis et al., 1985).

Aids-Related Complex (CDC Groups 3 and 4A–4E)

Earlier in the epidemic, AIDS-related complex or AIDS-related condition (ARC) was considered a significant aspect of the HIV disease spectrum because of its prevalence (Abrams, 1986, 1988). *Aids-related complex* is a term that was used to characterize persons with continuing, significant constitutional signs and symptoms, such as persistent fevers, persistent generalized lymphadenopathy, idiopathic thrombocytopenia purpura, chronic diarrhea, night sweats, and extreme fatigue, whose laboratory test findings indicated humoral and cell-mediated immune dysfunction. Despite these signs and symptoms, such persons lacked the diagnosis of an AIDS-index opportunistic infection or neoplasm (Ziegler & Abrams, 1985). As the natural history of HIV became better elucidated, the HIV classification system in Table 41–3 was created, and it recategorized persons with ARC into group 3 or group 4 (CDC, 1986). This HIV classification system eliminates the term *ARC* in the schema; nevertheless, its use continues in some clinical settings.

Diagnosis of AIDS (CDC Group 4)

An AIDS diagnosis represents the most serious pathophysiologic consequence in the spectrum of HIV disease. The sensitive laboratory methods discussed earlier to determine HIV infection have been invaluable in confirming the diagnosis of AIDS. These laboratory tests were unavailable early in the epidemic. The CDC revised the case definition of AIDS in 1987 to incorporate laboratory evidence of HIV infection. Table 41–5, reprinted from the *Morbidity and Mortality Weekly Report,* lists the diagnostic criteria for AIDS (CDC, 1987c).

MEDICAL MANAGEMENT

The goals of medical treatment to halt the effects of HIV are fourfold. The first goal is the early detection of persons infected with HIV. As discussed previously, the recent clinical trial that demonstrated the efficacy of zidovudine in delaying the onset of AIDS in persons who are asymptomatic but seropositive for HIV supports this goal (Volberding et al., 1990; NIAID, 1989). In addition, the CDC recommends primary prophylaxis against *P. carinii* pneumonia for persons without a history of it if they have evidence of severely decreased T4 (CD4) cell counts (less than 200/mm³) (CDC, 1989b). Finally, tuberculosis screening is recommended for all persons who are seropositive for HIV. If the individual has a reaction to purified protein derivative, it is recommended that tuberculosis prophylaxis be initiated to prevent reactivated disease (Jacobson, 1988).

The second goal is the continued development of safe and effective antiviral agents. Ongoing research continues to develop antiviral agents other than zidovudine that will act at various sites on the HIV molecule and at various stages in its replication (Yarchoan, Mitsuya, & Broder, 1988). Zidovudine (Retrovir), formerly known as azidothymidine or AZT, is the only antiviral agent for HIV infection that has been approved by the United States Food and Drug Administration. Zidovudine is a reverse transcriptase inhibitor

Table 41–5. 1987 REVISION OF CASE DEFINITION FOR AIDS FOR SURVEILLANCE PURPOSES

For national reporting, a case of AIDS is defined as an illness characterized by one or more of the following "indicator" diseases, depending on the status of laboratory evidence of HIV infection, as shown below.

I. **Without Laboratory Evidence Regarding HIV Infection**
   If laboratory tests for HIV were not performed or gave inconclusive results and the patient had no other cause of immunodeficiency listed in Section I.A below, then any disease listed in Section I.B indicates AIDS if it was diagnosed by a definitive method.
   A. **Causes of immunodeficiency that disqualify diseases as indicators of AIDS in the absence of laboratory evidence for HIV infection.**
      1. High-dose or long-term systemic corticosteroid therapy or other immunosuppressive/cytotoxic therapy less than 3 months before the onset of the indicator disease
      2. Any of the following diseases diagnosed less than 3 months after diagnosis of the indicator disease: Hodgkin's disease, non-Hodgkin's lymphoma (other than primary brain lymphoma), lymphocytic leukemia, multiple myeloma, any other cancer of lymphoreticular or histiocytic tissue, or angioimmunoblastic lymphadenopathy
      3. A genetic (congenital) immunodeficiency syndrome or an acquired immunodeficiency syndrome atypical of HIV infection, such as one involving hypogammaglobulinemia
   B. **Indicator diseases diagnosed definitively**
      1. Candidiasis of the esophagus, trachea, bronchi, or lungs
      2. Cryptococcosis, extrapulmonary
      3. Cryptosporidiosis with diarrhea persisting more than 1 month
      4. Cytomegalovirus disease of an organ other than the liver, spleen, or lymph nodes in a patient younger than 1 month of age
      5. Herpes simplex virus infection causing a mucocutaneous ulcer that persists longer than 1 month; or bronchitis, pneumonitis, or esophagitis for any duration affecting a patient older than 1 month of age
      6. Kaposi's sarcoma affecting a patient younger than 60 years of age
      7. Lymphoma of the brain (primary) affecting a patient younger than 60 years of age
      8. Lymphoid interstitial pneumonia and/or pulmonary lymphoid hyperplasia (LIP/PLH complex) affecting a child younger than 13 years of age
      9. *Mycobacterium avium* complex or *M. kansasii* disease, disseminated (at a site other than or in addition to the lungs, skin, or cervical or hilar lymph nodes)
      10. *Pneumocystis carinii* pneumonia
      11. Progressive multifocal leukoencephalopathy
      12. Toxoplasmosis of the brain affecting a patient older than 1 month of age

II. **With Laboratory Evidence of HIV Infection**
   Regardless of the presence of other causes of immunodeficiency (I.A.), in the presence of laboratory evidence for HIV infection, any disease listed above (I.B.) or below (II.B) indicates a diagnosis of AIDS.
   A. **Indicator Diseases Diagnosed Definitively**
      1. Bacterial infections, multiple or recurrent (any combination of at least two within a 2-year period), or any of the following types affecting a child younger than 13 years of age: septicemia, pneumonia, meningitis, bone or joint infection, or abscess of an internal organ or body cavity (excluding otitis media or superficial skin or mucosal abscesses), caused by *Haemophilus, Streptococcus* (including pneumococcus), or other pyogenic bacteria
      2. Coccidioidomycosis, disseminated (at a site other than or in addition to lungs or cervical or hilar lymph nodes)
      3. HIV encephalopathy (also called "HIV dementia," "AIDS dementia," or "subacute encephalitis due to HIV")
      4. Histoplasmosis, disseminated (at a site other than or in addition to lungs or cervical or hilar lymph nodes)
      5. Isosporiasis with diarrhea persisting longer than 1 month
      6. Kaposi's sarcoma at any age
      7. Lymphoma of the brain (primary) at any age
      8. Other non-Hodgkin's lymphoma of B-cell or unknown immunologic phenotype and the following histologic types:
         a. small noncleaved lymphoma (either Burkitt or non-Burkitt type)
         b. immunoblastic sarcoma (equivalent to any of the following, although not necessarily all in combination: immunoblastic lymphoma, large-cell lymphoma, diffuse histiocytic lymphoma, diffuse undifferentiated lymphoma, or high-grade lymphoma)
         Note: Lymphomas are not included here if they are of T-cell immunologic phenotype or their histologic type is not described or is described as "lymphocytic," "lymphoblastic," "small cleaved," or "plasmacytoid lymphocytic"
      9. Any mycobacterial disease caused by mycobacteria other than *M. tuberculosis,* disseminated (at a site other than or in addition to lungs, skin, or cervical or hilar lymph nodes)
      10. Disease caused by *M. tuberculosis,* extrapulmonary (involving at least one site outside the lungs, regardless of whether there is concurrent pulmonary involvement)
      11. *Salmonella* (nontyphoid) septicemia, recurrent
      12. HIV wasting syndrome (emaciation, "slim disease")
   B. **Indicator diseases diagnosed presumptively**
      In some situations, a patient's condition will not permit the performance of definitive diagnostic tests. In these situations, accepted clinical practice may be to diagnose the following presumptively based on the presence of characteristic clinical and laboratory abnormalities:
      1. Candidiasis of the esophagus
      2. Cytomegalovirus retinitis with loss of vision
      3. Kaposi's sarcoma
      4. Lymphoid interstitial pneumonia and/or pulmonary lymphoid hyperplasia (LIP/PLH complex) affecting a child younger than 13 years of age
      5. Mycobacterial disease (acid-fast bacilli with species not identified by culture), disseminated (involving at least one site other than or in addition to lungs, skin, or cervical or hilar lymph nodes)
      6. *Pneumocystis carinii* pneumonia
      7. Toxoplasmosis of the brain affecting a patient older than 1 month of age

III. **With Laboratory Evidence Against HIV Infection**
   With laboratory test results negative for HIV infection, a diagnosis of AIDS for surveillance purposes is ruled out unless:
   A. All other causes of immunodeficiency listed above in Section I.A are excluded; **AND**
   B. The patient has had either:
      1. *Pneumocystis carinii* pneumonia diagnosed by a definitive method; **OR**
      2. a. any of the other diseases indicative of AIDS listed above in Section I.B diagnosed by a definitive method **AND**
         b. a T-helper/inducer (CD4) lymphocyte count less than 400/mm³.

(From CDC. [1987]. Revision of the CDC surveillance case definition for acquired immunodeficiency syndrome. *MMWR, 36* [Suppl. 1] pp. 1–15.)

(Yarchoan et al., 1989). It inhibits HIV replication. The initial clinical trials of AZT in persons with severe ARC or AIDS demonstrated improved survival, temporary increase in CD4 cell counts, fewer opportunistic diseases, weight gain, and decreased viral load as measured by the p24 antigen test (Fischl et al., 1987). The initial recommended dose of 1200 mg/day was also associated with significant toxicities, especially severe anemia and neutropenia, which often resulted in its discontinuance (Richman et al., 1987). The recently reported clinical trial 019 demonstrated that AZT both delayed progression to AIDS in persons who were seropositive for HIV and had T4 (CD4) cell counts of less than 500 mm^3 and was efficacious and safer (fewer toxicities) at a dose of 500 mg/day (Volberding et al., 1990; NIAID, 1989). Because zidovudine may be carcinogenic, mutagenic, or both, its long-term safety is questionable. It has been suggested that zidovudine be given to individuals (e.g., health care workers who have sustained a significant exposure to HIV via needlestick injury) to prevent HIV infection at the time of exposure. The efficacy and safety of this practice are unknown (Yarchoan et al., 1989).

The third goal is to restore normal immune functioning. Clinical trials currently under way are attempting to find safe and effective immunotherapies (Lane & Fauci, 1985). Unfortunately, efforts to restore immune function in persons with AIDS, including bone marrow transplantation, have been unsuccessful to date (Holland et al., 1989).

Finally, the fourth goal is the early diagnosis and treatment of opportunistic infections, secondary cancers, and HIV-associated conditions.

Opportunistic Infections

According to the CDC, 86 per cent of all persons with AIDS presented initially with an opportunistic infection at the time of diagnosis. Of these, 64 per cent were diagnosed with *P. carinii* pneumonia; the remaining 22 per cent were diagnosed with other opportunistic infections. Five per cent of the patients who were diagnosed with AIDS presented with both *P. carinii* pneumonia and Kaposi's sarcoma; 14 per cent presented with only Kaposi's sarcoma (CDC, 1989c). In general, persons with one or more opportunistic infections have a worse prognosis than persons with only Kaposi's sarcoma. Recurrent or multiple opportunistic infections are also poor prognosticators (Volberding, 1985). Persons with opportunistic infections are more likely to be hospitalized for initial therapy (Arno & Hughes, 1986). Some opportunistic infections, such as *P. carinii* pneumonia, may be acutely life threatening and require immediate medical care.

Volberding (1985) has pointed out two confounding variables that complicate the medical management of the person with AIDS. First is the resistence of AIDS-associated opportunistic infections to conventional therapies, which means that patients with AIDS require longer courses of treatment than might be required for persons whose immune systems are not compromised. Second is the frequency of toxicities and complications related to treatment.

Glatt and colleagues (1988) identified six principles that influence the diagnosis and treatment of HIV-related infections. First, fungal, parasitic, and viral infections are rarely curable. Long-term suppressive therapy is usually required after the acute episode is controlled. Second, the majority of HIV infections are caused by the reactivation of previously acquired organisms and are not communicable. The only exceptions to this tenet are tuberculosis, herpes zoster, and perhaps salmonellosis. Third, multiple, concurrent infections are common. Fourth, certain fungal and parasitic infections are endemic to different locales. Therefore, travel history and place of origin may provide useful diagnostic information. Fifth, certain bacterial infections are now being recognized as HIV related, for example, pneumococcal pneumonia in young and middle-aged adults. Finally, HIV-associated infections are frequently severe, often disseminated, and characterized by a high density of organisms.

An understanding of the common opportunistic infections and malignancies associated with AIDS forms the physiologic basis of providing care to the person with AIDS. Table 41–6 lists the most prevalent opportunistic infections and associated conditions that are noted in persons with advanced HIV disease. It describes the signs and symptoms of these opportunistic infections, and it reviews diagnostic procedures and therapeutic measures for each infection or condition. Finally, it notes complications and concerns related to medical and nursing management. Not all of the opportunistic infections and HIV-associated conditions are included in this table. Table 41–7 outlines AIDS-related malignancies. The reader is directed to review articles to supplement and expand on the information provided in the tables (Armstrong et al., 1985; Broder, 1987; DeVita, Hellman, & Rosenberg, 1988; Glatt, Chirgwin, & Landesman, 1988; Sande & Volberding, 1988; Young, 1986).

Secondary Cancers

Forty per cent of AIDS cases reported early in the epidemic had a cancer diagnosis as their AIDS-qualifying condition. Secondary cancers now account for only about 20 per cent of cases as the AIDS-index diagnosis (Groopman, 1987). The most common AIDS-related malignancy is Kaposi's sarcoma, but this AIDS-related disease varies from its classic and endemic forms that are seen in non-HIV populations and has been coined *epidemic KS* (Safai, 1987). This multicentric tumor that originates in blood vessels accounted for almost 90 per cent of all AIDS-related malignancies (Volberding, 1986).

Non-Hodgkin's lymphoma, especially as a primary brain tumor, accounted for an additional 10 per cent (Groopman, 1987). AIDS-related non-Hodgkin's lymphoma staging has documented bone marrow and gastrointestinal tract involvement as well as nodal involvement (Levine, 1987). These two cancers are

Table 41–6. OPPORTUNISTIC INFECTIONS AND OTHER CONDITIONS FREQUENTLY NOTED IN ADVANCED HIV DISEASE

Candidiasis (Cello, 1988; Greenspan, Greenspan, & Winkler, 1988)
  Oropharyngeal
  Esophageal
  Perineal
Signs and Symptoms
1. Oropharyngeal lesions
    White, cottage cheese–like patches that can be scraped off
    Red flat lesions
    Pain
    Anorexia and dysphagia
2. Esophageal lesions
    Dysphagia
    Odynophagia
    Retrosternal burning
3. Perineal lesions
    Pain
    Pruritus
    Discharge
    Wet, desquamated, reddened lesions
Diagnosis
1. Oral, esophageal, perineal lesions are scraped for wet mount, cultured, and examined histologically for *Candida albicans*
2. Clinical examination of lesions may be sufficient to begin therapy
Therapy
1. Oral lesions:
    Clotrimazole troches orally five times per day for 14 days; long-term low-dose prophylaxis may be necessary
    Nystatin oral pastilles 5 times per day
    Ketoconazole 200 mg daily for 10–14 days in refractory, symptomatic cases
2. Esophageal lesions
    Ketoconazole 200 mg orally one to four times per day for 10–14 days
    Low-dose amphotericin B for refractory symptomatic cases
3. Perineal lesions
    Clotrimazole cream to affected areas two times per day
4. For extensive uncontrolled lesions or lesions not responsive to above
    Low-dose amphotericin B intravenous administration daily for 7–10 days
Complications and Comments
1. Long-term therapy often required owing to recurrence
2. Candidiasis qualifies as an AIDS index diagnosis if confirmed by biopsy (see Table 41–3)
Cryptococcosis (Grant & Armstrong, 1988)
  Meningitis
  Disseminated
Signs and Symptoms
1. Meningitis
    Fever
    Headache
    Nuchal rigidity often not seen
    Change in mental status
    Focal neurologic findings, e.g., seizures, photophobia, are uncommon
2. Disseminated cryptococcosis may occur with the following presentations:
    Pneumonia, pleural effusion, interstitial pneumonitis
    Lymphadenopathy
    Peritonitis
    Retinitis
    Arthritis
    Cutaneous lesions
    Myocarditis
    Prostatitis
Diagnosis
1. Identification of *Cryptococcus neoformans* organism in cerebrospinal fluid, blood, biopsy specimen, or body fluid
2. Detection of cryptococcal antigen in blood, cerebrospinal fluid, urine, or other body fluid
Therapy
1. Amphotericin B intravenous infusion: dose calculated by weight with/without flucytosine oral capsules: dose calculated by weight to potentiate amphotericin
    B; flucytosine alone generally *not* sufficient treatment
2. Therapy may have to be administered indefinitely to control fungal infection
3. Periodic spinal tap to ensure disappearance of organism and to determine efficacy of therapy
4. Fluconazole, an oral antifungal agent, is currently being evaluated for use in patients in whom amphotericin B treatment has failed
Complications and Comments
1. Disseminated disease process is common but not necessarily symptomatic
2. Flucytosine may cause neutropenia; may need to discontinue therapy
3. Therapy is not curative, but there may be marked clinical improvement; cultures and serologic tests may remain positive even after prolonged therapy
4. Despite the frequently indolent meningitis presentation, the overall mortality rate, even with treatment, exceeds 60%
5. Amphotericin B is associated with severe and multiple toxicities: fever, rigors, chills, nausea, vomiting, hematuria, and renal insufficiency
Cryptosporidiosis (Soave, 1988)
  Enteritis
Signs and Symptoms
1. Moderate to severe watery diarrhea up to 25 L per day, often explosive
2. Abdominal cramping, often after meals
3. Dehydration
4. Weight loss and wasting
5. Nausea and vomiting
6. Fever
7. Symptoms may vary in intensity
Diagnosis
1. Identification of *Cryptosporidium* organism in stool specimen by acid-fast stain
2. Identification of *Cryptosporidium* organism in gastrointestinal mucosa by biopsy

Table continued on following page

Table 41-6. OPPORTUNISTIC INFECTIONS AND OTHER CONDITIONS FREQUENTLY
NOTED IN ADVANCED HIV DISEASE *Continued*

Therapy
1. Currently no effective treatment
2. Symptomatic relief using antidiarrheal medications, including opiates
3. Temporary intravenous fluid replacement may be helpful in relieving dehydration
4. Experimental protocol:
   Octreotide acetate (Sandostatin) with total parenteral nutrition

Complications and Comments
1. Infection can be an extremely disabling problem and can cause significant nutritional deficiencies and life-threatening metabolic derangements
2. *Isospora belli,* another parasitic infection of the bowel, is clinically indistinguishable from *Cryptosporidium*
3. Persons with AIDS frequently have multiple, concurrent, enteric pathogens that can cause diarrhea

Cytomegalovirus (CMV) (Drew, Buhles, & Erlich, 1988)
   Chorioretinitis
   Enteritis
   Pneumonia

Signs and Symptoms
1.. Chorioretinitis
   Unilateral visual field loss, decreased visual acuity, or both
   Usually progresses to bilateral involvement
   Ophthalmologic exam; yellow or white exudates and hemorrhages
   May result in retinal detachment
2. Gastrointestinal
   Diarrhea
   Weight loss
   Anorexia
   Fever
   Abdominal pain
   Ulcerations in the esophagus, stomach, duodenum associated with pain
3. Pulmonary
   Respiratory distress: shortness of breath, dyspnea on exertion, nonproductive cough
   Lung examination frequently normal
4. Adrenalitis with adrenal insufficiency
   Orthostatic hypotension
   Weakness

Diagnosis
1. Identification of CMV inclusion bodies by histologic examination from biopsy and evidence of virus-mediated damage
2. Isolation of the virus cultured from throat washings, blood, and urine with evidence of disease

Therapy
1. Ganciclovir (DHPG) has recently received Food and Drug Administration approval for CMV retinitis. Its use for other CMV conditions is being evaluated
2. DHPG is administered by intravenous infusion:
   For induction therapy: dose 5 mg/kg bid over 1 hr for 2 weeks
   For maintenance therapy: dose 5–6 mg/kg for 5–7 days/week
   Dose may be reduced in renal insufficiency
3. Toxicities associated with DHPG: neutropenia (common), thrombocytopenia, confusion, dizziness, nausea, vomiting, and headache
4. Phosphoroformate (Foscarnet) is currently being evaluated for persons who show no clinical response to DHPG

Complications and Comments
1. CMV is a common latent herpesvirus in 40–60% of the general population; in homosexual men, approximately 95% have antibodies to CMV
2. CMV has been recovered from urine, semen, blood, and saliva, but its colonization does not always signify disease
3. CMV may itself be immunosuppressive and therefore may potentiate other opportunistic infections
4. DHPG is an analogue of acyclovir but is 50 times more active against CMV than acyclovir
5. CMV retinitis occurs in 25% of AIDS patients, usually later in the disease course

Herpes Simplex Virus (Drew, Buhles, & Erlich, 1988)
   Oral
   Perirectal

Signs and Symptoms
1. Oral lesions
   Occur in oral cavity or on lips
   Vesicles may coalesce and cause large areas of ulceration
   Lesions may spread into the esophagus, causing painful esophagitis
2. Perirectal lesions
   Large cutaneous lesions around the rectum
   Rectal pain
   Bleeding
   Discharge
3. Mucocutaneous genital lesions may occur but are less common than rectal lesions

Diagnosis
1. Lesions are scraped or biopsied and cultured for the virus by immunofluorescent techniques
2. Clinical inspection and presumptive diagnosis are often made to begin therapy

Therapy
1. Acyclovir 200 mg orally five times per day
2. Acyclovir intravenous therapy every 8 hours (dose calculated by weight) for 7 days
3. Prophylactic acyclovir orally three to five times per day to suppress recurrence

Complications and Comments
1. Disseminated herpes simplex virus is rare
2. Vesicles are highly contagious
3. Ulcerated perirectal lesions may require aggressive wound management
4. Pain may be a significant problem, requiring analgesia
5. Visible facial lesions can be disfiguring and stigmatizing

Herpes Zoster Virus (Drew, Buhles, & Erlich, 1988)
   Lesions
   Disseminated

Table 41–6. OPPORTUNISTIC INFECTIONS AND OTHER CONDITIONS FREQUENTLY
NOTED IN ADVANCED HIV DISEASE *Continued*

Signs and Symptoms
1. Lesions
   Occur along dermatomes (nerve pathways)
   Cutaneous lesions
   ● painful
   ● erythematous papules with or without vesicles
2. Disseminated
   Cutaneous vesicles on the hands and feet
   Possible neurologic dysfunction
Diagnosis
1. Clinical inspection is usually sufficient for diagnosis
2. Vesicles may be scraped and then cultured for the virus by immunofluorescent techniques, but it is rarely done
Therapy
1. High-dose acyclovir 600–800 mg orally five times per day OR
2. Acyclovir intravenous therapy 10–12 mg/kg every 8 hours for 7 days
3. Prophylactic acyclovir orally three to five times per day may be required indefinitely
Complications and Comments
1. Herpes zoster is reactivated; varicella (chickenpox) viral infection
2. Histologically, herpes zoster is indistinguishable from herpes simplex
3. Postherpetic neuralgia may occur after acute infection clears and is very painful
4. Narcotic analgesics are frequently required to control herpetic pain

HIV Encephalopathy (AIDS Dementia Complex) (Dilley & Boccellari, 1988; Holland & Tross, 1985; Price et al., 1988; Schofferman & Schoen, 1987)
Signs and Symptoms
1. Early Stage
   Cognitive: Decreased concentration, decreased memory, slowing mental function
   Behavioral: Personality change, social withdrawal and apathy, occasional agitation, and infrequent psychotic behavior
   Motor: Balance disturbance, clumsiness, leg weakness
2. Late Stage
   Global dementia: Limited speech; multiple neurologic abnormalities, including bowel and bladder incontinence; consciousness usually intact—vacant stare
       with virtual complete social withdrawal from caregivers
Diagnosis
1. Absence of concurrent illness, especially involving the central nervous system, must be ruled out by lumbar puncture, computed tomography (CT) or magnetic
   resonance imaging (MRI)
2. CT or MRI findings consistent with cortical atrophy, white matter abnormalities
3. Neuropsychiatric evaluation and neuropsychological testing essential to avoid misdiagnosing
Treatment
1. No definitive treatment to reverse condition
2. Zidovudine (AZT) has been shown to improve cognitive function. Discontinuance of this drug because of toxicities may result in rapid cognitive decline
3. Neuropsychotropics may be used carefully to reduce agitation or concurrent depression
4. Environmental adaptation to promote consistency and continuity
Complications and Comments
1. Progression or natural history not well defined
2. Variable changes in levels of orientation may be observed
3. Loss of developmental milestones in children

Mycobacterium Avium–Intracellulare (MAI) infection (Hawkins et al., 1986; Jacobson, 1988)
   Disseminated
Signs and Symptoms
1. Fevers
2. Drenching night sweats
3. Weight loss
4. Debilitation
5. Chronic diarrhea
6. Abdominal pain
7. Bone marrow infection
   Leukopenia
   Anemia
   Thrombocytopenia
8. Abnormal liver function tests
Diagnosis
1. Identification of MAI from cultures of blood, urine, stool, or sputum with evidence of infection or disease
2. Biopsy of bone marrow, lymph nodes, liver, spleen, and lung tissues and subsequent cultures of these tissues demonstrate MAI
Therapy
1. Frequent blood transfusions may be required as supportive therapy
2. Currently no effective therapy available
3. Various drug combinations have been tried but have shown limited success:
   Rifampin, ethambutol, amikacin
   Ethionamide, cycloserine, pyrazinamide
   Amikacin, ansamycin, clofazimine, ethambutol, ciprofloxacin
3. Experimental protocols:
   Liposome-encapsulated amphotericin
   Trimetrexate
   Trimethyl benzyl-piperazinyl rifamycin
Complications and Comments
1. MAI has been found in approximately 50% of AIDS patients autopsied
2. Often diagnosed after patient has other or multiple opportunistic diseases
3. Prognosis generally poor after diagnosis of disseminated MAI

Pneumocystis carinii Pneumonia (PCP) (CDC, 1989b; Hopewell, 1988; Masur & Kovacs, 1988)
Signs and Symptoms
1. Fever
2. Cough, nonproductive
3. Shortness of breath

Table continued on following page

Table 41–6. OPPORTUNISTIC INFECTIONS AND OTHER CONDITIONS FREQUENTLY
NOTED IN ADVANCED HIV DISEASE *Continued*

4. Tachypnea
5. Weight loss
6. Oral candidiasis, hairy leukoplakia, or both may be present
7. Dry crackles may be auscultated on lung examination; however, lung examination may show normal results

Diagnosis
1. Clinical examination and presumptive diagnosis may be followed by therapy, depending on severity of illness
2. Sputum induction, transbronchial lavage, or biopsy with identification of organism by histologic examination
3. Chest x-ray usually demonstrates symmetrical, diffuse, intersitial infiltrates, but 5–10% of AIDS patients have normal results on chest x-ray
4. Arterial blood gas determinations frequently indicate hypoxemia, the degree of which reflects the severity of lung involvement. Differences in oxygen saturation levels with exercise and at rest are common
5. Pulmonary function test values frequently are decreased, especially $D_{L_{CO}}$
6. Gallium scan may indicate nonspecific interstitial disease suggestive of, but not diagnostic for, PCP

Therapy
1. Trimethoprim-sulfamethoxazole by mouth or intravenously every 8 hours for 21 days; dose calculated by weight
2. Pentamidine isethionate therapy by intravenous infusion daily for 21 days; dose calculated by weight
3. Dapsone/trimethoprim orally
4. Primary or secondary prophylaxis for PCP:
   Trimethoprim-sulfamethoxazole orally bid
   Pentamidine isethionate inhaled 300 mg once per month
   Sulfadoxine and pyrimethamine orally one time per week
5. Experimental protocols include:
   Aerosolized pentamidine
   Clindamycin/primaquine orally
   Trimetrexate

Complications and Comments
1. PCP is the most frequent index diagnosis in AIDS; 60% of all patients have had PCP as their primary diagnosis; 20% more patients develop PCP later in the course of illness
2. Clinical presentation with PCP may be acute and fulminant but more often is indolent; with acute onset, patient may have severe respiratory distress and may require intubation and mechanical ventilation; with indolent presentation, mild symptoms may be present 1 to 2 weeks or months before diagnosis
3. Other concurrent pulmonary infections frequently coexist, e.g., CMV, cryptococcal or other viral or bacterial pneumonias, and Kaposi's sarcoma pulmonary lesions
4. Recurrent episodes of PCP infection are common; therefore, secondary PCP prophylaxis is recommended; primary prophylaxis is recommended for persons without a prior history of PCP and with a T4 (CD4) count of less than 200 mm³.

Toxoplasmosis (Israelski & Remington, 1988)
   Encephalitis
Signs and Symptoms
1. Fever
2. Headache
3. Lethargy
4. Confusion
5. Seizures
6. Cognitive impairment
7. Focal neurologic signs, e.g., hemiparesis, aphasia, ataxia, visual disturbance, or movement disorder

Diagnosis
1. Presumptive clinical diagnosis is usually made without invasive techniques; clinical diagnosis includes a CT scan or MRI that typically shows multiple bilateral enhancing mass lesions
2. Definitive identification of *Toxoplasma gondii* is made by brain biopsy and histologic examination of tissue but is rarely needed
3. Often empiric treatment is begun with documented central nervous system lesions, and lesions are reevaluated after 10 to 14 days with CT or MRI if no clinical improvement is noted

Therapy
1. After loading doses of pyrimethamine 50 mg orally every 12 hours for 2 days, pyrimethamine 75–100 mg orally one time per day; and sulfadiazine 6–8 gm/day in divided doses plus folinic acid 10–50 mg/day orally
2. Drugs currently being evaluated:
   Clindamycin
   Trimetrexate

Complications and Comments
1. Therapy usually continues indefinitely because of high probability of recurrence
2. *Toxoplasma gondii* also can be found in the stool of cats and in raw or undercooked meat
3. May be complicated by syndrome of inappropriate antidiuretic hormone secretion
4. *Toxoplasma* antibody titer may be useful screening tool, but it does not differentiate latent from reactivated disease

also reviewed later in this book. However, because of their frequency in AIDS, they are briefly reviewed in Table 41–7.

Other cancers noted in persons infected with HIV have included Hodgkin's disease; squamous cell cancers of the head, neck, or oral cavity; cervical cancer; and cloacogenic anorectal cancers (Donehower, 1987). These tumors will be discussed later in this volume. They may be associated with other risk factors (e.g., age, sex, sexual activity, or substance abuse) because their link in the HIV spectrum of disease has not been established (Daling et al., 1987).

An interesting observation noted in persons who develop AIDS-related cancers is the prevalence of specific herpes virus infections. Cytomegalovirus infec-

tion has been noted frequently in persons with Kaposi's sarcoma, and Epstein-Barr virus infection has been documented in persons with certain lymphomas (Groopman, 1987). It has been suggested that HIV has oncogenic potential. If this hypothesis is accurate, the incidence of other cancers may be expected to increase in AIDS patients (Donehower, 1987). Persons receiving cytotoxic cancer therapy for an AIDS-related cancer are at increased risk for developing an opportunistic infection (Groopman, 1987).

NURSING MANAGEMENT

The complex medical, social, and psychological issues that are linked to AIDS and the spectrum of HIV

Table 41–7. SECONDARY CANCERS IN HIV DISEASE

Kaposi's Sarcoma (KS) (Mitsuyasu, 1988a, 1988b; Mitsuyasu & Miles, 1987; Safai, 1987; Volberding, 1986)
    Vascular origin
    Multicentric at presentation
    Disseminated
Signs and Symptoms
1. Characteristic skin lesions
      Early lesions
      ● faint pink-to-bluish macular lesions
      ● large red-to-purple indurated plaques
      ● often found on the face or in the oral cavity
      ● do not blanch when pressed
      ● painless unless breakdown occurs or if located on the soles of feet
      Progressive lesions
      ● dark red-to-brown or blue nodules
      ● grow in size and coalesce
      ● found on all body surfaces
      ● may be associated pain
2. Disseminated lesions, advanced KS
      Widespread occurrence of lesions involving the skin, oral mucosa, lymph nodes, and visceral organs
      Edema due to lymphatic blockage present in extremities and face
      Pain may be associated with edema
      Respiratory distress due to pulmonary lesions
      Gastrointestinal symptoms due to lesions in gastrointestinal tract
Diagnosis
1. Identification of KS by biopsy of, e.g., skin lesion, lymph node, gut, bone marrow, and histologic examination
2. Validated staging system lacking
Therapy
1. Chemotherapy
      Vincristine, vinblastine, etoposide (VP-16), and doxorubicin have been used commonly
      Other chemotherapeutic agents have been used with some success
2. Radiation therapy
      Used for palliation of symptoms related to edema caused by lymphatic blockage
      To provide pain relief caused by bulky or obstructing oral or lower extremity lesions
      For cosmetic purposes
3. Biologic response modifiers
      Interferon-α has been approved for AIDS-related KS and has resulted in decrease of skin lesions; it is generally not efficacious for advanced disease
Complications and Comments
1. Before AIDS and epidemic KS:
      KS found primarily in elderly men of Italian or eastern European Jewish ancestry, young black African men and children, and patients receiving immunosuppressive therapy following transplant surgery
      Disease course indolent
      Improvement noted in transplant patients with removal of immunosuppressive therapy
2. KS considered a clinical marker for underlying immune deficiency in AIDS patients
3. Lesions generally do not ulcerate, although ulceration may occur
4. KS seen more frequently in homosexuals than in other patients with AIDS
5. Visible lesions can lead to social embarrassment and isolation
6. Approximately 50% of cases have gastrointestinal involvement; 10–20% have pulmonary involvement
7. Pulmonary KS associated with poor prognosis
AIDS-Associated Non-Hodgkin's Lymphomas (NHL) (Kaplan, 1988)
    Primary central nervous system
    Other extranodal disease
Signs and Symptoms
1. Primary central nervous system lymphoma
      Headache
      Cognitive impairment, e.g., confusion, lethargy, memory loss
      Focal neurologic deficits, e.g., gait disturbances, seizures, hemiparesis
2. Other extranodal disease presentations
      Bone marrow
      Rectal and other gastrointestinal
      Soft tissue
      Pulmonary
      Cardiac
3. May have history of persistent generalized lymphadenopathy
4. Nonspecific B symptoms; fever, night sweats, and weight loss are often present
Diagnosis
1. CT scan or MRI to identify lesions; lesions cannot be differentiated by CT scan or MRI from infectious mass lesions present with opportunistic infections
2. Biopsy and histologic examination alone confirm diagnosis of lymphoma
3. Grading and staging of disease influence treatment decisions and affect estimated prognosis
Therapy
1. Currently no effective treatment for primary central nervous system lymphoma
2. Chemotherapy and radiation protocols have been used; generally in central nervous system lymphoma, response is poor even in non-AIDS patients
3. Chemotherapy protocols used for other AIDS-NHL patients include CHOP, BACOP, and M-BACOD
Comments
1. Occasionally precedes or follows the diagnosis of KS
2. Often diagnosis is made coincidentally, without prodrome or autopsy
3. Generally occurs in more advanced HIV disease
4. Response and survival rates in other extranodal disease presentations have been directly related to prior HIV-related disease
5. Neutropenia following chemotherapy and other intercurrent opportunistic infections frequently limit or delay treatment

CHOP, cyclophosphamide, hydroxydaunorubicin (Adriamycin), vincristine (Oncovin), and prednisone; BACOP, bleomycin, doxorubicin, cyclophosphamide, vincristine, prednisone; M-BACOD, methotrexate, bleomycin, doxorubicin (Adriamycins), cyclophosphamide, vincristine, dexamethasone.

Box 41–2. BELIEFS ABOUT AIDS

STUDY

Flaskerud, J. H., & Rush, C. E. (1989). **AIDS and traditional health beliefs and practices of black women.** *Nursing Research, 38,* 210–215.

METHOD

A qualitative study used participant observation in small focus groups to verify and expand the health beliefs and practices reported in the literature and relate these to AIDS.

SAMPLE

Twenty-two black women, aged 27 to 68, Protestant, with 8 to 12 years of education: 36 per cent (n = 8) were married, and 36 per cent (n = 8) were separated or divorced.

FINDINGS

This study corroborated the sources of illness reported in the literature. AIDS was believed to be caused by lowered resistance, social conditions, and supernatural causes even though most women stated that the virus was transmitted through sexual contact and sharing needles. Lowered resistance was due to exposure to cold, lack of cleanliness, unsanitary conditions, and cyclic weaknesses, especially among women and children. Social conditions included a lack of AIDS education, a lack of accessible health care, and an initial belief that AIDS was a gay or white person's disease. The beliefs that homosexual behavior and intravenous drug use were unnatural acts and that AIDS was a plague that had been predicted in the Bible were the supernatural causes cited. AIDS prevention and treatment remedies included the use of laxatives and bathing after sex to rid the body of impurities, life-style moderation, and prayer or spiritual healing.

IMPLICATIONS FOR PRACTICE

Educational programs must reenforce positive health beliefs and practices, e.g., life-style moderation. Safe sex education might include bathing after intercourse but clarify that this practice alone will not prevent HIV transmission. Clinicians should assess client use of laxatives to manage the symptoms of fever or other respiratory symptoms. Antidiarrheal agents may be regarded as unhealthful.

---

disease present care-intensive challenges to nursing. Although the purpose of this chapter was to describe the pathophysiologic effects of HIV and AIDS and their treatment, no discussion of the human response to HIV can be concluded without some mention of the context within which this illness occurs (Herek & Glunt, 1988). At the same time, comprehensively reviewing the nursing management of HIV illness is beyond the scope of this chapter. Excellent references are included for further review (Donehower, 1987; Flaskerud, 1989; Gee & Moran, 1988; Grady, 1988; Lewis, 1988).

Wells (1987) poignantly described the complexities and challenges AIDS presents for nurses when he noted that nurses may find themselves in the "unthinkable position of not wanting to care for someone . . . [and be forced] to look at ourselves as individuals." Nurses' attitudes, values, and beliefs affect nursing practice. With the epidemic of HIV, nurses are forced to examine their attitudes, values, and beliefs regarding sexuality, intimacy, substance use, family, racial and ethnic populations, vulnerability, death and dying, and occupational risk. Each one of these topics is pro-

foundly complex. Taken together, they can be overwhelming.

Educational opportunities and supportive environments that encourage the expression of even unthinkable fears and concerns regarding HIV can help to dispel them (Pasacreta & Jacobsen, 1989). Given the volume of new information available regarding this epidemic, "keeping current" can be another challenge. No doubt, at the time you are reading this sentence, some information presented in this chapter has been challenged.

Literature sources for current, clinically relevant AIDS information include *The Morbidity and Mortality Weekly Report (MMWR),* a CDC publication that summarizes its HIV and AIDS reports approximately every 6 months; *New England Journal of Medicine; Lancet;* and *Annals of Internal Medicine.* Nursing journals such as *American Journal of Nursing, Nursing, Oncology Nursing Forum, Nurse Practitioner,* and *Journal of Continuing Education in Nursing,* among others, may be useful resources. An AIDS literature computer database (AIDSLINE) is also available as part of the MEDLARS system of databases based at the National Library of Medicine and available in many health sciences libraries. Local and state health departments as well as the CDC have current epidemiologic data. There is a national nursing specialty organization, Association of Nurses in AIDS Care (ANAC), whose mission is to provide support and information to its members.

Knowledge of the epidemiology, pathophysiology, and medical management of HIV disease can provide valuable basic information to nurses across practice settings. For example, sexually active adults and substance users are populations at greatest risk for acquiring and transmitting HIV (Box 41–2). Risk reduction and health promotion programs should be targeted to these groups. Nurses encounter these clients in all settings: in schools and at work, in acute care, and in outpatient and home settings. Pre- and post-HIV test counseling are specific early detection activities for HIV that nurses can perform or advocate that their clients have access to.

An understanding of the pathophysiology of HIV provides the basis for all nursing care. For example, nurses are not perceived as credible health educators or supportive counselors if they lack a basic understanding of how this virus affects the body and of its pathophysiologic sequelae. Expert symptom management requires this knowledge, as does the ability to coach and to support patients and their families through the long-term, variable, and uncertain HIV illness trajectory.

Finally, knowledge of the medical management of HIV is crucial: the diagnosis and treatment of HIV and diseases associated with it are core components of nursing care. Usually nurses are not only administering the relevant therapies but also monitoring the response to them and managing any associated toxicities. In addition, educating patients and their families regarding diagnostic procedures and treatment options supports a sense of personal control over this devastating illness.

In conclusion, the epidemic of HIV has affected and will continue to affect nursing and health care delivery well into the next decade. This epidemic has pointed out the inequities and inadequacies of health care delivery in the United States. It has challenged the values of health care providers and resulted in a reexamination of the ethical codes that ground professional relationships to society. Nurses influence the care of persons with HIV not only as practitioners but also as educators, as administrators, as researchers, and as policy makers (Bloch & Phillips, 1989; Grant & Armstrong, 1988; Halloran, Hughes, & Mayer, 1988).

References

Abrams, D. I. (1986). Lymphadenopathy related to the acquired immunodeficiency syndrome in homosexual men. *Medical Clinics of North America, 70,* 693–705.

Abrams, D. I. (1988). The pre-AIDS syndromes: Asymptomatic carriers, thrombocytopenic purpura, persistent generalized lymphadenopathy, and AIDS-related complex. In M. A. Sande & P. A.

Volberding (Eds.), *The medical management of AIDS* (pp. 91–102). Philadelphia: W. B. Saunders Co.

Armann, A. J. (1985). The acquired immunodeficiency syndrome in infants and children. *Annals of Internal Medicine, 103,* 734–737.

Armstrong, D., Gold, J. W., Dryjanski, J., Whimkey, E., Polsky, B., Hawkins, C. Brown, A. E., Bernard, E., & Kiehn, T. E. (1985). Treatment of infections in patients with the acquired immunodeficiency syndrome. *Annals of Internal Medicine, 103,* 738–743.

Arno, P. S., & Hughes, R. G. (1987, April). Local responses to the AIDS epidemic: New York and San Francisco. *New York State Journal of Medicine, 87* (5):264–272.

Bennett, J., & Gee, G., (1988). History and overview of HIV infection. In G. Gee & T. A. Moran (Eds.), *AIDS: Concepts in nursing practice* (pp. 3–24). Baltimore: Williams & Wilkins.

Bloch, D., & Phillips, T. (1989, November/December). Nurses develop AIDS action agenda. *American Nurse,* p. 27.

Bowen, D. L., Lane, H. C., & Fauci, A. S. (1985a). Immunologic features of AIDS. In V. DeVita, S. Hellman, & S. Rosenberg (Eds.), *AIDS: Etiology, diagnosis, treatment, and prevention* (pp. 89–109). Philadelphia: J. B. Lippincott Co.

Bowen, D. L., Lane, H. C., & Fauci, A. S. (1985b). Immunopathogenesis of the acquired immunodeficiency syndrome. *Annals of Internal Medicine, 103,* 704–709.

Brickner, P. W., Torres, R. A., Barnes, M., Newman, R. G., DesJarlais, D. C., Whalen, D. P., & Rogers, D. E. (1989). Recommendations for control and prevention of human immunodeficiency virus (HIV) infection in intravenous drug users. *Annals of Internal Medicine, 110,* 833–837.

Broder, S. (Ed.). (1987). *AIDS: Modern concepts and therapeutic challenges.* New York: Marcel Dekker, Inc.

Castro, K. G., Hardy, A. M., & Curran, J. W. (1986). The acquired immunodeficiency syndrome: Epidemiology and risk factors for transmission. *Medical Clinics of North America, 70,* 635–648.

Centers for Disease Control (CDC). (1981). Kaposi's sarcoma and pneumocystis pneumonia among homosexual men—New York City and California. *Morbidity and Mortality Weekly Report (MMWR), 30,* 305–308.

CDC. (1986). Classification system for HTLV-III/LAV infections. *MMWR, 35,* 334–338.

CDC. (1987a). Public Health Service guidelines for counseling and antibody testing to prevent HIV infection and AIDS. *MMWR, 36,* 509–514.

CDC. (1987b, August 21). Recommendations for prevention of HIV transmission in health-care settings. *MMWR, 36* (Suppl. 2), 1–18.

CDC. (1987c). Revision of the CDC surveillance case definition for acquired immunodeficiency syndrome. *MMWR, 36* (Suppl. 1), 1–15.

CDC. (1989a). Guidelines for prevention of transmission of human immunodeficiency virus and hepatitis B virus to healthcare and public safety workers. *MMWR, 38* (Suppl. 6), 1–37.

CDC. (1989b). Guidelines for prophylaxis against *Pneumocystis carinii* pneumonia for persons infected with human immunodeficiency virus. *MMWR, 38* (Suppl. 5), 1–9.

CDC. (1989c, October). *HIV/AIDS surveillance report—United States AIDS program through September, 1989.*

CDC. (1989d). Interpretation and use of the western blot assay for serodiagnosis of human immunodeficiency virus type 1 infections. *MMWR, 38* (Suppl. 7), 1–7.

CDC. (1989e). Sexually transmitted diseases treatment guidelines. *MMWR, 38* (Suppl. 8), vii–4.

CDC. (1990, February). *HIV/AIDS surveillance report,* 1–18.

Cello, J. P. (1988). Gastrointestinal Manifestations of HIV infection. In M. A. Sande & P. A. Volberding (Eds.), *The Medical Management of AIDS* (pp. 141–152). Philadelphia: W. B. Saunders Co.

Cohn, J. A. (1989). Virology, immunology, and natural history of HIV infection. *Journal of Nurse-Midwifery, 34,* 242–252.

Coolfont report: A PHS plan for prevention and control of AIDS and the AIDS virus. (1986). *Public Health Reports, 101,* 341–348.

Curran, J. W. (1985). The epidemiology and prevention of the acquired immunodeficiency syndrome. *Annals of Internal Medicine, 103,* 657–662.

Daling, J. R., Weiss, J. R., Weiss, N. S., Hislop, T. G., Maden, C., Coates, R. J., Sherman, K. J., Ashley, R. L., Beagrier, M., Ryan, J. A., & Corey, L. (1987). Sexual practices, sexually transmitted diseases, and the incidence of anal cancer. *New England Journal of Medicine, 317,* 973–977.

DeVita, V., Hellman, S., & Rosenberg, S. (Eds.). (1988). *AIDS: Etiology, diagnosis, treatment and prevention.* Philadelphia: J. B. Lippincott Co.

Dilley, J. W., & Boccellari, A. (1988). AIDS dementia complex: Diagnosis and management. *Focus, 3,* 1–3.

Donehower, M. G. (1987). Malignant complications of AIDS. *Oncology Nursing Forum, 14*(1), 57–64.

Drew, W. L., Buhles, W., & Erlich, K. S. (1988). Herpes virus infections: How to use ganciclovir. (DHPG) and acyclovir. In M. A. Sande & P. A. Volberding (Eds.), *The medical management of AIDS* (pp. 271–290). Philadelphia: W. B. Saunders Co.

Fauci, A. S., Macher, A. M., Longo, D. L., Lane, H. C., Rook, A. H., Masur, H., & Gellmann, E. P. (1984). Acquired immunodeficiency syndrome: Epidemiologic, clinical, immunologic, and therapeutic considerations. *Annals of Internal Medicine, 100,* 92–106.

Fischl, M. A., Richman, D. D., Grieco, M. H., Gottlieb, M. S., Volberding, P. A., Laskin, O. L., Leedom, J. M., Groopman, J. E., Mildvan, D., Schooley, R. T., Jackson, G. G., Durack, D. T., King, D. & the AZT Collaborative Working Group. (1987). The efficacy of azidothymidine (AZT) in the treatment of patients with AIDS and AIDS-related complex. *New England Journal of Medicine, 317,* 185–191.

Flaskerud, J. H. (Ed.). (1989). *AIDS/HIV infection: A reference guide for nursing professionals.* Philadelphia: W. B. Saunders Co.

Francis, D. P., Jaffe, H. W., Fultz, P. N., Getchell, J. P., McDougal, J. S., & Feorino, P. M. (1985). The natural history of infection with the lymphadenopathy-associated virus/human T-lymphotropic virus type III. *Annals of Internal Medicine, 103,* 719–722.

Francis, D. P., & Chin, J. (1986, August). *The prevention of AIDS in the United States.* Unpublished manuscript, pp. 12–18.

Friedland, G. H., & Klein, R. (1987). Transmission of the human immunodeficiency virus. *New England Journal of Medicine, 317,* 1125–1135.

Gallo, R. C., & Montagnier, L. (Eds.). (1988). AIDS in 1988. *Scientific American, 259*(4), 40–48.

Gee, G. S., & Moran, T. A. (1988). *AIDS: Concepts in nursing practice.* Baltimore: Williams & Wilkins.

Gerbert, B. (1988). Why fear persists: Health care professionals and AIDS. *Journal of the American Medical Association, 260,* 3481–3483.

Glatt, A. E., Chirgwin, K., & Landesman, S. H. (1988). Treatment of infections associated with human immunodeficiency virus. *New England Journal of Medicine, 318,* 1439–1448.

Grady, C. (Ed.). (1988). *Nursing Clinics of North America, 23*(4).

Grady, C. (1989). Acquired immunodeficiency syndrome: The impact on professional nursing practice. *Cancer Nursing, 12,* 1–9.

Grant, I. H., & Armstrong, D. (1988). Fungal infections in AIDS: Cryptococcosis. In M. A. Sande & P. A. Volberding (Eds.), *The medical management of AIDS,* (pp. 225–234). Philadelphia: W. B. Saunders Co.

Greenspan, J. S., Greenspan, D., & Winkler, J. R. (1988). Diagnosis and management of the oral manifestations of HIV infection and AIDS. In M. A. Sande & P. A. Volberding (Eds.), *The medical management of AIDS* (pp. 127–140). Philadelphia: W. B. Saunders Co.

Groopman, J. E. (1987). Neoplasms in the acquired immunodeficiency syndrome: The multidisciplinary approach to treatment. *Seminars on Oncology, 14,* 1–6.

Grossman, M. (1988). Children with AIDS. In M. A. Sande & P. A. Volberding (Eds.), *The medical management of AIDS* (pp. 319–330). Philadelphia: W. B. Saunders Co.

Halloran, J., Hughes, A., & Mayer, D. K. (1988). Oncology Nursing Society position paper on HIV-related issues. *Oncology Nursing Forum, 15,* 206–217.

Haseltine, W. A., & Wong-Staal, F. (1988). The molecular biology of the AIDS virus. *Scientific American, 259*(4), 52–62.

Hawkins, C. C., Gold, J. W., Whimkey, E., Kiehn, T. E., Brannon, P., Cammarata, R., Brown, A. E., & Armstrong, D. (1986). *Mycobacterium avium* complex infections in patients with the acquired immunodeficiency syndrome. *Annals of Internal Medicine, 105,* 184–188.

Herek, G. M., & Glunt, E. K. (1988). An epidemic of stigma: Public reactions to AIDS. *American Psychologist, 43,* 886–891.

Heyward, W. L., & Curran, J. W. (1989). The epidemiology of AIDS in the U.S. *Scientific American, 259*(4), 72–81.

Ho, D. D., Pomerantz, R. J., & Kaplan, J. C. (1987). Pathogenesis of infection with human immunodeficiency virus. *New England Journal of Medicine, 317,* 278–286.

Holland, H. K., Saral, R., Rossi, J. J., Donnenberg, A. D., Burns, W. H., Beschorner, W. E., Farzadegan, H., Jones, R. J., Quinnan, G. V., Vogelsang, G. B., Vriesendorp, H. M., Wingard, J. R., Zaia, J. A., & Santos, G. W. (1989). Allogeneic bone marrow transplantation, zidovudine, and human immunodeficiency virus type 1 (HIV-1) infection. *Annals of Internal Medicine, 111,* 973–981.

Holland, J. C., & Tross, S. (1985). The psychosocial and neuropsychiatric sequelae of the acquired immunodeficiency syndrome and related disorders. *Annals of Internal Medicine, 103,* 760–764.

Hopewell, P. C. (1988). Diagnosis of *Pneumocystis carinii* pneumonia. In M. A. Sande & P. A. Volberding (Eds.), *The medical management of AIDS* (pp. 169–180). Philadelphia: W. B. Saunders Co.

Israelski, D. M., & Remington, J. S. (1988). Toxoplasmic encephalitis in patients with AIDS. In M. A. Sande & P. A. Volberding (Eds.), *The medical management of AIDS* (pp. 193–212). Philadelphia: W. B. Saunders Co.

Jacobson, M. A. (1988) Mycobacterial diseases: Tuberculosis and *Mycobacterium avium* complex. In M. A. Sande & P. A. Volberding (Eds.), *The medical management of AIDS* (pp. 235–247). Philadelphia: W. B. Saunders Co.

Kaplan, L. D. (1988). AIDS-associated lymphomas. In M. A. Sande & P. A. Volberding (Eds.), *The medical management of AIDS* (pp. 307–318). Philadelphia: W. B. Saunders Co.

Lane, H. C., & Fauci, A. S. (1985). Immunologic reconstitution in the acquired immunodeficiency syndrome. *Annals of Internal Medicine, 103,* 714–718.

Levine, A. M. (1987). Non-Hodgkin's lymphomas and other malignancies in the acquired immunodeficiency syndrome. *Seminars in Oncology, 14,* 34–39.

Lewis, A. (Ed.). (1988). *Nursing care of the person with AIDS/ARC.* Rockville, MD: Aspen Publications.

Lifson, A., Bookbinder, S., Sheppard, H., Wilbur, J., Hessol, N., Mawle, A., Stanley, M., Hart, C., O'Malley, P., & Rutherford, G. (1989, June). *The natural history of HIV infection in a cohort of homosexual and bisexual men: Clinical manifestations 1978–1989* (abstract). V International Conference on AIDS, Montreal.

Lovejoy, N. C. (1988). The pathophysiology of AIDS. *Oncology Nursing Forum, 15,* 563–571.

Masur, H., & Kovacs, J. A. (1988). Treatment and prophylaxis of *Pneumocystis carinii* pneumonia. In M. A. Sande & P. A. Volberding (Eds.), *The medical management of AIDS* (pp. 181–192). Philadelphia: W. B. Saunders Co.

Mitsuyasu, R. T., & Miles, S. A. (1987). Biotherapy with interferon in AIDS-related Kaposi's sarcoma. *Oncology Nursing Forum, 14* (6, Suppl.), 27–31.

Mitsuyasu, R. T. (1988a). Kaposi's sarcoma in the acquired immunodeficiency syndrome. In M. A. Sande & P. A. Volberding (Eds.), *The medical management of AIDS* (pp. 291–306). Philadelphia: W. B. Saunders Co.

Mitsuyasu, R. T. (1988b). The role of alpha interferon in the biotherapy of hematologic malignancies and AIDS-related Kaposi's sarcoma. *Oncology Nursing Forum, 15*(Suppl. 6), 7–12.

National Institute of Allergy and Infectious Diseases (NIAID) Press Release—AZT/019, August 17, 1989.

Pasacreta, J. V., & Jacobsen, P. B. (1989). Addressing the need for staff support among nurses caring for the AIDS population. *Oncology Nursing Forum, 16,* 659–670.

Price, R. W., Sidtis, J. J., Navia, B. A., Pumarola-Stone, T., & Ornitz, D. B. (1988). AIDS dementia complex. In M. L. Rosenblum, R. M. Levy, & D. E. Bredesen (Eds.), *AIDS and the nervous system* (pp. 203–219). New York: Raven Press.

Project Inform. (1988). *Supplement on HIV testing.* San Francisco: Author.

Richman, D. D., Fischl, M. A., Grieco, M. H., Gottlieb, M. S., Volberding, P. A., Laskin, O. L., Leedom, J. M., Groopman, J. E., Mildvan, D., Hirsch, M., Jackson, G. G., Durack, D. T., Nusinoff-Lehrman, S., & the AZT Collaborative Working Group. (1987). The toxicity of azidothymidine (AZT) in the treatment of patients with AIDS and AIDS-related complex. *New England Journal of Medicine, 317,* 192–197.

Safai, B. (1987). Pathophysiology and epidemiology of epidemic Kaposi's sarcoma. *Seminars in Oncology, 14,* 7–12.

Sande, M. A., & Volberding, P. A. (Eds.). (1988). *The medical management of AIDS.* Philadelphia: W. B. Saunders Co.

Schofferman, J., & Schoen, K. (1987, October). AIDS-dementia syndrome. *Medical Aspects of Human Sexuality,* pp. 58–70.

Soave, R. (1988). Cryptosporidiosis and isosporiasis in patients with AIDS. In M. A. Sande & P. A. Volberding (Eds.), *The medical management of AIDS* (pp. 259–270). Philadelphia: W. B. Saunders Co.

Tindall, B., Cooper, D. A., Donovan, B., & Penny, R. (1988). Primary human immunodeficiency virus infection: Clinical and serologic aspects. In M. A. Sande & P. A. Volberding (Eds.), *The medical management of AIDS* (pp. 75–90). Philadelphia: W. B. Saunders Co.

Volberding, P. A. (1985). The clinical spectrum of the acquired immunodeficiency syndrome: Implications for comprehensive patient care. *Annals of Internal Medicine, 103,* 729–733.

Volberding, P. A. (1986). Kaposi's sarcoma and the acquired immunodeficiency syndrome. *Medical Clinics of North America, 70,* 665–675.

Volberding, P. A., Lagakos, S. W., Koch, M. A., Pettinelli, C., Myers, M. W., Booth, D. K., Balfour, H. H., Reichman, R. C., Bartlett, J. A., Hirsch, M. S., Murphy, R. L., Hardy, W. D., Soeiro, R., Fischl, M. A., Bartlett, J. G., Merigan, T. C., Hyslop, N. E., Richman, D. D., Valentine, F. T., Corey, L., & the AIDS Clinical Trials Group of the National Institute of Allergy and Infectious Diseases. (1990). Zidovudine in asymptomatic human immunodeficiency virus infection: A controlled trial in persons with fewer than 500 CD4-positive cells per cubic millimeter. *New England Journal of Medicine, 322,* 941–949.

Wells, R. (1987). A perspective of care. *International Nursing Review, 34*(3), 64–66.

Yarchoan, R., Mitsuya, H., Myers, C. E., & Broder, S. (1989). Clinical pharmacology of 3′-azido-2′,3′-dideoxythymidine (zidovudine) and related dideoxynucleosides. *New England Journal of Medicine, 321,* 726–738.

Yarchoan, R., Mitsuya, H., & Broder, S. (1988, October). AIDS therapies. *Scientific American, 259,* 110–119.

Young, L. S. (1986). Management of opportunistic infections complicating acquired immunodeficiency syndrome. *Medical Clinics of North America, 70,* 677–692.

Ziegler, J. A., & Abrams, D. I. (1985). The AIDS-related complex. In V. DeVita, S. Hellman, & S. Rosenberg (Eds.), *AIDS: Etiology, diagnosis, treatment, and prevention* (pp. 223–233). Philadelphia: J. B. Lippincott Co.

CANCER AS AN ILLNESS

42

Nursing Management of Persons at Risk for Cancer: Prototype—Cervical Intraepithelial Neoplasia

MARY RUBIN

The women who are at risk for cervical intraepithelial neoplasia (CIN) are basically healthy individuals who often are unaware of the precancerous condition. Women of all ages can develop CIN. Although it was once thought to be a clinical problem for older women, recent data reveal a disturbing rise in its incidence among adolescents (Sadeeghi, Hsieh, & Gunn, 1984; Spitzer & Krumholz, 1988). A young woman may, in fact, receive the news of an abnormal reading following her first Papanicolaou smear. For this reason, preventive health care measures should include encouraging sexually active adolescents to incorporate Papanicolaou smear screening into their health maintenance regimens.

Although the incidence of cervical cancer has decreased greatly over the past decade due to improved screening techniques, about 13,000 new cases still are reported each year (American Cancer Society, 1988). Unlike many other forms of cancer, cervical cancer has a reliable screening method for early detection. The Papanicolaou smear is not only effective in detecting invasive cancer but also highly sensitive in detecting the preinvasive state or CIN. When diagnosis occurs early, many options exist for early, conservative treatment and management of this condition, thus making possible prevention of cervical cancer.

This chapter presents background information concerning the development of CIN, reviews the risk factors associated with the disease, and explores the role the nurse plays in the management of these cases. Figure 42–1 shows the steps in the diagnosis, treatment, and follow-up of CIN and the many phases in which the nurse can intervene in the process.

DEFINITION OF THE PROBLEM

Precancer Phase

A woman's cervix has a zone of transformation (T zone) that undergoes maturation throughout her reproductive life. The T zone varies in shape and size and is predetermined during embryologic development. In most women, this zone is confined to the surface of the cervix. In some women, who had been exposed to diethylstilbestrol (DES) in utero, the T zone may extend into the vagina (Gasser, 1985). As the cells evolve from columnar epithelium to mature

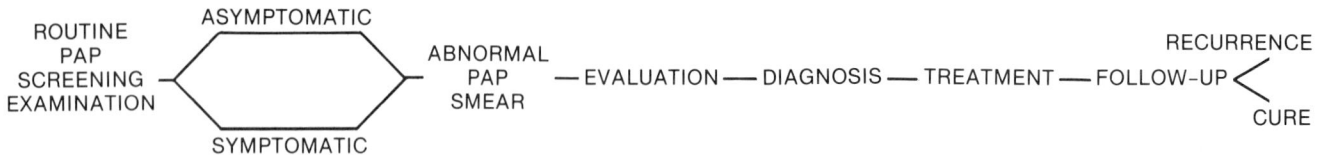

Figure 42–1. Trajectory of the diagnosis, treatment, and management of cervical intraepithelial neoplasia. *PAP,* Papanicolaou.

squamous epithelium by a process of squamous metaplasia, they are most susceptible to abnormal transition to the state of CIN (Atkinson & Ernst, 1987).

Figure 42–2 depicts the developmental process of cervical cells. The range of cells as observed by the cytologist on Papanicolaou smear may vary from normal to cancerous. The precancer phase of CIN is best viewed as a continuum from stages CIN 1 to CIN 3. With normal maturation, as seen in the first division in Figure 42–2, clearly distinguishable basal, parabasal, intermediate, and superficial cells develop from the basement membrane to the surface. During the development of CIN of increasing severity, a greater proportion of tissue depth from the basement membrane to the surface is composed of only basal cells. Because these cells often have larger nuclei and less cytoplasm, they are said to have a greater nuclear to cytoplasmic ratio. When these cells begin to develop beneath the basement membrane, either microinvasive cancer (1 to 3 mm) or invasive cancer (greater than 3 mm) is present (Ferenczy & Winkler, 1987).

In most cases a woman is not aware that she has this condition. Unless she has symptoms of vaginal discharge or vulvar warts, she would not expect the Papanicolaou smear to be anything but normal. At the time of the routine pelvic examination with Papanicolaou smear, the nurse can use this opportunity to begin to educate the woman about this smear and the range of possibilities for the laboratory reading. Many women know that a Papanicolaou smear is done to detect cancer, but most are unaware of the precancerous states that can also be present. Once the diagnosis is suspected from the cytology reading, the process of evaluation, treatment, and follow-up provides many opportunities for the nurse to play a significant role in teaching the woman about the disease and the regimen needed to return the cervix to a healthy state.

Risk Factors

A number of risk factors are associated with oncogenesis in cervical cells. No one factor is thought to be the cause of cervical cancer. The initial phase of the process, CIN, is a result of many co-factors interacting with the cervical cells over a period of time. Some of the risk factors associated with CIN are young age at first coitus, multiple partners, relations with male partners who have had multiple partners, smoking, and exposure to agents of sexually transmitted diseases

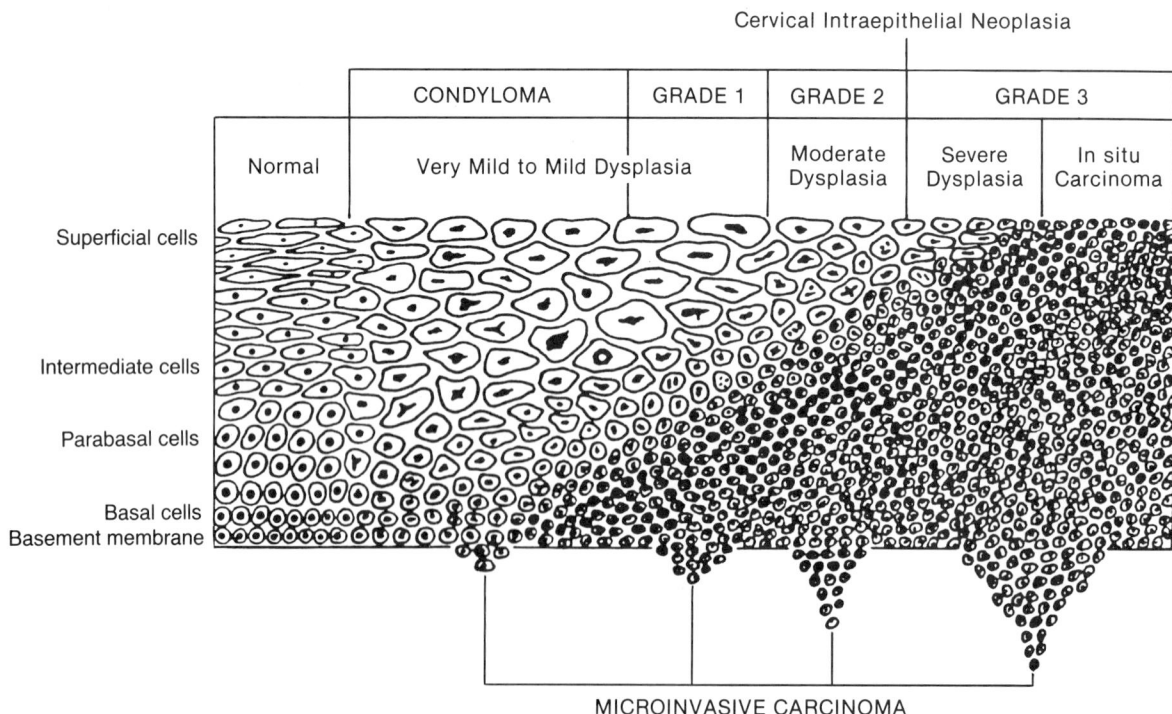

Figure 42–2. Developmental process of cervical intraepithelial neoplasia. (From Ferenczy, A. & Winkler, B. [1987]. Cervical intraepithelial neoplasia and condyloma. In R. Kurman [Ed.], *Blaustein's pathology of the female genital tract* [3rd. ed.]. New York: Springer-Verlag. Reproduced by permission.)

(STDs) such as herpes simplex virus (HSV), *Trichomonas,* and human papilloma virus (HPV), the cause of condylomas or venereal warts (Alexander, 1973; Brinton et al., 1987; Celentano, Klassen, Weissman, & Rosenshein, 1987; Hellberg, Nilsson, Haley, Hoffman, & Wynder, 1988; Noller et al., 1987). Although antenatal exposure to DES is associated with an increased incidence of clear cell adenocarcinoma of the cervix and vagina, thus far it has not been associated with an increased incidence of squamous cell cancer of the cervix. The risk is still unknown because these women are just now approaching the age range (youngest 17 years, oldest early 40s) at which an increased incidence of cervical cancer might be expected. It has, however, been found that DES daughters have a twofold higher incidence of CIN than unexposed women (Bornstein, Adam, Adler-Storthz, & Kaufman, 1987).

The patient's own immune system is also an important factor in the cancer formula. Persons who are immunosuppressed appear to be more susceptible to cervical abnormality, particularly to viral infections such as with HSV and HPV. Because of increasing evidence of the association of HPV with CIN and cancer, this virus is of particular concern. At least four of the 58 currently identifiable strains of HPV (types 16, 18, 31, and 35) have been linked to oncogenesis of cervical tissue (Sedlacek & Cunnane, 1987). With the increased incidence of HPV infections in actively maturing cervical epithelium of many young women, there is concern about the possibility of decreased transition time from CIN 1 to cancer in a younger population.

CASE PRESENTATION

Rose is a 20 year old gravida 1 para 0 therapeutic abortion 1 DES-exposed daughter who has been sexually active since age 16 years. She has been healthy and has had no major medical problems or surgery other than a therapeutic abortion at age 18 years. She has had regular pelvic examinations along with colposcopic evaluation since age 14 years, when her mother discovered that she had taken DES while pregnant with Rose.

During past evaluations, Rose has had several colposcopically directed biopsies from the wide developing transformation zone, the results of which were reviewed as normal squamous metaplasia. Her cytology readings until now have been consistent with that normal reading. Her sexual history includes three sexual partners since age 16 years. Initially, Rose had not used contraception consistently, and she became pregnant. Following the therapeutic abortion, she began taking oral contraceptives and has since used them as her mode of contraception. She has been treated in the past for both *Candida* and *Trichomonas* infections and currently has a Papanicolaou smear reading indicating CIN 1 and the presence of HPV. Her current sexual partner was not aware of the existence of HPV until Rose was evaluated and diagnosed. At that time it was recommended that her partner be evaluated by

a urologist or dermatologist, and evidence of HPV was found. He was treated with an application of 85 per cent trichloroacetic acid to the penile HPV. The incidence of penile cancer and other long-term effects for men with previous condyloma is not known.

Psychosocial Implications of DES Exposure

The psychosocial aspects of this case are multidimensional.

1. Rose had to face the fear of initial pelvic examination at a very young age. She not only had more frequent Papanicolaou tests than most young women her age, but also experienced a more lengthy examination because she had to undergo colposcopic evaluation and occasional biopsy of the cervix. Colposcopy is an examination of the cervix through an instrument called a colposcope (a microscope with a light source mounted on a stand, that provides a magnified view of the cervix). It is recommended for DES-exposed women and those with abnormal Papanicolaou smears. The trauma of this experience varies depending on the sensitivity of the examiners. The nurse present at these early examinations can be instrumental in preparing the young woman for the examination and providing support to her throughout the experience. Rose is understandably more accepting of the pelvic examination at age 20 than she was at age 14.

2. The fear of cancer was introduced to her at an early age. With all of the initial concern about the association between DES exposure and the development of clear cell adenocarcinoma of the cervix or vagina, Rose's sensitivity concerning the possibility of cancer in her lifetime was most assuredly heightened. No long-term data were available at that time and still are not concerning the increased risk of cancer for DES-exposed offspring in the future. The nurse working with Rose can assure her that, thus far, there has been no evidence of an increased incidence of any form of cancer for the DES daughters other than the early association with the clear cell cancer in a limited number of women. For the most part, this has been found on initial pelvic examination. Regular follow-up examinations will help to ensure that problems have not developed.

3. Anger is also among the emotions experienced by DES-exposed daughters. Many of the younger patients are angry at their mothers for having taken the medication and making this early pelvic examination necessary. As they become more aware of the known implications of the drug, such as the possibility of cancer or complications when they become pregnant, some women direct this anger at the physician for having given the medication and at the drug companies for having produced the medication. Litigation has sometimes been initiated by the women who are trying to affix the blame for their uncertain condition. The nurse can be supportive to the woman and allow her to express her anger and concerns while not taking sides in the placement of blame.

4. Uncertainty about the future is expressed by many of these women. Uncertainty results when one or more of the following dimensions is present: "(1) vagueness, (2) lack of clarity, (3) ambiguity, (4) unpredictability, (5) inconsistency, (6) probability, (7) multiple meaning, and (8) lack of information" (Norton, 1975). The unpredictability of developing cancer and the unknown degree of probability of impairment of reproductive function are sources of distress and contribute to Rose's perceived uncertainty. The nurse can be a valuable support person who allows the woman to express her feelings and evaluates her level of understanding about the condition. Because lack of information can also contribute to the uncertainty felt by the woman, providing her with current factual information about DES exposure can help to mitigate her distress. Patient information pamphlets and newsletters are available that give current information regarding these concerns (DES Action National, 1986; DES Action USA; U.S. Department of Health, Education, and Welfare, 1981).

Psychosocial Implications of the Diagnosis of CIN and HPV Infection

1. Women often react to the loss of their perceived wellness and the need for more frequent Papanicolaou smears along with colposcopic examinations. In addition, the regimen of treatment may require more time in the outpatient offices or even an admission to the hospital for more extensive treatment.

2. The woman often fears loss of fertility due to the treatment procedures. The DES-exposed daughters, as in Rose's case, already have great concern about future fertility due to their preexisting condition. The diagnosis of precancer of the cervix only adds to their level of anxiety.

3. Because of the association of CIN and HPV with possible progression to cervical cancer, the young woman is understandably concerned about her risk for cancer in the present and in the future.

4. Anger is also a factor with the diagnosis of CIN, especially when HPV infection as a sexually transmitted disease is part of the diagnosis. Most young women of Rose's age are not well informed about HPV and have not been using barrier methods of contraception to protect their susceptible transformation zone from exposure to all of the potential oncogenic agents implicated in the carcinogenesis of cervical tissue. Many have tried to be responsible by using oral contraceptives for prevention of pregnancy while being totally unaware of the risk to the cervix with each new sexual partner.

5. The woman can often feel quite depressed about the need for alteration in sexual activity throughout the evaluation and treatment phases for CIN and HPV. She may question her chances for "normal sexuality" in the future. She is often understandably concerned about informing her current partner about her diagnosis and the effect it will have on their relationship. She will need support in finding the right approach to discussing this information with her partner and in encouraging him to seek evaluation and treatment.

6. Coping with the uncertainty about the wellness of her body in the future and the return to a normal state of health are among the concerns faced by Rose and other women like her. Mishel (1981), as one of the early nurse researchers contributing to our understanding of uncertainty in illness, developed an uncertainty in illness scale (MUIS). She showed in her early work that the dimensions of ambiguity, vagueness, unpredictability, and lack of information are antecedents of uncertainty. Because many of the early CIN lesions are associated with HPV, the uncertainty factor is very real. The known association of HPV with precancerous and cancerous changes in the cervix, vagina, and vulva creates the climate for uncertainty for the future health in this group of women. Currently there is no specific "cure" for HPV infection, and factual information concerning the diagnosis is evolving. Methods of removing visible warts from the cervix, vagina, and vulva exist, such as cryosurgery, laser treatment, or chemical cautery, but none of the current methods of treatment totally eradicates the virus from the tissue. Therefore, visible warts often recur and abnormal Papanicolaou smears are found.

When counseling the woman about the diagnosis, the clinician conveys the areas of uncertainty about the diagnosis and lack of information regarding incubation period of the virus, routes of transmission, and cure. Implications of uncertainty in the diagnostic phase of a diagnosis may differ from those in the later stages of the condition. Mishel (1981) found that patients experienced greater uncertainty in their diagnostic work-up phase than did surgical patients or those who were chronically ill. It could be that patients with CIN and those with associated HPV infection experience different degrees of uncertainty as well as different dimensions of uncertainty in the route from diagnosis to follow-up (Box 42–1).

Ongoing research at many oncology centers will, it is hoped, provide answers concerning more definitive treatment in the near future. This information can be

---

Box 42–1. WOMEN'S CONCERNS AND COPING WITH ABNORMAL PAPANICOLAOU TEST RESULTS

As part of a broader study on women's concerns about abnormal Papanicolaou smears, Lauver and Rubin found that the questions and concerns of 118 women revealed aspects of uncertainty. Primary concerns were uncertainty about the purpose of the Papanicolaou smear and lack of knowledge about follow-up procedures being recommended. Later statements at the time of evaluation concerning thoughts and feelings about the diagnosis revealed ambiguity about the meaning of the results (e.g., is this cancer or something serious?).

(Lauver, D., & Rubin, M. [1991]. Women's concerns and coping with abnormal papanicolaou tests. *Journal of Obstetric, Gynecologic, and Neonatal Nursing.*)

conveyed to the patient in a sensitive manner to put the situation into proper perspective for her and provide the support she needs to cope with the uncertainty.

Little data-based knowledge exists to guide us in our nursing care of patients experiencing uncertainty. Mishel's refined perceived uncertainty model (1988) offers an avenue to understanding the consequences of uncertainty based on whether the uncertain event is perceived as a threat or an opportunity. Braden and Lynn (1987) showed a negative relationship between uncertainty and the variables of self-care, performance of role behaviors, and satisfaction with life in a group of patients treated for gynecologic cancer. Alteration in coping strategies and increased emotional distress were identified as consequences of uncertainty in subjects of a study evaluating uncertainty and distress in myocardial infarct patients (Chrisman et al., 1988). Additional research on the consequences of uncertainty in illness is needed.

MANAGEMENT AND TREATMENT OF CIN AND HPV INFECTION

Evaluation of an Abnormal Cytology Reading

The evaluation process often begins with a repeat Papanicolaou smear as a check on the original finding. The Papanicolaou smear was the initial screening technique to detect the presence of abnormal cells in the transformation zone. Figure 42–3 outlines the process of evaluation of CIN.

With the cytology diagnosis of CIN, the woman is most appropriately referred for colposcopic evaluation. The colposcope allows a specially trained physician or nurse colposcopist to evaluate the T zone more precisely for evidence of tissue patterns associated with the diagnosis on cytology. First the examiner inspects the vulva, vagina, and cervix grossly for signs of abnormality. Next, a 3 to 5 per cent acetic acid (vinegar) solution is applied to the cervix, and the most colposcopically abnormal areas are selected for biopsy. Not all of the details of the colposcopic appearance will be discussed in this chapter, but more information can be found in various colposcopy textbooks, such as those by Cartier (1977), Giuntoli, Atkinson, Ernst, Rubin, and Egan (1987), and Stafl and Kolstadt (1977). It is colposcopically directed biopsies that provide the histologic diagnosis necessary for decision making regarding treatment and management of HPV infection, CIN, and cancer. Many colposcopists agree that evaluation of the endocervical canal with endocervical curettage should be part of every colposcopy examination unless the woman is pregnant. An essential element of every colposcopic examination is being able to clearly visualize the squamocolumnar junction (SCJ). This is the critical border at which the developing squamous tissue of the T zone meets the original columnar epithelium. Unless it is well visualized, the examiner cannot be sure that a more serious lesion is not being missed in the endocervical canal.

Choices for Treatment and Management

The colposcopically directed biopsy will provide the necessary information for establishing an accurate diagnosis. The woman should be given instructions to expect minimal bleeding and to refrain from inserting anything into the vagina (i.e., douching, inserting tampons, or having intercourse) for 4 to 5 days after the biopsy. The choices for treatment and management once the diagnosis has been established by histologic sampling include cryosurgery, electrocautery, laser vaporization, cone biopsy, and hysterectomy. They are outlined in Table 42–1. Instructions after treatment can be addressed by the nurse in the treatment setting. Restrictions concerning intercourse vary; with cryosurgery and electrocautery, abstinence for 3 to 4 weeks is recommended. With laser vaporization and cone biopsy, 4 to 6 weeks is more appropriate. After hysterectomy, abstinence may be recommended for 6 to 8 weeks. Signs of infection such as purulent discharge or fever must be reviewed with the patient to decrease the complications of pyometritis.

NURSING INTERVENTIONS

Provide Factual Information About CIN and HPV Infection

Research by Lauver and Rubin (1991) has uncovered the need for information addressing various needs throughout the process of evaluation for CIN and HPV infection. The nurse must determine the woman's level of knowledge concerning the diagnosis. In addition, the nurse must be comfortable discussing the range of abnormality diagnosed on cytology so that any questions raised concerning causes of the Papanicolaou results, seriousness of the diagnosis, diagnostic implications, and procedures for follow-up can be answered. To supplement the explanations, the woman can be provided with factual information in patient education pamphlets.

Little information is available concerning women's reactions to the news of abnormal cytologic findings. Lauver and Rubin (1991) and Beresford and Gervaize (1987) found that hearing about abnormal Papanicolaou results often stimulates fear and anxiety. However, the degree of fear and anxiety reported differed in the two studies. Need for information surfaced as the predominant factor in Lauver and Rubin's study (1991), whereas emotional needs were the focus in Beresford and Gervaise's work (1987) (Box 42–2).

Colposcopy
Biopsy
ECC

Negative endocervical curettage
Squamocolumnar junction seen

Positive endocervical
curettage
Squamocolumnar junction not seen
Complex transformation zone
Unanswered CIN 3

Invasive cancer
on biopsy

Oncology work-up

No colposcopic
atypia

Cervical intraepithileal
neoplasia biopsy

Cone biopsy

Surgery,
radiation,
or both

Follow with
cytology
or
recolposcopy
in 4-6 months

Repeat
Pap smear
every 4 months × 1 year
plus
(Endocervical curettage)

Laser*

Hysterectomy

Cryosurgery*   Electrocautery*

Cone
biopsy

Repeat Pap smear
and
endocervical
curettage
in 4 months

Repeat Pap smear
every 6-12 months

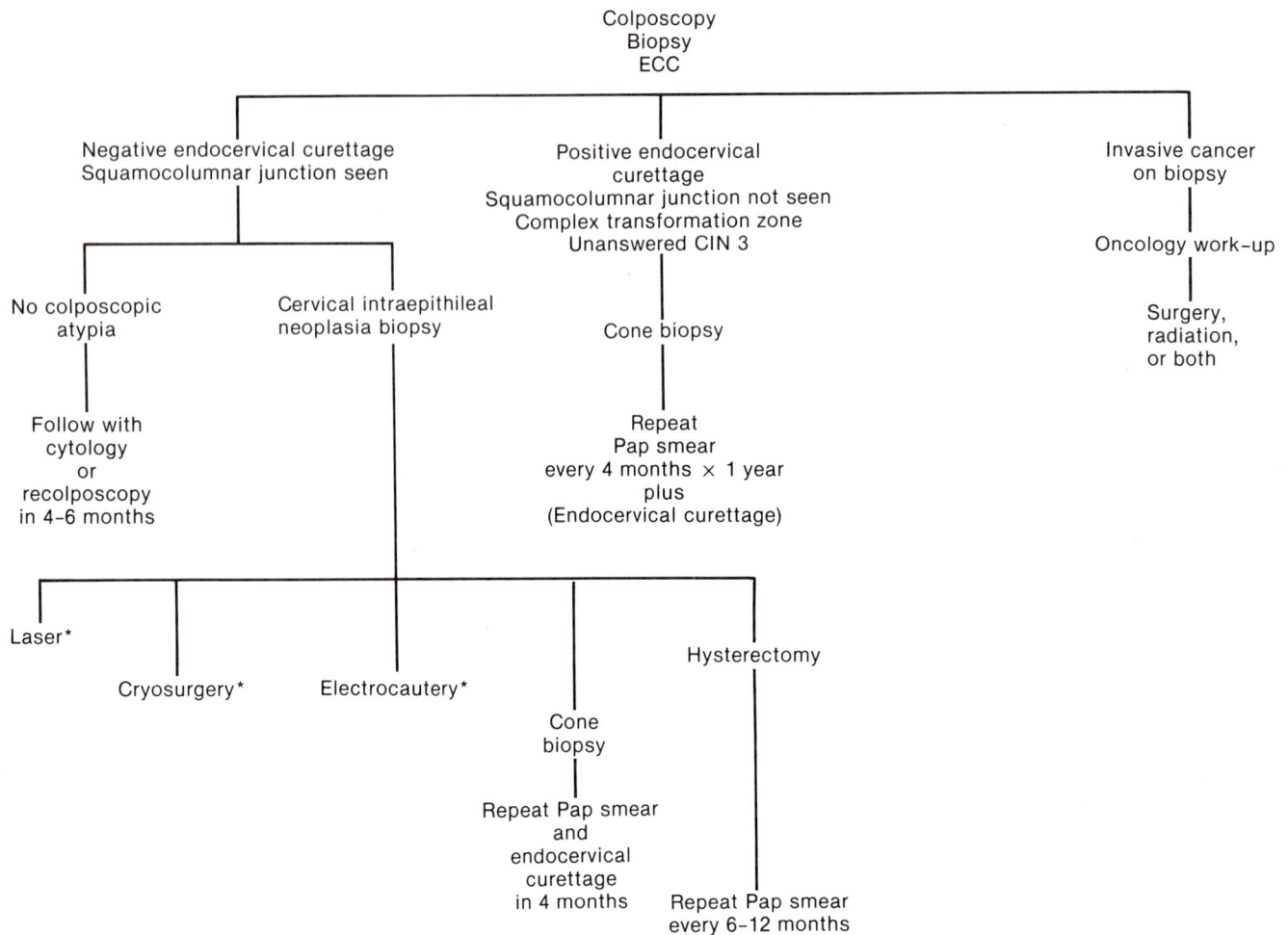

Figure 42–3. Management of cervical intraepithelial neoplasia. *ECC,* endocervical curettage; *Pap,* Papanicolaou.
*Repeat Papanicolaou smear every 4 months for 1 year. Recolposcopy plan.

Table 42–1. TREATMENTS FOR CERVICAL INTRAEPITHELIAL NEOPLASIA (CIN)

Treatment Method	Definition	Length of Time for Treatment	Characteristics	Disadvantages
Cryosurgery	Destruction of CIN by the use of a probe cooled with a refrigerant such as nitrous oxide	5–10 min	Office procedure Little or no discomfort No anesthesia required	Can cause: Narrowing of cervical os Profuse watery discharge for 3–4 weeks
Electrocautery	Destruction of CIN by use of a probe heated with an electric current	10–15 min (dependent on size of T zone)	May be done in office if area of CIN is not extensive	Can be painful May require local anesthesia
Laser vaporization	Destruction of CIN by use of a high-powered focused light beam	10–15 min (dependent on size of T zone)	May be done in office, short-stay operating room, or main operating room	Usually requires local or general anesthesia Risk of post-treatment hemorrhage
Cone biopsy	Use of a knife or laser beam to remove the entire T zone and the CIN surgically	20–30 min	Usually done in operating room More recently performed as office procedure	Requires general or regional anesthesia Risk of post-treatment hemorrhage Can cause narrowing of os or incompetent cervix
Hysterectomy	Use of surgery to remove CIN and the entire uterus	60–90 min	Requires operating room	Requires general or regional anesthesia

Box 42–2. THE EMOTIONAL IMPACT OF ABNORMAL PAPANICOLAOU SMEARS ON PATIENTS REFERRED FOR COLPOSCOPY

Beresford and Gervaise, in a Canadian colposcopy clinic, interviewed 50 women about their concerns. Interpreting open-ended questions, researchers found that more than half of the women expressed fear of cancer, of loss of reproductive or sexual function, and of the medical procedures they would undergo. Some expressed feeling loss of control of their good health and mood changes such as irritability and anger. Others reported behavior manifestations such as crying and weight changes.

(Beresford, J., & Gervaize, P. [1987]. The emotional impact of abnormal Pap smears on patients referred for colposcopy. *Colposcopy and Gynecologic Laser Surgery, 83,* 70–74.)

Clarify Management and Treatment Regimens for CIN and HPV Infection

In Rose's case, colposcopic abnormalities were present that were consistent with her cytologic reading of CIN 1 with presence of HPV. Refer to Figure 42–3 to see that because there was no evidence of cancer on her colposcopically directed biopsies, because the SCJ was seen in its entirety, and because the endocervical curettage was negative for CIN, the management regimen can be conservative with greater preservation of normal tissue. CIN 1 and HPV infection were confirmed by biopsy; therefore, most clinicians would recommend treatment. Rose had various options for treatment, including cryosurgery, electrocautery, and laser vaporization. In counseling her about the choices, the nurse should help her understand the advantages and disadvantages of each of the methods, as outlined in Table 42–1. Because Rose has a wide T zone due to her DES exposure and because she had colposcopic abnormality throughout the T zone, laser vaporization is probably the treatment of choice (Richart, 1987). It allows precise destruction of abnormal tissue under direct visualization with the colposcope. In addition, it heals with little scarring, often preserving the ability of the SCJ to be visualized. This may be important because the presence of HPV may cause recurrent abnormal cytologic findings, necessitating future evaluation of the T zone. If the SCJ has been driven into the endocervical canal during the healing process after treatment, choices for treatment in the future might have to be less conservative. When the woman is young and has not yet had children, the treatment method that is the most conservative and at the same time allows for the best results in destruction of CIN is the treatment of choice.

Reinforce Need for Regular Follow-up and Secondary Prevention

A critical aspect of early detection of CIN and HPV infection is the woman's understanding of the need for close follow-up. Many women think that the evaluation and treatment phase is the last step in the process. Part of a conservative treatment plan is the woman's cooperation in a regimen of regular follow-up. The woman needs to share in the responsibility for returning on a regular basis for repeat cytologic studies and occasionally colposcopy to ensure that progression to a more serious cervical condition does not go undetected.

Another aspect of secondary prevention is the woman's understanding of the need to protect the cervix from reexposure to the elements that contributed to the original abnormal transformation on her cervix. Incorporating barrier methods such as condoms into her sexual practices may help protect her from recurrence of abnormal cytology. Also, choosing a healthy life style with proper nutrition and adequate sleep and exercise will help her immune system to function optimally and add to her defense against recurrence (Rhude, Story, & Indman, 1987). If the patient smokes, she needs to be advised that data are beginning to show that women who smoke are more vulnerable to carcinoma of the cervix (Hellberg et al., 1988).

Provide Emotional Support

Many of the questions the patient asks, especially regarding HPV infections, as yet have no specific answers. The woman may have great anguish over carrying the virus and transmitting it to future partners. The young woman who is attempting to establish an identity and to cope with her own sexuality is now given an extra burden of increased concern for the health of future sexual partners. This responsibility is often quite overwhelming and can evoke great emotion. The nurse needs to be available to discuss these concerns. Even though there are often no definitive answers, allowing the woman to express her feelings and providing her with support may be enough to help her find a way to put things into proper perspective and cope with the uncertainty. On occasion the woman may need the expertise of a mental health professional to assist in resolving her feelings. Channels of communication can be kept open for the future so that if the woman wishes to discuss additional information or concerns, she can rely on the nurse as a valuable resource.

References

Alexander, R. E. (1973). Possible etiologies of cancer of the cervix other than herpesvirus. *Cancer Research, 33,* 1485–1496.

American Cancer Society. (1988). *Cancer facts and figures, 1988* (No. 5008-LE). New York: Author.

Atkinson, B., & Ernst, C. (1987). Cytology of the female reproductive tract. In C. Garcia, J. Mikuta, & N. Rosenblum (Eds.), *Current therapy in surgical gynecology* (pp. 28–34). Philadelphia: B. C. Decker, Inc.

Beresford, J., & Gervaize, P. (1987). The emotional impact of abnormal Pap smears on patients referred for colposcopy. *Colposcopy and Gynecologic Laser Surgery, 83,* 70–74.

Bornstein, J., Adam, E., Adler-Storthz, K., & Kaufman, R. (1987).

Development of cervical and vaginal squamous cell neoplasia as a late consequence of in utero exposure to diethylstilbestrol. *Obstetrical and Gynecological Survey, 43*(1), 15–21.

Braden, C. J., & Lynn, M. (1987, October). *Antecedents to and outcomes of uncertainty experienced in chronic illness.* Paper presented at Nursing Advances in Health: Model, Methods, and Application, ANA Council of Nurse Researchers 1987 International Nursing Research Conference, Washington, DC.

Brinton, L., Hamman, R., Huggins, G., Lehman, H., Levine, R., Mallin, K., & Fraumeni, J. (1987). Sexual and reproductive risk factors for invasive squamous cell cancer. *Journal of the National Cancer Institute, 79,* 23–30.

Cartier, R. (1977). *Practical colposcopy.* Basel, Switzerland: S. Karger.

Celentano, D., Klassen, A., Weissman, C., & Rosenshein, N. (1987). The role of contraceptive use in cervical cancer: The Maryland cervical cancer case control study. *American Journal of Epidemiology, 126,* 592–604.

Chrisman, N., McConnell, E., Pfeiffer, C., Webster, K., Schmitt, M., & Ries, J. (1988). Uncertainty, coping, and distress following myocardial infarction: Transition from hospital to home. *Research in Nursing and Health, 11,* 71–82.

DES Action National. (1986). *Reproductive outcomes in women exposed in utero to diethylstilbestrol: A review of the literature, 1978 to 1984.* New Hyde Park, NY: Long Island Jewish Medical Center.

DES Action National. (1986). *Reproductive outcomes in women exposed in utero to diethylstilbestrol.* San Francisco: Author.

Ferenczy, A., & Winkler, B. (1987). Cervical intraepithelial neoplasia and condyloma. In R. Kurman (Ed.), *Blaustein's pathology of the female genital tract* (3rd ed, pp. 177–217). New York: Springer-Verlag.

Gasser, R. F. (1985). The prenatal development of the cervix, vagina, and vulva. *Colposcopist, 17,* 1–10.

Giuntoli, R., Atkinson, B., Ernst, C., Rubin, M., & Egan, V. (1987). *Atkinson's correlative atlas of colposcopy, cytology, and histopathology.* Philadelphia: J. B. Lippincott Co.

Hellberg, D., Nilsson, S., Haley, J., Hoffman, D., & Wynder, E. (1988). Smoking and cervical intraepithelial neoplasia: Nicotine and cotinine in serum and cervical mucus in smokers and non-smokers. *American Journal of Obstetrics and Gynecology, 158,* 910–913.

Lauver, D., & Rubin, M. (1991). Women's concerns and coping with abnormal Papanicolaou tests. *Journal of Obstetric, Gynecologic, and Neonatal Nursing.*

Mishel, M. (1981). The measurement of uncertainty. *Nursing Research, 30,* 258–263.

Mishel, M. (1988). Uncertainty in illness. *Image, 20,* 225–232.

Noller, K., O'Brien, P., Melton, L., Offerd, J., Richart, R., Robboy, S., & Kaufman, R. (1987). Coital risk factors for cervical cancer. *American Journal of Clinical Oncology, 10,* 222–226.

Norton, R. N. (1975). Measurement of ambiguity tolerance. *Journal of Personality Assessment, 39,* 607–619.

Rhude, P., Story, B., & Indman, P. (1987, March-April). Venereal warts: The unmentionable STD. *Medical Self-Care,* pp. 52–53.

Richart, R. M. (1987). Causes and management of cervical intraepithelial neoplasia. *Cancer, 60,* 1951–1959.

Sadeeghi, S. B., Hsieh, E., & Gunn, S. (1984). Prevalence of cervical intraepithelial neoplasia in sexually active teenagers and young adults. *American Journal of Obstetrics and Gynecology, 148,* 726–729.

Sedlacek, T., & Cunnane, M. (1987). Condylomata acuminata: Diagnosis and management. *Postgraduate Obstetrics and Gynecology, 7,* 1–7.

Spitzer, M., & Krumholz, B. (1988). Pap smear screening for teenagers: A lifesaving precaution. *Contemporary Ob/Gyn, 31,* 33–42.

Stafl, A., & Kolstadt, P. (1977). *Atlas of colposcopy,* Baltimore: University Park Press.

U.S. Department of Health, Education, and Welfare. (1981). *Questions and answers about DES exposure before birth* (No. NIH 77-1118). Bethesda, MD: Public Health Service—National Institutes of Health.

CHAPTER 43

Nursing Management of Persons Treated for Cure: Prototype—Hodgkin's Disease

SHEILA B. BAEZ
MARYLIN J. DODD
JANET E. DiJULEO

Advances in the medical management of cancer have substantially increased client survival during the last two decades. More than 5 million Americans living today have a history of cancer, 3 million of them diagnosed 5 or more years ago. Most of these 3 million can be considered "cured," meaning they have no evidence of disease and the same life expectancy as a person who never had cancer (American Cancer Society [ACS], 1989). These numbers reflect the use of current diagnostic techniques, multimodality therapy, and the multidisciplinary team approach to the treatment of cancer.

This chapter uses a case presentation format to illustrate aspects of the cancer experience unique to persons being treated with curative intent. Hodgkin's disease is an excellent example of those cancers that have undergone a transformation in the past 20 years, having changed from a usually fatal disease to one that is cured frequently. Many of the problems, challenges, and stumbling blocks encountered by persons with Hodgkin's disease typify the experience of anyone being treated for "cure." The nursing interventions suggested, therefore, will, it is hoped, be applicable to an ever-growing segment of our cancer population.

FOCUS OF NURSING CARE

The needs of the person with cancer are different today from what they were 20 years ago, when long-term survival was rare. A need for support and sympathy has given way to a need for support, hope, and active interventions from cancer care professionals who approach the patient with curative intent. The focus of care has shifted from helping the patient and family deal with impending death to helping them cope with life and uncertainty (Lacher, 1986).

The process of surviving cancer has been divided into three phases or "seasons" by Mullen (1985), a cancer survivor and founder of the National Coalition for Cancer Survivorship. The initial season, *acute survival,* begins at the time of diagnosis and treatment. It is a time dominated by cancer treatments, when fear and anxiety are constant elements, and when patients are called on to confront their own mortality.

The second season, *extended survival,* begins on the completion of basic treatment when the patient enters a phase of watchful waiting. Psychologically, it is a time preoccupied by fear of recurrence. Physically, it is a time of diminished strength and of fatigue, as well as a time of coming to grips with altered body image.

The final season, termed *permanent survival,* is roughly equated with cure. Indelibly affected by the cancer experience, the cancer survivor remains at risk for problems with employment and insurance, as well as long-term effects of cancer treatments (Mullen, 1985).

Traditionally, cancer nurses have developed expertise in the physical and psychosocial care of persons undergoing cancer treatments or experiencing cancer recurrence and progression. As more people survive cancer for longer periods, however, the scope of cancer nursing practice has enlarged to include the psychological, social, and physical issues of survivorship. Today's 3 million cancer survivors make up a population about whom little is known, whose day-to-day reality may include late effects of treatment or disease-related disability, employment or insurance discrimination, and long-term monitoring for recurrence. As cancer survivors live out their normal life spans, they will be seen by nurses working in a variety of health care settings. These nurses need to be cognizant of the physical and psychosocial problems that warrant specialized health management in this patient population (Leonard & Waskerwitz, 1986).

CASE PRESENTATION

Diana, a 19-year-old college student, came to her family physician complaining of a sore throat and a lump in her neck of several weeks' duration. The lump did not respond to antibiotics so laboratory studies and a chest radiograph were obtained. Hemoglobin, hematocrit, platelet count, and white blood cell count were found to be within normal limits; skin tests were nonreactive. A chest radiograph was abnormal, revealing mediastinal lymphadenopathy. Subsequent lymph node biopsy of the left supraclavicular area revealed the presence of diagnostic Reed-Sternberg cells and was reported as indicative of nodular sclerosing Hodgkin's disease. Diana was then referred to a medical oncologist.

Further diagnostic studies and an in-depth history and physical examination were completed. Diana was questioned about the general symptoms that can occur with Hodgkin's disease. Although tiredness had been a problem, she denied experiencing any constitutional or "B" symptoms, including fevers, night sweats, or weight loss. Renal and liver function test results, including serum alkaline phosphatase level, were within normal limits. The erythrocyte sedimentation rate and serum copper level were elevated, however, reflecting active Hodgkin's disease. Diana denied having used oral contraceptives, which can falsely elevate serum copper levels. A computer tomographic (CT) scan of the chest delineated mediastinal involvement but showed no evidence of pleural effusion. A bipedal lymphangiogram was negative; however, a CT of the abdomen was positive for several large periaortic nodes.

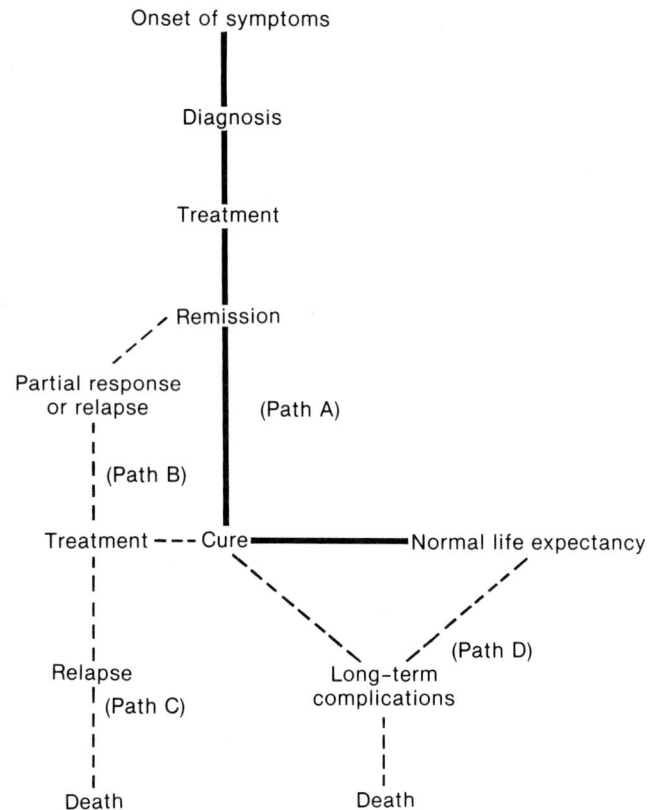

Figure 43–1. Disease trajectory for Hodgkin's disease.

A staging laparotomy was performed to confirm the presence of abdominal disease. The surgery included a careful exploration of the abdomen, removal of the spleen, and biopsy of the liver, lymph nodes, and bone marrow to obtain pathologic proof of Hodgkin's disease. An oopheropexy was performed to move the ovaries behind the uterus and, it was hoped, preserve normal ovarian function by shielding them from future exposure to therapeutic radiation. More than five splenic lesions and one positive periaortic node were found. The Ann Arbor Staging Classification was used to determine that Diana had Hodgkin's disease stage IIIA$_s$ (asymptomatic [A] involvement of lymph node regions on both sides of the diaphragm and the spleen [III$_s$]) (Dutcher, 1985).

The extensive splenic involvement (defined as five or more nodules visible in cut sections of spleen) with Hodgkin's disease necessitated a combined-method treatment approach. Radiation therapy combined with multidrug chemotherapy offered an 80 per cent chance of complete remission and probable cure. The treatment course, lasting 11 months, began with three cycles of multidrug chemotherapy. The MOPP regimen, consisting of mechlorethamine (nitrogen mustard), vincristine (Oncovin), procarbazine, and prednisone, was used. After a 1-month rest period, radiation therapy was administered to the dominant site of disease (e.g., supradiaphragmatic mantle). This was followed by a 1-month rest, an additional three cycles of MOPP chemotherapy, and lastly, radiation therapy to the anatomic area contiguous to active disease (e.g., the peri-aortic nodes).

Two years after completion of treatment, Diana continues to do well. She has graduated from college with a B.A. in accounting and is currently employed. She hopes to marry but worries about her ability to have children. The possibility of a second malignancy weighs heavily on her mind. The future, she states, still holds much uncertainty.

TRAJECTORY OF HODGKIN'S DISEASE

Hodgkin's disease can occur at any age, but in the United States it is seen most commonly in young adults aged 15 to 35 years, with a second peak in frequency during the age range from 50 to 60 years (Lacher, 1986). Fourteen per cent of the estimated 51,800 new cases of lymphoma occurring in the United States in 1989 were projected to be cases of Hodgkin's disease. This figure includes approximately 4200 men and 3200 women. The disease was expected to cause an estimated 1500 deaths (ACS, 1989).

The disease course for the majority of persons with Hodgkin's disease progresses in a predictable fashion from onset of symptoms and diagnosis, through treatment to remission, cure, and a normal life expectancy (Fig. 43–1, Path A). Patients with stage I and stage II (depending on presentation and specific histologic features) Hodgkin's disease have demonstrated a 90 per cent 4-year survival when treated with radiation therapy alone. Patients with stage III disease who received chemotherapy-radiotherapy regimens have an 80 per cent or better survival at 4 years. And, in stage IV disease, 4-year survivals of 79 per cent of patients treated with chemotherapy alone have been reported (Sullivan, Fuller, & Butler, 1984).

Patients who fail to achieve a complete remission or who experience relapses with Hodgkin's disease require repeated treatments with chemotherapy or radiation therapy (Path B). Combination chemotherapy offers an effective "salvage" treatment to patients with localized disease who develop recurrence after treatment with radiation therapy (Come & Mayer, 1983). Forty-five to 50 per cent of patients with advanced Hodgkin's disease will fail to achieve a complete response with initial multidrug chemotherapy or will have subsequent recurrence of tumors. Twenty-five per cent of these persons may be cured by subsequent chemotherapy (Santoro, Bonfante, & Bonadonna, 1982). Unfortunately, the remaining patients will experience repeated relapses (Path C) and will eventually succumb to their disease.

The diagnostic and therapeutic methods involved in the management of Hodgkin's disease can create a number of complications or side effects (Path D) (Boren & Sullivan, 1986). Detection and management of late effects of therapy are the focus of long-term follow-up.

APPROACHES TO NURSING CARE OF PERSONS BEING TREATED FOR CURE

Screening and Detection

Problem 1: Failure to Recognize the Importance of Early Diagnosis and Treatment in Potentially Curable Cancers

Diana was in the middle of final examinations when she first noticed the lump in her neck. She felt too pressured for time to get the lump checked at the college infirmary, and she made no connection between the lump and the lassitude and tiredness she had been experiencing for the last month. Rather, she blamed her tiredness on late night study habits and on anxiety about grades.

Several weeks later after Diana returned home for school break, her mother became concerned about the lump in her neck and about her daughter's lack of appetite and energy. The family practitioner was consulted, and antibiotics were ordered for a presumed localized infection. When the lump did not respond after 2 weeks of treatment, a biopsy of Diana's left supraclavicular area was performed in the day-surgery center at a local hospital. She was instructed on postoperative wound care by the nurses, and the biopsy site healed without complication.

Interventions

The American Cancer Society (ACS) has estimated that about 178,000 people with cancer would probably die in 1989 who might have been saved by earlier diagnosis and prompt treatment (ACS, 1989). Involvement of nurses in cancer detection has historically been minimal. They have contributed more over the past few years as a result of several trends, including the expansion of the nursing role in all health care settings, growth of the nurse practitioner role, and inclusion of physical assessment courses in nursing curricula. Today, cancer case finding is done by nurses who work in a variety of health care settings (Frank-Stromborg, 1981).

Besides actively participating in cancer screening, nurses are influencing the areas of prevention and detection of cancer by utilizing teaching and counseling skills more fully. Cancer nurses have studied attitudes of the public toward cancer and have attempted to obtain baseline data on present levels of knowledge about cancer (Brooks, 1979; Luther, Price, & Rose, 1982). Such information can be used to understand and influence behavior related to cancer and can result in a reduction of mortality and morbidity. Nurses have incorporated increased knowledge of cancer risk factors into the development of new public education programs. These programs emphasize the incorporation of cancer prevention behaviors and early detection techniques into life styles (Knopf & Morra, 1983; Knudsen, Schulman, Fowler, & Van den Hoek, 1984).

Nurses interact on a regular, intimate, and often influential basis with patients, relatives, and the general public (Brooks, 1979). By fostering open communications and through the provision of accurate information, emotional support, and counseling, nurses can have a major influence on attitudes of fear surrounding cancer detection and, it is hoped, help reduce delays in diagnosis.

Because nurses actively perform health screening, they should know the clinical manifestations of Hodgkin's disease and promptly refer the person with suspicious findings to the appropriate health care provider. Asking questions pertinent to the presentation of Hodgkin's disease will often help the patient recall significant signs and symptoms (Holcombe & Henderson, 1981).

Biopsy of a lymph node is necessary to obtain pathologic proof of the diagnosis of Hodgkin's disease. Patient and family education done in physicians' offices or day-surgery centers should inform the patient of what the biopsy procedure will entail, that it is usually done under local anesthesia, and that postoperative wound care includes wearing loose-fitting clothing over the surgical site and waiting until sutures are removed before bathing the area (Boren & Sullivan, 1986).

At diagnosis, the attitude of health professionals is of paramount importance. Because Hodgkin's disease is a relatively rare lymphoma, it is important that nurses be educated on the changing prognosis of the disease. Only by being aware of recent advances in the treatment of this and other curable cancers can the nurse provide a climate of realistic hope and support so important to patients and families during the stressful time surrounding biopsy and diagnosis (Koocher, O'Malley, Gogan, & Foster, 1980).

Continuing education classes for office and day-surgery nurses should be held on the latest developments in cancer treatment and should routinely include discussions on how to communicate with patients and families. Such classes might best be taught by oncology nurses with experience in counseling and treating these persons. After gaining an awareness that successful therapies are available, nurses will be able to confront their own dread of a cancer diagnosis honestly and without the fear that could impair communication with the patient and family (Koocher et al., 1980).

Problem 2: Anxiety and Emotional Distress Secondary to Cancer Diagnosis

Diana and her parents were informed by their family practitioner that the diagnosis of Hodgkin's disease, nodular sclerosing type, had been made. She sat down in private with them and discussed implications of the diagnosis and referral to an oncologist. In retrospect, Diana and her family stated that the attitude of hope and support they received from their doctor was crucial in facilitating their ability to cope at the time of diagnosis.

During the weeks that followed, Diana and her parents reacted to her diagnosis with varying degrees of shock and disbelief. Her father became extremely inquisitive about every aspect of the medical plan of care. Diana's mother seemed to be on the verge of emotional collapse. She cried frequently and rushed to meet Diana's every request. Diana remained aloof from her parents and seemed unwilling to show any emotion. She focused instead on details of tests and procedures.

Interventions

The diagnosis of cancer is emotionally disruptive to the patient and the family. When cancer is first suggested, they grow apprehensive because of assumptions that cancer is invariably lethal, painful, and debilitating and results in distancing from others (Stewart, 1980). Many of these misconceptions are based on inaccurate information or distorted stories and memories.

Once the diagnosis is confirmed, anticipatory fears of cancer are realized and often evolve into a period of crisis. Crisis has been defined as "a situation which the individual considers to be hazardous" (Rapoport, 1965). Crisis develops because a person's normal equilibrium is disrupted. Familiar problem-solving activities are not adequate and do not lead rapidly to the prior balanced state.

Self-questioning is common during the period after a cancer diagnosis as the patient and family members ask "Why me (us)?", "What did I (we) do to cause this to happen?" Their reactions to the diagnosis are a function of cultural (extrinsic) and familial (intrinsic) factors. The ability of the family to cope with the pressure, fear, disorganization, and disruption that accompany cancer will depend on how the family members functioned and related to one another in the past (Vettese, 1976). Assessment of intrafamilial coping and interactions can give some indication of the impact the cancer experience is having on family integrity (Welch, 1979).

The nursing goal during this period is to counter the emotional disorder being experienced by the patient and family. The general approach is to help the patient manage the crisis by considering one step at a time. Once diagnosis is made, verify that the patient and family are aware of treatment options. Act as an informed listener, helping people as they work to integrate the tremendous threat that cancer poses to their sense of well-being (Marino & Kouser, 1981).

As a result of delays in seeking health care and the frequent misdiagnosis of Hodgkin's disease (e.g., as adenitis or cat-scratch fever), weeks or months may elapse between onset of symptoms and institution of appropriate therapy. This delay can add to the anxiety on the part of patients or families, not only introducing fear that the disease has spread but also arousing guilt for causing the delay (Boren & Sullivan, 1986). Delays resulting from misdiagnosis may also be the focus of considerable anger toward the referring physician.

Nurses can help to alleviate some of this stress by encouraging the verbalization of feelings and providing the reassurance that delays in diagnosis and institution of appropriate therapy are common in Hodgkin's disease and are probably not the "fault" of the family or the physician (Caplan, 1964). It is helpful to explain that although in retrospect the diagnosis may seem obvious, the community physician had to rule out more probable causes of symptoms before initiating a frightening, costly, and time-consuming cancer work-up. The nurse should attempt to channel anger away from persons and redirect energies to the present (i.e., use constructive participation in patient's treatment) (Hall, Hardin, & Conatser, 1982). Additional guilt may stem from feelings that patients or their families have somehow caused the diagnosis by not caring adequately for themselves or by not handling stress properly (i.e., the so-called cancer personality) (Simonton, Mathews-Simonton, & Creighton, 1978). Again, nurses can help dispel these feelings by listening, reassuring the patient that the onset of disease was not anyone's "fault," and supplying consistent, truthful information.

Much of the anxiety and emotional distress associated with the diagnosis of Hodgkin's disease can be reduced by educating the patient and family about what the disease is, what tests will be done to determine its distribution in the body, and how it will be treated (Boren & Sullivan, 1986). Nurses working with Hodgkin's disease patients need to be aware of stage, histology, and prognosis of the individual patient, but in general they can be positive about excellent survival rates.

Regardless of the potential for cure, all persons with cancer must come to terms with the possibility of death (Mullen, 1985). Cooper, a 23-year-old social worker diagnosed as having Hodgkin's disease, wrote, "to the oncologist an 80% cure rate for Hodgkin's disease may look impressive. To the patient it may look more like a one in five chance of impending death" (Cooper, 1982).

Introducing patients currently undergoing treatment to someone who has successfully completed therapy has been employed to give evidence of cure. Establishing such a relationship early in the course of treatment opens a patient-to-patient communication channel that will facilitate coping throughout all phases of the disease process, regardless of eventual outcome.

Staging Work-up

Problem 1: Fear and Knowledge Deficit Concerning Staging Procedures

Diana's first visit to the cancer center passed in a blur. The family's collective anxiety level was very high. Diana relaxed somewhat after establishing a rapport with the oncologist. She also met briefly with the oncology nurse and was given an information packet about the cancer center and staff, a hospital map, and an educational booklet about Hodgkin's disease. The booklet briefly explained upcoming test procedures. The nurse reviewed important aspects of each test, focusing especially on the lymphangiogram and care of the resulting foot incision. She took several

minutes to complete a patient assessment and to explain that the tests would define the location of Hodgkin's disease in Diana's body.

Outpatient staging procedures, including the lymphangiogram, were scheduled. Throughout the testing period, Diana reread the information packet often as new questions came to mind or to recall details of what had been taught. She felt frustrated by an inability to concentrate, but she remembered the nurse had warned that anxiety often interferes with learning ability. Diana and her family members were grateful for the written information.

Diana was told that her Hodgkin's disease was clinical stage IIIA, and that a staging laparotomy would be needed to verify the extent of abdominal disease. She understood that this information was important to determine if treatment with chemotherapy would be necessary in addition to radiation therapy. The thought of chemotherapy frightened her.

Interventions

During the staging work-up, the patient and family are introduced to a team of cancer professionals who will provide support and consistency of care during the difficult days of treatment (Koocher & O'Malley, 1981). The nursing staff's involvement with the patient and family begins at this time. Their initial encounter with an informed, compassionate nurse lays the foundation for an ongoing trust relationship. This meeting is an ideal opportunity to obtain a complete nursing history or database. Tangible benefits include obtaining a complete health history and familiarizing the patient and family with the center and its policies. Just as important, a nurse-patient relationship is established that is based on an understanding of the patient and family system. Information is gained that will greatly facilitate design of an individualized plan of care (Hall et al., 1982).

A psychosocial assessment of the patient should be done that includes information about the nuclear and extended family and about prior experience with and reaction to stress and crises (Hall et al., 1982). It is important to find out what cancer means to the patient and family. It may represent loss of valued roles or, at the opposite extreme, an opportunity to use the sick role for secondary gain. An assessment should also be made of financial strengths and weaknesses. Information on employment status, insurance policies, or government agency funding provides the nurse with a picture of the stresses the patient and family may be experiencing. From this initial assessment, referrals may be made for social or psychological support services.

Success in the treatment of Hodgkin's disease is a function of providing the appropriate treatment for the precise anatomic extent of the disease (Dutcher & Wiernik, 1985). Nursing support is vital throughout the staging work-up phase. The nurse can be instrumental in helping the patient and family understand that staging procedures provide information that helps determine the best individualized treatment plan (Holcombe & Henderson, 1981).

Although many patients may be familiar with routine examinations, such as blood sampling or chest radiographs, more sophisticated tests, such as lymphangiograms, intravenous pyelograms, and CT scans, may create considerable anxiety. To relieve this anxiety and help patients participate in their own care, the nurse should explain the reasons for tests, the test procedures, and possible side effects. Written material, in simple terms, can clarify and reinforce information taught (Boren & Sullivan, 1986; Redman, 1980). Such material should include the day-to-day time frame for conducting tests and indicate what the patient can do to ensure their successful completion (Table 43–1). Repetition of a diagnostic test because of inadequate preparation creates undue patient tension. Adequately informing the patient better ensures that necessary tests will be completed successfully and reduces the length of this stressful and uncertain period.

A patient teaching booklet has been developed for Hodgkin's disease, which provides a comprehensive overview of the staging, treatment, and prognosis of the disease (Holcombe & Henderson, 1981). In addition, diagrams of lymph node chains and vital organ locations are included to illustrate and clarify areas of human anatomy poorly understood by the lay person (Fig. 43–2). This booklet is an invaluable resource to the nurse for the education of Hodgkin's disease patients and is an excellent model for the design of booklets for other cancer diagnoses.

Table 43–1. PATIENT TEACHING TOOL: LYMPHANGIOGRAM

Reason for the Test
A lymphangiogram is a routine staging procedure done to look for evidence of Hodgkin's disease in the abdominal lymph nodes, which usually cannot be felt.

Testing Procedure
This test involves the injection of an oil-based dye into the lymph system at the top of the feet. This is a minor surgical procedure that requires small incisions at the tops of the feet. The dye goes through the lymph system up the legs and into the abdominal lymph nodes. The dye can then be seen on x-ray films. The pattern of dye in the nodes helps determine if they might be involved with Hodgkin's disease. Thereafter, the response to treatment can be followed by periodic x-ray films of the abdomen.

Time Frame
The lymphangiogram takes several hours the first day, with follow-up x-ray films on the second day. The dye remains in the lymph nodes for months to more than a year.

Possible Side Effects
1. Urine and feet may have a bluish discoloration.
2. Allergic reaction to contrast dyes may occur.
3. Infection may occur at site of incision.
4. Pulmonary oil embolism may occur.
5. Fever occurs in 40 per cent of patients within 24 hr of injection.

What You Can Do to Ensure Successful Completion of the Test
1. Report any shortness of breath occurring after injection of dye.
2. Wear loose-fitting shoes to avoid irritating incision lines.
3. Do not immerse feet in water until the stitches have been removed.
4. Clean the incision line daily with alcohol.
5. Report any sign of redness or swelling.

(From Jacobs, C. [1979]. A patient teaching tool: Hodgkin's disease. *Cancer Nursing, 2,* 153–166. Reproduced by permission.)

Patient and family anxiety levels may adversely affect the ability to learn. Many patients are overwhelmed by the number of people with whom they come into contact during their initial cancer evaluation or by the amount of information given. Therefore, teaching may need to be repeated on several occasions and misinformation corrected whenever identified. Consistent follow-up is helpful.

The majority of patients being treated for Hodgkin's disease will complete the diagnostic and treatment phases of their illness as outpatients. To provide for stability and continuity of care, every effort should be made to assign one or two primary nurses to the patient (Holcombe & Henderson, 1981). This nurse should be present when the patient and family are given confirmation of a cancer diagnosis by the physician and during subsequent discussions about the stage and extent of disease and treatment recommendations. Having a member of the nursing staff present identifies the nurse as part of a support system on which the patient and family can draw after the physician has left the room (Hall et al., 1982). The same nurse should care for the patient during each office visit, performing a routine check-in and assessment, assisting the physician with procedures, doing patient and family teaching, and handling follow-up calls.

Problem 2: Developmental Problems Encountered by Young Adults with Cancer

Diana attended a local college but did not live at home. Feeling the need to establish independence from parents and to escape smothering maternal affection, she had moved to the college dormitory. After the staging laparotomy, however, Diana found she could not care for herself and returned home. Resuming dependence on her parents proved difficult to accept. Diana found that participating in a structured support group provided a welcomed opportunity to vent frustrations about her mother's way of doing things.

Interventions

Caring for the young adult with cancer poses a unique challenge to the nurse (Kane, 1981; Valentine, 1978). Both the age and the developmental stage of the patient influence how he or she will cope (see Chapter 7). Understanding the normal developmental tasks of young adulthood gives the nurse insight on how best to help patients and families deal with disruptions caused by cancer and treatment.

Impact of Cancer. When cancer is diagnosed, the ability of the young adult to perform developmental tasks may be altered. Specifically, the experience often affects the normal development of body image and self-concept, relationships with others, autonomy, and life direction (Blotcky, 1986; Valentine, 1978).

Being diagnosed as having a serious disease that requires long-term treatment results in the perception of being "different" or "abnormal" and often produces feelings of inferiority and lowered self-esteem (Cohen,

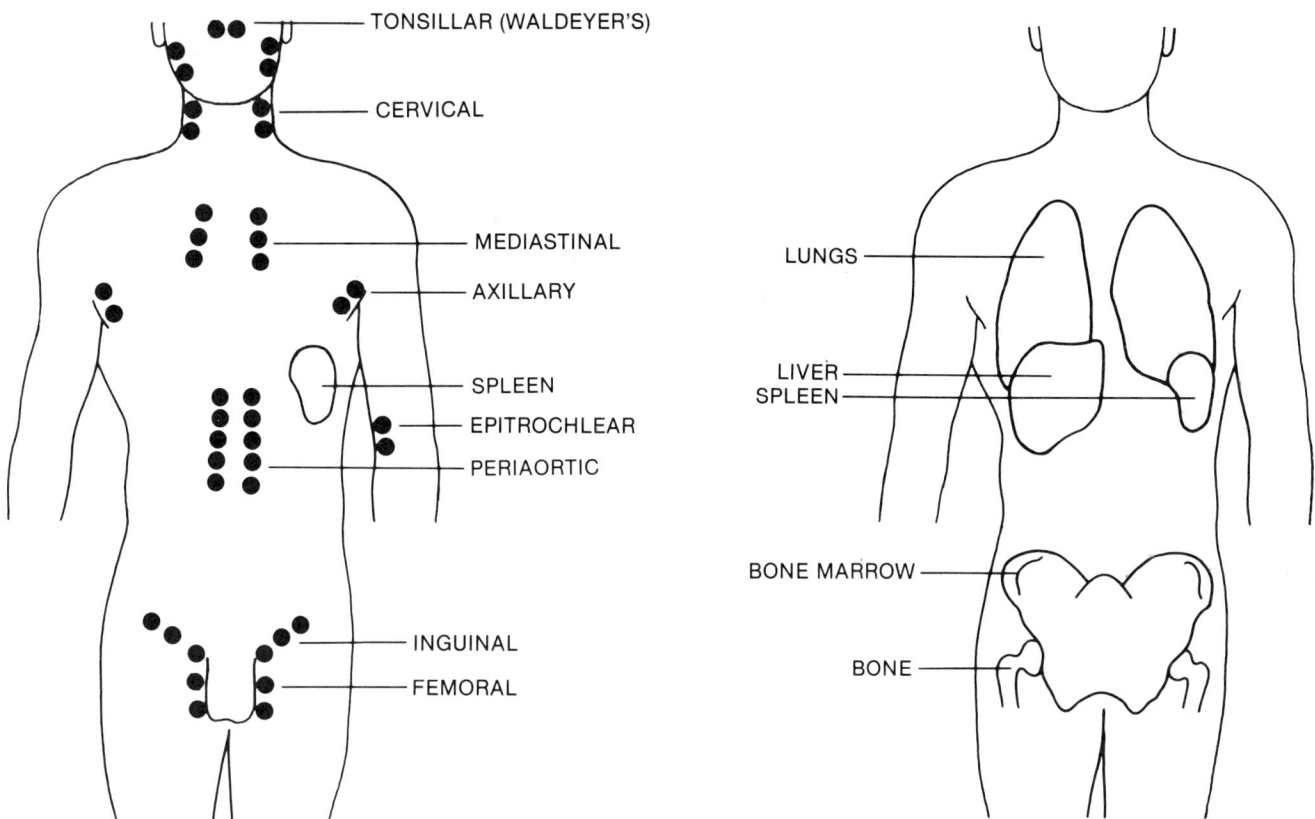

Figure 43–2. Patient teaching diagrams of lymph node chains and vital organ locations. (From Jacobs, C. [1979]. A patient teaching tool: Hodgkin's disease. *Cancer Nursing, 2,* 153–166.)

1986a). These negative feelings are compounded by physical changes resulting from the disease or treatment. Perception of the physical evidence of change varies with the individual patient, but it seems to be in direct proportion to the person's self-esteem before the diagnosis of cancer (Dunlop, 1982; Welch, 1979).

The impact of physical changes inherent to cancer therapies will also reflect on the life style of the young adult. Alopecia is interpreted as a loss of attractiveness or sex appeal. Social dating may be avoided for fear a wig will fall off (Valentine, 1978). Great stress may be placed on intimate relationships. Engaging in sex may be difficult when body image is threatened by surgery or chemotherapy. Nurses should reassure the young adult that some changes are temporary, such as tiredness or hair loss (Blotcky, 1986). The need to mourn permanent changes in physical appearance or reproductive potential should be supported, and verbalization of feelings of loss should be encouraged. The nurse should emphasize that the onset of disease has not changed the patient's worth as a person.

Feelings of low self-esteem coupled with fear of rejection by peers may inhibit involvement in social activities. Dunlop (1982) found that social isolation was a painful experience for the young adult. Absence from school or work results in feeling left out of the central topics of peer conversation and causes friends to feel awkward talking about these things around the sick person. A primary goal of the nurse is to help

normalize life, facilitating the return of the young adult to non-illness-related activities such as school, work, and church. The oncology nurse often provides school personnel with accurate medical information and an understanding of the psychosocial and educational implications of the disease (Blotcky, 1986).

Independence-dependence conflicts between parents and the young adult are intensified and complicated by cancer. The more independent the young adult was before cancer, the more difficult it is to move back home, accept care, ask for money, or be advised. Frustration at forced dependence may be expressed as moodiness, secretiveness, resentfulness, or rages and attacks (Delengowski & Dugan-Jordan, 1986; Dunlop, 1982). Physicians and nurses may be viewed along with parents as authority figures and may become targets of rebellion (Blotcky, 1986). Nonproductive struggles can be avoided if young adults are offered care options whenever possible (for example, the choice of vein for intravenous chemotherapy administration). Efforts to include the young adult in decision making help foster feelings of independence and control of the situation.

Young adults normally are concerned about the future direction of their lives. The young adult with cancer is concerned about how the disease will limit future possibilities (Blotcky, 1986). Nurses can help the patient make realistic plans for the future by discussing concrete options. Communicating specific information about sterility, sperm banking, pregnancy, and late effects of treatments clearly and sensitively is necessary if young adults are to make informed decisions.

Noncompliance. Occasionally the young adult or adolescent with cancer exhibits potentially life-threatening behavior such as noncompliance with the treatment regimen or outright treatment refusal. Although acceptance of therapy reflects recognition of its central role in recovery from cancer, treatment refusal has a multifactoral basis (Cohen, 1986b). The interacting elements include characteristics of the patient, the family, and the treatment. Whereas these factors are present, to a degree, in all young adults with cancer, they do not become significant until they actually do culminate in a patient's noncompliance (Olson, Kaufman, Ware, & Cheney, 1986). Patients who underestimate the seriousness of their diagnosis, who have elevated levels of anger or helplessness, or who have abnormally low levels of anxiety are more likely to be noncompliant. Others, who use denial as a coping mechanism, may focus on current problems and discomforts rather than on the future implications of treatment noncompliance. The threat of fatal disease may simply be too great for them to affirm by seeking and accepting treatment (Cohen, 1986b).

The presence of marital or familial difficulties, including a history of adolescent rebellious behavior or overinvolved or distant parents, may suggest future compliance problems (Olson et al., 1986). Family or personal religious beliefs that view God as the only legitimate provider or restorer of health may lead patients to refuse treatment (Cohen, 1986b). When treatment refusal is based on denial of the reality of the disease or on religious grounds, the nurse should ensure that the patient has an understanding of treatment objectives and has accurately interpreted the risks and consequences of actions. Suggestions that medical care augments but does not replace faith may provide validation that the health care team respects religious beliefs (Cohen, 1986b).

Increasing duration and complexity of treatment is associated with increased likelihood of noncompliance. A correlation is also seen between noncompliance, difficulty of medication schedules, and degree of side effects. Educational strategies have been shown to increase compliance (Olson et al., 1986). Reminder devices, such as stickers with medication instruction, or self-monitoring techniques, such as a diary, have been effective in facilitating compliance (Cohen, 1986b).

Dunlop (1982) states that prevention is the principal intervention to reduce noncompliance and other negative risk-taking behaviors. Early meetings are recommended between the treatment team and the young adult to develop a treatment schedule reflective of special events, school days, or work demands, in addition to clinic days and treatment cycles. Pertinent information about the disease, staging procedures, and treatment should be given and updated throughout the treatment course to enable the young adult to participate as a partner in the planning and decision-making process.

The maintenance of communication and mutual respect is difficult under circumstances such as noncompliance or refusal of treatment. The health care provider is challenged to respect the integrity of the young person with cancer and his or her perception of the problems and possible solutions (Cohen, 1986b). Providing a supportive atmosphere, rather than using scare tactics or blame, to identify reasons for noncompliance and ways to improve the situation is recommended. Developing a trust relationship with a counselor not on the oncology team, who represents an unbiased opinion, may help the young adult solve problems that seem personally insurmountable.

The oncology nurse is in a key position to help young adults deal with the psychosocial stresses of cancer. Young adults should be followed by a primary nurse, who can provide access to preventive interventions and early recognition of psychological difficulties (Blotcky, 1986). In a preventive model, the nurse acts as a guide and advocate for the young adult and family throughout the disease course, helping them to reach and maintain a reasonable level of adjustment (Drotar, Crawford, & Genofsky, 1984). By focusing on coping rather than on deficits or psychopathology, the nurse communicates a sense of hope or optimism to the patient. Such a perspective emphasizes the stressful yet manageable prospect of living with a chronic disease, and the young adult can perceive the illness as an opportunity for mastery and personal growth (Blotcky, 1986).

Nurses and other caregivers often identify with the young adult who is close to their own chronologic age (Valentine, 1978). Comments such as "What if it were me?" are common as staff members consider their own mortality. Caregivers caught in this dilemma are best cautioned that a decrease in therapeutic effectiveness may result if overidentification occurs. They may react with sympathy rather than empathy and allow their own needs to take precedence over those of the patient (Delengowski & Dugan-Jordan, 1986).

Treatment

Problem 1: Potential Inability to Cope with Aggressive Treatment Protocols and Related Side Effects

Diana became depressed with the start of chemotherapy. Body image changes were happening too fast: the abdominal scar made wearing a two-piece bathing suit embarrassing, and wearing a wig for extended periods proved to be itchy and uncomfortable. Anticipation of returning to school brought feelings of panic. Would everyone know about the cancer and treat her differently? Would people stare? How would she ever keep up with studies?

Diana met with the oncology nurse and social worker at the cancer center to plan how best to get through the first three cycles of chemotherapy. They suggested a reduced school class load and scheduled chemotherapy for Friday afternoons so that the weekend could be used to recover. Attendance at a structured cancer support group to meet others with similar concerns and problems was encouraged.

Nausea and vomiting occurred after chemotherapy administration. Antiemetics were somewhat effective in controlling this side effect, but they were accompanied by an annoying degree of sedation. Diana appreciated the amnesia that heavy sleep afforded, however. Granulocyte counts dropped below 1000/mm^3, forcing the modification of her chemotherapy dosage on two occasions. During these periods Diana practiced good preventive hygiene and avoided exposure to crowds. Fortunately, no infections developed.

Tiredness became a problem during radiation therapy. To cope with this symptom, Diana's class load at school was reduced further. Anorexia lingered for weeks. She lost a total of 10 lb while on treatment.

Within 6 months of starting treatment Diana's chest radiograph had returned to normal. A more positive emotional attitude enabled her to look hopefully toward the future.

Interventions

The acute phase of Hodgkin's disease is defined and dominated by cancer treatment and side effects. How people tolerate treatment is in large part a reflection of how they cope with the emotional stresses of the period.

Oncology nurses play an important role in support of patients and families through aggressive treatment protocols with curative intent. In addition to managing side effects associated with chemotherapy and radiotherapy, nurses facilitate the development of effective patient and family coping strategies. Coping has been defined as the (1) cognitive, emotional, and behavioral responses evoked in relation to a harm or threat, and aimed at problem solving and regulation of emotional distress; and (2) the balance of power in the interaction between harms or threats and the resources to counteract them (Derdiarian, 1987; Lazarus & Folkman, 1984).

How each patient and family copes with cancer treatment and side effects will vary depending on perceptions of the situation, personalities, and past experiences (Sidle, Adams, Cady, & Moos, 1969). Coping strategies commonly employed include (1) seeking information, (2) taking direct action, and (3) turning to others for help and support (Cohen, 1986a; Sidle et al., 1969; Weisman, 1979). Nursing interventions to facilitate these strategies are discussed in relation to the patient being treated for cure.

Seeking Information. Seeking information is a fundamental method of coping and takes place early in the coping process (Cohen & Lazarus, 1979). Efforts to gain intellectual mastery provide a measure of control for those feeling helpless in their circumstances. Although persons with cancer are better informed today about their diagnosis and prognosis (Souhami, 1978), additional information is needed about care and treatment to reduce fear and anxiety (Friedman, 1980). Nurses do a great service by interpreting treatment information and helping persons with cancer to understand and cope with the anticipated course of disease. Education of the person with cancer has been recognized as a component of oncology nursing practice (Johnson & Green, 1981). The *Standards of Oncology Nursing Practice,* coauthored by the members of Oncology Nursing Society and the American Nurses' Association (1987), lists the following measurable goals for information that the client will attain:

1. Describes the state of the disease and therapy at a level consistent with his or her educational and emotional status.

2. Participates in the decision-making process pertaining to the plan of care and life activities.

3. Identifies appropriate community and personal resources that provide information and services.

4. Describes appropriate actions for highly predictable problems, oncologic emergencies, and major side effects of the disease or therapy.

5. Describes the schedule when ongoing therapy is predicted.

Because the assimilation of information regarding cancer and treatments takes place over time (Hall et al., 1982), continuity of nursing care greatly facilitates comprehensive instruction. Besides providing initial teaching, the nurse should be available to reteach or correct misinformation if necessary. To tailor information and support to the individual patient, nursing assessment of the kind and extent of information needed is suggested. Assessment is enhanced by giving the patient permission and opportunity to express feelings and needs (Friedman, 1980).

Initial chemotherapy teaching should include an explanation of any proposed clinical trial, a broad overview of how chemotherapy works, and information on specific drugs, their administration schedules, expected toxicities, and techniques to manage side effects.

Radiation therapy teaching should include information on the purpose of therapy, the use of megavoltage equipment, the design of treatment fields, techniques, doses to be delivered, expected toxicities and how to manage them, and potential postradiation syndromes. Written material is a useful supplement to information given. Two patient teaching booklets—"Radiation Therapy and You" (86-2227) and "Chemotherapy and You" (86-1136)—developed by the National Cancer Institute (NCI) and available free of charge, help provide standardized information to each patient being treated.*

Treatment for Hodgkin's disease is usually begun immediately after the diagnostic and staging work-up. Chemotherapy is commonly initiated only 2 weeks after exploratory laparotomy and splenectomy. At the start of treatment, limited teaching of essential information about the purpose of treatments, side effects, and related management techniques is recommended. Information should be given simply and be expanded at subsequent visits. Jacobs and co-workers (1983) have demonstrated the benefits of education in persons with Hodgkin's disease (Box 43–1).

---

*Publications Order, Office of Cancer Communications, National Cancer Institute, Building 31, Room 10A24, Bethesda, MD 20892.

Box 43–1. EFFECTS OF CANCER EDUCATION AND PEER SUPPORT GROUPS ON PATIENT BEHAVIOR

The purpose of two controlled, prospective studies was to determine if psychological and social functioning could be enhanced in patients with Hodgkin's disease by either education or peer support groups. Eighty-one patients were evaluated with the Cancer Patient Behavior Scale before and after intervention. Patients in the education group received a printed booklet about Hodgkin's disease, which discussed diagnosis, staging, treatment methods, treatment problems, and prognosis. In addition, they received newsletters that contained information about latest advances in the treatment of Hodgkin's disease as well as a patient question-answer section. Group participants demonstrated a significant improvement in knowledge of Hodgkin's disease ($p < 0.01$) and experienced significant reduction in their extent of anxiety ($p = 0.02$) and treatment problems ($p = 0.009$). An improvement was shown in depression ($p = 0.10$) and in lessened life disruption ($p = 0.08$) compared with a control group. After participation in peer support groups, patients showed no improvement in tested areas of life functioning. The researchers believed that their educational intervention required minimal expense and professional involvement and therefore could be implemented widely.

Structured education programs designed to complement the informal teaching of health care providers are being implemented in increasing numbers for persons with cancer. Johnson (1982) studied the effects of a cancer education course and demonstrated an improvement in participant scores on three dependent variables: knowledge of cancer, anxiety, and meaningfulness in life. The significance of these results were used by the ACS to aid in the development of an ongoing cancer education program entitled "I Can Cope." Such programs provide information and support to persons in need of such services and have been well received by the public and health care providers alike (see Chapter 62).

Direct Action. The perception of being in control of a threatening situation, or of having the ability to influence the outcome, is likely to facilitate coping; whereas high levels of uncertainty can disrupt coping ability (Meichenbaum & Cope, 1978; Rotter, 1966). The end result of nursing's efforts to educate the patient about treatments and potential toxicities is that patients will understand what is happening to them and will know what direct actions they can take to minimize side effects.

Dodd (1982, 1983, 1984a, 1984b, 1987a, 1988a, 1988b) has extensively studied the performance of self-care behaviors (SCBs) by persons with cancer and has proposed that facilitating self-care in patients who are receiving chemotherapy and radiation therapy is essential to providing quality nursing care (Dodd, 1982). Orem (1980) defined self-care as "the practice of activities that individuals initiate and perform on their own behalf in maintaining life, health, and well-being." She emphasized the significant role of the nurse in helping patients meet self-care demands when actual or potential deficits exist (Orem, 1980).

The first of Dodd's self-care studies (1982) was undertaken to assess self-care activity and test methods for enhancing self-care. Persons receiving chemotherapy who were interviewed before the study intervention (n = 48) reported the occurrence of treatment side effects (mean, 7.69) and a need for action but initiated few SCBs (0.81). After being instructed on chemotherapy, potential side effects, and side effect management (SEM) techniques, the study group performed significantly more SCBs ($p < 0.01$) than the control group whose members received no information. In addition, the study group members initiated SCBs before their side effects became severe (Dodd, 1983).

Several longitudinal studies were completed by Dodd (1984a, 1984b, 1988b) to determine patterns of SEM. In the first of these studies (1988b), persons with breast cancer (n = 30) who were beginning adjuvant chemotherapy were taught to record SCBs in a log. Self-care behaviors were defined as any activity performed for the purpose of alleviating a side effect of chemotherapy. Results corroborated the earlier study: patients did not know which SCBs were helpful, and they often waited until side effects were severe before initiating self-care; some patients believed side effects were to be endured and were reluctant to complain about treatment; patients cited themselves as the most frequent source of information for their SCBs, whereas the nurse was infrequently cited (Dodd, 1988a, 1988b). In a secondary analysis of the data, this sample's *preventive* SCBs were found to be very low. Preventive activities are those initiated by the patient before the side effect is experienced. The average number of preventive activity was 0.09. Given that the average number of potential side effects from chemotherapy was 18, the lack of self-care activity was remarkable (Dodd, 1984b).

In the second longitudinal study (Dodd, 1984a), 30 persons receiving radiation therapy completed the SCB log. They reported having experienced an average of 3.3 side effects, yet initiated few (mean, 1.6) SCBs. In addition, they reported not knowing what SCBs to perform. Patients' preventive self-care activity was again very low.

Two final experimental studies were performed to test the effectiveness of providing SEM information proactively to persons initiating either radiation therapy (Dodd, 1987a) or chemotherapy (Dodd, 1988a, 1988b). In both studies, 60 patients were randomized into either experimental or control groups. Experimental group subjects received written information on SEM before development of any side effects. They were taught to record side effects and SCBs in the logs. The radiation therapy experimental group recorded side effects experienced in their SCB logs for the duration of their treatment (6 weeks). This group performed more selected SCBs than did controls ($p = 0.02$).

However, the three other SCB ratio scores (reflecting total SCB activity, effectiveness of activity, and overall management) were not significantly different, although all of the average ratio scores and preventive activity scores were higher for the experimental group (Dodd, 1987a). The persons receiving chemotherapy who also received SEM information scored significantly higher on all four of the SCB ratios (selected SCB activity, total activity, effectiveness of activity, and overall management) than did the control group. Similarly, the group that received SEM information performed significantly more preventive self-care activities than did controls (Dodd, 1988a, 1988b).

The major implication of these studies is that nurses need to increase efforts to facilitate patient's self-care activities and thus decrease the morbidity of cancer treatment. Dodd's book (1987b) represents a compilation of the information on chemotherapy, radiation therapy, and suggestions for self-care management of side effects used in her research (Table 43–2). This book provides the type of information frequently sought by patients and families to facilitate the process of coping.

Turning to Others for Help and Support. Showing a warm, interested concern for the person with cancer as an individual is an important approach to helping

Table 43–2. SELF-CARE BEHAVIORS: MANAGING CONSTIPATION

Description
Chemotherapy may diminish the nerve impulses to the intestines. These impulses are needed to move food through the intestines. Once the food has been broken down by digestion, the waste material (stool) may not move through the intestines as well as it did before chemotherapy.

Duration
Constipation caused by chemotherapy is temporary and is relieved when the therapy is completed. Within a week after the drug has been discontinued, normal bowel habits should have returned.

Self-Care Measures
- Eat high-fiber foods that include whole grain cereal, bran, raw fruits, vegetables, nuts, dried fruits, and raisins. Gradually add bran to the diet, starting with 2 teaspoons per day. Increase this amount gradually to 4 to 6 teaspoons; too rapid an increase can cause diarrhea. If chewing raw fruits and vegetables is a problem, try grating them.
- Eat fruits such as oranges, peaches, pears, and prunes.
- Drink plenty of fluids (e.g., 6 to 8 glasses a day).
- Exercise if physically able and walk as much as possible. If confined to bed, do bed exercises by contracting and relaxing different sets of body muscles.
- Take stool softeners and laxatives. If pain medicine is required—especially narcotics—take bulk-forming laxatives (e.g., Metamucil). Some laxatives when used continually can irritate the bowel, often making it difficult to regain normal bowel habits once chemotherapy or pain medicines are discontinued.
- Take enemas and suppositories if stool softeners and laxatives are not effective.

Consult Physician or Nurse:
- If no bowel movements have occurred for 3 or more days—for example, if the normal pattern is daily bowel movements and on the fourth day the bowels have not moved; or if the normal pattern is every 2 to 3 days and on the sixth day the bowels have not moved.

(Adapted from Dodd, M. J. [1987]. *Managing side effects of chemotherapy and radiation therapy: A guide for nurses and patients,* Norwalk, CT: Appleton & Lange.)

patients in coping. All persons with cancer need to feel that someone is available and willing to listen and is knowledgeable and understanding of what they are experiencing (Speese-Owens, 1981).

Nurses also provide support for persons with cancer by facilitating one-to-one contacts with others with similar diagnoses and by meeting with cancer groups to provide information and reassurance (Friedman, 1980). Support groups offer cancer patients an opportunity to verbalize fears and anxieties. They provide reservoirs of special information and coping techniques used successfully by group members to deal with common problems (Adams, 1979). Caplan and Killilea (1976) note that "those who have already successfully coped with a crisis can be the best sources of support."

Survivorship

Problem 1: Psychosocial Difficulties Encountered by Cancer Survivors

Diana was surprised to feel mixed emotions as the day for completion of treatment drew near. Although stopping chemotherapy and radiation therapy had been eagerly anticipated over the last year, the discontinuation of all therapy caused feelings of apprehension. Voicing these fears to the oncology nurse, Diana compared the cessation of treatment with the loss of a security blanket and wondered if "the doctors really knew what they were doing." The nurse empathized with Diana's feelings of uncertainty and assured her that the decision to stop treatment was not made randomly but was based on the prior treatment outcomes of hundreds of patients.

Diana attended a support group throughout the next year. She now had the energy to deal with emotions that had been kept submerged throughout treatment. The group gave her the social support and permission to express feelings of anger toward a physician who had not communicated openly and honestly and toward hospital departments that had not been efficient. The group also provided the opportunity to express gratitude for the support received from physicians and nurses and thankfulness at having achieved a complete remission. Fear of disease recurrence dominated Diana's conversation whenever she felt physically or emotionally "down." When feeling good, Diana expressed the desire to work as a volunteer and support others through treatment for Hodgkin's disease.

Interventions

The successful termination of cancer treatment does not necessarily signal an end to the difficulties and stresses faced by persons with cancer and their families. Survivors frequently find themselves at significant risk for physical and psychosocial sequelae. This risk arises from the late effects, or delayed physical complications of aggressive cancer treatment methods, the psychological fallout of living with a life-threatening illness (Cella & Tross, 1986; Lamsky, List, & Ritter-Sterr, 1986), and the practical consequences of having been labeled a patient with cancer.

Survival Research. The majority of cancer survival literature deals with the medical outcomes of disease and treatment. Considerably less information has been accumulated about long-term psychological adjustment of cancer survivors. Studies that have been conducted focus, for the most part, on developmental problems of the child surviving cancer (Koocher & O'Malley, 1981) and only recently have specifically addressed the quality of life of adult survivors (Cella & Tross, 1986; Fobair et al., 1986; Maher, 1982).

Cella and Tross (1986) compared the psychological adjustment of 60 young men who were Hodgkin's disease survivors with 20 age-matched healthy men. Assessment included objective self-report, projective testing, observer rating, and interview. Although no differences were found between cancer survivors and healthy controls on most measures, the survivors demonstrated significantly lowered intimacy motivation, increased avoidant thinking about illness, diminished work capacity, and illness-related concerns. Conversely, survivors were significantly more appreciative of life than controls (Cella & Tross, 1986).

Three studies by the ACS focused on work experiences of women after cancer treatment (Feldman, 1987). A total of 229 women were interviewed 1 to 5 years after diagnosis along with their physicians and employers (or, if of school age, their parents and principals). More than half of white-collar workers, more than 80 per cent of blue-collar workers, and more than half of young adult students reported problems related to cancer history. The researchers broke these problems down into three categories. The first, gross discrimination, included dismissal or demotion; denial of promotion or cost of living wage increase given to other employees; or termination or reduction of health insurance, retirement benefits, or modification of work conditions, with cancer given as the specified reason. The second category concerned workplace attitudes, including ostracism by fellow workers, superiors, or subordinates; overt hostility, consisting of mimicry of prosthetic devices or verbal cruelty about physical changes; or overly solicitous or protective behavior. The third category consisted of diverse personal attitudes brought to the workplace by the survivors, including uneasiness, anxiety, and anger.

Fobair and associates (1986) explored the long-term adjustment patterns of a large number of Hodgkin's disease survivors. The investigators found significant problems in areas of functioning, including marital and family relationships, employment, energy levels, and emotional well-being (Box 43–2). Several recommendations were made based on study findings.

1. Depression, feelings of social isolation and helplessness, and poorer social functioning may occur during treatment. Screening patients for depression, increasing staff sensitivity, and helping patients to cope with depression through the provision of group and individual counseling may help minimize this natural response to serious illness. Potential problems with energy return, activity level, and body image should be anticipated and addressed during treatment and the early follow-up period.

2. Advising patients of potential psychosocial hazards may reduce the impact of those problems experienced. Patient education materials should include the following information: the return to normal energy levels may take up to a year, and the rapidity of return is related directly to age, stage of disease, and intensity of treatment. Marital stress is common; therefore, couple therapy or other counseling is recommended if resentment, anger, or withdrawal by the spouse occurs.

3. Work-related problems occur often. Treatment staff can be of assistance in explaining to employers the nature and length of any limitations imposed by the illness and stressing the generally favorable prognosis for persons with Hodgkin's disease (Fobair et al., 1986).

Psychosocial Difficulties Experienced by Cancer Survivors. The psychosocial difficulties experienced after completion of treatment may come as a surprise to many cancer survivors. The concept of anomia has been used to analyze the special rehabilitative problems of persons with cancer (Maher, 1982). Anomia as defined by Maher is a "temporary state of mind, occasioned by a sudden alteration in one's life situation, and characterized by confusion and anxiety, uncertainty, loss of purpose, and a sense of separation from one's usual social support system." The degree to which recovery from cancer is viewed as anomic is related to the person with cancer's perception of his or her prognosis: the poorer the prognosis in his or her eyes, the greater the likelihood that a cure or remission will be viewed as unexpected and anomic. Maher compared their situation to that of persons who have had unanticipated good fortune: the positive implications of the event may be enormous, but there are certain negative elements as well.

In extensive interviews with persons recovering from cancer, Maher (1982) found that although individual experiences were highly variable, no recovery was devoid of unpleasant or negative elements, including (1) the withdrawal of the intensified social support that accompanied the diagnosis and early treatment, (2) ambivalence about discontinuation of treatment, (3) anxiety about disease recurrence, (4) adjustment to permanent disabilities resulting from the disease or its treatment, (5) the need to resume life-oriented modes of thought after a successful adjustment to the idea of death, (6) anger at perceived inadequacies in the handling of treatment, and (7) confusion about feelings of depression when the objective situation has improved.

Most people experience an outpouring of sympathy and support from family and friends during the acute phase of cancer treatment. As time goes on, however, sustainment of this level of support becomes difficult for those around the person with cancer (Welch, 1979). On completion of treatment, the survivor who is ambulatory and healthy looking is likely to be refused the

Box 43–2. PSYCHOSOCIAL PROBLEMS AMONG SURVIVORS OF HODGKIN'S DISEASE

Fobair and colleagues looked at the type and frequency of psychosocial difficulties found among 403 long-term survivors of Hodgkin's disease. The median duration of follow-up was 9 years. A self-administered questionnaire using standard survey items was used to collect data on disruption in three areas of life: sense of well-being, personal relationships, and employment.

Results indicate that 90 per cent of the survivors reported that energy had been affected adversely by treatment, and 37 per cent believed it had not yet returned to normal. Older patients and patients with advanced-stage (IIb, IIIb, IV) disease who received combined modality therapy took longer for energy to return. Patients with self-reported energy loss were more likely to be depressed. Activity level of 80 per cent of patients studied was affected adversely by treatment, with median time to resume normal activities estimated to be 8 months.

The effects of illness on personal relationships were examined. An evaluation of marital status revealed moderately high divorce rates (32 per cent). The issue of fertility after treatment was investigated, revealing that 32 per cent (130) of the 403 patients in the study tried to conceive after treatment. Of the 130 patients, 52 (40 per cent) were successful and delivered healthy children, whereas 78 (60 per cent) of the patients were unable to conceive. Those patients who had combined modality treatment were less likely to conceive children after treatment ($p = 0.007$). Twenty per cent of the sample indicated a decrease in sexual activity. Loss of energy and symptoms of depression were correlated significantly with decrease in sexual function.

Employment patterns favored men returning to work, and number of hours worked was highly correlated with less depression, younger age, and return of energy. Difficulties at work were reported by 42 per cent of the patients. These problems included denial of health insurance or other benefits, not being offered a job or promotion, termination of employment after therapy, conflicts with supervisors or co-workers, rejection by the military, and inability to obtain life insurance.

---

privileges of the sick role. Supportive energies and understanding on the part of others may be at their lowest level at the very time the survivor may be in greatest need of interpersonal support (Maher, 1982). In addition to family and friends, the health care team may be ready to close the file on this case. After the completion of treatment, oncology nurses and social workers tend to have a reduced role in providing the survivor and family with support and counseling. The resulting void leaves many persons with cancer to fend for themselves in a "healthy" world (Mullen, 1985). A growing number of groups and publications address the needs of cancer survivors. The National Coalition for Cancer Survivorship (NCCS), founded in 1986, is the umbrella group for cancer survivor organizations nationwide. The NCCS Charter describes the purpose and objectives of the group (Table 43–3). A National Cancer Survivors Day, the first Sunday in June, is sponsored annually by Cope Magazine* and the ACS. The support of such endeavors by physicians, nurses, and social workers, coupled with systematic referrals to support services early in the recovery process, may aid adjustment, relieve suffering, and stimulate the further development of survivor resources.

To continue Maher's analysis (1982), an anomic situation is characterized by confusion, anxiety, and uncertainty. Several aspects of the cancer survivor's situation cause insecurity, including the decision to stop treatment and fear of disease recurrence. The decision to stop treatment is not made with scientific certainty, but rather is based on a number of variables, especially the results of clinical trials. Knowledge of the inexact nature of decision making leaves many survivors with lingering doubts as to whether stopping

treatment was the right thing to do. Insecurity and anxiety about the possibility of disease recurrence dominates psychologically the period following cessation of treatment (Mullen, 1985). Koocher and O'Malley (1981) found that this uncertainty about duration of remission and ultimate outcome of disease, which they termed the "Damocles syndrome," produced anxiety, depressive mood and ideas, poor body image,

Table 43–3. NATIONAL COALITION FOR CANCER SURVIVORSHIP CHARTER

Preamble

Cancer is an unwelcome intruder in life. Yet cancer is also an inescapable part of many lives. From the time of its discovery and for the balance of life, an individual diagnosed with cancer is a survivor. Surviving is an enormously important, often difficult, always challenging human enterprise that involves the individual, the family, and the givers of care.

Mission Statement

The mission of the National Coalition for Cancer Survivorship (NCCS) is to communicate that there can be vibrant, productive life following the diagnosis of cancer; that millions of cancer survivors share a common, transforming experience that has impacted their lives with new challenges and enhanced potentials; and that these survivors, their families and supporters represent a burgeoning constituency and a powerful, positive force in society.

Objectives

The objectives of NCCS are

1. To serve as a clearinghouse for information, publications, and programs for the many organizations working on the issues of survivorship.

2. To provide a voice for the many common and recurring issues of those organizations reflecting the spirit, skills, and needs of the survivorship community.

3. To advocate the interests of cancer survivors to secure their rights and combat prejudice.

4. To promote the study of the problems and potentials of survivorship.

(From NCCS Newsletter, 1987, *1*[1]. Albuquerque: National Coalition for Cancer Survivorship. Address: National Coalition Cancer Survivorship, 323 Eighth Street S.W., Albuquerque, NM 87102.)

---

*Pulse Publications, Inc., P.O. Box 1677, Franklin, Tennessee 37065-1677.

and fear of recurrence. Increased fear of cancer recurrence has been found 3 years after cancer treatment in a group of 104 cancer survivors (Schmale et al., 1983). The task of coping with the uncertainty of a cure continues, on some level, for an indefinite period of time (Slaven, 1981).

Physical limitations resulting from cancer and treatment may range from decreased strength, fatigue, and exercise capacity to loss of a body part or change in appearance (Maher, 1982; Mullen, 1985). These consequences will temporarily or permanently make a difference in the life styles of survivors and involve some adjustment. Permanent disabilities will require adjustment that is both practical and emotional. Practically, survivors must cope with new daily tasks, which often take more time (e.g., colostomy care). Emotionally, these people must come to terms with the trauma of disfigurement or functional impairment. Anomia involves the rapid escalation of expectations in the face of the sudden removal of old limitations. Frustration and disappointment may occur as a result of the nonlinear quality of healing. Physical improvement generally comes in spurts, with occasional setbacks. The less prepared the cancer survivor is for such disappointments, the more severe the anomia is likely to be (Maher, 1982).

Loss of purpose, or indeterminancy, is another aspect of anomia. In the cancer survivor's case, indeterminancy is seen primarily in the inability to engage in meaningful future-oriented activity. "Make Today Count" is both a philosophy of life and the name of a support group for persons with cancer. The program is based on the theory that it is easier to face death if a person lives one day at a time, fully, without thinking of the future. This "live for today" philosophy is evident in a poem by Brenda Neal, a cancer survivor (Neal, 1985):

PRIORITIES

I'd rather live

with uncertainty

than a deferred pension plan.

I'd rather embrace the unknown,

dancing on the edge

of tomorrow

than worry about a future

that may never come.

I can plan my life away

saving for the proverbial

RAINY DAY,

but what do I do

in the meantime -

when the sun's shining?

In an apparent paradox, the more the person with cancer has learned to "live for today" during treatment, the more likely it is he or she may feel overwhelmed when faced with the prospect of tomorrow.

The period of adjustment after completion of cancer treatment includes some rethinking of treatment experiences. Negative feelings surface now, when there is the time and energy to handle them, rather than during the confusion and fatigue of the treatment period (Derdiarian, 1987). Maher (1982) found that lack of information was the most frequent complaint voiced: information about side effects to treatment, about alternative treatments available, and about ways to minimize side effects.

Depression is the final negative element of cancer recovery outlined by Maher (1982). Depression occurring as a result of frustration with disability or fear of recurrence is understandable to the person with cancer and others. Depression related to the fact of a cure may come as a painful shock, causing a sense of confusion and the feeling that one is reacting abnormally. Feeling depressed at the point of successful completion of treatment may be the most disorienting of the psychosocial difficulties described.

Problem 2: Late Effects of Cancer and Treatments

At 2 years after treatment, Diana has yet to experience any significant late effects of Hodgkin's disease or its treatment. Looking to the future, Diana should be able to bear healthy children. Because of her splenectomy, she will require antibiotic prophylaxis after each delivery. Most importantly, she should be able to live her normal life expectancy free of any second malignancy.

Interventions

Increasing attention has been paid in recent years to the identification and management of late sequelae experienced by survivors of cancer. These late effects can be defined as persistent adverse physical changes related to the disease process, therapy, or both (Cella & Tross, 1986; Leonard & Waskerwitz, 1986; Ruccione & Fergusson, 1984). Late effects have been identified only because greater numbers of people have survived cancer for longer periods. These adverse changes are of particular concern in the area of pediatric oncology, for which current estimates predict that approximately 60 per cent of all children with cancer will be cured (Meadows, Krejmas, & Belasco, 1980). Although children appear to tolerate the acute toxicities of treatment better than adults, maturing organs seem to be more vulnerable to the development of late toxicities (Bleyer, 1982).

Late effects differ from the acute toxicities of cancer treatment in their unpredictable nature of onset and extent. Many of these sequelae could not have been anticipated when treatment started. Although some effects are directly associated with certain treatment regimens, unique host and disease characteristics may interact with treatment factors in the causation of others (Ruccione & Fergusson, 1984). Two broad categories of late effects have been identified: disruption of organ function with or without anatomic abnormalities, and oncogenesis (D'Angio, 1978).

The growing numbers of cancer survivors are being seen by nurses working in a variety of health care settings. An awareness of the possible late effects of treatment is needed if these survivors are to be provided with the education and support demanded by these concerns (Leonard & Waskerwitz, 1986). Because they have no symptoms of the original cancer, some survivors may not be motivated to comply with long-term follow-up care. Others may not have sought health care because they did not know that ongoing medical problems they were experiencing were sequelae (Lansky et al., 1986). Patients and families often are distressed to learn that long-term problems may affect the health they have fought to regain.

Nursing interventions for late effects include evaluation, referral, and education. To conduct evaluations of cancer survivors, oncology nurses must have knowledge of sequelae that occur as late effects and what screening measures are indicated. A review of systems and physical examination should be based on the following: (1) diagnosis and sites of disease, (2) type and scope of cancer treatment, (3) age during treatment, and (4) current age and life style (Leonard & Waskerwitz, 1986). The actual management of specific sequelae often requires referral to another medical or nursing subspecialty. Patient education is a major nursing responsibility that involves orientation of cancer survivors and their families about the occurrence of and follow-up for late effects. Development of patient education materials is needed to help the nurse define and describe late effects (Leonard & Waskerwitz, 1986).

SUMMARY

This chapter has outlined aspects of nursing care unique to persons with cancer who are being treated with curative intent. Hodgkin's disease was used as a prototype throughout the cancer trajectory from screening and detection through survivorship. Recommendations made here will, it is hoped, be applicable to an ever-growing segment of the cancer population.

References

Adams, J. (1979). Mutual-help groups: Enhancing the coping ability of oncology clients. *Cancer Nursing, 2,* 95–98.

American Cancer Society. (1989). *Cancer facts and figures, 1989.* Atlanta: Author.

Bleyer, W. A. (1982). Delayed toxicities of chemotherapy on childhood tissues. *Frontiers of Radiation Therapeutics and Oncology, 16,* 50–54.

Blotcky, A. D. (1986). Helping adolescents with cancer cope with their disease. *Seminars in Oncology Nursing, 2,* 117–122.

Boren, H. A., & Sullivan, M. P. (1986). Hodgkin's disease. In M. J. Hockenberry & D. K. Coody (Eds.), *Pediatric oncology and hematology: Perspectives on care* (pp. 54–80). St. Louis: C. V. Mosby Co.

Brooks, A. (1979). Public and professional attitudes towards cancer: A view from Great Britain. *Cancer Nursing, 2,* 453–460.

Caplan, G. (1964). *Principles of preventive psychiatry.* New York: Basic Books.

Caplan, G., & Killilea, M. (1976). *Support systems and mutual help.* New York: Grune & Stratton, Inc.

Cella, D. F., & Tross, S. (1986). Psychological adjustment to survival from Hodgkin's disease. *Journal of Consulting and Clinical Psychology, 54,* 616–622.

Cohen, D. G. (1986a). Growing up differently. *Seminars in Oncology Nursing, 2,* 84–89.

Cohen, D. G. (1986b). Treatment refusal in adolescents. *Seminars in Oncology Nursing, 2,,* 112–116.

Cohen, F., & Lazarus, R. S. (1979). Coping with stress of illness. In G. C. Stone, F. Cohen, & N. E. Alder (Eds.), *Health psychology* (pp. 217–224). San Francisco: Jossey-Bass.

Come, S. E., & Mayer, R. J. (1983). Hodgkin's disease: Chemotherapy. In M. C. Brain & P. B. McCulloch (Eds.), *Current therapy in hematology–oncology, 1983–1984* (pp. 126–133). Philadelphia: B. C. Decker, Inc.

Cooper, A. (1982). Hodgkin's disease. *Lancet, 1,* 612–613.

D'Angio, G. T. (1978). Complications of treatment encountered in lymphoma-leukemia long-term survivors. *Cancer, 42,* 1015–1025.

Delengowski, A., & Dugan-Jordan, M. (1986). Care of the adolescent cancer patient on an adult medical oncology unit. *Seminars in Oncology Nursing, 2,* 95–103.

Derdiarian, A. (1987). Informational needs of recently diagnosed cancer patients, Part 1. *Cancer Nursing, 10,* 101–115.

DeVita, Y. T., Jaffe, E. S., & Hellman, S. (1985). Hodgkin's disease and the non-Hodgkin's lymphomas. In Y. T. DeVita, Jr., S. Hellman, & S. A. Rosenberg (Eds.), *Cancer: principles and practice of oncology* (2nd ed., pp. 1623–1709). Philadelphia: J. B. Lippincott Co.

DeVita, Y. T., Jr., Serpick, A. A., & Carbone, P. P. (1970). Combination chemotherapy in the treatment of advanced Hodgkin's disease. *Annals of Internal Medicine, 75,* 881–895.

Dodd, M. J. (1982). Assessing patient self-care for side effects of cancer chemotherapy. *Cancer Nursing, 5,* 447–451.

Dodd, M. J. (1983). Self-care for side effects of cancer chemotherapy: An assessment of nursing interventions. *Cancer Nursing, 6,* 63–67.

Dodd, M. J. (1984a). Patterns of self-care in cancer patients receiving radiation therapy. *Oncology Nursing Forum, 10*(3), 23–27.

Dodd, M. J. (1984b). Self-care for preventing side effects by breast cancer patients in chemotherapy. *Public Health Nursing, 1,* 202–209.

Dodd, M. J. (1987a). Efficacy of proactive information on self-care in radiation therapy patients. *Heart and Lung, 16,* 538–544.

Dodd, M. J. (1987b). *Managing side effects of chemotherapy and radiation therapy: A guide for nurses and patients.* Norwalk, CT: Appleton & Lange.

Dodd, M. J. (1988a). Efficacy of proactive information on self-care in chemotherapy patients. *Journal of Patient Education and Counseling, 11,* 215–225.

Dodd, M. J. (1988b). Patterns of self-care in patients with breast cancer. *Western Journal of Nursing Research, 10*(2), 7–14.

Drotar, D., Crawford, P., & Ganofsky, M. A. (1984). Prevention with chronically ill children. In M. C. Roberts & L. Peterson (Eds.), *Prevention of problems in childhood: Psychological research and applications* (pp. 232–265). New York: John Wiley & Sons.

Dunlop, J. G. (1982). Critical problems facing young adults with cancer. *Oncology Nursing Forum, 9*(3), 33–38.

Dutcher, J. P., & Wiernik, P. H. (1985). Hodgkin's disease. In P. H. Wiernik (Ed.), *Leukemias and lymphomas* (pp. 63–95). New York: Churchill Livingstone.

Erikson, E. H. (1963). *Childhood and society.* New York: Norton.

Feldman, F. L. (1987). Female cancer patients and caregivers: Experiences in the workplace. *Woman and Health, 11,* 137–153.

Fobair, P., Hoppe, R. T., Bloom, J., Cox, R., Yarghese, A., & Spiegel, D. (1986). Psychosocial problems among survivors of Hodgkin's disease. *Journal of Clinical Oncology, 4,* 805–814.

Frank-Stromborg, M. (1981). Nursing's contributions to case finding and early detection of cancer. In L. B. Marino (Ed.), *Cancer nursing.* St. Louis: C. V. Mosby Co.

Friedman, B. D. (1980). Coping with cancer: A guide for health care professionals. *Cancer Nursing, 3,* 105–110.

Hall, M., Hardin, K., & Conatser, C. (1982). The challenges of psychological care. In D. Fochtman & G. Y. Foley (Eds.), *Nursing care of the child with cancer.* Boston: Little, Brown & Co.

Havinghurst, R. J. (1972). *Developmental tasks and education* (3rd ed., pp. 83–93). New York: David McKay Co.

Holcombe, J., & Henderson, B. R. (1981). Nursing care of the patient with a disorder of the blood and blood-forming organs. In R. Bouchard-Kurtz & N. Speese-Owens (Eds.), *Nursing care of the cancer patient* (4th ed., pp. 215–248). St. Louis: C. V. Mosby Co.

Hoppe, R. T. (1983). Hodgkin's disease: Radiation treatment. In M. C. Brain & P. B. McCulloch (Eds.), *Current therapy in hematology-oncology, 1983–1984* (pp. 120–126). Philadelphia: B. C. Decker, Inc.

Jacobs, C. (1979). A patient teaching tool: Hodgkin's disease. *Cancer Nursing, 2,* 153–166.

Jacobs, C., Ross, R. D., Walker, I. M., & Stockdale, F. E. (1983). Behavior of cancer patients: A randomized study of the effects of education and peer support groups. *American Journal of Clinical Oncology, 6,* 347–350.

Johnson J. (1982). The effects of a patient education course on persons with a chronic illness. *Cancer Nursing, 5,* 117–123.

Johnson J., & Green, M. H. (1981). Client education: An integral part of cancer nursing. In L. B. Marino (Ed.), *Cancer nursing* (pp. 79–97). St. Louis: C. V. Mosby Co.

Kane, N. E. (1981). The young adult with cancer: A developmental approach. *Oncology Nursing Forum, 8*(3), 16–19.

Knopf, M. K., & Morra, M. E. (1983). Smokers, former smokers, and non-smokers: A correlation study of nurses in Connecticut. *Oncology Nursing Forum, 10*(4), 40–45.

Knudsen, N., Schulman, S., Fowler, R., & Van den Hoek, J. (1984). Why bother with stop smoking education for lung cancer patients. *Oncology Nursing Forum, 11*(3), 30–33.

Koocher, G., & O'Malley, J. E. (1981). *The Damocles syndrome: Psychosocial consequences of surviving childhood cancer.* New York: McGraw-Hill Book Co.

Koocher, G., O'Malley, J. E., Gogan, J. L., & Foster, D. J. (1980). Psychological adjustment among pediatric cancer survivors. *Journal of Childhood Psychology and Psychiatry, 21,* 163–173.

Lacher, M. J. (1986). Hodgkin's disease and other lymphomas. In A. I. Holleb (Ed.), *The American Cancer Society Book* (pp. 429–438). New York: Doubleday & Co.

Lansky, S. B., List, M. A., & Ritter-Sterr, C. (1986). Psychosocial consequences of cure. *Cancer, 58,* 529–533.

Lazarus, R. S., & Folkman, S. (1984). Coping and adaptation. In D. W. Gentry (Ed.), *The handbook of behavioral medicine* (pp. 282–325). New York: Guilford.

Leonard, M. A., & Waskerwitz, M. J. (1986). Late effects in adolescent survivors of childhood cancer. *Seminars in Oncology Nursing, 2,* 126–132.

Levinson, D. J. (1978). *The seasons of a man's life.* New York: Ballantine Books.

Luther, S. L., Price, J. H., & Rose, C. A. (1982). The public's knowledge about cancer. *Cancer Nursing, 5,* 109–116.

Maher, E. L. (1982). Anomic aspects of recovery from cancer. *Social Science Medicine, 16,* 907–912.

Marino, L. B., & Kooser, J. A. (1981). The psychosocial care of cancer clients and their families: Periods of high risk. In L. B. Marino (Ed.), *Cancer nursing* (pp. 53–66). St. Louis: C. V. Mosby Co.

Meadows, A. T., Krejmas, N. L., & Belasco, J. B. (1980). The medical cost of cure: Sequelae in survivors of childhood cancer. In J. van Eyes & M. P. Sullivan (Eds.), *Status of the curability of childhood cancers* (pp. 263–276). New York: Raven Press.

Meichenbaum, D., & Turk, D. (1978). The cognitive-behavioral management of anxiety, anger and pain. In P. O. Davidson (Ed.), *The behavioral management of anxiety, depression, and pain.* New York: Brunner/Mazel.

Meyer, V. (1973). The psychology of the young adult. *Nursing Clinics of North America, 8,* 5–17.

Mullen, F. (1985). Seasons of survival: Reflections of a physician with cancer. *New England Journal of Medicine, 313,* 271.

Neal, B. (1985). Priorities. *Living Through Cancer, 3*(5).

Olson, R., Kaufman, K., Ware, L., & Chaney, J. (1986). Compliance with treatment regimens. *Seminars in Oncology Nursing, 2,* 104–111.

Oncology Nursing Society and American Nurses Association. (1987). *Standards for oncology nursing practice.* Kansas City, MO: ANA.

Orem, D. E. (1980). *Nursing: Concepts of practice* (2nd ed.). New York: McGraw-Hill Book Co.

Rapoport, L. (1965). The state of crisis: Some theoretical considerations. In H. J. Parad (Ed.), *Crisis intervention: Selected readings* (pp. 22–31). New York: Family Service Association of America.

Redman, B. (1980). *The process of patient teaching in nursing* (4th ed.). St. Louis: C. V. Mosby Co.

Rotter, J. B. (1966). Generalized expectancies for internal versus external control of reinforcement. *Psychological Monographs, 80* 41–43.

Ruccione, K., & Fergusson, J. (1984). Late effects of childhood cancer and its treatment. *Oncology Nursing Forum, 11*(5), 54–64.

Santoro, A., Bonfante, V., & Bonadonna, G. (1982). Salvage chemotherapy with ABVD in MOPP-resistant Hodgkin's disease. *Annals of Internal Medicine, 96,* 139–143.

Schmale, A. H., Marrow, G. R., Schmitt, M. H., Adler, L. M., Enclow, A., Murawski, B. I., & Gates, C. (1983). Well-being of cancer survivors. *Psychosomatic Medicine, 45,* 163–169.

Sidle, A., Adams, J., Cady, P., & Moos, R. (1969). Development of a coping scale. *Archives of General Psychiatry, 20,* 226–232.

Simonton, O. C., Mathews-Simonton, S., & Creighton, J. (1978). *Getting well again.* Los Angeles: J. P. Tarcher, Inc.

Slaven, L. A. (1981). Evolving psychosocial issues in the treatment of childhood cancer. In G. P. Koocher & J. E. O'Malley (Eds.), *The Damocles syndrome: Psychosocial consequences of surviving childhood cancer* (pp. 1–30). New York: McGraw-Hill Book Co.

Smith, S., Cairns, M., & Sturgeon, J. (1981). Poor drug compliance in an adolescent with leukemia. *American Journal of Pediatric Hematology and Oncology, 3,* 297–300.

Souhami, R. L. (1978). Teaching what to say about cancer. *Lancet, 2,* 935–936.

Speese-Owens, N. (1981). Psychological components of cancer nursing. In R. Bouchard-Kurtz & N. Speese-Owens (Eds.), *Nursing care of the cancer patient* (pp. 45–60). St. Louis: C. V. Mosby Co.

Stewart, A. L. (1980). *Coping with serious illness: A conceptual overview.* Santa Monica, CA: Rand.

Sullivan, M. P., Fuller, L. M., & Butler, J. J. (1984). Hodgkin's disease. In W. W. Sutow & D. J. Fernbach (Eds.), *Clinical pediatric oncology* (pp. 416–451). St. Louis: C. V. Mosby Co.

Tester, W. J., Kinsella, T. J., Walker, B., Makuch, R. W., Kelley, P. A., Glatstein, E., & DeVita, V. T. (1984). Second malignant neoplasms complicating Hodgkin's disease: The National Cancer Institute experience. *Journal of Clinical Oncology, 2,* 762–769.

Valentine, A. S. (1978). Caring for the young adult with cancer. *Cancer Nursing, 1,* 385–389.

Vettese, J. (1976). Problems of the patient confronting the diagnosis of cancer. In J. W. Cullen (Ed.), *Cancer: The behavioral dimensions* (pp. 275–282). New York: Raven Press.

Waskerwitz, M. J., & Fergusson, J. H. (1986). Late effects of cancer treatment in children. In M. J. Hockenberry & D. K. Coody (Eds.), *Pediatric oncology and hematology: Perspectives on care* (pp. 469–492). St. Louis: C. V. Mosby Co.

Weisman, A. L. (1979). *Coping with cancer.* New York: McGraw-Hill Book Co.

Welch, D. (1979). Assessing psychosocial needs involve d in cancer patient care during treatment. *Oncology Nursing Forum, 6,* 12–18.

Wortman, C. B., & Dunkel-Schetter, C. (1979). Interpersonal relationships and cancer: A theoretical analysis. *Journal of Social Issues, 35,* 140–151.

CHAPTER 44

Nursing Management of Persons with Recurrent Disease: Prototype—Leukemia

BONNY JOHNSON

The experience of recurrent cancer constitutes for many people the most difficult and prolonged period of their disease. Living with the threat of or the reality of recurrent disease is common. In 1989, the American Cancer Society (ACS) estimated that 910,000 new cases of cancer would occur; approximately half this number of deaths were recorded, owing to recurrent or uncontrolled cancer. Taking into consideration those persons who are still alive with cancer from previous years, it can easily be imagined that up to 1.5 million Americans at any one time are living with cancer and the threat of its recurrence.

Leukemia has been selected as a prototype in this chapter for the patient experience of recurrence. Leukemia is a striking example of a malignant condition that, when it recurs, signifies that the best chance for cure has passed. In addition, persons with leukemia often experience more than one relapse, further taxing both physical and psychosocial resources over the course of the disease. Statistically, for 1989, the ACS estimated that 27,300 new cases of leukemia and 18,000 deaths from the disease would occur. Only 1800 of these new cases are childhood acute lymphoblastic leukemia (ALL), of which up to 75 per cent may be cured. For the remaining patients—adults with leukemia—5-year survival is approximately 30 per cent, and of those with acute nonlymphocytic leukemia (ANLL) (8000) the median survival is only 1 year.

Appropriate and helpful nursing management of persons with recurrent cancer relies on certain assumptions: (1) because no one can completely understand another person's experience of cancer, the best approach is one that is open and sensitive to each person's needs; (2) the response of each person to recurrence of disease varies tremendously; (3) a person's reaction to and ability to cope with recurrent cancer is modified by such factors as age, responsibility, family, social and work roles, and goals and hopes for the future. Knowledge of personal health and psychosocial history, as well as an understanding of the basic concepts that underlie the experience of coping with cancer, will provide a framework on which to organize a plan of care for persons during their illness.

DEFINITION OF PHASE

For the purpose of discussion, the terms *relapse, recurrence,* and *reappearance* of disease will be used interchangeably. Often, *relapse* refers to disease that worsens during treatment or to cases in which a complete remission was never truly achieved. *Recurrence* usually reflects a return of cancer (especially solid tumors or localized disease) after a period of time without evidence of disease. In either case, the person has already received primary treatment for cancer, and a recurrence indicates that more treatment is needed.

The significance of cancer recurrence, although it has received little attention in the literature, cannot be underestimated. The diagnosis of cancer is one of the greatest threats to life that anyone can experience. Implicit in this threat is the sense that the disease has ultimate control, and that "one's own body is destroying oneself" (Hersh, 1985). Recurrence after primary treatment, at the very least, reasserts that the disease is in control and signifies progression of the cancer. Abrams (1966) writes that this lack of personal control influences the verbal and nonverbal activity of the patient more than any other factor, especially as the disease progresses.

Schmale (1976) refers to recurrence as indicating that the disease is even more powerful than previously expected; whereas at diagnosis the hope that cure is possible successfully diminishes anxiety, the worst possibility (that cure is not possible) comes true at the time of recurrence. Weisman (1979b) described the change that occurs as when the "hope for cure" becomes the "struggle for existence." The person experiences to an even greater degree the "existential plight of cancer"—intense concern over life and death issues—which Weisman and Worden (1976) described as occurring at the time of diagnosis of cancer.

Although other recurrences and relapses may occur subsequently, none carries the surprise and shock of the first; responses to further setbacks may reflect increasing acceptance, changes in expectations, fatigue, and increasing pessimism. In addition, the ability to cope with multiple recurrences will be directly related to the success of the patient in coping with the diagnosis and first relapse. Therefore, knowledge of early coping strategies will help the nurse and patient or family understand ways of coping with the subsequent changes in disease status.

Case Presentation

Jill is a 32-year-old white woman diagnosed as having ANLL in November 1988. Her past medical history is significant for idiopathic thrombocytopenia purpura 9 years ago, which was treated with steroids, and, subsequently, with splenectomy. Jill continues to have mildly elevated liver function test results related to hepatitis from a blood transfusion several years ago. She has no other medical problems.

Jill came to medical attention in November 1988 with an upper respiratory tract infection that did not respond to antibiotic therapy and with easy bruisability. On the day before her first hospital admission, a complete blood count showed myeloblasts, and she was told that she probably had leukemia. The following day she was admitted because of increased menstrual flow, and "I was getting scared at home." She received one course of induction therapy consisting of daunorubicin, cytosine arabinoside, and thioguanine (DAT). Her hospitalization was complicated by fevers and disseminated intravascular coagulation (DIC), and she did not achieve a remission until she was given a second course of DAT. Jill was discharged the day before Christmas.

Jill has been married to Ed for 13 years, and they have a 2-year-old son, Will. They recently moved out of a mobile trailer, which had been their home for the past 2.5 years, to a two-bedroom apartment. Jill works part-time as a waitress, and Ed is a teacher at a nearby technical school.

Jill is one of four sisters; her parents are divorced and remarried. There is some role reversal between Jill and her mother, who lives nearby. Although she has accepted this role up to this point in her life, she now feels she does not want to spend her energy on this type of relationship. During hospitalization, she used a social worker to try to resolve this issue. Her relationship with her husband is strong, and their communication is open.

When Jill was discharged from the hospital, the major issue for her was to decide what type of treatment to take as consolidation therapy. Because complete remission had been difficult to achieve, she was given three options: (1) an allogeneic bone marrow transplant (one sister was an HLA-compatible donor); (2) an autologous bone marrow transplant, or (3) standard chemotherapy. Although Jill is an intelligent and active participant in her care, she found it very difficult to absorb the meaning of statistics when they had to be applied to her life.

Jill chose to undergo an autologous bone marrow transplant, which necessitated a long hospitalization at a large city hospital 2 hours' drive from her home. Her hospital course was smooth, although not without expected complications. Despite much teaching and successful learning about her treatment and care needs, Jill was surprised at how much more fatigued and anorectic she was compared with her experience of induction therapy. The bone marrow engraftment was only temporarily successful, as a bone marrow biopsy taken just before discharge revealed 15 per cent blasts and decreased number of megakaryocytes. Attempts to reinduce a remission with aggressive chemotherapy were successful, and Jill was discharged to continue maintainence treatment under the care of her local physician.

Jill went home 2 months after her admission. The issues for her at this time were to rejoin her family and regain control of her daily life activities. Her son was beginning to display signs of separation anxiety as a result of the long hospitalization, and she arranged her days around spending time with him. She has decided not to go back to work for the time being. Instead, she described needing to find a meaning of this illness in her life and felt it might be her calling to share the experience in some way. She has been asked to speak before the Leukemia Society of America (LSA), and she accepted.

Jill was recently readmitted to her local hospital for treatment of an upper respiratory tract infection. This forced her to confront the reality that "I have a long way to go before I'll feel like myself." She is now at home on antibiotic therapy and states that she does not have her usual energy. She has been told that maintenance therapy may hold off her disease for the near future, but she has not asked for, nor has she been given, a more specific prognosis.

Ed continues to work, while Jill has asked for and accepted help at home from her family, friends, and occasional home health aides. She experienced some difficulty with her mother's excessive need to be present initially and was helped by her nurse to compromise by enlisting her mother's help with cooking once a week. Although she appears to have accepted the fact that she does not have her usual energy, she feels she has been successful in reserving what little she has for her relationships with her husband and son. She admits that they have had little time for fun, and she and her husband would like to arrange a vacation alone together. She is only now considering what this illness has meant to him and seems to want to work on this concern.

DISEASE TRAJECTORY

Acute Nonlymphocytic Leukemia

Primary Treatment

The pathophysiology and treatment of leukemia are discussed in detail in Chapter 35. Jill's case presentation is useful in illustrating several points that make ANLL an instructive example for nurses caring for patients with recurrent cancer. Usually ANLL appears during the third decade of life, with symptoms that are insidious and vague, such as fatigue, anorexia, malaise, or infection that cannot be controlled with antibiotics. Wiernik (1985) states that 10 per cent of ANLL patients have an illness syndrome of pancytopenia that is not diagnosed as ANLL until months or years of progression toward unequivocal leukemia. The surprise of the diagnosis of ANLL in this setting may contribute to the level of distress experienced by the patient and family. Chekryn (1984) reports that the element of surprise is a major source of distress described by patients and spouses when cancer recurs, as the expectation was that the disease would be cured. Similarly, Weisman and Worden (1985–1986) found that patients who thought themselves to be at low risk for recurrence were more distressed when it occurred than those who expected it, and that few patients who developed recurrences before 1 year were surprised.

Primary treatment for ANLL is usually started immediately after diagnosis. Perhaps because of the aggressive approach of the therapy, an air of emergency results for both recipients and caregivers. By the time the diagnosis is made, any delay in cytotoxic therapy quickly results in a decline in the condition of the patient. Lengthy hospitalization is required, as several antitumor agents are given in sequence or together in treatment protocols that are designed to be non-cross-resistant in their mode of action. Because the most effective drugs for treatment of leukemia are bone marrow suppressive, and because the marrow is compromised by disease, the toxicity of induction therapy is much greater than for many cancers, including other leukemias. The result is a long period of induction chemotherapy and supportive care that may render the patient sicker than before treatment. The expected benefit from such aggressive therapy is, however, a complete remission and perhaps a cure.

Consolidation treatment may be used after the induction phase, once a complete bone marrow remission has been achieved (<5 per cent myeloblasts in the marrow by biopsy). This regimen may include two or three more cycles of the same drugs that were shown to be effective during induction or different agents entirely. For high-risk patients, such as Jill, who did not go into a complete remission easily, bone marrow transplant might be considered at this point.

In approximately 60 per cent of cases, patients with ANLL then experience a complete remission of several months to years, during which time they feel well. Although it is controversial, maintenance chemotherapy may be given for an additional 12 to 15 months beyond diagnosis. Maintenance therapy is generally well tolerated and can be given in an outpatient setting on a monthly schedule. The median remission duration for those who experience an initial complete remission is 1 to 1.5 years; more importantly, 25 per cent of these patients appear to be long-term survivors (>4 years in complete remission) (Wiernik, 1985).

Typical Course of Disease

Leukemia provides an example of a cancer that is no longer curable if it recurs. In addition, for most patients in complete remission, the fear of recurrence is ever present, and the likelihood of relapse is statistically probable. Relapse is usually heralded by subtle changes (e.g., thrombocytopenia) that reflect a return of blasts and concomitant suppression of normal marrow cells. Patients who require frequent blood tests and who undergo occasional marrow examinations await the results of these tests with anxiety and fear. In his book *Stay of Execution,* Stuart Alsop (1973) writes about frequently waiting for blood counts that "can spell life or death." In his words:

> A marrow test is an unpleasant experience, and a biopsy is more so. But neither is nearly so unpleasant as waiting for the results. . . . If I had had a lot of blasts in the peripheral blood, he [Dr.—] would have had no choice but to put me into chemotherapy right away. Otherwise, the blasts in the blood would have eaten away at the blood, crowding out the life-giving good cells, and they would thus have ensured death in a matter of weeks at the most.

Once a patient's ANLL has relapsed, subsequent complete remissions are infrequent and of brief duration (<6 months). For the most part, the patient remains in relapse, which may be partially controlled by ongoing treatment with anthracyclines or antimetabolites, or with more experimental drugs such as amsacrine (Legha et al., 1980) or mitoxantrone (Paciucci, Cutner, & Holland, 1984). Of greater importance during the period of recurrent disease is supportive care to prevent or minimize the symptoms of leukemia or the effects of treatment, such as infection, bleeding, anemia, or hyperuricemia (see Chapter 35), and to support the patient and family as they work psychologically at "managing the cancer" (Weisman, 1979a).

FRAMEWORK FOR RECURRENT CANCER EXPERIENCE

Definition

Weisman (1979a) was among the first researchers to examine the period of cancer recurrence within the context of four "psychosocial phases" encompassing the entire course of illness, from the "existential plight" at diagnosis to the period of deterioration and decline (Table 44–1). The purpose of defining the experience of cancer as a sequence of these four phases is to correlate psychosocial crises and needs with the clinical course of the patient so that the experience *as a whole* may be better understood and treated.

For the purposes of this discussion, the third phase, recurrence and relapse, encompasses the time from actual recurrence, including a period called "limbo," during which the status quo is maintained, to the time when the patient no longer expects treatment to change the ultimate course of disease.

The researchers (Weisman & Worden, 1976, 1985–1986; Weisman, 1979a) used emotional distress and coping patterns as two dependent variables in describing the impact of cancer diagnosis and recurrence. Figure 44–1 defines the level of vulnerability (to emotional distress) over the course of illness as related to a patient's higher or lower emotional distress level. The trends presented designate specific times when the nurse may expect the patient to demonstrate increased emotional vulnerability; they also indicate that whether patients are at lower or higher risk for distress, the distress they experience at the time of initial recurrence is greater than or equal to the level at the time of diagnosis. The "existential plight of cancer" therefore provides a framework for understanding the experience of recurrence. In addition, the research methodology used to describe the plight has been used to study patients with recurrent cancer (Weisman & Worden, 1985–1986).

The concept of existential plight is "a luckless predicament [experienced by almost all cancer patients] in which one's very existence seems endangered . . . [and] signifies an exacerbation [sic] of thoughts about life and death" (Weisman & Worden, 1976, p. 3). The intensity of this experience varies in degree and duration; it appears to be strongest during the first 3 to 4 months after diagnosis and may continue (throughout the course of illness) to a greater or lesser degree depending on the individual patient's experience. Patients must use new or different coping skills in resolving, controlling, or managing the anxiety resulting from these concerns about life and death, as well as other "predominant concerns," such as health, work, religion, family, friends, and self-appraisal (Weisman & Worden, 1976).

The level of emotional distress experienced at any point is referred to as vulnerability and is a function of the ability of the person to cope effectively. Thus with methods for measuring levels of psychosocial and emotional distress, Weisman and Worden (1985–1986) correlated "good coping" with lower levels of emotional distress and "bad coping" with higher levels. Ingredients of good coping included optimism, belief that treatment will help, and open communication with others. Poorer coping was demonstrated by persons who were more pessimistic in general, had marital problems, or had past regrets.

The patient who develops recurrent cancer experiences a secondary existential plight, operationally defined as higher levels of emotional or psychosocial distress, demanding renewed energies toward effective coping. One such coping strategy employed is anticipatory grieving in preparation for losses that include career plans and aspirations, personal relationships and self-image, and, more broadly, loss of control and loss of hope (Hersh, 1985; Barsevick & McCarthy, 1987). Chekryn (1984) found grief to be one of eight themes in the experience of cancer recurrence for patients and their spouses (Box 44–1). She described the grief to be for the loss of the "cured status" and emphasized the importance of acknowledgment and legitimization of the response. Grieving was also seen as a major behavioral response in leukemics by Sanders and Kardinal (1977) for both unresolved losses of the past and anticipation of future loss. The degree to which grief work for the past losses can be experienced and resolved will dictate the ability of the person to cope with future concerns. These researchers saw anticipatory grieving in the involvement of leukemia patients with each other. This involvement provided a means whereby they could more tolerably anticipate their own impending death by temporarily identifying with persons at more advanced stages of disease. Although Jill derived personal satisfaction from her work with the LSA, her need to share in another's experience of existential threat may safely allow her to grieve her own future loss.

Table 44–1. EXPECTATIONS AT SUCCESSIVE PSYCHOSOCIAL PHASES

	Existential Plight	Accommodation and Mitigation	Recurrence and Relapse	Deterioration and Decline
Aims	Cure	Surveillance	Control	Care
Impairment	Transient	Variable	Increased	Nearly total
Quality of life	Same or slight change	Variable	Definite limitation	Drastic reduction
Goals	No more disease	No more concerns	Respite and reprieve	Relief
Attitude	Optimistic	Optimistic	Guarded	Pessimistic or resigned
Time perspective	Ambiguous or open	Open	Cautious or restricted	Closed
Denial	Temporary	Mixed	Slight	Seldom
Coping	Active	Active	Mixed	Passive

(Reprinted by permission of the publisher from Weisman, A. D. [1979]. A model for psychosocial phasing in cancer. In *General hospital psychiatry* [pp. 187–195]. Copyright 1979 by Elsevier Science Publishing Co., Inc.)

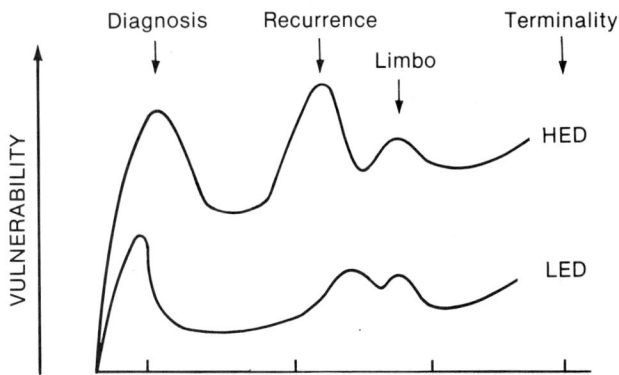

Figure 44-1. Variations in vulnerability levels during each phase of the cancer experience for higher emotional distress (HED) and lower emotional distress (LED) patients. (Reprinted by permission of the publisher from Weisman, A. D. [1979]. A model for psychosocial phasing in cancer. In *General hospital psychiatry* [pp. 187–195]. Copyright 1979 by Elsevier Science Publishing Co., Inc.)

Thus loss, as a concept, provides a useful guide in understanding changes that affect every aspect of life, for the patient with recurrent cancer experiences past, present, and future threats. Weisman and Worden (1976) emphasized that the threat is to both physical survival and life plans. It might be hypothesized that younger patients, or those at midlife, may experience a greater sense of loss and need for anticipatory grief than those in their later years. In a study of patients with recurrent cancer, Weisman and Worden (1985–1986) found that patients with Hodgkin's disease, a younger population, experienced greater existential concerns that persisted longer than other groups. In addition, those with more unresolved grief, or with regrets, may require support to accomplish their past grief work and move into anticipatory grieving (Derdiarian, 1984; Sanders & Kardinal, 1977; Scott, Goode, & Arlin, 1983). Coping strategies, such as redefinition and minimization (Weisman, 1979b), may help the patient and family change expectations of the future and experience less of a sense of loss.

Because of variations in experience of recurrent cancer from one patient-family unit to another, and even for one patient-family unit from day to day, Weisman (1979a) provided an organization of the concepts into a framework that may be applied to persons in various circumstances (adapted in Table 44–2).

An attempt has been made to juxtapose the patient's physical experience with his or her psychosocial expectations during this phase. From this perspective, nurses might be able to (1) view the spectrum of physical and psychosocial responses across areas of concern; and (2) predict, mitigate, or legitimize certain psychosocial responses related to specific physical changes, responses, and needs. In addition, the model may be useful as a guide for health care professionals to look at the way they respond to the physical and psychosocial needs of the ANLL patient and how responses influence patient behaviors.

Experiential Areas of Patients and Families

Control

The primary physical health objective for the patient and for the health care team at the onset and during the period of ANLL recurrence is to control the disease or to achieve another remission. For ANLL in particular, with its overriding importance of achieving remission, treatment must be aggressive to the point of being life threatening. Similarly, the patient requires sophisticated and intensive physical care and supportive treatment (e.g., protective isolation, blood component therapy, multiple and potentially toxic antimicrobial agents).

The intensity of the initial treatment for first ANLL recurrence may have the effect of asserting the power of the health care professionals and medical system at a time when the primary psychosocial aim of the patients is to be in control themselves. The ability to feel in control to some degree is necessary for effective coping, particularly as it allows the patient to manage panic, despair, and uncertainty and to tolerate the side effects of the disease and treatment. Thus when the *medical team* asserts control, the patient loses power

---

Box 44–1. CANCER RECURRENCE: PERSONAL MEANING, COMMUNICATION, AND MARITAL ADJUSTMENT

Although cancer recurrence is a common phenomenon, no known research has documented the psychosocial meaning of recurrence to the marital dyad. This article reports a descriptive correlational study about the meaning of cancer recurrence to patient and spouse and the communication they exchanged about it. Twenty-two subjects, 12 women with cancer recurrence and 10 spouses, participated in separate interviews and completed a standardized measure of marital adjustment.

Findings indicated that cancer recurrence posed individual and family hardships: difficulties with closure; uncertainty; grief; feelings of injustice, fear, and anger; existential concerns; a concern with coping; family impact; and an absence of communicated shared meaning between patient and spouse about the cancer recurrence. A substantial number of subjects stated they did not talk with their spouses about the recurrence. Furthermore, those who said they did talk about it did not share their spouse's meaning about the recurrence. Nevertheless, patients said they received a significant degree of support from spousal communication. The lack of a communicated shared meaning did not suggest dysfunction as measured by the marital adjustment scale. The findings suggest direction for nursing assessment and intervention.

(From Chekryn, J. [1984]. Cancer recurrence: Personal meaning, communication, and marital adjustment. *Cancer Nursing,* 7:491–498.)

Table 44–2. COMPARISON OF PHYSICAL AND PSYCHOSOCIAL EXPECTATIONS AT TIME OF RELAPSE OR RECURRENCE

	Physical	Psychosocial
Aims	Remission Symptom control	Control
Impairment	Variable Increased	Increased
Quality of Life	Reduced	Definite limitation
Goals	Cure or remission; prolonged survival	Respite and reprieve
Attitude	Cautious optimism	Guarded
Time Perspective	Limited	Cautious or restricted
Denial	Slight	Slight
Coping	Limited	Mixed

and high levels of emotional distress occur, which may or may not decrease as the patient regains control.

The ability to feel in control depends on the perception of having the power or the ability to influence or predict the future to some degree, or on both. Loss of control results in behaviors such as anger, hostility, withdrawal, and depression (Box 44–2) (Lewis, 1982). *Uncertainty,* reinforced by the experience of recurrence—and therefore the disease's power to control—becomes a major deterrent to a sense of power and control over one's life. Giacquinta (1977) described the family's experience when one member has cancer during the "living-dying" interval; learning to live with uncertainty about why the person got cancer, and not knowing how to help, can cause problems as the family members reorganize their roles and "frame memories."

Areas over which a patient may attempt to achieve control will vary according to physical capabilities and psychological needs. For example, if a remission is achieved after recurrence, patients may assert total control over their lives to the extent that they succeed in denying their illness and become noncompliant in areas of medical follow-up or acceptance of treatment (e.g., "The treatment is worse than the disease," so the treatment is rejected [Schmale, 1976]). On the other hand, patients whose physical status has deteriorated may derive sufficient sense of control by monitoring their own pain regimen, scheduling visitors, or planning their diet. Jill derived some degree of control by choosing to work with the LSA, and, later, by organizing those who helped her at home. Throughout her illness, she remained surprisingly able to identify those areas of her life to which she wanted to give her time and energy, as well as those persons who would be most helpful.

Level of Impairment

Disabilities or symptoms that adversely affect the daily functioning of anyone with recurrent cancer vary in both kind and degree. For the patient with recurrent ANLL, the severity of physical impairment may relate directly to the site of recurrence (e.g., bone, soft tissue, central nervous system) and to the degree of myeloblast proliferation. Of interest with regard to psychosocial response is the correlation researchers have drawn between emotional distress and physical distress (Weisman, 1985–1986). Although great variation has existed with regard to signs and symptoms of disease at the time of recurrence in the patient sample, the degree of disability and overall sickness has been predictive of level of distress regardless of other factors.

The concepts of grief and control already discussed apply to the experience of recurrent symptoms, as the patient must mourn the lessening or loss of a particular body function or capability. Similarly, loss of physical control results in a fear that control of the psychological and social aspects of life also will be lost (Barsevick & McCarthy, 1987), at least until the person adjusts to the change by redefining expectations of his or her capabilities and setting new goals in managing disabilities. All coping efforts, again, are toward decreasing the anxiety and distress caused by the change in physical status.

Box 44–2. THE RELATIONSHIP OF PERSONAL OUTCOME AND QUALITY OF LIFE IN TERMINAL ILLNESS

Within the theoretical framework of Rotter's Social Learning Theory and Seligman's Learned Helplessness, the investigator designed a study to test the relationship of experienced personal control and quality of life for patients with late-stage cancer. Quality of life was measured by Rosenberg's Self-Esteem Scale; the Lewis, Fusich, and Parsell Anxiety Scale; and the Crumbaugh Purpose-in-Life Test. Personal control was measured by the Health Locus of Control Scale (HCC). Fifty-seven patients with late-stage cancer responded to the four standardized measures during a one-time interview. Results of the study demonstrated that experienced personal control over life correlated significantly with self-esteem ($r = -0.33$, $p = 0.001$); purpose in life ($r = 0.45$, $p = 0.001$) and anxiety ($r = -0.30$, $p = 0.001$). The study offers preliminary evidence of the importance of experienced personal control over life as a meaningful and significant correlate of psychological well-being, a component of quality of life, in terminal patients with cancer.

(Data from Lewis, F. M. [1982]. Experienced personal control and quality of life in late-stage cancer patients. *Nursing Research, 31*:113–119.)

Quality of Life

How a patient judges his or her own quality of life may be viewed from both physical and psychosocial perspectives. Weisman's attempt (1979b) has been to combine the two arenas, because the effectiveness of coping (ability to manage emotional distress) depends so heavily on a person's tolerance of physical changes. In the setting of recurrent disease, the patient must deal with the appearance of new or recurrent symptoms, the physical stress of more aggressive treatment, and the inability to deny the limitations any longer— that therapy has failed and the disease has regained control. The individual patient's perception of limitations demands a renewed use of previously effective coping skills or a need to learn new strategies for mitigating anxiety, thereby improving overall quality of life.

Goals

Physically, the goals of the patient center on control of debilitating symptoms and influencing the course of the disease. However, expectations of treatment vary and range from hope for freedom from discomfort to hope for complete recovery. Interestingly, the goal of medical treatment, however improbable, may still be cure; the degree to which the curative intent of treatment results in denial of patient's rights or expectations must be examined by nurses and physicians. Inability of caregivers to recognize and legitimize valid coping strategies such as redefinition of goals, life-style readjustment, and expression of feelings will impinge on the patient's ability to actively participate and cooperate with treatment (Sanders & Kardinal, 1977).

Weisman (1979a) termed the necessary psychosocial goal at the time of recurrence *respite and reprieve*. Remembering that the overall expectations at this time, compared with those at diagnosis, are moderate in nature, and that both the physical and psychological stamina of the patient are taxed (especially after multiple recurrences), coping efforts are aimed at psychological comfort, reduction of anxiety to a tolerable level, learning to deal with the underlying fear and anxiety, and adjusting to the apparent changes in life style and social roles. Successful achievement of a sense of respite results in the period of "limbo" (Fig. 44–1), during which the intensity of earlier problems has abated. The preterminal problems are yet to come (Weisman & Worden, 1985–1986). The patient and family experience less emotional distress and demonstrate greater cooperation with the medical demands of treatment. Schmale (1976) wrote that the initial anxiety about dying abates and is replaced by a "strong sense of relief and a belief that everything is going to be all right . . . even when [the patient] has been told previously that treatment was palliative. . . ."

Attitude

The patient's attitude in both physical and psychosocial areas of concern during this period is guarded: guarded optimism that treatment will result in remission and continuing uncertainty that the disease will again gain control. This attitude may cause patients and families to seek out alternative, unproven treatments (Derdiarian, 1984) or agree to undergo medically sanctioned experimental therapy. Socially, and maladaptively, this guarded attitude may result in the patient's withdrawal or "passive surrender" (Scott et al., 1983). More typically, the patient assumes a more insular relationship with the family or close friends; in addition, relationships with others, both caregivers and acquaintances, change in style and kind.

Abrams (1966, p. 317) examined the patterns of communication among patients with early, advancing, and terminal cancer: "It is the stage [advanced] of guarded attitudes, circumlocution and verbal obliquity, but, to one who can follow the clues, it is, paradoxically, the most revealing stage." As the patient's perception of threat increases, his or her needs change, and communication may reach an impasse. Words used by medical professionals may take on what appears to be inappropriate significance (Abrams, 1966; Alsop, 1973; Schmale, 1976). Patients whose approach was direct become protectively "amnesic about the course of the illness" (Abrams, 1966); the overwhelming sense of dependence on medical success may enhance the patient's fear of abandonment by the physician.

Time Perspective

For the patient with recurrent cancer, time is of the essence. Although the average duration of first remission in ANLL is 1 year, once relapse occurs, the duration of each succeeding remission, if there is one, is approximately one half that of the previous remission. Psychologically, the realization of mortality and existential concerns are intensified by the knowledge that time is limited. Weisman and Worden (1985–1986) found that most people had resolved the critical emotional and social issues by the time of recurrence, and in the context of more limited time, could focus on health problems and increasing survival.

Denial

Denial is a temporary and necessary defense, which, when combined with other coping behaviors, provides the patient with relief while he or she works to resolve feelings of stress (Weisman, 1979a). The use of denial as a coping strategy appears to take on different roles at various times during the period of recurrence. In the face of high emotional distress, more denial may be necessary until the person's anxiety level can be tolerated. For example, Schmale (1976) attributed one patient's initial noncompliance with treatment to either his need to blame the physician for the recurrence or his inability to accept the change in health status. Exploration of alternative, unproven treatment methods may also constitute a form of denial.

As expectations for survival change, denial plays only a slight role as a coping mechanism (Weisman, 1979a). One important example of denial in this setting is termed "denial of implications" (Weisman, 1979b). Although patients may adjust to the demands of new treatment and appreciate the social supports that have worked in the past, their status as "recurrent cancer patients" means that they are never entirely free of concern. The inability to cope with the blunt reality of death without panic results in efforts to absorb the truth slowly, filtering the reality to make it more tolerable. In the case provided, Jill's comment that she does not yet feel "like myself again" would imply that she actually expects to reach that point. Alsop provides poignant personal examples of living with this constant concern, which he terms a "little pea of fear," or "background music" (Alsop, 1973).

> The conscious effort to close off one's mind, or part of it, to the inevitability of death plays a part, I suspect, in the oddly cheerful tone of much of what I've written in this book. . . . In this way the unbearable becomes bearable, and one learns to live with death by not thinking about it too much.

And further:

> A man can't be afraid all the time . . . when death is due to occur at some time in the fairly near but indefinite future . . . it is possible to forget about death for many hours at a time.

The Turnages (1976), in their personal account of living with cancer, *More Than You Dared to Ask*, describe the same "background music": "questions will haunt your subconscious for months—possibly years . . . [they] become your steady companions, prodding and shaking you."

Tolerance or Coping

From a physical standpoint, the person's ability to tolerate or cope with recurrent disease will vary, depending on the extent of recurrence and response to therapy. Over time, however, the patient becomes less able to recover from cytotoxic treatment as the ability to reconstitute normal bone marrow cells diminishes. Nutritional status wanes, and tolerance of side effects decreases. Similarly, frequency of crises, especially in the case of multiple relapses, causes fatigue for the patient, family, and health care team. Families, specifically, show fatigue when they become desensitized to the situation (Hersh, 1985). In addition, family members may demonstrate anger when their own needs are unmet (Giacquinta, 1977; Olsen, 1970). Specific coping skills may help the patient achieve relief at various times during this period or be ineffective at other times. Patients may vacillate between feelings of hope and despair or demonstrate varying degrees of cooperation and dependence or independence (Weisman, 1979a).

NURSING MANAGEMENT

Communication

The intensity of the experience of cancer for the person with recurrent cancer directly affects everyone involved in care. This, together with the variation in experience of cancer between individuals, requires nurses to maintain open lines of communication and to remain sensitive to changes in the needs of patient and family for information and support. A potential obstacle to this openness is the inability of the nurse to cope with the patient's change in health status and impending death. As one patient wrote: "You [the patient] are the constant reminder that everyone is mortal. They see in you their own fear of death" (Turnage, 1976, p. 26). Recognition of their own feelings of failure, guilt, and helplessness may allow nurses to resist avoidance behaviors and focus on the needs of the patient and family. Staff support systems, access to psychological consultation, group meetings, and multidisciplinary conferences may help maintain morale (Scott et al., 1983).

To be effective, communication must be sensitive and honest; as discussed, patients with recurrent cancer may have a greater need for facts about their disease (as compared with psychological issues), and they may attribute undue significance to specific words or information given. In addition, because the patient is now living with a constant degree of uncertainty, medical and nursing personnel can be a source of certainty and predictability. In her review of the family's experience of cancer, Northouse (1984) emphasized the need for families to obtain information for "intellectual mastery and control over the cancer process." The research of Lewandowski and Jones (1988) attempted to identify helpful nursing interventions in relation to three phases of living with cancer: initial, adaptation, and terminal. During the adaptation phase (a "sometimes lengthy period between diagnosis and cure"), the highest-ranked interventions related to relief of symptoms for the patient and securing information about his or her condition and treatment. These investigations conclude that over the course of illness, the family takes in information, changes, and grows, and "therefore nursing intervention aimed at teaching the patient with cancer and family must assume a priority position in the family's total care." Remembering this, nurses may be more supportive if they choose words carefully and focus on providing important and helpful information and on reinforcing positive aspects of therapy and positive behaviors of the patient (Abrams, 1966; Scott et al., 1983; Weisman & Worden, 1985–1986). Nurses should assess each patient for knowledge needs about prognosis and treatment, because this may be the area of greatest concern at the time of recurrence (Weisman and Worden, 1985–1986). On the other hand, the need to absorb information gradually during the early period of recurrence requires sensitivity about what information the patient and family really wants. As Turnage and Turnage (1976) state, "You are both surprised that you do not need all the details about the disease."

Support

In recognition of patients' potential fear of abandonment, nurses can provide not only companionship but also a link between the patient-family unit and other health professionals. This role may be as an advocate or as a referral agent when other professional help is needed (e.g., social services, psychiatry, home care, physical therapy). Blank, Clark, Longman, and At-wood (1989) identified perceived home care needs of eight outpatients and their eight caregivers; a primary need of both groups was for interpersonal support. Frank-Stromborg (1986) found social support groups to be highly significant in helping cancer outpatients to cope with their disease, specifically as these groups promote a feeling of health instead of sick-role behavior.

Assessment of the social supports available for each patient will dictate whether the nurse relies on existing family and friends to provide support or helps the patient and family seek out new sources of emotional support. The spousal relationship is an important support, whether or not open communication about the disease recurrence occurs (Chekryn, 1984).

The patient's behavior needs to be analyzed in terms of his important relationships, the roles within them, and issues to be resolved in each case. . . . People have contracts with others that determine behavior, decisions, and interactions. Understanding the nature of the unstated agreements between two people usually sheds light on one or the other's behavior (Scott et al., 1983, p. 204).

Knowledge that during recurrence, families tend to become more insular in relation to the outside world places the emphasis on these relationships for support. Northouse (1981) suggested that patients who have less support from their families have more difficulty adjusting and more fears of recurrence. Nurses can work with patients and families to make necessary decisions about care.

Revenson, Wollman, and Felton (1983) described a paradoxical relationship between supportive behaviors and adjustment to cancer. On the basis of interviews with 32 nonhospitalized adult cancer patients, they found that for patients *not* receiving treatment for cancer and for those with more physical limitations, higher levels of social support (e.g., providing warmth, advice, aid, or companionship) correlated with "increased negative affect, lowered self-esteem and mastery, and greater difficulty in acceptance of death." However, for patients undergoing therapy, supportive behaviors did not negatively affect adjustment to illness (Revenson et al., 1983). Although the authors are careful to note that support from family and friends is a necessary buffer to stress, they go on to explain that social support, when it is given unnecessarily or insensitively (to meet the needs of the provider, rather than those of the patient), results in "secondary victimization" of the person in need. Understanding this potential negative overtone to emotional support may help nurses recognize its occurrence and suggest different approaches to those involved. Whereas Jill was in a position of relative control in her life, her mother's overzealous help resulted in Jill's feeling like a child; making it possible for her to accept her mother's need to help required that she decide what that help would be.

Open-mindedness

As the patient with recurrent cancer works to cope with the change in his or her disease status, expressions of feelings—anger, passivity, fear, depression, grief—may be necessary at various times; resolution of these feelings requires that others acknowledge the right of the patient to feel them. If members of the medical and nursing profession can maintain open minds about the meaning of the experience to each patient, they can better work with the patient and family toward mitigating the distress caused by these feelings. This insight will depend on the degree of communication that occurs with both patients and families, as well as the amount of physical and emotional comfort afforded them.

Relinquishing Control

The issue of personal control assumes paramount importance in the setting of recurrent cancer, because the unpredictability and uncertainty imposed by the disease diminish the patient's sense of power. The ability of patients to maintain control requires that they feel some degree of hope, whether for remission or for symptom control. Nurses can help infuse feelings of hope by both managing symptoms effectively and explaining the plan of treatment in positive terms. Exploration for new, alternative treatment options may even be appropriate with patients and families when the existing treatment fails.

Nurses can help to restore control by contracting with patients concerning their treatment. Reinforcement of learning will assure the nurse that appropriate knowledge has been obtained and will also demonstrate to the patient that he or she has sufficient information to care for himself or herself.

Nurses and physicians may struggle for control themselves, especially in this setting, which engenders feeling of helplessness and frustration. Of special importance is the degree to which health professionals must make the transition from cure-oriented treatment to control of the cancer at the same time that the patient and family are attempting to make this change in their own expectations.

References

Abrams, R. D. (1966). The patient with cancer—his changing pattern of communication. *New England Journal of Medicine, 288,* 317–322.

Alsop, S. (1973). *Stay of execution.* Philadelphia: J. B. Lippincott Co.

American Cancer Society. (1989). *Cancer facts and figures 1989.* Atlanta: Author.

Barsevick, A. M., & McCarthy, P. R. (1987). The treatment/chronicity phase. In S. Groenwald (Ed.), *Cancer nursing: Principles and practice* (pp. 114–121). Boston: Jones and Bartlett, Publishers.

Blank, J. J., Clark, L., Longman, A. J., & Atwood, J. R. (1989). Perceived home care needs of cancer patients and their caregivers. *Cancer Nursing, 12,* 78–84.

Chekryn, J. (1984). Cancer recurrence: Personal meaning, communication, and marital adjustment. *Cancer Nursing, 7,* 491–498.

Derdiarian, A. (1984). Psychosocial variables in cancer management: Considerations for nursing management. In D. L. Vredevoe, A. Derdiarian, L. P. Sarna, M. Friel, & J. A. G. Shiplacoff (Eds.), *Concepts of oncology nursing* (pp. 36–50). Englewood Cliffs, NJ, Prentice-Hall, Inc.

Frank-Stromborg, M. (1986). Health promotion behaviors in ambulatory cancer patients: Facts or fiction? *Oncology Nursing Forum, 13,* 37–43.

Giacquinta, B. (1977). Helping families face the crisis of cancer. *American Journal of Nursing, 77,* 1585–1588.

Hersh, S. P. (1985). Psychologic aspects of patients with cancer. In V. T. DeVita, Jr., S. Hellman, & S. A. Rosenberg, (Eds.), *Cancer: Principles and practice of oncology* (2nd ed., pp. 2051–2066). Philadelphia: J. B. Lippincott Co.

Legha, S. S., Keating, M. J., Zander, A. R., McCredie, K., Bodey, G., Freireich, E. (1980). 4′(9-acridinylamino) methanesulfon-*m*-ansidide (AMSA): A new drug effective in the treatment of adult acute leukemia. *Annals of Internal Medicine, 93,* 17–21.

Lewandowski, W., & Jones, S. L. (1988). The family with cancer: Nursing interventions throughout the course of living with cancer. *Cancer Nursing, 11,* 313–321.

Northouse, L. L. (1981). Mastectomy patients and the fear of cancer recurrence. *Cancer Nursing, 4,* 213–220.

Northouse, L. L. (1984). The impact of cancer on the family: An overview. *International Journal of Psychiatry and Medicine, 14,* 215–243.

Olsen, E. H. (1970). The impact of serious illness on the family system. *Postgraduate Medicine, 47,* 169–174.

Paciucci, P. A., Cuttner, J., & Holland, J. F. (1984). Mitoxantrone as a single agent and in combination chemotherapy in patients with refractory acute leukemia. *Seminars in Oncology, 11*(Suppl. 1), 36–40.

Revenson, T. A., Wollman, B. A., & Felton, B. J. (1983). Social support as stress buffers for adult cancer patients. *Psychosomatic Medicine, 45,* 321–331.

Sanders, J. B., & Kardinal, C. G. (1977). Adaptive coping mechanisms in adult acute leukemia patients in remission. *Journal of the American Medical Association, 238,* 952–954.

Schmale, A. H. (1976). Psychological reactions to recurrences, metastases, or disseminated cancer. *International Journal of Radiation Oncology, Biology, and Physics, 1,* 515–520.

Scott, D. W., Goode, W. L., & Arlin, Z. A. (1983). The psychodynamics of multiple remissions in a patient with acute nonlymphoblastic leukemia. *Cancer Nursing, 6,* 201–206.

Turnage, M. N., & Turnage, A. S. (1976). *More than you dare to ask.* Atlanta: John Knox Press.

Weisman, A. D. (1979a). *Coping with cancer.* New York: McGraw-Hill Book Co.

Weisman, A. D. (1979b). A model for psychosocial phasing in cancer. In *General hospital psychiatry* (pp. 187–195). New York: Elsevier–North Holland.

Weisman, A. D., & Worden, J. W. (1976). The existential plight in cancer: Significance of the first 100 days. *International Journal of Psychiatry in Medicine, 7,* 1–15.

Weisman, A. D., & Worden, J. W. (1985–1986). The emotional impact of recurrent cancer. *Journal of Psychosocial Oncology, 3*(4), 5–16.

Wiernik, P. H. (1985). *Leukemias and lymphomas.* New York: Churchill Livingstone.

CHAPTER 45

Nursing Management of Persons with Progressive Disease: Prototype—Lung Cancer

ROSEMARY POLOMANO
MARY DEE McEVOY

LIVING-DYING INTERVAL OF LUNG CANCER
Acute Phase
Chronic Living-Dying Phase

Terminal Phase
SUMMARY

Each type of cancer is associated with a unique trajectory and, correspondingly, each trajectory elicits a variety of patient responses. Although strides have been made in the treatment of many cancers, resulting in longer disease-free survival periods, lung cancer remains associated with limited treatment options and a downward trajectory. This chapter reviews the nursing care of a disease with a downward trajectory using a case study method of a patient with lung cancer.

In 1990, the American Cancer Society (ACS) estimated that 157,000 new cases of lung cancer would occur in the United States, and that approximately 142,000 more deaths would occur from lung cancer than from any other type of cancer in 1990. Lung cancer is responsible for 35 per cent of cancer deaths in men and 20 per cent in women. In fact, the mortality rate from lung cancer has steadily risen over the past decade, whereas mortality rates for other common cancers have not changed appreciably. With the 5-year survival approaching 13 per cent and effective treatment options being limited, it is no surprise that persons diagnosed as having lung cancer experience a downward disease trajectory. Health professionals need to appreciate that care of patients with lung cancer often centers on supportive and terminal care. Numerous psychosocial responses accompany a diagnosis of lung cancer. First, it is well established that more than 80 per cent of all lung cancers are linked to cigarette smoking, especially in smokers with a history of 20 pack-years or more (Loeb et al., 1984). Tobacco labeling and promotion of smoke-free environments emphasize the strong association of smoking to lung cancer. The issue of guilt for patients who feel that they may have contributed to their disease must be addressed.

It is also well known among health professionals that effective screening techniques for lung cancer detection are not available. However, this fact is not understood by the public in general. Persons who have yearly physical examinations incorporating chest radiographs often have a false sense of security, believing that the prospect of facing lung cancer is removed if chest radiographs are negative. Not only is the diagnosis of lung cancer complicated by ineffective screening techniques; in addition, the signs and symptoms, which are often nonspecific and vague, lead to a diagnosis more frequently only in the advanced stages. Therefore, anger, a second common reaction, is expressed when a patient believe he or she has engaged in acceptable health practices with little or no benefit to overall survival. Lastly, fear and desperation are experienced and commonly associated with the gloomy prognosis, limited treatment options for a favorable outcome, and, more important, thoughts about experience of the effects of the cancer and cancer therapies.

Through a case study analysis, the initial responses to a diagnosis of lung cancer are viewed in the context of Pattison's (1977) clinical model of chronic illness. Complications of lung cancer are addressed, with careful consideration of the respiratory system. Nursing interventions are integrated throughout the text.

LIVING-DYING INTERVAL OF LUNG CANCER

The diagnosis of lung cancer, as with all cancer, often evokes insurmountable anxiety. Pattison (1976, 1977) delineates a clinical model descriptive of the clinical phases a person experiences once he or she learns that death from the disease is inevitable, called the *living-dying interval*. The living-dying interval is the time between the crisis knowledge of death and the point of death. Pattison (1977) describes the initial reaction to a life-threatening illness as a feeling of being immobilized, characterized by shock, disbelief, and the perception that life is standing still.

Using crisis theory proposed by Parad (1965), Pattison analyzes the experience of dying. He theorizes that the knowledge of death precipitates a crisis that by definition is not able to be solved—that is, death can be acknowledged but it cannot be solved. The problem of death is a new experience with which a person has no prior experience on which to draw. Each person's own death is unique, to be experienced only once. The experience of death is seen as a threat to one's goals. The crisis period is characterized by a tension that mounts to a peak and then falls, with peak anxiety occurring at a considerable time before death. The living-dying interval is composed of three phases: the acute phase, the chronic living-dying phase, and the terminal phase.

The acute phase is characterized by acute crisis anxiety as a reaction to the initial diagnosis of a condition that will probably end in death. It elicits feelings of anxiety, disorientation, helplessness, confusion, and bewilderment (Pattison, 1977).

Two experiences dominate the chronic living-dying period. The person struggles to cope with the illness and its subsequent problems and with the psychosocial responses to illness and impending death (Rands, 1984). Numerous problems are experienced during the long chronic phase, including remissions and relapses; increased financial, social, physical, and emotional pressures; long-term family disruption; periods of uncertainty; dilemmas about treatment choices; intensive treatment regimens and side effects; and progressive decline. In addition, amid all these concerns, the patient is also forced to integrate dying into his or her life circumstances.

The terminal phase is a short period, with an imprecise onset. It starts when the person begins to withdraw from the environment and concludes with actual death.

Although Pattison (1976, 1977) describes the living-dying interval predominantly in terms of the patient, other people interacting with the patient ultimately experience the same phases, albeit with varying degrees of intensity. In this chapter. Using the living-dying interval as a framework, the experience of the patient with lung cancer is discussed, moving through the acute phase to the chronic and terminal phases.

Acute Phase

The acute phase of the living-dying interval is characterized by acute anxiety brought on by the diagnosis of a disease that will ultimately be terminal. This is the period of peak anxiety.

Mr. M. is a 69-year-old man who consulted his local physician because of shortness of breath, dyspnea on exertion, a productive cough, a 10-pound weight loss over 2 months, slight facial plethora, distended neck veins, and edematous upper extremities. He reported a 40 pack-year smoking history. Because Mr. M. knew he was at risk for lung cancer, he had been following his physician's advice and had a yearly chest radiograph and physical examination. His last chest radiograph, just 6 months earlier, was reported as normal. However, over the last few weeks, he had become progressively distressed about the aforementioned symptoms.

Somewhat debilitated and distressed over experiencing anorexia, weight loss, and shortness of breath, Mr. M. was anxious to learn the cause of his symptoms. He was then informed by his local physician that his chest radiograph demonstrated a large mediastinal mass. Because his symptoms of superior vena cava syndrome (SVC) were striking and nearly 90 per cent of all SVC cases are related to cancer, Mr. M. was referred to a local cancer center.

Shocked by the probability of a malignant condition, Mr. M. went to the local cancer center accompanied by his wife. On arrival in the outpatient area, his symptoms of shortness of breath and facial plethora appeared more striking. The physician informed Mr. M. that this was a serious situation and obtained consent to perform an emergency bronchoscopy. Mr. M. tolerated the procedure well and was admitted for constant observation of further respiratory distress as the danger of tracheal compression was a major concern. The cytologic specimen of bronchial washings showed evidence of squamous cell carcinoma of the lung.

While Mr. M. was recuperating from his bronchoscopy, the physician approached Mr. and Mrs. M. to inform them that a diagnosis of lung cancer was confirmed and that the cancer probably extended outside the lung area. In total disbelief, Mr. M. responded, "How could this be? I just had a clean bill of health." The physician deferred giving any further information regarding long-term treatment options and focused on the immediate need for radiation treatments to the mediastinum. Radiotherapy was initiated at 300 cGy daily for 3 days to relieve the superior vena cava compression. During his radiotherapy, Mr. M. became very withdrawn, appeared extremely depressed, and refused to discuss the situation with his wife. Four days after radiotherapy and steroid therapy, the signs and symptoms of SVC subsided. Mr. M. was feeling better, with his appetite returning to normal, and was experiencing only minimal difficulty breathing. On this particular day, the nurse caring for Mr. M. found him in his room smoking a cigarette and crying. He responded "Well, I guess I got what I deserved. I knew all along that these darned cigarettes cause cancer, but I never thought it would happen to me. No sense in grieving now, the damage is done."

According to Pattison (1976, 1977), the acute phase of the living-dying interval is characterized by the anxiety related to the uncertain diagnosis accompanied by the potential that the condition will result in death. Research by Benedict (1989) confirms the presence of anxiety in patients with lung cancer. Benedict found that 34 per cent of her sample of 30 subjects reported anxiety. Mr. M., although experiencing vague symptoms, also had confidence in a good prognosis owing to his good results on yearly physical examinations. The diagnostic period was accentuated by referral to a distant medical center and the need to undertake an uncomfortable diagnostic procedure. These two additional burdens served to increase Mr. M.'s anxiety regarding his potential diagnosis. The anxiety experienced in the acute phase is heightened in patients with lung cancer because they must also confront the feelings of guilt that surround their diagnosis.

Patients who recognize that their personal behaviors

or habits could have contributed to the onset of this disease face a number of psychosocial problems in coping with their illness. Considerable research has documented the correlation of smoking with the development of lung cancer (Higgins, Maltan, & Wyndes, 1988; Wilcox et al., 1988). In addition, extensive literature on health promotion has addressed the physiologic basis for the causal link, the differences between active and passive smoking (Correa et al., 1983; Sandler et al., 1985), and behaviors of health professionals with regard to smoking and cessation of smoking (Garfinkle & Stillman, 1986; Knopf & Morra, 1983). However, information that addresses the guilt related to smoking is limited. Mumma and McCorkle (1982–1983) report on coping in patients with lung cancer and heart attacks. A structured interview with questions referring to the patient's condition, purpose of treatment, the future, death, and personal factors was conducted at 1 and 2 months after diagnosis. These researchers found that 31 of 65 lung cancer subjects viewed themselves as somewhat responsible for their disease, with 24 relating the cause to smoking.

Family members may also experience guilt, feeling that all would have been well if only they had been more aggressive in convincing the patient to quit. Alternatively, a spouse who also smokes, may feel that if he or she had quit smoking, perhaps the patient also would have stopped. It is important that family members understand and explore their own feelings so they may help the patient make an individual conscious choice to stop smoking.

Nurses can help family members explore their feelings about smoking by using broad statements such as, "You seem to have difficulty with Mr. M.'s smoking—how do you feel about that?" Statements such as these encourage family members to express their feelings of guilt or anger. Family members need to be able to express their feelings as well to understand the complexity of behavior change.

Anger frequently accompanies the anxiety of initial diagnosis. One of Mr. M.'s initial responses to his diagnosis of lung cancer was disbelief. "How could this be?" he verbalized to his nurse. "I went to the doctors every year and had my yearly chest x-ray; why didn't my doctor pick this up earlier?" Mr. M.'s reaction is a common one. Many patients who engage in what are considered good health practices may think cancel on their risk-taking habits and thus become angry or feel betrayed when they have relied too heavily on the yearly check-up. Feelings of guilt may exacerbate their anger about what they view as inadequate screening techniques.

Screening for lung cancer has been a subject of controversy for many years. At present the ACS does not recommend specific routine screening techniques for the early detection of lung cancer (ACS, 1980). The efficacy of lung cancer screening has not yet been determined, given the costs of routine tests to detect lung cancer and the disappointing benefits (Appenheimer, 1987). It is essential that the public realize that significant benefits may accrue from screening for some cancers, such as breast and colon, but not from others.

In addition, cessation of smoking must become recognized as the primary means of prevention of lung cancer.

The nurse must listen and allow the patient to express feelings of anger and disbelief. As mentioned earlier, Pattison (1977) stresses that patients behave very differently during the initial phase of diagnosis for a life-threatening illness. He cautions against trying to respond to all of these behaviors, for in time patients revert to more appropriate patterns of coping.

An acknowledgment of anger and an empathetic approach are necessary for patients to gain trust in caregivers and to foster a therapeutic relationship. After the initial reaction of anger, the nurse should take the opportunity to clarify the patient's misconceptions and to help the patient deal with the here and now and to refrain from continually reverting back to the past. Patient and family counseling may be necessary for patients who are unable to work through their anger and guilt. Research by Quinn, Fontana, and Reznikoff (1986) indicated that helping patients to feel less guilty may be worthwhile. In a study of coping strategies, they interviewed 60 male patients with lung cancer and their wives. They found a significant positive relationship between self-blaming denial—a situation in which people not only try to find a cause for their illness but also blame themselves for the cause—and greater psychological distress.

The need to undergo procedures to relieve the patient's symptoms often results in exacerbation of the psychosocial responses of guilt and anger. The acute phase in lung cancer may be relatively short, with movement into the chronic phase occurring relatively rapidly. Hence, feelings of anger and guilt may be observed in the chronic phase as well. As an example of this situation, Mr. M.'s symptoms relating to superior vena cava syndrome required prompt nursing management.

Chronic Living-Dying Phase

The chronic phase of the living-dying interval is the longest phase, requiring considerable adaptation on the part of the patient (Pattison, 1977). Feelings of anxiety wax and wane as the patient is confronted with the need to make decisions regarding treatment and with the need to manage symptoms brought on both by the disease itself and by the treatment. One of the major tasks for the patient during this phase is to integrate dying into his or her life style (Pattison, 1977). As the prospect of death becomes slowly recognized, frequently patients experience anticipatory grief.

Anticipatory grief is grief in anticipation of a loss (Weisman, 1972). This grief is beneficial in that it allows reality of the loss to be absorbed gradually; it allows the patient the opportunity to finish unfinished business, both physical and psychic; and finally, it allows the family and friends to begin to contemplate what life will be like without the one who dies. Both the dying person and family members experience anticipatory grief. Futterman, Hoffman, and Sabshin (1972) delineate five aspects of anticipatory grief, including acknowledgment that death is near, physical and psychological aspects of the grieving process, reconciliation, detachment, and memorialization. Although there is danger that the mourner will isolate the dying person, anticipatory grief can assist in the work of grief, which is discussed later.

McCorkle and Donaldson (1986) reported on grief in persons with newly diagnosed lung cancer and heart disease at 1 and 2 months after diagnosis. In a sample of 56 cancer patients and 65 heart attack patients, both groups report less grief at 2 months after diagnosis. The investigators theorize that 2 months may be an inadequate time period to absorb the reality of a life-threatening disease. However, a relationship between existential concerns and grief was reported, with both groups experiencing more grief with more existential concerns.

Feelings of fear and desperation accompany the chronic phase as patients attempt to live with lung cancer.

After the symptoms of SVC syndrome resolved, Mr. M. was then faced with the dilemma of how his lung cancer would be managed. He expressed his fears of not wanting to die in pain and that he wanted to spend the remainder of his life experiencing as little physical and emotional distress as possible in the comfortable surroundings of his home. Both he and his wife agreed that if treatment options for advanced squamous cell carcinoma offered little hope for long-term survival, Mr. M. would refuse further anticancer therapy. On the other hand, thoughts of doing nothing for his cancer continually plagued Mr. M. as he became preoccupied with the fear of eventually suffocating from the cancer in his lung. He continually queried the nurses with questions such as, "How will I die? Will I drown in my own secretions? What happens when the cancer fills my lungs?"

On the fifth day after Mr. M.'s admission to the hospital, after being somewhat protected from informational overload until he recovered from the symptoms of SVC syndrome, it was time for the physician to discuss treatment options with Mr. M. and his wife.

Treatment options, although varied and limited to specific histologic types, provide little hope for long-term survival or control of advanced lung cancer (Harwood, 1987). Feelings of desperation can overcome patients and families when they realize that treatment options are few and the results are often unfavorable. Patients frequently are confronted with the decision to accept, delay, or refuse treatment. Moreover, the ability to weigh the risks and benefits of treatment may be compromised by the patient's limited understanding of the significance of the side effects and the participation required to manage and deal with these effects. Hope and reassurance are possible if the effects of the disease and its treatment are manageable.

Keeping in mind the extent of Mr. M.'s lung cancer and the cell type, treatment options for palliation or control of symptoms were proposed. The physician informed Mr. M. that his tumor was inoperable. Mr. M., who had grasped the hope that the tumor could be removed surgically and was confident that this was the most effective treatment, was devastated by the

news. He was also informed that squamous cell carcinoma was relatively insensitive to chemotherapeutic agents and that the role of chemotherapy in the treatment of non-small-cell cancer of the lung is questionable. However, Mr. M.'s physician did stress the possible benefit of radiotherapy. O'Rourke and Crawford (1987) question the benefits of radiotherapy in asymptomatic patients because the overall prognosis is poor, time and financial investments are considerable, and systemic and local toxicities may compromise the quality of life. Nonetheless, Mr. M. was offered radiotherapy as a treatment option now or later if he so desired.

To help Mr. M. make an informed decision regarding radiotherapy as a treatment option, the nurse reviewed the major side effects of radiation therapy and mentioned ways in which Mr. M. could participate in his care to alleviate or manage these effects (see also Chapter 20).

Initially, the poor prognosis, limited treatment options, and anticipated downward trajectory make the experience of coping with lung cancer somewhat different from other cancers. Weisman and Worden (1976) reported greater emotional distress and existential concerns in patients with lung cancer than in patients with breast and colon cancers, Hodgkin's disease, and malignant melanoma within the first 100 days after treatment. The nurse must be particularly attentive to the early responses of patients with lung cancer in the initial phase of their disease. Helping patients to sort out their concerns and fears is of utmost importance in fostering adaptation and adjustment to illness.

Mr. M., after pondering the possibility of receiving radiotherapy, decided to go home to be with his family and to reconsider treatment at a later date. On the morning of discharge, the nurse caring for Mr. M. tried to assess his level of understanding of his condition. The nurse asked Mr. M. what was his biggest concern about going home. He responded "What happens if I get home and I can't breathe?" It seems that this was Mr. M.'s primary fear. Once again, the management of symptoms becomes a primary nursing responsibility.

The difficult, labored breathing termed *dyspnea* is commonly experienced and can potentially occur during almost any stage of lung cancer. It often results from problems of the lower respiratory tract. A variety of mechanisms that are commonly involved in dyspnea in patients with lung cancer are listed in Table 45–1. Coy and Kennelly (1980) report that from 15 to 40 per cent of newly diagnosed lung cancer patients experience dyspnea.

Because the lung is perceived as the major respiratory organ, having lung cancer often evokes considerable anxiety in the patient over the thought of not being able to breathe. Brown, Carrieri, Janson-Bjerklie, and Dodd (1986), using a sample of 30 patients with lung cancer who experienced shortness of breath, measured the severity of dyspnea using a Dyspnea Visual Analogue Scale. The categories *not breathless at all* and *extremely breathless* were the two anchors at opposite ends (Janssen-Bjerklie, Carrieri, & Hudes,

Table 45–1. COMMON CAUSES OF DYSPNEA ASSOCIATED WITH LUNG CANCER

Obstructed bronchi or trachea
Atelectasis
Pleural effusions
Superior vena cava syndrome
Radiation pneumonitis
Post-obstructive pneumonitis
Antineoplastic therapy
Pneumonias
Anxiety
Involvement of lung parenchyma by tumor
Persistent uncontrollable cough

1986). These investigators also used the American Thoracic Society (1978) Grade of Breathlessness Scale (GBS), a six-point instrument that measures dyspnea on a scale of 0 (no shortness of breath) to 5 (too breathless to leave the house). Both of these assessment tools provide a reliable means of measuring dyspnea experienced by patients with lung cancer.

Brown and colleagues (1986) also identified patient-oriented behaviors or activities that are effective in minimizing dyspnea (Table 45–2). These investigators also emphasized the need for patient education, because not one of their subjects reported receiving information from the nurse on how to manage dyspnea; the strategies they did use were believed to have been self-taught.

Nurses must recognize that the fear of dyspnea or of difficulty with breathing often becomes a major focus for patients with lung cancer. As 15 to 40 per cent of newly diagnosed patients have dyspnea and an estimated 70 per cent of all lung cancer patients in general experience dyspnea, it is the responsibility of the nurse to prepare patients and families to deal effectively with this symptom. Careful attention must be given to those who already have experienced dyspnea, particularly at the time of diagnosis, for their initial fear of dyspnea may be heightened. Table 45–3 outlines nursing care for patients with dyspnea.

Other symptoms have also been reported by persons with lung cancer. Benedict (1989) found that disability, physical pain, changed daily activities, and fatigue are related to patients' perceptions of high levels of suffering. In comparing 56 persons with lung cancer and 65 persons with myocardial infarction, McCorkle and Benoliel (1983) reported that cancer patients experienced significantly more distress than patients with heart disease. Symptoms reported included fatigue, pain, lack of appetite, and insomnia. Of particular interest is the report that increased symptom distress was associated with decreased probability of survival (Kukall, McCorkle, & Driever, 1986). Thus with Mr. M.'s multiple symptoms, the terminal phase was soon evident.

Terminal Phase

The terminal phase is marked by a short time period in which the person begins to withdraw (Pattison, 1977) and a shift in focus occurs from treatment to palliation.

The family realizes that death is inevitably near. This phase of the living-dying interval is characterized by symptom management and comfort as well as by grieving.

Frightened by the thoughts of not doing anything for his tumor, yet discouraged by the few benefits and increased side effects of treatment, Mr. M. decided to delay any further treatment. The nurse caring for Mr. M. initiated a referral to a local Community Health Nursing Agency.

Research by McCorkle and colleagues highlights the importance of home care (1989). They reported a clinical trial on the effect of three types of home care services—a specialized oncology home care program, standard home care, and office care—on the responses of patients with lung cancer (Box 45–1).

McCorkle (1984) stresses that in preparation for discharge, the nurse should realize the importance of anticipating problems and preparing patients and families to deal with them. The patient's current capabili-

Table 45–2. MANAGEMENT STRATEGIES FOR DYSPNEA USED BY A SAMPLE OF LUNG CANCER PATIENTS (N = 30)

Strategy	Number	Per Cent
Immediate Coping Strategies		
Positioning	14	46.7
Move slower	13	43.3
Use of an inhaler	4	13.3
Posture	3	10.0
Medicines	2	6.7
Pursed lip breathing	2	6.7
Long-Term Adaptive Strategies		
Activities of Daily Living (ADL)		
1. Assistance or transfer of ADLs to others	22	73.3
2. Changes in bathing	22	73.3
3. Changes in eating	20	66.7
4. Changes in dressing, grooming	17	56.7
5. Changes in living arrangements	2	6.7
General Activities		
1. Advanced planning of activities	29	97.6
2. Change in time of activities	29	97.6
3. Planned decrease or modified activities	29	97.6
Other Behaviors		
1. Breathing strategies (pattern with activities)	6	20.0
2. Avoid precipitants	5	16.7
3. Home remedies	2	6.7
4. Increased exercise	2	6.7
5. Increased ventilation (taking deep breaths)	2	6.7
6. Diversional activities	1	3.3
7. Protective behaviors	1	3.3
8. Relaxation techniques	1	3.3
Social Isolation	24	80.0
Emotional Strategies		
1. Accepts situation	23	76.6
2. Avoids being alone	16	53.3
3. Good attitude, stays in good frame of mind	15	50.0
4. Prayer, meditation	7	23.3
5. Avoids thinking about it	4	13.3
6. Eliminates stress	3	10.0
7. Conscious attempt to be calm	2	6.7
8. Affection from families	1	3.3

(From Brown, M., Carrieri, V., Johnson-Bjerklie, S., & Dodd, M. [1986]. Lung cancer and dyspnea: The patient's perception. *Oncology Nursing Forum, 13* [5], 22. Reproduced by permission.)

Table 45–3. NURSING INTERVENTIONS IN THE PATIENT WITH RESPIRATORY DYSFUNCTION

Assessment
  Auscultate breath sounds in all lung fields
  Assess patient for dyspnea, tachypnea, and cough
  Assess respiratory symmetry and use of accessory
  muscles
  Monitor temperature
  Note amount, color, consistency, and odor of secretions
  Assess skin color, temperature, and moisture
  Check blood pressure and heart rate
  Monitor respiratory rate
Management of respiratory distress
  Elevate the head of the bed
  Modify activity
  Apply humidification: vaporizer, face tent
  Turn, cough, and deep breathing exercises
  Administer O₂ as ordered
  NaHCO₃ mouth rinses or cleanse mouth with NaHCO₃-
  impregnated swabs
  Nasopharyngeal or oropharyngeal suctioning
  Fluids if tolerated
  Eliminate environmental irritating inhalants that may precipitate
  coughing
  Respiratory supportive measures
    Intermittent positive pressure breathing (IPPB) (if ordered)
    Pursed lip breathing
    Incentive spirometry
Administer medications to manage respiratory problems
  Tachypnea: small doses of morphine sulfate, by mouth, by
  rectum, or subcutaneously
  Increased secretions: scopolamine, atropine; avoid respiratory
  repressors (e.g., barbiturates, alcohol)
  Tenacious secretions: expectorants
  Hiccoughs: chlorpromazine suppository, 25 mg rectally every 8
  hr as needed; chlorpromazine tablets, 10 mg every 8 hr as
  needed
  Cough: antitussive preparations; codeine alone or in cough-
  suppressant preparations
Manage anxiety
  Administer antianxiety medications
    1. Benzodiazepines: lorazepam (Ativan), alprazolam (Xanax),
    diazepam (Valium)
    2. Phenothiazines: chlorpromazine (Thorazine),
    perchlorpromazine (Compazine)
    3. Butyrophenones: haloperidal (Haldol)
  Environmental intervention
    1. Decrease sensory stimuli (noise reduction, commotion from
    visitors)
    2. Provide mild distraction (music, touch, TV)
    3. Organize belongings and necessary items as patient wishes
  Administer medications promptly
  Minimize information

ties are determined, keeping in mind that these may rapidly change as the patient's condition deteriorates. A formula for discharge planning questions is given in Table 45–4 (White, 1987).

Shortly after Mr. M. returned home from the hospital, Mrs. M. noticed a significant decrease in his appetite, and he became disinterested in food. Since he entered the hospital just 3 weeks ago, Mr. M. experienced a 10-pound weight loss. Mrs. M. could hardly believe that such a considerable weight loss could occur in such a short period of time after the diagnosis of cancer. Fearful of further weight loss, she diligently tried to feed him, preparing all the foods he had liked in the past.

Knox (1983) emphasizes that anorexia can be one of the earliest signs of cancer. Furthermore, if it is persistent, marked tissue wasting can result, referred to as *cancer cachexia.* A variety of factors are likely to explain such disruptions in normal eating patterns and metabolic aberrations that eventually lead to pronounced weight loss. The multidimensional aspects of cancer cachexia are described by Buzby and Steinberg (1981) (Fig. 45–1). Certainly, cancer therapies are likely to produce nutritional problems, but in addition the tumor itself can cause anorexia. Theolodiges (1979) postulated that certain anorexigenic metabolites produced from the tumor exert a direct effect on the appetite center, the hypothalamus. Lindsey (1986) more specifically suggests that many of these products, such as lactate, peptides, and other biochemical substances, circulate and potentially interfere with normal central and peripheral mechanisms that regulate food intake. The pathophysiology of anorexia in cancer patients, although multifactorial, remains not fully understood (DeWys, 1977). However, it is important for nurses to identify all possible causes and to treat the symptoms to the extent that is possible.

Because Mr. M. was not receiving any cancer treatment, it was possible that the anorexia was a tumor-mediated response. Pain may also contribute to anorexia, but this was not a problem in this particular situation. It is more likely that fatigue, lack of exercise, and the psychological stress of coping with a sudden progressive illness confounded the problem of anorexia, and these factors should be included as contributing to the anorexia. Frustrated and distraught over her husband's inability to eat, Mrs. M. consulted the visiting nurse.

The visiting nurse offered some helpful suggestions to maximize Mr. M.'s food intake. First, an assessment of Mr. M.'s appetite patterns was recommended. Because Mr. M. reported that the early morning was the easiest time to eat—as many other patients do—small, frequent feedings in the morning were encouraged. "Why doesn't my husband like the foods that he has enjoyed all of his life?" Mrs. M. questioned. DeWys and Walters (1975) conclude that significant taste abnormalities exist among patients. They found an elevated taste threshold for sweets, specifically sucrose and an aversion to meats. Additionally, Vickers, Nielson, and Theologides (1981) observed specific food preferences among patients with cancer. According to their results, patients who experienced food aversions to red meats also found other protein foods, such as fish, poultry, and eggs, less appealing.

To combat the complex problem of anorexia, Grant (1986) offers some helpful suggestions to increase oral intake. Decreasing food portions and offering six small feedings can help reduce the loss of appetite associated with the appearance of large amounts of food. High caloric foods with nutritional value, such as milk shakes, and foods high in protein should be offered both at mealtimes and throughout the day. If patients have an aversion to meats, other sources of protein should be offered including cheeses, yogurt, and other dairy products. Caution should be exercised with the ingestion of dairy products if a lactose intolerance exists. Armed with the knowledge that food preferences can be a problem for patients experiencing

---

Box 45–1. A RANDOMIZED CLINICAL TRIAL OF HOME NURSING CARE FOR LUNG CANCER PATIENTS

A randomized clinical trial was conducted to assess the effects of home nursing care for patients with progressive lung cancer. One hundred sixty-six patients were assigned to either an oncology home care group (OHC) that received care from oncology home care nurses, a standard home group (SHC) that received ce fm egu me care nurses, or an office care group (OC) that received whatever care they eee ecept for home care. Patients were entered into the study 2 months after diagnosis and followed for 6 months. Patients were interviewed at 6-week intervals across five occasions. At the end of the study, there were no differences in pain, mood disturbance, and concerns among the three groups. There were significant differences in symptom distress, enforced social dependency, and health perceptions. The two home nursing care groups had less distress and greater independence 6 weeks longer than the office care group. In addition, the two home nursing care groups steadily reported worse health perceptions. Thus it was remarkable that the office care group, which indicated more symptom distress and social dependency with time, also indicated perceptions of improved health with time. These results suggest that home nursing care assists patients with forestalling distress from symptoms and maintaining their independence longer in comparison to no home nursing care. Home care may also include helping patients in acknowledging the reality of their situation.

(McCorkle, R., Benoliel, J., Donaldson, G., Georgiadou, F., Moinpour, C., & Goodell, B. [1989]. A randomized clinical trial of home nursing care for lung cancer patients. *Cancer, 64,* 1375–1382.)

---

anorexia, Mr. M.'s community health nurse instructed Mrs. M. in meal planning and choice of foods. The nurse provided some guidelines and listed foods to avoid, because Mr. M. had an aversion to meats. Cold foods were encouraged, and strong odors were to be avoided because they might suppress the appetite. The nurse reassured Mrs. M. that trial and error were required to find which foods were better tolerated than others. Once a particular food or foods seemed desirable, Mrs. M. was told to continue to serve the food(s). To increase Mr. M.'s appetite, mild exercise (if tolerated) and provisions for a relaxing environment at mealtimes were recommended. Liquid dietary supplements were offered, but Mr. M. refused to drink these.

Efforts to prevent further weight loss were unsuccessful, and Mr. M., in a matter of several weeks, lost an additional 15 pounds. Mrs. M. verbalized that she could no longer stand to watch her husband waste away to nothing and urged the nurse to intervene. "He

Table 45–4. DISCHARGE PLANNING QUESTIONS

1. Can the patient enter or leave the home safely? Are there stairs? How many?
2. Can the patient conduct activities of daily living independently? If not, who is available to help?
3. Will adaptive equipment be needed? Grab bars, shower bench, commode?
4. Do the patient and caregiver understand the medications, treatments, diet equipment?
5. Does the patient have enough supplies and medications to last until the first follow-up clinic appointment?
6. What health care professionals can the patient call on for advice?
7. Is referral to an outside agency needed?
8. How are services to be paid?
   Medicare, Medicaid, private insurance, or private pay? Are there any deductibles?
   What alternatives exist for the person who cannot afford to pay?
9. What other resources are available in the patient's local community? Churches, fraternal organizations, disease-related groups?

(Modified with permission from White, E. [1987]. Home care of the patient with advanced lung cancer. *Seminars in Oncology Nursing, 3,* 217.)

can't even take water anymore, his breathing is so bad," she exclaimed. Fry (1986) acknowledges that ethical difficulties arise for health professionals when the patient can no longer ingest nutrients and water to sustain life. If the patient is competent, his or her wishes should be considered before implementing artificial means to sustain nutrition or hydration. For this reason, the nurse arranged a meeting with Mr. and Mrs. M. and their two grown children. Mr. M. was encouraged to express his wishes. He looked at his wife and said, "I just can't eat anymore. I can hardly breath and it is difficult to swallow. My mouth is so dry." So that the family would also hear, the nurse asked Mr. M. what would make him more comfortable. "Just help me breath and make my mouth feel better," he said. The nurse assessed Mr. M. for signs of dehydration. Apparently he was voiding less and less each day. His skin turgor was poor, and his mouth was parched. Because Mr. M. had told his family that he did not want his suffering prolonged any longer than possible, the nurse asked Mr. M. if he just wanted to be made comfortable. The use of an intravenous infusion of fluids would relieve his dry mouth and dehydration. This infusion could be given intermittently whenever he wanted fluids. He agreed. The physician was notified of this request, and an infusion of dextrose and normal saline solution was given. The priorities of care shifted from a nutritional aspect to comfort measures. Mrs. M. was instructed to administer frequent mouth care. As mentioned earlier, efforts to relieve his dyspnea were implemented.

During the terminal phase of the patient's illness, both the patient and the family begin to experience grief. Grief is the process of psychological, social, and somatic reaction to the perception of loss (Rando, 1984). Rando further states that grief is manifested in all three realms (physical, psychological, and social), incorporates many changes, is a natural process, and is based on the person's unique perception of the loss. Thus people respond differently in the same situation.

Many authors have defined the process of grief, after the patient has died (Engel, 1964; Kübler-Ross, 1969;

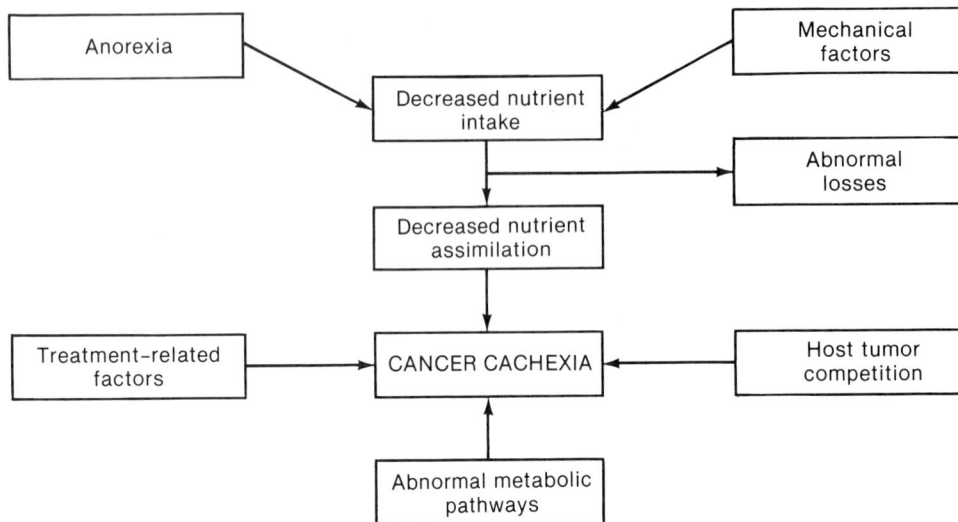

Figure 45–1. Factors contributing to the development of cancer cachexia. (From Buzby, G. P. & Steinberg, J. J. [1981]. Nutrition in cancer patients. *Surgical Clinics of North America, 61,* 693. Reproduced by permission.)

Lindemann, 1944; Parkes & Weiss, 1983; Worden, 1982). Bowlby (1980) and Parkes (1970) delineate four phases of grief:

1. Numbness.
2. Yearning and searching, in which the attempt is made to find and recover the lost person. This phase is characterized by anger, disbelief, and tension.
3. Disorganization and despair, in which depression takes over as the lost person is not recovered.
4. Reorganization, in which there is a return to past interests and the beginning of new relationships.

Physiologic reactions to grief are common. Examples include anorexia, sleeplessness, crying, exhaustion, nervousness, and shortness of breath (Rando, 1984).

It is clear that work is required to complete the phases of grief, as the person must simultaneously manage the physical manifestations resulting from grief. It is not surprising, then, that grief may become unresolved. Several authors describe the signs of unresolved grief (Lazare, 1979; Lindemann, 1944; Worden, 1982). Manifestations include hostility, agitated depression, self-accusation, guilt, random behavior, feeling that death occurred just yesterday regardless of the date, grief being triggered by minor events, radical changes in life style, and phobias about death. Rando

(1984) cautions that these symptoms may easily be present during acute grief. However, should they persist over time, the possibility of unresolved grief exists.

The purpose of intervention during grief after death is to facilitate the expression of emotions while helping the mourner through the phases of grief. Strategies suggested by Rando (1984) include the following:

1. Make contact with the bereaved. Although it may seem more natural to leave the mourner alone, it is crucial to make contact. This process will include reaching out in an active manner, such as telephoning, offering assistance, and being present emotionally.
2. Demonstrate verbally and nonverbally that it is acceptable to grieve.
3. Assess the mourner's response to grief. Useful questions include, "Can you tell me about the death? Tell me about your relationship, have you been through other bad times?
4. Treat the physical symptoms of grief.
5. Allow the bereaved to cry, talk, and review.
6. Help the mourner identify secondary losses and complete unfinished business.
7. Assist in the reinvestment in life.

As Mr. M. went home to die, gradually he became more and more lethargic. Through nursing manage-

---

Box 45–2. HOME NURSING INTERVENTIONS FOR DYING PATIENTS AND THEIR SPOUSES: HEALTH TRANSITIONS FOR THOSE LEFT BEHIND

The overall purpose of this controlled randomized clinical trial was to determine whether there were differences in the effect of home nursing care by specialized clinical nurse specialists (OHC), home care by standard home health nurses (SHC), and office care without home nursing care (OC) on the psychological symptoms, health perceptions, and grief responses of the spouses of patients with lung cancer over time. The trajectory of the patient's illness was a steady downhill course. Although 100 spouses were entered into the study, analysis was restricted to 47 spouses who completed one interview before the patient's death and at least one interview afterward. Our findings indicated that spouses experienced similar patterns of symptoms and decreased health perceptions prior to the death and after, regardless of the care received. The major difference in the patterns among the groups was the quickened recovery of the OHC group. We attributed this improved pattern to the nursing intervention of home care provided by specialized oncology nurses.

(Donaldson, G., McCorkle, R., Benoliel, J., Georgiadou, F., & Moinpour, C. [1990]. Home nursing interventions for dying patients and their spouses: Health transitions for those left behind. Manuscript submitted for publication.)

ment of his symptoms, he was able to obtain adequate pain relief, which helped reduce his fear of being dyspneic. Although acknowledging that caring for Mr. M. was difficult, Mrs. M. felt that it also helped her in the grieving process. Research has demonstrated that home nursing care provided to patients during their terminal illness benefits the family members after the death (Box 45–2).

SUMMARY

The downward trajectory of the person experiencing lung cancer has been presented through a case study approach framed within the context of the living-dying interval delineated by Pattison (1977). The psychosocial responses of guilt, anger, fear, and desperation have been highlighted as these are most acute in those who must confront the realization that their behavior may have been responsible for the occurrence of their disease. Symptom control related to the respiratory system is essential to increase the person's quality of life because dyspnea is prevalent in lung cancer. Finally, aspects of anticipatory grief and grief for the patient and family must be assessed.

References

American Cancer Society. (1980). Guidelines for the cancer-related checkup: Recommendations and rationale. *CA: A Cancer Journal for Clinicians, 30,* 191–240.

American Cancer Society. (1990). *Cancer facts and figures, 1990* (p. 9). New York.

American Thoracic Society. (1978). Recommended respiratory disease questionnaire for use with adults and children in epidemiological research. *Respiratory Disease, 118,* 7–53.

Appenheimer, A. (1987). Screening and diagnosis of cancer in office practice. *Primary Care, 14,* 255–269.

Benedict, S. (1989). The suffering associated with lung cancer. *Cancer Nursing, 12,* 34–40.

Bowlby, J. (1980). *Attachment and loss: Loss, sadness and depressions* (Vol. III). New York: Basic Books.

Brown, M., Carrieri, V., Janson-Bjerklie, S., & Dodd, M. (1986). Lung cancer and dyspnea: The patient's perception. *Oncology Nursing Forum, 13*(5), 19–24.

Buzby, G., & Steinberg, S. (1981). Nutrition in cancer patients. *Surgical Clinics of North America, 61,* 691–700.

Correa, P., Pickle, L., Fontham, E., Lin, Y.E., & Haenszel, W. (1983). Passive smoking and lung cancer. *Lancet, 2,* 595–597.

Coy, R., & Kennelly, G. (1980). The role of curative radiotherapy in the treatment of lung cancer. *Cancer, 45,* 678–702.

DeWys, W. (1977). Anorexia in cancer patients. *Cancer Research, 37,* 2354–2358.

DeWys, W., & Walters, K. (1975). Abnormalities of taste sensation in cancer patients. *Cancer, 36,* 1888–1896.

Engel, G. (1964). Grief and mourning. *American Journal of Nursing, 64,* 93–98.

Fry, S.T. (1986). Ethical aspects of decision making in the feeding of cancer patients. *Seminars in Oncology Nursing, 2,* 59–62.

Futterman, E., Hoffman, I., & Sabshin, M. (1972). Parental anticipatory mourning. In B. Schoenberg, A. Carr, D. Peretz, & A. Kutscher (Eds.), *Psychosocial aspects of terminal care* (pp. 243–272). New York: Columbia University Press.

Garfinkle, L., & Stillman, S. (1986). Cigarette smoking among physicians, dentists and nurses. *CA: A Cancer Journal for Clinicians, 36,* 3.

Grant, M. (1986). Nutritional intervention: Increasing oral intake. *Seminars in Oncology Nursing, 2,* 36–43.

Harwood, K. (1987). Non–small cell lung cancer: Issues in diagnosis, staging and treatment. *Seminars in Oncology Nursing, 3,* 183–193.

Higgins, I., Maltan, C., & Wynder, E. (1988). Lung cancer among cigar & pipe smokers. *Preventive Medicine, 17,* 116–129.

Janson-Bjerklie, S., Carrieri, V., & Hudes, M. (1986). The sensation of pulmonary dyspnea. *Nursing Research, 35,* 154–159.

Knopf, M., & Morra, M. (1983). Smokers, former smokers and nonsmokers: A correlation study of nurses in Connecticut. *Oncology Nursing Forum, 10,* 40–45.

Knox, L. (1983). Nutrition and cancer. *Nursing Clinics of North America, 18,* 97–109.

Kübler-Ross, E. (1969). *On death and dying.* New York: Macmillan.

Kukall, W., McCorkle, R., & Driever, M. (1986). Symptom distress, current concerns and mood disturbance after diagnosis of life-threatening illness. *Social Science and Medicine, 17,* 431–438.

Lazare, A., (1979). *Outpatient psychiatry: Diagnosis and treatment.* Baltimore: Williams & Wilkins.

Lindemann, E. (1944). Symptomatology and management of acute grief. *American Journal of Psychiatry, 101,* 141–148.

Lindsey, A. (1986). Cancer cachexia: Effects of the disease and its treatment. *Seminars in Oncology Nursing, 12,* 19–29.

Loeb, L., Ernster, V., Warner, K, Abbotts, J.E., & Laszio, J. (1984). Smoking and lung cancer: An overview. *Cancer Research, 44,* 5940–5958.

McCorkle, R. (1984). Home care for adults and children. In *Proceedings of the Fourth National Conference on Cancer Nursing, 1983* (pp. 28–35). New York: American Cancer Society.

McCorkle, R., & Benoliel, J. (1983). Symptom distress, current concerns and mood disturbance after diagnosis of life-threatening illness. *Social Science in Medicine, 17,* 431–438.

McCorkle, R., Benoliel, J., Donaldson, G., Georgiadou, F., Moinpour, C., & Goodell, B. (1989). A randomized trial of home nursing care for lung cancer patients. *Cancer, 64,* 1375–1382.

McCorkle, R., & Donaldson, G. (1986). Anticipatory grief in persons newly diagnosed with life-threatening disease. In McCorkle, R., Honladarom, G. (Eds.), *Issues and topics in Cancer Nursing* (pp. 207–225). Norwalk, CT: Appleton-Century-Crofts.

Mumma, C., & McCorkle, R. (1982–1983). Causal attribution and life-threatening disease. *International Journal of Psychiatry in Medicine, 12,* 311–319.

O'Rourke, M., & Crawford, J. (1987). Lung cancer in the elderly. *Clinics in Geriatric Medicine, 3,* 595–623.

Parad, H. (1965). *Crisis intervention: Selected readings.* New York: Family Services Association.

Parkes, C. (1970). Seeking and finding a lost object. *Social Science and Medicine, 4,* 187–201.

Parkes, C., & Weiss, R. (1983). *Recovery from bereavement.* New York: Basic Books.

Pattison, E. (1976). The dying experience: Retrospective analysis. In Schneidman, E. (Ed.), *Death: Current perspectives* (pp. 303–315). Palo Alto, CA: Mayfield.

Pattison, E. (1977). *The experience of dying.* Englewood Cliffs, NJ: Prentice-Hall, Inc.

Quinn, M., Fontana, A., & Reznikoff, M. (1986). Psychological distress in reaction to lung cancer as a function of spousal support and coping strategy. *Journal of Psychosocial Oncology, 4,* 79–86.

Rando, T. (1984). *Grief, dying and death: Clinical interventions for caregivers.* Champaign, IL: Research Press.

Sandler, D., Everson, R., Wilcox, A.E., & Browder, J. (1985). Cancer risk in adulthood from early life exposure to parents' smoking. *American Journal of Public Health, 75,* 487–492.

Theolodiges, A. (1979). Cancer cachexia. *Cancer, 43,* 2004–2012.

Vickers, Z., Nielson, S., & Theologides, A. (1981). Food preferences of patients with cancer. *Journal of the American Dietetic Association, 79,* 441–445.

Weisman, A. (1972). *On death and denying.* New York: Behavioral Publications.

Weisman, A., & Worden, J. (1976). The existential plight in cancer: Significance of the first 100 days. *International Journal of Psychiatry in Medicine, 7,* 1–15.

White, E. J. (1987). Home care of the patient with advanced lung cancer. *Seminars in Oncology Nursing, 3,* 216–221.

Wilcox, B., Wilcox, M., Schoenberg, J., Mason, T., Bill, J., & Sternhagen, A. (1988). Smoking and lung cancer. Risk as a function of cigarette tar content. *Preventive Medicine, 17,* 263–273.

Worden, J. (1982). *Grief counseling and grief therapy: A handbook for the mental health practitioner.* New York: Springer-Verlag.

CHAPTER 46

Nursing Management of Persons with Disease about Which Little Is Known: Prototype—AIDS

JUDITH M. SAUNDERS

A disease may occur infrequently but contain few mysteries to impede its diagnosis and treatment. In contrast, a disease such as AIDS may occur with such frequency that it is an epidemic yet continue to defy containment and prevention because critical disease features remain unknown. Poliomyelitis now occurs infrequently because the gradual accumulation of knowledge made possible its prevention. Poliomyelitis used to be dreaded as an illness that crippled adults and children, although tragedy was heightened because children most often were its victims. Once a disease is fully understood, clinicians and researchers have adequate information about risk factors, disease progression, etiology, effective treatment, and prevention (Box 46–1). For example, although Hansen's disease occurs infrequently in the United States, its risk factors, cause, treatment, and prevention are fairly well understood. Conversely, Alzheimer's disease occurs often among people older than 65 years, yet we are uncertain about risk factors and pathogenesis and cannot adequately treat or prevent this tragic illness.

AIDS is an excellent example of an illness about which little is known. The person with these types of illnesses, including AIDS, copes not only with the illness itself, but also with inconsistent and inadequate knowledge.

Since AIDS was first identified in 1981, major advances in knowledge have been achieved: the virus that causes the disease has been isolated; identified risk factors have been confirmed; the disease progression has been retarded; and methods of detecting infection with the virus have been refined (Cassileth & Berlyne, 1989). Yet critical features of this illness have

stayed elusive, and a diagnosis of AIDS has remained almost synonymous with a death sentence.

Using AIDS as a prototype of an illness about which little is known, this chapter explores the clinical impact of and the nursing care particular to those features of illnesses for which critical information components are missing or deficient (see Chapter 41 for a more complete discussion).

Box 46–1. COMPONENT OF DISEASE KNOWLEDGE

The following list contains the essential information we must have about a disease for adequate prevention, diagnosis, and treatment. The disease is well-known, scientifically and clinically, when all five factors are fully known. Most often, knowledge proceeds unevenly across the five factors. Sometimes diseases can be prevented before all mechanisms are fully known. Time and study are required to know about diseases, and if a disease is rare in occurrence, knowledge accumulation is hampered. Simply occurring in great numbers, such as epidemics, does not guarantee that barriers can be overcome in developing knowledge in all five components.

1. Know risk factors and those groups at risk for the disease
2. Know the usual progression of the disease
3. Identify the cause(s)
4. Develop treatments that either cure or minimize sequelae
5. Know how to prevent the illness and its spread, if contagious

CASE ILLUSTRATION

James, a 48-year-old federal employee, developed herpes zoster as the first in a series of illnesses that culminated after 3 months in a diagnosis of *Pneumocystis carinii* pneumonia. James and his lover, Mark, had been concerned about AIDS during this 3-month siege of illnesses, yet they were stunned at the actual diagnosis of AIDS. After James recovered from this initial, relatively mild episode of *P. carinii* pneumonia and returned to work, he found he did not have the energy to continue with his job. When James retired on medical disability, his brother and sister-in-law volunteered to supplement his monthly income. If they had not, James and Mark would have had money for only a marginal existence, because Mark's work as a medical records clerk was sporadic. James and Mark continued their lives with few outward changes after the diagnosis. Both preferred meeting friends in small groups for dinner or a movie rather than being involved with community activities. As James's energy diminished, they went out less often, and Mark assumed more of the routine chores around the house. James spent more time watching television and reading. It was 1985 and public awareness of AIDS was growing. James found that television and news articles portrayed AIDS through statistics rather than through its effect on people, which led to a public perception of AIDS as an impersonal and distant illness. James began writing letters to editors and attending meetings at which AIDS was discussed. He identified himself as a person with AIDS and spoke about how his own life was touched by AIDS. His goal was to give this illness a personal and immediate presence in his community. An unexpected benefit was that it provided him with a purpose in life.

A second major change for James was the way he and his gay family related to one another. James and Mark defined their gay family as each other, three other gay men who had been friends with James for more than 10 years, and two lesbians, also long-standing friends. This group was consistent with the way the gay family is defined by Keane and Rasi (1989). Soon after AIDS was diagnosed, James and his gay family were together for dinner. After dinner they began talking about what this family meant to them. They had always taken each other for granted and had never talked about the meaning these relationships held for them. As a result of this evening, James shifted his priorities to spend more time with people he loved.

James was relatively healthy during the next few months, although he continued to be troubled by severe fatigue, mild chronic diarrhea, oral candidiasis, and occasional vomiting. He adjusted his schedule to accommodate his low energy, while continuing to learn about AIDS and his treatment options and to write and speak about how AIDS had affected his life. After 8 months, he developed a second, more severe *P. carinii* pneumonia that was resistant to treatment, and he developed other complications: he was delirious for several days, and he began having severe headaches,

along with severe bouts of vomiting. Eventually he recovered from this episode of *P. carinii* pneumonia and the delirium. Although medications relieved the continuing headaches, the vomiting continued to be severe at times and unpredictable in onset and duration. Although she arranged consultations and ran many tests, his physician could not confirm the cause of either the headaches or the vomiting.

It was a year after he was diagnosed as having AIDS that James noticed the purple discoloration on his abdomen that he had feared might develop. Hoping it was a blood blister, James hesitantly showed the discolored area to his physician, who immediately biopsied the lesion. Pathology reports confirmed her fears—it was Kaposi's sarcoma. James's fatigue level mounted, but he continued to be able to do a few household chores and he accepted a few public speaking engagements. His symptoms gave evidence of steady disease progression. His vomiting increased in frequency; whatever he ate seemed to stimulate vomiting. Diarrhea, which used to be mild, was now often severe. The headaches intensified and interfered with his ability to concentrate and write, even when he had the energy. James was rehospitalized for nearly 2 months, yet the physician still could not confirm the cause of the vomiting. His nutritional status was stabilized when he was placed on total parenteral nutrition (TPN), and he remained on TPN the rest of his life. Mark would "hook James up to his gourmet dreams" each night so that his days were not encumbered with this procedure. James learned to live without tasting food. Still, he gradually became weaker. James died about 1.5 years after he had been diagnosed as having AIDS.

TRAJECTORY OF AIDS AS AN ILLNESS ABOUT WHICH LITTLE IS KNOWN

The function of a trajectory, or designated course of the illness, is to provide patients and staff with an explanation that can be used to develop plans for their current actions. Health care professionals must continually redefine the illness trajectory to modify and update plans. Formulating a trajectory is a process that staff members use even when it involves an illness with major limitations of knowledge about its course (Glaser & Strauss, 1965). Although its etiologic agent is known, AIDS differs from many traditional diseases because it represents a late manifestation of the human immunodeficiency virus (HIV) infection that will make the person susceptible to multiple opportunistic infections and diseases (Lovejoy, 1988; Redfield & Burke, 1988). The course of the disease is partially dependent on the particular constellation of diseases and opportunistic infections the person with AIDS develops.

Although the usual pattern of disease progression is considered in formulating a trajectory, other issues are also influential, such as life style (Mays & Cochran, 1987), treatment access and effectiveness (Gee, Wong, & Moran, 1989), co-factors (White, 1989), the patient's personal and social resources, and less tangible factors, such as age or general hardiness (Kobasa, 1985).

In Melville's short novel *Billy Budd, Foretopman,* Billy Budd is a conscripted sailor who symbolizes a "captive explorer," helpless to protest being taken away from his comfortable seaman's berth onto a navy warship (Melville, 1986). Thus began a journey that eventually eroded innocence and resulted in death and grief. People who have illnesses about which we know little and in which the stakes are high (such as a life-threatening illness) resemble "captive explorers." These people are pioneers not by choice for an illness that yields great discomfort during the progression toward death and grief or for testing treatment methods that promise little hope of cure. Most people with AIDS would choose to remain ordinary and obscure, not to be forced into the role of a captive explorer.

Plotting the trajectory of a captive explorer with a little-known illness involves making decisions from information that is incomplete, and often contradictory, at the same time as the patient is receiving treatments that are experimental. With AIDS, the captive explorer may hope to sight land before time runs out but can only see water in every direction. People with AIDS hope for vaccines, more effective and accessible treatments, and methods to strengthen immunity.

The specific features of the trajectory of an illness about which little is known that is explored in this chapter include the person's (1) anticipating and being confirmed in a diagnosis, (2) altered awareness, (3) knowledge imbalance, (4) seeking relief from symptom distress, (5) inadequate resources, (6) indecision about treatment, (7) responding to ethical problems, and (8) facing death prematurely.

Anticipating and Being Confirmed in a Diagnosis

AIDS is a disease that is transmitted by sexual contact or by exposure to body fluids in such a way that the AIDS virus is able to enter the blood stream. Many of those at greatest risk for AIDS—gay men and intravenous drug users—know of their vulnerability and have begun to confirm this susceptibility by being tested for infection with HIV. Persons who know they are HIV positive wonder *when* more often than *if* they will develop AIDS, the severe form of HIV infection (Moss et al., 1988). The lengthy incubation period after infection provides a long time for people to worry about developing AIDS, to monitor their T-cell counts, to examine their bodies for signs of illness, to experiment with ways to prevent or retard the course of the infection, and to hope for new discoveries (Mahar, 1989).

Other susceptible persons may not know that they are infected with HIV until AIDS has been diagnosed. When the source of their infection was a sexual partner whose high-risk activities were not known to them, the newly diagnosed person may feel betrayed by the partner and angry, as well as frightened and stunned by the diagnosis. More women are being diagnosed as having AIDS with the most rapidly growing source of infection for them being sexual contact, not IVDU (Coates et al., 1988; Shaw, 1988).

James knew he was at risk for AIDS because he had had casual sex with many partners before he met his life partner Mark. In 1985, when he developed AIDS, there was little benefit from being tested for HIV infection: drugs such as zidovudine and aerosol pentamidine were not yet used to retard the disease course or to prevent *P. carinii* pneumonia (Coates et al., 1988). He and Mark each decided not to be tested, but they watched themselves closely and tried to stay healthy. They regarded every sniffle or bout of influenza suspiciously and anxiously.

James learned that he had AIDS after 3 months of continuous illnesses. His initial response to the diagnosis of AIDS, relief at finally having his fear become real and valid, was similar to Palermino's description (1988) of his initial reaction to diagnosis. The waiting had ended, and James immediately started making changes in his life, saying, "I don't have time to waste now. Every minute has to count." He asked Mark to find them a new apartment, with lots of sun and flowers. James seemed to gain energy, although a more typical reaction to this diagnosis is temporary immobilization, anxiety, and depression. Pattison (1977) has described being diagnosed with a life-threatening condition as a crisis period that ushers in the living-dying interval, and the first phase of this interval is this initial awareness of the seriousness of the illness and its possible outcome. AIDS has been well publicized and is recognized by many people, but patients who are diagnosed as having other illnesses that we know little about, such as amyotrophic lateral sclerosis, might react by asking, "What is it?"

Distressing symptoms and altered immune status (determined by monitoring T-cell counts, for example) may alert the person to an impending AIDS diagnosis, but the actual diagnosis evokes many responses after the initial shock and numbness begin to recede. A common struggle is the fear of losing control. People commonly ask, "How can I retain my values and life style while this disease erodes my body and steals my strength?" Fear of losing control motivates some persons to consider plans for suicide (Palermino, 1988; Saunders & Buckingham, 1988). If assessment shows that suicide risk is low, the patient may benefit from discussion and exploration of alternative ways to maintain control besides suicide (Hall, Koehler, & Lewis, 1989; Saunders & Buckingham, 1988).

After the response of shock, numbness, and disbelief that characterizes immediate reactions, the person diagnosed as having AIDS must share the bad news with others. Mobilizing support is especially important when so much about the disease remains unknown except that death will result unless major breakthroughs occur quickly (Palermino, 1988).

Altered Awareness

Receiving a diagnosis of a life-threatening illness causes many persons to change their perspective on life and its daily demands (Palermino, 1988; Saunders, 1989). AIDS or its treatment may also cause changes in perception and meaning. Although people with life-threatening illnesses tend to notice changes in their bodies more than when they were well, this awareness is intensified when the particular illness is one about which so much is still unknown. Heightened awareness and increased scrutiny of body changes are more common in people with AIDS than is denial of new symptoms. Some people with AIDS also report existential changes that are recognized by an altered awareness of important relationships in their lives and a heightened sense how little time is left. A shift in priorities often occurs, resulting from the increased awareness of what provides pleasure (nature, people, music) and an impatience with pettiness and conflict. Not being able to control the length of time they live makes it more important to increase awareness of those things that add to the quality of their lives. James initiated changes in his life style that reflected this shift in priorities while he was still hospitalized after receiving a diagnosis of AIDS.

Two other common sources of altered awareness may occur in AIDS: AIDS dementia complex (ADC) and cytomegalovirus (CMV) retinochoroiditis. The onset of ADC often is insidious and the patient may not notice the initial symptoms. Early symptoms that reflect an altered awareness include forgetfulness, decreased attention span, confusion, and an unsteady gait and lack of coordination (Hall et al., 1989). In contrast, the onset of CMV retinitis may be rapid, and without treatment, blindness will ensue (McMahon & Coyne, 1989). Treatment, usually with gancyclovir, must be lifelong, or relapse will occur (McMahon and Coyne, 1989).

James developed some forgetfulness and decreased attention span, but his symptoms remained mild until he died, so he remained actively involved in decisions and self-care. He was more amused than embarrassed the time he went out with unmatched socks. He kept a notepad beside the telephone to record pertinent information from each phone call; this worked so well as a memory aid that he also carried a small notebook with him.

Altered awareness may result from physiologic changes that accompany the illness or its treatment or from a changed outlook on life that stems from having an illness about which little is known—especially if the illness is life-threatening.

Knowledge Imbalance

People with little-understood illnesses and their supportive others soon acquire a considerable knowledge of what is known about the illness and its treatment options. Not infrequently, they encounter health care workers who know less about the illness than they do. This quest for knowledge is one way that people with AIDS can reduce their uncertainty and strive for maintaining control. The patient's knowing more than

the health care professional can be awkward if the nurse or physician is not comfortable having the patient as teacher.

Information needs for a patient with HIV infection are extensive: chances of developing AIDS, co-factors associated with rapid progression, prevention of contagion to others, life-style changes that enhance immunity, and others (Moran, Lovejoy, Viele, Dodd, & Abrams, 1988; Vlahov, 1989) (Box 46–2). Although patients will ask health professionals for information, they will also seek information from alternative resources in their quest for strategies to maintain existing health, retard disease progression, treat illnesses, and manage symptoms (Cassileth & Berlyne, 1989).

James monitored his T-cell count closely and quickly sought out new information about drugs reputed to have some success in treating illnesses associated with AIDS. He stopped using alcohol and marijuana because he feared these would further depress his already compromised immune system. He attended a workshop conducted by Elisabeth Kübler-Ross and returned enthusiastic and determined to live each day to the fullest.

This search for knowledge about AIDS and its treatment has led people beyond the boundaries of traditional health care to alternate health care systems, as was also true for people with cancer (Cassileth & Berlyne, 1989; Irish, 1989). Alternative health measures explored by HIV-infected people vary in style, safety, and effectiveness; they include meditation, megavitamins, dietary supplements, major dietary shifts, acupuncture, bodily cleansing rituals such as colonic treatments, exercise programs, self-help support groups, and others (Cassileth & Berlyne, 1989; Irish, 1989; Moffat, Spiegel, Parrish, & Helquist, 1987; Van Ness, 1985). Patients with illnesses in which many features are unknown, who perceive traditional health care resources as incomplete or inadequate, will be more likely to turn to alternative resources.

Patients have learned of medicines used to treat AIDS in other countries that are not approved for use in the United States, and many have found access to these drugs via various routes (Shilts, 1987). This search for knowledge has led people with HIV disease to misinformation, as they search out the "latest word" from each other and from obscure sources (Bennett, 1988). When incorrect information is acted on without checking its accuracy, problems can occur.

Many measures promising to strengthen natural immunity and resistance may promote health by advocating proper diet, balancing exercise and rest, reducing stress, and promoting a positive self-image (Pender, 1987). Yet other promised cures may actually be harmful. Guidelines are sparse to help vulnerable patients detect those alternative health measures that may be dangerous, either inherently or potentially because they lure the patient away from effective treatment (Irish, 1989). Many resources exist to help people make positive life-style changes. One comprehensive resource designed to assist people who are concerned about AIDS to care for themselves is the book by Moffatt and co-workers (1987).

Box 46–2. INFORMATIONAL NEEDS OF HOMOSEXUAL MEN DIAGNOSED AS HAVING AIDS OR
AIDS-RELATED COMPLEX

This study elicited responses to six open-ended questions from 76 homosexual or bisexual men diagnosed as having AIDS or AIDS-related complex (ARC). The purpose of the study was to describe how well the medical community dealt with the patient's questions and sexuality. Patients also were asked how their health care providers could have been more helpful; what educational material regarding safe sex was most helpful; who gave them the materials; and finally, if they had changed their sexual behavior, who or what was responsible for the change. Their responses were coded by three masters' or doctorally prepared oncology nurses. Overall, the participants found the medical community did not help with their sexual needs; materials instead were obtained in the community or through gay organizations. In addition, participants felt they themselves were responsible for the changes in their behavior.

(From Moran, T. A., Lovejoy, N., Viele, C. S., Dodd, M. J., & Abrams, D. I. [1988]. Informational needs of homosexual men diagnosed with AIDS or AIDS-related complex. *Oncology Nursing Forum, 15*(3), 311–314.)

Seeking Relief from Symptom Distress

Techniques that measure symptom distress and that provide relief have increased in complexity and effectiveness in recent years. In illnesses for which so much is unknown, such as AIDS, the techniques that have been successful in providing relief for certain symptoms in other diseases or conditions may be less effective when used for the symptom distress of AIDS. Inability to relieve suffering may also cause nurses to feel their nursing care is ineffective. Rhodes and Watson (1987) assert that inadequate relief from symptom distress may result in the patient's withdrawal from potentially curative treatment and may impede self-care and independence.

Because AIDS may encompass many illnesses and opportunistic infections, individual patients may experience many diverse symptoms (McMahon & Coyne, 1989). Early symptoms of HIV infection include fatigue, night sweats, and swollen and painful lymph glands. As the infection progresses, nursing care will focus on specific illnesses and opportunistic infections.

Because patients are hospitalized briefly for the most acute conditions, most of the patients' care requirements will be met by the patient and the patient's personal support network in the home setting. Not only does the nurse need to develop skill in monitoring the patient for emerging problems, but also the patient and supportive others need to be taught self-monitoring, basics of health maintenance, procedures for symptom management, reportable signs and symptoms, effect and interactions of medications, and infection control measures (Muller, 1989).

Specific conditions, such as Kaposi's sarcoma, may present particular challenges to the nurse (Jacob, 1989). Most physical care requirements of patients with AIDS will draw knowledge and skills already highly developed among oncology nurses, such as symptom management and care of the immunocompromised client (Halloran, Hughes, & Mayer, 1988: McMahon & Coyne, 1989). Problems especially pronounced in people with AIDS include a lifelong schedule of medication, adverse neutropenic drug reactions, illegal drug use, and estrangement from family of origin (McMahon & Coyne, 1989). Nurses usually can apply knowledge and skills from clinical practice to problems associated with diseases about which little is known. Nurses should proceed cautiously and evaluate the results of their interventions carefully.

Inadequate Resources

AIDS has displaced cancer as the illness associated with social stigma. Whereas social support has the potential to buffer the ill effects of cancer, the stigma associated with cancer may stimulate others to avoid the patient, close off communication on important topics, and show other evidence of rejection (Dunkel-Schetter, 1984; Dunkel-Schetter & Wortman, 1982; Wortman, 1984).

An AIDS-related stigma (Herek & Glunt, 1988) has evolved because AIDS is a life-threatening, contagious illness and also because it is associated with gay men, intravenous drug users, minorities, prostitutes, and other "outsiders" (Saunders, 1989). Stigma is the driving force behind discrimination, resulting in social consequences that people with HIV disease experience: family estrangement, job loss, eviction, refusal of services, and denial of insurance (Saunders, 1989). Learning about the life styles of their patients can help nurses identify their own attitudes and can result in more personal and effective care (Saunders, 1988).

Many gay men have developed alternative families from among their friends and mates (Keane & Rasi, 1989), as was true for James and Mark. These gay families provide many functions usually filled by traditional families. When relationships with traditional families are intact, the gay and traditional families supplement each other as resources for the patient. Too often, however, strained relationships exist between intravenous drug users or gay men and their families. Intravenous drug users have not formed community resources and support networks among themselves that are characteristic of gay men and the gay community (Williams, 1988).

Fear of contagion is a component of AIDS-related stigma and a prominent reason why people avoid contact with a person who has AIDS. This fear was especially potent before educational campaigns weakened or dispelled myths. Early in this epidemic, many health care workers and the general public refused contact with people who were diagnosed as having AIDS: morgue staffs refused bodies; pathologists refused to perform autopsies; hospitals denied admission to patients with AIDS. Community resources cannot be developed adequately in an atmosphere of misinformation, stigma, and discrimination. Illnesses with many unknown elements may be particularly vulnerable to fear and misinformation that impede development of community resources. Shilts (1987) offered evidence that politics guided public health decisions and funding decisions nationally as well as in specific urban settings. He argued that delays by federal and public health officials in establishing resources to contain and treat this illness were directly linked to AIDS-related stigma.

The gay and lesbian community mobilized its resources for education and treatment and lobbied for adequate funding (Saunders, 1989). James traveled to Washington, DC, to appeal to congressional leaders for funding for research and treatment. Other patients with illnesses that we know little about also may become motivated to encourage development of funding to combat the illness as they simultaneously search for sufficient resources for their own survival.

Many community resources assist people with AIDS and their supportive others. Shanti is one example of a volunteer organization found in many cities in the United States that offers individual and group support. The National AIDS Hotline (1-800-342-AIDS), which operates 24 hr per day, can help identify local resources or answer specific questions about HIV infection. Many states also have AIDS hotlines, and local public health departments and gay and lesbian service centers also provide excellent information. Because most diseases that we know little about do not reach epidemic proportions, nurses and patients may have difficulty locating resources. Resources may be sparse because funding for developing and advertising resources is limited.

Indecision about Treatment

When treatments offer scant hope for cure and are known to entail painful or dangerous side effects, patients may have trouble deciding whether to accept the treatment offered. One person will decide to try all "reasonable offers" in the hope that something will work, whereas another person may decide that using such experimental treatment not only is dehumanizing but also offers little hope of benefit. Often the choice is not about accepting treatment generally, but rather about which combination of drugs can be used to advantage. Participating in treatment becomes the focus of long discussions between patients and supportive others. Even when the benefits seem to warrant the inherent risks, patients may hesitate to try a particular treatment because of its expense. Gee and colleagues (1989) present an excellent overview of medical treatments available and the nursing implications of these

treatments. As with AIDS, illnesses that we know little about often have experimental treatments for which the outcomes have not been fully determined.

Responding to Ethical Problems

Seropositivity not only is an indication that a person has been infected with HIV; it also is a pronouncement that the person has the capacity to infect others. The first problem the person confronts is whether to tell others. When contact with others is casual, the decision becomes a simple personal choice. If contact with others involved interactions that may have infected them, personal choice competes with a sense of responsibility to others. Disclosure of infection brings other questions, because AIDS is closely identified with a gay life style or intravenous drug use.

Persons who knew they were at risk for infection with HIV faced a similar ethical problem if they were involved in an active sexual relationship. Protecting one's privacy only becomes a problem when that privacy poses risks to others. Those at risk for AIDS need to consider carefully how they can engage in intimate relationships safely for themselves and for others.

People with AIDS have the right to refuse treatment that is life-sustaining or life-saving, as do patients with cancer or other diagnoses. They also have the right of access to treatment that is normally afforded others in similar circumstances. Ethical problems that influence the trajectory of people with AIDS involve actions of others, such as when health care providers refuse to provide care because the patient has AIDS. As health care professionals have learned more about AIDS and how to protect themselves, refusal to provide care has become rare (Jackson & Lynch, 1989; Koenig, 1988).

Already facing death from AIDS, some people consider suicide so that they can have control over a deteriorating quality of life. Some patients may simply want to explore suicide as an option with health care staff through discussions, whereas others may ask for help in carrying out their plans (Saunders & Buckingham, 1988). Attitudes about suicide in our society have become more tolerant in recent years, but moral and legal questions complicate any consideration of suicide (Saunders & Valente, 1988; Valente & Saunders, 1989).

Facing Death Prematurely

When grieving parents who attended a meeting of Compassionate Friends (a self-help group for bereaved parents) were asked what was the most difficult age for a child to die, their answers ranged from infancy to middle age. As the parents cited reasons to support their answers, it became clear that the worst age for a child to die was the age of the grieving parent's child at death. Perhaps there is no "correct age" to face death. Perhaps death always seems premature for the patient or family.

AIDS is a disease of young adults. Most people with AIDS in the United States are between the ages of 25 and 45 years (Howard & Curran, 1988). Young adults are busy planning and building for the future, so being diagnosed as having an illness that is a virtual death sentence is a contradiction to everything the young adult is poised to do. The young adult may bring the same intensity of search for meaning to dying that formerly characterized building for the future.

As people approach middle age, many have mellowed in their expectations and have begun to fine-tune a sense of obligation and responsibility. For the middle-aged person, death forces a reordering of obligations along with a commitment to fulfill responsibilities. James redirected his sense of responsibility and found meaning in making AIDS a human disease, not a series of statistics and sensational reports. His strong sense of obligation and responsibility was characteristic of his developmental age.

AIDS is a chronic disease that typically progresses slowly and steadily from exposure to death, perhaps over a 10-year period (Redfield & Burke, 1988). When the disease course follows a more acute trajectory, the patient may face death before developing a personal readiness.

Not all illnesses that we know little about have the same high fatality record as does AIDS. When the illness forces a "premature confrontation with death," the developmental age of the patient will influence the coping measures used.

DESCRIPTION OF NURSING PROBLEMS

AIDS is a chronic illness with the potential to affect every bodily system and to create psychosocial problems as well. The "captive explorer" who is diagnosed as having an illness with critical information elements that are unknown, or incompletely known, faces an almost overwhelming task in coping with the effects of the illness and in finding accurate sources of information. Conscientious health care professionals also may have difficulty locating credible and useful information about little-understood illnesses. A survey of 266 issues of five nursing journals (three general nursing journals and two cancer nursing journals) revealed that only eight articles were published about AIDS from 1982 to 1985: 20 additional articles were published between 1986 and September of 1987 (Saunders, 1987). Cancer nurses who turned to nursing literature had few references to help guide nursing care of their patients with AIDS before 1986. Fortunately, the situation has changed, and many excellent references have been developed.

Related Nursing Issues

Nursing care of patients who have an illness about which little is known will depend, in part, on the major features of that illness and its trajectory. In helping patients assimilate a diagnosis, the nurse will assess how well the patient copes with this stressful event and will be alert for any indication that the patient is overwhelmed and is in crisis. Crisis intervention techniques (e.g., involving significant others and increasing resources) can effectively reduce the feeling of being overwhelmed and can support caring. Because high anxiety interferes with the patient's ability to absorb information, the nurse should be supportive and accessible. By arranging frequent contacts with the patient during the early period after diagnosis, the nurse can provide continued opportunity for assessment while allowing the patient to voice concerns and questions as they arise.

With AIDS, patients may alter their perspective on life because they have an illness with no known cure. Nurses can encourage patients to explore their feelings and set new life goals and priorities. Some patients will benefit from referrals to supportive groups in which others are grappling with similar issues. Early detection of symptoms of ADC or CMV retinitis will facilitate effective treatment and initiation of nursing care measures to promote self-care (Hall et al., 1989, McMahon & Coyne, 1989).

One method that patients use to reduce the uncertainty of having an illness for which no treatment is optimal is to seek knowledge from a wide variety of resources. Patients may supplement traditional medical treatments with nontraditional therapies that are not familiar to many nurses. Nurses who keep communication open with their patients about these nontraditional therapies will be in a better position to evaluate the therapy effects. Irish (1989) discusses strategies to keep communication open and ways to evaluate potential harm of these unconventional therapies, and he describes some unconventional treatments.

Symptoms associated with illnesses that we know little about may respond to nursing interventions that have been effective with cancer patients, but they also may require modification or new approaches. Oncology nurses are very familiar with fatigue, and patients with AIDS respond well when cancer nurses apply proven methods, such as those described by McCorkle (1984). AIDS is an example of an illness for which nursing strategies used with cancer patients are effective sometimes, but not always. McMahon and Coyne (1989) provide an excellent discussion of symptom management strategies for people with AIDS, and they also highlight ways to modify these strategies if necessary.

Adequate matching of patients with resources depends on a careful assessment of the patient's needs and on the nurse's awareness of existing resources. Social service staff and clinical specialists in psychosocial oncology may be helpful in identifying existing support services. Some resources offer a service the patient needs, but the patient may be uncomfortable in that setting. For example, settings that are used primarily by gay men may not be acceptable to men or women who are not gay. Nurses can guide patients in developing self-care support groups to meet their own needs in areas without existing resources. Nurses also may direct efforts toward educating other professional colleagues and the public about resources that are needed by patients with illnesses that are not fully understood.

The ethical issues surrounding AIDS are complex for nurses and their patients (Koenig, 1988). After helping the patient think through health care values, choices, and potential risks, the nurse may need to consult an ethicist or other health care staff member if the patient continues in high-risk behaviors for self and others. Patients who discuss suicide require careful assessment to determine whether they need treatment for depression or assistance in exploring options to maintain control in a threatening situation. Nurses cannot legally or ethically help patients with suicide (Valente & Saunders, 1989). Another ethical issue is that about which so little is known may stimulate fear about safety precautions and how nurses can care for patients without undue personal risk. Under most circumstances, nurses have an ethical obligation to care for HIV infected patients (Halloran, Hughes, & Mayer, 1988; Koenig, 1988).

The nurse creates a safe interpersonal environment that allows patients to explore feelings and concerns related to their illness. It is important for the nurse to create opportunities for patients to discuss their feelings about death, yet it is equally important to allow patients to choose *not* to discuss their feelings or thoughts (Palermino, 1988). Patients have diverse affairs to organize, and their goals will vary. Listening and acknowledging the importance of patients' concerns will encourage them in their problem-solving efforts. Nurses who have reflected on their own concerns about death will be in a stronger position to help patients.

The Nurse's Role in Maintaining Hope

Patients can become discouraged when their questions repeatedly are answered with "I don't know." Nurses are challenged to help patients maintain hope despite knowledge gaps, symptoms that resist interventions, and living with an illness that has a high fatality rate. Studies have advanced our understanding of hope and provided us with tools to measure its presence (DuFault & Martocchio, 1985; Nowotny, 1989).

Hope is a multidimensional concept that brings together much more than a positive outlook on life (DuFault & Martocchio, 1985). Hope can be a general, positive outlook on life (general hope) or have a particular focus on specific objects, such as hope for pain relief or for a good night's sleep. DuFault & Martocchio (1985) identified five expectations that are associated with the hope object: (1) it may be improved, (2) what is lacking may be attained or received, (3) desired circumstances will occur, (4) currently valued objects may continue to be present in the future, and (5) unfavorable possibilities will not occur. Assessing these expectations may help the nurse identify statements by patients that are relevant to maintaining hope. For example, James reported that vomiting was distressing, and he hoped to reduce vomiting so that he could eat without precipitating these unpleasant episodes. Gradually this hope shifted to stopping the vomiting by not eating but maintaining good nutritional status with TPN.

Phillips (1989) asserts that caregivers as well as patients must maintain hope; sustaining hope is actually the basis of self-care. Having negative thoughts about their illness prompted adolescents with cancer to move toward hopefulness, whereas hopefulness was pivotal to being able to cope successfully with the problems of cancer and its treatment (Hinds & Martin, 1988). Although maintaining hope is usually thought of as important to a person's quality of life, it also may be important in keeping patients involved in activities that promote health and treat their illness.

Some patients will be able to maintain hope with little outside assistance, but many patients will benefit from carefully planned nursing interventions. Simply encouraging a patient to "stay in there and keep trying" is not effective when the patient's hope is weak. Having a framework of the multiple dimensions of hope will facilitate interventions that are matched to the specific needs of the patient (Saunders, 1989). Nowotny (1989) identified six dimensions of hope that closely parallel DuFault and Martocchio's (1985) dimensions of hope: confidence in the outcome; active involvement of the individual; perception of a potential future; spiritual beliefs; communication with others through thinking, feelings, or actions; and self-trust.

James had difficulty trusting himself, having confidence in the outcome, and perceiving the possibility of the future more than with other dimensions of hope. He wondered how he could make decisions that were best for him and for Mark. He eventually learned to shift his temporal orientation to shorter time frames and to link time with specific activities or goals.

When a person who customarily practices self-care withdraws and allows others to make decisions and apply procedures, the nurse will assess this behavioral change to determine if the patient is less hopeful. Behaviors from other dimensions of hopefulness will provide indicators of areas of intact hopefulness and areas in which assistance is needed. If both general and specific hope are impaired, the nurse will need to assess the patient for depression, because hopelessness is a symptom of depression (Saunders & Valente, 1988; Valente & Saunders, 1989).

References

Bennett, J. (1988). Helping people with AIDS live well at home. In C. Grady (Ed.), *AIDS Nursing Clinics of North America, 23,* 731–748.

Cassileth, B., & Berlyne, D. (1989). Counseling the patient who wants to try unorthodox therapies. *Oncology, 3,* 29–34.

Centers for Disease Control. (1989, April 14). Update: Acquired immunodeficiency syndrome—United States, 1981–1988. *Morbidity and Mortality Weekly Report, 38,* 229–236.

Coates, T. J., Stall, R. D., Kegeles, S. M., Lo, B., Morin, S. F., & McKusick, L. (1988). AIDS antibody testing. Will it stop the AIDS epidemic: Will it help people infected with HIV? *American Psychologist, 43,* 859–864.

Curran, J. W., Jaffe, H. W., Hardy, A. M., Morgan, W. M., Selik, R. M., & Dondero, T. J. (1988). Epidemiology of HIV infection and AIDS in the United States. *Science, 239,* 610–616.

DuFault, K., & Martocchio, B. (1985). Hope: Its spheres and dimensions. *Nursing Clinics of North America, 20,* 379–391.

Dunkel-Schetter, C. (1984). Social support and cancer: Findings based on patient interviews and their implications. *Journal of Social Issues, 40,* 77–95.

Dunkel-Schetter, C., & Wortman, C. B. (1982). The interpersonal dynamics of cancer. Problems in social relationships and their impact on the patient. In H. S. Friedman & M. R. DiMatteo (Eds.), *Interpersonal issues in health care* (pp. 69–100). New York: Academic Press.

Gallo, R. C., & Montagnier, L. (1988). AIDS in 1988. *Scientific American, 259,* 41–48.

Gee, G., Wong, R., & Moran, T. (1989). Current treatment strategies for HIV Infection. *Seminars in Oncology Nursing, 5,* 249–254.

Glaser, B. G. & Strauss, A. L. (1965). *Awareness of dying.* London: Weidenfeld & Nicolson.

Hall, J. M., Koehler, S. L., & Lewis, A. (1989). HIV-related mental health nursing issues. *Seminars in Oncology Nursing, 5,* 276–283.

Halloran, J., Hughes, A., & Mayer, D. K. (1988). Oncology Nursing Society position paper on HIV-related issues. *Seminars in Oncology Nursing, 15,* 206–217.

Herek, G. M., & Glunt, E. K. (1988). An epidemic of stigma. Public reactions to AIDS. *American Psychologist, 43,* 886–891.

Hinds, P. S., & Martin, J. (1988). Hopefulness and the self-sustaining process in adolescents with cancer. *Nursing Research, 37,* 336–340.

Howard, W. L., & Curran, J. W. (1988). The epidemiology of AIDS in the U.S. *Scientific American, 20,* 72–81.

Irish, A. (1989). Maintaining health in persons with HIV infection. *Seminars in Oncology Nursing, 5,* 302–307.

Jackson, M., & Lynch, P. (1989). Infection prevention and control in the era of the AIDS/HIV epidemic. *Seminars in Oncology Nursing, 5,* 236–243.

Jacob, J. L., Baird, B. F., Haller, S. & Ostchega, Y. (1989). AIDS-related Kaposi's sarcoma: Concepts of care. *Seminars in Oncology Nursing, 5,* 263–275.

Keane, M. W., & Rasi, R. A. (1989). Interacting with gay families. In J. B. Meisenhelder & C. L. LaCharite (Eds.), *Comfort in caring. Nursing the person with HIV infection* (pp. 43–52). Glenview, IL: Scott, Foresman & Co.

Kobasa, S. C. (1985). Stressful life events, personality, and health: An inquiry into hardiness. In A. Monat & R. S. Lazarus (Eds.), *Stress and coping: An anthology* (pp. 174–188). New York: Columbia University Press.

Koenig, B. A. (1988). Ethical and legal issues in the AIDS epidemic. In A. Lewis (Ed.), *Nursing care of the person with AIDS/ARC* (pp. 287–305). Rockville, MD: Aspen.

Lovejoy, N. C. (1988). The pathophysiology of AIDS. *Oncology Nursing Forum, 15,* 563–571.

Mahar, M. (1989, March 13). Pitiless scourge: Separating out the hype from hope on AIDS. *Barron's* (pp. 6–26).

Mays, V. M., & Cochran, S. D. (1987). Acquired immunodeficiency syndrome and black Americans: Special psychosocial issues. *Public Health Reports, 102,* 224–231.

McCorkle, R. (1984). Diagnostic reasoning in nursing care of advanced cancer patients in the home. In D. L. Carnevali, P. H. Mitchell, N. F. Woods, & C. A. Tanner (Eds.), *Diagnostic reasoning in nursing* (pp. 107–131). Philadelphia: J. B. Lippincott Co.

McMahon, K. M., & Coyne, N. (1989). Symptom management in patients with AIDS. *Seminars in Oncology Nursing, 5,* 289–301.

Melville, H. (1986). *Billy Budd and other stories.* New York: Penguin.

Moffatt, B., Spiegel, J., Parrish, S., & Helquist, M. (1987). *AIDS: A self-care manual.* (AIDS Project Los Angeles.) Santa Monica: IBS Press.

Moran, T. A., Lovejoy, N., Viele, C. S., Dodd, M. J., & Abrams, D. I. (1988). Informational needs of homosexual men diagnosed with AIDS or AIDS-related complex. *Oncology Nursing Forum, 15,* 311–314.

Moss, A. R., Bacchetti, P., Osmond, D., Krampf, W., Chaisson, R. G., Stites, D., Wilber, J., Allain, J., & Carlson, J. (1988). Seropositivity for HIV and the development of AIDS or AIDS related condition: Three year follow-up of the San Francisco General Hospital cohort. *British Medical Journal (Clinical Research), 296,* 745–750.

Muller, R. (1989). Patient teaching: Empowering for self-care. In J. B. Meisenhelder & C. L. LaCharite (Eds.), *Comfort in caring. Nursing the person with HIV infection* (pp. 225–254). Glenview, IL: Scott, Foresman & Co.

Nowotny, M. L. (1989). Assessment of hope in patients with cancer: Development of an instrument. *Nursing Research, 16,* 57–61.

Palermino, R. (1988). Psychosocial issues: One man's personal experience. In A. Lewis (Ed.), *Nursing care of the person with AIDS/ARC* (pp. 63–70). Rockville, MD: Aspen.

Pattison, E. M. (1977). *The experience of dying.* Englewood Cliffs, NJ: Prentice-Hall, Inc.

Pender, N. J. (1987). *Health promotion in nursing practice* (2nd ed.). Norwalk, CT: Appleton & Lange.

Phillips, J. (1989). Sustaining our hope. In J. B. Meisenhelder & C. L. LaCharite (Eds.), *Comfort in caring. Nursing the person with HIV infection* (pp. 31–40), Glenview, IL: Scott, Foresman & Co.

Redfield, R. R., & Burke, D. S. (1988). HIV infection: The clinical picture. *Scientific American, 259,* 90–98.

Rhodes, V. A., & Watson, P. M. (1987). Symptom distress—the concept: Past and present. *Seminars in Oncology Nursing, 3,* 242–247.

Saunders, J. M. (1987, September). Issues in treatment: Care of the person with AIDS. *Proceedings of the Fifth National Conference on Cancer Nursing.* New York: American Cancer Society.

Saunders, J. M. (1988). Intervening with gay and lesbian couples and cancer. In M. Leahey & L. M. Wright (Eds.), *Families and life-threatening illness* (pp. 326–345). Springhouse, PA: Springhouse Corporation.

Saunders, J. M. (1989). Psychosocial and cultural issues in HIV infection. *Seminars in Oncology Nursing, 5,* 284–288.

Saunders, J. M., & Buckingham, S. (1988) Suicidal AIDS patients. When the depression turns deadly. *Nursing, 18*(7), 59–64.

Saunders, J. M., & Valente, S. M. (1988). Cancer and suicide. *Oncology Nursing Forum, 15*(5), 575–581.

Shaw, N. (1988). Women. In A. Lewis (Ed.), *Nursing care of the person with AIDS/ARC* (pp. 39–42). Rockville, MD: Aspen.

Shilts, R. (1987). *And the band played on—politics, people and the AIDS epidemic.* New York: St. Martin's Press.

Valente, S. M., & Saunders, J. M. (1989). Dealing with serious depression in cancer patients. *Nursing, 19*(2), 44–47.

Van Ness, P. N. (1985). *Alternative and holistic health care for AIDS and its prevention: A sourcebook of descriptions, bibliography and practitioners in the Washington, DC–Baltimore, Maryland area.* Sponsored by the Whitman Walker Clinic.

Vlahov, D. (1989). AIDS: Overview, immunology, virology and informational needs. *Seminars in Oncology Nursing, 5,* 227–235.

White, K. (1989). Cofactors: Do they influence HIV infection and progression? *AIDS Patient Care, 3,*(3), 24–27.

Williams, A. (1988). Managing addictive behavior. In J. B. Meisenhelder & C. L. LaCharite (Eds.), *Comfort in caring. Nursing the person with HIV infection* (pp. 53–66). Glenview, IL: Scott Foresman & Co.

Wortman, C. B. (1984). Social support and the cancer patient: Conceptual and methodologic issues. *Cancer, 53*(Suppl. 10), 2339–2360.

MAJOR CLINICAL NURSING PROBLEMS

CHAPTER 47

Alterations in Nutrition

MARCIA GRANT
MARY E. ROPKA

Alterations in nutritional status associated with the cancerous disease itself as well as with the antitumor treatments are common in cancer patients. Although weight gain has been reported in a small select subpopulation of cancer patients, mainly breast cancer patients undergoing adjuvant therapy (Knobf, 1985), the majority of cancer patients with alterations in nutritional status experience anorexia, weight loss, cachexia, and malnutrition (Heber, 1989). Such nutritional alterations further compromise the patient's health when they cause disease and therapy complications or intolerances (Holroyde & Reichard, 1986). The potential life-threatening nature of this sequence of events is exemplified by serious secondary infections or an inability to complete essential cancer treatment. Approximately two thirds of those patients who die from cancer experience anorexia and weight loss before death (DeWys et al., 1980; Morrison, 1976).

SIGNIFICANCE OF NUTRITIONAL ALTERATIONS

Weight loss is an important clinical composite indicator of nutritional status: A loss of weight more than 5 per cent of total body weight in 4 weeks or more than 10 per cent in 6 months is considered severe (Blackburn & Harvey, 1980). Although such a significant weight loss may not in and of itself be dangerous, complications can occur when the weight loss is coupled with any other major stress, such as trauma, surgery, fever, or infection (Blackburn & Harvey, 1980).

Anorexia and cachexia can lead to compromised immune status as manifested by decreased macrophage mobilization, depressed lymphocyte function, and impaired phagocytosis (Shils, 1979). In such a compromised state, the patient is vulnerable to infections that may be life threatening. When the nutritional state is corrected, the immune state may also be reversed, improving the patient's response to disease and therapy (Kaminski, Nasr, Moss, Berger, & Sriran, 1982).

If anorexia and a subsequent malnutrition occur during cancer therapy, the effect may be disabling and may even interrupt the therapy (Costa & Donaldson, 1979). For example, radiation therapy for patients who lose significant amounts of weight may be discontinued before an adequate tumoricidal dose of radiation is administered (Copeland, Souchon, MacFadyen, Rapp, & Dudrick, 1977). Surgical patients with recent substantial weight loss may experience impaired wound healing (Ruberg, 1984). When the surgical procedure involves extensive resection of soft tissue, as with radical neck dissection, wound healing complications may occur (Copeland, et al., 1975). For patients receiving selected antitumor chemotherapy, nutritional compromise frequently occurs after other treatments associated with side effects such as nausea, vomiting, and mucosal ulcerations. In combination, these side effects can be dose limiting, thus decreasing the amount of chemotherapy that was administered to levels below therapeutic doses (Costa & Donaldson, 1979).

The most devastating nutritional consequence associated with cancer is cachexia, a profound systemic abnormality in host metabolism that is characterized by weakness, wasting, general depletion, redistribution of host components, hormonal aberrations, and progressive failure in vital function (Costa, 1977; Lindsey, Piper, & Stotts, 1982). Cachexia is a common occurrence in progressive malignancy and is seen in as many as two thirds of terminally ill cancer patients (Morrison, 1976). The prevalence of protein-calorie malnutrition in hospitalized cancer patients was examined by Nixon and colleagues (1980). In this cross-sectional study, a convenience sample of 54 consecutively admitted patients was examined. Patients with cancers from a variety of sites were included. Findings revealed a nearly universal occurrence of protein-calorie malnutrition, characterized by loss of adipose tissue, body mass, and skeletal muscle that varied unpredictably in extent among patients.

DeWys and co-workers (1980) described the nutritional problems in patients with cancer, focusing on both the frequency of weight loss in a variety of tumor types and the prognostic importance of weight loss before survival. Data were collected from 3047 patients enrolled in 12 chemotherapy protocols of the Eastern Cooperative Oncology Group (ECOG). Weight loss, defined both as (1) percentage loss when current weight is compared with the patient's weight before illness and (2) loss within the previous 6 months, was collected by patient interview. Results revealed that 46 per cent of the patients experienced no weight loss, 22 per cent demonstrated less than 5 per cent weight loss, 17 per cent experience a weight loss between 5 and 10 per cent, and 15 per cent experienced greater than 10 per cent weight loss. For nine of the 12 chemotherapy protocols, survival was significantly shorter in patients who had experienced weight loss when compared to those who had not lost weight. Furthermore, any occurrence of weight loss appeared to constitute the essential prognostic factor, not whether or not the patient dropped significantly below ideal body weight.

Nutritional alterations that occur in patients with cancer can lead to complications that interfere with patient progress and treatment. These alterations are found in a variety of patients who have cancer and may appear early in the course of the disease. Early recognition and aggressive management of these nutritional alterations is an important component of patient care.

PHYSIOLOGIC FEATURES OF NUTRITION

Provision of adequate nutrition at the cellular level involves a number of processes, including ingestion of food, digestion, absorption, elimination, and metabolism. Each of these processes provides critical components in the chain of events that maintains cellular nutrition. Digestion and absorption occur throughout the gastrointestinal tract. Accessory organs such as the liver and pancreas provide substances critical to both digestion and metabolism.

Ingestion

In health, control of food ingestion includes physiologic, psychological, and sociocultural factors (Fig. 47–1). A functional gastrointestinal tract is essential.

Physiologic Factors

Physiologic factors include central and peripheral components. The central components are located in the central nervous system and function as a central integrating and ingestion controlling center (DeWys, Costa, & Henkin, 1981). For example, the glucostatic hypothalamic dual center hypothesis predicts a central nervous system component with two centers: (1) the feeding center, which activates feeding, and (2) the satiety center, which inhibits feeding behavior. It has been hypothesized that the source of stimulation for

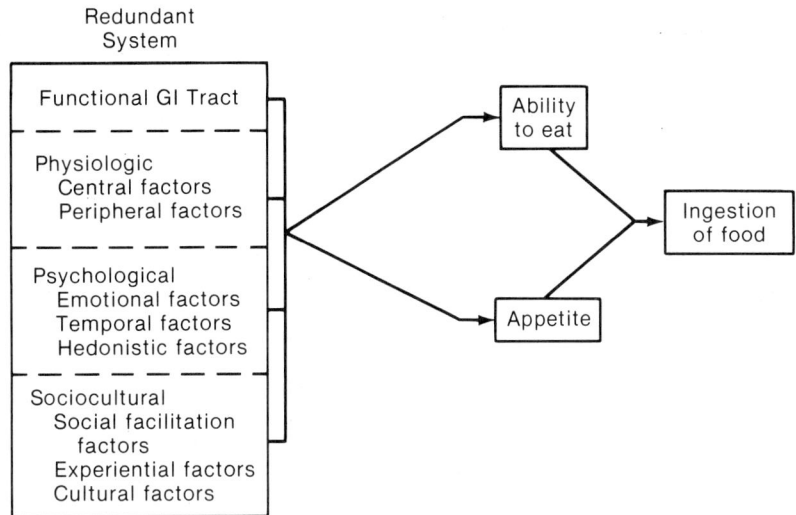

Figure 47–1. Food intake model. *GI,* gastrointestinal.

these centers is the blood glucose level (Mayer, 1955). Peripheral components include a system of sensors for taste and smell in the oronasal region (Rolls, 1981); a system of sensors that is primarily volumetric in the upper gastrointestinal tract (Davis & Campbell, 1973); and a system of sensors (for example, in the liver) that is responsive to changes in metabolites and hormones in the blood (DeWys et al., 1981).

Long-term controls over feeding behavior have also been identified and include the lipostatic theory, also known as the set point theory (Friedman & Stricker, 1976). According to this theory, when fat reserves are depleted, the satiety signal is decreased, and an increase in feeding behavior occurs. The thermostatic theory proposes a relationship between body temperature and feeding as demonstrated by studies of cold stressed rats who eat more and engage in more activity so as to generate heat through increased metabolism (Spector, Brobeck, & Hamilton, 1968). Another long-term control theory proposes a relationship between levels of circulating amino acids and food intake. In one study, animals reduced their intake of food when

their diet was low or devoid of a single amino acid or when there was an excess of one amino acid (Mellinkoff, Frankland, & Boyle, 1956).

Experimental studies have been conducted to test the physiologic factors of the system for maintaining dietary intake, but specific relationships between factors are not yet known. The system appears to be a multifactorial one, with no hierarchy yet described.

Psychological Factors

Psychological factors are influential in the control of dietary intake as well. Emotional states such as depression and anxiety have been known to result in decreased dietary intake (Beck, 1972). Stress has been associated with both decreases and increases in dietary intake, whereas other factors, such as time of day, have been associated with the initiation of feeding activity (Wooley et al., 1975). Other factors associated with food intake include the pleasure of good meals enjoyed in an ambient atmosphere (Wooley et al., 1975).

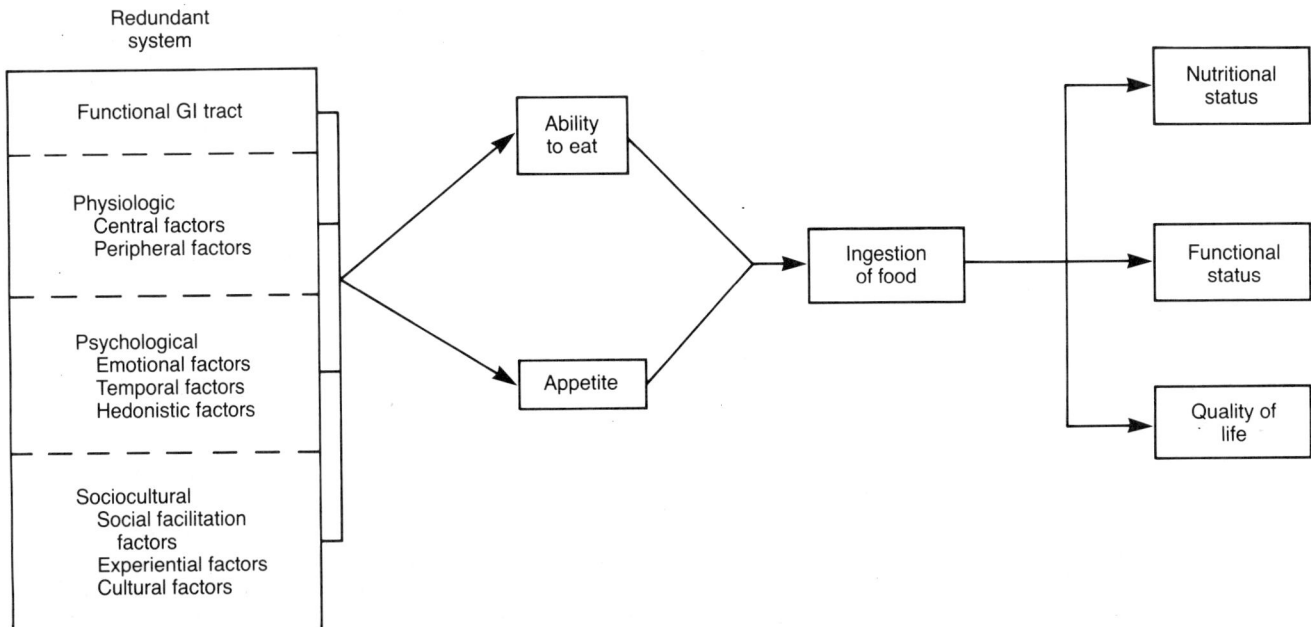

Figure 47–2. Impact of maintaining an Adequate Food Intake.

Sociocultural Factors

Sociocultural factors are influential in determining the environment for eating, the companions with whom people eat, and the specific types of foods that are prepared and eaten (Wooley et al., 1975).

The psychological and sociocultural factors influencing dietary intake have not been studied as extensively as the physiologic factors. The extent of their potential impact on feeding behavior is not yet known, nor is the influence of the combination of physiologic, psychological, and sociocultural factors.

In summary, the system for maintaining dietary intake appears to be one with built-in redundancy. That is, multiple factors initiate feeding behavior, but absence of one does not involve a breakdown in the system stimulating food intake. Thus an integrated approach to studying the phenomenon of eating disorders is needed. The result of maintaining adequate food intake is normal nutritional status (Fig. 47–2). The healthy animal eats to stay alive and functional. For humans, however, ingestion of food is heavily intertwined with social and pleasurable events. Thus ingestion of food not only is necessary for normal human growth and development but also provides pleasure and adds to the quality of life.

Digestion

The mouth, esophagus, stomach, small intestine, and large intestine form the major anatomic structures of the gastrointestinal tract. Normal oral status is reviewed in Chapter 48. The esophagus is a muscular, collapsible tube through which ingested food passes to the stomach. Although digestion begins in the mouth, it occurs primarily in the stomach and the small intestine. Other organs, namely the liver, gallbladder, and pancreas, facilitate digestion by secretion of enzymes and hormones. Enzymes contained in oral, gastric, and intestinal secretions initiate and aid the breakdown of ingested complex food substances into simpler components that are more readily absorbed, such as glucose, fatty acids, and amino acids.

Absorption

Absorption of digested food occurs predominantly in the small intestine. The intestinal rugae with their microscopic villi provide a large absorptive surface through which the end products of digestion can be absorbed into the blood stream and the lymphatics. Substances required immediately by cells move directly from the blood stream into the cellular structures. In contrast, excess substances such as simple sugars are primarily stored as glycogen in the liver, whereas fatty acids are deposited in fat cells located in various parts of the body. Some amino acids are deaminized in the liver, with the rest remaining in the blood stream for use as needed by various body cells.

Metabolism

Metabolism is the process by which energy is provided to drive the various vital body and cellular functions. This energy is provided as the digestive end products are used by various cells. Energy is used by cells to build tissue and secrete substances. The basal metabolic rate is defined as the amount of heat produced by the body 14 to 18 hr after the last meal in a room approximately at 22.5°C with the body at complete rest (Frohse, Brodel, & Schlossberg, 1985). This rate equals the energy requirements needed by the body for maintenance of vital functions, such as circulation, respiratory and digestive activities, and muscle tone.

OCCURRENCE OF NUTRITIONAL DEPLETION IN CANCER AND DURING CANCER TREATMENT

Factors influential in the occurrence of nutritional depletion in cancer patients may be divided into gastrointestinal dysfunction, central nervous system disturbances, peripheral factors, and psychosocial factors. Frequently several factors are involved simultaneously.

Dysfunctional Gastrointestinal Tract

Diminished dietary intake in cancer patients is related to abnormalities of digestion and absorption in the gastrointestinal tract. Two potential processes may occur. The first involves tumors that impinge directly on the gastrointestinal tract and acessory organs, such as the liver, and thus interfere with the normal movement of food through the gastrointestinal tract and with the digestion of food and absorption of digestive end products. The second involves changes within the gastrointestinal tract that are associated with malnutrition.

Tumors that arise in or impinge on the gastrointestinal tract may directly affect nutritional status by interfering with the ingestion, digestion, or absorption of food. Tumors located at different anatomic locations affect nutritional status differently. For example, the difficulty resulting from tumors of the head and neck is primarily one of mechanical interference with food intake and chewing that results in decreased food ingestion (Lawrence, 1979).

Tumors of the stomach may affect nutritional status by interfering mechanically with normal gastric function and by causing intragastric losses of blood and protein-rich fluid (Lawrence, 1979). Gastrectomy is the treatment of choice for most of the gastric cancers. Following gastrectomy, carbohydrate and protein digestion remain relatively intact as long as eating patterns are altered (small, frequent meals), but malabsorption of fat can occur (Lawrence, 1979). Although primary tumors of the small intestine are rare, metastases from other sites are not uncommon. Mechanical obstruction can occur. Loss of blood and protein-rich fluids into the intestinal lumen can result in severe nutritional depletion (Dickerson, 1983).

Tumors of the liver and the pancreas result in deficiencies in digestive enzymes and hormones, resulting in malabsorption of fat, protein, carbohydrates, vitamins, and minerals (Dickerson, 1983). Anorexia is a frequent complaint in patients with pancreatic cancer and leads to a progressive weight loss (Lawrence, 1979).

When the malnourished state is present for a sufficiently long period of time to cause changes in the small intestinal lining, a vicious cycle of further depletion may occur. The migrating cells of the intestinal villi are shed into the intestinal lining, carrying with them enzymes used in the digestion of food (Moog, 1981). When a malnourished state persists, changes in this lining occur that include decreases in numbers of villi and result in reduction of available intestinal enzymes so that malabsorption occurs (Dickerson, 1983). This is frequently referred to clinically as the smooth bowel syndrome.

In summary, when tumors involve the gastrointestinal tract and other digestive accessory organs, interference with the mechanical aspects of digestion and with the absorption of end products occurs, which can lead to nutritional depletion. A malnourished state further compromises nutritional status of the patient with gastrointestinal pathology.

Central Nervous System Disturbances

Evidence has been found that links nutritional depletion with disturbances in the central nervous system. One mechanism involves the hypothesis that as brain tryptophan levels increase, serotonin synthesis increases. Because high levels of brain serotonin can cause anorexia (Krause, Humphrey, von Meyenfeldt, James, & Fischer, 1981), patients with cancer may experience anorexia when increased levels of tryptophan are present. Increased levels of tryptophan and brain serotonin have been demonstrated in tumor-bearing rats (Krause et al, 1981; Nichols, Maickel, & Yim, 1983; Wesdorf, Krause, & von Meyenfeldt, 1983). The source of the tryptophan that leads to greater serotonin turnover has not been determined. It may be secreted by tumor tissue, but this has not been demonstrated. Other causes of central nervous system–related anorexia include the occurrence of distressing symptoms such as nausea, vomiting, and pain (Bernstein, 1986).

Early satiety is yet another general symptom that leads to decreased gastric emptying, slow peristalsis, and complaints of feeling of fullness. More than one of these central nervous system factors may be present at any one time, making it difficult to identify a clear cause for nutritional depletion.

Peripheral Factors

Peripheral factors originating in the oral-gustatory system have also been implicated in decreased intake experienced by cancer patients. Such disturbances include stomatitis or mucositis, xerostomia, taste and smell changes, and learned food aversions. Major research efforts have been undertaken regarding taste and smell changes and food aversions. Abnormalities of taste and smell have been observed in a variety of populations of patients with cancer. DeWys and Walters (1975) studied 50 patients with metastatic cancer who ranged in age from 16 to 79 years (median, 57 years). Decreased taste sensation was reported by 25 of the patients, and aversion to meat was reported by 16 of the patients. Patients with reported abnormal taste demonstrated increased incidence of weight loss.

In contrast, another study of taste thresholds in patients with esophageal cancer did not reveal the same pattern of taste changes (Kamath, Mams, Lad, Kohrs, & McGuire, 1983). Twelve patients with cancer were compared with a control group matched for age as well as for smoking and alcohol consumption. No significant difference in taste threshold changes was demonstrated. However, comparison with another control group of healthy nonsmokers showed marked differences. Thus, taste changes may be related to smoking and alcohol consumption, rather than to the existence of cancer.

Bernstein (1982) hypothesized that tumor growth may suppress appetite indirectly by causing learned food aversions. These aversions are learned because they are associated with unpleasant internal symptoms that ultimately result in decreased dietary intake. This hypothesis was first identified in Bernstein's studies of children and adults, followed by studies using an experimental animal model (Bernstein & Bernstein, 1981) (Box 47–1). Bernstein (1986) views these food aversions as a likely contributing factor to the occurrence of anorexia in patients with cancer who undergo cancer chemotherapy.

In 1982, Johnston and colleagues reported a study involving 31 patients receiving 6 weeks of primary radiation therapy for localized head and neck cancers. Patients whose mean age was 58 years, with a range of 40 to 79 years, rated each one of the following symptoms on separate 10-cm visual analogue scales, once a week during therapy and at 3 months and 6 months after therapy: ability to smell, dysgeusia, dysphagia for solids or liquids, appetite, fatigue, xerostomia, mouth or throat pain, and skin irritation. Twenty of the 31 patients (68 per cent) lost more than 5 per cent of their weight at presentation within 1 month of completing treatment, with weight losses ranging from 5.4 to 18.9 per cent. Some patients continued to lose weight up to 6 months after treatment. Analysis revealed that the symptom scores were worse for patients who had lost more than 5 per cent of their pretreatment weight within the first 4 weeks of radiation therapy. Xerostomia and dysphagia continued to increase up to the end of treatment and persisted for up to 6 months, whereas other symptoms decreased by the first follow-up visit. Each symptom became more severe during the treatment period.

Mossman and Henkin (1978) conducted a series of studies focusing on taste, smell, and salivary and ap-

---

Box 47–1. TASTE CHANGES DURING CHEMOTHERAPY ASSOCIATED WITH LEARNED FOOD AVERSIONS

The hypothesis that tumor growth may suppress appetite indirectly by causing learned food aversions was tested by Bernstein and Bernstein using an animal model and with children and adults. In the study of children, subjects were randomly assigned to an experimental group that was offered a novel flavor of ice cream before chemotherapy treatment. The control group was offered an equal time period of exposure to a toy. A second control group received neither exposure to the toy or the novel ice cream but received chemotherapy that was not associated with any gastrointestinal irritation. Food aversion testing was conducted 2 to 4 weeks later by offering patients a choice between eating the ice cream or playing with a game. The results indicated that the patients in the control group were three times more likely to choose the ice cream as patients in the experimental group. It appears that the children developed learned aversions to the ice cream when it was consumed before chemotherapy treatment that induced gastrointestinal discomfort. The study was repeated in an adult population with similar results. Food aversions are a likely contributing factor to the occurrence of anorexia in patients receiving chemotherapy.

(From Bernstein, I. L., & Bernstein, I. D. [1981]. Learned food aversions and cancer anorexia. *Cancer Treatment Reports, 65* [Suppl. 5], 43–47.)

---

petite changes in patients undergoing radiation therapy. A descriptive study of 27 patients with various cancers of the head and neck was composed of two study groups (Mossman & Henkin, 1978). In the first group (n = 9), all patients were tested 1 year after completion of radiation therapy, and all had persistent taste changes, six reported anorexia, and five had xerostomia. In the second group of subjects (n = 18), one had had taste changes before radiation therapy, and three had had anorexia before radiation therapy. During and after therapy, 12 of the 18 patients experienced taste loss, and 9 of the 18 patients experienced anorexia. Not all patients with taste changes experienced anorexia; however, all except one patient with anorexia experienced taste changes. The taste changes started 3 weeks after radiation therapy began; bitter and salt tastes showed the earliest and greatest impairment, and sweet taste the least.

Dental problems may occur in a variety of cancer populations but can be particularly important when found in patients already experiencing eating problems. Dental problems lead to nutritional disorders because they frequently result in patients' limiting their dietary selections, especially to diets low in protein and total calories.

Changes in Metabolic Requirements

If decreased food intake alone accounted for the nutritional depletion frequently observed in patients with cancer, provision of excess calories should reverse the depletion. Although such an approach is sometimes successful, a large number of patients with cancer lose weight out of proportion to their intake. Provision of adequate calories by oral, enteral, or parenteral routes does not change median survival rates of patients with advanced cancer (Heber et al., 1986; Heber, Chlebowski, Meguid, & McAndrew, 1986). Abnormalities in energy expenditure and in glucose, fat, and protein metabolism are hypothesized as additional factors that influence nutritional depletion in cancer patients (Heber, Chlebowski, Meguid, & McAndrew, 1986).

Although improvement in measurements of energy expenditure via metabolic bedside carts has resulted in increased data on patients with cancer, determination of metabolic expenditure has not yielded any results that can account for observed weight losses. Both heterogeneous and homogeneous populations of patients with cancer have been studied, with equivocal results (Bozzetti et al., 1983; Dempsey, et al., 1984). Some patients appear to be hypermetabolic, some have findings within normal limits, and some are hypometabolic. Comparisons with factors such as location of disease, extent of disease, and age have not revealed significant differences among these groups.

ALTERATIONS IN CARBOHYDRATE, FAT, AND PROTEIN METABOLISM

Marked changes in the metabolism of carbohydrate, fat, and protein have been demonstrated in patients with cancer.

Alterations in Carbohydrate Metabolism

Several abnormalities in glucose metabolism have been observed in cancer, including increased occurrence of amino acid derived from glucose production via gluconeogenesis. Brennan (1977) reported a case study of a patient with diffuse lymphoma who was not hypermetabolic from increased stress, exercise, or infection. The basal metabolic rate was minimally elevated at 115 per cent of the predicted normal level. Even when 3000 to 4000 calories of parenteral nutrition were administered daily, no weight gain was obtained. Brennan concluded that the tumor-bearing host appeared unable to conserve lean tissue and body protein even when starvation was reversed.

Two additional alterations are an increased cycling of energy-expensive lactate to glucose via the Cori cycle (Stein, 1978) and a slower decrease in blood glucose levels during glucose tolerance tests. The latter finding is consistent with data on impaired glucose tolerance or insulin resistance that has been revealed by several studies (Smith, Kisner, & Schein, 1980). In summary, alterations in carbohydrate metabolism occur in patients with cancer and may play a part in the occurrence of nutritional depletion during the course of cancer and cancer treatment.

Alterations in Fat Metabolism

Alterations in fat metabolism also have been observed in cancer. Tumor-bearing rats and mice lose more fat than controls (Lundholm, Edstrom, Ekman, Karlberg, & Schersten, 1981). However, this pattern has not been demonstrated consistently in humans. Nevertheless, profound wasting of body fat in cachectic persons occurs (Smith et al., 1980). A potential explanation for this wasting is the production by the tumor tissue of lipolytic substances that increase mobilization of fat.

Some studies have demonstrated the inability of the patient who has cancer to adapt to chronic starvation by utilization of fat stores (McAndrew, 1986). Instead, gluconeogenesis continues to occur from amino acid sources. The extent of depletion of fat store is also under study. Moore and co-workers (1963) conducted extensive body composition studies on one lymphoma patient and found that total body water was 77.5 per cent, suggesting that there was literally no body fat present. Similar results were achieved by Warnold, Lundholm, and Schersten (1978) who found that when contrasted to controls, patients with cancer exhibited diminished body fat in the presence of a relatively expanded extracellular water.

Alterations in fat metabolism have been demonstrated in cancer, but their exact mechanisms are not known.

Alterations in Protein Metabolism

Studies of altered protein metabolism in cancer revealed increased glucose-to-alanine conversion, increased alanine levels, and increased flux of alanine from the circulation (Waterhouse, Jeanpretre, & Keilson, 1979). These findings are consistent with the conversion of alanine to glucose via gluconeogenesis and illustrate the patient's inability during starvation to spare protein-derived glucose from being used as fuel.

Another study revealed a pattern that can be described as a remodeling of body protein (Carmichael, Clague, Keir, & Johnston, 1980). This study described whole body protein turnover, synthesis, and breakdown in 11 patients with colorectal carcinoma who had uniform dietary intake. Protein turnover increased with advancement of disease but was lower in anorectic patients, indicating expected adaptation to starvation. Increased body protein synthesis was also demonstrated. Although all patients were in positive nitrogen balance, anthropometric measurements indicated loss of host protein. The explanation offered for this finding was that there may be a translocation of protein from body muscle to more active sites of protein synthesis, such as in the tumor tissue itself.

In summary, one explanation of the nutritional depletion that occurs in patients with cancer focuses on alterations in energy expenditure and in carbohydrate, fat, and protein metabolism (Kurzer & Meguid, 1986; Lundholm, 1986). Findings demonstrate abnormalities, but patterns are not consistent and the degree of abnormality demonstrated does not account for the extent of weight loss that occurs in most patients (Kaempfer & Lindsey, 1986). It appears that although alterations in energy expenditure and carbohydrate, fat, and protein metabolism may account for some of the nutritional depletion seen in patients with cancer, decreases in dietary intake continue to play a major role in the continued and profound weight loss observed.

PSYCHOSOCIAL FACTORS INFLUENCING NUTRITIONAL DEPLETION

A number of psychosocial factors are thought to be associated with nutritional depletion in cancer patients. Documentation of these factors has been identified primarily through clinical experience and descriptive studies. In the work reported by Holland, Rowland, and Plumb (1977), three general areas of anorexia have been identified: (1) anorexia that is transient and related to the initial diagnosis, recurrence, or prognosis of disease; (2) anorexia related to cancer treatment; and (3) anorexia related to the disease.

In a descriptive study of 50 patients undergoing curative radiation therapy on a variety of anatomic sites, Peck and Boland (1977) conducted psychiatric interviews before and after therapy, focusing on patient attitude toward treatment and illness. Sixty per cent of the patients showed a significant degree of anxiety before treatment, and 80 per cent did so after completion of treatment. Such an emotional environment could compound decreased appetite and ingestion during and after cancer therapy. Other reports of psychosocial factors affecting appetite are primarily case reports (Peteet, Medeiros, Slavin, & Walsh-Burke, 1981) and clinical observations (Gormican, 1980).

Schmale (1979) proposed that a profound withdrawal state occurs in some patients who are extremely depressed. This state is accompanied by a radical decrease in dietary intake and a resulting weight loss.

Social factors related to nutritional depletion that are experienced by patients with cancer include cultural differences reflected in choices of food during hospitalization, absence of usual eating companions, and the inability to consume usual foods. For example, if the normal diet includes spicy, highly seasoned foods and the patient is undergoing treatment that leads to a sore, inflamed mouth, these foods are no longer tolerated.

Examination of factors influencing dietary intake and feeding behavior reveals a multifactorial, redundant model, composed of physiologic, psychological and sociocultural factors (Novin & VanderWeele,

1977; Toates, 1981). Interference with one of the factors may produce a temporary decrease in dietary intake, whereas interference with several of the factors over a period of time could result in devastating nutritional problems (Grijalva & Lindholm, 1982).

In patients with cancer, diverse physiologic and psychosocial factors influence food intake by decreasing dietary intake and increasing metabolic need. To prevent serious nutritional depletion, early and consistent interventions for the precipitating problems are needed. Although nurses' knowledge regarding what exact nutritional approaches are needed is incomplete, plans to help patients, especially those undergoing active treatment, must be comprehensive and individualized. One approach to the initiation of such a plan is to identify the major factors present and then plan interventions specific to each factor. The foundation needed to manage these problems is a thorough nutritional assessment.

ASSESSMENT AND MANAGEMENT OF NUTRITIONAL PROBLEMS

Nutritional Abnormalities in the Person with Cancer

Nutritional abnormalities in patients with cancer occur as a result of the tumor itself or as a consequence of the effects of various cancer treatment methods, including surgery, chemotherapy, radiation therapy, and immunotherapy, used alone or in combination.

Definition

Malnutrition, or nutritional depletion, occurs when provision of energy and nutrients is inadequate to sustain the functioning of all physiologic systems. Protein-calorie malnutrition has received the most attention, although deficiencies of many individual nutrients (including fluids and electrolytes, vitamins, minerals, and trace elements) have also been described. In addition to deficits, excesses of nutrients must also be considered in this age of macrobiotic diets, megavitamin therapy, and other nutritional fads.

Although much is written about malnutrition, the term is frequently not defined. *Malnutrition,* or *macronutrient deficiency(ies),* commonly observed in some patients with cancer may be categorized as adult marasmus (chronic depletion of muscle and fat), acute visceral attrition (kwashiorkor-like), or a combination of the two (protein-calorie malnutrition). Malnutrition occurs when intake of nutrients is inadequate, in terms of either quantity or quality, to meet metabolic needs.

The term *protein-calorie malnutrition,* also called *protein-energy malnutrition,* includes a wide spectrum of general nutritional conditions that range clinically from almost undetectable symptoms to frank starvation and kwashiorkor (Viteri & Torun, 1988). Protein-energy malnutrition results from a protracted period in which the patient fails to ingest or receive adequate amounts of energy and protein, resulting in a combination of marasmus and kwashiorkor (Holman, 1987). *Marasmus* occurs as a result of prolonged inadequate intake of energy sources during (metabolically) unstressed starvation. Marasmus is characterized by gradual wasting of body fat and skeletal muscle mass, with preservation of visceral proteins (serum albumin, transferrin, and prealbumin) and immunocompetence. The marasmic individual has minimal nutritional reserves and tolerates repeated or prolonged stress poorly (Grant, Custer, & Thurlow, 1981). *Kwashiorkor* is the term used for another type of malnutrition that occurs as a result of stressed starvation and an inadequate intake of protein relative to energy. Kwashiorkor is characterized by preserved anthropometric measurements, especially fat stores; low visceral protein levels (serum albumin, transferrin, and prealbumin); and measures that reflect impaired immunologic function, specifically impaired cell-mediated immunity. In addition, muscle wasting may occur after prolonged catabolic conditions. The person suffering from kwashiorkor may not appear overly thin because of the presence of edema. Frequently the patient with cancer experiences a combination of the two. Combined marasmus-kwashiorkor is characterized by skeletal muscle wasting; depletion of fat stores; low serum visceral protein concentrations, such as serum albumin and transferrin; and impaired immunocompetence. Persons with the combined form are at greatest risk of serious morbidity and mortality if nutritional support is not provided.

Causes of Malnutrition

Nutritional abnormalities that occur in the person with cancer can result from the tumor itself; from the various methods of antitumor therapy, such as surgery, radiation therapy, chemotherapy, and immunotherapy; or from the combined effects of both.

The degree of malnutrition that occurs is influenced by the anatomic site of the tumor; the extent of disease; and duration, amount, and combination of antitumor therapy. The frequency with which malnutrition is reported varies, but it tends to occur more commonly with tumors at certain sites, specifically tumors of the head and neck, central nervous system, gastrointestinal tract, and lung; in addition, highly malignant lymphomas also frequently are accompanied by malnutrition (Ollenschlager, Konkol, & Modder, 1988).

Surgery. Surgery is performed with both curative and palliative intent. Surgery can affect the development of malnutrition because of the normally expected increased metabolic demands that result simply from perioperative catabolism. Surgery is at times associated with undesirable prolonged periods (greater than 10 days) of inadequate nutritional intake resulting from preoperative diagnostic work-ups, surgery itself and its requisite healing period, or surgical complications. In addition, radical resection of specific anatomic sites is likely to impair the patient's ability to ingest, digest, or absorb nutrients, resulting in chronic nutritional consequences. These anatomic sites include the head and neck region and the gastrointestinal tract.

Radiation Therapy. Although radiation therapy has

desired therapeutic effects in that it kills tumor cells, it also causes changes in or destruction of normal cells. Radiation therapy, particularly of the oral cavity, pharynx, esophagus, and abdomen, is likely to result in impaired nutrition owing to decreased ability to ingest, digest, or absorb nutrients. Furthermore, this type of therapy contributes to symptoms such as anorexia, mucositis, and xerostomia that make it more difficult for people to eat. Radiation therapy factors that are reported to affect the development of nutritional problems include (1) the part of the body in the radiation field, (2) the intensity of the radiation tumor dose, (3) the time period over which radiation therapy is delivered, (4) the volume of tissue that receives radiation therapy, (5) the nutritional status of the patient when he or she begins radiation therapy, (6) the sensitivity of the tissue to radiation, and (7) the person's general physical and psychological status before treatment. Side effects and complications of radiation therapy may be fairly immediate, beginning as early as within 2 to 4 weeks after initiating radiation therapy or within 6 weeks after completing RT. Late effects of radiation therapy may be extensive and irreversible, occurring years after the culmination of radiation therapy.

Chemotherapy. Antitumor chemotherapy contributes to the development of malnutrition by interfering with the person's ability to ingest nutrients. As with radiation therapy, chemotherapy not only is therapeutic in that it kills tumor cells but it also can cause side effects and toxicities, such as taste changes, nausea, vomiting, stomatitis, anorexia, and diarrhea, which interfere with intake. In addition, the subsequent development of malnutrition impairs the digestive and absorptive abilities of the gastrointestinal tract, especially as a result of mucosal atrophy that further compromises the bowel's absorptive function and as a result of dysfunction of major organ systems such as the liver.

Nutritional Assessment in Cancer

Nutritional assessment is performed to determine a person's nutritional status or the degree to which his or her need for nutrients and energy is being met by present intake. Detection of protein-energy malnutrition has received the most attention, particularly among hospitalized patients. However, it is also important to consider vitamins, minerals, fats, and electrolytes. In addition to deficits, nutrient excesses are potential problems.

Goals of Nutritional Assessment

Nutritional assessment can be performed for a number of reasons, including: (1) to screen for persons with cancer who are *at high risk* for developing nutritional problems; (2) to identify those patients with *existing* nutritional abnormalities; (3) to determine nutritional *requirements* so that appropriate nutritional interventions can be prescribed; and (4) to follow *responses* to nutritional therapies. Determination of

which specific nutritional assessment methods are most appropriate must be made while considering the goal or goals of the nutritional assessment. The assessment goals most relevant for clinical purposes can be summarized either as approaches to evaluate current nutritional status or approaches to prescribe treatment and follow response to nutritional intervention.

Methods of Nutritional Assessment

Unfortunately, there is no simple direct method or single datum by which the nutritional status of a person can accurately be established. Instead, measures that are thought to reflect nutritional status indirectly are used. In addition, it is difficult to determine which of these single measures or combinations of measurements is most accurate because of the absence of a "gold standard" by which malnutrition can be determined and used for comparison. Furthermore, judgments regarding the presence or absence of malnutrition and the degree to which it exists are usually based on the comparison of a patient's results to standard values. The validity of existing standards that are used to categorize nutritional status is questionable. Finally, many of the potential measures thought to indirectly reflect nutritional status are useful for research and epidemiologic purposes but are not practical or effective for making clinical judgments about individual patients.

Individual Assessment Measures. Historically, the trends in nutritional assessment have gone full circle since the 1970s, when protein-energy malnutrition in hospitalized patients was first widely recognized. For many years before that time, nutritional assessment involved primarily "clinical judgment" based on the history and physical examination. In the 1970s, a number of investigators proposed more technical and quantitative methods for nutritional assessment that were believed to reflect nutritional status indirectly. They can be categorized into five main areas: (1) biochemical, (2) immune function, (3) anthropometric, (4) dietary intake, and (5) clinical observation.

Biochemical laboratory measures proposed to reflect nutritional status include serum albumin, serum transferrin, and serum prealbumin levels; nitrogen balance studies; and creatinine-height index.

Measures of *immune function* associated with nutritional status include anergy panels reflecting cell-mediated immunity and total lymphocyte counts. Particularly in the patient with cancer, alterations in immune function may result from the disease or its treatment rather than from nutritional factors. *Anthropometric measurements* involve skinfold (SF) measures at various anatomic sites, midarm muscle circumference (MAMC), and body weight (WT). Body weight can be considered (1) as an isolated measure; (2) in relation to height (weight for height); or (3) in comparison to ideal body weight (percentage IBW), to usual body weight (percentage UBW) for that person, or to prior weight (percentage weight change).

Dietary evaluation can include both an assessment of what the person actually eats and drinks and an evaluation of knowledge about nutrition. A number of approaches for assessing dietary intake can be employed such as: 24-hour recall; food frequency questionnaires; complete dietary histories; direct observation of food intake; or evaluation by the basic four food groups, dietary goals, or recommended dietary allowances. A comprehensive dietary history estimates whether the diet is sufficient, determines food preferences, evaluates current and previous dietary patterns, and provides information on social and economic factors influencing the person's ability to obtain and prepare food. A simple diet history provides a rough idea of the adequacy of intake by reviewing meal patterns, extent of "empty" calories consumed, and amount and type of snack foods and dietary supplements. Requesting the patient with cancer to maintain a diary of all intake for a limited period of time not only can be helpful in assessing what he or she is actually eating but also can provide motivation for the patient.

Finally, *clinical observation* involves evaluation of the person's physical condition; consideration of psychosocial factors, including the ability to obtain and prepare food; determination of socioeconomic status; review of current medications (including vitamins); and information regarding comorbidity or other current health problems in addition to the cancer.

Reduced Assessment Schemes. Instead of using all of these potential measures related to nutritional status, some investigators have attempted to develop reduced schemes, or combinations, of nutritional assessment measures that could be useful clinically. Because of the absence of a gold standard by which to establish malnutrition, the measures included in these reduced combinations have not been judged in terms of their ability to predict malnutrition per se; instead they have been judged by their ability to predict surrogate outcomes that are both associated with malnutrition and more easily determined, such as the surgical complications of delayed wound healing and infection, differences in tolerance for response to antitumor therapy, or survival. This is appropriate because the clinician is, after all, ultimately interested in what happens to the patient. The clinician wants to identify correctly those persons in whom nutritional intervention is indicated and for whom it will make a difference in terms of clinical outcomes.

One example of a reduced assessment scheme is the Prognostic Nutrition Index (PNI), developed by Buzby and colleagues (1980). The PNI is a statistical model developed to predict surgical morbidity and mortality from four selected nutritional parameters measured preoperatively. This method is not appropriate for following response to nutritional intervention. The PNI is calculated by the following formula: PNI = 158 − 16.60 (serum albumin level in grams [g] per 100 milliliters [ml]) − 0.78 (triceps skinfold thickness in millimeters [mm]) − 0.20 (serum transferrin level in milligrams [mg] per 100 ml) − 5.8 (cutaneous delayed hypersensitivity reaction to mumps virus, streptokinase-streptodornase, or *Candida*). The cutaneous delayed hypersensitivity skin tests were graded as 0

(nonreactive), 1 (< 5 mm induration), or 2 (≥ 5 mm induration). The investigators suggest that patients with a PNI of less than 40 per cent are at low risk for complications; a PNI of 40 to 49 per cent indicates intermediate risk; and a PNI ≥ 50 per cent reveals the high-risk category. Although this system was developed in patients undergoing gastrointestinal surgery, it has been evaluated in patients with other tumors (including those of the head and neck), who were also surgical candidates (Hooley, Levine, Floers, Wheeler, & Steiger, 1983). Patients assigned to the PNI high-risk category were far more likely than those in the other PNI categories to experience greater complications at a higher rate (Buzby, Mullen, Matthews, Hobbs, & Rosata, 1980; Goodwin & Torres, 1984; Hooley et al., 1983; Muller, Keller, Brenner, Walter, & Holzmuller, 1986).

General Management of Nutritional Problems

Two important considerations in approaching the management of nutritional alterations in the patient with cancer include (1) when does nutritional status make a difference in terms of clinical outcomes? and (2) who benefits from nutritional intervention, or when does nutritional intervention make a difference in clinical outcomes? For a number of years, it has been assumed that aggressive nutritional intervention would be good for every patient with cancer who was actively undergoing treatment. It is important to take a careful look at the answers to the foregoing questions both because of increasingly limited resources for patient care and because nutritional interventions themselves are not always benign or without risk.

Ollenschlager and colleagues (1988) state two general indications for intensive nutritional therapy. The first indication is *apparent malnutrition*, characterized by current body weight less than 90 per cent of IBW, weight loss greater than 10 per cent over 6 months or 5 per cent within 1 month, or serum albumin levels less than 3.5 g/100 ml. The second indication is *imminent malnutrition*, characterized by inadequate spontaneous oral intake less than 60 per cent of predicted nutrient requirements for more than 1 week, administration of intensive antineoplastic therapy, or sepsis.

The second important consideration in approaching the management of nutritional alterations in persons with cancer involves determining which patients actually will benefit from nutritional intervention. For example, this question has been considered regarding the administration of total parenteral nutrition (TPN) to patients with cancer who are receiving chemotherapy or radiation therapy or to patients undergoing surgery. Appropriate evaluation of the potential efficacy of nutritional intervention should also consider the degree of malnutrition that exists. Although it is generally agreed that nutritional supplementation does not improve morbidity and mortality of well-nourished individuals, it has not been clearly demonstrated that nutritional therapy enhances patient outcomes when malnutrition is indeed present. Preoperative or postoperative nutritional therapy, or both, resulted in improved complication or mortality rates in some studies when the nutritional intervention was limited to those patients who were "significantly malnourished" (Maillet, 1987).

Evidence for the efficacy of nutritional support by TPN in decreasing radiation therapy– or chemotherapy-associated morbidity and mortality is weak (Detsky, Baker, O'Rourke, & Goel, 1987). The American College of Physicians' (ACP) Clinical Efficacy Assessment Project is conducted to evaluate and provide information about the safety and efficacy of diagnostic and therapeutic methods and medical practices. A position paper resulting from this project was issued reflecting state-of-the-art knowledge obtained by a meta-analysis of 11 prospective controlled randomized trials of perioperative TPN. The individual studies included end points of iatrogenic complications from the TPN itself, complications from major surgery, and death. Only one of the original studies showed a statistically significant reduction in complications or fatality rates for patients treated with perioperative TPN. The authors of this position paper concluded that even though nutritional supplementation did not benefit those who were well nourished, it was possible that perioperative TPN may be helpful for three subgroups: (1) patients who are severely malnourished before undergoing major surgery; (2) patients who are well-nourished before surgery but who develop complications that are expected to result in a prolonged period of ileus or inadequate nutritional intake; and (3) patients who are well-nourished before undergoing surgery that usually results in prolonged periods of inadequate nutritional intake even if complications do not occur. These conclusions are further supported by the American Society of Parenteral and Enteral Nutrition (ASPEN) guidelines (1986) for use of TPN in hospitalized patients.

A similar ACP Clinical Efficacy Assessment Project position paper addressed the evidence for efficacy of nutritional supplementation by TPN to decrease morbidity and mortality during chemotherapy or combined chemotherapy and radiation therapy. A meta-analysis approach was used to pool the results of 12 prospective controlled randomized clinical trials whose outcomes included overall survival, short-term survival, tumor response, and treatment toxicity (McGeer, Detsky, & O'Rourke, 1990). This study recommended that the routine use of TPN for patients receiving chemotherapy should be strongly discouraged. The authors suggested that TPN may not be as detrimental to persons who were already malnourished, but the overall rate of complications from the TPN itself was indeed troubling.

Determining Energy and Protein Needs

Once it has been established that a patient requires nutritional intervention, the prescription must be based on individualized estimates of energy and protein re-

quirements. Overfeeding of carbohydrates may produce respiratory distress in patients with marginal pulmonary reserve or may produce hepatic steatosis. Inadequate provision of substrates may lead to suboptimal nitrogen retention and loss of lean body mass.

Energy Requirements. One pretreatment goal is the estimation of energy requirements to provide a nutritional regimen that replaces burned fuel and prevents loss of tissue mass. This is accomplished by estimating total caloric requirements on the basis of sex, height, weight, age, and disease state, or by measuring oxygen consumption and determining actual metabolic requirements. The precise metabolic effect of the presence of a tumor is still controversial, with some studies reporting hypermetabolism, some hypometabolism, and some no changes in metabolic rate (Knox, et al., 1983).

Energy expenditure estimates that provide a basis for determining caloric requirements can be obtained either by indirect calorimetry or by use of the Harris-Benedict formula (Harris & Benedict, 1979) to calculate basal energy expenditure. A third approach is utilization of a simple "kilocalorie per kilogram formula" to calculate estimated calorie needs. The goal in the metabolically stressed or catabolic patient is to maintain energy stores, whereas in the metabolically unstressed patient it is to replete existing deficits (Rombeau, Caldwell, Forlaw, & Guenter, 1989).

In indirect calorimetry, estimated energy expenditure is calculated by measuring respiratory gas exchange. This method is impractical for routine clinical use and finds its primary application in research.

The Harris-Benedict formula differs slightly according to the patient's sex. For men, the basal energy expenditure (BEE) is calculated as follows:

$$\text{BEE (men)} = 66.47 + (13.75) \text{ (weight in kg)} + (5.00) \text{ (height in cm)} - (6.75) \text{ (age in yr)}$$

For women, the BEE is calculated using the Harris-Benedict formula as follows:

$$\text{BEE (women)} = 655.096 + (9.56) \text{ (weight in kg)} + (1.85) \text{ (height in cm)} - (4.68) \text{ (age in yr)}$$

The BEE, also known as basal metabolic rate (BMR), can then be multiplied by an adjustment factor that reflects either activity level or metabolic stress level (or both), to determine an estimate of total energy needs. Factors for activity suggested by Long and colleagues (1979) are 1.2 for persons who are on bed rest and 1.3 for hospitalized but ambulatory patients. Injury factors are 1.2 for minor surgery, 1.2 to 1.7 for acute phase septic patients who are normotensive, 0.5 for acute phase septic patients who are hypotensive, and 1.0 for septic patients during the recovery phase (Rombeau, et al., 1989). In addition, the metabolic rate is elevated by fever, during which energy expenditure increases approximately 7 per cent for every degree of temperature above normal measured on the Fahrenheit scale or 13 per cent per degree of temperature elevation measured on the Celsius scale (Kinney

& Roe, 1962; Wilmore, 1977). For weight repletion, approximately 1000 calories per day should be added, for a total of 7000 calories per week.

The third method of estimating energy needs—which is by far the easiest to use in the clinical setting—is the kilocalorie per kilogram method. Daily calorie needs are determined by multiplying the current weight in kilograms by the suggested estimated kilocalorie levels. The suggested kilocalorie per kilogram levels vary slightly depending on the source, but are basically very similar. Recommendations for *maintenance* (anabolism) at rest range from 25 kcal/kg of current body weight per day for men and 20 kcal/kg of current body weight per day for women to a range of 30 to 35 kcal/kg of current body weight per day. Recommendations for *repletion* during catabolism are 40 to 50 kcal/kg of current body weight per day. Reports regarding hypermetabolism in patients with tumors have been inconsistent. These guidelines provide the average patient with 2000 to 2500 kcal/day for maintenance and with 3000 to 4000 kcal/day for repletion.

Protein Requirements. Requisite amounts of protein can be estimated from energy expenditure, such as from the Harris-Benedict formula. Nitrogen is used as a marker for protein, so that the two terms are used essentially interchangeably. When the calculated energy expenditure is used to form the basis of the protein requirement calculation, the suggested ratio of nitrogen in grams to calories is 1:300 for maintenance and 1:150 for repletion (Blackburn, Bistrian, & Miani, 1976). Alternatively, the actual mathematical conversion is 6.25 g of protein per 1 g of nitrogen (Rombeau et al., 1989). The recommended daily allowance (RDA) for protein is 0.6 to 0.8 g of protein/kg of body weight/day.

Nitrogen balance studies provide a means for verifying whether nitrogen intake is in balance with metabolic demands. They reflect the adequacy of protein supplied to maintain lean body mass. Nitrogen balance studies are useful both to determine a baseline index of protein status and as a measure of net changes in total body protein mass. Eight-five to 90 per cent of nitrogen is lost through urinary excretion of urea. In addition, a small constant amount is lost through the skin and feces. Nitrogen balance is calculated by the following formula:

$$\frac{\text{protein intake (g)}}{6.25} - \left(\begin{array}{l}\text{24-hr urinary urea nitrogen [g]} \\ + \text{ 4 g [estimate of fecal and} \\ \text{integumentary losses])}\end{array}\right)$$

The left part of this formula, protein intake in grams divided by 6.25, represents nitrogen intake in grams. Nitrogen balance studies can be particularly helpful when used intermittently to evaluate the protein intake of the critically ill patient receiving enteral or parenteral nutritional support. During treatment or recovery from illness, the daily goal is a positive nitrogen balance of 2 to 3 g.

Once the decision is made that a patient with cancer requires nutritional therapy, one of the first considerations is deciding what route should be used to deliver it. In general, the rule that guides this decision is, "If the gut works, use it." Nutritional repletion is more successful when delivered enterally than parenterally. In addition, the use of TPN involves a fairly high risk of complications and is expensive and relatively complicated to deliver.

Regardless of the route by which nutritional support is administered, assessment of the nutrition knowledge of the individual patient and his or her caregiver is essential. This includes understanding of the importance of adequate nutrition in maintaining or restoring health, knowing about proper dietary selection, and knowing how to manage cancer or treatment symptoms that potentially interfere with receiving adequate nutrition.

Increasing Oral Intake

Although the symptoms that result from the cancer or its treatment perhaps do not obviously appear to be directly related to nutrition, their management is very important because of the impact that these symptoms—such as pain, nausea, vomiting, dysphagia, odynophagia, taste changes, xerostomia, fatigue, respiratory distress, diarrhea, constipation, or depression and anxiety—can have on limiting the patient's ability to obtain, prepare, and receive adequate nutrition. This is especially true of nutrition by the oral route.

General measures that can help maintain adequate nutritional status involve (1) good oral hygiene; (2) moistening of the mouth with nonharmful agents; (3) careful dental evaluation to assess and correct gum disease, missing teeth, caries, poorly fitting dentures, and stomatitis; and (4) encouraging physical activity and exercise at a level appropriate for the patient.

In general, instruction regarding the importance of a high-protein, high-calorie intake is an essential beginning (Box 47–2). Involving the patient and family in planning or providing meals and snacks that are appealing may increase the likelihood that the patient will be able to consume more. Food preparation and presentation can also influence the ability to eat. Avoiding spicy or acidic foods and beverages and foods served at hot temperatures minimizes discomfort from stomatitis and oral lesions. Altering food texture may make it easier to chew or swallow when mastication or deglutition problems are present. When xerostomia (dry mouth) is a problem, serving foods with juices, liquids, gravies, or other sources of moisture may help. However, this comfort measure must be balanced with the need to avoid consumption of liquids or other foods that are devoid of nutritional value, sometimes referred to as consuming "empty calories." Nutritional approaches to decreasing diarrhea are discussed separately later in this chapter. Decreasing portions and increasing the frequency of eating by serving small, frequent meals, six or more times per day, instead of three large meals may be more effective for the person who has difficulty eating, especially in the presence of anorexia. In addition, when the ability to consume adequate amounts through normal dietary approaches is significantly limited, the use of supplements becomes essential. In reality, supplements may then become the

---

Box 47–2. INCREASING ORAL INTAKE IN CANCER PATIENTS

A quasi-experimental study of 41 patients with head and neck cancer was conducted to test the effects of a structured teaching program aimed at increasing oral intake during radiation therapy. Subjects were randomized to (1) an experimental group whose members were given individualized dietary caloric and protein intake requirements; an audiovisual program of usual diet intake problems occurring during therapy and the related self-care; a handout of the program contents; and a book, *Eating Hints,* published by the National Cancer Institute that contained recommendations for dietary intake and nutritious recipies or (2) a control group whose members received the usual care. A 3-day diet intake history was taken weekly during the study. For experimental patients, analysis of food intake, comparing it with recommended dietary intake, was conducted, and the information obtained was relayed to the patient to encourage adjustments in the diet as needed. Analysis included the impact of the program on anorexia, adequacy of oral intake, nutritional status including weight changes, functional status, and quality of life.

Results revealed that the experimental group had a possible vulnerability to nutritional problems during radiation therapy because of a history of significantly greater weight loss before treatment. Three experimental trends were (1) lower appetite scores, (2) higher caloric and protein intake, and (3) weight loss comparable with that in the control group.

The experimental group maintained dietary intake at a level higher than that of the control group despite the loss of appetite and ability to eat. It would appear that cancer and cancer treatment affect oral intake during radiation therapy, and a nutritional counseling program can be used to encourage increased oral intake.

(From Grant, M. [in press]. Patterns of anorexia in cancer patients. *Proceedings of the American Cancer Society First National Nursing Research Conference,* November-December, 1989.)

---

major source of nutrition, and the usual dietary intake of food and beverage becomes the "supplement."

Nutritional Supplements

Decisions regarding what supplements to use for oral or enteral nutritional support are based on many factors, both nutritional and practical. Nutritional supplements may be prepared at home, prepared institutionally, or purchased commercially. Commercially prepared products are advantageous in that they are convenient and their nutritional composition is known and standardized.

Nutritional formula products are classified as complete mixtures of nutrients; modular; or special, such as hepatic, renal, or pulmonary failure preparations. Modular products provide sources of either protein, carbohydrate as powder or liquid, or long- or medium-chain fatty acids alone or with carbohydrate. These products are usually low residue, unless specifically developed to provide residue, such as Enrich. Most nutritionally complete products deliver between 1 and 2 kcal/ml. Complete formulas that provide all essential nutrients, including carbohydrate, protein, fat, vitamins, and minerals, can contain lactose or be lactose free. Elemental diets usually are higher in osmolality and are less palatable, but they require less digestive and absorptive capabilities. The approximate compositions of selected commercially prepared defined-formula diets and modular supplements are given in Table 47–1 (Feldman, 1988; Paige, 1988).

Enteral Nutrition

When provision of nutrition is inadequate by the oral route because patients either cannot eat or will not eat but the gastrointestinal tract is functioning normally, the administration of nutritional support by

the enteral route is preferable to the parenteral route. Enteral nutrition promotes more efficient utilization of nutrients and better preservation of intestinal functioning than administration by the parenteral route (Goodwin & Wilmore, 1988). If the gastrointestinal tract is functioning, it is preferable that it be used because making use of this route is less expensive, has a lower potential for complications, and is generally easier to manage.

Indications for nasoenteric tube feeding are summarized in Table 47–2 (Feldman, 1988). Nasoenteric tube feedings are contraindicated when complete or incomplete gastric or intestinal obstruction is present, severe gastroesophageal reflux is a problem, or paralytic ileus occurs.

Enteral administration can be by bolus, intermittently by pump, or continuously by pump. Bolus feedings are much easier to provide as long as they are tolerated well and do not cause symptoms such as nausea, vomiting, discomfort, or diarrhea. Bolus feedings into the stomach may begin by introducing 50 to 100 ml of isotonic or slightly hypotonic formula every 3 hrs, increasing by 50 ml every one or two feedings up to a maximum of 250 to 300 ml every 3 to 4 hrs. This is then followed by an increase to full-strength solution.

When enteral feedings must be administered by pump instead of by bolus to minimize symptoms, administration of the enteral feedings entirely during the night or intermittently throughout any part of the day or night may be less disruptive to the patient's other activities, including simple ambulation. Enteral nutrition can be provided in any setting, including the home.

A number of anatomic locations are possible for insertion of gastric tubes for enteral feedings, including, but not limited to, (1) nasogastric intubation, (2) a gastrostomy tube placed surgically through the ab-

Table 47–1. APPROXIMATE COMPOSITION OF DEFINED-FORMULA DIETS AND MODULAR SUPPLEMENTS

Diet or Supplement	Caloric Density (kcal/ml)	Carbohydrate (g/L)	Carbohydrate Source	Fat (g/L)	Fat Source	Protein (g/L)	Protein Source	N/kcal Ratio	Osmolality (mOsm/kg)	Na (mEq/L)	K (mEq/L)
Whole Food Base											
Compleat B	1	120	Vegetables, fruit, maltodextrins, lactose, sucrose	40	Corn oil, milk	40	Beef, nonfat milk	1:156	390	52	33
Formula 2	1	123	Vegetables, fruit, lactose, sucrose, starch	40	Corn oil, egg yolk	38	Beef, nonfat milk, egg yolk	1:164	475	26	45
Vitaneed	1	130	Vegetables, fruit, maltodextrins, corn syrup solids	40	Soy oil, monoglycerides, diglycerides	35	Beef, calcium caseinate	1:179	400	24	32
Milk Base											
Nutri-1000	1	101	Corn syrup solids, sucrose, lactose	55	Corn oil, monoglycerides, diglycerides	40	Skim milk, sodium caseinate	1:156	500	23	39
Meritene Liquid	1	115	Corn syrup solids, sucrose, lactose	33	Corn oil, monoglycerides, diglycerides	60	Skim milk, sodium caseinate	1:104	600	40	43
Carnation Instant (powder)*	1	135	Corn syrup solids, sucrose, lactose	31	Milk fat	58	Milk, soy protein, sodium caseinate	1:107	600	40	70
Lactose-Free, Intact Protein											
Ensure	1.1	143	Corn syrup solids, sucrose	37	Corn oil	37	Soy protein, sodium and calcium caseinate	1:186	450	32	38
Ensure Plus	1.5	197	Corn syrup solids, sucrose	53	Corn oil	55	Soy protein, sodium and calcium caseinate	1:171	600	32	34
Sustacal Liquid	1	138	Corn syrup solids, sucrose	23	Soy oil	60	Soy protein, sodium and calcium caseinate	1:104	625	40	53
Enrich	1.1	162	Soy polysaccharide, sucrose, hydrolyzed corn starch	37	Corn oil	40	Soy protein, sodium and calcium caseinate	1:156	480	37	40
Isocal	1	130	Glucose, oligosaccharides, corn syrup solids	44	Soy oil, MCTs	34	Soy protein, sodium and calcium caseinate	1:183	350	23	33
Osmolite	1	144	Corn syrup solids	38	Corn oil, soy oil, MCTs	40	Soy protein, sodium and calcium caseinate	1:186	300	25	23
Nutri-1000 LF	1	101	Corn syrup solids, sucrose	55	Corn oil, soy oil, monoglycerides, diglycerides	38	Soy protein, sodium and calcium caseinate	1:164	380	31	38
Magnacal	2	250	Corn syrup solids, sucrose, maltodextrins	80	Soy oil, monoglycerides, diglycerides	70	Sodium and calcium caseinate	1:179	520	43	32

Precision Isotonic	1	144	Glucose oligosaccharides, sucrose	30	Soy oil, monoglycerides, diglycerides	29	Egg albumin solids, sodium caseinate	1:208	300	33	25
Precision HN	1	217	Maltodextrins, sucrose	1.3	Soy oil, MCTs, monoglycerides, diglycerides	44	Egg albumin solids	1:149	560	43	23
Chemically Defined											
Flexical	1	154	Sucrose, dextrins	34	Soy oil, MCTs, monoglycerides, diglycerides	23	Casein hydrolysate, amino acids	1:272	550	15	32
Nutramigen (powder)*	0.67	86	Sucrose, tapioca starch	26	Corn oil	22	Casein hydrolysate	1:284	440	14	17
			Glucose oligo- and polysaccharides, sucrose, hydrolyzed corn starch		Sunflower oil, MCTs		Whey solids, soy and meat protein hydrolysates, amino acids	1:149	460	17	30
Elemental											
Vivonex	1	226	Glucose oligosaccharides	1.4	Safflower oil	20	Amino acids	1:313	550	37	30
Vivonex HN	1	211	Glucose oligosaccharides	0.9	Safflower oil	43	Amino acids	1:149	810	34	18
Vipep	1	170	Corn syrup solids, sucrose, corn starch	25	Corn oil, MCTs	25	Amino acids, oligopeptides, polypeptides	1:250	520	33	22
Special Formula											
Amin-Aid	2	324	Maltodextrins, sucrose	70	Partially hydrogenated soy oil	19	Essential amino acids	1:643	900	<3	<3
Hepatic Aid	1.6	287	Maltodextrins, sucrose	36	Soy oil, lecithin, monoglycerides, diglycerides	43	Amino acids	1:240	900	0	0
Lofenalac	0.67	86	Corn syrup	27	Corn oil	22	Casein hydrolysate	1:284	920	14	17
Modular Supplements											
MCT Oil	8	0	—	933	MCTs	0	—	—	20	0	0
Microlipid	4.5	0	—	500	Safflower oil	0	—	—	32	0	0
Polycose Liquid	2	500	Glucose oligosaccharides	0	—	0	—	—	850	27	6
Sumacal Plus	2.5	625	Glucose syrup solids, maltodextrins	0	—	0	—	0	860	12	11
Controlyte (powder)*	2.1	298	Corn starch hydrolysates	100	Vegetable oil	0.2	—	—	590	2.5	0.5
EMF (liquid)	2 (protein)	0	—	0	—	500	—	—	690	106	10
Citrotein (powder)*	0.7	129	Sucrose, maltodextrins	2	Vegetable oil, monoglycerides, diglycerides	43	Egg solids	1:102	500	32	20

NOTE: Composition varies with individual lot and with flavoring. Osmolality is approximately one quarter greater than osmolarity.
*Reconstituted as recommended by manufacturer to give the stated caloric density.
MCTs, medium chain triglycerides.
(From Paige, D. M. [1988]. *Clinical nutrition* [2nd ed.]. St. Louis, C. V. Mosby Co.)

Table 47–2. INDICATIONS FOR NASOENTERIC
TUBE FEEDING

Severe protein or calorie malnutrition
Anorexia
Fractures or neoplasms of head and neck preventing oral intake
Neurologic or psychiatric disorders, preventing oral intake
Coma or depressed mental state
Serious illness with very high metabolic requirements (burns)
Enterocutaneous fistulas
Short bowel syndrome
Bowel preparation for surgery in seriously ill or malnourished
  patients
Crohn's disease
Type I glycogen storage disease
Chemotherapy or radiotherapy
Renal or hepatic failure

From Feldman, E. B. [1988]. *Essentials of clinical nutrition.*
Philadelphia: F. A. Davis. Reproduced by permission.)

dominal wall, (3) an endoscopically placed percutaneous endoscopically guided gastrostomy (PEG) tube, or (4) cervical feeding esophagostomy or pharyngostomy. Occasionally, an enteral feeding tube called a jejunostomy is inserted into the small intestine, in which case bolus feedings are not tolerated and a continuous infusion pump must be used. The development of pliable, small-caliber feeding tubes and defined-formula diets and modular products has increased the tolerance and attractiveness of enteral feeding as opposed to parenteral routes.

Selection of enteral feeding products depends on the mode of administration, the patient's underlying nutritional difficulty, the route and rate of administration, product osmolarity, and nutrient content of the feedings. Diverse defined-formula diets can be either chemically defined or elemental and are constituted by combining set amounts of individual nutrients in a fixed polymeric formula (see Table 47–1). None of the commercially prepared general-purpose defined-formula diets contains vitamin K, although they do contain other vitamins in fixed amounts. Even though trace elements are included, patients on long-term enteral feedings should be monitored periodically to make sure they are receiving adequate amounts.

Persons receiving enteral nutrition should be monitored for commonly occurring side effects, including nausea and vomiting, diarrhea, constipation, and metabolic complications. Tube feeding metabolic complications, listed in order of decreasing frequency, include hyperkalemia, hyponatremia, hypophosphatemia, overhydration, hyperglycemia, hyperphosphatemia, and zinc deficiency (Feldman, 1988).

Parenteral Nutrition

Utilization of the parenteral route for administering nutritional support is the least preferable. Because of the increased risk of mechanical, metabolic, or septic complications, the greater expense, and the potential difficulties in managing parenteral administration, especially by nonprofessionals, enteral approaches are preferred, regardless of whether they are delivered in the home or the institutional setting. If the gastrointestinal tract is functioning, it is always the route of choice for administration. Parenteral feeding is used when the gastrointestinal tract is inaccessible or not functioning, or when it is functioning but is not capable of absorbing sufficient nutrients to meet metabolic requirements.

Parenteral nutritional support can be administered either peripherally or through a central line. Peripheral venous cannulation is indicated when intravenous administration of nutrient solutions with low osmolality is planned for limited periods of time. Peripheral intravenous nutritional support is used most effectively for weight maintenance in nonhypermetabolic patients (BEE less than 1800 kcal/day), for maintenance before initiating central parenteral feeding, or for supplementing tube feedings; it also is used to limit protein breakdown in stable postoperative patients whose oral intake is expected to return to adequate levels within 10 days (Goodwin & Wilmore, 1988).

All essential nutrients, including water, energy, protein in the form of essential amino acids, essential fatty acids, minerals, electrolytes, trace minerals, and vitamins, must be provided by TPN (Table 47–3). Sixty to 80 per cent of the calories are supplied by the dextrose solution. Twenty per cent lipid emulsions provide 1.1 to 2.0 kcal/ml owing to their glycerol and lipid (9 kcal/g) content. Although the exact requirements in cancer patients are unknown, it is generally recommended that least 20 per cent of daily energy requirements be provided as lipid (Feldman, 1988).

Solutions infused through a peripheral vein must be of appropriate osmolarity to prevent venous sclerosis and thrombophlebitis. The total concentrations of glucose, amino acids, and electrolytes determine the osmolarity of the infusate.

Different types of needles may be inserted to provided venous access, such as a butterfly needle, an over-the-needle (OTN) cannula, a through-the-needle (TTN) cannula, or a drum catheter.

Administration of parenteral nutrition through a long-term venous access device—TPN—requires placement of a central venous line into the subclavian vein or an alternative anatomic site that can tolerate high-volume, high-osmolality infusions. A Hickman or a Broviac catheter may be inserted near the suprasternal notch to provide access to the subclavian vein. Triple-lumen catheters may be inserted when the central line is required for administration of medications, such as antitumor or antimicrobial chemotherapy.

Administration of nutrition support through a central line requires the use of an infusion pump. Selected drugs, such as vasopressors, antiarrhythmics, heparin, insulin, oxytocin (Pitocin), and various chemotherapeutic agents, may also be administered using these pumps. Infusion pumps are electronic devices that deliver fluid at a relatively constant, preset flow rate. Three types of infusion pumps are (1) peristaltic, (2) piston syringe, or (3) piston cylinder cassette pumps. Peristaltic pumps work by applying an external force to the tubing of the intravenous administration set. Accuracy of peristaltic pumps depends on a number of factors: speed of the rotor, length of the tubing segment between rollers, amount of deformation of the tubing

Table 47–3. DEVELOPING A PRESCRIPTION FOR TOTAL
INTRAVENOUS FEEDING

Tasks	Examples—How To; What
1. Determine IBW	106 + 8 × 6 = 48 154 lb = 70 kg
2. Determine fluid requirements and tolerances	2000–3000 ml = "maintenance" if normal kidneys 700 ml = gastrointestinal replacement 500 ml = increased insensible losses (tachypnea) 360 ml/°C = 3200–4200 ml
3. Determine protein requirement 0.8 g/kg for maintenance 1.5+ for anabolism extra for stress	2 g/kg IBW × 70 kg (maintenance, anabolism, stress) = 140 g
4. Determine energy requirements	20 kcal/kg IBW for maintenance/activity 15 kcal/kg IBW for anabolism—for maximum N balance 25–50% above BEE = 5 kcal/kg IBW for stress = 40–45 kcal/kg × 70 kg = 2800–3150 kcal/day
5. Determine desired percentage fat calories (usual 20%)	500 ml 10% lipid emulsion provides 550 kcal (= 20% of caloric needs) 12 hr = 40 ml/hr
6. Determine glucose calories IV = 3.4 kcal/g	2800 kcal total required 550 kcal from lipid = 2250 kcal from glucose divide by 3.4 kcal/g IV glucose = 662 g glucose
7. Order amino acid–glucose solution	2700–3700 ml, 662 g dextrose, 140 g amino acids/24 hr = 110–150 ml/hr

Task 8. Add electrolytes based on preexisting deficiencies or excess

	Electrolyte	Needs (anabolic + NG replacement)*/day	
8. Add electrolytes based on preexisting deficiencies or excess	100 { Na, mEq	60–200 + ~60 = 120–260	
	K, mEq	60–200 + ~6 = 66–206	
	Cl, mEq	80–120 + ~70 = 150–190	
	20 { Mg, mEq	8–20 + — = 8–20	
	P, mMol	13–26 + — = 13–26	
	Ca, mEq	10–20 + — = 10–20	

9. Add vitamins	10 ml MVI-12 added each day. Suspect deficiency water soluble vitamins, add extra vitamins B and C

Task 10. Add trace elements

10. Add trace elements	Mineral	Needs (anabolic + GI replacement)/day	
	Zn, mg	2.5–4.0 + 8.4 = 11–12	
	Cu, mg	0.5–1.5 + — = 0.5–1.5	
	Mn, mg	1–2 + — = 1–2	
	Cr, μg	10–20 + — = 10–20	
	Add each day		

11. Order monitoring

12. Order catheter care

13. Order physical therapy—needed to replete somatic muscle

IBW, ideal body weight; N, nitrogen; IV, intravenous; NG, nasogastric; MVI-12, multiple vitamin infusion; GI, gastrointestinal; BEE, basal energy expenditure.

*Mixture of bile and gastric juice.

(From Feldman, E. B. [1988]. *Essentials of clinical nutrition.* Philadelphia: F. A. Davis.)

with use, and internal diameter of the tubing. Piston syringe pumps involve a prefilled syringe that delivers fluid at a constant rate by a pump motor that drives the syringe plunger. These pumps are usually used when small amounts of fluid are to be delivered. In the piston cylinder cassette pump, a small-volume syringe located in the line between the bottle and the patient alternately fills by positive pressure and expels its contents. Meticulous central venous catheter care, which is usually provided by the nurse, is essential to prevent catheter-related infectious complications, especially in the immunocompromised cancer patient. In addition, the central catheter should not be used for administration of blood products or for blood sampling. "Piggybacking" medications through the catheter should be avoided.

SPECIAL PROBLEMS ASSOCIATED WITH NUTRITIONAL DEPLETION

Early Satiety

Definition

Early satiety is experienced as a feeling of fullness shortly after beginning to ingest a meal. It may be caused by tumor directly infringing on the upper gastrointestinal tract and decreasing the size of the meal that can be ingested. Other causes of early satiety are delayed gastric emptying and decreased peristalsis. Early satiety frequently is absent at breakfast, mild at lunch, and severe by dinnertime.

Management

Interventions for early satiety include providing the largest proportion of required calories and protein for breakfast, when early satiety is minimal. Frequent small meals may allow for ingestion of adequate calories and protein. "Empty calorie" foods, such as diet drinks, coffee, and tea, should be avoided, especially at mealtimes. Ideally, every mouthful ingested should provide the maximum calories and protein possible. Use of nutritional supplements for patients suffering from early satiety is recommended.

Nausea and Vomiting

Definition

Nausea and vomiting are common symptoms experienced by cancer patients. Associated causes include radiation to the brain or the total body, fluid and electrolyte imbalances, chemotherapy or analgesic side effects, uremia, intestinal obstruction, brain and hepatic metastases, infections, and septicemia (Donaldson, 1984; Eyre & Ward, 1984; Reuben & Mor, 1986).

Nausea is an extremely uncomfortable sensation experienced in the back of the throat and epigastrium, which generally ends with vomiting. It may be accompanied by pallor, cold clammy skin, increased salivation, faintness, tachycardia, and diarrhea. Frequently, decreased gastric activity accompanies nausea.

Vomiting is an involuntary reflex by which the contents of the stomach and the intestine are expelled.

Vomiting is immediately preceded by widespread autonomic stimulation resulting in tachypnea, copious salivation, dilation of the pupils, sweating, pallor, and rapid heartbeat (Nord & Sodeman, 1985).

Several types of vomiting occur in cancer patients. When associated with the administration of chemotherapy, vomiting varies, depending on the emetic potential of the medications administered (Table 47–4). Anticipatory nausea and vomiting (ANV) is a learned phenomenon that is stimulated by something that occurs in association with the true stimulant. Learned stimuli include thoughts, sights, tastes, and odors related to the treatment. Because ANV is a learned response, it occurs after the first chemotherapeutic dose has been administered. Occurrence of ANV may increase with each successive cycle of chemotherapy. Vomiting also occurs in association with radiation therapy, obstructions, infections, and intestinal inflammatory diseases.

Pathophysiologic Mechanisms

Nausea and vomiting occur after stimulation of a complex reflex coordinated by the vomiting center in the medullary lateral reticular formation (Sallan & Cronin, 1985). Neurologic stimulation may occur in one or more of several pathways. Pathways most frequently involved in cancer patients include the chemoreceptor trigger zone, which responds to circulating levels of chemicals; the vagal visceral afferents, which respond to gastrointestinal pathology; the sympathetic visceral afferents, which respond to hollow organ pathology; and the cerebral cortex and limbic system, which respond to stimuli from the senses, anxiety, pain, and increases in intracranial pressure (Yasko,

Table 47–4. EMETIC POTENTIAL OF COMMON CHEMOTHERAPEUTIC AGENTS

Mild/Rare	Moderate	Severe and Common
Asparaginase	Actinomycin	Carmustine
Busulfan	Cyclophosphamide	Cisplatin
Bleomycin	Daunorubicin	Cyclophosphamide*
Chlorambucil	Doxorubicin	Dacarbazine
Cytarabine	Methotrexate	Hydroxyurea*
Diethylstilbestrol	Mitomycin	Lomustine
Dromostanolone		Mechlorethamine
Etoposide		Methotrexate*
Floxuridine		Mitotane
Fluorouracil		Nitrogen mustard
Leuprolide		Pipobroman
Medroxyprogesterone		Plicamycin
acetate		Procarbazine
Megestrol		Streptozocin
Melphalan		Uracil mustard
Mercaptopurine		
Polyestradiol		
Tamoxifen		
Testolactone		
Thioguanine		
Thio-TEPA		
Vinblastine		
Vincristine		

*High dose.

(From Grant, M. [1987b]. Nausea, vomiting and anorexia. *Seminars in Oncology Nursing, 3,* 277–286.)

1985). Mediation of stimuli is carried out by a variety of neurotransmitters, such as acetylcholine, dopamine, and serotonin.

Management

Clinical assessment of nausea and vomiting begins with a description of the patterns of occurrence and severity. As the patient moves from the potential for nausea and vomiting to the occurrence of moderate and severe symptoms, the assessment changes (Table 47–5). Interventions for nausea and vomiting include both pharmacologic and nonpharmacologic approaches (Grant, 1987a). Medications used to prevent and control these symptoms differ and depend on the cause and severity of the symptoms. Selection of the most appropriate antiemetic regimen is related to the different mechanisms involved. The classes of medications used and their mechanisms of action, side effects, and specific examples are given in Table 47–6. Nonpharmacologic approaches include dietary interventions and behavioral interventions. These are summarized in Table 47–7.

Helping patients to control and manage the distress associated with nausea and vomiting is a challenging area of oncology nursing. Improvements in both pharmacologic and nonpharmacologic interventions have provided the oncology nurse with a beginning understanding of how to provide skilled nursing care for these problems. Continued testing and refinement of this care are needed to support the patient and improve the quality of life in this vulnerable population.

Taste and Smell Changes

Definition

Changes in taste and smell have been documented in studies of both humans and animals with cancer. Even though mechanisms for development of these abnormalities have been studied extensively, many questions persist. Taste abnormalities may involve the development of a taste aversion, learned taste preferences, or changes in taste acuity. Development of taste and smell changes in cancer patients may be associated with administration of chemotherapy, radiation therapy, or tumor growth. For example, the occurrence of side effects such as nausea and vomiting with administration of specific chemotherapeutic agents can result in aversions to foods ingested during the course of therapy. Aversions may be stronger and may occur more quickly if new or novel foods are ingested (Bernstein, 1982). Aversions may disappear on completion of the therapy and when tumor growth has been stopped.

Common taste changes include aversions to meat and meat products, increased tolerance for sweet substances, and avoidance of foods taken during the time immediately surrounding treatment. Variations occur with individual patients.

Table 47–5. NURSING CARE PLAN FOR THE PATIENT WITH POTENTIAL NAUSEA AND VOMITING

Assessment	Expected Outcomes	Interventions
Determine whether patient or family expects nausea and vomiting (N&V)	Expectations of patient or family are realistic	Determine whether patient has a high potential for N&V related to the disease present and and the treatment Teach patient or family what to expect regarding N&V
Determine what the patient or family believes about the occurrence of N&V	Myths about the occurrence of N&V need to be corrected	Describe the causes of N&V and its relationship to disease and treatment
Determine what coping patterns patient usually uses to manage stress and discomfort	Patient manages to cope effectively with N&V	Identify previous successful coping behaviors; encourage patient to use these behaviors to manage N&V
Determine the potential for N&V depending on the treatment or stage of disease	Prevent or minimize N&V	Administer antiemetic agents as prescribed to prevent occurrence; institute nonpharmacologic measures
Identify patterns of occurrence, amount of distress, and effectiveness of interventions	Provide the most effective management of N&V	Evaluate effectiveness of interventions, revising approaches to provide the most effective relief of N&V and the associated distresses
Evaluate dietary intake	Maintain nutritional status	Provide for oral intake during times of least N&V; have patient avoid foods high in fat Provide frequent small meals
Identify environment most conducive to eating	Maintain adequate nutritional intake	Avoid areas with strong odors; provide a clean, pleasant environment for meals

Management

Interventions for taste and smell changes generally are individualized to the specific patient. However, some general guidelines are recommended. Protein sources should be derived from bland protein foods, such as milk and milk products, fish, and chicken. Beef and pork tend to taste bitter and should be avoided. When the "sweet" threshold is elevated, foods that ordinarily are considered too sweet will be acceptable. Some patients add additional sugar to sweeten foods more; other patients have reported a decrease in sweet threshold and develop an intolerance for anything sweet. For these patients, complex carbohydrates can be substituted to meet needed energy and carbohydrate requirements.

If supplements are used, a taste test is advised. The patient can then select the supplement that tastes best. To avoid developing specific taste intolerances, favorite foods should be avoided during periods of nausea and vomiting. Also, substituted food, such as supplements introduced during radiation therapy, may become the target for development of taste aversions. If supplements are required, switching supplements may prove to be more successful for the patient.

Mood Changes

Definition

Changes in moods are common in cancer patients. Depression and anxiety may occur before the diagnosis is confirmed, after the diagnosis is made, during treatment, and at the time of recurrences. These mood states tend to be accompanied by decreases in food intake. Careful monitoring of the type and timing of dietary intake is an initial step in evaluating the seriousness of the mood on food intake.

Management

Improving the environment for eating and providing familiar foods and familiar settings can be used to make meals more appealing. Presence of friends or family members during mealtimes also makes the atmosphere more pleasant and homelike for the patient. Disruptive interactions with family members should be avoided, and the nurse may need to ask family members to leave if such a situation arises. Providing rest before mealtime may help the patient be better prepared for eating. A positive and supportive approach helps the depressed or anxious patient to ingest adequate calories and protein.

Dysphagia

Definition

Problems with swallowing can pose a severe threat to maintaining adequate nutritional status. *Dysphagia* is a term used to identify difficulty swallowing (as opposed to the term *odynophagia,* which refers to painful swallowing [Greenberger, 1986]). Dysphagia is particularly likely to occur as a result of the local effects of tumors of the head and neck or the esophagus, or secondary to treatment, especially with radiation therapy or surgical resection. Surgical excision of structures important to swallowing, such as the tongue, the soft or bony palate, the supraglottic larynx, or the esophagus, is particularly likely to result in dysphagia.

Types of dysphagia relate to the three phases of swallowing—oral, pharyngeal, and esophageal. *Transfer dysphagia* refers to problems in the delivery of a

Table 47–6. ANTIEMETICS USED FOR NAUSEA AND VOMITING IN CANCER PATIENTS

Pharmacologic Effects	Side Effects and Toxicities	Comments	Examples (including Routes and Common Dosages)
Anticholinergics Depress vestibular stimuli Suppress emetic center	Sedation	Effective in nausea and vomiting due to motion sickness	Scopolamine transdermal
Antihistamines Depress cerebral cortex Depress vestibular stimuli Inhibit histamine-mediated stimuli	Drowsiness (frequently a desired effect) Anticholinergic effects at high doses	Most effective in nausea and vomiting due to motion sickness Used primarily in combination antiemetic regimens	Diphenhydramine: PO, IM, IV, 25–50 mg
Barbiturates Depress CNS	Respiratory depression Somnolence	Action potentiated when administered with phenothiazines Used primarily in combination antiemetic regimens	Pentobarbital: PO, 100 mg Secobarbital PO, IV, 100 mg
Benzodiazepines Depress CNS Produce amnesic effects	Sedation	Sedation effects may compromise older patients and those with known respiratory difficulty Amnesic effects considered an advantage Used in combination antiemetic regimens	Lorazepam: IV, 0.05 mg/kg Diazepam: PO, 5 mg; IM, 2.5 mg
Benzoquinolizines Suppress CTZ Anxiolytic Anticholinergic activity	Sedation Hypersensitivity Rare hypotension	Clinical trials report controversial results on efficacy	Benzquinamide: IM, IV, 25–50 mg Trimethobenzamide: PO, 250 mg; IV, 200 mg
Butyrophenones Suppress CTZ Block dopamine-mediated stimuli Decrease vestibular stimuli Anxiolytic	Hypertension Extrapyramidal effects Sedation and somnolence Agitation and restlessness	Side effects partly controlled with diphenhydramine Tolerance develops after repeated doses	Haloperidol: PO, IM, 2–5 mg; IV, 2 mg Droperidol: IM, IV, 1–3 mg
Cannabinoids Anticholinergic activity Other unknown	Extrapyramidal effects, including ataxia, hallucinations, dysphoria, hypertension, euphoria, frank psychosis Somnolence	Side effects fewer in younger patients or experienced user Abuse potential	Marijuana cigarettes Delta-9-tetrahydrocannabinol: PO, 5–15 mg/M^2 Levonantradol: PO, 0.05–1.5 mg
Phenothiazines Suppress CTZ Block dopamine-mediated stimuli Depress emetic center Inhibit autonomic effects via the vagus nerve	Faintness, nasal stuffiness, dry mouth, palpitations, orthostatic hypotension, constipation Hypersensitivity Extrapyramidal effects Jaundice, blood dyscrasias	Diphenhydramine used for side effects Good for mild nausea Causes sedation	Prochlorperazine: PO, IM, IV, 10 mg; rectal, 25 mg Thiethylperazine: PO, IM, IV, rectal, 10 mg Chlorpromazine: PO, IM, IV, rectal, 12.5–50 mg Promethazine: PO, IM, IV, rectal, 25 mg
Steroids Possible prostaglandin inhibition	Lethargy Weakness Generalized swelling	Used primarily in combination antiemetic regimens	Dexamethazone: PO, 4–10 mg; IM, IV, 10–20 mg Methyl prednisone: IV, 250 mg
Substituted Benzamides Suppress CTZ Block dopamine-mediated stimuli Anticholinergic activity	Extrapyramidal effects such as anxiety, restlessness, dystonia	Side effects decreased in patients under 40 Side effects partly controlled with diphenhydramine	Metoclopramide: IV, 1–3 mg/kg

CNS, central nervous system; CTZ, Chemotactic trigger zone. (From Grant, M. [1987b]. Nausea, vomiting & anorexia. *Seminars in Oncology Nursing, 3,* 277–286.)

bolus of food or fluid from the mouth into the esophagus, involving dysfunction of the mouth or tongue, pharynx, or hypopharynx. Transfer dysphagia frequently results from neuromuscular incoordination of these areas. It may also be caused by carcinoma of the mouth, tongue, or hypopharyngeal region. Cricopharyngeal dysfunction is another common cause of transfer dysphagia. *Transport dysphagia* is an esophageal problem in which transport of the bolus down the body of the esophagus is altered. The presence of an extrinsic

Table 47-7. NONPHARMACOLOGIC INTERVENTIONS FOR NAUSEA AND VOMITING

Nutrition Interventions
Adjust time of eating to coordinate with periods of least nausea and vomiting
Avoid foods that precipitate nausea and vomiting (e.g., foods high in fat content, spicy foods, or foods patient associates with nausea and vomiting)
Provide foods that are bland, easily digestible, and still nutritious (e.g., crackers, baked and boiled foods, sodas, mild fruits and vegetables)
Use nutritional supplements to provide maximum calories and protein with a minimum of intake
Avoid favorite foods during periods of nausea and vomiting to avoid developing aversions to these foods
Provide small meals, pleasant environment, and good company during mealtimes
Behavior Interventions
Use distraction to decrease distress during periods of nausea and vomiting (e.g., music, television, radio)
Teach the patient behavior techniques (e.g., hypnosis, guided imagery, biofeedback, and progressive muscle relaxation)

or intrinsic lesion, such as a tumor or stricture, obstructing the esophageal lumen can cause transport dysphagia. Weak, absent, or disorganized peristaltic activity of the esophagus is another source of transport dysphagia. Finally, *delivery dysphagia,* or problems with bolus entry into the stomach, also can occur. Benign or malignant obstructing lesions, such as tumors or strictures, or lower esophageal sphincter dysfunction can produce this problem.

Management

Thorough assessment of potential or existing problems with dysphagia is an important first step, in addition to evaluation of the patient's current nutritional status. Signs and symptoms to observe for and report include (1) choking when swallowing liquids or solids; (2) drooling, regurgitation, or retention of food accompanying swallowing of liquids or solids; (3) food sticking in the pharynx or esophagus; (4) pain or discomfort when swallowing liquids or solids; (5) weakness of lips, tongue, or jaw; and (6) lesions in the oral cavity.

Some relatively simple interventions help minimize or eliminate dysphagia (Grady, Farnen, Ascheman, Passman, & Palazola, 1985). The patient should sit with his or her head elevated at least 45 degrees while eating or drinking and should maintain that upright position for 15 to 30 min after finishing. Six to eight frequent, small feedings are more desirable than three big meals. Milk products should be avoided if mucus is copious. When aspiration is feared or likely, suction apparatus should be readily available. When the oral musculature is defective, bites should make use of the strong side of the mouth. If propelling the bolus to the posterior part of the tongue is a problem, food should be placed on the posterior part of the tongue with a syringe or long-handled spoon.

The following swallowing exercise or technique is helpful to prevent aspiration: (1) flex the neck; (2) inhale; (3) place a small amount of food on the tongue; (4) consciously hold the breath while swallowing; (5)

exhale and gently cough or clear the throat; and (6) wait at least 30 seconds between swallows.

Dysphagia involving the oral musculature may be improved by providing semisolid foods (puddings, canned fruit, mashed potatoes) when chewing is impaired; by consuming thin, pureed foods; or by placing food on the posterior part of the tongue with a long-handled spoon (DeLisa, Miller, Melnick, Mikulic, & Gerber, 1985; Donoghue, 1988). Dysphagia involving the pharyngeal phase of swallowing may be minimized by alternating solids and liquids, making postural changes, or performing the swallowing exercises described earlier. Esophageal dysphagia may require use of food supplements or ultimately enteral nutritional support.

Malabsorption and Diarrhea

Definition

Expressed functionally, diarrhea is too much of a too loose or liquid stool. Tremendous variation exists as to what different people consider to be "normal" in terms of their usual bowel function. A change in bowel habits is implicit in the identification of diarrhea as a problem for the patient with cancer. Clinically, significant alterations in stool frequency, fluidity, or abnormal constituents herald diarrhea; however, stool weight greater than 300 g on the usual Western diet is an operational definition of diarrhea (Greenberger, 1986).

Pathophysiologic Mechanisms

Understanding of the potential pathophysiologic mechanisms of diarrhea is essential to its identification and management. Diarrhea can be classified according to one of three predominant mechanisms—secretory, osmotic, or mixed. Table 47-8 summarizes information regarding the three classifications of diarrhea mechanisms in terms of (1) actual pathophysiologic mechanism, (2) characteristics of the diarrhea and its fluid composition, and (3) cancer-related examples.

Etiology. Diarrhea that is specific to the person with cancer can result either from the tumor itself or from its treatment. Examples of conditions causing diarrhea that are directly tumor-related include carcinoma of the pancreas (osmotic, from inadequate digestive enzymes); carcinoid syndrome (secretory, from serotonin or prostaglandins); villous adenoma (secretory, from unidentified secretagogue); medullary carcinoma of the thyroid (secretory, from calcitonin or prostaglandins); tumors producing vasoactive intestinal peptide (VIP) (secretory, from VIP); Zollinger-Ellison syndrome (secretory, from gastrin); and tumors that infiltrate the small or large intestine (osmotic from decreased absorption of solutes).

Each of the modalities employed in cancer treatment—surgical resection, chemotherapy, radiation therapy to fields including the gastrointestinal tract, or immunotherapy—potentially involves anatomic or physiologic alterations that can lead to diarrhea (Cul-

Table 47–8. PATHOPHYSIOLOGIC MECHANISMS OF DIARRHEA

Type of Diarrhea	Mechanism	Characteristics and Composition	Cancer-Related Examples
Osmotic	Unabsorbable or poorly absorbable solute in gastrointestinal tract	24-hr stool volume usually <1 L Stool volume decreases when fasting Potassium lost in excess of sodium Net effect is water and potassium depletion rather than electrolyte depletion Stool pH acidic <7	Lactose intolerance Cathartics Postgastrectomy
Secretory	Increased secretory activity of gastrointestinal tract (absorption may be normal); also from inhibition of electrolyte and water absorption	24-hr stool volume usually >1 L (large stool volume) Stool volume does not decrease when fasting Sodium lost in excess of potassium Net effect is electrolyte depletion Stool pH neutral, 7	Non-beta islet cell tumors of pancreas Zollinger-Ellison syndrome Villous adenoma Medullary carcinoma of thyroid
Mixed	Hypermotility states involve increased rate of transit; osmotic effect of ingested solutes occurs from rapid intestinal transit and diminished net absorption	Variable	Cholinergic medication Carcinoid syndrome

(Adapted from Greenberger, N.J. [1986.] Gastrointestinal disorders: *A Pathophysiologic Approach* [3rd ed.]. Chicago: Year Book Medical Publishers.)

hane, 1983). When these treatments are used in combination, the results can be compounded. In addition, medications that are used to treat side effects of antitumor therapy, such as antacids, antibiotics, or colchicine, can also secondarily cause diarrhea. Lactose intolerance, occurring temporarily from radiation therapy or chemotherapy or permanently from surgical resection, can also cause diarrhea. Increased stress or anxiety can produce increased gastric motility that then results in diarrhea. Malnutrition itself can contribute to the occurrence of diarrhea as a result of decreased functioning absorptive surface in the intestine. Finally, supplemental feedings with products whose osmolality is high can produce an osmotic diarrhea.

Management

Thoughtful evaluation to determine the cause of the diarrhea, as well as confirmation of it as a problem, provides a firm foundation for planning interventions for the cancer patient (Davis, 1985). A careful and thorough history that includes review of signs and symptoms, medications, dietary and nutritional status, usual patterns of elimination, prior surgeries, and concurrent medical conditions is essential. Management may emphasize, but is not limited to, dietary and pharmacologic measures. Treatment of underlying conditions, such as pancreatic insufficiency, hyperthyroidism, or diabetes mellitus, is essential when they are thought to play a significant role.

Assessment should include consideration of (1) ability to care for oneself, including food acquisition and preparation; (2) tolerance of activity and exercise; (3) gastrointestinal discomfort; (4) family and support systems; (5) sources of stress and anxiety; (6) usual patterns of elimination; (7) pattern of diarrhea (onset, duration, amount, appearance, frequency); (8) associated symptoms (cramping, flatus, abdominal distention); (9) possibility of partial fecal obstruction; (10) nutritional status and requirements, including fluid and electrolyte balance; (11) dietary patterns; (12) sleep-rest patterns and level of fatigue; (13) perineal-perianal skin integrity; and (14) effect on usual life style (Ropka, 1985).

Interventions should be developed that (1) are based on information acquired from the assessment and (2) consider both the cause and pathophysiologic mechanism of the diarrhea. Providing the patient with appropriate information is particularly important.

Pharmacologic agents for control of diarrhea, such as Kaopectate (Upjohn), Lomotil (Searle), Immodium, low-dose codeine, or bulk-forming agents should be administered as directed. Patients should be cautioned to observe for side effects or toxicities of these medications and should be advised about what to report to their health care provider. Many antacids contain substances that work osmotically, such as magnesium. When antacids are required on a regular basis, their selection should include consideration of bowel status, avoiding antacids that contain magnesium if diarrhea is a concurrent problem.

Nutritional and dietary considerations are important in the management of diarrhea, both to decrease the occurrence of diarrhea and to ensure adequate nutritional status. They include the following: (1) eat low-residue foods that are high in protein and calories; (2) attempt small, frequent snacks rather than three large meals per day; (3) avoid foods that irritate or stimulate the gastrointestinal tract; (4) avoid extreme temperatures in foods or beverages; (5) eliminate foods that are highly spiced or greasy; (6) ensure adequate intake of uncarbonated fluids (2 to 3 quarts per day), best served at room temperature; (7) eliminate lactose-containing foods and beverages to prevent lactose intolerance; (8) utilize nutritional supplements to increase calorie and protein intake; (9) consider a liquid diet or enteral nutritional support if diarrhea becomes severe.

Local and systemic measures that will increase comfort are essential. Heat may be applied to the abdomen to relieve the discomfort of cramping. Substances that protect skin and mucous membranes and promote healing, such as A & D ointment, Desitin, or Nupercainal can be applied to the perirectal area. Local anesthetics, such as Tucks, may be used around the rectum. Sitz baths may provide further comfort. The rectal area and perineum should be gently and thoroughly cleaned, followed by careful drying after each bowel movement. Anal or rectal stimulation should be avoided.

Constipation

Definition

The occurrence of constipation is common in cancer patients. Prevention of this symptom by active management in vulnerable patients is of utmost importance. Constipation occurs when the stool becomes hard, dry, and difficult to pass, or when bowel movements are so infrequent that patients experience abdominal discomfort.

Etiology

Constipation in the cancer patient may occur as a result of decreased motility of the gastrointestinal tract, metabolic changes such as hypocalcemia, inadequate food intake, decreased exercise, and medications such as narcotics and vinca alkaloids. The environment of the cancer patient may have an effect on the occurrence of constipation because of hospital admission, the need for using a bedpan, a lack of privacy, and a change in normal daily routines.

Management

Management of constipation begins with a thorough assessment of the patient via a comprehensive history and physical examination. Evaluation should include a review of medications, diet, and liquid intake. Symptoms to look for include a distended abdomen with palpable colon, abdominal discomfort, hypoactive bowel sounds, and a history of no bowel movement for more than 2 days despite oral intake of food. A small amount of diarrhea may also be present, and hard stool may be palpable in the rectum.

Nutritional and dietary considerations effective in the treatment of constipation include increasing fluid intake to more than six glasses of water per day and increasing the fiber content of the diet. When pain medications are ordered, they should be accompanied by increased fluids, increased fiber, and specific medications such as Peri-Colace or Doxidan (Brooks, 1978; Portenoy, 1987). If fecal impaction is present, manual evacuation may be needed and can be preceded by a stool softener.

Patients and their families need to be educated to monitor bowel movements, maintain fluid intake, increase fiber sources, and avoid constipating foods such as dairy products and fried foods. The best approach to constipation is to identify a potential problem and vigorously implement approaches to prevent both constipation and impaction.

SUMMARY

Alterations in nutrition are common in cancer patients. They may occur at any stage of disease but are most common during treatment and when tumors are extensive. Anorexia and cachexia are frequently present in terminally ill patients. Skillful and creative nursing care is essential in individualizing approaches to maintaining patients' nutritional status.

References

American Society of Parenteral and Enteral Nutritional Board of Directors. (1986). Guidelines for use of total parenteral nutrition in the hospitalized patient. *Journal of Parenteral and Enteral Nutrition, 10,* 441–445.

Beck, A. (1972). *Depression: Causes and treatment.* Philadelphia: University of Pennsylvania Press.

Bernstein, I. L. (1982). Physiological and psychological mechanisms of cancer anorexia. *Cancer Research, 42,* 7155–7205.

Bernstein, I. L. (1986). Etiology of anorexia in cancer. *Cancer, 58*(Suppl. 8), 1881–1886.

Bernstein, I. L., & Bernstein, I. D. (1981). Learned food aversions and cancer anorexia. *Cancer Treatment Reports, 65*(Suppl. 5), 43–47.

Blackburn, G. L., Bistrian, B. R., & Miani, B. S. (1976). Nutritional and metabolic assessment of the hospitalized patient. *Surgical Clinics of North America, 56,* 1192–1225.

Blackburn, G. L., & Harvey, K. B. (1980). Clinical nutritional assessment of the hospitalized patient. In P. J. Garry (Ed.), *Human nutrition: Clinical and biochemical aspects* (pp. 15–26). Washington, DC: American Association for Clinical Chemistry.

Bozzetti, F., Pagnoni, A. M., & Del Vecchio, M. (1980). Excessive caloric expenditure as a cause of malnutrition in patients with cancer. *Surgery, Gynecology, and Obstetrics, 150,* 229–234.

Brennan, M. F., (1977). Uncomplicated starvation versus cancer cachexia. *Cancer Research, 37,* 2359–2364.

Brooks, F. (1978). *Gastrointestinal pathophysiology.* New York: Oxford University Press.

Buzby, G. P., Mullen, J. L., Matthews, D. C., Hobbs, C. L., & Rosata, E. F. (1980). Prognostic nutrition index in gastrointestinal surgery. *American Journal of Surgery, 139,* 160–167.

Carmichael, M. J., Clague, M. B., Keir, M. J., & Johnston, I. D. A. (1980). Whole body protein turnover, synthesis and breakdown in patient with colorectal carcinoma. *British Journal of Surgery, 67,* 736–739.

Copeland, E. M., MacFayden, B. V., MacComb, W. S., Guillamondegui, O., Jesse, R. H., & Dudrick, S. J. (1975). Intravenous hyperalimentation in patients with head and neck cancer. *Cancer, 35,* 606–611.

Copeland, E. M., Souchon, E. A., MacFadyen, V. V., Rapp, M. A., & Dudrick, S. J. (1977). Intravenous hyperalimentation as an adjunct to radiation therapy. *Cancer, 39,* 609–616.

Costa, G. (1977). Cachexia, the metabolic component of neoplastic diseases. *Cancer Research, 37,* 2327–2336.

Costa, G., & Donaldson, S. S. (1979). Current concepts in cancer: Effects of cancer and cancer treatment on the nutrition of the host. *New England Journal of Medicine, 300,* 1417–1474.

Culhane, B. (1983). Diarrhea. In J. M. Yasko (Ed.), *Guidelines for cancer care: Symptom management* (pp. 188–197). Reston, VA: Reston Publishing.

Davis, J. D., & Campbell, C. S. (1973). Peripheral control of meal size in the rat: Effect of sham feeding on meal size and drinking rats. *Journal of Comparative and Physiological Psychology, 83,* 379–387.

Davis, M. (1985). Bowel elimination, alterations in: Diarrhea. In J. C. McNally, J. C. Stair, & E. T. Somerville (Eds.), *Guidelines for cancer nursing practice* (pp. 239–242). Orlando, FL: Grune & Stratton, Inc.

DeLisa, J. A., Miller, R. M., Melnick, R. R., Mikulic, M. A., & Gerber, L. H. (1985). Rehabilitation of the cancer patient: Nutrition and glutition. In V. T. DeVita, Jr., S. Hellman, & S. A. Rosenberg (Eds.), *Cancer: Principles and practice of oncology* (2nd ed., pp. 2168–2169). Philadelphia: J. B. Lippincott Co.

Dempsey, D. T., Feurer, I. D., Knox, L. S., Crosby, L. O., Buzby, G. P., & Mullen, J. L. (1984). Energy expenditure in malnourished gastrointestinal cancer patients. *Cancer, 53,* 1265–1273.

Detsky, A. S., Baker, J. P., O'Rourke, D., & Goel, V. (1987). Perioperative parental nutrition: A meta-analysis. *Annals of Internal Medicine, 107,* 195–203.

DeWys, W. D., Begg, C., Lavin, P. T., Band, P. R., Bennett, J. M., Bertino, J. R., Cohen, M. H., Douglass, H. O., Engstrom, P. F., Ezdinli, E. Z., Horton, J., Johnson, C., Silverstein, N. M., Skeel, R. T., Sponzo, R. W., & Tormey, D. C. (1980). Prognostic effect of weight loss prior to chemotherapy in cancer patients. *American Journal of Medicine, 69,* 491–497.

DeWys, W. D., Costa, G., & Henkin, R. (1981). Clinical parameters related to anorexia. *Cancer Treatment Reports, 65*(Suppl. 5), 49–52.

DeWys, W. D., & Walters, K. (1975). Abnormalities of taste sensation in cancer patients. *Cancer, 36,* 1888–1896.

Dickerson, J. W. T. (1983). Nutrition of the cancer patient. In H. H. Draper (Ed.), *Advances in Nutritional Research* (pp. 105–131). New York: Plenum Press.

Donaldson, S. S. (1984). Nutritional support as an adjunct to radiation therapy. *Journal of Parenteral and Enteral Nutrition, 8,* 302–310.

Donoghue, M. (1988). Dysphagia. In S. B. Baird (Ed.), *Decision making in oncology nursing* (pp. 96–97). Toronto: B. C. Decker.

Eyre, H. . & Ward, J. H. (1984). Control of cancer chemotherapy-induced nausea and vomiting. *Cancer 54,* 2642–2648.

Feldman, E. B. (1988). *Essentials of clinical nutrition.* Philadelphia: F. A. Davis.

Friedman, M. I., & Stricker, E. M. (1976). The physiological psychology of hunger: A physiological perspective. *Psychological Review, 83,* 409–424.

Frohse, F., Brodel, M., & Schlossberg, L. (1985). *Atlas of human anatomy* (pp. 62–67). New York: Barnes and Noble.

Goodwin, C. W., & Wilmore, D. W. (1988). Enteral and parenteral nutrition. In Paige, D. M., Jacobson, H. N., Owen, G. M., Sherwin, R., Solomons, N., & Young, V. R. (Eds.), *Clinical nutrition* (2nd ed, pp. 476–503). St. Louis: C. V. Mosby Co.

Goodwin, W. J., & Torres, J. (1984). The value of the Prognostic Nutritional Index in the management of patients with advanced carcinoma of the head and neck. *Head and Neck Surgery, 6,* 932–937.

Gormican, A. (1980). Influencing food acceptance in anorexic cancer patients. *Postgraduate Medicine, 68,* 145–152.

Grady, R. P., Farnen, J., Ascheman, P., Passman, B., & Palazola, S. M. (1985). Nutrition, alteration in: Less than body requirements related to dysphagia. In J. C. McNally, J. C. Stair, & E. T. Somerville (Eds.), *Guidelines for cancer nursing practice* (pp. 239–242). Orlando, FL: Grune & Stratton, Inc.

Grant, J. P., Custer, P. B., & Thurlow, J. (1981). Current techniques of nutritional assessment. *Surgical Clinics of North America, 61,* 437–463.

Grant, M. (1987a). Nausea and vomiting. In Nursing Management of Common Problems. *Proceedings of the Fifth National Conference on Cancer Nursing,* American Cancer Society, September, pp. 16–24.

Grant, M. (1987b). Nausea, vomiting, and anorexia. *Seminars in Oncology Nursing, 3:*277–286.

Greenberger, N. J. (1986). *Gastrointestinal disorders: A pathophysiologic approach* (3rd ed.). Chicago: Year Book Medical Publishers.

Grijalva, C. V., & Lindholm, E. (1982). The role of the autonomic nervous system in hypothalamic feeding syndromes. *Appetite, 3,* 111–124.

Harris, J. A., & Benedict, F. G. (1919). *Biometric studies of basal metabolism in man.* Publication No. 279. Washington, DC: Carnegie Institute of Washington.

Heber, D. (1989). Metabolic pathology of cancer malnutrition. *Nutrition, 5,* 135–137.

Heber, D., Byerley, L. O., Chi, J., Grosvenor, M., Bergmon, R. N., Coleman, M., & Chlebowski, R. (1986). Pathophysiology of malnutrition in the adult cancer patient. *Cancer, 58,* 1867–1873.

Heber, D., Chlebowski, R. T., Meguid, M., & McAndrew, P. (1986). Malnutrition in cancer: Mechanisms and therapy. *Nutrition International, 2,* 184–187.

Holland, M. C. B., Rowland, J., & Plumb, M. (1977). Psychological aspects of anorexia in cancer patients. *Cancer Research, 37,* 2425–2428.

Holman, S. R. (1987). *Essentials of nutrition for the health professions.* Philadelphia: J. B. Lippincott Co.

Holroyde, C. P., & Reichard, G. A. (1986). General metabolic abnormalities in cancer patients: Anorexia and cachexia. *Surgical Clinics of North America, 66,* 947–956.

Hooley, R., Levine, H., Flores, T. C., Wheeler, T., & Steiger, E. (1983). Predicting postoperative head and neck complications using nutritional assessment: The Prognostic Nutritional Index. *Archives of Otolaryngology, 109,* 83–85.

Johnston, C. A., Keane, T. J., & Prudo, S. M. (1982). Weight loss in patients receiving radical radiation therapy for head and neck cancer: A prospective study. *Journal of Parenteral and Enteral Nutrition, 6,* 399–402.

Kaempfer, S. H., & Lindsey, A. M. (1986). Energy expenditure in cancer: A review. *Cancer Nursing, 9,* 194–199.

Kamath, S., Mams, P. B., Lad, T. E., Kohrs, M. B., & McGuire, W. P. (1983). Taste thresholds of patients with cancer of the esophagus. *Cancer, 52,* 386–389.

Kaminski, M. V., Nasr, N. J., Moss, A. J., Berger, R. L., & Sriran, K. (1982). Nutritional status, immunity and survival in neoplastic disease. *Nutritional Support Services, 2,* 7–13.

Kinney, J. M., & Roe, C. F. (1962). Caloric equivalent of fever. I. Patterns of postoperative response. *Annals of Surgery, 156,* 610–622.

Knobf, M. K. P. (1985). Weight gain and adjuvant chemotherapy. *Oncology Nursing Forum, 12*(6); 13–22.

Knox, L. S., Crosby, L. O., Feurer, I. D., Buzby, G. P., Miller, C. L., & Mullen, J. L. (1983). Energy expenditure in malnourished cancer patients. *Annals of Surgery, 197,* 152–162.

Krause, R., Humphrey, C., von Meyenfeldt, M., James, H., & Fischer, J. E. (1981). A central mechanism for anorexia in cancer: A hypothesis. *Cancer Treatment Reports, 65,* 15–21.

Kurzer, M., & Meguid, M. M. (1986). Cancer and protein metabolism. *Surgical Clinics of North America, 66,* 969–1001.

Lawrence, W., Jr. (1979). Effects of cancer on nutrition. *Cancer, 43* (Suppl.), 2020–2029.

Lindsey, A. M., Piper, B. F., & Stotts, N. A. (1982). The phenomenon of cancer cachexia: A review. *Oncology Nursing Forum, 9*(2), 38–42.

Long, C. L., Schaffel, N., Geiger, J. W., Schiller, W. R., & Blackmore, W. S. (1979). Metabolic response to injury and illness: Estimation of energy and protein needs from indirect calorimetry and nitrogen balance. *Journal of Parenteral and Enteral Nutrition, 3,* 452–456.

Lundholm, K., Edstrom, S., Ekman, L., Karlberg, I., & Schersten, T. (1981). Metabolism in peripheral tissues in cancer patients. *Cancer Treatment Reports, 65,* 79–83.

Lundholm, K. G. (1986). Body compositional changes in cancer patients. *Surgical Clinics of North America, 66,* 1013–1023.

Maillet, J. O. (1987). The cancer patient (pp. 243–264). In C. E. Lange (Ed.), *Nutritional support in critical care.* Rockville, MD: Aspen.

Mayer, J. (1955). Regulation of energy intake and body weight. The glucostatic theory and the lipostatic hypothesis. *Annals of the New York Academy of Sciences, 63,* 15–43.

McAndrew, P. (1986). Fat metabolism and cancer. *Surgical Clinics of North America, 66,* 1003–1012.

McGeer, A. J., Detsky, A. S., & O'Rourke, K. (1990). Parenteral nutrition in cancer patients undergoing chemotherapy: A meta-analysis. *Nutrition, 6,* 233–240.

Mellinkoff, S. M., Frankland, D., & Boyle, D. (1956). Relationship between serum amino acid concentration and fluctuations in appetite. *Journal of Applied Physiology, 8,* 535–538.

Moog, F. (1981). The lining of the small intestine. *Scientific American, 245*(5), 154–203.

Moore, F. D., Olesen, K. H., McMurrey, J. D., Parker, M. R., Ball, N., & Boyden, C. M. (1963). *The body cell mass and its supporting environment.* Philadelphia: W. B. Saunders Co.

Morrison, S. D. (1976). Theoretical review: Control of food intake in cancer cachexia: A challenge and a tool. *Physiology and Behavior, 17,* 705–614.

Mossman, K. L., & Henkin, R. I. (1978). Radiation-induced changes in taste acuity in cancer patients. *International Journal of Radiation Oncology, Biology, Physics, 4,* 663–670.

Muller, J. M., Keller, H. W., Brenner, U., Walter, M., & Holzmuller, W. (1986). Indications and effects of preoperative parenteral nutrition. *World Journal of Surgery, 10,* 53–63.

Nichols, M., Maickel, R. P., & Yim, G. K. W. (1983). Increased central serotonergic activity associated with nocturnal anorexia induced by Walker 256 carcinoma. *Life Sciences, 32,* 1819–1825.

Nixon, D. W., Heymsfield, S. B., Cohen, A. E., Kutner, M. H., Ansley, J., Lawson, D. H., & Rudman, D. (1980). Protein-calorie undernutrition in hospitalized cancer patients. *American Journal of Medicine, 68,* 683–690.

Nord, H. J., & Sodeman, W. A. (1985). The stomach. In W. A. Sodeman & T. M. Sodeman (Eds.), *Sodeman's pathologic physiology: Mechanisms of disease* (pp. 787–791). Philadelphia, W. B. Saunders Co.

Novin, D., & VanderWeele, D. A. (1977). Visceral involvement in feeding: There is more to regulation than the hypothalamus. *Progress in Psychological and Physiological Psychology, 7,* 193–241.

Ollenschlager, G., Konkol, K., & Modder, B. (1988). Indications for and results of nutritional therapy in cancer patients. *Recent Results in Cancer Research, 108,* 172–184.

Paige, D. M. (1988). *Clinical nutrition* (2nd ed.). St. Louis, C. V. Mosby Co.

Peck, A., & Boland, J. (1977). Emotional reactions to radiation treatment. *Cancer, 40,* 180–184.

Peteet, J. R., Medeiros, C., Slavin, L., & Walsh-Burke, K. (1981). Psychological aspects of artificial feeding in cancer patients. *Journal of Parenteral and Enteral Nutrition, 5,* 138–140.

Portenoy, R. K. (1987). Constipation in the cancer patient: Causes and management. *Medical Clinics of North America, 71,* 303–311.

Reuben, D. B., & Mor, F. (1986). Nausea and vomiting in terminal cancer patients. *Archives of Internal Medicine, 146,* 2021–2023.

Rolls, E. T. (1981). Central nervous system mechanism related to feeding and appetite. *British Medical Bulletin, 37,* 131–134.

Rombeau, J. L., Caldwell, M. D., Forlaw, L., & Guenter, P. A. (1989). *Atlas of nutritional support techniques* (p. 54). Boston: Little, Brown & Co.

Ropka, M. E. (1985). Nutrition. In B. L. Johnson & J. Gross (Eds.), *Handbook of oncology nursing* (pp. 185–227). New York: John Wiley.

Ruberg, R. L. (1984). Role of nutrition in wound healing. *Surgical Clinics of North America, 64,* 705–714.

Sallan, S. E., & Cronin, C. M. (1985). Nausea and vomiting. In V. T. DeVita, Jr., S. Hellman, & S. A. Rosenberg (Eds.), *Cancer: Principles and practice of oncology* (pp. 2008–2013). Philadelphia: J. B. Lippincott Co.

Schmale, A. H. (1979). Psychological aspects of anorexia: Areas for study. *Cancer, 43,* 2087–2092.

Shils, M. E. (1979). Principles of nutritional therapy. *Cancer, 143,* 2093–2102.

Smith, F. P., Kisner, D., & Schein, P. S. (1980). Nutrition and cancer: Prospects for clinical research. *Nutrition and Cancer, 2,* 34–39.

Spector, N. H., Brobeck, J. R., & Hamilton, C. L. (1968). Feeding and core temperature in albino rats: Changes induced by preoptic heating and cooling. *Science, 161,* 286–288.

Stein, T. P. (1978). Cachexia, gluconeogenesis and progressive weight loss in cancer patients. *Journal of Theoretical Biology, 73,* 51–59.

Toates, F. M. (1981). The control of ingestive behavior by internal and external stimuli—a theoretical review. *Appetite, 2,* 35–50.

Viteri, F. E., & Torun, B. (1988). Protein-energy malnutrition. In D. M. Paige, H. N. Jacobson, G. M. Owen, R. Sherwin, N. Solomons, & V. R. Young (Eds.), *Clinical nutrition* (2nd ed., pp. 531–546). St. Louis: C. V. Mosby Co.

Warnold, I., Lundholm, K., & Schersten, T. (1978). Energy balance and body composition in cancer patients. *Cancer Research, 38,* 1801–1807.

Waterhouse, C., Jeanpretre, N., & Keilson, J. (1979). Gluconeogenesis from alanine in patients with progressive malignant disease. *Cancer Research, 39,* 1968–1972.

Wesdorf, R. L. C., Krause, R., & von Meyenfeldt, M. F. (1983). Cancer cachexia and its nutritional implications. *British Journal of Medicine, 70,* 352–355.

Wilmore, D. W. (1977). *Metabolic management of the critically ill.* New York: Plenum.

Wooley, O. W., Bartoshuk, L. M., Cubanac, M. J. C., Ferstl, R., Gutezeit, G. W. R., McFarland, D. J., Oetting, M., Pudel, V. E., Rodin, J., & Simmons, F. J. (1975). Psychological aspects of feeding: Group report. In T. Silverstone (Ed.), *Appetite and food intake: Report of the Dahlem Workshop on Appetite and Food Intake* (pp. 285–312). Berlin: Abakon Verlagsyesellschoft.

Yasko, J. M. (1985). Holistic management of nausea and vomiting caused by chemotherapy. *Topics in Clinical Nursing, 7,* 26–38.

Alterations in Oral Status

RYAN R. IWAMOTO

Alterations that occur in the oral cavity of persons with cancer may be a result of the disease, the cancer treatment, or other factors affecting oral health. Damage to the oral mucosa is often inevitable with some cancer treatments. The pain and discomfort that accompany this side effect are frequently considered to be major problems for persons with cancer (Daeffler, 1980a). Oral hygiene measures may not prevent the damage caused by the local tissue effect of radiation therapy or the inhibition of cell replication due to chemotherapy (Daeffler, 1981). However, when oral care is provided systematically, infections and further damage to the oral mucosa can be prevented (Beck, 1979).

This chapter

- describes normal anatomy and physiology of the mouth;
- reviews various stressors, such as cancer treatments, on the oral mucosa;
- discusses the various oral care measures that have been studied and described; and
- describes nursing interventions for specific alterations in oral status.

ANATOMY AND PHYSIOLOGY OF THE MOUTH

The mouth is composed of the lips, buccal mucosa, gingiva, teeth, hard and soft palates, and tongue (Fig. 48–1). The epithelium of the oral mucosa is made up of stratified squamous cells. These cells have a high turnover rate of approximately 10 to 14 days. There are three types of oral mucosa: (1) the lining mucosa, which covers the labial and buccal regions, the soft palate, and the ventral side of the tongue, is a nonkeratinized epithelium; (2) the masticatory mucosa, which covers the gingiva and hard palate, is a keratinized epithelium; and (3) the specialized mucosa, which lines various areas of the oral cavity, contains the taste buds. The mucosa normally appears moist, soft, and pink. The oral mucosa serves as the first line of defense against infection and humidifies air as it is inhaled. The oral mucosa also facilitates ion exchange of sodium, potassium, chloride, and bicarbonate. Three pairs of salivary glands in the mouth, as well as other mouth glands, normally keep the mucous membranes moist and lubricate food for chewing and swallowing. The salivary glands also secrete the digestive enzymes ptyalin and amylase. The tongue is used for speech, chewing, and swallowing. Taste buds are located on the tongue as well as on the soft palate, glossopalatine arch, and posterior wall of the pharynx. The primary taste sensations are sweet, sour, salty, and bitter. An individual can perceive many different tastes that result from a combination of the different primary sensations.

STRESSORS IN THE ORAL CAVITY
General Stressors

There are many stressors in the oral cavity. Routine oral hygiene measures such as brushing and flossing

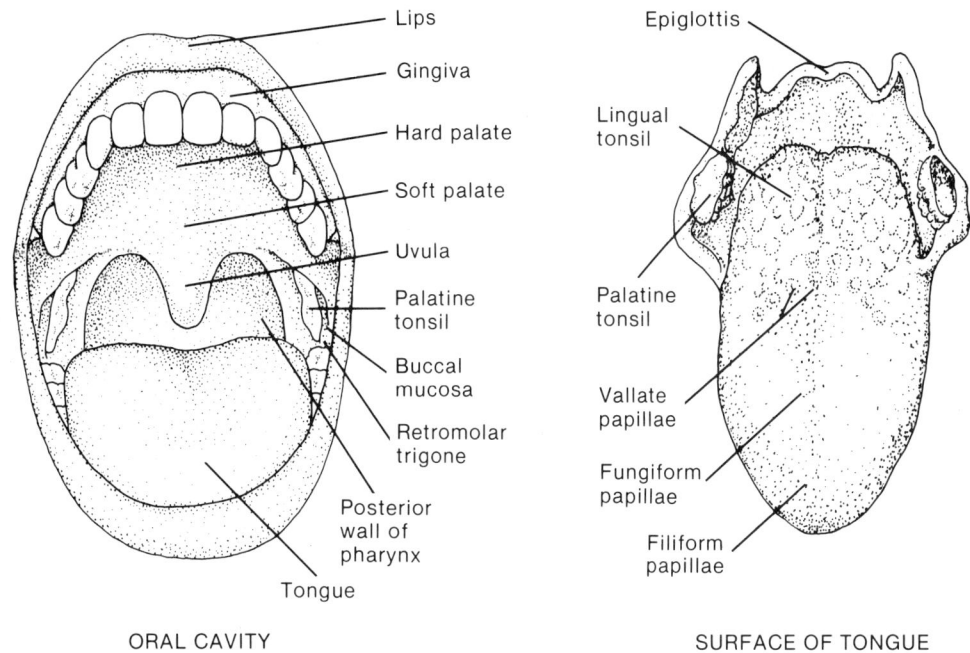

Figure 48–1. Anatomy of the mouth.

ORAL CAVITY

SURFACE OF TONGUE

can cause trauma to the tissues, which results in transient bacteremia. DeWalt and Haines (1969) evaluated the effect of specific stressors on normal oral mucosa. The stressors studied included oral breathing, continuous nasal oxygen, intermittent mechanical suction, and absence of oral intake. The subject in this investigation was studied for 5 hr. After 1 hr, significant changes in the mouth were seen. These changes included xerostomia, taste changes, pain, enlargement of the tongue papillae, edema, and hyperemia of the oral mucosa.

Poor oral hygiene habits and consumption of tobacco and alcohol can damage the oral mucosa. When mouth care is neglected, plaque, calculus, and debris collect around the teeth, causing irritation of the gingiva. This irritation develops into an inflammatory response, and the gingiva separates from the teeth and forms pockets. Debris and bacteria collect in these pockets, causing more inflammation and proliferation of bacteria (Daeffler, 1980a; Hickey, Toth, & Lindquist, 1982).

In persons with cancer, alterations in the oral status occur as a result of the disease, the treatment, or both (Fig. 48–2). Infiltration of the oral and pharyngeal mucosa by leukemias or lymphomas can cause gingival and tonsillar enlargement (Barrett, 1984b). These infiltrative lesions are exacerbated by local irritation and can lead to gingivitis (Segelman & Doku, 1977). The person frequently experiences pain and bleeding of mucosal tissues.

Nutritional deficiencies can cause a thinning of the oral mucosa, an inflammation of the tongue, and a decreased ability to repair tissues. Many factors lead to nutritional deficits in persons with cancer. The incidence of anorexia and cachexia is well documented. Nausea and vomiting from the treatment or the disease, gastrointestinal obstructions and malabsorption, fatigue, and depression are often experienced by persons with cancer and can lead to nutritional deficiencies. In addition, the oral complications as a result of cancer

or its treatment can further prevent the person from eating and drinking adequately.

Chemotherapy

The nonspecific effects of chemotherapy on highly proliferating cells can result in alterations of the oral mucosa (Barrett, 1984b; Carl, 1983; Peterson & Sonis, 1982). The antitumor antibiotics, such as dactinomycin, daunorubicin, doxorubicin, and bleomycin, as well as the antimetabolites, 5-fluorouracil and methotrexate, are known for their toxic effects on the oral mucosa. A number of abnormalities occur (Table 48–1).

Stomatitis

Stomatitis (also called mucositis) is a generalized inflammation of the oral mucosa that may range from

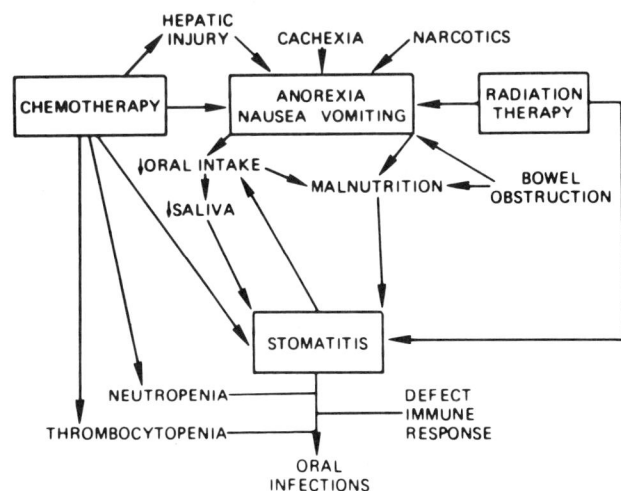

Figure 48–2. Interrelationships of factors contributing to alterations of oral status in persons with cancer. (From Daeffler, R. [1980]. Oral hygiene measures for patients with cancer. I. *Cancer Nursing, 3,* 348. Reproduced by permission.).

Table 48–1. ORAL COMPLICATIONS OF CHEMOTHERAPY

Stomatitis	Xerostomia
Infections	Neuropathy
Bleeding	Taste changes

mild erythema to severe ulceration. Approximately 40 per cent of persons receiving chemotherapy will develop some form of stomatitis (Peterson & Sonis, 1982). Chemotherapy interferes with cell production and maturation. Therefore, the basal cell layers of the oral mucosa are inhibited from replacing the superficial epithelium. The mucosa atrophies, which results in an inflammatory response—stomatitis (DeGregorio, Lee, & Ries, 1982). The development of stomatitis is varied and can occur on any mucosal surface, although ulceration usually occurs on nonkeratinized surfaces (Barrett, 1987; Hickey et al., 1982; Lindquist, Hickey, & Drane, 1978; Peterson & Sonis, 1982). Within 5 to 7 days of drug administration, changes in the oral mucosa are seen and may persist for 4 to 10 days (Daeffler, 1980a; Ostchega, 1980). Initially, the oral mucosa may have a slight burning sensation and erythema. This reaction may spontaneously resolve or progress to superficial epithelial desquamation, severe ulceration and pain, glossal edema, and secondary infections (Barrett, 1984b; Beck, 1979; Ketron, 1984; Segelman & Doku, 1977). In addition, any minor, local trauma can disrupt the remaining thin layer of mucosa, leading to further inflammation and ulceration.

These changes in oral status that result from chemotherapy correlate with the timing of myelosuppression (Hickey et al., 1982). Oral toxicity is observed 3 to 5 days before the initial drop in leukocyte counts following chemotherapy. The oral symptoms reach their most severe form before the peripheral granulocyte nadir. Subsequently, a complete resolution of stomatitis is found to occur 3 to 5 days before the full recovery of granulocyte counts.

Predisposing factors for stomatitis include poor oral hygiene, dental caries, improperly fitting dental prostheses, gingival diseases, chronic low-grade mouth infections, smoking and alcohol habits, and older age, which is accompanied by decreased salivary flow rates and mucosal atrophy (Daeffler, 1980a). A significant relationship has been noted between the presence of dental plaque and stomatitis (Lindquist et al., 1978). People with dental plaque who are receiving chemotherapy develop significantly more stomatitis for longer periods of time than people without dental plaque. Stomatitis is graded according to level of severity, as shown in Table 48–2 and Color Figure 6 (Barrett, 1984b; Hickey et al., 1982; Hyland, 1986; Lindquist et al., 1978).

Infections

Chemotherapy inhibits the primary and secondary immune responses to antigens. This immune deficiency combined with chemotherapy-induced leukopenia results in increased incidence of infections. The infections are usually those of gram-negative opportunistic bacteria, such as *Pseudomonas* and *Klebsiella, Enterobacter, Escherichia coli,* and the fungus *Candida* (Minah et al., 1986; Segelman & Doku, 1977). Persistent local oral infections can be transferred to the esophagus and stomach, become invasive, and lead to septicemia and death (Daeffler, 1980a; DePaola, Peterson, Leupold, & Overholser, 1983; Hickey et al., 1982).

The two normal host defenses against gram-negative bacteria that are weakened by chemotherapy and antibiotics are a lessening of oral secretions and an alteration of the interbacterial inhibition of normal oral flora. As a result, oral bacteria increase in number and pathogenicity. An in vitro study demonstrated that resident flora and gram-positive organisms were inhibited by chemotherapeutic agents to a greater degree than nonresident and gram-negative organisms (Harchar, 1981). Because chemotherapeutic agents diffuse into the oral tissues, the drugs may have a direct effect on the oral flora. Gram-positive infections may appear as dry, brownish-yellow, purulent, circular eruptions. Gram-negative infections appear as creamy white, glistening, nonpurulent ulcers (Clinical Practice Committee, 1982; Goodman & Stoner, 1985). These lesions are usually painful.

Candida is a common organism found in the mouth (Segelman & Doku, 1977). Candidiasis tends to occur in persons who have received intensive chemotherapy; experienced long periods of leukopenia and increased incidence of stomatitis; and received broad-spectrum antimicrobial therapy, steroid medications, or both (DeGregorio et al., 1982; Epstein, 1989). Manifestations and symptoms of candidiasis vary (Table 48–3). *Candida* usually appears as irregular, white plaques with multiple dome elevations; involves localized or large areas of the oral mucosa; and is usually preceded by stomatitis. Persons may notice a "dry," burning sensation or tenderness in their mouths that is unrelated to xerostomia (Cheater, 1985). *Candida* can be difficult to isolate and identify. Persons with oropharyngeal candidiasis are at significant risk of developing esophageal and systemic candidiasis.

Many studies have evaluated prophylaxis and treatment of candidiasis. Oral nystatin has not shown prophylactic efficacy against the incidence of localized or systemic candidiasis (Barrett, 1984a; DeGregorio et al., 1982). In addition, nystatin's ability to eliminate colonized *Candida* from the oropharynx is questionable (Barrett, 1984a). The use of topical and systemic amphotericin B has been reported to be effective in preventing and treating candidiasis (de Vries-Hospers, Mulder, Sleijfer, & Van Saene, 1982; DeGregorio et al., 1982). Ketoconazole was not significantly more or less effective than amphotericin B in preventing yeast colonization in neutropenic persons (Donnelly et al., 1984). However, prophylaxis tended to fail in persons treated with ketoconazole alone. Absorption of ketoconazole is dependent on gastric acidity. Therefore, antacids and medications that affect gastric secretions should be taken at least 2 hours after ketoconazole. Clotrimazole has been found to be effective in the treatment of oral candidiasis and may prevent the development of esophageal candidiasis (Quintiliani,

Table 48–2. NURSING CARE PLAN FOR A PATIENT WITH STOMATITIS

Assessment	Interventions	Expected Outcomes
Nursing Diagnosis: Alteration in Oral Mucous Membrane		
Grade 0:		
No stomatitis. Mucosa is moist, pink, and soft. No ulceration or lesions. No discomfort in mouth.	Instruct the client to stop smoking and reduce the intake of alcoholic beverages.	Minimization of mouth irritation.
	After each meal and at bedtime, brush teeth with dentifrice and floss (except during periods of thrombocytopenia and neutropenia). A plaque-disclosing dye can be helpful in identifying plaque to be removed by brushing or flossing. If client is edentulous, frequent oral irrigations should be performed.	Cleansing of oral cavity.
Grade I:		
Mild stomatitis. Whitish gingival area observable, or client mentions slight burning sensation or discomfort in oral cavity.	Every 2 hr, provide normal saline rinses. Brush teeth after meals and at bedtime using dentifrice if not irritating. Floss at least once a day (except during periods of thrombocytopenia and neutropenia).	Cleansing of oral cavity.
	Use an ice massage to the web between the thumb and index finger of the hand on the same side as the painful area in the mouth.	Reported to be an effective measure to reduce pain (see Box 48–2), possibly because of the intense peripheral stimulation that activates the brainstem inhibitory fibers (Howard-Ruben, 1984).
	Provide a soft, bland diet.	Less irritation to the oral tissues as result of a soft diet.
Grade II:		
Moderate stomatitis. Moderate erythema, shallow ulcerations, or white patches present. Client complains of pain but can continue to eat, drink, and swallow.	Every 1 to 2 hr, provide normal saline rinses. Brush teeth after meals and at bedtime using dentifrice if not irritating. Use Toothettes if toothbrushing is not tolerated. Floss once a day if tolerated (except during periods of thrombocytopenia and neutropenia).	Providing maximum oral care with least mucosal trauma.
	Topical anesthetics may be used if needed.	Decrease in pain.
	Provide a soft, bland diet, especially cool foods. A dietitian can help plan meals to meet the nutritional needs of the client.	Increase in comfort while eating and minimization of mucosal trauma. (Cool foods are better tolerated.)
Grade III:		
Severe stomatitis. Severe erythema, full thickness ulceration, mucosal necrosis, bleeding, white patches present. Client complains of severe pain and is unable to eat, drink, or swallow.	Every 1 to 2 hr, provide normal saline rinses. Toothbrushing and flossing may not be tolerated, so Toothette or gauze-wrapped finger is used to remove debris and plaque. Oral irrigations gently cleanse the mouth.	Providing maximum oral care with least mucosal trauma.
	An interim dental prosthesis to protect ulcerated mucosa and provide a surface for chewing has been described (DePaola, 1983). It is worn while eating and at night while sleeping.	Prosthesis allows for immediate comfort and function.
	Topical anesthetics and systemic analgesics may be used as needed.	Pain reduction.
	Topical thrombin may be used.	Topical thrombin may stop oral bleeding.
	Tube feeding or parenteral nutrition may be needed.	Nutritional status of client will be maintained.

Note: Following resolution of stomatitis, clients should again brush their teeth after each meal and at bedtime and floss once a day.

Owens, Quercia, Klimek, & Nightingale, 1984; Shechtman, Funaro, Robin, Bottone, & Cuttner, 1984). In addition, chlorhexidine mouth rinses have shown some effectiveness in modifying candidiasis (Weisdorf et al., 1989).

Herpetic stomatitis has a wide range of manifestations and severity (Barrett, 1984b; National Institutes of Health, 1989). Clusters of vesicles or lesions may appear within the oral cavity and extend over the lips. The person frequently experiences pain (Daeffler, 1981). The antiviral agent acyclovir is used for prophylaxis and treatment of oral herpes simplex infections (Barrett, 1984b).

The myelosuppressive and mucosal effects of che-

Table 48-3. CLINICAL MANIFESTATIONS OF CANDIDIASIS

Pseudomembranous (thrush)
White plaques on mucosa that can be wiped off
Atrophic
Erythema with few, if any, white plaques. May be accompanied by
angular cheilitis
Hyperplastic
Leukoplakia-like plaques that cannot be removed as a result of
invasion into epithelium

(Data from Epstein, 1989.)

motherapy can result in an acute exacerbation of preexisting periodontal disease (Peterson & Sonis, 1982; Williams, Peterson, & Overholser, 1982). Periodontal disease, which includes gingivitis and periodontitis, is an extremely prevalent chronic inflammatory disease of the supporting structures of the teeth (Carl, 1983; Hickey et al., 1982; Peterson & Sonis, 1982). A tenfold increase of bacterial and fungal organisms is seen with periodontitis (McElroy, 1984). The signs and symptoms of acute periodontal exacerbation are localized tenderness to palpation, temperatures higher than 38.3°C, and slight trismus (Segelman & Doku, 1977; Williams et al., 1982). However, during periods of leukopenia, oral infections may develop without these symptoms (Daeffler, 1980a).

The simple act of chewing can introduce thousands of potential pathogens into the blood stream around diseased periodontal tissues (McElroy, 1984). Chronic infections of dental pulp may become sources of systemic infection during myelosuppression (Peterson & Sonis, 1982). Although optimal therapy for pulp infection is controversial, elimination of the source of infection by tooth extraction or pulp extirpation may often be the treatment of choice. Tooth extractions performed during myelosuppression are managed carefully with antibiotic prophylaxis and platelet transfusions to minimize complications (Peterson & Sonis, 1982).

People with dentures are susceptible to infection while receiving chemotherapy. Although removing the dentures during chemotherapy can lead to decreases in self-esteem, chewing ability, and nutritional intake, a poorly fitting denture can lead to inflammation, ulceration, and secondary infections (DePaola et al., 1983).

Bleeding

Bleeding in the oral mucosa often occurs as a result of thrombocytopenia. The oral cavity may demonstrate an early warning of severe thrombocytopenia, because oral petechiae often precede skin bruising (Barrett, 1984b). The person experiences oozing of blood in the mouth, which causes intermittent blood clots to form and break away (Ostchega, 1980). These blood clots may be aspirated and cause choking. Prolonged and spontaneous bleeding occurs mainly in the gingival interdental areas and can increase the person's susceptibility to infection. Spontaneous gingival bleeding can occur when the platelet count falls below 15,000; it tends to be more severe in persons with preexisting

periodontal disease or poor oral hygiene (Carl, 1980; Peterson & Sonis, 1982). Petechiae and hematoma formation in the oral mucosa can occur when the platelet count falls below 20,000.

Xerostomia

Xerostomia related to chemotherapy has been reported (Carl, 1983; Peterson & Sonis, 1982). Doxorubicin hydrochloride has been noted for causing xerostomia by diminishing salivary gland activity (Ostchega, 1980). On examination, the oral membranes appear dry and atrophic. In severe cases of xerostomia, the tongue becomes heavily furred, and the oral mucosa and lips become cracked and painful. Xerostomia also occurs as a result of other medications taken by persons with cancer (Cheater, 1985). These classes of medications include phenothiazines, tricyclic antidepressants, antihistamines, anticholinergics, and antispasmodics. Xerostomia is temporary and is treated palliatively with saliva substitutes.

Neuropathy

Chemotherapy-induced neuropathy may affect the oral cavity (DePaola et al., 1983; Peterson & Sonis, 1982). The symptoms mimic those of odontogenic or periodontal origin. Vincristine sulfate has been reported to cause neuropathy of the trigeminal and facial nerves, which manifests as jaw pain, circumoral paresthesias, and weakness of the facial muscles (Carl, 1980).

Taste Changes

An unpleasant taste in the mouth has been reported anecdotally while cyclophosphamide is being administered or immediately following the infusion of the drug. Eating or smelling plain, white, soft mints during and after the infusion has been reported to be helpful in masking or eliminating the bad taste (Pehanrich, 1983).

Radiation Therapy

Radiation therapy to the head and neck region causes several alterations in the oral cavity (Table 48-4). A study evaluating nutritional compromise related to side effects of head and neck irradiation found that subjects lost between 1.3 to 7.5 per cent of their initial body weight during the course of therapy (Iwamoto, 1981). Although muscle mass was maintained, fat stores were lost. The subjects who had an adequate

Table 48-4. ORAL COMPLICATIONS OF RADIATION THERAPY

Stomatitis	Infections
Taste changes	Osteoradionecrosis
Xerostomia	Trismus
Caries formation	

amount of energy stores tended to be younger and to experience less stomatitis in spite of a decreased caloric intake and weight loss than did the subjects who were older and more nutritionally depleted. Taste changes were reported by 42 per cent of the subjects, and decreases in salivary flow rates were noted in 80 per cent of the subjects. The subjects who had adequate energy stores received a higher radiation dosage before their lowest salivary flow rate was reached; recovery to 80 per cent of their initial salivary flow rate was quicker for them than for the subjects who were nutritionally depleted.

Stomatitis

Stomatitis occurs as a result of hyperemia and edema of the mucosa, which can lead to the formation of ulcers. These ulcers can appear after the oral cavity has received 1000 cGy (1 to 2 weeks). The early changes in the mucosa occur as a result of the effect of radiation on the fine vasculature of the tissues, which leads to vascular congestion and increased capillary permeability (Beumer, Curtis, & Harrison, 1979). The mucosa becomes whitish, and then a pseudomembrane gradually forms (Color Figure 7). This membrane can slough off, leaving a reddish and friable underlying epithelium with ulcer formation. At 2500 cGy the entire mucosa may become involved (Carl, 1983). Severe stomatitis occurs with treatment of tumors of the nasopharynx, soft palate, floor of the mouth, and retromolar area. The severity of the reaction depends on the area and volume treated, the radiation dose, and the individual. Persons who have a compromised oral mucosa as a result of alcoholism and who continue to consume alcohol and tobacco will have the most severe mucosal changes (Beumer et al., 1979; Miller, Vergo, & Feldman, 1981). With high doses of radiation to the head and neck area, chronic ulcers may form.

The peak of symptoms occurs at 6000 to 7000 cGy and may persist for 2 to 3 weeks after the completion of therapy (Beumer et al., 1979; Carl, 1983). Mucosal reactions as a result of radiation therapy are frequently hastened or enhanced with concomitant chemotherapy (Hilderley, 1986). An increased mucosal reaction can also occur as a result of scatter radiation from large metallic tooth restorations to adjacent areas. The radiation oncologist may place a piece of gauze between the mucosa and tooth during treatment to minimize this reaction. In addition, a rest from radiation treatment is sometimes needed to allow the tissues to heal.

Edema of the buccal mucosa, submental, and submandibular areas of the mouth and tongue can occur. As a result, persons receiving head and neck irradiation may have difficulty with the fit of their dental prostheses, impaired salivary control, and speech problems. The acute symptoms of radiation-induced stomatitis resolve within a few weeks after treatment is completed. However, long-term mucosal effects may occur and may include a thinned, overlying epithelium as a result of decreased keratinization and a less vascular and more fibrotic submucosa (Bersani & Carl, 1983; Beumer et al., 1979).

Taste Changes

Taste changes as a result of head and neck irradiation often occur (DeWys & Walters, 1975). These changes can affect each of the primary taste sensations (Conger, 1973). Some people experience a decrease in all tastes, which has been termed *mouth-blindness* (McCarthy-Leventhal, 1959). A partial or complete taste loss may occur. In addition, unpleasant tastes are sometimes evident. An increased sensitivity for bitter tastes and a decreased sensitivity for sweet tastes are commonly noted. Changes in bitter and salty tastes occur earliest and last longest (Mossman & Henkin, 1978). A "burnt" or "bad" taste is noted by some people. As a result, these people find the taste of coffee and chocolate very unpleasant.

Degeneration and atrophy of the taste buds as well as damage to the microvilli of the taste cells are noted at 1000 cGy and can continue until the end of treatment (Beumer et al., 1979; Sullivan & Fleming, 1986). Although some return of taste may occur several months after treatment, some taste changes are permanent (Lowe, 1986). Mossman and associates (1982) reported that impairment of taste and salivary function persisted in some persons for up to 7 years after radiation therapy. The most commonly affected tastes were salty and bitter, and the least affected were sweet and sour. The presence of saliva may play an important role in regaining normal taste acuity.

Xerostomia

Xerostomia, or a decrease in saliva production, occurs when a dose range of 1000 to 2000 cGy is reached (Carl, 1983; Iwamoto, 1981; Kashima, Kirkhan, & Andrews, 1965). Saliva is important for taste as well as for chemical digestion. People with xerostomia have difficulty with speech, chewing, and swallowing. Increased friction with removable oral prostheses and problems with retention of the prostheses are also noted. The serous acinar cells of the parotid glands are more affected than the mucinous acinar cells. Therefore, the saliva flow rate decreases, and the saliva becomes viscous and ropey and adheres to the oral mucosa. Xerostomia is initially worse at night (especially in mouth breathers) and better during the day but eventually becomes a more persistent problem as treatment continues. The severity and chronicity of xerostomia is related to the type and dose of radiation, the area treated, and the age of the person. When the retromolar trigone, tonsils, soft palate, and nasopharynx are treated, severe xerostomia occurs. If the parotid and submandibular glands are within the treatment field, salivary gland function almost completely ceases (Carl, 1983). The parotid gland is less affected when the floor of the mouth and the base of the tongue are treated with radiation therapy, and an increase in saliva output can be noted 1 to 2 years after treatment (Beumer et al., 1979).

Xerostomia seldom reverses completely and remains a chronic problem in people who receive a cumulative dose of greater than 4000 cGy to the head and neck region. Although some persons have a subjective improvement in xerostomia, there usually is no measurable change (Dreizen, Brown, Daly, & Drane, 1977). Some improvement is noted in younger persons who are treated for Hodgkin's disease (Carl, 1980, 1983).

Caries

When xerostomia occurs, the pH of the saliva is lowered, and the saliva no longer acts as a buffering and lubricating agent. Therefore, an increase in caries formation is observed, and periodontal breakdown occurs (Karmiol & Walsh, 1975). This breakdown starts as a diffuse demineralization and can lead to progressive tooth decay with lessened capacity for repair and regeneration of the periodontium.

Caries occur first in the cervical areas of teeth, close to and below the margins of the gingiva (Carl, 1980). Teeth are at risk for caries if they lie within the treatment field. If the nasopharynx and posterior soft palate are being treated, the teeth in these areas are especially vulnerable to caries development. A rampant form of caries occurs secondary to xerostomia (Dreizen et al., 1977). In addition, a shift in the oral flora composition to increased numbers of cariogenic bacteria occurs. This shift is long-lasting and is seen up to 4 years after therapy (Beumer, 1979).

Infections

Stomatitis, poor oral hygiene, broken teeth, faulty restorations, and periodontal disease contribute to persistent oral infections in persons with head and neck cancer (Lowe, 1986). Oral candidiasis frequently occurs during radiation therapy to the head and neck region. The tongue, buccal mucosa, and mucosal surfaces beneath dentures are prime sites for infection (Beumer et al., 1979). In addition, an increase in enteric bacteria is observed in the mouth as a result of xerostomia and increased age (Bernhoft & Skaug, 1985).

Osteoradionecrosis

All persons who receive head and neck irradiation are susceptible to osteoradionecrosis. The potential for osteoradionecrosis lasts a lifetime and can be evident several months to years after therapy is completed (Levin & Ferris, 1980). Poor oral hygiene and continued use of mouth irritants such as alcohol and tobacco are major contributing factors in the development of osteoradionecrosis (Dreizen et al., 1977). Osteoradionecrosis is progressive and irreversible and occurs more frequently in the mandible than in the maxilla, because the blood supply in the mandible is less profuse than it is in the maxilla (Wescott, 1985). The marrow becomes acellular and avascular, with increased fibrosis and fatty degeneration. Therefore, the bone structure is unable to respond to trauma or infection (Beumer

et al., 1979). These changes are subclinical effects that are neither felt right away by the person nor seen by the clinician. However, with severe osteoradionecrosis, the person experiences pain, trismus, fistula formation, and pathologic fractures with loss of tissue and bone (Carl, 1980).

Osteoradionecrosis tends to occur in persons who have chronic and advanced periodontal disease and is frequently preceded by periodontal infections associated with teeth within the treatment field (Carl, 1980). Conservative treatment of teeth, with the retention of as many teeth as possible, is performed before the start of radiation therapy. However, to avoid potential complications, partial or full-tooth extractions are done for people who are unmotivated or unable to perform oral hygiene or who have unrestorable teeth (Carl, 1980; Miller et al., 1981; Ritchie, Brown, Guerra, & Mason, 1985; Wescott, 1985). Extractions and restorations need to be done 10 to 14 days before the start of radiation therapy to allow for healing (Lane & Forgay, 1981; Wescott, 1985).

Following head and neck irradiation, trauma in the oral cavity, such as extraction of teeth, oral surgery, and denture irritation, must be avoided (Miller et al., 1981). Tooth extraction and periodontal surgery can be the initiating factor in tissue breakdown. When osteoradionecrosis occurs, treatment involves gentle debridement with salt and soda rinses, antibiotic packs, and systemic antibiotic therapy. Hyperbaric oxygen has been used alone or in combination with surgery to improve tissue healing (Hart & Mainous, 1976; Mansfield, Sanders, Heimbach, & Marx, 1981; Ritchie et al., 1985; Westcott, 1985).

Trismus

Trismus is a disturbance due to myositis of the muscles of mastication and occurs with unpredictable frequency and severity. As a result of fibrosis, trismus can become a chronic problem (Miller et al., 1981). The mouth opening may be restricted to 10 to 15 mm, which impairs chewing and oral access. Trismus occurs when the temporomandibular joint and masticatory muscles are within the treatment field. This treatment field is used for tumors in the nasopharynx, retromolar areas, and posterior palate. Trismus tends to be more severe when surgery and radiation therapy are combined (Bersani & Carl, 1983; Beumer et al., 1979).

Treatment for trismus involves the repetition of jaw exercises and the use of dynamic bite openers, which can increase the mouth opening by 10 to 15 mm. Early exercizing of the mandible can lessen the severity of trismus in persons at high-risk for this problem (Beumer et al., 1979). Exercises help to decrease fibrosis of the muscles and increase the mouth opening (Table 48–5).

Surgery

Surgery to the head and neck region disrupts the oral mucosa when the tumor and surrounding struc-

Table 48–5. EXERCISES FOR TRISMUS

1. Open mouth as wide as possible 20 times in succession three times a day.
2. Place heels of both hands under jaw, push up with hands while stretching mouth open. The pressure provides resistance to the mandible as it opens and thereby strengthens the muscles.
3. Place middle and index finger on mandibular teeth and thumb on maxillary teeth. Use fingers in twisting motion to pry the mouth open. Hold open as wide as possible for 2 seconds, then relax. Repeat ten times with the right hand and then repeat with the left hand. Repeat the entire sequence four times a day.

(Data from Ritchie, Brown, Guerran, & Mason 1985; Sullivan & Fleming, 1986.)

tures are removed. Complications may develop during and after surgery. Indications for oral surgery include fractures, hemorrhage, and orofacial abscesses, which can lead to airway obstruction. For the person who requires oral surgery for infectious complications during myelosuppression, preoperative, intraoperative, and postoperative care and planning can avert complications. Difficulty with speech, chewing, and swallowing are common problems after hemimandibulectomy or glossectomy. If the muscles of mastication have been surgically manipulated, fibrosis may occur, leading to trismus.

ORAL CARE

Systematic performance of oral care is most effective in minimizing the destructive effects of cancer therapy on oral mucosa (Box 48–1) (Beck, 1979; Carl, 1983; Dudjak, 1985). The process of providing oral care itself improves the general condition of the mouth (Van Drimmelen & Rollins, 1969). Passos and Brand (1966) found that improved oral conditions were evident the longer oral care was provided. Regardless of the agent used, oral status improved when the person resumed oral feedings.

The purpose of oral care is to provide a comfortable and functional mouth, which is necessary for nutrition and communication, and to prevent infections (Daeffler, 1981). This is accomplished by keeping the oral mucosa and lips clean, soft, moist, and intact. As a result, the reservoir of pathogens in the mouth is reduced. Irritants that could further damage the oral mucosa are minimized to prevent hemorrhage, periodontal disease, and caries. Oral pain and discomfort are relieved to enhance oral intake, and the oral cavity is kept aesthetically clean and fresh (Daeffler, 1981; Hickey et al., 1982; McElroy, 1984).

Hickey and co-workers (1982) described other benefits of oral care, including minimizing treatment delays, decreasing length of hospitalization as a result of lessened complications, decreasing cost, and reducing staff time needed to manage complications.

Hart and Rasmussen (1982) reported that although most nurses identified the need to prevent stomatitis to maintain comfort and nutrition and to minimize infections, there was a lack of consistency in the assessment and provision of care.

Assessment

Oral care starts with assessment. By carefully and systematically inspecting the person's mouth, the nurse can detect alterations in oral status and provide early interventions. An individualized assessment is needed, because perceptions and symptoms vary greatly from person to person (Daeffler, 1981). This assessment includes an initial history, which evaluates oral hygiene habits (flossing and brushing), history of gingivitis, use and fit of oral prosthesis or dentures, other sources of irritation and infection, and previous complications with cancer therapy. The initial assessment should be done before the start of treatment (Beck, 1979; Hyland, 1986; Ostchega, 1980; Williams et al., 1982). An examination of the oral cavity is necessary at least daily once treatment has started, and twice a day during periods of myelosuppression (Barrett, 1984b; Beck, 1979; Ostchega, 1980). Observations and changes in oral status should be recorded.

The equipment used in an examination includes gloves, pen-sized flashlight, and tongue blades. All mucosal surfaces within the oral cavity should be examined: hard and soft palates, buccal mucosa, dorsal and ventral surfaces of the tongue, gingiva, lips, and

---

Box 48–1. SYSTEMATIC ORAL CARE PROTOCOL IMPROVES ORAL STATUS AFTER CHEMOTHERAPY

A systematic oral care protocol was evaluated to determine its efficacy in minimizing or preventing stomatitis in patients who had recently received chemotherapy. Parameters included general physical condition, condition of the oral tissues, and oral perceptions. This protocol included a thorough inspection and assessment of the mouth, with specific interventions being dependent on the condition of the tissues.

The control group of patients (n = 25) was evaluated every other day for a 25-day period. Twenty-two treated patients were then similarly evaluated for another 25-day period.

The condition of the oral tissues in the treated patients was better than that in the control group (p < 0.01). The incidence of oral infections was 32 per cent in the treated group as compared with 48 per cent in the control group.

Interestingly, in spite of the poor condition of the oral tissues in the control group, the perceptions of control group patients were not significantly different from those of the patients in the treated group. This finding reinforces the need for a nursing assessment of the oral tissues to detect changes early and provide prompt interventions. Patients may not complain until the stomatitis is severe.

(From Beck, S. [1979]. Impact of systematic oral care protocol on stomatitis after chemotherapy. *Cancer Nursing, 2,* 185–199.)

tonsillar fossa. Moisture, color, and texture of the mucosa and debris in the oral cavity are assessed during the examination (Beck, 1979; Schweiger, Lang, & Schweiger, 1980). Teeth are evaluated for color, shine, and debris. The amount of saliva as well as the perception of changes in taste, voice, and comfort is noted.

Several assessment tools have been published (Table 48–6). The Oral Assessment Guide (OAG), as described by Eilers and colleagues (1988), was developed to help standardize the assessment of the mouth, voice, and swallowing ability. Based on clinical experience, expert panel review, and review of other oral assessment tools, the OAG defines three levels of descriptors for each of eight categories (see Color Figure 8). High reliability of 0.912 among raters was established by registered nurses who were trained in the use of the tool.

A pilot study using the OAG with 20 subjects who were undergoing bone marrow transplantation concluded that the tool was useful in quantifying changes in the oral cavities of these patients. There was a high level of compliance by nurses using the tool. The OAG is used to communicate changes in the oral cavity and to determine and plan interventions.

An examination by a dentist is important before the start of cancer therapy (Hickey et al., 1982; Ketron, 1984; Lowe, 1986; National Institutes of Health, 1989). The dentist performs a clinical examination to evaluate the condition of the teeth and surrounding structures, identify possible foci of infection, and correct oral and dental problems (Carl, 1983; Lowe, 1986). The dentist also evaluates whether teeth should be extracted before starting radiation therapy to the head and neck region. The dentist is able to perform initial dental prophylaxis: scaling to remove tartar and polishing of teeth (Lowe, 1986; Williams et al., 1982).

The correlation between the presence of dental plaque and the development of stomatitis during chemotherapy is high. Lindquist and colleagues (1978) found that people who received dental scaling and

prophylaxis as well as oral hygiene instructions before chemotherapy experienced less stomatitis with shorter duration of symptoms than did those who had oral hygiene instructions but did not receive dental scaling. Dental prophylaxis also decreased the incidence of oral infections (Hickey et al., 1982). There was no increase in the systemic sequelae (fever and bacteremia) as a result of oral and dental care, and no correlation was seen between the severity and duration of stomatitis and the dose of chemotherapy. Therefore, dental care before chemotherapy can help to reduce the incidence of oral complications.

For the person about to start head and neck irradiation, the dentist can provide initial fluoride therapy and instruct the person on the procedure for daily fluoride applications (Lowe, 1986). Oral radiographs are not contraindicated before, during, or after radiation therapy. When a full series of radiographs is done, no area of the mouth receives a dose of more than 1 cGy (Levin & Ferris, 1980).

Careful assessment of denture use is necessary to reduce the oral complications that can occur in the edentulous person (Bernhoft & Skaug, 1985). The denture wearer's mouth is inspected for signs of irritation. Dentures also need to be evaluated for stability, retention, and occlusion (DePaola et al., 1983). Unstable or unretentive dentures can cause tissue irritation or ulceration. Xerostomia may also cause problems with denture retention. Almost all persons with dentures report that their dentures do not seem to fit so well shortly after chemotherapy has started or on withdrawal of chemotherapy (DePaola et al., 1983). The cause of this phenomenon is unknown. However, if they are used with care, well-fitted and tolerated dentures do not have to be temporarily discontinued (Bernhoft & Skaug, 1985). After cancer therapy, denture construction for edentulous persons should be delayed until epithelialization is complete (DePaola et al., 1983).

Intervention

The frequency of oral care is determined by the medical condition of the person and the status of the oral tissues. Oral care should be done at least after each meal and at bedtime. In addition, oral care before meals helps to freshen the mouth and stimulate the appetite (Beck, 1979). For those patients who have mild stomatitis (grade I), care is given at least every 2 hr. For those with moderate-to-severe stomatitis (grades II and III), oral care should be done at least every 1 to 2 hr (Lane & Forgay, 1981). Beck (1979) found that systematic care minimized oral complications in persons receiving chemotherapy regardless of their hydration status. DeWalt (1975) demonstrated that although daily improvement in oral tissues is seen with oral care, the tissue responses to oral care are not cumulative over a long period of time. Further, omission of oral care for 2 to 6 hr can nullify the past benefits of care (DeWalt, 1975; Ginsberg, 1961). Ginsberg (1961) studied the oral care of persons in acute

Table 48–6. ORAL ASSESSMENT TOOLS AND METHODS

Source	Tools and Methods
Ginsberg, 1961	Description of oral assessment
Passos & Brand, 1966	Guide for numerical rating of the condition of the mouth
Van Drimmelen & Rollins, 1969	Guide for numerical rating of the condition of the mouth (adapted from Passos & Brand, 1966)
DeWalt, 1975	Schematic presentation of dependent variables, tools for data collection, methods of measurement, and ratings
Beck, 1979	Oral exam guide; oral perception guide
Schweiger, Lang, & Schweiger, 1980	Oral assessment
Ostchega, 1980	A guide to assessing and treating chemotherapy's oral complications
Daeffler, 1981	Process standard for oral care
Allbright, 1984	Description of specific problems and suggested interventions
Goodman & Stoner, 1985	Assessment
Eilers, Berger, & Petersen, 1988	Oral assessment guide

renal failure. In that study, all mouth care equipment or procedures improved oral status, and complications were avoided when mouth care was provided at specified intervals and was specific to the person's individual needs.

While a person is undergoing cancer therapy, meticulous denture cleansing habits are needed (DePaola, 1983). Daily mechanical cleansing with a denture brush and an antimicrobial detergent such as chlorhexidine gluconate should be performed. Soft liners may be used to improve the stability of dentures. These liners are changed daily to minimize microbial growth. Dentures should be removed while sleeping and at other times to allow the mucosa to rest. Dentures should be soaked overnight, and the oral mucosa may be rinsed with chlorhexidine gluconate (Bernhoft & Skaug, 1985). If a person is unable to wear dentures because of pain, stomatitis, or bleeding, the dentures should be stored in a denture cup that contains a solution of Efferdent (Warner-Lambert Co., Morris Plains, NJ), Kleenite (Richardson-Vicks, Inc., Wilton, CT), or water (Cunningham, 1984). This solution should be changed daily. Before placing the dentures in the mouth, it is important to rinse the dentures well with water.

Cunningham (1984) cautions against the use of dentures that are in poor repair or are more than 5 years old. In addition, if the neutrophil count is less than or equal to 1000, the platelet count is less than or equal to 50,000, and no other pathology is present, the prostheses should only be worn for meals.

Instruments for Oral Care

The instruments used in oral care help remove debris and stimulate the gingiva. The following is a review of the various instruments for oral care.

Periodontal disease is prevented by removing plaque from teeth. Plaque is best removed with toothbrushing and flossing (Beck, 1979; Williams et al., 1982). A small, soft, nylon-bristled toothbrush effectively removes debris and stimulates gingival tissue. The Bass technique of brushing used in combination with flossing is the most effective method in minimizing the accumulation of plaque (Carl, 1983). The toothbrush is held at a 45-degree angle at the junction of the gingival margin and teeth and is moved in short, horizontal strokes. The teeth should be brushed for at least 3 to 4 min (Bersani & Carl, 1983). Unwaxed dental floss is used once a day in conjunction with tooth brushing to remove dental plaque and debris (Ostchega, 1980). Although toothbrushing and flossing are the most effective means of removing debris and plaque, they are contraindicated during periods of severe stomatitis, neutropenia, and thrombocytopenia (platelet count less than 20,000) because of the potential for bleeding, bacteremia, fungemia, and septicemia (Daeffler, 1981; Williams et al., 1982).

During periods of thrombocytopenia and neutropenia, Toothettes are more appropriate to use. Toothettes are sponge-tipped applicators that are less trau-matic to gingival tissues but are also less effective than a toothbrush in removing plaque and debris (Daeffler, 1981). Toothettes are useful for stimulating gingival tissue. Unflavored Toothettes are recommended because the flavoring and dentifrice that is sometimes applied to the Toothette can further irritate the mucosa. For severe discomfort, a piece of gauze wrapped around the finger is useful and less painful to remove debris (Allbright, 1984; Williams et al., 1982).

A gavage bag or gravity drip container with tubing is sometimes used to gently remove crusts and debris from the mouth. A red rubber-tipped catheter can be connected to the tubing to facilitate irrigation. A 500-ml normal saline intravenous solution bag with tubing attached to an 18-gauge angiocatheter can also be used to gently irrigate the mouth (Mosco, 1986). A bulb syringe can serve the same purpose (Daeffler, 1980b).

The power spray or Water Pik (Teledyne Water Pik, Fort Collins, CO) used at a low-pressure setting is helpful in removing debris. Hickey and co-workers (1982) reported that although water lavage did not alter the duration and severity of stomatitis, it did decrease oral debris and saliva viscosity and gave the person a sense of cleanliness. However, some question exists about whether such a power spray causes a transient septicemia (Daeffler, 1981). An atomizer may be used for mouth care (Pegram, 1983). A small portable air compressor is connected to an atomizer with a long nozzle tip. The atomizer is filled with normal saline or other solution and delivers a fine mist to the oral tissues without damaging them. People report a soothing effect on dry, inflamed, and ulcerated tissues. Suction equipment should be available for people who are at risk for aspiration.

Agents for Oral Care

The ideal mouthwash removes debris and moistens and softens the mucosa. The different agents used in oral care have three main purposes: to clean and remove debris, to lubricate and moisturize the oral mucosa, and to control pain (Table 48–7). Combination solutions are available that incorporate two or three different agents to provide optimal oral care. Passos and Brand (1966) described the optimal oral hygiene measure as one that is mechanically or chemically to clean the oral cavity without altering the properties and functioning of the mouth. In addition, this oral hygiene measure would leave the mucosa moist and lubricated.

Cleansing Agents

Cleansing agents provide mechanical or chemical washing action that removes loose debris and softens and removes mucous crusts. Normal saline acts as a palliative agent to aid granulation (Daeffler, 1980b). Saline is economical, readily available, and least damaging of the agents. A normal saline solution can be made with 1 teaspoon of salt mixed in 1 L of water. Daeffler (1980b) and Segelman and Doku (1977) sug-

Table 48–7. AGENTS FOR ORAL CARE

Agents	Comments
Cleansing	
Normal saline	Economical, available, least irritating
Sodium bicarbonate	Decreases odors, buffers acidity, dissolves mucin
Hydrogen peroxide	Germicidal, mechanical cleansing, debriding. Use diluted solution and follow with normal saline or water rinse. Aspiration precautions with foaming action
Commercial mouthwashes	Avoid mouthwashes containing alcohol, oils, astringents, antiseptics, and flavorings
Chlorhexidine gluconate	Antimicrobial: decreases dental plaque and gingival inflammation. Bitter taste, tooth staining
Lubricating	
Saliva substitutes	Decreases pain, dryness; protects mucosa
Lemon-glycerin	Mouth irritant, decalcifies teeth
Water-soluble lubricant, lanolin	Lip emollient; if petrolatum used, avoid aspirating
Pain Control	
Coating	
Kaopectate, milk of magnesia, Orabase	Covers ulcerated mucosa; temporary pain relief; may dry mucosa
Sucralfate	Binds to exposed mucosa for pain relief and protection
Hydroxypropyl cellulose film former (Zilactin)	Binds to oral mucosa forming protective coating; transient stinging with gel application
Vitamin E	Anecdotal reports of pain control; heals stomatitis
Topical Anesthetic	
Lidocaine viscous	Transient pain relief; interferes with gag reflex when swallowed
Dyclonine hydrochloride	Transient pain relief; useful in persons with xerostomia; aspiration precautions if swallowed
Cocaine solution	Transient pain relief; monitor central nervous system effects; tachycardia
Combination mouthwashes	Usually contains nonsteroidal anti-inflammatory agent in addition to topical anesthetic
Systemic	
Narcotic medications	For severe pain; taken 30–60 min before meals and as needed
Nonsteroidal anti-inflammatory agents	
Other	
Topical thrombin	To control minor bleeding
Fluoride	To prevent caries; apply to debris-free teeth after thorough mouth care
Allopurinol	To minimize chemotherapy-induced stomatitis
Antibiotic mouthwashes	For prophylaxis and treatment of oral infections such as candidiasis and gram-negative opportunistic organisms

gest the use of normal saline for persons with leukemia because it is not irritating or harmful to the mucosa. Sterile saline is used if the person is neutropenic or if ulcers are present. However, normal saline does not effectively remove hardened mucus, debris, or crusts.

Sodium bicarbonate is used as a cleansing agent and helps to decrease odor and relieve pain (Daeffler, 1980b). This agent also helps to buffer acidity in the mouth and dissolve mucin (Cheater, 1985). Sodium bicarbonate may be used after meals for general care and every 2 hours when ulcerations are present (Barrett, 1984b). A combination mouthwash of "salt and soda" is described in the literature (Daeffler, 1980b; Ritchie et al., 1985; Sullivan & Fleming, 1986; Wescott, 1985). Salt and sodium bicarbonate in a 1:1 ratio is mixed in warm water (one-half to 1 teaspoon of each in a L of water) and used every 3 to 4 hours. This mouthwash is able to clean and lubricate tissues and provide moderate local pain control (Daeffler, 1980b).

Hydrogen peroxide is a germicidal solution that is used for its mechanical cleansing, debriding, and effervescence (Daeffler, 1980b; Lowe, 1986). Passos and Brand (1966) evaluated the use of milk of magnesia, aromatic mouth wash, and hydrogen peroxide for oral care of persons who had had surgery. Although there was no significant difference in the efficacy of the three agents, hydrogen peroxide tended to maintain and improve mouth condition. However, hydrogen peroxide can also damage exposed bone, and caution must be used when ulcers or fresh granulation surfaces are present, because the solution tends to break down this tissue (Daeffler, 1980b; Passos & Brand, 1966). It is also irritating to the tongue and buccal mucosa. Elongation of the filiform and foliate papillae of the tongue has been noted (Segelman & Doku, 1977; Tombes, 1987). The elongated papillae serve as an excellent matrix for candidiasis. Therefore, hydrogen peroxide should be used with caution (Segelman & Doku, 1977). The efficacy and safety of long-term use of hydrogen peroxide has been questioned (Amigoni, Johnson, & Kalkwarf, 1987; Weitzman, Weitberg, Niederman, & Stossel, 1984). Cells are damaged when they are exposed to a high concentration of oxidants. With long-term use, peroxide may function as a co-carcinogen (Weitzman et al., 1984). Caution must be observed when a person has a compromised cough reflex because of the foaming action of hydrogen peroxide. The person who is unable to cough may have a problem with aspirating the foam (Daeffler, 1980b). Fungal adherence may be increased with the use of hydrogen peroxide (Tombes, 1987). Superinfections may occur as the normal oral flora balance is disturbed. In some people, oral use of hydrogen peroxide also causes nausea and subjective feelings of thirst and dryness of the mouth.

Hydrogen peroxide 3 per cent should only be used if mechanical cleansing action is essential and should be diluted to one-fourth strength (Daeffler, 1980b; Goodman & Stoner, 1985; Lowe, 1986). Use of hydrogen peroxide must be followed with a normal saline or water rinse. Suction equipment should be readily available for people who are unable to tolerate the foaming action of this agent.

Hogan (1983) found that a refrigerated solution of hydrogen peroxide provided a numbing anesthetic effect. She suggests that the cold solution can cause vasoconstriction and help stop bleeding secondary to severe stomatitis, thrombocytopenia, or both. The preference for half-strength hydrogen peroxide versus baking soda and water has been evaluated in persons receiving head and neck irradiation (Dudjak, 1985). These investigators found that half-strength hydrogen peroxide was less irritating to use than baking soda and water.

Commercial mouthwashes should be avoided because they often contain oils, astringents, and antiseptics. These can lead to drying, irritation, erythema, ulceration, and epithelial sloughing (Bernstein, 1978; Bersani & Carl, 1983; Cheater, 1985; Daeffler, 1980b; Sullivan & Fleming, 1986).

Chlorhexidine is an antimicrobial agent used to help decrease dental plaque and gingival inflammation. Investigations of the prophylactic use of chlorhexidine gluconate in preventing or decreasing oral complications have had conflicting results. In a double-blind, placebo-controlled study, McGaw and Belch (1985) found the mouth rinse provided good control of plaque and gingival inflammation with decreased severity and duration of mucositis in 16 leukemic patients undergoing remission-induction therapy. In contrast, Weisdorf and co-workers (1989) in a double-blind, placebo-controlled trial of chlorhexidine gluconate in bone marrow transplant recipients (n = 100) found trends toward improved oral hygiene in the treated group but no significant difference in mucositis.

Lubricating Agents

Lubricating agents such as saliva substitutes contain methyl cellulose. Some saliva substitutes contain ptyalin, a salivary enzyme, and fluoride to prevent caries (Beumer et al., 1979). These lubricating agents help to decrease oral discomfort and buffer the hyperacidity that occurs with xerostomia (Bernhoft & Skaug, 1985; Cheater, 1985). Saliva substitutes lubricate and protect the denture-supporting tissues and increase bonding of the prosthesis to the mucosa.

Lemon-glycerin solutions and swabs have been studied for their use as oral care agents (Daeffler, 1980b; Van Drimmelen & Rollins, 1969; Wiley, 1969). Glycerin has a drying effect as it absorbs water and irritates the mucosa. The acidity of the lemon can decalcify teeth, reduce the buffering capacity of saliva, and be painful on broken mucosal surfaces (Wiley, 1969). Therefore, lemon-glycerin swabs should be avoided.

Moi-Stir (Kingswood Laboratories, Inc., Carmel, IN) is one type of saliva substitute that was compared with lemon-glycerin swabs for effect on oral status in a study by Poland (1987). The subjects tended to prefer Moi-Stir over lemon glycerin, and on examination, the measures of oral status (dryness, etc.) improved with Moi-Stir and worsened with lemon glycerin.

A thin layer of water-soluble lubricant or lanolin applied to sore, dry, and cracked lips helps to lubricate and soften them. These agents prevent evaporation and drying. If petrolatum is used, caution must be taken against aspirating the lubricant (Daeffler, 1980b).

Pain Control Agents

Pain control agents are divided into three general categories. The first category includes agents that coat or cover the painful areas of the mucosa, the second category includes the topical anesthetic agents, and the third category includes the systemic analgesics.

Coating Agents. Kaopectate (Upjohn Co., Kalamazoo, MI), milk of magnesia, and Orabase (Colgate-Hoyt Laboratories, Canton, MA) help to coat painful mucosal areas. The pectin in Kaopectate coats the denuded areas of the mucosa to prevent further irritation (Segelman & Doku, 1977). Milk of magnesia has been used to coat the mucosa and is reported to decrease acidity, dissolve mucin, and stimulate saliva (Cheater, 1985; Daeffler, 1980b). Milk of magnesia also exerts an osmotic effect, can dry the mucosa, and should not be used if a person has xerostomia. Orabase is a protective paste that is composed of gelatin, pectin, and carboxymethyl cellulose in a hydrocarbon gel. This odorless and tasteless paste is applied to ulcerations and provides temporary relief of pain (Daeffler, 1980b).

Sucralfate suspension is a compound of sulfated sucrose and aluminum hydroxide that has been used for gastric and duodenal ulcers. This agent forms an adhesive substance that binds to exposed mucosa and forms a protective barrier that promotes healing of ulcerated tissues. Anecdotal reports of the use of sucralfate suspension for chemotherapy-induced oral stomatitis described mouth ulcers that were healed within 2 to 3 days of use, enabling tolerance of oral nutrition (Ferraro & Mattern, 1984; Wilkes, 1986). A randomized, double-blind study of 48 children and adolescents who received remission-induction chemotherapy for leukemia revealed that subjects who used sucralfate reported less oral pain than those who used placebo (58 per cent and 25 per cent, respectively, reported no discomfort; p = 0.06). Observers also noted more moderate to severe mucositis in the placebo group (38 per cent) than in the treated group (12 per cent). However, there was no difference in the maximal subjective and objective mucositis scores. In addition, the incidence of infection was similar in both groups. The investigators did not find objective evidence of healing or lessening of stomatitis in the treated group.

Hydroxypropyl cellulose film former (Zilactin, Zila Pharmaceuticals, Phoenix, AZ) binds to oral mucosal surfaces, which provides a protective coating and leads to pain relief. With application of the gel, there is a transient stinging sensation as the gel dries and forms a film. Investigators have found this product protects areas of ulcerations from irritation associated with food intake (Rodu & Russell, 1988).

The use of vitamin E has been reported anecdotally

to be beneficial in controlling pain and promoting healing of oral stomatitis (Hogan, 1984; Oncology Staff Nurses, 1982).

Topical Anesthetic Agents. Topical anesthetic agents numb the oral mucosa. Lidocaine viscous is frequently used 15 to 20 min before meals to provide comfort during meals. The anesthetic effect is brief, and some people find the taste of lidocaine unpleasant (Daeffler, 1980b). If swallowed, lidocaine viscous may also interfere with the pharyngeal stage of swallowing (Daeffler, 1981). Dyclonine hydrochloride has been reported to be an effective topical anesthetic agent that is especially effective for people with xerostomia (Daeffler, 1980b; Lowe, 1986; Segelman & Doku, 1977). This agent takes 10 min before onset of effects and lasts for approximately 1 hour.

Gentzsch (1983) described the use of a dilute solution of cocaine to control pain associated with stomatitis. People used this solution every 2 to 3 hours around the clock and had a significant reduction in oral pain without tachycardia, central nervous system effects, or alterations in taste.

Combination mouthwashes of topical anesthetics, diphenhydramine, and milk of magnesia or Kaopectate have been reported (Beck, 1979; Carter, 1986; Hilderley, 1986; Segelman & Doku, 1977; Wescott, 1985). A nonsteroidal anti-inflammatory agent is frequently included in the mouthwash to decrease inflammation and provide topical as well as systemic (peripheral) relief of pain (Beck, 1979).

Innovative strategies to administer these agents have been reported. Carter (1986) described administering 5 ml of a mixture of equal parts of dyclonine hydrochloride and diphenhydramine over crushed ice in a 30-ml medicine cup. The person sips this mixture 30 min before meals and as needed. The analgesia that is provided with the agents is enhanced by the cold temperature of the solution.

Anesthetic sprays may provide topical relief of pain. However, caution must be used in administering these sprays because of the damage that can be done to inflamed mucosa (Daeffler, 1981).

Systemic Analgesic Agents. Systemic analgesics may sometimes be necessary for severe oral discomfort and should be taken about 30 to 60 min before meals. These analgesics include nonsteroidal anti-inflammatory agents as well as narcotic medications (Schubert & Newton, 1987).

Other Agents

A variety of other agents are used to control oral complications such as bleeding, caries, and infections. Topical thrombin has been described in the literature for controlling minor, persistent oral bleeding (Barrett, 1984b; Carl, 1983; Peterson & Sonis, 1982; Preston, 1983). The medication is applied with a cotton-tipped applicator or gauze to the affected area every 4 hr and as needed. Bleeding is stopped with as few as two applications (Peterson & Sonis, 1982).

Daily fluoride treatments are important to prevent caries when xerostomia occurs as the result of radiation

therapy to the head and neck region. Fluoride acts by incorporating into the enamel and dentin, thereby remineralizing the teeth and preventing caries formation (Beumer et al., 1979; Lowe, 1986). In addition, fluoride may inhibit plaque formation and decrease the number of cariogenic organisms in the mouth (Lowe, 1986). Dreizen and colleagues (1977) reported that in a 3-yr follow-up study, fluoride was effective in protecting high-risk persons who received head and neck irradiation from developing xerostomia-related caries regardless of the sucrose content of their diet. They found that oral hygiene alone was not adequate to prevent dental decay. Caries occurred and progressed rapidly in persons not using fluoride. In addition, when fluoride was added to the oral hygiene program for these persons, ongoing caries were stopped, and new developments were prevented.

A 1 per cent sodium fluoride or 0.4 per cent stannous fluoride gel is used. For people with good oral hygiene practices and minimal xerostomia, the fluoride gel or special toothpaste may be applied on the teeth with a toothbrush (Carl, 1983; Sullivan & Fleming, 1986). For others, custom-made fluoride carriers or trays are used. The gel is placed within the trays, which are then fitted over the teeth. The trays remain on the teeth for 5 to 10 min and then are removed (Sullivan & Fleming, 1986; Wescott, 1985). The person may expectorate the excess fluoride but may not eat, drink, or rinse his or her mouth for 30 min following the fluoride application. To be effective, the fluoride treatment needs to be done on debris-free teeth following thorough mouth care (Carl, 1980, 1983; Dreizen et al., 1977; Lowe, 1986; Sullivan & Fleming, 1986). If tooth decay occurs in spite of the daily use of fluoride, the fluoride treatments are then applied twice a day (Ritchie et al., 1985). For persons who have xerostomia as a result of irradiation to the head and neck region, the fluoride treatments need to be continued indefinitely to prevent caries (Sullivan & Fleming, 1986; Westcott, 1985).

An evaluation of six patients found allopurinol rinses helpful in minimizing chemotherapy-induced stomatitis (Clark & Slevin, 1985). Because the medication is diluted and spit out after use, there are minimal systemic effects. One interesting effect of using allopurinol mouth rinse was a reported improvement in taste alterations in two patients studied.

Antibiotic mouthwashes are used to prevent and treat oral infections due to *Candida* species and gram-negative opportunistic organisms. Frequently, anti-inflammatory agents and antihistamines are used in combination with antibiotic mouth rinses to provide symptomatic relief of the infection.

CLIENT NEEDS AND NURSING INTERVENTIONS

Stomatitis

Assess the person's willingness and competence to perform mouth care. Instruct the client to stop smoking and reduce the intake of alcoholic beverages to minimize mouth irritation. Interventions for stomatitis vary depending upon the degree of tissue damage. See Table 48–2 and Box 48–2 for a description of the levels or grades of stomatitis and the related nursing interventions.

Leukemic Infiltration of Gingival Tissues

Nursing interventions are palliative. Frequent warm saline rinses five to six times a day will help to keep the mouth clean until the oral cavity and blood counts improve (Bersani & Carl, 1983; Segelman & Doku, 1977). Dietary modifications to a soft, bland diet may be necessary if chewing is difficult. If hemorrhage occurs, utilize nursing interventions for bleeding that are listed in the following section.

Bleeding

Monitor platelet counts. For persons who have thrombocytopenia, the risk of bleeding in the oral cavity is always present. Provide systematic mouth care. Utilize bleeding precautions by reducing or eliminating mouth irritants such as ill-fitting dentures or retainers. These dental prostheses should be removed at least 8 hr daily. Orthodontic bands and wires are also mechanical irritants and can traumatize the oral mucosa and precipitate periodontal infections (Carl, 1983). Although plaque control is important to maintain a healthy gingiva, toothbrushing and flossing should be discontinued if the platelet count falls below 20,000. A Toothette or gauze-wrapped finger may be useful to remove debris and plaque from teeth surfaces.

If active bleeding occurs, gently irrigate the oral cavity with normal saline to identify the areas that are bleeding. A periodontal dressing pack may be applied to exert pressure to the bleeding site (Carl, 1980; Wescott, 1985). Bleeding usually stops within a few minutes. During this time, the person should not smoke or suck on straws, because the clot can be dislodged. A soft diet should be provided to reduce the trauma of chewing. Topical thrombin may be helpful to stop persistent, mild bleeding.

If thrombocytopenia is anticipated during the course

of therapy, a dentist should examine the person before starting therapy and between courses of treatment to evaluate oral status, eliminate sharp or rough tooth margins, modify ill-fitting dentures, and provide dental prophylaxis and scaling (Barrett, 1984b; Hickey et al., 1982).

Infections

Intensive oral hygiene before and after myelosuppressive therapy has been found to be helpful in preventing infections (Peterson & Sonis, 1982). Monitor neutrophil counts; anticipate complications as the neutrophil count decreases. Inspect the mouth twice a day for local signs of an infection: erythema, pain, plaque formation, and candidiasis. Observe for systemic effects such as fever, increased pulse, and malaise. Culture suspicious mouth lesions. Administer antibiotics as prescribed. If an oral fungal infection develops in a person who wears dentures, the dentures should be removed during the administration of topical antibiotics (Barrett, 1984b). Continue with mouth care and maintain cleanliness of instruments used in the mouth.

Taste Changes

Assess changes in taste perception. Assess which foods have altered or disagreeable tastes and which foods taste the same. It is important to remember that "taste" is influenced by many factors, including color and smell of food, emotional state of the person, and learned responses (Gallucci & Iwamoto, 1981). Modification of these factors can improve the appetite. Adding herbs, seasonings, sauces, or sugar can improve the taste of foods and enhance their palatability. Varying the temperatures of food and presenting foods with different textures can be helpful. Marinating and cooking meats in sweet sauces help to disguise the unpleasant tastes many people experience (Strohl, 1984). Cold cooked chicken, eggs, mild-flavored fish, and cheeses are frequently preferred over meats as sources of protein. Some people have reported that certain foods have little taste or may taste odd, but that sweet- and sour-flavored foods are palatable. Sweet and sour salad

---

Box 48–2. DENTAL PAIN CONTROLLED WITH ICE MASSAGE OF THE HAND

Forty patients with acute dental pain participated in a study to determine the efficacy of pain control with ice massage of the web between the thumb and index finger of the hand (Hoku point). Ice massage was provided by ice cubes inserted into wet gauze and gently massaged on the skin around the Hoku point of the hand on the same side as the painful region of the mouth. The massage was continued until the patient stated that the area felt numb or after a period of 7 min, whichever occurred first. The control group received tactile massage of the Hoku point alone or with the explicit suggestion that the massage was intended to alleviate their pain.

The ice massage decreased the intensity of pain by 50 per cent or more in 90 per cent of subjects in the experimental group, whereas tactile stimulation alone or with the added suggestion decreased the intensity of pain by 50 per cent or more in only 20 per cent of subjects in the control group. Ice massage of the Hoku point may provide additional pain control for patients with stomatitis.

(From Melzack, R., Guité, S., & Gonshor, A. [1980]. Relief of dental pain by ice massage of the hand. *Canadian Medical Association Journal, 122,* 189–191.)

dressings have been used to enhance the flavor of foods other than salads (Strohl, 1984). The sense of taste and smell are closely interrelated. With cancer therapy, the sense of smell is frequently less affected than that of taste. Some people have found that sniffing food before placing it in their mouths gives them a "taste" of the food. Mouth care before and after meals is especially important to refresh and clear the mouth of residual tastes. Since taste changes can last for several years after the course of treatment is completed, assessment for taste alterations and their effect on nutritional status should be done with each follow-up visit (Strohl, 1983).

Xerostomia

Saliva substitutes are convenient although temporary palliative measures to relieve xerostomia. Approximately 2 ml of the solution will provide some relief. Sugarless gum or mints can help to stimulate saliva production in persons with low salivary flow rates (Cheater, 1985; Lowe, 1986; Sullivan & Fleming, 1986). Increasing fluid intake can help relieve dryness and moisten the mouth. People frequently carry containers of water, iced tea, or other liquids to use as needed. For people with xerostomia without oral inflammation or pain, carbonated drinks such as cider or apple juice with soda or lemonade can be especially enjoyable. Some find sucking on ice chips helpful. Eating fresh fruits such as melons or grapes is well tolerated. Dry foods and foods that require an increased amount of saliva for chewing should be avoided. Foods need to be softened or moistened with gravy to make swallowing easier. Fluids should accompany meals and snacks. Mouth care itself stimulates saliva flow and should be performed before and after meals. Evaluate medications for anticholinergic side effects, which diminish saliva flow. Lip care needs to be provided with an emollient.

Papain, the proteolytic enzyme found in papayas and used in meat tenderizers, may assist in dissolving and breaking up thick, ropey oral secretions (Larsen, 1982). Eating fresh papayas or drinking papaya juice may be recommended before meals. Papain can also be purchased over the counter. The patient holds the enzyme in the mouth for about 10 min before meals. An alternative method is to swab the oral cavity with meat tenderizer before meals.

A major consequence of xerostomia is dental caries. The gingival areas and crevices need to be kept free of debris and plaque to prevent dental decay and periodontal disease (Carl, 1980). Mouth care with toothbrushing and flossing and daily use of fluoride should be maintained (Dreizen et al., 1977). Follow-up appointments with the dentist every 2 to 3 months are important for an evaluation of oral care, fluoride use, prosthesis fit, periodontal disease, and osteoradionecrosis.

SUMMARY

Alterations in the mouth as a result of cancer or its treatment can result in pain, increased susceptibility to serious infection, and compromised nutritional status. Nurses are in a vital position to assess high-risk persons for early symptoms and provide care to prevent or minimize these problems. Teach the patient and the family about oral complications that may occur as a result of cancer therapy. Instruct the patient on ways to examine the mouth, what signs and symptoms to monitor and report, and how to perform mouth care. Emphasize the importance of regular and systematic mouth care to prevent or minimize oral complications. With consistent application of oral care, further damage to the oral mucosa can be prevented, pain can be relieved or minimized, and tolerance and response to treatment can be improved.

References

Allbright, A. (1984). Oral care for the cancer chemotherapy patient. *Nursing Times, 80,* 40–42.

Amigoni, N. A., Johnson, G. K., & Kalkwarf, K. L. (1987). The use of sodium bicarbonate and hydrogen peroxide in periodontal therapy: A review. *Journal of the American Dental Association, 114,* 217–221.

Barrett, A. P. (1984a). Evaluation of nystatin in prevention and elimination of oropharyngeal *Candida* in immunosuppressed patients. *Oral Surgery, 58,* 148–151.

Barrett, A. P. (1984b). Oral mucosal complications in cancer chemotherapy. *Australia and New Zealand Journal of Medicine, 14,* 7–12.

Barrett, A. P. (1987). Clinical characteristics and mechanisms involved in chemotherapy-induced oral ulceration. *Oral Surgery, Oral Medicine, Oral Pathology, 63,* 424–428.

Beck, S. (1979). Impact of a systematic oral care protocol on stomatitis after chemotherapy. *Cancer Nursing, 2,* 185–199.

Bernhoft, C-H., & Skaug, N. (1985). Oral findings in irradiated edentulous patients. *Internal Journal of Oral Surgery, 14,* 416–427.

Bernstein, M. L. (1978). Oral mucosal white lesions associated with excessive use of Listerine mouthwash. *Oral Surgery, 46,* 781–785.

Bersani, G., & Carl, W. (1983). Oral care for cancer patients. *American Journal of Nursing, 83,* 533–536.

Beumer, J., Curtis, T., & Harrison, R. E. (1979). Radiation therapy of the oral cavity: Sequelae and management, Part I. *Head and Neck Surgery, 1,* 301–312.

Carl, W. (1980). Dental management of head and neck cancer patients. *Journal of Surgical Oncology, 15,* 265–281.

Carl, W. (1983). Oral complications in cancer patients. *American Family Physician, 27,* 161–170.

Carter, P. (1986). Pain relief for mucositis. *Oncology Nursing Forum, 13,* 88.

Cheater, F. (1985). Xerostomia in malignant disease. *Nursing Mirror, 161,* 25–27.

Clark, P. I., & Slevin, M. L. (1985). Allopurinol mouthwashes and 5-fluorouracil induced oral toxicity. *European Journal of Surgical Oncology, 11,* 267–268.

Clinical Practice Committee. (1982). Guidelines for nursing care of patients with altered protective mechanisms. *Oncology Nursing Forum, 9*(1), 68–73.

Conger, A. (1973). Loss and recovery of taste acuity in patients irradiated to the oral cavity. *Radiation Research, 53,* 338–347.

Cunningham, M. (1984). Dental prosthetics: Physical and microbial insults. *Oncology Nursing Forum, 11,* 78.

Daeffler, R. (1980a). Oral hygiene measures for patients with cancer. I. *Cancer Nursing, 3,* 347–356.

Daeffler, R. (1980b). Oral hygiene measures for patients with cancer. II. *Cancer Nursing, 3,* 427–432.

Daeffler, R. (1981). Oral hygiene measures for patients with cancer. III. *Cancer Nursing, 4,* 29–35.

Davis, J. C. (1981). Soft tissue radiation necrosis: The role of hyperbaric oxygen. *HBO Review, 2,* 153–167.

DeGregorio, M. W., Lee, W. M. F., & Ries, C. A. (1982). *Candida* infections in patients with acute leukemia: Ineffectiveness of nystatin prophylaxis and relationship between oropharyngeal and systemic candidiasis. *Cancer, 50,* 2780–2784.

DePaola, L. G. (1983). The use of an interim protective prosthesis during cancer chemotherapy. *Journal of Prosthetic Dentistry, 49,* 527–528.

DePaola, L. G., Peterson, D. E., Leupold, R. J., & Overholser, C. D. (1983). Prosthodontic considerations for patients undergoing cancer chemotherapy. *Journal of the American Dental Association, 107,* 48–51.

De Vries-Hospers, H. G., Mulder, N. H., Sleijfer, D. T., & Van Saene, H. K. F. (1982). The effect of amphotericin B lozenges on the presence and number of *Candida* cells in the oropharynx of neutropenic leukemia patients. *Infection, 10,* 71–75.

DeWalt, E. M. (1975). Effect of timed hygienic measures on oral mucosa in a group of elderly subjects. *Nursing Research, 24,* 104–108.

DeWalt, E. M., & Haines, A. K. (1969). The effects of specified stressors on healthy oral mucosa. *Nursing Research, 18,* 22–27.

DeWys, W., & Walters, K. (1975). Abnormalities of taste sensation in cancer patients. *Cancer, 36,* 1888–1893.

Donnelly, J. P., Starke, I. D., Galton, D. A. G., Catovsky, D., Goldman, J. M., & Darrell, J. H. (1984). Oral ketoconazole and amphotericin B for the prevention of yeast colonization in patients with acute leukemia. *Journal of Hospital Infection, 5,* 83–91.

Dreizen, S., Brown, L. R., Daly, T. E., & Drane, J. B. (1977). Prevention of xerostomia-related dental caries in irradiated cancer patients. *Journal of Dental Research, 56,* 99–104.

Dudjak, L. A. (1985). The effects of two oral care protocols on mucositis due to head and neck radiation. *Oncology Nursing Forum, 12*(suppl.); Abstract No. 194.

Eilers, J., Berger, A. M., & Petersen, M. C. (1988). Development, testing and application of the oral assessment guide. *Oncology Nursing Forum, 15,* 325–330.

Epstein, J. B. (1989). Oral and pharyngeal candidiasis. *Postgraduate Medicine, 85,* 257–269.

Ferraro, J. M., & Mattern, J. Q. A. (1984). Sucralfate suspension for stomatitis. *Drug Intelligence and Clinical Pharmacy, 18,* 153.

Gallucci, B. B., & Iwamoto, R. R. (1981). Taste alterations in patients with cancer. *Nursing Care of the Cancer Patient with Nutritional Problems: Report of the Ross Oncology Nursing Round Table,* pp. 40–46.

Gentzsch, P. (1983). Control of pain associated with stomatitis. *Oncology Nursing Forum, 10,* 78.

Ginsberg, M. K. (1961). A study of oral hygiene nursing care. *American Journal of Nursing, 61,* 67–69.

Goodman, M. S., & Stoner, C. (1985). Mucous membrane integrity, impairment of: Stomatitis. In J. C. McNally, J. C. Stair, & E. T. Somerville, (Eds), *Guidelines for cancer nursing practice* (pp. 178–182). Orlando: Grune & Stratton, Inc.

Harchar, M. A. J. (1981). *The effect of five chemotherapeutic agents and nystatin on normal oral and skin flora and on common pathogenic organisms.* Unpublished master's thesis, University of Washington, Seattle, WA.

Hart, C. N., & Rasmussen, D. (1982). Patient care evaluation: A comparison of current practice and nursing literature for oral care of persons receiving chemotherapy. *Oncology Nursing Forum, 9,* 22–27.

Hart, G. B., & Mainous, E. G. (1976). The treatment of radiation necrosis with hyperbaric oxygen. *Cancer, 37,* 2580–2585.

Hickey, A. J., Toth, B. B., & Lindquist, S. B. (1982). Effect of intravenous hyperalimentation and oral care on the development of oral stomatitis during cancer chemotherapy. *Journal of Prosthetic Dentistry, 47,* 188–193.

Hilderley, L. (1986). Relieving radiation esophagitis. *Oncology Nursing Forum, 13,* 71.

Hogan, C. (1983). Oral hygiene. *Oncology Nursing Forum, 10,* 69.

Hogan, C. (1984). Vitamin E for stomatitis. *Oncology Nursing Forum, 11,* 69.

Howard-Ruben, J. (1984). Controlling pain from stomatitis. *Oncology Nursing Forum, 11,* 92.

Hyland, S. (1986). Selecting a tool for measuring stomatitis. *Oncology Nursing Forum, 13,* 119–120.

Iwamoto, R. R. (1981). *The nutritional status of patients with head and neck cancer receiving radiation therapy.* Unpublished master's thesis, University of Washington, Seattle, WA.

Karmiol, M., & Walsh, R. (1975). Dental caries after radiotherapy of the oral cavity. *Journal of the American Dental Association, 91,* 838–845.

Kashima, H. K., Kirkhan, W. R., & Andrews, R. J. (1965). Postirradiation sialadenitis. *American Journal of Roentgenology, Radium Therapy, and Nuclear Medicine, 94,* 271–291.

Ketron, F. R. (1984). Chemotherapy: Oral hygiene measures for resulting stomatitis. *Journal of Tennessee Dental Association, 64,* 36–38.

Lane, B., & Forgay, M. (1981). Upgrading your oral hygiene protocol for the patient with cancer. *The Canadian Nurse, 77,* 27–29.

Larsen, G. L. (1982). Rehabilitation for the patient with head and neck cancer. *American Journal of Nursing, 82,* 119–122.

Levin, A. C., & Ferris, G. M. (1980). The treatment of post-radiation therapy patients. *Florida Dental Journal, 51,* 41–44.

Lindquist, S. F., Hickey, A. J., & Drane, J. B. (1978). Effect of oral hygiene on stomatitis in patients receiving cancer chemotherapy. *Journal of Prosthetic Dentistry, 40,* 312–314.

Lowe, O. (1986). Pretreatment dental assessment and management of patients undergoing head and neck irradiation. *Clinical Preventive Dentistry, 8,* 24–30.

Mansfield, M. J., Sanders, D. W., Heimbach, R. D., & Marx, R. E. (1981). Hyperbaric oxygen as an adjunct in the treatment of osteoradionecrosis of the mandible. *Journal of Oral Surgery, 39,* 585–589.

McCarthy-Leventhal, E. (1959). Post-radiation mouth blindness. *Lancet, 2,* 1138–1139.

McElroy, T. H. (1984). Infection in the patient receiving chemotherapy for cancer: Oral considerations. *Journal of the American Dental Association, 109,* 454–456.

McGaw, W. T., & Belch, A. (1985). Oral complications of acute leukemia: Prophylactic impact of a chlorhexidine mouth rinse regimen. *Oral Surgery, Oral Medicine, and Oral Pathology, 60,* 275–280.

Melzack, R., Guité, S., & Gonshor, A. (1980). Relief of dental pain by ice massage of the hand. *Canadian Medical Association Journal, 122,* 189–191.

Miller, E. C., Vergo, T. J., & Feldman, M. I. (1981). Dental management of patients undergoing radiation therapy for cancer of the head and neck. *The Compendium of Continuing Education, 2,* 350–356.

Minah, G. G., Rednor, J. L., Peterson, D. E., Overholser, C. D., DePaola, L. G., & Suzuki, J. B. (1986). Oral succession of gram-negative bacilli in myelosuppressed cancer patients. *Journal of Clinical Microbiology, 24,* 210–213.

Mosco, M. (1986). Oral irrigation tips. *Oncology Nursing Forum, 13,* 88.

Mossman, K., Shatzman, A., & Chencharick, J. (1982). Long-term effects of radiotherapy on taste and salivary function in man. *International Journal of Radiation Oncology, Biology and Physics, 8,* 991–997.

Mossman, K. L., & Henkin, R. T. (1978). Radiation-induced changes in taste acuity in cancer patients. *International Journal of Radiation Oncology, Biology and Physics, 4,* 663–670.

National Institutes of Health. (1989). Oral complications of cancer therapies: Diagnosis, prevention, and treatment. *Consensus Development Conference Statement, 7*(7), 1–11.

Oncology Nursing Society, Clinical Practice Committee. (1982). Guidelines for nursing care of patients with altered protective mechanisms. *Oncology Nursing Forum, 9,* 68–73.

Oncology Staff Nurses. (1982). Stomatitis treatment. *Oncology Nursing Forum, 9*(4), 65.

Ostchega, Y. (1980). Preventing and treating cancer chemotherapy's oral complications. *Nursing 80, 10,* 47–52.

Passos, J. Y., & Brand, L. M. (1966). Effects of agents used for oral hygiene. *Nursing Research, 15,* 196–202.

Pegram, S. (1983). Atomizer helps mouth care. *Oncology Nursing Forum, 10,* 59.

Pehanrich, M. (1983). A tip for the taste buds . . . *Oncology Nursing Forum, 10,* 60.

Peterson, D. E., & Sonis, S. T. (1982). Oral complications of cancer chemotherapy: Present status and future studies. *Cancer Treatment Reports, 66,* 1251–1256.

Poland, J. M. (1987). Comparing Moi-stir to lemon-glycerin swabs. *American Journal of Nursing, 87,* 422–424.

Preston, F. A. (1983). Management of oral bleeding caused by thrombocytopenia. *Oncology Nursing Forum, 10,* 59.

Quintiliani, R., Owens, N. J., Quercia, R. A., Klimek, J. J., & Nightingale, C. H. (1984). Treatment and prevention of oropharyngeal candidiasis. *American Journal of Medicine, 76,* 44–48.

Ritchie, J. R., Brown, J. R., Guerra, L. R., & Mason, G. (1985). Dental care for the irradiated cancer patient. *Quintessence International, 16,* 837–842.

Rodu, B., & Russell, C. M. (1988). Performance of a hydroxypropyl cellulose film former in normal and ulcerated oral mucosa. *Oral Surgery, Oral Medicine, Oral Pathology, 65,* 699–703.

Schubert, M. M., & Newton, R. E. (1987). The use of benzydamine HCl for the management of cancer therapy-induced mucositis: Preliminary report of a multicentre study. *International Journal of Tissue Reactions, 9,* 99–103.

Schweiger, J. L., Lang, J. W., & Schweiger, J. W. (1980). Oral assessment. How to do it. *American Journal of Nursing, 80,* 654–657.

Segelman, A. E., & Doku, H. C. (1977). Treatment of the oral complications of leukemia. *Journal of Oral Surgery, 35,* 469–477.

Shechtman, L. B., Funaro, L., Robin, T., Bottone, E. J., & Cuttner, J. (1984). Clotrimazole treatment of oral candidiasis in patients with neoplastic disease. *American Journal of Medicine, 76,* 91–94.

Shenep, J. L., Kalwinsky, D. K., Hutson, P. R., George, S. L., Dodge, R. K., Blankenship, K. R., & Thornton, D. (1988). Efficacy of oral sucralfate suspension in prevention and treatment of chemotherapy-induced mucositis. *Journal of Pediatrics, 113,* 758–763.

Strohl, R. (1983). Taste sensations after radiation therapy. *Oncology Nursing Forum, 10,* 80.

Strohl, R. (1984). Understanding taste changes. *Oncology Nursing Forum, 11,* 81–84.

Sullivan, M. D., & Fleming, T. J. (1986). Oral care for the radiotherapy-treated head and neck cancer patient. *Dental Hygiene, 60,* 112–114.

Tombes, M. E. (1987). *The effects of hydrogen peroxide rinses on normal oral mucosa.* Unpublished master's thesis, University of Washington, Seattle, WA.

Van Drimmelen, J., & Rollins, H. F. (1969). Evaluation of a commonly used oral hygiene agent. *Nursing Research, 18,* 327–332.

Weisdorf, D. J., Bostrom, B., Raether, D., Mattingly, M., Walker, P., Pihlstrom, B., Ferrieri, P., Haake, R., Goldman, A., Woods, W., Ramsay, N. K. C., & Kersey, J. H. (1989). Oropharyngeal mucositis complicating bone marrow transplantation: Prognostic factors and the effect of chlorhexidine mouth rinses. *Bone Marrow Transplantation, 4,* 89–95.

Weitzman, S. A., Weitberg, A. B., Niederman, R., & Stossel, T. P. (1984). Chronic treatment with hydrogen peroxide: Is it safe? *Journal of Periodontology, 55,* 510–511.

Wescott, W. B. (1985). Dental management of patients being treated for oral cancer. *CDA Journal, 13,* 42–47.

Wiley, S. B. (1969). Why glycerol and lemon juice? *American Journal of Nursing, 69,* 342–344.

Wilkes, G. M. (1986). Sucralfate suspension for mucositis. *Oncology Nursing Forum, 13,* 71–72.

Williams, L. T., Peterson, D. E., & Overholser, C. D. (1982). Acute peridontal infection in myelosuppressed oncology patients: Evaluation and nursing care. *Cancer Nursing, 5,* 465–467.

CHAPTER 49

Alterations in Protective Mechanisms: Hematopoiesis and Bone Marrow Depression

DOUGLAS HAEUBER
JUDITH A. SPROSS

Hematopoiesis is a term used to describe the process of proliferation, differentiation, and maturation of blood cells. Although the process has been increasingly well defined through experimental research, much of what is known about human hematopoiesis remains speculative. Not all aspects of hematopoiesis observed in animal models have been confirmed in humans. The process of blood cell formation described here represents what has been demonstrated in humans plus what is likely to be true in humans on the basis of studies using animal models. This chapter describes normal hematopoiesis, alterations in hematopoietic processes caused by cancer or cancer treatment and other factors, and nursing assessment and care of persons who are at risk for or have cancer-related bone marrow depression. To help the reader, Table 49–1 provides a list of related abbreviations.

ORGANS OF HEMATOPOIESIS

Bone Marrow

The organs of hematopoiesis include the bone marrow, spleen, and lymphoid tissues. The bone is the principal site for production of blood cells. From birth until about the age of 4 years, most bones are involved in hematopoiesis. By the age of 18 years, much of the marrow has been replaced by fat cells, so that hematopoietic marrow is only found in the vertebrae, ribs, skull, pelvis, and proximal epiphyses of the femur and humerus. The distribution of active bone marrow in adults is illustrated in Figure 49–1. In the elderly the proportion of fatty marrow increases so that only half of the ribs and sternum are sites of hematopoiesis.

Physiologic function of bone marrow depends on a number of factors, including the availability of selected micronutrients, a specialized microenvironment, normal stem cell function, regulation by specific hematopoietic and other hormones, and feedback inhibition from cell production (Gordon & Barrett, 1985). The reticular cells and stroma, which contain macrophages and fat cells, provide a hematopoietic inductive microenvironment (HIM), which is essential to blood cell production. The exact nature of HIM in humans is unclear. The marrow is also richly innervated, suggesting one mechanism by which the marrow may be activated on demand. These nerves may influence blood flow in the marrow and cellular release by responding to changes in intramedullary pressure and to extramedullary influences.

Spleen

The spleen contains both lymphoid and reticuloendothelial components. The spleen is an "early re-

Table 49–1. ALTERATIONS IN PROTECTIVE MECHANISMS: HEMATOPOIESIS AND BONE MARROW DEPRESSION

Abbreviation	Description
BFU	Burst-forming unit
BMD	Bone marrow depression
BRM	Biologic response modifiers
CCI	Corrected count interval
CFC	Colony-forming cell
CFU	Colony-forming unit
CMI	Cell-mediated immunity
CSF	Colony-stimulating factor
DIC	Disseminated intravascular coagulation
Eo	Eosinophil
EPO	Erythropoietin
GCP	Granulocytopenia
G-CSF	Granulocyte colony-stimulating factor
GEMM	Granulocyte, erythroid, monocyte, megakaryocyte
GM-CSF	Granulocyte-monocyte colony-stimulating factor
HI	Humoral immunity
HIM	Hematopoietic micro environment
IFNs	Interferons
IL 2	Interleukin 2
IL 3	Interleukin 3
MAB	Monoclonal antibodies
Mk	Megakaryocyte
NK	Natural killer (cells)
PCM	Protein-calorie malnutrition
PgE	Prostaglandin E
PT	Prothrombin time
PTT	Partial thromboplastin time
RBC	Red blood cells
RES	Reticuloendothelial system
RT	Radiation therapy
TNF	Tumor necrosis factor
TNI	Total nodal irradiation
WBC	White blood cells

sponder" to infection; it is a site of antibody and opsonin activity (opsonins prepare foreign material for phagocytosis). Other functions include phagocytosis, storage of platelets (20 to 30 per cent of total platelet mass), iron metabolism, and mechanical filtration of cellular and noncellular debris.

Lymphoid Tissue

Lymph nodes are collections of lymphocytes, plasma cells, and macrophages existing in chains along the course of large blood vessels throughout the body. They drain regional tissue and empty into large, efferent lymph channels, clearing foreign material from the blood. Solitary lymph nodules found in certain parts of the body (such as the Peyer's patches of the ileum) produce a local response to antigen.

NORMAL HEMATOPOIETIC PROCESSES

Normal hematopoiesis results in the production of white cells, platelets, and red cells, and the processes of proliferation, differentiation, and maturation are mediated by various humoral factors. Predominant among these are the expanding set of so-called hematopoietic growth factors, also known as colony-stimulating factors (CSFs) or poietins. A schematic outline of marrow cell kinetics that illustrates the continuum

of proliferation and differentiation of both stem cells and the factors that mediate the process is given in Figure 49–2.

The stem cell is the keystone of bone marrow hematopoiesis. Several specific stem cells have been identified, and these are named according to their degree of differentiation and maturation (Erslev & Weiss, 1983). *Pluripotential* stem cells, the youngest and most "primitive," are capable of extensive, possibly lifelong self-renewal and of differentiation to all cell lineages, both myeloid and lymphoid (Queensberry, 1983). This concept of self-renewal (or stem cell immortality) is important when the effects of cancer treatment on bone marrow and people's ability to

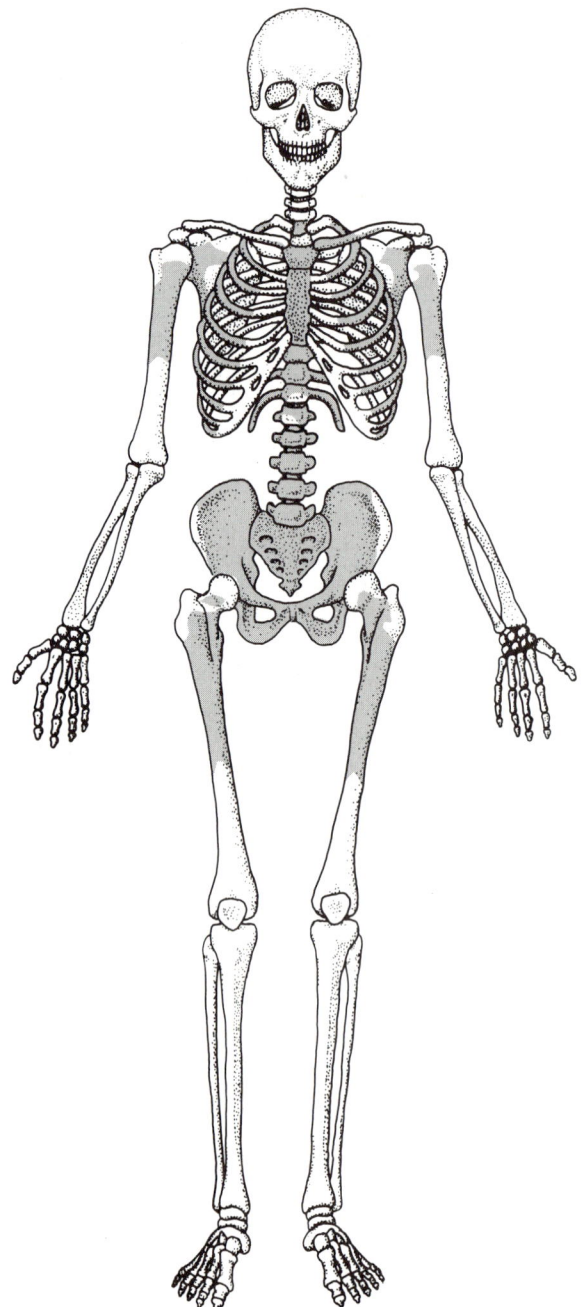

Figure 49–1. Distribution of active bone marrow in a normal adult. The striped portion represents the area of active marrow.

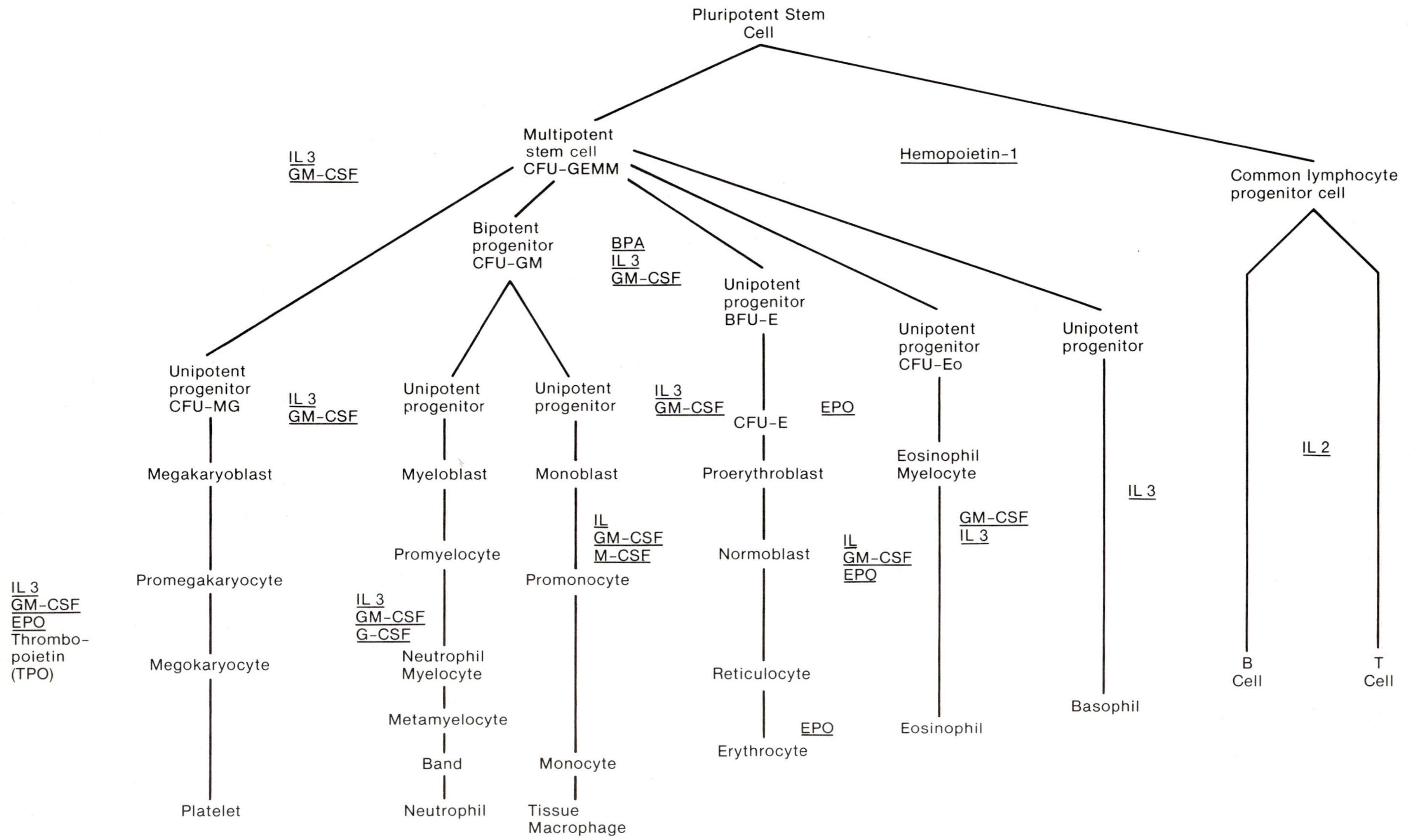

Figure 49–2. Schematic of marrow cell kinetics, proliferation, and differentiation. Factors mediating cell differentiation are italicized. CFU, colony-forming unit; GEMM, granulocyte, erythroid, monocyte, megakaryocyte; Eo, eosinophil; CSF, colony-stimulating factor; IL, interleukin; G-CSF, granulocyte colony-stimulating factor; GM-CSF, granulocyte-macrophage colony-stimulating factor; M-CSF, macrophage colony-stimulating factor; BPA, burst-promoting activity; EPO, Erythropoietin; BFU-E, burst-forming unit-erythroid; CFU-E, colony-forming unit-erythroid; CFU-GM, colony-forming unit-granulocyte-monocyte.

761

recover bone narrow function after cytotoxic treatment are considered. One explanation of this concept hypothesizes a "stem cell niche," in which one daughter cell remains, retaining its capacity for self-renewal, while the other daughter cell leaves the niche to enter the HIM of the marrow. On being exposed to the various influences in HIM, including growth factors, this daughter cell is induced to further divide and gradually loses its capacity to self-replicate as it proceeds to differentiate (Schofield, 1978).

Multipotential stem cells are characterized by limited self-renewal capability. These cells, like pluripotential stem cells, are not irreversibly committed to a single cell lineage, but they are more differentiated than pluripotential stem cells. The best example of a multipotential stem cell is the CFU-GEMM. (The term *colony-forming unit* or *colony-forming cell* [CFU or CFC] with the name of a cell line describes a specific stem cell or progenitor cell). CFU-GEMM is capable of differentiating to a more mature progenitor cell in any one of the following cell lines: *granulocyte*, *erythroid*, *monocyte*, or *megakaryocyte*. These cells provide offspring that are better differentiated and more responsive to poietins. *Bipotential* cells are progenitor cells capable of limited self-renewal and of differentiation to two cell lines. *Unipotential* cells are progenitor cells capable of limited self-renewal and of differentiation to one cell line (e.g., CFC-Eo [eosinophil]; CFC-Mk [megakaryocyte]). The progeny of these various progenitor cells are termed *precursor* cells; they are incapable of self-renewal and are morphologically recognizable as members of a single cell line.

Another important element in the process of normal hematopoiesis is a set of growth factors termed CSFs. These are highly specific proteins or cytokines that stimulate progenitor and precursor cells to differentiate and mature. Hematopoiesis is dependent on their presence. As with other cytokines, CSFs seem to act on target cells via receptors on cell membranes. The different distribution of specific receptors explains responsiveness to various CSFs. Numerous types of CSFs have been identified. Some, such as multi-CSF, interleukin 2 (IL 2), and GM-CSF, seem to affect more than one cell line. Others, such as G-CSF and erythropoietin, are specific to a particular cell line or a group of precursor cells.

HEMATOPOIESIS

Leukopoiesis

The major function of white blood cells (WBCs) is to defend the host against infection. Circulating WBCs are classified as granulocytes or agranulocytes. Each of these two groups is further divided into specific cell types. These cells and their functions are listed in Table 49–2. WBCs are responsible for both cell-mediated immunity (CMI) and humoral immunity (HI). Cell-mediated immunity refers to immune defenses that rely on a direct cellular activity (e.g., phagocytosis by a neutrophil); HI refers to immune defenses that

Table 49–2. FUNCTIONS OF GRANULOCYTES AND MONOCYTES

Cell Type	Function
Granulocyte	
Neutrophil	Phagocytosis, random locomotion, chemotaxis, killing microorganisms, pus formation, lysosome production
Basophil	Releases histamine, heparin, and enzymes in acute inflammation; may prevent clot formation and growth
Eosinophil	Phagocytosis and elaboration of enzymes in allergic reactions; may contribute to fibrin clot digestion; detoxify foreign protein
Monocytes-macrophages	
Blood (free)	Phagocytosis of microorganisms, tumors, cellular debris
Tissue (fixed; also called histiocytes)	Phagocytosis of microorganisms, tumor, cellular and noncellular debris; mediate lymphocyte antibody activity; filtration of particles

rely on an indirect cellular activity (e.g., the elaboration of antibody by B lymphocytes).

Leukopoiesis or *granulopoiesis* refers to the development, differentiation, and maturation of granulocytes and monocytes. *Lymphopoiesis* is the term used to describe the process for lymphocytes. The developmental sequence for these processes is illustrated in Figure 49–2.

The production and release of granulocytes and monocytes is mediated by various CSFs and influenced by the presence of infection and inflammation and by exercise, stress, and glucocorticoids. The interaction between infection and the increased production of neutrophils has not been clearly defined. It seems to involve a feedback loop in which the presence of endotoxins and other bacterial byproducts causes increased production and release of CSFs by macrophages and endothelial cells, which in turn leads to the proliferation and release of neutrophils from the marrow. In addition, another humoral agent, neutrophil-releasing factor, has been postulated. There is probably a negative arm of the feedback loop in which the presence of mature neutrophils causes certain subpopulations of monocytes to release prostaglandin E (PgE), which has an inhibitory effect on the neutrophil population. Various populations of lymphocytes, such as natural killer (NK) cells, are also involved in this process.

The multipotential progenitors of granulocytes are GEMM-CFC or granulocyte-monocyte colony-forming cells (GM-CFC). During the proliferation stages, these cells divide and differentiate to myeloblasts, promyelocytes, and myelocytes. As these cells mature they become metamyelocytes, bands, and finally neutrophils, basophils, or eosinophils. *Neutrophils* are the first line of defense against infection. They constitute 50 to 70 per cent of the total WBC count. Immature neutrophils are referred to as bands or segmental forms because of the nature of their nuclei. The normal value is 3 per cent of the WBC count. *Left shift* is a term used to describe an increase in the percentage of neutrophils and bands (immature neutrophils) in response to infection. When an infection occurs, the level of circulating neutrophils increases through processes described earlier.

In addition to their presence in the marrow, granulocytes exist in the blood stream as a circulating pool, where they have a lifespan of about 12 hr. They are quite mobile and can be attracted to the site of infection by a process called chemotaxis. Once there, they are capable of becoming attached to vessel endothelial cells (marginating) and can enter the tissues by diapedesis. In cancer patients, depressed neutrophil counts are often associated with cancer therapies or infiltration of bone marrow by cancer.

Less is known about *basophils* than about the other granulocytes. They are not phagocytic. The granules in the basophils are related to the granules in mast cells and, therefore, these two cell lines are usually discussed together. In fact, debate continues on whether basophils are precursors of mast cells. *Mast cells* play a role in allergies, anaphylactic shock, and regulation of blood flow. Elevations of basophils are associated with some cancers, with postsplenectomy states, and with estrogen use but their numbers seem unaffected by infection. Basophils constitute up to 1 per cent of total WBC count. *Eosinophils* detoxify foreign protein. They control the effects of mast cells and neutralize the products of mast cells. Their numbers become elevated in drug reactions (e.g., codeine), with steroid use, and in some cancers (e.g., Hodgkin's disease). These cells account for 2 to 4 per cent of the WBC count. *Monocytes* (see Table 49–2) are active as mechanical barriers against organisms and play a role—already described—in the neutrophil feedback loop. Fixed monocytes *(macrophages)* are found in the spleen, lymph nodes, bone marrow, liver capsule, and adrenals. In addition to their phagocytic activities, macrophages influence antibody synthesis by lymphocytes. They are sensitive to steroids and elevations in their numbers occur in persons with chronic infections, in those recovering from infection, and in those with neutropenia.

Lymphopoiesis

Although the development of lymphocytes occurs separately from that of other blood cell lineages, research indicates that like other cell lines, the lymphoid line has its origin in the pluripotential stem cells discussed earlier. At some early point after the initial division of the pluripotential stem cell into daughter cells, the lymphoid line follows a separate course, influenced by some of the same CSFs (e.g., interleukin 3 [IL 3] or multi-CSF) as well as by different ones [IL 2].

Development of lymphocytes depends on the migration of bone marrow precursors to specialized sites in the mononuclear phagocyte system (MPS) (formerly termed the reticuloendothelial system or RES), where further proliferation and differentiation occur. This sequence is illustrated in Figure 49–2. The lymphocyte stem cell gives rise to at least two types of cells: the T lymphocytes, which mature under the influence of thymic endothelium (a thymopoietin has been postulated), and the B lymphocytes, which differentiate and mature in the MPS in response to a postulated B-cell growth factor.

Each of these cell groups has a variety of functions (Table 49–3). Primarily they enable the immune system to distinguish self from nonself or foreign antigens and to respond to foreign antigens. These cells are responsible for the "memory" of the immune system, so that when exposed to the same antigen in the future, a quicker response can be mounted. T cells have both regulator and effector functions in the immune system. They are the primary effectors of CMI and immunoregulation. They mediate delayed cutaneous hypersensitivity reactions and transplant rejection. They seem to orchestrate the overall immune response to specific antigen as well as provide immunosurveillance against cancer. T cells protect against fungi and viruses and respond to bacterial diseases that have an insidious onset.

Lymphocytes are mobile and long-lived. Their life span may be measured in terms of years. They recirculate by passing from the thoracic duct into the blood stream, which carries the cells to lymph nodes; these cells can also be transported to lymph nodes through lymphatic drainage. Lymphocytes constitute 20 to 40 per cent of the total WBC count; elevations in their numbers are seen in viral infections, and lymphopenia is often associated with the acquired immune deficiency syndrome (AIDS).

Thrombopoiesis

The processes by which platelets (thrombocytes) develop and mature are less well defined than those for leukocytes and erythrocytes (see Fig. 49–2). However, there does appear to be a growth factor, thrombopoietin, specific to the megakaryocytic line. Under the influence of this stimulus, the line differentiates in

Table 49–3. FUNCTIONS OF LYMPHOCYTES

Cell	Function
Lymphocytes	
B cells (humoral immunity)	Complement fixation
Plasma cell	Antibody production
Memory cell	"Remembers" antigen
T cells (cellular immunity)	
Null cells (natural killer [NK] and killer [K] cells)	Produce lymphokines; destroy cells directly or indirectly
Helper cells	Mediate antibody production by B cells; promote T-cell activity
Suppressor cells	Diminish B- and possibly T-cell activity; mediate both cellular and humoral immunity
Memory cells	Recognize and respond to previously encountered antigens

the following pattern: CSF-megakaryocyte (CSF-Mk), promegakaryoblast, megakaryoblast, promegakaryocyte, megakaryocyte, and platelet. Normal platelet values range from 150,000 to 400,000 per mm³. Platelets, which are nonnucleated fragments of megakaryocytes, survive in the circulation for 7 to 10 days. They are responsible for clot formation and maintaining integrity of vascular endothelium by attaching to one another and adhering to blood vessel walls. Platelets are also a source of phospholipids for the clotting system and for plasma proteins.

Erythropoiesis

Red blood cells (RBCs) are derived from the pluripotential stem cells by way of a unipotential stem cell called the burst-forming unit (BFU-E [erythroid]) (Queensberry, 1983). Under the influence of a growth factor called burst-promoting activity (BPA), BFU-E gives rise to CFC-E, a more differentiated progenitor cell of the erythroid line. This group of progenitor cells in turn is influenced by one of the earliest identified of the hematopoietic growth factors, erythropoietin (EP). Both in vitro and in vivo studies suggest that EP accelerates RBC production by inducing the CFU-Es to differentiate into proerythroblasts. Ninety per cent of EP production occurs in the kidneys. The remaining 5 to 10 per cent of extrarenal EP appears to be made in the liver. The primary factor influencing the production of EP is tissue oxygenation—cellular hypoxia initiates its production. Prostaglandin E and prostacyclin are also thought to influence renal EP. Although it appears that EP is the predominant influence on the erythroid line, there is evidence that other growth factors, such as GM-CSF and G-CSF, may be involved in this process as well. On the basis of in vitro studies, EP also seems to influence the progressive differentiation and proliferation of various erythroid precursor cells, including basophils, erythroblasts, polychromatic erythroblasts, and the immediate precursors of RBCs, marrow, and blood reticulocytes. Red blood cell production and metabolism require vitamin B_{12} and folic acid.

The major function of RBCs is to transport hemoglobin, which carries oxygen from lungs to tissues. Other functions include eliminating carbon dioxide, hemoglobin synthesis and maintenance, membrane maintenance, and buffering the blood (Erslev, 1983). The normal values for RBCs range from 4.2 to 5.4 million/ml in women and from 6 to 6.2 million/ml in men.

PATHOPHYSIOLOGIC EFFECTS OF CANCER AND CANCER THERAPY ON HEMATOPOIESIS

Normal hematopoiesis is often disrupted in the cancer patient. In addition to having had marrow replaced by tumor, the patient often experiences bone marrow toxicity from chemotherapy, radiation therapy, and surgery. When caring for persons with cancer, the nurse needs to be alert to these and other factors (e.g., nutrition, age) that may alter bone marrow function.

Tumor Effects

Cancer may affect hematopoiesis directly or indirectly. Invasion and replacement of the bone marrow by tumor is called myelophthisis. Cancer cells compete with normal hematopoietic cells for nutrients and destroy hematopoietic cells. Anemia, thrombocytopenia, granulocytopenia, and impaired NK cell activity may result (Beck, 1985; Bull, DeVita, & Carbone, 1975; Sarzotti, Baron, & Klingoll, 1987; Schlicter & Harker, 1974). Acute leukemias pack the marrow, creating pancytopenia, which places the patient at risk for multiple complications from bone marrow depression (BMD).

Cancer can alter hematopoiesis and immune regulation whether or not marrow invasion occurs (Bull et al., 1975). Hodgkin's disease causes a defect in CMI by disrupting T-cell function, mobility, distribution, and the ratio between helper and suppressor T cells (Bull et al., 1975; Gupta, 1986; Harris & Copeland, 1974). Multiple myeloma causes defects in humoral immunity (Gupta, 1986; Jacobson & Zolla-Pazner, 1986).

Roth (1983) has proposed four possible mechanisms of tumor-related immunosuppression. These include

1. An increase in the number or proportion of immunosuppressive cells.

2. Elevated plasma levels of circulating antigen-antibody complexes.

3. Increased levels of acute phase reactants with immunosuppressive properties (e.g., serum lipoproteins).

4. An unidentified humoral factor secreted by tumors that is immunosuppressive.

Chemotherapy

The treatment most often associated with hematologic toxicity and marrow suppression is chemotherapy. The degree to which a patient experiences marrow suppression after chemotherapy depends on the agents used; the doses, schedules, and routes of administration; previous antineoplastic treatment; concomitant adjuvant therapy; and factors such as age, nutritional status, and tumor type and stage.

The hematologic toxicity of chemotherapy varies widely. Acute chemotherapy-induced myelosuppression is usually caused by the destruction of the proliferating progenitors (CFU-GM, BFU-E, and so forth) of mature cells. As progenitor cells are destroyed, preexisting mature cells are cleared at the end of their natural cycles, and the nadir of a person's blood cell counts occurs. Differences in lengths of the life cycle of blood cells account for the high incidence of granulocytopenia and thrombocytopenia.

Antineoplastic agents that are phase specific are

myelosuppressive because of their impact on proliferating progenitor cells, which are in active phases when drugs are administered, but they do not destroy cells in the resting phase. Agents that are phase nonspecific destroy cells in the resting phase and can have a delayed, prolonged, and cumulative myelosuppressive effect. This is a consequence of the damage they do to nonproliferating stem cells, which are essential in the marrow response to a challenge such as chemotherapy. The relative degrees of myelosuppression of specific agents are listed in Table 49–4.

Use of combinations of chemotherapeutic agents and sequencing may complicate myelosuppression. For example, neither cisplatin nor mitomycin C is very myelosuppressive when used as a single agent, but in a population of esophageal cancer patients who received these drugs in combination, nearly half developed severe hematologic toxicity (Stoll, Lanin, & Engstrom, 1985). Other factors may influence the degree, severity, and duration of BMD. These factors include liver and kidney function, the presence of effusions, and exposure to other nonantineoplastic drugs that interact synergistically with the chemotherapeutic agents (e.g., nitrosoureas and cimetidine) (Kirschner & Preisler, 1985). In patients with malignant effusions, drugs may accumulate and slowly be released into the circulation—a factor that may delay BMD, prolong it, or make it more severe.

In addition to acute bone marrow toxicity, chemotherapy has delayed and long-term effects on the bone marrow. Late effects include marrow failure secondary to atrophy and fibrosis or the appearance of second tumors. Several possible explanations for these late effects of chemotherapy have been postulated (Abrams, 1983; Frisch, Bartl, & Chaichuk, 1986; Hardy & Balducci, 1985; Kovacs et al., 1985; Lohrman, 1984). There may be a decrease in the size of the

pluripotential stem cell compartment. In this compartment there may be a shift from younger to older stem cells with an accompanying diminished capacity for self-renewal. Three changes in the bone marrow seem to occur in the chemotherapy-treated patient (Frisch et al., 1986). Initially, there is a hyper- or normocellular state with a large degree of ongoing phagocytosis. Then the marrow enters a stage characterized by edema, inflammation, and decreased hematopoietic activity. Finally, the marrow becomes hypocellular with small islands of normal hematopoiesis. Yeomans (1987) has delineated the myelodysplastic states that can result from the third stage.

Lithium carbonate causes granulocytosis, and this has led investigators to make attempts to ameliorate BMD by administering this drug during chemotherapy treatment courses; the results have been equivocal (Abrams, 1983; Horns, Schirer, Stanley, & Greenberg, 1984; Richtman, Makii, Weiser, & Herbst, 1984). Rescue regimens have been used with certain drugs to reduce bone marrow and epithelial toxicity. An effort has also been made to capitalize on the so-called rebound-overshoot phenomenon, in which marrow elements proliferate more rapidly after certain chemotherapy agents are administered. Theoretically, a patient's marrow could be primed by the administration of a small dose of one agent in preparation for the chemotherapy regimen (Abrams, 1983; Braun & Harris, 1985), but results of trials have been less than promising. Autologous marrow transplants are another intervention used to overcome otherwise mortal hematologic toxicity of high-dose chemotherapy or radiation therapy (see Chapter 27).

Testing of a new approach to the problem of BMD has recently begun in clinical settings. This involves the administration of CSFs or hematopoietic growth factors. The most commonly used of the CSFs are granulocyte colony-stimulating factor, (G-CSF), granulocyte-macrophage colony-stimulating factor (GM-CSF), and erythropoietin.

These naturally occurring hormone-like substances stimulate one or more of the cell lines in the hematopoietic system, inducing proliferation and differentiation. Although their presence in the body has been known for some time, advances in genetic engineering have allowed them to be produced in "industrial" quantities and have led to clinical testing of the agents. Thus far four primary patient populations have been targeted:

- cancer patients experiencing blood count nadirs owing to antineoplastic treatments
- bone marrow transplant patients
- persons with myelodysplastic syndromes
- persons with AIDS

Side effects appear to be limited, and clinical results have been encouraging. Further advances in the application and the identification of other CSFs, such as a factor affecting platelet production, are promising areas of research (Haeuber & DiJulio, 1989).

Table 49–4. DRUG CLASS OR COMPOUND AND DEGREE AND DURATION OF MYELOSUPPRESSION

Drug or Drug Class	Degree of Suppression*	Nadir of Myelosuppression (Days)	Duration of Marrow Recovery (Days)
Anthracycline	III	8–13	21–24
Vinca alkaloids	I–II	4–8	7–21
Mustard alkylator			
Nitrogen mustard	III	7–14	28
Antifolates	III	7–14	14–21
Antipyrimidines	III	7–14	22–24
Antipurines	II	7–14	14–21
Podophyllotoxins	II	8–14	22–28
Alkylators	II	10–21	18–40
Nitrosoureas	III	28–60	35–85
Miscellaneous†			
Busulfan	III	11–30	24–54
Cisplatin	I	14	21
Dacarbazine	III	21–28	28–35
Hydroxyurea	II	7	14–21
Mithramycin	I	5–10	10–18
Mitomycin	II	28–42	42–56
Procarbazine	II	25–36	35–60
Razoxane (ICRF)	II	11–16	12–25

*I, mild; II, moderate; III, severe (based on common dose schedules).
†Agents differing from their class of compounds.
(From Hoagland, H. [1982]. Hematologic complications of cancer chemotherapy. *Seminars in Oncology, 9,* 95–102. Reproduced by permission.)

Radiotherapy

The effects of radiotherapy on bone marrow and immunity are similar to those of chemotherapy. Certain factors are present in radiotherapy that determine the degree of risk for BMD. Although total radiation doses and fractionation schedule are important, the most significant factor is the volume of productive marrow in the treatment field (see Fig. 49–1). The volumes of bone marrow in several typical fields are listed in Table 49–5. Radiation to sites that include major blood vessels and lymphatic channels is toxic to lymphocytes. For this reason, mediastinal radiotherapy can be more immunosuppressive than radiotherapy to other sites.

Radiotherapy is not as destructive to progenitor cells as chemotherapy but is much more damaging to cells in the G_0 phase. Therefore, radiotherapy has a greater impact on pluripotential stem cells. Except for total nodal or total body irradiation, radiotherapy does not usually cause the nadirs in blood counts seen with chemotherapy. This is because radiation treatment is a local therapy that leaves substantial amounts of marrow intact and able to compensate for the damage to the irradiated marrow (unless compromised by prior radiotherapy or prior chemotherapy). Irradiated marrow recovers through a twofold process: (1) migration of stem cells from unirradiated marrow to the treated area; and (2) conversion of mesenchymal cells in the haversian canal of the cortex of irradiated bone into actively proliferating cells (Rubin & Scarantino, 1978). An intact marrow stroma is vital to maintain a suitable environment for stem cell seeding and hematopoiesis. However, unlike chemotherapy, radiotherapy has a clear, negative effect on stromal elements, causing disruption of the sinusoidal architecture, fibrosis, and necrosis (Fliedner, Northdurft, & Clavo, 1986). The estimate of the upper limit of radiation doses above which marrow regeneration will not occur owing to stromal damage varies from 3000 centigrays (cGy) (rad) (Rubin, 1984) to 4000 to 5000 cGy (Fliedner et al., 1986).

The destruction of the marrow microenvironment and the fact that radiotherapy is most damaging to the pluripotential stem cell pool that is not actively proliferating account for the potential long-term effects of this therapy. Residual effects include hypoplasia or aplasia of certain marrow segments and a propensity to various myelodysplastic syndromes. As a result, the radiotherapy patient may be relatively intolerant of further antineoplastic therapy, such as chemotherapy. The peripheral blood counts, although providing essential data to determine the timing and scheduling of chemotherapy and the type of supportive care a patient requires, are unreliable indicators either of the functional status of the marrow or of its ability to tolerate additional antineoplastic therapy (Fliedner et al., 1986; Rubin & Scarantino, 1978; Schofield, 1986). It is apparent that the volume of marrow irradiated is as important as the therapeutic dose in determining future treatment tolerance.

In addition to radiotherapy's effects on neutrophils, platelets, and RBCs, it is significantly more lymphocytotoxic than chemotherapy. The most significant effects occur when large parts of the lymphoid system are included in the treatment field, as in the case of total nodal irradiation (TNI) for Hodgkin's disease or radiotherapy to the chest with its large volume of circulating blood and lymph (Blomgren et al., 1981; Dickinson & Stone, 1981; DuBois & Serrou, 1981).

The precise effects of radiotherapy on lymphocytes have not been determined, but it is agreed that in radiation-induced lymphopenia the T-cell subset is particularly affected (DuBois & Serrou, 1981). Delayed-hypersensitivity immune responses are more depressed than antibody responses to antigen. Evidence of continued immunosuppression persists for 6 months to 2 years after treatment (Blomgren et al., 1981; McLaren et al., 1981; Wara, Wara, & Amman, 1981). It should be noted that although research has repeatedly confirmed these immunosuppressive effects, a clear link between the effects of radiotherapy on the immune system and clinical effects such as increased susceptibility to infection has not been established (Davies, Wallis, & Peckham, 1981; Tubiana, Arriagada, & Sarragin, 1986).

Chemotherapy and radiotherapy have synergistic effects on bone marrow. In general, chemotherapy should precede radiotherapy. The impact of chemotherapy on proliferating progenitor cells often causes an overshoot or rebound effect during the recovery period, which is believed to provide a buffer against effects of radiotherapy especially as the latter tends not to be as cytotoxic to rapidly proliferating cells. When radiotherapy is administered first, as the marrow responds to the insult with increased proliferation and circulation of stem cells, bone marrow is more vulnerable to the impact of chemotherapy on dividing cells.

Surgery

One of the earliest articles to suggest that surgery could be immunosuppressive appeared in 1958 (Buinoukos, McDonald, & Cole, 1958). Since then, numerous studies have reinforced this conclusion. The ad-

Table 49–5. ESTIMATED PERCENTAGE OF BONE MARROW VOLUME IN SELECTED RADIATION TREATMENT FIELDS

Disease	Radiotherapy Technique	Percentage of Marrow in Field
Hodgkin's disease	Total nodal irradiation	60–70
	Extended field	40–50
	Segmental field	20–25
Non-Hodgkin's lymphoma	Total body irradiation	100
	Extended field	40–50
Leukemias	Cranial and spinal	25–40
Breast cancer	Chest wall	15–20
Pancreas	Abdominal	15–20

(Adapted with permission from Ruben, P., & Scarantino, C. [1978]. The bone marrow organ: The critical structure in radiation-drug interactions. *International Journal of Radiation Oncology, Biology, Physics, 4,* 3–23. Copyright 1978, Pergamon Press plc.)

ministration of anesthesia and the trauma and stress of surgery can be immunosuppressive (Cole, 1985). Because surgery is a common method of therapy for cancer patients, it is important to review this information briefly.

Most studies of immunosuppression in surgical patients indicate that the most important effects are on CMI as measured by delayed hypersensitivity skin test responses. Hjortso and Kehlet (1986) found that 24 patients undergoing abdominal surgery had significantly weaker skin test responses than 16 control subjects. The degree of immunosuppression also correlated with serum albumin level, suggesting a possible nutritional component. When serial skin response to antigen was tested preoperatively and postoperatively in 100 surgical patients, a diminished immune response occurred (Riboli, Terrizi, Arnulfio, & Bertoglio, 1984). These authors found that a suppressed immune response peaked on the third postoperative day and that recovery occurred between the seventh and tenth postoperative days. Among cancer patients in the sample, the depressed immune response was more severe and prolonged with a lower recovery plateau. Before surgery, cancer patients did not have significantly lower scores. Another study found that humoral immunity also is diminished in surgical patients, especially among those who were anergic by skin test before surgery (Nohr, Christov, Broadhead, & Meakins, 1983). Yoshihara, Tanaka, and Orita (1986) found that NK cell activity is reduced in the postoperative period and suggested that surgical effects on immune response could be due to depression of lymphocyte blastogenesis or leukocyte migration inhibition. They also postulate that depressed NK activity may enhance metastatic seeding during the postoperative period.

Possible effects of a depressed immune response after surgery include increased risk of infection, septicemia, and increased mortality. Because surgery is a common intervention in cancer patients, it is important to be aware of potential surgically induced immunosuppression during the postoperative period and of the prolonged recovery time that may be needed for cancer patients to return to a normal immunologic state.

Biotherapy

Biotherapy, or the use of biologic response modifiers (BRMs), has been called the "cancer treatment modality of the future" (Mayer, 1987). These agents, including interferons (IFNs), tumor necrosis factor (TNF), monoclonal antibodies (MAB), and IL 2, exert potentially therapeutic effects through several possible mechanisms: (1) exerting a direct antitumor effect; (2) restoring, augmenting, or otherwise modulating the patient's immune system; and (3) demonstrating other biologic effects, such as interference with tumor cells' ability to metastasize (see Chapter 23) (Abernathy, 1987).

Experience is too limited to be able to define the nature and severity of toxicities associated with specific BRMs. Certain side effects are clearly associated with selected BRMs, such as the constitutional symptoms associated with IFN administration, including fever, chills, myalgia, fatigue, and weakness (Irwin, 1987).

Considering that the mechanism of action of BRMs is to modulate the immune system, the potential for hematologic toxicity is apparent. In fact, those agents with which there is the most experience (IFNs and MABs) do demonstrate hematologic toxicities. Abundant evidence exists that IFN therapy causes a reversible fall in WBCs, and with continued treatment a patient may experience a mild anemia, thrombocytopenia (TCP), and lymphopenia (Fischl, 1986; Quesada, Talpaz, Rios, Kurzrock, & Gutterman, 1986). The hematologic effects are severe enough to warrant caution when IFN is given in conjunction with chemotherapy. Monoclonal antibody infusions have been associated with a substantial decrease in WBCs (reversible). One study found that patients who evidenced a decline in WBCs greater than 25 per cent tended to manifest other side effects, such as fever, rigors, and chills (Dillman, Beauregard, Halpern, & Clutter, 1986).

The mechanisms by which the BRMs cause their hematologic effects continue to be the subject of speculation. Some authorities maintain that the pattern of hematologic toxicity of IFN indicates a sequestration process, in which the release of blood components from the marrow is blocked (Kirkwood & Ernstoff, 1984; Scott, 1983). On the other hand, results of some in vitro studies indicate that, additionally, the proliferation of hematopoietic progenitor cells (GM-CFC, BFU-E, GEMM-CFC) is inhibited by exposure to IFN (Contino, Testa, & Dexter, 1986). Given the complexity of these systems, there is undoubtedly more than one mechanism of action. These reports suggest that nurses should monitor hematologic status of patients undergoing BRM therapy (see Chapter 23).

Aging

Cancer is a disease of the elderly. Considering the myelosuppressive nature of antineoplastic treatments, it is essential to be aware of age changes that occur in the hematopoietic and immune systems. Platelets do not appear to be affected by aging (Williams, 1983). However, if, as some researchers suggest, there is an overall age-related diminution in hematopoietic reserve, effects on platelets would be expected as well. There is conflicting evidence regarding changes in the leukocyte count and the ability of aged persons to mount an adequate leukocyte response to infection (Lipschitz, Mitchell, & Thompson, 1981; Williams, 1983). Investigators in one study found that a healthy elderly population had an increased incidence of leukopenia and neutropenia (Lipschitz et al., 1981).

Anemia seems to be a fairly common change in the elderly (Williams, 1983). Lipschitz and co-workers (1981) found mild anemia in 21 per cent of women and 34 per cent of men in a study of 222 healthy elderly persons. They were unable to identify a cause for the condition. They concluded that anemia and concomitant leukopenia and neutropenia may represent an overall reduction in hematopoietic reserve and an increased susceptibility to stresses on the hematopoietic system. Similarities between hematopoietic changes associated with aging and protein-calorie malnutrition have been observed (Lipschitz & Udupa, 1986).

The most active research regarding aging and hematopoietic function has focused on changes in the immune system. Although there are some contradictory conclusions, aging seems to be accompanied by defects in delayed hypersensitivity response and in cytotoxic T-cell generation as well as by diminished quality and quantity of antibody responses to antigen (Weksler, 1981; Weksler, Hansman, & Schwab, 1984). Many of the changes that occur seem to be related to alterations in T-lymphocyte function. This may be an outcome of involution of the thymus and decreased thymic hormone production. One result of changing T-cell function is a diminished production of the lymphokine IL 2, which is necessary for amplification of the effector cells' response to antigen (Thoman, 1985; Trofatter, 1986). There may also be a disruption in the ratio of T-helper to T-suppressor cells, which could account in part for the increased numbers of autoantibodies found in the elderly (Weksler et al., 1984). The most important conclusion is that aging may be a factor in the inability of a patient's hematopoietic system to withstand the substantial stress of cancer and its treatment.

Nutrition

Nutrition is a very important factor in determining a person's hematologic and immunologic status. The connection between nutritional intake and anemia from deficiencies of such nutrients as iron, folate, and vitamin B_{12} is well known (Beck, 1988; Fairbanks & Beutler, 1983; Oski, 1983). A relationship also exists between nutrition and immunity. It has long been recognized that an increased risk of infection occurs among persons suffering from protein-calorie malnutrition (PCM) (Corman, 1985); PCM causes lymphopenia, cutaneous anergy, diminished levels of complement, and a diminution of certain immunoglobulins (Corman, 1985). As in the case of aging, T cells and CMI are substantially more affected by malnutrition than B cells are (Law, Dudrick, & Abdou, 1973). Levy (1982) argues that malnutrition also impairs the killing activities of neutrophils and macrophages and that there is decreased production of lymphokines and chemotactic factors.

Harvey, Bothe, and Blackburn (1979) observed that PCM is the most common secondary diagnosis among cancer patients. In their study of malnourished cancer patients, they found a much higher mortality rate among patients who remained anergic as a result of malnutrition. Balducci and Hardy (1985) found that myelotoxicity caused by chemotherapy and radiotherapy is enhanced by the protein deprivation of cancer cachexia. They note that malnutrition in humans is accompanied by marrow suppression and a diminished granulocyte reserve and that in protein-deprived mice, the concentration of pluripotential hematopoietic stem cells is decreased. There is no convincing evidence that nutritional support in the form of hyperalimentation will prevent or even ameliorate antineoplastic therapy–induced myelotoxicity. However, Balducci and Hardy (1985) asserted that patients will better tolerate cytotoxic therapy if they are nutritionally supported because side effects other than BMD may impair nutrition (e.g., nausea, vomiting, anorexia, and mucositis).

Psychoneuroimmunology

Specific associations between psychological states and disease have been identified (e.g., stress and hypertension). Within the last 10 years, increasing attention has been directed toward an apparent relationship between stress and infectious diseases, autoimmune disorders, and cancer. This field of investigation, psychoneuroimmunology, postulates essential interconnections among the central nervous system (CNS) and the neuroendocrine and immune systems.

Increasing evidence from clinical, epidemiologic, and experimental studies suggests that the psychological state of persons can affect their immune systems. Given the multiplicity of physiologic, financial, social, and emotional pressures experienced by cancer patients, it is important that this factor be considered in assessing overall risk of hematopoietic or immune system compromise. Irwin and Anisman (1984) proposed a schematic framework indicating some of the interconnections with which psychoneuroimmunology is concerned.

The evidence for these interrelationships comes from animal and human research. Often the conclusions are regarded as tenuous. Part of the problem has to do with the complexity of systems involved, both singly and as a network. In general, research in psychoneuroimmunology has moved from clinical and epidemiologic studies that attempted to retrospectively relate illness with the occurrence of previous stressful events to more carefully controlled and precisely defined experimental studies with animals (Borysenko & Borysenko, 1982; Riley, 1981) and humans (Dorian, Keystone, Garfinkel & Brown, 1981; Palmblad, Petrini, Wasserman, & Akerstadt, 1979; Palmblad et al., 1976). In addition, studies have been conducted of persons who have demonstrated compromised immune function during or after the experience of naturally stressful events in their lives, such as bereavement (Bartrop, Luckhurst, Lazarus, Kiloh, & Penny, 1977; Schiffer, 1983).

One of the direct links between the CNS and the immune system is thought to be hormonal, products of the hypothalamic-pituitary-adrenal axis. Stein, Schiavi, and Camerino (1976) demonstrated that certain types of electrolytic lesions to the hypothalamus alter the extent to which experimental animals experience anaphylaxis and delayed hypersensitivity reactions. Among possible hormonal mediators, corticosteroids in rodents and cortisol in humans were thought

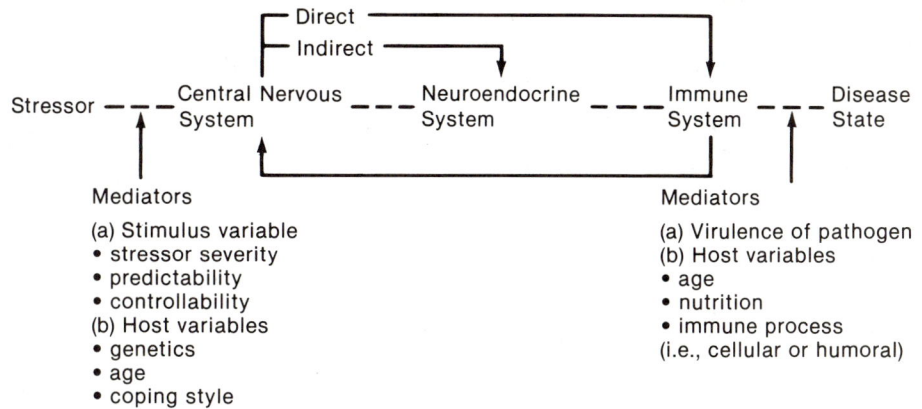

Figure 49–3. Proposed interconnections among psychoneuroimmunologic variables. (Redrawn with permission from Irwin, J., & Anisman, H. [1984]. Stress and pathology: Immunological and central nervous system interactions. In C. L. Cooper [Ed.], *Psychosocial stress and cancer* [p. 94]. New York: John Wiley & Sons.)

to be instrumental in depressing immune responses, as they were known to be lymphocytotoxic and were released during a response to stress. However, the role of cortisol in immunosuppression in humans has come into question, owing partly to the development of increasingly sensitive hormonal assays that have identified a plethora of substances that seem to interact in the complicated process of neuroendocrine-mediated immune alterations (Borysenko & Borysenko, 1982). Some of the hormones involved in this process seem to be somatotropin, prolactin, thyrotropin, thyroxine, and endorphins (Blalock, 1989; Borysenko & Borysenko, 1982; Monjan, 1981).

The possibility that a direct link exists between the CNS and the immune system has been suggested by the finding in certain animal species of neural innervation of lymphoid tissues, such as the spleen and thymus (Bullock, 1985), and by the presence of receptors for neurotransmitters on lymphocytes (Ader, 1985; Baker, 1987; Hall & Goldstein, 1981; Locke, 1982).

Some of the factors that may be involved in the response of the immune system to stress are identified in Figure 49–3. They include the actual or perceived severity of the stressor, its predictability, and its controllability (Irwin & Anisman, 1984; Stein, 1985). Other factors that may be involved include the duration and chronicity of the stressor (Baker, 1987; Sklar & Anisman, 1979) and patients' coping ability. In an

excellent review of the field of psychoneuroimmunology, Locke (1982) suggests that coping ability may be central to maintenance of immunocompetence under stressful circumstances. If this is the case, the role of health care professionals in providing support to cancer patients through such techniques as visualization, guided imagery, and relaxation therapy may be important in maintaining the integrity of the immune system.

OVERVIEW OF NURSING ASSESSMENT

The initial assessment of the person at risk of BMD should be comprehensive and includes the health history, physical examination, and laboratory tests. Subsequent assessments may be targeted to the specific hematopoietic impairment. A thorough health history is essential to determining potential or existing BMD, identifying needs for patient education related to BMD, and planning and implementing preventive and therapeutic nursing interventions. No clear data are available on the relationship between the number of risk factors for BMD and the severity of BMD, although the authors' clinical experiences suggest that patients with several risk factors may experience more severe BMD. When taking the health history, risk factors that may predate the diagnosis of cancer as well as those that are associated with cancer therapy

Table 49–6. THE HEALTH HISTORY: RISK FACTORS FOR BONE MARROW DEPRESSION (BMD)

Before Cancer Diagnosis and Treatment

Family history of myeloproliferative or hematologic disease, diabetes, cancer

History negative for chickenpox

Immunizations (types, dates, responses)

Environmental or occupational exposures to hematotoxic substances (for example, benzene, chloramphenicol, radiation)

Other medical problems (for example, other immunosuppressive illnesses such as diabetes, infectious diseases, and their therapies [include type, date, duration of therapy]; surgeries; steroid or other immunosuppressive therapies)

Psychosocial history: major life stressor(s), stress-related illnesses: substance abuse; usual coping style; sources of support; recent losses; learning style; sleep patterns

Sexual history and hygiene; number of partners, history of sexually transmitted diseases and therapy; usual sexual practices

Nutritional history: recent weight loss, diet history

Elimination patterns: positive history of constipation, urinary tract infections

Activity pattern

History of splenectomy

Immunosuppressive therapies and patterns of bone marrow toxicity

Therapies or hospitalizations for BMD complications (for example, transfusions, antimicrobial therapies, life support)

Types of bone marrow toxicity (infection or sepsis [source], bleeding, severe anemia)

Responses to BMD: effects on work and home life, activity level

Patient or family response to therapy and complications

and its complications can be identified. Elements of the health history essential to evaluating actual or potential BMD are found in Table 49–6. Although the focus of this section is generalized BMD, nurses should be aware that splenectomized patients present special problems. First, variation in WBC counts are often seen and several serial counts may be needed to evaluate so-called abnormal findings. Second, this population has a greater risk of abrupt and severe infection owing to loss of the spleen's filtering function (Crosby, 1983).

The history gives nurses an idea of factors that may influence or complicate a patient's response to bone marrow toxic therapy. Table 49–7 highlights physical examination findings that may be associated with BMD (Spross, 1985). Risk factors for specific complications of BMD are listed in Table 49–8.

A variety of diagnostic tests can help the nurse assess potential or existing BMD. The complete blood count (CBC), differential count, and platelet count are key laboratory values for evaluating BMD in a person with cancer. Normal values for these tests are given in Table 49–9. The blood for these studies may be obtained by venipuncture or fingerstick. Values of particular interest are the WBC count, hemoglobin (Hg), hematocrit (Hct), platelets, and the granulocyte count (polymorphonuclear leukocytes, segmental forms, and bands). These tests are monitored to assess bone marrow response to treatment and to modify therapy as needed. BMD may be significant enough to warrant postponement or discontinuation of therapy or dose reduction. The frequency with which this is monitored depends on the specific therapeutic regimen (see Chapter 21). Other diagnostic tests and the information they provide are listed in Table 49–10.

COMPLICATIONS

Having discussed normal hematopoiesis, pathophysiologic changes in this process, and general assessment of a person with potential or actual BMD, it is important to look at the potential complications of BMD and describe the nursing care of persons experiencing these complications. The most serious complications of BMD are infection and bleeding. Nurses play a critical role in prevention and early detection of these complications. Anemia associated with cancer-related BMD rarely presents significant clinical problems. In studies examining nursing interventions with patients undergoing chemotherapy, Dodd (1983) found that patients who had both drug information and information about self-management strategies had less severe complications and sought medical care earlier than those who did not receive this systematic information.

Clinical Problem: Infection

Infection is the most common cause of morbidity and mortality in patients with cancer. Risk of infection is correlated with severity and duration of granulocytopenia (GCP). In addition, extremes of age, compromised host defense, and colonization with potential pathogens increase the risk of serious infection in persons with cancer.

In the cancer patient with GCP, infection may be difficult to assess because the usual response to infection, neutrophil mobilization, does not occur. The nurse has an important role in prevention and detection of infection and in monitoring the patient's responses to preventive and therapeutic interventions.

Prevention

Persons with cancer may have several coexisting risk factors for infection, as is clear from the discussion of bone marrow pathophysiology. Identification of risk factors from history, laboratory values, and clinical examination directs the nursing care plan. Prevention strategies are focused on patient education, avoiding damage to host defenses, bolstering host defenses, reducing acquisition of new potential pathogens, and

---

Table 49–7. PHYSICAL EXAMINATION OF THE CLIENT WITH ACTUAL OR POTENTIAL BONE MARROW DEPRESSION

General condition
  Age (very old and very young at higher risk), fatigue (may be a sign of anemia), malaise (may be a sign of infection), cachexia
Skin and mucous membranes
  Open lesions, excoriated skin, pressure areas, mucositis, petechiae, ecchymoses, swelling, tenderness, biopsy sites; skin test results (anergy or negative responses to purified protein derivative [PPD], Dichloronitrobenzene [DCNB], streptokinase-streptodornase [SKSD] indicate diminished cellular immunity)
Head, Eyes, Ears, Nose, Throat
  Headache, visual changes, pupillary changes, pain, tenderness, exudate, enlarged lymph nodes
Cardiopulmonary
  Respiratory rate, pattern, breath sounds (wheezing, consolidation), quantity and quality of sputum, pain, shortness of breath, use of accessory muscles, tachycardia, activity intolerance
Gastrointestinal
  Pain, bleeding, diarrhea, character of stool, constipation, ascites, character of vomitus
Genitourinary
  Dysuria, bleeding, exudate (color, quantity, quality); character of menses; dyspareunia; pelvic examination
Central Nervous System
  Headache, visual changes, change in level of consciousness, cognition, dizziness
Musculoskeletal
  Inspect and palpate reported areas of tenderness (hemarthroses may occur in acute leukemia)

Baseline and changes in systems should be evaluated.

Table 49–8. RISK FACTORS FOR SPECIFIC COMPLICATIONS OF BONE MARROW DEPRESSION

Infection
Abnormal function of phagocytes (e.g., acute leukemia)
Insufficient phagocytes (e.g., postchemotherapy granulocytopenia)
Abnormal antibodies (e.g., multiple myeloma)
Insufficient antibody (e.g., protein malnutrition)
Absent or damaged mechanical barriers (e.g., splenectomy)

Bleeding
Abnormal function of platelets (e.g., idiopathic thrombocytopenia)
Insufficient platelets (e.g., hemorrhage)
Defect in intrinsic or extrinsic clotting system (e.g., liver dysfunction due to metastases)

Anemia
Abnormal function of RBCs (e.g., RBC dysfunction)
Insufficient RBCs (e.g., postchemotherapy anemia)

suppressing colonizing organisms (Tables 49–11 and 49–12) (Pizzo & Young, 1985).

The importance of patient and family education cannot be overemphasized. It is helpful to teach the patient as well as a family member or significant other. Patients undergoing active bone marrow suppressive therapy may be too ill or stressed to absorb or process information given to them that might be life saving. Patients may remember side effects of therapy, such as hair loss or nausea and vomiting, but forget that therapy may cause life-threatening infection or bleeding. Nurses must attempt to evaluate whether learning took place.

Risk reduction may involve changing lifelong habits (such as stopping the use of enemas or suppositories for chronic constipation), changing jobs, or obtaining temporary disability leave to avoid exposure to potential pathogens. Total protected environment and oral nonabsorbable antibiotics have been studied to see if risk and severity of infection can be reduced. Conclusions from these studies suggest that these measures, which are quite expensive, should be used only in patients undergoing high-risk therapies, such as high-dose chemotherapy or bone marrow transplantation.

Early Detection

Because infection is the leading cause of morbidity and mortality in cancer patients, early detection is essential, particularly in the patient with GCP. Levels of risk associated with specific granulocyte values are given in Table 49–13. An undetected, untreated infection often ends in death for the febrile cancer patient with GCP (Pizzo & Young, 1985). Early detection of infection in febrile patients with cancer is complicated by a number of factors. Fever may result from tumor, chemotherapeutic and antimicrobial drugs, and transfusions.

In the patient with GCP, fever most often has an infectious cause. The absence of sufficient, functional neutrophils in GCP means the clinician is unlikely to observe classic signs and symptoms of infection (e.g., no pus in lesions or urine). Fever in the nonneutropenic patient can be evaluated according to general medical principles, but the urgency with which fever in GCP must be addressed is such that Pizzo and Young (1985) recommend that institutional criteria and policies should be established and adhered to to minimize infection-related morbidity. Such a policy and criteria for fever work-up in patients with granulocytopenia are outlined as follows: Any patient with a granulocyte count less than 1000 cells/mm³ who has a single temperature elevation above 38.3° C or two or more elevations above 38° C will have a fever work-up. The fever work-up includes two sets of preantibiotic blood cultures, chest radiograph, and cultures of sputum, urine, wound, and other accessible sites suggestive of infection. If blood is drawn for culture from a vascular access device or indwelling Silastic catheter, additional blood for cultures must be obtained from a peripheral vein. Once the fever work-up is completed, a regimen of empiric antibiotics is usually begun without waiting for culture results. Once culture and sensitivity test results are known, therapy can be adjusted to treat the identified organisms.

Early detection of infection, especially in hospital-

Table 49–9. NORMAL VALUES FOR SELECTED PERIPHERAL BLOOD TESTS (CBC, DIFFERENTIAL, PLATELETS) AND CALCULATION FOR ABSOLUTE GRANULOCYTE COUNT

Normal laboratory values			
Hemoglobin:	men	14–16.5 g/dl	
	women	12–16 g/dl	
Hematocrit:	men	42–51%	
	women	37–47%	
Platelets		145,000–364,000 per mm³	
White blood count		5000–10,000 per mm³	

	Normal Percentage of WBCs	Absolute Cell Count
WBC differential count		
Lymphocytes	15–52	720–5600
Segmental forms (neutrophils, polymorphonuclear leukocytes)	35–73	1680–7884
Bands	0–11	0–1188
Monocytes	2–14	96–1512
Eosinophils	0–5	0–540
Basophils	0–2	0–216

Absolute granulocyte count (AGC):
   AGC is the percentage of segmental forms plus bands multiplied times the WBC:
   % segmental cells + % bands × WBC = AGC

Table 49–10. DIAGNOSTIC TESTS USEFUL IN EVALUATING ACTUAL OR POTENTIAL BONE MARROW DEPRESSION

Diagnostic Test	Information Provided
Bone marrow biopsy or aspirate	Evidence of replacement of marrow by cancer
	Evidence of bone marrow recovery
	Response of myeloproliferative cancer to therapy
Radiographs	Evidence of infection
Cultures	Type, site of infection, and antimicrobial sensitivities
Serum total protein and albumin levels	Protein stores (hematopoietic cells and an intact immune system need protein; depressed levels reflect an added risk of infection)
Skin testing	Evidence of anergy reflects an inability to mount an effective immune response

ized patients with GCP, depends on astute nursing care. Nurses' sustained contact with patients enables them to detect subtle and overt changes in their conditions that suggest infection. In addition to monitoring temperatures, daily assessment of high-risk areas is vital. High-risk areas include axillae, oral cavity, perineum (particularly anorectal area), intertriginous areas, and existing wounds or other integumentary changes (e.g., ingrown toenail). Anorectal pain in GCP may be the first sign of a perirectal infection. This symptom may precede objective findings by 2 to 10 days. Neutropenic enterocolitis occurs in persons with severe GCP and is characterized by diffuse abdominal cramping and distention, fever, bloody diarrhea, and decreased or absent bowel sounds. An ingrown toenail or periodontal infection may evolve into a serious infection. Obstructive pneumonia can occur in patients with lung tumors. In some patients, pain or tenderness may be the only initial sign of infection. High-risk sites should be inspected at least daily in persons who are hospitalized. Some patients may simply have changes in personality and behavior or hypotension in the absence of a fever, which may signal a serious infection. For outpatients, they and their families must be taught to have a high index of suspicion for infections when such changes occur and should know how to contact the oncologist or oncology nurse. Visiting nurse referrals for such patients should include clear information on the patient's level of risk, parameters to be monitored, and reportable signs and symptoms. The importance of a timely response to fever in the cancer patient

Table 49–11. CONTENT FOR PATIENT EDUCATION REGARDING PREVENTION AND EARLY DETECTION OF INFECTION

Self-inspection of high-risk areas for signs of infection
Temperature-taking
Self-care of vascular access devices and other invasive equipment
Functions of white blood cells (WBCs)
Reportable signs and symptoms
Hygiene (skin, oral, sexual)
Prevention of exposure to communicable diseases
Expected time of WBC nadir
Self-monitoring for superinfection when on antibiotics
Health-promoting self-care practices (good nutrition, sleep, stress reduction techniques)

Table 49–12. STRATEGIES FOR INFECTION PREVENTION IN THE IMMUNOCOMPROMISED CANCER PATIENT

Bolster Host Defenses
- Rapid remission induction
- Balanced, nutritional diet
- Administer prescribed vaccines
- Administer prescribed immunomodulators
- Administer prescribed leukocytes
- Transfusions
- Encourage use of stress-reduction techniques

Avoid Damage to Body Barriers
- Avoid invasive procedures (rectal thermometers and medications; urinary catheters)
- Initiate pulmonary toilet and other measures to prevent bedrest complications for immobilized patients or those with limited mobility

Reduce Acquisition of New Potential Pathogens
- Meticulous handwashing
- Cooked food diet for granulocyte counts < 500 cells/mm³
- No humidifiers
- No cut flowers in room
- Avoid exposure to communicable infections
- Monitor environment for risk factors (e.g., inadequate housekeeping)
- Inspect biopsy sites, sites of venous access devices (VADs)
- Maintain asepsis when caring for patients with VADs, other invasive devices, and wounds
- Maintain total protected environment procedures when prescribed

Suppress Colonizing Organisms
- Administer prescribed antimicrobials; monitor serum levels; monitor patients on antimicrobials for superinfection
- Monitor patient compliance with self-administration of antimicrobial drugs

(Adapted from Pizzo, P. A. & Schimpff, S. C. [1983]. Strategies for the prevention of infection in the myelosuppressed or immunosuppressed cancer patient. *Cancer Treatment Reports,* The National Cancer Institute, Bethesda, Maryland. *67,* 223–234.)

with GCP or BMD cannot be overemphasized. Hours can mean the difference between life and death, between easily treated infections and sepsis.

Treatment

Common sites of infection and treatments are found in Table 49–14. Medical therapy of infections consists primarily of antibiotics and supportive therapy (Box 49–1). A decision tree that illustrates the usual medical approach to the febrile neutropenic patient is illustrated in Figure 49–4. Granulocyte transfusions are rarely used. Their efficacy in prophylaxis has not been established; therapeutically, they seem to improve survival in patients with prolonged, severe GCP (<500 cells/mm³ for longer than 30 days). Donor availability also is a limiting factor.

Although antipyretics are often used to bring tem-

Table 49–13. RISK OF BACTERIAL INFECTION ASSOCIATED WITH GRANULOCYTOPENIA

Absolute Granulocyte Count	Risk of Bacterial Infection
1500–2000 per mm³	Not significant
>1000 per mm³	Minimal
>500 per mm³	Moderate
<500 per mm³	Severe

(From Brandt, B. [1984]. A nursing protocol for the client with neutropenia. *Oncology Nursing Forum, 11* [2], 24–28. Reproduced by permission.)

Table 49–14. INFECTIONS IN CANCER PATIENTS AND USUAL THERAPY

Pathogen	Sources	Common Sites	Presentation	Treatment
Bacteria				

Pseudomonas	Multiple	Wounds
		GI tract
		GU tract
		Lung
			Purulence
			Enterocolitis
			UTI
			Pneumonia
				Carbenicillin, ticarcillin,
				  gentamicin
				  tobramycin

Klebsiella	Multiple	Lung	Pneumonia	Gentamicin,
				  tobramycin, amikacin,
				  cephalothin

Escherichia coli	Multiple	GI tract
		GU tract
		Bone
		Wounds
		Blood
			Enterocolitis
			UTI
			Osteomyelitis
			Purulence
			Sepsis
				Ampicillin, carbenicillin,
				  cephalosporins,
				  gentamicin

Staphylococcus	Multiple	Lung Bone GI tract CNS Wounds	Pneumonia Osteomyelitis Enterocolitis Meningitis Purulence	Methacillin, oxacillin, nafcillin
Fungi				

Candida	Normal flora	GI tract
		Lung
		GU tract
			Thrush, esophagitis
			Pneumonia
			UTI, vaginitis
				Amphotericin B,
				  miconazole,
				  clotrimazole, nystatin

Cryptococcus	Soil, pigeon feces	Lung CNS	Pneumonia Meningitis	Amphotericin B, 5-fluorocytosine

Aspergillus	Air, building materials,
	  pigeon feces
		Lung	Bronchopneumonia	Amphotericin B,
				  nystatin, 5-
				  fluorocytosine

Viruses				

Herpes simplex,
  type 1
	Oral secretions	Upper GI
		  tract
		Skin
		CNS
			Stomatitis, esophagitis
			Eczema
			Encephalitis
				Idoxuridine, vidarabine,
				  acycloguanine,
				  adenine, arabinoside,
				  Burow's solution

Cytomegalovirus	Normal flora, blood
	  products
		Lung
		CNS
			Pneumonia
			Encephalitis
				Cytarabine, adenine,
				  arabinoside

Varicella zoster	Person-to-person
	  transmission
		Skin	Shingles	Corticosteroids, local
				  anesthetics,
				  cytarabine, adenine,
				  arabinoside

Protozoa				

Pneumocystis	Normal flora, person-to-
	  person transmission
		Lung	Pneumonia	Pyrimethamine,
				  sulfadiazine,
				  trimethoprim,
				  sulfamethoxazole

Toxoplasma gondii	Oocytes in cat feces,
	  inadequately cooked
	  meat or blood
	  products
		Disseminated	Chills, fever,
			  diaphoresis,
			  encephalitis,
			  pericarditis
				Pyrimethamine,
				  sulfadiazine

GI, gastrointestinal; GU, genitourinary; CNS, central nervous system; UTI, urinary tract infection; UGI, urogenital infection.
(From Ellerhorst-Ryan, J. M. [1985]. Complications of the myeloproliferative system: Infection and sepsis. *Seminars in Oncology Nursing, 1*, 244–250. Reproduced by permission.)

peratures down, at least one investigator recommends against using antipyretics when temperature is below 105° C in the patient with GCP (Cunha, 1985). Fever maximizes host defenses by several mechanisms: inhibition or destruction of microorganisms; diminishing certain trace elements, which further inhibits replication of microorganisms; increased production of antiviral interferons; and increased mobility and phagocytosis of polymorphonuclear leukocytes. Cunha (1985) identifies three situations in which physicians might consider antipyretics in the febrile patient with GCP: (1) if the patient is particularly uncomfortable; (2) if the temperature is 105° C or above; and (3) if the patient has serious cardiopulmonary disease that might be exacerbated by the fever. Prolonged fever in persons with limited ability to ingest food and fluid may in-

crease the risk of metabolic complications from dehydration and malnourishment.

Clinical Problem: Thrombocytopenia

Thrombocytopenia, a reduction in the number of circulating platelets, is relatively common in persons with cancer. It may be a disorder of production, distribution, or destruction (Burstein & Harker, 1981; Handin, 1985). Perhaps the most common cause of TCP among cancer patients is a disorder of production involving decreased megakaryocytopoiesis. This may be due to marrow replacement by tumor or to an acute or delayed effect of chemotherapy or radiotherapy.

The most common disorder of distribution that oc-

Box 49–1. EVIDENCE FOR EARLY EMPIRIC ANTIBIOTIC THERAPY FOR THE CANCER PATIENT WITH GRANULOCYTOPENIA

Pizzo, P. A., Robichaud, K. J., Welsey, R., & Conners, J. P. (1982). **Fever in the pediatric and young adult patient population: A prospective study of 1001 episodes.** *Medicine, 61,* 153–165.

This 1982 study demonstrates the importance that a descriptive study can have in the management of the patient with cancer. Pizzo and his colleagues examined the cause of fever in granulocytopenic versus nongranulocytopenic patients to determine appropriate therapies for two populations exhibiting similar signs and symptoms. In particular, they sought a rationale for the implementation of antibiotic therapy and prophylaxis for the cancer patient.

Among the most interesting results of this comprehensive 5-year study were the following:
1. Sixty per cent of fevers in nongranulocytopenic patients were due to noninfectious causes—for example, administration of specific chemotherapeutic agents.
2. An infectious cause was discovered in only 17 per cent of nongranulocytopenic patients and those were usually minor in nature.
3. In contrast, evidence of infectious causes was present in more than 50 per cent of granulocytopenic patients, even though an etiologic agent could be identified (i.e., by culture) in only one half.

On the basis of these results, the authors concluded that although the focus of assessment and treatment of the febrile nongranulocytopenic patient should be noninfectious causes of fever, the use of early empiric antibiotic therapy should be utilized in all granulocytopenic cancer patients who become febrile. Additionally, the authors noted that the one exception to this rule of thumb in nongranulocytopenic patients is those patients whose granulocyte count is falling rapidly subsequent to chemotherapy. This group's risk is equal to that of patients who are already granulocytopenic. As a consequence of this and similar studies, early initiation of empiric antibiotic therapy has become standard treatment in granulocytopenic cancer patients and in those who are becoming granulocytopenic.

---

curs in cancer patients is hypersplenism, in which more than the usual 20 to 30 per cent of platelets are sequestered in the spleen and not available in the circulation. If this type of TCP disorder is suspected, the spleen should be carefully assessed for splenomegaly, because the absence of a palpable spleen will rule this out (Schlichter & Harker, 1974).

Several disorders of destruction may cause TCP in the person with cancer, including coagulopathies (e.g., disseminated intravascular coagulation [DIC]) (Alfrey, White, & Zelnick, 1984), tumor effects that may release factors that activate coagulation (Schlichter & Harker, 1974), and effects of infection in which bacterial endotoxins and leukocyte response to them can enhance platelet consumption (Schlichter & Harker, 1974). Considering the treatment-induced GCP that often accompanies TCP, the patient is highly susceptible to infection and its effects on platelets (Schiffer, 1983). Certain drugs (e.g., salicylates) also affect platelets by interfering with megakaryocytopoiesis, inducing an immune TCP, or altering platelet function, all of which can exacerbate a thrombocytopenic disorder.

Estimates of the incidence of TCP in different tumor populations range from 4 to 39 per cent (Alfrey et al., 1984). It occurs most often in patients with hematologic cancers; however, it also occurs with solid tumors that invade the marrow, particularly breast, prostate, and lung cancers (Alfrey et al., 1984). The first clinical report of association between TCP and increased risk of bleeding appeared in 1962.

The role that nurses play in clinical assessment of the patient with TCP and in patient education is an important one. A person's risk of bleeding cannot be determined solely from the platelet count. Other factors that influence this risk include the presence of infection; potential sources of bleeding; the direction in which the platelet count is moving; and the cause of TCP. The interaction of TCP and infection has been discussed. Potential bleeding sites may be observable (e.g., wounds or the site of an invasive procedure) or hidden (e.g., necrotic tumor masses, mucositis, or intracranial bleeding). The direction in which the platelet count is moving is significant because a patient is at greater risk for hemorrhage when the count is still falling than when it is rising, even when the absolute number is the same. The reason appears to be related to the fact that the platelets in circulation when the count is returning to normal tend to be younger and larger and therefore clot more effectively (Aderka, Praff, Santo, Weinberger, & Pinkhas, 1986; Graze, 1980; Welch, 1978). Treatment-induced TCP tends to be of shorter duration and is associated with less risk of bleeding than that resulting from a myelophthisic marrow (Aderka, et al., 1986).

Serial platelet values are an important part of the clinical assessment of the person with potential or existing TCP. A grading system developed at University of California, Los Angeles, uses the following values to assess risk of bleeding in TCP patients, with 0 being normal, and 4 indicating the most risk (Bick, 1985):

$0 = 100,000$ platelets/mm^3
$1 = 75,000$ to $100,000$ platelets/mm^3
$2 = 50,000$ to $75,000$ platelets/mm^3
$3 = 25,000$ to $50,000$ platelets/mm^3
$4 = $ less than $25,000$ platelets/mm^3

Unless there are other predisposing factors (e.g., infection), a patient with more than 50,000 platelets/mm^3 is thought to have a slight risk of hemorrhage. In fact, a count of 50,000 platelets is often considered to be the level at which invasive procedures such as bronchoscopy and endoscopy can be performed with minimal risk (Dutcher, 1986). The risk of spontaneous hemorrhage is much greater when the count is fewer than 20,000/mm^3. However, spontaneous hemorrhage may occur at values higher than that when other factors

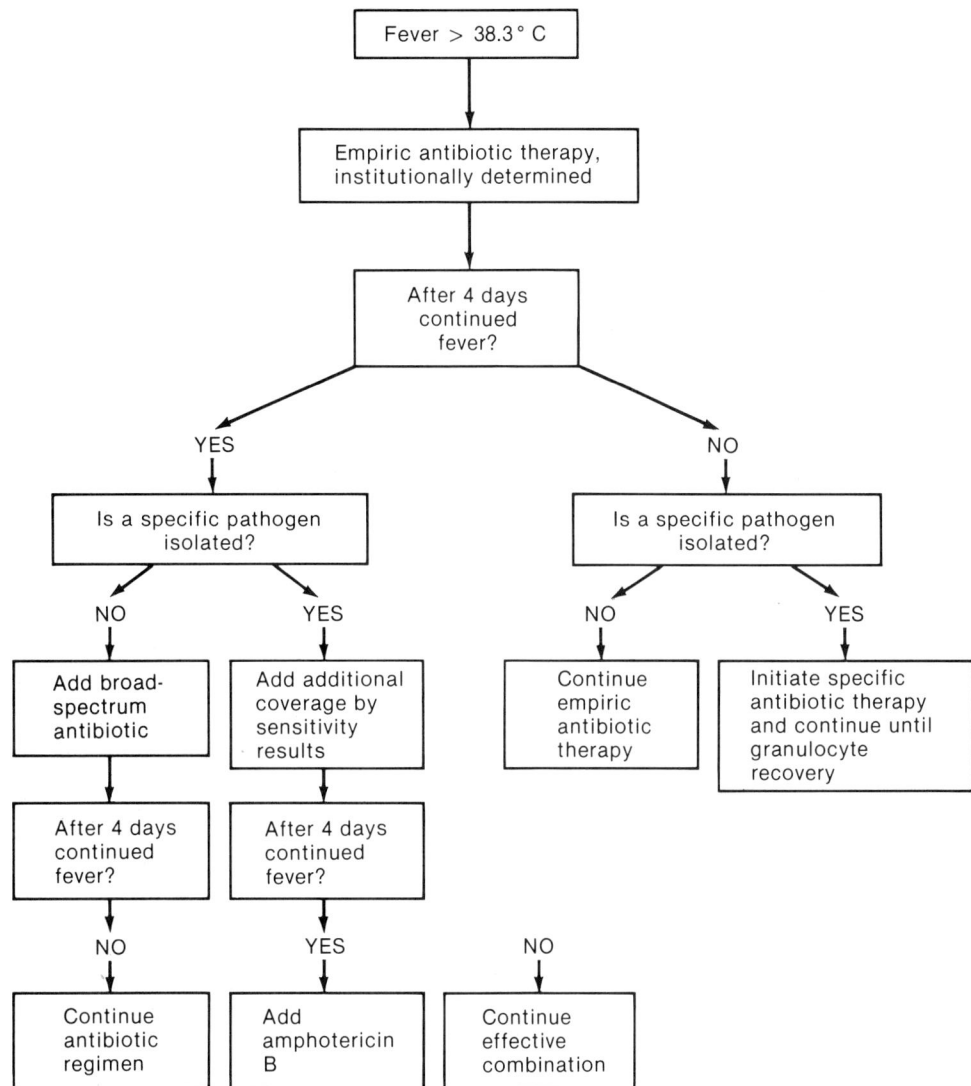

Figure 49–4. One example of antibiotic management of fever in the patient with granulocytopenia.

compromise platelet production or function (such as infection, fever). In addition to platelet count, the nurse should monitor the CBC and measures of coagulation such as prothrombin time (PT), partial thromboplastin time (PTT), bleeding time, and DIC screens when indicated.

Physical assessment of the person with TCP should be thorough. Bleeding may occur in any organ; however, sites in which it may be life-threatening are priorities for assessment. These include the brain, the respiratory system, and the gastrointestinal system. Reportable neurologic observations include history of a recent fall or blow to the head, headache, blurred vision, pupillary changes, and changes in mental status such as confusion or disorientation. Respiratory bleeding may be heralded by hemoptysis or by changes in respiratory status, such as congestion or wet cough. Hematemesis or blood in the stool may signal gastrointestinal tract hemorrhage. All gastrointestinal output, including emesis, nasogastric tube drainage, and stool should be checked by guaiac test for blood. Changes in vital signs such as hypotension and tachycardia may be the nurse's first clue to a spontaneous hemorrhage.

Depending on the acuteness of the patient's condition, physical assessment and vital signs should be done every shift or more often.

Other areas that may require daily or more frequent assessment include the skin, mucosa, and eyes. Petechiae, purpura, and easy bruising are hallmarks of a low platelet count and changes in the number or extent of such signs should be followed closely by head-to-toe inspection. A careful oral assessment should be done to detect petechiae or hemorrhagic blebs on the palate or oral mucosa as well as for bleeding from sites of mucositis. Occurrence and duration of epistaxis should be documented. Retinal hemorrhage may also occur.

In addition to assessment and monitoring, the nurse may use preventive interventions. The nurse can ensure that other providers know the patient's condition so that invasive procedures that may cause bleeding (such as enemas and biopsies) are avoided—or, in the case of important, invasive diagnostic procedures, that preprocedure or postprocedure interventions (e.g. platelet transfusion; pressure to venipuncture sites) are initiated. Constipation, nausea, and vomiting are clinical events that increase intracranial pressure and may precipitate bleeding in a person at risk. Interventions to prevent these problems are essential in the patient with TCP. Menstrual bleeding in women with TCP should be monitored (e.g., by counting pads); administration of hormones to inhibit menses may be needed to minimize profound blood loss. Patient education information for TCP is found in Table 49–15.

The treatment of choice for TCP (usually at levels less than 20,000 platelets per mm³) is platelet transfusion. Some clinicians maintain that patients will tolerate a platelet count of 10,000 to 20,000 if there is no evidence of bleeding (Aderka et al., 1986). Usually six to eight units of platelets are transfused depending on the initial degree of TCP and the patient's weight. One unit of platelets is the number of platelets obtained from 500 ml of whole blood. The response or "bump" obtained by a patient after transfusion is determined by a 1-hr posttransfusion platelet count. The corrected count increment (CCI) is calculated as follows:

$$\text{Observed increment} \times \frac{\text{body surface area (m}^2)}{\text{number of platelets transfused} \times 10^{11}}$$

The usual expected increase is 5000 to 10,000 platelets/mm³ unit transfused. If the increment is substantially lower than this, the patient is likely to be alloimmunized—that is, to have developed antibodies against histocompatibility locus antigens (HLA) transfused with the platelets. Dutcher (1986) found that patients without antibodies had an average 1-hr CCI of 16,100 platelets/mm³ compared to 5600 for those who were alloimmunized. A small 1-hr CCI indicates alloimmunization, whereas a decreasing 24-hr CCI usually indicates other processes that shorten platelet survival time, such as infection, fever, coagulopathy, or hepatosplenomegaly.

The question of whether the process of alloimmunization is enhanced by multiple transfusions has been addressed by Dutcher (1986). She found that there does not appear to be a relationship between the number of platelet transfusions and subsequent alloimmunization because some patients were sensitized after only two transfusions whereas others were not sensitized despite multiple transfusions. Dutcher concluded that alloimmunization does not depend on a dose-response relationship but rather on the immunologic responsiveness of the patient.

If the patient does develop a sensitivity to random platelets, it becomes necessary to find donors whose platelets are as closely matched in terms of HLA antigens as possible. In some cases, a family member

Table 49–15. CONTENT OF PATIENT EDUCATION REGARDING THROMBOCYTOPENIA (TCP)

- Function of platelets and normal laboratory values
- Pathophysiology of TCP and expected course of recovery
- Reportable signs and symptoms of bleeding
- Preventive measures (e.g., eliminating environmental hazards; using an electric razor instead of a safety razor)
- Avoiding invasive procedures (e.g., enemas, suppositories)
- Development of a bowel maintenance program
- Prophylactic antiemetics for nausea and vomiting
- Avoidance of drugs that impair platelet function

may be able to give multiple units through plateletpheresis. In other situations, a match that is close will have to suffice.

Clinical Problem: Neutropenia

Case Study

Neutropenia is possibly the most problematic aspect of myelosuppression, whether the marrow failure is due to antineoplastic treatment, disease extension, or other causes. Appropriate and timely supportive care of the febrile neutropenic patient is essential and may involve standard antibiotic therapy, the use of controversial approaches, such as granulocyte transfusions, and, more recently, the administration of hematopoietic CSFs. The following case study of a patient who is neutropenic as a result of an unusual illness, myelodysplastic syndrome (MDS) or preleukemia, illustrates clearly how these various therapeutic approaches can be employed in conjunction and in succession to carry a patient through an infectious event.

Mr. O. is a white man in his late seventies who is married and has several grown children. He lives with his wife, who is suffering from a chronic mental illness. His past medical history is significant for a hernia repair, several episodes of diverticulitis, and an episode of cholecystitis. During a routine physical examination, it was discovered that Mr. O. was leukopenic (WBC = 1500), mildly anemic (Hgb = 11.1), and somewhat thrombocytopenic (platelets = 128,000). A bone marrow biopsy at the time indicated early MDS. Initially, treatment was begun with folate and vitamin B₆, although later this was stopped when his counts seemed to be normalizing.

Later Mr. O. became febrile and had abdominal cramping and pain. This initially was thought to be another episode of diverticulitis, but with conservative treatment the situation only worsened. Mr. O. was hospitalized owing to increasing fever and hypotension and was diagnosed as having septicemia from *Pseudomonas aeruginosa* infection. He was found to have an impacted gallstone as well as an anal fissure. At this admission, Mr. O. was neutropenic with a total WBC count of 400. He was treated with antibiotics and, because he was a poor surgical candidate, with a medication to dissolve the gallstone. After a month-long hospitalization, Mr. O. was discharged home.

Several months later, the patient was enrolled in a study of the use of the colony-stimulating factor rhG-CSF for treatment of persons with MDS. At the time Mr. O. began the protocol, his total WBC was 1500 (absolute neutrophil count [ANC] = 75), hematocrit was 32.5, reticulocytes made up 0.6 per cent of the total, and platelets numbered 139,000. The results of a bone marrow biopsy at the time were consistent with MDS. During the 2 months that Mr. O. was being treated with G-CSF (at four escalating dose levels), he remained consistently neutropenic and was hospitalized for 1 week owing to an infectious episode related to his rectal fissure. At the end of the study, Mr. O.'s blood counts did show some slight evidence of responding to the highest dose of the growth factor. Results were as follows: WBC = 1.1 (ANC = 253); hematocrit = 27.1; platelets = 187,000, and reticulocytes = 3.7 per cent. A bone marrow biopsy at the time demonstrated a modest degree of enhanced myeloid maturation.

Six weeks later, Mr. O. was offered, and accepted, the option of continuing to be treated with G-CSF for an extended period of up to 6 months. Therapy was initially begun at the highest dose level reached during the earlier phase of the study. Mr. O.'s counts were as follows: WBC = 1.5 (ANC = 375); hematocrit = 31.0; platelets = 136,000; and reticulocytes = 1.1 per cent. At the end of 2 weeks of treatment, when his WBC count had fallen to 0.6 with an ANC of 8, Mr. O. was again admitted to the hospital with *Pseudomonas* sepsis, which was treated with antibiotics. At this time, his daily dose of the growth factor was nearly doubled.

Mr. O.'s blood counts continued their lackluster response to the treatment with G-CSF for almost a month, when they began to demonstrate some improvement. By 7 weeks into the therapy, his counts were as follows: WBC = 1.8 (ANC = 1044); hematocrit = 33.8; platelets = 163,000; and reticulocytes = 1.4 per cent. For the first time in many months, Mr. O. was not absolutely neutropenic. With a daily maintenance dose of rhG-CSF at 5 μg/kg, Mr. O. remained nonneutropenic. At the end of 6 months when, in accordance with the study protocol, he ceased being treated with the growth factor, his counts were as follows: WBC = 4.2 (ANC = 2898); hematocrit = 37.4; and platelets = 175,000. A bone marrow biopsy showed no evidence of leukemic blasts and once again demonstrated enhanced myeloid maturation.

After he left the study protocol, Mr. O.'s blood counts began the descent that is commonly seen in studies of CSFs when the marrow stimulant is no longer being administered. In the middle of April, when Mr. O. had once again become absolutely neutropenic with an ANC < 500, rhG-CSF was reinitiated at the previous dose. About a week later, Mr. O. was readmitted to the hospital with a cellulitis of the right groin and of the left anterior tibia and temperature spikes to about 39° Centigrade. His admission blood counts were WBC = 0.5 (ANC = 80); hematocrit = 28.7; and platelets = 99,000. Blood cultures were no surprise, revealing growth of *Pseudomonas aeruginosa* yet again. An antibiotic regimen was initiated, which included cetazidime, gentamicin, and cefazolin sodium (Kefzol). Over the course of this hospitalization, which lasted 3 weeks, the antibiotic regimen underwent various transformations until finally tobramycin and imipenem were settled on as most effective. In addition, probably owing to the lengthy course of antibiotics, metronidazole (Flagyl) had to be added for treatment of diarrhea after a positive clostridium difficile titer was noted.

Six days into the hospitalization, as the areas of cellulitis continued to extend despite aggressive antibiotic therapy, the decision was made to utilize gran-

ulocyte transfusions despite their well-known attendant risks. For 10 days, the patient was treated with WBC transfusions after premedication with diphenhydramine (Benadryl) and hydrocortisone. In addition, after 8 days of hospitalization, with a WBC count of 0.6 and an ANC of 192, the rhG-CSF dose was doubled to 10 μg/kg/day. This step was undertaken only after a dermatology consultation indicated that the skin lesions were not vasculitis and a bone marrow biopsy demonstrated that leukemic transformation had not occurred, both of which are potential complications of therapy with rhG-CSF.

Finally, 11 or 12 days into the hospitalization, the patient demonstrated both systemic and local improvement, having become afebrile and reporting less pain at the sites of cellulitis. Both areas for the first time showed evidence of regression. The patient continued to be neutropenic with a WBC count of 1.2 and an ANC of 144. After some debate, in part because the patient was becoming somewhat depressed at his continued hospitalization, a decision was made to discharge Mr. O. on a 7-day course of oral ciprofloxacin despite his continued neutropenia. His counts, after some fluctuations, seemed to be improving. On discharge, Mr. O.'s WBC count was 2.3; his ANC was 253; his hematocrit was 43.2 (he received 3 to 4 units of packed RBCs during the hospital course); and his platelet count was 116,000. A week later, Mr. O. was doing well with WBC count = 2.3; ANC = 575; hematocrit = 39.1; and platelets = 72,000. The last-mentioned platelet count was mysterious and was a source of serious concern. Unfortunately, Mr. O.'s marrow disorder allows no respite from medical or personal vigilance. See also Box 49–2.

Clinical Problem: Anemia

Anemia is a common condition in cancer patients. Dutcher (1986) estimated that it occurs in 50 per cent of cancer patients. Usually anemia is relatively mild and does not require treatment. In more severe cases intermittent transfusion is required. Several mechanisms underlie anemia: hypoproliferation, ineffective erythropoiesis, and hemolysis (Hillman & Finch, 1985). Most anemias in cancer patients result from one of the first two mechanisms. The most frequent cause of anemia in cancer patients is a poorly understood condition called *anemia of chronic disease*, a hypoproliferative state (Cartwright, 1966; Dutcher, 1986). This type of anemia is rarely debilitating or progressive and does not require treatment as the hematocrit value usually remains above 30 per cent. Although the mechanisms underlying the development of anemia are not well defined, it has been speculated that anemia is part of a "hematologic stress syndrome" (Erslev, 1983a). It is characterized by a shortened RBC life span, disturbed iron metabolism, and deficient compensatory increase in the rate of RBC production (Cartwright, 1966, 1971; Erslev, 1983).

Although the anemia of chronic disease does not imply marrow invasion by tumor, myelophthisis can

---

Box 49–2. FUTURE MANAGEMENT OF MYELOSUPPRESSION WITH COLONY-STIMULATING FACTOR

Antman, K., et al. (1988). **Effects of recombinant human granulocyte-macrophage colony-stimulating factor on chemotherapy-induced myelosuppression.** *New England Journal of Medicine, 319,* 593–598.

This research study is representative of a number of articles that have begun to report on efforts to utilize colony-stimulating factors (CSFs) in managing the hematopoietic suppressive effects of antineoplastic treatments. These agents offer a range of exciting possibilities in application to cancer patients.

Antman and co-workers used granulocyte-macrophage colony-stimulating factor (GM-CSF) to try to prevent or ameliorate the marrow nadirs of 16 adults being treated for sarcoma with chemotherapy (doxorubicin, dacarbazine, and ifosfamide). They compared the nadirs of the same patients receiving two cycles of the chemotherapy course before and after a course in which they received GM-CSF. They found that the duration of neutropenia was 3.5 days after chemotherapy combined with GM-CSF treatment, compared with 7.4 days for chemotherapy without GM-CSF.

This study and others demonstrate the important role CSFs can play in decreasing marrow-suppressive effects of anticancer treatments, consequently making it possible for patients to receive higher doses and to complete rigorous courses of therapy. To this point, these studies share a significant limitation. Although most of them demonstrate that CSFs do stimulate marrow activity, they have yet to make the connection between this increased activity and the clinically more important end results, decreased frequency of complications such as infection.

---

cause anemia, either by itself or in conjunction with anemia of chronic disease (Bulin, 1974; Hillman & Finch, 1985; Laszlo, 1983). Myelophthisis is a hypoproliferative state because replacement of marrow by tumor causes a decrease in both stem cells and erythroid precursor cells. The severity of this anemia depends on the extent of the primary disease, and although the patient can be supported with transfusion, the therapy of choice is to control the cancer. Acute or insidious blood loss can aggravate hypoproliferative anemia.

Antineoplastic therapies can also cause hypoproliferative anemia because the erythrocyte line recovers more slowly than other cell lines. Thus some chemotherapy schedules that are planned primarily around the granulocyte and platelet counts can lead to a chronic anemia. The erythroid line also can be involved in the prolonged or delayed pancytopenia caused by certain drugs, which strongly affect pluripotential stem cells (Dutcher, 1986).

Ineffective erythropoiesis is associated with nutritional deficiencies, particularly of iron, vitamin B_{12}, and folate (Hillman & Finch, 1985). This may be a significant problem in persons with cancer cachexia and anorexia.

The classic symptoms reported by the person with anemia include fatigue, lassitude, and weakness; palpitation, dyspnea, increased sweating, and pounding headache also may occur. Other symptoms associated with anemia may be anorexia or other gastrointestinal tract disturbances owing to diminished oxygen supply to this system and insomnia, decreased concentration, and confusion. All of these symptoms may be exacerbated in the elderly, who may have preexisting age-related or pathologic cardiovascular conditions. In general, most persons can tolerate a hematocrit reading that falls to 25 per cent or greater before experiencing significant symptoms. In addition to eliciting patients' subjective symptoms, the examiner should pay particular attention to two features in the client with anemia: color of skin and mucous membranes and cardiovascular status (Maxwell, 1984). Examination of mucous

membranes is particularly important in clients whose skin color precludes adequate assessment. Other areas that may demonstrate the pallor of anemia are the nailbeds, the conjunctivae, and palmar creases of the hands. In severe anemia, patients may have evidence of increased cardiac output, such as tachycardia, powerful apical impulses, and murmurs that result from increased contractile force and blood turbulence (Hillman & Finch, 1985).

In addition to assessing the foregoing symptoms, laboratory evaluation includes at least a CBC and may also require other tests, such as for plasma iron, total iron binding capacity, and serum ferritin. The reticulocyte count is an indicator of RBC turnover and marrow response to anemic conditions. The mean corpuscular volume (MCV) and mean corpuscular hemoglobin (MCH) are useful indicators of impaired hemoglobin synthesis. A peripheral blood smear may reveal changes in RBC shape and characteristics indicative of particular types of anemic disorders. Finally, a bone marrow aspirate and biopsy may be performed after an abnormal blood smear to further define abnormal morphology as well as indicate decreased overall marrow cellularity owing to neoplastic or fibrotic processes (Hillman & Finch, 1985).

It is preferable to attend to the underlying cause of anemia (e.g., with radiation or chemotherapy); when that is not possible the anemia itself is treated. Patients may also require supportive packed cell transfusions while undergoing marrow suppressive therapy to keep the hematocrit level above 25%. The indications, process, and hazards of transfusion therapy are discussed elsewhere (see Chapter 26). A number of potential hazards exist, including transfusion reactions, circulatory overload (especially in the elderly and those with cardiac disorders), alloimmunization to HLA antigens, and the contraction of non-A, non-B hepatitis or AIDS. The risks of acquiring AIDS from blood transfusions have received much attention in the last several years. Recent estimates of these risks are on the order of 5 to 10 per cent for hepatitis and approximately 1 in 250,000 for AIDS (Bove, 1987). These risks have led to the increased use of direct donor transfusions and the practice of storing one's own blood for future use. Clearly, this approach is not feasible for many cancer patients.

In addition to medical therapy of anemia, the nurse should teach the client self-care measures to manage symptoms of anemia. The most significant intervention would be related to energy conservation and pacing activities. These interventions are described in Chapter 58.

SUMMARY

This chapter has described the physiology of hematopoiesis, cancer-related pathophysiology of BMD, and nursing assessment and interventions. Complications of BMD may be life threatening. Astute nursing care involving early identification of risk factors, preventive interventions, patient education, early detection and reporting of signs and symptoms of complications, and supportive care through BMD complications can make the difference between life or death and comfort or discomfort in the person with actual or potential BMD.

References

Abernathy, E. (1987). Biotherapy: An introductory overview. *Oncology Nursing Forum, 14* (Suppl.), 13–15.

Abrams, R. A. (1983). Hematopoietic dysfunction resulting from antineoplastic therapy: Current concepts and potential for management. In D. J. Higby (Ed.), *Supportive care in cancer therapy* (pp. 169–198). Boston: Martinus Nijhoff Publishing.

Ader, R. (1985). Behaviorally conditioned modulation of immunity. In R. Guilleme, M. Cohn, & T. Melnechuk (Eds.), *Neural modulation of immunity* (pp. 55–66). New York: Raven Press.

Aderka, D., Praff, G., Santo, M., Weinberger, A., & Pinkhas, J. (1986). Bleeding due to thrombocytopenia in acute leukemias and reevaluation of the prophylactic platelet transfusion policy. *American Journal of Medical Sciences, 291*, 147–151.

Alfrey, C. P., Jr., White, M. R., & Zelnick, P. W. (1984). Abnormalities of white blood cells, platelets, and hemostasis. In F. E. Smith & M. Lane (Eds.), *Medical complications of malignancy* (pp. 207–218). New York: John Wiley & Sons.

Antman, K. S., Griffin, J. D., Elias, M. D., Socinski, M. A., Ryan, L., Cannistra, S. A., Oette, D., Whitley, M., Frei, E. III, & Schnipper, L. E. (1988). Effect of recombinant human granulocyte-macrophage colony stimulating factor on chemotherapy-induced myelosuppression. *New England Journal of Medicine, 319*, 593–598.

Baker, G. H. B. (1987). Psychological factors and immunity. *Journal of Psychosomatic Medicine, 12*, 1–10.

Balducci, L., & Hardy, C. (1985). Cancer and malnutrition—a critical interaction: a review. *American Journal of Hematology, 18*, 91–103.

Bartrop, R. W., Luckhurst, E., Lazarus, L., Kiloh, L. G., & Penny, R. (1977). Depressed lymphocyte function after bereavement. *Lancet, 1*, 834–836.

Beck, W. S. (1983). The megaloblastic anemias. In W. J. Williams, E. Beutler, A. J. Erslev, & M. A. Lichtman (Eds.), *Hematology* (pp. 434–465). New York: McGraw-Hill Book Co.

Beck, W. S. (1985). Normocytic anemias. In W. S. Beck (Ed.), *Hematology* (pp. 43–57). Cambridge, MA: MIT Press.

Bick, R. L. (1985). *Disorders of hemostasis and thrombosis: Principles of clinical practice.* New York: Thieme.

Blalock, E. (1989). A molecular basis for bidirectional communication between the immune and neuroendocrine systems. *Physiological Reviews, 69*, 1–32.

Blomgren, H., Baral, E., Jarstrand, C., Petrini, B., Strender, L. E., Wallgren, A., & Wasserman, J. (1981). Effect of external radiation therapy on the peripheral lymphocyte subpopulation. In J. B. DuBois, B. Serrou, & C. Rosenfeld (Eds.), *Immunopharmacologic effects of radiation therapy* (pp. 299–319). New York: Raven Press.

Borysenko, M., & Borysenko, J. (1982). Stress, behavior and immunity: Animal models and mediating mechanisms. *General Hospital Psychiatry, 4*, 59–67.

Bove, J. R. (1987). Transfusion-associated hepatitis and AIDS: What is the risk? *New England Journal of Medicine, 317*, 242–245.

Braun, D. P., & Harris, J. E. (1985). Effects of cytotoxic chemotherapy on immune function in cancer patients. *Cancer Treatment Symposium, 1*, 19–25.

Buinoukos, P., McDonald, G., & Cole, W. (1958). Role of operative stress on the resistance of the experimental animal to inoculated cancer cells. *Annals of Surgery, 148*, 642–648.

Bulin, N. J. (1974). Anemia of cancer. *Annals of the New York Academy of Sciences, 230*, 209–211.

Bull, J. M., DeVita, V. T., & Carbone, P. P. (1975). In vitro granulocyte production in patients with Hodgkin's disease and lymphocytic, histiocytic and mixed lymphomas. *Blood, 45*, 833–842.

Bullock, K. (1985). Neuroanatomy of lymphoid tissue: A review. In R. Guilleme, M. Cohn, & T. Melnechuk (Eds.), *Neural modulation of immunity* (pp. 111–142). New York: Raven Press.

Burstein, S. A., & Harker, L. A. (1981). Quantitative platelet disorders. In A. L. Bloom & D. P. Thomas (Eds.), *Hemostasis and thrombosis* (pp. 279—300). Edinburgh: Churchill Livingstone.

Cartwright, G. E. (1966). The anemia of chronic disorders. *Seminars in Hematology, 3*, 351–375.

Cartwright, G. E. (1971). Annotation: The anemia of chronic disorders. *British Journal of Haematology, 21*, 147–152.

Cole, W. H. (1985). The increase in immunosuppression and its role in the development of malignant lesions. *Journal of Surgical Oncology, 30*, 139–144.

Contino, L. H., Testa, N. G., & Dexter, T. M. (1986). The myelosuppressive effect of recombinant interferon (gamma) in short-term and long-term marrow cultures. *British Journal of Haematology, 63*, 517–524.

Corman, L. C. (1985). The relationship between nutrition, infection and immunity. *Medical Clinics of North America, 69*, 519–531.

Crosby, W. H. (1983). Structure and function of the spleen. In W. J. Williams, E. Beutler, A. J. Erslev, & M. A. Lichtman (Eds.), *Hematology* (pp. 89–97). New York: McGraw-Hill Book Co.

Cunha, B. A. (1985). Significance of fever in the compromised host. *Nursing Clinics of North America, 20*, 163–170.

Davies, A. J. S., Wallis, V. J., & Peckham, M. J. (1981). Suppression of the immune response by ionizing radiation. In J. B. DuBois, B. Serrou, & C. Rosenfeld (Eds.), *Immunopharmacologic effects of radiation therapy* (pp. 1–6). New York: Raven Press.

Dickinson, J. P., & Stone, J. (1981). Immunodepression during long-term follow-up of post-mastectomy patients treated with conventional or modified x-ray or electron regimens. In J. B. DuBois, B. Serrou, & C. Rosenfeld (Eds.), *Immunopharmacologic effects of radiation therapy* (pp. 231–240). New York: Raven Press.

Dillman, R. O., Beauregard, J. C., Halpern, S. E., & Clutter, M. (1986). Toxicities and side effects associated with intravenous infusions of murine monoclonal antibodies. *Journal of Biological Response Modifiers, 5*, 73–84.

Dodd, M. (1983). Self-care for side effects in cancer chemotherapy: An assessment of nursing interventions. Part II. *Cancer Nursing, 6*, 63–67.

Dorian, B. J., Keystone, E., Garfinkel, P., & Brown, G. (1981). Immune mechanisms in acute psychological stress. *Psychosomatic Medicine, 43*, 84 (Abstract).

DuBois, J. B., & Serrou, B. (1981). Effects of ionizing radiation on cell-mediated immunity in cancer patients. In J. B. DuBois, B. Serrou, & C. Rosenfeld (Eds.), *Immunopharmacologic effects of radiation therapy* (pp. 275–299). New York: Raven Press.

Dutcher, J. P. (1986). Platelet and granulocyte transfusions in cancer patients. In P. K. Ray (Ed.), *Advances in immunity and cancer therapy* (vol. 2, pp. 211–249). New York: Springer-Verlag.

Erslev, A. J. (1983a). Anemia of chronic disorders. In W. J. Williams, E. Beutler, A. J. Erslev, & M. A. Lichtman (Eds.), *Hematology* (pp. 522–528). New York: McGraw-Hill Book Co.

Erslev, A. J. (1983b). Production of erythrocytes. In W. J. Williams, E. Beutler, A. J. Erslev, & M. A. Lichtman (Eds.), *Hematology* (pp. 365–375). New York: McGraw-Hill Book Co.

Erslev, A. J., & Weiss, L. (1983). Structure and function of the marrow. In W. J. Williams, E. Beutler, A. J. Erslev, & M. A. Lichtman (Eds.), *Hematology* (pp. 75–83). New York: McGraw-Hill Book Co.

Fairbanks, V. F., & Beutler, E. (1983). Iron deficiency. In W. J. Williams, E. Beutler, A. J. Erslev, & M. A. Lichtman (Eds.), *Hematology* (pp. 466–489). New York: McGraw-Hill Book Co.

Fischl, M. A. (1986). Patient tolerance to interferon: Clinical and laboratory assessments. *Medical Clinics of North America, 70*, Suppl., 41–45.

Fliedner, T. M., Northdurft, W., & Clavo, W. (1986). The development of radiation late effects to the bone marrow after single and chronic exposure. *International Journal of Radiation Biology, 49*, 35–46.

Frisch, B., Bartl, R., & Chaichuk, S. (1986). Therapy-induced myelodysplasia and secondary leukemia. *Scandinavian Journal of Haematology, 36* (Suppl. 45), 38–47.

Gordon, M., & Barrett, A. (1985). *Bone marrow disorders: The biological basis of clinical problems.* Oxford: Blackwell Scientific Publishers.

Graze, P. R. (1980). Bone marrow failure: Management of anemia, infections and bleeding in the cancer patient. In C. M. Haskell (Ed.), *Cancer treatment.* Philadelphia: W. B. Saunders Co.

Gupta, S. (1986). Abnormality in immunoregulating cells in human malignancies. In P. K. Ray (Ed.), *Advances in immunity and cancer therapy* (vol. 2, pp. 131–154). New York: Springer-Verlag.

Haeuber, D., & DiJulio, J. (1989). Hematopoietic colony stimulating factors: An overview. *Oncology Nursing Forum, 16*, 247–255.

Hall, N. R., & Goldstein, A. L. (1981). Neurotransmitters and the immune system. In R. Ader (Ed.), *Psychoneuroimmunology* (pp. 521–543). New York: Academic Press.

Handin, R. I. (1985). Hemorrhagic disorders. II: Platelets and purpura. In W. S. Beck (Ed.), *Hematology.* Cambridge, MA: MIT Press.

Hardy, C., & Balducci, L. (1985). Hematopoietic alterations of cancer. *American Journal of the Medical Sciences, 90*, 196–205.

Harris, J., & Copeland, D. (1974). Impaired immunoresponsiveness in tumor patients. *Annals of the New York Academy of Sciences, 230*, 56–85.

Harvey, K., Bothe A., Jr., & Blackburn, G. (1979). Nutritional assessment and patient outcome during oncological therapy. *Cancer, 43*, 2065–2069.

Hillman, R. S., & Finch, C. A. (1985). *Red cell manual* (5th ed.). Philadelphia: F. A. Davis Co.

Hjortso, N. C., & Kehlet, H. (1986). Influence of surgery, age and serum albumin on delayed hypersensitivity. *Acta Chirurgica Scandinavica, 152*, 175–179.

Horns, R. C., Jr., Schirer, S. L., Stanley, L., & Greenberg, P. L. (1984). Lithium treatments in adults with acute myeloid leukemia receiving chemotherapy. *Medical and Pediatric Oncology, 12*, 169–172.

Irwin, J., & Anisman, H. (1984). Stress and pathology: Immunological and central nervous system interactions. In C. L. Cooper (Ed.), *Psychosocial stress and cancer* (pp. 93–147). New York: John Wiley & Sons.

Irwin, M. M. (1987). Patients receiving biological response modifiers: Overview of nursing care. *Oncology Nursing Forum 14* (Suppl.), 32–37.

Jacobson, D. R., & Zolla-Pazner, S. (1986). Immunosuppression and infection in multiple myeloma. *Seminars in Oncology, 13*, 282–290.

Kirkwood, J., & Ernstoff, M. (1984). Interferons in the treatment of human cancer. *Journal of Clinical Oncology, 2*, 336.

Kirschner, J. J., & Preisler, H. D. (1985). Bone marrow toxicity of antitumor agents. In D. J. Higby (Ed.), *The cancer patient and supportive care* (pp. 1–30). Boston: Martinus Nijhoff Publishing.

Kovacs, C. J., Johnke, R. M., Emma, D. A., Scarantino, C. W., Brindle, M. T., Pogrove, R. M., & Evans, M. J. (1985). Residual Adriamycin (Adr)-induced hematopoietic damage: A consideration for subsequent radiotherapy. *International Journal of Radiation Oncology, Biology, and Physics, 11*, 1955–1961.

Laszlo, J. (1983). Anemia associated with marrow infiltration. In W. J. Williams, E. Beutler, A. J. Erslev, & M. A. Lichtman (Eds.), *Hematology* (pp. 522–528). New York: McGraw-Hill Book Co.

Law, D. K., Dudrick, S. J., & Abdou, N. J. (1973). Immunocompetence of patients with protein-calorie malnutrition: The effects of nutritional depletion. *Annals of Internal Medicine, 79*, 545–550.

Levy, J. (1982). Nutrition and the immune system. In D. P. Stites, J. D. Stobo, H. H. Fudenberg, & J. V. Wells (Eds.), *Basic and clinical immunology* (pp. 297–305). Los Altos, CA: Lange Medical Publications.

Lipschitz, D. A., Mitchell, C. O., & Thompson, C. (1981). The anemia of senescence. *American Journal of Hematology, 11*, 47–54.

Lipschitz, D. A., & Udupa, K. B. (1986). Age and the hematopoietic system. *Journal of the American Geriatric Society, 34*, 448–454.

Locke, E. (1982). Stress, adaptation, and immunity: Studies in humans. *General Hospital Psychiatry, 4*, 49–58.

Lohrman, H. P. (1984). The problem of permanent bone marrow damage after cytotoxic drug treatment. *Oncology, 41*, 180–184.

Maxwell, M. (1984). When the cancer patient becomes anemic. *Cancer Nursing, 7*, 321–326.

Mayer, D. (1987). Foreword. *Oncology Nursing Forum, 14* (Suppl.), 2.

McLaren, J. R., Olkowski, Z., Skeen, M., McConnell, F., Benigno, B., Mansour, K., Nixon, D., Shah, N., & Eells, R. (1981). Responses of immune parameters to irradiation of patients with head and neck, bronchogenic, and uterine cervical cancers and to subsequent immunotherapy. In J. B. DuBois, B. Serrou, & C. Rosenfeld (Eds.), *Immunopharmacologic effects of radiation therapy* (pp. 253–274). New York: Raven Press.

Monjan, A. A. (1981). Stress and immunologic competence: Studies in animals. In R. Ader (Ed.), *Psychoneuroimmunology* (pp. 185–228). New York: Academic Press.

Nohr, C. W., Christou, N. V., Broadhead, M., & Meakins, J. L. (1983). Failure of humoral immunity in surgical patients. *Surgical Forum, 34*, 127–129.

Oski, F. A. (1983). Anemia related to nutritional deficiencies other than vitamin B_{12} and folic acid. In W. J. Williams, E. Beutler, A. J. Erslev, & M. A. Lichtman (Eds.), *Hematology* (pp. 532–537). New York: McGraw-Hill Book Co.

Palmblad, J., Petrini, B., Wasserman, J., & Akerstadt, T. (1979). Lymphocyte and granulocyte reactions during sleep deprivation. *Psychosomatic Medicine, 41*, 273–279.

Palmblad, J., Cantell, K. Strander, H., Troberg, J., Karlsson, C. S., Levi, L., Granstrom, M., & Unger, P. (1976). Stressor exposure and immunological response in man: Interferon-producing capacity and phagocytosis. *Journal of Psychosomatic Research, 20*, 193–199.

Pizzo, P. A., Robichaud, K. J., Welsey, R., & Conners, J. P. (1982). Fever in the pediatric and young adult population: A prospective study of 1001 episodes. *Medicine, 61*, 153–165.

Pizzo, P. A., & Young, R. C. (1985). Infections in the cancer patient. In V. T. DeVita, Jr., S. Hellman, & S. A. Rosenberg (Eds.), *Cancer: Principles and practice of oncology* (pp. 1963–1998). Philadelphia: J. B. Lippincott Co.

Queensberry, P. J. (1983). Hematopoietic stem cells. In W. J. Williams, E. Beutler, A. J. Erslev, & M. A. Lichtman (Eds.), *Hematology* (pp. 129–142). New York: McGraw-Hill Book Co.

Quesada, J. R., Talpaz, M., Rios, A., Kurzrock, R., & Gutterman, J. U. (1986). Clinical toxicity of interferons in cancer patients: A review. *Journal of Clinical Oncology, 4*, 234–243.

Riboli, E. B., Terrizi, A., Arnulfio, F., & Bertoglio, S. (1984). Immunosuppressive effect of surgery evaluated by the multitest cell-mediated immunity system. *Canadian Journal of Surgery, 27*, 60–63.

Richtman, C. M., Makii, M. M., Weiser, P. A., & Herbst, A. L. (1984). The effect of lithium carbonate on chemotherapy-induced neutropenia and thrombocytopenia. *American Journal of Hematology, 96*, 313–323.

Riley, V. (1981). Psychoneuroendocrine influences on neoplasia. *Science, 212*, 1100–1109.

Roth, J. (1983). Tumor-induced immunosuppression. *Surgery, Gynecology, Obstetrics, 156*, 233–240.

Rubin, P. (1984). Late effects of chemotherapy and radiation therapy: A new hypothesis. *International Journal of Radiation Oncology, Biology, and Physics, 10*, 5–34.

Rubin, P., & Scarantino, C. W. (1978). The bone marrow organ: The critical structure in radiation-drug interaction. *International Journal of Radiation Oncology, Biology, and Physics, 4*, 3–23.

Sarzotti, M., Baron, S., & Klingoll, G. R. (1978). EL-4 metastases in spleen and bone marrow suppress the NK activity generated in these organs. *International Journal of Cancer, 39*, 118–125.

Schiffer, C. A. (1983). Platelet transfusion therapy for patients with cancer. In D. J. Higby (Ed.), *Supportive care in cancer therapy* (pp. 45–62). Boston: Martinus Nijhoff Publishing.

Schleifer, S. J., Keller, S. E., Camerino, M., Thornton, J. C., & Stein, M. (1983). Suppression of lymphocyte stimulation following bereavement. *Journal of the American Medical Association, 250*, 374–377.

Schlicter, S., & Harker, L. (1974). Hemostasis in malignancy. *Annals of the New York Academy of Sciences, 230*, 252–261.

Schofield, R. (1978). The relationship between the spleen colony-forming cell and the haematopoietic stem cell: A hypothesis. *Blood Cells, 4*, 7–25.

Schofield, R. (1986). Assessment of cytotoxic injury to bone marrow. *British Journal of Cancer, 53* (Suppl. VII), 115–125.

Scott, G. M. (1983). The toxic effects of interferon in man. In I. Gresser (Ed.), *Interferon* (pp. 85–114). London: Academic Press.

Sklar, L., & Anisman, I. (1979). Stress and coping factors influence tumor growth. *Science, 205*, 513–515.

Spross, J. (1985). Alteration in protective mechanisms. In B. Johnson & J. Spross (Eds.), *Handbook of oncology nursing*. New York: John Wiley & Sons.

Stein, M. (1985). Bereavement, depression, stress, and immunity. In R. Guilleme, M. Cohn, & T. Melnechuk (Eds.), *Neural modulation of immunity* (pp. 29–44). New York: Raven Press.

Stein, M., Schiavi, R., & Camerino, M. (1976). Influence of brain and behavior on the immune system. *Science, 191*, 435–440.

Stoll, D. B., Lavin, P. T., & Engstrom, P. F. (1985). Hematologic toxicity of cisplatin and mitomycin in combination for squamous cell carcinoma of the esophagus. *American Journal of Clinical Oncology, 8*, 231–234.

Thoman, M. L. (1985). Role of interleukin-2 in the age-related impairment of immune function. *Journal of the American Geriatrics Society, 33*, 781–787.

Trofatter, K. E. (1986). Immune responses and aging. *Clinical Obstetrics and Gynecology, 29*, 384–396.

Tubiana, M., Arriagada, R., & Sarragin, D. (1986). Human cancer natural history, radiation-induced immunodepression and postoperative radiation therapy. *International Journal of Radiation Oncology, Biology, and Physics, 12*, 477–485.

Wara, W., Wara, D., & Amman, A. J. (1981). Immunosuppression and reconstitution after radiation therapy. In J. B. DuBois, B. Serrou, & C. Rosenfeld (Eds.), *Immunopharmacologic effects of radiation therapy* (pp. 219–229). New York: Raven Press.

Weksler, M. (1981). The senescence of the immune system. *Hospital Practice, 16* (10), 53–64.

Weksler, M. E., Hansman, P. B., & Schwab, R. (1984). Effects of aging on the immune response. In D. P. Stites, J. D. Stobo, H. H. Fudenberg, & J. V. Wells (Eds.), *Basic and clinical immunology* (pp. 302–310). Los Altos, CA: Lange Medical Publications.

Welch, D. (1978). Thrombocytopenia in the adult with acute leukemia. *Cancer Nursing, 1*, 463–466.

Williams, W. J. (1983). Hematology in the aged. In W. J. Williams, E. Beutler, A. J. Erslev, & M. A. Lichtman (Eds.), *Hematology* (pp. 47–53). New York: McGraw-Hill Book Co.

Yeomans, A. C. (1987). Myelodysplastic syndromes: A preleukemic disorder. *Cancer Nursing, 10*, 32–40.

Yoshihara, H., Tanaka, N., & Orita, K. (1986). Suppression of natural killer cell activity by surgical stress in cancer patients and the underlying mechanisms. *Acta Medica Okayama, 40*, 113–119.

CHAPTER 50

Alterations in Comfort: Pain

NESSA COYLE
KATHLEEN M. FOLEY

Early and aggressive management of pain is among the highest priorities for the nurse when working with cancer patients. Unrelieved pain can strip people of their dignity; make them wish for an early death; destroy a family's ability to remain with the patient; and leave the staff feeling angry, ineffectual, and frustrated. Paradoxically, the patient may be blamed in some way if the pain remains severe despite the unstinting efforts of staff and family.

More than 70 per cent of patients could have their pain controlled satisfactorily by pharmacologic approaches alone (Ventafridda, Tamburini, & De Conno, 1985; Ventafridda, Tamburini, & Caraceni, 1987), and the combination of drugs with other methods could control most of the remaining 30 per cent. However, estimates from the World Health Organization (1986) and other sources suggest that cancer pain treatment is often inadequate (Aitken-Swan, 1959; Bonica, 1984; Coyle, Adelhardt, Foley, & Portenoy, 1990; Dant & Cleeland, 1982; Donovan, Dillon, & McGuire, in press; Foley, 1985a; Parks, 1978). To improve this situation the complex nature of pain must be addressed and barriers to appropriate pain management defined and corrected (Wisconsin Cancer Pain Initiative, 1988). Nurses have both the opportunity and the responsibility

to play a significant role in these areas (NIH Consensus Development Conference, 1987).

PREVALENCE OF PAIN IN CANCER PATIENTS

Data describing the incidence, prevalence, and severity of pain in the cancer population suggest that moderate to severe pain is experienced by one third of patients in active therapy and by 60 to 90 per cent of patients with advanced disease (Table 50–1). However, most of these surveys were carried out within large inpatient cancer centers, and the extent of the problem in small community hospitals or for patients being cared for at home is not known. Personal communication with home care nurses suggests the problem may be even greater.

This chapter provides a basic review of the cause of pain in the cancer patient, explores psychosocial factors influencing the pain experience, discusses general principles in the assessment of pain with application of measurement tools to evaluate pain and pain relief, and reviews a variety of approaches to the management of pain.

Table 50–1. EPIDEMIOLOGY OF CANCER PAIN

Author(s)	Patient Population	Stage of Disease	Medical Care System	Survey Method	Prevalence of Pain (%)
Cartwright, Hockey, & Anderson (1973)	215 adults	Far advanced cancer	Inpatients and outpatients, England	Reports of surviving spouses	87
Foley (1979)	156 adults and children	Early and advanced cancer	Cancer hospital, USA	Chart review of analgesic use	29
Foley (1979)	397 adults:				
	358 cases	Early and advanced cancer	Cancer hospital, USA	Patient interview	38
	39 cases	Far advanced cancer	Cancer hospital, USA	Patient interview	60
Haram (1978)	607 adults	Far advanced cancer	Hospice, England	Patient interview	66
Molinari (1979)		Far advanced head and neck cancer	NCI, Milan, Italy	Patient interview	50
Norton & Lack (1986)	100 adults	Far advanced cancer	Hospice, USA	Patient interview	75
Pannuti, Rossi, & Marroro (1980)	284 adults	Far advanced cancer	Oncology service, Italy	Patient interview and follow-up	64
Rubin, Rogers, & Foley (1987)	53 children	All stages	Inpatient cancer hospital, USA	Patient interview	47
Trotter, Scott, & Macbeth (1981)	237 adults	Far advanced cancer	Outpatient oncology service, England	Patient interview	72
Twycross & Fairfield (1982)	500 adults	Far advanced cancer	Hospice, England	Analgesic use	80
Wilkes (1974)	300 adults	Far advanced cancer	Hospice, England	Patient interview	58

(Adapted from Foley, K. M., & Sundaresan, N. [1985]. Management of cancer pain. In V. T. DeVita, Jr., S. Hellman, & S. A. Rosenberg, [Eds.], *Cancer: Principles and practice of oncology,* [vol. 2, 2nd ed., p. 1941]. Philadelphia: J. B. Lippincott Co. Reproduced by permission.)

CAUSE OF PAIN IN CANCER PATIENTS

Definition of Pain

Pain has been defined as "an unpleasant sensory and emotional experience associated with actual or potential tissue damage or described in terms of such damage" (Merskey, 1986). Pain is a subjective experience and may be either acute or chronic. The signs of *acute pain* parallel those of anxiety, with hyperactivity of the autonomic nervous system. A well-defined pattern of onset occurs with evidence of tissue damage. As tissue healing takes place, the pain resolves. In *chronic pain,* the signs frequently parallel those of depression. The autonomic nervous system adapts, and the objective signs that are seen in acute pain are no longer present. The best measure of pain is the patient's report. Chronic pain draws attention to itself by its persistence. Suffering associated with the meaning of this pain may be profound.

Major Pain Types

Acute and chronic pain may be associated with somatic pain, visceral pain, and neuropathic pain (Payne, 1987).

Somatic Pain

Somatic pain occurs as a result of activation of nociceptors (sensory receptors) in cutaneous and deep tissues. The pain is described by the patient as gnawing and aching, and it is usually constant and well localized. This is the most common type of pain experienced by cancer patients, and it is frequently associated with tumor metastasis to the bone, postsurgical incisional pain, and myofascial or musculoskeletal pain. Prosta-

glandin synthesis is thought to be important in the mechanism of tumor growth and pain in bone metastasis (Ferreira, Nakamura, & Castro, 1978; Mundy & Spiro, 1981). Corticosteroids and nonsteroidal antiinflammatory drugs (NSAIDs), which inhibit prostaglandin synthesis, decrease bone pain and may decrease tumor growth in bone (Brodie, 1974; Mundy & Spiro, 1981; Vane, 1971). These drugs therefore play a significant role in the management of bone pain, along with the opioids.

Visceral Pain

Visceral pain results from activation of nociceptors in the cardiovascular and respiratory systems and in the gastrointestinal and genitourinary tracts. Injury that causes pain in cutaneous tissue, such as cutting, burning, or crushing, does not usually result in visceral pain. Stimuli necessary to produce visceral pain include irritation of the mucosal and serosal surfaces, torsion and traction of the mesentery, contraction of a hollow viscus, and impaction (Leek, 1972). Similar stimuli are necessary to produce pain in the bladder and ureters. Unlike somatic pain, visceral pain is poorly localized, is frequently referred to a cutaneous site distant from the lesion, and may be associated with tenderness in the referred cutaneous site. Examples of referred pain are right shoulder pain from liver metastasis and abdominal or leg pain that may occur in the setting of prostate cancer. Visceral pain is described by the patient as "deep," "squeezing," or "pressure." When the pain is acute or signals bowel obstruction, associated symptoms such as nausea, vomiting, and diaphoresis may be present. Visceral pain usually responds well to the opioid drugs.

Neuropathic Pain

Neuropathic pain results from neural injury, either peripheral or central (Payne, 1987; Tasker 1984; Tasker, Tsudn, & Hawrylshyn, 1983; Wall, 1984). The injury may result from tumor invasion, surgery, radiation therapy, chemotherapy, or other factors. Examples of neuropathic pain include metastatic or radiation-induced brachial or lumbar plexopathies, epidural spinal cord compression, postherpetic neuralgia, and painful vincristine and cisplatin neuropathies. Pain resulting from neural injury usually seems unfamiliar to the patient and often burning or stabbing in quality (Tasker, 1984; Tasker et al., 1983). Neurologic deficits may also be present.

Neuropathic pain appears to be less responsive to the opioid drugs than somatic or visceral pain. Combining an opioid with adjuvant drugs such as a tricyclic antidepressant or anticonvulsant is often more effective (Foley, 1985c; Portenoy, 1987b).

Common Pain Syndromes and Sites of Pain

In many patients with advanced disease, the pain originates from multiple sites and sources (Table 50–2). Each type of pain needs a careful systematic evaluation for appropriate management. The pattern of pain a patient describes frequently is characteristic of

Table 50–2. CAUSES OF PAIN IN 100 CANCER PATIENTS

	Number of Pains*		
	Male	Female	Total
Caused by Cancer (67%)			
Bone	30 (16)	28 (15)	58 (31)
Nerve compression	24 (16)	32 (15)	56 (31)
Soft tissue infiltration	21 (19)	14 (12)	35 (31)
Visceral involvement	15 (15)	18 (16)	33 (31)
Muscle spasm	9 (7)	5 (4)	14 (11)
Lymphedema	—	4 (3)	4 (3)
Raised intracranial pressure	—	2 (2)	2 (2)
Myopathy	—	2 (1)	2 (1)
	99 (42)	105 (49)	204 (91)
Related to treatment (5%)			
Postoperative	1 (1)	7 (6)	8 (7)
Colostomy	1 (1)	1 (1)	2 (2)
Nerve block	—	2 (1)	2 (1)
Postoperative adhesions	1 (1)	—	1 (1)
Postradiation fibrosis	—	1 (1)	1 (1)
Esophageal	—	1 (1)	1 (1)
	3 (3)	12 (9)	15 (12)
Associated pains (6%)			
Constipation	6 (6)	5 (5)	11 (11)
Capsulitis of shoulder	1 (1)	3 (3)	4 (4)
Bedsore	—	1 (1)	1 (1)
Postherpetic neuralgia	—	1 (1)	1 (1)
Pulmonary embolus	1 (1)	—	1 (1)
Penile spasm (catheter)	1 (1)	—	1 (1)
	9 (9)	10 (10)	19 (19)
Unrelated pains (22%)			
Musculoskeletal	19 (10)	24 (17)	43 (27)
Osteoarthritis	2 (1)	2 (2)	4 (3)
Migraine	1 (1)	1 (1)	2 (2)
Miscellaneous	6 (5)	10 (8)	16 (13)
	28 (15)	37 (24)	65 (39)
TOTAL	**138**	**165**	**303 (100)**

*Figures in parentheses indicate number of patients in this category, as distinct from number of pains.

(Adapted from Twycross, R. G., & Fairfield, S. [1982]. Pain in far advanced cancer. *Pain, 14,* 303–310.)

a particular pain syndrome. Therefore, knowledge of the more common pain syndromes and listening to the patient as the expert on his or her pain are essential first steps in management.

The most common pain syndromes found in cancer patients fall into four major categories: pain associated with direct tumor involvement of pain-sensitive structures, such as bone, nerve, and hollow viscus; pain associated with cancer therapy, such as surgery, chemotherapy, and radiation therapy; pain associated with immobility; and pain unrelated to cancer or to its treatment (Coyle & Foley, 1987; Foley, 1985; Foley, 1987; Portenoy, 1987c). The common pain syndromes associated with cancer and its treatment are outlined in Tables 50–3 and 50–4.

Epidural Spinal Cord Compression

Epidural spinal cord compression, in which pain is the presenting complaint in 96 per cent of patients, requires special emphasis. Paraplegia can result if the early signs and symptoms of cord compression are not recognized and appropriate treatment carried out. Epidural cord compression occurs in about 5 to 10 per cent of patients with cancer. Although any patient may develop this neuro-oncologic complication, it is more commonly seen in patients with cancer of the lung, prostate, and breast (Kanner, Martini, & Foley, 1981; Posher, 1987). Spinal cord damage results from compression by tumor in the epidural space or from direct invasion of the cord. Pain may be present for days or weeks before other neurologic signs and symptoms appear. The pain is of two types. *Local pain,* which occurs near the site of the involved vertebral body, is described by the patient as dull, aching, and constant. This pain is made worse by lying down and may be relieved by sitting or standing. *Radicular pain* is more common when the cervical or lumbosacral spine is involved. Cervical and lumbosacral radicular pain is usually unilateral, whereas thoracic radicular pain is usually bilateral. The patient frequently describes this pain as constricting, band-like, as though he or she were "in a cast," and radiating around the abdomen or chest. If left untreated, neurologic signs and symptoms progress to include weakness, sensory changes, and bowel and bladder dysfunction. Once neurologic symptoms other than pain occur, rapid progression to complete paraplegia may occur over a period of hours or days (Posner, 1987).

The prognosis depends on the neurologic status of the patient when treatment is started. Patients who are ambulatory usually remain so, whereas those who are not rarely regain function after treatment. The natural history of untreated epidural cord compression illustrates the need for careful attention to the patient's complaint of pain and early diagnosis of the cause of pain, so that appropriate management can be instituted.

PSYCHOSOCIAL FACTORS INFLUENCING THE PAIN EXPERIENCE

Both psychosocial and physiologic variables have a major impact on the pain experience (Ahles, Blan-

Table 50–3. PAIN ASSOCIATED WITH DIRECT TUMOR INVOLVEMENT

Direct Tumor Involvement	Signs and Symptoms
Tumor infiltration of bone	
Base of skull syndrome (Greenberg, Deck, & Vikram, 1981):	Pain may precede neurologic signs and symptoms by weeks or months
1. Jugular foramen metastases	Occipital pain, referred to vertex of head; pain exacerbated by movement; tenderness over the occipital condyle; depending on nerves involved, may include hoarseness, dysarthria, dysphagia, neck and shoulder weakness, ptosis
2. Clivus metastases	Vertex headache exacerbated by neck flexion; lower cranial nerve dysfunction begins unilaterally, progresses to bilateral dysfunction
3. Sphenoid sinus	Severe bifrontal headache (radiates to both temples); intermittent retro-orbital pain; nasal stuffiness, fullness in head
Vertebral body syndromes	Pain is an early symptom
1. Odontoid process (Greenberg et al., 1981): C1 involvement may result in pathologic fracture, subluxation, and spinal cord or brain stem compression	Severe neck pain radiating over posterior aspect of the skull and vertex; pain exacerbated by flexion; progressive sensory and motor signs begin in upper extremities; pain localized to adjacent paraspinal area
2. C7-T1 (Cascino, Kori, & Krol, 1985; Kanner, Martini, & Foley, 1982a; Kori, Foley, & Posner, 1981): Tumor spread may be hematogenous or along nerves from tumor originating in brachial plexus or paravertebral space to contiguous vertebral body and epidural space	Constant dull ache, radiating to both shoulders; tenderness on percussion over spinous process at this level; radicular pain, usually unilateral in posterior arm, elbow, and ulnar aspect of hand; ptosis and miosis (Horner's syndrome)
3. L1 (Greenberg et al., 1981):	Dull, aching, mid-back pain; exacerbated by lying or sitting, relieved by standing; pain—radiating, girdle-like band anteriorly or to both paraspinal and lumbosacral areas; may be referred to sacroiliac joint or superior iliac crest
Sacral syndrome (Jackel, Young, & Foley, 1985): Most frequent in patients with gynecologic, genitourinary, or colonic cancers	Aching pain in low back or coccygeal area; insidious onset; exacerbated by lying or sitting, relieved by walking; increasing pain with perianal sensory loss; bowel, bladder dysfunction; impotence
Tumor infiltration of nerve (Gilbert, Kim, & Posner, 1978; Posner, 1987):	
Epidural spinal cord compression: Neurologic symptoms vary with site of disease; considered a medical emergency	Severe neck and back pain is initial symptom in 96% of patients; motor weakness-paraplegia; sensory loss varies with level; loss of bowel and bladder function
Peripheral nerve proximal infiltration: occurs from paravertebral or retroperitoneal tumor	Constant burning pain; hypoesthesia and dysesthesia in area of sensory loss, early symptom
Plexus	
1. Brachial plexopathy (Cascino et al., 1985; Kanner, Martini, & Foley, 1982b; Kori et al., 1981): Associated with lung (Pancoast) and breast cancer and lymphoma	Pain radiating to ipsilateral shoulder and posterior aspect of arm and elbow (C8-T1 distribution); pain and paresthesias in fourth and fifth fingers, may precede objective clinical signs by weeks or months; paresthesias progress to numbness, weakness, C7-T1 distribution
2. Lumbar plexopathy (Jackel et al., 1985): Result of extension of genitourinary, gynecologic, and colonic cancer	Pain in L1-L3 distribution radiates to anterior portion of thigh or groin; pain in L5-S1 distribution radiates down posterior aspect of leg to the heel; paresthesias are followed by numbness and dysesthesias; progressive motor and sensory loss in plexus distribution
3. Sacral plexopathy (Jackel et al., 1985): Occurs most frequently in patients with colonic, genitourinary, and gynecologic cancers	Pain dull, aching, midline; sensory loss beginning in perianal area; sensory findings are at first unilateral; progression to bilateral sacral sensory loss and autonomic dysfunction; impotence, bowel and bladder dysfunction; patient unable to lie or sit down
Root	
1. Leptomeningeal metastases (Olson, Chernik, & Posner, 1978): Result of tumor infiltration of the leptomeninges with or without invasion of the parenchyma of the nervous system	Pain occurs in 40% of patients; may be constant headache with or without stiff neck; may be localized low back and buttock pain

(Adapted with permission from Coyle, N., & Foley, K. M. [1987]. Prevalence and profile of pain syndromes in cancer patients. In D. B. McGuire, & C. H. Yarbro [eds.], *Cancer pain management* (pp. 32–33). Orlando, Fl: Grune & Stratton, Inc.)

chard, & Ruchdeschel, 1983; Beecher, 1956; Cleleand, 1984; Coyle et al., in press). These are reviewed within the context of general psychosocial variables, profiling the cancer patient with pain and looking at the effect of environmental setting on pain management.

Profile of Patients with Cancer Pain

The pain of cancer is experienced not only as the response of an organism to tissue damage, but also as the response of a person with a life trajectory of pain and pleasure and of present and future hopes and despair. This may be described as the "suffering" component of cancer pain and is tightly woven into the pain experience. Within this framework, patients with cancer pain can be categorized within five groups, as outlined in Table 50–5.

Patients with Acute Cancer-Related Pain

The first group includes those patients with acute cancer-related pain. The pain may be associated with

Table 50–4. PAIN SYNDROMES ASSOCIATED WITH CANCER THERAPY

Syndromes	Signs and Symptoms
Postsurgical Syndromes:	
Postthoracotomy (Foley, 1985b; Kanner, Martini, & Foley, 1981, 1982b): Caused by injury to intercostal nerves	Constant pain in distribution of intercostal nerve; occurs 1–2 months post surgery; pain—band-like in area of sensory loss; occasional intermittent shock-like pains; dysesthesias in the scar area with hyperesthesias in the surrounding area; pain worse with movement; may develop frozen shoulder
Postmastectomy (Foley, 1985b; Granek, Ashikari, & Foley, 1984): Caused by interruption of intercostobrachial nerve (T1–T2)	Pain in posterior aspect of arm and axilla, radiates to anterior part of chest wall; pain starts 1–2 months after surgery; pain tight and constricting; no associated lymphedema; pain worse on movement; may result in frozen shoulder
Radical neck dissection (Foley, 1985b): Caused by injury or interruption of cervical nerves	Constant burning sensation in area of sensory loss; may be dysesthesias and intermittent shock-like pain (unpleasant tingling and stinging)
Phantom limb syndrome (Foley, 1985b; Sherman, Sherman, & Parker, 1984);	Two types: (1) Phantom pain identical in nature to preoperative pain; (2) stump pain from traumatic neuroma
Postchemotherapy Syndromes (Foley, 1985b; LeQuesne, 1984; Young & Posner, 1980):	
Peripheral neuropathy associated with symmetric polyneuropathy from Vinca alkaloid treatment	Painful dysesthesias; localized to feet and hands; pain increased by superficial stimuli; resolves with reduction in chemotherapy
Steroid pseudorheumatism (Foley, 1985b; Rotstein & Good, 1957): Caused by steroid withdrawal	Diffuse myalgias and arthralgias; muscle and joint tenderness; no inflammatory signs; generalized malaise and fatigue; disappears if steroids are resumed
Aseptic necrosis (Ihde & DeVita, 1975) of the femoral head and less frequently of humeral head (complication of steroid therapy—more common in patients with Hodgkin's disease)	Shoulder or hip pain
Postherpetic neuralgia (Portenoy, Duma, & Foley, 1986; Price, 1982): Herpes zoster infection occurs in areas of tumor or of radiotherapy—more common in patients who develop the infection after age 50 years	Pain with three distinct components: either all three or only one may be present; continuous burning in area of sensory loss; intermittent and shock-like pain; painful dysesthesias.
Postradiation Syndromes (Foley, 1985b, 1987; Kori, Foley, & Posner, 1981):	
Radiation fibrosis of brachial and lumbar plexus (may occur 6 months to 20 years after radiotherapy)	Numbness or paresthesias of the hand; lymphedema in arm; radiation skin changes; induration of supraclavicular and axillary areas; motor weakness, deltoid and biceps muscles; C5, C6 distribution; progression of signs leading to painful, swollen, useless arm
Radiation myelopathy (Jellinger & Sturm, 1971; Palmer, 1972; Stoll & Andrews, 1966): (pain early symptom in 15% of patients)	Pain may be localized to area of spinal cord damage or referred to distant site; dysesthesias below level of cord lesion
Radiation-induced secondary tumors (Foley, Woodruff, & Ellis, 1979) occurring 4–20 yr after radiation	Painful enlarging mass in previously irradiated area

(Adapted with permission from Coyle, N., & Foley, K. M. [1987]. Prevalence and profile of pain syndromes in cancer patients. In D. B. McGuire, & C. H. Yarbro (Eds.), *Cancer pain management* (pp. 34–35). Orlando, Fl: Grune & Stratton, Inc.)

tumor growth or with cancer therapy. Patients with acute tumor-related pain may have first sought medical attention because of pain or have had their first cancer recurrence heralded by pain. For this group of patients, uncertainty and fear color any recurrent pain symptoms even if unrelated to their cancer.

Those patients whose acute pain is related to cancer

Table 50–5. TYPES OF PATIENTS WITH PAIN FROM CANCER

> Acute cancer-related pain
>> Associated with the diagnosis of cancer
>> Associated with cancer therapy
> Chronic cancer-related pain
>> Associated with tumor progression
>> Associated with cancer therapy
> Preexisting chronic pain and cancer-related pain
> A history of drug addiction and cancer-related pain
>> Actively involved in illicit drug use
>> In methadone maintenance program
>> With history of past drug abuse
> Dying patients with cancer-related pain

(Adapted with permission from Foley, K. M. [1985a]. The treatment of cancer pain. *New England Journal of Medicine, 313,* 84–95.)

therapy (e.g., postoperative pain or pain secondary to mouth ulcerations from chemotherapy) do not have quite the same uncertainty and fear. The potential for pain associated with a particular treatment method may have been explained to the patient, and in the patient's and staff's minds, it may be seen as a necessary part of getting well. The difference for the patient and staff in dealing with acute pain related to disease progression and acute pain related to disease treatment is the meaning of the pain.

Patients with Chronic Cancer-Related Pain

The second group includes patients with chronic cancer-related pain. As with the acute pain group, the pain may be associated with disease progression or with its treatment. In patients with chronic pain associated with tumor progression, the escalating pain is caused by tumor infiltration of pain-sensitive structures. Suffering plays a major role in the "total" pain these patients experience, and both physiologic and psychological fatigue is common. These factors must be addressed if therapy is to be adequately managed.

Chronic pain may also be associated with cancer treatment (e.g., postmastectomy, postthoracotomy, and phantom limb pain). The cause of the pain may be secondary to nerve injury and development of a traumatic neuroma. It is essential that the cause of the pain be explained to the patient and family as being unrelated to tumor progression. This has a major effect on the patient's psychological state. Methods of treatment of this type of pain concentrate on physical therapy and the use of the cognitive behavioral approaches.

Patients with Preexisting Chronic Pain and Cancer-Related Pain

The third group includes patients with a history of chronic pain unrelated to cancer, who then develop cancer and have cancer-related pain. These patients already have a compromised functional and psychological state because of their previous chronic pain. With the added stress of cancer and its accompanying pain, the risk is high for further psychological and functional deterioration. Early identification of this group of patients enables appropriate supportive intervention.

Patients with a History of Drug Abuse and Cancer-Related Pain

The fourth group includes patients with a history of drug abuse who develop cancer-related pain. Three subgroups of patients can be identified within this heading. These are (1) patients who are actively using street drugs, (2) patients who are in methadone maintenance programs, and (3) patients who have not used illicit drugs for many years.

Persons in the first subgroup strain the resources of the most sophisticated pain management team and require tight controls on the way their analgesics are dispensed; they also need intensive ongoing support if they are discharged back into the community. Because these patients frequently interact with a number of physicians and nurses, staff manipulation may be an issue. One physician, knowledgeable in pain management and symptom control, should be identified as the person to adjust analgesics and write all prescriptions, and one experienced oncology or hospice nurse should be identified as the person to organize and coordinate the patient's plan of care. Communication among members of involved disciplines on an inpatient and outpatient basis is essential and usually is facilitated by the nurse. Consultation may be sought from persons familiar with working with the addict population.

The second and third subgroups (persons in methadone maintenance programs, or those who have not used drugs for many years) do not present a management problem if the following issues are recognized. First, these patients may be at high risk for recidivism because of the stress of cancer and pain. Alternative behavioral ways of dealing with stress must be taught to the patient and support networks set up both in the hospital and community. Second, patients in methadone maintenance programs have become used to narcotics and may require a larger amount of opioid analgesics to control their pain than would "normally" be anticipated. This reflects tolerance and not drug abuse. Third, multidisciplinary staff conferences are essential at the unit level, so that nurses and doctors have an opportunity to explore their own attitudes and concerns about prescribing or administering a narcotic agent to a patient with a history of drug abuse. Unless these steps are taken, this group of patients is extraordinarily vulnerable to having the pain poorly managed.

Patients with Pain Who Are Dying

Patients with cancer and pain who are dying constitute the fifth group. The primary focus of care is comfort, and treatment is no longer directed toward curing the disease. At no time is pain more destructive than in the dying patient. Families are left with a lasting memory of the pain of the person's death, which is difficult to erase. Both pain and suffering must be vigorously addressed in the dying patient through consistent, competent, compassionate support and appropriate analgesic titration. Families and nurses sometimes worry about giving that last injection before the patient dies and wonder if it contributed to the patient's death (Foley, 1988). That fear may result in a patient's having to suffer unnecessary pain. There are several ways to handle the situation: first, by reinforcing the fact to both staff members and family that the patient is dying of cancer and will die in the near future of his or her disease regardless of whether analgesics are administered. The difference might be whether the person dies in pain or is relatively comfortable. If staff members continue to be uneasy about administering adequate amounts of narcotics to control the dying patient's pain, especially when respirations may be slowing, using a continuous intravenous infusion to administer the analgesic may alleviate the problem and ensure that the patient receives adequate pain relief.

Environmental Settings and Their Influence on Pain Management

The environment within which the patient with cancer pain receives care affects both response to pain management and adequacy of pain control (Melzack, Ofiesh, & Mount, 1983; Morris et al., 1986). For example, staff members on critical care units have a different set of priorities than those working on units with dying patients. A study by Melzack and colleagues (1983) examined the adequacy of pain control in two groups of terminally ill cancer patients, one in a standard hospital environment, the other in a palliative care unit within the same institution. Although morphine administration was titrated in a similar manner in both settings to control pain, the patients being cared for in the palliative care unit obtained a significantly greater level of pain relief. This was attributed to the psychological impact of the unit on the patient and family through its focus on comfort, care, and attention to individual worries and concerns.

Professional variables also affect adequacy of pain management. These include the knowledge of pain control and the nurse's and patient's cultural backgrounds, social class, and age (Angell, 1982; Boyd & Pilowsky, 1966; Bonica, 1985; Charap, 1987; Levin, Cleeland, & Dar, 1985; Marks & Sachar, 1973; Parks, 1978; Rankin & Snider, 1984; Wisconsin Cancer Pain Initiative 1988; Zborowski, 1952). Nurses and doctors not infrequently expect disease processes to be associated with a specific level of pain. Patients whose pain experience falls outside the expected norm may be disbelieved about their pain and frequently have a disorganizing effect on the staff. The result may be the staff's labeling the patient uncooperative and demanding. Conflict between patients and staff members most frequently centers on ethical issues, such as those involving belief in the patient's pain and administering adequate doses of narcotic analgesics to relieve the pain, based not on "hard data" but on the patient's word.

ASSESSMENT OF PAIN

Knowledge of the basic anatomy and physiology underlying pain, as well as an awareness of common pain syndromes, multiple sites of pain, and profiles of patients with cancer-related pain, is a necessary background to the nursing assessment of the pain complaint. It is important to remember that pain is a symptom, not a diagnosis. Pain perception is not merely a reflection of the amount of tissue damage a patient sustains but also a complex state determined by many factors, including age, sex, cultural and environmental influences, and multiple psychological variables. All of these factors must be explored if the pain assessment is to be complete. The assessment is ongoing and is based on a careful medical and psychosocial history and on examining the site of the pain and potential pain referral sources. Many patients, particularly those with chronic pain of unknown origin, have a history of adversary relationships with doctors and nurses, relating to perceived failure to believe in the severity of the patient's pain on the patient's own word and to conflicts concerning the use of narcotic analgesics. Belief in the patient's pain and acknowledgment of the devastating effect that pain can have on the lives of both the patient and the family are critical not only to the assessment of pain but also to its management.

The Pain History: General Principles

Current Pain Complaints

The general principles involved in taking a pain history are outlined in Table 50–6. The first step is to take a careful history of the current pain complaints. As outlined previously, patients frequently have more than one site and source of pain. Each needs to be

Table 50–6. THE PAIN HISTORY: GENERAL PRINCIPLES FOR THE ONCOLOGY NURSE

Believe the patient's complaint
Take a careful history of the complaint of pain and place it temporally in the patient's cancer history
Assess the psychological and social factors confounding the pain complaint
Examine the site of pain and possible referred sites
Ensure ongoing assessment of the patient's pain and effectiveness of pain relief measures

evaluated to ensure appropriate management. Included are the onset of the pain, its site and characteristics, the referral patterns, exacerbating and relieving factors, and any associated symptoms.

Onset

The onset (temporal classification) of the pain includes questions relating to when the pain started, how long the person has had pain, and what were the precipitating events. The patient's responses indicate to the nurse whether the pain is acute or chronic and whether the probable cause is the disease, the treatment, or neither the disease nor its treatment.

Site(s)

The site(s) (topographic classification) of the pain may be best illustrated by the patient's demonstrating on his or her body, or on the nurse interviewer's body, where the focus of the pain is felt and its pattern of radiation to other areas. Another useful approach is for the patient to use a body chart (Fig. 50–1) and shade in each area of pain. Knowledge of referral patterns are important because referred pain sites are tender to touch and may be misinterpreted as the source of the pain. For example, referred pain in the arm or leg is often the first sign of brachial plexus or lumbar plexus tumor infiltration, respectively.

Characteristics

Characteristics of the pain are learned by asking the patient to describe it. For example, is it sharp, shooting, burning, aching, or throbbing? These characteristics help answer the question of whether the pain is somatic, visceral, or neuropathic in origin. Severity and pattern of the pain are also included in the assessment: is it mild, moderate or severe; is the pain constant or intermittent; is there a cyclic pattern, with changes in the pain occurring throughout the day and over time?

Exacerbating and Relieving Factors

Exacerbating and relieving factors of pain are frequently recognized by patients and either used or avoided in the attempt to control pain. The nurse obtains this information not only as additional data for understanding the source of the pain but also as support for effective patient-initiated pain management ap-

Back   **Front**

Right   **Left**   **Left**   **Right**

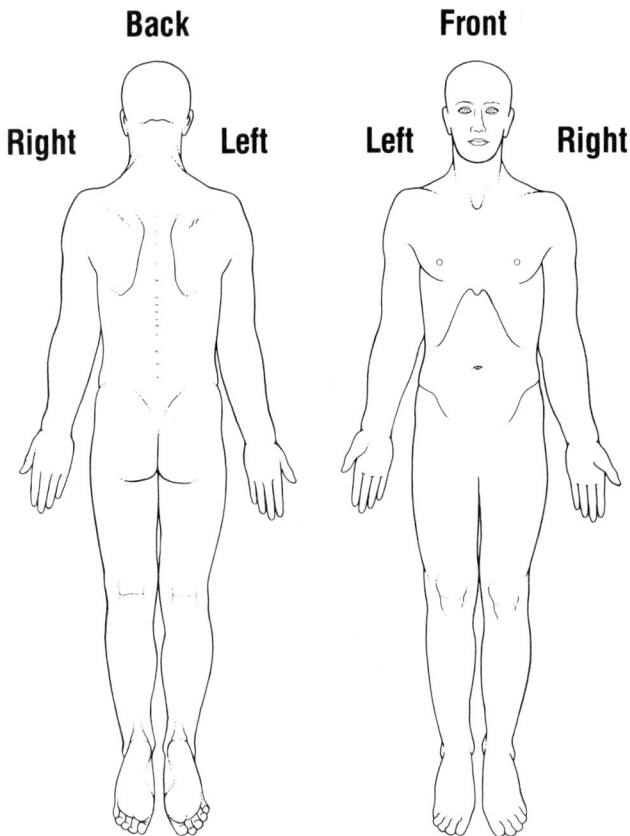

Figure 50–1. Body chart. The patient indicates on the body chart the different sites of pain.

proaches. Depending on the site and suspected source of the pain, relevant questions are asked. For example, questions may deal with whether the pain occurs on swallowing, on straining when having a bowel movement, or when taking a variety of body positions, such as lying, sitting, or standing. A survey of breakthrough pains (defined as a transient flare of severe pain on a background of moderate pain or less) reported that 63 per cent of patients experienced this type of pain during a 1-day period (Portenoy & Hagen, in press). It is not unusual for patients to say that their pain becomes worse when they are anxious, and that when their pain is not controlled they become both anxious and depressed. This is important information when teaching patients the effect of mood and emotions on pain tolerance.

Associated Symptoms

Associated symptoms occurring on a background of pain require critical attention, as they may signal an acute complication in the patient. For example, a patient with advanced colonic cancer and chronic abdominal pain who develops obstipation with associated nausea and vomiting needs an immediate medical evaluation to rule out obstruction. A second example, in which the effects of body position on the cancer patient's pain and the associated symptoms suggest a diagnosis, is the patient with epidural cord compression. In this case the nurse elicits a history of severe

back pain that worsens when lying in bed, and becomes better when walking around, and is associated with bowel and bladder dysfunction. In such patients the effects of rapid medical intervention, often using a combination of high-dose steroids and radiation therapy to prevent paraplegia, are positive (Posner, 1987).

Psychosocial History

After eliciting a careful history of the present pain complaint, the next step is to obtain a psychosocial history. This will provide information about how pain influences the patient's day-to-day living and psychological and social functioning. It is also important that the nurse direct questions toward the patient's previous experience with both pain unrelated to cancer and to cancer-related pain. Questions are aimed at gaining an understanding of the place of anxiety and depression in the patient's pain complaint. What does the pain signify to the patient, and what does the patient most fear? Does the patient have difficulty in sleeping, and does the pattern of insomnia reflect depression, anxiety, and/or poorly controlled pain? Past and current stressors in the patient's and family's lives are also explored. Questions are asked about how the person has dealt with stress in the past, so that appropriate behavioral techniques can be taught or reinforced (Donovan, 1987; Meinhardt & McCaffery, 1983).

Past Pain Relief Management Approaches

The nature and effectiveness of past pain relief management approaches the patient has undergone are reviewed. These include chemotherapy, surgery, radiation therapy, and behavioral modification techniques. Special attention is given to the analgesic history. Questions are asked about the current analgesic regimen, including the drug(s), route of administration, dose, time interval between doses, effectiveness of pain relief, and side effects, if any, such as sedation, nausea, constipation, or feeling "mentally hazy." Questions are also asked about prior exposure to narcotics on the part of the patient, family, or friends. Fears and misconceptions concerning the use of narcotics for pain frequently surface at this time, and unless they are dealt with in an open and forthright manner, they will interfere with the appropriate use of these drugs.

Examining the Site of Pain and Possible Referral Sites

Examining the site of pain and possible referral sites is part of the nursing assessment. This examination may substantiate the clinical history with additional data, but findings may appear essentially normal despite a patient's complaint of pain. A critical factor for the nurse to remember is that normal results on physical examination do not negate a patient's pain complaint.

MEASUREMENT TOOLS TO EVALUATE PAIN AND PAIN RELIEF MEASURES

Pain by its nature is a subjective experience. A problem arises when doctors and nurses, who are used to basing their treatment decisions on objective data, are asked to base their decisions to a large part on the patient's verbal report of pain and pain relief. If the patient is given tools to translate the subjective experience of pain into a more objective form, communication between the patient, doctor, and nurse is enhanced. Asking the patient standardized questions also lessens the likelihood that valuable information will be omitted.

A variety of instruments are available to evaluate pain and the effectiveness of pain relief measures. Some, because of their length and complexity, are more suitable for research purposes than for clinical use (McGuire, 1984; Syrjala, 1987). The McGill Pain Questionnaire is the most widely used of such tools (McGuire, 1984a; Melzack, 1975). To address the need for a more concise clinical tool, useful for the often fatigued patient with advanced cancer, Daut, Cleeland, and Flannery (1983) developed the Brief Pain Inventory. This tool evaluates the following dimensions: history of pain; site of pain; intensity of pain; medications and treatments used to relieve pain; relief obtained; and the effects of pain on mood, activities, and interpersonal relationships. The tool has been found to be useful, valid, and reliable. More recently attempts have been made to assess "quality of life" as an outcome measure in the management of cancer pain. (Ferrell, Wisdom, & Wenzl, 1989).

Assessment and reassessment of the patient in pain is an ongoing process. New pains develop, and old pains disappear. Levels of distress also may vary. These changing parameters must be monitored by the nurse on a regular basis and are a useful measure of the effectiveness of pain management techniques. The Memorial Pain Assessment Card, designed specifically to assess the effectiveness of a particular analgesic dose for a particular patient, is now being evaluated for use in this more global way (Fishman et al., 1987). This is a simple self-rating instrument consisting of a verbal pain rating scale and three visual analog scales that measure pain intensity, pain relief, and mood. This instrument takes less than 30 seconds for the patient to complete, and can therefore be administered as frequently as necessary to measure a patient's response to therapy (Fig. 50–2).

Two other simple measures frequently used in the clinical setting to evaluate the effectiveness of a treatment approach are numerical estimates (0 = no pain, and 10 = the worst possible pain) and categoric scales (none, mild, moderate, and severe). Documenting the amount of pain relief a patient is receiving is a critical part of assessment.

MANAGEMENT OF PAIN

The management of pain flows directly from its assessment. Inadequate assessment of pain usually results in inadequate pain relief. Because of the multidimensional nature of both pain and suffering in the cancer patient, a multidisciplinary approach is most effective (NIH Consensus Development Conference, 1987; Cleeland, Rotondi, & Brechner, 1986; Coyle, 1989; Coyle et al., in press; Foley, 1985). As patient advocate, the nurse frequently coordinates such a multidisciplinary approach for the patient and family and must therefore be familiar with the various pain management techniques used (Coyle, 1989a,b). The following discussion addresses principles of drug therapy, anesthetic approaches, neurosurgical approaches, neuroaugmentative approaches, behavioral approaches, and continuity of care. Not included are treatments directed against the disease process itself—for example, radiation therapy, chemotherapy, and surgery. However, such treatments, especially radiation therapy, may have a dramatic effect on relieving pain.

Drug Therapy: Basic Principles

Drug therapy is the mainstay of cancer pain treatment and includes the use of nonnarcotic agents, narcotics, and adjuvant drugs. Each is selected on the basis of the cause and severity of the pain, the metabolic state of the patient, and the person's response to the drug.

Nonnarcotic Analgesics (Nonsteroidal Anti-Inflammatory Drugs)

Nonnarcotic analgesics have four major pharmacologic properties: analgesic, antipyretic, antiplatelet, and anti-inflammatory. They have a peripheral site of action and produce analgesia by inhibiting prostaglandin synthetase (Kantor, 1982; Vane, 1971). Prostaglandins sensitize peripheral nerve endings to the pain-producing effects of chemical substances such as bradykinin. Nonsteroidal anti-inflammatory drugs are most effective in treating mild to moderate pain when an inflammatory component is present. In the patient with cancer, they are frequently used in combination with a narcotic. Unlike the narcotic drugs, the NSAIDs have a *ceiling effect* (a dose beyond which added analgesia is not obtained) but do not produce tolerance, physical dependence, or psychological dependence (Coyle, 1987; Foley, 1985; Kantor, 1982). The major adverse effects of this class of drugs are hematologic (e.g., interference with platelet aggregation), gastrointestinal (e.g., dyspepsia and ulcer formation), hypersensitivity reactions (e.g., severe breathing restriction and hives), and renal (e.g., edema and renal insufficiency) (American Pain Society, 1989). Prostaglandins mediate these adverse effects. The most commonly used NSAIDs are ibuprofen (Motrin), fenoprofen (Nalfon), diflunisal (Dolobid), and naproxen (Naprosyn). Choline magnesium trisalicylate, a less widely known anti-inflammatory drug, does not interfere with platelet aggregation and is therefore especially useful for patients with decreased blood counts

Figure 50–2. Memorial pain assessment card, *front* (*1* and *4*) and *back* (*2* and *3*). The card is folded along the broken line, and each measure is presented to the patient separately in the numbered order. *(1)* Visual analog scale (VAS) pain intensity; *(2)* Modified Tursky pain descriptors scale; *(3)* VAS pain relief; *(4)* VAS mood (From Fishman et al. [1987]. The Memorial Pain Assessment Card: A valid instrument for the assessment of cancer pain. *Cancer, 60,* 1151–1157.)

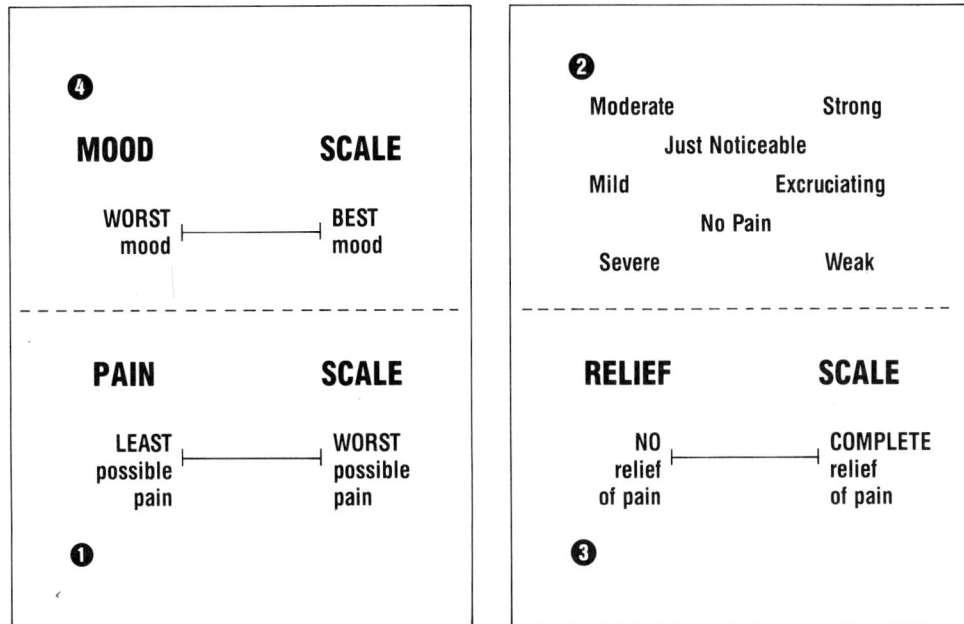

❹

MOOD   SCALE

WORST |————————| BEST
mood   mood

- -

PAIN   SCALE

LEAST |————————| WORST
possible   possible
pain   pain

❶

❷

Moderate   Strong
Just Noticeable
Mild   Excruciating
No Pain
Severe   Weak

- -

RELIEF   SCALE

NO |————————| COMPLETE
relief   relief
of pain   of pain

❸

(Cohen, Thomas, & Coen, 1978). Acetaminophen, although lacking anti-inflammatory effects, is also helpful in managing pain in this group of patients. The major adverse effect of acetaminophen is hepatotoxicity, and this drug must therefore be used with caution in patients with severe liver dysfunction (Kantor, 1982).

Narcotic Analgesics

Narcotic analgesics produce their analgesic effects by binding to the opiate receptors at the peripheral and central nervous systems and altering the perception of pain (Jaffe & Martin, 1980). Misconceptions concerning tolerance, physical dependence, and psychological dependence (addiction) by doctors, nurses, and patients are a major reason for the undertreatment of cancer pain (Charap, 1987; Foley, 1988, 1989; Marks & Sachar, 1973; Watt-Watson, 1987; Wisconsin Cancer Pain Initiative, 1988).

Tolerance. Tolerance means that a larger dose of a drug is needed to maintain the same effect (Coyle, 1987; Foley, 1988). It may occur in any patient receiving narcotic analgesics on a regular basis and is related to dose, frequency of administration, and route of administration. The first sign of the development of tolerance is the patient's complaint that the analgesic effect of the drug does not last as long, and the pain starts returning after, for example, 2.5 hr instead of 3 hr. In the cancer patient, increasing analgesic requirements are frequently associated with progressive disease (Coyle, Adelhardt, & Foley, 1988; Coyle et al., 1990; Foley, 1985a). Lack of understanding of tolerance by doctors and nurses reinforces two basic patient fears: (1) that they have become addicted to the drugs, and (2) that if "too much" of the drug is used now, when they "really need it," the medication will not work.

The effects of tolerance in the patient with chronic cancer pain can be minimized by using a combination of narcotic and nonnarcotic drugs and by switching to an alternative narcotic (cross-tolerance is not complete among narcotics), starting at one half to one third of the equianalgesic dose of the previous drug (American Pain Society, 1989; Foley, 1985a).

Physical Dependence. Physical dependence is an altered physiologic state occurring in patients who use opioid drugs on a long-term basis (American Pain Society, 1989; Coyle, 1987; Jaffe, 1980). If the drug is stopped abruptly, the patient exhibits signs of withdrawal but without exhibiting drug-seeking behavior unless specifically related to pain. Signs of abrupt opioid withdrawal in the tolerant patient include anxiety, alternating hot flashes and cold chills, salivation, lacrimation, rhinorrhea, diaphoresis, piloerection, nausea, vomiting, abdominal cramping, and insomnia. The time course of the withdrawal syndrome depends on the half-life of the drug. For example, in drugs with a short half-life, such as morphine or hydro-morphone (Dilaudid), symptoms may occur within 6 to 12 hr of stopping the drug and be most severe after 24 to 72 hr. In drugs with a long half-life, such as levorphanol (Levo-Dromoran) and methadone (Dolophine), the symptoms may not occur for several days (American Pain Society, 1989; Foley & Inturrisi, 1987). Gradual reduction of the opioid drug in the tolerant patient who no longer has pain will prevent the withdrawal syndrome. An appropriate tapering schedule is suggested by the American Pain Society (1989): On days 1 and 2, give one fourth of the previous 24-hr opioid dose in divided doses. Then decrease the dose by 75 per cent every 2 days until a daily dose of 10 to 15 mg of intramuscular morphine equivalents is reached. The patient is kept on this dose for 2 days, after which the drug can be stopped. A suggested alternative approach is to switch the patient to oral methadone at 25 per cent of the equianalgesic dose of the previous drug, and then proceed in the outlined manner.

The use of an antagonist such as naloxone in the drug-tolerant patient will precipitate acute withdrawal symptoms unless carefully titrated (American Pain Society, 1989; Foley & Inturris, 1987). Patients to whom this has happened describe the sensation as feeling as if they had been plugged into a live electric socket, and pain recurs promptly. Such patients may become extremely fearful of falling asleep, fearing a repeat of the abrupt awakening with excruciating pain. Being "sleepy" (sedated) and the precipitation of the acute withdrawal syndrome become tightly linked in these patients' minds. If a drug overdose is suspected in a tolerant patient, a dilute solution of naloxone should be used (0.4 mg in 10 ml of normal saline solution) (American Pain Society, 1989; Foley & Inturrisi, 1987). This may be administered by intravenous push every 2 min until the patient becomes responsive. As the half-life of naloxone is considerably shorter than that of the majority of the opioid drugs, an intravenous infusion of naloxone, carefully titrated to respirations and level of pain, may be the safest approach once the patient has become responsive. In the comatose patient, an endotracheal tube should be inserted before the administration of naloxone to prevent aspiration.

Psychological Dependence. Psychological dependence ("addiction") is defined as a pattern of compulsive drug use characterized by a continued craving for a narcotic and the need to use the narcotic for effects other than pain relief (Jaffe, 1980). Drug-seeking behavior is characteristic, the person using any means to obtain the drug. Psychological dependence is rare in cancer patients (Macaluso, Weinberg, & Foley, 1988; Porter & Jick, 1980), but it is frequently cited as the reason why doctors underprescribe narcotics, why nurses administer smaller amounts than are prescribed or at longer time intervals than are appropriate, and why patients are reluctant to take adequate amounts of a narcotic to control their pain.

Narcotic analgesics are classified according to their ability to bind to opiate receptor sites and produce analgesia. Agonist drugs, such as morphine and methadone, bind to the opiate receptor sites and produce analgesia in this way (Jaffe & Martin, 1980). Drugs of the antagonist variety such as naloxone block the effect of morphine and similar drugs at the receptor level (Jaffe & Martin, 1980). Mixed agonist-antagonist drugs, such as pentazocine (Talwin), nalbuphine, and butorphanol, have analgesic properties but may produce withdrawal symptoms when administered to the narcotic-tolerant patient (Houde, 1979). For this reason, opioids of the mixed agonist-antagonist variety are infrequently used for cancer patients. Other disadvantages are that, with the exception of pentazocine, these drugs are available only in parenteral form and that oral pentazocine is available only in combination with naloxone, aspirin, or acetaminophen. This group of drugs also produces psychotomimetic effects in the patient (visual hallucinations, delusions, vivid daydreams, and feelings of unreality) when larger doses are given (Houde, 1979).

Guiding Principle. The following principles guide the oncology nurse in the use of narcotic analgesics to manage cancer pain (Table 50–7):

Table 50–7. PRINCIPLES TO GUIDE THE ONCOLOGY NURSE IN THE USE OF NARCOTIC ANALGESICS TO MANAGE CANCER PAIN

Select a drug appropriate to the patient's level of pain, previous analgesic history, metabolic state and extent of disease
Know the pharmacology of the selected drug(s):
  (a) Drug class (agonist, agonist-antagonist, antagonist)
  (b) Duration of analgesic effects
  (c) Pharmacokinetic properties of the drug(s)
  (d) Equianalgesic doses for the drug and its route of administration
Know the difference and clinical significance among tolerance, physical dependence, and psychological dependence
Suggest a route or routes of drug administration geared to the patient's needs (i.e., to maximize the analgesic effects and reduce adverse effects)
Administer the analgesic(s) on a regular basis; make sure "rescue" doses are available
Use drug combinations to provide added analgesia (e.g., NSAIDs)
Avoid drug combinations that increase sedation without enhancing analgesia (e.g., most phenothiazines)
Anticipate and treat side effects:
  (a) Respiratory depression (not usually a problem in the tolerant patient)
  (b) Nausea and vomiting
  (c) Sedation
  (d) Constipation
  (e) Urinary retention
  (f) Multifocal myoclonus
Prevent and treat acute withdrawal:
  (a) Taper drugs slowly
  (b) Use diluted doses of naloxone (0.4 mg in 10 ml of saline) to reverse respiratory depression in the tolerant patient
Respect individual differences in pain and response to therapy

1. Select a drug appropriate to the patient's level of pain, previous analgesic history, extent of disease, and metabolic state. For mild to moderate pain not adequately controlled with nonnarcotic drugs alone, an oral narcotic such as codeine, oxycodone, or propoxyphene, is an appropriate choice. For the patient with moderate to severe pain, morphine, hydromorphone, levorphanol, or methadone should be selected. In the metabolically unstable patient, a drug with a short half-life, such as hydromorphone or morphine, is preferable to a drug with a long half-life, such as methadone or levorphanol. Once an analgesic has been selected, the patient should be given an adequate trial of the drug before switching to an alternative agent. An adequate trial means that the dose of the drug should be gradually increased until there is adequate pain relief or limiting side effects. If limiting side effects occur, switching to an alternative drug is appropriate.

2. Know the pharmacology of the selected drug. Pharmacologic information needed includes the type of drug, the onset of effect, the time to peak effect, the duration of effect, the half-life of the drug and relationship to analgesia, and the equianalgesic dose of the drug in relation both to other drugs and to routes of administration.

Identifying the type of drug alerts the nurse to the inappropriate selection of a mixed agonist-antagonist type drug such as pentazocine, in a narcotic AGONIST–dependent patient; this may precipitate withdrawal. Knowledge of the onset, peak, and duration of analgesic effects of the drug in relation to the route of administration enables the nurse to ensure that the

Table 50–8. PLASMA HALF-LIFE FOR NARCOTIC
ANALGESICS

Drug	Plasma Half-Life (hr)
Morphine	2–3.5
Meperidine	3–4
Methadone	15–30
Levorphanol	12–16
Heroin*	0.05
Hydromorphone	2–3
Pentazocine	2–3
Nalbuphine	5
Butorphanol	25–3.5
Codeine	3
Propoxyphene	12

*Biotransformed to acetylmorphine and morphine (Foley & Inturrisi, 1987).

drugs are administered at appropriate time intervals for maximum analgesic effectiveness. Drugs administered by the oral or rectal route usually have a slower onset of action and a longer duration of effect than those administered parenterally. For example, an oral dosing regimen is frequently at 3- to 4-hr time intervals, whereas an intravenous bolus regimen may provide the patient with analgesia only for 1 to 2 hr. Because of this difference in onset of action and peak effect in drugs administered by the parenteral and oral routes, patients may become anxious and pain may be initially less well controlled if a change from parenteral to oral dosing is made abruptly. Instead, half the drug should be administered parenterally and half given (in equianalgesic dose) orally, with both doses being administered at the same time. The parenteral drug is then slowly decreased as the oral dose is increased. A successful switch from the parenteral to oral route of drug administration may take several days to a week and should not be hurried. The nurse becomes the patient's advocate in this respect.

The plasma half-life of a narcotic analgesic has important ramifications for the nurse, especially during the titration phase, or if the patient is elderly or

Table 50–9. ANALGESICS BOTH NARCOTIC AND NONNARCOTIC, COMMONLY USED ORALLY FOR MILD TO MODERATE PAIN

Drug	Equianalgesic Dose* (mg)	Starting Oral Dose Range (mg)	Comments	Precautions
Nonnarcotics				
Aspirin	650	650	Often used in combination with narcotic-type analgesics	Renal dysfunction; avoid during pregnancy, in hemostatic disorders and in combination with steroids
Acetaminophen	650	650	Like aspirin	
Ibuprofen (Motrin)	ND	200–400	Higher analgesic potential than aspirin	Like aspirin
Fenoprofen (Nalfon)	ND	200–400	Like ibuprofen	Like aspirin
Diflunisal (Dolobid)	ND	500–1000	Longer duration of action than ibuprofen; higher analgesic potential than aspirin	Like aspirin
Naproxen (Naprosyn)	ND	250–500	Like diflunisal	Like aspirin
Morphine-like agonists				
Codeine	32–65	32–65	"Weak" morphine; often used in combination with nonnarcotic analgesics; biotransformed, in part to morphine	Impaired ventilation; bronchial asthma; increased intracranial pressure
Oxycodone	5	5–10	Shorter acting; also in combination with nonnarcotic analgesics (Percodan, Percocet) which limits dose escalation	Like codeine
Meperidine (Demerol)	50	50–100	Shorter acting; biotransformed to normeperidine, a toxic metabolite	Normeperidine accumulates with repetitive dosing causing CNS excitation; not for patients with impaired renal function or receiving monoamine oxidase inhibitors
Propoxyphene HCl (Darvon) Propoxyphene napsylate (Darvon-N)	65–130	65–130	"Weak" narcotic; often used in combination with nonnarcotic analgesics; long half-life biotransformed to potentially toxic metabolite (norpropoxyphene)	Propoxyphene and metabolite accumulate with repetitive dosing; overdose complicated by convulsions
Mixed agonist-antagonist				
Pentazocine (Talwin)	50	50–100	In combination with nonnarcotics; in combination with naloxone to discourage parenteral abuse	May cause psychotomimetic effects; may precipitate withdrawal in narcotic-dependent patients

ND, not determined; CNS, central nervous system.
For these equianalgesic doses (see also Comments) the time of peak analgesia ranges from 1.5 to 2 hr and the duration from 4 to 6 hr. Oxycodone and meperidine are shorter-acting (3 to 5 hr) and diflunisal and naproxen are longer-acting (8 to 12 hr).
*These are the recommended starting doses from which the optimal dose for each patient is determined by titration and the maximal dose limited by adverse effects.
(From Foley, K. M., & Inturrisi, C. E. [1987]. Analgesic drug therapy in cancer pain principles and practice. *Medical Clinics of North America, 71*, 210–211. Reproduced by permission.)

Table 50-10. NARCOTIC-TYPE ANALGESICS COMMONLY USED FOR MODERATE TO SEVERE PAIN

Drug	Equianalgesic Intramuscular Dose* (mg)	Intramuscular Oral Potency	Starting Oral Dose Range (mg)	Comments	Precautions
Morphine-like agonists					
Morphine	10	3–6	30–60	Standard of comparison for narcotic type analgesics	Lower doses for aged patients and those with impaired ventilation, bronchial asthma, increased intracranial pressure, liver failure
Hydromorphone (Dilaudid)	1.5	5	4–8	Slightly shorter acting HP intramuscular dosage form for tolerant patients	Like morphine
Methadone (Dolophine)	10	2	10–20	Good oral potency; long plasma half-life	Like morphine; may accumulate with repetitive dosing causing excessive sedation
Levorphanol (Levo-Dromoran)	2	2	2–4	Like methadone	Like methadone
Oxymorphone (Numorphan)	1		See Comments	Not available orally	Like IM morphine
Heroin	5	(6–10)	Not recommended	Slightly shorter acting; biotransformed to active metabolites (e.g., morphine); not available in United States	Like morphine
Meperidine (Demerol)	75	4	Not recommended	Slightly shorter acting; used orally for less severe pain	Normeperidine (toxic metabolite) accumulates with repetitive dosing causing CNS excitation; not for patients with impaired renal function or receiving monoamine oxidase inhibitors†
Codeine	130	1.5	See Comments	Used orally for less severe pain	Like morphine
Mixed agonist-antagonists					
Pentazocine (Talwin)	60	3	See Comments	Used orally for less severe pain; mixed agonist-antagonist; less abuse liability than morphine; included in Schedule IV of Controlled Substances Act	May cause psychotomimetic effects; may precipitate withdrawal in narcotic-dependent patients; not for myocardial infarction†
Nalbuphine (Nubain)	10		See Comments	Not available orally; like intramuscular pentazocine but not scheduled	Incidence of psychotomimetic effects lower than with pentazocine
Butorphanol (Stadol)	2		See Comments	Not available orally; like IM nalbuphine	Like intramuscular pentazocine
Partial Agonists					
Buprenorphine (Buprenex)	0.4		See Comments	Not available orally; sublingual preparation not yet in the United States; less abuse liability than morphine; does not produce psychotomimetic effects	May precipitate withdrawal in narcotic-dependent patients

CNS, central nervous system; HP, high potency.

For these equianalgesic intramuscular doses (see also Comments) the time of peak analgesia in nontolerant patients ranges from ½ to 1 h and the duration from 4 to 6 h. The peak analgesic effect is delayed and the duration prolonged after oral administration.

*These doses are recommended starting in doses from which the optimal dose for each patient is determined by titration and the maximal dose limited by adverse effects.

†Irritating to tissues on repeated administration.

(From Foley, N. M., & Inturrisi, C. E. (1987). Analgesic drug therapy in cancer pain principles and practice. *Medical Clinics of North America, 71,* 210–211. Reproduced by permission.)

experiences metabolic changes (Table 50–8). Side effects may occur as the plasma level rises toward steady state. The full therapeutic effect of a drug cannot be assessed until steady state is reached. This occurs after about four to five half-lives of a drug (conversely, this is also the time it takes for almost complete elimination of a drug from the body after the drug is discontinued). Repeated dosing with a drug of a short half-life, such as morphine or hydromorphone, approaches steady state within 24 hr, whereas a drug with a long half-life, such as methadone, may take 4 to 5 days or longer (Ettinger, Vitale, & Trump, 1979). Because of the concern that side effects may occur days after dosing is begun as plasma levels rise, drugs with a long half-life such as methadone should be administered initially on an "as needed" basis (every 2 to 3 hr). After several days, the patient's 24-hr drug requirement is established and that dose can be divided into equal parts and administered at time intervals of anywhere from 3 to 8 hr, depending on the patient's response. This approach, although controversial, minimizes the risk of accumulation in the plasma and oversedation during the titration period.

One of the most common reasons for undermedication of patients with pain is lack of attention to equianalgesic drug doses when switching from one drug to another or when changing routes of drug administration. For example, when a patient is receiving parenteral morphine sulfate, 10 mg every 4 hr, to control pain and is now able to take oral drugs, three to six times that amount may be required for the patient to receive equivalent analgesic effects. This is the result of first-pass liver metabolism. The nurse must be mindful of each drug's oral-parenteral equianalgesic ratio (Tables 50–9 and 50–10). Because cross-tolerance among narcotics is not complete, when switching from one narcotic to another narcotic the nurse may administer anywhere from one half to one quarter the equianalgesic dose and obtain equivalent pain relief (Coyle, 1987; Foley, 1985a). When methadone is to be the new drug, clinical experience has shown that the equianalgesic dose decrement may be even greater.

3. Administering analgesics on a regular basis is the accepted approach in the management of chronic cancer-related pain. The dosing intervals depend on the time action curve of the drug and are usually every 3 to 4 hr. Patients receiving controlled-release morphine preparations have a dosing interval of from 8 to 12 hr (Lapin, Portenoy, Coyle, Houde, & Foley, 1989). Because episodes of breakthrough or pain are common in the cancer patient (Portenoy & Hagen, in press), "booster" or "rescue" doses must also be made available. These booster doses are allowed at 1- to 2-hr intervals and are equivalent to the 1-hr milligram dose the patient is receiving (e.g., if a patient is receiving 60 mg of analgesic morphine every 4 hr for pain, a rescue dose would be 15 mg every hr or 30 mg every 2 hr). The number of booster doses a patient requires in a 24-hr period is used as a guide to titrate the patient's around-the-clock dosing regimen. Standard exceptions to the around-the-clock dosing regimen for chronic cancer pain patients are during the initial titration period of methadone (Coyle, 1987; Ettinger, Vitale, & Trump, 1979) or when the patient's medical or mental status makes such an approach unwise. The nurse frequently is the person who makes this judgment.

4. Choosing a combined drug approach is based on an understanding of the characteristics of the patient's pain and action of the selected drug(s). Sometimes analgesia is enhanced using this approach, without the need to increase the narcotic dose. Such drug combinations include a narcotic plus a nonnarcotic such as aspirin or acetaminophen (given at the same time). This type of combination may be particularly effective for bone pain. Tricyclic antidepressants, such as amytriptyline, may similarly increase pain relief, particularly when a neuropathic component is present (Foley, 1985c; France & Krishnan, 1988; Portenoy, 1987b; Portenoy, Duma, & Foley, 1986; Price, 1982; Walsh, 1983). This drug is usually given at night in doses much smaller than those used for depression. For cancer patients with a sharp shooting component to the neuropathic pain, the addition of an anticonvulsant such as carbamazepine can be very effective (Foley, 1985c; Molinari, 1979; Portenoy, 1987b; Swerdlow, 1984). Other adjuvant analgesics include antihistamines (Stambaugh & Lane, 1983), the phenothiazine methotrimeprazine (Beaver, Wallenstein, Houde, & Rogers, 1966) (other phenothiazines neither relieve pain nor potentiate opioid analgesia [Foley, 1985a]), and amphetamines (Bruera, Roca, & Cedars, 1985). Steroids can have a dramatic effect in reducing bone or nerve compression pain (Foley, 1981, 1985a; Gilbert, Kim, & Posner, 1978) and may also be introduced into an analgesic regimen when the narcotic has not brought the pain under adequate control. By carefully monitoring the patient's pain relief and side effects of the drug combinations, the nurse ensures appropriate adjustment of these combination regimens.

5. Gearing the route of administration to the patient's needs is critical for the cancer patient (Coyle et al., 1990). During the course of the disease, the patient may develop the need for oral, rectal, subcutaneous, intravenous, epidural, or intrathecal routes of drug administration (Coyle et al., 1990; Scheidler, 1987). There may be episodes of severe pain in which rapid relief is necessary, or nausea and vomiting may occur and a route other than the oral route is required. The patient may have obstruction, be without venous access, and require long-term parenteral pain management in the home. Selection of a particular route depends on patient need, appropriate drug availability, and practicality of the approach. Although the oral route remains the route of choice for the majority of patients, a rapidly evolving technology has facilitated the alternative routes. Selection criteria for the various routes of narcotic administration are outlined in Table 50–11.

Patient-controlled analgesia is becoming increasingly popular in some institutions for the management of postoperative pain, and the acute pain associated with severe stomatitis after bone marrow transplantation has been managed using this technique (Chapman & Hill, 1989). PCA enables patients to administer the drug themselves and titrate the analgesic within preset parameters. Patient-controlled analgesia for chronic cancer pain management is a useful approach for selected patients.

6. The appropriate treatment of adverse effects is essential, because these adverse effects may limit a

Table 50–11. ROUTE OF DRUG ADMINISTRATION

Route	Patient Selection Criteria	Advantages	Disadvantages	Comments
Oral	• Route of choice • Mild to severe pain • Most common reasons for oral route failure: 　1. Amount given not sufficient for severity of pain 　2. Equianalgesic ratios not adhered to when switching from parenteral to oral route 　3. Parenteral to oral change made too quickly 　4. Drug administered at intervals too long for time action curve of the drug	• Most acceptable to patients • Simple • Noninvasive • Longer duration of effect than parenteral route • Tolerance develops less rapidly than with parenteral routes • Controlled-release preparations of morphine available and can be given at 8- to 12-hr intervals • Preparations available in liquid form	• Drug subjected to first-pass liver metabolism • Onset of action slower than parenteral route • Absorption affected by stomach emptying time, presence of food, gastrointestinal mobility	• Patients with diarrhea may not absorb the analgesic and require an alternative route
Sublingual, Buccal, Rectal	• Mild to moderate pain • Unable to tolerate oral route (e.g., nausea, vomiting) • Unable to swallow (e.g., head and neck cancer, esophageal disease)	• Avoids need for repeated injections • Easy to administer • Drug not subject to first-pass liver metabolism • Rectal route, longer duration of effect than oral	• Unpalatable taste (sublingual and buccal) • Limited drugs available for sublingual and buccal routes • Rectal route unacceptable to some patients • Tissue irritation (rectal) • Onset of action similar to oral (rectal)	• Hypodermic, tablets, and oral solutions have been used as sublingual and buccal preparations with varying effect • Narcotics available in suppository form are morphine, hydromorphone (Dilaudid), and oxymorphone (Numorphan) • Suppositories contraindicated in patients with a platelet count of 50 or below
Subcutaneous (intermittent, infusion) and Intramuscular	• Moderate to severe pain • Unable to tolerate the oral route • Obstruction • Malabsorption problem • Postoperative period	• Intravenous access not required • Subcutaneous route can be continuous or intermittent • Onset of action more rapid than oral route • Drug not subject to first-pass liver metabolism • Family can learn administration techniques, both continuous infusion and intermittent injections	• Absorption variable, depending on muscle, fat, and blood supply • Peaks and troughs unless continuous subcutaneous infusion • Duration of action shorter than oral route (intermittent intramuscular-subcutaneous) • Patient may be dependent on others to administer the analgesic on time (intermittent intramuscular-subcutaneous)	• Intermittent injections contraindicated in patients with a platelet count of 50 or below • Meperidine (Demerol) should not be used for continuous subcutaneous infusions as it is a tissue irritant • Continuous subcutaneous infusion is the method of choice in patient with obstruction being cared for at home • A variety of portable pumps are available for continuous subcutaneous infusion use
Intravenous (bolus infusion)	• Severe pain (rapid control needed) • Dying patient with rapidly escalating pain • Postoperative period • Children unable to take oral medications • Alternative routes ineffective	• Bioavailability 100% • Rapid onset of action (10–15 min) • Can be given by bolus or continuous infusion • Variety of access ports available • Milligram dose of drug administered not limited by volume requirement	• Need for intravenous access • Short duration of effect with bolus • Rapid development of tolerance • "Bolus" effect with intermittent injections • Hospital constraints: 　1. Patient on intravenous narcotic infusion must be monitored in an intensive care unit 　2. Nurses not permitted to administer intravenous narcotic bolus	• ⅓ of patients on intravenous infusions do not get adequate pain relief despite titration to unacceptable side effects • Intravenous narcotics do not guarantee adequate pain relief

Table 50–11. ROUTE OF DRUG ADMINISTRATION *Continued*

Route	Patient Selection Criteria	Advantages	Disadvantages	Comments

Epidural (ED) and Intrathecal (IT)	• Not clearly established
	• Pain due to tumor infiltration of bone, nerve or hollow viscus below T6 (midline sacral or perineal pain)
	• Opiate naive, unable to tolerate side effects of narcotics by other routes
	• Elderly patient, unable to tolerate side effects of narcotics by other routes
		• Selective activation of spinal opiate receptors so that analgesia may be achieved with fewer side effects
		• Smaller dose of opioid required than when given by alternative route (e.g., dose for opiate-naive patient: IT morphine = 0.5–1.0 mg; ED morphine = 5–10 mg)
			• Adverse effects similar to those after systemic administration
			• Onset of analgesia occurs later than intravenous route (30–60 min with morphine)
			• Rapid development of tolerance (IT morphine requirement can increase over 4–6 months to 100–150 mg/day; these doses are close to maximum that can be infused at a rate of 2–3 ml/day; solubility of morphine is 60 mg/ml)
			• Respiratory depression occurs both early (after 1–2 hr) and late (after 6–24 hr)
			• Adverse effects include facial pruritus and urinary retention (15%)
				• Epidural opioids are administered by intermittent injections or continuous infusion (the family can be taught to do this)
				• Intrathecal opioids are usually administered via an implanted catheter and subcutaneous reservoir by continuous infusion (an RN or MD will fill this q2–3 weeks)
				• A patient who is tolerant to narcotics by the oral or parenteral route will also be tolerant to narcotics by the IT or ED route
				• To determine the dose for IT morphine:
				  a. Administer via lumbar puncture 1 mg IT for each 10 mg given intramuscularly q4h given systemically
				  b. Titrate slowly for adequate pain relief (assessed as 50% pain relief over 8 hr)
				  c. This dose provides the basis for calculating the initial morphine infusion; clinical experience indicates this should be 2–3 times the bolus dose of morphine delivered over the next 24 hr
				  d. If the initial infusion rate provides inadequate analgesia, the dose can be increased by 50 to 100% (cerebrospinal fluid elimination half-life of morphine is about 2 hr; it takes 8 to 10 hr to reach steady state; therefore, it is important to assess the effect of each infusion rate over at least a 24-hr period before dose escalation)

patient's ability to increase his or her narcotic intake and achieve adequate pain relief. The most common adverse effects include sedation, respiratory depression, nausea and vomiting, urinary retention, constipation, and central nervous system hyperactivity (Foley & Sunderesan, 1985; Kantor, Hopper, & Laska, 1981; Portenoy, 1987a).

Sedation occurs most commonly during the titration period of a drug, especially if the drug has a long half-life, such as methadone or levorphanol. If sedation persists a variety of strategies are available to the nurse: (1) the dose given at one time may be reduced while at the same time shortening the interval between doses; (2) the opiate may be changed to one with a shorter half-life, so that incomplete cross-tolerance allows reduction in drug intake by as much as 50 per cent; (3) an amphetamine may be added to the patient's regimen to counteract the sedative effects of the narcotic. The appearance of sedation in a patient previously stabilized on a narcotic regimen for pain is rarely caused by the narcotic alone. Usually, something has happened to the patient metabolically or other drugs with sedative qualities have been introduced to the patient's regimen—for example, cimetidine, barbiturates, or anxiolytics.

Respiratory depression, the most feared adverse effect of the narcotic drugs, occurs infrequently in cancer patients who have been using these drugs on a long-term basis. The risk is greater if the patient changes metabolically or no longer has pain. Therefore ongoing monitoring by the nurse of the patient receiving long-term narcotic is essential. Respiratory depression occurs most commonly in the nontolerant patient after acute administration of a narcotic and is associated with other signs, such as sedation and mental cloudiness. Usually the patient becomes increasingly difficult to arouse before respiratory depression occurs. If respiratory depression does occur, the use of the narcotic antagonist naloxone has been described. Because naloxone is a short-acting drug, repeated administrations may be required, including the use of an intravenous drip (see pp. 791–792).

Nausea and vomiting result from the action of morphine-like drugs on the medullary chemoreceptor trigger zone. The incidence of nausea and vomiting increases in the ambulatory patient, suggesting a vestibular component. Tolerance develops to these side effects with repeated administration of the drug. Nausea with one narcotic does not mean that the patient will become nauseated on all such drugs. An antiemetic, or an antiemetic histamine such as hydroxyzine (Vistaril), given on a regular basis, is helpful while tolerance is developing. If nausea persists, an alternative narcotic may be used or other sources of nausea sought.

Constipation is an expected effect of the use of narcotic analgesics. It occurs because of the interaction of the narcotic with opiate receptors within the gastrointestinal tract. This results in dry stool and delayed peristalsis. Consequently, any patient started on a narcotic regimen should, at the same time, be started on a bowel regimen. Included in this regimen should be a stool softener, and cathartic; in addition, attention must be paid to diet (Portenoy, 1987a). Unless constipation is managed appropriately, it can become the overriding factor in a patient's life, even greater than pain.

Central nervous system hyperactivity may complicate the long-term use of any of the narcotic analgesics, especially with high repetitive doses. The risk is increased in patients with liver or kidney dysfunction. The patient may develop myoclonus, which, if severe, would warrant switching to an alternative narcotic. The long-term use of meperidine and propoxyphene in high repetitive doses places the patients at risk for seizures. Meperidine is contraindicated in the management of chronic cancer-related pain (Kaiko, Foley, & Brabinski, 1983).

An increase in smooth muscle tone, resulting in increased sphincter tone and urinary retention, may occur with the use of morphine-like drugs. This is frequently a dose-related phenomenon and may necessitate switching to an alternative narcotic at a decreased dose.

7. The development of tolerance has been discussed in detail previously. When adjusting a narcotic analgesic regimen, the nurse must clearly understand the concept of incomplete cross-tolerance.

8. The effect of abruptly stopping narcotic analgesics in a patient who has been using them chronically may be the precipitation of the withdrawal syndrome. A tapering schedule for narcotic analgesics has been outlined previously.

9. Respecting individual differences among patients is paramount if the nurse is to believe the patient's complaint of pain (Box 50–1). Patients react differently to analgesics, and the patient is the one who can judge the effectiveness of an analgesic regimen and then tell the nurse. Using the tools described previously, specific questions need to be asked: Is the amount of drug given at one time adequate for satisfactory pain relief? (If not, increase the dose by 50 per cent.) Does the amount of drug administered to the patient at one time give satisfactory pain relief, but the pain comes back before the next dose is due? (If so, decrease the time interval between doses.) Are the side effects of the drug unacceptable to the patient? (If so, treat the side effects appropriately, or switch to an alternative analgesic or route of drug administration.)

If the patient is on an around-the-clock dosing regimen and is experiencing inadequate pain relief, it is important to make sure that the patient is actually receiving the drugs prescribed at the time intervals prescribed before changing the regimen. Personally checking the patient's medication card (for inpatients) or reviewing in detail how the outpatient is actually taking the drugs is essential. After this review, appropriate adjustments in the patient's regimen can be made.

10. The use of placebos to assess whether pain is "real" has no place in the management of cancer-related pain. The placebo response is a powerful clinical tool built on trust between the patient, nurse, and doctor. Misuse of such a positive and powerful patient response can have a devastating effect on the nurse-patient relationship and disrupt subsequent efforts at pain control.

Adjuvant Analgesics

Adjuvant analgesics are a third group of drugs used to treat patients with pain. This group includes several different categories of drugs including tricyclic antidepressants, anticonvulsants, phenothiazides, and corticosteroids. These drugs produce analgesia in certain painful states by mechanisms not directly related to the opiate receptor system.

Tricyclic antidepressants (e.g., amitriptyline, imipramine, desipramine) are frequently used to treat pain with a neuropathic component (Portenoy, 1987b; Portenoy, Duma, & Foley, 1986). This pain is often described by patients as having a dysesthetic burning

---

Box 50–1. INTEGRATING NURSING RESEARCH WITH CLINICAL PRACTICE

STUDY

Coyle, N., Adelhardt, J., Foley, K. M., & Portenoy, R. K. (1990). **The character of terminal illness in the advanced cancer patient: Pain and other symptoms during the last four weeks of life.** *Journal of Pain and Symptom Management.* 5, 88–93.

SAMPLE

Ninety consecutive patients who had been followed through the Supportive Care Program of the Pain Service, Memorial Sloan-Kettering Cancer Center, during their last 4 weeks of life.

METHOD

A retrospective chart review was carried out. Complaints of pain and other symptoms were tabulated from these records at time intervals of 4 weeks, 3 weeks, 2 weeks, and 1 week before death. Patterns of opioid use and routes of drug administration were examined at the same times and 24 hr prior to death. Suicidal ideation and requests for euthanasia at any point during the patients' course were also recorded.

FINDINGS

Tremendous variability was seen in the patients' opioid requirements during the last 4 weeks of life, ranging from 7 to 35,164 mg morphine equivalents intra in 24 hrs. Fifty-three patients (59 per cent) required more than one route of drug administration during this period. Four weeks before death, 64 patients (71 per cent) described three or more symptoms distressing enough to interfere with activity. Fatigue, weakness, sedation, and cognitive impairment were the most prevalent symptoms. Eighteen patients (20 per cent) acknowledged suicidal ideation, whereas an additional four patients had a specific plan for suicide. Four patients requested euthanasia, each in response to a symptom that was not well controlled.

SIGNIFICANCE

The persistence of symptoms and the fluctuations in both their severity and impact on the patient and family mandate continuity of care with ongoing monitoring, adjustment of treatments, and family support.

---

quality and may be associated with surgical trauma, radiation therapy, chemotherapy, and infiltration of the nerve by tumor. The mechanism of action of the tricyclic antidepressants is believed to involve enhancement of the descending pain modulation system by blocking the reuptake of serotonin and norepinephrine.

Anticonvulsants (phenytoin, carbamazepine, sodium valproate, clonazepam) are useful in treating paroxysmal lancinating pain arising from peripheral nerve damage (Portenoy, 1987b; Swerdlow, 1984). This pain is frequently described by patients as having a sharp, shooting component. Examples are postherpetic neuralgia or glossopharyngeal neuralgia. The mechanism of action is believed to be suppression of spontaneous neuronal firing.

Phenothiazides, with the exception of methotrimeprazine, do not relieve pain or enhance opioid analgesia. Methotrimeprazine may be useful in the management of the patient who is highly tolerant to opioids or experiences dose-limiting side effects. It lacks both the respiratory depressant and constipating effects of the opioids. The drug also has anxiolytic and antiemetic properties (American Pain Society, 1989; Beaver et al., 1966). This drug, however, is only available in

parenteral form and has significant orthostatic and sedative side effects.

Corticosteroids have specific and nonspecific effects in the management of acute and chronic cancer pain (American Pain Society, 1989; Foley, 1985a; Posner, 1987). They may directly lyse some tumors (e.g., lymphoma) and ameliorate painful nerve or spinal cord compression by reducing edema in tumor and nervous tissue.

As previously noted, it is common for patients with cancer to have a variety of pains with differing etiologies. Management may therefore comprise a combination of opioid drugs, nonsteroidal antiinflammatory drugs, and adjuvant drugs. Ongoing monitoring for the desired effects and adverse effects is an important nursing function, especially in these often very ill cancer patients whose metabolic state may be changing frequently.

ANESTHETIC APPROACHES

Anesthetic approaches are most useful in treating patients with well-defined localized pain (Cousins &

Bridenbough, 1988; Ferrar-Brechner, 1989; Swerdlow, 1987). Short-acting and long-acting anesthetics are used for temporary and diagnostic nerve blocks, whereas phenol, alcohol, and freezing cryoprobe are the common neurolytic approaches for permanent blocks. The limitation of these procedures is that each peripheral nerve subserves sensory function over multiple levels, requiring multiple nerves to be blocked for adequate pain control. The use of an autonomic nerve block, such as the celiac plexus block, to manage midabdominal pain associated with cancer of the pancreas can be very successful and is often considered the procedure of choice for such patients (Leung, Bowen-Wright, & Aveling, 1983).

Epidural and intrathecal nerve blocks with neurolytic agents can produce motor weakness and autonomic dysfunction. However, intermittent or continuous epidural infusions of local anesthetics have been used for management of severe pain associated with lumbosacral plexus or sacral lesions without interruption of motor or autonomic function. Sometimes this approach is used to give the patient a "drug holiday," allowing a temporary reduction in the amount of systemic opioids the patient requires, while still maintaining adequate pain control. It is imperative the nurse recognize the differences in site of action, effect, and adverse effects of intrathecal and epidural opioids and epidural local anesthetics. These are outlined in Table 50–12.

Two anesthetic approaches used to manage the patient with diffuse pain are a chemical hypophysectomy and intermittent inhalation therapy of nitrous oxide. Chemical hypophysectomy, which involves the injection of alcohol into the sella turcica under radiologic guidance, is used to control pain in patients with widespread metastatic disease (Levin & Ramirez, 1984). The result in some patients can be dramatic. Nitrous oxide is most useful in managing acute incident pain, especially in the patient with advanced cancer who is comfortable at rest but not on movement (Fosburg & Crone, 1983). It is also a useful tool for managing procedure-related pain.

Trigger point injections may be useful for almost 15 per cent of cancer-related pains reported to be musculoskeletal in origin (Travel & Simons, 1983; Twycross & Lack, 1983). A focal injection of saline solution or local anesthetic is made into a painful muscle, often providing dramatic relief. When relief is temporary, further blocks may relieve pain for longer periods of time.

NEUROSURGICAL PROCEDURES

Cordotomy and the placement of epidural and intrathecal or intraventricular catheters are the most common neurosurgical procedures for pain relief (Sunderesan, DiGiacinto, & Hughes, 1988). A cordotomy involves the interruption of the anterolateral spinothalamic tract in the cervical or thoracic region. It may be performed by an open surgical approach or by a percutaneous stereotactic procedure. This technique is most useful in managing unilateral pain below the waist. Initial complications in a small percentage of patients include paresis, ataxia, and urinary dysfunction. Although initial pain relief from cordotomy occurs in 70 to 90 per cent of patients, this levels to 80 per cent in 3 months, and at the end of 1 year, about 40 per cent of patients report a return of pain (Levin & Ramirez, 1984; Sunderesan et al., 1988). After both open or percutaneous cordotomy, pain may be "unmasked" on the opposite side of the body. Other pains throughout the body may also become unmasked, leaving the patient as dysfunctional as before. Informed consent means the patient and family are made aware of the potential for these various occurences; otherwise high unfulfilled expectations of total and permanent pain relief may trigger a major depression (Coyle et al., in press).

A phenomenon that is beginning to be recognized clinically is the depression that occurs in patients who receive complete pain relief after a neuroablative procedure, such as a cordotomy. Pain has left abruptly, and suddenly the implication of having advanced disease is the overwhelming force (Coyle et al., in press). The oncology nurse plays a major role in working with these patients and families both before and after such procedures.

NEUROAUGMENTATIVE APPROACHES

Neuroaugmentative techniques include counterirritation (for example, systematic rubbing of a painful part, or applying alternating heat and cold), transcutaneous nerve stimulation, acupuncture, dorsal column stimulation, and deep brain stimulation. Such approaches are thought to provide pain relief by activating endogenous pain-modulating systems (Albe-Fessard, Condes-Lara, & Sanderson, 1984). The most commonly used neuroaugmentative approaches for cancer patients are counterirritation and transcutaneous nerve stimulation. These approaches are most effective for nerve injury pain (including deafferentation pain and postherpetic neuralgia). Frequently they are used in combination with other pain management techniques.

BEHAVIORAL APPROACHES

Behavioral interventions are particularly helpful to the patient in developing a sense of mastery over incident pain and procedure-related pain. A sense of uncertainty and loss of control can overwhelm a patient, increasing the suffering and level of pain. This model suggests that pain and suffering, although tightly intermeshed, are not the same phenomenon, and that both need to be targeted to manage a patient's "total" pain (Ahles et al., 1983; Coyle, 1989a; Coyle et al., in press; Fishman & Loscalzo, 1987; McGuire, 1987).

The assessment phase, as in the general pain assessment, is the first step in these therapeutic interventions. During the process of discussion with the nurse, the

Table 50–12. SPINAL OPIOID ANALGESIA AND EPIDURAL LOCAL ANESTHETICS: DIFFERENCES IN SITE OF ACTION, EFFECTS, AND ADVERSE EFFECTS

	Selection Criteria	Patient Contraindications	Target Site	Mechanism of Action	Desired Effect	Adverse Effects
Epidural Local Anesthetics	• Regional analgesia for patients with intractable pain or unacceptable side effects from opioids • Regional analgesia for patients tolerant to spinal opioid drugs; local anesthetics used for 1–2 weeks to give opioid "drug holiday" • Regional analgesia selected as approach of choice for pain management	• Local infection • Coagulation disorders • Low platelet count	• Nerve rootlets bathed in cerebrospinal fluid, and paravertebral nerves	• Blockade of sodium channels in peripheral nerve subserving pain transmission (high concentrations produce motor, sensory, and autonomic or blockade)	• Analgesia with minimal to no clinical effect on other sensory, autonomic, or motor functions (lidocaine acts in 5–10 min and lasts for 1–2 hr; bupivacaine acts in 10–20 min and lasts for 4–8 hr)	*Adverse Effects not Reversed by Naloxone:* • Vascular uptake may cause central nervous system and cardiac toxicity *Signs:* lightheadedness, perioral numbness, tinnitus, followed by twitching, convulsions, respiratory depression, coma and shock *Nursing Precautions:* Because toxicity usually occurs from inadvertent intravascular injection, aspirate catheter before each injection; know early signs, and stop the injection if they occur • Motor blockade leading to weakness • Complete sensory blockade leading to loss of function • Inhibition of sympathetic outflow leading to hypotension *Nursing Precautions:* Because dehydration predisposes to this, patients usually have an intravenous line running; monitor the blood pressure and keep the patient in bed for 20–30 min after the injection • A high cervical block can cause respiratory depression • Tachyphylaxis (less of effect to a given dose of local anesthetics) can occur over several days

Table continued on following page

Table 50–12. SPINAL OPIOID ANALGESIA AND EPIDURAL LOCAL ANESTHETICS: DIFFERENCES IN SITE OF ACTION, EFFECTS, AND ADVERSE EFFECTS *Continued*

	Selection Criteria	Patient Contraindications	Target Site	Mechanism of Action	Desired Effect	Adverse Effects
Spinal Opioids	• Pain below the midthoracic level; usually midline sacral and perineal pain • Postoperative pain, epidural opioids selected as approach of choice (abdominal or thoracic surgery)	• Local infection • Coagulation disorders • Low platelet count	• Dorsal horn of the spinal cord	• Activation of opioid receptors in dorsal horn • Rostral redistribution and activation of supraspinal opioid sites • Systemic uptake and distribution of drug through vasculature • Lipid solubility largely determines drug distribution in cerebrospinal fluid (e.g., slow tissue uptake of hydrophilic morphine leads to large rostral redistribution)	• Analgesia without significant motor, sensory, or autonomic effects	*Adverse Effects Reversed by Naloxone:* • Increased adverse effects in nontolerant patients (e.g., postoperatively), large dose, high catheter placement, sudden Valsalva • Acute (1–3 hr) and delayed (8–24 hr) respiratory depression • Nausea, vomiting • Urinary retention (15%) • Pruritus

patient gradually develops an awareness of the multidimensional nature of the pain and suffering. Through keeping a pain diary or by noting the fluctuating levels of the pain, the patient begins to recognize the relationship of stress and anxiety to increased pain. In the next step, the patient learns self-monitoring, so that signs of stress are recognized. During this phase, patients pay attention to their "internal dialogue" and learn to recognize dysfunctional statements in relation to pain, such as "this pain is killing me, it will never go away, and there is nothing I can do about it." Instead the patient learns to say, "the pain is terrible, it has been terrible in the past and got better, it will get better this time, this is what I must do...." In other words, the patient has moved from a noncoping to a coping statement. Frequently patients believe that the presence of pain implies danger of immediate harm and become emotionally aroused by that perception. Although this arousal is useful in the presence of acute pain, it serves no useful purpose in the presence of chronic cancer-related pain. The behavioral techniques most helpful to this group of patients are focused breathing, muscle relaxation, and guided imagery (Adler & Hemmeler, 1984; Fishman & Loscalzo, 1987).

CONTINUITY OF CARE AND SUPPORTIVE CARE

Patients with cancer pain are an extremely vulnerable group. Symptoms may change rapidly and require immediate intervention to prevent further escalation. In a system in which multiple physicians and other health care workers are involved with the patient and family, fragmentation of care and confusion over responsibility for a particular symptom is common. This problem is exacerbated when the patient's care involves both the community and the hospital setting (Coyle, 1989a).

Continuity of care and supportive care with a multidisciplinary team approach is increasingly being recognized as an integral part of the care of a patient with chronic pain and cancer. A variety of models of continuing care have been developed. Such models include (1) hospice, which may consist of home care with brief periods of hospitalization for symptoms poorly controlled at home or institutional care away from the hospital environment; (2) palliative care service within a general hospital, in which the resources of the hospital are readily available to the patient, family, and community; (3) the use of a mobile van unit directed by the staff of a general hospital, in which frequent team visits are used to provide care for extremely ill and dying patients at home; and (4) a supportive care model, which can be developed as part of a pain service within a comprehensive cancer center and which attempts to integrate family and community resources to provide the patient with continuity of care from home to hospital.

In few areas has the emerging role of the clinical nurse specialist had a greater impact on patient care than in pain management and supportive care (Coyle, 1989a, 1989b; Coyle & Portenoy, 1990). These are areas of fundamental concern to the quality of life of patients with cancer. Nursing advances over the past decade in both clinical practice and research provide hope for the future.

References

An NIH Consensus Development Conference (1981). The integrated approach to the management of pain. *Journal of Pain and Symptom Management, 2,* 35–41.

Adler, R. H., & Hemmeler, W. (1984). Psychological treatment modalities for pain in cancer patients. *Recent Results of Cancer Research, 89*, 195–200.

Ahles, T. A. (1987). Psychological techniques for the management of cancer-related pain. In D. B. McGuire & C. H. Yarbro (Eds.), *Cancer pain management* (pp. 245–588). Orlando, Fl: Grune & Stratton, Inc.

Ahles, T. A., Blanchard, E. B., & Ruchdeschel, J. C. (1983). The multidimensional nature of cancer-related pain. *Pain, 17*, 277–288.

Aitken-Swan, J. (1959). Nursing of the late cancer patient at home: The family's impressions. *Practitioner, 183*, 64–69.

Albe-Fessard, D., Condes-Lara, M., & Sanderson P. (1984). Neural mechanisms of pain: Tentative explanation of the special role played by the areas of paleospinothalamic projection in patients with deafferentation pain syndromes. In L. Kruger & J. C. Liebeskind (Eds.), *Advances in pain research and therapy* (vol. 1, pp. 167–182). New York: Raven Press.

American Pain Society. (1989). *Principles of analgesic use in the treatment of acute pain and chronic cancer pain: A concise guide to medical practice* (2nd ed.). Skokie, IL: Author.

Angell, M. (1982). The quality of mercy. *New England Journal of Medicine, 306*, 98–99.

Arner, S. (1982). The role of nerve blocks in the treatment of cancer pain. *Acta Anaesthesiologica Scandinavica, 74*, 104–108.

Beaver, W. T., Wallenstein, S. M., Houde, R. W., & Rogers, A. (1966). A comparison of the analgesic effects of methotrimeprazine and morphine in patients with cancer. *Clinical Pharmacology and Therapeutics 7*, 436–446.

Beecher, H. K. (1956). Relationship of significance of wound to the pain experienced. *Journal of the American Medical Association, 161*, 1609–1613.

Bond, M. R., & Pilowsky I. (1966). Subjective assessment of pain and its relationship to the administration of analgesics in patients with advanced cancer. *Journal of Psychosomatic Research, 10*, 203–208.

Bonica, J. J. (1984). Management of cancer pain. *Recent Results in Cancer Research, 89*, 13–27.

Bonica, J. J. (1985). Treatment of cancer pain: Current status and future needs. In H. L. Fields, R. Dubner, & F. Cervero (Eds.), *Advances in pain research and therapy* (vol. 2, pp. 589–599). New York: Raven Press.

Brodie, G. N. (1974). Indomethacin and bone pain. *Lancet, 1,* 1160.

Bruera, E., Carrara S., & Roca, E. (1986). Double-blind evaluation of the effects of mazindol on pain, depression, anxiety, appetite, and activity in terminally ill cancer patients. *Cancer Treatment Reports, 70*, 295–298.

Bruera, E., Roca, E., & Cedaro, L. (1985). Action of methylprednisolone in terminal cancer patients: A prospective randomized double-blind study. *Cancer Treatment Reports, 69*, 751–754.

Carson, B. S. (1987). Neurologic and neurosurgical approaches to cancer pain. In D. B. McGuire & C. H. Yarbro (Eds.), *Cancer pain management* (pp. 223–243). Orlando, Fl: Grune & Stratton, Inc.

Cartwright, A., Hockey, L., & Anderson, A. B. M. (1973). *Life before death.* London: Routledge and Kegan Paul.

Cascino, T. L., Kori, S. H., & Krol, G. (1985). CT scanning of the brachial plexus in patients with cancer. *Neurology, 35*, 8–14.

Catalano, R. B. (1987). Pharmacologic management and treatment of cancer pain. In D. B. McGuire & C. H. Yarbro (Eds.), *Cancer pain management* (pp. 151–201). Orlando, Fl: Grune & Stratton, Inc.

Chapman, C. R., & Hill, H. F. (1989). Prolonged morphine administration and addiction liability: Evaluation of 2 theories in a bone marrow transplantation unit. *Cancer, 63*, 1636–1655.

Charap, A. D. (1987). The knowledge, attitudes and experience of medical personnel treating pain in the terminally ill. *Mt. Sinai Journal of Medicine, 45*, 561–580.

Cleeland, C. S. (1984). The impact of pain on the patient with cancer. *Cancer, 54*, 2635–2641.

Cleeland, C. S., Rotondi, A., & Brechner, T. (1986). A model for the treatment of cancer pain. *Journal of Pain and Symptom Management, 1*, 209–216.

Cohen, A., Thomas, G. B., & Coen, E. E. (1978). Serum concentration, safety and tolerance of oral doses of choline magnesium trisalicylate. *Current Therapy Research, 23*, 358–364.

Cousins, M. J., & Bridenbough, P. O. (1988). *Neural blockade* (2nd ed.) Philadelphia: J. B. Lippincott Co.

Coyle, N. (1987). Analgesics and pain: Current concepts. *Nursing Clinics of North America, 22*, 727–741.

Coyle, N. (1989a). Continuity of care for the cancer patient in pain. *Cancer, 63*, 2289–2293.

Coyle, N. (1989b). The role of the nurse in pain management. In K. M. Foley & R. Payne (Eds.), *Current therapy of pain* (pp. 63–69). Toronto: B. C. Decker.

Coyle, N., Adelhardt, J., & Foley, K. M. (1988). Disease progression and tolerance in the cancer pain patient. *Journal of Pain and Symptom Management, 3*, Abstract No. 58.

Coyle, N., Adelhardt, J., Foley, K. M., & Portenoy, R. K. (1990). Character of terminal illness in the advanced cancer patient: Pain and other symptoms in the last 4 weeks of life. *Journal of Pain and Symptom Management, 5*, 83–93.

Coyle, N., & Foley, K. M. (1987). Prevalence and profile of pain syndromes in cancer patients. In D. B. McGuire & C. H. Yarbro (Eds.), *Cancer pain management* (pp. 21–46). Orlando, Fl: Grune & Stratton, Inc.

Coyle, N., & Portenoy, R. K. (1990). Advances in cancer pain management. In P. Ashwanden, A. Belcher, A. Hubbard, R. Moskewitz, & N. Riese (Eds.), *Oncology nursing: Advances in treatment and trends into the twenty-first century.*

Daut, R. L., & Cleeland, C. S. (1982). The prevalence and severity of pain in cancer. *Cancer, 50*, 1913–1918.

Daut, R. L., Cleeland, C. S., & Flannery R. C. (1983). Development of the Wisconsin Brief Pain Questionnaire to assess pain in cancer and other diseases. *Pain, 17*, 197–210.

Donovan, M. I. (1987). Clinical assessment of cancer pain. In D. B. McGuire & C. H. Yarbro (Eds.), *Cancer pain management* (pp. 105–131). Orlando, Fl: Grune & Stratton, Inc.

Donovan, M. I., Dillon, P., & McGuire, L. (1987). Incidence and characteristics of pain in a sample of medical-surgical inpatients. *Pain, 30*, 69–78.

Ettinger, D. S., Vitale, P. J., & Trump, D. L. (1979). Important clinical pharmacologic considerations in the use of methadone in cancer patients. *Cancer Treatment Reports, 63*, 457–459.

Ferreira, S. H., Nakamura, M., & Castro, M. S. A. (1978). The hyperanalgesic effects of prostacylin and prostagladin E2. *Prostaglandins, 16*, 31–37.

Ferrell, B. L., Wisdom, C., & Wenzl, C. (1989). Quality of life as an outcome variable in the management of cancer pain. *Cancer, 60*, 2321–2327.

Ferrer-Brechner, T. (1989). Anesthetic techniques for the management of cancer pain. *Cancer, 63*, 2343–2347.

Fishman, B., & Loscalzo, M. (1987). Cognitive behavioral intervention in management of cancer pain: Principles and applications. *Medical Clinics of North America, 71*, 271–287.

Fishman, B., Pasternak, S., Wallenstein, S. L., Houde, R. W., Holland, J., & Foley, K. M. (1987). The Memorial Pain Assessment Card: A valid instrument for the assessment of cancer pain. *Cancer, 60*, 1151–1157.

Foley, K. M. (1979). Pain syndromes in patients with cancer. In J. J. Bonica & V. Ventafridda (Eds.), *Advances in pain research and therapy* (vol. 2, pp. 59–75). New York: Raven Press.

Foley, K. M. (1981). Analgesic management of bone pain. In L. Weiss & H. A. Gilbert (Eds.), *Bone metastasis* (pp. 348–368). Boston: G. K. Hall.

Foley, K. M. (1985a). The treatment of cancer pain. *New England Journal of Medicine, 313*, 84–95.

Foley, K. M. (1985b). Control of pain in cancer. In P. Calabresi, P. Schein, & S. Rosenberg (Eds.), *Medical oncology: Basic principles and clinical management of cancer* (p. 1393). New York: Macmillan.

Foley, K. M. (1985c). Adjuvant analgesic drugs in cancer pain management. In G. M. Aronoff (Ed.), *Evaluation and treatment of chronic pain.* (pp. 425–434). Baltimore: Urban and Schwarzenberg.

Foley, K. M. (1987). Pain syndromes in patients with cancer. *Medical Clinic of North America, 71*, 169–184.

Foley, K. M., & Inturrisi, C. E. (1987). Analgesic drug therapy in cancer pain: Principles and practice. *Medical Clinics of North America, 71*, 207–232.

Foley, K. M. (1988). Controversies in cancer pain management. *Cancer, 63*, 2257–2265.

Foley, K. M. (1989). The decriminalization of cancer pain. In S. Hill (ed.), *Advances in pain research and therapy: The management of pain in a drug oriented society* (pp. 5–18). New York: Raven Press.

Foley, K. M., & Sundaresan, N. (1985). Management of cancer pain. In V. T. DeVita, Jr., S. Hellman, & S. A. Rosenberg (Eds.), *Cancer: Principles and practice of oncology* (vol. 2, 2nd ed., p. 1941). Philadelphia: J. B. Lippincott Co.

Foley, K. M., Woodruff, J., & Ellis, F. (1979). Radiation-induced malignant and atypical schwannomas. *Annals of Neurology, 7,* 311–318.

Fosburg, M. T., & Crone, R. K. (1983). Nitrous oxide analgesia for refractory pain in the terminally ill. *Journal of the American Medical Association, 250,* 511–513.

France, R. D., & Krishnan, K. R. R. (1988). Psychotrophic drugs in chronic pain. In R. D. France & K. R. R. Krishnan (Eds.), *Chronic pain* (pp. 323–374). Washington, DC: American Psychiatric Press.

Gilbert, R. W., Kim, J. H., & Posner, J. B. (1978). Epidural spinal cord compression from metastatic tumor: diagnosis and treatment. *Annals of Neurology, 5,* 40–51.

Granek, I., Ashikari, R., & Foley, K. M. (1984). The post-mastectomy pain syndrome. *Procedure of the American Society of Clinical Oncology, 3,* 122.

Greenberg, J. S., Deck M. D. F., & Vikram, B. (1981). Metastases to the base of the skull: Clinical findings in 43 patients. *Neurology, 31,* 350–357.

Haram, B. J. (1978). *Facts and Figures in the Management of Terminal Disease* (pp. 12–18). London: Edward Arnold Press.

Houde, R. W. (1979). Analgesic effectiveness of the narcotic agonist-antagonists. *British Journal of Clinical Pharmacology, 7,* 297S–308S.

Ihde, D. C., & DeVita, V. (1975). Osteonecrosis of the femoral head in patients with lymphoma treated with intermittent combination chemotherapy (including corticosteroids). *Cancer, 36,* 1585–1588.

Jackel, K. A., Young, D. F., & Foley, K. M. (1985). The natural history of lumbosacral plexopathy in cancer. *Neurology, 35,* 8–15.

Jaffe, J. H. (1980). Drug addiction and drug abuse. In L. S. Goodman & S. Gilman (Eds.), *The pharmacolgic basis of therapeutics* (6th ed., pp. 535–584). New York: Macmillan.

Jaffe, J. H., & Martin, W. R. (1980). Opioid analgesics and antagonists. In L. S. Goodman & S. Gilman (Eds.), *The pharmacologic basis of therapeutics* (6th ed., pp. 494–534). New York: Macmillan.

Jellinger, K., & Sturm, K. W. (1971). Delayed radiation myelopathy in man. *Journal of Neurological Sciences, 14,* 389–408.

Kaiko, R. F., Foley, K. M., & Brabinski, P. Y. (1983). Central nervous system excitory effects of meperidine in cancer patients. *Annals of Neurology, 13,* 180–185.

Kanner, R. M., Martini, N., & Foley, K. M. (1981). Epidural spinal cord compression in pancoast syndrome (superior pulmonary sulcus tumor): Clinical presentation and outcome. *Annals of Neurology, 10,* 77.

Kanner, R. M., Martini, N., & Foley, K. M. (1982a). Incidence of pain and other clinical manifestations of superior pulmonary sulcus (Pancoast tumors). In J. J. Bonica & V. Ventafridda (Eds.), *Advances in pain research and therapy* (pp. 27–38). New York: Raven Press.

Kanner, R. M., Martini, N., & Foley, K. M. (1982b). Nature and incidence of post-thoracotomy pain. *Proceedings of the American Society of Clinical Oncology, 1,* 52.

Kantor, T. G. (1982). The control of pain by nonsteroidal anti-inflammatory drugs. *Medical Clinics of North America, 66,* 1053–1059.

Kantor, T. G., Hopper, M., & Laska, E. (1981). Adverse effects of commonly ordered oral narcotics. *Journal of Clinical Pharmacology, 21,* 1.

Kori, S., Foley, K. M., & Posner, J. B. (1981). Brachial plexus lesions in patients with cancer: Clinical findings in 100 cases. *Neurology, 31,* 45–50.

Lapin, J., Portenoy, R. K., Coyle, N., Houde, R. W., & Foley, K. M. (1989). Guidelines for use of controlled-release oral morphine. *Cancer Nursing, 12,* 202–208

Leek, B. F. (1972). Abdominal visceral receptors. In E. Neil (Ed.), *Handbook of sensory physiology* (vol. 3, pp. 113–160). Berlin: Springer-Verlag.

LeQuesne, P. M. (1984). Neuropathy due to drugs. In P. J. Dyck, P. K. Thomas, & E. H. Lambert (Eds.), *Peripheral neuropathy* (Vol. 2, 2nd ed., pp. 2126–2179). Philadelphia: W. B. Saunders Co.

Leung, J. W., Bowen-Wright, M., & Aveling, W. (1983). Celiac plexus block for pain in pancreatic cancer and chronic pancreatitis. *British Journal of Surgery, 70,* 730–732.

Levin, A. B., & Ramirez, L. L. (1984). Treatment of cancer pain with hypophysectomy: Surgical and chemical. In C. Bebedetti, C. R. Chapman, & G. Moricca (Eds.), *Advances in pain research and therapy* (vol. 7, pp. 631–647). New York: Raven Press.

Levin, D. N., Cleeland, C. S., & Dar, R. (1985). Public attitudes towards cancer pain. *Cancer, 56,* 2337–2339.

Macaluso, C., Weinberg, D., & Foley, K. M. (1988). Opioid abuse and misuse in a cancer pain population. *Journal of Pain and Symptom Management, 3,* Abstract No. S24.

Marks, R. M., & Sachar, E. J. (1973). Undertreatment of medical inpatients with narcotic analgesics. *Annals of Internal Medicine, 78,* 173–181.

McGuire, D. B. (1984a). Assessment of chronic pain in cancer inpatients using the McGill Pain Questionnaire. *Oncology Nursing Forum, 11,* 32–37.

McGuire, D. B. (1984b). Selecting an instrument to measure cancer-related pain. *Oncology Nursing Forum, 11,* 85–87.

McGuire, D. B. (1987). The multidimensional phenomenon of cancer pain. In D. B. McGuire & C. H. Yarbro (Eds.), *Cancer pain management* (pp. 1–20). Orlando, Fl: Grune & Stratton, Inc.

Meinhardt, N. T., & McCaffery, M. (1983) *Pain: A nursing approach to assessment and analysis.* Norwalk, CT: Appleton-Century-Crofts.

Melzack, R. (1975). The McGill Pain Questionnaire: Major properties and scoring methods. *Pain, 1,* 277–299.

Melzack, R., Ofiesh, J. B., & Mount, B. M. (1982). The Bromptom's mixture: Effects on pain in cancer patients. In A. Ajemian & B. M. Mount (Eds.), *The R. V. H. manual of palliative care* (pp. 167–171). Salem, NH: Ayer Company.

Merskey, H. (1986). Classification of chronic pain: Description of chronic pain syndromes and definitions of pain terms. *Pain, 3*(Suppl.), S1–S225. Abstract No. s217.

Molinari, R. (1979). Therapy of cancer pain in the head and neck. In J. J. Bonica & V. Ventafridd (Eds.), *Advances in pain research and therapy* (vol. 2, pp. 131–138). New York: Raven Press.

Morris, J. N., Mor, V., Goldberg, R. J., Sherwood, S., Greer, D. S., & Hiris J. (1986). The effect of treatment setting and patient characteristics on pain in terminal cancer patients: A report from the National Hospice Study. *Journal of Chronic Diseases, 39,* 27–35.

Mundy, G. R., & Spiro, T. P. (1981). The mechanism of bone metastasis and bone destruction by tumor cells. In L. Weiss & H. A. Gilbert (Eds.), *Bone metastasis* (p. 65). Boston: G. K. Hall.

Norton, W. S., & Lack, S. A. (1980). Control of symptoms other than pain. In R. G. Twycross & V. Ventafridda (Eds.), *The continuing care of patients with terminal cancer* (pp. 167–178). Oxford: Pergamon Press.

Olson, M. E., Chernik, N. L., & Posner, J. B. (1978). Infiltration of the leptomeninges by systemic cancer: A clinical and pathological study. *Archives of Neurology, 30,* 122–137.

Pagni, C. A. (1984). Role of neurosurgery in cancer pain: Reevaluation of old methods and new trends. In C. Benedetti, C. R. Chapman, & G. Moricca (Eds.), *Advances in pain research and therapy* (vol. 7, pp. 631–647). New York: Raven Press.

Palmer, J. J. (1972). Radiation myelopathy. *Brain, 95,* 109–122.

Pannuti, E., Rossi, A. P., & Marroro, D. (1980). Natural history of cancer pain, in continuing care of terminal patients. In *Proceeding of the International Seminars of Continuing Care of Terminal Cancer Patients* (pp. 75–89). New York: Pergamon Press.

Parks, C. M. (1978). Home or hospital? Terminal care as seen by the surving spouse. *Journal of the Royal College of General Practitioners, 28,* 19–30.

Payne, R. (1987). Anatomy, physiology and neuropharmacolgy of cancer pain. *Medical Clinics of North America, 71,* 153–155.

Portenoy, R. K. (1987a). Constipation in the cancer patient: Causes and management. *Medical Clinics of North America, 71,* 303–311.

Portenoy, R. K. (1987b). Drug treatment of pain syndromes. *Seminars in Neurology, 7,* 139–149.

Portenoy, R. K. (1987c). Cancer pain: Epidemiology and syndromes. *Cancer, 63,* 2298–2307.

Portenoy, R. K., Duma, C., & Foley, K. M. (1986). Acute herpetic and postherpetic neuralgia: Clinical features and current management. *Annals of Neurology, 20,* 651–664.

Portenoy, R. K., & Hagen, N. A. (in press). Breakthrough pain: Definition and management. Pain.

Porter, J., & Jick, H. (1980). Addiction rate in patients treated with narcotics [letter]. *New England Journal of Medicine, 302,* 123.

Posner, J. B. (1987). Back pain and epidural spinal cord compression. *Medical Clinics of North America, 71,* 185–205.

Price, R. W. (1982). Herpes zoster: An approach to systemic therapy. *Medical Clinics of North America, 66,* 1105–1118.

Rankin, M., & Snider, B. (1984). Nurses' perception of cancer pain. *Cancer Nursing, 1,* 149–155.

Rotstein, J., & Good, R. A. (1957). Steroid pseudorheumatism. *Archives of Internal Medicine, 99,* 545–555.

Sheidler, V. R. (1987). New methods in analgesic delivery. In D. B. McGuire & C. H. Yarbro (Eds.), *Cancer pain management* (pp. 203–222). Orlando, Fl: Grune & Stratton, Inc.

Sherman, R. A., Sherman, C. J., & Parker, L. (1984). Chronic phantom and stump pain among American veterans: Results of a survey. *Pain, 18,* 83–95.

Stambaugh, J. E., Jr., & Lane, C. (1983). Analgesic efficacy and pharmacokinetic evaluation of meperidine and hydroxyzine, alone and in combination. *Cancer Investigation, 1,* 111–117.

Stoll, B. A., & Andrews, J. T. (1966). Radiation-induced peripheral neuropathy. *British Medical Journal, 1,* 834–837.

Sunderesan, N., DiGiacinto, G. V., & Hughes, J. E. O. (1988). Neurosurgery in the treatment of cancer pain. *Cancer, 63,* 2365–2377.

Swerdlow, M. (1984). Anticonvulsant drugs and chronic pain. *Clinical Neuropharmacology, 7,* 51–82.

Swerdlow, M. (1987). Role of chemical neurolysis and local anesthetic infiltration. In M. Swerdlow & V. Ventafridda (Eds.), *Cancer pain* (pp. 105–128). Lancaster, England: M.T.P. Press.

Syrjala, K. L. (1987). The measurement of pain. In D. B. McGuire & C. H. Yarbro (Eds.), *Cancer pain management* (pp. 133–150). Orlando, Fl: Grune & Stratton, Inc.

Tasker, R. (1984). Deafferentation. In P. D. Wall & R. Melzack (Eds.), *Textbook of pain* (pp. 119–132). New York: Churchill Livingstone.

Tasker, R. R., Tsudn, T., & Hawrylshyn, P. (1983). Clinical neurophysiological investigation of deafferention pain. In J. J. Bonica, U. Lindblom, & A. Iggo (Eds.), *Advances in pain research and therapy* (vol. 5, pp. 713–138). New York: Raven Press.

Thomas, J. E., Cascino, T. E., & Earle, J. D. (1985). Differential diagnosis between radiation and tumor plexopathy of the pelvis. *Neurology, 35,* 1–7.

Travel, J. G., & Simons, D. G. (1983). *Myofascial pain and dysfunction: The trigger point manual.* Baltimore: Williams & Wilkins.

Trotter, J. M., Scott, R., & Macbeth, F. R. (1981). Problems of the oncology outpatient: Role of the liaison health visitor. *British Medical Journal, 282,* 122–124.

Twycross, R. G. (1974). Clinical experience with diamorphine in advanced malignant disease. *International Journal of Clincial Pharmacology, Therapy, and Toxicology, 8,* 184–198.

Twycross, R. G., & Fairfield, S. (1982). Pain in far advanced cancer. *Pain, 14,* 303–310.

Twycross, R. G., & Lack, S. A. (1983). Home care. In R. G. Twycross & S. A. Lack (Eds.), *Symptom control in far advanced cancer: Pain relief* (pp. 297–324). London: Pittman.

Vane, J. R. (1971). Inhibition of prostaglandin synthesis as a mechanism of action for aspirin-like drugs. *Nature: New Biology, 231,* 232–235.

Ventafridda, V., Tamburini, M., & Caraceni, A. (1987). A validation study of the WHO method for cancer pain relief. *Cancer, 59,* 850–856.

Ventafridda, V., Tamburini, M., & DeConno, F. (1985). Comprehensive treatment in cancer pain. In H. L. Fields, R. Dubner, & F. Cervero (Eds.), *Advances in pain research and therapy* (vol. 9, pp. 617–628). New York: Raven Press.

Wall, P. D. (1984). Mechanisms of acute and chronic pain. In J. J. Bonica, U. Lindblom, & A. Iggo (Eds.), *Advances in pain research and therapy* (vol. 5, pp. 95–104). New York: Raven Press.

Walsh, T. D. (1983). Antidepressants and chronic pain. *Clinical Neuropharmacology, 6,* 271–295.

Watt-Watson, J. H. (1987). Nurses' knowledge of pain issues: A survey. *Journal of Pain and Symptom Management, 2,* 207–211.

Wilkes, E. (1974). Some problems in cancer management. *Proceedings of the Royal Society of Medicine, 67,* 23–27.

Wisconsin Cancer Pain Initiative. (1988). The cancer pain problem: Wisconsin's response. A report on the Wisconsin Cancer Pain Initiative. *Journal of Pain and Symptom Management, 3,* s2–s5.

World Health Organization. (1986). *Cancer pain relief* (p. 1). Geneva: Author.

Young, D. F., & Posner, J. B. (1980). Nervous system toxicity of chemotherapeutic agents. In P. J. Vinken & G. W. Bruyn (Eds.), *Handbook of clinical neurology* (pp. 91–129). Amsterdam: North-Holland.

Zborowski, M. (1952). Cultural components in response to pain. *Journal of Social Issues, 8,* 16–30.

CHAPTER 51

Alterations in Patient Coping

ANNE JALOWIEC
SUSAN DUDAS

THE STRESS OF CANCER

It is widely acknowledged that cancer is one of the most feared and stressful of all diseases. Therefore, cancer is a severe threat not only to the physical welfare of patients but also to their psychological well-being, and it can cause such reactions as anxiety, depression, despair, helplessness, guilt, and anger (Weisman, 1979). Until fairly recently, much of the literature on cancer had emphasized coping with the stress of impending death; however, with improvements in treatment methods and increased survival rates, the focus has now changed to coping with cancer as a chronic disease. Coping can be defined simply as using various behavioral and cognitive means to deal with the physical and psychological threats imposed by a stressful situation—in this case cancer.

The importance of coping in the cancer experience is reflected in the identification of coping as one of the ten standards for cancer nursing as developed by the Oncology Nursing Society (1979). This standard is stated as follows: While living with cancer, the client and family manage stress within their physical, psychological, and spiritual capabilities and their value systems. The applicable nursing diagnosis is ineffective coping. Populations at risk for ineffective coping are persons who have diagnostic work-ups and receive a positive diagnosis of cancer, those undergoing initial treatment for cancer, persons with relapse or unsuccessful treatment of cancer, and those under stress because of perceived vulnerability to cancer (Doublsky, 1985).

Cancer patients have to cope with a wide variety of stressors, including loss of function in numerous body systems, pain, nausea and vomiting, anorexia, fatigue, mutilation and disfigurement, decreased mobility, social isolation, uncertainty regarding the future, loss of self-esteem, fear of death and dying, loss of control over one's own body and over numerous aspects of daily living, adjusting to the hospital environment, fear of dependency, need to understand new medical terms, dealing with a variety of health care providers, sexual problems, strained interpersonal relationships, diminished work capacity or loss of job, cognitive impairment, financial problems, inability to perform various social roles, and fear of recurrence of the cancer (Table 51–1) (Burish, Meyerowitz, Carey, & Morrow, 1987; Stoll, 1986). Obviously, some of these stressors may be more dominant at certain stages of the illness than at others, and they may vary in their intensity depending on the individual characteristics of both the person and the situation.

This chapter therefore focuses on a domain very salient to nursing—that of patient coping with the stresses of cancer. Included in this discussion of the various aspects of coping as related to cancer are (1) an overview of conceptual models and assessment techniques relevant for oncology nursing, (2) a review of enabling and hindering factors in coping with cancer, and (3) a description of nursing interventions that can promote more effective ways for the patient to cope with the stresses of this illness. The aim is to foster in the oncology nurse an appreciation for the complexity and the primacy of the coping process in cancer patients.

MODELS OF STRESS AND COPING

An overview is given of three major models of stress and coping that have relevance for oncology nursing:

Table 51–1. POTENTIAL STRESSORS FOR CANCER PATIENTS

Pain
Anorexia, nausea, vomiting
Fatigue
Mutilation or disfigurement
Decreased mobility
Loss of function in body systems
Social isolation
Uncertainty regarding the future
Loss of self-esteem
Fear of death and dying
Loss of control over body functions
Loss of control over activities of daily living
Adjusting to hospital environment
Fear of dependency
Understanding new medical terms
Dealing with numerous health care providers
Sexual problems
Strained interpersonal relationships
Diminished work capacity or loss of job
Financial problems
Inability to perform social roles
Cognitive impairment
Fear of recurrence of cancer

(Data from Burish, Meyerowitz, Carey, & Morrow, 1987; Stoll, 1986.)

Selye's physiologic model, Lazarus's psychological model, and Weisman's cancer-specific model.

Selye's Physiologic Model of Stress

Selye (1957) was the first to popularize a physiologic model of stress, which evolved largely as a result of animal research and was based on stimulus-response theory. Selye labeled the stress response as the general adaptation syndrome. It has three stages: alarm, resistance, and exhaustion. During the alarm stage, physiologic mechanisms in the body are mobilized so that the person can deal with whatever is threatening homeostasis. During the resistance stage, the person is adapting to the stressor and is trying to return to a state of equilibrium. The stage of exhaustion occurs when the stressor is overwhelming in intensity or duration and the person no longer has the resources to handle the situation; this eventually causes a breakdown in body systems. Of particular importance to oncology is the accumulating evidence that prolonged or excessive stress results in the depression of the immune system, which increases the likelihood of tumorigenesis, thus prompting investigators to question the role that stress plays in the causation of cancer (Campbell & Cohen, 1985).

The stress response results in the activation of many body systems, most notably the pituitary, hypothalamus, adrenals, and sympathetic nervous system, with the subsequent secretion of many hormones and chemicals (e.g., epinephrine, norepinephrine, cortisol) that prepare the body to function at a high level of intensity. Asterita (1985) notes that the stress response is composed of more than 1400 physiochemical changes, which are initiated by the nervous system and then carried out by neuroendocrine mechanisms. (See Asterita's text [1985] for a comprehensive discussion of the physiology of stress.)

Selye (1957) postulated that the same type of stress reaction occurs in response to *any kind* of stressor; however, Mason (1975) later found varying hormonal profiles in persons exposed to different types of physical stressors (heat, cold, exercise). In addition, other research (e.g., Frankenhaeuser [1980]) has suggested that different patterns of hormonal, autonomic, and cardiovascular reactivity occur during active coping with an aversive situation than those that occur in passive avoidance or feeling helpless. These newer data therefore raise some questions about the nonspecificity of the stress response as postulated by Selye.

Although Selye's original model of stress is undergoing some modification, the overall physiologic model of stress still has relevance for oncology nursing because it helps nurses understand the enormous physiologic burden imposed on the body by the psychological stress of illness.

Lazarus's Psychological Model of Stress and Coping

The model of stress and coping proposed by Lazarus and developed by him and his associates (Lazarus, 1966; Lazarus & Folkman, 1984) offers a generic framework for understanding the adaptation process and is the predominant paradigm in general use today. Lazarus's theory is primarily psychological and is based on a transactional model that focuses on the relationship between the person and the environment. Unlike a stimulus-response model (which flows in only one direction), the transactional model allows for reciprocal feedback pathways between the person and the environment (Lazarus & Folkman, 1984); hence this model is more reflective of what actually transpires during the process of coping with stress.

Lazarus and Folkman (1984, p. 141) define coping as "constantly changing cognitive and behavioral efforts to manage specific external and/or internal demands that are appraised as taxing or exceeding the resources of the person." Therefore, coping is seen as effortful, dynamic, cognitively mediated, and process oriented. Within Lazarus's framework, coping serves two main functions: managing the problem or stressful situation (problem-focused) and regulating the emotional distress arising from the situation (emotion-focused).

Central to Lazarus's theory is cognitive appraisal, which gives every situation a special meaning for each person. Lazarus and Folkman (1984) identified three main types of cognitive appraisal that take place during the adaptation process: primary appraisal, secondary appraisal, and reappraisal. Primary appraisal refers to a person's evaluation of what a particular situation means to that person's well-being; in other words, is the situation stressful, benign, or neutral? If a situation is appraised as stressful, it can be seen as harmful, threatening, or challenging. (This difference in perception of the situation is important because some research [Kobasa, 1979] has suggested that people who appraise a stressful situation as challenging do better than persons who see the situation as threatening or harmful.) Secondary appraisal concerns the person's evaluation of what can be done in a particular situation (i.e., coping options). Reappraisal is simply a reevaluation of a previous situation based on new incoming information.

Lazarus and Folkman (1984) identified many person-related and situation-related factors as influencing cognitive appraisal. Person-related factors include various commitments, values, beliefs, attitudes, and goals that the person has, whereas situation-related factors include newness of the situation, predictability of the event, likelihood of occurrence of the event, temporal uncertainty, imminence and duration of the event, situational ambiguity, and timing of the event within the developmental life cycle. Each of these factors can influence the stress and coping process and thus result in different patterns of adaptational outcomes.

Lazarus's theory of stress and coping can therefore be seen as having special relevance for oncology nursing because it is a transactional model that allows for feedback between the person and the environment; it places primary emphasis on the particular meaning of a situation to the individual; it takes into consideration the many person-related and situation-related factors that can affect the stress and coping process; and it focuses on the dynamic nature of adaptation. The dynamic nature of stress and coping is especially germane to oncology patients because they must constantly cope with the many different demands of their illness as it progresses and as new therapies are tried. Thus Lazarus (1987) notes that any time nurses are examining the coping process in cancer patients, they should identify very specifically what the patient is actually having to cope with at that point and how the coping process is changing over time.

Weisman's Cancer-Specific Model of Stress and Coping

The model of stress and coping developed by Weisman (1979, 1984a, 1984b) is based on extensive work with cancer patients. He identified four psychosocial stages in coping with cancer, each with differing characteristics, concerns, and implications for interventions. These stages are existential plight, accommodation and mitigation, recurrence and relapse, and deterioration and decline. Such a staging typology allows identification of problems specific to each stage, determination of interventions appropriate for the different stages, and identification of patients at high risk for extreme distress at each stage. It also provides a framework for comparing patients both within and across the various stages.

The first stage, existential plight, is characterized by acute distress at having the diagnosis of cancer confirmed; at this time patients are preoccupied with thoughts of death and dying but attempt to actively cope with this new threat to their well-being. Therefore, during this first stage, patients need accurate information, candor, warm support from significant others, and an optimistic attitude (Weisman, 1984b).

The second stage, accommodation and mitigation, begins when patients return to their normal routines, resume previous social roles, and attempt to get on with the business of living. Because patients are trying to resume previous duties and responsibilities, they may encounter many new problems during this stage as they try to accommodate the demands of their illness to the demands of normal, everyday routines. This second stage is both a period of trying to regain equilibrium and a time of surveillance during which patients need information on monitoring for further problems and need professionals who are readily available to answer questions as they arise (Weisman, 1984b). At this time, patients also benefit from ongoing interaction with mutual support groups whose members have similar problems and concerns.

Although Weisman views prolonged remission or apparent cure as falling within the second stage, he does not seem to take adequate account of the specific needs of *long-time* survivors of cancer. Needs of this group vary depending on many factors, including functional disabilities resulting from cancer treatment and insecurity associated with the fear of cancer recurrence (Welch, Follo, & Nelson, 1982). This fear may persist for many years after remission or cure. Thus an intervening stage between stages 2 and 3 should be developed so that this typology more accurately reflects reality and therefore would be more useful.

Stage 3, recurrence and relapse, ensues when patients experience a return of their cancer, either while still undergoing treatment or long after treatment has been terminated. This is a difficult period during which patients experience depression, pessimism, renewed preoccupation with death and dying, feelings of helplessness, and disenchantment with treatment methods. Patients also tend to be more guarded and cautious at this time and seem to feel as if they are in limbo (Weisman, 1984b). Because they realize that fewer options are now open to them and less time is left than they originally thought, patients often become more compliant. Previous expectations for a cure of the cancer are now reduced to a hope to merely control the disease process and to have periods of respite from the symptoms (Weisman, 1984b). Weisman (1984b) notes that little research has been done on this third stage, so it is hard to identify appropriate interventions, except for the obvious need to determine which treatment method might now be indicated and the need to manage and control symptoms. In addition, it would seem that patients need encouragement and support so that they can regain their previous outlook for a useful and productive life.

Stage 4, deterioration and decline, is characterized by palliative care rather than curative treatments, as the patient's condition deteriorates and quality of life diminishes. For some patients, this stage comes on abruptly; for others it is more insidious. A unique characteristic of this stage is a relentless need to take care of unfinished business (Weisman, 1984b). During this time patients also become pessimistic and resigned to their fate; long for relief of symptoms; and become exhausted, apathetic, and withdrawn. They become more egocentric and thus less concerned with what is going on around them. During this stage patients need symptom control, comfort, and a warm and caring attitude, plus practical help with planning for the future needs of their family after their death (Weisman, 1984b). This stage, of course, ends with the death of the patient.

Weisman (1979, 1984a) also identified 15 major coping styles that patients use to handle the stresses of cancer. These are rational inquiry, mutuality, affect reversal, suppression, displacement, confrontation, redefinition, passive acceptance, impulsivity, consideration of alternatives, tension reduction, disengagement, projection, compliance, and moral masochism. These 15 coping styles are described in Table 51–2.

In addition, Weisman (1979, 1984a) proposed what he called *countercoping* strategies used by health professionals to help patients cope more effectively. Countercoping is seen as complementing the patient's coping efforts by strengthening good strategies and minimizing harmful ones. Weisman identified four countercoping tasks: clarification and control, collaboration, directed relief, and cooling off. The types of interventions that exemplify each countercoping task are given in Table 51–3.

The extensive work done by Weisman on the coping process in cancer patients has much applicability for oncology nursing. Weisman's model can prove useful for nurses in understanding what the cancer patient is experiencing, in anticipating the needs of patients at various stages of the illness trajectory, and in planning for holistic cancer care.

Table 51–2. COPING STYLES USED BY CANCER PATIENTS

Coping Style	Description
Mutuality	Share concern; talk to other people
Confrontation	Take firm action; confront the problem
Redefinition	Focus on positive aspects of situation
Displacement	Keep busy; distract yourself with activities
Suppression	Try to forget; put things out of your mind
Disengagement	Withdraw into isolation; get away from problem
Projection	Blame someone or something else for problem
Impulsivity	Do something reckless or impractical
Rational inquiry	Seek information; get guidance
Affect reversal	Laugh it off; make light of situation
Passive acceptance	Submit to the inevitable; resign yourself
Tension reduction	Find an escape with such things as drink or drugs
Moral masochism	Blame yourself; atone for wrongdoings
Cooperative compliance	Seek direction; do what you're told
Consideration of alternatives	Review alternatives; consider consequences

(Adapted with permission from Weisman, A. D. [1984]. *The coping capacity: on the nature of being mortal.* New York: Human Sciences Press. Originally appeared in Weisman, A. D. [1979]. *Coping with cancer* [p. 15]. New York: McGraw-Hill Book Co.)

Table 51–3. COUNTERCOPING TASKS AND REPRESENTATIVE INTERVENTIONS

Countercoping Task	Interventions
Clarification or control	Directly confront problem
	Provide reliable and accurate information
	Reduce problem to manageable size
	Consider feasibility or consequences of options
Collaboration	Share concern without sharing distress
	Appropriately refer problems to others
	Discourage hasty actions
	Share your understanding of problem
Directed relief	Encourage expression of pent-up feelings
	Permit temporary avoidance and distraction
	Encourage previously successful diversions
	Allow ventilation of doubt and confusion
Cooling off	Modulate tendencies for emotional extremes
	Promote self-esteem and confidence
	Emphasize rational and prudent actions
	Share silence as needed

(Adapted with permission from Weisman, A. D. [1984]. *The coping capacity: on the nature of being mortal.* New York: Human Sciences Press. Originally appeared in Weisman, A. D. [1979]. *Coping with cancer* [p. 109]. New York: McGraw-Hill Book Co.)

CLINICAL ASSESSMENT OF COPING BEHAVIOR

Nurses have increasingly incorporated assessment of the coping behavior and adaptive potential of clients into their clinical practice, using both formal tools and less structured assessment approaches (Miaskowski & Nielsen, 1985; Welch et al., 1982). To determine which patients are at risk for ineffective coping, nurses need to identify specific stressors in the patient's life, assess the patient's perception of those stressors and attributional beliefs about their causes, and evaluate the available coping resources and social support systems. Psychosocial adjustment can be further assessed by obtaining information on the patient's previous ways of dealing with stress, the patient's perception of illness, and prior relationships with people who had cancer (Welch et al., 1982). The last-mentioned factor can exert either a positive or a negative influence on the patient's outlook on the diagnosis, depending on the types of experiences the patient has had with other cancer patients. Such an assessment should also include information on family history, interpersonal relationships, and the patient's expectations of nursing care.

Further, Weisman (1976) suggested that by listening well and learning to ask tactful questions, health professionals can better elicit information on the patient's psychological status. The use of open-ended questions can also provide an elaboration of the patient's views and emotional states, so that psychosocial vulnerability can be recognized and appropriate interventions instituted.

These assessment techniques are necessary to obtain information on the patient's available coping strategies and to determine the patient's problem-solving ability. These aspects are then incorporated into the nursing care plan, so that appropriate interventions can be planned to allay the patient's anxiety, decrease stress, and facilitate more effective ways for coping with the stresses of cancer.

Three methods of assessing coping behavior, which would be useful for both oncology nursing practice and research, are described in more detail: Lazarus's Ways of Coping Checklist, the Jalowiec Coping Scale, and Weisman's coping interview.

Lazarus's Ways of Coping Checklist

The Ways of Coping Checklist was developed by Lazarus (a psychologist) (Lazarus & Folkman, 1984) and is the most commonly cited coping tool in the general stress and coping literature today (original version: Lazarus, 1977; most recent version: Lazarus & Folkman, 1984). The tool lists 66 coping strategies that are rated on a four-point scale to indicate the extent of use of each strategy. The coping strategies are rated in response to a particular situation described on another tool that elicits information on the stressful event. The items on Lazarus's scale are classified into eight types of coping behavior: confrontive, distancing, self-control, seeking social support, accepting responsibility, escape-avoidance, planful problem solving, and positive reappraisal (Folkman, Lazarus, Dunkel-Schetter, Delongis, & Gruen, 1986).

The Jalowiec Coping Scale

The Jalowiec Coping Scale (JCS) was developed by a nurse (Jalowiec, 1987) and has been used extensively in nursing research (original version: 1977; revised version: 1987). The JCS lists 60 coping strategies that are classified into eight types of coping behavior: confrontive, evasive, optimistic, fatalistic, emotive, palliative, supportant, and self-reliant. The coping strategies are rated on frequency of use and also on degree of effectiveness, both on four-point scales. Coping strategies are rated in response to the stressful situation under study as listed at the top of the tool.

Weisman's Coping Interview

Weisman (a psychiatrist) (1979) did not develop a formal coping tool per se, but uses a coping interview to elicit information on the problems and concerns of the cancer patient, what the patient is doing about the problems, and who the patient turns to for help. The predominant concerns identified by cancer patients through these interviews fall into seven categories: health, self-appraisal (as self-esteem, proficiency, approval), work and finances, relationships with family, relationships with friends, religion, and concerns about death.

On the basis of these interviews, Weisman (1979) identified the 15 major coping styles used by cancer patients to deal with these concerns, as listed previously in Table 51–2. Persons who cope well with cancer, according to Weisman, are those who confront reality,

Table 51–4. CHARACTERISTICS OF GOOD CANCER COPERS

Confront reality
Consider alternatives
Avoid excessive denial
Communicate openly with others
Self-reliant but accept help when offered
Make use of available resources
Flexible
Realistically hopeful
Try to maintain morale and self-esteem
Focus on problem solving when appropriate
Focus on problem redefinition when situation not
   amenable to problem solving

(Data from Weisman, 1979).

consider alternatives, focus on problem solving when the situation is amenable to problem solving but turn to problem redefinition when it is not, avoid excessive use of denial, communicate openly with significant others, are largely self-reliant but can accept help when it is offered, make use of available resources, are flexible and realistically hopeful, and try to maintain morale and self-esteem (Table 51–4).

Weisman (1979) also uses a scale that indicates how vulnerable the cancer patient is to high emotional distress by rating the person on the following 13 characteristics: hopelessness, turmoil, frustration, depression, powerlessness, anxiety, exhaustion, worthlessness, abandonment, denial, truculence (positive versus negative attitudes toward care providers), repudiation of significant others, and time perspective. On the basis of the results from this scale, Weisman (1979) identified the following correlates of vulnerability for high emotional distress in cancer patients: pessimism; psychiatric history; high anxiety; low ego strength; prior marital problems; low socioeconomic status; alcohol abuse; multiple-problem background; poor problem-solving techniques; little or no church attendance; many physical symptoms and concerns; advanced stage of cancer; expectation of little support from others; regrets about the past; sees the doctor as less helpful; feels like giving up; and uses more of the coping strategies related to suppression, fatalism, disengagement, projection, and moral masochism (Table 51–5). The oncology nurse can use this vulnerability profile as an assessment checklist to identify patients who are at high risk for suffering extreme emotional distress from having cancer.

Cancer patients are especially prone to high emotional distress at certain times in the illness process. These have been identified as the time of diagnosis or recurrence of the disease, after loss of a bodily function or part, when repeated complications occur, when effective treatments have been exhausted, and when social support fails (Lee, 1986). Therefore, health care providers need to monitor cancer patients vigilantly for increased distress at these times.

ENABLING AND HINDERING FACTORS IN PATIENT COPING

Reports in the literature have indicated that many coping factors can influence adjustment to cancer;

Table 51-5. CORRELATES OF VULNERABILITY FOR HIGH EMOTIONAL DISTRESS IN CANCER PATIENTS

Pessimism or fatalism
High anxiety
Low ego strength
Psychiatric history
Low socioeconomic status
Marital problems
Alcohol abuse
Multiple-problem background
Poor problem-solving techniques
Little or no church attendance
Multiple physical symptoms
Advanced stage of cancer
Numerous concerns
Expectation of little social support
Has regrets about the past
Sees doctor as less helpful
Feels like giving up
Uses more suppression and disengagement
Uses more projection
Uses more self-blame

(Adapted with permission from Weisman, A. D. [1979], *Coping with cancer* [p. 67]. New York: McGraw-Hill Book Co.)

some coping activities facilitate the adaptation process (enabling factors), whereas others hinder it. Enabling factors include social support, control, hardiness, positive appraisal, hopefulness, humor, positive comparisons, religiosity, healthy self-esteem, good body image, information seeking, open communication, social skills, and problem-solving ability (Table 51–6). In contrast, coping factors that hinder adaptation include denial, avoidance, helplessness, powerlessness, hopelessness, despair, depression, erosion of autonomy, isolation, withdrawal, fear, anger, hostility, guilt, blaming others, wishful thinking, and noncompliance (see Table 51–6). Selected factors are discussed next.

Enabling Factors in Coping with Cancer

Social Support

Ample evidence has documented the essential importance of an adequate social support system when trying to cope with almost any formidable stressor, including serious illness (Cohen & Syme, 1985; Dun-

kel-Schetter, 1984; Saunders & McCorkle, 1987; Weisman, 1979; Wortman & Dunkel-Schetter, 1987). Social support can include both formal and informal systems of support and can emanate from a diversity of sources, such as spouse, parents, children, siblings, relatives, friends, supervisors and co-workers, clergy, teachers, counselors, health care providers, and members of self-help groups with the same type of problem. Social support systems can provide help of many different kinds to stressed persons. This help can come in the form of providing an avenue for the ventilation of feelings; affirming the person's importance and place in the world; encouraging the open expression of thoughts and feelings (especially negative ones); acknowledging the appropriateness of a person's interpretation of events; providing feedback on the person's behavior; having someone to confide in; supplying needed information and advice; acting as an advocate for the person; and providing more tangible types of support, such as materials, money, and physical help with chores and responsibilities (Table 51–7) (Cohen & Syme, 1985; Wortman & Dunkel-Schetter, 1987).

Social support can facilitate adaptation by altering the use of coping strategies, by influencing the occurrence and appraisal of stressful events, by enhancing the motivation for health-promoting behaviors, by increasing self-esteem and altering mood states, and by synergistically interacting with other resources that promote adaptation (Wortman & Dunkel-Schetter, 1987). Hence, social support may have both direct and indirect (i.e., buffering or mediating) effects.

Some researchers have questioned whether it is the actual provision of social support that has the salutary effect, or whether stressed persons just have to *feel* that there are people available to help them if they ever need it, whether or not they actually use the help (Wortman & Dunkel-Schetter, 1987). Therefore, the way that social support is assessed may vary widely, ranging from counting the person's significant others, to obtaining the person's perception of available support, to finding out who would be there to help in various situations, to determining who has actually provided support of different kinds in specific situations, or to assessing the person's satisfaction with the extent of support available or provided.

Evidence abounds in the literature on the beneficial

Table 51-6. ENABLING AND HINDERING FACTORS IN COPING WITH CANCER

Enabling Factors	Hindering Factors
Social support systems	Denial
Perception of control	Avoidance
Hardiness	Helplessness
Humor	Powerlessness
Positive appraisal	Hopelessness or
Hopefulness	despair
Positive comparisons	Depression
Religiosity	Guilt
Self-esteem	Erosion of autonomy
Information seeking	Isolation or withdrawal
Open communication	Wishful thinking
Social skills	Anger or hostility
Problem-solving ability	Blaming others
	Noncompliance

Table 51-7. WAYS IN WHICH SOCIAL SUPPORT HELPS IN COPING

Provides avenue for ventilation of feelings
Affirms person's importance
Encourages open expression of negative feelings
Provides feedback on behavior
Provides confidante
Supplies information
Provides advice
Acts as advocate for person
Supplies tangible materials
Provides financial aid
Provides help with duties or responsibilities
Acknowledges appropriateness of personal interpretation of events

(Data from Cohen & Syme, 1985; Wortman & Dunkel-Schetter, 1987.)

impact of social support in promoting various types of positive outcomes in cancer patients; only a few of the findings are cited here. A longitudinal study reported a significant association between social involvement and survival 20 years later in breast cancer patients (Funch & Marshall, 1983). Dunkel-Schetter (1984) noted that support was positively related to various measures of psychological well-being. Similarly, breast cancer patients who believed they had more social support were found to be better adjusted emotionally on the basis of both physician and patient ratings (Lichtman, Wood, & Taylor, 1982). Enhanced self-esteem and greater feelings of self-efficacy in dealing with illness also were reported by cancer patients who participated in support-promoting interventions (Gordon et al., 1980). Additional evidence on the utility of social support for coping with cancer can be found in the articles by Follick, Smith, and Turk (1984), Saunders and McCorkle (1987), Wortman and Dunkel-Schetter (1987), and Young (1986).

Thus the evidence is overwhelming that patients who are able to maintain close relationships with family and friends, despite their illness, are more likely to cope effectively with cancer. Hence, it is imperative that the nurse help cancer patients to mobilize their social supports by including significant others in the plan of care and by informing patients of the various types of programs available that have supportive functions.

Programs have been designed to provide more formal types of support groups for patients with various kinds of cancer, thereby supplying both educational and psychosocial resources to help patients and families cope more effectively. Peer groups with similar cancer experiences, such as mastectomy patients and Reach to Recovery, have proved useful primarily as a function of modeling—that is, as a method of learning better ways to cope by sharing and knowing someone else who has successfully coped with cancer (Adams, 1979). "WE CAN" weekends, a family-oriented program for persons experiencing the crisis of terminal illness, have been designed to help cancer patients and their families improve problem-solving techniques, strengthen self-esteem, and increase interactional skills (Lane & Davis, 1985). This program also tries to combat the social isolation that often occurs in families unable to cope with the reality of the cancer diagnosis.

Although most writers overwhelmingly laud the beneficial effects of social support, Wortman and Dunkel-Schetter (1987) and Tilden and Galyen (1987) remind us that social support can also have negative aspects, which can then increase stress rather than buffer it. For example, social support can have a negative impact when a person's privacy is invaded, when promises are made that are not kept, when unwelcome or misleading advice is offered, when the other person discourages compliance with the treatment regimen, when a feeling of extreme dependency is created, or when the other person extracts more from the relationship than is given in return. Hence, some social relationships can cost more than any positive benefits that might be gleaned from the association. Therefore, oncology nurses need to be cautious in evaluating the quality and adequacy of social support systems of their cancer patients. Just because a patient has a large network of significant others, it should not be taken for granted that the person is deriving solely positive benefits from that network.

Control

Writers have for a long time promulgated the beneficial impact of the factor of control on the stress and coping process (Fisher, 1986; Langer, 1983; Lefcourt, 1982; Strickland, 1978; Wallston & Wallston, 1981). Langer (1983) points out that control is such a primary and motivating force in life that it is perceived even in situations that are determined by chance (such as lotteries), and that people selectively filter information that enhances their perception of control. The concept of control is often seen as the opposite of learned helplessness (Seligman, 1975) and is related to the concepts of self-efficacy (Bandura, 1977), learned resourcefulness (Rosenbaum, 1983) and causal attribution (Weiner, 1972).

Most of the work on control evolved from Rotter's concept (1966) of internal versus external locus of control. Persons with an internal locus of control feel that they themselves can influence and control the events in their lives, whereas persons with an external locus of control feel that their lives are controlled by others. Thus it is usually thought that having personal control over a situation reduces feelings of threat and helplessness and gives a person a sense of mastery over the situation, thereby leading to better adaptational outcomes. Much research has supported this view, both generally and in relation to cancer patients (Langer, 1983; Lefcourt, 1982; Lewis, 1982; Marks, Richardson, Graham, & Levine, 1986; Padilla & Grant, 1985; Strickland, 1978; Taylor, Lichtman, & Wood, 1984). For example, both Lewis (1982) and Padilla and Grant (1985) reported that cancer patients who felt that they had more personal control over their illness also had a higher quality of life.

It is hypothesized that the impact of locus of control on adaptation operates partially through cognitive appraisal of the situation and partially via coping behavior. Hence, having an internal versus an external control orientation has been found to affect how persons view a situation and therefore how they choose to cope with it. For example, persons with an internal locus of control have been noted to use the following types of coping behavior: more task-centered and less emotion-centered coping strategies (Anderson, 1977), more constructive and fewer aggressive and self-blame strategies (Brissett & Nowicki, 1973), more direct-action types of coping behavior and less suppression-related coping (Parkes, 1984), and more information-seeking types of coping behavior (Wallston & Wallston, 1981). Overall, then, research seems to indicate that persons with an internal locus of control show a preference for constructive coping strategies that work toward altering the stressful situation, whereas those with an external locus of control prefer more palliative types of coping behavior. Knowing that a cancer patient has an internal locus of control has relevance for anticipating the types of coping behavior that may be displayed by such patients, and it also has implications for the teaching and promotion of more action-oriented coping skills.

Folkman and Lazarus (1980) found that persons used more problem-focused coping if they felt they had some control over health-related situations, but they used more emotion-focused coping if they felt little or no control. Therefore, if nurses encourage cancer patients to control as many aspects of their disease and treatment regimen as possible, they can promote the greater use of problem-oriented coping strategies that can lead to more successful resolution of the problems encountered during illness. Moreover, because patients' feelings of personal control are sometimes eroded by the lack of improvement in their condition, nurses need to constantly reinforce patients' efforts to exert control to foster confidence in their ongoing ability to maintain control over their lives (Marks et al., 1986). Silberfarb and Greer (1982) hypothesized that patients' feelings of reduced control may partly account for the increasing popularity of less orthodox treatments for cancer (e.g., mental imagery). Therefore, nurses should reinforce patients' control efforts by encouraging an active role in the treatment process, by letting patients know what alternatives they have related to the many aspects of the treatment regimen, by allowing and promoting decision-making, by providing the information necessary for sound decision-making, and by giving positive feedback on patients' appropriate efforts to control their environment (Table 51–8) (Dennis, 1987; Lewis, 1982; Marks et al., 1986).

What was originally thought to be a simple concept of control has now been shown to be a complex phenomenon that can have varying implications for the adaptation process. Thus Rotter's concept (1966) of dichotomous control has now evolved into a multidimensional conceptualization. For example, Wallston, Wallston, and De Vellis (1978) extended Rotter's idea

Table 51–8. WAYS TO INCREASE PATIENT'S PERCEPTION OF CONTROL

Encourage problem-solving behavior
Foster confidence in ability to control situation
Encourage information-seeking behavior
Let patient know what to expect
Encourage active role in treatment program
Inform patient of alternatives or options
Allow decision making in care
Provide necessary information for decision making
Promote self-care activities
Identify personal assets that facilitate control
Identify elements in environment conducive to control
Discourage excessive or inappropriate dependency
Give positive feedback on appropriate efforts to control environment
Encourage action-oriented coping activities when appropriate to situation
Encourage cognitive control activities when behavioral control not possible
Help patient differentiate between controllable versus uncontrollable situations
Help patient identify things he or she wants to control versus things the patient does not wish to control

of internal and external control in the health arena by postulating that external control has two discrete aspects: powerful others and chance. Therefore, although internal or personal control is still believed to be the most beneficial, control by other persons (such as health care professionals) is viewed as better than feeling that events are due to chance or fate or luck— that is, totally random and thus having no potential at all for control.

Averill (1973) too identified three kinds of control, although his dimensions dealt with different types of control activities, as opposed to Rotter's idea (1966) of different loci of control. Averill's dimensions were cognitive control (interpreting events), decisional control (choosing from alternative options), and behavioral control (engaging in direct action on the environment). Using Averill's classification, Dennis (1987) found that hospitalized patients (including cancer patients) attached the utmost importance to having cognitive control over surgery, treatment, and necessary life-style changes. Furthermore, possession of information was critical for cognitive control; therefore, Dennis saw the need for facilitating the flow of information between caregiver and patient so that the patient can exercise sufficient cognitive control over the illness. Dennis also found that of the different types of patients studied, cancer patients were the ones who wanted most to exert decisional control; it was believed that they wanted this control because they had to cope with more noxious types of experiences.

Thompson (1981) later built on Averill's (1973) classification with a four-category typology of control: cognitive, behavioral, informational, and retrospective (the last category meaning that the person decided after the fact that he or she could have controlled the situation and therefore should be able to do so in the future). Each dimension of control can have varying effects; therefore, not all types of controlling efforts may be equally successful in moderating stress. After reviewing the literature, Thompson concluded that cognitive control has the most consistent success in moderating stress, both before and after the stressful event, whereas informational control does not have a beneficial impact in all circumstances. Thompson further stated that the effect of retrospective control was largely unknown at that time, and that behavioral control probably works better for anticipatory coping rather than for reactive coping after the stressful event has occurred.

Taylor, Lichtman, & Wood (1984) tested the varying effects of Thompson's four types of control (1981) on adjustment to breast cancer. Consistent with Thompson's hypothesis, Taylor and co-workers found that cognitive control showed the strongest relationship to adjustment. Behavioral control showed the next strongest relationship, even though this study dealt more with reactive coping than with anticipatory coping. No significant relationships were found between adjustment and either informational or retrospective control. It should be pointed out that informational control was operationalized in Taylor and colleagues' study as information-seeking behavior (contacts with books, media, other patients, and so forth), not as the amount of accurate information that the patient actually had. It is also interesting to note that a curvilinear (albeit nonsignificant) relationship was found between informational control and adjustment; therefore, those patients who sought out either a few or many sources of information were more poorly adjusted than those who sought out a moderate number of sources. Thus too few sources may leave the patient lacking in information, and too many sources may leave the patient feeling confused or overloaded; both instances could lead to decreased ability to control the situation.

Taylor and co-workers (1984) also found that both personal control and control by other persons (e.g., the physician) were highly correlated with better adjustment to the illness. With cancer patients, the strong belief in the control by others is understandable given the patient's reliance on other persons and on the success of the treatment regimen. This study points out the importance of examining the various aspects of control and their subsequent implications in a specific illness population; therefore, control should not be treated as a unitary concept with the same impact on all persons.

To increase the complexity of the phenomenon of control even more, the following issues have been raised (Fisher, 1986; Langer, 1983). First, what is the more salient element: veridical (real) control or merely the perception of control? Second, do all people *want* to control all aspects of their life (e.g., some people gladly relinquish control of certain things, such as fixing their car)? Third, do people *expect* to have control over all things in their life? Fourth, what happens when a person tries to control something but does not have the necessary skills for controlling it (e.g., intelligence, knowledge, material and financial resources, stamina)? Each of these issues has relevance for the impact of control on the lives of cancer patients and needs to be taken into consideration by oncology nurses. It should also be kept in mind that, depending on the operation of these issues in a particular situation, control can be more stress inducing than stress alleviating, especially in relation to the questions of desired control and the necessary skills to control. In this regard, Dennis (1987) points out that nurses should not insist that patients control things that they are not equipped to handle, nor should they deprive patients of controlling-type coping strategies if patients desire them.

Hardiness

Related to the factor of control is the concept of hardiness, which was developed by Kobasa in her work on stress and illness in business executives (Kobasa, 1979; Kobasa, Maddi, & Kahn, 1982). She found, both retrospectively and prospectively, that executives who experienced a large number of stressful events but who possessed this hardiness factor, were less prone to illness than executives who were exposed to high stress but did not possess hardiness. Kobasa conceptualized hardiness as a stress-moderating personality style composed of three essential characteristics: commitment, challenge, and control. Thus hardy persons feel committed to something that is important in their lives (as work or family), and therefore they feel that their lives are meaningful; they feel challenged rather than threatened by change, stress, and problems; and they feel that they have some control over their lives and their environment. Underlying all of this is a pervasive optimistic bent that hardy persons feel they will be successful in whatever dealings they have with the world. Therefore, hardiness moderates stress by influencing both the cognitive appraisal of stressful situations and the choice of coping strategies.

Kobasa's initial findings on the positive effects of hardiness in executives have since been replicated with other populations; for example, with lawyers (Kobasa, 1982), nurses (Keane, Ducette, & Adler, 1985), diabetic patients (Pollock, 1986), and cancer patients (Lee, 1983). In diabetic patients, Pollock (1986) reported that hardiness was related to better adaptation to the illness in both the physiologic and psychosocial domains. Lee (1983) found that cancer patients who remained active despite their illness and adjusted well to the stresses of having cancer possessed the quality of hardiness. Furthermore, hardiness also went hand-in-hand with a strong will to survive in cancer patients. It should be noted, however, that Lee specified the critical attributes of hardiness as endurance, strength, boldness, and control, which are somewhat different from Kobasa's dimensions (1979).

Identifying a patient with cancer as hardy can allow nurses to anticipate the patient's reactions to cancer and treatment and to plan patient care more effectively. For example, hardy patients with cancer might need to be given more latitude in decision making regarding their illness and treatment because they tend to be more independent and assertive (Lee, 1983). In the same vein, it is important to keep hardy patients actively involved in what is going on, because they tend to feel a deep commitment to what they value in life. These hardy patients might also seem to have a higher pain threshold owing to their need to control their environment (Lee, 1983). Because hardy persons like a challenge, it is wise to phrase information regarding cancer and treatment so that the patient sees that such factors can also help to foster development and inner growth. Furthermore, hardy cancer patients might be expected to be efficient problem solvers, to feel that they can handle almost anything, and to tend to see things in a positive light.

On the other hand, oncology nurses should keep in mind Lee's warning (1983) that hardiness could also possibly have negative effects on cancer patients because the strong sense of independence and personal control in hardy persons may cause them to ignore professional advice regarding treatment. It is also important to remember Pollock's finding (1986) that hardiness did not have a stress-moderating impact in arthritic patients because of insufficient control over their pain; this point can have implications that the stress-buffering effect of hardiness could be less in cancer patients who have severe and unrelenting pain.

Hopefulness

A feeling of hope is paramount for patient adjustment to cancer and indeed for survival itself; in fact, hope is probably the single most important factor needed for living with cancer (Weisman, 1979). Hope enables patients to cope with problems in ways that make possible the desired outcomes. Thus hope can figure prominently in the dynamics of self-fulfilling prophecies, for being hopeful may cause goals to be realized owing merely to the fact that people work harder toward those goals when they are motivated by hope (Smith, 1983).

Nurses can bolster the patient's sense of hope by communicating confidence in the efficacy of therapy, by helping patients identify those aspects of life that are important to them and therefore worth living for, by helping patients develop an awareness of the small things in life that can be enjoyed, by setting realistic goals that will promote a sense of accomplishment and thereby generate further hope when they are attained, by being enthusiastic in interactions with the patient, and by helping patients to incorporate religion and humor into their lives (Table 51–9) (Hickey, 1986; Roberts, 1986). When patients can no longer realistically hope for a long life or for a cure from cancer, hope can then be redirected toward short-term, more tangible goals, such as a week with less suffering or a chance to see spring come again, or ultimately a hope for a comfortable death (Hickey, 1986).

Information Seeking

An important enabling factor in coping with cancer is that of seeking information. For example, information-seeking behavior was significantly correlated with less distress and better social adjustment in breast cancer patients (Orr, 1986), and patients who received systematic information on chemotherapy drugs and side effects were able to undertake more self-care (Dodd, 1984). Encouraging the patient to seek accurate information also will facilitate development of the patient's decision-making abilities. Patient education materials often reinforce the idea that the patient is responsible for asking questions if he or she wants more information; therefore, patients should be advised that they are free to ask direct questions about any aspect of their illness. Detailed information about cancer and its treatment is needed to reduce the uncertainty inherent in the cancer experience and to

Table 51–9. WAYS TO BOLSTER HOPE IN CANCER PATIENTS

Encourage setting of realistic goals
Give positive feedback on small successes in goals
Communicate confidence in efficacy of treatment
Enhance patient's self-esteem
Help patient identify things in life worth living for
Help patient become aware of small things in life to enjoy
Be enthusiastic in patient interactions
Help patient utilize religion for coping
Use humor as appropriate to the situation
Redirect hope as necessary to short-term goals

(Data from Hickey, 1986; Roberts, 1986.)

allow the patient to feel a sense of control over the situation (Mishel, Hostetter, King, & Graham, 1984). However, it is important to evaluate how much information is desired by the patient; some patients may not want detailed information at certain times because it may be overwhelming and thus may interfere with their ability to cope (Weisman, 1984a). Facilitating patient acquisition of needed information about the illness and about how to cope with the cancer experience is the basis for various educational programs offered to patients with cancer (e.g., the American Cancer Society program I Can Cope) (Johnson, 1982).

Problem-Solving Ability

Problem-solving ability is a necessary prerequisite for adequately coping with any serious illness, especially cancer (Cohen & Lazarus, 1979; Moos, 1986). For example, Scott, Oberst, and Bookbinder (1984) found that men with genitourinary cancer who had better problem-solving ability were able to cope more effectively with their cancer, as measured by resolution of cancer-related problems and less dysphoria. Patients at risk for ineffective coping by virtue of few problem-solving skills can be taught to accurately identify problems and to consider choices for handling stressful situations. Sobel and Worden (1981) have demonstrated that problem-solving behavior can be taught systematically. Points covered in their problem-solving approach are defining the highest priority problems; identifying the patient's feelings, thoughts, and behaviors in response to those problems; relaxing before confronting the problem; taking into consideration all possible solutions; identifying the advantages and disadvantages of all options; and choosing the best solution.

Hindering Factors in Coping with Cancer

Denial

Denial has long been considered one of the worst things to do when trying to cope with a stressful situation, especially a situation as serious as a life-threatening illness. However, denial is not an all-or-none phenomenon, for many cancer patients show some degree of denial, which may fluctuate during various phases of their illness (Hughes, 1986a). In addition, patients may show acceptance of some aspects of their illness but reject other aspects; for example, patients may acknowledge that they indeed have cancer but may ignore certain evidence indicating that the cancer is incurable. Accordingly, Weisman (1979) has identified three orders of denial in cancer patients. First-order denial is repudiation of the diagnosis itself. Second-order denial is dissociation of the diagnosis from its therapeutic implications. Third-order denial is renunciation of deterioration and decline in status. Using Weisman's classification, Orr (1986) found that breast cancer patients who used first-order denial showed poorer adjustment, whereas those using second-order denial were better adjusted. Because denial is not a unitary concept, what the patient is specifically denying and to what extent denial is operating in a particular situation can have quite different implications for that person's physical and psychological well-being.

Extremes in denial have been shown to be an obstacle in adjusting to the many demands of the cancer experience. For example, excessive denial has been associated with indifference toward serious symptoms, delay in seeking treatment, noncompliance with therapeutic regimens, nonuse of existing resources for information and support, blaming others for self-induced problems associated with the illness, and poorer long-term adjustment to cancer (Hughes, 1986a; Weisman, 1979).

Although, as already noted, denial has long been considered a hindering factor in coping with a serious illness, more recent research (Lazarus, 1983; Lazarus & Folkman, 1984) suggests that the role of denial is more complicated than was originally thought. Therefore, denial may in fact be beneficial at some points in the coping process. For example, denial of the seriousness of the illness when the person first learns of a diagnosis of cancer can often give the person time to get used to the idea of being ill; therefore, the person can have some breathing space to muster the energy and resources needed to cope with the problems that will follow. Also, denial that he or she is going to die soon from the cancer may allow the person to keep living life as fully as possible and not dwell morbidly on what is to come. In addition, denial has been found in some studies to be associated with less depression, lower levels of both physiologic and psychosocial disruption, and, surprisingly, with increased rates of survival in cancer patients (Greer, Morris, & Pettingale, 1979; Katz, Weiner, Gallagher, & Hellman, 1970). Denial does cause problems, however, when it interferes with taking the necessary steps to see a doctor, continue treatment, or make plans for the future that might be indicated (e.g., to plan for the financial welfare of dependent children). Therefore, denial might indeed work well in the short run in handling the distress associated with cancer and treatment, but it is not as effective in the long run for resolving problems and for adjusting to the demands of the illness.

As Weisman (1979, p. 46) points out so well, "the proper balance between denial and acceptance cannot be packaged into the proper dosage for everyone." Therefore, nurses should not make snap judgments that denial is bad for all cancer patients at all times. Too often in the past, nurses have believed that it was their responsibility to make sure the patient accepted the stark reality of the situation so that they could help prepare the person to die in the right way. However, knowing what is now known about denial, nurses should instead examine the particular characteristics of a patient's situation and see if denial might not in fact be doing the patient some good, at least for the time being.

Helplessness or Powerlessness

Patients with serious illnesses often experience a sense of helplessness and powerlessness related to the loss of both physiologic control over their body and psychological control over the events in their life as well as to the loss of control over their environment (Miller, 1983; Roberts, 1986). Contributing to helplessness in cancer patients are feelings of uncertainty, ambiguity, indecisiveness, despair, and the expectation that nothing can be done to change the ultimate outcome of the situation (Stoner, 1985). The phenomenon of *learned helplessness* was first identified by Seligman (1975) as a precipitating factor in depression. The cancer experience too readily fosters learned helplessness because of its devastating implications for the patient's welfare, its chronic nature, the recurring acute episodes, the need for long-term adherence to a treatment regimen, the debilitating side effects associated with treatment methods, and the patient's previous experiences with others who have died from cancer.

Observing patients for vulnerability during crucial periods of their illness is useful for detecting signs of helplessness that require treatment. Interventions recommended for preventing or relieving helplessness include setting realistic goals, sharing information about what can be expected, pointing out varying degrees of success achieved by therapy (no matter how small), helping the patient accept a realistic explanation of why uncontrollable events have occurred, identifying elements in the patient's environment that are more conducive to control, allowing patients to make decisions about different aspects of their care, and eliminating any activities that encourage undue or inappropriate dependency and diminish control (Roberts, 1986; Stoner, 1985).

Hopelessness and Depression

Along with helplessness, feelings of hopelessness have also been identified as one of the major characteristics of depression (Beck, 1967). The uncertainty so prevalent in the cancer experience may be detrimental to keeping the patient hopeful and involved in treatment plans. Therefore, perceived unpredictability concerning the course and outcome of an illness has been shown to have a strong negative effect on the patient's attitude and adjustment during diagnosis and treatment. For example, uncertainty has been associated with a loss of motivation, sadness, depression, fatalism, passivity, giving up, poor expectations about the future, and a pervasive pessimistic attitude (Mishel, Hostetter, King, & Graham, 1984; Roberts, 1986). Hopeless and depressed persons also display a sense of worthlessness and lowered self-esteem; therefore, they feel that they do not matter at all and should not be bothered with.

Hopelessness can be detected through an assessment of patients' lack of self-esteem and of their unrealistic or distorted negative expectations about the future. Using a tool such as the Beck Depression Inventory (Beck, Ward, Mendelson, Mock, & Erbrugh, 1961) early in a cancer treatment program can detect those persons needing structured positive experiences to foster more optimistic attitudes and feelings of personal control. Positive and control-promoting experiences are necessary to counteract these patients' expectations that nothing they do can change the outcome of their cancer situation. Otherwise, the feelings of hopelessness and depression can prove to be a monumental impediment to adjustment because of the immobilizing effect on patient progress in all aspects of treatment (Hughes, 1986b). In fact, a long-term study on breast cancer even showed that those patients who felt hopeless, helpless, and depressed had lower rates of survival at both 5 (Greer et al., 1979) and 10 years after testing (Pettingale, 1984); the same was found in patients with testicular cancer after a 7-year period (Edwards, DiClemente, & Samuels, 1985).

In identifying depression, the nurse should keep in mind that sometimes it is hard to sort out some of the physical symptoms of depression (e.g., anorexia, fatigue, weight loss, sleep disturbance) from symptoms of the cancer itself or from side effects of therapy. Therefore, assessing the presence of the psychological concomitants of depression (hopelessness, helplessness, worthlessness, despair) is important in differentiating symptoms attributable to organic and therapeutic causes from those resulting from depression.

Anger and Hostility

Anger or hostility may be a generalized response to cancer not specifically directed toward anyone or anything in particular, or it may be focused on someone specific or on some particular aspect of the disease or therapy (Roberts, 1986). Feelings of anger may also be accompanied by a sense of frustration and unfairness at being stricken with cancer. Persons who especially tend to display feelings of anger and hostility are those who have followed all the precautionary measures that are promulgated as protective against serious illness (e.g., eating right, exercising, avoiding known carcinogens, and living life in moderation) but nonetheless develop cancer. Conversely, anger directed inwardly might be found in persons who failed to heed the advice of the health community and subsequently developed cancer—for example, those who continued to smoke despite warnings from health care providers. In addition, people who have been very active and athletic before the diagnosis of cancer also might become angry at the thought of the dependency enforced by chronic illness. Thus anger sometimes serves to mask the feelings of powerlessness that patients with serious illness often experience (Roberts, 1986).

The persistence of anger in patients with cancer can lead to a diversion of energy away from constructive coping with illness-related problems to inappropriate blaming of others for existing problems; it also can cause significant others to shy away from contact with the patient, thereby adding the problem of social isolation. Patients therefore need to be helped to identify the reasons for and objects of their anger, to learn to express anger in nondestructive ways, and

then be helped to redirect hostile feelings into more constructive channels (Roberts, 1986). The patient also needs to know that anger is a normal reaction to cancer.

Health professionals have long held the belief that repressed anger is more dangerous than ventilated anger; this led to the development of various cathartic techniques, both verbal and physical, for promoting the expression of anger. However, ventilatory techniques for handling anger have been found to be more effective when they are combined with cognitive restructuring techniques in which the person is taught to reinterpret feelings and events in a new light (Murray, 1985). Although most health professionals see anger as an undesirable reaction to stress (often because the patient seems more difficult to handle), it should be pointed out that two studies (Derogatis, Abeloff, & Melisaratos, 1979; Greer et al., 1979) have indicated that breast cancer patients who expressed anger and hostility (i.e., displayed a fighting spirit) had better survival rates. Therefore, "getting up the patient's dander" may help by stimulating the emotional energy needed to motivate the patient to deal with problems more actively, rather than handling problems with passive avoidance or a feeling of helplessness.

METHODS FOR PROMOTING EFFECTIVE PATIENT COPING

A primary role for oncology nurses is to facilitate a functional coping process in patients under their care; therefore, nurses should help patients to use their coping abilities more effectively (McNally, Stair, & Somerville, 1985). The need for periodic alterations and adjustments in coping should be kept in mind and monitored because of the chronic nature of cancer with its recurring acute episodes. Further, nurses need to recognize the uniqueness of the individual cancer patient and to encourage and support those constructive coping activities that seem to work best for that patient. For cancer patients with a nursing diagnosis of ineffective coping, Doublsky (1985) suggests that nurses focus on stressors and responses to them during therapeutic interactions and also try to reinforce positive self-care behaviors. For those persons with severely impaired coping and incapacitating psychoemotional behaviors, Doublsky recommends setting limits while at the same time showing positive acceptance of the patient, as well as collaborating with mental health workers to develop individualized therapeutic plans. For the more severe case of ineffective coping, referral to a professional counselor is the appropriate nursing intervention.

In addition to verbal communication with cancer patients about coping strategies, written materials can be used to teach patients new coping skills. Carey and Jevne (1986) have developed an effective teaching program for postmastectomy patients to help them cope with breast cancer. The program includes specific guidelines on dealing with emotions, handling changes in family roles and relationships, encouraging family involvement in care, dealing with problems in sexuality, discussing cancer with other patients, communicating with physicians and family, and developing specific coping skills. The educational materials also advise patients to help friends and family to be comfortable with the cancer diagnosis by giving accurate information without dwelling on the matter and by sharing their feelings and needs.

This teaching program indicates that it helps the patient to know that denial, anger, frustration, guilt, worry, depression, sadness, and fear are all normal reactions to cancer. Suggestions are offered to patients for dealing with these emotions by distracting themselves through activity, by talking with someone with whom they feel comfortable, by solving everyday problems as they arise and not letting them build up, and by learning specific relaxation techniques. For example, to handle anger in an appropriate way without alienating needed social support resources, Carey and Jevne (1986) advise that patients write down their feelings, confide in someone they feel close to, and even hang up some sort of punching bag to serve as a tension-release mechanism. Furthermore, patients are encouraged to use all the support resources they can muster. Other useful suggestions, such as considering a shift in or reduction of responsibilities for a period of time if feeling tired or overwhelmed, are also provided in this helpful educational program.

To enable health care providers to facilitate patients' coping by accomplishing the countercoping tasks of clarification, collaboration, relief, and cooling off, Weisman (1976, 1979, 1984b) suggests the following activities appropriate for nurses: clarify problems for the patient, help patients maintain control by encouraging them to exercise whatever options they have available to them, try to discourage emotional extremes by offering a willing and noncritical ear so that patients can relieve pent-up tensions without fear of retribution, redirect the patient to more constructive channels for releasing anxiety, reduce the problem to manageable size, share concern but without further aggravating the patient's feelings of anxiety, discourage hasty actions, and at times just be comfortable with sharing periods of silence with the patient (see Table 51–3). In these sometimes small but nonetheless effective ways, the nurse can promote the patient's positive adaptation to the stresses of cancer.

In addition, nurses should encourage patients to take advantage of the many resources available for cancer patients, such as the multiple services offered by the American (and regional) Cancer Society and often by local hospitals and community groups. Patients need to be provided with timely information on all such resources. While still hospitalized, patients should be given for future reference a list of the addresses and phone numbers of important local agencies that can serve their many needs. However, it should be kept in mind that patients might not be ready to avail themselves of certain resources when they first learn of them; therefore, patients need to be reminded on an ongoing basis of current resources available in the area, either through newsletters, phone calls, posted notices, pamphlets, or meetings. Any such protocol for informing patients should be systematized so that the distribution of information is not happenstance and left to serendipity.

Patients should also be advised of the various support groups available for cancer patients generally and for their specific type of cancer or operation, such as ostomy patients, laryngectomy patients, and mastectomy patients. Patients should be encouraged to attend such meetings with a partner or friend, so that they can link up with the appropriate self-help support groups available in their area. Again, patients may not be ready for this immediately, so they need to be reminded later that such groups exist and how to contact them.

Furthermore, patients should be informed of the diversity of cognitive and behavioral methods available for controlling the extreme emotional distress and various other problems associated with cancer. These methods include the following: progressive relaxation, meditation, biofeedback, hypnosis, stress inoculation training, systematic desensitization, mental imagery, and various kinds of cognitive restructuring (thought-changing) techniques. (Interested readers are referred to Feuerstein, Labbe, & Kuczmierczyk [1986] and Lazarus & Folkman [1984] for an overview of these techniques.) Not all patients may be attuned to using such techniques, nor do all patients benefit equally from them; nevertheless, patients should be apprised of the existence of such methods for handling tension and anxiety. Preliminary studies (Cunningham, 1986) do indicate that some of these methods also seem useful for controlling the pain of cancer and the nausea and vomiting associated with chemotherapy.

Some programs have combined several of the aforementioned cognitive approaches for use with cancer patients; examples are the Exceptional Cancer Patient Program in New Haven (a combination of meditation and mental imagery) and the Cancer Self-Help Program in Toronto (a combination of relaxation, meditation, mental imagery, and cognitive self-help techniques) (Cunningham, 1986). So far, the results of studies on the efficacy of many of the approaches already mentioned have been either equivocal or positive but not replicated. Moreover, some approaches have not been tested systematically. Because many of these methods are fairly new (or at least not yet widely used) and are still undergoing development and implementation, it is too early to say which of these cognitive approaches will prove to be the most fruitful for cancer patients.

SUMMARY

Owing to the complexity of the coping process and to the magnitude and diversity of stressors with which patients with cancer have to deal, oncology nurses have a substantial challenge facing them if they are to help their patients cope more effectively with their illness and its treatment. The oncology nurse is indeed one of the most significant professional support systems available to the patient with cancer because the nurse has the most frequent contact with the patient, possesses the critical skills and knowledge for facilitating the adaptive process in patients with cancer, and is wholeheartedly invested in the premise of holistic cancer care. Therefore, no nursing care plan should be without specific goals and activities directed toward helping the patient with cancer achieve the highest adaptive level possible in dealing with illness and its treatment.

References

Adams, J. (1979). Mutual-help groups: Enhancing the coping ability of oncology clients. *Cancer Nursing, 2,* 95–98.

Anderson, C. R. (1977). Locus of control, coping behaviors, and performance in a stress setting: A longitudinal study. *Journal of Applied Psychology, 62,* 446–451.

Asterita, M. F. (1985). *The physiology of stress.* New York: Human Sciences Press.

Averill, J. (1973). Personal control of aversive stimulation and its relation to stress. *Psychological Bulletin, 80,* 286–303.

Bandura, A. (1977). Self-efficacy: Toward a unifying theory of behavioral change. *Psychological Review, 84,* 191–215.

Beck, A. T. (1967). *Depression: Clinical, experimental and theoretical aspects.* New York: Harper & Row Publishers, Inc.

Beck, A. T., Ward, C. H., Mendelson, M., Mock, J., & Erbaugh, J. (1961). An inventory for measuring depression. *Archives of General Psychiatry, 4,* 561–571.

Brissett, M., & Nowicki, S., Jr. (1973). Internal versus external control of reinforcement and reaction to frustration. *Journal of Personality and Social Psychology, 25,* 35–44.

Burish, T. G., Meyerowitz, B. E., Carey, M. P., & Morrow, G. R. (1987). The stressful effects of cancer in adults. In A. Baum & J. E. Singer (Eds.), *Handbook of psychology and health. Vol. 5: Stress* (pp. 137–173). Hillsdale, NJ: Erlbaum.

Campbell, P. A., & Cohen, J. J. (1985). Effects of stress on the immune response. In T. M. Field, P. M. McCabe, & N. Schneiderman (Eds.), *Stress and coping* (pp. 135–145). Hillsdale, NJ: Erlbaum.

Carey, R. L., & Jevne, R. (1986). Development of an information package for post-mastectomy patients on adjuvant therapy. *Oncology Nursing Forum, 13*(3), 78–83.

Cohen, F., & Lazarus, R. S. (1979). Coping with the stresses of illness. In G. C. Stone, F. Cohen, & N. E. Adler (Eds.), *Health psychology: A handbook* (pp. 217–254). San Francisco: Jossey-Bass.

Cohen, S., & Syme, S. L. (Eds.). (1985). *Social support and health.* New York: Academic Press.

Cunningham, A. J. (1986). Psychological self-help by cancer patients. In B. A. Stoll (Ed.), *Coping with cancer stress* (pp. 131–142). Dordrecht, Netherlands: Martinus Nijhoff.

Dennis, K. E. (1987). Dimensions of client control. *Nursing Research, 36,* 151–156.

Derogatis, L. T., Abeloff, M. D., & Melisaratos, N. (1979). Psychological coping mechanisms and survival time in metastatic breast cancer. *Journal of the American Medical Association, 242,* 1504–1508.

Dodd, M. J. (1984). Measuring informational intervention for chemotherapy knowledge and self-care behavior. *Research in Nursing and Health, 7,* 43–50.

Doublsky, J. (1985). Ineffective individual coping. In J. C. McNally, J. C. Stair, & E. T. Somerville (Eds.), *Guidelines for cancer nursing practice* (pp. 62–65). Orlando, FL: Grune & Stratton, Inc.

Dunkel-Schetter, C. (1984). Social support and cancer: Findings based on patient interviews and their implications. *Journal of Social Issues, 40,* 77–98.

Edwards, J., DiClemente, C., & Samuels, M. L. (1985). Psychological characteristics: A pretreatment survival marker of patients with testicular cancer. *Journal of Psychosocial Oncology, 3,* 79–94.

Feuerstein, M., Labbe, E. E., & Kuczmierczyk, A. R. (1986). *Health psychology: A psychobiological perspective.* New York: Plenum.

Fisher, S. (1986). *Stress and strategy.* Hillsdale, NJ: Erlbaum.

Folkman, S., & Lazarus, R. S. (1980). An analysis of coping in a middle-aged community sample. *Journal of Health and Social Behavior, 21,* 219–239.

Folkman, S., Lazarus, R. S., Dunkel-Schetter, C., DeLongis, A., & Gruen, R. J. (1986). Dynamics of a stressful encounter: Cognitive appraisal, coping, and encounter outcomes. *Journal of Personality and Social Psychology, 50,* 992–1003.

Follick, M. J., Smith, T. W., & Turk, D. C. (1984). Psychosocial adjustment following ostomy. *Health Psychology, 3,* 505–517.

Frankenhaeuser, M. (1980). Psychobiological aspects of life stress. In S. Levine & H. Ursin (Eds.), *Coping and health* (pp. 203–223). New York: Plenum.

Funch, D. P., & Marshall, J. R. (1983). The role of stress, social support and age in survival from breast cancer. *Journal of Psychosomatic Research, 27,* 77–83.

Gordon, W. A., Freidenbergs, I., Diller, L., Hibbard, M., Wolf, C., Levine, L., Lipkins, R., Ezrachi, O., & Lucido, D. (1980). Efficacy of psychosocial intervention with cancer patients. *Journal of Consulting and Clinical Psychology, 48,* 743–759.

Greer, S., Morris, T., & Pettingale, K. W. (1979). Psychological response to breast cancer: Effect on outcome. *Lancet, 2,* 758–787.

Hickey, S. S. (1986). Enabling hope. *Cancer Nursing, 9,* 133–137.

Hughes, J. (1986a). Denial in cancer patients. In B. A. Stoll (Ed.), *Coping with cancer stress* (pp. 63–70). Dordrecht, Netherlands: Martinus Nijhoff.

Hughes, J. (1986b). Depression in cancer patients. In B. A. Stoll (Ed.), *Coping with cancer stress* (pp. 53–62). Dordrecht, Netherlands: Martinus Nijhoff.

Jalowiec, A. (1987). *Changes in the revised Jalowiec Coping Scale.* Unpublished manuscript, Loyola University of Chicago.

Johnson, J. (1982). The effects of a patient education course on persons with a chronic illness. *Cancer Nursing, 5,* 117–123.

Katz, J. L., Weiner, H., Gallagher, T. F., & Hellman, L. (1970). Stress distress and ego defenses: Psychoendocrine response to impending breast tumor biopsy. *Archives of General Psychiatry, 23,* 131–142.

Keane, A., Ducette, J., & Adler, D. (1985). Stress in ICU and non-ICU nurses. *Nursing Research, 34,* 231–236.

Kobasa, S. C. (1979). Stressful life events, personality, and health: An inquiry into hardiness. *Journal of Personality and Social Psychology, 37,* 1–11.

Kobasa, S. C. (1982). Commitment and coping in stress resistance among lawyers. *Journal of Personality and Social Psychology, 42,* 707–717.

Kobasa, S. C., Maddi, S. R., & Kahn, S. (1982). Hardiness and health: A prospective study. *Journal of Personality and Social Psychology, 42,* 168–177.

Lane, C. A., & Davis, A. W. (1985). Implementation: WE CAN weekend in the rural setting. *Cancer Nursing, 8,* 323–328.

Langer, E. J. (1983). *The psychology of control.* Beverly Hills, CA: Sage.

Lazarus, R. S. (1966). *Psychological stress and the coping process.* New York: McGraw-Hill Book Co.

Lazarus, R. S. (1983). The costs and benefits of denial. In S. Breznitz (Ed.), *Denial of stress* (pp. 1–30). New York: International Universities Press.

Lazarus, R. S. (1987, May). *Stress and coping in health and illness: Implications for expert nursing practice.* Paper presented at the Stress, Coping, and Caring Conference, University of California, Berkeley.

Lazarus, R. S., & Folkman, S. (1984). *Stress, appraisal, and coping.* New York: Springer-Verlag.

Lee, H. J. (1983). Analysis of a concept: Hardiness. *Oncology Nursing Forum, 10*(4), 32–35.

Lee, M. S. (1986). Monitoring of coping. In B. A. Stoll (Ed.), *Coping with cancer stress* (pp. 113–121). Dordrecht, Netherlands: Martinus Nijhoff.

Lefcourt, H. M. (1982). *Locus of control: Current trends in theory and research* (2nd ed.). Hillsdale, NJ: Erlbaum.

Lewis, F. M. (1982). Experienced personal control and quality of life in late-stage cancer patients. *Nursing Research, 31,* 113–119.

Lichtman, R. R., Wood, J., & Taylor, S. (1982, August). *Close relationships after breast surgery.* Paper presented at the annual meeting of the American Psychological Association, Washington, DC.

Marks, G., Richardson, J. L., Graham, J. W., & Levine, A. (1986). Role of health locus of control beliefs and expectations of treatment efficacy in adjustment to cancer. *Journal of Personality and Social Psychology, 51,* 443–450.

Mason, J. W. (1975). Emotion as reflected in patterns of endocrine integration. In L. Levi (Ed.), *Emotions: Their parameters and measurement* (pp. 143–181). New York: Raven Press.

McNally, J. C., Stair, J. C., & Somerville, E. T. (Eds.). (1985). *Guidelines for cancer nursing practice.* Orlando, FL: Grune & Stratton, Inc.

Miaskowski, C. A., & Nielsen, B. (1985). A cancer nursing assessment tool. *Oncology Nursing Forum, 2*(6), 37–42.

Miller, J. F. (1983). *Coping with chronic illness: Overcoming powerlessness.* Philadelphia: F. A. Davis Co.

Mishel, M. H., Hostetter, T., King, B., & Graham, V. (1984). Predictors of psychosocial adjustment in patients newly diagnosed with gynecological cancer. *Cancer Nursing, 7,* 291–299.

Moos, R. H. (Ed.). (1986). *Coping with life crises: An integrated approach.* New York: Plenum.

Murray, E. J. (1985). Coping and anger. In T. M. Field, P. M. McCabe, & N. Scheiderman (Eds.), *Stress and coping* (pp. 243–261). Hillsdale, NJ: Erlbaum.

Oncology Nursing Society. (1979). *Outcome standards for cancer nursing practice.* Kansas City, MO: American Nurses' Association.

Orr, E. (1986). Open communication as an effective stress management method for breast cancer patients. *Journal of Human Stress, 12,* 175–185.

Padilla, G. V., & Grant, M. M. (1985). Quality of life as a cancer nursing outcome variable. *Advances in Nursing Science, 8*(1), 45–60.

Parkes, K. R. (1984). Locus of control, cognitive appraisal, and coping in stressful episodes. *Journal of Personality and Social Psychology, 46,* 655–668.

Pettingale, K. W. (1984). Coping and cancer prognosis. *Journal of Psychosomatic Research, 28,* 363–364.

Pollock, S. E. (1986). Human responses to chronic illness: Physiologic and psychosocial adaptation. *Nursing Research, 35,* 90–95.

Roberts, S. L. (1986). *Behavioral concepts and the critically ill patient* (2nd ed.). Norwalk, CT: Appleton-Century-Crofts.

Rosenbaum, M. (1983). Learned resourcefulness as a behavioral repertoire for the self-regulation of internal events: Issues and speculations. In M. Rosenbaum, C. M. Franks, & Y. Jaffe (Eds.), *Perspectives on behavior therapy in the eighties* (pp. 54–73). New York: Springer-Verlag.

Rotter, J. B. (1966). Generalized expectancies for internal versus external control of reinforcement. *Psychological Monographs, 80*(609).

Saunders, J. M., & McCorkle, R. (1987). Social support and coping with lung cancer. *Western Journal of Nursing Research, 9,* 29–42.

Scott, D. W., Oberst, M. T., & Bookbinder, M. I. (1984). Stress-coping response in genitourinary carcinoma in men. *Nursing Research, 33,* 325–329.

Seligman, M. E. P. (1975). *Helplessness: On depression, development, and death.* San Francisco: W. H. Freeman.

Selye, H. (1957). *The stress of life.* London: Longmans, Green.

Silberfarb, P. M., & Greer, S. (1982). Psychological concomitants of cancer: Clinical aspects. *American Journal of Psychotherapy, 36,* 470–478.

Smith, M. B. (1983). Hope and despair: Keys to the socio-psychodynamics of youth. *American Journal of Orthopsychiatry, 53,* 388–399.

Sobel, H. J., & Worden, J. W. (1981). *Helping cancer patients cope: A problem-solving intervention for health care professionals.* New York: BMA Audio Cassettes, Guilford Publishers.

Stoll, B. A. (Ed.). (1986). *Coping with cancer stress.* Dordrecht, Netherlands: Martinus Nijhoff.

Stoner, C. (1985). Learned helplessness: Analysis and application. *Oncology Nursing Forum, 12*(1), 31–35.

Strickland, B. R. (1978). Internal-external expectancies and health-related behaviors. *Journal of Consulting and Clinical Psychology, 46,* 1192–1211.

Taylor, S. E., Lichtman, R. R., & Wood, J. V. (1984). Attributions, beliefs about control, and adjustment to breast cancer. *Journal of Personality and Social Psychology, 46,* 489–502.

Thompson, S. C. (1981). Will it hurt less if I can control it? A complex answer to a simple question. *Psychological Bulletin, 90,* 89–101.

Tilden, V. P., & Galyen, R. D. (1987). Cost and conflict: The darker side of social support. *Western Journal of Nursing Research, 9,* 9–18.

Wallston, K. A., & Wallston, B. S. (1981). Health locus of control scales. In H. M. Lefcourt (Ed.), *Research with the locus of control construct. Vol. 1: Assessment methods* (pp. 189–243). New York: Academic Press.

Wallston, K. A., Wallston, B. S., & DeVellis, R. (1978). Development of the Multidimensional Health Locus of Control Scales. *Health Education Monographs, 6,* 161–170.

Weiner, B. (1972). *Theories of motivation.* Chicago: Rand McNally.

Weisman, A. D. (1976). Early diagnosis of vulnerability in cancer patients. *American Journal of the Medical Sciences, 271,* 187–196.

Weisman, A. D. (1979). *Coping with cancer.* New York: McGraw-Hill Book Co.

Weisman, A. D. (1984a). *The coping capacity: On the nature of being mortal.* New York: Human Sciences Press.

Weisman, A. D. (1984b). A model for psychosocial phasing in cancer. In R. H. Moos (Ed.), *Coping with physical illness. Vol. 2: New perspectives* (pp. 107–122). New York: Plenum.

Welch, D., Follo, J., & Nelson, E. (1982). The development of a specialized nursing assessment tool for cancer patients. *Oncology Nursing Forum, 9*(1), 37–44.

Wortman, C. B., & Dunkel-Schetter, C. (1987). Conceptual and methodological issues in the study of social support. In A. Baum & J. E. Singer (Eds.), *Handbook of psychology and health. Vol. 5: Stress* (pp. 63–108). Hillsdale, NJ: Erlbaum.

Young, S. (1986). The exceptional cancer patient support group: Coping with cancer. *Journal of Holistic Nursing, 4*(1), 6–13.

CHAPTER 52

Alterations in Body Image

NANCY BURNS
BARBARA C. HOLMES

The theory of body image has been used commonly, in nursing and other disciplines, in efforts to explain the nature and behavior of the person. Body image changes probably occur in most individuals with cancer, and if these changes are not effectively integrated with the self system, they can greatly diminish the quality of life. Nursing actions, based on a thorough knowledge of body image theory, may be able to facilitate healthy management of body image changes by the person with cancer, the family, and the patient's social system. This chapter explores the theoretic notions of body image; presents current knowledge from measurement and research related to body image; and explores the health consequences of alterations in body image. The nursing care of persons who are at risk of, or who experiencing, difficulty in integrating body image changes within their self structure is discussed within a nursing process framework.

THE DEVELOPMENT OF THEORETIC THOUGHT ABOUT BODY IMAGE

The recognition of body image as a mental construct first became apparent through the reported experiences of phantom body parts after amputations. The inability of persons with amputated limbs to perceive their bodies as they actually existed stimulated attempts to explain the phenomenon by scientists from a variety of disciplines. Freud (1961 [1927]), in developing his psychoanalytic theory, referred to body image phenomenon, which he considered to be an element of the ego, as "body-ego." Freud explained the emergence of the body-ego primarily in terms of stages of sexual development. Head (1920), a neurologist, explained body image in terms of brain and neurologic function. From this perspective, the body image develops from infancy as a result of sensory experiences and motor activities. As a portion of the body moves, the person relates both the new position of the body part and the sensation of moving it to the overall posture of the body. These experiences are accumulated, stored in the sensory cortex of the brain, and integrated with present experiences to result in the body image, which operates outside of consciousness. The body image allows the person to relate the posture of the body to objects in the environment (Jacobson, 1964). This perspective of body image includes four elements: awareness of parts of the body, perception of the relative size of parts of the body, awareness of positions of body parts, and sensation related to body parts (Arseni, Botez, & Maretsis, 1966).

Schilder (1935) built on Head's theory to include the person's personal investment in various body parts and environmental influences as factors influencing body image. He expanded Head's postural image to include sensations from the skeleton, muscles, nerves, and viscera in adding to the image of the body. Schilder proposed that people form a picture of their body appearance within their minds. This picture includes interpersonal, environmental, and temporal factors. People's views of their bodies are, in part, determined by the perceptions of their bodies by other persons in their environment, which are communicated to them. Schilder believed that people not only perceive a body image but express a body image. Several theorists suggest that the body and its parts are viewed by the self, or the ego, as an object (Johnson, 1976; Metcalfe & Fischman, 1985; Schilder, 1935). From this perspective, the body is viewed as a thing apart from the ego. Szasz (1957) also proposed that, with maturity, came an increasingly complex body-ego integration.

Fisher (1968, 1970, 1973) suggests that there are several elements of body image: body boundary (or border), body awareness, and meanings the person places on various body parts. Fisher has developed instruments to measure each of these three elements of body image; his research indicated that they are not correlated. Fisher also found that the body image boundary may extend beyond the person to include clothing, jewelry, and even such things as the car the person drives (Crumbaugh, 1968). The space around the person and the belongings within that space may be considered part of the body image (Fisher, 1970, 1973; Horowitz, 1966). The degree of perceived vulnerability of the body or particular parts of the body is also a part of body image. Schain and Howards (1985) included two parts of the "body self": the functional self (what I can do) and the aesthetic self (what I look like).

The body image develops gradually as the person matures (Anthony, 1971; Erikson, 1963). Erikson (1963, 1980) has described the gradual development of the body image during childhood, using Freud's perspective of the body as primarily a sexual entity. This development perspective is commonly used in nursing (Blaesing & Brockhaus, 1972; Dempsey, 1972; Murray, 1972a,b). Derogatis (1980) disagrees with this point of view and proposes that body image and sexuality are separate but related elements that influence a person's identity.

From experiences that begin in childhood, persons learn to place different values on various parts of their body (Fisher, 1968, 1970, 1973; Fry, 1980). Many persons learn to view parts of their body as dirty. Dirtiness carries with it a feeling of disgust (Kubie, 1937). It is often not acceptable to touch these parts of the body or look at them. Other body parts are highly valued and may be highlighted by body posture. Hair styling, cosmetics, and clothing may be selected to proudly display these body parts. The valuing of particular body parts varies to some extent from one person to another, from one culture to another, and from one period of time to another (Mead, 1934; Pricer, 1986; Quinn, 1984; Schonfeld, 1963).

Body image is related to self-esteem, self-concept, and identity (Mathes & Kahn, 1975; Rubin, 1968). High self-esteem is a feeling of worthiness. Body image and self-esteem have been found to be highly correlated. Individuals who have poor body image also tend to have low self-esteem. Self-concept has been defined as the composite of all the feelings a person has about the self. From this point of view, body image and self-esteem are considered elements of self-concept. Others consider the four concepts as separate but constantly interacting. Schain and Howards (1985) suggest that there are four components of self-concept: (1) the body self, (2) the interpersonal self (the interaction between self and others), (3) the achieving self (goals and aspirations), and (4) the identification self (values, ethics, beliefs, spiritual behavior, and ethnic views). Self-concept and identity are sometimes viewed as interchangeable concepts. Tabachnick (1967) suggests that identity has two elements: (1) social definition, which defines the relationship with the outside world, and (2) self-realization, which reflects inner autonomy and is manifested by adherence to personal goals. Problems arise when the balance between these two elements of identity is disrupted (Weigert & Hastings, 1977).

MEASURING AND STUDYING BODY IMAGE

Numerous instruments have been developed to measure body image or specific dimensions of body image (Table 52–1). The most frequently used instrument is the Body Cathexis Scale developed by Secord and Jourard (1953). For more information about this scale, see Box 52–1. Many of the instruments have interesting potential for increasing understanding of body image.

A burst of research activity related to body image occurred in the 1960s and early 1970s. Some of these studies indicated that evaluations of body appearance and attractiveness of others were closely related to expectations of their performance and judgments of their worth (Berscheid, Walster, & Gohrnstedt, 1972; Dion, Berscheid, & Walster, 1972; Dipboye, Fromkin, & Wiback, 1975; Doúty, Moore, & Hartford, 1974; Efran, 1974; Landy & Sigall, 1974). These judgments of others based on their appearance begin in childhood (Richardson, Goodman, Hastorf, & Dornbusch, 1961) and seem to be so ingrained that Fisher (1973) believes it is not possible to change them.

In recent years, studies have moved from defining body image to examining the dynamics of body image in persons with birth defects, obesity, injuries, or surgery (Boren, 1985; Boren & Meell, 1985; Denning, 1982; Dropkin, 1979a; 1979b, 1981, 1985; Hoover, 1984; Kalick, Goldwyn, & Noe, 1981; Lewis, 1978; Orbach & Tallent, 1965; Piff, 1986; Polivy, 1974). In the area of cancer, women with mastectomies have been the most frequently studied. Twenty years ago, studies indicated serious, unresolved body image problems in women who had undergone a radical mastectomy. More recent studies, however, do not bear out these findings (Andersen & Jochimsen, 1985; Krouse & Krouse, 1981; Morris, Greer, & White, 1977; Polivy, 1977; Ray, 1977; Renneker & Cutler, 1952; Sanger & Reznikoff, 1981). Krouse and Krouse (1981) suggest that older studies used a case study approach and interpreted the results within psychodynamic theories, assuming that the most serious threat to body image occurred because of the sexual symbolism of the breast. More recent studies, using repeated measure designs that follow the subjects over a 1- to 5-year period, have been able to describe a process of body image change. The results indicate that body image changes do not occur immediately but appear 2 to 6 months later (Krouse & Krouse, 1981; Polivy, 1977). Three fourths of women integrate these changes by 1 year after surgery (Morris et al., 1977; West, 1977).

Three factors may be involved in the different findings of more recent studies. First, the treatment (and prognosis) have changed. Overall, breast cancer is being identified earlier, and surgery tends to be more conservative, which results in less impact on body function. Surgical treatment is often accompanied by chemotherapy or radiation, or both. Second, psychosocial care after mastectomy has improved greatly over

Table 52–1. BODY IMAGE MEASUREMENT METHODS

Author	Measure	Studies in Which Measure Is Used
Secord (1953)	Word association procedure using homonyms	Sanger & Reznikoff (1981)
Osgood, Suci, & Tannenbaum (1957)	Body Attitude Scale	Collingwood & Willett (1971)
Secord & Jourard (1953)	Body-Cathexis Scale	Mahoney (1974), Bille (1977), Baxley, Erdman, Henry, Roof (1984), Schwab, Harmeling (1968), Wagner, Bye (1979), Sanger, Reznikoff (1981), Ray (1977), Gerard (1982)
Fisher & Cleveland (1968)	Body Boundary Scale	Sewell & Edwards (1980)
Fisher & Cleveland (1968)	Body Awareness Scale	Sewell & Edwards (1980)
Fisher & Cleveland (1968)	Body Values Scale	Sewell & Edwards (1980)
Fisher & Cleveland (1968)	Rorschach method of measuring body boundaries	Fisher (1967), Sanger & Reznikoff (1981)
Schwab & Harmeling (1968)	Body-Image Test	
Rosen & Ross (1968)	Satisfaction with Body Appearance	Lerner, Karabenick, & Stuart (1973)
Rosen & Ross (1968)	Importance of Body Parts	Lerner, Karabenick, & Stuart (1973), Mahoney (1974)
Rosen & Ross (1968)	Importance of Body Parts in Evaluating Attractiveness of Others	Lerner, Karabenick, & Stuart (1973)
Berscheid, Walster, & Gohrnstedt (1972)	Body Image Questionnaire	Polivy (1977), Krouse & Krouse (1981), Krouse & Krouse (1982)
Tzeng (1975)	Present Body Image	Tzeng (1977), Champion, Austin, & Tzeng (1982)
Tzeng (1975)	Ideal Body Image	Tzeng (1977), Champion, Austin, & Tzeng (1982)
Allebeck, Hallberg, & Espmark (1976)	Direct measure of body image by television apparatus	
McCloskey (1976)	Body Image Assessment Tool	
Derogatis & Melisaratos (1979)	BODY (subscale of DSFI)	Andersen & Jochimsen (1985)
Schlacter (cited in Fawcett & Frye [1980])	Topographic device to measure perceived body space	Fawcett & Frye (1980), Fawcett & Chodil (1978)
Kurtz (cited in Fawcett & Frye [1980])	Body Attitude Scale	
Baird (1985)	Baird Body Image Assessment Tool	
deHaes, van Oostrom, & Welvaart (1986)	Impact of Illness on Body Image	

DSFI, Derogatis Sexual Functioning Inventory.

the last 20 years, which could perhaps have affected the severity of body image changes. Third, precision and objectiveness of measurement of body image in studies have improved, allowing more accurate interpretation of findings.

Of importance is the need to identify those persons at risk of being unsuccessful in integrating body image changes. Depression and emotional lability before the surgery may be predictive of poor adjustment in the following year (Morris et al., 1977). Those patients who experienced phantom breast syndrome also may have greater problems integrating an altered body image (Christensen, Blichert-Toft, Giersing, Richardt, & Bechmann, 1982). Persons who are dissatisfied with many body parts rather than just those affected by the illness also tend to have difficulty integrating an altered body image. This negative feeling toward the whole body can be related to high levels of emotional distress (Kolb, 1959; Leonard, 1972; Schwab & Harmeling, 1968).

Women with gynecologic surgery for cancer, who are frequently used as a comparison group in studies of women with mastectomies, experience much greater difficulty integrating an altered body image than women with mastectomies. Although the appearance of the body does not change after gynecologic surgery, its functioning may have changed in ways that are important to these people. Alopecia has also been associated with negative scores on body image scales (Baxley, Erdman, Henry, & Roof, 1984; Wabrek & Gunn, 1984; Wagner & Bye, 1979).

HEALTH CONSEQUENCES OF ALTERATIONS IN BODY IMAGE

An alteration in body image occurs over time, to some extent is an unconscious process, and needs to be integrated within the self system. This process requires emotional energy, which could otherwise be invested in other pursuits. Reality, for that person, has changed, and uncertainty has increased. To some, it must seem as if their personal world is being torn asunder (Hart & Kenney, 1981). The process of restructuring the body image may involve changing (1) the image of the body contained within the brain, (2) body posture, (3) body movement, and (4) body function. The person must then determine the personal meaning of the body alteration and evaluate the reaction of members of his or her social support system to the body change. All of these changes must then be integrated within the self structure, with an image of, acceptance of, and love of "this is who I am."

Studies seem to indicate that success in achieving total integration of an altered body image may be related to body image, self-esteem, self-concept, and identity before the alteration of body image (Carter, 1980; Champion, Austin, & Tseng, 1982; Dropkin,

---

Box 52–1. THE BODY-CATHEXIS SCALE

Secord and Jourard define body-cathexis as "the degree of feeling of satisfaction or dissatisfaction with the various parts or processes of the body" (p. 343).

The first part of the scale consists of a listing of 46 parts of the body and body functions. Examples of items are hair, ears, energy level, profile, skin texture, sex activities. Each item is followed by a scale of 1 through 5. The numbers represent the following feelings:

1. Have strong feelings and wish change could somehow be made.
2. Don't like, but can put up with.
3. Have no particular feelings one way or the other.
4. Am satisfied.
5. Consider myself fortunate.

The second part of the scale consists of 55 items representing conceptual aspects of the self. Examples of these items are first name, life goals, general knowledge, sensitivity to opinions of others, happiness. These items are rated using the scale described above.

These scales are scored separately by summing the ratings for each item and dividing by the number of items in that part of the scale. This provides a summed score for each person on these two parts of the scale.

Secord and Jourard also report development of a homonym test, which consists of 75 homonyms, some of which have meanings pertaining to the body and some of which do not. Many of the homonyms have meanings pertaining to pain, disease, or bodily injury. Neutral homonyms are interspersed within the list "for purposes of disguise." This test is scored by totaling the number of body responses to the 75 homonyms.

In addition, an anxiety indicator score is obtained, which is scored differently for male and female subjects. Eleven items for which cathexis was most negative for men are summed for men and the eleven items that were most negative for women are summed for women.

Reliabilities for the various scales are moderately high, ranging from 0.63 to 0.92.

Some indications of validity are provided by significant intercorrelations among the various parts of the scale. Concurrent validity is demonstrated by significant correlations between each of the parts of the Body-Cathexis scale and the Maslow Test, which measures insecurity.

The Body-Cathexis scale has been used in many studies examining body image (see citations in Table 52–1).

The scale is useful for appraising the feelings of a person toward his or her body. It could be used to identify persons at high risk for difficulty in managing an alteration in body image or as a measurement tool for research.

(Secord, P. F., & Jourard, S. M. [1953]. The appraisal of body-cathexis: Body-cathexis and the self. *Journal of Consulting Psychology, 17,* 343–347.)

1983; Paine, Alves, & Tubino, 1985; Rosen & Ross, 1968). Because many of the studies have been retrospective and thus have not measured these concepts before the body altering event, there is no clear understanding of how low values on these concepts before the event are associated with inability to integrate a changed body image within the self system. In addition, the effect of such factors as coping skills and effective social support systems before and after a body altering event has not been studied (Brown & Bjelic, 1977).

However, it is clear that failure to integrate a changed body image is associated with long-term depression, difficulty with interpersonal interactions, withdrawal from social interaction, and, overall, a lower quality of life (Beardslee & Sperhac, 1978; deHaes, van Oostrom, & Welvaart, 1986; Krouse, 1985; Krouse & Krouse, 1981, 1982; Ray, 1977; Sewell & Edwards, 1980). This outcome can be life threatening for persons with cancer in that these persons may choose not to continue treatment. The body image change seems to be even more important than life itself. The depression, lack of energy, and overwhelming changes in view of self leave little strength for participating in the fight for life. From the research, it would appear that these consequences are experienced to some degree by about 25 per cent of persons who have a major body alteration (Andersen & Jochimsen,

1985; Polivy, 1974; Schwab & Harmeling, 1968; Scott, 1983).

NURSING ACTIONS RELATED TO PERSONS EXPERIENCING ALTERED BODY IMAGE

It would appear that nurses could influence the outcome of altered body image at two points: (1) during the process of the initial body image changing event, and (2) during the process of integrating the body image into the self structure. The nurse could influence the changing body image through helping the patient think through the meaning of the change, through proposing alternative meanings not considered by the patient, through role modeling healthy responses to the change, through providing positive feedback as a person in the environment reacting to the change, by helping family members and social support system members to examine the meaning of the changes, and by communicating acceptance of the changes to the patient (Hurley, Meyer-Ruppell, & Evans, 1983). Because this process seems to occur over a 2- to 6-month period, ideally, availability of nursing care should extend over this period of time, at least intermittently. Little research has been conducted to determine the effectiveness of interventions during the short period of hospitalization. A few studies do indicate that programs designed to increase knowledge of the body change and how to manage it do make a difference in the person's success in integrating the altered body image (Capone, Good, Westie, & Jacobson, 1980).

CANCER SITUATIONS IN WHICH BODY IMAGE MAY BE ALTERED

The knowledge that a person has cancer affects body image before the initiation of treatment or the obvious changes caused by progression of the disease. The person feels a higher degree of vulnerability, a decreased awareness of what is happening within his or her body, and a decreased power to control these little-understood changes. An anticipation of overwhelming changes in the body, which no personal action can prevent, affects the patient. Following this realization, the person is confronted with major assaults to body image as the consequence of necessary treatments for the cancer and of progression of the disease. Although some body image changes are related to total body function, others differ with the cancer site and treatment choice (Christian, 1982; Clark, 1977; Murray, 1980).

The more obvious alterations in body structure have received the most attention in the literature. This includes cancers of the head and neck (Tierny, 1975), breast (Carroll, 1981; Christensen et al., 1982; deHaes et al., 1986; Gerard, 1982; Kennerly, 1977; Knobf, 1985; Krouse & Krouse, 1981; Miller & Graham, 1975; Morris, 1979; Polivy, 1977; Ray, 1977; Sanger & Reznikoff, 1981; Schain, 1985; Schain et al., 1983; Scott, 1983; Scott & Eisendrath, 1985–1986); reproductive organs (Capone et al., 1980; Krouse, 1985; Sewell & Edwards, 1980), and those involving ostomies (Gallagher, 1972; Riches, 1983). The serious threats to body image caused by such cancers as skin cancer, lung cancer, upper gastrointestinal tract cancers, hepatocarcinoma, leukemia, and lymphomas have not been addressed very extensively in the literature.

Side effects of current treatment methods used in care of the cancer patient can also produce body image changes. The most obvious of these are the mutilating effects of surgery, such as experienced by breast and gynecologic cancer patients. However, any cancer that requires surgery will affect body image. Radiotherapy often leads to such consequences as skin changes, alopecia, vaginal stenosis, changes in bowel habits, changes in urinary frequency, pain, fatigue, nausea and vomiting, and infection. Each of these has an effect on body image. Chemotherapy also produces severe adverse reactions, including stomatitis, nausea and vomiting, alopecia, neurotoxicity, hemorrhaging, infection, fatigue, skin changes, diarrhea, sexual dysfunction, and respiratory dysfunction, all of which alter body image (Baxley, Erdman, Henry, & Roof, 1984;

Beardslee & Miller, 1981; Beardslee & Neff, 1982; Griffiths, 1980).

The cancer process itself produces body image changes as the patient copes with pain, fatigue, weakness, susceptibility to infection, spinal cord compression, septic shock, weight gain, and weight loss (Olson, 1967). The person may be more distressed over the body changes caused by the cancer than by the threat to survival. Because of the nurse's more immediate concern with the patient's survival and comfort, patient difficulties related to body image changes may not be noted or may be discounted. The nurse may not be able to understand how the patient could focus on body image in the midst of a life-threatening crisis when for the patient it may be the most important concern. The focusing of the patient on body image change may be due to denial of impending death, a need for control, or simply that body image is truly the most pressing concern at that time. Although the nurse must continue to address survival and comfort, additional nursing measures must be implemented concurrently to help the patient in managing the alteration in body image.

DETECTING ALTERATIONS IN BODY IMAGE

Because changes in body image apparently do not occur until 2 to 6 months after the actual change in the body, it is not realistic to assess for changes in the body image immediately after diagnosis or surgery. However, it is important for the nurse to make a judgment about the patient's capacity for effectively integrating the body image change when it occurs. Therefore, the initial assessment will be of such factors as self-esteem, self-concept, general coping skills, family dynamics, and social support systems. One purpose of the assessment is to identify patients who are at high risk of experiencing difficulty in managing a body image change. Another purpose is to gather information that can be used to provide guidance to the patient in planning strategies to facilitate effective management of the body image change when it occurs (Norris, 1978).

The body image change generally occurs at a time in which accessibility to nursing care is diminished. If the patient is receiving adjuvant therapy, the nurses in the outpatient clinic or physician's office will have the most contact during this critical period. If the patient does not have contact with the nurse, ideally the patient should have been given a source of referral for nursing care before discharge. Then, if problems related to body image emerge, a source of nursing care will be available. The clinical nurse specialist on the oncology unit would be a logical source for this nursing care or for further referral.

In assessing body image changes or risk, the nurse must be aware of both verbal and nonverbal messages the patient is communicating. Rarely will the patient clearly verbalize his or her feelings about the changes that have occurred. In fact, he or she may not be consciously aware of many of these feelings. Cues that patients are experiencing difficulties in dealing with body image changes include changes in patient approaches to their bodies; avoidance of discussion of any possible changes; emphatically discussing the positive aspects while denying or ignoring the negative aspects; displaced anger at staff members or family; depression; and overcompensation, indicated by a desire to help other patients with similar problems when they have not yet resolved their own problems.

It is also important to gather information about the patient from other health professionals. Interaction with nurses who cared for the patient during periods of hospitalization can provide valuable information. Information can come from a variety of sources, including housekeepers, physical therapists, respiratory therapists, and other persons in contact with the patient. Cues gathered by various members of the health care team will provide a much clearer picture of the patient's situation from which to develop effective interventions.

Generally the period from 2 to 6 months after diagnosis of cancer is a time of ongoing treatment or follow-up. It is during this time that patient concerns regarding body image changes emerge. Although sometimes the patient expresses concerns during interaction with the nurse, it may be necessary for the nurse to reintroduce the topic of body image changes. Ongoing contact with other nurses who have previously cared for the patient will enable the nurse to determine what information the patient was given previously, so that the information can be reinforced and expanded. The nurse can also obtain information about the patient's previous coping strategies. Carroll (1981) presents variables likely to influence the patient's perception of the crisis initiated by body image change. These include demographic information, patient expectations, importance of body parts, physical and psychological association of the body part, cultural-social information, perception and quantity of available help, attitudes toward the physician, general health status before the diagnosis, and dream content since diagnosis (Wilbur, 1980).

Open-ended questions can be used to determine the patient's perception of the impact of the cancer experience on his or her life. This can lead to questioning that can stimulate the patient to evaluate the effectiveness of current coping techniques. Questions that have been found to be useful include the following: "What does this diagnosis of cancer mean to you?" "How is it affecting your life?" "How do you feel you are coping with it?" Concurrently with questioning the patient, the nurse can judge whether the patient is avoiding conversation about the impact of the cancer, or, conversely, is intellectualizing the impact. In some cases the patient may expend more energy in wanting to help other patients with similar concerns than in discussing personal concerns.

The types of questions asked of the patient depend on the quality of the nurse-patient relationship. If a working therapeutic relationship has been established, the nurse can proceed with more probing questions (Bard & Sutherland, 1955; Knobf, 1985). Otherwise, relationship-establishing strategies must precede questioning.

The nurse begins by providing factual information, followed by asking questions that require cognition on the part of the patient. Only then does the nurse progress to questions requiring an emotional response on the part of the patient.

Comments and questions that focus directly on the body image changes can be used at this time. These should relate to the patient's particular situation and may include such comments as the following: "Frequently patients are hesitant to resume social relationships after a mastectomy [or colostomy, or head and neck surgery]. Although I see you as being the same person you were, how are you feeling about these changes in your life?" The nurse may share examples of questions previously asked by other patients with the patient. These may include "Will my husband still want me?" "Should I keep my scar covered during intimate times?" "Should I encourage my spouse to touch the altered part?" "What do I tell my children?" (Lamb & Woods, 1981).

Body image changes that affect internal organs, excluding the reproductive organs, or that are caused by symptoms mentioned in the previous section (fatigue, pain, and so forth) are frequently ignored because they are not directly associated with a visual change in the patient's body. In assessing the patient, these aspects must be included. The nurse should question the patient about thoughts or feelings related to the removal of internal organs, such as fears that the patient may have about the removal of the pancreas. Feelings about the self may also be influenced by experiences such as fatigue, pain, or hemorrhaging. Patients may express feelings of lowered self-esteem because of inability to perform tasks in the previous manner.

INTERVENTIONS THAT FACILITATE HEALTHY RESPONSE TO BODY IMAGE CHANGES

Immediately after the body changing event, the patient usually is not concerned with body image changes. This time is more consumed with task-oriented concerns such as physical healing and the struggle for survival. Only after these immediate concerns are addressed will the patient then turn toward the threat to body image initiated by these changes in his or her body.

The first and most important element for effective interventions for managing body image changes is the establishment of a trust relationship between the nurse and the patient. Maximum effectiveness can be achieved through a nurse-patient relationship that is initiated at the time of diagnosis and continues through the period of integration of the altered body image, which, if successful, can be expected to occur between 1 and 2 years later. Effective nursing interventions focus on education, support, counseling, and referral. Within a trust relationship, the more delicate issues of body image changes can be explored (Bard & Sutherland, 1955; Donovan & Girton, 1984; Marten, 1978; Riddle, 1972; Roback, Kirshner, & Roback, 1981–1982).

Initial interventions with a patient in the early stages of treatment for cancer should include educational preparation for the impending body image change. The nurse needs to be knowledgeable about the specific body image changes associated with the patient's situation. Explanation of impending events related to the cancer process and its treatment and the expected impact on body image can be helpful. The nurse should emphasize that reactions to these changes are commonly experienced by patients with the particular diagnosis. Providing information about these changes will set the groundwork for further nurse-patient discussions at a later time.

This also is an ideal time to inform the patient of the availability of peer support groups. The patient needs reinforcement that his or her concerns are normal. To provide effective referral, the nurse must be aware of community resources for peer support. The American Cancer Society, local cancer treatment centers, and local hospitals usually have information about these groups. In some areas of the country, the American Cancer Society's Reach to Recovery and Dialogue programs have peer support groups as part of their services. The United Ostomy Association and the Lost Chord Club also may provide peer support groups.

If the patient does not respond to the nurse's introduction of the topic, the nurse needs to let the patient know that it is permissible to initiate the topic any time he or she chooses. Also, the nurse should reintroduce the topic periodically, to provide the patient with many opportunities to discuss concerns. It is important to implicitly give permission to discuss the topic but not to force discussion. The patient's not responding to the nurse's cues does not necessarily imply lack of integration of body image changes. Some patients are able to integrate the body image changes from their own mental health base and personal resources. This is confirmed by observation of healthy adaptation to the alteration (i.e., touching the altered site, open discussion about the altered body part).

The nurse must also act as advocate in ensuring that the best possible care is given to the alteration site itself to minimize the severity of the body image change. This includes input regarding proper use of equipment (correct bagging techniques of ostomies, correct wound care) and observation of early breakdown of the healing process (early signs of infection, improper suture care, drainage amounts). The knowledgeable, experienced nurse cannot assume that these potential problems will be managed effectively by the physician or the other members of the health care team.

Body image changes frequently are not addressed by the nurse because of time constraints. Dealing with body image changes requires additional time commitment on the part of the nurse that usually is not reflected in the amount of nursing care hours designated in patient classification systems. With a shortage of qualified nurses doing patient care, this aspect frequently gets put on the back burner in favor of "measurable" nursing tasks. A nurse functioning in an expanded role is more likely to have the time necessary for providing these interventions. However, the cost effectiveness of these interventions needs to be documented before institutions or agencies will commit the time required for the care.

Frequently the alteration is so obvious that the nurse assumes that the patient is dealing with it. For example, so much information about breast disease and alteration has been published in the lay press that the nurse may assume that the patient is "educated" about the potential emotional responses to loss of a major body organ.

Body image changes are sometimes not addressed because of the nurse's personal discomfort in dealing with the situation. In addition to knowledge about body image theory, the nurse must have worked through personal dilemmas related to body image (MacElveen-Hoehn & McCorkle, 1985).

Besides expediting assessment, open-ended questions can be used as an intervention. The questioning also serves as permission granting to the patient to talk about the subject. It can be a starting point for family intervention. The inclusion of the family or significant others in assessment and intervention should be decided on in conjunction with the patient. The patient should be allowed to determine when the family is brought into the discussions about the alteration and may need assistance from the nurse in sharing fears or hopes with the family.

If numerous opportunities for the patient to ask questions are provided, repeated explanations of body function changes are possible. This often leads to discussion involving problem-solving techniques, coping options, and evaluation.

EVALUATING THE INTEGRATION OF BODY IMAGE CHANGES

The outcomes of nursing care related to body image changes have not been examined, either clinically or through research. Because of this lack of knowledge, it is difficult to judge the effectiveness of nursing care in this area. Nurses who are actively involved in evaluating interventions for body image changes are doing so from an anecdotal, intuitive perspective. Developing a body of knowledge related to body image changes requires an understanding of desired outcomes. Because the manifestation of these outcomes typically do not occur until many months after the nursing intervention, measuring these outcomes at the present time may not be feasible from a clinical practice perspective. The nurse may not even be in contact with the patient in any manner by the time the changes occur. In terms of nursing practice, it is important that the effectiveness of nursing interventions to facilitate the integration of altered body image be demonstrated.

This can be accomplished only through research. The first step in this endeavor must be to identify measurable, desirable outcomes. These outcomes come from common sense and the nurse's observations of characteristics of patients who have successfully achieved a reintegrated body image. Although it is not certain which outcomes are actually associated with an improvement in body image, the observed outcomes will provide a starting point for research. The second step will require longitudinal studies in which the relationship between nursing interventions and desired outcomes is examined. This requires the development of clearly defined nursing interventions and multiple studies in which their effects on specific outcomes are tested. The third step will be to develop a predictive model of the impact of the nursing interventions. This step is dependent on the identification of effective nursing interventions and outcomes associated with improved body image. Many studies demonstrating a predictable outcome from a specific nursing intervention are needed. With this information, the nurse can use a specific nursing intervention with greater confidence that the desired outcome will be achieved.

From clinical practice we know that there are some patients who are unable or unwilling to incorporate the body image change and thus could be classified as a high-risk group. Within this high-risk group will be some persons who, because of their mental health status, are unable to incorporate the body image change, and other persons who prefer the secondary gains of a poor body image to the benefits of successfully integrating the body image change. Through research, a profile of persons who are unsuccessful in reintegrating altered body image will emerge. This profile can then be used to identify high-risk patients and to determine appropriate nursing interventions.

Recognizing that none of this research has begun, we would like to propose some outcomes which, from our clinical experience, seem to be associated with effective integration of an altered body image.

- Resumption of former life style, including relationships, employment, style of dress
- Verbalization of concerns about body image changes
- Manifestation of healthy coping ability
- Ability to touch, look at, reveal altered body site
- Ability to incorporate necessary changes to allow activity (work, play, sex) to be satisfying
- Change in dream content to reflect reintegration of altered body image
- Incorporation of altered body part as part of the "me" identity
- Evidence of high self-esteem
- Ability to discuss and consider reconstruction
- Willingness to resume sexual relations

Alteration in body images, if not effectively integrated within the self system, can greatly diminish the quality of life. Immediate commencement of concentrated research efforts directed toward identifying appropriate nursing intervention to facilitate the altered body image is of utmost importance. This presents an excellent opportunity for collaboration between nurse clinicians and nurse researchers. Once the knowledge derived from investigational studies is available, patients will benefit immensely from the scientifically based nursing interventions of the skilled professional nurse.

References

Allebeck, P., Hallberg, D., & Espmark, S. (1976). Body image—an apparatus for measuring disturbances in estimation of size and shape. *Journal of Psychosomatic Research, 20,* 583–589.

Andersen, B. L., & Jochimsen, P. R. (1985). Sexual functioning among breast cancer, gynecologic cancer, and healthy women. *Journal of Consulting and Clinical Psychology, 53,* 25–32.

Anthony, E. J. (1971). The child's discovery of his body. In C. B. Kopp (Ed.), *Readings in early development* (pp. 402–424). Springfield, IL: Charles C Thomas.

Arseni, C., Botez, M. I., & Maretsis, M. (1966). Paroxysmal disorders of the body image. *Psychiatric Neurology, 151,* 1–14.

Baird, S. E. (1985). Development of a nursing assessment tool to diagnose altered body image in immobilized patients. *Orthopaedic Nursing, 4*(1), 47–54.

Bard, M., & Sutherland, A. M. (1955). Psychological impact of cancer and its treatment: IV. Adaptation to radical mastectomy. *Cancer: Diagnosis, Treatment, Research, 8,* 656–672.

Baxley, K. O., Erdman, L. K., Henry, E. B., Roof, B. J. (1984). Alopecia: Effect on cancer patients' body image. *Cancer Nursing, 7,* 499–503.

Beardslee, C., & Miller, S. (1981). Reactions of an adolescent girl during the initial period of treatment of a neoplastic disease. *Maternal-Child Nursing Journal, 10,* 175–183.

Beardslee, C., & Neff, J. A. (1982). Body related concerns of children with cancer as compared with the concerns of other children. *Maternal-Child Nursing Journal, 11,* 121–134.

Beardslee, C., & Sperhac, A. (1978). Reaction formation in a preadolescent girl. *Maternal-Child-Nursing, 7,* 31–40.

Berscheid, E., Walster, E., & Gohrnstedt, G. (1972). Body image: A Psychology Today questionnaire. *Psychology Today, 6*(2), 58–66.

Berscheid, E., Walster, E., & Gohrnstedt, G. (1973). The happy American body: A survey report. *Psychology Today, 7*(6), 119–131.

Bille, D. A., (1977). The role of body image in patient compliance and education. *Heart and Lung, 6,* 143–148.

Blaesing, S., & Brockhaus, J. (1972). The development of body image in the child. *Nursing Clinics of North America, 7,* 597–607.

Boren, J. A., (1985). Adolescent adjustment to amputation necessitated by bone cancers. *Orthopaedic Nursing, 4*(5), 30–32.

Boren, J. A., & Meell, H. (1985). Adolescent amputee ski rehabilitation program. *Journal of the Association of Pediatric Oncology Nurses, 2,* 16–23.

Brown, A., & Bjelic, J. (1977). Coping strategies of two adolescents with malignancy. *Maternal-Child Nursing Journal, 6,* 77–85.

Cantor, R. C. (1980). Self-esteem, sexuality and cancer-related stress. *Frontiers of Radiation Therapy Oncology, 14,* 51–54.

Capone, M. A., Good, R. S., Westie, K. S., & Jacobson, A. F. (1980). Psychosocial rehabilitation of gynecologic oncology patients. *Archives of Physical Medicine and Rehabilitation, 61,* 128–132.

Carroll, R. M., (1981). The impact of mastectomy on body image. *Oncology Nursing Forum, 8*(4), 29–32.

Champion, V. L., Austin, J. K., & Tzeng, O. (1982). Assessment of relationship between self-concept and body image using multivariate techniques. *Issues in Mental Health Nursing, 4,* 299–315.

Christensen, K., Blichert-Toft, M., Giersing, U., Richardt, C., & Bechmann, J. (1982). Phantom breast syndrome in young women after mastectomy for breast cancer. *Acta Chirurica Scandinavica, 148,* 351–354.

Christian, B. J. (1982). Immobilization: Psychological aspects. In C. Norris (Ed.): *Concept clarification in nursing* (pp. 341–356). Rockville, MD: Aspen Systems.

Clark, C. C. (1977). *Nursing concepts and processes* (pp. 399–419). Albany, NY: Delmar.

Collingwood, T. R., & Willett, L. (1971). The effects of physical training upon self-concept and body attitude. *Journal of Clinical Psychology, 27,* 411–412.

Crumbaugh, J. (1968, July). The automobile as part of the body-image in America. *Mental Hygiene,* pp. 349–350.

deHaes, J. C. J. M., van Oostrom, M. A., Welvaart, K. (1986). The effect of radical and conserving surgery on the quality of life of early breast cancer patients. *European Journal of Surgical Oncology, 12,* 337–342.

Dempsey, M. O. (1972). The development of body image in the adolescent. *Nursing Clinics of North America, 7,* 609–615.

Denning, D. C., (1982). Head and neck cancer: Our reactions. *Cancer Nursing, 5,* 269–273.

Derogatis, L. R. (1980). Breast and gynecologic cancers: Their unique impact on body image and sexual identity in women. *Frontiers of Radiation Therapy Oncology, 14,* 1–11.

Derogatis, L. R., & Melisaratos, N. (1979). The DSFI: A multidimensional measure of sexual functioning. *Journal of Sex and Marital Therapy, 5,* 244–281.

Dion, K., Berscheid, E., & Walster, E. (1972). What is beautiful is good. *Journal of Personality and Social Psychology, 24,* 285–290.

Dipboye, R. L., Fromkin, H. L., & Wiback, K. (1975). Relative importance of applicant sex, attractiveness, and scholastic standing in evaluation of job applicant résumés. *Journal of Applied Psychology, 60,* 39–43.

Donovan, M. I., & Girton, S. E. (1984). *Cancer care nursing* (2nd ed., pp. 479–356). Norwalk, CT: Appleton-Century-Crofts.

Douty, H. I., Moore, J. B., & Hartford, D. (1974). Body characteristics in relation to life adjustment, body-image and attitudes of college females. *Perceptual and Motor Skills, 39,* 499–521.

Dropkin, M. J. (1979a). Compliance in postoperative head and neck patients. *Cancer Nursing, 2,* 379–384.

Dropkin, M. J. (1979b). Compliant behavior and changed body image. *American Journal of Nursing, 79,* 1249.

Dropkin, M. J. (1981). Changes in body image associated with head and neck cancer. In L. B. Marino (Ed.), *Cancer nursing* (pp. 560–581). St. Louis: C. V. Mosby Co.

Dropkin, M. J. (1983). Body image reintegration and coping effectiveness after head and neck surgery. *The Journal, 2,* 7–16.

Dropkin, M. J. (1985). Rehabilitation after disfigurative facial surgery. *Plastic Surgical Nursing, 5,* 130–134.

Efran, M. G. (1974). The effect of physical appearance on the judgment of guilt, interpersonal attraction, and severity of recommended punishment in a simulated jury task. *Journal of Research in Personality, 8,* 45–54.

Erikson, E. J. (1963). *Childhood and society* (2nd ed.) New York: W. W. Norton & Co.

Erikson, E. J. (1980). *Identity and the life cycle.* New York: W. W. Norton & Co.

Fawcett, J., & Chodil, J. J. (1980). The topographical device: Development and research. In E. Bauwens (Ed.), *Research for clinical nursing: Its strategies and findings* (Monograph Series 1979: Three). Indianapolis, IN: Sigma Theta Tau.

Fawcett, J., & Frye, S. (1980). An exploratory study of body image dimensionality. *Nursing Research, 29,* 324–327.

Fisher, S. (1967). Motivation for patient delay. *Archives of General Psychiatry, 16,* 676–678.

Fisher, S. (1968). *Body image and personality.* New York: Dover Press.

Fisher, S. (1970). *Body experience in fantasy and behavior.* New York: Appleton-Century-Crofts.

Fisher, S. (1973). *Body consciousness: You are what you feel.* Englewood Cliffs, NJ: Prentice-Hall, Inc.

Fisher, S., & Cleveland, S. (1968). *Body image and personality.* New York: Dover.

Freud, S. (1961). *The ego and the id* (vol. 1). London: Hogarth. (Original work published 1927).

Fry, W. (1980, December). A gift of mirrors: An essay in psychological evolution. *North American Review,* pp. 53–58.

Gallagher, A. M. (1972). Body image changes in the patient with a colostomy. *Nursing Clinics of North America, 7,* 669–679.

Gerard, D. (1982). Sexual functioning after mastectomy: Life vs. lab. *Journal of Sex and Marital Therapy, 8,* 305–315.

Griffiths, S. S. (1980). Changes in body image caused by antineoplastic drugs. *Issues in Comprehensive Pediatric Nursing, 4,* 17–27.

Hart, L. K., & Kenney, C. K. D. (1981). Loss of identity control. In L. K. Hart, J. L. Reese, & M. O. Fearing (Eds.), *Concepts common to acute illness* (pp. 9–30). St. Louis: C. V. Mosby Co.

Head, H. (1920). *Studies in neurology.* London: Oxford.

Henker, F. O., III. (1979). Body-image conflict following trauma and surgery. *Psychosomatics, 20,* 812–820.

Henker, F. O., III. (1982). Body image in obstetrics and gynecology. *Obstetrics and Gynecology Annual, 11,* 341–348.

Hoover, M. L. (1984). The self-image of overweight adolescent females: A review of the literature. *Maternal-Child Nursing Journal, 13*(2), 125–137.

Horowitz, M. J. (1966). Body image. *Archives of General Psychiatry, 14,* 456–460.

Hurley, M., Meyer-Ruppel, A., & Evans, E. (1983). Emma needed more than standard teaching. *Nursing, 13*(3), 62–64.

Jacobson, E. (1964). *The self and the object world.* New York: International Universities Press.

Johnson, J. L. (1976). A research brief: The sexual concerns of the cancer patient and his or her spouse. *Counseling and Values, 20,* 186–188.

Kalick, S. M., Goldwyn, R. M., & Noe, J. M. (1981). Social issues and body image concerns of port wine stain patients undergoing laser therapy. *Lasers in Surgery and Medicine. 1,* 205–213.

Kennerly, S. L. (1977). Breast cancer: Confronting one's changed image. "What I've learned about mastectomy." *American Journal of Nursing, 77,* 1430–1432.

Knobf, M. K. T. (1985). Primary breast cancer: Physical consequences and rehabilitation. *Seminars in Oncology Nursing, 1,* 214–224.

Kolb, L. C. (1959). Disturbances of the body-image. In S. Arieti (Ed.), *American handbook of psychiatry* (vol. I, pp. 749–769). New York: Basic Books, Inc.

Krouse, H. J. (1985). A psychological model of adjustment in gynecologic cancer patients. *Oncology Nursing Forum, 12*(6), 45–49.

Krouse, H. J., & Krouse, J. H. (1981). Psychological factors in postmastectomy adjustment. *Psychological Reports, 48,* 275–278.

Krouse, H. J., & Krouse, J. H. (1982). Cancer as crisis: The critical elements of adjustment. *Nursing Research, 31*(2), 96–101.

Kubie, L. S. (1937). The fantasy of dirt. *Psychoanalytic Quarterly, 6,* 388–425.

Lamb, M. A., & Woods, N. F. (1981). Sexuality and the cancer patient. *Cancer Nursing, 4,* 137–144.

Landy, D., & Sigall, H. (1974). Beauty is talent: Task evaluation as a function of performer's physical attractiveness. *Journal of Personality and Social Psychology, 29,* 299–304.

Leonard, B. J. (1972). Body image changes in chronic illness. *Nursing Clinics of North America, 7,* 687–695.

Lerner, R. M. Karabenick, S. A., & Stuart, J. L. (1973). Relations among physical attractiveness, body attitudes, and self-concept in male and female college students. *The Journal of Psychology, 85,* 119–129.

Lewis, C. W. (1978). Body image and obesity. *Journal of Psychiatric Nursing and Mental Health Services. 16,* 22–29.

MacElveen-Hoehn, P., & McCorkle, R. (1985). Understanding sexuality in progressive cancer. *Seminars in Oncology Nursing, 1,* 56–62.

Mahoney, E. R. (1974). Body-cathexis and self-esteem: The importance of subjective importance. *Journal of Psychology, 88,* 27–30.

Marten, L. (1978). Self-care nursing model for patients experiencing radical change in body image. *Journal of Obstetric, Gynecologic and Neonatal Nursing, 7*(6), 9–13.

Mathes, E. W., & Kahn, A. (1975). Physical attractiveness, happiness, neuroticism, and self-esteem. *Journal of Psychology, 90,* 27–30.

McCloskey, J. C. (1976). How to make the most of body image theory in nursing practice. *Nursing, 6*(5), 68–72.

Mead, G. H. (1934). *Mind, self, and society,* Chicago: University of Chicago Press.

Metcalfe, M. C., & Fischman, S. H. (1985). Factors affecting the sexuality of patients with head and neck cancer. *Oncology Nursing Forum, 12*(2), 21–25.

Miller, S. J., & Graham, W. P., III. (1975). Breast reconstruction after radical mastectomy. *American Family Physician, 11,* 97–101.

Morris, T. (1979). Psychological adjustment to mastectomy. *Cancer Treatment Reviews, 6,* 41–61.

Morris, T., Greer, J. S., & White, P. (1977). Psychological and social adjustment to mastectomy: A two-year follow-up study. *Cancer, 40,* 2318–2387.

Murray, J. B. (1980). Psychosomatic aspects of cancer: An overview. *The Journal of Genetic Psychology, 136,* 185–194.

Murray, R. L. E. (1972a). Body image development in adulthood. *Nursing Clinics of North America, 7,* 617–630.

Murray, R. I. E. (1972b). Principles of nursing intervention for the adult patient with body image changes. *Nursing Clinics of North America, 7,* 697–707.

Norris, C. M. (1978). Body image—its relevance to professional nursing. In C. E. Carlson & B. Blackwell (Eds.), *Behavioral concepts and nursing interventions* (2nd ed., pp. 5–36). Philadelphia, J. B. Lippincott Co.

Olson, E. V. (1967). The hazards of immobility. *American Journal of Nursing, 67,* 780–797.

Orbach, C. E., & Tallent, N. (1965). Modification of perceived body and of body concepts. *Archives of General Psychiatry, 12,* 126–135.

Osgood, L., Suci, G., & Tannenbaum, D. (1957). *The measurement of meaning.* Urbana: University of Illinois Press.

Paine, P., Alves, E., & Tubino, P. (1985). Size of human figure drawing and Goodenough-Harris scores of pediatric oncology patients: A pilot study. *Perceptual and Motor Skills, 60,* 911–914.

Piff, C. (1986). Facing up to disfigurement. *Nursing Times, 82*(34), 16–17.

Polivy, J. (1974). Psychological reactions to hysterectomy: A critical review. *American Journal of Obstetrics and Gynecology, 118,* 417–426.

Polivy, J. (1977). Psychological effects of mastectomy on a woman's feminine self-concept. *The Journal of Nervous and Mental Disease, 164,* 77–87.

Price, B. (1986). Body image: Keeping up appearances. *Nursing Times, 82*(40), 58–61.

Quinn, M. (1984). Facts, fallacies and femininity. *Nursing Mirror, 159,* 16–18.

Ray, C. (1977). Psychological implications of mastectomy. *British Journal of Social and Clinical Psychology, 16,* 373–377.

Renneker, R., & Cutler, M. (1952). Psychological problems of adjustment to cancer of the breast. *Journal of the American Medical Association, 148,* 133–138.

Richardson, S. A., Goodman, N., Hastorf, A. H., & Dornbusch, S. M. (1961). Cultural uniformity in reaction to physical disabilities. *American Sociological Review, 26,* 241–247.

Riches, D. (1983). Nursing Mirror clinical forum. 8. Stoma care: Will I have to wear braces? *Nursing Mirror, 157,* vi–viii.

Riddle, I. (1972). Nursing intervention to promote body image integrity in children. *Nursing Clinics of North America, 7,* 654–661.

Roback, H. B., Kirshner, H., & Roback, E. (1981–1982). Physical self-concept changes in a mildly facially disfigured neurofibromatosis patient following communication skill training. *International Journal of Psychiatry in Medicine. 11,* 137–143.

Rosen, G. M., & Ross, A. O. (1968). Relationship of body image to self-concept. *Journal of Consulting and Clinical Psychology, 32,* 100.

Rubin, R. (1968). Body image and self-esteem. *Nursing Outlook, 16,* 20–23.

Sanger, C. K., & Reznikoff, M. (1981). A comparison of the psychological effects of breast-saving procedures with the modified radical mastectomy. *Cancer, 48,* 2341–2346.

Schain, W. S. (1985). Breast cancer surgeries and psychosexual sequelae: Implications for remediation. *Seminars in Oncology Nursing, 1,* 200–205.

Schain, W. S., Edwards, B. K., Gorrell, C. R., de Moss, E. V., Lippman, M. E., Gerber, L. H., & Lichter, A. S. (1983). Psychosocial and physical outcomes of primary breast cancer therapy: mastectomy vs. excisional biopsy and irradiation. *Breast Cancer Research and Treatment, 3,* 377–382.

Schain, W. S., & Howards, S. S. (1985). Sexual problems of patients with cancer. In DeVita, V. T., Jr., Hellman, S., & Rosenberg, S. A. (Eds.), *Cancer: Principles and practice of oncology* (2nd ed., pp. 2066–2082). Philadelphia: J. B. Lippincott Co.

Schilder, P. (1935). *The image and appearance of the human body. Studies in the constructive energies of the psyche.* London: Kegan Paul.

Schonfeld, W. A. (1963). Body-image in adolescents: A psychiatric concept for the pediatrician. *Pediatrics, 3,* 845–855.

Schwab, J. J., & Harmeling, J. D. (1968). Body image and medical illness. *Psychosomatic Medicine, 30,* 51–61.

Scott, D. W. (1983). Quality of life following the diagnosis of breast cancer. *Topics in Clinical Nursing, 4*(4), 20–37.

Scott, D. W., & Eisendrath, S. J. (1985–1986). Dynamics of the recovery process following initial diagnosis of breast cancer. *Journal of Psychosocial Oncology, 3*(4), 53–67.

Secord, P. (1953). Objectification of word association procedures by the use of homonyms: A measure of body cathexis. *Journal of Personality, 21,* 479–495.

Secord, P. F., & Jourard, S. M. (1953). The appraisal of body-cathexis: Body-cathexis and the self. *Journal of Consulting Psychology, 17,* 343–347.

Sewell, H. H., & Edwards, D. W. (1980). Pelvic genital cancer: Body image and sexuality. *Frontiers in Radiation Therapy Oncology, 14,* 35–41.

Silberfarb, P. M. (1977–1978). Psychiatric themes in the rehabilitation of mastectomy patients. *International Journal of Psychiatry in Medicine, 8,* 159–167.

Szasz, T. S. (1957). *Pain and pleasure.* New York: Basic Books, Inc.

Tabachnick, N. (1967). Self-realization and social definition: Two aspects of identity formation. *International Journal of Psychoanalysis, 48,* 68–75.

Taylor, S. E., Lichtman, R. R., Wood, J. V., Bluming, A. Z., Dosik, G. M., & Leibowitz, R. L. (1985). Illness-related and treatment-related factors in psychological adjustment to breast cancer. *Cancer, 55,* 2506–2513.

Tierny, E. A. (1975). Accepting disfigurement when death is the alternative. *American Journal of Nursing, 75,* 2149–2150.

Tzeng, O. C. S. (1975). Differentiation of affective and denotative meaning systems and their influence in personality ratings. *Journal of Personality and Social Psychology, 32,* 978–988.

Tzeng, O. C. S. (1977). Individual differences in self conception. A multivariate approach. *Journal of Perceptual and Motor Skills, 45,* 1119–1124.

Wabrek, A. J., & Gunn, J. L. (1984). Sexual and psychological implications of gynecologic malignancy. *Journal of Obstetric, Gynecologic, and Neonatal Nursing, 13,* 371–376.

Wagner, L., & Bye, M. G. (1979). Body image and patients experiencing alopecia as a result of cancer chemotherapy. *Cancer Nursing, 2,* 365–369.

Weigert, A. J., & Hastings, R. (1977). Identity loss, family and social change. *American Journal of Sociology, 82,* 1171–1185.

West, D. W. (1977). Social adaptation patterns among cancer patients with facial disfigurement resulting from surgery. *Archives of Physical Medical and Rehabilitation, 58,* 473–479.

Wilbur, J. (1980). Sexual development and body image in the teenager with cancer. *Frontier in Radiation Therapy Oncology, 14,* 108–114.

CHAPTER 53

Alterations in Sexuality and Sexual Functioning*

MARGARET A. LAMB

Cancer affects all aspects of a person's life. Most people diagnosed with cancer have concerns about the sexual ramifications of their illness as well as the proposed treatment for their disease (Glasgow, Halfin, & Althausen 1987; Lamb & Woods, 1981; Smith, 1989).

In 1990 approximately 1,040,000 people will be diagnosed as having cancer (American Cancer Society, 1990). More than 5 million Americans who are alive today have a history of cancer. Often health professionals focus on the disease process and its treatment. They may neglect the issue of sexuality because of a lack of information regarding the impact of the disease and its treatment on sexual functioning as well as a generalized feeling of discomfort discussing these issues with clients. This chapter outlines current knowledge regarding the impact of cancer and its treatment on sexual functioning, discusses the psychosocial factors that affect sexual functioning, enhances the practitioner's skills in the assessment and management of alterations in sexual functioning, addresses the special prob-

lems associated with alterations in sexual functioning, and presents related issues and concerns.

SEXUAL FUNCTIONING

General Considerations

Sexuality is a multidimensional, complex phenomenon involving biologic, psychological, interpersonal, and behavioral dimensions. The World Health Organization's Report on Education and Treatment in Human Sexuality (1975) asserts that sexual health is the integration of the somatic, emotional, intellectual, and social aspects of sexual being in ways that are positively enriching and that enhance personality, communication, and love. A wide range of "normal" sexual functioning exists within the population. This spectrum could include the ability to maintain interpersonal relationships to the ability to sustain the closeness of an intimate, sexually active relationship.

Psychosocial Aspects of Sexuality

Optimal sexual functioning relies on the integration of key biopsychosocial components. The psychosocial

*Supported by the National Institutes of Health, National Center for Nursing Research Service Award 1 F31 NR06316-01A1, and The American Cancer Society, Pre-Doctoral Scholarship Program.

elements involved in sexual functioning vary, depending on the developmental stage of the individuals involved. The young adult faces an array of intimacy issues, including learning to give and receive love, choosing whether or not to marry, and choosing a marital or sexual partner or partners (Woods, 1990). In adulthood, the majority of clients will focus on the capacity to give and receive gratification in a stable relationship. This capacity is not only centered around the physiologic aspects of sexuality, to be discussed subsequently, but the individual's concept of self as a sexual being and his or her sex role. Older adults often focus on the critical task of resolving feelings of self-esteem and despair (Woods, 1990). This task includes acceptance of one's life cycle and the social factors that accompanied it. These include emancipating adolescent children, achieving a career peak, and accommodating aging parents. During the later years, from retirement to death, sexual activity and interest persist. Sexual functioning is dependent on relatively good health and an interested and interesting partner. Aging persons may find it necessary to nurture one another, to cope with bereavement and widowhood, and to find new meaning in life (Woods, 1990).

Physiologic Aspects of Sexuality

The psychosocial aspects of sexual functioning are complemented by the biologic components. The human sexual response cycle comprises two principle physiologic changes: vasocongestion and myotonia. Vasocongestion is the congestion of blood vessels, usually venous, and myotonia refers to increased muscular tension (Woods, 1990). These physiologic changes are dependent on an intact neurologic system and an appropriate hormonal milieu.

An accurate assessment of sexual dysfunctions is based on a basic understanding of the normal occurrences in the sexual response cycle. Interventions are used to alleviate or minimize the identified causes of sexual dysfunctions.

Many dysfunctions can be caused by physiologic, psychological, or social variables or a combination of several factors. The discussion of physiologic factors is followed here by the psychosocial implications of cancer and its treatment.

The four major stages in the human sexual response cycle are excitement, plateau, orgasm, and resolution (Masters & Johnson, 1966). Excitement is characterized by the onset of erotic feelings and the attainment of erection in men and vaginal lubrication in women. Plateau is a more advanced stage of excitement in which the sex glands become more engorged and undergo positional changes. A number of extragenital conditions also occur, including color change, respiration shifts, and generalized increase in arousal. Orgasm is experienced as the most intense and pleasurable aspect of the sexual response cycle. The male experiences expulsive contractions of the entire length of the penile urethra. Semen is rhythmically expelled from the erect penis. At the onset of ejaculation, the internal bladder sphincter closes, preventing retrograde ejacu-

lation into the bladder. Women experience orgasm as rhythmic contractions of the circumvaginal and perineal muscles and of the swollen tissues of the orgasmic platform. The *orgasmic platform* refers to the vasocongestion of the outer third of the vagina and the labia minora. Resolution is marked by a return to normal of the genital and extragenital responses to sexual stimulation.

Sexual dysfunction occurs in the areas of desire (interest), arousal (excitement), and orgasm (tension release) (Woods, 1990). The fourth stage mentioned, resolution, is not associated with sexual dysfunction because it refers to the gradual return to the prearousal state. Physical, psychological, social, and environmental factors may cause these dysfunctions. Neoplastic disease can cause both biologic alterations and psychosocial sequelae that can affect sexuality negatively. The remaining sections of this chapter address (1) the biologic effects of cancer and its treatment that may interfere with sexual expression; (2) the psychosocial effects that the diagnosis of cancer may have on the client and partner; (3) the assessment and management of sexual dysfunctions related to neoplastic disease; and (4) the special problems associated with alterations in sexual functioning.

PATHOPHYSIOLOGIC FACTORS LEADING TO ALTERATIONS IN SEXUAL FUNCTIONING

Cancers of the Genitourinary Tract: Female

Women who have been diagnosed with genitourinary cancer often harbor fears regarding the impact of the disease process and the suggested treatment on sexual functioning (Jusenius, 1981; Smith, 1989) (see Chapters 32 and 34). Many women newly diagnosed with gynecologic cancer report a significant decrease in sexual activity and satisfaction (Box 53–1) (Andersen, 1987, Harris, Good, & Pollack, 1982; Jenkins, 1988). Gynecologic malignancies inherently affect body parts that are involved in sexual acts. The four most common types of gynecologic malignancies, in order of their occurrence, are endometrial cancer, cervical cancer, ovarian cancer, and cancer of the vulva.

Endometrial Cancer

Abnormal vaginal bleeding is the most common symptom associated with endometrial cancer. Abnormal vaginal bleeding can hinder sexual relations because either the client or the partner may feel that vaginal bleeding is aesthetically unappealing. Fear of increased bleeding, spread of the disease, or pain can also negatively affect sexual relations. Most patients diagnosed with endometrial cancer are in the early stages of the disease. The standard surgical procedure is abdominal hysterectomy with bilateral salpingo-oophorectomy. Zussman and colleagues (1981) found

Box 53–1. SEXUAL CHANGES AFTER TREATMENT FOR GYNECOLOGIC CANCER

Jenkins, B. (1988). **Patients' report of sexual changes after treatment for gynecologic cancer.** *Oncology Nursing Forum, 15*(3), 349–354.

The sexual changes experienced by 20 sexually active women following surgical and radiotherapy treatment for endometrial and cervical cancer were researched. In response to a mailed questionnaire, statistically significant negative changes were shown in four indicators of sexual function. These indicators were (1) frequency of intercourse, (2) orgasm, (3) feelings of desire, and (4) enjoyment. Fifty-nine per cent of the women reported no sexual counseling before or after treatment. Most of those who did receive sexual information reported that this information was given by the radiotherapist. No sexual counseling was given by nurses. Eighty-eight per cent of these women wanted sexual discussions initiated by the physician or the nurse.

that 33 to 46 per cent of women reported decreased sexual response after hysterectomy-oophorectomy. Pelvic irradiation for endometrial cancer may be employed in both early and late stages of the disease. Pelvic irradiation can cause vaginal thinning, dryness, and stenosis (Andersen, 1985). All of these side effects can occur and may persist as chronic problems. Sexuality will be altered as a result of these problems unless interventions to prevent or minimize them are employed.

Cancer of the Cervix

Cancer of the cervix is the second most common form of gynecologic cancer. Women who present with early cervical cancer are generally asymptomatic, whereas those who present with advanced disease often experience postcoital bleeding, pelvic or sciatic pain, and a thin watery discharge. All of these symptoms are likely to inhibit sexual relations (Andersen, Lachenbruch, Anderson, & DeProsse, 1986). The treatment options employed for women diagnosed with cervical cancer vary, depending on the stage of the disease. Radical hysterectomy has been associated with diminished or completely disrupted sexuality in the range of 6 to 19 per cent (Andersen, 1985). Pelvic irradiation for cancer of the cervix has been associated with a 66 per cent rate of sexual dysfunction (Bertelsen, 1983). Pelvic exenteration may be employed for the treatment of locally persistent or recurrent cervical cancer. Because of the removal of the vaginal canal as well as the introduction of other profound anatomic changes, sexual activity is profoundly affected by this surgery (Andersen, 1985; Andersen & Hacker, 1983b; Jusenius, 1981; Lamb, 1985; Schrover & Fifer, 1985; Wabrek & Gunn, 1984).

Pelvic exenteration may be accompanied by vaginal reconstruction to facilitate healing and continued sexual intercourse (Andersen, 1985, 1987; Andersen & Hacker, 1983b). Women who have undergone creation of a neovagina following exenteration have reported two outcomes related to sexual functioning: 57 per cent stated that the reconstruction had been a success and that they were able to continue satisfactory sexual relations; 43 per cent reported disruption in the frequency of sexual activity, dissatisfaction with the variety of the activity or with their ability to become aroused, or dissatisfaction with the neovagina itself (the length was too short; the cavity was too large; there was a chronic discharge; intercourse was painful) (Andersen & Hacker, 1983b). Continued surgical adaptations accompanied by better sexual counseling and follow-up are needed to improve the positive response rates.

Cancer of the Ovary

Ovarian cancer is the third most frequently diagnosed gynecologic malignancy. The symptoms most commonly associated with cancer of the ovary are anorexia, weight loss, increased abdominal girth, change in bowel function, and vague abdominal pain. These symptoms may affect sexual activity but are commonly insidious in onset and are often associated with late-stage disease. Although no studies of the sexual functioning of patients with ovarian cancer have been done to date, one can extrapolate data from studies done with women who have undergone abdominal hysterectomy and bilateral salpingo-oophorectomy. Adjuvant chemotherapy is routinely prescribed after surgery for women with ovarian cancer. This chemotherapy can have devastating effects on body image, self-image, and sexuality. Side effects include alopecia, anorexia, weight loss, lethargy, and bone marrow depression. Patients with end-stage ovarian cancer often experience a prolonged terminal stage. Many experience repeated bouts of intestinal obstruction, abdominal ascites, cachexia, pleural effusion, and sepsis. Any one of these late-stage symptoms can profoundly affect the ability to express physical love.

Cancer of the Vulva

Vulvar cancer is most commonly treated with radical vulvectomy and bilateral groin node dissection. This procedure has a tremendous impact on body image and sexual functioning (Andersen, 1985; Andersen & Hacker, 1983a; Andreasson, Moth, Jensen, & Bock, 1986; Jusenius, 1981; Lamb, 1985; Moth, Andreasson, Jensen, & Bock, 1983). Fifty per cent of women no longer attempted coitus after the operation and more than two thirds of the women who did make coital attempts experienced pain and some degree of sexual dysfunction (Moth et al., 1983). Andersen and Hacker (1983a) found that, despite the fact that intercourse remained possible, sexual functioning underwent a major disruption after radical vulvectomy. These findings were confirmed by a study in Denmark (Andreasson et al., 1986) in which half of all of the participants had experienced both sexual dysfunction and psychological problems following radical vulvectomy surgery.

Cancer of the Bladder

Bladder carcinoma is the most frequent malignant tumor of the urinary tract. This disease occurs more commonly in the male population with a ratio of 2:1, males to females (Rubin, 1983). One of the more commonly prescribed treatment options for cancer of the bladder is radical cystectomy. Little information has been reported regarding female sexual functioning after radical cystectomy. Schrover and colleagues (1984) found that women who are sexually active before undergoing radical cystectomy can resume a satisfying sex life with appropriate counseling. Vaginal dryness, tightness, and pain were experienced by all women on initial coital attempts. Most couples were able to overcome these difficulties with the use of vaginal hormone cream, vaginal dilation, and Kegal exercises to help the women become aware of muscle tension in the pelvic floor that may contribute to coital pain. All women who made the effort to resume sexual activity experienced a complete recovery in their ability to achieve orgasm.

Cancers of the Genitourinary Tract: Male

Men who have been diagnosed with genitourinary tract cancer often have sexual difficulties related to the disease itself as well as to the treatments prescribed (Shipes & Lehr, 1982). Sexual disturbances can result in an inability to attain an erection, an ejaculation, or both. These disturbances can result from both physiologic as well as psychological sequelae. The most common genitourinary cancers of the male population are cancer of the prostate, bladder, and testis (see Chapter 32).

Prostate Cancer

The sexual dysfunctions associated with cancer of the prostate have been studied widely (Spengler, 1983). Sexual difficulties may arise from even a diagnostic biopsy of the prostate gland. Approximately 24 per cent of open perineal biopsy patients and 32 per cent of the transurethral resection patients reported erectile failure (Andersen, 1985). The treatment for cancer of the prostate varies with the age of the patient, the extent of the disease, and the patient's preference. The current treatment options include irradiation (both external and interstitial implant), radical prostatectomy, oral estrogens, or bilateral orchiectomy. Radiation therapy to the prostate and surrounding tissues can result in erectile difficulties in 37 per cent of the population (Andersen, 1985). Fibrosis of the pelvic vasculature or damage to the pelvic nerves is believed to be the cause of these difficulties (Bachers, 1985). The impotence associated with definitive radiation for cancer of the prostate is usually insidious in onset and permanent in nature (Shipes & Lehr, 1982). The incidence of sexual dysfunction is much higher in patients who undergo a radical prostatectomy. Diminished or complete erectile failure is seen in up to 90 per cent of this population, whereas ejaculation difficulties, with or without some degree of erectile failure, are seen in 78 per cent of the population (Andersen, 1985). Postoperative impotency has been diminished recently by a nerve-sparing technique described by Shapiro (1987). Oral estrogens, bilateral orchiectomy, or both are currently used to treat metastatic or extensive disease. Of patients who reported erectile difficulties, 47 per cent were treated with orchiectomy alone, 22 per cent with estrogen alone, and 73 per cent with the combined treatment (Andersen, 1985). Gynecomastia is a common occurrence in men treated with estrogen, but this side effect has not been directly correlated with sexual dysfunctions.

Cancer of the Bladder

Sexual dysfunction related to the treatment of bladder cancer is dependent on the stage and subsequent treatment of the disease. The treatment of superficial bladder cancer (transurethral resection, intravesicle chemotherapy, or fulguration) usually does not result in organic dysfunction. However, repeated cystoscopies can result in a temporarily diminished desire for sex and transient pain during erection and ejaculation (Schrover, Von Eschenbach, Smith, & Gonzalez, 1984). More advanced bladder cancer is treated with either definitive irradiation or radical cystectomy, which usually results in sexual dysfunctions similar to those reported for the surgery and radiation used to treat cancer of the prostate (Andersen, 1985). However, an additional consideration for patients undergoing cystectomy is the necessary formation of an ostomy. Self-esteem and body image can be profoundly affected by the presence of the appliance (Shipes, 1987). Enterostomal therapists play a crucial role in the couple's adaptation to this surgery.

Cancer of the Testes

Testicular cancer, although rare, is the number one cause of death from cancer in men between the ages of 20 and 40 (Wujcik, Carbonnell, Taseff, Sciarra, & Isaac, 1986). A unilateral inguinal orchiectomy, with the preservation of the disease-free testicle, maintains both organic sexual function and fertility. However, the loss of a testis can be devastating to a young man's self-image. Retroperitoneal lymphadenectomy may be used as both a diagnostic and a therapeutic tool. This surgical procedure can sever the nerves that are necessary for seminal emissions, thus decreasing the amount of ejaculate during orgasm (Bachers, 1985). Patients who require bilateral orchiectomy experience a decrease in sexual desire because of lowered levels of serum testosterone as well as an alteration in secondary sex characteristics. The effect of combined chemotherapy and surgery on the sexuality of men with testicular cancer was studied by Brenner and colleagues (1985). Only 11 per cent of the patients sampled reported normal ejaculation following combined treatment. However, no long-term effects on sexual desire were observed. Schrover and co-workers (1986) studied the sexual difficulties experienced by men who had received radiotherapy for testicular cancer. Low rates of sexual activity were reported by 19 per cent of the respondents, low sexual desire by 12 per cent, erectile dysfunction by 15 per cent, difficulty reaching orgasm by 10 per cent, and premature ejaculation by 14 per cent. The two most frequently reported problems were reduced intensity of orgasm (33 per cent) and decrease in seminal volume (49 per cent).

Cancers of Other Related Systems

Breast Cancer

The diagnosis of breast cancer and the subsequent surgical removal of a breast are major fears among American women (Walbroehl, 1985). Although the trend in recent years has been to offer alternative forms of treatment, any therapy involving the breasts is often viewed as disfiguring. The type of treatment options available are dependent on the histologic type of lesion and the extent of the disease (see Chapter 33). Treatments for breast cancer include mastectomy (either simple, modified radical, or radical), lumpectomy, radiation therapy, and chemotherapy. General disruption of sexual activity, reduced frequency of intercourse, or orgasmic difficulties are estimated to occur in 21 to 39 per cent of all breast cancer patients, regardless of the treatment employed (Andersen, 1985). Body image disruption is believed to be the major factor involved in the sexual difficulties of breast cancer patients (Beckmann, Blichert-Toft, & Johansen, 1983; Golden, 1983).

Reconstructive surgery following mastectomy is done on a much more frequent basis today. Little research to date has evaluated the effectiveness of reconstructive surgery in lessening the sexual disruptions previously reported. Sexual dysfunction following mastectomy has been reported in the range of 23 to 37 per cent (Schain, 1985). In addition, 36 per cent of the partners of mastectomy patients have noted a negative impact on sexuality related to the disease and subsequent treatment (Wellisch, 1985). Breast conservation through lumpectomy and adjuvant irradiation is becoming a more common practice, when feasible. The impact of this form of treatment on sexual functioning has not yet been studied extensively. Schain (1985) is currently examining the effect of this form of treatment on the partner. Clinical impressions to date have revealed some dysfunctions immediately following therapy with a gradual return to near normal function over time. Chemotherapy is often used adjuvantly and palliatively in the treatment of breast cancer. The side effects of chemotherapy can themselves cause disruptions in sexual relationships. Hormonal manipulations, as a result of either chemotherapy or oophorectomy, can cause menopausal symptoms, which can also interfere with sexual expression.

The overall psychological impact of breast cancer on relationships is considerable. Both the patient and her sexual partner can experience temporary or permanent sexual difficulties. Wellisch (1985) described five important variables that influence the impact of breast cancer on a marital relationship. (1) the status of the relationship before the cancer developed; (2) the longevity of the marriage; (3) the stage of the breast cancer, especially as this influences the treatment required; (4) the point in the course of the illness; and (5) the interpersonal skills of the partners. Nursing care directed toward the impact of the treatment for breast cancer on sexuality should include educational information, support, and counseling. Three nursing care plans developed by Schwarz-Applebaum and colleagues (1984), designed specifically for couples, are shown in Tables 53–1, 53–2, and 53–3.

Cancer of the Head and Neck

Head and neck cancer does not directly affect the sexual functioning of the client. Rather, the disease and its treatment are often severely disfiguring and thus cause a dramatic alteration in body image. Facial disfigurement can cause sexual difficulties for both the patient and the sexual partner (Metcalfe & Fischman, 1985) (see Chapter 36). Few studies have been done that directly address the impact of head and neck cancers on sexual functioning. The direct and indirect sexual implications of radiation therapy and chemotherapy for patients with head and neck cancer are addressed by Shipes and Lehr (1982). The only known direct effect of radiation therapy is a decrease in sexual desire. The indirect effects include sore, dry mouth, drooling, nausea and vomiting, loss of taste and smell, hoarseness, and malaise. Chemotherapeutic agents have also been associated with side effects that inhibit sexual functioning. These include alopecia, nausea and vomiting, diarrhea, constipation, mucositis, altered sense of taste and smell, and erectile problems. In addition, many men report fever, weakness, and fatigue associated with bone marrow suppression. Permanent or temporary sterility, a decrease in sex drive, and alterations in secondary sex characteristics such as hair distribution, voice changes, and breast development have also been noted (Shipes & Lehr, 1982). Strategies and interventions need to be identified through research that will assist couples in coping with the sexual disruptions associated with this group of diseases (Metcalfe & Fischman, 1985).

Cancers Affecting the Nervous System

Colorectal Cancers

Colorectal cancers and their treatment can produce major effects related to sexual dysfunction (see Chapter 33). Sexual ramifications of colorectal cancer include those related to the formation of an ostomy or those related to neurologic deficits (Shipes, 1987). Nursing assessment and interventions related to ostomy and possible sexual dysfunction are discussed under

Text continued on page 840

Table 53–1. NURSING CARE PLAN: SEXUALITY AND MODIFIED RADICAL MASTECTOMY

Assessment	Interventions	Expected Outcomes
Nursing Diagnosis: Potential change in sexual self-concept due to loss of breast		
Initiate discussion of sexuality at admission; reinforce throughout hospitalization and at postsurgical follow-up visits	Initiate discussion of sexuality Explore the degree of importance of breasts in client's sexual self-concept Discuss relative importance of other areas influencing expression of sexual self-concept (health, energy, etc.)	Client discusses personal view of importance of breasts to sexual self-concept; client states ways to enlist support systems in maintaining sexual self-concept
Begin discussion at admission; expand topic throughout hospitalization	Give adequate time for grieving for loss of breast	
Initiate discussion of appearance of incision before first dressing change; assess readiness to look at incision with each check of wound	Assess readiness to look at incision: • initiate discussion of appearance of incision • draw line picture of surgical area • help patient look at area with mirror	Client describes appearance of incision
Discuss progress in viewing incision at postsurgical follow-up visits	• help patient look at actual incision when ready	Client describes plans to look at incision and chest wall and shares feelings about appearance of incision
	Explore possibility of health changes that may occur after modified radical mastectomy (temporary decrease in energy level, temporary difficulty performing routine household duties, changes in arm and hand, changes in range of motion of affected arm and shoulder, numbness or pulling in incision area with healing, decreased sensation in pectoral area and inner aspect of arm, phantom breast sensation, change in sleep patterns).	
Nursing Diagnosis: Potential diminished self-concept because of limited information about ways to enhance postoperative appearance		
Begin discussion before discharge; clarify concerns at postsurgical follow-up visits	Discuss breast prostheses: • when to purchase, relative to period of wound healing • importance of weight, consistency, size, and contour of prosthesis in promoting good posture and carriage • advantages and disadvantages of different types of prostheses • cost and possibility of insurance coverage • availability of different prostheses in geographical area (use current listings from Reach to Recovery in all of the above) Explore option of Reach to Recovery visit: • check with local unit of Reach to Recovery to determine options for referral initiation	Client lists important variables in choice of a prosthesis, taking her life style into account; client states plan for purchase of prosthesis (e.g., timing of purchase, various places to purchase prosthesis, etc.)
	Discuss attractive clothing options emphasizing remaining body strengths • need for wide shoulder straps and arm holes to prevent pressure on affected arm • wear opaque night gowns, ruffles at neckline to disguise operative area • emphasize other body parts with cut of clothing	Client describes ways to use clothing to enhance appearance
Discuss at postsurgical follow-up visit at least 4 weeks after surgery	• use of waterproof skin tone cosmetics to disguise mastectomy scar (if desired after wound has healed)	
Initiate discussion before hospital discharge	Discuss mechanics of how to get into clothing already owned: • insert affected arm first into over-the-head clothing • use of zipper pull for items with back zippers • how to fasten bra with one hand or fasten it in front and turn bra around Discuss breast reconstruction alternatives (as appropriate to client interest): • breast mound will have normal contour underneath clothing • varying importance of construction of new nipple to self concept • no fear of shifting an external prosthesis with vigorous activity including sports	Client can dress herself by discharge and describes methods to use when dressing in clothing owned before surgery
Nursing Diagnosis: Possible reluctance to adopt positive health habits because of fear of discovery of malignancy in the other breast and limited information		
	Reaffirm importance of monthly Breast Self Examination (BSE) Teach technique of BSE (as indicated) according to the normal tissue textures on unoperated breast, palpation of local incision, axilla, ribs, and intercostal area on operated side	Every month, client performs BSE on unoperated breast and examines operated side
	Teach avoidance of compressive forces on affected arm to decrease risk of lymphedema: • no blood pressure measurements on affected arm • carry heavy loads with other arm Teach avoidance of skin trauma to minimize risk of local infection: • no injections on affected arm • protect affected arm from burns and cuts	Client lists precautions to prevent injury to affected arm
	Encourage annual mammogram	Client has annual mammogram
	Encourage follow-up at scheduled postsurgical clinic visits	Client attends scheduled appointments at postsurgical follow-up clinic appointments

Table 53–1. NURSING CARE PLAN: SEXUALITY AND MODIFIED RADICAL MASTECTOMY *Continued*

Assessment	Interventions	Expected Outcomes
Nursing Diagnosis: *Potential for diminished involvement in relationships because of fear of rejection*		
Discuss before discharge and reinforce throughout postsurgical follow-up visits	Discuss importance to self-concept of maintaining involvement in previous activities Explore fears of mutilation and unacceptability and other concerns that might limit involvement in relationships Discuss need for others to have time to become accustomed to changes in client's body Discuss likelihood for a single woman to be reluctant to enter new sexual relationships (as appropriate to situation) Encourage recognition of client's assets List possible ways to promote resumption of former life style Role play situations likely to be encountered in establishing relationships	Client verbalizes risk for temporary disruption in former activities and states ways to promote resumption of life style
Nursing Diagnosis: *Possible reluctance to participate in sexual intercourse after hospital discharge because of fear of disruption of surgical incision and pain*		
Initiate discussion before discharge from hospital; reassess and continue teaching at postsurgical follow-up visits; include partner in discussion, if possible	Explore whether this is an issue for client: • whether partner is available • whether concerns exist about resuming intercourse Discuss client's usual methods of sexual expression and importance of breasts in sexual stimulation Reaffirm need for frank discussion between sexual partners and need of time for partner to become accustomed to changes in appearance of surgical area Discuss possibility that client may project own feelings onto partner Teach methods to decrease pain in surgical area or affected arm (if applicable): • use of warm soaks • warm tub baths • pain medication before intercourse • massage Explore alternate sexual positions that may be acceptable to client and partner: • male astride with small pillow over incision • female astride and supported with pillows to lessen pressure on affected arm • side lying with affected arm down and creative use of pillows to lessen pressure on affected arm • rear entry approach with woman lying on pillows to decrease pressure on affected arm	Client verbalizes methods to facilitate intercourse that are acceptable to herself and her partner Client reports satisfactory experience of intercourse or sexual expression Client discusses and role plays ways to express mutual fears and concerns about sexual intercourse with partner
Nursing Diagnosis: *Possible reluctance to participate in sexual intercourse because of fear of rejection by partner*		
Discuss before discharge from hospital and reinforce at postsurgical follow-up visits	Explore whether this is an issue for client Encourage honest sharing of concerns and feelings between partners Encourage rapid return to previous pattern of sexual activity and maintenance of usual patterns of modesty (as acceptable to client and partner) Assess desire for temporary options to decrease confrontation with partner during intercourse: • use of night bra • undress before partner does • sexual intercourse in the dark • use of alternate sexual positions Discuss client's and current or future partners' needs to have time to become accustomed to loss of breast and appearance of incision: • be patient with self and partner(s) • realize concerns may surface initially or resurface weeks or months after the surgery Encourage seeking professional assistance if partners cannot achieve mutually satisfying experiences	Client discusses concern about partner's reaction to changed appearance and plans ways to help partner become accustomed to changed appearance
Nursing Diagnosis: *Potential reluctance for partner to participate in sexual intercourse because of misconceptions about cancer and about own reaction*		
Discuss with client early in course of recovery and explore with partner or client at follow-up visits	Discuss appearance of incision with partner Reaffirm that partner's response is important to woman's self-esteem Reaffirm need for closeness and expression of caring; involve partner in touching, stroking arm, and the like Explore misconceptions about cancer etiology: • cancer is not contagious • aggressive sexual play does not cause cancer Encourage frank sharing of concerns between partners Emphasize pleasuring of partner focusing on other mutually pleasurable areas of woman's body	Client or partner describes mutually satisfactory sexual expression

(Modified with permission from Schwarz-Appelbaum, J., Dedrick, J., Jusenius, K., & Kirchner, C. W. [1984]. Nursing care plans: Sexuality and treatment of breast cancer. *Oncology Nursing Forum, 11* [6], 16–24.)

Table 53–2. NURSING CARE PLAN: SEXUALITY AND TYELECTOMY WITH EXTERNAL BEAM RADIATION AND/OR IRIDIUM IMPLANTATION

Assessment	Interventions	Expected Outcomes
Nursing Diagnosis: Potential for threatened self-concept due to changes in irradiated breast tissue and tyelectomy scar		
Initiate assessment and teaching before therapy	Explore client's self-concept and importance of breasts	Client discusses possibility of changes in breasts
Monitor change throughout therapy and in follow-up radiation therapy clinic visits	Assess breast tissue before therapy	Client discusses importance of these changes to her self-concept
	Describe changes that can occur in appearance of irradiated breast: • change in skin color • altered consistency or texture • possible change in size of irradiated breast • possible diminished sensation or tingling in irradiated breast Review radiation treatment side effects: • skin reactions (erythema, dry or moist desquamation) • fatigue • cough secondary to pneumonitis • dry throat	
	Mention specific precautions to minimize skin reactions: • keep treatment field dry • wash treatment field only with water or mild cleansing agents (mild soaps, diluted hydrogen peroxide, saline) • avoid rubbing, friction, heat, cold, chemical irritants (perfume, laundry detergents, creams, deodorants, tape, dressings, direct sunlight exposure) Review expected skin reactions at various radiation levels Assist in managing side effects as they occur	Client lists precautions to minimize radiation skin reactions
Nursing Diagnosis: Possibility of diminished involvement in sexual relationships due to treatment logistics, fatigue, and concerns about being radioactive		
Initiate discussion prior to therapy; monitor throughout therapy	Assess effect of therapy on sexual relationships Reaffirm importance of continued involvement in relationships Clarify misconceptions about radioactivity	Client defines ways radiation therapy can affect involvement in current relationships and activities
	Explore methods to promote resumption of activities and provide adequate rest: • mobilization of existing support systems (e.g., household or child care assistance, transportation resources) • temporary rearrangement of schedules • allowance for naps or rest periods as necessary	Client states plans to continue involvement in relationships and activities or to modify life style
Nursing Diagnosis: Possible change in satisfaction with intercourse and foreplay because of change in breast tissue and breast sensation		
Initiate discussion before therapy	Discuss importance of breasts in foreplay and intercourse	Client discusses possibility of changes in breast tissue and breast sensation
Continue monitoring throughout follow-up radiation therapy clinic visits	Discuss possible changes in breast tissue and breast sensation that may have an effect on satisfaction with intercourse and foreplay: • change in skin color • altered consistency or texture • possible change in size of irradiated breast • possible diminished sensation or tingling in irradiated breast	Client lists ways to achieve pleasuring that are acceptable to both client and sexual partner
	Investigate ways to facilitate pleasuring using remaining body strengths (e.g., stimulation of other breast or thigh stimulation) Role play ways for client and partner to discuss effects of radiation therapy and determine mutually acceptable methods of pleasuring Determine whether alternative pleasuring activities are acceptable to client and partner	
Nursing Diagnosis: Possible reluctance of partner to engage in intercourse, foreplay, (or both) because of concerns about radiation exposure or changes in breast tissue		
Initiate discussion before therapy	Reaffirm importance of closeness and intercourse in relationship	Client and partner reestablish mutually acceptable patterns of sexual functioning
Whenever possible, include partner in discussions during follow-up radiation therapy clinic visits	Assess whether misconceptions about radiation therapy or changes in breast tissue or both have influenced partner's enthusiasm for intercourse Encourage honest sharing of concerns and feelings between partners Assure partner that there is no residual radioactivity after radiation therapy treatment Teach partner about potential change in breast tissue Discuss alternatives in pleasuring	Client and partner identify areas of concern with sexual functioning and discuss ways to continue to demonstrate affection and caring and to achieve mutually acceptable pleasuring

(Modified with permission from Schwarz-Appelbaum, J., Dedrick, J., Jusenius, K., & Kirchner, C. W. [1984]. Nursing care plans: Sexuality and treatment of breast cancer. *Oncology Nursing Forum, 11* [6], 16–24.)

Table 53–3. NURSING CARE PLAN: SEXUALITY AND ADJUVANT CHEMOTHERAPY CONSISTING OF CYCLOPHOSPHAMIDE (CYTOXAN), METHOTREXATE, AND 5-FLUOROURACIL (CMF)

Assessment	Interventions	Expected Outcomes
Nursing Diagnosis: *Potential alteration of sexual self-concept because of weight gain and alopecia*		
Before initiating chemotherapy, teach likelihood of gaining weight and experiencing alopecia Reinforce teaching during therapy	Teach client potential for weight gain and alopecia Weigh at each clinic visit Encourage exercise Promote calorie reduction within the framework of a well-balanced diet Encourage reducing nausea by eating small quantities of carbohydrates to reduce excessive weight gain Encourage client to purchase wig, scarves, turbans within 2 weeks of initiating therapy: • wigs should allow for air circulation • scarves and turbans should be cotton, not polyester • a written prescription for a wig may help with insurance reimbursement	Client verbalizes signs and symptoms of chemotherapy that affect sexual self-concept immediately after teaching and 1 week after instruction Client maintains weight within 5–10 lbs. of baseline
Nursing Diagnosis: *Potential for temporary or permanent amenorrhea because of ovarian suppression*		
Start teaching before initiating chemotherapy	Emphasize to premenopausal clients that resumption of normal menses may take variable lengths of time after completion of chemotherapy Identify high-risk clients for permanent infertility (age 40 and over): • explore options for child rearing, if appropriate (e.g., adoption, surrogate motherhood) Teach client importance of using birth control during active therapy and for at least 12 months after therapy Discuss decision-making concepts related to pregnancy (if applicable)	Client verbalizes that CMF chemotherapy may affect fertility Premenopausal client verbalizes risks associated with becoming pregnant during adjuvant chemotherapy
Nursing Diagnosis: *Occurrence of menopausal symptoms usually associated with aging (e.g., hot flashes, decreased or absent vaginal secretions) because of ovarian suppression*		
Use as prescribed by physician if hot flashes become problematic	Explore use of Bellergal-5 to control hot flashes Instruct client in use of water-soluble vaginal lubricant if vaginal secretions are decreased (e.g., K-Y Jelly)	
Nursing Diagnosis: *Potential disruption of sexual relationships because of depression or global anxiety regarding cancer and therapy resulting from cyclic nature of treatment*		
Initiate teaching before chemotherapy; continue to reinforce throughout treatment	Assess client's understanding of disease and treatment goals; clarify misconceptions Encourage client to verbalize concerns, involve appropriate support services Reaffirm importance of client resuming pretreatment life style	Client verbalizes signs and symptoms of CMF chemotherapy that affect sexual relationship and verbalizes ways to counter these Client verbalizes that partner is supportive
Nursing Diagnosis: *Possible reluctance to engage in sexual intercourse because of decreased libido, fatigue, hormonal changes, dyspareunia, and changed amount of vaginal secretions*		
Initiate teaching when chemotherapy is started Continue to reinforce during subsequent cycles of chemotherapy	Teach use of intervals between chemotherapy for greatest sexual activity to optimize energy level Instruct client to monitor daily energy patterns and to use time of highest energy for sexual activity Recommend male astride position to conserve client's energy Teach methods to counter vaginal dryness: • water-soluble vaginal lubricants (e.g., K-Y Jelly) • increase time or change pattern of foreplay to increase natural vaginal secretions Avoid excessive douching or perfumed douches to decrease risk of vaginal dryness or irritation or disruption of normal vaginal flora	Immediately after teaching and 1 week after initial chemotherapy treatment, client verbalizes signs and symptoms of chemotherapy that may affect sexual functioning Client verbalizes that a personally acceptable level of sexual activity is possible while proceeding with treatment regimen Client does not complain of dyspareunia

Table continued on following page

Table 53–3. NURSING CARE PLAN: SEXUALITY AND ADJUVANT CHEMOTHERAPY CONSISTING OF CYCLOPHOSPHAMIDE (CYTOXAN), METHOTREXATE, AND 5-FLUOROURACIL (CMF) *Continued*

Assessment	Interventions	Expected Outcomes
Assess vaginal secretions at each treatment cycle (if oral mucositis is present, there may be other mucosal involvement)	Teach client to report increased vaginal secretions or alteration in vaginal discharge; if symptomatic, nurses should: • check temperature • culture • if yeast present, use antifungal agents as prescribed by physician (e.g., nystatin (Mycostatin), ketoconazole, yogurt) • reinforce that saliva and vaginal secretions may transmit infection	Client uses appropriate regimen as instructed for candidiasis

Nursing Diagnosis: Possibility that partner feels unable to help a loved one through crisis because of knowledge deficit concerning cancer and fear of causing infection in a potentially immunosuppressed person

Initiate discussion with partner before beginning chemotherapy or early in the course of treatment	Assess partner's understanding of disease and treatment goals; clarify misconceptions	Partner verbalizes potential effects of chemotherapy on sexual relationship
	Offer partner time to express concern without presence of client Offer partner concrete suggestions on ways for him to support client: • exercise together • plan recreational activities during treatment rather than postponing until treatment stops • encourage open expression and willingness to listen • household demands should be consistent with client's energy level	Partner is able to state two ways he can concretely support client through treatment

(Modified with permission from Schwarz-Appelbaum, J., Dedrick, J., Jusenius, K., & Kirchner, C. W. [1984]. Nursing care plans: Sexuality and treatment of breast cancer. *Oncology Nursing Forum, 11* [6], 16–24.)

"Special Problems Associated with Alterations in Sexual Functioning." The neural disruption is associated with anterior and posterior resection. The parasympathetic nerve damage associated with abdominal-perineal resection for cancer of the rectum results in erectile impotence in 50 to 100 per cent of the patients (Grunberg, 1986). Ejaculation is lost in 50 to 75 per cent of patients who undergo abdominoperineal resection (Dobkin & Broadwell, 1986), and 25 per cent report an inability to penetrate the vagina (La Monica, Audisio, Tamburini, Filberti, & Ventafridda, 1985). Reduction in sexual desire has also been reported for both men (32 to 59 per cent) and women (28 per cent) who have undergone surgical resection for colorectal cancer (Andersen, 1985). Twenty-one per cent of this same female population reported genital numbness and dyspareunia. In addition to the pathophysiologic basis for sexual disruptions, altered body image and self-esteem on the part of the patient can affect sexuality negatively. The partner also may harbor fears and misconceptions that will result in sexual difficulties.

Central Nervous System Tumors

Both primary and metastatic lesions arising in the central nervous system can affect sexual desire and functioning (see Chapter 39). Sexual function is dependent on cortical influences, peripheral nerves, autonomic pathways, spinal cord pathways, and reflex centers (Woods, 1990). Thus pathologic lesions involving any of these structures may lead to sexual dysfunction. Scant research has been done on the impact of central nervous system tumors and sexual function. It

is possible, however, to extrapolate from the immense body of knowledge on patients with spinal cord injuries and with lesions involving the brain. Much of this literature has involved male patients, probably because more males have spinal cord injuries and because women are assumed to accept more readily a passive sexual role. An intact pathway from the cortex to the sex organ is not necessary for certain components of the human sexual response cycle, for example, attainment of erection and ejaculation. Rather these functions are mediated by spinal cord reflexes. The important factor to consider is the level of the injury and the degree of interruption of nerve impulses. Sexual gratification can be experienced from feelings other than those emanating from the sex organs. A thorough assessment followed by individualized interventions can optimize sexual functioning in the client with tumors of the nervous system.

Table 53–4 contains a summary of the effects of various cancer on sexuality, including sexual function, fertility, body image, and partners.

Changes in Hormonal Environment and Vasculature

An appropriate hormonal milieu and adequate vasculature to the sex organs is necessary for sexual functioning. Many cancers and treatments affect either or both of these components. A decrease in the amount of circulating estrogen, through surgical removal of the ovaries or chemical suppression by chemotherapy, can result in vaginal dryness, thinning, and other meno-

Table 53–4. EFFECTS OF CANCER ON SEXUALITY, INCLUDING SEXUAL FUNCTION, FERTILITY, BODY IMAGE, AND PARTNERS

Site	Dysfunction Organic	Dysfunction Psychological	Effect on Fertility	Altered Body Image	Impact on Partner	Comments
Cervix	Treatment of in situ with cone biopsy will not cause dysfunction; radical hysterectomy will shorten the vagina by one third to one half; this may be appreciable but usually is not	Sometimes	No, with cone·biopsy for in situ stages; yes, with hysterectomy, radiotherapy, or both	Sometimes	Sometimes (partner may feel he can "catch" cancer or be affected by its treatment, especially by radiotherapy)	Radiotherapy to the pelvis will cause thickening of the vagina and may cause stenosis, and/or fistula formation, or both
Endometrial	Total abdominal hysterectomy with pelvic node dissection usually causes no dysfunction; radiotherapy to the pelvis will cause thickening of the vagina if it is included in the fields	Sometimes	Yes, with either radiotherapy or surgery	Sometimes	Sometimes	Because of lack of literature on female sexual response, it is very difficult to determine difference between physical and emotional dysfunction
Ovary	In premenopausal women, bilateral oophorectomy will result in menopausal symptoms	Sometimes	Yes (except with cases with unilateral oophorectomy)	Sometimes	Sometimes	
Vulva	Simple vulvectomy can result in introital stenosis; radical vulvectomy includes removal of the clitoris	Usually	No; patient is often postmenopausal	Most often	Usually	Radical vulvectomy can cause a decrease in range of motion of lower extremities.
Breast	The absence of foreplay using nipple stimulation for arousal may cause some difficulties	Usually	None	Usually	Usually	If oophorectomy and hormonal manipulations are utilized, this can affect all aspects of sexuality
Prostate	Total prostatectomy results in impotence; simple prostatectomy usually results in retrograde ejaculation	Usually	Usually	Usually	Usually	Bilateral orchiectomy or hormonal manipulations can result in decreased libido and sexual responsiveness; if estrogen treatment is initiated, gynecomastia may result
Testicular	Nerve damage due to retroperitoneal lymph node dissection usually results in retrograde ejaculation and can cause impotence	Usually	Sometimes, if unilateral; always, if bilateral; suggest utilization of sperm bank before chemotherapy and retroperitoneal lymph node dissection	Yes	Usually	Hormonal aberration (especially decrease in androgen) will cause a decrease in libido and may cause impotence, retarded ejaculation, and a decrease in sexual responsiveness
Bladder	Local—seldom; in males, radical cystectomy involves removal of bladder, urethra, and prostate . . . therefore, he is impotent. In females, cystectomy usually includes urethra, uterus, and anterior vagina	Usually	Always with radiotherapy; this cancer is most common in older men	Yes (patients usually have urinary conduit with a stoma)	Usually	

Table continued on following page

Table 53–4. EFFECTS OF CANCER ON SEXUALITY, INCLUDING SEXUAL FUNCTION,
FERTILITY, BODY IMAGE, AND PARTNERS *Continued*

| Site | Dysfunction | | Effect on Fertility | Altered Body Image | Impact on Partner | Comments |
	Organic	Psychological				
Colon and Rectum	Usually; nerve damage in males negatively effects erectile ability	Usually; esp. with formation of an ostomy	None; except with radiotherapy and chemotherapy	Yes (if colostomy formed)	Sometimes	Women sometimes have a hysterectomy with the operative procedure
Leukemia	The disease process and associated blood counts with chemotherapy may affect ability to have an erection	Sometimes	Chemotherapy affects sperm count and ova maturation rebound after cessation of treatment	Usually	Usually	Extensive fatigue often diminishes sex drive and function
Hodgkins	The disease process and the effects of the therapy may decrease sexual drive and ability	Sometimes	Yes, with radiotherapy to the pelvis without shielding of the gonads; chemotherapy will decrease sperm and ova maturation	Usually	Usually	Patients on chemotherapy alone should be using some form of contraception; the effect on the sperm counts and ova maturation by chemotherapy is not totally understood

NOTE: Chemotherapy, radiation, and analgesics are all associated with generalized feelings of malaise. This can have a profound effect on the feelings of self-esteem, self-worth, sexuality, and libido. All these factors should be taken into consideration when assessing the sexual needs and problems of cancer patients and their families.

(From Lamb, M., & Woods, N. F. [1981]. Sexuality and the cancer patient. *Cancer Nursing, 4,* 137–144. Reproduced by permission.)

pausal symptoms (Andersen, 1985). Men treated with estrogen experience gynecomastia and a decrease in libido (Schrover et al., 1984). A decrease in the amount of circulating androgens, through surgical removal or chemical suppression, can also result in a decrease in sexual drive and feminization in males (Schrover, Gonzales, & von Eschenbach, 1986). Hormonal replacement may be indicated or contraindicated, depending on the reason for the suppression. Patients with hormonally dependent tumors may have their systemic hormonal environment intentionally altered, or this alteration may have been an inadvertent effect of therapy. Interventions, therefore, may be either an adaptation to or a correction of the hormonal imbalance.

A decrease in the vasculature to the genitals can also interfere with sexual functioning. In the male, this decrease can result in an inability to attain or maintain an erection (Schrover et al., 1986). In the female, it will result in vaginal dryness, thinning, and dyspareunia (Andersen, 1985). The etiologic factors associated with an alteration in genital vasculature include (1) direct tumor compression of the vessels supplying the genitals, (2) surgical disruption of the genital vasculature, and (3) vascular fibrosis as a result of radiation therapy. This vascular compromise can be temporary or permanent; often the onset is insidious in nature, especially if the cause is tumor compression or radiation fibrosis. Treatments may be employed to correct the deficiency in vascularization, but correction is not always possible. Interventions aimed at adaptation to the resulting dysfunction may be the option of choice. These interventions may include use of a water-soluble lubricant if vaginal dryness is a problem or insertion of a penile implant if erectile disruption is the resulting problem.

PSYCHOSOCIAL FACTORS INFLUENCING SEXUAL FUNCTIONING

Psychological Factors

The psychological factors that often affect sexuality include (1) alteration in body image, (2) diminished self-esteem, (3) role change, (4) attitudes, (5) beliefs and misconceptions, and (6) anxiety or depression. Any one or combination of these factors can affect the sexual functioning of the patient with cancer. Difficulties can occur at any point in the continuum of cancer care: during diagnosis, work-up, treatment, or follow-up or during the stage of progressive or terminal disease, should this be the outcome. The client with cancer, the partner, or both can manifest sexual difficulties that are related to their psychological responses. The emphasis of this chapter is on the direct effect of these psychological responses on sexual functioning.

Body Image and Self-Esteem

Body image can be viewed as a component of self-esteem (Derogatis, 1980). Self-esteem can be defined simply as the reputation we have of ourselves. The process of giving and receiving sexual pleasure is closely connected to a sense of safety, in both our person and our body (Cantor, 1980). Living with cancer produces changes in self-esteem, some transient, some permanent. These changes are based on both an immediate reality as well as an anticipation of possible further changes. Self-esteem can be affected negatively by cancer, with or without apparent changes in body image, which, in turn, may contribute to feelings of sexual inadequacy (Cooley & Cobb, 1986a, 1986b; Foltz, 1987). If in addition to altered self-esteem, the patient must adjust to changes in physical appearance, sexual functioning can be compromised further.

The identification and remediation of the patient's impoverished self-esteem, body-image disturbance, and sexual disruption are key goals of cancer care (Schain, 1980; Wood & Tambrink, 1983). An assessment of self-esteem can be achieved during an informal discussion and should be conducted at repeated intervals throughout the cancer continuum. This information will be essential in identifying and correcting sexual dysfunctions related to alterations in self-esteem. Efforts should be made directly, through counseling and behavior modification, to build self-esteem to a level compatible with a feeling of being worthwhile (Enelow, 1975).

Anxiety and Depression

Anxiety and depression are the two most common affective disruptions among patients with cancer (Andersen, 1985). Clinical depression can be diagnosed in 17 to 25 per cent of the hospitalized cancer population (Petty & Noyes, 1981). Anxiety about the future occurs at critical periods for patients with cancer: at diagnosis, at evidence of recurrence, and during the side effects of therapy. Both anxiety and depression have profound effects on sexual functioning (Wise, 1978).

A decrease in sexual interest, libido, and activity are all results of depressive and anxious states (Mims & Swenson, 1980). Depression and anxiety have both been associated with erectile dysfunctions; anxiety has been associated with premature ejaculation (Woods, 1990). Interventions are aimed at alleviating the anxiety and depression.

Role Changes

Social role refers to the patterns of behavior shared by individuals who occupy a certain position or fulfill a certain function in society (Enelow, 1975). Each individual may occupy a variety of social and cultural roles. Parent, wife, husband, financial provider, and homemaker are a few of the many roles that may be transiently or permanently affected by cancer and cancer treatment. During illness, some roles are relinquished and assumed by others. Role reversals are sometimes necessary (Johnson, 1986). A person's identity and sense of worth may be threatened when role changes occur. The shifting roles within families of cancer patients should be taken into account when considering the possible etiologic factors associated with sexual dysfunctions. For example, the role of the sexual partner may no longer be compatible with that of the man who is no longer the financial supporter of the family; by contrast, a women may no longer feel like a wife and sexual partner if her husband must participate in her physical care.

Attitudes, Beliefs, and Misconceptions

The attitudes and beliefs of a person with cancer regarding cancer and its treatment often affect sexual functioning. Attitudes and beliefs are formed over time and are based on previous experience as well as on formal and informal education. In our society, many beliefs and attitudes regarding cancer are incompatible with normal sexual functioning. Cancer is often viewed as a "punishment" for past deeds, either real or fantasized (Cantor, 1980; Sewell & Edwards, 1980). Some patients may harbor misconceptions regarding the etiology of cancer and the impact that it may have on their own as well as their partner's sexual functioning. Fear of contagion is another misconception of some patients (Golden & Golden, 1980). Many people fear that they can "give" cancer to or "get" cancer from their loved ones through close physical contact, especially through sexual intercourse. A frank and open discussion between client and caregiver will often uncover the attitudes, beliefs, and misconceptions that can have a negative effect on sexual functioning. Education regarding the etiology, treatment, and long-term effects of cancer and its treatment on sexuality is an integral part of the holistic care of the cancer patient. Dispelling myths and misconceptions is a part of this educational process.

Social Factors

Social factors that affect the sexual functioning of the patient with cancer include (1) availability of a sexual partner; (2) evidence of anxiety or depression on the part of the partner; (3) effect of role changes on the partner; and (4) partner's attitudes, beliefs, and misconceptions. Patients who do not have a sexual partner may have difficulties establishing an intimate relationship. The stress of cancer can often cause a fragile relationship to deteriorate. People who, at the time of diagnosis, are single, widowed, or divorced often state that it is difficult to initiate an intimate relationship. Many factors may account for this phenomenon: fear of rejection due to the diagnosis or possible alteration in body image; inability to meet available people socially because of prolonged treatments and convalescence; and uncertainty about the future.

The partner, too, is vulnerable to similar psychological factors that may impede normal sexual expression, such as anxiety, depression, guilt, and misconceptions. Anxiety and depression on the part of the partner will have detrimental effects on sexuality, similar to those experienced by the patient with these affective disorders. The partner may feel that the cancer patient is too sick for sexual activity or may feel guilty about making sexual overtures to someone who is experiencing the trauma of cancer diagnosis and treatment.

Partners also may fear that the cancer is contagious or that the treatment will somehow affect them. Some spouses fear that the patient's radiation treatments will render the patient either temporarily or permanently radioactive. Other partners may have difficulty adjusting to the altered physical appearance of the patient. Role changes affect the partner in the same manner as they affect the patient. For example, the partner may not be able to switch roles easily from that of caregiver to that of sexual partner. Because of the variety of social factors to be considered, individualized interventions should be planned for the couple with sexual dysfunctions during the period of cancer care.

Environmental Factors

Two main environmental factors that may impede sexual expression are (1) hospitalization, with its inherent lack of privacy and traditional views of the patient as an asexual being, and (2) alterations in the home environment that often lead to a decrease in the privacy necessary for intimate relations to occur. The hospital setting is notorious for the lack of quiet, uninterrupted time. Most patients are placed in semiprivate rooms and are monitored constantly by physicians, nurses, and other health care professionals. Visiting hours may or may not be structured, thereby further diminishing available time alone. Recently some hospitals have initiated policies to allow for private, uninterrupted time; however, this is an exception rather than a rule. Nurses can take an active role in policy setting to allow for intimate time in the hospital setting. This will serve to validate the humanness of their patients as well as to offer holistic care.

The home setting is sometimes altered to allow for convalescent, progressive, or terminal care. This alteration is rarely conducive to intimate relationships. A hospital bed in the family living area or first-floor den will not provide the privacy necessary for sexual activity. Couples should be encouraged to negotiate with family members, friends, and members of the health care team for private time on a regular basis. Whether or not they choose to use this time for sexual activity is not an issue. The availability of this time will allow for some degree of spontaneity and closeness otherwise lost owing to the hectic surroundings.

ASSESSMENT AND MANAGEMENT OF ALTERATIONS IN SEXUAL FUNCTIONING

Sexual Assessment

Assessment of sexual health begins with a sexual history and is supplemented by data regarding the person's general health, such as that obtained from a physical examination or a general health history (Lamb & Woods, 1981). The literature contains a number of articles that address sexual assessment, many of which are specific to cancer patients (Chapman & Sughrue, 1987; Greenberg, 1984; Lamb & Woods, 1981;

MacElveen-Hoehn, 1985). The following is a brief sexual assessment that can be easily incorporated into a more general nursing assessment:

> Has being ill interfered with your being a (husband, father, wife, mother)?
> Has your illness changed the way you see yourself as a man/woman?
> Has your illness affected your sexual function? (Lamb & Woods, 1981)

The first question relates to sexual role, the second pertains to self-image, and the last addresses sexual function. Often it is necessary to ask only the first or second question, because the client will open up and freely discuss data related to the third item. If the discussion of the answers to these questions uncovers a specific sexual problem, a more in-depth assessment may be necessary. This would include the onset and course of the problem, the client or couple's ideas about what may have caused the problem and its persistence, the solutions that have been attempted to date, the solutions that are acceptable (sexual counseling, exploring alternate forms of sexual gratification), and the goals of an attempted treatment plan. A physical examination, not necessarily specific to sexual function, will also shed light onto potential sexual problems. Dyspnea on exertion, range of motion difficulties, vaginal stenosis detected during an internal pelvic examination are all examples of physical limitations that may impede sexual functioning.

It is easy to reflect on such findings and incorporate them into a sexual assessment question. An example of this might be, "Does your difficulty breathing interfere with your sexual relations with your wife/husband/ partner?" Similar information gained from the patient's records can be incorporated into the sexual history, "Often when blood counts are low, energy level is reduced. Many people find that this interferes with their sexual desire. Have you experienced this?"

To assess the sexual health of oncology patients effectively, the nurse must first be comfortable with the topic of sexuality. Comfort with self as a sexually expressive human being will convey comfort to others (Fetter, 1987). Personal beliefs and attitudes regarding sexuality are also major factors that may influence sexual assessment. Several studies have addressed the sexual attitudes held by professional nurses caring for oncology patients (Box 53–2) (Fisher, 1983, 1985; Fisher & Levin, 1983; Williams, Wilson, Hongladarom, & McDonell, 1986; Wilson & Williams, 1988). Insufficient knowledge and a discrepancy between affective responses, which indicated comfort with sexuality issues, and behavioral items, which indicated actual involvement with sexual concerns, were discovered. The need for further sexual education for oncology nurses was identified. Education for oncology nurses can be gained informally via discussions with peers and consultants with expertise in the area of human sexuality. Formal training can be gained through in-service presentations, workshops, or sexual attitude reassessment programs. Individualized knowledge can be achieved by keeping abreast of the new developments

---

Box 53–2. NURSES' ATTITUDES TOWARD SEXUALITY

Wilson, E., & Williams, H. A. (1988). **Oncology nurses' attitudes and behaviors related to sexuality of patients with cancer.** *Oncology Nursing Forum, 15*(1), 49–53.

This descriptive study explored the attitudes of 937 oncology nurses toward sexuality in cancer patients. The analysis of the responses to a mailed questionnaire revealed a positive relationship between attitudes toward sexuality in patients with cancer and number of nursing care practices related to alterations in sexuality. Nurses with more years of experience and more education reported more nursing practices related to the sexual issues of their clients. Lack of knowledge was frequently cited as a reason for not addressing sexual concerns. There was an overall lack of awareness of the presence and needs of individuals with a homosexual orientation. Nursing rounds and continuing education were two ways that were cited to increase nurses' knowledge of and comfort with discussing these issues.

---

within the field by attending conferences and reading journals and textbooks.

The ease of obtaining a sexual history can be enhanced by using several simple techniques; ensuring privacy and confidentiality, allowing ample, uninterrupted time, and maintaining a nonjudgmental attitude. A discussion of sexuality early in one's association with the client will legitimize sexuality as a important aspect of health care and ensure that it is an appropriate topic for concern in the nurse-client relationship. Anxiety will be reduced by moving from less sensitive to more sensitive topics. Use of language that is understandable to the client is essential. However, the use of slang or street language may be uncomfortable for the professional nurse; therefore, defining terms early in the discussion will alleviate this potential problem.

Certain communication techniques incorporated into the interview may also be helpful. Using open-ended questions, questions referring to frequency rather than occurrence, and "unloading" questions are specific examples of such techniques. An example of an open-ended question might be, "Some women are concerned that the removal of the uterus will decrease their sexual pleasure. Do you have this concern?" A question that refers to frequency rather than occurrence is, "How often do you have sexual intercourse" as opposed to "Do you have sexual intercourse?" "Unloading" the question refers to statement such as, "Some men masturbate on a regular basis, whereas others seldom or never masturbate. How often do you masturbate?" Finally, asking the client if he or she has any questions at the end of the assessment will convey a willingness to explore further those issues that were brought up during the assessment.

Interventions

The literature contains many articles that address sexual rehabilitation and interventions. Some focus on

cancer patients in general (Adams, 1980; Chapman & Sughrue, 1987; Enelow, 1975; Lamb & Woods, 1981; MacElveen-Hoehn, 1985; Smith, 1989; Von Eschenbach & Schrover, 1984) and others discuss specific subgroups of oncology patients (Bachers, 1985; Capone, Westie, & Good, 1980; Cooley & Cobb, 1986a, 1986b; Donahue, 1978; Golden, 1983; Grunberg, 1986; Metcalfe & Fischman, 1985; Schain, 1985; Schrover & Fife, 1985; Schwarz-Appelbaum, Dedrick, Jusenius, & Kirchner, 1984; Shipes & Lehr, 1982). The specific sexual needs or concerns of the client dictate the approach and content of the discussion. These needs and concerns can be either current or anticipated. The American Cancer Society has published two comprehensive booklets to assist cancer patients to adapt to the sexual changes that take place during cancer therapy: *Sexuality and Cancer: For the Woman Who Has Cancer, and Her Partner,* and *Sexuality and Cancer: For the Man Who Has Cancer, and His Partner.*

Intervention can be approached in many fashions. The P-LI-SS-IT model provides four levels of intervention (Annon, 1974). P-LI-SS-IT is an acronym for permission, limited information, specific suggestion, and intensive therapy. The first three levels are considered brief therapy and the fourth is intensive therapy.

Permission. Permission to discuss sexual concerns and problems is the initial step of intervention. Open communication regarding sexuality is essential for the subsequent components of the intervention process. Often patients want to know whether their sexual practices are normal or acceptable. This includes both actual sexual behaviors as well as thoughts, desires, and dreams. Concerns may also develop about becoming sexually aroused at what is thought to be inappropriate times for example, while the partner is hospitalized. Permission includes reassuring the patient and partner regarding all components of sexuality.

Limited Information. The second level of treatment is referred to as limited information. This level includes the first level, permission, but, in addition, gives specific information that addresses sexual concerns, myths, misconceptions, and questions that have arisen. Included in this level are basic facts on the appropriateness of sexual activity at this point, on the possibility of contagion or exacerbation of the malignancy. False assumptions about loss of sexual function and concerns about fertility are addressed. Providing anticipatory guidance regarding what to expect as a result of disease and treatment is included in this discussion.

Specific Suggestions. If the problem requires more than permission and information, the third level, specific suggestions, is initiated. This level of counseling attempts to help the couple directly to change behavior to reach a stated goal. Before embarking, the professional should have obtained a sexual problem history, as outlined previously. A clearly stated goal is also a requisite for the third level. The resultant plan will include specific activities for the couple. Usually, the couple is seen on several occasions. The subsequent sessions are used to assess progress and address related concerns. Specific suggestions usually pertain to the areas of communication, symptom management, and alternate physical expression.

Communication between partners should be fostered. This includes candid discussions regarding their emotional response to the disease and treatments, their fears and concerns, as well as their development of active listening skills. Symptom management is essential to optimize sexual expression. Cancer and its associated treatments often cause nausea and vomiting, weight loss, pain, fatigue, shortness of breath, and range of motion difficulties. The management of all of these symptoms may be necessary. Alternate physical expression is necessary if sexual disruption is due to organic changes. If intercourse is difficult or impossible, the couple will have to explore or expand alternate forms of expressing physical love. A thorough discussion of the couple's values and attitudes should be done before initiating alternative suggestions. There are many ways of stimulating and giving sexual pleasure: hugging, fondling, caressing, cuddling, kissing, and hand holding. Genital intercourse is only one way of expressing physical love. Sexual gratification may be derived from manual, digital, and oral stimulation. Intrathigh, anal, and intramammary intercourse are also options if the female partner is unable to continue to experience vaginal penetration (Fisher, 1983).

Intensive Therapy. Intensive therapy can be instituted if adequate progress is not being made or if the couple has long-standing sexual or marital problems. At this point, the couple is referred to a professional who has received advanced training in sex therapy. This person may be a nurse, social worker, psychiatrist, psychologist, or sex therapist (Schain, 1981).

SPECIAL PROBLEMS ASSOCIATED WITH ALTERATIONS IN SEXUAL FUNCTIONING

Cancer and cancer care often have symptoms or side effects that can negatively affect sexual functioning. This section addresses specific interventions for the most commonly experienced problems associated with cancer and its treatment. These problems include fertility concerns, range of motion difficulties, ostomy formation, nausea and vomiting, pain, fatigue, shortness of breath, and coping with progressive or terminal illness.

Fertility Concerns

Clients diagnosed with cancer during their childbearing years often have concerns regarding their future ability to parent children (Chapman, 1982; Kaempfer, 1981; Kaempfer, Hoffman, & Wiley, 1983; Kaempfer & Major, 1986; Kaempfer, Wiley, Hoffman, & Rhodes, 1985; Yarbro & Perry, 1985). Surgery, radiation, and chemotherapy have all been demonstrated to cause sterility. The topic of permanent or temporary sterility should be discussed before the onset of treatment. The client or couple's attitudes and values regarding future childbearing should be explored thoroughly. Once the assessment has been completed, preventive measures and procreative alternatives

should be discussed and planned. Examples of preventive measures are surgical relocation of the ovaries before pelvic irradiation or shielding of the gonads during radiation therapy. If preventive measures are not feasible, procreative alternatives can be suggested, such as contributing sperm to a sperm bank before treatment, artificial insemination, in vitro fertilization and embryo transfer, or adoption.

Storing sperm in a sperm bank is a reproductive option that should be considered when counseling male cancer patients. The banking of sperm offers the client protection from the mutagenic and antifertility effects of cancer therapy (Kaempfer, 1981). The preserved sperm can then potentially be used in subsequent artificial insemination or in vitro fertilization, as indicated. The issues related to this procedure for male cancer patients are still evolving. These issues include appropriateness of the candidate, costs, collection and storage procedures, legal considerations, and ethical issues (Kaempfer, 1981; Kaempfer et al., 1983, 1985). The American Fertility Society (1608 13th Avenue South, Birmingham, AL 35256) provides publications pertaining to infertility and lists of human semen cryobanks in the United States and facilities involved in in vitro fertilization and embryo transfer.

Artificial insemination is the next logical step after banking sperm and determining the appropriate time for conception. Artificial insemination is a procedure that usually occurs in an outpatient setting. Once the approximate date of ovulation is determined, usually via recording of basal body temperature and monitoring of cervical mucosa characteristics, the insemination is scheduled. Two inseminations are done per ovulation cycle. Six to 12 cycles of insemination are often required before pregnancy occurs (Kaempfer et al., 1983).

In vitro fertilization and embryo transfer is yet another evolving option for couples who anticipate or are actually experiencing infertility problems. An indepth discussion of this procedure is unwarranted in this text. However, to briefly summarize the ovaries are continually monitored via periodic ultrasound to determine the appropriate time for laparascopic attainment of the ovum. Once the ripe follicles are obtained, they are mixed with the partner's semen in a culture dish, which is then incubated for 36 to 40 hours. The resultant embryo is then transferred into the uterus, and, if pregnancy occurs, it is established within 2 weeks (Kaempfer et al., 1985). A number of issues must be considered by the couple considering this procreative alternative. The overall success rate of in vitro fertilization and embryo transfer is quite low. The costs of the procedure, which is not customarily covered by insurance, are exorbitant. The cost factor alone often leaves this option available to a very few. Finally, this procedure has been found to be quite emotionally taxing. Often an exploration of the couple's coping abilities is determined before initiation into the program (Kaempfer et al., 1985). All of these factors should be taken into account by the couple considering this option.

Range of Motion Difficulties

The progression of the cancer as well as the surgical procedures utilized to treat it may leave the patient with limited range of motion (Chapter 54). The emphasis of this discussion is on interventions to optimize the sexual functioning of clients with range of motion difficulties. Suggestions to minimize these effects are to (1) experiment with different positions, (2) use pillows to support body weight, (3) employ relaxation techniques or massage, (4) use warm baths or hot or cold soaks to affected areas before intercourse, (5) use medications (sparingly), and (6) explore alternate ways of expressing physical love.

Ostomy

The presence of an ostomy may affect sexual expression. Education, both before and after surgery, can prevent or minimize the detrimental effects that the presence of an ostomy may have on sexuality (Penninger, Moore, & Frager, 1985; Shipes, 1987; Stadil, 1983). Specific interventions are dependent on the patient's particular type of ostomy. Patients with continent ostomies can plan their sexual activity, remove the appliance, and cover the stoma before initiating sexual relations. If the appliance cannot be removed safely, the patient can empty the appliance before initiating intercourse, use a cover or a body stocking to conceal the appliance, or turn the appliance to the side (if the ostomate is in the dependent position). If the appliance is in the way, explore alternate positions; if a leak occurs, continue sexual play in the shower. The United Ostomy Association (36 Executive Parl, Suite 120, Irvine, CA 92714; (714)660–8624) has published several booklets that deal specifically with the sexual concerns of ostomates: *Sex, Courtships and the Single Ostomate; Sex, Pregnancy and the Female Ostomate;* and *Sex and the Male Ostomate.*

Nausea and Vomiting

Nausea and vomiting are frequently associated with cancer treatments. These side effects can interfere directly with sexual functioning. Numerous drug and nondrug approaches have been recommended for control of nausea and vomiting (see Chapter 47). Antiemetics are often used; however, they may interfere with sexual function because of their sedative effects. Articles have been published on patient control of nausea and vomiting. If this can be done, alternate nondrug methods to control these symptoms should be explored. These include (1) recalling past strategies that were successful in controlling nausea and vomiting; (2) eating foods that are cold or at room temperature; (3) eating small, frequent meals (especially refraining from large meals before sexual play); (4) avoiding foods with strong odors; (5) avoiding sights, sounds, and smells that stimulate nausea; (6) using relaxation or distraction techniques; (7) providing for fresh air (an open window), and (8) timing sexual activities around periods of nausea (if known).

Pain

Sexual arousal is often impaired by the presence of pain. The goal of pain therapy is to relieve pain or discomfort without hindering sexual responsiveness. The use of pain medication may decrease libido or interfere with erectile ability (Lamb & Woods, 1981). Experimenting with alternate forms of pain management, other than medication, should be explored. Relaxation techniques, such as guided imagery, may be helpful. Romantic music can be employed both for mood setting and for distraction and relaxation. Sexual activity itself is a form of distraction. Biofeedback, self-hypnosis, and application of hot and cold packs to the affected areas may substantially alleviate discomfort. The couple should be encouraged to experiment: to discover and use the most comfortable positions. The creative use of pillows should also be suggested. Massage can be both therapeutic in reducing pain as well as an arousal technique. Pain medication should be used sparingly, if at all. Finally, alternate ways of expressing physical love should be explored if the couple's traditional methods of sexual gratification are no longer feasible because of discomfort.

Fatigue

Methods to minimize exertion are necessary if fatigue is a limiting factor in sexual activity. Providing time for rest before and after intercourse is often sufficient to minimize the detrimental effects of a decrease in available energy. Other suggestions include (1) avoid the stress of consuming heavy meals or alcohol before intercourse, (2) avoid extremes in temperature, (3) experiment with positions that require minimal exertion (male client-female astride, female client-male astride, side lying); (4) take timing into consideration (intercourse in the morning rather than at night), and (5) periodically delegate or delay household tasks such as child care and meal preparation to conserve energy for intimate relations.

Shortness of Breath

Sexual activity can be directly impaired by dyspnea (Welch-McCaffrey, 1983). The fear of potential dyspnea itself is often a deterrent to initiating sexual play. The use of a water bed to accentuate physical movements during sexual activity can be suggested. In addition, keeping the affected partner's head and upper torso raised (via the use of pillows) will also encourage adequate oxygenation. Pulmonary hygiene before sexual activity may also be of benefit. Finally, the affected partner should be encouraged to assume a more passive role and a dependent position during sexual activity.

SUMMARY AND CONTINUING AREAS OF CONCERNS AND ISSUES

Cancer and the therapies employed to combat it often result in a compromise of quality of life. To minimize the adverse effects of these diseases and their treatments on those affected, clinicians should address the real or potential alterations in sexual functioning that occur. The more than 5 million Americans alive today who have a history of cancer should be seen as holistic beings whose needs, hopes, and concerns are the same as all others. The ramifications of withholding sexual information from clients with cancer can be profound. A little investment on the nurse's part to provide information and support can make a significant difference in the couple's ability to adjust to changes in sexual functioning (Smith, 1989).

The difficulties of a team approach in this domain are apparent. Confusion may arise as to which care provider (primary care nurse, clinical nurse specialist, physician, social worker, or others) has counseled the client or couple regarding sexual concerns. What information has been given, in what depth, to whom (client, partner, or both), regarding which actual or potential problems, and how to avoid or minimize these effects are just a few of the issues that surface. Nurses should take a leading role in the assessment and remediation of clients' concerns regarding the sexual ramifications of their disease and resultant treatments.

The sexual dysfunctions resulting from cancer are becoming less unknown and mysterious. As research in this field continues, the sexual dysfunctions experienced by oncology patients are becoming more delineated, and interventions are being explored to prevent or minimize the adverse sexual sequelae of cancer and its treatment.

References

Adams, A. K. (1980). The sex counseling role of the cancer clinician. *Frontiers of Radiation Therapy and Oncology, 14,* 66–78.

Amercian Cancer Society. (1990). *Cancer facts and figures—1990.* New York: Author.

Andersen B. L. (1987). Sexual functioning complications in women with gynecologic cancer: Outcomes and directions for prevention. *Cancer, 60* (Suppl.), 2123–2128.

Andersen, B. L. (1985). Sexual functioning morbidity among cancer survivors. *Cancer, 55,* 1835–1842.

Andersen, B. L. (1987). Sexual functioning complications in women with gynecologic cancer: Outcomes and directions for prevention. *Cancer, 60* (Suppl.), 2123–2128.

Andersen, B. L., & Hacker, N. F. (1983a). Psychosexual adjustment after vulvar surgery. *Obstetrics and Gynecology, 62,*457–462.

Andersen, B. L., & Hacker, N. F. (1983b). Psychosexual adjustment following pelvic exenteration. *Obstetrics and Gynecology, 61,* 331–338.

Andersen, B. L., Lachenbruch, P. A., Anderson, B., & DeProsse, C. (1986). Sexual dysfunction and signs of gynecologic cancer. *Cancer, 57,* 1880–1886.

Andreasson, B., Moth, I., Jensen, S. B., & Bock, J. E. (1986). Sexual function and somatic psychic reactions in vulvectomy-operated women and their partners. *Acta Obstetrica et Gynecologica Scandinavica, 65,*7–10.

Annon, J. S. (1974). *The behavioral treatment of sexual problems.* Honolulu: Mercantile Printing.

Bachers, E. S. (1985). Sexual dysfunction after treatment for genitourinary cancer. *Seminars in Oncology Nursing, 1,* 18–24.

Beckmann, J., Blichert-Toft, M., & Johansen, L. (1983). Psychological effects of mastectomy. *Danish Medical Bulletin, 30*(Suppl. 2), 7–10.

Bertelsen, K. (1983). Sexual dysfunction after treatment for cervical cancer. *Danish Medical Bulletin, 30*(Suppl. 2), 31–34.

Brenner, J., Vugrin, D., & Whitmore, W. F. (1985). Effect of treatment on fertility and sexual function in males treated with metastatic nonseminomatous germ cell tumors of the testis. *American Journal of Clinical Oncology, 8,* 178–182.

Cantor, R. C. (1980). Self-esteem, sexuality and cancer-related stress. *Frontiers in Radiation Therapy and Oncology, 14,* 51–54.

Capone, M. A., Westie, K. S., & Good, R. S. (1980). Sexual rehabilitation of the gynecologic cancer patient: An effective counseling model. *Frontiers in Radiation Therapy and Oncology, 14,* 123–129.

Chapman, J., & Sughrue, J. (1987). A model for sexual assessment and intervention. *Health Care for Women International, 8,* 87–99.

Chapman, R. M. (1982). Effect of cytotoxic therapy on sexuality and gonadal function. *Seminars in Oncology, 9,* 84–94.

Cooley, M. E., & Cobb, S. C. (1986a). Sexual and reproductive issues for women with Hodgkin's disease. Overview of issues. *Cancer Nursing, 9,* 188–193.

Cooley, M. E., & Cobb, S. C. (1986b). Sexual and reproductive issues for women with Hodgkin's disease. Application of the PLISSIT model. *Cancer Nursing, 9,* 248–255.

Derogatis, L. R. (1980). Breast and gynecologic cancers. *Frontiers in Radiation Therapy and Oncology, 14,*1–11.

Dobkin, K. A., & Broadwell, D. C. (1986). Nursing considerations for the patient undergoing colostomy surgery. *Seminars in Oncology Nursing, 2,* 249–255.

Donahue, D. C. (1978). Sexual rehabilitation of gynecologic cancer patients. *Medical Aspects of Human Sexuality, 2,* 51–52.

Enelow, A. J. (1975). Psychosocial rehabilitation for cancer patients. *Frontiers in Radiation Therapy and Oncology, 10,* 178–182.

Fetter, M. P. (1987). Reaching a level of sexual comfort. *Health Education, 18,* 6–8.

Fisher, S. G. (1983). The psychosexual effect of cancer and cancer treatment. *Oncology Nursing Forum, 10*(2), 63–67.

Fisher, S. G. (1985). The sexual knowledge and attitudes of oncology nurses: Implications for nursing education. *Seminars in Oncology Nursing, 1,* 63–68.

Fisher, S. G., & Levin, D. L. (1983). The sexual knowledge and attitudes of professional nurses caring for oncology patients. *Cancer Nursing, 6,* 55–61.

Foltz, A. T. (1987). The influence of cancer on self concept and quality of life. *Seminars in Oncology Nursing, 3,* 303–312.

Glasgow, M., Halfin, V., & Althausen, A. F. (1987). Sexual response and cancer. *CA: A Cancer Journal for Clinicians, 37,* 322–332.

Golden, J. S., & Golden, M. (1980). Cancer and sex. *Frontiers in Radiation Therapy and Oncology, 14,* 59–65.

Golden, M. (1983). Female sexuality and crisis of mastectomy. *Danish Medical Bulletin, 30*(Suppl. 2), 13–16.

Greenberg, D. B. (1984). The measurement of sexual dysfunction in cancer patients. *Cancer, 53*(Suppl.), 2281–2285.

Grunberg, K. J. (1986). Sexual rehabilitation of the cancer patient undergoing ostomy surgery. *Journal of Enterostomal Therapy, 13,* 148–152.

Harris, R., Good, R. S., & Pollack, L. (1982). Sexual behavior of gynecologic cancer patients. *Archives of Sexual Behavior, 11,* 503–510.

Jenkins, B. (1988). Patients' report of sexual changes after treatment for gynecologic cancer. *Oncology Nursing Forum, 15*(3), 349–354.

Johnson, J. (1986). Sexual concerns of the cancer patient. *Nursing Republic of South Africa Verpleging, 1*(10), 24–25.

Jusenius, K. (1981). Sexuality and gynecologic cancer. *Cancer Nursing, 4,* 479–484.

Kaempfer, S. H. (1981). The effects of cancer chemotherapy on reproduction: A review of the literature. *Oncology Nursing Forum, 8*(1), 11–18.

Kaempfer, S. H., Hoffman, D. J., & Wiley, F. M. (1983). Sperm banking: A reproductive option in cancer therapy. *Cancer Nursing, 4,* 31–38.

Kaempfer, S. H., & Major, P. (1986). Fertility considerations in the gynecologic cancer patient. *Oncology Nursing Forum, 13*(1), 27.

Kaempfer, S. H., Wiley, F. M., Hoffman, D. J., & Rhodes, E. A. (1985). Fertility considerations and procreative alternatives in cancer care. *Seminars in Oncology Nursing, 1*, 25–34.

Lamb, M. (1985). Sexual dysfunction in the gynecologic oncology patient. *Seminars in Oncology Nursing, 1*, 9–17.

Lamb, M., & Woods, N. F. (1981). Sexuality and the cancer patient. *Cancer Nursing, 4*, 137–144.

LaMonica, G., Audisio, R. A., Tamburini, M., Filberti, A., & Ventafridda, V. (1985). Incidence of sexual dysfunction in male patients treated surgically for rectal malignancy. *Diseases of the Colon and Rectum, 23*, 937–940.

MacElveen-Hoehn, P. (1985). Sexual assessment and counseling. *Seminars in Oncology Nursing, 1*, 69–75.

Masters W., & Johnson, V. (1966) *Human sexual response.* Boston: Little, Brown & Co.

Metcalfe, M. C., & Fischman, S. H. (1985). Factors affecting the sexuality of patients with head and neck cancer. *Oncology Nursing Forum, 12*(2), 21–25.

Mims, F. H., & Swenson, M. (1980). *Sexuality: A nursing perspective.* New York: McGraw-Hill Book Co.

Moth, I., Andreasson, B., Jensen, S. B., & Bock, J. E. (1983). Sexual function and somatopsychic reactions after vulvectomy. *Danish Medical Bulletin, 30*(Suppl. 2), 27–30.

Penninger, J. I., Moore, S. B., & Frager, S. R. (1985). After the ostomy: Helping your patient reclaim his sexuality. *RN, 48*(4), 46–50.

Petty, F., & Noyes, R. (1981). Depression secondary to cancer. *Biologic Psychiatry, 16*, 1203–1220.

Rubin, P. (Ed). (1983). *Clinical oncology: A multidisciplinary approach.* New York: American Cancer Society.

Schain, W. S. (1980). Sexual functioning, self-esteem and cancer care. *Frontiers in Radiation Therapy and Oncology, 14*, 12–19.

Schain, W. S. (1981). Role of the sex therapist in the care of the cancer patient. *Frontiers in Radiation Therapy and Oncology, 15*, 168–183.

Schain, W. S. (1985). Breast cancer surgeries and psychosexual sequelae: Implications for remediation. *Seminars in Oncology Nursing, 1*, 200–205.

Schrover, L. R., & Fife, M. (1985). Sexual counseling of patients undergoing radical surgery for pelvic or genital cancer. *Journal of Psychosocial Oncology, 3*(3), 21–41.

Schrover, L. R., Gonzales, J., & von Eschenbach, A. C. (1986). Sexual and marital relationships after radiotherapy for seminoma. *Urology, 27*, 117–123.

Schrover, L. R., von Eschenbach, A. C., Smith, D. B., & Gonzales, J. (1984). Sexual rehabilitation of urologic cancer patients: A practical approach. *CA: A Cancer Journal for Clinicians, 34*(2), 66–73.

Schwarz-Appelbaum, J., Dedrick, J., Jusenius, K., & Kirchner, C. W. (1984). Nursing care plans: Sexuality and treatment of breast cancer. *Oncology Nursing Forum, 11*(6), 16–24.

Sewell, H. H., & Edwards, D. W. (1980). Pelvic genitial cancer: Body image and sexuality. *Frontiers of Radiation Therapy and Oncology, 14*, 35–41.

Shapiro, E. (1987). Modified surgery curbs dysfunction. *Cope, 1*(10), 52.

Shipes, E. (1987). Sexual functioning following ostomy surgery. *Nursing Clinics of North America, 22*, 303–310.

Shipes, E., & Lehr, S. (1982). Sexuality and the male cancer patient. *Cancer Nursing, 5*, 375–381.

Smith, D. B. (1989). Sexual rehabilitation of the cancer patient. *Cancer Nursing, 12*, 10–15.

Spengler, A. (1983). Radical prostatectomy and sexuality. *Sexuality and Disability, 6*, 155–166.

Stadil, F. (1983). Intestinal stomas. *Danish Medical Bulletin. 30*(Suppl. 2), 35–37.

von Eschenbach, A. C., & Schrover, L. R. (1984). The role of sexual rehabilitation in the treatment of patients with cancer. *Cancer, 54*(Suppl.), 2662–2667.

Wabrek, A. J., & Gunn, J. L. (1984, Nov./Dec.). Sexual and psychological implications of gynecologic malignancy. *JOGN Nursing*, pp. 371–376.

Walbroehl, G. S. (1985). Sexuality in cancer patients. *American Family Physician, 31*, 153–158.

Welch-McCaffrey, D. (1983). Dyspnea and sexual intercourse. *Oncology Nursing Forum, 10*(1), 80.

Wellisch, D. K. (1985). The psychologic impact of breast cancer on relationships. *Seminars in Oncology Nursing, 1*, 195–199.

Williams, H. A., Wilson, M. E., Hongladarom, G., & McDonell, M. (1986). Nurses' attitudes toward sexuality in cancer patients. *Oncology Nursing Forum, 13*(2), 39–43.

Wilson, M. E., & Williams, H. A. (1988). Oncology nurses' attitudes and behaviors related to sexuality of patients with cancer. *Oncology Nursing Forum, 15*(1), 49–53.

Wise, T. N. (1978). Sexual functioning in neoplastic disease. *Medical Aspects of Human Sexuality, 12*, 16–31.

Wood, J. D., & Tombrink, J. (1983). Impact of cancer on sexuality and self image: A group program for patients and partners. *Social Work in Health Care, 8*(4), 45–54.

Woods, N. F. (1990). *Human sexuality in health and illness.* 3rd Edition. St. Louis: C. V. Mosby Co.

World Health Organization. (1975). Education and treatment in human sexuality: The training of health professionals, Report of a WHO meeting. Technical report series no. 572. Geneva: Author.

Wujcik, D., Carbonell, M. A., Taseff, L., Sciarra, L., & Isaac, E. (1986). Managing the patient with testicular cancer. *Nursing 86, 16*(8), 42–45.

Yarbro, C., & Perry, M. C. (1985). The effect of cancer therapy on gonadal function. *Seminars in Oncology Nursing, 1*, 3–8.

Zussman, L., Zussman, S., Sunley, R., & Bjornson, E. (1981). Sexual response after hysterectomy-oophorectomy: Recent studies and reconsideration of psychogenesis. *American Journal of Obstetrics and Gynecology, 140*, 725–729.

CHAPTER 54

Alterations in Mobility

KARIN DUFAULT
SHARON CANNELL FIRSICH

Alterations in mobility present some challenging problems to the nurse caring for the person with cancer. Although they are less obvious than such problems as nutrition and pain, alterations in mobility may profoundly affect the quality of life for the person and family as they deal with the disease and its treatment (McNally, Stair, & Somerville, 1985). In this chapter the interaction between normal physiology and mobility is examined, after which some of the psychosocial factors that affect and are affected by mobility are discussed. Information related to management of specific nursing diagnoses and some of the common problems of cancer-related immobility also are presented.

THE INTERACTION OF NORMAL PHYSIOLOGY AND MOBILITY

Effects of Position and Weight Bearing

The maintenance of normal muscle and bone strength and structure is partially dependent on weight bearing and normal levels of activity. Both weight bearing and normal mobility help to maintain the balance between bone formation and resorption and muscle mass and strength (Potter & Perry, 1985). The effect of position on mobility is usually produced by limitation of position, which prevents weight bearing or full muscle use, thereby decreasing joint motion and muscle strength.

The direct effect of position and weight bearing is of greatest importance for mobility of the musculoskeletal system, but it is also important to keep in mind the other physical functions that are influenced by mobility: metabolic, respiratory, cardiovascular, integumentary, and eliminative (originally described by Olson in 1967 [Box 54–1 and Table 54–1]).

Metabolic functions undergo changes as the metabolic rate is decreased. Tissue atrophies and protein catabolism increases, bone demineralization begins, alteration in the exchange of nutrients occurs, and gastrointestinal disturbances develop (Olson, 1967). *Respiratory* changes then occur, partly as a direct effect of the immobility, partly as an effect of the metabolic changes. Hemoglobin decreases, lung expansion decreases, and generalized muscle weakness and stasis of secretions develop. The major changes in cardiovascular functioning are orthostatic hypotension, increased cardiac workload, and thrombus formation. Immobility has its greatest effects on the integrity of the *skin* of elderly people with altered sensory or motor function and nutritional or metabolic changes—a fair description of many persons with cancer. Any one of these factors puts the person at risk for alterations in skin integrity (Olson, 1967). In the *eliminative* processes, several changes relate to altered mobility: urine retention, renal calculi, and urinary tract infections

---

Box 54-1. CLASSIC ARTICLE: "THE HAZARDS OF IMMOBILITY," EDITED BY E. OLSON

In April, 1967, in the *American Journal of Nursing* a series of articles was published that changed immeasurably the way in which nurses thought about immobility and its effect on the people for whom they were caring. With co-authors Lida F. Thompson, Joyce McCarthy, Bonnie Jean Johnson, Ruth E. Edmonds, Lois M. Schroeder, and Mildred Wade, Edith Olson presented a comprehensive look at the effects of immobility. Effects on cardiovascular, respiratory, gastrointestinal, motor, and urinary function were examined in detail. Additionally, effects on metabolic and psychosocial equilibrium were presented. The studies are thoroughly referenced and conclusions were drawn. Nursing implications were then offered in each area.

This series of articles grew out of a symposium presented by these authors at the annual meeting of the Colorado Nurses' Association in the Spring of 1966, and these authors have continued to make many contributions to nursing and nursing literature over the years.

Any nurse interested in the problems of immobility will do well to thoroughly study this series. It truly deserves the designation "classic."

---

may result, and constipation becomes a common problem.

Effects of Muscle and Joint Movement

The general body effects of position and weight bearing on immobility have been discussed, but the specific effects of decreased muscle and joint use also need to be considered. Normal range of motion can be maintained only with full use and normal activity. With increasing age, range of motion, particularly in the spine, tends to decrease even in persons without actual disease conditions, although these changes are extremely variable from person to person.

The mechanical effect of muscle and, indirectly, joint movement is part of the body's mechanism for maintaining adequate venous return. Alterations result in increased venous stasis and increase the threat of thrombus formation.

Skin integrity is protected indirectly with normal mobility of the muscles and joints, as the maintenance of venous return helps prevent stasis and edema. In addition, normal movement prevents undue pressure on any particular area of the skin, again helping to guard against the dangers that pressure and ischemia present to the skin.

It is clear how important normal mobility is to the maintenance of the integrity of physical functioning. When the effects of disease, treatment, and aging are considered, they must be viewed within the context of these interactions of activity and normal systemic functioning (Gregor, McCarthy, Chwirchak, Meluch, & Mion, 1986).

PATHOPHYSIOLOGIC FACTORS THAT INTERFERE WITH MOBILITY IN THE PERSON WITH CANCER

Effect of Disease Process and Treatment

Alterations in mobility stemming from the disease process may be categorized as either structural or functional. In structural effects there is actual disease involvement of the mobilizing body parts themselves (e.g., bones, muscle, nerves, or connective tissue). These structural changes may be due to destruction of tissue, or they may be a result of pain or edema in the body part, which then leads to alterations in the mobilizing structures themselves. In functional effects, the altered mobility is an indirect effect, such as fatigue or altered mental status, that has been produced by the disease process. The alteration means that, initially, at least, there is no damage to the mobilizing structures, but because the person is unable to use those structures normally, owing to the absence of strength, coordination, and so forth, the lack of use results in structural changes, as discussed earlier.

The disease process may have a direct effect on mobility, but an equal problem may be the effect of

Table 54-1. POTENTIAL EFFECTS OF IMMOBILITY

Physiologic
Metabolic
  Reduced metabolic rate
  Reduced adrenal corticoids
  Stress reactions
Cardiovascular
  Orthostatic hypotension
  Increased workload
  Thrombus formation
Skin
  Decubitus ulcers
Respiratory
  Decreased respiratory movement
  Stasis of secretions
  Oxygen–carbon dioxide imbalance
Musculoskeletal
  Osteoporosis
  Contractures
Urinary
  Urinary tract stones
Gastrointestinal
  Ingestion
  Elimination
    Suppression of defecation
    Constipation
Psychosocial
Altered perceptions
Altered social roles
Altered mood states
Developmental
Delayed achievement of developmental tasks
Regression to previous developmental level

the treatment. Again this may be structural: surgery, radiation, and even chemotherapy may cause actual changes in the body parts that are necessary for mobility. In addition, these same treatment methods may cause various effects that indirectly produce a functional loss of mobility: pain, fatigue, and weakness all may at some time be part of the person's daily life and have a profound effect on the ability to be normally mobile.

Effect of Lymphedema

Lymphedema may be produced in the person with cancer by the disease itself, with malignant involvement of lymph nodes or surrounding structures causing obstruction of lymph flow and preventing the movement of these osmotically active materials back into the systemic circulation (Kneisl & Ames, 1986). This same effect may be produced by surgery or radiation during or subsequent to the treatment process as healing and fibrosis occur. Obviously, the location of the alteration will be the most important determinant of the effect on mobility (Porth, 1986). Lymphedema, although a less common cause of lower extremity immobility in cancer survivors, is still a relatively common problem in the arms of women with radical or modified radical mastectomies. Even with less extensive breast surgery, both discomfort and decreased mobility may result in the affected arm when the patient undergoes lymph node dissection or radiation. It is important to keep in mind that in chronic edema the tissue spaces become stretched so that less filtration pressure is needed to maintain the edema. This stretching then makes permanent correction of the edema difficult (Porth, 1986). Prevention of extensive edema that may threaten mobility of any body part then becomes an important goal of posttreatment nursing care. Treatment with radiation or surgery is sometimes helpful in relieving the obstruction that is causing the edema.

Effect of Tumor Involvement of the Bone

Characteristically, the person with a primary bone tumor has a painful mass. This pain often is not actually of immobilizing degree at the outset but may cause alteration in normal mobility as the person's usual activities begin to be curtailed owing to pain (Price & Wilson, 1986). Because primary lesions of the bone most commonly occur in children and young people, often in the bones of the extremities, the effect of increasing disease and subsequent treatment on mobility is likely to be profound. As pain increases, mobility becomes much more limited.

Treatment is most commonly surgical and is certain to produce some modification in mobility; in addition, often some alteration will be permanent. Cryosurgery, radiotherapy, and chemotherapy may also be used at some stages of treatment and may produce either temporary or permanent alteration in mobility of the affected part. Again, treatment may cause additional pain and fatigue, which compound the total physical impact and further decrease the person's mobility. Secondary use of radiation therapy, chemotherapy, or surgery may be helpful in reducing pain and therefore increasing mobility. Both the presence of metastatic tumor and its treatment have some of the same effects on mobility as those of primary bone tumor in that bone pain will probably occur, with its immobilizing effect, and again treatment may produce side effects that compound the immobilization.

Additional threats to mobility often are present for the person with bony metastasis. The population with metastatic disease is likely to be an older group than that of patients with primary disease, so that mobility is already threatened, either from the aging process itself or from other systemic disease. Usually these people have been treated, or the disease itself may have resulted in immobilizing residual effects. Treatment options may be limited because of the previous treatment. In metastatic disease the extremities are less likely to be affected, and the bones of the spine, rib cage, and pelvis are more commonly involved. Tumor in these locations often has a profound effect on the person's ability to be normally mobile, whether because of pain at the site or because of weakened bone structure, which may result in pathologic fractures.

Effect of Spinal Cord Compression

Some primary spinal cord tumors may cause alteration in central nervous system function. These are often relatively slowly progressive, and the neurologic deficits appear later in the course of disease because the spinal cord is able to adapt to the compression (Price & Wilson, 1986). With metastatic lesions, however, neurologic change is often rapid and progressive. Because of the anatomic structure of the spine, symptoms generally begin well below the site of the lesion, and the level of impairment ascends as the compression increases and deeper cord levels are affected. Cord compressions can also disturb the patient's sense of position, producing ataxia with its resultant disturbance of mobility. Metastatic tumors are likely to be extradural, and pain—either localized or radicular—is often the first symptom (Price & Wilson, 1986). The localized pain tends to be increased by movement and is particularly immobilizing. Actual compression of the spine may come from encroachment of the tumor, collapse of the vertebral column, or hemorrhage from the tumor. Once the compression begins it rapidly becomes total—paresthesia and sensory loss progress to irreversible paraplegia unless decompression can be accomplished (Price & Wilson, 1986). Decompression is most likely to be surgical, although radiation and chemotherapy may also be employed in this urgent situation. Fortunately, early recognition and management of the problem can prevent these serious effects. This makes the nursing responsibilities of assessment and rapid diagnosis of altered sensation and functioning critical.

Effect of Central Nervous System Involvement

Because of the diversity of brain tumors it is difficult to generalize about their effect on mobility. Altered mobility observed in persons with brain tumors most often is related to treatment effects occurring after the surgery, radiation therapy, or chemotherapy used to treat the primary lesion. This treatment may cause alteration in mobility because of sided weakness or seizures, just as the disease itself may. In addition, as is true for countless situations, the direct effects of either the treatment or the disease itself, such as pain and fatigue, may have considerable effect on the ability of the person to be normally mobile.

PSYCHOSOCIAL FACTORS THAT INTERFERE WITH MOBILITY IN THE PERSON WITH CANCER

Besides the pathophysiologic features that alter the ability of a person with cancer to be freely mobile, numerous psychosocial factors influence mobility. Some are described by Olson (see Table 54–1). One manner of examining the psychosocial factors is to consider patterns of activities of daily living, of general life style, and of coping.

Patterns of Activities of Daily Living

The degree of functional independence experienced by a person may influence both the responses to changes in mobility and the changes themselves. Functional independence encompasses the wide range of activities engaged in by persons during the course of a 24-hr day and are often described as activities of daily living and self-care. Activities of daily living capabilities often are considered in the light of whether the person is independent in bed, in the home, or in the community.

Among the activities that are examined to determine functional independence are the following: (1) bathing, (2) communicating, (3) exercising, (4) grooming, (5) dressing, (6) eating, (7) bed and hygiene activities, (8) mobility, (9) transferring, (10) recreation, (11) socializing, (12) homemaking, (13) sexual activities, (14) avocational activities, and (15) vocational activities (Chiou & Burnett, 1985; Martin, Holt, & Hicks, 1980). A study by Chiou and Burnett (1985) indicated the importance of patients' values as they relate to specific activities of daily living. The value placed on the activity was an important factor to consider in identifying rehabilitation goals in this study, which involved stroke patients. The relative value of the activities that indicated functional independence for the person with

cancer may also have a bearing on the response of the person to alteration in self-care and more specifically to alterations in mobility. Awareness of the degree to which alterations in mobility interfere with the functional independence activities of greatest value to the person can provide insights into understanding the real impact of the changes. The understanding can guide nursing interventions as they relate both to mobility and to enhancement of the other significantly valued activities of daily living. Among the most highly valued activities of daily living are those related to mobility.

Decreased mobility and activities of daily living ranked highest of rehabilitation problems identified in cancer patients in several studies (Cancer Rehabilitation Coordination Team, 1978; Donovan & Girton, 1984; Lehmann, DeLisa, & Warren, 1978).

General Life-style Patterns

Life-style patterns represent a complex outcome of many personal, interpersonal, environmental, and societal factors, which arise not only from the person's present situation but also from his or her life history and heredity. Carnevali and Patrick (1979) defined life style as the totality of a person's approach to living. It incorporates such characteristics as preferences for independence or dependence, high or low stress levels, spontaneity and change or structure and regularity, extroversion or introversion, rapid or slow pace, and high or low physical activity. The preferences translate into observable behaviors in approaching routine as well as unusual events.

Health professionals have focused attention on identifying elements of healthy and unhealthy life-style patterns. Major determinants of health include (1) nutrition, (2) physical fitness, (3) psychosocial stressors, (4) stress management or reduction, and (5) sense of purpose and will. Other important dimensions of life style include the relationship network and the strength of the family structure, cultural variables, and economic and educational factors.

The Health Hazard Appraisal by Milsum (1980) is one instrument for examining life style in an effort to promote health by preventing death and disability attributable to reducible risk. Three patterns are characterized: sedentary, middle-aged workers whose risk is two or more times the average risk for disease; persons who have an aggregate risk somewhat above average and whose appraised age is perhaps up to 5 years above actual age; and persons living at very low risk and for whom the emphasis is on the desirability of maintaining and improving the present good status.

It can be hypothesized that the healthier the life style (before and during the cancer course), the more likely that a person will possess the physical, psychological, social, and spiritual resources to cope with the effects resulting from the diagnosis of cancer, including alterations in mobility. Understanding the general life-style patterns of the person with cancer and the family can further the understanding of the impact that altered mobility has and the potential problems it imposes on the person as well as of the coping resources available to deal with the changes.

Coping Patterns

Coping has been described by Lazarus and Launier (1978) as "efforts, both action oriented and intrapsychic, to manage (i.e., master, tolerate, reduce, minimize) environmental and internal demands, and conflicts among them, which tax or exceed a person's resources." Weisman (1979), in speaking of coping with cancer, states that coping is "what one does about a problem in order to bring about relief, reward, quiescence, and equilibrium." Coping functions with a problem-solving focus when efforts are made to cope with the stress itself by dealing with obstacles and opportunities in the environment and in oneself. Coping functions with an emotion focus when efforts are made to regulate the emotional stress and distress palliatively.

The Omega Project at Massachusetts General Hospital (1974–1979) provided descriptions of how cancer patients cope or fail to cope. Weisman and Worden (1977) identified the factors associated with patients who are at high risk of emotional distress (vulnerability) and the coping strategies that are most likely to be ineffective. These factors include the following:

- Marital problems
- Living alone
- Economic marginality
- Alcohol abuse
- Multiple problems in family of origin
- Lack of church affiliation
- Psychiatric history
- Suicidal ideation
- Low ego strength
- High anxiety level
- Pessimistic attitude
- Advanced stage of cancer
- Multiple reported symptoms
- Multiple current concerns and problems of all types with poor resolution
- Little help or support expected or received
- Health professionals seen as unhelpful or unconcerned
- Use of coping strategies of (1) suppression and passivity, (2) isolation and withdrawal, (3) blaming others, and (4) blaming self

The greater the number of high-risk factors present, the greater the risk of suffering distress and failing to cope with the stressors of the diagnosis and treatment of cancer. In addition to determining the least effective coping strategies, the researchers identified the most effective categories (Table 54–2).

The three most effective coping strategies evident in Weisman and Worden's study—that is, those that relieved distress and resolved the problem—were confrontation, redefinition, and cooperative compliance. A conclusion drawn by Weisman and Worden (1977)

Table 54–2. COPING STRATEGIES

Seek more information (rational inquiry)
Share concern and talk with others (mutuality)
Laugh it off; make light of situation (affect reversal)
Try to forget; put it out of your mind (suppression)
Do other things for distraction (displacement or redirection)
Take firm action based on present understanding (confront)
Accept but find something favorable (redefine or revise)
Submit to the inevitable; fatalism (passive acceptance)
Do something, anything, however reckless or impractical (impulsivity)
Consider or negotiate feasible alternative (if x, then y)
Reduce tension with excessive drink, drugs, danger (life threats)
Withdraw into isolation; get away (disengagement)
Blame someone or something (externalize or project)
Seek direction; do as you are told (cooperative compliance)
Blame yourself; sacrifice or atone (moral masochism)

(Data from Weisman, 1979.)

was that the dividing crux between good copers and bad copers is the difference between resourcefulness and rigidity and between constructive optimism versus a pessimism that expects replication of earlier defeats.

By taking time to discover people's past patterns of coping with stress, health professionals can better help persons who are experiencing the new stress of living with alterations of immobility. Other information that is important includes the patient's available coping resources, including problem-solving skills; energy; health; morale; and social, spiritual, and economic support systems; and the person's perceptions of stressors (as harm, threat, or challenge), their interpretation of events, and their general beliefs and specific beliefs about causes. It is possible that use of a person's least effective coping strategies can lead to the depression, apathy, hopelessness, and helplessness that results in decreased physical activity and greater immobility than his or her physical condition would suggest. By the same token, a person's psychosocial response to physiologically imposed immobility may be depression, negative behavioral changes, changes in sleep-wake cycles, decreased problem-solving ability, loss of interest in surroundings, increased isolation, and sensory deprivation depending on the coping resources and abilities (see Table 54–1). Use of more effective coping strategies and resources results in a more positive picture, in which alterations in mobility are seen as one more challenge to be overcome or adapted to achieve yet other goals or to ensure fulfillment of treasured hopes.

PROCESS OF ASSESSMENT IN THE DIAGNOSTIC PROCESS

Assessment of the Problem

The nurse will need to assess the level of mobility in managing the care of any client using the theoretic framework with which the nurse is most comfortable. Within that assessment, certain patterns must be discerned if an adequate nursing diagnosis is to be made. The Standards for Oncology Nursing Practice (American Nurses' Association & Oncology Nursing Society

[ANA-ONS], 1987) point out the nurse's responsibility to collect data in a systematic and continuous fashion. Nursing data need to be gathered regarding both the level of mobility and the potential for sequelae related to immobility. The data collected must be both objective and subjective (ANA-ONS, 1987).

The two aspects of data gathering—history and physical assessment—must be attended to. There are many indexes for measuring the activities of daily living—probably the most useful way to examine the alteration in mobility. Because more than 43 different indexes have been developed, few of which have been documented empirically, it is difficult for the nurse to find a generally accepted means of evaluating the patient's level of activity (Feinstein, Joseph, & Wells, 1986). Probably the two most commonly used scales are the Karnofsky Scale (Table 54–3) and the Barthel Index (Table 54–4). Although few scales have been developed specifically for oncology patients, the existing scales often have useful approaches for the nurse's consideration in assessment of the patient with a problem of immobility (Gulick, 1986; Robinson, 1986; Williams, 1986).

Having developed the initial database that allows assessment of the person's present level of mobility and the potential for sequelae secondary to that level of mobility, the nurse is ready to move on to the identification of actual or potential health problems and formulate the nursing diagnoses on which the care plan can be built (Table 54–5).

Defining the Characteristics of the Problem

The accepted nursing diagnosis for alterations in mobility is mobility, impaired physical—related to alterations in lower limbs or alterations in upper limbs

Table 54–3. PATIENT PERFORMANCE RATING (KARNOFSKY)

Able to carry on normal activity; no special care	100	Normal; no complaints; no evidence of disease
	90	Able to carry on normal activity; minor signs or symptoms of disease
	80	Normal activity with effort; some signs or symptoms of disease
Unable to work; able to live at home; cares for most personal needs; a varying amount of assistance is needed	70	Cares for self; unable to carry on normal activity or to do active work
	60	Requires occasional assistance but is able to care for most needs
	50	Requires considerable assistance and frequent medical care
Unable to care for self; requires equivalent of institutional or hospital care; disease may be progressing rapidly	40	Disabled; requires special care and assistance
	30	Severely disabled; hospitalization is indicated although death not imminent
	20	Very sick; hospitalization necessary
	10	Moribund; fatal processes progressing rapidly
	1	Unconscious
	0	Dead

(Data from Chang & Hawes, 1983.)

Table 54–4. BARTHEL INDEX

Independent		Dependent		
Intact	Limited	Helper	Null	
10	5	1	1	Drink from cup; Feed from dish
5	5	3	0	Dress upper body
5	5	2	0	Dress lower body
0	0	−2	0	Don brace or prosthesis
5	5	0	0	Groom
4	4	0	0	Wash or bathe
10	10	5	0	Bladder continence
10	10	5	0	Bowel continence
4	4	2	0	Care of perineum, use of cloth at toilet
15	15	7	0	Transfer, chair
6	5	3	0	Transfer, toilet
1	1	0	0	Transfer, tub or shower
15	15	10	0	Walk on level 50 yards or more
10	10	5	0	Up and down stairs, 1 flight
15	5	0	0	Wheelchair 50 yards/if not walking
				Barthel Total Score

(Data from Jacelon, 1986.)

(Carpenito, 1987). The major characteristics that must be present are the inability to move purposefully within the environment, including bed mobility, transfers, and ambulation or the inability to move because of imposed restrictions (e.g., bed rest, mechanical devices). Clearly these major characteristics are not uncommon in oncology patients in various stages of disease and treatment. Minor characteristics that may be present are range of motion limitations, limited muscle strength or control, and impaired coordination. Information gathered from the assessment process should allow the nurse to identify which of these defining characteristics are present or are realistic potentials for a given client.

Etiologic and Risk Factors Related to the Problem

Because the diagnostic process allows the nurse to put in rational order the quantities of information accumulated in the database, it is necessary to look beyond the major and minor characteristics of the problem to examine etiologic and contributing factors as it is toward these factors that nursing interventions are likely to be addressed. For impaired physical mobility, these factors fall into four categories: pathophysiologic, treatment related, situational, and maturational. The *pathophysiologic* factors may relate to neuromuscular impairment or to musculoskeletal factors. The *treatment-related* factors may be associated with activity restrictions such as bed rest, physical changes such as amputation, or mechanical devices. *Situational* factors are personal or environmental and may consist of such things as pain or trauma. Finally, *maturational* developmental factors involve primarily the very young or the very elderly and their limitations such as lack of balance in the toddler or cautious gait in the elderly with failing eyesight (see Table 54–1).

Having carefully examined the factors that contribute to defining the problem, the nurse is ready to

Table 54–5. FOCUSED ASSESSMENT CRITERIA

Subjective Data
History of systemic disorders
  Neurologic
  Cardiovascular
  Musculoskeletal
  Respiratory
  Debilitating diseases
History of symptoms that interfere with mobility
  Symptoms
    Pain
    Muscle weakness
    Fatigue
  Criteria
    Onset
    Duration
    Location
    Description
    Frequency
    Precipitated by what?
    Relieved by what?
    Aggravated by what?
History of recent trauma or surgery
Current drug therapy
  Pain
  Sedative
  Laxatives
  Chemotherapy
Objective Data
Dominant hand
Motor function
  Right arm
  Left arm
  Right leg
  Left leg
Mobility
  Ability to turn self
  Ability to sit
  Ability to stand
  Ability to transfer
  Ability to ambulate
Weight bearing (assess right and left sides)
  Gait
  Assistive devices
  Restrictive devices
  Range of motion (shoulders, elbows, arms, hips, legs)
Endurance
  Assess
    Resting pulse, blood pressure, respirations
    Blood pressure, respirations, and pulse after activity
    After activity, assess for the presence of indicators of hypoxia
Peripheral circulation
  Capillary refill time
  Skin color, temperature, and turgor
  Peripheral pulses

address the planning and implementation of care for the patient with altered mobility. Nursing care interventions are related to other nursing diagnoses that affect or are affected by altered mobility. The following section addresses in more detail the nursing care related to some specific problems of mobility.

MANAGING SPECIFIC PROBLEMS OF MOBILITY

Activity Intolerance

Activity intolerance (the state in which the person experiences an inability, physiologically and psychologically, to endure or tolerate an increase in activity) is a commonly occurring problem for the person experiencing cancer or cancer treatment and is directly related to the impairment of physical mobility. The causative factors may relate to fatigue or problems with oxygen transport. When these factors have been adequately identified for the patient, nursing action can be taken (see Table 54–5). In focusing the assessment data (both subjective and objective), it is helpful first to examine factors that increase fatigue, then to examine the effects of fatigue on the activity level, and then to examine the actual response to activity. It is here that the use of an activity index such as the Karnofsky Scale (see Table 54–3) or Barthel Index (see Table 54–4) can be useful.

After the assessment data are focused, it is possible to examine the results and decide which contributing factors (such as inadequate sleep or rest periods, pain, medications, daily schedule, and lack of incentive) are variably amenable to nursing action. The daily schedule and rest periods require creative problem solving with client, family, and caregivers all involved so that a satisfactory schedule can be developed. Pain management is not discussed here because it is covered extensively elsewhere in this book (see Chapter 50), but it is crucial to the achievement of optimal activity levels for the person. Further treatment, such as surgery, radiation therapy, and chemotherapy, will at times be indicated to reduce pain and allow increased mobility. Medications sometimes interfere with sleep management for the person with activity intolerance—either because side effects of medication make adequate sleep difficult or because the scheduling of medications interferes with the sleep cycle. Usually with consideration of the goal (to increase sleep and rest, thereby increasing activity tolerance), it is possible to modify medication schedules to reduce, if not eliminate, the negative effect of the medication regimen on sleep pattern. The lack of incentive may present the greatest challenge to the nurse in motivating the client to increased levels of activity. Although it is difficult to find research documentation for many of the nursing interventions used in this challenging problem, empirically it has been found helpful to make contracts with the client about activity; identify progress; and consider concrete incentives, such as behavioral or physical rewards.

Factors other than disease or treatment also may affect activity tolerance. Age, physical strength, and cardiopulmonary status are all factors that may be of significance in altering the activity tolerance (Kozier & Erb, 1987).

Having attempted management of the person's activity intolerance, it is essential then to evaluate, both subjectively and objectively, the response to those nursing interventions that were utilized, using both the outcomes designed with the plan and reassessment of the original measures to indicate the progress or lack of progress. The results of this kind of systematic evaluation allow for a decision to discontinue ineffective interventions or increase effective interventions on the basis of clearly identified phenomena rather than subjective impressions.

Alteration in Activities of Daily Living and Self-Care

The success of persons in maintaining functional independence while coping with cancer depends in part on the effectiveness and efficiency of their mobility. When the ability to move around is compromised, so too may be initiative, self-confidence, and motivation to be involved in the activities that had significance to daily life. An essential step in caring for the cancer patient with alterations in mobility is to learn from the patient what the status of his or her mobility is in relationship to usual activities of daily living and customary life style (Williams, 1986). What activities can or cannot be done independently? Which activities require assistance? Which activities are of greatest significance to the person, and which do the family consider most important? Has the patient given up some activities and at what price? Have frequency, duration, and regularity of the activities been changed because of mobility alterations? How is the family affected by the changes? What are the safety concerns related both to the alteration in mobility and the alteration in activities of daily living? One of the most obvious associations between altered mobility and activities of daily living is the fact that most activities of daily living ordinarily occur in certain places within the home, workplace, or community. If a person is unable to walk to the usual setting for whatever reason, independently or with assistance, other modes of getting there must be used, such as wheelchair or lift. Otherwise, the activity must be performed wherever the person might be spending the majority of time, such as in bed. The extent to which this is a significant deviation from what has been normal to the person's life style may indicate the difficulty of adapting to the change (Carnevali, 1985). Limitations of physical movement of the upper extremities, such as with lymphedema or pathologic fractures, also affect the ability to perform self-care activities.

Another factor to be assessed is whether the process leading to the alteration in mobility is the same process directly affecting alteration in the self-care ability. For example, if spinal cord compression damage is the cause of the alteration in mobility, it may also be the direct cause of deficits in other personal self-care abilities, such as toileting, depending on the level of spinal cord involved. Compensating for the mobility change would not necessarily correct the self-care deficit and would call for additional nursing interventions that targeted the neurologic problems. Pain may be another type of limitation on both mobility and self-care ability.

The assessment also includes objective data in the form of observing mobility factors in relationship to performance of specific activities of daily living. For purposes of this discussion, selected activities of self-care relating to feeding, bathing, toileting, and dressing are presented.

The ability to feed oneself may be affected by the partial or complete incapacity to sit up, one dimension of mobility, that could arise from central nervous system involvement; bone tumors; fractures; fatigue; or ingestion of narcotics, sedatives, or tranquilizers. Nursing interventions can be directed toward understanding the causes of the incapacity to sit up and providing the necessary assistance to place the patient in the most appropriate position for eating that is not contraindicated. Assistive and supportive devices should be used to foster maximum independence for the patient and to provide support and avoid injury for caregiver.

In some instances a client will have a missing or disabled upper limb that will limit self-feeding. The eating environment should allow sufficient time for eating with adequate supervision and assistance necessary for relearning and adapting. Teaching the use of adaptive devices such as plate guards, utensils with large handles, and rocker knives will also foster independence.

The ability to bathe and groom, toilet, and dress oneself in the usual manner may be related to the ability to sit up, stand, transfer, position, or ambulate independently. Often the person suffering from alterations in mobility is capable of performing the activity once correctly positioned to do so. Nursing actions are directed at enhancing mobility whenever possible by physically supporting the person, using appropriate aids, minimizing environmental barriers, protecting from physical harm, providing privacy, and encouraging muscle strengthening exercises to prevent further loss and restore function. Collaboration with other members of disciplines involved in rehabilitation, such as physical and occupational therapists, is critical. Nurses provide assistance in a timely manner with the other self-care activities as needed until the person is able to resume self-care and teach family members how to best foster independence in the patient while at the same time helping in those areas in which the patient is dependent on others to successfully complete the task. The personal care activities of daily living are essential to maintain healthy skin, teeth, alimentary tract, and mucous membranes; to maintain continence; to prevent infection; to promote self-esteem; and to preserve self-concept.

Alteration in Bowel Elimination

Probably the most significant interaction between mobility and bowel elimination is the tendency to constipation when mobility is seriously limited (Kozier & Erb, 1987). If the person reports hard stools fewer than three times weekly and complains of difficulty moving the bowels and also is immobile, it is likely that the two are at least partially related. A therapeutic bowel regimen will need to be instituted until or unless the immobility problem can be resolved. Corrective measures should include evaluation of the diet with an attempt to increase the fiber. Bran should be used moderately at first, but fresh fruits and vegetables can be encouraged to an amount equal to 800 g per day (4 to 5 servings). Encourage the client to identify fruits and foods that have laxative effects. Fluid intake should total at least 2 L daily, with the emphasis on water or fruit juices, not on caffeine drinks. Warm water should be drunk in the morning to stimulate the gastrocolic reflex. Activity or even range of motion exercises are often helpful. Establish a regular time for elimination using the client's normal pattern as much as possible with relation to time, place, position, and equipment. Privacy is extremely important to many people. It may be necessary to use suppositories, stool softeners, or mild laxatives. Constipation should be treated early and consistently for the immobilized person so that it can be managed with the most physiologic and least irritating measures. When the patient is neutropenic or thrombocytopenic it is particularly important to use care in managing constipation to prevent trauma to the rectal area. Diarrhea as an alteration in bowel elimination may present a problem for the client in that immobility may be increased by the fear of increasing diarrhea ("every time I move, I have another stool"). This is obviously best dealt with by managing the diarrhea effectively, to allow mobility to return to optimal levels.

Alteration in Peripheral Tissue Perfusion

One of the classic problems associated with immobility is the development of peripheral thromboses, which present the nursing problem of altered peripheral tissue perfusion. The primary nursing concern here is a preventive one to keep this a potential problem rather than an actual one. When immobility is added to the tendency toward increased clotting often present in persons with cancer (Price & Wilson, 1986), the person is at considerable risk for development of thromboses. Having established that the potential for this problem exists, the nurse will be watchful that blood pressure is maintained at optimum levels to allow adequate tissue perfusion—whether this is a problem of cardiac output or of peripheral circulation—especially as it is affected by the sympathetic nervous system. In addition, cellular perfusion, which is vulnerable to obstruction and changes in oxygen level of the circulating blood, must be maintained. Position and mobility have important effects on the optimal maintenance of tissue perfusion. Antiembolic stockings should be used by these patients. Range of motion exercises at least every shift with arm and leg exercises every 1 to 2 hr should be a part of the plan of care. If the person has a problem of immobility that decreases general activity or promotes obstruction of circulation, it is incumbent on the nurse to be alert to means of minimizing the circulatory compromise that may result, thereby minimizing the potential problem. It is also important to realize that the thrombocytopenic patient may need guidance in the kind and amount of activity that is safe.

Impairment of Skin Integrity

The major defining characteristics of the nursing diagnosis relating to the potential impairment of skin integrity are that the person reports fatigue and inability to move or turn and is on imposed bed rest or is immobile. Obviously the person with cancer who has altered physical mobility is at high risk for this nursing diagnosis. When the contributing factors of impaired oxygen are added, the risk becomes even greater. In assessing clients for particular risk, the oncology nurse will watch for skin deficits such as dryness, edema, thinness, or obesity and for impaired oxygen transport as in anemia or edema. Irritants such as radiation therapy, incontinence, nutritional deficits, systemic problems such as infection or liver failure, and sensory deficits present particular hazards as well.

Once the person is known to either have an active problem with impaired skin integrity or be at high risk, the nurse's activity will center on trying to reduce the contributing factors involved. Obviously attempts will be made to increase mobility to the greatest extent possible because this is one of the cardinal factors. In addition, careful management of incontinence, positioning, nutrition, and skin surveillance will be essential if the skin integrity problems are to be minimized. Protective devices will be needed, such as special mattresses and beds, as will skin care regimens. Consultation with an enterostomal skin care therapist is appropriate. Health teaching may be an important part of the management of this problem, especially if the person is being cared for at home. Evaluation of the management of impairments in skin integrity must assess both the repair and healing that occur and the success in preventing new problems.

Alteration in Meaningfulness— Powerlessness

Alterations in mobility and the subsequent experience of dependence can lead to a perceived lack of personal control over one's life, accompanied by apathy, anger, or depression. Each change that threatens the patient's normal life style, creates dependence, threatens adequacy and competence, and removes the person from the decision-making process at any level can bring varying degrees of helplessness and powerlessness and the sense that external forces are controlling. The powerlessness may be manifested by physical findings such as facial flushing or pallor, rapid or bounding pulse, increased blood pressure, sweating, trembling, restlessness, sleep disturbances, changes in eating habits, irritability, demanding behavior, or avoiding or leaving situations.

Powerlessness is a subjective state and therefore requires validation on the part of the person experiencing it. An assessment should include the person's usual level of control and decision making and the effects that losing control produces. By asking the patient questions related to decision-making patterns, role responsibilities, perceptions of control, and personal fears, subjective data will be obtained that will contribute to the nursing assessment of the patient's sense of potential or actual powerlessness. By observing the patient's manner of participation in activities of daily living or information seeking and responses to limits placed on decision making and self-control, the nurse can identify the factors contributing to the sense of powerlessness and provide opportunities for patient involvement in decision making that can be followed consistently by all caregivers.

Carpenito (1987) pointed out that health care providers' routines are among the factors that can contribute to feelings of powerlessness. She advocated that patients be allowed to manipulate surroundings, such as deciding what is to be kept where; that the daily plan of activities be discussed, with the patient making as many decisions as possible about it; that patients' decisions be respected and followed once given options; and that specific choices be recorded on the care plan to ensure that all staff members will acknowledge the person's preferences. Promises must be kept and opportunities provided for the patient and family to express feelings and participate in care.

Maternalism or paternalism on the part of health professionals needs to be recognized and dealt with, and each health care professional should share actions that he or she discovered to be preferred by the patient. Realistic areas of control can be identified, paving the way for future control (hopes and goals). Enhancing problem-solving skills is also strongly indicated. Helping the person suffering from powerlessness due to altered mobility to interact with others who have also experienced a similar reaction in similar circumstances and were able to regain a sense of meaning, mastery, and power could also be extremely beneficial.

Alteration in Emotional Integrity— Grieving

The grieving process is a normal and expected response to a significant loss of something valued. Losing one's ability to be mobile is in itself a significant loss of freedom and control, which may precipitate yet other losses for the person with cancer. Becoming unable to move may result in loss of ability to perform other activities of daily living independently; loss of body image, self-esteem, and self-identity; loss of social contacts; loss of employment; loss of stable income; and loss of ability to perform usual roles, to name but a few (Baird, 1985). Altered mobility also may herald for the person with cancer the progression of disease and with it the anticipated loss of a personal future and of life itself, with all its associated grief. The family experiences the grieving process along with the patient.

Understanding the typical phases of grief described by researchers (Bowlby, 1961; Peretz, 1970; Worden, 1982) provides a framework for identifying behaviors that most people are likely to display or express. Common grief reactions include shock and disbelief, yearning and protest, disorganization and despair, reorganization and restitution, and resolution. Grief work involves (1) facing pain with all the sorrow and distress that that entails and recognizing the full reality of what is happening as a normal part of life, and (2) permitting emotional expression of the full range of feelings.

Nursing interventions are directed toward helping the patient and family to express the grief, to describe the meaning of the losses, to competently move through the grieving process with a sense of realistic hope, and to experience the losses as a potential for personal growth. To do so, many of the same strategies as those described in the section on coping are used.

Although most persons are successful in completing grief work, some exhibit signs that the normal grief process has been seriously delayed or disrupted (Peretz, 1970). Psychiatric intervention is required when one or more of the following characteristics are present: (1) extreme depressive reaction, (2) psychotic break with reality, (3) suicidal tendencies, and (4) substance abuse. The goal of psychotherapy is to transform pathologic grief states to forms of mourning that proceed to resolution.

Sensory-Perceptual Alteration—Visual, Kinesthetic

Alterations in mobility can result in a decrease in the amount, pattern, and interpretation of incoming stimuli of a physiologic, sensory, motor, and environmental nature, particularly if the person is bedbound. Lack of communication and lack of touch contact may occur when the person affected by restrictions on mobility has relied on relationships outside the home as the primary source of input. Loved ones and acquaintances may be reluctant to maintain contact because of their own sense of helplessness, not knowing what to say or do to be of assistance in the situation.

Decreased mobility also may result in decreased physiologic function of the respiratory, renal, cerebral, circulatory, and sensory systems, which alter sensory-perceptual function. Immobility also may interfere with sleep-rest cycles and with fluid, electrolyte, and nutritional balances, all of which may influence the ways in which the environment is sensed and perceived. In addition, all of these changes may be accompanied by fear of the unknown and potential and actual losses of control, income, familiar persons, objects, and surroundings. Heightened anxiety, depression, fatigue, and boredom contribute to a dulling of sensory responses.

Nursing action can be directed toward manipulating the environment to provide adequate and significant sensory stimulation and toward teaching the patient and family to do likewise. Attention needs to be paid to identifying stimulation, activity, and diversion that are meaningful to the patient. The nurse can assess the environment and make alterations so that color, lighting, sound, and windows are used to make a pleasant, interesting, and inviting environment. Availability of radio, television, and reading materials can help maintain interest in the outside world and provide both entertainment and topics for conversation with others. Active diversions with others (both within the environment in which the person is receiving care and outside it) that do not depend on intact mobility skills can enhance sensory stimulation and decrease the sense of isolation that sensory deprivation fosters. Meaningful human interaction and the sense of value and comfort that comes from it are probably the greatest protectors against sensory-perceptual alterations.

This section has dealt with the interaction of a number of nursing problems resulting from altered physical mobility. It is vital for the nurse to recognize and deal with these problems concurrently if the client is to reach optimal levels of mobility and if unnecessary complications are to be prevented.

MANAGING SPECIAL PROBLEMS OF MOBILITY

Lymphedema

With improved surgical techniques and less extensive mastectomy surgery, lymphedema is not as common a problem as it was in the past, but it still does occur and may be of sufficient degree to alter mobility for the patient. The woman with axillary lymph node dissection for breast cancer and the man with prostate cancer or penectomy and groin node dissection most commonly experience this problem. Any time lymph node dissection has occurred or tumor has interfered with lymphatic circulation, the patient has a potential problem. Physically, the problem in mobility usually occurs because of tissue edema that is secondary to obstruction, whether it is caused by scar tissue or by tumor. The edema must be minimized because it tends to become chronic once it is established in the tissue. Ironically, some of the measures used to reduce edema, such as elevation of the part or elastic bandaging, also tend to reduce mobility so it is important to strike a balance between one treatment and another to maintain maximum range of motion.

Collateral lymphatic drainage usually develops throughout the first 3 to 4 weeks after surgery. Prevention of edema by elevation of the part, massage and exercise to encourage circulation and maintenance of function, and prevention of infection are particularly important during the first 3 months after surgery. If a problem with edema continues despite these conservative measures, an elastic sleeve or stocking may be used. A pneumatic pump attached to such a support may also be useful in reducing edema and allow the client to be more comfortable and more mobile. The physical therapist may be an important resource at this point. Client teaching should include avoiding blood pressure measurement, injections, blood drawing, contact with abrasive or irritating materials, and lifting or carrying heavy objects with the affected limb.

Because the problem of lymphedema tends to increase immobility, and because immobility may increase the lymphedema for the person subject to such a problem, it is important that the nurse take early and vigorous action to assist in managing this uncommon but significant problem.

Bone Tumors

Because two major symptoms of bone tumors—pain and impairment of function—directly affect mobility,

it is not surprising that these tumors present a particular challenge to nursing care with respect to mobility (Porth, 1986).

Management of pain is obviously a high priority if the person is to increase mobility successfully. This subject is covered in detail in Chapter 50, but the nurse should keep in mind that the nonsteroidal anti-inflammatory drugs (NSAIDs) alone or with narcotic pain medications may be most helpful for the person with bone involvement. Additionally, radiation therapy may be necessary to reduce tumor bulk and pain. Nonchemical means of pain management, such as diversion and imaging, may be of particular significance and activity itself may be an adjunct in pain management.

Pathologic fractures present a special problem for mobility in the person with bone tumors. In most cases the fracture treatment methods are similar to those for other fractures, but the complexity of managing pathologic fractures is greater because of the underlying disease process. The effect of the fracture and its treatment will depend largely on the location of the tumor. Sometimes amputation is necessary and presents its own problems for mobility (Farrell, 1986).

The treatment of bone tumors, whether by surgery, radiation therapy, or chemotherapy, will usually increase mobility and decrease pain. At times these treatments negatively affect mobility by increasing pain, fatigue, and strength. Because primary bone tumors are more likely to occur in young people, often these patients have the advantage of youthful resiliency of tissue and spirit. However, this is likely to be combined with the typical impatience of youth. All of these can be assets for the nurse working with these clients if managed wisely. Conversely, the management of metastatic bone tumor often presents real challenges because the person is likely to be older, has other disease or treatments as part of the history, and may focus on many other things besides regaining mobility. In any event, it is likely to require imaginative and careful symptom management on the part of the nurse for the client to achieve optimal mobility when bone tumors are present.

Spinal Cord Compression

Spinal cord and nerve root compression of whatever cause (primary spinal cord tumors; metastases from lung, breast, prostate, and kidney; or lymphoma and multiple myeloma) constitutes an oncologic emergency. The characteristic initial symptom in 90 per cent of patients is pain and discomfort in the form of thoracolumbar back pain, often in a belt-like distribution and frequently extending to the groin or legs. Lower extremity weakness is evident in approximately 76 per cent of patients (Klein, 1985). The weakness, reflex alterations, or paralysis results from upper or lower motor neuron damage.

Unfortunately, the condition often is not recognized until paraplegia is established. The symptoms of muscular weakness, tiredness, and heaviness of the extremities and sensory paresthesia are too often ignored by the patient, physicians, and nurses. When paraplegia or quadriplegia becomes manifest, recovery to a good level of function is unusual.

To prevent devastating complications, it is essential to provide careful nursing assessment and patient teaching emphasizing timely reporting of signs and symptoms related to potential spinal cord compression for those at risk. Other symptoms related to spinal cord compression include constipation and urinary retention with overflow incontinence, altered gait, ataxia, loss of muscle tone and decreased sensation in the extremities.

Early diagnosis and treatment can lead to complete restoration of function. Treatment may involve an emergency decompression laminectomy, adrenocorticosteroids, radiation therapy, or chemotherapy, depending on tumor sensitivities and previous treatment. If the condition progresses without treatment or with unsuccessful treatment, irreversible paralysis occurs below the level of the spinal cord compression. The degree of compression will have a direct effect on the patient's mobility or immobility status and on the nursing measures taken to prevent loss of function, restore function, compensate for and adapt to permanent loss of elements of mobility, and prevent or minimize further complications arising from impaired mobility. In addition to other interventions, safety measures must be implemented for persons whose ambulatory ability is compromised, such as use of assistive devices; handrails; appropriately adapted chairs and furnishings; clear, wide passageways; and elimination of environmental barriers to activity.

When symptoms have had a rapid onset and treatment does not have the desired effect, patients can experience significant depression because life styles are abruptly disrupted and body integrity is threatened. The emotional and financial impact for the patient and family is important for health professionals to identify and acknowledge so appropriate interventions can be used to strengthen coping resources.

Amputation

Lower extremity amputations have a more direct effect on general mobility than do upper extremity amputations but the general problems are similar: adapting to a prosthesis, making necessary modifications in activities of daily living, and maintaining a positive attitude toward the rehabilitation process. Because of the belief of some health care personnel as well as lay people that rehabilitation is pointless in cancer, particularly metastatic cancer, this process may be particularly challenging for the oncology nurse. If the nursing care of the person with an amputation secondary to malignancy is to be effective, this challenge must be met. It is important to keep in mind that amputation is rarely used alone and the person is almost always treated with some combination of chemotherapy or radiation therapy. These treatments may

have other implications for the client's mobility (Farrell, 1986).

Additional problems of immobility are often present because of the other risk factors common to the person with cancer. These have been discussed previously but deserve highlighting—for example, the problem of trying to help the person with a lower extremity amputation to ambulate when the pain level is high, the energy level low, and the incentive to achieve mobility limited. If the oncology nurse has limited experience in working with patients who have an amputation, it is wise to consult colleagues experienced in orthopedic nursing, rehabilitation nursing, and physical therapy and to refer to related references in the literature. One of the most important areas for the nurse to keep in mind in nursing the person with an amputation is the alteration in body image and self-concept. That person has often had many other assaults on body image during the diagnostic and treatment process. Because amputation for cancer diagnoses is used almost exclusively for primary bone tumors this group presents somewhat different nursing concerns from the person with metastatic bone tumor, who will be treated with radiation or chemotherapy. Problems with upper extremity amputations most commonly relate to retraining the person both for working with a prosthetic limb and for managing activities of daily living in a new manner. Planning for rehabilitation is essential and begins, as always, with the beginning of treatment.

Central Nervous System Tumors

The final special problem of mobility to be discussed is that of central nervous system tumors, another potential oncologic complication that can result in a neurologic emergency. Space-occupying brain malignancies can be primary tumors, but most often they result from arterial metastases from cancers of the lung, breast, prostate, and colon, malignant melanoma, lymphoma, and leukemia. Neurologic symptoms are related to the location and size of the cancer, the extent of local compression and destruction of brain tissue by the mass and edema, and the degree of increased intracranial pressure or obstruction to the normal flow of cerebrospinal fluid.

Mobility may be particularly affected with parietal lobe involvement because sensorimotor function is under parietal control and may be manifested by weakness, atrophy, clumsiness, dysdiadochokinesis, and independent movements unrecognized by the patient. Cerebellar dysfunction can decrease mobility by reducing muscle coordination and ataxia resulting from compression of motor tracts. Frontal (precentral) lobe involvement may result in weakness, hemiparesis, disturbed gait, automatism, rigidity, tonic spasms of toes, and seizures, all of which can affect mobility. Occipital lobe damage may cause visual damage that likewise influences mobility.

The initial treatment of primary tumors is often surgical excision, with removal limited by the location and invasiveness of the cancer. Because most of the malignant brain tumors, both primary and metastatic, are radiosensitive, radiation therapy generally is indicated. Researchers are hopeful that radiation therapy of metastatic disease to the brain may be improved through using radiosensitizers and improved use of computed tomography (CT) and magnetic resonance imaging (MRI) to guide therapy. Local or systemic chemotherapy has been more effective to date for metastatic tumors than for primary tumors, although continued clinical investigations hold greater promise (Kornblith, Walker, & Cassady, 1982).

Ultmann and Phillips (1982) identified factors that must be considered when determining appropriate treatment for patients with brain metastasis. When the general condition of the patient seems to indicate treatment of the central nervous system lesion, these investigators consider the following factors to determine the type of local treatment to be employed (namely, surgery, radiation therapy, chemotherapy, or a combination):

1. Number of lesions
2. Location of lesions
3. Primary site
4. Patient age and general functional condition
5. Status of other metastatic disease and the primary tumor
6. Relative radioresponsiveness and radiocontrollability
7. Interval between treatment of the primary lesion and development of brain metastases

Nursing care of the patient with alterations in mobility related to central nervous system tumors and their treatment includes careful monitoring and reporting of existing or new symptoms, helping with mobility, and intervening to protect from injury, as previously described in other parts of this chapter. Assessment includes observations of any evidence of increased intracranial pressure and sensory changes as well as motor function and muscular strength of extremities. Activity tolerance and unsteady gait also need to be assessed with each contact, recording ataxia and subjective indications of weakness and fatigue (Chernecky & Ramsey, 1984).

As is true in the case of nursing care of persons with spinal cord tumors, significant nursing energies are devoted to dealing with the psychosocial and emotional impact of central nervous system tumors. Interventions are directed toward issues relating to the sense of loss of control, loss of body integrity, threats to hope, and fears associated with dying. Patient and family education concerning understanding the illness and its signs and symptoms, determining their impact on daily life, and identifying ways to enhance the quality of remaining life are extremely important.

SUMMARY

Nursing care for the person with cancer who has problems of altered mobility is indeed a challenging process. Although the nursing techniques are not unique, the specialized knowledge and skills of the oncology nurse must be used to their fullest. What is unique is the importance of careful diagnosis of the problem so that nursing care is in the truest sense of the word individualized. When a problem exists, only actions carefully designed to reduce the particular contributing factors for that specific problem will be maximally effective. Probably this is the reason why much of the nursing research that has been done in this area has focused on assessment and diagnosis. It is to be hoped that work will soon begin that examines the efficacy of various care techniques related to increasing mobility. Only then can selection of nursing interventions rely more on research-documented evidence of effectiveness and less on empirical experience and exchange of ideas. The latter remains a rich source of information for the oncology nurse, however, and cooperation among specialists in rehabilitation, orthopedic, and neurologic nursing is vital for the optimum care of the person with a problem of physical mobility.

References

American Nurses' Association & Oncology Nursing Society. (1987). *Standards for oncology nursing practice.* Kansas City, MO: American Nurses' Association.

Baird, S. (1985). Development of a nursing assessment tool to diagnose altered body image in immobilized patients. *Orthopaedic Nursing, 4,* 47–54.

Bowlby, J. (1961). Processes of mourning. *International Journal of Psychoanalysis, 42,* 317–340.

Cancer Rehabilitation Coordination Team. (1978). *Final report to National Cancer Institute.* Unpublished document, University of Pittsburgh, School of Health-Related Professionals.

Carnevali, D. (1985). A daily functional health status perspective for nursing diagnosis and treatment in critical care nursing. *Heart and Lung, 14,* 437–443.

Carnevali, D. L., & Patrick, M. (1979). *Nursing management for the elderly.* Philadelphia: J. B. Lippincott Co.

Carpenito, L. J. (1987). *Nursing diagnosis: Application to clinical practice* (2nd ed.). Philadelphia: J. B. Lippincott Co.

Chang, S. K., & Hawes, K. A. (1983). The adequacy of the Karnofsky rating and global adjustment to illness scale as outcome measures in cancer rehabilitation and continuing care. In P. F. Engstrom, P. N. Anderson, & L. E. Mortenson (Eds.), *Advances in cancer control: Research and development* (pp. 429–443). New York: Alan R. Liss, Inc.

Chernecky, C. C., & Ramsey, P. W. (1984). *Critical nursing care of the client with cancer.* Norwalk, CT: Appleton-Century-Crofts.

Chiou, I. L., & Burnett, C. N. (1985). Values of activities of daily living. *Physical Therapy, 65,* 902–906.

Donovan, M. I., & Girton, S. (1984). *Cancer care nursing.* Norwalk, CT: Appleton-Century-Crofts.

Farrell, J. (1986). *Illustrated guide to orthopedic nursing* (3rd ed.). Philadelphia: J. B. Lippincott Co.

Feinstein, A. R., Joseph, B. R., & Wells, C. K. (1986). Scientific and clinical problems in indexes of functional disability. *Annals of Internal Medicine, 105,* 413–420.

Gregor, S., McCarthy, K., Chwirchak, D., Meluch, M., & Mion, L. C. (1986). Characteristics and functional outcomes of elderly rehabilitation patients. *Rehabilitation Nursing, 11*(3), 10–14.

Gulick, E. E. (1986). The self-assessment of health among the chronically ill. *Topics in Clinical Nursing, 8*(1), 74–82.

Jacelon, C. S. (1986). The Barthel index and other indices of functional ability. *Rehabilitation Nursing, 11*(4), 9–11.

Klein, P. W. (1985). Neurological emergencies. *Seminars in Oncology Nursing, 1,* 278–284.

Kneisl, C. R., & Ames, S. W. (1986). *Adult health nursing: A biopsychosocial approach.* Menlo Park, CA: Addison-Wesley Publishing Co.

Kornblith, P. L., Walker, M. D., & Cassady, J. R. (1982). Neoplasms of the central nervous system. In V. T. DeVita, Jr., S. Hellman, & S. A. Rosenberg (Eds.), *Cancer: Principles and practice of oncology*. Philadelphia: J. B. Lippincott Co.

Kozier, B., & Erb, G. (1987). *Techniques in clinical nursing: A nursing process approach*. Menlo Park, CA: Addison-Wesley Publishing Co.

Lazarus, E. S., & Launier, R. (1978). Stress-related transactions between person and environment. In L. A. Pervin & M. Lewis (Eds.), *Perspectives in international psychology* (pp. 287–322). New York: Plenum.

Lehmann, J., DeLisa, J. A., & Warren, C. G. (1978). Cancer rehabilitation: Assessment of need, development and evaluation of a model of care. *Archives of Physical Medicine and Rehabilitation, 59*, 410–419.

Martin, N., Holt, N. B., & Hicks, D. (1980). *Comprehensive rehabilitation nursing*. New York: McGraw-Hill Book Co.

McNally, J. C., Stair, J. C., & Somerville, E. T. (1985). *Guidelines for cancer nursing practice*. Orlando, FL: Grune & Stratton, Inc.

Milsum, J. H. (1980). Lifestyle changes for the whole person: Stimulation through health hazard appraisal. In P. O. Davidson & S. M. Davidson (Eds.), *Behavioral medicine: Changing health lifestyles*. New York: Brunner/Mazel.

Olson, E. (1967). The hazards of immobility. *American Journal of Nursing, 67*, 780–797.

Peretz, D. (1970). Reaction to loss. In B. Schoenberg, A. C. Carr, D. Peretz, & A. H. Kutscher (Eds.), *Loss and grief: Psychological management in medical practice*. New York: Columbia University Press.

Porth, C. M. (1986). *Pathophysiology: Concepts of altered health states* (2nd ed.). Philadelphia: J. B. Lippincott Co.

Potter, P. A., & Perry, A. G. (1985). *Fundamentals of nursing: Concepts, process, and practice*. St. Louis: C. V. Mosby Co.

Price, S. A., & Wilson, L. M. (1986). *Pathophysiology: Clinical concepts of disease processes* (3rd ed.). New York: McGraw-Hill Book Co.

Robinson, B. E. (1986). Validation of the functional assessment inventory against a multidisciplinary home care team. *Journal American Geriatric Society, 34*, 851–854.

Ultmann, J. E., & Phillips, T. L. (1982). Treatment of metastatic cancer. In V. T. Devita, Jr., S. Hellman, & S. A. Rosenberg (Eds.), *Cancer: Principles and practice of oncology*. Philadelphia: J. B. Lippincott Co.

Weisman, A. D. (1979). *Coping with cancer*. New York: McGraw-Hill Book Co.

Weisman, A. D., & Worden, J. W. (1977). *Coping and vulnerability in cancer patients: A research report*. Cambridge, MA: Shea Brothers.

Williams, A. J. (1986). Self-care model: An assessment tool based on Orem's theory. *Nursing Success Today, 3*(7), 26–28.

Worden, J. W. (1982). *Grief counseling and grief therapy: A handbook for the mental health practitioner*. New York: Springer Publishing Co.

55

Complications of Advanced Disease

CYNTHIA CHERNECKY
RUTH L. KRECH

ANATOMIC AND PHYSIOLOGIC FEATURES

Definition of Advanced Disease

Advanced disease is defined as at least one acute organ dysfunction caused by either metastasis or cancer treatment that results in a client's need for comprehensive management in an intensive care environment. This condition differs from metastasis alone, a single oncologic emergency, and any other circumstance that does not involve acute organ dysfunction *and* does not require comprehensive intensive care.

This chapter focuses on nursing care of the individual who experiences complications of advanced disease. The first section discusses vital organ functions. The second section includes scientific knowledge about the pathophysiologic and interfering factors that lead to advanced disease and are caused by metastases and sequelae of therapies. The third section of this chapter addresses associated nursing diagnoses and interventions. The final section covers special problems related to advanced disease.

Normal Function of Body Organs

Knowledge of the normal function of six specific organs provides the foundation for understanding the concept of advanced disease.

1. The brain is the primary center for regulating and coordinating body activities. This includes analytical thought, memory, behaviors, and communication.
2. The heart provides force so blood can be propelled through the vascular system.
3. Bones provide body support and organ protection and play an active role in the formation of blood cells.
4. The lungs exchange carbon dioxide for oxygen in the blood.
5. The liver serves many functions, but in this chapter it is viewed as a return site for blood from the intestines and spleen on its way to being returned to the systemic circulation.
6. The kidney provides for regulation of extracellular fluid, electrolyte balances, and excretion of urine.

PATHOPHYSIOLOGY AND INTERFERING FACTORS LEADING TO ADVANCED DISEASE

Dysfunctions in one vital organ generally lead to subsequent dysfunctions in other vital organs because the vital organs function interdependently. For example, a problem in the heart will decrease the amount of blood flow to the lungs. Consequently, there will be less oxygenated blood delivered to the other organs, thereby reducing their efficiency. The subsequent discussion delineates examples of specific vital organ metastases and cancer treatment–related sequelae.

Vital Organ Metastasis

Brain

Two per cent of all cancers are primary brain tumors, and 15 per cent of all cancer clients develop neurologic symptoms from advanced disease (Posner, 1979). For common sites associated with brain metastasis, see Table 55–1. The most common site of metastasis in the brain occurs in the frontal lobe. Although less common, metastases to the temporal, parietal, and occipital lobes occur with similar frequency. The brain stem is the least likely site for metastasis (Vieth & Odom, 1965). Figure 55–1 demonstrates metastatic lesions with surrounding edema in both the frontal and parietal lobes on computed tomography (CT) scan.

Generalized signs and symptoms of brain metastasis include headache, loss of motor function, impaired mentation with lethargy, seizures, sensory loss, and increased intracranial pressure (Table 55–2). These signs and symptoms result in deficits in the following four areas: cognition, mobility, activities of daily living, and bladder and bowel control. The latter three areas are quite manageable on a general medical-surgical division. However, a deficit in cognition, known as neuropsychiatric syndrome, presents an acute situation in which the need for nursing care is greatly increased.

Neuropsychiatric syndrome can be manifested in several ways, ranging from acute anxiety disorders and personality changes to depressed consciousness, stupor, and coma (Billings, 1985). Astute nursing assessment is imperative because this syndrome can appear suddenly. Once the presence of neuropsychiatric syndrome is ascertained, general management can be initiated, including orientation, hygiene, safety and suicide precautions, and constant monitoring of vital

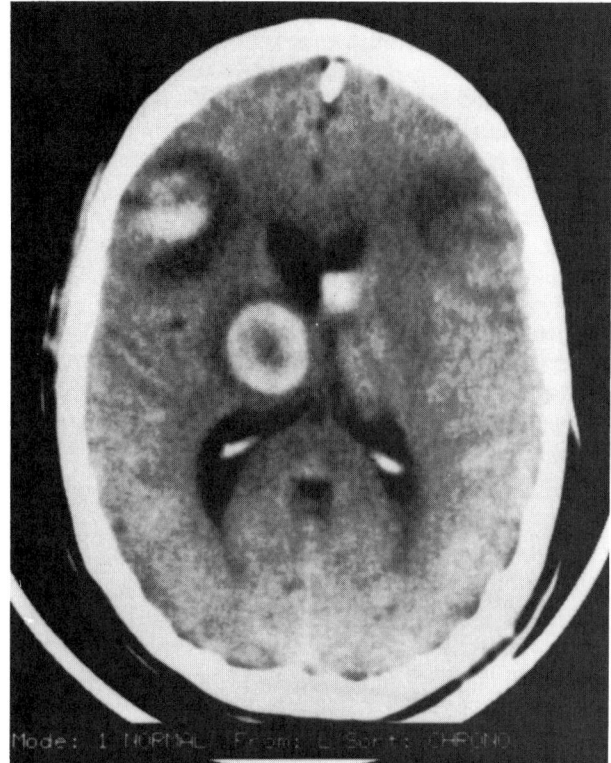

Figure 55–1. Brain metastasis of frontal and parietal lobes with accompanying edema surrounding frontal lobe tumor as seen on computed tomographic scan.

signs. Discussion, explanations, and support should be given to family members because the sudden onset of this syndrome is frightening.

Heart

Another facet of advanced disease is heart involvement. Metastases to the heart, specifically the pericardium, occur in 5 to 10 per cent of all clients with cancer (Hanfling, 1960). Although cardiac metastasis can occur through any of the defined modes of metastases (see Chapter 14), blood-borne and lymphatic metastases are most common. These two patterns of metastases probably account for the fact that cardiac metastasis is almost always accompanied by metastasis to other organs (Bisel, Wroblewski, & LaDue, 1953). Cancers associated with heart metastasis are identified in Table 55–1.

Table 55–1. TYPES OF CANCERS THAT METASTASIZE TO FIVE SPECIFIC VITAL ORGANS

Brain	Heart	Bone
Lung	Lung	Lung
Breast	Breast	Breast
Melanoma	Melanoma	Prostate
Renal cell	Acute leukemia	Melanoma
	Lymphoma	Lymphoma
	Gastrointestinal	Kidney
		Thyroid
		Bladder
		Cervix
		Endometrium
		Pancreas
		Gastrinoma

Lung	Liver
Breast	Ovary
Lymphoma	Endometrium
Leukemia	Breast
Mesothelioma	Colon
Ovary	Gastric
Genitourinary	Pancreas
Gastrointestinal	Lymphoma
Melanoma	Multiple myeloma
Sarcoma	Melanoma

Table 55–2. SIGNS AND SYMPTOMS OF INCREASED INTRACRANIAL PRESSURE (ICP)

1. Decreased level of consciousness
2. Pupil dilation; occurs on the same side as the tumor
3. Increased systolic blood pressure and widening pulse pressure followed by a sharp drop in blood pressure
4. Bradycardia followed by a sharp tachycardia
5. Simultaneous bradycardia and increased systolic blood pressure*
6. Decreased respiratory rate
7. Papilledema only when increased ICP develops slowly
8. Hyperreflexia
9. Gait impairment

*Early significant finding.

Metastasis to the pericardium results in the accumulation of fluid in the pericardial sac. This sac is elastic and may stretch to accommodate as much as 1 liter of fluid before cardiac decompensation occurs (Pursley, 1983). This results in a syndrome known as pericardial effusion, which, if ignored, can progress rapidly into cardiac tamponade (see Chapter 57). If cardiac tamponade can be avoided, the mean survival rate of clients with pericardial effusion alone is 9 to 13 months (Smith, Lane, & Hudgins, 1974). Because of the potential morbidity associated with the progression of pericardial effusion, a thorough knowledge of the signs and symptoms is imperative. These include dyspnea, cough, nausea, vomiting, epigastric abdominal pain, hepatomegaly, leg edema, and neck vein distention.

Management of undiagnosed pericardial effusion includes treatment of the symptoms, such as providing oxygen for dyspnea, and direct bolstering of the body's hemodynamic compensatory responses with intravenous fluids and vasopressors. The most important method of management includes frequent monitoring of the client's heart rate, electrocardiogram, blood pressure, and changes in or additions to the aforementioned symptoms. Once a definitive diagnosis has been made, pericardial effusion can be treated with a pericardiocentesis, chemotherapy to the pericardial cavity, or external beam radiation to the heart.

Bone

The third vital organ identified in advanced disease is the skeletal system or bones. Metastasis to the bone occurs in 70 per cent of all clients with cancer (Jaffe, 1958) (see Table 55–1). One of the most sensitive diagnostic tests in the determination of bone metastasis is the bone scan. Figure 55–2 illustrates bone metastasis to the ribs, shoulder, humerus, and lumbar spine. Bone metastasis, which deossifies and softens bones, itself is not lethal. However, the resulting pain, neurologic deficits, and immobility can significantly decrease a client's quality of life. The quality of life can be further compromised by the occurrence of a pathologic fracture.

Pathologic fractures occur in 8 per cent of all clients with cancer (Faehnrich, 1983). Although symptoms may vary according to the location of the fracture, there are guidelines for assessment that apply to any location. These include inspection of the bones for swelling, erythema, abnormal joint position, or curvature; palpation of the joints and bones to detect pain, tenderness, change of temperature, or grating during movement; and evaluation of neurologic function distal to the affected area (Faehnrich, 1983).

More specifically, pathologic fractures occur most commonly in the spine, ribs, long bones (Fig. 55–3), and sternum. Metastases primarily affect the thoracic and lumbar regions of the spine. Signs and symptoms of spinal involvement include progressive numbness, weakness, muscle wasting, and bladder and bowel incontinence. Pathologic rib fractures can occur as a result of a simple cough or sneeze. The only sign of a

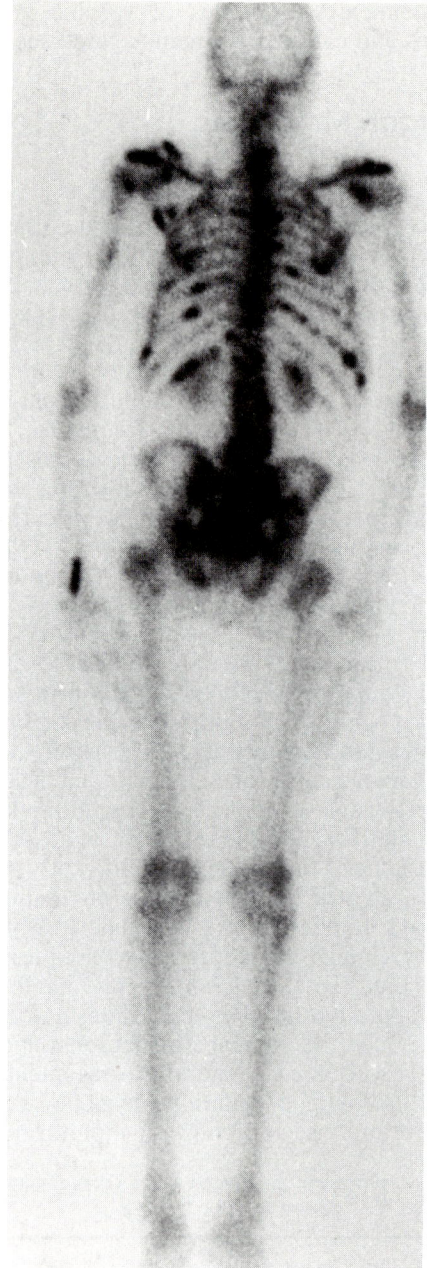

Figure 55–2. Bone scan shows metastatic lesions of ribs, shoulder, left humerus, and lumbar spine.

rib fracture is pain, aggravated by breathing, which is not relieved by rest. Pathologic fractures of the long bones may be prevented by prophylactic internal fixation. Such surgery results in an increased survival rate when compared with that of attempts to correct these fractures after they occur (Chernecky & Ramsey, 1984; Lancaster et al., 1988) (Box 55–1). The least frequent site for metastasis is the sternum. However, when fractures occur here, they heal slowly and cause more disfigurement.

Management of pathologic fractures generally focuses on pain control, palliative chemotherapy, and localized radiation therapy. Localized radiation is either partially or completely effective in the treatment of bone pain in 73 to 96 per cent of clients (Gilbert et

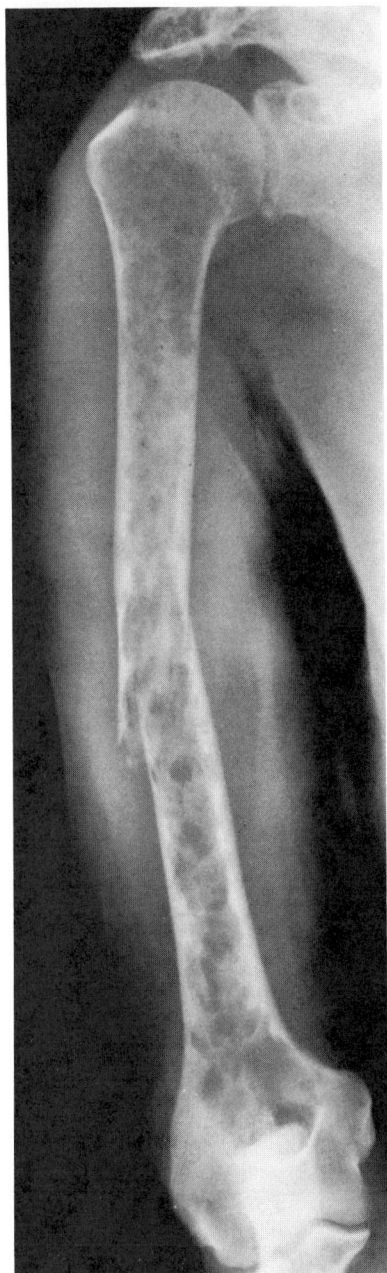

Figure 55–3. Plain film of humerus reveals diffuse bone metastasis and a pathologic fracture.

al., 1977). Nevertheless, when possible, prevention of pathologic fractures is the ideal type of management. This can be accomplished by using principles of anatomy and physiology when caring for clients with bone metastases. Specific interventions are addressed in the nursing diagnosis portion of this chapter.

Lung

Lung metastasis, which is the second most common site of metastasis, occurs in 29 per cent of all clients with cancer (Willis, 1967) (Fig. 55–4). The most frequent complication of advanced disease in the lungs is malignant pleural effusion. In fact, almost 50 per cent

of all pleural effusions are caused by cancer (Harper, 1979) (see Table 55–1).

Pleural effusion is an exudative process in which irritation of the pleural membrane by cancer cells results in an increased production of fluid in the interpleural space (Chernecky & Ramsey, 1984). In Figure 55–5, the left lung is 75 per cent filled with fluid, resulting in a drastic decrease in lung expansion. Normally, the space between the visceral and parietal pleura contains 5 to 15 ml of fluid. However, when cancer cells create overproduction and underabsorption, the interpleural space can contain more than 500 ml of fluid (Chernow & Sahn, 1977). Although approximately 25 per cent of clients with pleural effusion present with no symptoms, signs and symptoms for those with as much as 300 ml of interpleural fluid include dyspnea, pain, and hypoxia. For those with more than 300 ml of fluid in the interpleural space, signs and symptoms become more severe. These include tachycardia, tachypnea, asymmetric bulging of the intercostal spaces, diminished or absent breath sounds, and mediastinal shift.

Goals of management of malignant pleural effusion include treatment of both the symptoms and the cause (metastasis). Selection of the treatment depends on the prognosis and the present condition of the client. There are three basic treatment methods: surgical pleurectomy, needle thoracentesis, and chest tube insertion. Surgical pleurectomy is reserved for clients who are good surgical risks because the procedure has a 10 per cent mortality rate (Martini, Bains, & Beattie, 1975). Needle thoracentesis and chest tube insertion relieve symptoms, but additional procedures such as sclerosis or pleurodesis (Wood, Gillis, Blumgart, 1976) (Box 55–2) are required for control of pleural effusion (Table 55–3). Once treatment for pleural effusion has been implemented, ongoing nursing assessment of respiratory status is imperative.

Liver

One of the most common phenomenon of advanced disease is metastatic liver involvement (see Table 55–1). This has a most profound impact on survival rates. For example, mean survival rates of clients with liver metastasis range from 1.4 months for clients with widespread metastasis to 16.7 months for clients with minimal disease (Wood et al., 1976). A CT scan can evaluate liver metastasis (Fig. 55–6).

A complication of advanced disease to the liver that may decrease the length of survival time is malignant ascites. Two types of ascites are related to liver metastasis: malignant chylous ascites and malignant clear ascites.

Malignant chylous ascites occurs because of an obstruction in the lymphatics. Consequently, the fluid is turbid milky or creamy due to the presence of lymph. This type of ascites occurs most frequently as a result of lymphoma (Mauch, 1982).

Malignant clear ascites occurs as a result of a hypoalbuminemia-induced reduction in the plasma oncotic pressure. In this situation, the protein in the ascitic

---

Box 55–1. PATHOLOGIC FRACTURES OF THE HUMERUS

STUDY

Lancaster, J. M., Koman, L. A., Gristina, A. G., Rovere, G. D., Poehling, G. G., Nicastro, J. F., & Adair, D. M. (1988). **Pathologic fractures of the humerus.** *Southern Medical Journal, 81,* 52–55.

SAMPLE

Fifty-two subjects with 57 actual or impending pathologic fractures of the humerus. The median age of the subjects was 62 yr, and 71 per cent had diagnoses of breast cancer or multiple myeloma. All subjects were expected to live at least 6 weeks.

MEASURES

A four-point rating system (excellent, good, fair, poor) for pain relief and function was used to compare nonoperative care to three types of internal fixations (Küntscher rod, Rush rod, Neer endoprosthesis) of pathologic fractures. Local irradiation was used in six of seven nonoperative cases and in 25 of 45 cases after surgery.

FINDINGS

Those patients who were treated nonoperatively had fair to poor pain relief and poor function. Those patients whose fractures were stabilized with the Küntscher rod and Rush rods had excellent to good pain relief and good function. Those whose fractures were stabilized with the Neer endoprosthesis had good pain relief and good function.

LIMITATIONS

The review of pain relief and function was done retrospectively. Thus the researchers made the assumption that the procedures caused the good pain relief and function. This conclusion would be more strongly demonstrated if the study had been designed prospectively.

fluid is greater than the serum protein, and additional fluid is drawn into the abdominal cavity (Mauch, 1982).

General signs and symptoms of malignant ascites include abdominal distention, shortness of breath, and nausea. Although malignant chylous ascites may cause a rise in temperature, a diagnostic paracentesis and fluid culture should be performed to determine the type of malignant ascites.

In terms of management of malignant ascites, it should be noted that repeated paracentesis of abdominal fluid has not been effective in reducing ascites. Instead, this technique results in protein loss and risks fluid deprivation. Several therapies are effective, however, in relieving ascites (Table 55–4).

Sequelae of Therapies

As described earlier, the effects of metastasis on the vital organs result in many complications of advanced disease. In addition, therapies for cancers can lead to critical complications. This section discusses complications associated with drug toxicities, radiation therapy, and bone marrow transplantation.

Drug Toxicities

Drug toxicities affect four major organs: heart, lung, liver, and kidney (Table 55–5). For example, chemotherapy-induced heart toxicities cause heart enlargement, which develops into congestive heart failure and pulmonary hypertension (Chernecky & Ramsey, 1984). In the lungs, antineoplastic agents damage the alveolar epithelium and the basement membrane, which decreases the amount of collagen secreted. The result is fibrosis with impaired gas exchange (Wickham, 1986). The effects of chemotherapy on the liver range from increased level of hepatic enzymes seen with high doses of the drugs to hepatic fibrosis associated with long-term therapy, although the etiology is unknown (Chabner & Myers, 1982). Each of the aforementioned types of toxicities is not uncommon in cancer therapy, but kidney toxicity is a more common cause of advanced disease and is discussed in more detail.

Drug-related kidney toxicity occurs when the chemotherapeutic agents cause direct damage to the glomerulus, tubules, or both. In addition, drugs can cause indirect damage through vascular changes. The risk of such damage increases when combination drug regimens are used (Hickey, 1986).

The signs and symptoms of kidney toxicity mimic

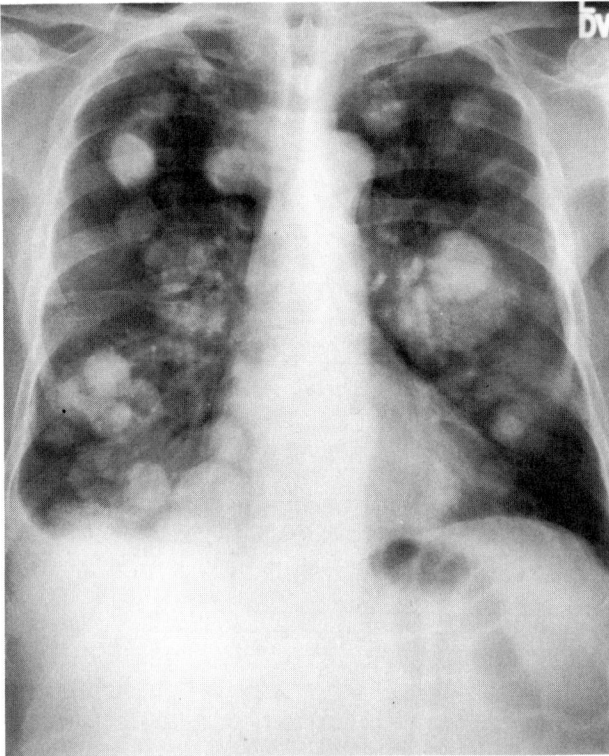

Figure 55–4. Anterior-posterior view of chest radiograph shows multiple bilateral metastatic lesions.

those of renal failure. They include increased blood urea nitrogen and creatinine values, decreased urinary output, fluid retention, pulmonary rales, nausea, vomiting, edema, and pruritus. In addition, the client should be monitored for metabolic acidosis and cardiac dysrhythmias.

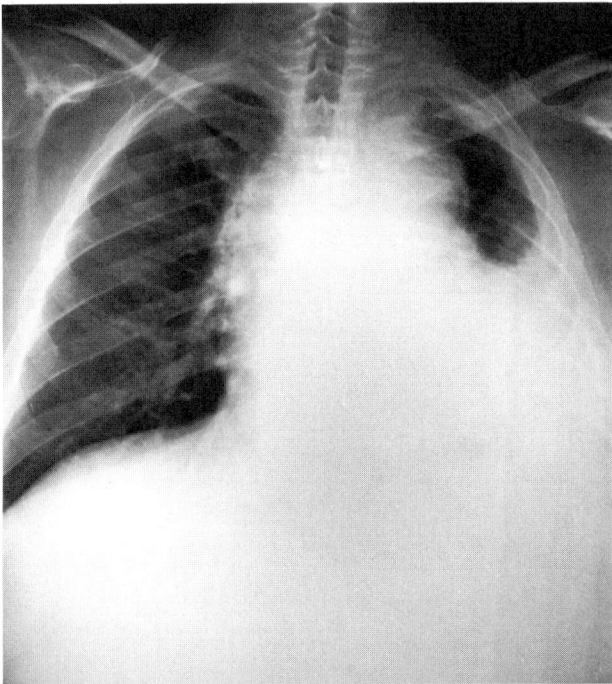

Figure 55–5. Anterior-posterior view of chest radiograph. Left lung space is 75 per cent replaced by fluid, as indicated by the total whitening of left lower lobes.

Management of chemotherapy-induced kidney toxicity would include efforts to prevent renal toxicity such as to administer diuretics and hydration before, during, and after drug administration. Of course, even though prevention efforts are employed, it is not always possible to avoid renal failure, and the client may progress into chronic renal failure. In this instance dialysis would be indicated.

Radiation

Unlike systemic chemotherapy, external radiation–induced advanced disease is site specific. That is, the areas of the body receiving the radiation will be the areas in which potential complications can occur. For example, radiation to the head and neck area may cause nausea, taste changes, and stomatitis. Although symptoms such as these are quite manageable, the consequences of radiation to the bowel are potentially fatal.

For clients whose cancer extends through the bowel wall, surgery alone is insufficient. Initially, radiation offers further control of the cancer with minimal danger of complications. However, with 5000 rads or greater, the client has a 10 per cent chance of developing bowel adhesions, bowel obstruction, or fistulization (Sugarbaker, Macdonald, & Gunderson, 1982). Six to 12 months after therapy, the bowel may become increasingly friable, eliminating the possibility of further surgical intervention. The outcome is malabsorption and paralytic ileus with concomitant bowel necrosis.

Signs and symptoms of this outcome include gas, abdominal distention, abdominal pain, and absent bowel sounds. Unfortunately, this syndrome is not curable. Instead, management focuses on symptom relief, such as nasogastric tube insertion and pain control measures.

Bone Marrow Transplantation

The third therapeutic sequela that is likely to cause advanced disease is bone marrow transplantation. This therapy is generally used to treat leukemias, although it is being used experimentally on some solid tumors such as lung cancer, breast cancer, and melanoma. (Schryber, Lacasse, & Barton-Burke, 1987). Bone marrow transplantation has one major complication: graft-versus-host disease (GVHD) (see Chapter 27).

Graft-versus-host disease occurs when the donor T cells proliferate and attack various cells in the already compromised host. The four grades of GVHD are distinguished by the degree of organ involvement, with grade 1 involving only a skin rash and grade 4 involving multiorgan failure and extreme decrease in clinical performance. In addition, GVHD can be either acute, with an onset of 7 to 14 days, or chronic, with an onset of 2 to 12 months after bone marrow transplantation.

Graft-versus-host disease involves multiple organ failure, which includes (1) the skin, with associated rash, sloughing, and turning bronze in color; (2) gastrointestinal tract dysfunction, including nausea, pai and malabsorption; (3) liver dysfunction, includi

---

Box 55–2. EFFECT OF CLIENT POSITIONING FOLLOWING PLEURODESIS

STUDY

Lorch, D. G., Gordon, L., Wooten, S., Cooper, J., Strange, C., & Sahn, S. A. (1988). **Effect of patient positioning on distribution of tetracycline in the pleural space during pleurodesis.** *Chest, 93,* 527–529.

SAMPLE

Five subjects, aged 32 to 73, with recurrent, symptomatic, malignant pleural effusions. Three subjects had lung cancer, one had non-Hodgkin's lymphoma, and one had adenocarcinoma of unknown origin. All subjects had an expected survival of several months.

MEASURES

After the subjects' pleural drainage decreased and effusions were absent on chest radiographs, tetracycline was radiolabeled and inserted through subjects' chest tubes. Scintigraphic imaging was done immediately after tetracycline instillation before patient rotation. Repeat images were obtained at 30 and 120 min as patients were rotated through six positions.

FINDINGS

Four of the five subjects exhibited dispersement of the tetracycline throughout the pleural space before any position changes. The fifth subject, who had a hydropneumothorax and a trapped lung, revealed slight improvement of the dispersion of tetracycline with rotation. Thus for most patients with malignant pleural effusion, tetracycline pleurodesis can be well achieved without patient rotation. This adds to the comfort of the client and frees staff from implementing a rigorous client rotation schedule.

LIMITATIONS

The images demonstrated immediate tetracycline dispersion, yet all subjects were rotated in spite of this finding. The study would be stronger with a control group of subjects who were not rotated so that the interval images could be compared. Additionally, a larger sample and homogeneity of subjects would add strength to the study.

---

jaundice and hemorrhage; and (4) bone marrow dysfunction, including pancytopenia and infection.

Unfortunately, GVHD occurs to some degree in 50 to 70 per cent of all bone marrow transplantation clients (Chernecky & Ramsey, 1984). Management includes symptom control only.

PROCESS OF ASSESSMENT AND MANAGEMENT OF ADVANCED DISEASE

Assessment and management of advanced disease is a complex process. Taking into account the anatomic and pathophysiologic factors and therapeutic sequelae

already presented, the nurse has a basis on which to assess and care for clients with advanced disease. This portion of the chapter focuses on extending data collection, through physical assessment and diagnostics, and culminates in the presentation of selected nursing

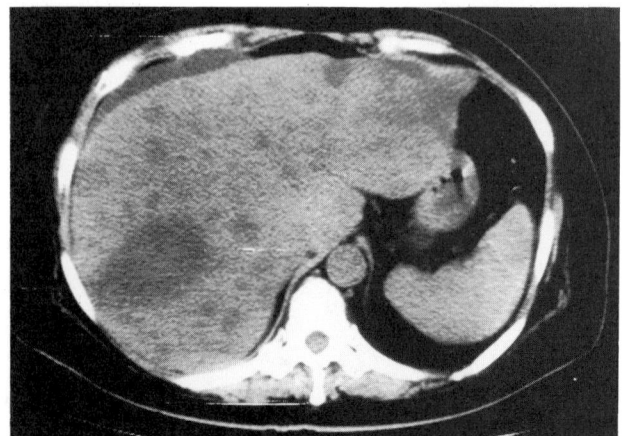

Figure 55–6. Computed tomographic scan shows an enlarged liver with widespread metastasis, as evidenced by the darker irregularly shaped areas of gray.

Table 55–3. AGENTS INSERTED INTO THE PLEURAL SPACE TO CONTROL PLEURAL EFFUSION

Radioactive Isotopes	Chemotherapeutic Agents	Sclerosing Agents
Gold	Bleomycin	Talc
Phosphorus	Cyclophosphamide	Tetracycline
Yttrium	(Cytoxan)	
Yttrium gold	5-fluorouracil	
	Nitrogen mustard	
	Thiotepa	

Table 55–4. THERAPIES FOR MALIGNANT ASCITES

Systemic chemotherapy	Use the chemotherapy protocol for the primary cancer
Intraperitoneal radiation	Chromic phosphate or gold
Intraperitoneal chemotherapy	Bleomycin, 5-fluorouracil, nitrogen mustard, or thiotepa; this therapy is not effective in chylous ascites
Surgery	LeVeen or Denver shunts; these shunts are used for palliation to relieve pressure; they may remain open from a few days to 3 yr with 50 per cent functioning for at least 1 yr (Spiro, 1983).

diagnoses and interventions for the client with advanced disease.

Physical Assessment, Laboratory Values, and Diagnostic Tests of Vital Organs

Physical assessment serves as a device for detecting abnormalities that may be life threatening and for identifying signs that may suggest complications of advanced disease. Additional sources of data are necessary to complete the process of assessment. These sources include laboratory values and diagnostic tests. Assessment for advanced disease, including all three aspects of data collection, is presented in Table 55–6.

Nursing Diagnoses and for Interventions for Advanced Disease

The establishment of a database leads to the next phase of the nursing process: formulation of the nursing

Table 55–5. DRUGS THAT ARE TOXIC TO VITAL ORGANS

Heart	Lung	Kidney
Amphotericin B	Adenine	Amikacin (Amikin)
Daunorubicin	arabinoside	Aminoglycosides
Doxorubicin	(Ara-A)	• Gentamicin*
(Adriamycin)	Bleomycin	• Kanamycin*
Cyclophosphamide	Busulfan	• Neomycin†
(Cytoxan) acts	Carmustine	• Streptomycin*
synergistically with	Chloramphenicol	• Vancomycin
doxorubicin	Cyclophosphamide	Amphotericin B
	Methotrexate	Carmustine (BCNU)*
Liver	Mitomycin	Cephaloridine
Amphotericin B	Procarbazine	Cisplatin†
Chlorambucil	Colistin sulfate	Colistin sulfate
(Leukeran)	(Polymixin) is	(Polymixin B)
Cyclophosphamide	associated with	Cyclophosphamide
Cytosine arabinoside	respiratory arrest	Hydroxyurea
(Ara-C)		L-asparaginase
Griseofulvin		Lomustine (CCNU)*
L-asparaginase		Methotrexate—high
Methotrexate		dose†
Pyrazinamide		Mithramycin†
		Mitomycin C†
		Semustine
		(MeCCNU)*
		Streptozocin†
		Vinblastine

*High risk of nephrotoxicity with long-term use.
†High risk of immediate nephrotoxicity.

care plan. Neither the nursing diagnoses (Kelly, 1985) nor the associated interventions are intended to be all inclusive. As each client differs, so will his or her care plan. Thus the subsequent care plans should serve only as guidelines for care plan formulation of clients with advanced disease.

Brain: Alteration in Thought Processes

The client shows evidence of impaired thought processes related to decreased level of consciousness and impaired judgment resulting from neuropsychiatric syndrome.

Nursing interventions:

1. Assess level of consciousness every 2 to 4 hr.

2. Assess for increased intracranial pressure (see Table 55–2) every hour or with each client contact.

3. Check vital signs every 1 to 2 hr.

4. Take safety precautions: padded side rails, soft restraints, bed in lowest position, call light within easy reach.

5. Reorient the client to time, place, and reason for hospitalization with each client contact.

6. Explain the client's condition to the client and the client's family with each contact. Assist them in asking questions and expressing concerns about the present and future.

Heart: Decreased Cardiac Output

The client experiences altered cardiac output (decreased) that is related to dyspnea, tachycardia, neck vein distention, and epigastric or abdominal pain that results from pericardial effusion.

Nursing interventions:

1. Assess respiratory rate, heart rate, and blood pressure every 15 to 30 minutes and record pulse pressure.

2. Assess neck vein distention with head of bed elevated up to 60 degrees every hour.

3. Assess electrocardiogram for a decrease in QRS voltage, electrical alternans, and dysrhythmias.

4. Monitor intake and output every hour.

5. Auscultate heart and lung sounds every 2 hr.

6. Administer oxygen as prescribed.

Bone: Impaired Physical Mobility

The client has impaired physical mobility related to pain, numbness, weakness, and bladder and bowel incontinence resulting from pathologic fractures.

Nursing interventions:

1. Palpate bones for tenderness and crepitus every 4 hr.

2. Assess alignment of bones every hour.

3. Position the client using techniques of proper body alignment associated with comfort and support of wasted limbs.

4. Measure respiratory rate and quality every 4 hr.

5. Monitor intake and output every 8 hr, noting continence.

Table 55–6. ASSESSMENT FOR ADVANCED DISEASE

Organ/Problem	Physical Assessment	Lab Values	Diagnostics
Brain/neuropsychiatric syndrome	Personality changes Decision making Math computations Level of consciousness Seizure activity Increased intracranial pressure (Table 55–2)	Phenobarbital Phenytoin (Dilantin)	Computed tomography brain scan Magnetic resonance imaging of brain
Heart/pericardial effusion	Respiratory rate Liver palpation Neck vein distention Heart rate Blood pressure Heart sounds	Arterial blood gases	Electrocardiogram Echocardiogram Chest radiograph
Bone/pathologic fractures	Pain Respiratory rate Assess extremities: ● motor function ● tactile perception ● muscle strength ● bowel and bladder control	Calcium Phosphorus	Radiograph of bone Bone scan
Lung/pleural effusion	Heart rate Respiratory rate Breath sound Lung symmetry	Arterial blood gases Fluid cytology	Thoracentesis Chest radiograph Pulmonary function test
Liver/malignant ascites	Respiratory rate Abdominal girth Bowel sounds Abdominal palpation	Fluid cytology Albumin Fluid carcinoembryonic antigen	Paracentesis Computed tomography scan of liver
Kidney/renal failure	Lung sounds Palpation for edema	Blood urea nitrogen Arterial blood gases Creatinine Specific gravity of urine Electrolytes	Electrocardiogram Intravenous pyelogram

6. Splint the client within the draw sheet when transfering.

7. Medicate around the clock for pain.

8. Schedule passive and active range of motion exercises, taking into account a client's pain and ability.

9. Encourage isometric exercises when range of motion exercises are contraindicated.

Lung: Impaired Gas Exchange

The client experiences impaired gas exchange related to dyspnea, hypoxia, absent breath sounds, and altered arterial blood gases resulting from pleural effusion.

Nursing interventions:

1. Auscultate breath sounds every 2 hr. Do not expect to hear a friction rub because fluid separates the pleura.

2. Inspect thorax for symmetry of respiratory movement, use of accessory muscles, and tracheal position every 2 hr.

3. Measure blood pressure and heart rate every 2 hr.

4. Monitor intake and output every 4 hr.

5. Elevate head of bed to 60 degrees for comfort.

6. Assess respiratory rate every 30 min.

7. Administer oxygen as prescribed.

8. Medicate for pain, anxiety, or both.

Liver: Altered Nutrition

The client shows effects of altered nutrition—less than body requirements—related to abdominal disten-

tion, hypoalbuminemia, shortness of breath, and nausea resulting from malignant ascites.

Nursing interventions:

1. Monitor intake and output every 4 hr.

2. Measure abdominal girth daily.

3. Record blood pressure, heart rate, and respirations every 2 hr.

4. Monitor serum albumin levels and serum and urine osmolality.

5. Restrict sodium intake.

6. Restrict fluids to less than 1500 ml per day.

7. Weigh daily.

8. Assist the client to a high Fowler's position to ease respirations.

9. Perform skin care every 4 hr.

Kidney: Impaired Skin Integrity

The client experiences alteration in skin integrity related to fluid retention, edema, and increased blood urea nitrogen level resulting from chemotherapy-induced renal failure.

Nursing interventions:

1. Monitor intake and output every hour.

2. Weigh the client at the same time every day.

3. Record blood pressure, heart rate, and respiratory rate every 2 hr.

4. Turn and position the client every 2 hr.

5. Massage bony prominences and apply lotion to skin every 4 hr.

6. Provide hyperalimentation as prescribed.
7. Restrict dietary protein intake.

SPECIAL PROBLEMS RELATED TO ADVANCED DISEASE

Although it would seem as though the complications of advanced disease are serious in and of themselves, several problems must not be ignored. These include drainage odor, hope, and suicidal ideation.

Drainage Odor

In advanced disease in which metastases are extensive, it is not unusual to encounter direct invasion of cancer cells into the epithelium. This phenomenon occurs most commonly from primary cancers of the breast, stomach, head and neck, lung, uterus, ovary, and colon, as well as from melanoma and lymphoma. This type of metastasis causes loss of vascularity with ultimate necrosis and infection. The result is a purulent, friable, malodorous lesion (Foltz, 1980).

Because cure of these lesions is rare, the problem most significant to the client is odor. The offensive smell is noticed not only by family, hospital staff, and other visitors, but also by the client. Although others may not say anything, the client, aware of the odor, feels embarrassed, and may withdraw socially.

Management of these odors offers relief of one of the many problems a client with advanced disease must face. Initial management should always include wound cleansing and debridement; however, these measures alone are rarely effective. Some commercial products are available to apply on dressings such as Nilodor, Tap-a-Drop, Puri-Clens, Ostozyme, and Banish-ItQ but often these products produce odors that are equally distressing to the client (Foltz, 1980). One of the most effective methods of odor control is irrigation with room-temperature yogurt or buttermilk and normal saline. Odiferous wounds, irrigated with these products at least four times a day on a regular basis, become nonproblematic within 4 days (Welch, 1981). A second effective method is to mix a 6-g packet of Bard absorptive dressing with 10 ml of sterile water and 10 ml of Puri-Clens (Sweed Co.) and place this mixture in the wound, followed by a sterile dressing, twice a day. Although aerosols should not be used exclusively, commercial room deodorizers, such as Hexon odor antagonist, may be helpful.

Hope

"Hope is a multidimensional dynamic life force characterized by a confident yet uncertain expectation of achieving a future good which, to the hoping person, is realistically possible and personally significant" (DuFault & Martocchio, 1985). For any client with cancer, hope is an important concept. Usually the hope is for a cure or remission so that a "normal" life style can be resumed. However, when a complication occurs, whether it is the first indication or a later indication of advanced disease, the hope for cure is shattered.

It is the responsibility of nurses to help such clients and their families understand that hope is not lost. Although nurses must acknowledge the fact that cure is no longer a realistic possibility, other hopes may be kept alive. Nurses can encourage a hopeful attitude by helping clients and their families develop an awareness of life, identify reasons for living, establish support systems, incorporate religion or humor, and set realistic goals (Hickey, 1986). Nurses must emphasize that although hopes may change in focus and direction, there is never "no hope."

Suicidal Ideation

The final special problem associated with advanced disease is suicidal ideation. Suicide is 1.3 times higher in men with cancer and 1.9 times higher in women with cancer than in the general population. Cancers associated with suicide attempts include leukemia and breast, head and neck, lung and upper gastrointestinal tract cancers (Kline, 1984).

Suicide attempts arise in an effort to gain control over a situation in which there is no perceived control. Signs and symptoms include verbalization of the intention and the means with which to act on that intention, loss of hope, and loss of interest in any specific aspect of life.

Nursing management of the client with suicidal ideation includes constant assessment and observation because clients generally leave "clues." The nurse should also be available to assist in channeling aggressive feelings into constructive behaviors, fostering feelings of control, and finding hope and meaning in life. In addition to caring for the client, nurses should be attentive to the needs of the family by offering explanations and support. It is also appropriate when such a situation arises to consult a psychiatric mental health clinical nurse specialist.

SUMMARY

This chapter delineated specific complications of advanced disease according to the vital organs and the pathophysiology involved. In addition, this chapter presented guidelines for nursing management in terms of assessment, nursing diagnoses, and nursing interventions. Finally, three special problems associated with advanced disease and its management were described with subsequent guidelines for nursing management.

Advanced disease is a complex phenomenon, and it often mandates decisions that will result directly in life or death. This chapter has focused on aggressive management of complications of advanced disease. However, advanced disease itself is not curable, and management of such complications has limitations. It is vital for caregivers to consider the goals of the client and family as well as the goals of aggressive management when complications are imminent. Potential risks and benefits of interventions should always be examined carefully to ensure the client maximum quality of life as he or she defines it. When there is agreement among all parties that aggressive management is no longer appropriate, invasive, disturbing interventions such as measurements of abdominal girth or frequent monitoring of vital signs should be minimized or eliminated and palliative management should be implemented (see Chapter 28).

References

Billings, J. A. (1985). *Outpatient management of advanced cancer.* Philadelphia: J. B. Lippincott Co.

Bisel, H. F., Wroblewski, F., & LaDue, J. S. (1953). Incidence and clinical manifestations of cardiac metastases. *Journal of the American Medical Association, 153,* 712–715.

Chabner, B. A., & Myers, C. E. (1982). Clinical pharmacology of cancer chemotherapy. In V. T. DeVita, Jr., S. Hellman, & S. A. Rosenberg (Eds.), *Cancer: Principles and practice and oncology* (pp. 156–197). Philadelphia: J. B. Lippincott Co.

Chernecky, C. C., & Ramsey, P. W. (1984). *Critical nursing care of the client with cancer.* East Norwalk, CT: Appleton-Century-Crofts.

Chernow, B., & Sahn, S. A. (1977). Carcinomatosis involvement of the pleura: An analysis of 96 patients. *American Journal of Medicine, 63,* 695–702.

DuFault, K., & Martocchio, B. C. (1985). Hope: Its spheres and dimensions. *Nursing Clinics of North America, 20,* 379–391.

Faehnrich, J. (1983). When pathologic fractures threaten. *RN, 46*(11), 34–37.

Foltz, A. T. (1980). Nursing care of ulcerating metastatic lesions. *Oncology Nursing Forum, 7*(2), 8–13.

Gilbert, H. A., Kagan, A. R., Nussbaum, H., Raoarstatzman, J., Chan, P., Allen, B., & Forsythe, A. (1977). Evaluation of radiation therapy for bone metastases: Pain relief and quality of life. *American Journal of Roentgenology, 129,* 1095.

Hanfling, S. M. (1960). Metastatic cancer of the heart. *Circulation, 22,* 474–481.

Harper, G. R. (1979). Pleural effusions in cancer. *Clinical Cancer Briefs, 1*(2), 1–8.

Hickey, S. S. (1986). Enabling hope. *Cancer Nursing, 9,* 133–137.

Jaffe, W. L. (1958). *Tumors and tumerous conditions of the bones and joints.* Philadelphia: Lea & Febiger.

Kelly, M. A. (1985). *Nursing diagnosis source book: Guidelines for clinical application.* E. Norwalk, CT: Appleton-Century Crofts.

Kline, P. M. (1984). Suicidal ideation. In C. C. Chernecky & P. W. Ramsey, (Eds.), *Critical nursing care of the client with cancer* (pp. 272–276). East Norwalk, CT: Appleton-Century-Crofts.

Lancaster, J. M., Koman, L. A., Gristina, A. G., Rovere, G. D., Poehling, G. G., Nicastro, J. F., & Adair, D. M. (1988). Pathologic fractures of the humerus. *Southern Medical Journal, 81,* 52–55.

Lorch, D. G., Gordon, L., Wooten, S., Cooper, J., Strange, C., & Sahn, S. A. (1988). Effect of patient positioning on distribution of tetracycline in the pleural space during pleurodesis. *Chest, 93,* 527–529.

Lydon, J. (1986). Nephrotoxicity of cancer treatment. *Oncology Nursing Forum, 13*(2), 69–77.

Martini, N., Bains, M. S., & Beattie, E. J. (1975). Indications for pleurectomy in malignant effusions. *Cancer, 35,* 734–738.

Mauch, P. M. (1982). Treatment of malignant ascites. In V. T. DeVita, Jr., S. Hellman, & S. A. Rosenberg (Eds.), *Cancer: Principles and practice of oncology* (pp. 156–197). Philadelphia: J. B. Lippincott Co.

Posner, J. B. (1979). Neurological complications of systemic cancer. *Medical Clinics of North America, 63,* 783–800.

Pursley, P. (1983). Acute cardiac tamponade. *American Journal of Nursing, 83,* 1414–1418.

Rosetti, A. C. (1985). Nursing care of the patients treated with intrapleural tetracycline for control of malignant pleural effusion. *Cancer Nursing, 8,* 103–109.

Schryber, S., Lacasse, C. R., & Barton-Burke, M. (1987). Autologous bone marrow transplantation. *Oncology Nursing Forum, 14*(4), 74–80.

Smith, F. E., Lane, M., & Hudgins, P. T. (1974). Conservative management of malignant pericardial effusion. *Cancer, 33,* 47.

Spiro, H. M. (1983). *Clinical gastroenterology* (3rd ed.). New York: Macmillan.

Sugarbaker, P. H., Macdonald, J. S., & Gunderson, L. L. (1982). Colorectal cancer. In V. T. DeVita, Jr., S. Hellman, & S. A. Rosenberg (Eds.), *Cancer: Principles and practice of oncology* (pp. 643–723). Philadelphia: J. B. Lippincott Co.

Vieth, R. G., & Odom, G. L. (1965). Intracranial metastases and their neurosurgical treatment. *Journal of Neurosurgery, 23,* 375–383.

Welch, L. B. (1981). Simple new remedy for the odor of open lesions. *RN, 44*(2), 42–43.

Wickham, R. (1986). Pulmonary toxicity secondary to cancer treatment. *Oncology Nursing Forum, 13*(5), 69–76.

Willis, R. A. (1967). *Pathology of tumors.* London: Appleton-Century-Crofts.

Wood, C. B., Gillis, C. R., & Blumgart, L. H. (1976). A retrospective study of the natural history of patients with liver metastasis from colorectal cancer. *Clinical Oncology, 2,* 285.

CHAPTER 56

Supportive Care of the Dying Patient

JOYCE ZERWEKH

"Birth is a fatal disease."

—Woody Allen

TRANSITION

The transition from active treatment to supportive care of the dying patient involves a major turning point in philosophy and action. On ceasing to try to rescue the perishing, one is then free to care for the dying (Ramsey, 1970). Unfortunately, care of the dying is impaired by a profound reluctance to speak the truth about medical limitations and a profound trust that technology can reverse end-stage disease one more time.

What are the costs of denial of death for the individual and society? For the individual and loved ones, the cost is denial of choice when the reality of death has not been acknowledged, and aggravation of physical and emotional suffering when comfort is not emphasized and grief is not permitted. For society, the cost of trying to rescue the perishing dominates our national health care budget: nearly one third of Medicare expenses pays for terminal care (Torrens, 1985).

Nurses can promote up-front decision making in that transition between living and dying. As colleagues on the health care team, it is vital to insist on open discussion and decisions regarding the continuance of active treatment and the relief of suffering. By what logic is therapy continued? Is there a reasonable chance of benefit? What are the hardships for the person? Nurses witness these hardships and likewise must bear witness to them when the health care team is making decisions. Burdens of treatment are weighed against all known benefits or lack thereof. In oncology, the move from active treatment that can significantly pro-

long life or offer a cure to palliative treatment that comforts the terminally ill is often a continuum, so that there is not a definite point when a patient is treated as living one day and dying the next. The fully informed patient lives with a foot in each world—that of the living and that of those preparing to die. Contemporary American secular ethicists emphasize that the patient's self-determination should be a predominant ethical concern. "The last few days and hours of life comprise a vital time of partnership between the dying person and those, including helping professionals, who would provide vigil and comfort at his or her side" (Blues & Zerwekh, 1984).

PATHOPHYSIOLOGY OF MULTIPLE ORGAN FAILURE

Many changes near the time of death are predictable, and anticipating them can help prepare the dying person and family to manage. Infection, organ failure, pulmonary or myocardial infarction, hemorrhage, or extensive carcinomatosis have been identified as major processes underlying cancer death (Inagaki, Rodriguez, & Bodey, 1974). The closer the moment of death, the more likely are common pathophysiologic events. The progression from innumerable preterminal disease processes to final cardiopulmonary arrest can be conceptualized as a journey down a tunnel that is wide at the top but becomes steeper and narrower with "a gradually diminishing number of possible conditions, any and all of which will lead to a relatively limited pathophysiologic 'common pathway of death' " (Younger, 1987). This terminal common pathway will eventually include cardiopulmonary failure and often renal or hepatic failure, or both. The human responses to this predictable multisystem failure include nursing diagnostic focus on impaired physical mobility, nutrition and fluid balance, thought processes, comfort, gas exchange and airway clearance, and then impending death.

The heart may fail because of myocardial damage or the workload imposed by preterminal pathologic conditions, such as pulmonary lesions, pericardial or myocardial metastases, anemia, sepsis, or brain herniation onto the medulla. Common causes of pulmonary failure include pulmonary lesions, pneumonia, pulmonary infarct, pulmonary edema, pulmonary effusion, or brain herniation. The hypoxemia and reduced perfusion of vital organs that accompany cardiopulmonary failure cause marked loss of capacity for mobility, eating or drinking, and mentation or consciousness. Comfort is impaired because of edema or ascites, acute air hunger due to impaired gas exchange or ineffective airway clearance, and feeling apprehensive until consciousness is lost. Death is impending as the blood pressure drops, peripheral cyanosis deepens, periods of apnea lengthen, and accumulating pulmonary and pharyngeal secretions produce a death rattle (Blues & Zerwekh, 1984).

Hepatic and renal failure are frequently associated events in death due to cancer. Hepatic metastases may eventually diminish liver function so that ammonia and other metabolites correlated with the development of hepatic encephalopathy are not detoxified. Reduced synthesis of albumin and reduced detoxification of aldosterone and antidiuretic hormone produce extravascular fluid accumulation, and resistance to blood flow into the liver forces fluid into the peritoneal cavity. Renal failure occurs with hypovolemia reducing renal perfusion with renal malignancy. Retention of sodium causes peripheral and pulmonary edema. Azotemia and metabolic acidosis occur owing to failure to excrete nitrogenous waste and hydrogen ions. These pathophysiologic events contribute to a remarkably common nursing diagnostic pattern. Again, capacity for mobility, nutrition absorption, and thought are impaired by accumulating toxic metabolites. Comfort is threatened by fluid build-up in the lungs, abdomen, and periphery.

HUMAN MORTALITY

Human Process

Institutional dying has only recently become the norm in Western society. In contrast, throughout human history, death occurred in one's own bed at home. These times should not be idealized without a recognition that such dying was premature by contemporary standards and generally without symptomatic relief. However, death in the past was a familiar crisis that people learned early *to face and to survive*. The sanitized and invisible contemporary pattern of dying does not permit the development of emotional and cognitive coping skills that until recently were a "given" in human experience. Nursing dying people and their loved ones involves recapturing the best of the past by helping people see death as a normal part of the life cycle, a phase that is extremely difficult but over which they have choices and some control.

Humanization instead of medicalization of dying involves a major shift in paradigm in which primary attention is given to the human experiences and choices of the person who is dying. Concern moves away from disease and technologic maintenance of failing systems. Open communication and participation are facilitated in contrast to withholding of information and withdrawal that result when dying is perceived as unspeakable defeat. In the midst of loss rests the paradoxical opportunity for growth and discovery of life and its meanings. The road to discovery is made more difficult by episodes of suffering, but we become stronger and wiser by consciously traveling together along it.

Switching Goals

Even when the expected outcome is death, nursing and medical practices too often continue unchanged, as if the expected outcome were life. Unfortunately for patient well-being, the difference between goals and interventions that support a comfortable dying and those that restore, resuscitate, and rehabilitate the living are striking. It is essential that the nurse take the lead in setting *conscious* deliberate goals to comfort individual and family members and respect their choices. Contrast, for instance, the automatic nursing rituals of putting someone in a chair, forcing fluids, drawing blood, monitoring many body functions, and administering drugs that no longer work. Particularly in the nursing home setting, every effort must be made to instruct aides and practical nurses to shift their energies toward comforting (see Chapter 28 for further discussion of palliative support).

Dying as an Individual Process

A person copes with dying as he or she has coped with living; the wise will be wise and the difficult stay difficult. "Those who are not informed about their life-threatening situation are wrongly denied their right to choose the way they will end their lifetime" (Blues & Zerwekh, 1984). Given adequate information appropriate to their individual circumstances, the responses to news of a limited life expectancy are as varied as people themselves. People who have been living with cancer and multiple treatment methods have already been living with a cloud over their heads. They have experienced many discomforts and inconveniences as their life has been increasingly medicalized. Body appearance and functions have changed. Roles and relationships have been altered. In short, they have already grieved many losses in grieving for the death of their familiar selves.

When the decision is made that no further treatment will stop the spread of cancer, normal coping mechanisms include initial shock and denial, which then is followed by varying degrees and expressions of denial, bargaining, sadness, and raging. The process is not linear but cyclic along a continuum. Thus it is not surprising to listen to a patient planning a funeral service one minute and a fishing trip for the following summer the next minute. Some patients who pass through these cycles in which they face multiple losses, including their own deaths, will experience times of plateau and eventually resolution. People cope with this final loss as they have coped with other losses and changes in their lives. Coping patterns are predicted by these past events as well as by cultural heritage. (See Chapter 10 for further discussion of responses to grief and Chapter 6 for an exploration of cultural impact.) To understand individual reaction, also remember that the grieving process is superimposed on normal development tasks, which are discussed in Chapter 7. Consider, for instance, the demands imposed by the conflicting grieving, developmental, and cultural tasks on a Japanese-American businessman, who is married, the father of two children, and dying of acute lymphocytic leukemia.

Normalizing is a basic strategy for individuals and families facing a terminal illness (Strauss, 1975). People do not wish to live every moment around the reality of dying. They normalize by discounting seriousness, drawing attention away from the disease, and trying to live life as usual. Some may do this until symptoms "flood" all activity and interaction.

Nursing diagnoses focus first on identifying individual strengths and then building on them. The patient's strengths should be defined precisely in diagnostic statements focusing on areas such as positive self-concept, positive body image, adequate self-esteem, satisfactory social interaction, effective crisis resolution, and effective individual coping (Houldin, Saltstein, & Ganles, 1987). Nurses should anticipate that the patient will face progressive impairments with anxiety, fear, anticipatory grieving, hopelessness, powerlessness, deficient knowledge, disturbance in self-concept, altered sexuality, and impaired social interaction.

Interventions to support the dying person are never standardized and are always relevant to specific nursing diagnoses. However, generic approaches for all people who are losing themselves include a strong affirmation of their personhood: strengthening and validating their identity, translating medical and nursing information to whatever is relevant for their everyday living and planning, and fostering choices about how to live and die (Zerwekh, 1983b). Family caregivers and hospice nurses have identified the paramount needs of the dying person to be respect for their wishes, control of discomfort, open communication with professional caregivers, and normal family relationships (Garland, Bass, & Otto, 1984).

People with chronic low self-esteem, depression, and feelings of powerlessness conceive of themselves as losers, and now they are facing life's final set of losses. A change in old self-defeating patterns is uncommon because of the energy and concentration required. Nevertheless, clients can be assisted to assume more personal power over their last days if the nurse will clarify and encourage each choice and praise each victory. If patients wish, they can be helped to cognitively rehearse a decision that they want to assert within the family or health care system. Our beliefs influence their beliefs about whether they are able to choose the final times in their lives.

Dying as a Family Process

All families face the same tasks. In even the most functional situations, the demands during this transitional time are tremendous. All must witness their loved one's physical and emotional suffering, grieve in their own way, manage everyday life, and learn to function without the loved one. Central family members must assume the caregiver role and gradually assume the responsibilities of the dying person. Caring for the dying person is balanced precariously with the needs of others; household economic survival and everyday tasks must continue. A history of open family communication, skill in problem solving, and ability to accept help from others and plan ahead enable the smoothest transitions. Stetz has described the caregiving demands experienced by spouses of dying cancer patients (Box 56–1).

As with the individual, generic interventions with the family foster strengths and family identity, provide information, and advocate the making of choices. The process of negotiating shared goals with several family members and the person who is dying is complex indeed. The nurse synthesizes client goals, individual family member goals, and the whole range of possible nursing goals to develop a working focus (Blues & Zerwekh, 1984). The goals of the family may occasionally take precedence over the goals of the client. For instance, promises to honor a person's wish to die at home may have to be altered if he or she becomes disoriented and incontinent. In this case, the needs of exhausted family caregivers may override earlier promises. The ultimate well-being of those who survive is a foremost family nursing concern.

Children in families in which a member is dying need special attention. Assessment should consider development stage and family roles. Until about 5 years of age, death is seen as reversible, and separation and abandonment are the central issues. While experiencing the sickness and death of a loved one, children must be understood in terms of what is normal for their age group. They need age-appropriate information, opportunities to express their feelings and thoughts, chances to be involved without inappropriate responsibility, chances to be playful and carefree at times, and knowledge of how their life in the family will continue. The school-aged child's predisposition to magical thinking and the adolescent's period of rebellion tend to foster a legacy of self-blame and guilt after the death (Blues & Zerwekh, 1984). Open, honest communication is the best prevention.

For some people, pets are important members of the family system, perhaps the most significant other in the person's life. Those with close attachments to

---

Box 56–1. CAREGIVING DEMANDS DURING ADVANCED CANCER: THE SPOUSE'S NEEDS

STUDY

Stetz, K. M. (1987). **Caregiving demands during advanced cancer: The spouse's needs.** *Cancer Nursing, 10,* 260–268.

PROBLEM

This study questioned the level of disability of those receiving home care, the caregiving demands reported by spouses, whether the demands varied with level of disability, and whether men and women report different demands.

DESIGN

The design was descriptive and cross-section. Sixty-five spouses of people with advanced cancer who were receiving care from a home health agency were interviewed at home using Stetz's Experience of Caregiving Interview. Transcriptions of their audiotaped responses to an open-ended question regarding situations that were difficult for them were content analyzed to define categories of caregiving demands. Physical disability was rated by the investigator using the Zubrod scale (a modification of the Karnofsky). Based on the caregiver's report and observation of the patient, a rating of 4 was given for complete disability and 0 for full activity.

SUMMARY AND INTERPRETATION

Forty-four of the caregivers were women; the median age was 69.5 years. Of the patients, 95.4 per cent had metastatic disease and progressive health deterioration; they were predominantly bedbound. Nine mutually exclusive caregiving demand categories were identified from the caregivers' reports and included the following: managing physical care, treatment, and imposed changes (69 per cent); managing household and finances (39 per cent); standing by (39 per cent); alterations in spouse's well-being and living patterns (22 per cent); constant vigilance (18 per cent); unmet health care system expectations (16 per cent); cancer itself (13 per cent); anticipating the future (9 per cent); and alterations in relationship with spouse (7 per cent). The frequent demands of standing by require nursing guidance to watch and cope with an uncontrollable situation rather than try to alter it. The infrequent reporting of demands of cancer itself, worry about the future, and alterations in spousal relationship are in contrast to common nursing assumptions; individualized assessment is essential.

Demands changed with level of disability. The three top caregiving demands stayed the same when Zubrod scores indicated severe disability of 3 and 4. When the disability was less and the Zubrod score was 2, the second most frequent demand was unmet expectations from the health care system and alteration in spouse's well-being. Demands also varied according to sex of caregiver. Men reported managing household and finances as their second most frequent demand, whereas women reported standing by as the second most frequent. Men need nursing assistance to develop different resources that were unfamiliar to their traditional role.

---

their beloved animals should be given every opportunity to have them present and placed comfortably on the bed, chair, or nearby floor. So close are some human-animal bonds that family members should understand that the pet will most likely grieve after the death.

A wide repertoire of nursing interventions is commonly needed to support family coping: these include active listening, resource identification, problem solving, advocacy, networking, coordination of health team and helpers, participation in family conferences, negotiation, values clarification, conflict resolution, referral, assistance with realistic limit setting, and grief counseling (Blues & Zerwekh, 1984). Therapeutic demands become more complex with dysfunctional family coping. Small realistic goals and structured expectations are vital. These therapeutic demands often come from needy families that bring out unhealthy rescuing impulses, tempting nurses to take on more and more of their burdens. Thus their feelings of helplessness and resentment are reinforced, and the nurse's own

resources are overwhelmed. They also may try to draw the nurse into their interpersonal conflicts and persuade the nurse to take sides against other family members or professional colleagues.

The strategy for nurses must be instead to assess the family system, set therapeutic boundaries, mediate conflicts, and help patients and family members to identify and build on their own strengths. Nurses are often preoccupied with pathology and dysfunction, but weaknesses are not a foundation for building; strengths are such a foundation. For instance, a young black family, newly "born again," believes the man of the family is healed, with his advanced bowel cancer slowly reabsorbing, despite a total bowel obstruction and a need for continuous total parenteral nutrition and morphine drips. He performs an amazingly normal parenting role, taking his 2-year-old son to the zoo and coaching his wife during childbirth. Is this family "ineffectively coping" with "dysfunctional grieving" or are its members hardy survivors struggling to normalize their lives within a belief system that gives them meaning and purpose?

Dying as a Spiritual Process

The spirit might be described as the central vitality in a person's soul. It is the nonphysical force that gives meaning and integrity to life and can be expressed in religious beliefs or anything that provides transcendent meaning. The spiritual comprises a person's relations to things larger than the self—causes, principles, art, history, higher forces, values, or the supernatural (Amenta & Bonnet, 1986).

As death draws near, the ordinary material preoccupations of everyday living and conventional medicine become irrelevant. Nurses who are busy with medical and nursing rituals should ask themselves about the relevance of their agendas. What do they matter? Facing the loss of self, loved ones, and known reality, the patient is struggling to find meaning and hope. What really matters for this person who will soon no longer be among the living? Take time to discover this person's story and struggles. The language of spiritual distress may include themes of estrangement from others and from God, blame of self and others, hatred of self and others, expression of anguish, wish for more faith and experience of God, or desire for specific religious practices.

The nurse's paramount responsibility is to listen, diagnose distress of the human spirit, and affirm the ultimate importance of spiritual concerns at the end of life. Although nurses should never impose their own beliefs on others, they may at times find that authentic dialogue requires a sincere sharing of their own personal meanings. Victor Frankl, the psychiatrist who survived the Nazi death camps, says that meaning can be found in recognizing the goodness of individual life accomplishments, experiencing ultimate truth or good, and turning a personal tragedy into a triumph (Amenta & Bonnet, 1986). If the nurse can remain present beside a dying person, that compassionate presence converts the experience into a triumph of love and human community. In the end, only ultimate realities are significant.

Where Death Will Occur

People should die where they choose, where they feel secure and comforted. For those with loving families whose members are capable of caregiving, that place will generally be at home. Home is familiar; life can be normalized; loved ones can actively participate; and closure of relationships is possible. However, dying at home becomes strenuous and stressful with an extended and unpredictable disease course, a physically and emotionally exhausted caregiver, a limited or absent personal support network, and nonsupportive health professionals. The absolute components of adequate home care include available health professionals who support home care and possess palliative care

expertise, available homemaking and personal care assistance, and loved ones who can respond to basic needs when the dying person can no longer manage alone (Zerwekh, 1989). Home hospice programs focus on the quality of life of the whole family. Psychosocial and spiritual dimensions of care are actively included. The terminal course of events is anticipated, and preparations are made for expert management of terminal symptoms. See Chapter 71 for a discussion of hospice philosophy and programs. Most people must still rely on conventional home health programs, with their narrow definitions of "homebound" and "skilled nursing." This nation needs a whole new community nursing infrastructure that recognizes the continuous needs for sustaining the chronically ill and those who are dying at home.

Alternatives to dying at home are narrower than in the past. Hospitalization under Medicare's Diagnosis-Related Groups does not permit admission for terminal care; brief stabilization of a medical problem such as pain, dehydration, or dyspnea is permitted, but then the person must be discharged. Nursing home placement is often the only option for dying, but nursing home costs must be paid out of pocket by the family or by Medicaid when the individual has become impoverished. In 1986, Medicare paid less than 2 per cent and private insurance less than 1 per cent of nursing home bills (Pear, 1987).

Decisions about the place of death should be discussed as early as possible. The public and health professionals need to understand the present constraints of hospital and home health services. A family needs to plan ahead by examining carefully all possible financial resources: individual and family assets, provisions and limitations of Medicare, and private insurance. Decisions should be determined by client and family wishes, known financial resources, and available community services. To maximize autonomy, every effort should be made for the person to live the last moments in a place of choice.

ASSESSMENT AND MANAGEMENT OF THE PERSON FACING IMMINENT DEATH

Assessment: Focusing on Comfort

When the desired outcome is comfort and death according to the patient's own preferences, the focus of nursing assessment is attention to the expression of subjective experience. Our clients are the only experts in what they are experiencing and desiring. Suffering cannot be confirmed by a blood level or scanned by the most sensitive machine. We know our pain with the greatest certainty, yet the pain of another is immediately in doubt (Scarry, 1985). Contemporary Americans desire privacy and liberty over community so that little is shared of emotional experience to appreciate another's suffering. Nurses are tempted to focus priorities on the "real" problems we want first to solve rather than the lived experience our client needs to share. Thoughtful assessment attends first to the client's expression of distress, validating it as a first priority for action. Occasionally a client's need for control will be stronger than the desire for comforting intervention. This wish is seldom expressed directly but can be discovered through repeated failure to adhere to palliative measures.

Assessment of persons who are dying systematically considers physical, psychosocial, and spiritual dimensions. However, a deliberate strategy should be pursued to collect only information that is useful for palliative purposes. The question should always be asked, How will having this information assist in providing comfort and meeting the client's expressed wishes? Hesitate before proceeding with exhaustive questions, invasive or hurtful procedures, or any assessment that may be needlessly intruding on the last remaining weeks of life. Is this blood draw, that rectal exam, the proposed bone scan really going to help comfort the person or fulfill a final wish? In general, new discomforts should be investigated to determine any cause that could be reversed. However, a thorough investigation should be bypassed when the burdens of diagnosis outweigh any palliative benefit, such as when death is imminent within days.

Anticipatory Guidance

An essential strategy is to prevent the recurrent physical and emotional crises that can be anticipated with progressive loss of function and likely complications of the disease course. In critical care units, equipment and drugs are on hand and consultants are on call for anticipated complications. Families of persons who are dying at home should be similarly ready to manage predictable problems. They should be able to say, "We were expecting this and we are prepared." Such anticipatory guidance is most likely to succeed when it matches a family style that copes by problem solving and planning ahead; it will be least successful with people who have lived their lives from crisis to crisis.

Managing Common Physical Responses to Dying

The nursing diagnostic categories that are anticipated during the final common pathophysiologic events should be reviewed when death approaches. This section addresses nursing care in situations of impaired mobility and progressive self-care deficits, impaired nutrition and fluid balance, alterations in elimination, deterioration in thought processes, alterations in comfort due to pain and ineffective gas exchange or airway clearance, and impending death.

Mobility and progressive self-care deficits are inevitable with a progressive downhill course, unless death occurs suddenly before this stage is reached. Client and family need to prepare for the day when the person is first chairbound and then bedbound. Goals focus on client choice. Does he or she wish to remain active and provide self-care as long as possible? Anticipation of increasing dependency is highly threatening, and acceptance of it is tantamount to accepting defeat, so intense grieving is to be expected. For instance, the home nurse's "practical" proposal to rent a hospital bed or plan for nursing home placement if there is no primary caregiver may be met with resistance. A variety of strong emotional reactions is normal.

Alterations in nutrition, fluid balance, and elimination are predictable. In the National Hospice study of 1119 patients (Wachtel, Allen-Masterson, Reuben, Goldberg, & Mor, 1988), the following symptoms were common in advanced cancer: anorexia (90 per cent), weight loss (84 per cent), constipation (52 per cent), and nausea or vomiting (44 per cent). Every effort should be made to provide adequate nutritional intake for the dying person who wishes to eat. However, food and fluid are essential when the anticipated outcome is living, but they are not essential for a comfortable dying. When a dying person can no longer eat or drink, the decision neither to force food or fluids orally nor to initiate tube or intravenous feeding is a torturous one for family and health care providers. Food and fluid are so closely linked with love and sustenance that well-meaning loved ones and professionals often *force* them on dying people against their wishes. This happens even though nutrition and fluid serve no purpose for people with advanced multisystem failure and may result in needless suffering. Tubes and infusions cause discomfort at the insertion site and divert energy from the person to the technology (Zerwekh, 1987b).

Hydrating a person with cardiopulmonary, renal, or hepatic failure can contribute to pulmonary edema and accumulating pharyngeal secretions, increase peripheral edema and ascites, increase the edema layer around tumors, result in vomiting of the increased gastric fluid volume when the intestine is blocked, and increase urine volume that requires catheterization because of patient weakness (Zerwekh, 1983a). The main complaint of dehydrated hospice patients who are near death is dry mouth, which can be relieved by good oral hygiene. The choice to use alimentation or intravenous hydration must be made individually with careful consideration of their usefulness or uselessness in restoring life or providing comfort or discomfort. When hardships outweigh benefits, who would ask a dying person to endure added useless suffering (Younger, 1987)? The nurse is mediator and fosters making conscious value judgments, clarifying positions, and making decisions within the family and the health care team.

In managing *nausea and vomiting* for the dying, comfort again and not better nutrition is the goal. Scheduled antiemetics used in combination are the most effective. In contrast to the parenteral route employed during chemotherapy, the person dying at home or in a nursing home is medicated using the rectal and oral routes, which require higher doses. Vomiting due to an inoperable malignant bowel obstruction is managed with stool softeners and metoclopramide to promote stomach emptying and small bowel peristalsis when obstruction is incomplete. Complete obstruction is managed with narcotics to slow the cramping of peristalsis and with antiemetics (Blues & Zerwekh, 1984). Dehydration reduces vomiting. A nasogastric tube is chosen only if the person prefers that to vomiting.

As mobility and intake of fiber and fluids diminish and narcotics slow peristalsis, *constipation* is prevented by regular concurrent administration of stool softener (docusate sodium) and bowel stimulants (senna or bisacodyl). Assessment and preventive bowel regimens are essential to avoid inflicting unnecessary discomfort. Stool will accumulate in the bowel despite minimum food intake. When constipation is present, bisacodyl suppositories or saline cathartics (milk of magnesia) may be helpful. To remove impacted stool, multiple oil retention enemas followed by soapsuds should be tried. Administer a narcotic and topical anesthetic before any manual disempaction.

Alterations in thought processes are inevitable with developing hypoxia, azotemia, hepatic encephalopathy, cerebral lesions, drug side effects, depression, and fever. Impairments range from diminishing attention and problem solving to disorientation and hallucinations to dropping level of consciousness before death. In the National Hospice Study, full mental capacity was reported intact in 50 per cent of patients within 4 to 6 weeks of death; complete incapacity was present in 12 per cent during the final 2 weeks (Wachtel et al., 1988). Loss of one's "mind" is a dreaded event for the dying. Management includes reversing any processes that can be reversed, readjustment of drug regimens, haldoperidol for acute disorientation, dexamethasone for cerebral edema, oxygen for hypoxia, and human presence to assure safety and orientation. Because level of orientation and consciousness fluctuate as death approaches, family and professionals should be prepared for periods of lucidity alternating with dysfunction.

Seizures are a very unusual but dreaded complication at the end of life. When the client is at home and the terminal course makes seizures likely, the family must be taught what to expect and how to manage. A number of drugs may be needed to be titrated to achieve control: anticonvulsants, barbiturates, and steroids to reduce intracranial pressure. The rectal route is effective in the administration of barbiturates (pentobarbital sodium suppositories) and phenytoin sodium. Suppositories should be considered instead of injections when the seizure-prone patient can no longer swallow.

Alterations in comfort are to be expected as death draws near. *Pain* is by no means inevitable in terminal cancer. Incidence of pain in the National Hospice Study was reported as 60 per cent (Wachtel et al., 1988). In terminal disease, the incidence of pain varies according to the primary and metastatic sites, with the highest incidence occurring when bone is involved.

Management of cancer pain is discussed at length in Chapter 51. Although a variety of therapeutic methods may be useful, the foundation of low technology terminal pain control is human presence and medication.

If the patient can swallow, long-acting morphine is recommended, 30 or 60 mg tablets (MS Contin or Roxanol SR are the drugs of choice) every 8 to 12 hr. When swallowing becomes a problem, concentrated liquid morphine (Roxanol solution, 20 mg/ml) or sublingual morphine tablets work well (Lattanzi-Licht, 1989). Sublingual or buccal morphine may be given regularly every 4 hr with doses equivalent to the parenteral rather than the oral route, because the morphine is directly absorbed into the blood stream. Breakthrough pain is well managed by immediate absorption through the oral mucosa rather than by resorting to injections (Enck, 1988). Rectal suppositories are another possibility and can be administered every 4 hr; dosage is equivalent to that for oral medication, and absorption through rectal blood vessels is reliable (Ellison & Lewis, 1984). Continuous *subcutaneous* morphine or hydromorphine infusions are an appropriate intermediate technology measure to maintain a constant level of narcotic in the blood stream without the costs and complications associated with the intravenous route (Coyle, Mauskop, Maggard, & Foley, 1986).

Higher technology routes for narcotic administration (intravenous, epidural, Ommaya reservoir) may be indicated when simpler routes are ineffective, but they do exact greater burdens (financial, medical and nursing management needed, potential for complications, and degree to which they preoccupy care). Whenever nurses can intervene in selecting pain control measures, the benefit and burdens should be brought out. Often a technology is chosen without deliberation because of current medical fascination with its use rather than its being most appropriate to achieve a particular person's comfort.

Alteration in comfort because of the dyspnea associated with impaired gas exchange or airway clearance is a highly distressing terminal problem (64 per cent of the National Center Study patients experienced dyspnea) (Wachtel et al., 1988). It is expertly managed by ensuring the presence of a caregiver, an upright position or a position of comfort, a supply of oxygen or other means of providing a sensation of circulating air, medication, and sometimes relaxation techniques. To control impending dyspneic attacks, morphine and tranquilizers are used. Morphine is administered sublingually or parenterally in doses titrated to aid in respiratory distress. It lowers awareness of muscle exertion, reduces anxiety, decreases ventilatory drive because of reduced demands on respiratory muscles, and reduces venous return and therefore pulmonary edema (Zerwekh, 1987a). Likewise, diphenhydramine and hydroxyzine, 25 to 100 mg intramuscularly, are effective in interrupting the vicious cycle of respiratory distress by reducing the associated anxiety. Family members at home should be taught how to administer the medications, which may be prepared in advance for emergency use. Pulmonary and pharyngeal secretions in the dehydrated patient may be reduced by the use of atropine, 0.4 to 1.0 mg administered sublingually, subcutaneously, and intramuscularly. Suctioning rarely is comforting at the end of life, but it is sometimes necessary because of the presence of an artificial airway. Meditation, relaxation, and visualization also have been used to slow the breath.

Impending Death

Death is impending as fluid intake becomes minimal, urine output is scant or absent, level of consciousness drops, blood pressures slides, peripheral cyanosis deepens, apneic periods lengthen, and pulmonary and pharyngeal secretions rattle (Blues & Zerwekh, 1984, pp. 178–186). Just as a midwife assists during the labor before birth, the nurse assists in the labor before death by explaining and normalizing each occurrence, offering comfort measures, and enhancing the humanity of the participants. The progress of events is explained as natural and predictable: "Her breath is slowing now. This is what we've been expecting. She can't speak to us anymore. That is the part of the natural anesthesia that always happens." Although the dying person is usually no longer able to participate, the nurse constantly reminds those gathered that everything spoken may be heard by the dying person. The timing of death remains uncertain, which is exhausting for family and those who would like to be present at the time of death. Nurses can try to help loved ones recognize that it is the lifelong relationship rather than the presence at the actual moment of death that is important. Guilt can be overwhelming when death occurs while a family member is out for a cup of coffee! Midwives say that we give birth most easily by relaxing and letting go, and so it is with death. If any of life's unfinished business can be resolved by loved ones saying what remains unsaid, asking for or offering forgiveness and love, such expressions should be fostered. Resolution of specific business matters or spiritual reconciliation may be needed.

Through words and guidance, the nurse is able to express a reverence for the awesome moment that is in process, that mysterious final passage. The mystical dimension of all the world's great religions emphasizes fostering a special consciousness at the end of life. For those with a specific religious identity, special prayers, meditations, reading of scriptures, and gathering of believers may be necessary at the bedside. Medical and nursing rituals are no longer of any import.

When death occurs at home (Zerwekh, 1989), the nurse helps family members prepare for what is ahead by knowing how to diagnose death and whom to call. Physician, coroner, funeral home, and sometimes police will have to be notified. Different regulations prevail in different areas, and the only way to prevent crises is to *negotiate in advance* with the different organizations involved. A respected funeral director in the community can be a vital partner in this understanding. The family must particularly understand the implications of calling the emergency telephone number 911, which will activate resuscitation procedures. Sometimes people take such action because of fear or ambivalent goals, but ways should be sought to circumvent the resulting purposeless technologic disaster. At home and in the nursing home and hospital, *do not resuscitate* orders must be clarified and well documented.

Following Death

After death has occurred, the family should be encouraged to do what feels comfortable and appropriate to their beliefs. Some people will choose to touch and speak to their loved one. Through touching and perhaps bathing the body, the nurse present at the time of death can model this as a normal way of working through the finality of death and saying goodby. Verbal and nonverbal expression will range from silence and withdrawal to wailing and rending of garments. The nurse advocates for the family to stay with the body as long as they wish and intervenes to prevent the rapid removal to morgue or mortuary. In anticipation of death, it is extremely valuable to help the family prepare a checklist of whom to call and what arrangements to make immediately after the death.

Bereavement places survivors at significantly higher risk of physical and emotional dysfunction. Recognizing this, bereavement services have been an essential component of hospice care. The Medicare hospice benefit requires that bereavement care be provided, but it does not reimburse for these services. Commonly, follow-up includes telephone calls, visits, or both by the nurse or separate bereavement time. Lattanzi-Licht's study of 268 bereavement programs (1989) noted a remarkable lack of definition of service components and lack of time and personnel. There is a demonstrated need for setting of clear goals and systematic assessment of high-risk family members to define priorities for care (Lattanzi-Licht, 1989). The nurse who works with many people who are dying brings a holistic understanding of the family to the assessment of those who may be at risk for dysfunctional grieving. Nurses who see only a few dying people or are especially involved with a family may choose to make bereavement contacts at the funeral or the family home. However, nurses are advised to continually question whether these contacts are healing for themselves and for family members. As the number of deceased patients reaches into the hundreds or thousands, most nurses choose to direct their attention to those living with cancer and to refer high-risk survivors to bereavement services.

LOOKING INTO THE FACE OF DEATH: THE COMPASSIONATE CAREGIVER

A nurse's patients keep dying; how can the nurse continue to care about them? Each person must find a balance. Awareness of self is the fulcrum. This can be a lifelong pursuit of self-discovery and a growing clarity about personal needs and agendas. Perhaps the nurse's choice of this work is not accidental; it may have a purpose that may be discovered as life unfolds. One challenge is not to impose one's own needs on patients

---

Box 56-2. PREPARING NURSES FOR CARE OF THE DYING

STUDY

Degner, L. F., & Gow, C. M. (1988). **Preparing nurses for care of the dying: A longitudinal study.** *Cancer Nursing, 11,* 160–169.

PROBLEM

This study addressed the question of whether a required clinical and classroom course on care of the dying could be demonstrated to be more effective preparation than a curriculum lacking a systematic death and dying coursework and practicum.

DESIGN

The longitudinal quasiexperiment studied an experimental group of junior baccalaureate nursing students who took a required eight-credit palliative nursing course, a control group of nursing students at another university that nonsystematically integrated death education, and a control group of nonnursing students. The dependent variables were death anxiety, measured by the Collett-Lester scale, and attitudes toward care of the dying, measured by the Winget scale. Subjects were queried at pretest before their junior year to obtain background information, death experience, and Collett-Lester and Winget scores. Two posttests were completed, one at the end of the junior year (a total sample of 306) and another 1 yr after graduation (a total sample of 170). The first posttest included completion of the two scales; the second posttest included completion of the two scales and participation in a semistructured interview that elicit nurses' experiences with care of the dying and recommendations regarding educational preparation to provide that care.

SUMMARY AND INTERPRETATION

Unfortunately, the three groups were not comparable at pretest. The experimental group began with a significantly higher level of death anxiety, which was then reduced close to the nursing control group level at both posttests. Statistical analysis did demonstrate this reduction to be an effect of the educational program. The experimental group was older and more experienced with death, which was attributed to the enrollment of registered nurses among them. Likewise, the experimental group began with and maintained better attitudes toward the dying. Both groups had parallel improved attitudes, which were attributed to maturation, at the time of the first posttest. At the second posttest, neither variable was demonstrated to have been affected by the palliative nursing class. One year after graduation, the experimental group reported more approach behavior in caring for those who were dying and a feeling of competence to provide care and more openness to discussion of death and dying issues. The investigators are currently developing a behavioral measure of these caregiving variables. When interviewed, the new graduates believed that nursing education should include coursework to help them examine their own feelings and those of patient and family. They strongly recommended supervised student practice to care for a dying person in both hospital and home. If death education is required in schools of education, it is proposed that this will increase graduate nurse approach behavior in care of the dying.

---

in ways that diminish their well-being. For instance, in situations of great suffering in which nurses face a bottomless pit of needs, they should beware of initiating *rescuing* responses that place them in the position of beneficent givers and the clients in the position of helpless victims (Steiner, 1974). Empowering others assumes that they have the potential to assume responsibility and build on their strengths. In the end, they see themselves as strong rather than seeing nurses as the source of the strength that brought them through (Zerwekh, 1983b).

"Give from your own excess, not from your essence" (Blues & Zerwekh, 1984). Consider ways to bring joy into life so that ways can be found to face death and despair. Association with good people and exposure to beauty are important and life-affirming.

Perhaps some of the following self-care plans may

be relevant and helpful to the oncology nurse. Explore spiritual teachings and practice. Find meaning in great literature, art, music, nature, and the everyday experience of love. Reexamine the ways in which denial, distancing, and materialism may hinder an authentic existence. Beware of overextension. Set limits on commitments, keep life uncluttered with things and activities, and establish boundaries between personal and public life, as needed (Blues & Zerwekh, 1984). And finally, consider the seasons of life: periods of plunging in to comfort the comfortless and make just the inequities and periods of personal renewal and reintegration. When energy and enthusiasm lessen, practice self-anticipatory guidance by developing a self-care plan before burnout.

Degner and Gow have studied the effectiveness of an undergraduate palliative nursing course to prepare graduates to work with dying people and their families (Box 56–2). The chapters in Unit XI discuss professional support for the oncology nurse.

References

Amenta, M. O., & Bonnet, N. L. (1986). *Nursing care of the terminally ill.* Boston: Little, Brown & Co.

Baines, M., & Ford, G. (1984). Practical care of the terminally ill patients. *Midlands Medicine, 17,* 17–21.

Blues, A., & Zerwekh, J. (1984). *Hospice and palliative nursing care.* Orlando, FL: Grune & Stratton, Inc.

Coyle, N., Mauskop, A., Maggard, J., & Foley, L. (1986). Continuous subcutaneous infusions of opiates in cancer patients with pain. *Oncology Nursing Forum, 13*(4), 53–57.

Ellison, N. M., & Lewis, G. O. (1984). Plasma concentrations following single doses of morphine sulfate in oral solution and rectal suppository. *Clinical Pharmacy, 3,* 614–617.

Enck, R. E. (1988). Mucosal membranes as alternative routes for morphine sulfate administration. *American Journal of Hospice Care, 5*(6), 17–18.

Garland, T. N., Bass, D. M., & Otto, M. E. (1984). The needs of hospice patients and primary caregivers. *American Journal of Hospice Care, 1*(3), 40–45.

Houldin, A. D., Saltstein, S. W., & Ganles, K. M. (1987). *Nursing diagnosis for wellness.* Philadelphia: J. B. Lippincott Co.

Inagaki, J., Rodriguez, M. D., & Bodey, M. D. (1974). Causes of death in cancer patients. *Cancer, 33,* 568–573.

Lattanzi-Licht, M. E. (1989). Bereavement studies: Practice and problems. *The Hospice Journal, 5,* 1–28.

Pear, R. (1987, September 13). Crisis is predicted in care of elderly. *New York Times,* p. 1.

Pitorak, E. F., & Drauss, J. C. (1987). Pain control with sublingual morphine. *American Journal of Hospice Care, 4*(2), 39–41.

Ramsey, P. (1970). *The patient as person: Explorations in medical ethics.* New Haven, CT: Yale University Press.

Scarry, E. (1985). *The body in pain: The making and unmaking of the world.* New York: Oxford University Press.

Steiner, C. (1974). *Scripts people live: Transactional analysis of life scripts.* New York: Bantam Books.

Strauss, A. (1975). *Chronic illness and quality of life.* St. Louis: C. V. Mosby Co.

Torrens, P. R. (Ed.) (1985). *Hospice programs and public policy.* Chicago: American Hospital Association.

Twycross, R. (1983). *Symptom control in far advanced cancer: Pain relief.* London: Pitman Publishing.

Wachtel, T., Allen-Masterson, S., Reuben, D., Goldberg, R., & Mor, V. (1988). The end stage cancer patient: Terminal common pathway. *The Hospice Journal, 4*(4), 43–80.

Younger, S. J. (1987). Do not resuscitate orders: No longer secret but still a problem. *Hastings Center Report, 17,* 24–33.

Zerwekh, J. V. (1983a). The dehydration question. *Nursing 83, 13,* 46–51.

Zerwekh, J. V. (1983b). Empowering the no longer patient. *Washington State Journal of Nursing, 54*(2), 12–17.

Zerwekh, J. V. (1987a). Comforting the dying, dyspneic patient. *Nursing 87, 17,* 66–69.

Zerwekh, J. V. (1987b). Should fluid and nutritional support be withheld from terminally ill patients? *American Journal of Hospice Care, 4*(4), 37–38.

Zerwekh, J. V. (1989). Home care of the dying. In I. Martison & A. Widmer (Eds.), *Home health care nursing* (pp. 217–236). Philadelphia: W. B. Saunders Co.

CHAPTER 57

Oncologic Emergencies

CHRISTINE MIASKOWSKI

OBSTRUCTIVE EMERGENCIES
Superior Vena Cava Syndrome
Intestinal Obstruction
Third Space Syndrome
METABOLIC EMERGENCIES
Syndrome of Inappropriate Antidiuretic
   Hormone Secretion
Hypercalcemia

Septic Shock
Disseminated Intravascular Coagulation
INFILTRATIVE EMERGENCIES
Neoplastic Cardiac Tamponade
Spinal Cord Compression
Carotid Artery Rupture
SUMMARY

Recent advances in the treatment of malignant disease have resulted in many patients' being cured of their initial disease. When the disease recurs, however, it can be associated with or manifest itself as a life-threatening emergency. In other cases, the malignancy may appear initially as a medical emergency. In either case, the occurrence of oncologic emergencies is becoming more frequent in clinical practice. Careful assessment of the oncology patient is essential to diagnose emergency conditions early and initiate treatment promptly. This prompt recognition and immediate treatment can halt the progression of the oncologic emergency and often reverse potentially disabling side effects.

This chapter on oncologic emergencies is divided into three sections. The first section reviews the obstructive emergencies: superior vena cava (SVC) syndrome, intestinal obstruction, and third space syndrome. The second portion of the chapter deals with the major metabolic emergencies: the syndrome of inappropriate antidiuretic hormone (SIADH) secretion, hypercalcemia, septic shock, and disseminated intravascular coagulation (DIC). The final section concentrates on the infiltrative emergencies and covers neoplastic cardiac tamponade, spinal cord compression, and carotid artery rupture. For each oncologic emergency, the anatomy and physiology of the syndrome are reviewed briefly; the pathophysiologic mechanism is explained; the assessment and management of the oncologic emergency are discussed; and a list of actual and potential nursing diagnoses the patient may experience is presented.

OBSTRUCTIVE EMERGENCIES

Cancer can obstruct major organs, blood vessels, and lymphatic channels. When obstruction occurs, a backup occurs in the flow of blood or body fluids through the channel that is involved. The major obstructive emergencies associated with malignant disease are SVC syndrome, intestinal obstruction, and third space syndrome.

Superior Vena Cava Syndrome

The superior vena cava is a thin-walled, low-pressure blood vessel that lies within the confined, rigid space of the mediastinal cavity. This blood vessel collects blood from the venous vessels that drain the head and neck and the upper thoracic cavity. Because the mediastinum is a rigid anatomic structure that includes the trachea, the vertebral column, the sternum and ribs, and the lymph nodes, there is little room to expand and accommodate the growth of neoplastic tissue. The growth of a tumor within the mediastinal cavity results in compression of the superior vena cava as well as other blood vessels and organs.

Four mechanisms underlie the development of SVC syndrome. The superior vena cava can be occluded by an extrinsic mass. Occlusion of the superior vena cava can occur as a result of tumor invasion into the vessel wall. A third mechanism can involve the obstruction of the vessel lumen by a neoplastic thrombus. The final mechanism may involve the occlusion of the vessel by thrombus formation on an intravascular catheter.

Eighty to 90 per cent of the cases of SVC syndrome occur from malignant disease. The most common cancers that can cause this syndrome are bronchogenic carcinoma and lymphomas. This oncologic emergency can be observed with metastatic disease from the esophagus, colon, testes, and breast.

The primary signs and symptoms result from the obstruction of blood flow in the venous system of the head, neck, and upper trunk. The severity of symptoms depends on the rapidity, degree, and location of the obstruction and whether collateral circulation has developed. Initial symptoms occur in the early morning hours and include periorbital and conjunctival edema, facial swelling, and tightness of the shirt collar (Stoke's sign). These symptoms disappear within a few hours when the patient assumes an upright position and drainage from the face can occur.

As the obstruction worsens, the nurse should assess the patient for the following signs and symptoms: fullness of the arms; swelling of the fingers and hands; difficulty removing rings; erythema of the face, neck, and upper trunk; and epistaxis. Late symptoms of this syndrome include distention of the veins of the thorax and upper extremities, dysphagia, cough, dyspnea, tachypnea, hoarseness, cyanosis, and intracranial hypertension. In the acute, emergency situation, obstruction of the superior vena cava leads to a decrease in venous return with a marked reduction in cardiac output and a decrease in cerebral perfusion. Patients present with respiratory difficulty, hypotension, and mental status changes.

The primary form of treatment for SVC syndrome is radiation therapy. For bronchogenic carcinoma the usual dose is 4000 to 6000 rads over a 5- to 7-week period; for malignant lymphoma the dose is approximately 2000 to 4000 rads. Radiation therapy may be initiated before a tissue diagnosis is confirmed to relieve the acute symptoms. Chemotherapy may be administered concurrently with the radiation therapy. The usual agents used are cyclophosphamide (Cytoxan), methotrexate, and nitrogen mustard (Chernecky & Ramsey, 1984).

Supportive care during treatment is of primary importance. Maintenance of a patent airway or relief of airway obstruction is a major objective. Oxygen therapy may be required if the patient is hypoxic. Diuretics may be used to relieve the swelling, but they must be used with extreme caution because they can further compromise venous return to the heart. Steroids may be administered to improve the patient's condition by decreasing the amount of inflammation. In some cases, heparin may be used to minimize or prevent further thrombus formation.

The major potential and actual nursing diagnoses for SVC syndrome as well as the associated nursing interventions are listed in Table 57–1. Special emphasis must be placed on supporting the patient through an extremely frightening situation.

Intestinal Obstruction

An intestinal obstruction can involve either the large or the small intestine. The clinical picture as well as therapeutic interventions depends on the nature of the tumor and the site and degree of obstruction. An intestinal obstruction means that the bowel content cannot pass normally to the rectum. Any type of obstruction will interfere with normal peristaltic activity. Normal peristalsis is brought about by the electrical conduction of contractile stimuli from one bowel segment to the next. Within the normal bowel, there is a gradient of rhythmic, intrinsic activity that decreases from the mouth to the anus. An obstruction to the

Table 57–1. ACTUAL AND POTENTIAL NURSING DIAGNOSES FOR THE OBSTRUCTIVE EMERGENCIES

Superior Vena Cava Syndrome
Decreased cardiac output
  Monitor vital signs
  Assess for pulsus paradoxus
  Monitor intake and output
  Measure central venous pressure or other hemodynamic parameters
  Maintain bed rest
Ineffective breathing pattern
  Assess respiratory status
  Monitor arterial blood gases
  Administer oxygen as necessary
  Provide respiratory support (e.g., intubation, tracheostomy) as needed
Decreased cerebral perfusion
  Assess mental status
  Teach patient ways to decrease intracranial pressure
  Promote venous drainage from the head
Severe anxiety
  Explain all procedures
  Medicate for pain as necessary
  Utilize relaxation techniques
  Place patient close to nurse's station
  Schedule frequent visits
Alteration in skin integrity
  Perform skin assessment
  Avoid tight or abrasive clothing
  Elevate extremities to promote venous return
Intestinal Obstruction
Fluid volume deficit
  Assess hydration status
  Monitor intake and output
  Administer intravenous hydration
Alteration in comfort
  Maintain patency of intestinal tube
  Medicate for pain as needed
Alteration in nutrition, less than body requirements
  Assess for protein-caloric malnutrition
  Consider intravenous alimentation
Third Space Syndrome
Loss phase
  Potential for fluid volume deficit
    Monitor intake and output to determine when the patient begins to increase urine output
    Assess renal function (blood urea nitrogen, creatinine)
    Monitor vital signs
    Monitor for signs and symptoms of hypovolemia
    Administer intravenous fluids and plasma proteins
Reabsorption phase
  Fluid volume excess
    Monitor intravenous hydration
    Monitor for signs and symptoms of hypervolemia
    Weigh patient daily

flow of gastric contents can lead to life-threatening pathophysiologic changes (Fig. 57–1).

The etiology of small bowel obstruction is primarily nonmalignant. Ninety per cent of all small bowel obstructions result from adhesions following abdominal surgery. Only 10 to 20 per cent of all small bowel obstructions are the result of malignant disease. Primary tumors of the small intestine account for only 1 to 3 per cent of the small bowel obstructions. Histologically, these tumors can be carcinoid, adenocarcinomas, sarcomas, lymphomas, or melanomas. The remaining small bowel obstructions that occur as a result of malignant disease arise from metastatic tumors of the colon-rectum, ovary, or cervix. The majority of large bowel obstructions (90 per cent) occur as a result

Intestinal Obstruction

↓

Interruption of Normal Peristalsis

↓

Intestinal Stasis

↓ accumulation of intestinal juices, gases, and bacterial growth

Compensatory Increase in Peristaltic Activity

↓

Increased Venous Pressure, Edema of the Bowel, Anoxia of the Bowel Wall

↓

Peritonitis

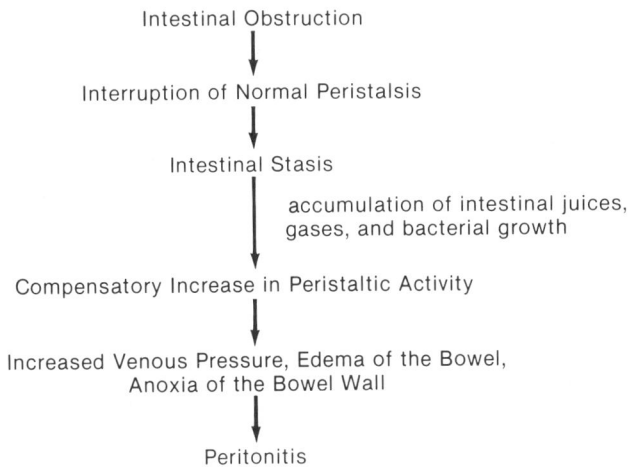

Figure 57–1. Consequences of an obstruction to the flow of gastric contents.

of malignant disease. The primary cancers that produce large bowel obstructions are adenocarcinomas. In addition, metastatic disease arising from ovarian or cervical tumors or from lymphomas can obstruct the large intestine.

The signs and symptoms of small and large bowel obstruction are listed in Table 57–2. A thorough abdominal assessment must be performed and should include a history of pain, vomiting, and frequency of bowel movements and an abdominal examination to evaluate for distention, palpable masses, and the quality and duration of bowel sounds.

The primary goals of medical therapy are to relieve the distention, correct the fluid imbalance, and, if possible, remove the obstruction. Patients will be treated initially with a nasogastric or long intestinal tube in an effort to achieve decompression. Vigorous hydration will be instituted that includes the replacement of electrolytes. If the lesion is resectable, surgery will be performed. The type of surgery performed (i.e., a resection and end-to-end anastamosis or a resection and colostomy) depends on the location and degree of the obstruction.

The major potential and actual nursing diagnoses for intestinal obstruction as well as the associated

Table 57–2. ASSESSMENT PARAMETERS FOR SMALL AND LARGE BOWEL OBSTRUCTION

Small Bowel Obstruction	Large Bowel Obstruction
Colicky pain, early in the obstruction	Crampy, lower abdominal pain
As obstruction progresses, pain becomes mild, nonlocalized, and a steady discomfort	
Obstipation	Alternating diarrhea and constipation
Distention	Marked distention
Vomiting begins early	Vomiting occurs late
Fever	
Leukocytosis	
Signs of hypovolemia	
Bowel sounds for both small and large bowel obstruction: Proximal to the obstruction they are high-pitched and hyperactive Distal to the obstruction they are diminished or absent	

nursing interventions are listed in Table 57–1. Special emphasis must be placed on assessing the patient for signs and symptoms of strangulation or perforation, which can occur acutely. If the character of the patient's pain changes and becomes more intense and continuous and abdominal girth decreases, strangulation should be suspected. If the patient develops rebound tenderness and bowel sounds stop abruptly, bowel rupture and associated peritonitis may have occurred. The physician should be notified immediately if either of these conditions is evident.

Third Space Syndrome

Third space syndrome is the shift in fluid from the vascular to the interstitial space owing to lowered plasma proteins; increased capillary permeability; or lymphatic blockage secondary to trauma, inflammation, or disease. Normally, body fluids are contained within three compartments: the vascular space, the intracellular space, and the interstitial space or third space. Fluid and particulate matter including plasma proteins are exchanged at the level of the capillary membrane. Fluid equilibrium is maintained at the level of the capillary membrane by a series of opposing pressures. Changes in pressures at the capillary membrane, increased capillary permeability, lowered plasma proteins, or changes in the integrity of the lymphatic system are the most common etiologic factors that produce a sequestering of fluid into the third space or interstitial space (Twombly, 1978).

Generalized third space syndrome is most commonly seen in oncology patients who have undergone major surgical procedures (e.g., abdominoperineal resection, pelvic exenteration) or who are in septic shock. Third space syndrome is divided into two phases: the loss phase and the reabsorption phase. The nursing assessment and management of the patient is dependent on the phase of the syndrome.

The loss phase typically occurs immediately after surgery and is usually self-limited to 48 to 72 hr. The phase is characterized by a shift in fluid from the vascular space to the interstitial space. Patients present with signs and symptoms of hypovolemia. The patient must be monitored for hypotension, tachycardia, low central venous pressure, decreased urine output, and an increased urine specific gravity. During the loss phase, the patient's fluid intake exceeds total output by a ratio of 3:1. Active treatment, during this phase of the syndrome, involves the replacement of fluid and electrolytes as well as plasma proteins. The infusion of plasma proteins will increase the plasma colloid oncotic pressure and "pull" fluids from the interstitial into the vascular space. Diuretics may be prescribed to remove the excess fluid that is being reabsorbed.

As the patient begins to recover and the inflammation begins to subside, the patient enters the reabsorption phase. The injured tissue heals, the damaged capillaries begin to repair, and normal permeability returns. In addition, the degree of lymphatic blockage decreases as collateral lymphatics develop. After surgery, plasma proteins begin to return to normal levels. The end result is that capillary pressures return to normal and the fluid within the interstitial space begins to be reabsorbed. The reabsorption phase is characterized by a shift in fluid from the interstitial space into the vascular space. The hallmark sign that the patient is entering the reabsorption phase is a marked increase in urine output (i.e., greater than 200 ml/hr). The major problem that can occur is hypervolemia. The patient should be monitored for hypertension, tachycardia, elevation in central venous pressure, weight gain, rales, dyspnea, and jugular venous distention. The primary treatment is to reduce the amount of intravenous hydration and monitor the patient's fluid balance.

The major potential and actual nursing diagnoses for the two phases of third space syndrome as well as the associated nursing interventions are listed in Table 57–1. The patient must be closely monitored for signs and symptoms of hypovolemia and hypervolemic shock.

METABOLIC EMERGENCIES

Malignant disease can cause metabolic abnormalities by producing ectopic hormones that affect specific target tissues and initiate an associated list of signs and symptoms, or it can produce major derangements in all metabolic pathways. The major metabolic emergencies associated with malignant disease include the SIADH secretion, hypercalcemia, septic shock, and DIC.

Syndrome of Inappropriate Antidiuretic Hormone Secretion

Normally, antidiuretic hormone (ADH) is released from the posterior pituitary gland when the plasma osmolality increases or the plasma volume decreases. The hormone acts on the collecting ducts of the kidney, causing a reabsorption of water and a concentrated and decreased urine volume. Antidiuretic hormone is normally released by pain, stress, trauma, hemorrhage, and certain drugs (Yasko, 1983).

The SIADH secretion is a syndrome of hypotonicity of plasma and hyponatremia that results from the aberrant production or sustained secretion of ADH (vasopressin). Inappropriate secretion is defined as secretion that continues in the face of hypotonicity of plasma. Cancer is the most frequent cause of the SIADH secretion. The type of cancer most frequently associated with the syndrome is carcinoma of the lung. Other types can include cancer of the pancreas, duodenum, brain, esophagus, colon, ovary, prostate, bronchus, and nasopharynx, and acute and chronic leukemia, mesothelioma, reticulum-cell sarcoma, Hodgkin's disease, thymoma, and lymphosarcoma. It has been shown that these cancers have the ability to synthesize, store, and release ADH. In addition, certain cancer chemotherapeutic agents can produce this syndrome.

Vincristine and cyclophosphamide have been shown to stimulate the release of excess amounts of ADH (Chernecky & Ramsey, 1984).

The signs and symptoms of the SIADH secretion are listed in Table 57–3. The signs and symptoms are reflective of water intoxication. This syndrome induces profound neurologic symptoms and should not be mistaken for a psychosis. Once the syndrome has been diagnosed, the treatment depends on the severity of the patient's symptoms. Initial treatment may simply involve water restriction. In severely symptomatic patients, 3 per cent sodium chloride solution will be administered.

The major potential and actual nursing diagnoses for the SIADH secretion as well as the associated nursing interventions are listed in Table 57–4.

Hypercalcemia

Calcium is the fifth most abundant cation in the body. Ninety-nine per cent of the body's calcium is in an insoluble form in the skeleton. The remaining 1 per cent is freely exchangeable calcium. Ionized calcium is the calcium of physiologic importance and is maintained within a very precise range. The two hormones that regulate serum calcium levels are parathyroid hormone and calcitonin. The release of parathyroid hormone results in an increase in serum calcium levels. Calcitonin release produces a decrease in serum calcium levels.

Several mechanisms are postulated to produce hypercalcemia in patients with cancer. Hypercalcemia can occur in the presence of bony metastasis. It is believed that the cancer produces a diffusible substance that causes bone resorption of calcium. The tumors most frequently associated with hypercalcemia and bony metastasis are located in the breast, bronchus, kidney, thyroid, ovaries, and colon. The second explanation for hypercalcemia is that certain tumors are suspected of producing excess amounts of parathyroid hormone. The tumors implicated in excess parathyroid hormone secretion are those associated with hyperne-

Table 57–3. ASSESSMENT PARAMETERS FOR SIADH SECRETION

Physical Assessment
Absence of edema
Serum sodium of less than 110 mEq/L
   Personality changes
   Weight gain
   Weakness
   Anorexia, nausea, and vomiting
   Lethargy
   Seizures
   Coma
Laboratory Assessment
Hyponatremia
Serum osmolality of less than 280 mOsm/kg
Decreased blood urea nitrogen and creatinine
Increased urinary excretion of sodium (>20 mEq/L)
Increased urine osmolality
Hypokalemia
Hypocalcemia

Table 57–4. ACTUAL AND POTENTIAL NURSING DIAGNOSES FOR METABOLIC EMERGENCIES

SIADH Secretion
Fluid volume excess
  Monitor laboratory data
  Perform neurologic assessment
  Restrict fluids as prescribed
  Administer 3% sodium chloride as prescribed
Hypercalcemia
Fluid volume deficit
  Administer intravenous hydration
  Monitor intake and output
  Assess hydration status
  Check urine specific gravity
Potential for decreased cardiac output
  Monitor vital signs
  Assess for electrocardiogram changes associated with
    hypercalcemia
Potential for injury and decreased activity tolerance
  Institute safety measures
  Perform neurologic assessment
  Encourage mobility to prevent bone resorption of calcium
Septic Shock
Fluid volume deficit
  Administer intravenous hydration
  Monitor intake and output
  Assess hydration status
  Check urine specific gravity
Potential for decreased cardiac output
  Monitor vital signs and hemodynamic parameters
  Titrate vasopressor therapy as prescribed
Potential for alteration in renal tissue perfusion
  Monitor intake and output
  Monitor renal function (blood urea nitrogen, creatinine)
Potential for alteration in cerebral tissue perfusion
  Perform neurologic assessment
  Administer oxygen as prescribed
Disseminated Intravascular Coagulation
Alteration in tissue perfusion
  Assess patient for evidence of clotting
  Administer oxygen as prescribed
  Administer adequate hydration for renal perfusion
Potential for injury
  Assess patient for evidence of bleeding
  Initiate bleeding or thrombocytopenia precautions
  Control active bleeding
  Administer platelets and transfusions as prescribed
Alteration in comfort
  Assess patient's degree of discomfort
  Administer analgesics as needed

phromas; squamous cell carcinoma of the lung; squamous cell carcinoma of the head and neck, cervix, penis, and esophagus; lymphomas; and leukemia. It should be noted that two other phenomena can contribute to and worsen hypercalcemia. These are immobility and dehydration (Lind, 1985).

The signs and symptoms of hypercalcemia reflect the importance of calcium in the physiologic functioning of all of the body's major organ systems. The severity of symptoms often correlates with the serum calcium level. Neuromuscular symptoms can include apathy, depression, malaise, fatigue, and profound muscle weakness. Cardiovascular effects are manifested on the electrocardiogram as shortening of the Q-T interval and prolongation of the P-R interval. The kidney attempts to remove excess levels of calcium, and symptoms of polyuria and nocturia are present. The gastrointestinal system is also affected. The patient can present with anorexia, nausea and vomiting, and abdominal pain. The gastrointestinal symptoms can progress to ileus and obstipation.

Treatment of hypercalcemia is focused on enhancing renal excretion of calcium and decreasing bone resorption of calcium. Increased renal excretion of calcium is accomplished through the use of intravenous hydration with normal saline and the administration of calciuretic diuretics. The rate of intravenous hydration and the dose of furosemide or ethacrynic acid prescribed is based on the serum level of calcium and the severity of the symptoms exhibited by the patient. To decrease bone resorption of calcium, drug therapy is initiated.

Mithramycin, a chemotherapeutic antibiotic, is often used. Effects of the drug are seen within 24 to 48 hr, and the effects may last up to 7 days. The major toxicities associated with mithramycin therapy are thrombocytopenia, hepatocellular necrosis, and hemorrhage. The second drug used in the management of hypercalcemia is calcitonin. This drug also inhibits bone resorption of calcium. The major side effect associated with calcitonin is nausea and vomiting. A third drug that is used with extreme caution in managing hypercalcemia is intravenous phosphate. The primary mechanism of action of this drug is to precipitate calcium into the bone. The danger, however, is that extraskeletal calcifications can occur in the heart and kidney and produce serious and sometimes fatal consequences (Lind, 1985).

The major potential and actual nursing diagnoses for hypercalcemia as well as the associated nursing interventions are listed in Table 57–4.

Septic Shock

Septic shock is the major form of distributive shock caused by a massive overwhelming infection throughout the entire body. It is the major cause of death in patients with cancer, particularly patients with leukemia and lymphoma. Shock is basically a disease of the cell. Normal cellular metabolic processes are disrupted in the shock state. This disruption results in deleterious consequences in every major organ system. The overall mechanism underlying septic shock is the death of bacteria. The death of the organism results in the release of endotoxins, which produce numerous effects.

Septic shock is divided into two phases. The first phase is referred to as *warm shock*. The release of endotoxins results in the secretion of various vasoactive substances. These vasoactive substances produce dilation of the venous and arterial systems. The release of endotoxin and the subsequent dilation of the arteries and veins result in a series of signs and symptoms including mental confusion, chills and fever, flushed and warm skin, tachycardia, tachypnea, and decreased PO_2. If the disease is not treated, the patient will progress into the second phase of the shock state, called *cold shock*. At this point, more endotoxin is released, which stimulates the release of histamine and bradykinin. These two substances are potent vasodilators that produce a series of reactions, including an increase in capillary permeability; a decrease in circulating blood volume, which results in a decrease in cardiac ouput; and a decrease in tissue perfusion. The patient in cold shock will exhibit the following signs and symptoms: cold skin, peripheral edema, tachycardia, hypotension, tachypnea, pulmonary congestion, hypoxemia, oliguria, and metabolic acidosis (Lamb, 1982).

The treatment of septic shock is summarized by the acronym VIP. *V* = Ventilate. Patients in septic shock require oxygen. If the patient's respiratory status is compromised, mechanical ventilation may be required. *I* = Infuse. The patient in septic shock is usually hypotensive. Crystalloid solutions as well as colloid solutions must be infused to maintain an adequate blood pressure. *P* = Perfusion. Cardiac output needs to be maintained, usually with pressor therapy. Dopamine is the vasopressor drug that is used most commonly because it will improve cardiac output and maintain renal perfusion. The mainstay of treatment for septic shock is antibiotic therapy. Antibiotics are prescribed empirically in patients with septic shock. The usual treatment regimen includes a penicillin, an aminoglycoside, and a cephalosporin.

The major potential and actual nursing diagnoses for septic shock as well as the associated nursing interventions are listed in Table 57–4.

Disseminated Intravascular Coagulation

Disseminated intravascular coagulation (DIC) is an alteration in the normal clotting mechanism that manifests itself as diffuse clotting occurring simultaneously with hemorrhage (Yasko & Schafer, 1983). The normal clotting cascade is a tightly controlled homeostatic mechanism, which protects the body when injury has occurred. The intrinsic and extrinsic pathways of the clotting cascade are illustrated in Figure 57–2.

Disseminated intravascular coagulation is seen not as a primary disorder but as a secondary complication that requires some type of triggering event. In patients with a cancer diagnosis, DIC has been associated with intravascular hemolysis from transfusion reactions; overwhelming viral or bacterial sepsis and shock, particularly from gram-negative sepsis; and release of thrombin from malignant cells (e.g., acute myelogenous leukemia, melanoma, or cancer of the lung, stomach, colon, breast, ovary, and prostate) (Yasko & Schafer, 1983).

The pathophysiologic mechanisms involved in DIC are pictured in Figure 57–3. The excessive conversion of prothrombin to thrombin and the generation of fibrin clots result in soluble clot deposition in tissue capillaries. This fibrin deposition impedes blood flow and can result in tissue hypoxia and necrosis. As the excessive clotting proceeds, normal homeostatic controls cannot maintain an adequate supply of platelets, clotting factors, and fibrinogen. In addition, fibrin split products—natural anticoagulants that are produced as part of the normal clotting cascade—begin to accumulate, and the patients has a tendency to hemorrhage.

Patients must be observed for evidence of bleeding and clotting. The most prominent signs of bleeding are petechiae, ecchymosis, and prolonged bleeding from injection sites. The skin, gingiva, conjunctiva, and retina should be examined carefully. In addition, patients should be monitored for episodes of epistaxis; bleeding from old injection sites; bleeding from incision sites; intestinal bleeding; and signs and symptoms of a major internal hemorrhage, including hypotension, tachycardia, decreased hematocrit levels, and markedly reduced urine output. Patients have a tendency to develop clots in the microcirculation of organs with the highest blood flow (e.g., kidney, central nervous system, and skin). Assessments should be made for hematuria, changes in mental status, and acrocyanosis (i.e., generalized sweating, with cold, mottled fingers and toes). The patient's coagulation profile, including prothrombin time, partial thromboplastin time, fibrinogen level, platelet count, and fibrin split products, must be monitored.

The primary treatment of DIC is to remove the precipitating factor or underlying cause, which may be difficult if the precipitating factor is the patient's cancer. The major intervention involves the administration of heparin. The rationale for this treatment is that heparin inactivates thrombin, which will inhibit the clotting process and thereby inhibit fibrinolysis. This series of reactions, in effect, stops the DIC cycle. The remaining medical interventions are supportive in nature and include platelet transfusions and interventions to prevent shock and acidosis. The major potential and actual nursing diagnoses for DIC as well as the associated nuring interventions are listed in Table 57–4.

INFILTRATIVE EMERGENCIES

Cancers can infiltrate major organs and produce devastating, life-threatening sequelae. The major infiltrative emergencies discussed in this section are neoplastic cardiac tamponade, spinal cord compression, and carotid artery rupture.

Neoplastic Cardiac Tamponade

The pericardium is a double-walled sac that surrounds the heart and the great vessels. It contains a visceral layer that directly lines the surface of the heart and an outer layer—the parietal layer—which is made of fibrous tissue and can move freely. The pericardial cavity lies between the two layers and contains approximately 25 to 35 ml of serous fluid. The pericardium provides a frictionless sac for the contractions of the heart and supports the heart in a stable position.

Neoplastic cardiac tamponade results from an accumulation of fluid in the pericardial sac; from a significant constriction of the pericardium by tumor; or from

NORMAL CLOTTING MECHANISM

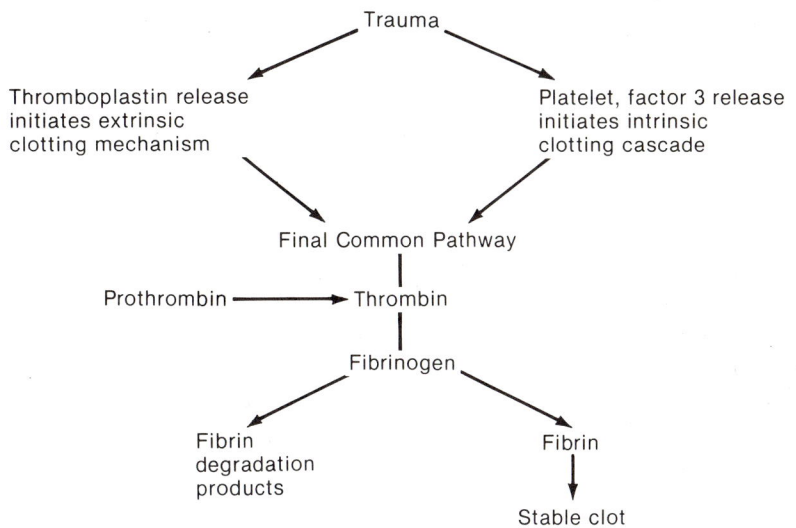

Trauma

Thromboplastin release
initiates extrinsic
clotting mechanism

Platelet, factor 3 release
initiates intrinsic
clotting cascade

Final Common Pathway

Prothrombin ⟶ Thrombin

Fibrinogen

Fibrin
degradation
products

Fibrin

Stable clot

Figure 57–2. The intrinsic and extrinsic pathways of the clotting cascade.

postirradiation pericarditis, which is indirectly related to the cancer (Theologides, 1978).

The signs and symptoms exhibited by the patient are extremely variable. The severity of symptoms depends on the rapidity of the development of the tamponade. The patient can exhibit any or all of the following symptoms: extreme anxiety and agitation, an oppressive feeling over the precordium, dyspnea and tachypnea, cough, dysphagia, hiccups, hoarseness, nausea and vomiting, perfuse perspiration, changes in level of consciousness, tachycardia, jugular venous distention, pulsus paradoxus, or distant or muffled heart sounds. The patient's electrocardiogram may show electrical alternans (Theologides, 1978).

Emergency management of the acutely ill patient involves rapid diagnosis and treatment with a pericardiocentesis to remove the fluid, as illustrated in Figure 57–4. The patient may require supportive therapy, including oxygen, intravenous hydration, and administration of pressor therapy. After the acute treatment, the patient may undergo surgery for a pericardial window or for placement of an indwelling pericardial catheter.

The major potential and actual nursing diagnoses for neoplastic cardiac tamponade as well as the associated nursing interventions are listed in Table 57–5.

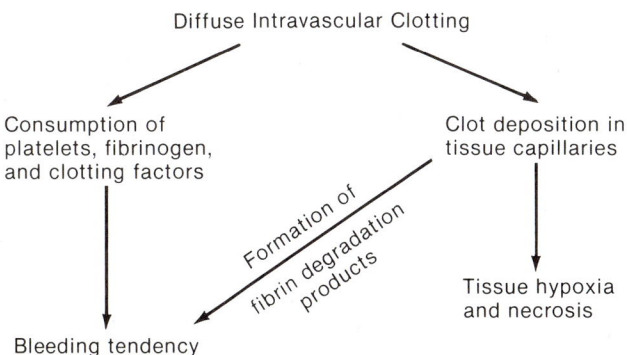

Diffuse Intravascular Clotting

Consumption of
platelets, fibrinogen,
and clotting factors

Clot deposition in
tissue capillaries

Formation of fibrin degradation products

Tissue hypoxia
and necrosis

Bleeding tendency

Figure 57–3. Pathophysiologic mechanisms in disseminated intravascular coagulation.

Spinal Cord Compression

Spinal cord compression develops in approximately 1 to 10 per cent of cancer patients. This oncologic emergency requires prompt diagnosis, evaluation, and treatment if permanent neurologic sequelae are to be prevented. Spinal cord compression can occur as a result of direct extension of the tumor from the paravertebral nodes to the spinal cord or from metastatic disease to the vertebral column. Seventy per cent of all cord compressions occur in the thoracic area. Tumors with the highest incidence of cord compression in the thoracic area are lung, breast, kidney, prostate, lymphoma, myeloma, melanoma, and gastrointestinal. Twenty per cent of all cord compressions occur in the lumbosacral area. Tumors with the highest incidence of cord compression in this area are gastrointestinal, melanoma, lymphoma, myeloma, kidney, prostate, breast, and lung. Finally, 10 per cent of cord compressions occur in the cervical area. Tumors that produce the highest incidence of cervical cord compressions in this area are lung, breast, melanoma, lymphoma, kidney, and myeloma (Bruckman & Blooment, 1978).

The signs and symptoms of cord compression vary, depending on the location and degree of the infiltration. The hallmark symptom is pain, which is usually located over the site of the cord compression. The pain typically worsens when the patient moves, coughs, sneezes, or performs a Valsalva maneuver. As the cord compression progresses, the patient experiences motor weakness followed by sensory changes. Late signs and symptoms of spinal cord compression are associated with autonomic dysfunction and include bowel and bladder dysfunction.

The medical management depends on the patient's primary tumor, the level of the blockage, the rapidity of onset of symptoms, the degree and duration of the blockage, and the patient's general condition. In general, a laminectomy is performed in patients with rapidly progressing or acutely severe neurologic deficits. Following surgery, the patient receives radiation

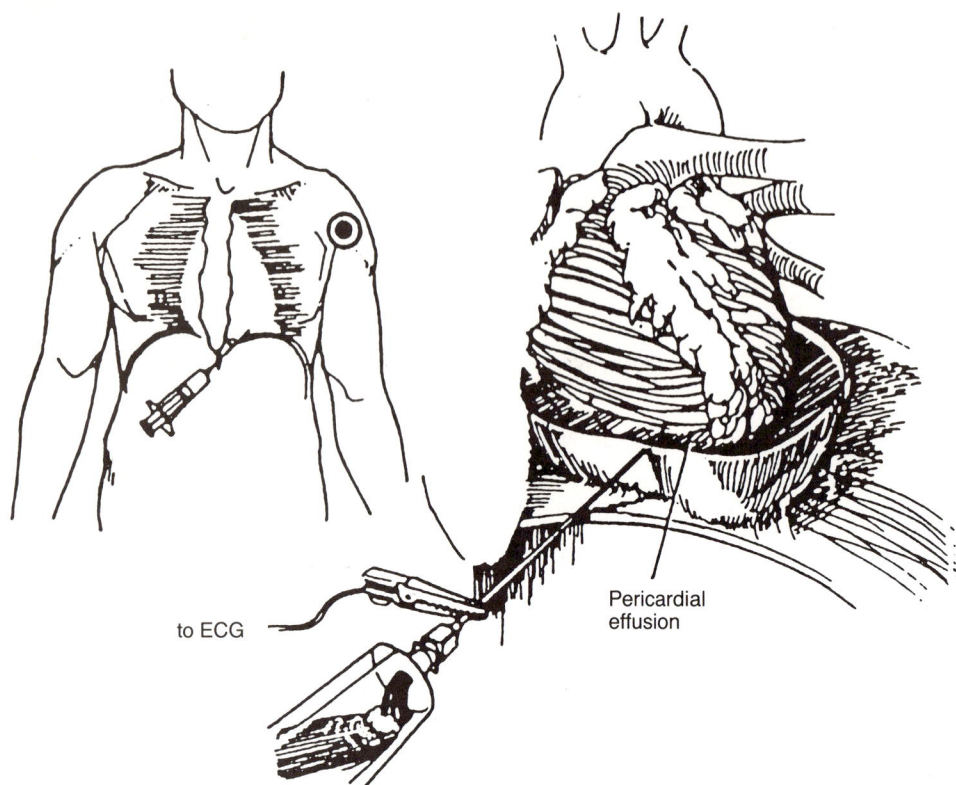

Figure 57–4. Emergency management of neoplastic cardiac tamponade with a pericardiocentesis to remove the fluid. (With permission from Adria Laboratories [1987]. *Understanding and Managing Oncologic Emergencies [p. 28]*. Dublin, Ohio: Adria Laboratories.)

to ECG

Pericardial effusion

therapy. Radiation therapy, as a single agent, is used in patients with minimal or slowly progressing symptoms or in patients who have an incomplete block on myelogram. Emergency management before surgery or radiation therapy includes intravenous administration of high doses of steroids. The optimal dose has not been determined. Many neurologists prescribe 100 mg/day of dexamethasone for 3 days (Bruckman & Blooment, 1978).

The major potential and actual nursing diagnoses for spinal cord compression as well as the associated nursing interventions are listed in Table 57–5.

Carotid Artery Rupture

Rupture of the carotid artery occurs most frequently in patients with head and neck cancers. The etiologic factors include invasion of the arterial wall by tumor or erosion of the arterial vessels after surgery or radiation therapy.

In general, minor oozing is evident at the site of the invasive lesion before the true emergency situation. Attempts to control bleeding locally are rarely successful, because the site is usually at the base of infected necrotic tumor and the bleeding is from branches of the external carotid artery. In the case of a carotid artery "blowout," treatment involves direct finger pressure over the bleeding site. The patient then receives adequate hydration and blood and blood products and is stabilized hemodynamically before surgery. The surgery involves ligation of the carotid artery above and below the site of rupture and excision of the necrotic segment (Howland & Carlon, 1985).

The major potential and actual nursing diagnoses for carotid artery rupture as well as the associated nursing interventions are listed in Table 57–5.

Table 57–5. ACTUAL AND POTENTIAL NURSING DIAGNOSES FOR INFILTRATIVE EMERGENCIES

Neoplastic Cardiac Tamponade
Decreased cardiac output
   Monitor vital signs and hemodynamic parameters
   Monitor for pulsus paradoxus
   Monitor electrocardiogram for electrical alternans
Potential for alteration in cerebral tissue perfusion
   Perform neurologic assessment
   Administer oxygen as prescribed
Spinal Cord Compression
Pain
   Perform a pain assessment
   Administer analgesics as prescribed
   Utilize nonpharmacologic strategies to decrease pain
Potential for alteration in mobility
   Perform a neurologic assessment
   Institute safety measures
Potential for alteration in skin integrity
   Perform skin assessment
   Institute preventive skin care measures
Carotid Artery Rupture
Potential for decreased cardiac output
   Monitor vital signs and hemodynamic parameters
   Administer intravenous fluid and blood as prescribed
Potential for alteration in cerebral tissue perfusion
   Perform a neurologic assessment
   Institute safety measures

SUMMARY

The occurrence of an oncologic emergency in a patient with cancer can be an extremely frightening situation. The patient may associate the emergency situation with the recurrence of tumor and feel overwhelmed and unable to cope. In additon, the family may be equally alarmed at the patient's dramatic change in condition. Nursing interventions must focus on assisting the patient and family to cope with the emergency situation. Many times patients will be in an unfamiliar environment if they require attention in the intensive care unit. Oncology nurses must ease the transition for the oncology patient in the critical care environment.

The incidence of oncologic emergencies will increase as patients live longer with their disease. Oncology nurses must take an active role in assessing the patient for signs and symptoms that warn of a potential emergency situation and take steps to treat the condition before such a situation occurs to avoid serious and often deleterious consequences.

References

Bruckman, J. E., & Blooment, W. D., (1978). Management of spinal cord compression. *Seminars in Oncology, 5,* 135–140.

Chernecky, C. C., & Ramsey, P. W. (1984). *Critical nursing care of the client with cancer.* Norwalk, CT: Appleton-Century-Crofts.

Howland, W. S., & Carlon, G. C. (Eds.). (1985). *Critical care of the cancer patient.* Chicago: Year Book Medical Publishers.

Lamb, L. (1982). Think you know septic shock? *Nursing 82, 12,* 34–43.

Lind, J. M. (1985). Ectopic hormonal production: Nursing implications. *Seminars in Oncology Nursing, 1,* 251–258.

Theologides, A. (1978). Neoplastic cardiac tamponade. *Seminars in Oncology, 5,* 181–190.

Twombly, M. (1978). The shift into the third space. *Nursing 78, 8*(6), 38–41.

Yasko, J. M. (1983). Syndrome of inappropriate antidiuretic hormone secretion. In J. M. Yasko (Ed.), *Guidelines for cancer care: Symptom management* (pp. 362–366). Reston, VA: Reston Publishing Co.

Yasko, J. M., & Schafer, S. L. (1983). Disseminated intravascular coagulation. In J. M. Yasko (Ed.), *Guidelines for cancer care: Symptom management* (pp. 324–329). Reston, VA: Reston Publishing Co.

CHAPTER 58

Alterations in Energy: The Sensation of Fatigue

BARBARA F. PIPER

ANATOMIC AND PHYSIOLOGIC FEATURES

Fatigue is a universal experience that is relieved usually by a good night's sleep. However, for many cancer patients, fatigue is not dissipated so easily. It becomes a chronic, unpleasant sensation that no longer protects the individual from overwork or exhaustion (Piper, 1986). Various theories have been proposed to explain how fatigue may occur (Cameron, 1973; Ciba Foundation Symposium, 1981; Grandjean, 1970; Morris, 1982). The actual mechanisms that produce fatigue, even at the muscle level, remain controversial (Roberts & Smith, 1989). Thus surprisingly little is known about fatigue that can guide nursing care (Piper, Lindsey, & Dodd, 1987).

Contributing Factors

Lack of Multidisciplinary Collaboration

Several factors have contributed to this lack of knowledge about fatigue. One of these relates to the number of different disciplines that have investigated fatigue, such as psychology (Grandjean, 1970), muscle physiology (Gibson & Edwards, 1985; Roberts & Smith, 1989), ergonomics, the discipline that examines industrial environments and worker fatigue (Kogi,

Saito, & Mitsuhashi, 1970; Komoike & Horiguchi, 1971; Saito, Kogi, & Kashiwagi, 1970; Yoshitake, 1969, 1971, 1978), nursing (Cimprich, 1990; Davis, 1984; Haylock & Hart, 1979; Jamar, 1989; Piper et al., in review; Putt, 1977; Rieger, 1987; Rhodes, Watson, & Hanson, 1988; Rhoten, 1982; Wickham et al., 1990), and medicine (Atkinson, 1985; Rose & King, 1978). This interest of different disciplines has led to many different definitions and perspectives in the literature that make it difficult to review findings from various studies and determine what is useful to nursing practice. In addition, one discipline's findings may not always be published in another discipline's journals; thus collaborative, multidisciplinary studies have not been conducted. This lack of communication and collaboration among the disciplines hinders knowledge development and may lead the naive reader to conclude that each discipline is studying a different type of fatigue. In reality, each discipline is contributing additional knowledge about the construct called *fatigue*.

Different Types of Fatigue

Many different types or classification systems for fatigue can be found in the literature. Muscle physiologists consider fatigue to be *central* when central nervous system mechanisms are involved and *peripheral* when peripheral nervous system mechanisms are involved (Gibson & Edwards, 1985). Central fatigue may be caused by lack of motivation, impaired transmission down the spinal cord, and impaired recruitment of motor neurons (Gibson & Edwards, 1985). It also may be caused by " . . . an exhaustion or malfunctioning of brain cells in the hypothalamic region" (Poteliakhoff, 1981, p. 94). In contrast, peripheral fatigue may be due to impaired functioning of the peripheral nerves, neuromuscular junction transmission, or fiber activation (Poteliakhoff, 1981). Figure 58–1 illustrates this classification system and the sites of impairment that may produce fatigue in healthy subjects. Little is known about how these normal physiologic mechanisms may be affected by abnormal processes such as cancer or other disease states. It may be possible that both central and peripheral mechanisms may be involved when a person experiences chronic fatigue.

Another classification system found in the literature categorizes fatigue as being *normal, pathologic, situational,* or *psychological* in its origins (Kellum, 1985). None of these classification systems is as helpful to guide nursing practice as is the *acute* and *chronic* model for fatigue that characterizes symptoms by their duration (Bartley & Chute, 1947; Piper, 1988). The literature suggests that differences may exist between these two states (Bartley & Chute, 1947; Cameron, 1973; McFarland, 1971; Muncie, 1941; Poteliakhoff, 1981; Potempa, Lopez, Reid, & Lawson, 1986; Riddle, 1982; Roberts & Smith, 1989). These differences and additional ones (Piper, 1988a) are summarized in Table 58–1.

Acute fatigue protects the individual from overwork or exhaustion; chronic fatigue may no longer perform this function and may serve no purpose (Riddle, 1982). Its actual function is unknown. Causes of acute fatigue usually are identifiable (Riddle, 1982) and involve a single mechanism. Often acute fatigue is related to some form of exertion or activity. In contrast, chronic fatigue may involve multiple (Riddle, 1982) and additive causes (Rockwell & Burr, 1977) that may not be easily identifiable or related to activity.

Acute fatigue is perceived as normal or expected tiredness. Symptoms are localized usually to a specific body region (Riddle, 1982), such as tired eyes, arms, or legs. Chronic fatigue is perceived as abnormal or excessive and is described as a more generalized, whole body response (Cameron, 1973; Poteliakhoff, 1981). In an analysis of self-care behavior logs (Piper & Dodd, 1987) that were completed by chemotherapy and radiation therapy patients, 30 patients or 36 per cent (total n = 84) experienced fatigue. The most common words used by patients to describe this sensation were "generalized tiredness" or "unusual or extreme fatigue." "Very low energy" was used also but to a lesser extent (Piper & Dodd, 1987). For many patients, chronic fatigue is described as a totally overwhelming experience; patients feel that they must give into it when it occurs and hope that it will dissipate soon. One radiation therapy patient described pulling over to the side of the road while she was driving because of feeling extremely fatigued. She had to sit in her car for 3 hours before the sensation lessened and she could safely resume driving.

Acute fatigue is rapid in onset, of short duration—days or weeks—and intermittent. Chronic fatigue has a longer, more insidious onset usually (Rockwell & Burr, 1977) that has a cumulative effect (Bartley & Chute, 1947; McFarland, 1971). When a threshold point is reached (Rockwell & Burr, 1977), the person realizes that the fatigue is unusual. It persists over time, lasts for more than 1 month (Potempa et al., 1986), and is constant or recurrent. Acute fatigue usually is dissipated by a good night's sleep. Chronic fatigue may not be resolved so easily (Bartley & Chute, 1947; Cameron, 1973; McFarland, 1971), and a combination of approaches may be needed to lessen the sensation (Piper, 1986; Riddle, 1982). Research approaches are needed to determine whether these differences actually exist, and if these states can coexist within one individual, as may occur when cancer patients experience acute and chronic forms of pain.

Lack of Nursing Studies

Another factor contributing to the lack of knowledge about fatigue is the paucity of nursing studies that addresses fatigue in patients with cancer. In the past 11 years, only eight nursing studies have been conducted that address fatigue as their primary focus (Cimprich, 1990; Davis, 1984; Haylock & Hart, 1979; Jamar, 1989; Piper et al., in review; Piper, Lindsey, et

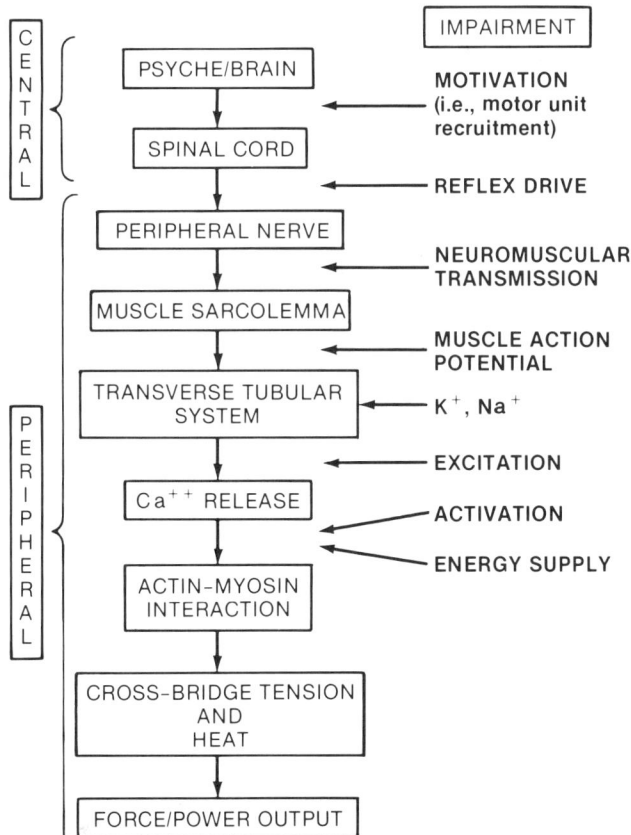

Figure 58–1. Central and peripheral model for fatigue. (Adapted with permission from Gibson, H., & Edwards, R. H. T. [1985]. Muscular exercise and fatigue. *Sports Medicine*, 2:121.)

Table 58–1. ACUTE AND CHRONIC FATIGUE MODEL: DISTINGUISHING CHARACTERISTICS

Characteristic	Acute Fatigue	Chronic Fatigue
Purpose/Function	Protective	Unknown, may no longer be protective
		May be nonfunctional
Population at Risk	Primarily healthy individuals	Primarily clinical populations
Etiology	Usually identifiable	May not be identifiable
	Usually involves a single mechanism or cause	Usually multiple and additive causes
	Often experienced in relation to some form of activity or exertion	Often experienced with no relation to activity or exertion
Perception	Normal, usual	Abnormal, unusual
	Expected/anticipated with respect to specific activities or forms of exertion	Excessive or disproportionate to past experience
	Primarily localized to a specific body part or system	Generalized, whole body-mind sensation
	Pleasant or unpleasant	Unpleasant
Time Dimension:		
Onset	Rapid	Insidious, gradual
		Cumulative
		Threshold model
Duration	Short; days or weeks	Long; persists over time
		More than 1 month
Pattern	Intermittent/sporadic	Constant/recurrent
Relief Dimension	Usually alleviated by a good night's sleep, adequate rest, proper diet, exercise program, or stress management techniques	Not completely dispelled by these methods
		A combination of approaches may be needed
	Resolves quickly	Does not resolve quickly
Impact on Activities of Daily Living and Quality of Life	Minor, minimal	Major

(From the American Cancer Society Monograph [1988]. *Nursing management of common problems: Fatigue in patients* [p. 26]. Reprinted with permission.)

al., 1989; Rieger, 1987; Wickham, 1990). From these and other nursing studies, it is clear that nurses are interested in the acute *and* chronic effects of fatigue in healthy and ill populations and in identifying subjective and objective fatigue indicators.

Lack of Concept Clarification

Frequently, concepts such as *malaise* and *weakness* are used interchangeably with fatigue as if they have the same meanings. This lack of distinction hinders knowledge development. Clinically, it is important to distinguish these concepts from one another, because nursing management depends on accurate assessment and diagnosis of patient problems, and nursing management may vary (Piper, Lindsey, & Dodd, 1987).

PATHOPHYSIOLOGIC MECHANISMS OF FATIGUE IN CANCER PATIENTS

Fatigue Framework

Many factors can cause fatigue in healthy and ill populations. In the following sections, a framework is presented that synthesizes the fatigue literature for the purpose of guiding nursing practice and research (Piper, Lindsey, & Dodd, 1987) in this pervasive phenomenon (Fig. 58–2). Using this framework, the nurse can begin to assess possible causes of fatigue in a specific patient situation and select an appropriate intervention to test. When fatigue becomes a chronic sensation, management may become more complex, and a combination of strategies may be needed. Mech-

anisms most likely to be associated with or to cause fatigue in patients with cancer are highlighted.

Manifestations of Fatigue

In the center of the framework are the subjective (perceptual) and the objective (physiologic, biochemical, and behavioral) indicators of fatigue that have been reported. Sign and symptom patterns may vary according to the primary cause of the fatigue, such as stimulation or overwork of a specific muscle group, type of occupational activity, or emotional depression (Piper, 1986; Saito et al., 1970). When fatigue becomes a chronic sensation, a combination of mechanisms may be involved. Further research is needed to clarify these relationships. Currently, the best way to assess and measure fatigue in clinical populations is to determine the person's own perception of the fatigue experience (Piper, Reiger et al., 1989). Fatigue is a subjective feeling of tiredness, influenced by circadian rhythm and other factors and varying in duration, unpleasantness, and intensity (Piper, 1986).

Mechanisms of Fatigue

Because changes in biologic and psychosocial patterns can influence signs and symptoms of fatigue, it is important for the nurse to assess whether changes in preexisting patterns have occurred as a result of illness or treatment. These patterns surround the center of the framework in Figure 58–2.

Accumulation of Metabolites. Accumulation of various metabolites has been associated with fatigue. Whether these products cause fatigue or merely par-

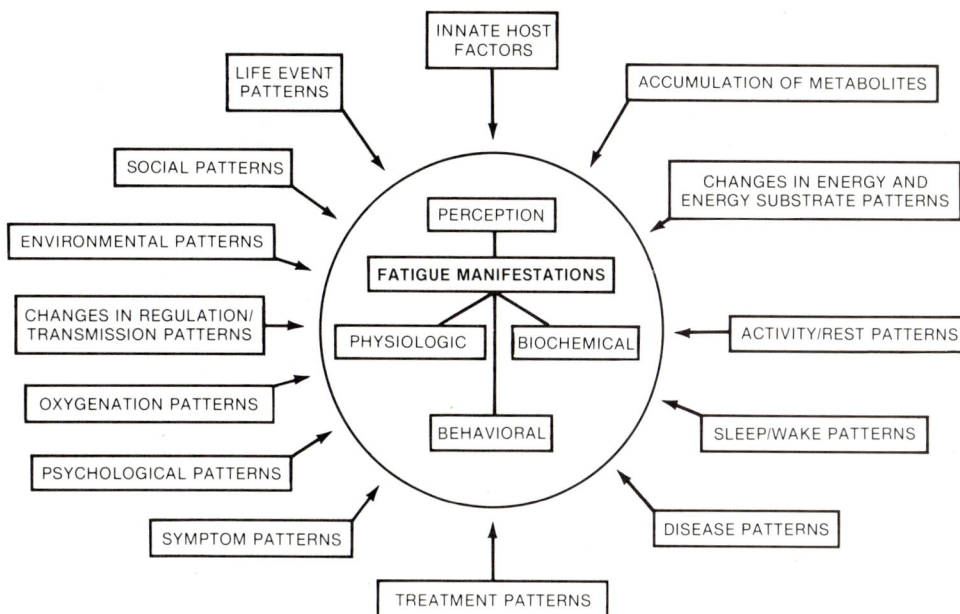

Figure 58–2. Fatigue framework in healthy and clinical populations. (Redrawn with permission from Piper, B. F., Lindsey, A. M., & Dodd, M. J. [1987]. Fatigue mechanisms in cancer patients: Developing nursing theory. *Oncology Nursing Forum, 14*[6]:18.)

allel its occurrence remains unknown. In cancer patients, the accumulation of lactate (Burt, Aoki, Gorschboth, Brennan, 1983; Gold, 1974; Morris, 1982), hydrogen ions (Karlsson, Sjodin, Jacobs, & Kaiser, 1981; Miller et al., 1988; Nakamura & Schwartz, 1972), and cell destruction end products (Haylock & Hart, 1979) are likely mechanisms. Continuous muscle work is known to produce an accumulation of lactic acid that can contribute to decreased muscle strength (Burt et al., 1983). In cancer patients, marked increases in Cori cycle activity and lactate production have been reported (Burt et al., 1983; Gold, 1974). The reason for this accelerated cycling is unknown (Gold, 1974).

Another possibility is that fatigue may be associated with changes that result from hydrogen ions that are produced as lactate accumulates (Karlsson et al., 1981). Hydrogen ions are thought to impede muscle force by decreasing the number of calcium ions that are bound to troponin during excitation-coupling. This reduces the number of actin-myosin interactions and results in decreased force (Nakamura & Schwartz, 1972) (see Fig. 58–1).

Fatigue may be caused by the accumulation of cell destruction end products and toxic metabolites in the blood that inhibit normal cell functioning when cells undergo lysis (Haylock & Hart, 1979). Increasing fluid intake in these patients may promote more rapid dilution and excretion of these substances and thus prevent fatigue.

Changes in Energy and Energy Substrate Patterns. Changes in energy production and substrates can profoundly influence human performance and development of fatigue. Changes in energy patterns are common in cancer patients and may result from abnormalities in energy expenditure, cancer cachexia, anorexia, infection (Straus et al., 1985; Valdini, 1985), fever (Edwards et al., 1972), and imbalances in thyroid hormones (Axelrod et al., 1983).

Activity and Rest Patterns. Activity and rest patterns can play significant roles in the prevention, cause, and alleviation of fatigue. Negative changes in activity patterns are common in cancer patients (Fernsler, 1986; Fobair et al., 1986; Frank-Stromborg & Wright, 1984). Whether fatigue is the underlying cause of these changes is unknown. How systematic changes in activity and rest patterns may affect fatigue positively also needs investigation.

Sleep and Awake Patterns. The relationship between sleep disorders (Hauri, Silverfarb, Oxman, & O'Leary, 1985) and fatigue should be examined.

Disease Patterns. Commonly, fatigue precedes, accompanies, or follows many adult and pediatric malignancies (Waskerwitz & Leonard, 1986). How fatigue patterns vary prospectively by disease type, site, and extent is unknown. In one retrospective study, patients with Hodgkin's disease indicated that energy levels may take 1 to 5 years following treatment to return to normal (Fobair et al., 1986). Rapidity of energy return was " . . . inversely related to age, stage of disease, and intensity of treatment" (Fobair et al., 1986, p. 812).

Treatment Patterns. Various medical treatments are associated with fatigue. Fatigue is reported to be a pervasive and distressing occurrence in chemotherapy patients. Anemia, cell destruction end products, and nausea and vomiting may be contributing factors (Piper, Lindsey, & Dodd, 1987). Because fatigue can be caused by disorders in neurotransmission, it is hypothesized that drugs that cross the blood-brain barrier or have neurotoxicities may be more likely to produce fatigue than other agents (Piper, Lindsey, & Dodd, 1987). Anecdotally, patients receiving vinca alkaloid chemotherapy report peripheral fatigue symptoms, such as leg and knee tiredness, and central symptoms, such as an inability to concentrate or to think clearly (see Fig. 58–1). Neurotoxicity is dose limiting for vincristine and is found at high doses for vinblastine. When these drugs have been used in combination, signs of neurotoxicity, insomnia, and weakness are reported (Stewart, Maroun, Lefebvre, & Heringer, 1986). Whether this class of agent is associated with a higher incidence of fatigue than other drug classifications remains to be investigated. Because many agents are used in combination drug protocols, it may be difficult to isolate the fatigue produced by one drug from that produced by another (Piper, Lindsey, & Dodd, 1987).

Fatigue Patterns. Frequently, fatigue patterns reflect chemotherapy treatment patterns. For example, some chemotherapy patients may report a "biphasic" fatigue pattern (Spross, 1987, p. 76). In these patients, fatigue occurs on day 1 of each treatment cycle, may last 1 to 4 days (corresponding to stress, antiemetic, and chemotherapy effects), and recurs during the nadir of each cycle (when bone marrow suppression is anticipated to be the greatest) (Spross, 1987). Patients may report both a cumulative effect over successive treatment cycles and improved energy levels between cycles (Meyerwitz, Watkins, & Sparks, 1983). More emotional distress and disruption in self-care abilities may be associated with the more long-term side effects of tiredness and weakness than from the more acute side effects, such as nausea and vomiting (Nerenz, Leventhal, & Love, 1982; Rhodes, Watson, & Hanson, 1988). Boxes 58–1, 58–2, and 58–3 summarize findings from three recent nursing studies that have investigated fatigue patterns in patients receiving chemotherapy (Jamar, 1989; Piper, Friedman et al., in review; Rhodes et al., 1988).

Fatigue is common in patients undergoing radiation therapy (Haylock & Hart, 1979; King, Nail, Kreamer, Strohl, & Johnson, 1985; Kobashi-Schoot, Hanewald, Van Dam, & Bruning, 1985) and seems to coincide with treatment patterns (Haylock & Hart, 1979; Spross, 1987). In one classic radiation therapy study, mean fatigue scores were increased significantly from first to last treatment day, were consistently lower on Sundays, and were higher in patients who underwent the lengthiest treatment regimens (Haylock & Hart, 1979). Another study followed patients weekly during treatment and monthly for 3 months after treatment (King et al., 1985). Fatigue patterns reported in this study are summarized by treatment site in Table 58–2.

Fatigue is common and often dose limiting in patients treated with biologic response modifiers (Davis, 1984; Piper, Rieger et al, 1989). It is not clear how fatigue may be caused by these agents, but because anorexia, weight loss, and fatigue form a constellation of symptoms in these patients, a combination of mechanisms, particularly central neurophysiologic mechanisms, are likely (Piper, Rieger et al., 1989). Fatigue patterns also may vary by diagnosis and by type and dose of biologic response modifier (Davis, 1984; Piper, Rieger et al., 1989; Rieger, 1987).

Box 58–1. FATIGUE IN WOMEN WITH OVARIAN CANCER RECEIVING CHEMOTHERAPY

STUDY

Jamar, S. C. (1989). **Fatigue in women receiving chemotherapy for ovarian cancer.** In S. G. Funk, E. M. Tornquist, M. T. Champagne, L. A. Copp, & R. A. Wise (Eds.), *Key aspects of comfort: Management of pain, fatigue and nausea* (pp. 224–233). New York: Springer.

SAMPLE

Sixteen Caucasian females, stage I to IV ovarian disease.

MEASURES

Pearson-Byars Fatigue Feeling Tone Checklist; Symptom Distress Scale; Profile of Mood States, short form; semi-structured interview.

FINDINGS

Fatigue was worse during the first week following chemotherapy; subsided during the next 2 to 3 weeks only to return during the first week of each subsequent cycle. Symptoms included "weak in the body," "sick to my stomach," "weary talking," and "sleepy." Twelve out of the 16 had to give up or change their activities because of fatigue. There was a negative correlation between subjective fatigue and hematocrit levels. Women who were single parents or without home care assistance had higher levels of fatigue.

LIMITATIONS

Small sample size at different stages and cycles of chemotherapy; one time interview and measurement.

Box 58–2. FATIGUE IN WOMEN WITH BREAST CANCER RECEIVING CHEMOTHERAPY

STUDY

Piper, B. F., Friedman, L., Hartigan, K., Post, B., Smith, J., Coleman, C. A., Gilman, N., Dodd, M. J., Lindsey, A. M., & Paul, S. (in review). **Fatigue in women with breast cancer receiving chemotherapy.**

SAMPLE

Thirty-seven Caucasian women with stage II breast cancer receiving C.M.F. chemotherapy on a 21-day treatment cycle.

MEASURES

Piper Fatigue Scale, Fatigue Symptom Checklist, Profile of Mood States; day 1 of each treatment cycle, and at nadirs, days 10/14 (time 1 to 4).

FINDINGS

Decreased appetite and performance status; increased need to sleep and nap more. Whole-body tiredness was the only symptom reported by 50 per cent or more of the women over all four time periods. Total mood disturbance scores and fatigue were greatest on day 1 of the second chemotherapy cycle, suggesting that the beginning of this cycle may be a particularly vulnerable period for these women. An inverse relationship between anemia and subjective fatigue was demonstrated.

LIMITATIONS

Convenience sample: Results cannot be generalized to other populations.

Box 58–3. FATIGUE IN CHEMOTHERAPY PATIENTS

STUDY

Rhodes, V. A., Watson, P. M., & Hanson, B. M. (1988). **Patients' descriptions of the influence of tiredness and weakness on self-care abilities.** *Cancer Nursing, 11,* 186–194.

SAMPLE

Twenty cancer outpatients; status post an average of six cycles of chemotherapy at first interview; 11 patients completed second interview.

MEASURES

Telephone interviews conducted by research assistant.

FINDINGS

Tiredness and weakness were the symptoms that most interfered with self-care abilities. Activities that were effective in treating these symptoms were planning and scheduling activities (spreading out activities over 1 wk versus doing them in 1 day, getting extra sleep, scheduling naps or rest periods, keeping busy); decreasing nonessential activities (housework, gardening, cooking, social activities); increasing dependence on others (obtaining assistance with cooking, cleaning, shopping, work).

LIMITATIONS

Retrospective; unclear how sample was selected from larger study sample; small sample size; no tiredness or weakness definitions provided or sample demographics (e.g., stage and type of disease or type of therapy).

Table 58–2. FATIGUE PATTERNS OVER TIME IN RADIATION THERAPY PATIENTS ACROSS TREATMENT SITES

Subjective Dimension	Site of Radiation Therapy			
	Chest (N = 15)	Head and Neck (N = 25)	Genitourinary (N = 26)	Gynecologic (N = 30)
Temporal				
Onset/course	1st wk: 60% 3rd wk: 93% 3 mo posttreatment: 46%	Increased steadily to a peak the last wk of treatment: 68% 1–3 mo posttreatment: 39%	Increased steadily to 5th week: 72% 1st mo posttreatment: 58% 3 mo posttreatment: 32%	Increased steadily to 5th wk: 72% 1st mo posttreatment: 58% 3 mo posttreatment: 32%
Pattern	Intermittent to continuous as treatment progressed Intermittent after treatment ended; Worse in afternoon	1st 4 wk, periodic; last 2 wk continuous Worse in afternoon and evening	1st 4 wk, periodic; last 2 wk, a few reported continuous Worse in afternoon	1st 4 wk, periodic; last 2 wk a few reported continuous Worse in afternoon
Intensity/ Severity	Consistent A little to moderately bad	Moderately bad to quite bad	Moderately bad	Moderately bad
Relief	Resting or sleeping in the afternoon helpful	Increase rest by planning daily afternoon nap; Go to bed early	Increase rest by an afternoon nap	Increase rest by an afternoon nap

(Data from King, Nail, Kreamer, Strohl, & Johnson, 1985.)

Fatigue may result from surgery (Rhoten, 1982; Rose & King, 1978) and diagnostic testing (King et al., 1985). It is likely that several mechanisms may interact or be synergistic in producing fatigue in surgical patients (Piper, Lindsey, & Dodd, 1987). Anxiety and test preparation and duration most likely influence fatigue during diagnostic testing. The nurse plays an important role in the prevention and alleviation of fatigue in these patients by reducing anxiety and by providing adequate rest periods (Piper, Lindsey, & Dodd, 1987).

Symptom Patterns. Other symptoms (Brown et al., 1986; Norris, 1982) may precede, accompany, or follow fatigue, such as pain, nausea, or diarrhea. Assessment and control of these symptoms may reduce or prevent symptoms of fatigue in cancer patients. Nursing needs to address the interrelationships between fatigue and other symptoms (Piper, Lindsey, & Dodd, 1987).

Oxygenation Patterns. Any factor that alters or interferes with the ability to obtain or maintain adequate oxygen levels in the lungs or blood, such as anemia, can influence fatigue (Piper, Lindsey, & Dodd, 1987).

Changes in Regulation/Transmission Patterns. Fluid or electrolyte imbalances or changes in neurohormone levels (Akerstedt, Gillberg, & Witterberg, 1982; Arendt, Borbely, Franey, & Wright, 1984) can potentially affect neurotransmission and muscle force, resulting in fatigue, sleep disorders, or altered biorhythms. Also, some reports suggest specific abnormalities in muscle electrophysiology and enzyme activity in some patients with cancer (Bruera et al., 1988).

PSYCHOSOCIAL FACTORS INFLUENCING FATIGUE

Psychological Patterns

Several psychological patterns, such as usual response to stressors (coping strategies), depression, anxiety, degree of motivation, and beliefs and attitudes, may influence fatigue in cancer patients (Bukberg, Penman, & Holland, 1984; Petty & Noyes, 1981; Proctor, Kernahan, & Taylor, 1981; Wittenborn & Buhler, 1979). For example, tiredness, fatigue, and sleep disturbances are common symptoms of depression (Wittenborn & Buhler, 1979). Depending on the study, moderate to severe depression may range from 17 to 42 per cent in hospitalized cancer patients (Bukberg et al., 1984; Petty & Noyes, 1981). Depression, lethargy, and somnolence may be related also to cranial radiation therapy, suggesting a centrally mediated mechanism for both fatigue and depression (Proctor et al., 1981).

Attitudes can influence behaviors. Chronic, unrelenting fatigue can lead to a loss of hope and a desire to escape. Chronic fatigue can prevent the person from engaging in the kinds of valued activities that give meaning to life. As a consequence, the person may lose the desire to go on living (Piper, 1986; Piper, Lindsey, & Dodd, 1987).

Other Related Patterns

Other factors that may contribute to fatigue include environmental patterns, such as noise (Piper, Lindsey, & Dodd, 1987), temperature, and allergens; social patterns, such as perceived social support, cultural beliefs, and economic factors; life-event patterns, such as the common transitional events associated with growth and development; and innate host factors, such as age, sex, genetic makeup (e.g., type of muscle fibers and their predisposition to fatigue) (Karlsson et al., 1981), and unique biorhythms.

ASSESSMENT AND MANAGEMENT OF FATIGUE

Assessment

To design an effective plan of care, the nurse should perform a thorough assessment of all subjective and objective data that may influence fatigue for that individual. Frequently, family members may be more sensitive than the patient to changes in the patient's usual pattern of fatigue and its impact.

Subjective data should include an assessment of usual patterns of functioning and possible changes that have occurred as a result of illness or treatment. When assessing the patient's perception, it is important for the nurse to remember the differences that may exist between acute and chronic fatigue states and the multidimensionality of the fatigue experience. Engel and Morgan (1973) suggest that the following dimensions of a symptom need to be assessed: symptom location, pattern, intensity, onset, and duration; aggravating and alleviating factors; and associated symptoms. Additional information should be collected about the person's perception of the meaning of fatigue; how distressing it is (Rhodes & Watson, 1987); and the physical, emotional, and mental symptoms experienced (Piper, Lindsey, & Dodd et al., 1989). Having the person maintain a daily fatigue diary for 1 week often reveals previously unrecognized patterns of fatigue (Piper, 1986).

Physical examination, laboratory data, and the patient's past and present medical history may reveal coexisting diseases, such as hypertension or diabetes, that may be contributing to the fatigue (Kellum, 1985). Because many medications are known to produce sedation or fatigue as a side effect, such as antiemetics, analgesics, and antihypertensives, it is important for the nurse to assess the patient's current medication history (Kellum, 1985). This should include information about prescription and nonprescription drugs; vitamin, caffeine, and alcohol intake (which disrupts rapid eye movement sleep); and other social or "recreational" drug use.

Behaviorally, the nurse needs to assess for any changes in the patient's physical appearance; performance status; and ways of moving, talking, or interacting that may indicate the presence of fatigue (Rhoten, 1982). Environmental factors such as heat or noise (Putt, 1977) need to be assessed. Frequently, assistive devices or furniture rearrangement may prevent needless expenditure of energy.

Nursing Diagnoses

The North American Nursing Diagnosis Association (NANDA) has accepted fatigue for clinical testing as a nursing diagnosis (Piper, 1989), which should stimulate further research into this sensation.

Many people assume that fatigue is tied to some form of activity, exertion, or ability to perform. In patients with cancer, there may be other reasons as well. Viewing fatigue from this limited perspective may lead to an ineffective plan of care. For example, chronically fatigued patients who have cancer may have multiple causes for their fatigue, such as radiation therapy, anxiety about cancer, anorexia, and insomnia. This type of diagnosis will require a more complex

intervention plan than if the problem were assessed from an activity dimension alone.

Measurement of Fatigue

Multidimensionality

Fatigue is a complex sensation that consists of subjective and objective dimensions (Piper, Lindsey, & Dodd, 1987). Subjective indicators are key to the understanding of how fatigue may vary between healthy and ill populations. The subjective dimension of fatigue has been measured primarily as the unidimensional feeling of tiredness (Heuting & Sarphati, 1966; McCorkle & Young, 1978; Pearson, 1957; Pearson & Byars, 1956). It has been only recently that fatigue, like pain, has been conceptualized and measured as a multidimensional construct using the statistical procedures of factor and key cluster analyses. (Kinsman & Weiser, 1976; Piper, Lindsey, et al., 1989; Yoshitake, 1969, 1971, 1978). In healthy subjects, symptoms seem to cluster around factors such as general fatigue (which includes tiredness), mental fatigue, and localized fatigue.

Subjective Dimension

Several instruments exist that measure subjective fatigue. Pearson and Byars (1956, 1957) developed a ten-item scale that measures the subjective feeling of tiredness (Table 58–3). This instrument has been used in numerous pilot investigations and in five patient studies (Davis, 1984; Freel & Hart, 1977; Hart, 1978; Haylock & Hart, 1979; Reiger, 1987). Instrument limitations include item colloquialism, unidimensionality, and lack of reliability and validity estimates to indicate that this instrument, originally designed to measure tiredness in airmen, measures tiredness in patient populations. One investigator has reported difficulties in using this instrument with some cancer patients (Rieger, 1987). It may perform better in clinical populations if it is investigator- rather than self-administered.

Numerous studies have been conducted by members

Table 58–3. CONTENT OF THE PEARSON-BYARS FATIGUE FEELING TONE CHECKLIST

Content
Very lively, extremely tired, quite fresh, slightly pooped, extremely peppy, somewhat fresh, petered out, very refreshed, fairly well pooped, ready to drop

3-Point Rating Scale
Less than, equal, more than

(Based on Pearson, R. G., & Byars, G. E. [1956]. *The development and validation* of a checklist for measuring subjective fatigue [p. 16]. Randolph AFB, TX: Texas School of Aviation Medicine, USAF.)

Table 58–4. FATIGUE SYMPTOM CHECKLIST

General Feelings of Incongruity
1. Feel heavy in the head
2. Feel tired in the whole body
3. Feel tired in the legs
4. Give a yawn
5. Feel the brain hot or muddled
6. Become drowsy
7. Feel strained in the eyes
8. Become rigid or clumsy in motion
9. Feel unsteady while standing
10. Want to lie down

Mental Fatigue
11. Find difficulty in thinking
12. Become weary while talking
13. Become nervous
14. Unable to concentrate
15. Unable to have an interest in thinking
16. Become apt to forget things
17. Lack self-confidence
18. Anxious about things
19. Unable to straighten up in posture
20. Lack patience

Specific Feelings of Incongruity
21. Have a headache
22. Feel stiff in the shoulders
23. Feel a pain in the waist
24. Feel constrained in breathing
25. Feel thirsty
26. Have a husky voice
27. Have dizziness
28. Have a spasm of the eyelids
29. Have a tremor in the limbs
30. Feel ill

(From Yoshitake, H. [1971]. Relations between the symptoms and the feeling of fatigue. *Ergonomics, 14*:177. Reproduced by permission.)

of the Japanese Industrial Research Committee on Fatigue that validate the Fatigue Symptom Checklist in Japanese workers (Kogi et al., 1970; Komorke et al., 1971; Saito et al., 1970; Yoshitake, 1969, 1971, 1978). This instrument contains 30 fatigue symptoms arranged in a checklist format so that the presence or absence of the symptom can be indicated. Findings from these studies suggest that there are three dimensions or subscales to the instrument: general feelings of incongruity, mental fatigue, and specific feelings of incongruity. These dimensions and their representative items are shown in Table 58–4.

Although this instrument has been used in clinical studies, it is not clear how the items on this instrument were developed originally or whether this instrument is appropriate to use with different cultures or with different clinical populations (Varrichio, 1985). The items need to be refactored to see if similar factors are found in the cancer population.

A new instrument that measures subjective fatigue, the Piper Fatigue Scale (PFS), has been tested and shows good reliability and validity estimates with radiation (Piper, Lindsey, & Dodd et al., 1989) and chemotherapy populations (Piper, Friedman et al., in review). The revised scale measures four dimensions of fatigue: temporal (relating to the timing, onset, and duration of the fatigue), severity (relating to intensity, distress, and degree of interference in activities of daily living), sensory (relating to the physical, emotional,

and mental symptoms of fatigue), and affective (relating to the emotional meaning of the fatigue). The PFS contains 41 visual analogue scale items plus three open-ended items that assess perceived causes of fatigue, relief measures, and associated symptoms. The instrument is available from the author for further clinical testing.

Subjective fatigue has been measured as a component of several instruments designed to measure other phenomena. These include the Symptom Distress Scale (McCorkle & Young, 1978); the Adapted Symptom Distress Scale (Rhodes, Watson, & Johnson, 1984); and the Profile of Mood States, or POMS (McNair, Lorr, & Droppleman, 1971).

Objective Dimension

A variety of *physiologic indicators* have been used to measure fatigue. These include melatonin, a neurotransmitter (Akerstedt et al., 1982; Arendt et al., 1984); the electromyogram (Malmquist, Ekholm, & Lindstrom, 1981); and heart rate and oxygen consumption (Burton, 1980). Other indicators that might be studied include rates and degrees of anemia and changes in levels of blood glucose, thyroid hormones, serum electrolytes, and temperature. An inverse relationship between the physiologic indicator anemia and subjective fatigue has been documented in patients with ovarian (Jamar, 1989) and breast cancers (Piper, Friedman et al., in review).

Several *biochemical indicators* have been studied. These include hydrogen ions or pH changes (Karlsson et al., 1981; Nakamura & Schwartz, 1972), muscle biopsies, magnetic resonance spectroscopy (Miller et al., 1988), lactate, and pyruvate (Rennie, Johnson, Park, & Sularman, 1973). The existence of a fatigue receptor has been postulated also (S. Lehman, personal communication, August 1986).

Nurses have attempted to identify *behavioral indicators* of fatigue (Freel & Hart, 1977; Putt, 1977; Rhoten, 1982). Rhoten developed an observational checklist to measure fatigue in five postoperative patients (Table 58–5). Categories include *general appearance,* and the subcategories of physical appearance,

Table 58–5. CATEGORIES AND SUBDIVISIONS OF THE RHOTEN OBSERVATIONAL CHECKLIST: BEHAVIORAL INDICATORS OR CORRELATES

General Appearance
  Physical appearance
  Coloring
  Breathing

Communication
  Eyes
  Facial expression
  Speech

Activity
  Movements
  Ambulation
  Posture
  Food and fluid intake

Attitude

(Data from Rhoten, 1982.)

coloring, and breathing; *communication,* with the subcategories of eyes, facial expression, and speech; *activity,* with the subcategories of movements, posture, ambulation, and food intake; and *attitudes.* Although this instrument has not been tested in other fatigue studies, it, and other instruments similar to it, warrant further investigation. Other investigators have examined relationships between symptoms of fatigue and performance behaviors in card sorting and bicycling activities (Freel & Hart, 1977; Heuting & Sarphati, 1966; MacVicar & Winningham, 1986; Pearson & Byars, 1956; Putt, 1977).

Empirical Fatigue Studies

To determine what is known about patterns of fatigue in clinical populations, the four nursing studies that have used the same subjective fatigue instruments, the Pearson-Byars Fatigue Feeling Scale (PBS), and the Japanese Industrial Fatigue Symptom Checklist (FSCL) were analyzed for their findings (Davis, 1984; Freel & Hart, 1977; Hart, 1978; Haylock & Hart, 1979).

Multiple sclerosis patients experience more severe feelings of fatigue generally, as measured by the PBS, than do healthy controls (Freel & Hart, 1977; Hart, 1978). In patients with cancer, feelings of fatigue increase over time in those who are being treated with either radiation therapy (Haylock & Hart, 1979) or interferon-α_2 therapy (Davis, 1984). When the factor of generalized feelings of incongruity on the FSCL is analyzed, the symptoms of wanting to lie down and tiredness in the body or legs are common findings. Impatience is a consistent finding in the mental fatigue category, and stiff shoulders and headaches are common in the specific incongruity category.

Management of Fatigue

Goals

Balancing energy intake with energy output (Levine, 1973) and believing that "Energy can be mobilized for healing . . . " (Meleis, 1986, p. 6) are essential assumptions and beliefs that underlie all nursing care. *Energy conservation* requires assessment of the person's current energy status, the energy-depleting factors that can and cannot be controlled, and the anticipated energy costs of various activities. All decisions about energy-conserving methods must be weighed against the negative consequences of increased patient dependence (Morris, 1982). The nurse recognizes also that what constitutes rest for one person may not constitute rest for another (Piper, 1986).

Effective energy utilization is needed to regenerate or maintain energy reserves. Activities should be encouraged to maintain and build on current levels of functioning (Morris, 1982). It is important for the nurse to teach patients to think about their energy stores as a bank. Deposits and withdrawals must be planned on a daily and weekly basis to ensure participation in valued activities. New goals or activities may need to be considered for those that no longer can be achieved (Morris, 1982).

Energy restoration can occur through efforts that conserve energy, promote energy expenditure (Morris, 1982), enhance nutritional status, and reduce the negative impact of physical and emotional stressors. In some patients, the goal to restore energy levels to pre-illness states may be unreasonable. Patients, nurses, and family members need to remember this to avoid setting unrealistic expectations or goals for themselves or others.

Interventions

Management of fatigue involves a wide range of nursing activities that span the treatment continuum, from preventing chronic fatigue (Kellum, 1985; Piper, 1986) and screening those who may be at high risk for it to tailoring therapies to fit the different etiologies and initiating referrals on the patient's behalf.

Unfortunately, no fatigue interventions that have been tested in cancer patients can be recommended to guide nursing practice at this time. Anecdotal and case study reports abound, particularly in the drug treatment realm. Clearly there is a need for nurses to test fatigue interventions once existing patterns of fatigue can be documented. Tables 58–6, 58–7, and 58–8 summarize data from the 11 best-designed studies that have investigated the effects of drug therapies, exercise, and rest on reports of subjective fatigue.

Five studies have examined the relationship between administered medications and fatigue (see Table 58–6); three have examined the relationship between exercise and fatigue; and three have addressed rest patterns. There is the suggestion from the MacVicar study that, at least in stage II breast cancer patients who are receiving chemotherapy, fatigue may be lessened by a supervised exercise program (MacVicar & Winningham, 1986).

Until additional studies can be conducted that test specific interventions in patients with cancer, those who have the disease may be our best teachers. Table 58–9 summarizes preliminary data on patient responses (Piper, Lindsey, Dodd, et al., 1989) to the question: "What do you believe most directly contributes to or causes your fatigue?" The responses are listed in descending order of frequency. Average respondents identified more than one reason for their fatigue. Changes in psychological patterns were the most common, with stress being the most frequent cause identified. This points out the importance of using the nursing strategies of therapeutic listening, counseling, and patient education to reduce anxiety and increase a patient's sense of control. One woman described how she avoided becoming unnecessarily fatigued by asking the receptionist to schedule tests only during the last 2 weeks of her treatment cycles when she was feeling better (Piper, 1987). This also gave her a sense of control, which is an important aspect of fatigue management (Kellum, 1985).

The nurse's role in controlling or preventing symp-

Table 58–6. DRUG STUDIES

Author(s) and Purpose	Subjects and Procedures	Major Findings
Ellis & Nassar, 1973		
To determine if injections of vitamin B_{12} improve the well-being and perception of tiredness in patients who are experiencing fatigue but do not have a deficiency of the vitamin.	14 patients and hospital staff with fatigue for which no organic cause could be found Crossover within subject design with random allocation of double-blind 5 mg hydroxycobalamin and placebo, both intramuscularly	All criteria including energy item showed a trend in favor of the B injections, but only improvement in well-being and happiness were statistically significant
Hicks, 1964		
To determine the effect of oral tablets of potassium and magnesium salts of aspartic acid on neuromuscular (chronic) fatigue, strength, and physical activity	145 office patients Double-blind study for 18 months, then code was broken	46% received Spartase (n = 66) 85% of these (n = 56) had a positive effect
McAdoo, Doering, Kraemer, Dessert, Brodie, & Hamburg, 1978		
To determine the effects of gonadotropin-releasing hormone (GNRH) given intravenously on human mood behavior, and other psychological parameters.	12 healthy male paid volunteers Double-blind random assignment design	There was a significant decrease in self-perceived fatigue and drowsiness as measured by the POMS and Aitkon scales apparent 6 hr after GNRH
Murray, 1985		
To characterize fatigue in multiple sclerosis patients and to evaluate the effects of various drug therapies on fatigue	40 patients were selected for the amantidine double-blind cross-over study; 32 completed the study (6 wk on the drug or placebo, followed by a 1-wk rest, followed by the drug or placebo)	Overall improvement was seen in 62.5% of patients on amantidine and 21.8% on placebo
Potempa, 1986		
To determine if perceptions of fatigue, rate of perceived exertion (RPE), and graded exercise performance differ among mildly hypertensive men.	19 stage I and II white male hypertensives	There were no significant differences between mean RPE scores from placebo to drug nor between drug treatment phases Fatigue subscale of the POMS did not appear valid or reliable for study
	Double-blind randomized cross-over design	Maximal exercise time did not vary significantly

toms related to medical therapies is important also. Skin reactions (see Table 58–9) and other symptoms, such as pain, shortness of breath, and headaches, were frequent causes of fatigue in these patients.

Table 58–10 summarizes patient responses, again in descending order of frequency, to a question asking what they did to relieve their fatigue (Piper & Dodd, 1987; Piper, Lindsey, & Dodd et al., 1989). Clearly, there is value in finding out what patients perceive will work for them. Distraction techniques included going to work, taking car rides, and listening to tapes or soft music.

One patient stated that chanting helped her to become distracted from her disease and other stressors that she experienced during the day. She would feel "re-energized" after these activities. Going to church sometimes had the same effect for her (Piper, 1987). Testing the efficacy of specific distraction therapies that have proven effective in pain patients on patients with fatigue is one approach to consider.

SPECIAL PROBLEMS RELATED TO FATIGUE

Quality of Life Issues

Fatigue can influence the quality of a person's life negatively by interfering in abilities to perform the kinds of activities and roles that give meaning and value to life. Chronically fatigued individuals may not have the same energy reserves that they once had. As a consequence, fewer activities are undertaken, and those that are performed may take longer to do and may require more effort. Because many of these changes can have negative effects on a person's life style and self-esteem, several quality-of-life instruments contain at least one item on fatigue (Frank-Stromborg, 1984; Grant, Padilla, Presant, Lipsett, & Runa, 1983).

Decreased Mobility

Fatigue can both result from and lead to decreased mobility and functional status (Davis, 1984). Prolonged inactivity and fatigue can cause decreased muscle strength, weakness, and loss of endurance. These changes can lead to a circular pattern of increased immobility, decreased activity tolerance, increased fatigue, and additional complications (Winningham, MacVicar, & Burke, 1986).

Decreased Self-Care

A person may become so fatigued and weak that performing the basic activities of daily living, such as

Table 58–7. EXERCISE STUDIES

Author(s) and Purpose	Subjects and Procedures	Major Findings
MacVicar & Winningham, 1986 Evaluate the effect of a progressive, 10 wk, 3 times/wk interval-training, cycle-ergometric exercise protocol on the physical and psychologic responses of breast cancer patients (functional capacity and mood states)	Ten women with breast cancer, receiving chemotherapy, without cardiovascular disease, and not on doxorubicin (Adriamycin)-containing regimens Six exercising, healthy, age-matched controls	Exercising cancer patients demonstrated increases in oxygen uptake, vigor-activity, and decreases in total mood disturbance scores Decreased fatigue scores were reported for the exercising groups; an increased score was reported in the nonexercising patient group
Pardue, 1984 Determine changes in fatigue and energy expenditure in chronic obstructive pulmonary disease patients who participate in a pulmonary rehabilitation program	82 chronic obstructive pulmonary disease patients 15-session, 5-wk outpatient course with classes held for 2 hr, 3 days/wk, consisting of didactic and practical applications (breathing, retraining, paced walking, individual exercise programs, energy conservation activities, relaxation training, etc.)	All subjects experienced significantly less fatigue following the rehabilitation program; the mean difference was greatest for the severe chronic obstructive pulmonary disease group and least for the moderate group Mental and physical symptoms were reported less frequently than were symptoms of general tiredness and decreased exercise tolerance; these symptoms improved as a result of the program
Thayer, 1987 To compare self-rated energy, tiredness, and tension effects of a common sugar snack versus a rapid 10-min walk	18 undergraduate students Random assignment of sugar snack (1.5 oz. candy) versus walk (10 min breathing deeply, swinging arms freely) over 12 experimental days in a 3-wk period of time	Majority of subjects felt increased energy for at least 20 min; less energy was perceived at 1 and 2 hr after eating a snack. Authors concluded that a 10-min rapid walk raises energy faster and to a greater degree than the sugar snack and avoids the unpleasant correlate of increased tension from the sugar snack

Table 58–8. REST STUDIES

Author(s) and Purpose	Subjects and Procedures	Major Findings
Altieri, 1984 Determine adequate rest periods after activities of daily living during the immediate post–myocardial infarction (MI) period	10 male MI patients 8–20 days after infarction ($\bar{x}$ = 13.5 days) Rest defined as the amount of time needed for 90% of the patients pressure rate product (peak systolic blood pressure × heart rate) to return to baseline	Adequate rest periods: After showering, 30.5 min After stair climbing, 7 min After walking, 10 min Showering required greater use of arm work than either stair climbing or walking; therefore greater blood pressure and heart rate changes were found with this activity, requiring a greater rest period for recovery
Bruya, 1981 Determine the effects of planned rest periods versus no planned rest periods following specific nursing care activities on intracranial pressure in intensive care unit patients	20 patients; 17 were male Mean age: 33 yr (males); 36 yr (females) 10 min of uninterrupted rest between nursing activities of vital signs, hyperventilation, suction, oral care, and bed, bath and hygiene routines for experimental group; 10 min of rest only after all three activities for control group	10-min rest periods did not effect intracranial pressure as anticipated; increased intracranial pressure was reported during the rest periods 10-min rest periods may be an insufficient time period to provide "rest" What constitutes rest needs to be determined, because rest may be more than simply being left alone
Daiss, Bertelson, & Benjamin, 1986 Investigate the effects of nap taking and resting on performance and mood	94 male and female university students in a sleep laboratory Habitual nappers and non-nappers (½–2 hr 3 times/wk) were randomly assigned to each of three groups: napping, resting in bed without falling asleep, or watching a neutral videotape (control group)	Sleep itself may not be the critical variable; rather the act of lying down and relaxing may help in decreasing negative affect Nap taking may provide an outlet for daily stress, which may influence mood states

Table 58–9. PERCEIVED CAUSES OF FATIGUE IN CANCER PATIENTS

Psychological Patterns	Sleep/Wake Patterns
• Stress	• Insomnia
• Worry	**Disease Patterns**
• Depression	• Cancer
• Anxiety	• Other
• Emotional strain	**Other Patterns**
Treatment Patterns	• Symptoms
• Radiation	• Environment
• Surgery	• Nutrition
• Chemotherapy	• Innate host factors
• Medical	
Activity/Rest Patterns	
• Work	
• Everyday activities	
• Hospital/RT travel	

(From Piper, B. F. [1989]. Fatigue: Current bases for practice. In S. G. Funk, E. M. Tornquist, M. T. Champagne, L. A. Copp, & R. A. Weise [Eds.], *Key aspects of comfort: Management of pain, fatigue, and nausea* [p. 196]. New York: Springer. Reproduced by permission.)

bathing, dressing, and eating, becomes too much of an effort without additional assistance from others. Helping people decide what is most important for them to do on their own can assist in maintaining independence and self-respect for as long as possible.

Social Isolation

As a person becomes increasingly more fatigued, the desire to engage in social activities and interactions declines. Increased physical dependence can lead to further declines in social activities, which can result in social isolation for both the patient and the family caregiver.

Role Changes and Family or Caregiver Fatigue

As chronic fatigue begins to alter what patients can do for themselves, family members or caregivers begin to assume many of the roles previously performed by patients. These increased physical and emotional demands on the family member can lead to caregiver role fatigue (Goldstein, Regnery, & Wellin, 1981).

Table 58–10. MEASURES USED BY CANCER PATIENTS TO RELIEVE FATIGUE

Activity/Rest Patterns	Sleep/Wake Patterns
• Rest	• Sleep
• Nap	**Other Patterns**
• Alter activities	• Nutritional
• Sit/lie down	• Environmental
• Read	• Social
• Walk/exercise	• Symptoms
Psychological Patterns	
• Distraction	
• Relaxation	

(From Piper, B. F. [1989]. Fatigue: Current bases for practice. In S. G. Funk, E. M. Tornquist, M. T. Champagne, L. A. Copp, & R. A. Weise [Eds.], *Key aspects of comfort: Management of pain, fatigue, and nausea* [p. 197]. New York: Springer. Reproduced by permission.)

Depression

As a result of the changes mentioned earlier, loss of self-esteem, depression, and loss of hope can occur. A person may not have the desire to fight the disease, participate in treatment, or go on living. Maintaining hope, fighting disease, and participating in treatment protocols take energy. For chronically fatigued individuals, it simply may take too much energy—energy that they may no longer have or want to expend—to go on living.

Negative Treatment and Disease Outcome

Three studies suggest that the presence of fatigue as measured by one subscale on the POMS (Levy, Herberman, Maluish, Schlien, & Lippman, 1985; Temoshok, 1987) or by one item on the Symptom Distress Scale (Kukell, McCorkle, & Driever, 1986) at diagnosis may predict a negative outcome in breast cancer (Levy et al., 1985), lung cancer (Kukell et al., 1986), and malignant melanoma patients (Temoshok, 1987). The POMS fatigue-inertia subscale scores predicted nodal status in breast cancer patients with a 71 per cent degree of accuracy (Levy et al., 1985); higher scores were associated also with an unfavorable outcome and shorter survival time in malignant melanoma patients (Temoshok, 1987). In lung cancer patients, increased fatigue and symptom distress scores were " . . . associated with an increased risk of death . . . [and] with a decreased probability of survival over time" (Kukell et al., 1986, p. 101). Although future studies are needed to validate these findings with repeated measures over time, nurses clearly need to recognize the importance of *early* recognition and treatment of acute fatigue before it becomes chronic fatigue.

SUMMARY

This chapter summarizes what is known about fatigue in patients with cancer to guide current nursing practice. Oncology nurses have a major role in recognizing and treating this pervasive, distressing, and perhaps life-threatening sensation. Much work needs to be done to document patterns of fatigue in specific cancer populations and to test various interventions. Only through a collaborative network of oncology nurses and nurse researchers can the care given to the chronically fatigued cancer patient be improved.

References

Akerstedt, T., Gillberg, M., & Witterberg, L. (1982). The circadian covariation of fatigue and urinary melatonin. *Biological Psychiatry, 17,* 547–554.

Alteri, C. A. (1984). The patient with myocardial infarction: Rest prescriptions for activities of daily living. *Heart and Lung, 13,* 355–360.

Arendt, D., Borbely, A. A., Franey, C., & Wright, J. (1984). The effects of chronic, small doses of melatonin given in the late afternoon on fatigue in man: A preliminary study. *Neuroscience Letters, 45*, 317–321.

Atkinson, H. (1985). *Women and fatigue.* New York: G. P. Putnam's Sons.

Axelrod, L., Halter, J. B., Cooper, D. S., Aoki, T. T., Roussell, A. M., & Bagshaw, S. L. (1983). Hormone levels and fuel flow in patients with weight loss and lung cancer. Evidence for excessive metabolic expenditure and for an adaptive response mediated by a reduced level of 3,5,3'-triiodothyronine. *Metabolism, 32*, 924–937.

Bartley, S. H., & Chute, E. (1947). *Fatigue and impairment in man.* New York: McGraw-Hill Book Co.

Brown, M. L., Carrieri, V., Janson-Bjerklie, S., & Dodd, M. J. (1986). Lung cancer and dyspnea: The patient's perception. *Oncology Nursing Forum, 13*(5), 19–24.

Bruera, E., Brenneis, C., Michaud, P. I., Jackson, R. N., & MacDonald, (1988). Muscle electrophysiology in patients with advanced breast cancer. *Journal of the National Cancer Institute, 80*, 282–285.

Bruya, M. A. (1981). Planned periods of rest in the intensive care unit: Nursing care activities and intracranial pressure. *Journal of Neurosurgical Nursing, 13*, 184–194.

Bukberg, J., Penman, D., & Holland, J. C. (1984). Depression in hospitalized cancer patients. *Psychosomatic Medicine, 46*, 199–212.

Burt, M. E., Aoki, T. T., Gorschboth, C. M., & Brennan, M. F. (1983). Peripheral tissue metabolism in cancer-bearing man. *Annals of Surgery, 198*, 685–691.

Burton, R. R. (1980). Human responses to repeated high G simulated aerial combat maneuvers. *Aviation, Space, and Environmental Medicine, 51*, 1185–1192.

Cameron, C. (1973). A theory of fatigue. *Ergonomics, 16*, 633–648.

Ciba Foundation Symposium 82. (1981). *Human muscle fatigue: Physiological mechanisms.* London: Pittman Medical.

Cimprich, B. (1990). Attentional fatigue in the cancer patient. *Oncology Nursing Forum, 17*(2, Suppl.), 218. (Abstract 321A)

Daiss, S. R., Bertelson, A. D., & Benjamin, L. T., Jr. (1986). Napping versus resting: Effects on performance and mood. *Psychophysiology, 23*, 82–88.

Davis, C. A. (1984). Interferon-induced fatigue. *Oncology Nursing Forum, 11*(Suppl.). (Abstract No. 72)

Edwards, R. H. T., Harris, R. C., Hultman, E., Kaijser, L., Koh, D., & Nordesjo, L. O. (1972). Effect of temperature on muscle energy metabolism and endurance during successive isometric contractions, sustained to fatigue, of the quadriceps muscle in man. *Journal of Physiology, 220*, 335–352.

Ellis, F. R., & Nasser, S. (1973). A pilot study of vitamin B12 in the treatment of tiredness. *British Journal of Nutrition, 30*, 277–283.

Engel, G. L., & Morgan, W. L. (1973). *Interviewing the patient.* Philadelphia: W. B. Saunders Co.

Fernsler, J. (1986). A comparison of patient and nurse perceptions of patients' self-care deficits associated with cancer chemotherapy. *Cancer Nursing, 9*, 50–57.

Fobair, P., Hoppe, R. T., Bloom, J., Cox, R., Varghese, A., & Spiegel, D. (1986). Psychosocial problems among survivors of Hodgkin's disease. *Journal of Clinical Oncology, 4*, 805–814.

Frank-Stromborg, M. (1984). Selecting an instrument to measure quality of life. *Oncology Nursing Forum, 11*(5), 88–91.

Frank-Stromborg, M., & Wright, P. (1984). Ambulatory cancer patients' perception of the physical and psychosocial changes in their lives since the diagnosis of cancer. *Cancer Nursing, 7*, 117–130.

Freel, M. I., & Hart, L. K. (1977). *Study of fatigue phenomena of multiple sclerosis patients* (USDHEW Grant No. 5R02-NU-00524-02). University of Iowa: Division of Nursing.

Gibson, H., & Edwards, R. H. T. (1985). Muscular exercise and fatigue. *Sports Medicine, 2*, 120–132.

Gold, J. (1974). Cancer cachexia and gluconeogenesis. *Annals of the New York Academy of Sciences, 230*, 103–110.

Goldstein, V., Regnery, G., & Wellin, E. (1981). Caretaker role fatigue. *Nursing Outlook, 29*, 24–30.

Grandjean, E. P. (1970). Fatigue. *American Industrial Hygiene Association Journal, 30*, 401–411.

Grant, M. M., Padilla, G. V., Presant, C., Lipsett, J., & Runa, P. (1983). *Proceedings of the Fourth National Conference on Cancer Nursing.* New York: American Cancer Society.

Hart, L. K. (1978). Fatigue in the patient with multiple sclerosis. *Research in Nursing & Health, 1*, 147–157.

Hauri, P., Silverfarb, P., Oxman, T., & O'Leary, P. (1985). Sleep in cancer patients. *Sleep Research, 14*, 237. (Abstract)

Haylock, P. J., & Hart, L. K. (1979). Fatigue in patients receiving localized radiation. *Cancer Nursing, 2*, 461–467.

Heuting, J. E., & Sarphati, H. R. (1966). Measuring fatigue. *Journal of Applied Physiology, 50*, 535–538.

Hicks, J. T. (1964). Treatment of fatigue in general practice: A double blind study. *Clinical Medicine, 71*, 85–90.

Jamar, S. C. (1989). Fatigue in women receiving chemotherapy for ovarian cancer. In S. G. Funk, E. M. Tornquist, M. T. Champagne, L. A. Copp & R. A. Weise (Eds.), *Key aspects of comfort: Management of pain, fatigue and nausea* (pp. 224–228). New York: Springer.

Karlsson, J., Sjodin, B., Jacobs, I., & Kaiser, P. (1981). Relevance of muscle fiber type to fatigue in short intense and prolonged exercise in man. In Ciba Foundation Symposium 82, *Human muscle fatigue: Physiological mechanisms* (pp. 59–74). London: Pittman Medical.

Kellum, M. D. (1985). Fatigue. In M. M. Jacobs & W. Geels (Eds.), *Signs and symptoms in nursing: Interpretation and management* (pp. 103–118). Philadelphia: J. B. Lippincott Co.

King, K. B., Nail, L. M., Kreamer, K., Strohl, R. A., & Johnson, J. E. (1985). Patients' descriptions of the experience of receiving radiation therapy. *Oncology Nursing Forum, 12*(4), 55–61.

Kinsman, R. A., & Weiser, P. C. (1976). Subjective symptomatology during work and fatigue. In E. Simonson & P. C. Weiser (Eds.), *Psychological aspects and physiological correlates of work and fatigue* (pp. 336–405). Springfield, IL: Charles C. Thomas.

Kobashi-Schoot, J. A. M., Hanewald, G. J. F. P., Van Dam, F. S. A. M., & Bruning, P. F. (1985). Assessment of malaise in cancer patients treated with radiotherapy. *Cancer Nursing, 8*, 306–313.

Kogi, K., Saito, Y., & Mitsuhashi, T. (1970). Validity of three components of subjective fatigue feelings. *Journal of the Science of Labor, 46*, 251–270.

Komoike, Y., & Horiguchi, S. (1971). Fatigue assessment on key punch operators, typists, and others. *Ergonomics, 14*, 101–109.

Kukell, W. A., McCorkle, R., & Driever, M. (1986). Symptom distress, psychosocial variables, and survival from lung cancer. *Journal of Psychosocial Oncology, 4*(1/2), 91–104.

Levine, M. E. (1973). *Introduction to clinical nursing* (2nd ed.). Philadelphia: F. A. Davis Co.

Levy, S. M., Herberman, R. B., Maluish, A. M., Schlien, B., & Lippman, M. (1985). Prognostic risk assessment in primary breast cancer by behavioral and immunological parameters. *Health Psychology, 4*, 99–113.

MacVicar, M. G., & Winningham, M. L. (1986). Promoting functional capacity of cancer patients. *The Cancer Bulletin, 38*, 235–239.

Malmquist, R., Ekholm, I., Lindstrom, L., Petersen, I., & Örtengren, R. (1981). Measurement of localized muscle fatigue in building work. *Ergonomics, 24*, 695–709.

McAdoo, B. C., Doering, C. H., Kraemer, H. C., Dessert, N., Brodie, H. K. H., & Hamburg, D. A. (1978). A study of the effects of gonadotropin-releasing hormone on human mood and behavior. *Psychosomatic Medicine, 40*, 199–209.

McCorkle, R., & Young, K. (1978). Development of a symptom distress scale. *Cancer Nursing, 1*, 373–377.

McFarland, R. A. (1971). Understanding fatigue in modern life. *Ergonomics, 14*, 1–10.

McNair, D. M., Lorr, M., & Droppleman, L. F. (1971). *Profile of mood states.* San Diego: Education and Industrial Testing Service.

Meleis, A. I. (1986). Theory development and domain concepts. In P. Moccia (Ed.), *New approaches to theory development* (p. 6). New York: National League for Nursing.

Meyerwitz, B. E., Watkins, I. K., & Sparks, F. C. (1983). Quality of life for breast cancer patients receiving adjuvant chemotherapy. *American Journal of Nursing, 83*, 232–235.

Miller, R. G., Boska, M. D., Moussaui, R. S., Carson, P. J., & Weiner, M. W. (1988). ^{31}P nuclear magnetic resonance studies of high energy phosphates and pH in human muscle fatigue: Comparison of aerobic and anaerobic exercise. *Journal of Clinical Investigation, 81*, 1190–1196.

Morris, M. L. (1982). Tiredness and fatigue. In C. M. Norris (Ed.), *Concept clarification in nursing* (pp. 263–275). Rockville, MD: Aspen Systems Corporation.

Muncie, W. (1941). Chronic fatigue. *Psychosomatic Medicine, 3,* 277–285.

Murray, T. J. (1985). Amantidine therapy for fatigue in multiple sclerosis. *Le Journal Canadien Des Sciences Neurologiques, 12,* 251–254.

Musci, E. (1983). *Relationship between family coping strategies and self-care during cancer chemotherapy.* Unpublished doctoral dissertation, University of California, San Francisco, School of Nursing.

Nakamura, Y., & Schwartz, S. (1972). The influence of hydrogen ion concentration on calcium binding and release by skeletal muscle sarcoplasmic reticulum. *Journal of General Physiology, 59,* 22–32.

Nerenz, D. R., Leventhal, H., & Love, R. R. (1982). Factors contributing to emotional distress during cancer chemotherapy. *Cancer, 50,* 1020–1027.

Norris, C. M. (1982). Synthesis of concepts: Evolving an umbrella concept-protection. In C. M. Norris (Ed.), *Concept clarification in nursing* (pp. 385–403). Rockville, MD: Aspen Systems.

Pardue, N. H. (1984). *Energy expenditure and subjective fatigue of chronic obstructive pulmonary disease patients before and after a pulmonary rehabilitation.* Unpublished doctoral dissertation, Catholic University, Washington, DC.

Pearson, R. G. (1957). Scale analysis of a fatigue checklist. *Journal of Applied Psychology, 41,* 186–191.

Pearson, R. G., & Byars, G. E. (1956). *The development and validation of a checklist for measuring subjective fatigue* (pp. 56–115). Randolph AFB, TX: Texas School of Aviation Medicine, USAF.

Petty, F., & Noyes, R., Jr. (1981). Depression secondary to cancer. *Biological Psychiatry, 16,* 1203–1221.

Piper, B. F. (1986). Fatigue. In V. K. Carrieri, A. M. Lindsey, & C. W. West (Eds.), *Pathophysiological phenomena in nursing: Human responses to illness* (pp. 219–234). Philadelphia: W. B. Saunders Co.

Piper, B. F. (1987). [Perceptions of fatigue in cancer patients who are receiving radiation and chemotherapy: A qualitative study]. University of California, San Francisco, School of Nursing. Unpublished S214A data.

Piper, B. F. (1988). Fatigue in cancer patients: Current perspectives on measurement and management. Fifth National Conference on Cancer Nursing. *Monograph on nursing management of common problems: State of the art.* New York: American Cancer Society.

Piper, B. F. (1989). Fatigue: Current bases for practice. In S. G. Funk, E. M. Tornquist, M. T. Champagne, L. A. Copp, & R. A. Wiese (Eds.), *Key aspects of comfort: Management of pain, fatigue and nausea* (pp. 187–198). New York: Springer.

Piper, B. F., & Dodd, M. J. (1987). [Fatigue analysis of chemotherapy and radiation therapy self-care behavior logs]. University of California, School of Nursing, Department of Physiological Nursing. Unpublished data.

Piper, B. F., Friedman, L., Hartigan, K., Post, B., Smith, J., Coleman, C. A., Gilman, N., Dodd, M. J., Lindsey, A. M., & Paul, S. (in review). Fatigue in women with breast cancer receiving chemotherapy.

Piper, B. F., Lindsey, A. M., & Dodd, M. J. (1987). Fatigue mechanisms in cancer patients: Developing nursing theory. *Oncology Nursing Forum, 14*(6), 17–23.

Piper, B. F., Lindsey, A. M., Dodd, M. J., Ferketich, S., Paul, S. M., & Weller, S. (1989). The development of an instrument to measure the subjective dimension of fatigue. In S. G. Funk, E. M. Tornquist, M. T. Champagne, L. A. Copp, & R. A. Weise (Eds.), *Key aspects of comfort: Management of pain, fatigue and nausea* (pp. 199–208). New York: Springer.

Piper, B. F., Rieger, P. T., Brophy, L., Haeuber, D., Hood, L. E., Lyver, A. & Sharp, E. (1989). Recent advances in the management of biotherapy-related side effects: Fatigue. *Oncology Nursing Forum, 16*(Suppl.).6, 27–34.

Poteliakhoff, A. (1981). Adrenocortical activity and some clinical findings in acute and chronic fatigue. *Journal of Psychosomatic Research, 25,* 91–95.

Potempa, K., Lopez, M., Reid, C., & Lawson, L. (1986). Chronic fatigue. *Image, 18,* 165–169.

Proctor, S. J., Kernahan, J., & Taylor, P. (1981). Depression as component of post-cranial irradiation somnolence syndrome [Letter to the editor]. *The Lancet, 1,* 1215–1216.

Putt, A. M. (1977). Effects of noise on fatigue in healthy middle-aged adults. *Communicating Nursing Research, 8,* 24–34.

Rieger, P. T. (1987). Interferon-induced fatigue: A study of fatigue measurement. Sigma Theta Tau International 29th Biennial Convention Book of Proceedings. (Abstract A163)

Rennie, M. J., Johnson, R. H., Park, D. M., & Sularman, W. R. (1973). Inappropriate fatigue during exercise associated with high blood lactates. *Clinical Science, 45,* 5.

Rhodes, V. A., & Watson, P. M. (1987). Symptom distress—the concept: Past and present. *Seminars in Oncology Nursing, 3,* 242–247.

Rhodes, V. A., Watson, P. M., & Hanson, B. M. (1988). Patients' descriptions of the influence of tiredness and weakness on self-care abilities. *Cancer Nursing, 11,* 186–194.

Rhodes, V. A., Watson, P. M., & Johnson, M. H. (1984). Development of reliable and valid measures of nausea and vomiting. *Cancer Nursing, 6,* 33–41.

Rhoten, D. (1982). Fatigue and the postsurgical patient. In C. M. Norris (Ed.), *Concept clarification in nursing* (pp. 277–300). Rockville, MD: Aspen Systems.

Riddle, P. K. (1982). Chronic fatigue and women: A description and suggested treatment. *Women and Health, 7,* 37–47.

Roberts, D., & Smith, D. J. (1989). Biochemical aspects of peripheral muscle fatigue. *Sports Medicine, 7,* 125–138.

Rockwell, D. A., & Burr, B. D. (1977). The tired patient. *Journal of Family Practice, 5,* 853–857.

Rose, E. A., & King, T. C. (1978). Understanding postoperative fatigue. *Surgery, Gynecology, and Obstetrics, 147,* 97–101.

Saito, Y., Kogi, K., & Kashiwagi, S. (1970). Factors underlying subjective feelings of fatigue. *Journal of Science and Labour, 46,* 205–224.

Spross, J. A. (1987). Fatigue. In S. B. Baird (Ed.), *Decision making in oncology nursing* (pp. 76–77). Philadelphia: B. C. Decker.

Stewart, D. J., Maroun, J. A., Lefebvre, B., & Heringer, R. (1986). Neurotoxicity and efficacy of combined vinca alkaloids in breast cancer. *Cancer Treatment Reports, 70,* 571–573.

Straus, S. E., Tosato, G., Armstrong, G., Lawley, T., Preble, O. T., Henle, W., Davey, R., Pearson, G., Epstein, J., Brus, I., & Blaese, M. (1985). Persisting illness and fatigue in adults with evidence of Epstein-Barr virus infection. *Annals of Internal Medicine, 102,* 7–16.

Temoshok, L. (1987). In Consultation: Discussion of psychosocial factors related to outcome in cutaneous malignant melanoma: A matched samples design. *Oncology News/Update, 2*(3), 6–7.

Thayer, R. E. (1987). Energy, tiredness, and tension effects of a sugar snack versus moderate exercise. *Journal of Personality and Social Psychology, 52,* 119–125.

Valdini, A. F. (1985). Fatigue of unknown etiology—a review. *Family Practice, 2,* 48–53.

Varrichio, C. G. (1985). Selecting a tool for measuring fatigue. *Oncology Nursing Forum, 12*(4), 122–123; 126–127.

Waskerwitz, M. J., & Leonard, M. (1986). Early detection of malignancy: From birth to twenty years. *Oncology Nursing Forum, 13*(1), 50–57.

Wickham, R., Blesch, K., Paice, J., Harte, N., Barry, S., Purl, S., Mooney, M., Cahill, M., Kopp, P. & Manson, S. (1990). *Oncology Nursing Forum, 17*(2 Suppl.), 146. (Abstract 35A)

Winningham, M. L., MacVicar, M. G., & Burke, C. A. (1986). Exercise for cancer patients: Guidelines and precautions. *The Physician and Sportsmedicine, 14,* 125–134.

Wittenborn, J. R., & Buhler, R. (1979). Somatic discomforts among depressed women. *Archives of General Psychiatry, 36,* 465–471.

Yoshitake, H. (1969). Rating the feelings of fatigue. *Journal of the Science of Labour, 45,* 422–432.

Yoshitake, H. (1971). Relations between the symptoms and the feeling of fatigue. *Ergonomics, 14,* 175–186.

Yoshitake, H. (1978). Three characteristic patterns of subjective fatigue symptoms. *Ergonomics, 21,* 231–233.

COMMUNICATION, COLLABORATION, AND EDUCATION

CHAPTER **59**

Interpersonal Communication Systems

LAUREL L. NORTHOUSE
PETER G. NORTHOUSE

Communication is a major concern for individuals living with cancer. These individuals have reported communication problems with health professionals (McIntosh, 1974; Mitchell & Glicksman, 1977) and with significant others, such as family and friends (Gordon et al., 1977; Hinton, 1981; Peters-Golden, 1982). To cope with the disease, patients must be able to communicate effectively with nurses, physicians, family, friends, and others who are important to them. Communication is an essential element in the overall treatment process and the critical factor in helping patients maintain productive relationships (Brewin, 1977; Cooper, 1982; Harker, 1972).

This chapter provides information that will help nurses understand and improve their ability to communicate with patients who have cancer. It begins with a discussion about the importance of communication in cancer nursing, and then provides a theoretic orientation to nurse-patient communication. The final section analyzes several specific communication concerns that confront patients and nurses during the cancer experience.

Given the importance of communication for nurses and patients, this chapter attempts to answer the following questions: What are the central elements of effective communication in the oncology setting? What obstacles between nurses and patients make effective communication difficult? How can oncology nurses become aware of patients' communication concerns and thereby help them adjust to their illness? What communication strategies can be used to enhance the effectiveness of nurse-patient communication?

THE IMPORTANCE OF COMMUNICATION IN CANCER NURSING

Evidence is accumulating that effective interpersonal relationships help people cope with cancer. Investigators have reported that supportive interpersonal relationships are associated with better survival rates (Weisman & Worden, 1975), higher levels of psychosocial adjustment (Bloom, 1982; Northouse, 1988; Vachon, 1986), and fewer fears of recurrence (Northouse, 1981). Within supportive relationships, communication plays a major role in helping patients cope with the effects of cancer. Through effective communication with others, patients disclose feelings, ventilate fears, and assert control in areas related to their illness.

Although interpersonal relationships are important during the cancer experience, patients have reported difficulty communicating with others about their illness. The majority of breast cancer patients in a study by Peters-Golden (1982) reported that their interactions with others became strained after the cancer diagnosis; they often felt misunderstood, received false optimism, and were avoided. Gordon and colleagues (1977) found that the lack of open family communication was a major problem cited by a sample of 136 cancer patients. Similarly, Meyerowitz, Watkins, and Sparks (1983) found that patients who were receiving adjuvant chemotherapy for breast cancer reported conflicts and negative changes in their relationships with family and friends. Cancer patients also have reported that communicating with health professionals is a problem (Quint, 1963). In one study, nearly half the patients said they did not discuss their problems with a nurse (Frank-Stromborg & Wright, 1984). Among the reasons given by patients for limited nurse-patient communication were a general lack of contact with nurses and the perception that nurses were "too busy."

Although effective communication is important to patients with cancer, it is equally important to oncology nurses. Many of the nurse's daily activities require effective communication. Obtaining accurate information, providing health education, answering questions, and giving support to patients are just a few of the many nursing activities that are communication intensive. In addition, the nurse frequently serves as a patient advocate or as an intermediary with other professionals. Interacting with family members is yet another activity that requires effective interpersonal communication on the part of oncology nurses.

Although nurses recognize the importance of communication in nursing care, they often have difficulty engaging in effective therapeutic communication with patients. One major problem confronting them is that they have little time to simply interact and "be with" clients. Typically, their supportive communications must be abbreviated and fit in between many other physical tasks that occur simultaneously. In addition, they sometimes lack the communication skills necessary to deal with the complex interpersonal issues that arise during the cancer experience. Perhaps it is not surprising that oncology nurses have reported the need for further education in communication (Craytor, Brown, & Marrow, 1978).

A THEORETICAL ORIENTATION TO NURSE-PATIENT COMMUNICATION

Before discussing the specific communication concerns of nurses and patients with cancer, it is important to clarify exactly what communication means and to describe the theoretic assumptions that underlly the communication process.

Interpersonal Communication Defined

Communication in oncology nursing settings is a complex and multifaceted process. Although the word *communication* is used often in a general way to describe a variety of events, it actually refers to an identifiable process that has specific characteristics. Because language is something people learn when they are young, they believe wrongly that effective communication is a simple, easily performed, straightforward process. In fact, effective communication is just the opposite; it is a process that demands a great deal of skill.

Interpersonal communication is the process whereby two individuals interact and share information according to a common set of rules (Northouse & Northouse, 1985). The process occurs through the use of symbolic behavior—through language. It is an ongoing process, and it involves human attitudes and feelings as well as information. Interactions between the patient with cancer and the nurse take place on many levels, including verbal and nonverbal, intentional and unintentional, content-oriented and relationship-oriented, nondirective and goal-directed, and humorous and serious. In a sense, interpersonal communication is the vehicle that connects nurse and patient. It allows them to express their thoughts and feelings with each other and to collaborate in meeting goals.

Assumptions about Interpersonal Communication

In studying how people communicate with each other, researchers have found that several general properties form the basis for the fundamental assumptions of human communication (Berlo, 1960; Knapp & Miller, 1985; Watzlawick, Beavin, & Jackson, 1967). These assumptions govern as well as explain communication that occurs in the oncology setting.

Assumption One: Interpersonal Communication Is a Process

To many people, the word *communication* triggers an image of one person sending a message to another person. This image is based on a linear approach to communication, which has also been referred to as the "hypodermic needle" model of communication; that is, person A instills a message into person B (Fig. 59–1). Communication is unidirectional, with one person directly influencing a second person through the use of specific messages. One problem with the linear approach is that it is too restrictive. Communication is more than a simple, one-way, or linear event; it is an ongoing, continuous, dynamic, and ever-changing process.

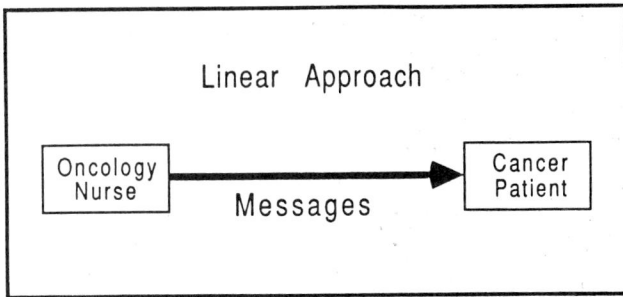

Figure 59–1. Linear approach to nurse-patient communication.

The assumption that communication is a process is an important one, because it emphasizes the complexity of interpersonal communication in the oncology setting. The assumption directs individuals to analyze factors that affect the nurse as well as the patient and to examine how the ongoing interchange between the two will vary, depending on the nature of their relationship and the situation. During communication, the communication skills, attitudes, knowledge, social system, and culture of both the nurse and the patient influence the interaction simultaneously. Analysis of the impact of a single message created by one person and sent to another is important; however, analysis of communication as a process is even more important, because it provides a richer understanding of how messages interact with and are mediated by many other variables involved in the communication process.

Assumption Two: Interpersonal Communication Is Transactional

To say communication is transactional means that both individuals in an interaction affect and are affected by each other. Communication involves reciprocal influence; each individual is both a source and a receiver at the same time. While constructing a message for a patient, the nurse is receiving cues simultaneously from the patient that influence how the message is formulated. A transactional approach emphasizes the simultaneous interplay between the sender and receiver of a message (Fig. 59–2).

From a transactional perspective, each individual perceives the other in the context of what occurs in the interaction. For example, if a nurse chooses to be

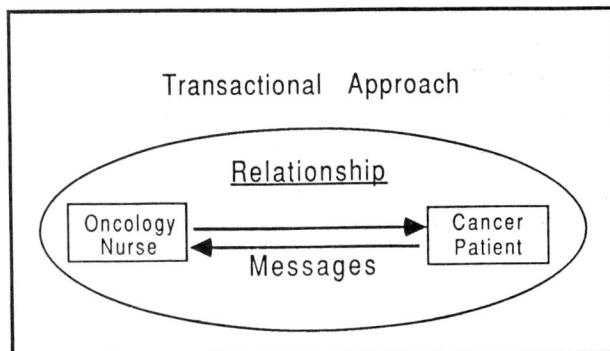

Figure 59–2. Transactional approach to nurse-patient communication.

dominant with a patient, it may be because the nurse desires to be dominant in general, or it may be because the nurse picks up cues from the patient indicating a preference to be submissive. In other words, the nature of the interaction can be influenced by the desires of the nurse or the patient, by each person's perceptions of the other person's desires, or by both factors working together simultaneously.

In the oncology setting, the transactional assumption helps explain the unique relationship that a nurse establishes with each patient. Each nurse brings a different set of experiences into the oncology setting, and these experiences influence the type of relationships the nurse develops with patients. Similarly, each patient experiences cancer in a unique way, which has a significant effect on the kinds of relationships the patient wants to have with health care staff. Therefore, the communication patterns that develop are constructed mutually by nurse and patient.

Assumption Three: Interpersonal Communication Is Multidimensional

When interpersonal communication takes place, it occurs on primarily two levels; that is, it is multidimensional. One level can be characterized as the *content dimension,* the other, as the *relationship dimension* (Watzlawick, Beavin, & Jackson, 1967). In interpersonal communication, these two dimensions are inextricably bound together. The content dimension of communication refers to the words, language, and information in a message; the relationship dimension refers to the aspect of a message that defines how participants in an interaction are connected to each other.

To illustrate the content and relationship dimensions, consider the following hypothetical statement made by a patient with cancer to a nurse: "Please change my nausea medication. The drug I've been taking isn't working." The *content* dimension of the message refers to the patient's desire to have the medication changed. The *relationship* dimension refers to how the patient and the nurse are affiliated. It includes the patient's attitude toward the nurse, the nurse's attitude toward the patient, and their feelings about each other. It is the relationship dimension that implicitly suggests how the content dimension should be interpreted, because the content alone can be interpreted in many ways. The exact meaning of the message emerges for the nurse and patient as a result of their interaction. If a caring relationship exists between the two, the nurse will probably interpret the content ("Please change my nausea medication. The drug I've been taking isn't working.") as a helpful suggestion from a patient who wants to be involved in his or her own care. However, if the relationship between the nurse and the patient is distant or strained, the nurse may interpret the content of the message as an inappropriate suggestion by an uninformed patient. These two interpretations illustrate how the meaning of a message is not in words alone but in how the giver and the receiver interpret the message in the context of their relationship.

In oncology settings, the implication of this assumption is that nurses need to be aware of *how* they communicate with patients in addition to *what* they communicate. In a study of helpful and unhelpful communication in cancer care, Thorne (1988) found that unhelpful communication was associated with a lack of concern toward the patient on the part of the nurse or physician. Because of the uncertain and threatening nature of cancer, it is important for health care providers to establish supportive and nurturing relationships with patients (McCorkle, 1981). Communicating both positive and negative information successfully is easier in the context of a caring relationship. For example, when telling patients about the possibility of adverse side effects of a certain chemotherapy regimen, nurses need to be sensitive to how they provide the information. The better the relationship between nurse and patient, the less threatening the information is likely to be to the patient. In other words, communication is more likely to be effective if the nurse pays equal attention to the content and the relationship dimensions of the message.

Before leaving the discussion of the multidimensionality of interpersonal communication, some attention needs to be given to the contribution of its nonverbal dimensions. Some investigators have estimated that 65 to 70 per cent of the meaning in a message is transmitted nonverbally (Birdwhistell, 1970); others have estimated that more than 90 per cent of the meaning of a message is accounted for by nonverbal aspects (Mehrabian, 1971). Nonverbal communication is relevant especially in the oncology setting, because patients and family members pay close attention to the nonverbal expressions of health care professionals to supplement the verbal communication they receive. In addition, patients commonly believe that important information is often "leaked" through nonverbal channels (Friedman, 1979); therefore, patients often scrutinize health care staff carefully to determine whether they are being completely honest. In addition to providing information, nonverbal communication such as touch, can provide patients with psychosocial support. McCorkle and Hollenbach (1983) reported that touch had a positive effect on the self-concept, level of depression, and overall hospital stay of patients undergoing a bone marrow transplant. Hospital staff, on the other hand, rely heavily on patients' nonverbal cues to assess their needs accurately. These cues help staff members interpret and validate the verbal messages patients express.

COMMUNICATION ISSUES CONFRONTING NURSES AND PATIENTS IN CANCER CARE

In attempting to understand communication issues in nurse-patient relationships, it is important to assess these issues from the perspectives of both patient and nurse, because each brings a unique set of concerns to the relationship. An analysis of the research literature suggests that, for patients, the major communication issues are related to maintaining a sense of control, seeking information, disclosing feelings, and searching for meaning (Northouse & Northouse, 1987), whereas the primary communication issues for nurses center on imparting information, communicating hope, and dealing with emotions.

Issues Confronting Patients

Maintaining a Sense of Control

The single most important problem confronting cancer patients is loss of control (Byrne, Stockwell, & Gudelis, 1984; Fiore, 1979; Maguire, 1985; Northouse & Wortman, 1990; Schmale et al., 1983; Speigel, 1979; Trillin, 1981)—a feeling of powerlessness resulting from the inability to predict or have an impact on events surrounding the illness. Control issues are pronounced for cancer patients because of the clinical dimensions of the disease. Cancer carries with it a high degree of uncertainty about its cause, diagnosis, treatment, and prognosis. Patients in remission experience uncertainty about the possibility of recurrence (Harker, 1972; Mullan, 1984; Northouse, 1981; Peters-Golden, 1982; Schmale et al., 1983). In addition, the impact of the uncertainty is heightened, because cancer is often regarded as more threatening than other diseases (Brewin, 1977; Mishel, Hostetter, King, & Graham, 1984; Peters-Golden, 1982).

What are the implications of the control issue for patients' communication needs? Foremost is their need to experience an interpersonal environment that is predictable. They need contexts that allow them to regain a sense of communication competence. By promoting consistent patterns of interaction with patients, nurses can enhance patients' sense of control. Patients who are communicated with and treated in predictable ways will feel more competent about how they are handling their illness. Allowing a patient to communicate with the same nurse over the course of illness is one way of enhancing patients' sense of control. Similarly, attempts to establish routine procedures so that the same ones are followed with patients during repeated visits (e.g., taking temperatures, weighing patients, drawing blood) fosters a sense of stability. The purpose of such efforts is to give patients a sense of mastery over their environment.

In addition to providing a predictable environment, nurses can help patients gain a sense of personal control over their own internal response to the illness experience by communicating in ways that help patients to preserve a reasonable degree of emotional balance and to prepare for an uncertain future (Moos & Tsu, 1977). Although patients may not be able to control their illness, they can control, or have an impact on, their response to the illness through the messages, and therefore meanings, they give themselves about their circumstances. Nurses contribute to these meanings through their interactions with patients. For example, a newly diagnosed cancer patient expressed great relief when a nurse told him that it was normal to have irrational reactions to the diagnosis of cancer. This information confirmed for the patient that events were not out of control—that he was still in charge of what was happening.

Another aspect of control that is important for nurses to consider is that cancer patients wish to have a sense of control in their relationships with health care providers, family members, and others. Some patients want to be dominant toward providers; others want providers to be dominant. Both perspectives indicate a desire to influence the provider-patient relationship. One major way that patients influence such relationships is to control their communication with others. By controlling what they talk about and how they talk about it, they may feel more in control of their relationships. For example, a patient may want to talk about the illness in a special way and, to that end, may force others to adapt to these expectations. Similarly, patients may want family members to play certain specific roles toward them and, as a result, communicate in ways that get family members to exhibit these roles. In other words, some patients attempt to satisfy their need for control by trying to control others.

Each patient is different, and each has an individual way of communicating. The challenge for nurses is to communicate with each patient in a way that gives the patient a sense of control. Above all, nurses must respond to patients in ways that allow patients to set the pace for the communication.

Obtaining Information

In the last three decades, dramatic shifts have occurred in the amount of information providers give patients with cancer. In the early 1960s, physicians often did not inform these patients of their diagnosis (Oken, 1961); by the late 1970s, this pattern had been reversed (Novack et al., 1979). Despite this shift toward more open communication, however, acquiring sufficient medical information remains a primary concern for patients with cancer (Morrow, Hoaglund, & Carpenter, 1983).

Obtaining information is important for patients who have cancer because it reduces their uncertainty concerning the illness. It gives them a framework for interpreting life-threatening events (Janis, 1958) and helps them feel that their responses to the uncertainties surrounding the illness are reasonable and normal (Buckalew, 1982; Dunkel-Schetter & Wortman, 1982). Waitzkin and Stoeckle (1972) go so far as to say that communicating information about illness can improve patients' physiologic and psychological responses to therapy.

Given that information is important for patients, the following questions frequently confront oncology nurses: How much information do patients want? What kind of information is most important to them? When is it appropriate not to give information? Obviously,

there are no easy or completely correct answers to these questions.

Cassileth and her associates (1980) studied the amount of information preferred by patients with cancer and found that most patients wanted maximum amounts of information. Those who sought detailed information tended to be younger, better educated, and more recently diagnosed than patients who avoided information (Box 59–1). Other investigators have corroborated the finding that age is the critical factor in the amount of information desired (Derdiarian, 1986; Hopkins, 1986).

The kind of information patients want has been of interest to researchers also. Derdiarian (1986, 1987) studied the information needs of patients with cancer in four categories: disease, personal, family, and social. Of these four types of information, patients gave the highest rank to the need for information about the disease. They were interested especially in obtaining information about treatments and prognosis. The importance of disease-related information to patients with cancer was reported also by Cassileth and colleagues (1980), who found that more than 50 per cent of the patients in their study wanted information about the side effects of treatments, treatment outcomes, the extent of disease, the potential for cure, and their day-to-day progress.

Although patients usually perceive information as beneficial, some investigators have expressed the concern that information can disrupt mechanisms of denial and lead to loss of hope and depression (Bloom, Ross, & Burnell, 1978; Brewin, 1977; Kellerman, Rigler, Siegel, & Katz, 1980; McIntosh, 1974; Weisman & Worden, 1976), especially in patients who have extensive cancer. For example, Hopkins (1986) found that patients with advanced cancer sought less information than did patients with more limited disease, and she attributed this difference to the protective defense of avoidance. Similar results were reported by Gotay

---

Box 59–1. PATIENTS' INFORMATION PREFERENCES

This study examined the attitudes of 256 patients with cancer about their information and participation preferences in health care decisions. Patients completed the Information Styles Questionnaire and the Beck Hopelessness Scale. Results indicated that patients who wanted to participate in treatment decisions were younger and better educated than those who wanted medical staff to make treatment decisions. In addition, patients who wanted as much information as possible about their illness were significantly younger than those who wanted minimal or only positive information. Furthermore, patients who preferred active involvement in their care and who wanted as much information as possible were more hopeful than patients who preferred less involvement and less information.

(Reproduced, with permission, from: Cassileth, B. R., Zupkis, R. Y., Sutton-Smith, K., & March, Y. [1980]. Information and participation preferences among cancer patients. *Annals of Internal Medicine, 92,* 832–836.)

(1984), who compared groups of early- and late-stage cancer patients and their mates and found that information seeking was a more common coping mechanism in the early-stage group. Patients with advanced cancer used avoidance and denial relatively often. Because information can function both positively and negatively for patients, the challenge for oncology nurses is to assess each patient's unique needs for information and attempt to provide the amount and kind of information that will be most effective for that patient.

Disclosing Feelings

Another communication issue of concern to patients with cancer is self-disclosure, the process whereby one individual communicates personal information, thoughts, and feelings to others. Disclosing feelings is of critical importance for several reasons (Silver & Wortman, 1980). First, it allows catharsis, the draining of emotional tension and anxiety that often accompanies a cancer diagnosis. Second, it allows patients to receive feedback from others that their reactions to cancer are normal, which in turn lessens anxiety and tension associated with these reactions. Third, it facilitates problem solving and enables patients to view their situation from a more meaningful perspective.

Although disclosing feelings appears to help patients adjust to their illness, often they feel inhibited (Spiegel, 1979). For example, in a study of 256 patients with cancer, only 52 per cent of the patients told their friends and neighbors about the diagnosis; 32 per cent had told only their most intimate friends; and 16 per cent did not reveal the diagnosis to friends (Cassileth et al., 1980). In a study of patients undergoing radiation therapy, the majority of the patients reported that they wished they could discuss their situation more openly with someone (Mitchell & Glicksman, 1977).

Disclosure is often a problem for patients because other people may avoid them or prefer not to discuss sensitive illness-related issues with them. In a study by Byrne, Stockwell, and Gudelis (1984), adolescent patients reported that their friends stayed away after hearing about the diagnosis. Similarly, 52 per cent of the breast cancer patients in Peters-Golden's study (1982) said that others avoided them. The patients who did discuss the illness with others reported that the interactions were frequently uncomfortable. When others tried to cheer them up, this forced cheerfulness often made the patients feel less normal and hindered them from revealing their true feelings (Box 59–2).

What strategies can nurses and other health professionals use to help cancer patients disclose their feelings? First, they need to assess and adapt to each patient's unique preferences for disclosure. As Bradac, Tardy, and Hosman (1980) pointed out, different people have different styles of disclosure. Thus some patients may be able to share information, worries, and concerns about their illness without hesitation, whereas others may rely heavily on one or two family members and prefer not to disclose feelings to friends or health professionals.

A second factor to consider is the nature of the relationship between participants. Patients will feel more comfortable about disclosing their feelings within an established nurse-patient relationship. It is unrealistic to expect them to disclose personal feelings to nurses or other professionals with whom they have little contact. Therefore, nurses need to focus on increasing their relationship-oriented rather than task-oriented time with cancer patients. In addition, attention also needs to be directed toward assigning the same nurse to the same patient over an extended period.

A third important factor is the setting of the interaction. Fast-paced oncology units, which provide little privacy, are noisy, and are characterized by frequent interruptions, inhibit patients from disclosing their feelings. Thus nurses need to establish within units a private, confidential environment that allows for the expression of feelings.

Searching for Meaning

A fourth concern confronting cancer patients is dealing with existential questions about the meaning of cancer and its impact on their lives. Cancer can disrupt virtually all aspects of the patient's life—everyday activities, short- and long-term goals, and the sense of worthiness and competence (Cantor, 1978). Everyone needs to view life as existentially meaningful, and cancer undermines this effort.

Communicating with patients about their efforts to find meaning and purpose is particularly important, because an increased sense of meaning appears to be related positively to satisfactory adjustment and coping (Silver & Wortman, 1980). Individuals who find personal meaning and value in their existence are better able to confront their circumstances (Frankl, 1963; Jourard, 1971; Spiegel, Bloom, & Yalom, 1981; Weisman & Worden, 1976). For example, Speigel, Bloom, and Yalom (1981) assessed the psychological benefits of support groups for 86 patients with metastatic carcinoma and found that supportive, direct confrontation with life-and-death issues resulted in a sense of mastery rather than demoralization. In addition, they found that patients who received support felt less isolated, helpless, and worthless. Similarly, Weisman and Worden (1976) found that cancer patients who coped well accepted their diagnosis and treatment with little equivocation, talked with others to clarify their plight, and exhibited a more favorable attitude toward their illness.

The critical factor in helping patients with their struggles about meaning is effective interpersonal communication. Communication with others is the vehicle and the medium patients use to sort out, analyze, and clarify questions about meaning. In a study of two support groups composed of adolescent oncology patients, Byrne, Stockwell, and Gudelis (1984) found that all the group members struggled with questions such as "Why me? Why did I get cancer?" and with the development of a life-and-death philosophy. Within the context of the group, patients were able to interact with one another and sort out their existential concerns. On the basis of 4 years of experience with a

---

Box 59–2. SOCIAL SUPPORT FOR BREAST CANCER PATIENTS

This study explored the social support perceived by 100 breast cancer patients and the support anticipated by 100 cancer-free individuals. Only 50 per cent of the breast cancer patients reported that they received adequate amounts of support to meet their needs. Seventy-two per cent of the women reported being treated differently after their cancer diagnosis and cited problems with feeling misunderstood, feared, or avoided. When the disease-free individuals were asked about their response to the breast cancer patients, the majority reported that they would feel sorry for them, would go out of their way to cheer them up, or would avoid the person with cancer. These individuals also expressed discomfort about the "correct" way of interacting with cancer patients, afraid at times that they would say the wrong thing to patients. Peters-Golden contends some of the difficulties encountered by cancer patients result from a lack of fit between the interaction and support needs of cancer patients and the type of interaction and support provided by people without cancer.

(From Peters-Golden, H. [1982]. Breast cancer: Varied perceptions of social support in the illness experience. *Social Science and Medicine, 16,* 483–491. Reproduced by permission.)

---

therapy group for patients with metastatic carcinoma, Yalom and Greaves (1977) concluded that patients were helped by discussing existential issues. They found a greater sense of meaning and fulfillment the more they were able to move away from morbid self-absorption and into extending themselves to others. Further evidence for the significance of communication was provided by Johnson (1982), who found that patients with cancer who participated in a patient education course reported a greater sense of meaning in their lives.

Issues Confronting Nurses

Although interpersonal communication is a transactional process, little research has been conducted on the problems confronting nurses as they communicate with patients with cancer. Most studies have focused on the patient half of the nurse-patient relationship. From the nurse's perspective, there are three issues of concern: imparting information, communicating hope, and dealing with emotions.

Imparting Information

Imparting information is an important aspect of the health professional's role, yet it is seldom an easy task. Many factors make imparting information a more complex process for professionals than it appears initially. First, patients have different levels of comprehension (Greenwald & Nevitt, 1982), different levels of competence (Schoene-Seifert & Childress, 1986), and, as discussed earlier, different preferences for information. Professionals should take these individual differences into consideration when imparting information. Second, information-giving sessions typically occur within a short time period (Blanchard, 1983). This leaves little opportunity for questions, clarification, or even assessment of the extent to which the patient understands the information. Third, nurses' and patients' perceptions of what kind of information patients need can differ. For example, Lauer, Murphy, and Powers (1982) studied nurses' and patients' ranking of patients' educational needs and found that patients ranked information about "minimizing side effects" as their major need, whereas nurses ranked "dealing with feelings" as the patients' most important need. This example of discrepant perceptions highlights the difficulty and complexity of imparting information. Professionals need to be certain that they are addressing the patient's real informational needs, not simply projecting their own perceptions of those needs onto patients.

Nurses, in particular, face another problem in imparting information; often, they are not perceived as a legitimate source of information for patients. For years, when patients and family members asked a nurse for information about such basic facts as their blood pressure or temperature, the nurse told them to ask the physician. This practice distorted the patient's perceptions of nurses as legitimate providers of information. Although nurses' attitudes have changed and most nurses now recognize that it is within the scope of nursing practice to provide information, some evidence suggests that patients' and family members' perceptions of the nurse have not changed. For example, Dyck and Wright (1986) reported that the majority of family members of cancer patients in their study did not perceive the nurse as having a major information-giving role, and 27 per cent still believed that releasing information was contrary to the nurse's code of ethics and beyond the nurse's scope of practice. Some subjects reported that they hesitated to ask nurses for information because it would put the nurses in an awkward position. Patients perceive the physician to be the primary source of information about disease and treatment issues and less frequently cite the nurse (Dodd, 1982; Frank-Stromborg & Wright, 1984).

What strategies can the nurse use to facilitate imparting information to cancer patients and their families? First, nurses need to recognize the legitimacy of their role in providing patients with information, not only about actual and potential problems associated with cancer, but also about ways to alleviate or prevent potential problems (American Nurses Association, 1980). Next, nurses need to educate patients and family members that nurses are available to provide not only comfort and support, but also information that will enable patients to better understand and cope with their illness. Furthermore, given the hesitancy of some patients to seek information from nurses, nurses need to assume more responsibility for initiating discussions with patients and seeking out their questions about the illness. Finally, assessing patients for the amount and kind of information they want as well as for the degree to which they understand the information previously provided is an important aspect of imparting information.

Communicating Hope

Because fear and uncertainty accompany a cancer diagnosis, communicating hope is another critical task facing nurses who work with cancer patients. Hope enables patients to move away from feeling weak and vulnerable and to function as fully as possible within the limits of their circumstances (Miller, 1985). Hope is fostered in patients through nurturing interactions with health professionals and others. It is provided by communicating in ways that enable patients to have positive expectations about their future, even though they face uncertain situations (Brewin, 1977; Holland, 1977; Nowotny, 1989). It also involves communicating in ways that help patients to feel inspirited (Jourard, 1971), maintain their morale, and maximize their courage (Brewin, 1977).

In recent years there has been a growing interest in the role of hope in adjustment to cancer (Baird, 1989; Herth, 1989; Hinds & Martin, 1988; Mishel et al., 1984; Nowotny, 1989; Owen, 1989; Schmale et al., 1983). Hinds and Martin (1988) studied the development of hopefulness in adolescents with cancer and found that it was a self-sustaining process that could be influenced by others, such as nurses. To achieve hopefulness in the face of health threats, adolescents went through four sequential phases: cognitive discomfort, distraction, cognitive comfort, and personal competence. Stoner and Kaempfer (1985) studied the impact of life expectancy (prognostic) information on patients' level of hope and found that patients who did not recall receiving prognostic information had more hope than patients who did recall receiving such information. Mishel and associates (1984) found a strong relationship between optimism and adjustment to illness in women with gynecologic cancer. Women who were pessimistic about their situation lacked confidence in the health care system and experienced more psychological distress. In contrast to Stoner and Kaempfer's findings, women in the Mishel and associates study who had more information about their illness were more optimistic than women with less information. In a qualitative study of staff and cancer patients on a radiation therapy unit, Buehler (1975) found that patients live on a hope-doubt continuum that is strongly influenced by staff communication. Staff in this study maintained an idealogy of hope exemplified by the message "we can help you," which they readily communicated to patients. The staff's hope was based on optimism about new advances in cancer research, new treatment methods, increased survival rates, and growing cooperation among cancer specialists.

What happens when health professionals fail to foster hope in cancer patients? Some reports suggest that patients may seek alternative or unorthodox methods of cancer treatment. For example, Holland (1981) contended that cancer patients who participated in a national study of Laetrile did so because they often felt that their physicians believed nothing more could be done for them. Physicians working with patients who had recurrent and disseminated cancer failed to communicate a sense of hope. Perceiving the physicians' attitude of hopelessness, patients sought alternative methods that at least offered some hope. Dunphy (1976) suggested that cancer patients' interest in Laetrile was related in part to the fact that professionals did not always inform patients that even in hopeless situations, arrests or remissions could occur.

Although hope appears to be essential for cancer patients, nurses and other health professionals hesitate to communicate hope at times for several reasons. First, some professionals believe that fostering hope in patients whose disease is extensive simply encourages denial and prevents patients from facing up to the seriousness of their illness. Although research indicates that selective denial may be a useful mechanism for protecting patients from hopelessness (Brewin, 1977; Cassileth et al., 1980; Wool & Goldberg, 1986), some professionals still view denial as maladaptive. Second, some professionals believe that they are being deceptive or providing false reassurance when they foster hope in patients who have a life-threatening disease. In an era of informed consent and malpractice suits, professionals tend to emphasize definitive disease-related information. Third, some professionals still equate hope with cure; thus they have difficulty offering hope to patients with extensive disease or to those receiving palliative treatments. Clearly, to communicate hope, professionals need to recognize that hope means the ability to maintain morale and courage (Brewin, 1977), not just the ability to eradicate disease.

To communicate hope, nurses and other health professionals need effective communication strategies. Miller and Knapp (1986) asked a sample of 60 ministers and 43 hospice workers to rate the appropriateness of seven different communication strategies used by caregivers in interactions with patients with cancer (Box 59–3). The respondents gave the highest ranking to the communication strategy called "Be Reflexive," which involved listening to the patient and "being there." This strategy was rated as the most important one during various time periods and across all emotional states. The communication strategy that received the second highest rating was "Be Demonstrative" (e.g., show affection), followed by "Be Definitive" (e.g., provide information). The communication strategy that received the lowest ranking was "Be Upbeat," which referred to focusing on happy, cheerful things and avoiding discussion of the illness. This study highlighted that communication that reflects the patient's feelings and allows the patient to control the agenda of the conversation was rated the most effective.

Other strategies help to maintain hope also. Miller (1985) suggested that nurses help patients focus on the moment, review their assets, maintain important rela-

---

Box 59–3. COMMUNICATION STRATEGIES WITH CANCER PATIENTS

Investigators asked 60 ministers and 43 hospice volunteers to rate the appropriateness of seven communication strategies used by caregivers in their interactions with dying cancer patients. Subjects rated the communication strategy called "Be Reflexive" (e.g., listen, be there) as the most appropriate strategy and the communication strategy called "Be Upbeat" (e.g., focus on cheerful topics) as the least appropriate strategy. Subjects also rated the appropriateness of each strategy across three stages of dying. Although "Be Reflexive" was rated as the most important strategy during each phase of dying, "Be Definitive" (e.g., provide information) and "Be Demonstrative" (e.g., show affection) were rated as important during the initial and middle phases of dying. "Be Demonstrative" was also rated important during the final phase of dying. When caregivers were asked to give advice to others on the best way to interact with dying patients, caregivers said to accept the patient, be honest and realistic, respond naturally, show emotional commitment, be with the patient as often as possible, and say little and listen.

(From Miller, Y. D., & Knapp, M. L. [1986]. The post-nuntio dilemma: Approaches to communicating with the dying. In *Communication yearbook* [Vol. 8, pp. 723–738]. Beverly Hills, CA: Sage Publications. Reproduced by permission.)

---

tionships, and monitor signs of progress. Hickey (1986) encouraged nurses to foster hope by helping patients develop short-term, realistic, attainable goals. Patients with cancer, she suggested, have many interests but have difficulty planning because of the disease. Similarly, Owen (1989) encouraged nurses to help patients set temporary goals that will enable patients to cope with changing treatments or prognoses. Brewin (1977) contended that regardless of the prognosis, it is important for health care providers to give patients reassurance and encouragement, even if they have to focus on a narrow area such as symptom relief. Communicating to patients that they are not alone in their struggles facilitates hope also. No matter what their circumstances, patients need to know there is hope.

According to Holland (1977), another communication strategy for building hope is to offer a rational perspective of cancer. When health care providers express an attitude and a philosophy that cancer is treatable, they help patients to act rationally and to feel less anxious. Hope is provided by offering a rational course of action that reduces shock, fear, and anxiety.

Dealing with Emotions

A third issue confronting oncology nurses is dealing with the tremendous array of emotions that surround the cancer experience. Cancer generates high levels of helplessness, fear, anger, and sadness in both patients and nurses. For the patient, these emotions emerge from the reality of having the disease. For the nurse, they arise out of the day-to-day stress of watching patient suffering and attempting to alleviate that suffering. Nurses in one study reported that dealing with patients' feelings and managing their own feelings about cancer were formidable tasks (Craytor et al., 1978).

What difficulties do nurses encounter as they try to deal with patients' emotions? One difficulty is that they have their own fears about cancer, which can interfere with their ability to discuss and assuage patients' fears (Paulen & Kuenstler, 1978; Vachon, Lyall, & Freeman, 1978). In addition, they often feel overwhelmed when patients express strong emotions, such as anger

and despair. Nurses in one study said they lacked the interpersonal and communication skills needed to handle the complex feelings expressed by cancer patients (Vachon et al., 1978). Furthermore, nurses feel frustrated and anxious when they cannot answer difficult, existential questions, such as "Why did I get cancer?" or "How long will I live?" (Paulen & Kuenstler, 1978).

Some evidence indicates that nurses use avoidance behaviors at times in attempting to deal with their feelings about cancer. Avoidance behaviors can take many forms; the most obvious one is to avoid spending time with patients. Quint (1965) found that nurses used nonverbal gestures that made it difficult for patients to initiate discussions or interrupted patients when the content of the conversations began to make them feel uncomfortable. Using linguistic analysis techniques, Mood and Lakin (1979) found that nursing personnel engaged in avoidance by substituting pronouns such as *it* for negatively charged words such as *death*. Although such avoidance behaviors may help the nurse cope with anxiety initially, they are less useful in helping to resolve the deeper emotional issues experienced by both patients and nurses.

Although oncology nurses have difficulty at times dealing with their emotions, they are often in a position to deal with patients' feelings. Not only are they in close physical proximity to patients on a continual basis, but they are perceived by patients as the member of the health care team who is most likely to deal with emotional concerns. In a study by Karani and Wiltshaw (1986), patients identified the nurse as the professional most likely to help them with concerns about sexuality, fears about their illness, and the impact of the illness on the lives of family members. Similarly, patients in a study by Frank-Stromborg and Wright (1984) reported that their interactions with the nurse provided them with emotional support.

If nurses are the professionals who are expected to deal with feelings, what communication strategies can help them to do so? First, because research suggests that the emotional profile of patients with cancer corresponds more closely to a stressed but normally functioning population than to a psychiatric population (Cassileth, Lusk, Miller, Brown, & Miller, 1985; Plumb & Holland, 1977), supportive rather than psychoanalytic techniques seem warranted. Listening appears to be among the most important supportive strategies available. Although active listening is often underrated, cancer patients identify listening consistently as one of the more important caring behaviors a nurse can demonstrate toward them (Larson, 1984). Listening enables patients to ventilate, which in turn allows them to get a better grip on their own circumstances. Some clinicians believe that discussions about feelings should be introduced gradually (Wool & Goldberg, 1986). For example, they suggest starting with a factual question, such as "What symptom did you notice first?" then moving to questions about feelings, such as "How do you feel about your illness?" or "What effect is your illness having on your family?" Finally, the importance of the nurse's supportive presence cannot be overstated. The cancer literature is replete with personal accounts about the great value of "standing by" and "being with" patients. Patients often are helped by having another person who will tolerate their fear, uncertainty, anger, and discomfort (Wool & Goldberg, 1986).

SUMMARY

Effective interpersonal communication is essential for cancer patients and nurses. It is instrumental in helping patients cope with their fears and uncertainty about the disease, and it provides nurses with a central means for providing support as well as accomplishing health-related goals. Communication between nurse and patient is not simple; it is a complex process that involves an awareness of the many factors that affect both participants simultaneously. Effective communication depends on what is communicated (the content dimension) as well as how it is communicated (the relationship dimension).

Because communication is a transactional process, communication issues must be assessed from the perspectives of both the patient and the nurse. For patients, four concerns emerge: maintaining a sense of control; obtaining information that will reduce their uncertainty; disclosing feelings that will help them ventilate, solve problems, and receive feedback and support; and searching for meaning. Communication with supportive others enables patients to achieve a sense of mastery, obtain the information they need, disclose their feelings, and analyze and clarify the existential impact of cancer on their lives.

Nurses bring a different set of concerns and responsibilities to the nurse-patient interaction. First, they must deal with the questions of what and how much information to give patients. Second, they must determine how to communicate hope in ways that will encourage patients to function as fully as possible within the limits of their circumstances. Third, they must work through their own feelings about cancer as well as respond to patients' fears and anxieties.

Effective interpersonal communication is not a panacea for all of the problems nurses confront in the oncology setting. However, it is an important aspect of high-quality cancer care. Through an awareness of the many complex communication issues that exist in the oncology setting, nurses can help patients and family members cope with the impact of cancer.

References

American Nurses Association. (1980). *Nursing: A social policy statement*. Kansas City, MO: Author.

Baird, S. (1989). Why hope now? *Oncology Nursing Forum, 16*(1), 9.

Berlo, D. K. (1960). *The process of communication*. New York: Holt, Rinehart & Winston.

Birdwhistell, R. L. (1970). *Kinesics and context*. Philadelphia: University of Pennsylvania Press.

Blanchard, C. G., Ruckdeschel, J. C., Blanchard, E. B., Arena, J. G., Saunders, N. L., & Malloy, E. D. (1983). Interactions between oncologists and patients during rounds. *Annals of Internal Medicine, 99*, 694–699.

Bloom, J. R. (1982). Social support, accommodation to stress and adjustment to breast cancer. *Social Science and Medicine, 16*, 1329–1338.

Bloom, J. R., Ross, R. D., & Burnell, G. (1978). The effect of social support on patient adjustment after breast surgery. *Patient Counseling and Health Education, 2*, 50–59.

Bradac, J. J., Tardy, C. H., & Hosman, L. A. (1980). Disclosure styles and a hint at their genesis. *Human Communication Research, 6*, 228–238.

Brewin, T. B. (1977). The cancer patient: Communication and morale. *British Medical Journal, 2*, 1623–1627.

Buckalew, P. G. (1982). On the opposite side of the bed: A nurse clinician's experiences with anxiety during chemotherapy. *Cancer Nursing, 5*, 435–439.

Buehler, J. A. (1975). What contributes to hope in the cancer patient? *American Journal of Nursing, 75*, 1353–1356.

Byrne, C. M., Stockwell, M., & Gudelis, S. (1984). Adolescent support groups in oncology. *Oncology Nursing Forum, 11*(4), 36–40.

Cantor, R. C. (1978). *And a time to live: Toward emotional well-being during the crisis of cancer*. New York: Harper & Row, Publishers.

Cassileth, B. R., Lusk, E. J., Miller, D. S., Brown, L. L., & Miller, C. (1985). Psychosocial correlates of survival in advanced malignant disease? *New England Journal of Medicine, 312*, 1551–1555.

Cassileth, B. R., Zupkis, R. Y., Sutton-Smith, K., & March, Y. (1980). Information and participation preferences among cancer patients. *Annals of Internal Medicine, 92*, 832–836.

Cooper, A. (1982). Disabilities and how to live with them—Hodgkin's disease. *Lancet, 1*, 612–613.

Craytor, J. K., Brown, J. K., & Morrow, G. R. (1978). Assessing learning needs of nurses who care for persons with cancer. *Cancer Nursing, 1*, 211–220.

Derdiarian, A. K. (1986). Informational needs of recently diagnosed cancer patients. *Nursing Research, 35*, 276–281.

Derdiarian, A. K. (1987). Informational needs of recently diagnosed cancer patients. Part II. Method and description. *Cancer Nursing, 10*, 156–163.

Dodd, M. (1982). Assessing patient self-care for side effects of cancer chemotherapy—Part I. *Cancer Nursing, 5*, 447–451.

Dunkel-Schetter, C., & Wortman, C. B. (1982). The interpersonal dynamics of cancer: Problems in social relationships and their impact on the patient. In H. S. Friedman & M. R. DiMatteo (Eds.), *Interpersonal issues in health care* (pp. 69–100). New York: Academic Press.

Dunphy, J. E. (1976). On caring for the patient with cancer. *New England Journal of Medicine, 295*, 313–319.

Dyck, S., & Wright, K. (1986). Family perceptions: The role of the nurse throughout an adult's cancer experience. *Oncology Nursing Forum, 12*(5), 53–56.

Fiore, N. (1979). Fighting cancer—one patient's perspective. *New England Journal of Medicine, 300*, 284–289.

Frankl, Y. (1963). *Man's search for meaning: An introduction to logotherapy*. New York: Simon & Schuster.

Frank-Stromborg, M., & Wright, P. (1984). Ambulatory cancer patients' perceptions of the physical and psychosocial changes in their lives since the diagnosis of cancer. *Cancer Nursing, 7,* 117–130.

Friedman, H. S., (1979). Nonverbal communication between patients and medical practitioners. *Journal of Social Issues, 35,* 1–11.

Gordon, W., Friedenbergs, I., Diller, L., Rothman, L., Wolf, C., Ruckdeschel-Hubbard, M., Ezgchi, O., & Gerstman, L. (1977). *The psychological problems of cancer patients: A retrospective study.* Paper presented at the American Psychological Association Meeting. San Francisco, CA.

Gotay, C. C. (1984). The experience of cancer during early and advanced stages: The views of patients and their mates. *Social Science and Medicine, 18,* 605–613.

Greenwald, H. P., & Nevitt, M. C. (1982). Physician attitudes toward communication with cancer patients. *Social Science and Medicine, 16,* 591–594.

Harker, B. L. (1972). Cancer and communication problems: A personal experience *Psychiatry in Medicine, 3,* 163–171.

Herth, K. A. (1989). Relationship between level of hope and level of coping response and other variables in patients with cancer. *Oncology Nursing Forum, 16*(1), 67–72.

Hickey, S. S. (1986). Enabling hope. *Cancer Nursing, 9,* 133–137.

Hinds, P., & Martin, J. (1988). Hopefulness and the self-sustaining process in adolescents with cancer. *Nursing Research, 37,* 336–339.

Hinton, J. (1981). Sharing or withholding awareness of dying between husband and wife. *Journal of Psychosomatic Research, 25,* 337–343.

Holland, J. C. (1977). Psychological management of cancer patients and their families. *Practical Psychology, 9,* 14–18.

Holland, J. C. (1981). Patients who seek unproven cancer remedies: A psychological perspective. *Clinical Bulletin, 11,* 102–105.

Hopkins, M. B. (1986). Information-seeking and adaptational outcomes in women receiving chemotherapy for breast cancer. *Cancer Nursing, 9,* 256–262.

Janis, I. L. (1958). *Psychological stress.* New York: John Wiley & Sons.

Johnson, J. L. (1982). The effects of a patient education course on persons with a chronic illness. *Cancer Nursing, 5,* 117–123.

Jourard, S. M. (1971). *The transparent self* (2nd ed.). New York: Van Nostrand Reinhold.

Karani, D., & Wittshaw, E. (1986). How well informed? *Cancer Nursing, 9,* 238–242.

Kellerman, J., Rigler, D., Siegel, S. E., & Katz, E. R. (1980). Disease-related communication and depression in pediatric patients. *Journal of Pediatric Psychology, 2,* 52–53.

Knapp, M. L., & Miller, G. R. (1985). *Handbook of interpersonal communication.* Newbury Park, CA: Sage Publications.

Larson, P. J. (1984). Cancer nurses' perceptions of caring. *Cancer Nursing, 9,* 86–91.

Lauer, P., Murphy, S., & Powers, M. (1982). Learning needs of cancer patients: A comparison of nurse and patient perceptions. *Nursing Research, 31,* 11–16.

Maguire, P. (1985). The psychological impact of cancer. *British Journal of Hospital Medicine, 34,* 100–103.

McCorkle, R. (1981). Communication approaches to effective cancer nursing care. In L. B. Marino (Ed.), *Cancer nursing* (pp. 405–419). St. Louis: C. V. Mosby Co.

McCorkle, R., & Hollenbach, M. (1983). Touch and the acutely ill. Paper presented at the Johnson and Johnson Pediatric Round Table #10: Touch. Key Largo, FL.

McIntosh, J. (1974). Processes of communication, information seeking and control associated with cancer: A selective review of the literature. *Social Science and Medicine, 8,* 167–182.

Mehrabian, A. (1971). *Silent messages.* Belmont, CA: Wadsworth.

Meyerowitz, B. E., Watkins, I., & Sparks, F. (1983). Quality of life for breast cancer patients receiving adjuvant chemotherapy. *American Journal of Nursing, 83,* 232–235.

Miller, J. F. (1985). Inspiring hope. *American Journal of Nursing, 85,* 22–25.

Miller, V. D., & Knapp, M. L. (1986). The *post nuntio* dilemma: Approaches to communicating with the dying. In *Communication yearbook* (Vol. 8, pp. 723–738). Beverly Hills, CA: Sage Publications.

Mishel, M., Hostetter, T., King, B., & Graham, V. (1984). Predictors of psychosocial adjustment in patients newly diagnosed with gynecological cancer. *Cancer Nursing, 7,* 291–299.

Mitchell, G. W., & Glicksman, A. S. (1977). Cancer patients: Knowledge and attitudes. *Cancer, 40,* 61–66.

Mood, D. W., & Lakin, B. A. (1979). Attitudes of nursing personnel toward death and dying: 1. Linguistic indicators of avoidance. *Research in Nursing and Health, 2,* 53–60.

Moos, R. H., & Tsu, V. D. (1977). The crisis of physical illness: An overview. In R. H. Moos (Ed.), *Coping with physical illness* (pp. 3–21). New York: Plenum Medical Book.

Morrow, G. R., Hoaglund, A. C., & Carpenter, P. J. (1983). Improving physician-patient communications in cancer treatment. *Journal of Psychosocial Oncology, 1,* 93–101.

Mullan, F. (1984). Re-entry: The educational needs of the cancer survivor. *Health Education Quarterly, 10,* 88–94.

Northouse, L. L. (1981). Mastectomy patients and the fear of cancer recurrence. *Cancer Nursing, 4,* 213–220.

Northouse, L. L. (1988). Social support in patients' and husbands' adjustment to breast cancer. *Nursing Research, 37,* 91–95.

Northouse, L. L., & Wortman, C. B. (1990). Models of helping and coping in cancer care. *Patient Education and Counseling, 15,* 49–64.

Northouse, P. G., & Northouse, L. L. (1985). *Health communication: A handbook for health professionals.* Englewood Cliffs, NJ: Prentice-Hall, Inc.

Northouse, P. G., & Northouse, L. L. (1987). Communication and cancer: Issues confronting patients, health professionals and family members. *Journal of Psychosocial Oncology, 5*(3), 17–46.

Novack, D. H., Plumer, R., Smith, R. L., Ochitill, H., Morrow, G. R., & Bennett, J. M. (1979). Changes in physicians' attitudes toward telling the cancer patient. *Journal of the American Medical Association, 241,* 897–900.

Nowotny, M. L. (1989). Assessment of hope in patients with cancer: Development of an Instrument. *Oncology Nursing Forum, 16*(1), 57–61.

Oken, C. (1961). What to tell cancer patients. *Journal of the American Medical Association, 86,* 86–94.

Owen, D. C. (1989). Nurses' perspectives on the meaning of hope in patients with cancer: A qualitative study. *Oncology Nursing Forum, 16*(1), 75–79.

Paulen, A., & Kuenstler, T. M. (1978). Learning to discuss the unmentionable. *Cancer Nursing, 1,* 197–199.

Peters-Golden, H. (1982). Breast cancer: Varied perceptions of social support in the illness experience. *Social Science and Medicine, 16,* 483–491.

Plumb, M. M., & Holland, J. (1977). Comparative studies of psychological function in patients with advanced cancer. I. Self-reported depressive symptoms. *Psychosomatic Medicine, 39,* 264–291.

Quint, J. C. (1963). Impact of mastectomy. *American Journal of Nursing, 63,* 88–92.

Quint, J. C. (1965). Institutionalized practices of information control. *Psychiatry, 28,* 119–132.

Schmale, A. H., Morrow, G. R., Schmitt, M. J., Adler, L. M., Enelow, A., Murawski, B. J., & Gates, C. (1983). Well-being of cancer survivors. *Psychosomatic Medicine, 45,* 163–169.

Schoene-Seifert, B., & Childress, J. F. (1986). How much should the cancer patient know and decide? *CA: A Cancer Journal for Clinicians, 36,* 85–94.

Silver, R. L., & Wortman, C. B. (1980). Coping with undesirable life events. In J. Garber & M. E. P. Seligman (Eds.). *Human helplessness: Theory and applications* (pp. 279–341). New York: Academic Press.

Spiegel, D. (1979). Psychological support for women with metastatic carcinoma. *Psychosomatics, 20,* 780–787.

Spiegel, D., Bloom, J. R., & Yalom, I. (1981). Group support for patients with metastatic cancer. *Archives of General Psychiatry, 38,* 527–533.

Stoner, M. H., & Kaempfer, S. H. (1985). Recalled life expectancy information, phase of illness and hope in cancer patients. *Research in Nursing & Health, 8,* 269–274.

Thorne, S. (1988). Helpful and unhelpful communications in cancer care: The patient perspective. *Oncology Nursing Forum, 15*(2), 167–172.

Trillin, A. A. (1981). Of dragons and garden peas. *New England Journal of Medicine, 304,* 699–701.

Vachon, M. L. (1986). A comparison of the impact of breast cancer and bereavement: Personality, social support and adaptation. In S. Hobfoll (Ed.), *Stress, social support and women* (pp. 187–204). New York: Hemisphere.

Vachon, M. L. S., Lyall, W. A., & Freeman, S. J. J. (1978). Measurement and management of stress in health professionals working with advanced cancer patients. *Death Education, 1,* 365–375.

Waitzkin, H., & Stoeckle, J. D. (1972). The communication of information about illness: Clinical, sociological and methodological considerations. *Advances in Psychosomatic Medicine, 8,* 180–215.

Watzlawick, P., Beavin, J., & Jackson, D. D. (1967). *Pragmatics of human communication.* New York: W. W. Norton.

Weisman, A. D., & Worden, J. W. (1975). Psychosocial analysis of cancer deaths. *Omega, 6,* 61–75.

Weisman, A. D., & Worden, J. W. (1976). The existential plight in cancer: Significance of the first 100 days. *International Journal of Psychiatry, 7,* 1–15.

Wool, M. S., & Goldberg, R. J. (1986). Assessment of denial in cancer patients: Implications for intervention. *Journal of Psychosocial Oncology, 4*(3), 1–14.

Yalom, I. D., & Greaves, C. (1977). Group therapy with the terminally ill. *American Journal of Psychiatry, 134,* 396–399.

CHAPTER 60

Helping Families Respond to Cancer

JUDITH L. JOHNSON
CHERYL ANN LANE

Promoting family health requires concomitant consideration of two factors: the effect of an illness on the family and the influence of family dynamics on the problems precipitated by that illness (Antonovsky, 1979). The family is the group with whom the patient has had the earliest, longest, and closest contact (Hsu, 1985). A cancer diagnosis is a threat to the family. Regardless of the intensity or nature of the presenting problems, cancer consistently disrupts the family's patterns of daily living. Disintegration rather than integration is created in nearly every family when cancer is diagnosed (Bruhn, 1977). For this reason, cancer care must become family focused (Tringali, 1986). Nurses should understand family structure, theory, dynamics of interaction, and cultural influences. With this knowledge, they can plan and implement ways to facilitate a family's adaptation to living with the ramifications of a cancer diagnosis.

This chapter outlines ways in which cancer affects the family, addresses cultural differences among families, and presents theoretic models for understanding family communication. The final sections provide practical guides for assessing families and planning strategies that facilitate family adaptation.

IMPACT OF CANCER ON THE FAMILY

The family is the first line of defense in support of the patient. With a diagnosis of cancer, however, the entire family may be in crisis (Christ, 1983; Gray-Price & Szczesny, 1985). In caring for persons with cancer, interventions for improving coping strategies must be evaluated not only for the person with the cancer but also for that person's family (Northouse, 1984; Oberst & James, 1985). What may be optimal for the patient may be devastating for the family (Eliopoulos, 1981). The key to this situation is to assist the family in maintaining its identity and the integrity of its members (Lovejoy, 1986; Northouse, 1984).

Family Coping Mechanisms

Geary (1979) has described five coping mechanisms commonly used by families who have a family member experiencing a health crisis. These include, first, minimization or attempting to downplay the significance of an event by acting inappropriately cheerful or nonchalant or by blocking information so that it cannot be understood. Second, intellectualization is employed through the development of an overly rational attitude and the deemphasis of any feeling about the experience. Third, families of patients in crisis use repetition. This can take the form of asking the same question over and over or restating information. Fourth, within the family, one member is often designated as the "strong" one. It is up to this person to support the other family members. The fifth behavior documented is the determination to "be there." Vigils are kept even when the health and well-being of family members are being sacrificed to achieve the vigil. These five behaviors are all attempts at coping and dealing with the crisis experience (Geary, 1979).

Points of Crisis

The cancer itself is a source of stress, but in addition, according to Giacquinta (1977) and Christ (1983), several specific points of crisis occur along the continuum of the illness. Diagnosis is the first point, followed by the beginning of treatment with its subsequent physical reactions. Failure to respond to therapy is a crisis point, as is reaching the end of the treatment protocol. If the patient develops a recurrence of cancer or if research protocols are begun, interpersonal chaos occurs. The final points of crisis include the discontinuation of active treatment and, finally, terminal illness (Christ, 1983). Each crisis point is experienced as personally disorienting and as an assault on the integrity of the entire family unit (Giacquinta, 1977).

Impact on Family Communication

Cassileth and Hamilton (1979) have identified ways in which cancer imposes on family communication, family direction, and interaction outside of the family. These include threatening or disrupting patterns of interaction, disturbing future plans, and altering external reference groups.

Threatening or Disrupting Patterns of Interaction

Roles and relationships of family members can either intensify or disintegrate. Some families have clearly defined roles for their members, whereas others have a free-for-all type of structure. One frequent role change that occurs following diagnosis is that duties and responsibilities are taken away from the sick family member and assumed by another. The result often is that one person feels a sense of loss and the other feels burdened by the added responsibilities.

Communication is a key factor in a family's adaptation to cancer. Who tells whom "the news"? The pattern of previous family sharing of sorrow, fear, and anger will be invoked in determining the way members share their feelings about the cancer diagnosis. Frequently people want to protect children from these anxiety-producing feelings and will choose not to tell them, at least during the initial phase of the illness. Many families are good at communicating information to one another but need encouragement to express their emotional needs. This is understandable, given the intense and fragile nature of these emotions. When the patient is the one who directs the flow of family communication, an even bigger change is created in the ways family members talk to one another.

Disturbing Future Plans

The roller-coaster effect of cancer makes it difficult for families to plan for the future. It creates an environment of uncertainty. A number of studies report that a major problem for families in learning to adapt to cancer is learning to live with an unknown future. The potential for recurrence creates considerable uncertainty in the minds of both patient and family members. Setting goals and having dreams for the future gives families a sense of specific purpose, direction, and uniqueness. These goals may be temporarily or permanently disrupted when a member has cancer. Displacement of plans causes varying levels of frustration, anger, and grief that are hard for family members to cope with.

Altering External Reference Groups

The work setting provides individuals with an important identity outside of the family. Cancer frequently impinges on a person's capacity to work, which in turn alters work relationships with fellow employees. Family members also report changes in their work environment, some noting that they were treated with overconcern from co-workers and others experiencing a total lack of interest or acknowledgement that they were having a family crisis. It appears that family members, along with the patient, experience the social stigma attached to cancer.

Members of extended families may also feel the impact of the cancer. They may now need to play a vital role in the daily lives of the nuclear family unit, whereas before the illness, their involvement may have been more limited. Grandparents may have to perform the parent role and respond to grandchildren who are acting out in response to parental absence. When family members are separated by distance, information may have to be conveyed and critical decisions made via telephone, severely limiting opportunity for family discussion, personal touch, and support.

Reference groups are also created by a cancer diagnosis. Doctors, nurses, social workers, and other patients on the same treatment schedules become familiar names and faces. These new people assume great importance for cancer families. Trips to the doctor and clinic are frequent and time-consuming events that dominate family life and conversation.

CULTURAL FACTORS THAT AFFECT FAMILY COMMUNICATIONS

When considering the uniqueness of others, nurses must not negate their own personal uniqueness. Everyone brings into a relationship a cultural heritage, conditional values, assumptions, and perceptions of reality; any of these can become the basis for cultural conflict (Marsella & Pedersen, 1981). Cultural factors influence assessment of needs and professional deportment in a therapeutic environment, as well as interpersonal relationships and perceptions of reality.

The most obvious source of culturally based misunderstanding is verbal language, but nonverbal behavior must also be considered. When communicating, the appropriateness of a message and whether it is heard correctly can be enhanced or diminished by a gesture, too much or too little eye contact, body language, and voice intonation. The importance of these aspects of communication varies among cultural, racial, and ethnic groups. Professionals establishing therapeutic relationships with minority clients often do not understand the importance of cultural differences (Sue, 1981) and camouflage their lack of knowledge by denying the existence or importance of these differences. This attitude ignores the uniqueness and individuality of each person and may be perpetuated so that the professional can avoid confronting sensitive racial and cultural issues. Although a professional can empathize with clients, empathy alone is not enough for the promotion of understanding. Nurses who work with families from minority groups must possess both insight and sensitivity. Misunderstandings that originate from cultural differences affect both verbal and nonverbal communication and can easily lead to alienation, inability to develop trust and rapport, or both (Marsella & Pedersen, 1981).

Cultural groups require patterns of interaction that are congruent with the life experiences of the members. Nurses can deal with these differences in interaction patterns by

- having a clear knowledge of minority group cultures and experiences (Marsella & Pedersen, 1981)
- not trying to solve cultural conflicts but instead making it more acceptable for members of minority groups to be part of two cultures (Sue, 1981)
- not holding rigid beliefs about and expectations of people who are culturally different (Marsella & Pedersen, 1981)

Cultural differences can undermine a well thought out therapeutic plan by eroding the most basic method of exchange—interpersonal communication. To determine the influence culture has on communication, the meaning of family and the predominant communication styles, values, customs, morals, and rituals must be explored. The meaning of illness and death is also of significance, but not much data have been amassed in this area. Each cultural, racial, or ethnic group has its own understanding of methods of interacting with health care professionals. To establish therapeutic relationships with those of different cultural origins, Rogers states that

> We need to know how the roles are modified as the family confront problems and how social control in the family operates as each person tries to change or reinforce the deviant or customary behavior. . . . we need . . . techniques for measuring these explicit and implicit interpersonal arrangements and processes that define the family as a social institution (Padilla & Ruiz, 1973, p. 45).

Axelson (1985, p. 287) states that "structured interpersonal relations vary with cultural heritage and traditions and have been shown to influence behavior." These opinions provide the basis for defining communications and health in the following cultures: Asian American, native American, black American, Hispanic and other Spanish-speaking American, and Appalachian Anglo-American.

Asian American

The Asian family has a strong sense of family orientation and belonging. Family members depend on one another for physical and emotional support. Their love is communicated through their actions, not through their words. Some Asian-American families are described as being enmeshed, overprotective, and rigid, which can lead to a lack of ability to resolve internal conflicts. Because Asian culture does not encourage the verbalization of emotions, conflict is not confronted directly. When confrontation does occur, it usually results in outbursts of anger, denial, or withdrawal. The only occasion on which Asians—in particular, Asian females—are expected to demonstrate emotion of any sort is at a funeral, during which they are expected to express grief by crying loudly. Communication of emotions or affection or divulgence of psychological problems overtly at any other time is believed to damage internal organs and to endanger health (Hsu, 1985).

To encourage an Asian American to share feelings is perceived as a lack of respect for the individual's integrity and will decrease the nurse's effectiveness and credibility. In communicating with members of this culture, a more logical, straightforward, structured approach is best (Marsella & Pedersen, 1981).

Communication is enhanced when the nurse is comfortable and effective in the use of silence. Silence is traditionally viewed as a sign of politeness and respect, especially when working with elders. Direct eye contact indicates lack of respect and should therefore be avoided.

The nuclear family structure is likened to a tower: the mother is the center, the father stands to the side, and all the children are at the base. The vertical relationship between parent and child is primary, with the relationship between mother and child being the closest. The relationship between husband and wife is horizontal, the same as sibling to sibling, and these relationships are considered to be secondary. The children in Asian families, although very close to their parents, characteristically do not have a very strong coalition with one another (Hsu, 1985). The Chinese hold that kinship bonds are stronger than marital bonds, as evidenced by the Chinese maxim, "Siblings are hands and feet while wives are only clothes," indicating that the wife is disposable but one must never sever one's limbs. Loyalty to the family of origin is stronger than loyalty to the marital relationship.

Times of crisis are often viewed as times of opportunity. The character for crisis in the Chinese language also means opportunity; therefore, the individual uses inner strength to face the situation.

The predominant religions of the traditional Chinese-American family are Buddhist and Taoist (Dillard, 1983). Illness is viewed as a trial to aid in the development of the person's soul. In times of health crisis, the Buddhist priest is the preferred person for counseling. There are special holy days throughout the year when patients may elect not to have medical or surgical treatment. If death occurs, last-rite chanting is performed at the bedside of the deceased soon after the death.

Native American

A native American is a person who is genetically one fourth or more American Indian (Bureau of Indian Affairs, 1986). The belief system of native Americans is manifested in the following four values:

- God is a benevolent force.
- The self is understood by observing nature.
- Relationships with others emphasize interdependence and sharing.
- The world is interconnected according to the same process and relationship that can be observed in nature (Avelson, 1985).

Indians respect all things, living and dead. They view the universe holistically and believe in equality, not supremacy (Sue, 1981).

Kinship relationships are valued highly. In one Indian language *piyospaye* means "extended family." During a time when assistance from a health care professional is required, individuals may feel more at ease and be more receptive if another Indian is allowed to sit with them and give an impression of the non-Indian. Indians have great trust in one another (Padilla & Ruiz, 1973). Trust and understanding are two of the most valued human attributes in the Indian culture.

There are numerous cultural differences between the native American and the Anglo. In fact, Sue (1981) states that "no two races could so grossly differ in value systems. . . ." Many of these differences can lead to ineffective communication and lack of understanding (Table 60–1). Traditional methods of counseling, such as psychoanalysis, group therapy, and Gestalt approaches, are not conducive to building a relationship of trust with a native American. These approaches are thought to be too confrontive and controlling and may actually infringe on or deny individuals their rights. Native Americans have a more nonverbal, almost passive posture, and even the most understanding of health care professionals may be met with resistance over differences in interpretation of eye contact, intonation, and idle comments. Suggestions can be interpreted as orders because the health care professional is viewed as an authority figure (Richardson, 1981).

When working with native Americans, it is best to assume the attitude of an attentive listener. These are people who communicate subtly with their body language, eyes, and tone of voice; clues will often be

Table 60–1. DIFFERENCES IN INDIAN AND ANGLO VALUES

Indians	Anglos
1. Happiness—this is paramount! Be able to laugh at misery; life is to be enjoyed	1. Success—generally involving status, security, wealth, and proficiency
2. Sharing—everything belongs to others, just as Mother Earth belongs to *all* people	2. Ownership—indicating a preference to own an outhouse rather than to share a mansion
3. Tribe and extended family first, before self	3. "Think of Number One!" syndrome
4. Humble—causing Indians to be passive-aggressive, gentle head hangers, and very modest	4. Competitive—believing "If you don't toot your own horn then who will?"
5. Honor your elders—they have wisdom	5. The future lies with the youth
6. Learning through legends; remembering the great stories of the past, that's where the knowledge comes from	6. Learning is found in school; get all the schooling that you possibly can because it can't be taken away from you

(From Richardson, E. H. [1981]. Cultural and historical perspectives in counseling American Indians. In D. W. Sue [Ed.], *Counseling the culturally different* [pp. 225–227]. New York: John Wiley & Sons, Inc. Reproduced by permission.)

missed (Richardson, 1981). The tone of the relationship should be casual and natural without concentrating on being effective, establishing priorities, or setting goals. Direct comments reduce suspicion.

Loud, overbearing, inquisition-like mannerisms are offensive to Indians and may make them feel subservient, thus eliminating any chance of rapport. Silences during conversations are characteristic. Attitudes of competition should be avoided (Sue, 1981).

Staring should be avoided, especially when talking about intimate aspects of life. The American Indian uses peripheral vision to avoid making direct eye contact, which is considered a hostile act. When speaking of intimacies, the American Indian may wish to sit beside rather than across from the health care professional (Sue, 1981).

When dealing with illness, each tribe has different practices, which can vary from a traditional Anglo approach to magic and herbal medicine. Medicine men, shamans, and conjurers use symbolic actions against illness and disease. In some tribes, such as the Navaho, protection is sought from superhuman powers despite the evidence of modern ideas. There is still a strong belief in ghosts.

Interactions are most effective when the culture is respected. Be reticent, humble, soft spoken and sensitive to the Indian's frame of reference.

Black American

Black culture is a people-oriented rather than an object-oriented culture that emphasizes humanism and the beauty of diversity (Smith, 1981). Within the black family, the female plays a significant role. She is seen as warm, accepting, and self-sacrificing and usually occupies the favored position in the family. Typically, children go to their mother when they seek permission for something, and the mother, in turn, speaks to the father on their behalf. The father makes the final decision. Children are taught early that family matters are not discussed with outsiders. To do so is a violation of family ethics. Resistance will most likely occur if a health care professional attempts to obtain information or discuss family-related matters with a child.

Religion plays an important role in the family value system (Dillard, 1983). It is believed that a strong faith will see a person through difficult times, including illness. Blacks characteristically turn to their church instead of to health care professionals for release from psychological stress (Wegmann, 1988). Blacks are members of most mainstream religions, with Christianity playing a central part in developing solidarity among blacks (Dillard, 1983).

Some blacks, however, are Black Muslims, a religion that generally adheres to Muslim tenets with an overlay of antagonism toward whites, especially Christians and Jews. Black Muslims do not participate excessively in any activity and always maintain personal habits of cleanliness. The religion prohibits the use of alcoholic beverages and the eating of pork and other traditional foods of black Americans. In times of health crisis, faith healing is not acceptable except to lift the patient's morale.

Much can also be learned about black culture by exploring black history, black humor with its paradoxes, as well as black literature and music. The arts have historically been the method through which blacks expressed their desires in life (Smith, 1981).

When communicating with black individuals, it is prudent to affirm their blackness and to use it as a means of validating their self-identity (Smith, 1981). When black Americans speak, they stand much closer to their listeners than Anglos are comfortable standing. Eye contact is not considered to be necessary to indicate attentiveness: being in the same room or in close proximity to another person is sufficient. Blacks make greater eye contact when speaking than when listening. They also tend to have greater body activity when speaking, which may be misinterpreted as a sign of aggression (Sue, 1981).

Hispanic and Other Spanish-Speaking American

The typical Hispanic family structure consists of an authoritarian father and a submissive mother, who is dominated by her husband. Males are believed to be supreme intellectually, socially, and biologically (Padilla & Ruiz, 1973). Children have a strong sense of being loved and are given indulgent affection (Dillard, 1983). Male children have more freedom than female children, who tend to be overprotected by their fathers. Hispanic families have strong kinship ties, and extended family members have rights, privileges, and duties (Madsen, 1969).

In addition to the bloodline kinship ties, a sacred relationship exists between a child and godparent. The responsibilities of this relationship are not only spiritual but also economic (Dillard, 1983; Keefe, Padilla, & Carlos, 1978). In times of crisis, stress, or serious illness, the extended family is the main source of support. Familial integration is measured by mutual aid. A patient may wish to return to familiar surroundings, such as an old neighborhood to seek solace. Culturally, this practice is considered to be one of the most adaptive responses to stress (Padilla & Ruiz, 1973).

A Spanish-speaking person stands close to others when speaking, avoids eye contact, and uses physical expressions such as kissing or bowing when greeting others (Vess, Moreland, & Schwebel, 1985).

The three prime sources of cultural conflict between Spanish-speaking individuals and Anglo health care professionals are language barriers, class-bound values, and culture-bound values (Marsella & Pedersen, 1981; Ruiz, 1981). In communicating with a Spanish-speaking person, cultural conflicts can be due to language barriers. Terminology used by the Anglo may also be misunderstood by Hispanics because of the effect produced by accent on clarity of speech. Confusion is created because some words, phrases, or expressions cannot be translated directly from one language to another.

Class-bound value conflicts are the result of health care professionals operating from within a middle-class value system. Nonphysician health care professionals are primarily middle-class Americans. A portion of the Hispanic population consists of immigrants who are financially compromised. In communicating, care should be taken to have a complete understanding of patients' priorities and basic needs to avoid imposing middle-class priorities where they are inappropriate.

Culture-bound values should not be used to evaluate what is normal and abnormal. Returning to the solace of an old neighborhood may be judged as escapism, regression, or denial by one culture but may be viewed as appropriate and adaptive behavior by another (Marsella & Pedersen, 1981).

Appalachian Anglo-American

The economically deprived area along the Appalachian mountains of Alabama, Georgia, Kentucky, Maryland, Mississippi, New York, North Carolina, Ohio, Pennsylvania, South Carolina, Tennessee, Virginia, and all of West Virginia is known as Appalachia. Eighteen million people live in this region, 90 per cent of them are white, and the main sources of livelihood are mining and farming.

Within Appalachia, there are two types of family systems: traditional and contemporary. The traditional family is held together primarily by standards of obligation, even though affection can and does exist. The wife is subordinate to the husband's authority, but there is a move toward a more equalitarian relationship. Children are raised with a strict hand; fear is used as the primary method to control children's behavior. In spite of the strict discipline, the relationship between child and parent is close but interdependent. Children remain close emotionally and physically to their parents throughout their entire life (Dillard, 1983).

When working with the traditional family, much of the communication should be directed to the husband, who will, in turn, communicate with his wife and children. If the patient is elderly, the children will be readily available to help out. Because life is viewed somewhat fatalistically within the traditional family system, compliance with health care measures may be a problem. These people believe that they are powerless to change or control their lives and therefore tend to let nature take its course.

The contemporary Appalachian family stresses closeness instead of obligation. They are not as dependent on kin. The grown children of a contemporary family do not necessarily live close by, so contact with them may have to be made by telephone or audio tape when a parent is critically or terminally ill. Members of the contemporary family strive to improve their lives, thus increasing the possibility of compliance in the area of medical care.

Although handicapped by poor education and limited marketable employment skills, members of this culture value wisdom, direction, and security, which they believe come from family life. Family solidarity, individualism, pride, and loyalty are emphasized. Making provisions for psychological services in the Appalachian area is almost impossible. Patients look to their families for psychological support. Outside professionals are viewed as intruders (Axelson, 1985; Dillard, 1983).

When trying to support and communicate with a patient or family member, the educational level of the individual should be assessed before explanations, information, or instructions are given. This will increase the likelihood of understanding.

Appalachians communicate in a manner similar to other middle-class Anglos. Barriers to verbal interaction include dialect, vocabulary, and expression. The literal translation of a sentence often has a different and even opposite meaning. Appalachian Anglo-Americans speak slowly and often punctuate their speech with long silences. Verbal aggression may cause a female to withdraw and a male to become hostile. When speaking, Appalachians do not make direct or constant eye contact, believing that it is more polite to shift the eyes (Dillard, 1983). This population might be described as people of few words and more action. The words they do use are simple, and their speech contains few qualifiers, adjectives, and adverbs, particularly when dealing with feelings (Axelson, 1985) (Table 60–2).

THEORETIC FOUNDATIONS FOR UNDERSTANDING FAMILY COMMUNICATIONS

Families vary widely in their communication styles. Consideration of various theoretic models will lend an

Table 60–2. ATTITUDINAL CONTRASTS BETWEEN TRAINED PROFESSIONALS AND MOUNTAINEERS

Trained Professionals	Appalachian Mountaineers
Taught to relate impersonally and to deal with others on an objective basis. The trained professional learns how to act as a "doctor," "lawyer," or other role.	For mountaineers, impersonality is odd. They are brought up to act person-to-person; to be treated as a role is a dehumanizing and demoralizing thing.
A professional's aloof objective approach could precipitate a suspicious reaction from mountaineers, which in response can prompt the doctor (or other professional) to think the mountaineer is just stupid or uncooperative.	If a mountaineer cannot penetrate the aloof "shell" of the professional, he or she tends to become suspicious.
Status roles may play a part in the professional/mountaineer relationship. One's sense of being is concerned with status in the predominant society.	In the old mountain society, there is no class structure or struggle. Underground in a coal mine, everybody is the same.
Professional people have organized life styles. Professionals are trained for order and punctuality. They think things can be arranged. Planning is essential and foremost.	Mountaineers have less ordered life styles. For them, life flows more naturally. They're not planners; they keep things "loose."
Professionals optimistically compete with life through striving to master and control imperfections in others and in life conditions.	Mountaineers have a more relaxed attitude toward life. They approach life with contentment and take it as it comes. Some might call this "fatalism." However, given a situation in which advancement and the opportunity to change things were nonexistent, it would not be fatalism, but realism.

(From Axelson, J. A. [1985]. *Counseling and development in a multicultural society* [p. 53]. Monterey, CA: Brooks/Cole. Originally appeared as Lewis, H. [1979]. *Trained professionals and mountaineers: Cross-cultural contrasts*. Presentation given at Northern Illinois University, September 24, Adapted by permission.)

understanding to these differences. Theory ultimately provides the structure from which a therapeutic intervention is derived (Baruth & Huber, 1984).

Psychoanalytic Theory

Psychoanalytic theory focuses on defense mechanisms, or attempts by the individual to prevent ego disorganization, and unconscious intrapsychic conflicts. Families experiencing a chronic or terminal illness may become handicapped by latent emotional problems, unresolved conflicts, or both. These can be brought to consciousness because the demands imposed by the family's health crisis jeopardize the mobilization of positive coping strategies. The defense mechanisms most frequently activated in a crisis by the unconscious intrapsychic mechanisms are denial, displacement, reaction formation, regression, and sublimation (Baruth & Huber, 1984).

Social Learning Theory

Social learning theorists propose that family members train one another. The present, not the past, is emphasized. Positive coping behaviors are reinforced. Collaboration and negotiation of changes necessitated by the diagnosis of cancer are taught through behavior exchange, communication enhancement, problem solving, and contracting (Baruth & Huber, 1984).

Systems Theory

A less fragmented and more encompassing approach to the family in crises is evident in systems theory. Relationships are seen as systems in themselves and as subsets of a greater system that extends into the community. The marital subsystem is held as the key to family functioning. Applications of system theory are Bowen's theory, problem solving theory, and family system theory.

Bowen's Theory

A strategy often used by families dealing with death and dying is called *triangulation* (Bowen, 1978). The crisis creates a situation in which family members are unable to communicate effectively. Therefore, a third person becomes involved to help maintain the relationship by mediating or deflecting. The tension is reduced, but this arrangement can be dangerous if the third person is a professional who is only temporarily involved with the family. When another family member is placed in this position, it is called *family projection process*. For example, a mother and father can focus on the "behavior problem" of a healthy child so that they do not have to deal with their feelings regarding a terminally ill child. Bowenian theorists are concerned with a person's degree of differentiation of self. Minuchin (1974), like Bowen, states that all families are somewhere on a continuum between emotional stick-togetherness, which results in family members having difficulty achieving independence, and differentiation. In a crisis, a differentiated person may react initially with emotion but will recover quickly because of an ability to distinguish between emotion and intellect (Bowen, 1978). The lower the level of differentiation, the less able are persons to determine what they believe, how they feel, or how they evaluate a situation apart from the beliefs of others in the family system.

The nurse who chooses to apply Bowen's theory encourages differentiation slowly by exploring how the individual feels, believes, and evaluates the situation rather than allowing him or her to accept the position assumed by the family. This is achieved through defining, clarifying, keeping the self detriangulated, teaching, and helping the person to make "I" statements (Geary, 1979).

Problem Solving Theory

Haley espouses problem solving theory as a systems approach to understanding marital and family crisis situations. Relationships by definition are a struggle for power and control through the messages exchanged, and control is often achieved through the exhibition of symptoms (Baruth & Huber, 1984). The power relationship must be clarified by teaching awareness of the true intentions of individuals who attempt to gain control by allowing these individuals to be involved in change or to accept their behavior. Within the family, the power hierarchy may be determined by age, sex, intelligence, history, function, or interest (Baruth & Huber, 1984).

A relationship is defined by levels of communication, including messages that are overt or covert and situations that are handled by establishment of explicit or implicit rules. Rule setting is an important domain of marital power and control (Baruth & Huber, 1984). Rules can protect a family member in one set of circumstances and cause difficulty in another. Covert rules about open expression of feelings, such as fear or anger, could have profound effects on a family's coping behavior during the period of illness.

Being present, implicit labeling, and paradoxical interventions are done to help partners see and understand their situation in a different light. Implicit labeling does not require overt behavior changes, whereas paradoxical interventions are explicit techniques that require behavior change; these changes are usually in the form of disobeying the professional's instructions. To obey the professional would give power to the professional; to disobey the professional usually changes the behavior in a positive sense. The confusion caused by the paradox initiates a move toward more adaptive functioning (Geary, 1979).

Family Systems Theory

McCubbin cites the works of Burr (1973) and Hill and Hansen (1964) in stating that strong relationships within the family system serve to buffer the stressors in life. Families that maintain open communication, are flexible, are able to negotiate, and are mutually involved in decision making during times of crisis are more likely to be psychologically and emotionally healthy. The adjustment process may be seriously affected if communication lines are closed, creating an atmosphere of a conspiracy of silence (Vess et al., 1985).

As a system, every family adopts its own unique way of structuring roles, relationships, and responsibilities to direct family life. These features are linked to a family's stage of development. In working with a family to enhance communication, the nurse should make an effort to understand the family's roles and rules that guide day-to-day activities. The sick person can become sicker or the well person can become sick as a secondary gain tactic in response to role changes (Bruhn, 1977). This pattern serves as an attention-getting mechanism, especially if someone feels overshadowed or overburdened.

Nye (1976) has identified eight primary roles in the family system: provider, housekeeper, child care, child socialization, sexual, recreational, therapeutic, and kinship. Each family member assumes a certain number of these roles. The communication sent to and from the individual in any of these roles is often centered around the holder's identity with the role. Cancer frequently alters persons' abilities to fulfill their assigned roles and therefore affects the content, quality, and quantity of communication. How a family accommodates to role shifts depends on the number and nature of the roles held by the patient, the availability and ability of other family members to assume the roles, and the accessibility of external support and resources for the individual assuming a new role and the person having to relinquish the role (Nye, 1976). Role and responsibility changes often leave the involved persons feeling a sense of personal loss or inadequacy.

Olsen (1970) stresses that families who make a good adjustment to illness have a clear separation of generations; flexibility within and between roles; direct and consistent communication; and, above all, tolerance for individual differences. When a family member becomes ill, it is essential to view the family as a whole rather than to think in terms of interactions between two or more members. It is helpful to examine theoretic models of family interaction to appreciate the manner in which families function.

FAMILY ASSESSMENT

Doing a family assessment is valuable because of the wide variation among individuals, families, and cultures. Because there is no one right way for a family to act or respond in time of crisis, more emphasis should be placed on assessing the family in a continuous systematic manner (Martocchio, 1985; Olsen, 1970). Assessment data provides the health care team with valuable information on family structure, expectations, and previous crisis experience. Because treatment continues over months and years, a plan for helping families can be established and reassessed on a regular basis.

Information relevant to the family's perception of the illness, the threat it presents, the resources available, and the family's past experiences of a similar nature enables the health care team to assist the family more fully. The team determines what information the family needs to maximize communication and coping skills and to anticipate the types of resources and support needed in the future.

Framework for Assessment

Hill and Hansen (1964) developed a framework for family assessment in chronic illness that is an excellent resource. This framework explores four factors that influence a family's ability to cope (Table 60–3). It may take more than one interview to complete the assessment form, but the format provides a consistency in the data-gathering process that is directed at the family as a unit of care.

Table 60–3. FACTORS INFLUENCING FAMILY COPING

Characteristics of the Illness
What is the family's understanding of the diagnosis?
What is the perceived degree of pain, disability, or threat to life?
What is understood about treatment and related side effects?
What belief is held regarding prognosis and potential for regaining health?

Perceived Threat to Family Relationships, Status, and Goals
How does the family define roles, relationships, and communication patterns?
What are the decision-making patterns before and after the illness?
What are the family goals, and how are they affected by the illness?
How do individual members feel about changes created by the illness?

Available Resources
What financial resources are available if income is threatened?
What are the family's support resources: relatives, friends, community support groups, and so forth?

Past Experiences with Similar Situations
What coping strategies has the family used in past crises?
What is the cancer history of the family, and what were experiences coping with cancer like for the family?

(Data from Hill & Hansen, 1964.)

Components That Affect Family Care

Belcher (1987) has also outlined components of family care that could serve as an assessment tool for establishing a database. This comprehensive guide addresses the interactive aspects of family care, including the meaning of cancer, the emotional impact of cancer on relationships, cancer's impact on roles, and the enhancement of strengths that help families cope. Collecting data on a family's coping strengths provides clues for planning helpful interventions throughout the continuum of care.

Screening Questionnaires

FAPGAR

The Family APGAR or FAPGAR is a brief screening questionnaire designed to gather data on the patient's view of the functional integrity of his or her family. Smilkstein (1984) defines five basic components of family functioning that must be considered when evaluating the family's overall state of health: *adaptation*—how assistance is received; *partnership*—how communication and problem solving are used in decision making; *growth*—how flexible the family is in regard to role change and nurturing; *affection*—how intimacy and emotional interaction are shared; and *resolve*—how time, space, and money are allocated among family members. Five questions are used to provide qualitative measurements of a family member's satisfaction with each of these components.

Family Inventory of Life Changes

The positive relationship between life events and illness has been set forth by Holmes and Rahe (1967). This same concept can rightly be extended to family health and illness. The linkage between stress-illness research and family stress theory is predicated on understanding the family as a system. Life events, both normative and situational, that are experienced by any single member or by the family as a whole add together to determine the impact of life changes. It is expected that a decline in family functioning will correlate negatively with a cumulative number of family life changes (McCubbin & Patterson, 1987).

The Family Inventory of Life Events and Changes, or FILE, is designed to assess the accumulation of life events experienced by a family (McCubbin & Patterson, 1987). This 71-item, self-report instrument is designed for adult members of the family unit. It asks them to check all events experienced by any member of the family over a period of 1 yr. Comparative norms have been established for families over the seven stages of the family life cycle. An individual family score, when compared with the norm in the appropriate stage, provides a means of classifying the family into a high-stress, moderate-stress, or low-stress group.

Wegmann (1988) describes several other instruments designed to assess family stress and coping. These objective measures can be used appropriately on a routine basis for gathering assessment data. They provide a numerical measurement of a family's resources and strengths and stressors already present, and they are good at forecasting families that may be at high risk for stress. An anticipatory plan of care can be derived from this type of approach to doing a family assessment.

FAMILY-CENTERED PROGRAMS

Family assessment is the initial step in identifying a family's needs, stressors, and strengths. Assessment data can be utilized in determining ways and means for assisting families to cope with cancer throughout the continuum of care (Welch-McCaffery, 1983). This translates into having services that extend from simply being available for understanding, support, and affirmation (Lovejoy, 1986; Mayer, 1986) to providing programs specifically designed to encompass the entire family unit. Criteria that promote families utilizing positive coping skills need to be incorporated into the design of family-centered programs. These criteria are the following:

- Improving problem-solving techniques used by families
- Strengthening families' interactional skills
- Increasing family members' sense of self-esteem

Resources, institutional support, financial constraints, and family receptivity are factors that must be considered when selecting type, format, and frequency of programs. Services should be designed so they are available when families want to use them.

Family Conferences

Family conferences should be held periodically throughout the continuum of care. These conferences should be scheduled in advance, open to all family members including the patient, held in a prearranged space that accommodates all family members and guarantees privacy, and conducted by the physician and other health care team members. This type of structured exchange between physicians and families promotes more accurate communication about the status of the family member's cancer and the treatment options. Family members can come prepared with questions, be given an opportunity to clarify certain points of concern, and collectively discuss the presenting problems in the presence of a third party, the health care team.

Conference audio tapes allow family members to replay the conference at a later date. Recall is frequently incomplete or in error, especially at stressful times. The tape is a tool for providing family education and promoting communication. For the absent family member, perhaps someone who lives at a distance, the audio tape is a way to hear the same explanations and information as those members who attended the conference.

Video Visits

Video visits can be conducted in the patient's hospital room or at a family gathering. It is a means for family members to share and express their love and concern more visually. Videotaping can be very poignant during the terminal phase of illness, when the patient has limited energy and the family visits are restricted because of time or distance. The playing of a video tape can close the gap between the patient and the extended family. It is also a historical document and may become a treasured family possession in future years.

Support Programs

Support can come from others who have experienced the same situation. In peer support groups, patients and their families not only exchange practical information and approaches to the numerous problems that must be faced but also offer emotional support (Kemler, 1985). Numerous groups exist nationally; Candlelighters, Make Today Count, and programs for ostomates and laryngectomees are well known examples. The process that takes place in a support group affirms to the members that they are sharing a specific journey.

Another means of support is offered through one-to-one visitation programs, such as the American Cancer Society programs of CanSurmount and Reach to Recovery. Volunteers, who are cancer survivors, visit newly diagnosed patients or patients facing the same surgery to provide support, reassurance, and living testimony that people do survive cancer. This type of one-to-one support offers an outlet for patients and family members to voice their fears and concerns to someone who has been there.

Retreat Programs

Getting away together can be structured as a therapeutic intervention for families. It gives them the time and freedom to confront problems posed by a cancer diagnosis.

We Can Weekend is an example of a program purposely designed to bring families together (Johnson & Norby, 1981). This program is based on the simple premise that every cancer family member can be actively involved in the restoration process. Family members are encouraged to see that in striving to regain balance in family life, it is helpful to learn about facts and feelings surrounding cancer. The program design is flexible enough to include all ages of children and is directive in discussing cancer and its ramifications. It provides a broad selection of educational activities and promotes communication within the family regarding members' feelings about cancer. The long-range goal of the We Can Weekend is to help families utilize positive skills for coping with cancer in their family.

Up to 18 families go to a retreat-type setting for a weekend accompanied by a staff of approximately 20 health professionals. The selected site offers classrooms and sleeping and eating facilities and a gymnasium, swimming pool, and large outdoor recreation area. Art, movement, and music activities are integrated throughout the 2 days to create an atmosphere of group togetherness and sensitivity. This program first began at North Memorial Medical Center in Minneapolis in 1978 and now is available in a number of sites in the United States (Lane & Davis, 1985).

Because family needs are continually changing, family-centered interventions must be flexible if they are to meet the needs of family members. Creativity and sensitivity are keys to designing and promoting family interventions.

This chapter has provided a rationale for why cancer care needs to be expanded to include all family members. Nurses must develop the skills to assess and plan strategies for meeting family needs throughout the continuum of care. They are the key people in guiding cancer families toward the establishment of healthy patterns of coping during the crisis and recurrent times of stress created by a cancer diagnosis.

References

Antonovsky, A. (1979). *Health, stress and coping.* San Francisco, CA: Jossey-Bass.

Axelson, J. A. (1985). *Counseling and development in a multicultural society.* Monterey, CA: Brooks/Cole Publishing Co.

Baruth, L. G., & Huber, C. H. (1984). *An introduction to marital theory and therapy.* Monterey, CA: Brooks/Cole Publishing Co.

Belcher, A. (1987). Communicating with the patient and family/significant others. In C. Ziegfeld (Ed.), *Core curriculum for oncology nursing* (pp. 347–350). Philadelphia: W. B. Saunders Co.

Bowen, M. (1978). *Family therapy in clinical practice.* New York: Jason Aronson.

Bruhn, J. G. (1977). Effects of chronic illness on the family. *Journal of Family Practice, 4,* 1057–1060.

Bureau of Indian Affairs, Department of the Interior. (1986). *American Indians today.* Washington, DC: U.S. Government Printing Office.

Burr, W. F. (1973). *Theory construction and the sociology of the family.* New York: John Wiley & Sons, Inc.

Cassileth, B. R., & Hamilton, J. (1979). The family with cancer. In Cassileth, B. R. *The cancer patient: Social and medical aspects of care* (pp. 233–247). Philadelphia, Lee & Febiger.

Christ, G. H. (1983). A psychosocial assessment framework for cancer patients and their families. *Health and Social Work, 8,* 57–64.

Dillard, J. M. (1983). *Multicultural counseling. Toward ethnic and cultural relevance in human encounters.* Chicago: Nelson-Hall.

Eliopoulos, C. (1981, April). Chronic care and the elderly: Impact on the client, the family and the nurse. *Topics in Clinical Nursing,* pp. 71–83.

Geary, M. C. (1979, March). Supporting family coping. *Supervisor Nurse,* pp. 52–60.

Giacquinta, B. (1977). Helping families face the crisis of cancer. *American Journal of Nursing, 77,* 1585–1587.

Gray-Price, H., & Szczesny, S. (1985, April). Crisis intervention with families of cancer patients: A developmental approach. *Topics in Clinical Nursing,* pp. 58–70.

Green, C. P. (1986). Changes in responsibility in women's families after the diagnosis of cancer. *Health Care for Women International, 7,* 221–239.

Hill, R., & Hansen, D. A. (1964). Families under stress. In H. T. Christensen (Ed.), *Handbook of marriage and the family* (pp. 782–819). Chicago: Rand McNally & Co.

Holmes, T. H., & Rahe, R. H. (1967). The social readjustment rating scale. *Journal of Psychosomatic Research, 11,* 213–218.

Hsu, J. (1985). The Chinese family: Relations, problems and therapy. In W-S Iseng & D. Y. H. Wu (Eds.), *Chinese culture and mental health* (pp. 95–105). New York: Academic Press.

Johnson, J. L., & Norby, P. A. (1981). We Can Weekend: A program for cancer families. *Cancer Nursing, 2,* 23–28.

Keefe, S. E., Padilla, A. M., & Carlos, M. L. (1978). Emotional support systems in two cultures: A comparison of Mexican Americans and Anglo American. Rockville, MD: National Institute of Mental Health.

Kemler, B. (1985). Family treatment in the health setting: The need for innovation. *Social Work in Health Care, 10*(4), 45–53.

Lane, C., & Davis, A. (1985). Implementation: We Can Weekend in the rural setting. *Cancer Nursing, 8,* 323–328.

Lewis, R., Ellison, E., & Woods, N. (1985). The impact of breast cancer on the family. *Seminars in Oncology Nursing, 1,* 206–213.

Lovejoy, N. (1986). Family response to cancer hospitalization. *Oncology Nursing Forum, 13*(2), 33–37.

MacVicar, M. G., & Archbold, P. (1976). A framework for family assessment in chronic illness. *Nursing Forum, 15,* 180–194.

Madsen, W. (1969). Mexican-Americans and Anglo-Americans: A comparative study of mental health in Texas. In S. C. Plog & R. B. Edgerton (Eds.), *Changing perspectives in mental illness.* New York: Holt, Rinehart & Winston, Inc.

Marsella, A. J., & Pedersen, P. B. (Eds.). (1981). *Cross-cultural counseling and psychotherapy.* New York: Pergamon Press.

Martocchio, B. (1985). Family coping: Helping families help themselves. *Seminars in Oncology Nursing, 1,* 292–297.

Mayer, D. (1986). Cancer patients' and families' perceptions of nurse caring behaviors. *Topics in Clinical Nursing, 7,* 63–69.

McCubbin, H., & Patterson, J. (1987). File, family inventory of life events and changes. In H. McCubbin & A. Thompson (Eds.), *Family assessment inventories for research and practice* (pp. 81–100). Madison: University of Wisconsin Press.

Minuchin, S. (1974). *Families and family therapy.* Cambridge: Harvard University Press.

Northouse, L. (1984). The impact of cancer on the family: An overview. *International Journal of Psychiatry in Medicine, 14,* 215–242.

Nye, P. Z. (1976). *Role structure and analysis of the family.* Beverly Hills, CA: Sage Publications.

Oberst, M. T., & James, R. A. (1985, April). Going home: Patient and spouse adjustment following cancer surgery. *Topics in Clinical Nursing,* pp. 46–57.

Olsen, E. H. (1970). The impact of serious illness on the family system. *Postgraduate Medicine, 2,* 169–174.

Padilla, A. M., & Ruiz, R. A. (1973). *Latino mental health.* Rockville, MD: National Institute of Mental Health.

Richardson, E. H. (1981). Cultural and historical perspectives in counseling American Indians. In D. W. Sue (Ed.), *Counseling the culturally different* (pp. 224–237). New York: John Wiley & Sons, Inc.

Ruiz, R. A. (1981). Cultural and historical perspectives in counseling Hispanics. In D. W. Sue (Ed.), *Counseling the culturally different* (pp. 191–195). New York: John Wiley & Sons, Inc.

Smilkstein, G. (1984). The physician and family function assessment. *Family Systems Medicine, 2,* 263–278.

Smith, E. J. (1981). Cultural and historical perspectives in counseling blacks. In D. W. Sue (Ed.), *Counseling the culturally different* (pp. 156–173). New York: John Wiley & Sons, Inc.

Sue, D. W. (Ed.). (1981). *Counseling the culturally different.* New York: John Wiley & Sons, Inc.

Tringali, C. (1986). The needs of family members of cancer patients. *Oncology Nursing Forum, 13*(4), 65–70.

Vess, J. D., Moreland, J. R., & Schwebel, A. I. (1985). An empirical assessment of the effects of cancer on family role functioning. *Journal of Psychosocial Oncology, 3,* 1–16.

Wegmann, J. (1988). Selecting a tool for measuring coping. In M. Frank-Stromborg (Ed.), *Instruments for clinical nursing research.* East Norwalk, CT: Appleton & Lange.

Welch-McCaffery, D. (1983). When it comes to cancer: Think family. *Nursing 83, 12,* 32–35.

CHAPTER 61

Developing Strategies for Public Education in Cancer

JAYNE I. FERNSLER

The impetus for public education in cancer was launched in 1913 by a small group of physicians and laypersons, who met to discuss cancer concerns and organized the American Society for the Control of Cancer, later called the American Cancer Society (ACS) (American Cancer Society [ACS], 1987a). Since that time, many others have become involved in public education efforts: health care professionals; social scientists; behavioral scientists; communications specialists; federal, state, and local governmental agencies; and the general public. Now the general public expects to receive information about cancer. Those who read newspapers and magazines, watch television, or listen to the radio are exposed to cancer information almost daily. The openness and eagerness with which many people seek information about cancer is in itself evidence of the progress that has been made in public cancer education since 1913. Despite this progress, there is still a segment of the population that is untouched or unmotivated by the usual media. Educators must continue to try new approaches to reach both the seekers and nonseekers of information.

DEFINING PUBLIC EDUCATION

In the preceding paragraph the words *public education* and *information* are used interchangeably. Although much of the literature in public cancer education does not differentiate between education and information specifically, most educators agree that imparting information is part of but not the whole of education. According to the Oncology Nursing Society (ONS) Education Committee (1983), education is a process that results in the acquisition of knowledge and skills and changes in behavior or attitudes. Although not explicit, this definition is implied in the stated aim of the ACS's public education programs: to provide people with information about cancer and what they can do to protect themselves in terms of health practices and life styles (ACS, 1990). The ACS believes that public education involves a two-way interaction between teacher and learner.

Van Parijs's (1986) international review of public education in primary and secondary cancer prevention included four types of programs designed for different goals: to increase public awareness of cancer, to change risk behavior, to teach self-examination techniques, and to promote early detection in the community. Van Parijs does not differentiate between public information and public education but discusses the uses and limitations of mass communication for raising the public's awareness about cancer. Griffiths (1981) maintains that both public information and education are the preferred means for changing human behavior. Public information disseminated through mass media may begin the process of individual decision making by promoting awareness. Interactive-type education programs reinforce the initial information and further promote behavior change.

MAJOR INITIATIVES IN PUBLIC EDUCATION

A number of organizations, including hospitals, health maintenance organizations, and voluntary health agencies, are concerned with the provision of cancer education to the public. This section focuses on

ACS MEMBERSHIP BOARD AND COMMITTEE STRUCTURE

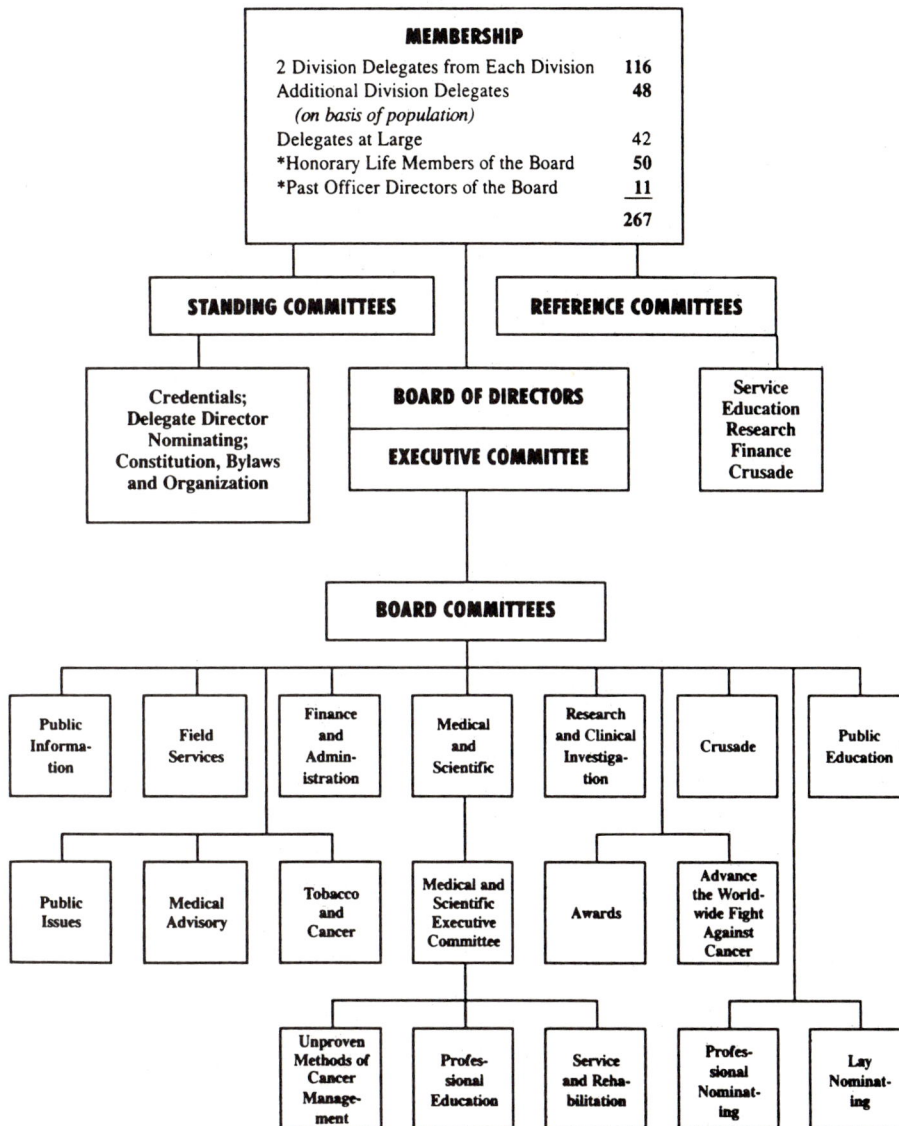

MEMBERSHIP	
2 Division Delegates from Each Division	116
Additional Division Delegates	48
(on basis of population)	
Delegates at Large	42
*Honorary Life Members of the Board	50
*Past Officer Directors of the Board	11
	267

STANDING COMMITTEES

REFERENCE COMMITTEES

Credentials;
Delegate Director
Nominating;
Constitution, Bylaws
and Organization

BOARD OF DIRECTORS

EXECUTIVE COMMITTEE

Service
Education
Research
Finance
Crusade

BOARD COMMITTEES

Public Information

Field Services

Finance and Administration

Medical and Scientific

Research and Clinical Investigation

Crusade

Public Education

Public Issues

Medical Advisory

Tobacco and Cancer

Medical and Scientific Executive Committee

Awards

Advance the Worldwide Fight Against Cancer

Unproven Methods of Cancer Management

Professional Education

Service and Rehabilitation

Professional Nominating

Lay Nominating

*As of date of publication; elected annually—number varies.

The Medical and Scientific Committee and its Executive Committee function through several major subcommittees in addition to those shown and through other subcommittees that may be established from time to time.

Figure 61–1. American Cancer Society membership board and committee structure. (From Fernsler, J. I. [1987]. *American Cancer Society factbook for health professionals* [3076–PE, p. 7]. New York: American Cancer Society. Reproduced by permission.)

those that are the most salient to nursing: the ACS, the National Cancer Institute (NCI), and the ONS. Considerable discussion is devoted to ACS and NCI because of the wide scope and availability of their programs and their evaluation efforts, and because nurses are likely to get involved in these activities.

The American Cancer Society

Purpose

The ACS was the first national organization to make a major commitment to educate the public about cancer. The commitment to public education is evident in the original organizational mission statement to "disseminate knowledge concerning the symptoms, treatment, and prevention of cancer; to investigate conditions under which cancer is found; and to compile statistics in regard thereto" (ACS, 1987a). Today the purposes of the ACS have expanded to further encompass public education. This purpose is addressed by a major committee within the ACS structure (Fig. 61–1), the Public Education Committee. Communication to the public at large concerning ACS and its programs is coordinated by another major committee, the Public Information Committee. The overall organizational structure of ACS is discussed in Chapter 83.

Structure

The national Public Education Committee is composed of volunteers who develop plans, guidelines, and materials for use at the division and unit levels of the organization (Table 61–1). Because educational approaches and materials are required for both adult and youth populations (Fig. 61–2), there are two separate subcommittees. Additional advisory and planning groups, consisting of unit, division, and national volunteers and staff, are formed on an ad hoc basis to address various tasks, such as planning a national meeting, developing specific materials, and forming focus groups. Consequently, although priorities for public education are initiated at the national level, the organizational structure allows for two-way communication between levels of the organization.

The ACS divisions are mandated by charter standards to have standing public education committees

Table 61–1. ACS PLANNING MATERIALS FOR USE AT DIVISION AND LOCAL LEVELS

Working Smart to Save More Lives
Public Education Materials
A Public Education Planning Guide for ACS Unit Volunteers
American Cancer Society Plan for the Youth Education Program
Managing Public Education in Your Unit
What Is P-A-C-E
Working with Other Health Agencies
Employee Education Program Handbook
Handbook for Colleges and Universities Program
Reaching Youth Outside the Classroom
Handbook on Schools Program
Clubs and Organizations Handbook

(Data from American Cancer Society. Reproduced by permission.)

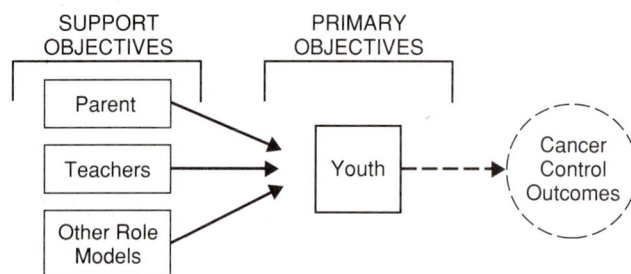

Figure 61–2. American Cancer Society (ACS) Youth Education Program. An excellent example of the type of planning material developed by the Youth Education Subcommittee. The plan includes a conceptual model for identifying objectives for the youth program, as shown in the figure. Criteria for developing objectives are based on the potential impact, trends, and resources of ACS programs and the relationship of the ACS's objectives to the nation's health objectives. Specific objectives are listed for each of five priority program areas: substance abuse, nutrition and eating patterns, cancer early detection, cancer the disease, and the environment. Guidelines for implementing and evaluating the plan are included along with an extensive bibliography. (From Fernsler, J. I. [1987]. *American Cancer Society plan for the youth education program* [0200.8–LE]. New York: American Cancer Society. Reproduced by permission.)

(ACS, 1983). Divisions, in turn, set standards for public education in the units. At a minimum, units must have written program objectives for public education (N. Lins, personal communication, August 31, 1987).

Program Planning, Implementation, and Evaluation

The focus of the ACS public education program is primary and secondary prevention of cancer: primary prevention through behavior change or reinforcement in relation to known risk factors and secondary prevention through scheduling regular cancer-related physical examinations and taking prompt action in the event that cancer signs or symptoms occur (Table 61–2). Consequently, although the ACS has literature about many cancer sites, their programs focus on information and behaviors related to high-incidence cancers that are mostly preventable or curable: colon and rectum, lung, breast, uterus, oral cavity, and skin. Priority is given to the first four sites, because primary prevention or early detection of these cancers results in a significant decrease in mortality (ACS, 1990).

The underlying assumption of the ACS approach to public education is that behavior change occurs over time, beginning with the acquisition of knowledge that a specific behavior is required for prevention or early detection of cancer (Fig. 61–3). Knowledge leads to awareness of one's own susceptibility as well as what action to take in relation to it. Education strategies are designed to help individuals at each step of the behavior change model from awareness to adoption of behavior to maintenance of the desired behavior. The ACS's ten recommended strategies for facilitating behavior change (Table 61–3) are congruent with standard principles of teaching and learning.

Educational methods are designed for use with both

Table 61-2. CANCER FACTS AND FIGURES 1990

Prevention

Primary Prevention Refers to Steps that Might be Taken to Avoid Those Factors that Might Lead to the Development of Cancer

Smoking	Cigarette smoking is responsible for 85% of lung cancer cases among men and 75% among women—about 83% overall. Smoking accounts for about 30% of all cancer deaths. Those who smoke two or more packs of cigarettes a day have lung cancer mortality rates 15 to 25 times greater than nonsmokers.
Sunlight	Almost all of the more than 600,000 cases of non-melanoma skin cancer diagnosed each year in the US are considered to be sun-related. Recent epidemiologic evidence shows that sun exposure is a major factor in the development of melanoma and that the incidence increases for those living near the equator.
Alcohol	Oral cancer and cancers of the larynx, throat, esophagus, and liver occur more frequently among heavy drinkers of alcohol.
Smokeless Tobacco	Use of chewing tobacco or snuff increases risk of cancer of the mouth, larynx, throat, and esophagus and is highly habit forming.
Estrogen	For mature women, estrogen treatment to control menopausal symptoms increases risk of endometrial cancer. Use of estrogen by menopausal women needs careful discussion by the woman and her physician.
Radiation	Excessive exposure to ionizing radiation can increase cancer risk. Most medical and dental x-rays are adjusted to deliver the lowest dose possible without sacrificing image quality. Excessive radon exposure in homes may increase risk of lung cancer, especially in cigarette smokers. If levels are found to be too high, remedial actions should be taken.
Occupational Hazards	Exposure to several different industrial agents (nickel, chromate, asbestos, vinyl chloride, etc.) increases risk of various cancers. Risk from asbestos is greatly increased when combined with cigarette smoking.
Nutrition	Risk for colon, breast, and uterine cancers increases in obese people. High-fat diets may contribute to the development of cancers of the breast, colon, and prostate. High-fiber foods may help reduce risk of colon cancer. A varied diet containing plenty of vegetables and fruits rich in vitamins A and C may reduce risk for a wide range of cancers. Salt-cured, smoked, and nitrite-cured foods have been linked to esophageal and stomach cancer. The heavy use of alcohol, especially when accompanied by cigarette smoking or chewing tobacco, increases risk of cancers of the mouth, larynx, throat, esophagus, and liver. (See above.)

Secondary Prevention Refers to Steps to be Taken to Diagnose a Cancer or Precursor as Early as Possible After It Has Developed

Colorectal Tests	The American Cancer Society recommends three tests for the early detection of colon and rectum cancer in people without symptoms. The digital rectal examination, performed by a physician during an office visit, should be performed every year after the age of 40; the stool blood test is recommended every year after 50; and the proctosigmoidoscopy examination should be carried out every 3 to 5 years, based on the advice of a physician.
Papanicolaou (PAP) Test	For cervical cancer, women who are or have been sexually active, or have reached age 18 years, should have an annual PAP test and pelvic examination. After a woman has had three or more consecutive satisfactory normal annual examinations, the PAP test may be performed less frequently at the discretion of her physician.
Breast Cancer Detection	The American Cancer Society recommends the monthly practice of breast self-examination (BSE) by women 20 years and older as a routine good health habit. Physical examination of the breast should be done every three years from ages 20 to 40 and then every year. The ACS recommends a mammogram every year for asymptomatic women age 50 and over, and a baseline mammogram between ages 35 and 39. Women 40 to 49 should have mammography every 1 to 2 years, depending on physical and mammographic findings.

(From American Cancer Society. [1990]. *Cancer facts and figures—1990* [5008-LE, p. 18]. Atlanta: Author. Reproduced by permission.)

adult and youth audiences. Most programs for adults include a talk, an audiovisual presentation, and a discussion. Youth programs are frequently presented by positive role models such as peers, parents, teachers, and media celebrities. Prepared ACS materials, designed for specific age groups, are available for teachers. Guidelines for selecting techniques and tools to match the target audience and the setting for a program are presented in Table 61-4.

Implementation of public education programs occurs primarily at the unit level of the ACS. Although unit public education committees vary in size and composition, depending on the geographic areas they serve, they should have at least an adult and a youth subcommittee and, if appropriate and feasible, subcommittees

for developing a speakers' bureau and for organizing programs in clubs and organizations, the workplace, home and neighborhood, and other health agencies. Volunteer planners who develop the overall program plan, recruit and train volunteers, and in general enforce ACS policies and procedures constitute the public education committee. Volunteer doers are recruited for their special knowledge and expertise in reaching specific target audiences, such as employees in the workplace, smokers, adults in clubs and organizations, and children in schools. Volunteers, such as nurses, business executives, former smokers, school teachers, clergy, and representatives from minority groups, are needed to tailor programs to meet the educational needs of specific groups. Programs are

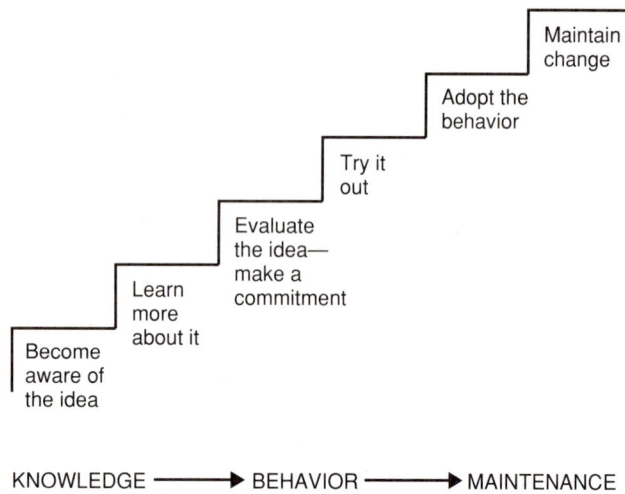

Figure 61–3. How people make decisions and change health habits. (From Fernsler, J. I. [1987]. *A public education planning guide for ACS unit volunteers* [p. 18]. New York: American Cancer Society. Reproduced by permission.)

usually initiated by volunteers approaching the target groups but may be, and frequently are, requested by the groups themselves.

The ACS uses three types of evaluation to monitor its public education program: process, impact, and outcome. *Process evaluation,* conducted at the unit level, is concerned with whether programs are being implemented as planned and whether the target audience is satisfied with them. Program Activities Report is the formalized system for reporting the number of people reached, the program topic, and the setting. Participant satisfaction is assessed immediately after a program via a brief questionnaire or several weeks later via a follow-up postcard.

Impact evaluation, performed at the national level, is concerned with changes in knowledge, attitudes, and behaviors as a result of the educational program (ACS, 1987b). Table 61–5 illustrates findings from one of

many surveys and studies sponsored by the ACS. A complete list of these studies is available from each ACS division office (ACS, 1987c).

Outcome evaluation, also performed primarily at the national level, is concerned with trends and changes in cancer morbidity and mortality. Data for this type of evaluation are gathered at the local, regional, and national level. The national ACS compiles the data and distributes it to ACS divisions (ACS, 1987b).

The National Cancer Institute

Purpose

The purpose of the NCI with regard to public education is to inform the public about prevention, early detection, and treatment of cancer (National Cancer Institute [NCI], 1988e). The Office of Cancer Communications (OCC) is the organizational component of the NCI that is responsible for public education as well as patient, family, and professional education. This section focuses on the public education component of the program.

Structure

The OCC has three major branches (Fig. 61–4). Established in 1977, the Information Projects branch is responsible for developing, promoting, and evaluating education and information programs for the public (NCI, 1988c). The Reports and Inquiries branch handles all public inquiries, including telephone inquiries received through the Cancer Information Service. Public interest in cancer care is reflected in the more than 350,000 requests for information that are processed by this branch each year (NCI, 1988e). The Information Resources branch produces NCI publications and distributes both OCC-developed and other cancer-related publications. In fiscal year 1986, more

Table 61–3. STRATEGIES FOR FACILITATING BEHAVIOR CHANGE

1. *Use messages tailored to the people you're trying to reach.* Attempt to see the world through their eyes and use words and examples that are familiar and meaningful to them.
2. *Give them the information they need.* There are a lot of ACS programs ready to help you.
3. *Give them specific messages about what you want them to do.* For example, set a date to stop smoking, practice BSE once a month. ACS booklets and films will help.
4. *Keep fear at a moderate level—neither too low nor too high.* Research shows that if people are too afraid, they become immobilized, but if they have no fear, they remain unconcerned. ACS public education materials have been developed carefully to strike the right balance.
5. *Involve them.* When people are involved actively in the learning process, they are more likely to recall the information and demonstrate the needed skills. Anything you can do to increase involvement will enhance learning. For example, ask the audience to list their reasons for quitting or to share ways they have to cut down on dietary fat.
6. *Show them how to do it.* Often, people are motivated to change, but they need to be shown how. For example, demonstrate the proper breast self-examination technique. Have a cooking demonstration of low-fat, high-fiber recipes. Show people how to get ready to quit smoking.
7. *Build their confidence that they can take action successfully.* If people slip up, let them know they haven't failed. This is especially true in the areas of smoking cessation and dietary change, where habits are complex and new habits must be practiced over and over.
8. *Show your target audience that you believe in them.* Let them know they have your support. That can make a difference.
9. *Reinforce the message.* Because behavior change is a long-term process, it's important to get back to people. The more you interact with a given group of people, the more likely it is that their behavior will change.
10. *Use more than one educational method to reach your target audience.* Consider using a combination of educational methods. This will give you the best chance for success.

(Adapted with permission from American Cancer Society. [1987]. *A public education planning guide for ACS unit volunteers* [pp. 18–20]. New York: Author.)

Table 61–4. THE ACS EDUCATION PLANNING SYSTEM—SELECTING THE TOOLS FOR PUBLIC EDUCATION

	Lecture	Audio-Visual Aids	Discussion	Individual Instruction	Demonstration & Skill-building	Role Playing	Inquiry Learning	Modeling	Behavior Modification	Institutional Change
Who										
Youth										
● Disadvantaged and blue collar	●	●●●	●●●	●●●	●●●	●●●	●●	●●●	●●●	●●●
● Middle class and higher	●●	●●	●●●	●●	●●●	●●●	●●●	●●●	●	●●
Adults										
● Disadvantaged	●	●●	●●●	●●●	●●●	●●●	●	●●●	●●	●
● Blue collar	●●	●●	●●●	●●●	●●●	●●●	●	●●●	●●	●●●
● White collar	●●●	●●	●●●	●●●	●●	●●	●	●●	●●●	●●
● Employed in home	●●●	●●●	●●●	●	●●●	●	●	●●	●●	●
● Retired	●●●	●●●	●●●	●●	●●●	●	●	●●●	●●●	●
Where										
● Worksite	●●	●●●	●●●	●	●●●	●●	●	●●●	●●	●●●
● Healthsite	●●	●●	●●●	●●●	●●	●	●	●	●●	●●●
● School	●●●	●●●	●●●	●●●	●●●	●●●	●●●	●●●	●●	●●
● Community	●●●	●●●	●●●	●●	●●	●	●	●●	●●	●●
What										
● Awareness	●	●●	●●●	●	●			●●●	●	●●
● Attitudes	●●	●●●	●●●	●●●	●●	●●	●●●	●●●	●●●	●●
● Knowledge	●●●	●●●	●●●	●●●	●●●	●●	●●●	●●●	●●	●●
● Behavior	●●	●●	●●●	●●●	●●●	●●●	●●●	●●●	●●●	●●●

Each "bullet" is a point. For each technique you are considering, count the points that apply to the *who, where,* and *what.* Your goal is to make sure that each public education event is worth at least 50 points. First you choose the place to reach a particular group. Then you select the techniques that will achieve the best learning payoff. In general, choose the three-point techniques for public education for a particular audience in a particular place.

(From American Cancer Society. [1987]. *A public education planning guide for ACS unit volunteers.* New York: Author. Reproduced by permission.)

than 16 million publications were distributed either directly by mail or indirectly through health care facilities, schools, professional meetings, supermarkets, and discount stores (NCI, 1988d).

Programs

The Information Projects branch has two major public education foci: breast cancer education and cancer prevention awareness. Targeted for all women older than 18 years, the Breast Cancer Education Program is designed to improve women's knowledge, attitudes, and practices related to breast cancer. The intended outcome is twofold: early detection of breast cancer through increased detection practices and re-

Table 61–5. KNOWLEDGE OF CANCER'S WARNING SIGNALS

	Percent of Population		
	1966 (%)	1978 (%)	Change (%)
A lump or thickening in the breast or elsewhere	87	85	−2
Unusual bleeding or discharge	77	70	−7
A change in a wart or mole	76	68	−8
A sore that does not heal	77	67	−10
Persistent cough or continuing hoarseness	53	65	+12
A change in bowel or bladder habits	55	59	+4
Persistent indigestion or difficulty in swallowing	42	46	+4

(From American Cancer Society. [1979]. *Public attitudes toward cancer and cancer tests* [3322–PE, p. 95]. New York: Author. Reproduced by permission.)

duced delay in seeking medical help for symptoms of breast cancer, and improved ability to deal with breast disease. Specific public education programs and materials for this program are listed in Table 61–6. Materials are also available for patients, health professionals, and program planners (NCI, 1988a).

Launched in March, 1984, the Cancer Prevention Awareness Program is a massive public education effort that was designed to contribute to the NCI's year 2000 goal—to reduce cancer mortality by 50 per cent (NCI, 1986). Although the program is targeted to the general public and focuses on seven modifiable cancer risk factors, blacks are targeted as the subgroup and tobacco and nutrition as the risk factors that have the greatest potential for reducing mortality. The program objectives are to improve the public's knowledge, attitudes, and behaviors regarding cancer prevention. The message is that one can control one's risk for cancer by taking specific actions (Table 61–7).

Mass media and individual and organizational intermediaries are the NCI's vehicles for communicating educational messages to the public. The OCC develops and distributes public service announcements, live announcer copy, modular program kits, and information kits to radio and television stations, news directors, and contacts in the print media. To reinforce the message and to reach a more specific target audience, the media campaign is conducted in waves and may feature positive role models, such as celebrities. For example, the media wave to reach blacks featured messages from Aretha Franklin and Roosevelt Grier.

Intermediaries are individual health professionals

National Cancer Institute
Office of Director

Office of Program Planning and Analysis

Office of Administrative Management

Office of Cancer Communications

Office of International Affairs

Office of Associate Director
Associate Director for Cancer Communications

Information Projects Branch

Reports and Inquiries Branch

Information Resources Branch

Health Promotion Section

Patient Education Section

Reports Section

Public Inquiries Section

Document Reference Section

Graphics/Audiovisual Section

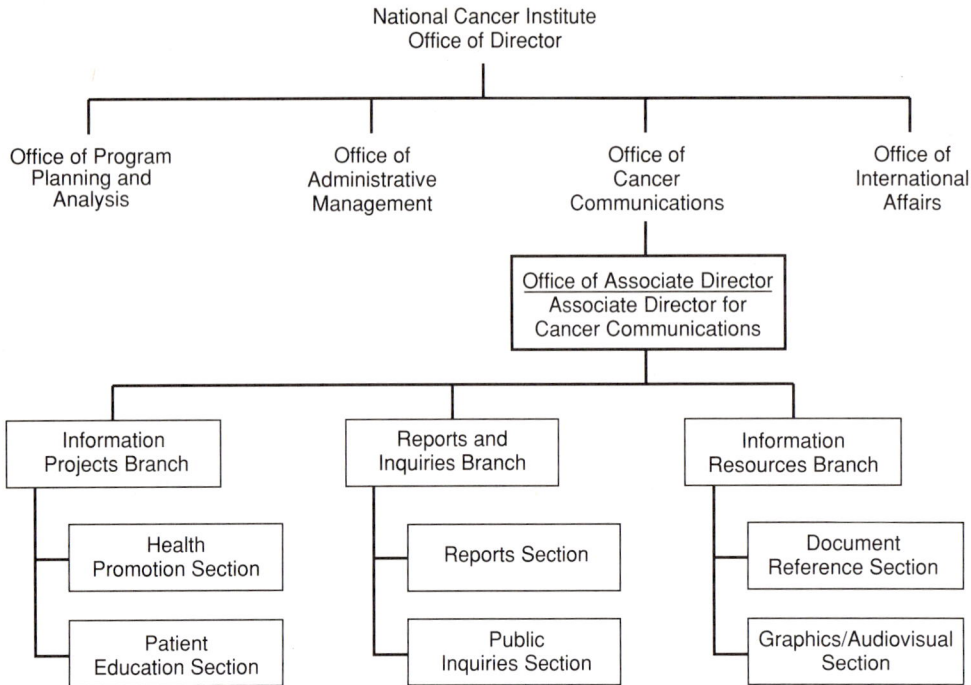

Figure 61–4. Office of cancer communications of the National Cancer Institute.

Table 61–6. BREAST CANCER EDUCATION PROGRAM, PUBLIC EDUCATION PROGRAMS, AND MATERIALS

"Breast Cancer: We're Making Progress Every Day"
This public education program (formerly entitled "Progress Against Breast Cancer") is designed for use by businesses, service clubs, religious organizations, unions, and other interest groups. Program materials include the following:
- a slide/tape or videocassette program providing an overview of the progress being made in breast cancer detection, diagnosis, treatment, and breast reconstruction;
- a pamphlet, "Breast Cancer: We're Making Progress Every Day," for each member of the audience, which summarizes the information contained in the program and contains step-by-step instructions on how to perform breast self-examination (BSE);
- two posters for display;
- a "User's Guide" to help those organizing the program;
- a print ad featuring movie critic Gene Shalit's review of the program;
- the *Breast Cancer Digest.*

"Breast Exams: What You Should Know"
Describes a variety of breast cancer screening methods including physical examination, mammography, and BSE. Also available in Spanish.

"Questions and Answers about Breast Lumps"
Discusses some of the most common noncancerous lumps, diagnostic procedures, treatment, and cancer risks.

"If You've Thought about Breast Cancer"
Written by Rose Kushner, this booklet contains information about symptoms of breast cancer, detection, diagnosis, treatment, rehabilitation, breast reconstruction, and other information helpful to breast cancer patients and their families.

"Breast Cancer: We're Making Progress Every Day"
Summarizes current information about breast cancer, including risks and signs of the disease; mammography, biopsy, and treatment options; breast reconstruction; and rehabilitation. An illustrated guide for BSE is included also. This pamphlet is a revised version of "Progress Against Breast Cancer."

"What You Need to Know about Cancer of the Breast"
This pamphlet discusses symptoms, diagnosis, rehabilitation, emotional issues, and questions to ask a doctor.

(Data from National Cancer Institute, 1988.)

and organizations, such as clubs, churches, voluntary agencies, and health agencies, that interact with the public and, therefore, can impart cancer prevention information directly to them. Titled "Partners in Prevention," this approach was launched through a series of workshops held for selected intermediaries throughout the country. A list of materials available for Partners in Prevention is included in Table 61–8. Other materials specific to tobacco and nutrition are also available to the public and to health professionals (NCI, 1987c).

Recruitment of leaders of black civic groups and professional organizations into Partners in Prevention has led to the development of the Joint Health Venture, a special effort to reach the black population. Organizations participating in this venture include the National Medical Association, National Urban League, National Football League, Shriners, National Black Nurses' Association, National Council of Negro Women, and selected national black sororities. The focus of the message to blacks is that cancer is preventable and that one's risk can be reduced by adopting certain behaviors. A booklet titled "Good News for Blacks about Cancer," a speaker's kit, and media

Table 61–7. STEPS INDIVIDUALS CAN TAKE TO CONTROL THEIR OWN RISK FACTORS

- Avoid tobacco in all forms.
- Include foods high in fiber daily (fruits, vegetables, and whole-grain breads and cereals).
- Choose foods low in fat.
- Consume alcoholic beverages moderately, if at all.
- Avoid unnecessary x-rays.
- Know and follow health and safety rules at your workplace.
- Avoid too much sunlight: wear protective clothing and use effective sunscreens.
- Take estrogens only as long as necessary.

(Data from National Cancer Institute, 1987.)

Table 61–8. KEY PROGRAM MATERIALS FOR PARTNERS IN PREVENTION (PIP)

Update:
A periodic communication to PIP members describing current cancer prevention program information from NCI, and national, state, and local cancer-related efforts of public, private, and voluntary organizations across the United States. Each issue of *Update* summarizes a major element of the prevention program and describes new NCI publications.

The Cancer Prevention Catalog:
Describes NCI cancer prevention publications.

Partners in Prevention Speaker's Kit on Cancer Prevention:
A modular kit designed to help health professionals make informed and effective presentations on cancer prevention and risk reduction. It contains a 20-min script, a script outline, an accompanying slide presentation, background and resource materials, and sample NCI cancer prevention publications. The kit is available at no cost, on a 1-month loan basis.

The Cancer Prevention Resource Directory:
A comprehensive guide to cancer prevention programs and materials at the federal, national, state, and local levels.

Partners in Prevention: Case Studies of Cancer Prevention in the Community:
Describes and analyzes the impact of the workshops on four CIS offices and affiliated organizations within their regions. This new report documents the importance of the commitment and continuity of CIS staff members to the level, duration, and success of follow-up activities.

(Data from National Cancer Institute, 1987.)

materials have been developed to facilitate dissemination of the message.

Implementation of the Cancer Prevention Awareness Program was preceded by extensive research and planning. Literature was reviewed in relation to the seven selected cancer risk factors; public knowledge, attitudes, and practices related to cancer and models of health education, communication, and marketing. Other recent prevention-oriented, health promotion campaigns were reviewed. Focus groups and special work groups were conducted to develop appropriate messages and strategies for a variety of audiences (NCI, 1987b). In addition, before launching the Cancer Prevention Awareness Program, the NCI conducted a national telephone survey to obtain baseline data on public knowledge, attitudes, and practices related to cancer prevention and risk (NCI, 1984).

Evaluation

The NCI monitors its public education activities through formative and impact evaluation. Formative evaluation is used in planning, designing, and pretesting materials and messages. The 1983 telephone survey on public knowledge, attitudes, and practices was used to identify the public's cancer information needs. A similar survey conducted in 1985, 1 year after the Cancer Prevention Awareness Program was implemented, revealed positive changes in the public's knowledge, attitudes, and behaviors (NCI, 1987a) and provided a rationale for revising materials and making future program plans. Periodic random sample telephone surveys are planned to identify changes in the public's knowledge, attitudes, and behavior over time.

Another type of formative evaluation—psychographic audience segmentation—is used to provide the

NCI with additional information on target audience subgroups. Using the psychographic technique, responses to questionnaires are sorted to group the audience according to values and attitudes. Both messages and media can then be designed for specific subgroups (NCI, 1988b).

Impact evaluation is conducted to evaluate the effectiveness of programs. Indirect measures of the influence of media campaigns include the number and type of public inquiries made to the Cancer Information Service, the number of requests for materials, the number of public service announcements made on radio and television, and the amount of exposure of the program in the print media. The effectiveness of the NCI's message in changing public knowledge, attitudes, and behaviors related to cancer prevention is measured through evaluation of specific programs and through periodic national surveys by the NCI and other government and private organizations (NCI, 1988b).

The Oncology Nursing Society

One of the goals of the ONS is to provide cancer education to the general public as well as to nurses. The Education Committee of the society developed *Outcome Standards for Public Cancer Education* (Oncology Nursing Society Education Committee, 1983, 1989) in the belief that the public should be educated about cancer and that nurses are responsible for educating them. The target audience is all people in the community, and the major objective is to inform them about their options related to prevention, early detection, rehabilitation, and living with cancer.

The ONS suggested that the following assumptions be considered when planning a public education program (Oncology Nursing Society Education Committee, 1983):

All individuals are at risk for developing cancer at some point in their lives.

Certain individuals possess a higher risk for developing cancer by virtue of their genetic background and/or environmental exposure.

Cancer control activities are influenced by political, social, cultural, and economic factors.

Active participation by the public in the educational process enhances learning.

Public education influences the public's knowledge, skills, and attitudes about risk factors related to carcinogens.

Health care needs and cancer risk factors identified by health care providers may differ from those perceived by the public.

Individuals come to learning situations with certain knowledge and beliefs about cancer which affect their learning.

Educational strategies must reflect the culture and ethnic diversities of the public.

These assumptions are inherent in the ONS revised standards and in the society's efforts to enhance public education in cancer nursing practice. Nurses are encouraged to submit abstracts of public education projects for either oral presentations or exhibition at the

ONS annual congress. Projects that reflect the assumptions are viewed favorably by the Education Committee. In addition, through funding from an NCI grant, the ONS conducted regional workshops to teach minority nurses how to develop and implement public education programs about cancer prevention and detection in their communities. As part of the evaluation of the project, minority nurses who participated in the workshops are now reporting their public education activities to the ONS.

The ONS's most recent initiative with regard to public education is the establishment of an award to support and recognize excellence in patient or public education. The award is presented annually to a nurse member of the society who is involved in creative programming that reflects the society's educational standards.

The Oncology Nursing Foundation, an ONS-related organization devoted to funding education and research, has a goal related to educating the general public about cancer and cancer care also. The foundation addresses this goal through a yearly request for proposals for public cancer education. The first such RFP was awarded in 1987 for a project to educate black women about the early detection of breast cancer.

In summary, the ONS's goal for public education is broad. The organization fosters public education indirectly by educating nurses and by providing a forum for them to share information about public education. The ONS also provides standards for nurses to use when developing or evaluating public education programs. The Oncology Nursing Foundation provides limited funding for public education projects.

Involvement of Nurses in Public Education

Nurses can be pivotal in public cancer education. They constitute the largest group of health professionals involved in cancer care, and they practice in a variety of settings where they interact with the public. In addition, nurses are often approached informally by friends and neighbors who want special information about cancer. Consequently, most nurses have target audiences readily available to them.

Nursing education prepares nurses to teach both patients and the public. Many nursing curricula are organized around a framework of health maintenance and wellness. Students in such programs learn skills in these areas in the community. One recently graduated baccalaureate nurse was recognized nationally for her proposed public awareness program about testicular self-examination (Carlin, 1986). The proposal included a stepwise procedure for implementing the program at the grassroots, county, state, and national levels.

Clinical experience prepares nurses to teach also. Greene (1986) states that by virtue of their contact with patients and families, nurses know the devastating effects of cancer and the value of early detection. She states also that nurses know how to communicate with people in appropriate language. Consequently, nurses who have been in practice for many years can bring a wealth of knowledge and experience to a teaching-learning situation.

Both ACS and NCI identify nurses as important volunteers or intermediaries in their goals to educate the public about cancer prevention and detection. Nurses can influence the public as role models and as health educators (NCI, 1987c). Their activities may be local, state, regional, or national in scope. Such activities have the potential to broaden nurses' skills, while empowering the public with useful information. Thus nurses' involvement in public education is mutually beneficial to nurses and society.

The nature and degree of an individual nurse's involvement in public education may depend on his or her employer, flexibility in work schedule, preparation and experience, and commitment to teaching others. A nurse's involvement may vary from leading an employee smoking cessation program at lunchtime to chairing an ACS committee that markets public education to potential audiences and develops policies and procedures for training and certifying speakers. Some institutions encourage their nurse employees' involvement in ACS public education efforts, whereas others appeal directly to the public with their own health education and prevention programs. In either situation, a nurse's participation may be limited by other demands of the job.

When the ONS board of directors asked members to report their activities with regard to cancer prevention and early detection, nursing students, practitioners, administrators, and educators responded with a variety of educational activities. The nurses reported both formal and informal teaching that was not necessarily part of their job descriptions. Specific examples of activities included informal teaching at exhibit sites in hospitals as well as in the community; making formal presentations as volunteers in cancer-related groups, such as a local ONS chapter, ACS, or NCI; answering cancer information calls; and assisting with screening and detection programs (Nevidjon, 1986).

PROGRAM DEVELOPMENT

Nurses are accustomed to using the nursing process in clinical practice. A similar systematic process is used in developing educational programs, regardless of the intended audience (professionals, patient, public). This section highlights public education program development from a nursing perspective. There is a detailed description of the stages of program development—assessment, planning, intervention, evaluation—in Chapter 62.

Setting Priorities

Nurses set priorities daily, because rarely are they able to do all that they think should be done in a clinical situation. Setting priorities in public education, as in clinical practice, is a safeguard against dissipating energy and resources by trying to do everything. Priority setting involves asking What are the greatest public education needs in this situation? Both ACS and NCI use national primary and secondary survey results to answer the question. At the local level, nurses can assess needs through observations made in clinical practice; data from the hospital or state tumor registry; and requests for information from family, friends, and neighbors. For example, through one or more of these methods the nurse may discover a plethora of cases of newly diagnosed, advanced breast cancer in women under the age of 30. This discovery, viewed in the appropriate context, may indicate an immediate need to educate young women about breast self-examination (BSE) and breast cancer.

Nurses in primary care settings, such as health maintenance organizations and physicians' offices, have special opportunities to assess the public's need for cancer information. They see both well and sick people and have the opportunity to assess changes in their knowledge and health behaviors over time. So-called noncompliant behaviors with regard to a health maintenance program may signal the need for education.

Formulating Objectives

Objectives are written in terms of what the learner is able to do at the completion of an educational program. Categories and components of objectives are discussed in Chapter 62. Objectives are useful to the teacher and the learner because they tend to keep both focused on the topic. Limiting objectives can be difficult, because one tends to think that the learner needs to know all about the topic. In the case of the previously described need to educate young women about BSE and breast cancer, the most important objectives are that women correctly perform BSE monthly and consult a physician immediately if they discover any signs of cancer. These objectives are realistic and measurable through return demonstration and follow-up. According to the ACS stepwise model of behavior change (see Fig. 61–3), however, women must first become aware of BSE and evaluate the practice before they try it.

The ONS public education standards (Oncology Nursing Society Education Committee, 1983, 1989) have been useful for program planning because they provide behavioral objectives or criteria for each area of content or each standard related to public education. Nurses in one hospital used the standards as a framework for developing the purpose, content, plans, and evaluation of a multidisciplinary cancer fair (Vega, 1985).

Developing a Budget

Public cancer education can be done relatively inexpensively if existing resources are tapped. For example, a program to educate young women about BSE and breast cancer could be coordinated with the local ACS Public Education Committee; local schools, colleges, and universities; and the county health department. With the support of experienced staff within these agencies, a nurse could coordinate the program and recruit other nurses as volunteer BSE instructors. Materials and equipment could be provided free of charge by the sponsoring organizations and by the NCI (see Table 61–6). Nevertheless, the nurse coordinator or the coordinating team should prepare a list of potential expense items, such as travel, postage, printing, educational pamphlets, audiovisual equipment, breast models, and posters. The sponsoring organizations should decide before the program who will assume the cost of items, such as postage, if follow-up information is requested from the women. Although including prepaid postage may seem expensive, it is cost effective in terms of enhancing the response rate from participants (Elwood, Erickson, & Lieberman, 1978).

Large-scale public education programs combined with screening involve the added expense of equipment, space for screening, laboratory costs, record keeping, and follow-up. These items should be given careful consideration when considering whether to screen as well as to educate the target audience. Depending on the nature of the program and the proposed activities, funding could be requested from the Oncology Nursing Foundation or the ACS Cancer Control Grant Program (ACS, 1986).

Selecting Methodologies

One method of promoting awareness and motivation among the target audience is to involve representatives of the group in program planning. Carlin (1986) reported success with soliciting artwork, from male high school students, for the cover of a pamphlet on testicular cancer and testicular self-examination. A similar approach could be used to involve high school and college females in developing materials for a BSE education program. Because the aim of the program is to encourage young women to adopt a behavior, the planners should consider the strategies listed in Table 61–3. The merit of using several methodologies is illustrated in Table 61–4. In this situation, a combination of lecture, audiovisual aids, discussion, demonstration, and return demonstration would be most effective.

Rutledge and Davis (1988) have identified factors that promote women's compliance with monthly BSE. Many of these factors can be addressed by nurses who teach BSE (Box 61–1).

Strategies for Hard-to-Reach Populations

Nurses are creative in reaching people who are outside the mainstream. One nurse, an ACS volunteer and patient education coordinator and outreach nurse

---

Box 61–1. BREAST SELF-EXAMINATION (BSE) COMPLIANCE AND THE HEALTH BELIEF MODEL

In this descriptive study, compliance with recommendations for BSE was examined within the framework of the Health Belief Model. A total of 248 women (ages 18 to 75) from YWCAs, industrial sites, and a university completed a 28-item questionnaire about health beliefs, breast cancer, and their self-reported practice of BSE. Of the sample, 31 per cent did not practice BSE, 15 per cent practiced monthly or more, and 54 per cent practiced less than monthly. Multiple regression analysis revealed that significant predictors of compliance were having a reminder, encouragement of family or friends, confidence in ability to perform BSE, younger age, physician interest in BSE compliance, disagreement that BSE causes unnecessary worry, and concern about breast cancer. Nurses should address these factors when teaching BSE by suggesting specific reminder cues, including family or friends in the teaching, providing opportunity for supervised practice of BSE, attending to the special needs of older women, and tempering the emphasis on all women's susceptibility to breast cancer with factual information about the availability of conservative surgery for lesions that are detected early and reconstructive surgery when the breast cannot be spared.

(From Rutledge, D. N., & Davis, G. T. [1988]. Breast self-examination compliance and the Health Belief Model. *Oncology Nursing Forum, 15*[2], 175–179.

---

in a small eastern community hospital, identified a need for breast cancer education among Amish women. An acquaintance of the nurse arranged her initial entry into the Amish community. She first observed the operation of an immunization clinic, which was held monthly by the public health department in the home of an Amish family. The Amish had agreed somewhat reluctantly to allow the clinic after an outbreak of whooping cough in their community. Then, with the help of a retired surgeon and a midwife who were familiar with the Amish community, a radiologic technologist, a volunteer, and a secretary, the nurse organized and implemented a BSE teaching and screening program in an Amish home.

The group planned strategies to accommodate the Amish values of privacy and simplicity. Registration and history taking was handled individually in a private room. Women in similar age groups were taught about breast cancer and BSE in groups of four. Posters were used in lieu of slides or a film because there was no electricity in the home. Advertising of the program was limited to posters placed in Amish homes, where church services are held, and in several Amish stores. Women who required mammograms were taught about the procedure by the radiologic technologist. These women were also given slips that permitted them to have mammograms done for $40.00 at a local radiology center on the days when the Amish generally go to town.

The best strategy for reaching selected populations is to consult them throughout program development. Then plan the program to accommodate their values and needs. For example, in working with Japanese-Americans, American Indians, and Hispanics, whose identity is strongly linked to the family unit, program planners should emphasize family roles and responsibilities rather than individual decision making regarding health habits. This approach fosters trust and understanding between educators and the target audience, essential ingredients for effective communication (Kagawa-Singer, 1987).

Blacks constitute the largest minority population that could benefit significantly from education about cancer prevention and early detection. Educational efforts must avoid stereotyping individuals within this population, while acknowledging their general mistrust of professional health care, which has resulted from years of discrimination and segregation (Guillory, 1987). Black clergy and the church are avenues for reaching a large portion of the black audience. In Delaware, gospelizing has been an effective medium for promoting cancer education and awareness among the black population in both urban and rural settings. This medium is unique; it appeals to individuals from a variety of socioeconomic and educational levels, including the illiterate.

Evaluation

Several types of evaluation were discussed previously in this chapter and are discussed in Chapter 62. Evaluation is the most troublesome component of public education, even when desired outcomes are specified clearly during the planning stage. Changes in people's knowledge, attitudes, and behaviors occur over time and may not be attributable to a single educational intervention. Unplanned news events may confound evaluation efforts by prompting people to take action such as participating in a screening program (Fink et al., 1978). However, such events tend to have a short-lived effect on people's behavior. Even when well-planned educational messages, interspersed with televised news, are effective in promoting the public's awareness, public compliance with follow-up screening behaviors may be low (Winchester et al., 1980).

When dealing with hard-to-reach populations, such as the Amish community that was described previously, standards for judging program effectiveness may have to be modified. For example, about half of the Amish women who were advised to have mammograms actually had them done. By usual standards, this response indicates a low compliance rate. Nevertheless, with this population, it represents a positive outcome of the program. Another positive outcome was that the providers were invited to repeat the program in other homes in the Amish community, and several of the women have maintained contact with the nurse coordinator. The long-term impact of the program will be evaluated through clinical observation and surveillance of the tumor registry data.

FUTURE DIRECTIONS FOR PUBLIC CANCER EDUCATION

Some years ago Butler and Paisley (1977) observed that public cancer education programs were generally lacking in appropriate application of social science principles and evaluation design. They made ten major recommendations, which have, for the most part, been considered in the public education programs of ACS and NCI. In the future, as both agencies intensify their efforts to reach nonseekers of information, particularly the socioeconomically disadvantaged and the illiterate, marketing and evaluation techniques will become even more crucial.

Continued and strengthened interagency cooperation and coordination will be needed to ensure broader coverage of the population while eliminating costly duplication of effort. One example of this cooperative effort is the recent activity by NCI and ACS to educate professionals as well as the public about available clinical trials. Another example is the proposed American Stop Smoking Intervention Study (ASSIST), which will be a combined effort of ACS, NCI, and regional as well as local coalitions working toward a smoke-free environment (ACS, 1988). In addition, alternative methods must be found to facilitate program implementation at the local level. ACS, NCI, and ONS all are attempting to address this need through regional committees or workshops. Educational approaches will need to be sensitive to the rapidly expanding elderly sector of the population.

IMPLICATIONS FOR CANCER NURSING PRACTICE

The time is right for nurses to expand their involvement in public cancer education. The public need exists, resources are available from the ACS (see Tables 61–1 to 61–4 and Figs. 61–2 and 61–3) and the NCI (Tables 61–6 to 61–8), and the standards for such activity are delineated by the ONS. Working collaboratively with other health care professionals, nurses have the potential to contribute significantly to the goal of reducing morbidity and mortality from cancer.

References

American Cancer Society. (1983). *Major policies* (1048–A). New York: Author.

American Cancer Society. (1986). *Policies governing the cancer control grants program of the American Cancer Society.* Atlanta: Author.

American Cancer Society. (1987a). *American Cancer Society factbook for health professionals* (3076–PE). New York: Author.

American Cancer Society. (1987b). *A public education planning guide for ACS unit volunteers.* New York: Author.

American Cancer Society. (1987c, August) *Circular letter* (PE–29). New York: Author.

American Cancer Society. (1988, December). *Memo to division executives* (DE–81). Atlanta: Author.

American Cancer Society. (1990). *Cancer facts and figures—1990* (5008–LE). Atlanta: Author.

Butler, M., & Paisley, W. (1977). Communicating cancer control to the public. *Health Education Monographs, 5,* 5–24.

Carlin, P. J. (1986). Testicular self examination: A public awareness program. *Public Health Reports, 101,* 98–102.

Elwood, T. W., Erickson, A., & Lieberman, S. (1978). Comparative educational approaches to screening for colorectal cancer. *American Journal of Public Health, 68,* 135–138.

Fink, R., Roeser, R., Venet, W., Strax, P., Venet, L., & Lacher, M. (1978). Effects of news events on response to a breast cancer screening program. *Public Health Reports, 93,* 318–327.

Greene, P. E. (1986). The role of the American Cancer Society in public education. *Seminars in Oncology Nursing, 2,* 206–210.

Griffiths, W. (1981). Can human behavior be modified? *Cancer, 47,* 1221–1225.

Guillory, J. (1987). Ethnic perspectives of cancer nursing: The black American. *Oncology Nursing Forum, 14*(3), 66–69.

Kagawa-Singer, M. (1987). Ethnic perspectives of cancer nursing: Hispanics and Japanese-Americans. *Oncology Nursing Forum, 14*(3), 59–65.

National Cancer Institute. (1984). *Cancer prevention awareness survey, management summary* (NIH Pub. No. 84–2676). Washington, DC: U.S. Government Printing Office.

National Cancer Institute. (1986). Cancer control objectives for the nation: 1985–2000 (NIH Pub. No. 86–2880). *NCI Monographs, 2,* 3–11.

National Cancer Institute. (1987a). *Cancer prevention awareness survey wave II management summary* (NIH Pub. No. 87–2908). Washington, DC: U.S. Government Printing Office.

National Cancer Institute. (1987b, October). *OCC planning board presentation: Cancer prevention awareness program.* Bethesda, MD: NCI Office of Cancer Communications.

National Cancer Institute. (1987c). *The cancer prevention awareness program: A program description.* Bethesda, MD: NCI Office of Cancer Communications.

National Cancer Institute. (1988a, January). *Breast cancer education program summary. NCI information programs.* Bethesda, MD: NCI Office of Cancer Communications.

National Cancer Institute. (1988b, January). *Evaluation. NCI information programs.* Bethesda, MD: NCI Office of Cancer Communications.

National Cancer Institute. (1988c, January). *Information projects branch NCI information programs.* Bethesda, MD: NCI Office of Cancer Communications.

National Cancer Institute. (1988d, January). *Publications. NCI information programs.* Bethesda, MD: NCI Office of Cancer Communications.

National Cancer Institute. (1988e, January). *Public response programs. NCI information programs.* Bethesda, MD: NCI Office of Cancer Communications.

Nevidjon, B. (1986). Cancer prevention and early detection: Reported activities of nurses. *Oncology Nursing Forum, 13*(4), 76–80.

Oncology Nursing Society Education Committee. (1983). *Outcome standards for public cancer education.* Pittsburgh: Oncology Nursing Society.

Oncology Nursing Society Education Committee. (1989). *Standards of oncology education: Patient/family and public.* Pittsburgh: Oncology Nursing Society.

Rutledge, D. N., & Davis, G. T. (1988). Breast self-examination compliance and the Health Belief Model. *Oncology Nursing Forum, 15*(2), 175–179.

Van Parijs, L. (1986). Public education in cancer prevention. *Bulletin of the World Health Organization, 64,* 917–927.

Vega, T. (1985). Outcome standards for public cancer education: The foundation for community education programs. *Oncology Nursing Forum, 12*(5), 66–67.

Winchester, D. P., Shull, J. H., Scanlon, E. F., Murrell, J. V., Smeltzer, C., Vrba, P., Iden, M., Streelman, D. H., Magpayo, R., Dow, J. W., & Sylvester, J. (1980). A mass screening program for colorectal cancer using chemical testing for occult blood in the stool. *Cancer, 45,* 2955–2958.

CHAPTER 62

Developing Strategies for Patient Education in Cancer

MARION E. MORRA

As a concept, patient education has evolved over time and continues to change. The surge of interest in the subject in the last 15 years has its roots in the fundamental shifts in the health care field and in society. A growing consumer interest in self-help and a more demanding attitude toward health care services have accelerated the acceptance of patient and family education. Today many hospitals, health departments, medical centers, health maintenance organizations, and physician office practices have departments that specialize in the field; some are even marketing and charging for their patient education services.

DEFINING PATIENT EDUCATION

Patient education has been defined in many ways, ranging from the simple to the complex. Johnson and Blumberg (1984) developed one definition that applied specifically to cancer: "A series of structured or non-structured experiences which are designed to assist patients to cope *voluntarily* with the immediate crisis response to their diagnosis, with long-term adjustments and with symptoms; gain needed information about sources of prevention, diagnosis and care; and develop needed skills, knowledge, and attitudes to maintain or regain health status."

This definition can be augmented by the Oncology Nursing Society's (ONS) outcome criteria (American Nurses' Association & Oncology Nursing Society, 1987), which provide a foundation for action by specifying the following anticipated knowledge levels by a patient or family member:

- Describes the state of the disease and therapy at a level consistent with his or her educational and emotional status

- Participates in the decision-making process pertaining to the plan of care and life activities
- Identifies appropriate community and personal resources that provide information and services
- Describes appropriate actions for highly predictable problems, oncologic emergencies, and major side effects of the disease or therapy
- Describes the schedule when ongoing therapy is predicted

In addition, the need for and the right to information are covered in many of the other ONS standards. Several other groups, including the American Medical Association (1985) and the Joint Commission of Accreditation of Hospitals (1987), have endorsed the need for patient education, especially in the inpatient and outpatient settings (Box 62–1).

Theories of Patient Education

Many facets of patient education contribute to its complexity. Some are rooted in the field of behavior change. Others are based in educational theories and practices, especially those for educating adults. Several of the theories and models, such as Maslow's hierarchy of needs, the Andragogy approach, the health beliefs model, and the PRECEDE model are covered elsewhere in this book (see Chapters 7 and 15).

The ONS has established a specific set of standards for cancer patient education, using the following basic assumptions:

- Application of the patient education process can have a positive influence on patient knowledge, skills, attitudes, and behaviors, all of which are instrumental in promoting a sense of control.

Box 62–1. MEETING-SELF CARE NEEDS: PATIENT GUIDELINES AND NURSING REFERENCE GUIDES FOR COMMON CLINICAL PROBLEMS

Early patient discharge, the nursing shortage, and high outpatient volume reduce the time available for patient education. Yet care complexity has increased the amount of information that is required to manage care at home. The Nursing Committee of the Yale Comprehensive Cancer Center (YCCC) generated common care standards for cancer patients so that patients seen by different disciplines (e.g., medical oncology, radiation therapy, gynecologic oncology, surgical oncology) would be given similar care and information.

After reviewing available materials, patient care guidelines for symptom control (beginning with ten common clinical problems) and nursing reference guides (to support the interventions proposed for symptom management) were developed. Nurses, using a common format, developed the guidelines based on current literature, to assist patients in self-care activities for constipation, diarrhea, nausea and vomiting, taste change, low platelet count, low white blood cell count, alopecia, fatigue, and oral care. The patient information, written at a sixth-grade level, answers four basic questions: What is it, what are its common causes, what can I do and when should I call the doctor? The nursing guidelines provide the knowledge base for symptom management and identify possible causes of the problem, intervention rationales, and potential complications.

A questionnaire and a five-point scale were developed to evaluate practicality, accuracy, and usefulness of the materials. The ten self-care guidelines were evaluated by a group of patients (n = 21); the ten accompanying nursing reference guides were evaluated by a group of nurses (n = 21). Both groups came from one inpatient and two outpatient settings at the YCCC, two community oncologists' offices, and one community nursing association. Patients found the self-care guidelines easy to understand (100 per cent), believable (100 per cent), at their level ("for someone like me"— 94 per cent), useful and informative (100 per cent), and containing new information (74 per cent). Patients also commented that they liked the self-care guidelines because they were brief, concise, clear, informative, and told them what to look for and what to do. On the rating scale, patients rated them as practical, encouraging, comforting, well done, informative, and the right length.

The nurses evaluated the nursing reference guide as easy to understand (100 per cent), sufficient to support the intervention (100 per cent), appropriate for the generalist nurse (74 per cent), and appropriate for the oncology nurse (69 per cent). On the rating scale, they judged the guides to be practical, comforting, encouraging, well done, informative, and useful. They also commented that the strength of the guides included their specific nursing interventions, comprehensiveness, potential causes and monitoring for potential problems, rationale for interventions, and use as a quick reference.

This approach to meeting self-care needs assists patients and families in problem assessment and management at home while maintaining quality nursing interventions in the context of increased care complexity and a nursing shortage.

(Adapted from Moore, J., & Knobf, T. [1988]. Meeting self-care needs: Patient guidelines and nursing reference guides. *Oncology Nursing Forum, 15* [Suppl.], 162.)

- Individuals learn differently because of unique cognitive, affective, and psychomotor abilities.
- Individuals come to learning situations with certain knowledge, attitudes, expectations, and beliefs about cancer that affect their ability to learn.
- Learners should be included in all phases of their educational experience to maximize their ability to meet their learning needs.
- Health care needs identified by the nurse may be different from the needs and wants of the learner.
- When differences in educational needs exist, learners' perceived needs must be considered and given priority in the overall educational plan.
- The learning environment should provide comfort, mutual trust, respect, freedom of expression, and acceptance of differences.
- Time must be allowed for learning to take place.
- It cannot be assumed that learning has occurred because a learner has been given instruction (Oncology Nursing Society, 1982).

The Essentials of Patient Education

A good reporter always asks six essential questions—who, what, when, where, why, and how. These questions are identical to those of interest to an investigator in the field of patient education.

Who Teaches. Many teachers, serving different purposes and filling different needs, are involved in programs of education for patients with cancer. They range from physicians and nurses to social workers and dietitians, family members and friends, pharmacists and physical therapists, former patients and volunteers, and information specialists and patient educators. Nurses, however, with their knowledge of the patient and the treatment, and with their special relationships with patients, have the potential to be among the most significant of the teachers. Although some nurses may also have the title of patient educator, every nurse can have a role in patient teaching.

Why Teach. The reasons for teaching range widely. Mazzuca (1982) found that patient education was successful in altering compliance and in improving physiologic progress and health outcomes. Also, a growing body of evidence suggests that knowledge and hopefulness go hand in hand. Cassileth and colleagues (1980) reported that patients who want as much information as possible, good and bad, are significantly more hopeful than those who prefer a minimal amount or only positive reports. Mischel and co-workers

(1984), who studied patients who had gynecologic cancer, found that women who know the details of the illness are more likely to have hope, which supports Cassileth's findings.

In addition, because nurse practice acts in some states now designate patient teaching as a nursing function, patient education has become not only a professional responsibility but a legal one as well. In many cases, patient education responsibilities are also delineated in position descriptions.

When to Teach. Teaching may take place at any time. However, learning happens only when the learner is ready. In education terms, this is known as the *teachable moment,* that is, the moment a learner makes a statement, asks a question, or otherwise seeks further knowledge. For patients who have cancer, the teachable moment is of major importance.

A patient in great stress is not in a learning mode. At these times, the nurse must tailor the program, helping the patient learn essential things—those that will most assist the patient in meeting current basic needs and in becoming comfortable, psychologically and physically, with the situation at hand. Periods of stress come at many and varying points in a patient's life: at diagnosis, beginning of treatment, ending of treatment, and recurrence. Because these factors affect learning, planning the timing for teaching must be part of the process.

Where to Teach. The when and where of teaching are closely related. Teaching may happen anywhere a person who is ready to learn comes into contact with the person or object who has the needed information. This can be in a structured or an unstructured situation. It can be in a clinic or hospital, in a doctor's office, or in a patient's home. It can happen face to face or over a telephone, in a group, or on a one-to-one basis.

What to Teach. What will be taught depends on an assessment of patient and family needs; these needs are the basis for writing teaching objectives. The American Hospital Association (1978) outlines five major categories of learning objectives for patient education programs:

- Facts and theories include learning and recall of information that has concrete references, such as names, amounts, terms, and definitions.
- Visual identification focuses on learning to use visual cues to discriminate one visual element from another, such as color and appearance.
- Principles and concepts include comprehending and applying the relationships among biologic events, the meaning of roles, or the principles that pertain to body system functions.
- Perceptual motor skills encompass performing tasks by using instruments.
- Attitudes, opinions, and motivations include influencing or changing behavior or course of action.

How to Teach. Approaches to teaching vary, but as with most other nursing processes, patient education consists of four stages: assessment, planning, intervention, and evaluation. It is helpful to use this systematic approach whether the teaching takes place in an inpatient or outpatient setting, in a classroom or a patient's home, or on a one-to-one basis or in a self-learning mode.

THE STAGES OF PATIENT EDUCATION

The Assessment Stage

The depth and breadth of assessment depends on the kind of patient education being planned. Planning the entire patient education program for a clinic will require a much broader understanding of the field than will developing a single patient booklet. However, whatever the type of patient education being envisioned, it is essential to make the assessment complete, accurate, and based on information from the learner, because the effectiveness of the end product depends on what information is gathered during this time.

This phase of work identifies and clearly defines the problem that needs to be addressed. Methods and tools for carrying out needs assessment vary from the simple to the complex (Table 62–1). Several models have been developed that can be used to carry out this stage. An example, using the competency model, is shown in Figure 62–1.

When working on a short-term, face-to-face communication problem, reviewing the patient's chart, nursing plans, and protocols; getting information from other health team members or journals; and talking with the patient and family will probably constitute the assessment. Because educational needs change, assessment must be done at various times during the diagnosis and treatment process, especially for one-on-one communications.

If a new patient education piece is planned, a review of the literature; an extensive search for existing materials; interviews with health care professionals; discussions with former patients, patients, and family members; and a structured questionnaire or survey may be necessary. The "Patient Education" feature that appears monthly in *Oncology Nursing Forum* gives

Table 62–1. NEEDS ASSESSMENT TOOLS AND METHODS

Methods	• Interview with patient, former patient, or family member
	• Observation
	• Group discussion
Tools	• Patient care records
	• Surveys
	• Nursing care plans
	• Questionnaire or checklist
	• Literature review
	• Search for existing materials
More Complex Tools	• Delphi II
	• Matrix assessment
	• Pyramid assessment
	• Card sort
	• Performance appraisal
	• In-basket
	• Role playing

(Adapted with permission from Frank-Stromborg, M. [1984]. Developing patient education material. *Oncology Nursing Forum, 11* [6], 70–72.)

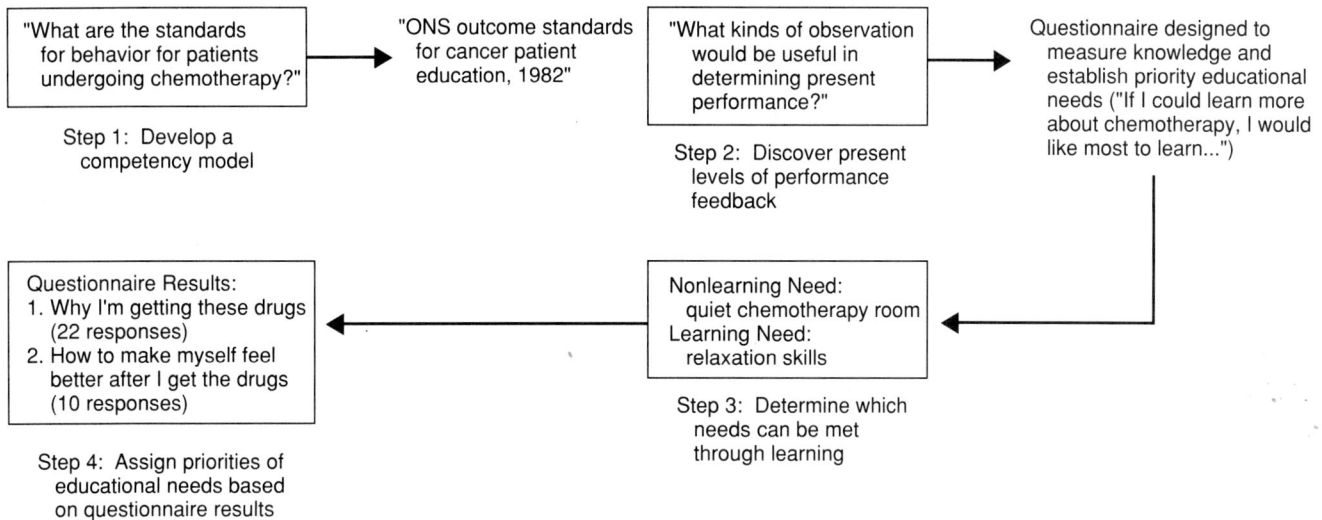

Figure 62–1. Conducting a needs assessment based on a competency model method. (From Frank-Stromborg, M. [1984]. Developing patient education material. *Oncology Nursing Forum, 11* [6], 70–72. Reproduced by permission.)

many examples of questionnaires that have been used in the assessment phase. Table 62–2 presents one example of a simple instrument that can be used to assess need for radiation therapy information. If a major hospital-wide or community-wide program is being planned, the PRECEDE model will be a helpful guide (Green, Kreuter, Deeds, & Partridge, 1980).

Table 62–2. EXAMPLE OF AN ASSESSMENT QUESTIONNAIRE FOR A RADIATION BOOKLET

The radiation departments want to develop an information booklet for patients receiving radiation therapy to the colon and rectum. We want the booklet to fit the needs of the patient. Please take a few minutes to answer the following questions. Circle the number that best fits how you feel about the following questions.
1 = not important to me
2 = important to me
3 = very important to me

1. How does radiation work?	3	2	1
2. What are the most common fears people have about radiation?	3	2	1
3. Will radiation affect how I heal?	3	2	1
4. Are there fertility problems associated with radiation?	3	2	1
5. Why do I need a full bladder when I receive radiation?	3	2	1
6. How may I improve my nutrition while receiving radiation?	3	2	1
7. Why might diarrhea happen?	3	2	1
8. How can I change my diet if diarrhea happens?	3	2	1
9. Why do skin changes happen?	3	2	1
10. How do I take care of my skin during radiation?	3	2	1
11. How do I take care of my skin if it is sensitive to radiation?	3	2	1
12. Why might I get nauseated?	3	2	1
13. How can I manage nausea?	3	2	1
14. What side effects won't I get?	3	2	1
15. Why do I need to have blood drawn?	3	2	1
16. What problems may happen after radiation is completed?	3	2	1

ANY OTHER QUESTIONS THAT ARE IMPORTANT TO YOU?

(From Witt, M. E. [1987]. Questions on colon and rectum radiation therapy. *Oncology Nursing Forum, 14*[3], 79. Reproduced by permission.)

During this phase, a selection process also occurs. The information is sorted, categorized, verified, and analyzed; what is not pertinent or needed should be discarded.

The final phase of the assessment stage is to write a short statement in the form of goals and objectives based on assessment that indicates the most important elements of the patient education project or program.

Most educational objectives consist of three parts: behavior (what the patient or family will be able to do at the end of the teaching sessions), context (under what circumstances they will be able to do it), and performance (how well the patient or family member will be able to execute it). The objectives are written using an action verb (such as *explain, state,* or *list*) and one task to be accomplished. They should be precise, learner-centered, and measurable.

Some Assessment Stage Problems

Establishing the Need. It is essential to establish whether there is indeed a need for the project. For instance, many booklets are available at present for patients undergoing chemotherapy, but it is not clear whether all the booklets are needed. Indeed, some of those published are not written as well nor do they give as much information as *Chemotherapy and You: A Guide to Self-Help During Treatment* (National Cancer Institute, 1987), which is available to anyone free of charge.

In the assessment phase, these questions should be asked: Why do we want to pursue this project? Is the need perceived by the patients and families or only by the caregivers? If a very similar product already exists, is it possible to use it as is; obtain permission to reprint it using another organization's name, either alone or in conjunction with the original sponsor; or augment it with another piece that elaborates on an area or areas currently seen as deficient?

Deciding What the Person Needs to Know and When. Understanding who needs to know what and

Table 62–3. KNOWLEDGE NEEDS OF THE PERSON LIVING WITH CANCER

Cancer—the illness	Coping responses
Description	Identifying, exploring, expanding
Symptoms	**Resources**
Detection	Community, hospital, private
Prevention	**Modification of life style**
Symptoms of recurrence	Role
Treatment of recurrence	Energy
Myths and untruths	Sexuality
Cancer—my illness	Body image
Specific type of cancer	Employment
Usual course	Nutrition
Metastasis	Stress
Prognosis	**Remission or recovery**
Diagnostic tests	Meaning of remission
Cancer—the treatment	How to deal with fears of
Surgery, chemotherapy,	recurrence
radiation	How to live with a chronic illness
Side effects	
Treatment of side effects	
Health care system	
How it works	
How to manage it	
Feelings	
Identifying, expressing,	
understanding	

(From Fredette, S. L., & Beattie, H. M. [1986]. Living with cancer: A patient education program. *Cancer Nursing, 9,* 308–316. Reproduced by permission.)

when is probably the most difficult part of the assessment process. One of the ONS patient education standards (1982) notes that learning needs should be assessed by a combination of methods: by asking specific questions about what patients know and need to know, by reviewing records, and by interviewing other health professionals to determine that information. There is no standard amount of information that all patients wish to have, but there has been some research on the knowledge needs of persons with cancer (one study is shown in Table 62–3). Messerli and colleagues (1980), in another study, reported that 86 per cent of mastectomy patients had questions concerning their treatment that they did not ask. Morra (1985), in analyzing calls received by the Cancer Information Service in Connecticut (1-800-4-CANCER), found that patients sought information early in the process, beginning with symptoms and diagnostic tests and continuing fairly steadily through treatment issues. Relatives and friends, however, seemed to enter the picture later on and ask more questions about treatment than any other issue.

When producing a product for wide distribution, the specific needs and wants of all individuals will not be known. It is important, however, to be sensitive to several factors: that patients and family members may have different needs at different times, that different people have different needs, and that physical and psychological states affect learning. Other groups of patients may be encountered, including those who do not want to be reached or who know what to do but are not doing it.

Understanding the Level of Information Needed. Two information levels must be considered: the depth of information of interest to the patient and family and the education level for which the product is being produced.

Cooper (1984), for example, in her research with lung cancer patients and their spouses, reported that nearly half of the spouses wanted more in-depth information than they had received from the doctor about the patient's condition, the probable course of the disease, and the use of chemotherapy.

Most health education materials are written to appeal to a broad spectrum of people. During the assessment process, it is important to get as detailed a picture as possible of the potential or target audience (Table 62–4). In a hospital setting, some demographic information about the patient population can be obtained from the social service department or from long-range planning personnel. At a voluntary agency, administrative personnel should be able to provide some clues about the people being served. Town or city planning departments have a wealth of information from the United States Bureau of the Census, many times broken down into block-by-block areas. Census information provides many population statistics including those on education, functional literacy, occupation, ethnic background, religion, and income.

The Planning Stage

During this stage, the planning of the specific items—what, how, when, and where the education will take place—is undertaken, based on the statement of goals and objectives written earlier. In addition, outcome criteria will be written so that evaluation can be accomplished. Factors that affect learning—the different needs of different people—must also be sorted out.

Factors That Affect Learning

Physical Status. Distressing physical factors affect a person's concentration and learning ability. Many patients with cancer have physical problems as a result of their disease or its treatment. The problems can include pain, nausea, fatigue, fever, lack of sleep, and side effects of medication. In addition, many patients

Table 62–4. SEGMENTING TARGET AUDIENCES

Sex
Race
Age
Education
Income
Marital status
Geographic locale
Psychographics
• Personality
• Life style
• Health care usage patterns
• Risk factors
• Perceptions of health problem
• Benefits sought from adopting more healthy behavior

(From National Cancer Institute. [1983]. *Making PSAs work: A handbook for health communications professionals* [NIH Publication No. 83-2485]. Bethesda, MD: U.S. Department of Health and Human Services.)

lack the energy to learn. For example, someone who has just returned from having a difficult set of radiographs taken probably does not have the energy to participate in a learning session.

Environmental Factors. Distractions make learning difficult. Distractions are many, in inpatient or outpatient settings. Television and radio programs, visitors to other patients in the room, and procedures being done to another patient are all distractions to learning.

Emotional Responses. Charged emotions—either sad or happy—hinder learning. Patient and family members are dealing with an illness that evokes a number of emotional responses, including fear, anxiety, worry, grief, anger, and guilt. Different emotions can be present at any time during the illness. For instance, the shock of the cancer diagnosis can immediately close one's mind·to other information. Or the decision that chemotherapy will be the treatment of choice can raise the level of anxiety. Patients and families may need time to assimilate the reality of their situation before teaching can begin.

People have different styles of coping with charged emotional environments. In most cases, a person's coping style during illness is similar to that person's normal coping style. People who are usually information seekers will also be interested in finding out details about their disease and its treatment. Those who usually refuse information or deflect it to family members will probably follow that course during illness.

Different Needs of Different People

People at different stages of life need different approaches, especially the young and the old. What will work for an 8 year old will probably not work for an 18 year old or an 80 year old.

Children Whose Parents Have Cancer. It is not just the patient with cancer who has information needs. All who are connected with the patient's world—be they children, parents, brothers and sisters, neighbors, or business colleagues—have a desire to know. Children are similar to other relatives in that they need to have the illnesses and treatments explained in a way they can understand. Graphic illustrations are often necessary.

Older People with Cancer. Older people need special attention. However, when planning patient education for older persons, it is important to understand that all older people are not alike in their needs. An active 60 year old has different informational needs from a bedridden 85 year old. Hearing and vision may be problems for some older patients. Messages may need to be both oral and written, using bigger type. Long sentences and fast speech should be avoided.

Many older people believe in cancer myths, and more than 50 per cent of the older people surveyed through a Fox Chase Cancer Center program believed cancer treatments were worse than the disease (Wilson et al., 1984). Issues such as these need to be taken into consideration when discussing treatment with older people. The elderly may also need to be taught

to ask questions of doctors, because many are afraid to question authority.

Minority and Ethnic Groups. Special planning is essential for target audiences consisting of minority and ethnic groups. The needs of these groups, which vary from setting to setting, were discussed in Chapter 61. Because these groups usually have different interests and needs as well as different health communication problems and attitudes, special programs and materials must be designed. Additional attention must be given to the attitudes and demeanor of the staff delivering the programs because these can have a major impact on the success of the educational effort.

Different Needs at Different Times

The information needs of patients and families vary. What they need to know during the diagnostic and treatment stages is quite different from what they need to know during the posttreatment, rehabilitation, and recurrence phases.

Diagnosis. Anyone who has worked with patients who have cancer and their families understands the fears and anxiety present during the crisis period while the disease is being diagnosed. The entire experience is new and fraught with fears and emotions, frightening procedures, and unfamiliar surroundings. Basic facts are badly needed, such as descriptions of which tests will be performed, what they consist of, how long they last, and what information they yield. Patients and families need information about the kinds of doctors who perform the tests and how the tests are interpreted. They need some understanding of the sequence of events and time factors involved. Information about the part of the body affected, the disease itself, and, especially, the medical terms frequently used is necessary so that intelligent questions can be asked of the health care team. Patients and families require materials to help them deal with the reality of the cancer diagnosis and information on how to be partners with the health care professionals who will be treating them. In general, both patients and families need as much information as they wish to have.

Treatment. Treatment stimulates an entirely new set of concerns. Information on type of cancer, its staging, typical patterns of growth and spread, and different kinds of treatment is important during this time. As noted by Crosson (1984), patients need to learn the following to make an informed choice regarding treatment:

- Rationale for why the suggested therapy is the treatment of choice
- Facts about how the treatment will affect the cancer
- Timetable and sequence of events
- Potential side effects, body alterations, or life-style changes and how to best cope with them
- Prognosis
- Techniques or routine needs for continuing care

This is also the time for patients and family members to consider second opinions—whether to have them and how to accomplish them without creating problems with physicians. Most patients are anxious about whether the treatment is the "right" one and whether it is being done at the "best" place. Some patients will question whether they wish to have treatment at all. If the patient decides to enter a clinical trial, information on many facets of this process, including informed consent, may be needed (Bujorian, 1988). Because much of cancer treatment has shifted from an inpatient to an outpatient operation and because patients need more self-care information, this stage presents important challenges (Villejo, Flynn, Klucharich, & Plummer, 1988).

Depending on the treatment recommended, patients and family members require specific information about the treatment itself, tailored to the treatment stage. Patients and family members also need to be taught ways to manage side effects and how to adjust normal routines to the treatment cycle. At this time, the realization of the diagnosis becomes a critical issue, as patients and family members begin long-term treatments.

Survivors. According to Mullan (1984), a doctor, cancer survivor, and founder of the National Coalition for Cancer Survivorship, education could play a role in several areas for patients who have completed their treatments and who are resuming active lives:

- Fear of recurrence: Patients need information about the cancer in question, follow-up requirements, and danger signs to watch for and reassurance that the fear of recurrence is an expected part of the recovery process.
- Living with compromise: Patients who have lost a visible body part or have had a body function compromised need clear, accurate, and candid information and reassurance that it is not unusual to feel remorse and bitterness because of this compromise or loss.
- Long-term living: Patients need help in understanding some of the long-term issues, including employment and insurance discrimination as well as the need for medical follow-up and observation.

Recurrence or Advanced Cancer. Dealing with recurrence and advanced cancer is difficult for both patients and families. In addition to the issues discussed for other phases, these patients usually have more acute physical difficulties that affect their ability to learn—restlessness, fever, infection, and pain—and myriad psychological problems, including uncertainty, grief, fear, and anger. Patients and family members must also deal with the issue of dying.

At this time, most families need practical information about providing physical care, such as feeding, administering medications, recognizing emergency symptoms, and identifying community resources. They also need help in dealing with their emotions; assistance with referrals to people who can help them with this issue can be helpful. Information to help them minimize financial and legal problems is also essential. During this phase of illness, many patients and families

are interested in learning about additional treatment options, such as finding places where investigational treatments are being done. In this precarious stage, information about treatment using unproven methods is often sought.

Outcome Criteria

The planning stage is the time to determine the outcome objectives by which the project will be evaluated. Frank-Stromborg (1985) outlined possible outcome areas to consider:

- Cognitive skills (learning evaluation): What new skills were learned or changed?
- Attitudes (reaction evaluation): How well did the participants like the program?
- Psychomotor skills (behavior evaluation): Have self-care behaviors occurred as a result of the patient education project?
- Cost-benefit analysis (results evaluation): What are the tangible results of the patient education experience?
- Patient improvement or change (results evaluation): What are the tangible results showing that the patient's quality of life improved?

When considering outcome areas, the planner must decide which ones can be evaluated—both in a practical sense as well as in an economic one—by reviewing the program objectives written during the assessment stage. The evaluation process itself is discussed in greater detail later in this chapter.

The Intervention Stage

The more care given to the assessment and planning stages, the easier implementation planning will be. The main issues of this stage are choosing the learning activities and selecting (and producing if necessary) the instructional media. Because people learn in different ways and the activities and media have different uses, it is usually necessary to incorporate one or more of the techniques and one or more media in teaching (Table 62–5).

Learning Activities

Learning activities are many and varied.

Lecture. A lecture is used to transmit information or illustrate principles. It can be used to transmit information in a short time to a large group. However, because it does not involve the listeners as active participants, it needs to be reinforced with additional learning activities.

Demonstration. Demonstration—telling the patients what to do and showing them how to do it—is particularly useful for teaching new skills, because it uses more than one of the senses. However, demonstration can be labor intensive because a staff person is usually needed to teach the skill, unless a video tape is used.

Table 62–5. TECHNIQUES FOR PRESENTING INFORMATION TO PATIENTS AND FAMILIES

1. *Present the most important material first.* The first material presented is best remembered. People also remember best the information they believe is most important.
2. *Offer information.* Do not wait for patients to ask. Sense concerns and doubts and respond to them. Make it easy for the person to start a conversation. Open the door by asking a question such as, "Would you like to talk about it?" or "Is there anything going on right now you'd like to talk about?"
3. Combine *sight and sound when presenting materials.* Eighty-five per cent of all information stored in a listener's brain has been received visually. Use printed explanations to accompany what is said. Remember that people respond to different methods of presenting printed material. Take advantage of the different ways people learn: questions and answers, pictures, charts, questions to ask, scoring quizzes; they reinforce one another.
4. *Ask patients and family members what they want to know about their illness.* Research has shown that people remember the information they are interested in knowing.
5. *Categorize.* Tell people the categories that will be discussed with them and then repeat that information. "I'm going to tell you what is wrong with you, what the treatment will be, and what sort of side effects you might expect." Then go back to each category and give the specific information. "This is what is wrong with you," and so on. People recall more facts when this technique is used.
6. *Don't be afraid to repeat information.* Patients forget about one third of what is said to them. Their recall of instructions and advice specifically is less than 50 per cent. Older patients forget more than younger ones. A person's intelligence seems to show no relation to an ability to recall and remember.
7. *Give information in small amounts whenever possible.* The proportion of information forgotten increases with the amount of information presented.
8. *Involve family members and supportive friends in the decision making as early as possible.* Ask what information they desire. The family needs to understand how and when they will be kept up to date with the patient's illness and course of treatment. Give them your telephone number and those of other appropriate places to call. Encourage them to actively support the patient's and the health professional's efforts.
9. *Try to give information when people are relatively calm.* Recall of information is related to level of anxiety and is poorest when anxiety is particularly high or low and best when anxiety is moderate. Because cancer is continually ranked by patients as the "most serious," "most stressful," and "most feared" disease, it is important to let people get over the initial shock before giving detailed information.
10. *Speak plainly and use short sentences.* Don't speak "medicalese." Remember that "palpate" and "palliate" are not household words, no matter what the age or education of your patient. In addition, older people (and many cancer patients fall into this group) commonly have more vision and hearing problems and find long sentences, rapid speech, and unfamiliar terms hard to understand.
11. *Ask for questions.* Open the door by encouraging patients and family members from the beginning to write down questions as they think of them for members of the health professional team to answer. Help them understand that team members expect questions, no matter how simple or complex they might be. Stress that there is no such thing as a "stupid" question if it is something that is bothering the patient.
12. *Help the patient and relatives understand from the beginning that there are choices.* Some are simple, such as choosing the time for outpatient treatment. Others are more complex, such as choosing among different therapies. However, there are choices, and if the patients are not involved, someone else is making the choices.
13. *Be responsive to even the most searching and difficult questions,* such as the value of second opinions or alternative treatments. Answer them freely and fully. Make it known that seeking a second opinion is an accepted practice and that the majority of physicians respect an individual's right to further consultation.
14. *Encourage patients and family members to ask the physician questions that only the physician can answer.* Older patients particularly have problems asking questions of physicians. Encourage them to write down the answers and keep them in a notebook or tape record them for review when they get home and for future reference. Suggest that patients bring someone with them when they have medical appointments. Different people hear different things.
15. *Ask questions.* Ask patients to repeat what has been told to them or to explain the meaning of what has been said. Document this for the record to share with other health care providers.
16. *Use silence.* Do not try to keep the conversation moving. A long pause will allow the questions or comments that will advise in which direction to go next.
17. *Take time to sit down.* Patients perceive a visit in which a health professional sits down as much longer than when the person is standing. Sitting close to the bed or at a patient's level adds warmth to the visit.
18. *Maintain eye contact.* It signals that a person is willing to talk. Not looking at a person means a conversation is not welcome.
19. *Watch your body language.* Patients are very sensitive to facial expressions, nuances of your body positions, and nervous habits. You do not seem open to conversation if you are tapping your fingers or looking at your watch every few seconds.
20. Finally, *do not worry about not saying the right thing.* In our discussion with patients and families it is clear that the simple, sincere gesture of one person reaching out to another communicates comfort, hope, and support. You, the nurse, are in a unique position to offer it.

(Adapted with permission from Morra, M. E. [1985]. Making choices: The consumers' perspective. *Cancer Nursing, 8*[Suppl. 1], 54–59.)

Table 62–6. LEARNING ACTIVITY AND OBJECTIVES

Learning Activity	Learning Objective				
	Learning Facts, Theories	Learning Visual Identifications	Comprehending and Applying Facts, Principles, and Concepts	Performing Perceptual Motor Skills	Influencing Attitudes, Opinions, and Motivations
Lecture	High	Low	Low	*Low	Medium-Low
Discussion	Medium	Low	Medium	*Low	High-Medium
Inquiry-oriented discussion	Medium	Medium-Low	High-Medium	Low	High
Independent study units	High	Medium	Medium	Medium	Medium-Low
Demonstration	High	*High	High	High	Low
Practice	Medium	Medium	High	*High	Medium-Low

*High, most effective; High, very effective; Medium, adequately effective; Low, not effective; *Low, least effective.
(Adapted with permission from American Hospital Association. [1978]. *Media Handbook: A guide to selecting, producing and using media for patient education programs*. Chicago: Author. Copyright 1978 by the American Hospital Association.)

Table 62–7. ANALYSIS OF INSTRUCTION MATERIALS

Media	Best Suited For	Problem Areas
Drawings, illustrations, or photographs	Reinforcement of verbal messages; for individuals or small groups	Usually expensive
Models, simulations, or real objects	Small-group teaching; interactive teaching	Usually expensive; often not portable
Exhibits and displays	Presenting one subject in a limited space	Usually expensive; difficult to transport
Programmed materials	Patients who can actively participate	Must be well designed to be effective
Printed materials	One-to-one or group situations	Depends on ability to reach
Audio materials	Those with low reading abilities or hearing dysfunctions	No visuals
Slides or overhead transparencies	Materials that change frequently or are used in different sequences; adaptable to individual or group study	Dark room needed
Filmstrips, films, or video tapes	Motion that should be shown	Not easily changed or adapted; special equipment needed

(Data from American Hospital Association, 1978.)

Table 62–8. INSTRUCTIONAL MEDIA AND LEARNING OBJECTIVES

Instructional Medium	Learning Objective				
	Learning Facts, Theories	Learning Visual Identifications	Comprehending and Applying Facts, Principles, Concepts	Performing Perceptual Motor Skills	Influencing Attitudes, Opinions, and Motivations
Drawings, illustrations, or photographs	Medium	High	High	Medium	Medium
Models, simulations, or real objects	Low	High	Medium	High	Low
Exhibits and displays	Medium	High	Medium	Low	Medium
Programmed materials	High	Low	High	Low	Medium
Printed materials	High	Low	High	Low	Medium
Audio recordings	High	Low	Low	Medium	Medium
Slides or overhead transparencies	Medium	High	Medium	Low	Low
Filmstrips, films, or video tapes	Medium	High	High	High	High

(Adapted with permission from American Hospital Association. [1978]. *Media Handbook: A guide to selecting, producing and using media for patient education programs*. Chicago: Author. Copyright 1978 by the American Hospital Association.)

Discussion. Discussion involves the participants and allows for free interchange of ideas. In many cases, a discussion is more helpful than a lecture because it can be used for one-on-one teaching as well as small group instruction. It requires more teaching skill than does a lecture.

Independent Study. Self-learning techniques of all kinds are becoming more popular as staff time becomes increasingly scarce. Patients can proceed at their own pace with the material and can review it as necessary. It can be used at the patients' convenience with minimal staff time needed for teaching.

Practice. In teaching a new skill, practice is an essential basic activity and usually follows a demonstration. Because it must be evaluated to ensure that the correct skills are being learned, it can be labor intensive.

Table 62–6 outlines the effectiveness of various learning activities in meeting the basic objectives of patient education programs.

Selecting Materials

The next step in the process is to select the learning materials. Each medium has different characteristics.

Drawings, Illustrations, and Photographs. This category can include graphs, charts, full-color drawings, and photographs. They are available in black and white and color, can be of varying sizes and sophistication, and can be useful to reinforce visually what is being heard orally.

Models, Simulators, and Real Objects. Three-dimensional models of body parts, equipment simulators (such as breast self-examination models), and real objects (such as irrigation equipment for colostomies) are informative when a skill needs to be taught and when demonstrations are being used.

Exhibits and Displays. Exhibits and displays usually combine several media—photographs, illustrations, models, and printed matter. They can be employed in many different locations and usually can stand alone without staff.

Programmed Materials. In this age of self-care, materials in which the learner controls the timing and results have taken on a larger role. Teaching machines, programmed texts, and computers allow patients and families to learn at their own rates and at their own convenience.

Printed Materials. Booklets, brochures, textbooks, handouts, research reports, and newspaper and magazine articles can usually supplement verbal information.

Audio. Audio cassette tapes are the most common form of this medium, because they are cheaper and more easily produced and stored than are records. They can be used to describe procedures and techniques as well as to record conversations with health professionals. These are frequently combined with visual materials.

Slides, Overhead Diagrams, and Transparencies. Each of these media has its own uses, problems, and advantages. All are employed more often with large groups than for individual teaching. Overheads are best used in small groups when action, such as writing on the diagrams, is important.

Filmstrips, Films, and Video Tapes. Video tapes have become the medium of choice, and, with the availability of home video cassette recorder units, have become a major teaching tool for patient and family education.

A variety of teaching methods and materials are needed to attract and keep the learner interested. People learn in different ways, so it is helpful to present materials using more than one method. In *Choices* (Morra & Potts, 1987), for instance, the same material is presented in question-and-answer format as well as in a chart and a drawing. Tables 62–7 and 62–8 analyze the aspects of instructional materials.

Sources of Educational Materials

As stated earlier, before considering the production of original patient education materials, it is wise to determine whether something appropriate is already available. In most cases, it is less expensive and easier to use existing materials than to produce new ones. There are several sources to check for materials: agencies (including the American Cancer Society, the Leukemia Society of America, and the American Lung Association), governmental institutions (such as the National Cancer Institute, state and local health departments), and private companies (such as pharmaceutical or hospital equipment firms). A call to the Cancer Information Service (1-800-4-CANCER) is a good starting point.

When considering material that is already available, it is necessary to determine whether it fits into the planned objectives and intended audience. It is also important to know whether the material has been pretested and evaluated.

Production of Patient Education Materials

The production of original patient education materials takes time, thought, planning, and money. To ensure that the final product is useful, many of the steps already discussed must be carried out:

- A literature review must be completed.
- A target audience must be defined.
- An educational level must be delineated.
- Measurable objectives must be written.
- A medium must be chosen.

When these steps are complete, a communications strategy can be formulated, giving the project's objectives, the target audiences to be reached, the information to be communicated, the strategy for the message, and the media to be used to reach the audience. Carefully planning the communications strategy will help in actually writing the materials.

Writing and production planning, the next steps to be accomplished, will be facilitated by following basic

Table 62–9. PRINCIPLES FOR PRODUCING PATIENT EDUCATION MATERIAL

1. Direct your copy to one person, using action verbs.
2. Use short words, short sentences, and short paragraphs.
3. Be sure to use a headline. On average, five times as many people read headlines as read body copy.
4. Write headlines that tell the story in a few words. Headlines with fewer than ten words get more readership than those with more.
5. Find bright, colorful nouns and vigorous active verbs for headlines. Headlines that promise the reader a benefit, contain news, or offer helpful information attract above-average readership.
6. Choose large-size type, especially if patients are older.
7. Use uppercase and lowercase letters. THEY ARE EASIER TO READ THAN ALL CAPITALS.
8. Try to keep your finished columns 3 to 4 inches wide. Most people are used to reading newspaper columns or magazine columns and find longer lines hard to read.
9. Set a key paragraph in boldface type for attention. Italics and underlining can also be used to highlight essential facts.
10. Use white space around text blocks to emphasize importance.
11. Add a subhead every 2 to 3 inches if your body copy runs more than several inches long.
12. Make use of illustrative materials. Clip art and graphics can enhance your work with little cost. Before-and-after pictures or pictures of end results increase readership.
13. Write a caption for every illustration, graph, or chart. More people read the captions under illustrations than read the body copy.
14. Use black type on a white background. It is easier to read than white type on a black or other dark background.
15. If you have unrelated facts, number them and set them in a list form.

Table 62–10. THE LANGUAGE OF PRINTING

Alignment	How text lines up on a column, such as flush right and flush left
Blow up	To enlarge photo or artwork
Body copy	Text
Bold face	Type that is darker than regular body type
Bullet	A round dot usually put in the margin to call attention; comes in various sizes
B/W	Short for black and white
Caption	Words used under a photo or illustration
Clip art	Artwork that can be cut out of a specially designed book to use in one's own work
Copy	Text
Crop	To eliminate unwanted parts of illustrations or photographs; this is not done by cutting the photograph but by marking so that only the main subject is enlarged
Desktop publishing	The use of a computer program and printer to prepare your own material for reproduction
Double-sided	A publication that is printed on both sides of the page
Dummy	Diagram of proposed layout
Facing pages	The two pages that face each other when the booklet is open. The even-numbered page is on the left and the odd-numbered page is on the right
Flush left/right	Vertical placement of right type; flush right means every line ends at the right-hand margin and thus forms a straight vertical line from top to bottom
Glossy	Shiny finish; photos can be ordered with a glossy finish
Graphics	The use of art work, either lettering or pictures
Italic	Letters that slant forward at a fixed angle
Justified	Spacing out type so that all lines in text are of equal length; all margins are even; also called flush left and flush right
Layout	Arrangement of text and artwork on a page
Margins	The white space on either side and at the top and bottom of the text
Paste-up	The results of pasting text and art on a sheet of paper; the final product will be reproduced from it
Ragged margins	Arrangement of type so that all lines are not even with the right or left margin; also known as staggered right or left
Reduce	To make a graphic smaller
Reverse	The opposite of the normal appearance, such as white type on a black background
Rub-on letters	Alphabets printed on backing sheets from which they can be transferred letter by letter to another surface, such as paper; available in various sizes and colors; arrows, stars, bullets, pointing fingers, and the like are also available; also called transfer letters, dry transfer letters, or by their trade names, such as Presstype and Letraset
Sans serif	Type style without horizontal bars on tops and bottoms of capital letters and extenders of lower-case letters
Serif	Type style with tiny horizontal bars on tops and bottoms of capital letters and extenders of lower-case letters
Subhead	Two- to six-word summary of an important or interesting point within the immediately following section of the story; used to break up a column of type
Two color	The use of two colors in printing; for instance, black text and red headlines is considered two-color printing
Typeset	Type that is set using a typesetting machine
White space	Blank space around copy

(Adapted with permission from Morra, M. E. [1984]. How to plan and carry out your poster session. *Oncology Nursing Forum, 11*[2], 52–57.)

guidelines for producing patient education materials (Tables 62–9 and 62–10).

The draft materials should be thoroughly pretested. Readability testing (Table 62–11 shows a sample readability test) should be carried out as a first step in pretesting draft manuscripts (National Cancer Institute, 1989). If the material is written at too high an educational level, rewriting must be done, substituting shorter, more understandable sentences to bring it down to a level that the target audience can comprehend. For example, *salient* can be changed to *main*, *accomplish* to *carry out*, *cessation* to *stop*, *fundamental* to *basic*. The material should also be tested on small groups of persons typical of the target audience.

The Evaluation Stage

Evaluation can take many forms—simple or complex, relatively inexpensive or costly. Evaluation is usually carried out to learn whether a program has been successful and to determine how to improve it, if necessary. Some projects are evaluated to satisfy institutional requirements or to justify the project's existence.

Types of Evaluation

There are three major types of evaluation: formative, summative, and outcome.

Table 62–11. HOW TO DO A SMOG READABILITY TEST

1. Use the whole text of the material that is being tested.
2. Count off three sets of ten consecutive sentences, one set near the beginning, one set in the middle, and one set near the end of the text.
3. Circle all the words in these 30 sentences that have three or more syllables (see NOTES below for guidelines).
4. Total the number of words circled to get a "total word count."
5. Use the conversion table below to find the approximate grade level.

NOTES
• If a word is repeated, it is counted each time it is used.
• Hyphenated words are counted as one word.
• Numbers should be pronounced to determine syllables.
• Proper nouns are counted.
• Abbreviations are read as if they were not abbreviated.

| | SMOG Conversion Table | |
Total Word Count	Approximate Grade Level (plus or minus 1.5 grades)
0–2	4
3–6	5
7–12	6
13–20	7
21–30	8
31–42	9
43–56	10
57–72	11
73–90	12
91–110	13
111–132	14
133–156	15
157–182	16
183–210	17
211–240	18

(Adapted from National Cancer Institute. [1989]. *Making health communication programs work* [NIH Publication No. 89–1493]. Bethesda, MD: U.S. Department of Health and Human Services.)

Formative Evaluation. Also known as process evaluation, formative evaluation is usually employed in early stages to help form or shape the program or during the project to help improve it as it goes along. It tests whether the goals are being met and the program is moving in the desired direction.

Summative Evaluation. Also known as impact evaluation, summative evaluation is usually gathered after the program is complete or at specific intervals, such as annually, to measure effectiveness and costs.

Outcome Evaluation. The third level of evaluation, outcome, uses mortality and morbidity for outcome indicators. This is a long-range undertaking with large population samples and is beyond the range of most patient education efforts.

Evaluation Steps

Typically, evaluation includes taking the following steps (National Cancer Institute, 1982):

• Determine evaluation needs
• Formulate evaluation questions
• Select evaluation design and data collection and analysis method
• Design and test instruments
• Collect data
• Analyze data
• Report data

The criteria for determining outcome of objectives have been described earlier. There are many methods of collecting data (Table 62–12). A survey conducted by the National Cancer Institute's Office of Cancer Communications of 609 institutions reporting inpatient cancer education activities found that patient satisfaction questionnaires and attendance counts at educational sessions were the most frequently used evaluation methods. More than half of the programs instituted some form of follow-up of patients, with the majority using short-term personal surveys. Approximately one quarter of the programs were measured by both pre- and posttests. The report concluded that although most cancer education programs were attempting some form of evaluation activities, the methods used reflected an early stage of development. Most evaluations focused on patient satisfaction and attendance as indicators of success, and only a small portion were able to determine patient behavior change (National Cancer Institute, 1982).

In most cases, the importance of evaluation is its use to improve the program or the project. A feedback loop is an essential part of the program with insights fed back into the program itself; revisions based on the results of the evaluation are made on the original project, and additional evaluations are conducted on the newly designed effort.

Patient education is a complex, ongoing process. Its theories are based in the fields of behavioral change and education. Four stages are essential for the teaching process: assessment, planning, intervention, and evaluation.

Table 62–12. METHODS FOR COLLECTING DATA IN EVALUATION PROCESS

Method	Advantage	Disadvantage	Types
Paper and pencil	Self-administered; anonymity easier to ensure; can administer to large groups; inexpensive.	Answers given do not ensure corresponding behavior; requires reading skill and ability to concentrate; skills required to construct written tests are complex; does not allow follow-up queries or clarification of answers; if tests used, must have reliability and validity.	*Questionnaires*—most frequently used; can elicit feelings about program or knowledge acquired in program. *Tests*—test questions are compatible with objectives of program; typically a pre- and posttest is given; can be standardized or tailor-made tests. *Rating Scale*—patient is asked to check the amount or degree of some factor.
Observation	Involves watching a patient's activities or behaviors in an objective, analytic manner.	Difficulties with validity and reliability: *Validity*—did the behavior observed occur because it was being observed? *Reliability*—was the behavior observed repeatedly performed? Observation requires skill.	*Direct observation* *Return demonstration* *Anecdotal notes* in nursing notes and progress notes (chart audit). *Skills checklist*
Verbal conversations	Allows flexibility; can provide in-depth information; can involve patient and support system; provides immediate feedback to evaluator.	Prevents anonymity; patient may give answers to please interviewer; if not goal directed can provide useless data; usually one-to-one; requires tact on interviewer's part.	*Methods* *Interview* *Guided question-answer session* *Interdisciplinary conference*

(From Frank-Stromborg, M. [1985]. Evaluating patient education material. *Oncology Nursing Forum, 12*[1], 65–67. Reproduced by permission.)

Many factors affect learning, especially for those who are patients with cancer, such as physical status, emotional responses, and stage of disease. These patients and their families have different needs for information at different times during their cancer experiences. Nurses can be effective teachers, helping patients and their families understand specific information, particularly during the periods of diagnosis and treatment. This information can allow patients and family members to become partners with their health care professionals and to help them gain some control over their lives during a stressful and confusing time.

References

American Hospital Association. (1978). *Media handbook: A guide to selecting, producing and using media for patient education programs.* Chicago: Author.

American Medical Association. (1985). *Statement on patient education.* Chicago: Author.

American Nurses' Association & Oncology Nursing Society. (1987). *Standards for oncology nursing practice* (p. 11). Kansas City, MO: American Nurses' Association.

Bujorian, G. A. (1988). Clinical trials: Patient issues in the decision-making process. *Oncology Nursing Forum, 15,* 779–783.

Cassileth, B. R., Zupkis, R. V., Sutton-Smith, K., & March, V. (1980). Information and participation preferences among cancer patients. *Annals of American Medicine, 92,* 832–836.

Cooper, E. T. (1984). A pilot study on effects of the diagnosis of lung cancer on family relationships. *Cancer Nursing, 7,* 301–308.

Crosson, K. (1984). Cancer patient education: What, where and by whom? *Health Education, 10* (Suppl.), 19–29.

Frank-Stromborg, M. (1985). Evaluating patient education material. *Oncology Nursing Forum, 12*(1), 65–67.

Green, L. W., Kreuter, I. W., Deeds, S. G., & Partridge, K. B. (1980). *Health education planning: A diagnostic approach.* Palo Alto, CA: Mayfield Publishing Co.

Johnson, J. L. B., & Blumberg, B. D. (1984). A commentary on cancer patient education. *Health Education Quarterly, 10,* 7–18.

Joint Commission on Accreditation for Hospitals. (1987). *Accreditation manual for hospitals.* Chicago: Author.

Mazzuca, S. A. (1982). Does patient education in chronic disease have therapeutic value? *Journal of Chronic Disease, 35,* 521–529.

Messerli, M. L., Garamendi, C., & Romano, J. (1980). Breast cancer: Information as a technique of crisis intervention. *American Journal of Orthopsychiatry, 50,* 728–731.

Mischel, M. H., Hosletter, T., King, B., & Graham, V. (1984). Predictors of psychosocial adjustment in patients newly diagnosed with gynecological cancer. *Cancer Nursing, 7,* 291–299.

Morra, M. E. (1985). Making choices: The consumer's perspective. *Cancer Nursing, 8* (Suppl. 1), 54–59.

Morra, M. E., & Potts, E. (1987). *Choices: Realistic alternatives in cancer treatment.* New York: Avon Books.

Mullan, F. (1984). Re-entry: The educational needs of cancer survivor. *Health Education Quarterly, 10* (Suppl.), 88–94.

National Cancer Institute. (1982). *Adult patient education in cancer.* Bethesda, MD: U.S. Department of Health and Human Services.

National Cancer Institute. (1987). *Chemotherapy and you: A guide to self-help during treatment* (NIH Publication No. 88-1136). Bethesda, MD: U.S. Department of Health and Human Services.

National Cancer Institute. (1989). *Making health communication programs work* (NIH Publication No. 89-1493). Bethesda, MD: U.S. Department of Health and Human Services.

Oncology Nursing Society. (1982). *Outcome standards for cancer patient education.* Pittsburgh, Author.

Villejo, L., Flynn, V., Klucharich, S., & Plummer, A. (1988). Strategies for cancer patient education: Overcoming barriers. *Cancer Bulletin, 40,* 365–369.

Wilson, C. M., Rimer, B. K., Bennett, D. J., Engstrom, P. F., Kane-Williams, E., & White, J. (1984). Educating the older patient: Obstacles and opportunities. *Health Education Quarterly, 10* (Suppl.), 76–87.

CHAPTER 63

Consultation and Collaboration Among Health Care Providers

FRANCES MARCUS LEWIS

Consultation and *collaboration* are catch words in our nursing vocabulary. Like *primary nursing, prescriptive authority,* or *nursing diagnosis,* they conjure up images of what is good and what is valued. They also smack of high status, positive self-esteem, and power. Consultation or collaboration is doing what is important and visionary. But what does it mean to consult or to collaborate? This chapter presents the essential positive and negative characteristics of both consultation and collaboration, viewing them on a continuum of involvement, each with its own essential properties and phases.

Both consultation and collaboration have consequences for the patient, the nurse, and the health care system, including other providers. This chapter explores these consequences. Much of our knowledge of the processes of consulting and collaborating is obscured by reports of those who have experienced only positive consequences (Baldwin, 1978; Bergstrom et al., 1984; Bishop, 1981; Coleman, Patrick, Eagle, & Hermaline, 1979; Cook, 1979; Peznecker, Draye, & McNeil, 1982; Poulin, Clifford, & McClure, 1981; Singleton, Edmunds, Rapson, & Steele, 1982; Wessell, 1981). Peznecker and McNeil (1979), for example, highlighted the positive aspects, mutual support, and the smooth and rapid process with which they collaborated on a nursing research project. Mauger and Huggins (1980), in another example, described a grant-supported project that facilitated collaborative research

in nursing education in the South. They noted the grant's achievements as well as the benefits of the support network that evolved as a result of the collaboration. What is needed, however, is an analysis of the process of consultation and collaboration so that both positive and negative outcomes can be understood.

DEVELOPMENT OF TERMS

Definitions

To collaborate is to work in conjunction with another or others; to cooperate (Oxford English Dictionary, 1971). The term derives originally from the Latin *collaborare,* meaning "to work together" (*col,* "together"; *aboarare,* "to work"). Implicit in the definition is the achievement of some common aim or goal (Baker, 1981; England, 1986; Engstrom, 1984; Komfled-Jacobs & Karshmer, 1977; Schumaker & Gross, 1980). To consult is to seek advice or guidance from another; to confer or to deliberate together (Oxford English Dictionary, 1971). The term derives from the Latin *consultum,* meaning "to take or ask counsel." Implicit in the definition is that the consultant has expertise that will advance the client's knowledge (Anders, 1978; Glaser, 1977; Maddux, 1955; Termini & Ciechuski, 1981). The process of advancing the client's knowledge involves a functional process of steps and phases. Merely being an expert in a body of knowledge is not enough to claim to be a consultant; a specialist is not automatically a consultant (Norris, 1977; Nuckolls, 1977; Oda, 1982; Pati, 1980).

Distinctions Between Terms

Collaboration, unlike consultation, involves ongoing participation in the implementation of activities related to a joint problem-solving process. Individuals who collaborate "roll up their sleeves" to do the work together and do not stop until the work is completed and the goal or aim is accomplished.

In contrast to collaboration, consultation can be limited to a short-term interaction in which the consultant advises, instructs, or otherwise provides essential information to others (Termini & Ciechuski, 1981; Virden & Chater, 1979). Ongoing involvement and direct participation in implementation are not part of the definition of consultation. Even when a consultant advises on all aspects of an activity, from goals through evaluation, the consultant is not directly involved in implementing the advice. Others do that. When implementation is involved, the consultant becomes a collaborator. A consultant draws the road map; a collaborator helps build the road.

From the previous definitions it is clear that consultation and collaboration differ in degree of involvement. For example, a hospital wants to build an acute care cancer unit, but the administration needs expert opinion on the critical features of the unit. They retain an oncology nurse clinical specialist to consult with them on the important characteristics of such a unit. The consultant, an expert in the literature and experienced in clinical practice, summarizes these features for them in a series of 2-day presentations over a period of 3 months.

The hospital administration realizes, however, that merely knowing the critical features of the unit will not be enough to make the unit acceptable to either house staff, attending physicians, or nursing staff. The administration wants to have representatives from these three professional groups collaborate in tailoring the unit's features to the hospital's unique setting and patient population. Representatives from the three professional groups agree to collaborate on assisting in the development and implementation of the unit. They find themselves in an extended series of planning meetings and working sessions with architects and hospital administrators; they become involved in such activities as patient and community surveys. They roll up their sleeves together to achieve a common goal: the successful development and implementation of a cancer care unit. They utilize the "road map" the consultant developed for them, but even more, they actively participate in implementing and tailoring the recommendations.

Critical Features of Consultation and Collaboration

There are four attributes of consultation and collaboration: conjoint problem solving, task interdependency, shared record keeping, and accountability (Lewis, 1985). Research by Weiss and David (1985) is the only known instrument development study in the area (Box 63–1).

Conjoint Problem Solving

Conjoint problem solving is the most critical component of consultation and collaboration. It involves joint determination and participation in the problem-solving process from the formation of goals to the establishment of criteria against which goal achievement is to be evaluated (Daniels & Bosch, 1978; Lamb & Napodano, 1984; Mailick & Ashley, 1981; Yaste, 1985). The problem and its solution are jointly determined (Tyler, Tamulerich, & Good, 1982).

Typically in a consultation, only selected aspects of a project or a patient-related issue are handled through a conjoint problem-solving process. More typically, the consultant is asked to focus on a specific aspect of a patient's situation, for example, the nursing management of pain.

In collaboration, conjoint problem solving is further characterized by a spirit of induction and mutual inquiry and discovery. Ideas are integrated and result in a new assessment, defined problem, or plan of action (Box 63–2) (Lamb & Napodano, 1984). The contributions of all members are equally valued, and the group process reflects an egalitarian exchange among all members. An individual's expertise and not some preconceived status ordering determines when and what he or she contributes (Bales, 1953; Feiger & Schmitt, 1979). Roles in a collaborative group are also often freely exchanged, and sharp boundaries between disciplines often fade.

Task Interdependence

Task interdependence is the second attribute of consultation and collaboration and reflects the interdigitation of effort required to achieve the goals and objectives. Total autonomy is antithetical to consultation and collaboration. At a minimum, a consultation results in a more informed plan of action. With collaboration, some component of the problem-solving process, for example, the goals or the means to achieve them, has been directly negotiated. Collaborators do not merely "do their own thing" and let others know what they have done. Rather plans to achieve the goals are worked out, and roles are linked so that the activities and practices result in the attainment of goals. For example, a physician might collaborate with a nurse about managing a family's anxiety during the induction phase of a bone marrow transplantation. Together they decide that both the mother and the father need separate and direct informational and coping support. The plan is for the nurse to offer both the mother and the father cognitive-behavioral tips that they can use to cope with the anxiety caused by the upcoming events. The physician's role is to interpret the lab tests and the events surrounding the transplant induction.

Box 63–1. MEASURE OF COLLABORATIVE PRACTICE

Before this study, there was no known standardized measure of collaborative practice with tested reliability and validity. The purpose of the study was to test the validity and reliability of a self-report measure of collaborative practice that assesses the degree to which the interactions of nurses and physicians facilitate synergistic patient care. Ninety-five nurses and 94 physicians completed the scales. Two relevant factors emerged in the instrument's analysis: direct assertion of professional expertise or opinion and classification of mutual responsibilities (nine-item nurse scale) and acknowledgment of nurses' contribution to patient care and consensus development with nurse (ten-item physician scale). Alpha coefficients were 0.80 and 0.84 for the scales, respectively. Six-week test and retest reliability was significant for both scales.

(Weiss, S. J., & David, H. P. [1985]. Validity and reliability of the collaborative practice scales. *Nursing Research, 34,* 299–305.)

Shared Record Keeping

Shared record keeping is the third important property of consultation and collaboration (Devereaux, 1981a, 1981b). Such records formalize the exchanges among the participants as well as link them to one another (Bergman & Fritz, 1981). Ideally, these written records make explicit the recommendations from the consultant and the goals, process, and outcome of the collaborators. Informality has little place here; quick exchanges in the hall or over the telephone do not adequately anchor either a consultant's recommendations or a collaborator's exchanges.

Nursing's unfortunate preoccupation with team meetings has emphasized inappropriately the importance of such meetings at the expense of the written word. Clearly what is needed is a better balance: team meetings among collaborators should be coupled with written documentation of the goals, progress, and outcomes of their joint efforts.

Accountability

Accountability is the process of making visible to relevant others the goals, process, cost, and outcomes of those things for which one is responsible (Batey & Lewis, 1982; Lewis & Batey, 1982). Both consultation and collaboration have an accountability component.

PROCESSES OF COLLABORATION AND CONSULTATION

Collaborative structures are not naturally occurring phenomena. They cannot be isolated from what already exists; they must be developed. Building collaborative arrangements requires resources and commitment. Positive thinking is not enough; building and sustaining requires action as well (Goodstein, 1978; Grubb, 1979; Kramer, 1977).

Fundamental to the resources component are the people, particularly those in positions of formal power who ultimately decide on the allocation of institutional resources. The go-getters in the front line who want to collaborate are naive if they think they alone have the resources to make it succeed on a long-term basis.

There may be resistance to the proposed collaborative arrangement. Resistance can come from those who are comfortable with the status quo. Fear, disinterest, or ignorance may breed such resistance. Elitist factions are another potential barrier; they may resist the initiation of a collaborative arrangement. Inherent in such a faction's beliefs is the erroneous and often self-inflated view that what is to be known is already known and nothing is to be gained by integrating the views and activities of others (Eiduson, 1964).

The relevant people or those who represent them must be involved in the early stages of collaborative arrangements. Relevance is determined by who has

Box 63–2. NURSE-PHYSICIAN COLLABORATION

Although collaboration between nurses and physicians is a highly valued activity, to date there has been little, if any, examination of the types of patient-provider interactions that result in the initiation of collaboration between nurses and physicians. The purpose of this study was to assess the types of patient-provider interactions that result in the initiation of collaboration between nurses and physicians and the degree to which collaboration occurs once it is initiated. Data were obtained from both provider self-reports and observers measuring the collaborative activities of two primary care teams, each composed of one internist and one nurse practitioner. Results revealed that 4.8 per cent of patient-provider interactions from Team 1 and 8.1 per cent of such reactions from Team 2 resulted in an interaction between nurse and physician. All but one of these interactions were initiated by the nurse. Five of the 22 nurse-physician interactions were coded as collaborative; the most common areas of collaboration were in joint problem definition and joint planning of care. The study raises serious concern over the absence of collaboration initiated by a physician.

(Lamb, G. S., & Napodano, R. J. [1984]. Physician-nurse practitioner interaction patterns in primary care practices. *American Journal of Public Health, 74,* 26–29.)

the power to facilitate as well as to impede the collaboration (Poulin et al., 1981). The engineers who will build the collaborative system should be selected carefully. These engineers, for example, staff nurses or clinical specialists, should be keenly aware of the reasons for which the agency wants to collaborate as well as the available and long-range resources that the agency is committing to the effort. The appointed engineers also need to have a keen vision and commitment to the mission of the organization. This vision will militate against cooptation, pressures toward consensus, or passive adoption of the views of others.

Goals and objectives for the collaboration must be focused, informed, and realistic. Why is collaboration sought? Toward what broad goals or more focused objectives is the group aiming? Pious hopes or wishes do not serve well in building collaborative arrangements. Clear and potentially attainable goals for the collaboration provide an initial basis on which to target work with others and also help participants bond to the collaborative process. This bonding can help sustain the building efforts and help participants get through any initial difficulties.

Agency priorities should not compete with establishing collaborative arrangements. If this seems likely, the timing of initiating the collaboration should be reconsidered. Ultimately, competing priorities can cause resources to be channeled elsewhere; at a minimum, the groundbreaking activities to initiate the collaboration could be aborted, and everyone will be frustrated.

Organizational resources and support structures are essential for maintaining a viable and successful arrangement (Loomis & Krone, 1980a, 1980b). Merely wanting to collaborate is not enough; the promise of ongoing resources must be present. Collaborative activities should not be tacked on to an already full workload or done after hours as extra work. If truly valued by the organization, hours spent in collaborative activities are consonant with hours spent elsewhere on the job.

In maintaining a collaborative system, issues of equity often arise. Is the workload equally distributed? Are all parties involved being equally or fairly credited with their respective contributions? In short, are things working out in both the short range and the long range for those involved? Martyrdom is not part of collaborating. If the scales feel unbalanced in terms of the distribution of the workload, the problem should be discussed with the collaborators. Long-term imbalances result in instability and resentment.

Phases in the Process of Consultation

The process of consultation has seven phases or stages: initiation, contracting, diagnostic analysis, goal setting, action plans, cycling feedback, and termination (Manksch, 1981; Nuckolls, 1977; O'Connor & Carr, 1981; Oda, 1982; Williamson, 1981). These phases roughly parallel three phases of the nursing process: assessment, diagnosis, and evaluation (Oda, 1982).

Underlying the entire consultative process is the sensitive attention to consultation as an interpersonal process; substantive exchange is only part of it. Rather, the consultant is constantly cycling information and feedback about the client's response and context to better serve the situation's needs.

Initiation

This phase of consultation involves the initial contact and entry of the consultant. Such entry heralds the person's or agency's desire for change or for an altered plan of action. Information of an increasingly sensitive nature is offered to the consultant; the disclosure process begins here and often continues throughout the consultant-client relationship.

Contracting and Diagnostic Analysis

These steps in consultation may occur sequentially or concurrently. Contracting involves the development of realistic activities or goals that both the consultant and the client offer to achieve with each other. Sometimes such contracting is done after a diagnostic analysis of the problem has occurred; sometimes contracting is done in broad strokes before the diagnostic analysis. For many, contracting is more an implicit than an explicit process.

Diagnostic Analysis

This analysis involves the determination of the problem—its scope, components, and ramifications. Often such activity is carried out during early periods of exchange but may be increasingly refined as more sensitive information is disclosed by the client. Ideally, this phase is not rushed because it is the basis for further work and major planning. Over time and with experience a consultant learns both to gather finer-tuned information and to organize it in increasingly sophisticated ways that best help the client. The obvious is instead relinquished for the most discriminating type of information, much like an expert clinician relinquishes attention to the unimportant and focuses instead on the definitive issues that need management (Benner, 1984).

Goal Setting

An explicit part of a consultation, goal setting makes clear the targets to be attained and helps arrange activities into a sequence to reach the desired ends. These goals link explicitly with the diagnosed problems or issues in the previous phase.

Action Plans

These plans are sequenced activities that become the routes to achieving the goals that were established in the goal-setting phase. Their actual delivery is the responsibility of the client; the consultant advises on them. If implementation is involved, the consultant becomes a collaborator.

Cycling Feedback

This phase of consultation involves an evaluation of the goals, process, cost, or outcomes recommended by the consultant. Its level of formality may vary; full-blown quality assurance or outcome evaluations may be involved (Green & Lewis, 1986). Alternatively, cycling feedback may be a relatively informal looking back at what was and what might have been. Regardless of its level of formality, a responsible consultant is invested in knowing about the results, how the outcomes compared with the recommended plan, and what results were attributed to the implemented plan.

Termination

An explicit part of a consultation, termination might be a short conference, a lengthy meeting, or a celebration. It may also involve more than one interchange. Sometimes it is linked to the cycling feedback phase. Regardless of its length or its degree of formality, it is critical to the process of consultation. If consultation is accepted as an interpersonal process in the area of the consultant's specialized knowledge, then termination involves both termination in the substantive area as well as in the interpersonal area. Ultimately, planned termination is an affirming exchange.

CONSEQUENCES OF CONSULTATION AND COLLABORATION

Managing Tension and Scarce Resources

Tension

Whether heightened or reduced, tension may be a consequence of either consultation or collaboration (Pelz, 1967; Petersen, 1981). It is not a matter of whether tension occurs; it is only a matter of when it occurs. This tension arises from four areas: differing values, task ambiguity, differing expectations, and allocation of scarce resources.

Differing Values

Value differences may precipitate tension. Values dominated by a biomedical tradition of illness causality, for example, are very different from those related to a perceptual or personal view of illness. Values will affect goals for treatment and service and pervade the activities of both the consultant and the collaborators.

Task Ambiguity

Ambiguous tasks can cause tension. When it is not clear what or how something should be done or who should do it, there will be tension. The participants find themselves struggling to sort out what each should be doing. Inefficiency often occurs; unnecessary repetition of work sometimes occurs.

Differing Expectations

Differences among the participants' expectations can produce tension. If one collaborator favors a particular course of action but another thinks it not feasible, there will be tension. Pious hopes sometimes substitute for achievable objectives, which, in turn, result in frustration for those involved.

Allocation of Scarce Resources

How to allocate scarce resources can cause tension. Ultimately, this amounts to an allocation of personnel, space, facilities, time, money, or future resources. Even when goals and objectives can be agreed on, allocating the resources to reach the goals may produce tension.

Given that tension is a concomitant of collaboration, the management of tension or conflict should be direct. Some people experience tension as a personal failure; this attitude is indeed naive, given that tension arises from many sources and not the "failure" of any single individual. When tension is experienced, it should be made an explicit item for discussion. Potential causes of the tension should be explored by the participants, and these causes should relate to the structural features of the consultative or collaborative arrangements, not to the personalities of the participants. Personality theory has no place in the matter.

Causes of the tension can be explored by asking and answering the following questions: Is the tension a matter of task ambiguity; does everyone know what he or she is to do to achieve the goals? Is the scope and intent of the collaborative or consultative arrangement clear to those involved? Are there agreed on expectations for the consultation or the collaboration? When expectations differ, can these differences be directly negotiated? When resource allocation is the source of contention, decisions about allocations should be made explicit for all to view and evaluate. Budget, personnel, and time are all important commodities that are legitimate matters around which there can be discussion.

Tension, although typically a pejorative term, can pique the participants (Pelz, 1967; 1976). It can bring about a direct negotiation of differences and an explicit working through of the issues around which the conflict is generated (Hinshaw, Chance, & Atwood, 1981; Gibeau, 1977). As Pelz (1967) noted, participants can be effective when faced with environmental demands, including the maintenance of divergent viewpoints in their associates. Ultimately the tension issue is probably a question of tolerable amount or a balance between demand and security (Pelz, 1967, p. 160).

ALTERNATIVE MODELS OF COLLABORATION

Collaborative arrangements can assume five alternative models or forms: the constant contributor model, the unification model, the pontification model, the declarative model, and the skill-based model (Lewis, 1985).

Constant Contributor Model

The constant contributor model of collaboration was developed by Loomis's team and is a solid example of a collaborative model. Its initial application occurred with nursing research projects in Michigan, in which university-based researchers and agency-based clinicians participated in joint research projects. Loomis's interest was in diminishing the differences between agency-based and university-based nursing research. Ideally, agency-based research needed to be more generalizable and less situation specific (Hinshaw et al., 1981). At the same time, university-based research needed to be more relevant to practice. To protect the contributions from each group during the conduct of the research, Loomis argued for equal contributions from all participants at each stage of the research process (Loomis, 1982; Loomis & Kroner, 1980a). There was to be a constant and equal contribution by all participants from statement of the research problem through data analyses and dissemination of results.

Declarative Model

The declarative model is commonly observed in physician-nurse collaborative systems. It is based on the authority of those participating to declare that they are operating in a collaborative system; they merely declare by fiat that collaboration is occurring. This model is often part of the personal testimonies of nurses who want others to believe that they participate in collaborative systems in which their contributions are valued and esteemed and in which they have formal power.

Sadly enough, the declarative model is mostly, if not totally, an illusion. Collaboration is not really occurring; nurses merely want it to be. The declarative model is often falsely represented in systems in which individuals are physically brought together to work in groups or teams. On close inspection of the group process, however, these team meetings are often dominated by a select few. There is limited, if any, evidence of conjoint problem solving, inductive spirit, joint explorations, or shared solutions. Participants in such systems may confuse what is with what they want it to be; illusion replaces reality.

Pontification Model

The pontification version of a collaborative model involves participants in a system characterized by the domination of only a few members who unilaterally declare or pontificate about what should be done and how it should be done. As in the declarative model, participants think they are collaborating because they get caught up in the illusion. Interpersonal exchange in such a model is characterized by rigid and permanent status hierarchies. Those at the top initiate and control the direction, scope, and implementation of activities. Both the way in which the problem, task, or project is conceived and the way it is worked through are established by the most powerful members. Debate, as well as discussion, rarely if ever occurs (Mauger & Huggins, 1980). Acts of deference are often subtle but a constant part of the group process; those in less powerful positions offer little more than head nodding or compliments. Those at the top pontificate—lay forth with bombastic vigor—what is and what should be.

Unification Model

The unification model of collaboration involves the formalized linking of groups or agencies; convergence or coalescence structurally connects those involved, for example, through budget and personnel (Styles, 1984). These linkages are part of the permanent structures of the agencies and pervasively influence the type and scope of exchanges. Because they are formal arrangements, they are not carried out merely at the whim of the unique personalities of the individuals occupying certain positions. Rather they are part of the job descriptions and lines of authority of the involved agencies.

Early examples of the unification model are represented in the joint appointment movement in nursing. Nurses often unconditionally valued the importance of these formal and long-term unification models and what they potentially offered the discipline. Currently, many examples of the unification model of collaboration operate between diploma schools and educational settings. Unification, it is believed by those involved, helps aging or partially limited agencies convert to an educational process within the mainstream of higher education and yet still utilize existing resources in the hospital-based programs (Styles, 1984, p. 23).

Skill-Based Model

This final model of collaboration, the skill-based model, builds on the best of all the critical attributes of collaboration. The key aspect of the model is the belief by all participants that every collaborator has a valued and esteemed set of contributions to make. This belief translates into an assumption that each person possesses a special and somewhat unique set of skills, a knowledge base, and a collection of experiences that are ultimately valued and esteemed by everyone. These skills are then shared with the other collaborators as the task or project requirements demand.

In the skill-based model an observer would see equally distributed rates of exchange and contributions from the members—indicators of equal status and shared power among all the members (Feiger & Schmitt, 1979; Lamb & Napodano, 1984). There would be conjoint problem solving, a spirit of induction and mutual discovery, task interdependency, and accountability. An example of a skill-based model of collaboration was offered by Hongladarom's team in the development and implementation of a multistate continuing education program for oncology nurses within community hospital settings (Hongladarom, 1983; Hongladarom, Lewis, Landenburger, & McCorkle, 1986).

SUMMARY AND FUTURE DIRECTIONS IN COLLABORATION AND CONSULTATION IN ONCOLOGY NURSING

Five features characterize consultation and collaboration: conjoint problem solving, task interdependency, shared record keeping, and accountability. These dimensions make consultation and collaboration a reality in a service setting. Phases in the consultation process involve initiation, contracting and analysis, goal setting, action plans, cycling feedback, and termination. Although both consultation and collaboration provide mechanisms that facilitate the best possible service, these processes have negative as well as positive consequences associated with their implementation, including those related to differing values and task ambiguity. Finally, five types of collaborative models are proposed that distinguish among alternative forms of collaboration: the constant contributor model, the declarative model, the pontification model, the unification model, and the skill-based model.

No doubt new practice structures will arise in the future within oncology nursing. These structures will reflect advanced clinical practice and clinical expertise (Suppers, Yarbro, & Mayer-Scogna, 1979), community-based programs, creative combining of oncology clinicians with nurse practitioners and area-wide home care services (Gibeau, 1977), third-party payment direct to oncology nursing specialists and nurse cancer counselors, and advanced roles in research (Felton & McLaughlin, 1976; Gortner, 1979; Mood & Parzuchowski, 1987; Singleton et al., 1982) and in primary health promotion and disease prevention (Henderson, Lewis, Thompson, & Wooldridge, 1990). All these roles potentially involve both consultative and collaborative activities between oncology nurses and other professional disciplines. However, nurses must take an active or proactive lead in developing and sustaining these new arrangements (Squyres, 1980). A proactive stance would help protect the nurse's role as patient advocate; would protect against another discipline's cooptation of nursing's practice goals and priorities; and would protect against inequity. Nurses have too long been passive in these areas as a collective group; new zeal and attention to these matters is needed.

References

Anders, R. L. (1978). Program consultation by a clinical specialist. *Journal of Nursing Administration, 8*(11), 34–38.

Baker, C. M. (1981). Moving toward interdependence: Strategies for collaboration. *Journal of Nursing Administration, 11*(4), 34–39.

Baldwin, A. C. (1978). Mental health consultation in the intensive care unit: Toward greater balance and precision of attribution. *Journal of Psychiatric Nursing and Mental Health Sciences, 16*(2), 17–21.

Bales, R. F. (1953). The equilibrium problem in small groups. In T. P. Parsons, R. F. Bales, & E. A. Shils (Eds.), *Working papers in the theory of action* (pp. 111–161). Glencoe, IL: The Free Press.

Batey, M. V., & Lewis, F. M. (1982). Clarifying autonomy and accountability in nursing service. Part 1. *Journal of Nursing Administration, 12*(9), 13–18.

Benner, P. (1984). *From novice to expert.* Menlo Park, CA: Addison-Wesley Publishing Co.

Bergman, A. S., & Fritz, G. F. (1981). Psychiatric and social work collaboration in a pediatric chronic illness hospital. *Social Work in Health Care, 7*, 45–55.

Bergstrom, N., Hansen, B. C., Grant, M., Hanson, R., Kubo, W., Padilla, G., & Wong, H. L. (1984). Collaborative nursing research: Anatomy of a successful consortium. *Nursing Research, 33*, 20–25.

Bishop, B. (1981). A case for collaboration. *Nursing Outlook, 29*, 110–111.

Boettcher, E. G. (1978). Nurse-client collaboration: Dynamic equilibrium in the nursing care system. *Journal of Psychiatric Nursing and Mental Health Services, 16*(12), 7–15.

Coleman, J. V., Patrick, D. L., Eagle, J., & Hermaline, J. A. (1979). Collaboration, consultation and referral in an integrated health-mental health program at an HMO. *Social Work in Health Care, 5*, 83–96.

Cook, R. L. (1979). Physician-nurse collaboration: A nurse's perspective. *Aviation Space and Environmental Medicine, 50*, 1179–1181.

Daniels, M. S., & Bosch, S. J. (1978). School health planning: A case for interagency collaboration. *Social Work in Health Care, 3*, 457–467.

Devereaux, P. M. (1981a). Essential elements of nurse-physician collaboration. *Journal of Nursing Administration, 11*(5), 19–23.

Devereaux, P. M. (1981b). Nurse/physician collaboration: Nursing practice consideration. *Journal of Nursing Administration, 11*(9), 34–39.

Eiduson, B. T. (1964). Intellectual inbreeding in the clinic? *Amer Journal of Orthopsychiatry, 34*, 714–721.

England, D. A. (1986). *Collaboration in nursing.* Rockville, MD: Aspen Publishers, Inc.

Engstrom, J. L. (1984). University, agency, and collaborative models for nursing research: An overview. *Image, 16*(3), 76–80.

Feiger, S. M., & Schmitt, M. H. (1979). Collegiality in interdisciplinary health teams: Its measurement and its effects. *Social Science and Medicine, 13A*, 217–229.

Felton, G., & McLaughlin, F. E. (1976). The collaborative process in generating a nursing research study. *Nursing Research, 25*, 115–120.

Gibeau, J. L. (1977). Education and consultation on mental health in long term care facilities: Problems, pitfalls, and solutions: The art of consultation—construction of a two way street versus the road not taken. *Journal of Geriatric Psychiatry 10*(2):163–171.

Glaser, E. M. (1977). Consultation in institutions for child development. *Journal of Applied Behavioral Science, 13*, 89–109.

Goodstein, L. D. (1978). *Consulting with human service systems.* Reading, MA: Addison-Wesley Publishing Co.

Gortner, S. R. (1979). Researchmanship: The competitors. *Western Journal of Nursing Research, 1*, 330–333.

Green, L. W., & Lewis, F. M. (1986). *Evaluation and measurement in health education and health promotion.* Palo Alto, CA: Mayfield.

Grubb, L. L. (1979). Nurse-physician collaboration. *Supervisor Nurse, 10*(3), 16, 19–21.

Henderson, M., Lewis, F. M., Thompson, B., & Wooldridge, J. (1990). *Test of a telephone intervention for blue collar smokers.* Grant/Contract No. 88-2245-20, Cancer Communication Systems Research, National Cancer Institute, September 1987 to August 1990.

Hinshaw, A. S., Chance, H. C., & Atwood, J. (1981). Research in practice: A process of collaboration and negotiation. *Journal of Nursing Administration, 11*(2), 33–38.

Hongladarom, G. (1983). A mobile cancer nursing outreach program: Assumptions and realities. *Cancer Nursing, 6,* 49–54.

Hongladarom, G., Lewis, F. M., Landenburger, K., & McCorkle, R. (1986). A community-based cancer nursing continuing education program. In R. McCorkle & G. Hongladarom (Eds.), *Issues and topics in cancer nursing.* Norwalk, CT: Appleton-Century-Crofts.

Komfled-Jacobs, G., & Karshmer, J. F. (1977). A collaborative model for university nursing education and agency staff development. *Journal of Psychiatric Nursing and Mental Health Services, 15*(11), 15–22.

Kramer, J. R. (1977). Education and consultation on mental health in long-term care facilities: Problems, pitfalls, and solutions: A process approach to staff training and consultation. *Journal of Geriatric Psychiatry, 10,* 197–213.

Lamb, G. S., & Napodano, R. J. (1984). Physician-nurse practitioner interaction patterns in primary care practices. *Amer Journal of Public Health, 74,* 26–29.

Lewis, F. M. (1985). *Collaboration: Alternative models and consequences* (keynote address). American Nurses' Association. Atlanta, GA.

Lewis, F. M., & Batey, M. V. (1982). Clarifying autonomy and accountability in nursing service. Part II. *Journal of Nursing Administration, 12*(10), 10–15.

Loomis, M. E. (1982). Resources for collaborative research. *Western Journal of Nursing Research, 4,* 65–74.

Loomis, M. E., & Krone, K. P. (1980a). Collaborative research development. *Journal of Nursing Administration, 10*(12), 32–35.

Loomis, M. E., & Krone, K. P. (1980b). Practice-relevant research development. In *New directions for nursing in the '80's* (pp. 111–122). Kansas City, MO: American Nurses' Association.

Maddux, J. F. (1955). Consultation in public health. *American Journal of Public Health, 45,* 1424–1430.

Mailick, M. D., & Ashley, A. A. (1981). Politics of interprofessional collaboration: Challenge to advocacy. *Social Casework, 62,* 131–137.

Mauger, B. L., & Huggins, K. (1980). Developing and implementing collaborative nursing education research in the South. *Nursing Research, 29,* 189–192.

Mauksch, I. G. (1981). Nurse-physician collaboration: A changing relationship. *Journal of Nursing Administration, 11*(6), 35–38.

McKenna, P. M. (1981). Role negotiation: A strategy for facilitating an interprofessional health care team. *Nursing Leadership, 4*(4), 23–28.

Mood, D. W., & Parzuchowski, J. (1987). *Locus of control, desire for control, and preference for information in patients with cancers of the head and neck: A pilot study.* Southwest Oncology Group (SWOG): 8633.

Norris, C. M. (1977). A few notes on consultation in nursing. *Nursing Outlook, 25,* 756–761.

Nuckolls, K. B. (1977). The consultation process: A reciprocal relationship. *MCN: American Journal of Maternal Child Nursing, 2,* 11–16.

Oberst, M. T. (1980). Nursing research: New definitions, collegial approaches. *Cancer Nursing, 3,* 459.

O'Connor, C. E., & Carr, S. (1981). Interdisciplinary collaboration between nursing and dental hygiene: Clinical care for the elderly. *Journal of Gerontological Nursing, 7,* 233–235.

Oda, D. S. (1982). Consultation: An expectation of leadership. *Nursing Leadership, 5,* 7–9.

Oxford English Dictionary. (1971). New York: Oxford University Press.

Pati, B. (1980). Nursing consultation: A collaborative process. *Journal of Nursing Administration, 10*(11), 33–37.

Pelz, D. C. (1967). Creative tensions in the research and development climate. *Science, 157*(3785), 160–165.

Pelz, D. C. (1976). Environments for creative performance within universities. In S. Messick & Associates, *Individuality in learning* (pp. 229–247). San Francisco: Jossey-Bass Publishers.

Petersen, M. B. H. (1981). The centralized education and nursing departments: Collaboration or collision? *Journal of Continuing Education in Nursing, 12*(6), 18–21.

Peznecker, B., Draye, M. A., & McNeil, J. (1982). Collaborative practice models in community health nursing. *Nursing Outlook, 30,* 298–302.

Peznecker, B. L., & McNeil, J. (1979). Collaborating on a service and education project. *Washington Nurse, 9,* 8–10.

Poulin, M. A., Clifford, J. C., & McClure, M. L. (1981). Working together: A positive experience in service-education collaboration. *Journal of Nursing Administration, 11*(11–12), 44–48.

Schumaker, D., & Gross, V. (1980). Toward collaboration: One small step. *Nursing and Health Care, 1,* 183–185.

Singleton, E. K., Edmunds, M. W., Rapson, M. F., & Steele, S. (1982). An experience in collaborative research. *Nursing Outlook, 30,* 395–401.

Squyres, W. D. (Ed.) (1980). *Patient education: An inquiry into the state of the art.* New York: Springer.

Styles, M. M. (1984). Reflections on collaboration and unification. *Image, 16,* 21–23.

Suppers, V., Yarbro, C. H., & Mayer-Scogna, D. (1979). Nursing intervention in clinical research: A model program of nursing contributions to a cooperative study group. *Oncology Nursing Forum, 6*(4), 26–27.

Termini, M., & Ciechuski, M. A. (1981). The consultation process. *Issues in Mental Health Nursing, 3*(1–2), 77–78.

Tyler, F. B., Tamulerich, M., & Good, P. (1982). A collaborative continuing education model. *Journal of Continuing Education in Nursing, 13,* 10–13.

Virden, S., & Chater, S. (1979). Curriculum consultation. *Nursing Leadership, 2*(3), 13–17.

Weiss, S. J., & David, H. P. (1985). Validity and reliability of the collaborative practice scales. *Nursing Research, 34,* 299–305.

Wessell, M. L. (1981). Learning about interdisciplinary collaboration. *Journal of Nursing Education, 20*(3), 39–44.

Willcocks, A. (1979). Weakness of consultation. *Health and Social Service Journal, 89*(4639), 481.

Williamson, J. A. (1981). Mutual interaction: A model of nursing practice. *Nursing Outlook, 29,* 104–107.

Yaste, C. K. (1985). *Collaborative practice in acute care settings: A descriptive study.* Unpublished master's thesis, University of Washington, Seattle.

64

Issues and Strategies in Professional Education

JUDITH A. PAICE
MARILEE I. DONOVAN

Only 25 years ago, the continued education of professional nurses was a rare and haphazard process. In 1967, a National Advisory Commission on Health Manpower recommended that a system be established to aid health practitioners in maintaining continued competence (Wilk, 1986). In 1971, "professional obsolescence" was identified as a key health concern in a report entitled *Licensure and Related Health Personnel Credentialing* (Wilk, 1986). Also in 1971, California became the first state to pass legislation requiring evidence of continuing education for nursing relicensure. In 1974, the American Nurses' Association (ANA) House of Delegates voted in support of mandatory education for relicensure. This chapter addresses the broad area of continuing education for professional nurses; institutional in-service training, self-learning activities, and certification are viewed as major subsets of continuing education. This chapter explores the development of continuing education in nursing, the role of continuing education, the variety of means available for providing continuing education, ways to motivate the learner, the process of certification, and future trends in the continuing education of cancer nurses.

THE ROLE OF CONTINUING EDUCATION AND STAFF DEVELOPMENT

Competent Delivery of Care

The goal of continuing education in nursing is to ensure the continued competent delivery of profes-

sional nursing care. Continuing education is expected to accomplish two related goals: improve the quality of nursing care and improve the status of the patients served (Greaves & Loquist, 1983). This broad area of professional education includes orienting new employees, assessing the expertise of staff in relevant skill areas, ensuring that the knowledge and skills of staff are up to date, cross-training and retraining of staff as patient populations change, providing the means to learn new skills as practice changes (e.g., computer skills, discharge planning), and providing the opportunity to develop expertise. Baird (1986) clearly expresses the magnitude of this task: "to modify the content for new students seems a far easier task than developing effective ways to ensure an updated knowledge base for those nurses already in practice."

Education Standards for Nurses

Regulatory agencies have recognized the need for continual learning by establishing standards related to the education of practicing nurses. Standard V, "Nursing Services," of the Joint Commission on the Accreditation of Health-Care Organizations, requires appropriate training and education for the responsibilities assumed by the caregiver (Joint Commission, 1982). The ANA and specialty organizations have established standards that require continuing evidence of professional competence (American Nurses' Association [ANA], 1984). The publications by the ANA's Division of Medical-Surgical Nursing Practice and the Oncology

Nursing Society (ONS)—*Outcome Standards for Cancer Nursing Practice* and *Standards for Oncology Nursing Practice*—and the ONS's *Outcome Standards for Cancer Nursing Education* specifically address the need for nurses involved in cancer care to have the necessary knowledge to provide that care (ANA & ONS, 1979, 1987; ONS, 1982). Recently, the litigious atmosphere in the United States has added an additional reason for providing effective continuing education: Management may now be held liable if an individual in its employ fails to practice competently (Scirma, 1987).

Responsibility for Continuing Education

Many nurses believe that their continuing education is solely the responsibility of their employers. Hopkin and Perlich (1985) suggest that one of the current unresolved conflicts in continuing education is related to who is primarily responsible for the ongoing development of health professionals—the health care agency or the professionals themselves? It appears that many *share* responsibility for the continued competent performance of all professional nurses: health care agencies, colleges and universities, professional organizations, *and* professional nurses themselves. Health care agencies and schools of nursing have primary responsibility for education essential to the provision of safe care *(what must be known)*. Knowledge and skills that enhance patient care or promote health maintenance or self-care activities are jointly the responsibility of the practitioner and the health care agency *(what is useful to know)*. And the knowledge and skills that are of general interest, that enhance professional development, or that enrich the learner are primarily the responsibility of the professional *(what is nice to know)*.

In addition to meeting the overall goal of continuing education, institutional continuing education (staff development) must be consistent with the mission of the institution or agency. Continuing cancer nursing education must also be consistent with the philosophy of cancer care within the health care agency and cancer unit and must address the ANA-ONS's *Outcome Standards for Cancer Nursing Practice* (ANA & ONS, 1979).

What Education Can and Cannot Do

Cost-containment efforts, coupled with the growing nursing shortage, demand that priorities be set and adhered to. Mundinger (1978) identified three levels of priorities within which educational offerings fit: to ensure safe care, to improve health outcomes, and to maintain health and promote self-care. When it is necessary to make the difficult decisions caused by the need to set priorities and to recognize limitations of resources and time, it is beneficial to consider what education can and cannot do. Too often an educational intervention is attempted when the problem is not a knowledge deficit. Studies of educational outcomes have demonstrated that competency (the accurate

knowledge) does not necessarily translate into competent performance (the practice of the knowledge or skill) (Griffith, 1981; Martin, McNeal, Kronenfeld, & Wheeler, 1986; Warmuth, 1987). This lack of competent performance may be a result of motivational deficits, supervisory deficits, peer group pressure, resource deficits, and the like. Education will not correct any of these problems.

Education has often been used as a reward or a diversion; the nurse who has performed exceptionally well is sent to an educational offering, or the nurse who is "burning out" is given an "education day" to recuperate. Peters and Austin (1985) stress that most companies do not pay enough attention to their employees, do not sufficiently reward innovation and risk-taking, and do not demonstrate enough respect for the persons who do the work of the organization. However, one must consider seriously whether education is the most effective, appropriate, and cost-effective method of addressing these needs.

Translating Knowledge into Expertise

In her exploration of the process by which nurses move from novice to expert practitioners, Benner (1984) stresses that expertise is the result of experience in making decisions within a particular context about the qualitative distinctions between similar and dissimilar cases. Expertise cannot be taught in the way education is usually approached; a nurse must *develop* expertise. However, a strong background in the biologic and behavioral bases of clinical practice is an essential tool for the development of expertise. These sciences can be taught. Specialization and subspecialization expedite the development of expertise because they narrow the focus of nurses and help them learn to interpret clinical situations, make discretionary judgments, and assume the risks inherent in expert practice.

One response to the reduced length of stay in hospitals and the nursing shortage is an increased emphasis on standardization (standardized care plans, policies, and procedures). Benner suggests that standardization inhibits the development of context-dependent decision making and discretionary judgment, which are marks of an expert practitioner. Interestingly, Benner also notes that educational strategies that enhance the integration of the novice practitioner (clear objectives, specific knowledge, abstract principles and theoretical models, and precise procedures) delay or prevent the development of advanced levels of practice. We concur with Benner's conclusions. Experienced nurses seldom rely on policies, procedures, or rules in making judgments. When an expert nurse says, "I think Mr. D. is 'going bad,'" it is unwise to ignore that intuition whether or not it can be explained.

EDUCATIONAL STRATEGIES

Health care organizations are responsible for providing the education necessary to deliver competent nursing care. A variety of strategies are available, in addition to the traditional staff development lecture, for ensuring that all staff receive the necessary information: teleconferencing, video teleconferencing, computer-assisted instruction, self-instructional packages, contract learning, and gaming and simulation.

Teleconferencing

Teleconferencing connects participants at various sites through a telephone or satellite system. Individuals who are geographically distant can then have access to continuing education comparable to that received by nurses throughout their region without having to spend time and money on travel and lodging. This relatively new method of instruction offers interactive learning by way of multiple media: audio, audio and video, or computer. Audio teleconferencing transmits the instructor's voice over a telephone line to speaker systems at different locations. Participants at various sites can communicate verbally with one another and with the presenter (Treloar, 1985). West Virginia University, the Hawaii Unit of the American Cancer Society, and Boston University, in cooperation with the Dana Farber Cancer Center, are examples of institutions that have developed effective teleconferencing activities in cancer nursing.

Video Teleconferencing

Audio and visual transmission joins viewers and presenters. Video cameras focus on the speaker during the presentation and on the audience during the question-and-answer sessions, allowing interaction between presenter and participants. The origination site and distant sites are often public or private television studios or teleconferencing facilities at universities, hospitals, or hotels. This sophisticated technology and the complex equipment employed to use it require consultation with media specialists and large initial expenditures (Limon, Spencer, & Henderson, 1985). If others have already established the system, cancer nursing organizations may have to pay only for the network time. Dartmouth Medical School, the University of Vermont Cancer Center, and a network of community hospitals supported monthly cancer nursing conferences from 1976 through 1982 as part of a federal breast cancer project. Audience members could comment and ask questions. Presentations were rotated so that nursing groups at each center shared responsibility for content preparation and presentation. Because the system was already in place, the cost of the video teleconferencing was limited to the cost of network time. The effectiveness and cost-benefit analysis of this approach have not yet been studied systematically.

Computer-Assisted Instruction

One area of unlimited, and to date largely unrealized, potential in continuing education and staff development is computer-assisted instruction (CAI). The reduced cost of computer hardware and greater availability of commercial software programs have made microcomputers more accessible to institutions and individuals (Brisson, 1985). Greater exposure to these systems, now beginning at the elementary education level, will ensure acceptance and reduce fear related to operating these devices.

The interactive nature of this instructional strategy and the ability of the learner to determine a pace suitable to an individual learning style provide a learning tool appropriate to the nurse as an adult learner. Few CAI packages specific to oncology nursing content are currently available. Only two programs related to oncology nursing are identified by the National League for Nursing (Bolwell, 1987). Much of oncology nursing continuing education content is appropriate to computer-based instruction, for example, site-specific disease information, symptom management strategies, and simulation techniques for advanced skills such as the care of venous access devices. A limitation of computer-based education is that it requires the regular availability of programming assistance to update content. Therefore, rapidly changing content areas should be avoided. As more nurses become computer competent, this may become less of a problem.

Self-instructional Modules

Using self-instructional modules includes setting specific objectives, taking pre- and post-tests, and studying content that allows the learner to meet the objectives in an independent manner. Self-paced programmed instruction (one type of self-instructional program) was found to be superior to standard lecture format when learning gains were evaluated (Guimei, 1977). This method of instruction is more appropriate for the adult learner because it allows learners to pursue the content at their own speed and to emphasize their own needs.

Greater learning was demonstrated using a self-instructional format than was achieved using standard lectures in eight of ten modules that were part of a hospital orientation program (Rufo, 1985). This approach allows independent orientation and frees the staff development educators from giving repetitive, time-consuming lectures. Cancer nursing content that is necessary to prepare staff nurses for employment on oncology units can be delivered using this format. The orientation to the Johns Hopkins Cancer Center is primarily self-instructional. Benefits of this approach include the return of the clinical nurse specialists from the classroom to the bedside and the immediacy of orientation (new staff are not required to wait until the next orientation is scheduled).

Preceptorship

A novice clinician enters the practice setting without fully developed problem-solving and clinical skills. Preceptorship, as a means of orienting new nurses, is an effective method to advance clinical competency (Everson, Panoc, Prat, & King, 1981). The specific needs of the new employee and of the unit can be addressed in the individualized education provided by precepting. The use of preceptors is well suited to orientation to oncology units, where new employees with varied backgrounds must achieve specific skills and develop a specialty practice. Mentorship, an extension of the preceptor role, supports not only knowledge and skill acquisition but also role development (Atwood, 1979).

Preceptorship and mentorship require skills not traditionally taught in undergraduate programs, and new preceptors require orientation to the role (Piemme, Tack, Kramer, & Evans, 1986). Such a program has been successfully implemented at the Clinical Center, National Institutes of Health. Only experienced staff should be considered for preceptor roles. The responsibilities and accomplishments of the preceptor must be evaluated and acknowledged during performance reviews if this role is to be credible and to develop in the system.

The combination of self-instructional packages and preceptorships has the potential for being the most individualized, effective, and cost-efficient orientation package. Evaluation of these strategies has not been carried out in a systematic manner.

Contract Learning

This approach involves an agreement between the educator and the learner involving learning activities. These contracts may be formal or informal, structured or unstructured, and written or verbal. Successfully used to promote patient education and compliance, contracts are now used in continuing education efforts. These agreements identify the objectives, content, methods of learning, and sequence of the learning activities based on the needs of the learner (Eagleton, 1984).

Gaps and Contracts is a technique that requires learners to identify gaps in their knowledge or in institutional practice (Donovan, Wolpert, & Yasko, 1981). The contract is then developed as a means to correct those inadequacies. The participants in a 48-hour oncology continuing education program offered semiannually at Rush–Presbyterian–St. Luke's Medical Center in Chicago (Table 64–1) use this technique to meet the needs of their practice settings. Each participant develops a contract that identifies a gap in nursing knowledge specific to his or her clinical unit and also a strategy to correct the deficiency. The unit managers and the continuing education course directors collaborate with the nurse and cosign the contract. Unit or departmental staff development programs, posters, and patient teaching booklets are some of the creative products of these contracts. The staff nurse unable to attend the continuing education offering and the patients on the clinical units benefit in a very concrete and measurable way from the education of one particular staff nurse.

Table 64–1. OUTLINE FOR ONCOLOGY COURSE FOR NURSES

Introduction to Course
The Disease: Cancer
Epidemiology, prevention, detection
Carcinogenesis and metastasis
Diagnosis and staging
Treatment
Chemotherapy
Surgical oncology
Radiation oncology
An integrative approach
Common Tumors and Symptom Management
Alterations in protective mechanisms: leukemia
Alterations in protective mechanisms: skin cancer
Self-care deficit: central nervous system tumors
Paraneoplastic syndromes
Breast cancer
Gynecologic and genitourinary cancer
Alterations in self-concept: sexuality
Alterations in comfort: pain
Alterations in elimination: gastrointestinal cancers
Alteration in nutrition
Head and neck cancers
Lung cancer
Ineffective airway clearance: pleural effusion
Additional Psychosocial Issues
Grief work
Role playing: support
Patient teaching
Discharge planning

Simulation

The simulation of skills is a well-recognized means of learning. Supervised practice of psychomotor skills, such as urinary catheterization and medication administration, is common at the undergraduate level. This is an effective teaching strategy when errors in technique may result in morbidity or mortality for the client (Burns, 1984). Oncology applications include procedures related to maintenance of infusion pumps, cannulation of vascular access devices, chemotherapy administration, teaching of breast or testicular self-examination, and other advanced skills. Simulation can also be applied to psychosocial skills, specifically to assessment and intervention. For instance, role playing patient, family, and health professional responses to the dying process of a simulated patient can help develop understanding of the different perspectives of the individuals involved and the conflicts likely to arise.

Gaming, or competitive simulation, is an activity initially employed by social scientists to explore coalitions between players. It was later used by military and business organizations to mimic the competition seen in these roles. Gaming has been utilized as an evaluation tool to measure nursing practice after completion of a continuing education course (Burns, 1984). Clinical knowledge and decision-making skills related to oncology nursing practice can be readily applied to this evaluative technique. However, developing clinical practice–relevant games is a time-consuming process.

MOTIVATION OF THE LEARNER

The process of continuing professional education can be fostered by creative learning strategies. The learner must, however, be motivated to participate in these activities for learning to occur. Although nurses agree on the need for continuing education, very few voluntarily participate. Mandatory continuing education for nurses, currently adopted in ten states, attempts to guarantee competent nursing care by ensuring maintenance of nursing knowledge. The involuntary nature of this legislation presumes that nurses will not attend continuing education programs without external pressure. Indeed, a study by Millonig (1985) concluded that nurses were motivated to participate in continuing education activities for reasons related to professional advancement (e.g., recognition of superiors, excellent performance review, promotion, merit increase) and external expectations (e.g., legislation, certification) (Box 64–1).

Mandatory Continuing Education

Controversy exists regarding the merits of mandatory continuing education. The results of studies that examined nurses' attitudes toward mandatory continuing education vary from overwhelming support to formidable opposition. Common perceptions of proponents include the assurance of quality patient care by mandating all nurses to participate in continuing education. Opponents frequently cite the lack of accessibility, the poor quality, and the expense of educational offerings and the lack of empirical evidence that continuing education has a positive effect on patient care.

Negative Influences on Motivation

Welch (1980) contends that the greater concern is the lack of recognition by nurses of the need for an updated knowledge base. She sees the following three categories as factors that influence negatively the nurse's motivation for pursuing continuing education.

Problems Related to Nursing Leadership

Clinical role models who demonstrate the value of continuing education are lacking. Few incentives for

attending educational programs (particularly monetary support and paid educational days to attend conferences) exist.

Problems Involving Continuing Education Departments

Educational programs are often developed by educators with little regard for the needs of the individual nurse learner.

Problems Resulting from the Absence of Socialization for Lifelong Learning

Nurses do not expect to need to continue their learning. Even those nurses who expect to continue their learning often expect that the cost and effort will be borne by their employers rather than by them.

Creating an environment conducive to participation in continuing education is imperative. Health care organizations should provide paid leaves of absence as well as full or partial registration reimbursement for programs that have *direct relevance* to the practice of the nurse. Although the direct and indirect costs are high (Table 64–2), Rufo (1985) claims that support of continuing education is cost effective because of the greater job satisfaction and improved retention of staff. Of the 92 participants who attended the 48-hour cancer nursing course at Rush–Presbyterian–St. Luke's Medical Center between 1983 and 1985, 75 per cent remain with the institution as of July 1987. Professional rewards for continuing education (via formal courses or independent learning packages) are essential. For instance, performance reviews should strongly acknowledge participation in continuing education and should question nonparticipation. Offering exposure to nurses in advanced practice roles, such as oncology clinical specialists, can provide the role modeling and encouragement to inspire nurses to attend continuing education.

CERTIFICATION

Professional organizations can motivate their members to pursue an advanced knowledge base by offering

---

Box 64–1. MOTIVATIONS OF NURSES WHO PARTICIPATE IN CONTINUING EDUCATION

In an attempt to identify factors contributing to the attendance of registered nurses in continuing education programs, Millonig studied 350 randomly selected full-time registered nurses in eight metropolitan hospitals. A two-part questionnaire was administered. The questionnaire consisted of questions requesting demographic information and an instrument that examined the reasons why individuals participate in learning activities (the Education Participation Scale.)

The findings indicated that registered nurses attend continuing education programs to seek professional advancement (to obtain higher job status, earn a degree or certificate, keep up with the competition). External expectations, such as compliance with the recommendations of a superior, contributed to attendance at continuing education activities.

According to Millonig, nursing administrators must reward nurses who participate in continuing education. Millonig claimed that support of continuing education is cost effective because participation in continuing education will ensure competence in clinical practice and more cost-effective care delivery.

(From Millonig, V. L. [1985]. Motivational orientation toward learning after graduation. *Nursing Administration Quarterly, 9*, 79–86. Reproduced by permission.)

Table 64–2. AREAS OF COST TO CONSIDER IN COST ANALYSES

	EXAMPLE 1: 100 registered nurses attend a 1-day cancer nursing seminar		EXAMPLE 2: 25 staff nurses attend a 1-day inservice on AIDS	
	No. 1: national keynote speaker No. 2: regional speaker No. 3: local speaker Lunch on own		All planners and speakers are institutional employees; half are nurses and half are physicians	
	No. 4: regional speaker — No. 1: national speaker No. 5: local speaker — No. 7: regional speaker No. 6: local speaker — No. 8: local speaker			
Development Costs				
Salaries of Planners	Three planners met four times for 1 hr each time (1 hr × 4 × three persons × average salary + fringe benefits)	$246	Two planners met for 2 hr once and 1 hr once (3 hr × 2 × average salary + fringe benefits)	$123
Salaries of Those Producing Materials	Coordinator contacts speakers, writes letters of confirmation, designs brochure, applies for continuing education units (24 hr × average salary + fringe benefits)	$491	Coordinator contacts speakers, arranges for room, equipment, develops handouts (8 hr × average salary + fringe benefits)	$164
	Secretary obtains mailing list, addresses and mails brochures, helps coordinator with planning materials, prepares handouts (20 hr × average salary + fringe benefits)	$232	Secretary types, duplicates, and collates handouts (16 hr × average salary + fringe benefits)	$186
Supplies and Equipment	2000 brochures, mailing list	$1200	25 posters generated on office computer and duplicated and distributed	$2
Contracted Services	Rental of videotaping equipment to produce tape for speaker no. 3	$50		
	Illustrator, preparation of slides and overhead transparencies	$300	Preparation of slides, transparencies	$0–300
	Printing of handout materials 120 packets (25 pages + folder)	$240	Printing of handout material 25 packets (25 pages + folder)	$53
Room and Building Costs	General overhead is seldom considered		General overhead is seldom considered	
Other	Postage and long-distance telephone calls	$315		
Operating Costs				
Salaries of Support Personnel	Set-up charge	$100	Two maintenance workers to set up and dismantle room (2 × 2 hr × average salary + fringe benefits)	$31
	Secretary to register, assist on day of seminar (9 hr × average salary + fringe benefits)	$105	Secretary to assist on day of program (9 hr × average salary + fringe benefits)	$105
Salaries of Educators	Honorarium for keynote speaker (No. 1)	$500	Salaries of local speakers (4 hr by physician, 4 hr by registered nurse × average salary + fringe benefits)	$280
	Honoraria for three regional speakers (Nos. 2, 4, and 7) ($100/each)	$300		
	Salaries of local speakers (Nos. 3, 5, 6, and 8) (1 day each × average salary + fringe benefits)	$508		
	Salary of coordinator to attend and evaluate (1.5 days × salary + fringe benefits)	$246	Salary of coordinator to attend and evaluate (1.5 days × salary + fringe benefits)	$246
	Salary of planning committee to attend (2 × 8 hr × average salary + fringe benefits)	$328	Planning committee members are educators (above)	
	Salaries of 100 nurses to attend (100 × 1 day × average salary + fringe benefits)	$12,900	Salaries of 25 nurses to attend (25 × 1 day × average salary + fringe benefits)	$3,225
Equipment	Rental of overhead and slide projector, VCR and TV	$0–100	Rental of overhead and slide projector	$0–25
Room and Building	Rental of conference room	$250	General overhead is generally not considered	
Food	Coffee, rolls, soft drinks	$350	Coffee, rolls, soft drinks	$30–150
Travel	Keynote speaker (airfare + per diem)	$310	—	
	Mileage costs for regional speakers	$75		
Total Costs		$19,146		$4890

certification within that specialty. The nurse is acknowledged for possessing expertise beyond that required for nursing licensure (McCorkle, 1984). Quality is also ensured for patients who receive nursing care from certified specialists (ANA, 1987). Professional regulation of nursing practice ensures competency based on professional standards. This competency is demonstrated by certification.

Oncology Certified Nurse

The ONS identified the benefits of certification and formed the Oncology Nursing Certification Corporation (ONCC) to coordinate the certification process in oncology nursing. A nurse who successfully demonstrates general competency within the specialty is designated an Oncology Certified Nurse (OCN) (Moore, Hogan, Longman, McNally, & Piper, 1982). Future certification may focus on subspecialties within oncology nursing. However, generalist oncology competency must first be demonstrated before developing credentials for subspecialization within specialty fields (Scofield, 1986).

Certification, therefore, serves as a means to promote continuing professional education and growth within oncology nursing as well as a way to indicate expertise to the consumer of nursing services (patients, families, and health care institutions and agencies). The many tools that have been developed for certification examination preparation (books, video tapes, curriculum outlines) can also serve as methods for continuing education.

FUTURE ISSUES AND TRENDS

The cost effectiveness of continuing education, the roles of staff development educators, and the demonstration of the efficacy of continued education (including demonstration of the impact of education on clinical practice) are areas for research and development in the future.

Cost Effectiveness

Cost containment has already produced changes in the type and amount of continuing education available. The primary mission of the care delivery system determines much of the education that is available. Reductions in staff development departments and nursing shortages in all areas limit the time that can be devoted to staff development. The cost-benefit ratio has not been well established for alternative educational methods such as internships, self-learning modules, computer-assisted instruction, or satellite networks. Cost analyses such as those described by Boston (1986), Hast (1986), del Bueno and Kelly (1980), or Kelly (1985) are becoming increasingly more necessary (see Table 64–2). Jazwiec (1987) suggests that cost studies should also include the productivity of the educators

or staff development department. She suggests such productivity measures as hours of preparation per hour of class, direct versus indirect program costs, cost per participant, and hours of instruction delivered per month.

Evaluating the Impact of Continuing Education

Although several methods of evaluating the impact of continuing education have been suggested, most educational programs continue to receive nothing more than a satisfaction evaluation. Research has most often demonstrated the effectiveness of education in increasing knowledge (Donovan et al., 1981; Rufo, 1985; Warmuth, 1987). Three recent studies of the impact of continuing education on nursing practice are described later. Warmuth (1987) reported on a process for evaluating the impact of education on the thinking, judging, evaluating, and performing aspects of practice. Participants in a continuing education program were contacted 6 months after the program and asked how they had used the course content in their practice. Twenty-nine nurses described 142 different ways in which they had used the content of the continuing education program. The findings of this study were remarkably similar to the findings of a study reported by Donovan and colleagues (1981) (Box 64–2).

Cook and Cohen (1986) asked the participants in a diabetes patient education training program to write a "commitment to change" plan. The overall success rate was 59 per cent at 6 months. For the least complex plans related to evaluation and selection of teaching materials, the success rate was 79 per cent.

Factors That Affect the Application of Continuing Education

Individual Performance. If continuing education in nursing is to accomplish the primary goal of ensuring the competent delivery of professional nursing care, educators must be more sensitive to the factors that affect whether an educational experience has a lasting influence on performance. The failure of knowledge to be translated into changes in the practice of the individual or of the group has now been documented (Valanis & Shortridge, 1987).

Valanis and Shortridge (1987) reported that there was an inverse correlation between years of exposure to antineoplastic agents and use of protective behaviors. Reasons given for not using protection were inconvenience, unavailability, deemed unnecessary, and not convinced of the danger. Only 5 per cent of the 632 ONS member nurses surveyed were unaware of the current information regarding the hazards of handling antineoplastic agents. Therefore, although 95 per cent had the knowledge, many were not practicing in accordance with this knowledge.

Group Behavior. When one nurse attends a continuing education program and is expected to return to

---

Box 64–2. FORMAL COMMITMENT TO CHANGE IMPROVES OUTCOME

A technique called *Gaps and Contracts* was developed by faculty members at the University of Pittsburgh to assist nurses in implementing new learning in the practice setting. Participants attended a 10-day cancer nursing workshop. On the first day of the workshop, learners were encouraged to identify gaps that existed between ideal nursing care and care given in their institution.

On the eighth day of the workshop, participants organized the identified gaps according to patient need, agency need, personal abilities, and available resources. With the assistance of the faculty members, each participant developed a strategy to eliminate the gap. This plan was documented in a letter to the participant's immediate supervisor—the "contract"—on the last day of the workshop. In all, 251 nurses wrote 450 contracts.

At 6 months, 153 (56 per cent) of the participants had successfully completed their contracts. The Gaps and Contracts strategy allows workshop participants to implement material learned during continuing education programs. This process also provides a mechanism for evaluating the effect of continuing education on nursing practice and patient care.

(From Donovan, M., Wolpert, P., & Yasko, J. [1981]. Gaps and contracts. *Nursing Outlook, 29*, 467–471. Reproduced by permission.)

---

the practice setting and to improve the practice of several peers, the situation is even more complex. Seldom have mechanisms been implemented to ensure that the education of one staff nurse is translated into the education of many and the improvement of patient care. When a single person (or a few persons) is (are) sent to a continuing education offering, specific objec-tives need to be established for the improvement of patient care relative to the attendance at the educa-tional offering. For instance, a nurse who attends a workshop on pain should do so because it has been established that pain assessment on the unit is ineffec-tive. The nurse selected to attend the educational program should be chosen because of interest in the topic and ability to improve patient care as a result of attendance. On returning from the program, the nurse should present a plan for improving the assessment of pain and develop a method for evaluating the improve-ment in patient care.

Table 64–3. FACTORS THAT AFFECT WHETHER AN EDUCATIONAL PROGRAM HAS A LASTING EFFECT ON PERFORMANCE

Characteristic	Typical Variables
Program	Relevance of topic, organization of program, setting, enthusiasm of teacher, correlation with learner's expectations and needs, perceived value, involvement of learner
Professional (learner)	Motivation, previous education, learning style and match with method of presentation, specialization, attitudes toward change, level of risk taking, degree to which information seeking is a natural behavior, capacity for innovation
Proposed changes	Complexity; how much help will be needed to accomplish the change; perceived benefit; how compatible is the change with past experience, values, and needs of the learner; is change able to be tested on a small scale first; will the results be visible?
Social system of the professional (many believe this is the single most important factor)	What are the norms regarding risk and innovation, openness of communication and willingness to collaborate, support from legitimate authority, perceived expertise of the change agent, capacity of reward systems to support change, availability of necessary resources?

SUMMARY

In developing or evaluating the appropriateness of an educational program, studies of the process by which innovations become part of practice suggest four areas of importance: the characteristics of the program itself, the characteristics of the learner, the behavioral change desired, and the social system of the profes-sional involved as learner (Table 64–3). Educators must develop and implement educational programs that address this lack of behavioral change associated with attendance at continuing education programs. The problems related to the implementation of innovation should be assessed systematically, and strategies should be developed to ensure that the factors associated with the program, the learner, the process of change, and the system enhance learning and application rather than detract from this process. A commitment of many professionals (learners as well as educators) will be necessary if the outcome of continuing education is to become the measurable improvement in patient care.

References

American Nurses' Association. (1984). *Standards for continuing education in nursing*. Kansas City, MO: Author.
American Nurses' Association. (1987). *The scope of nursing practice*. Kansas City, MO: Author.
American Nurses' Association and Oncology Nursing Society.

(1979). *Outcome standards for cancer nursing practice.* Kansas City, MO: American Nurses' Association.

American Nurses' Association and Oncology Nursing Society. (1987). *Standards for oncology nursing practice.* Kansas City, MO: American Nurses' Association.

Arneson, S. W. (1985a). Iowa nurses' attitudes toward mandatory continuing education. *Journal of Continuing Education in Nursing, 16,* 7–12.

Arneson, S. W. (1985b). Iowa nurses' attitudes toward mandatory continuing education: A two year follow-up study. *Journal of Continuing Education in Nursing, 16,* 13–18.

Atwood, A. H. (1979). The mentor in clinical practice. *Nursing Outlook, 27,* 714–717.

Baird, S. B. (1986). Issues in staff development: An administrator's view. In R. McCorkle & G. Hongladarom (Eds.), *Issues and Topics in Cancer Nursing.* E. Norwalk, CT: Appleton-Century-Crofts.

Benner, P. (1984). *From novice to expert.* Menlo Park, CA: Addison-Wesley.

Bolwell, C. (1987). *Directory of educational software for nursing.* New York: National League for Nursing.

Boston, C. M. (1986). Justifying costs for continuing nursing education departments. *Nursing Economics, 4*(2), 83–85.

Brisson, C. J. (1985). Computer applications in nursing continuing education. *Nursing Clinics of North America, 20,* 505–515.

Burns, K. A. (1984). Experience in the use of gaming and simulation as an evaluation tool for nurses. *Journal of Continuing Education in Nursing, 15,* 213–217.

Cervero, R. M. (1985). Continuing professional education and behavioral change: A model for research and evaluation. *Journal of Continuing Education in Nursing, 16,* 85–88.

Cook, S., & Cohen, R. M. (1986). Evaluating a workshop model for improving diabetes patient education programs: Is it really successful? *The Diabetes Educator, 12,* 48–50.

del Bueno, D. J., & Kelley, K. (1980). How cost effective is your staff development program? *Nurse Educator, 5,* 12–17.

Donovan, M., Wolpert, P., & Yasko, J. (1981). Gaps and contracts. *Nursing Outlook, 29,* 467–471.

Eagleton, B. (1984). Contract learning: An effective teaching-learning strategy. *Focus on Critical Care, 11,* 18–23.

Everson, S., Panoc, K., Prat, P., & King, A. M. (1981). Precepting as an entry method for newly hired staff. *Journal of Continuing Education in Nursing, 12,* 22–26.

Greaves, P. E., & Loquist, R. S. (1983). Impact evaluation: A competency-based approach. *Nursing Administration Quarterly, 7,* 81–86.

Griffith, W. S. (1981). Developing a valid data base for continuing education in the health sciences. *Mobius, 1,* 83–91.

Guimei, M. K. (1977). Effectiveness of a programmed instruction module on oral contraceptives. *Nursing Research, 26,* 452–455.

Hast, A. S. (1986). An approach to cost-effective education in the critical care setting. *Critical Care Education, 6,* 86–89.

Hopkin, L., & Perlich, L. (1985). An approach to funding nursing continuing education conferences. *Nursing Economics, 3,* 33–39.

Jazwiec, R. M. (1987). Economics, productivity and effectiveness. *Journal of Continuing Education in Nursing, 18,* 8–13.

Joint Commission for the Accreditation of Hospitals. (1982). *Accreditation manual for hospitals* (p. 119). Chicago: Author.

Kelly, K. J. (1985). Cost benefit and cost effectiveness analysis: Tools for the staff development manager. *Journal of Nursing Staff Development, 1,* 9–15.

Limon, S., Spencer, J. B., & Henderson, F. E. (1985). Video-teleconferencing by nurses for nurses. *Nursing and Health Care, 6,* 313–317.

Martin, D., McNeal, B., Kronenfeld, J., & Wheeler, F. (1986). The impact of professional education on nursing behavior in the practice setting. *Journal of Continuing Education in Nursing, 17,* 40–42.

McCloskey, J. (1984). Influence of rewards and incentives on staff nurse turnover rates. *Nursing Research, 23,* 247–249.

McCorkle, R. (1984). What certification is all about. *Oncology Nursing Forum, 11,* 12–13.

Millonig, V. L. (1985). Motivational orientation toward learning after graduation. *Nursing Administration Quarterly, 9,* 79–86.

Moore, P., Hogan, C., Longman, A., McNally, J., & Piper, B. (1982). Report of the task force on certification in oncology nursing. *Oncology Nursing Forum, 9,* 75–80.

Moskowitz, R. Z. (1985). Long-term continuing education programs in cancer nursing. *Oncology Nursing Forum, 12,* 92–93.

Mundinger, M. (1978). CE: Current contradictions in inservice. *Nursing Administration Quarterly, 2,* 65–71.

Oncology Nursing Society. (1982). *Outcome standards for cancer nursing education—fundamental level.* Pittsburgh, PA: Author.

Peters, T., & Austin, N. (1985). *A passion for excellence.* New York: Warner Books.

Piemme, J. A., Tack, B. B., Kramer, W., & Evans, J. (1986). Developing the nurse preceptor. *Journal of Continuing Education in Nursing, 17,* 186–189.

Rufo, K. (1985). Effectiveness of self-instructional packages in staff development activities. *Journal of Continuing Education in Nursing, 16,* 80–84.

Scirma, D. (1987). Assessing staff competency. *Journal of Nursing Administration, 17,* 41–45.

Scofield, R. (1986). Why a generalist exam in a specialty area. *Oncology Nursing Forum, 13,* 89.

Trammell, D. B. (1984). Educational preparation: Its effect on selection and degree of involvement in continuing education activities. *Journal of Continuing Education in Nursing, 16,* 223–226.

Treloar, L. L. (1985). Facts about teleconferencing for staff development administrators. *Journal of Continuing Education in Nursing, 16,* 47–52.

Valanis, B., & Shortridge, L. (1987). Self-protective practices of nurses handling antineoplastic drugs. *Oncology Nursing Forum, 14,* 23–27.

Warmuth, J. F. (1987). In search of the impact of continuing education. *Journal of Continuing Education in Nursing, 18,* 4–7.

Welch, D. (1980). The real issues behind providing continuing education in nursing. *Journal of Continuing Education in Nursing, 11,* 17–22.

Wilk, J. (1986). From continuous education to continuous learning: Moving toward accountability. *Journal of Continuing Education in Nursing, 17,* 16–18.

CHAPTER 65

Cancer Nursing Education Today

ROSE F. McGEE
JANE C. CLARK

By most standards, cancer nursing education is a relatively new field of study. Before 1940 the literature reflected limited concern with preparation for oncology nursing, yet cancer nursing education has experienced an orderly progression that originated in health care agencies, spread to undergraduate education programs, and was refined further in master's and doctoral programs. The newness of the field does not detract from the impressive strides made nor from the exciting potential for the future. Educators today are faced with challenges in undergraduate education to prepare the generalist and in graduate education to prepare the specialist. Issues related to faculty, students, and curriculum development, implementation, and evaluation are discussed in the following sections. Strategies to address selected issues for the present and future are explored.

FACULTY

Two issues recur in oncology nursing with respect to faculty: educational preparation and maintenance of clinical competency. Faculty preparation encompasses three areas of expertise: education, research, and practice.

Education

During the 1950s and 1960s, nurse educators in oncology were prepared primarily through continuing education programs (Hilkemeyer, 1985). During the 1970s, a cadre of qualified faculty emerged. Two factors contributed to this emergence: the clinical master's program in oncology and the increased number of nurses completing doctorates. These doctorates were primarily in education rather than in philosophy.

The pros and cons of the educational doctorate and diversity of doctoral preparation have been debated (Norris, 1985; Werley & Newcomb, 1983). Some nurse leaders propose that the structured, task-oriented approach of the educational major inhibited creative conceptualization and socialization in the field of nursing. The diversity of preparation is evidenced in oncology faculty today. The 1990 *Oncology Nursing Forum* listing of graduate oncology nursing programs reveals that the coordinators of the programs were prepared as follows: 9 Ed.Ds, 19 Ph.Ds, 8 nursing doctorates, and 6 master's degrees (Hinds, 1989). This diversity of preparation may contribute to variability in the quality of programs or may provide depth and breadth of conceptualization because of the varied educational degrees represented.

Research

The decade of the 1970s was termed by Benoliel (1983, p. 263) as the era in which "nursing came of age as a discipline," noting that graduate study brought nurses into contact with new ideas, with the methods of science, and with the opportunity to tie clinical observations to established bodies of knowledge. These exposures allowed master's prepared nurses to frame questions of interest within the context and framework of organized science. The questions formulated at the master's level formed the basis for movement into doctoral study. The ranks of doctorally prepared nurses increased, and specialization at the doctoral level was initiated. Doctorates in oncology created concern among some nurse leaders. Norris (1985, p. 10) stated "some faculty members will become so expert and so specialized that few, if any, other faculty members will understand their areas of expertise."

As educators, doctorally prepared faculty are prepared to assist students at all levels in formulating questions that contribute to the conceptualization of oncology nursing as a whole. The cumulative impact of these contributions is that oncology nursing is building an impressive foundation for quality nursing care.

Practice

In the emerging years of the specialty, educators were chosen because of clinical expertise. As these educators pursued doctoral study, many had less time to devote to maintaining clinical competency. This deficit was countered, to some extent, by the growing number of master's prepared nurses who served as clinical preceptors and assisted in role socialization of graduate students; however, the availability of clinical nurse specialists was not the answer to the lack of clinical competency among faculty. The development of the professional doctorates in nursing (D.N.S. and D.N.Sc.) helped to rectify the problem of clinical expertise at the doctoral level. In addition, creative approaches to attaining and maintaining clinical competence, such as joint appointments, unification models, and faculty practice, have been instigated.

STUDENTS

Dramatic changes in the profile of nursing students during the last decade include decreasing numbers of traditional applicants and increasing numbers of older, culturally diverse, and part-time students. In addition, admissions to both undergraduate and graduate nursing

programs have decreased. Although data exist to document these changes in nursing in general, cumulative data on the profile and number of students who choose oncology nursing are lacking.

Recruitment of Undergraduate Nursing Students to Oncology

With trends such as shifts in care from cancer centers to community hospitals, inpatient to outpatient settings, acute to long-term care, and treatment to prevention and early detection, one may infer that the need for oncology nurses prepared at the undergraduate level will continue to increase. Therefore, a key issue in oncology nursing education is the recruitment and retention of qualified oncology nurse generalists. Strategies that have been implemented to recruit students to oncology nursing are presented in Table 65–1. Although many of these strategies have been implemented over time, minimal evaluation data have been presented in the literature regarding the effectiveness of the programs in recruiting student nurses to oncology.

Limited data are available to determine the number of oncology nurse generalists in practice and to chart trends over time. In a 1977 membership survey conducted by the Oncology Nursing Society (ONS) (Miller & Herbst, 1978), 94 per cent of the respondents (n = 511) were prepared at the undergraduate level (Table 65–2). However, data from the ONS membership profile in 1990 indicate only 82 per cent (n = 13,166) of members were prepared at the undergraduate level.

Questions raised from the data include the following: Is the ONS membership representative of oncology nurses in general? Was the 1977 survey data representative of nurses in oncology at that time? Is ONS successful in recruiting the oncology nurse generalist to membership? Are the changes in percentage of undergraduate members reflective of an increase in the educational attainment of the oncology nurse? Answers to these questions are not available from current data sources.

Recruitment of Oncology Nurses to Graduate Programs

The second issue related to oncology nursing education is the recruitment of oncology nurses to graduate

Table 65–1. STRATEGIES TO RECRUIT STUDENT NURSES TO ONCOLOGY

Summer work-study programs	Memorial Sloan-Kettering Hospital
	M.D. Anderson Hospital
	Fox Chase Cancer Center
	National Cancer Institute
Role practicum in oncology	
Independent study in oncology	
Student involvement in volunteer and professional oncology organizations	American Cancer Society Oncology Nursing Society
Media appeals on oncology nursing	American Cancer Society Oncology Nursing Society
Student nurse conferences	American Cancer Society

Table 65–2. EDUCATION PROFILE OF ONS MEMBERSHIP (1977–1990)

Level of Education	ONS Membership Survey 1977 (n = 511)	ONS Membership Profile 1990 (n = 16,002)
AD/AA	42 (8%)	3208 (20%)
Diploma	243 (48%)	3584 (22%)
Baccalaureate	193 (38%)	6374 (40%)
Master's	29 (6%)	2627 (16%)
Doctorate	5 (<1%)	125 (1%)

programs. The ONS membership profile provides conservative estimates of the applicant pool for graduate study at the master's and doctoral levels (see Table 65–2). Traditional master's programs have been targeted for nurses prepared at the baccalaureate level. However, with the recent emphasis on educational mobility in nursing, several alternatives to traditional graduate study have been developed.

R.N.-M.N. programs have been designed to allow the nurse with a diploma or an associate degree to enter a master's programs after completing the necessary prerequisites without earning a baccalaureate degree. Curricula limit the repetition of courses required at the baccalaureate and master's levels. Several R.N.-M.N. programs offer specialization in oncology nursing.

Other curricula have been developed, such as generic master's programs with an oncology nursing option. These programs are designed for students with undergraduate degrees in other disciplines. Each strategy has implications for oncology nurse educators to ensure that specialty content and role socialization as a specialist are not compromised.

Changing Profile of Students

Students in nursing in general are older, more culturally diverse, and more likely to be enrolled in part-time study than were nursing students in the past. These changes in the profile of students present the nurse educator with a series of unique challenges.

Increased Part-time Enrollment

Changes in the nursing student profile and diminished financial support for nursing education have contributed to an increase in the proportion of part-time students enrolled in both undergraduate and graduate nursing programs. Data from the 1989 ONS membership profile indicate that 2798 (21 per cent) members were enrolled in undergraduate or graduate programs. The number of members enrolled part-time was four times greater than the number enrolled full-time. Issues related to the effects of part-time study in oncology nursing education include development of flexible schedules for both classroom and clinical experiences, role socialization, attainment of clinical competencies, maintenance of curricular integrity, and student satisfaction with the educational process.

Age of Applicants

Older students present a challenge to the oncology nurse educator in terms of evaluating learning needs and capitalizing on previous education and experience. Mast and Van Atta (1986) described four assumptions about adult learners that are applicable to curriculum planning, recruitment, and retention of nursing students in general and older applicants in particular (Table 65–3). These assumptions imply that those undergraduate and graduate oncology programs that are more flexible; use a variety of learning strategies; and foster collegiality among students, faculty, and clinical preceptors will be more successful in recruiting and retaining adult learners.

Increased Cultural Diversity

The need to recruit socioeconomically disadvantaged students to oncology nursing is imperative, based on findings by the American Cancer Society (ACS) (1986), which demonstrate that differences in cancer incidence, morbidity, and mortality are influenced significantly more by socioeconomic status than by race. Other studies have indicated that the most effective health care educator and provider for the socioeconomically disadvantaged individual is someone from the same status or culture. Unfortunately, data are not available on the cultural diversity of nurses currently in oncology care or in graduate programs in oncology nursing. In addition, no systematic assessment of oncology nursing curricula has been conducted to ensure that the specific needs of culturally diverse students and care recipients are identified and met.

The critical issues facing oncology nurse educators include how to recruit and retain additional students from various socioeconomic and cultural backgrounds and how to foster a teaching and learning environment

Table 65–3. STRATEGIES TO RECRUIT AND RETAIN OLDER STUDENTS

Assumption	Strategy

Adult learners see themselves as self-directing and responsible	Collegial relationships between students and faculty
	Self-directed and self-paced learning activities:
	    Computer-assisted instruction
	    Learning modules
	Preceptorships with clinical experts

Adult learners have a wealth of experience that serves as a resource for themselves and others	Diagnostic evaluation of student learning needs Seminar, peer teaching, volunteer activities, group activities
Adult learners are motivated to learn by what is perceived as applicable in their lives	Joint faculty-student practice Preceptor-student clinical experience Clinical objectives based on clinical nurse specialist role components
Adult learners focus on problem solving rather than abstract content	Joint faculty-student problem solving Research and teaching assistant roles for students

that is sensitive to the cognitive and affective needs of the respective social or cultural groups. The National League for Nursing (NLN) (National League for Nursing, 1977) published guidelines to address the recruitment and retention of high-risk disadvantaged and minority students. Strategies include increased financial assistance, access to supportive services, application of theoretic and practice concepts among populations from diverse cultural and economic backgrounds, employment of faculty of varied cultural backgrounds, and faculty development programs based on the needs of both students and clients from multicultural backgrounds (Louie, 1985).

Funding

Funding is and will continue to be an issue facing oncology nurse educators and students. Financial assistance for oncology nursing education has increased steadily since the passage of the National Cancer Act (1970). As oncology nursing was incorporated into graduate nursing programs, students became eligible for funding through the Division of Nursing and the National Cancer Institute Research Grants.

In addition to federal funding, private and professional organizations budgeted monies for oncology nursing education. In 1981 the ACS funded ten scholarships for master's students in oncology nursing. Based on the overwhelming number of applications received, the number of scholarships was increased to 20 in 1982. By 1990, a total of 219 master's students had been named as national ACS scholarship recipients. During the same time period, the ONS and the Oncology Nursing Foundation (ONF) established scholarships for undergraduate and graduate study.

As the number of oncology nurses enrolled in doctoral study increased, the ACS responded by establishing doctoral scholarships in oncology nursing in 1986. By 1990, 19 doctoral scholarships in oncology nursing had been awarded by the ACS. Funding for predoctoral and postdoctoral education in oncology nursing also has been allocated by the NCI.

However, even with the funding described, many students lack the necessary financial support. Selection criteria for many scholarships and grants-in-aid require full-time student status, thus limiting accessibility to funding for part-time students. Schools of nursing and service agencies have an opportunity to collaborate to identify funding sources for part-time students, especially those employed as registered nurses in health care agencies (Table 65–4).

Table 65–4. HEALTH CARE AGENCY STRATEGIES TO FUND NURSING EDUCATION

Courtesy scholarships
Educational loan programs
Tuition reimbursement
Flexible work hours
  Job sharing
  Baylor plan
  12-, 10-, and 8-hr workdays

CURRICULUM

Curriculum is influenced by characteristics of society and of the subject matter (Hunkins, 1980). Changes in oncology curricula can be attributed to the fact that oncology nursing education has been formulated within the context of rapid changes in the characteristics of the population served, in the treatment of cancer, in the system providing the care, and in the requirements of external accrediting and professional organizations.

Changes in Populations Served

Changes in the populations served focus on the extremes of the age spectrum. First, the young are surviving cancer at a much higher rate. Increased survival and extensive problems of survivorship have contributed to the increasing complexity of pediatric oncology. In addition, the percentage of aged in the United States population is increasing. The median age of cancer incidence is 65.4 years, and approximately 50 per cent of all cancers occur in the elderly (Weinrich & Nussbaum, 1984). Therefore, the needs of the elderly have been addressed as a subspecialty or as a content area in the curriculum by some educators.

The second change in the population served is the emphasis on human rights. The "Patient's Bill of Rights," introduced by the American Hospital Association in 1973, is representative of the impact of the human rights movement on health care. The hospice movement is another example of changes with respect to humanization in care (Corless, 1983). The combined influence of the expectation that observance of patient rights would contribute to more effective patient care and the commitment to patient, rather than physician advocacy, expressed in the revised *Code of Ethics for Nurses* (Davis, 1983), makes human rights an important content area in nursing curricula. Another impact on curriculum is the need to include content on bioethics. Informed consent, euthanasia, and the right to die are but a few of the recurring issues in oncology that involve biomedical ethics.

Changes in Cancer Treatment

Medical, scientific, and technologic advances in cancer treatment and supportive care have increased patient survival and influenced their quality of life (Hilkemeyer, 1985). These advances have, in turn, resulted in the crowding of undergraduate and graduate curricula or the lengthening of programs. Neither strategy is facilitative, because the former leads to high stress among students and the latter impedes doctoral study.

The complexity of cancer care has had other effects on oncology education. First, the demand for specialists has exceeded the capacity of traditional educational programs to meet the need (Craytor, 1985). A positive outcome of this situation has been the support of cancer nursing education and continued recommendations for federal support of graduate study, in particular, as evidenced by the Institute of Medicine Study (Institute of Medicine, Division of Health Care Services, 1983). A negative outcome has been the attempts by other professions to solve the nursing shortage, the most notable being the Registered Care Technician (RCT) proposal by the American Medical Association (AMA).

The number of oncology graduate programs listed in the *Oncology Nursing Forum* increased from 16 in 1981 to 42 in 1990. A negative outcome has been the tendency for schools of nursing to "get on the band-wagon," irrespective of the availability of qualified faculty to teach the specialty content. This tendency seemed particularly evident subsequent to the initiation of the ACS graduate scholarships in 1981. The number of programs listed in the *Oncology Nursing Forum* increased from ten to 33 between 1981 and 1983.

A study conducted by Yasko (1983) of 185 oncology clinical nurse specialists revealed extreme variability in master's level curricula. The majority of respondents reported a lack of theoretic content (69 per cent) or planned clinical experience in oncology (61 per cent). Planned contact with a clinical nurse specialist role model in the master's curriculum was reported by only 40 per cent, and 29 per cent of the sample reported having no content on the clinical nurse specialist role components.

Changes in Survival Patterns

In the 1930s, fewer than one in five people with cancer were alive 5 years after treatment, but currently one in three survives more than 5 years. This change in survival broadens the scope of cancer nursing to include both the acute and chronic phases of disease in hospitals, homes, outpatient clinics, and long-term facilities (Grant & Padilla, 1985). Teaching cancer as a chronic illness has required oncology nursing to become more family focused. The distribution of patients throughout the health continuum and the broadened focus of care have resulted in oncology specialties being developed within a range of educational tracks varying from critical care to community health.

Changes in the Health Care System

The hospice movement is a change in the system that has had an impact on oncology nursing education. The hospice movement is one that implies humanistic, self-determined care (McCabe, 1982). Nurses have provided leadership in hospice care and have gained immeasurably from the involvement. Symptom management strategies have been tested in the home in an environment of high independence and interdependence. These conditions have facilitated autonomy and accountability in nursing practice and have served to enlighten the public regarding the role of the nurse.

The impact of the recent trend of earlier discharge of patients with high acuity, initiated as a result of

prospective reimbursement (McCorkle & Germino, 1984), has not been fully realized in education at this time. Meeting the needs of high acuity patients in both the hospital and the home are issues that are of major concern in oncology care. Oncology nursing practices, such as consultative services to hospitals and home care agencies, have been developed to bridge the service gap. Meeting high acuity needs in the home may force educational programs to be more practitioner oriented. Both of these trends seem to be manifest in the role changes reported in the 1977 ONS membership survey and the 1990 ONS membership profile (Table 65–5).

Influence of Accrediting and Professional Organizations

The NLN accreditation, the ONS development of standards, and the Oncology Nursing Certification Corporation (ONCC) certification are three external influences that have had an impact on oncology nursing curriculum development. These organizations have provided resources to educators and established standards that protect consumers.

The NLN influences specialty education by requiring that the undergraduate program prepare generalists and the graduate program prepare specialists. The NLN criteria influence undergraduate education also by requiring the integration of research at this level. This requirement influences the success of the undergraduate who enters oncology nursing and needs the research background to understand treatment protocols and cooperative research studies.

At the graduate level, the NLN criteria require adequate clinical resources and faculty preparation for specialty tracks. One way that faculties have eluded this criterion to some degree is to identify oncology as a subspecialty within a medical-surgical or related track. Thus faculty members are required to be prepared at the generalist versus specialist level. The subspecialty track may be a means to recruit specialty students to programs that do not have faculty prepared in the specialty. Conversely, teaching oncology as a subspecialty of other tracks can be an efficient and effective strategy, if the goals are to broaden the base

Table 65–5. POSITION PROFILE OF ONS MEMBERS (1977/1990)

Position	ONS Membership Survey 1977 (n = 511)	ONS Membership Profile 1990 (n = 16,002)
Staff nurse	77 (15%)	7427 (45%)
Head nurse	51 (10%)	1749 (11%)
Clinician	44 (9%)	1140 (7%)
Nurse practitioner	0 (0%)	154 (1%)
Clinical nurse specialist	115 (23%)	1361 (8%)
Educator	35 (7%)	872 (6%)
Supervisor	21 (4%)	553 (3%)
Director	16 (3%)	732 (4%)
Researcher	20 (4%)	326 (2%)
Consultant	0 (0%)	126 (1%)
Other	132 (26%)	1394 (8%)

of preparation and to facilitate role socialization across subspecialty areas.

The NLN does not accredit doctoral programs in nursing; therefore, this level of education does not have the advantage of the peer review required at the undergraduate and master's levels. Some nurse educators lament this lack of standardization of doctoral programs and the resultant variability in quality. The assurance of quality of doctoral programs with a specialty in oncology is an unresolved issue among oncology nursing educators.

The majority of nurses caring for cancer patients are doing so because of the high incidence of the disease rather than because they chose oncology as a specialty. The quality of the fundamental and continuing education programs that prepare these nurses varies considerably. In 1982, the ONS developed the *Outcome Standards for Cancer Nursing Education—Fundamental Level* to address this problem. The document was designed to be used by educators in generic programs, instructors in continuing education programs, and individuals in assessing cancer nursing knowledge (Oncology Nursing Society, 1982).

Indirectly, the standards of practice developed jointly by the American Nurses' Association (ANA) and ONS for adult oncology nurses and by the ANA and Association of Pediatric Oncology Nurses (APON) for pediatric oncology nurses influence education. Graduates are expected to have the educational foundation to develop the level of expertise specified in the standards; therefore, educators in graduate programs are constrained to ensure achievement of the fundamental standards at the undergraduate level and preparation for certification at the graduate level.

Certification of oncology nurses was begun in 1986 by the ONCC. The *Core Curriculum for Oncology Nursing,* developed by a task force of the ONS Education Committee, serves as the basis for the examination. This text also serves as a reference for educators in determining the content of academic courses (Ziegfeld, 1987).

UNDERGRADUATE INFLUENCES

Impact of the Integrated Curriculum

The integrated undergraduate curriculum in nursing prompted nurse educators to reevaluate the meaning of nursing, delineate recurring themes in nursing, and develop new strategies to transmit nursing knowledge (Pennington, 1986). The impact of the integrated curriculum on specialty nursing is not known, but speculation has been rather extensive. By definition, integration appears to be the antithesis of specialization. Torres (1974, p. 2) defined integration as "blending the nursing content in such a way that the parts of specialties are no longer distinguishable."

On the other hand, the curriculum model that was replaced by the integrated curriculum was the medical model. The argument that the integrated curriculum had resulted in "integrating out" specialty content has been countered with the argument that the medical model "integrated out" nursing content (Torres, 1974).

The search for common concepts diminished the specialty content included in undergraduate programs. Traditionally, cancer nursing has been taught in a limited number of hours of didactic instruction within a medical-surgical rotation, and clinical experience with cancer patients may or may not have been planned concurrently. The integrated approach focused on broad concepts, applicable to many patient situations, thereby making the concurrent study of specialty content and clinical assignment less critical to learning. In addition, the focus on general versus specific knowledge provided the student a knowledge base that was not outdated quickly.

With all of the changes incurred with the integrated curriculum, oncology nursing content and experience in the undergraduate curriculum varied extensively across programs (Kruse, 1986). The prevalence of cancer is such that only the rare undergraduate student finishes a program without caring for a cancer patient. If specific knowledge does, in fact, counter negative attitudes, then the integrated curriculum allows little or no time to dispel the myths and negativism associated with cancer; therefore, recruitment to oncology practice may have been curtailed.

The national ONS issues a call for educational abstracts in conjunction with the annual ONS congress. Assuming that the topics addressed in these abstracts are a reflection of the issues in oncology education, the authors reviewed ONS educational abstract topics from 1982 to 1987 and found attitudes toward oncology to be a dominant concern. Strategies designed to lessen negative attitudes toward oncology mentioned in these abstracts include competency-based preceptorships to orient professional oncology nurses, work-study programs for senior baccalaureate students, multistate student nurse conferences, microcomputer clinical simulations, graduate nursing electives, nurse internships, and statewide comprehensive continuing education programs. The development of instruments to measure changes in attitude was addressed as well (Longman & Verran, 1987).

The question of effect of education on attitudes has been addressed directly among oncology educators. In one study, graduate students (Piper, Moore, & Dodd, 1985) demonstrated significant changes in cognitive scores with respect to cancer during graduate study but no significant changes in attitudes. Pessimism about cancer, in general, was found by Whelan (1984) in a study of American and British nurses. The pessimism toward cancer in general did not correspond with attitudes toward particular cancers. The researcher speculated that these differences may have been related to both cultural and educational differences among the two groups.

In contrast, Fanslow (1985) found more positive attitudes toward cancer and cancer therapies than expected. Studying a sample of 400 nurses, the mean attitude score was 3.66 on a Likert scale, which ranged from negative (1) to positive (5). Baccalaureate graduates had the highest attitude scores, followed by master's, associate degree, and diploma graduates, respectively; but these differences were not statistically significant. However, statistically significant differences were found between nurses' attitudes toward skills and oncology knowledge and beliefs. In this study, nurses were reported to have a positive attitude related to oncology-based knowledge, but a negative attitude toward cancer care.

Influence of Professional and Accrediting Organizations

Although disagreement persists among professional groups in terms of definition of the "nurse generalists" (Reed & Hoffman, 1986), consensus seems evident that undergraduate education prepares the generalist and that graduate education prepares the specialist. With the implementation of the 1978 NLN criterion that research should be a component of baccalaureate education, consensus has evolved as well regarding the teaching of research at both levels of education. The issues that result from these two areas of content specification are methods to standardize outcome objectives for each level and teaching strategies to achieve the objectives. The publication of the *Standards of Oncology Nursing Education: Generalist and Advanced Practice Levels* (Oncology Nursing Society, 1989) and the ACS-ONS *The Master's Degree with a Specialty in Oncology Nursing: Role Definition and Curriculum Guide* (American Cancer Society/Oncology Nursing Society, 1988) are evidence of professional commitment to standardization within the generalist and advanced levels. The need to determine effective teaching strategies in oncology nursing is evident in a review of ONS educational abstracts and the *Oncology Nursing Forum*. The oncology nursing literature was replete with evidence of innovative approaches to teaching oncology nursing. However, the issue of determining the "fit" between the level of content, the particular teaching strategy, and the achievement of outcome objectives was not addressed.

The concern for leveling of content in educational programs has been accompanied by a concern for appropriate recognition for the expertise of oncology nurses. The development of the oncology certification examination introduced another level of practice in oncology, namely, the registered nurse with oncology experience.

GRADUATE INFLUENCES

Two issues in oncology nursing are specific to graduate education: clinical specialization and expected outcome behaviors of the research component of the graduate program.

Clinical Specialization

The NLN (National League for Nursing, 1985) specified that the purpose of master's education is to prepare clinical specialists (advanced nurse practitioners), teachers, supervisors, and administrators whose special knowledge and skills are required to meet current and future nursing needs of the nation. One issue that has been debated in oncology is the level at which oncology specialization should be taught, that is, as an oncology specialty track or as a subspecialty of a broader tract. In a survey of graduate oncology programs (Piemme, 1985) 30 per cent (n = 30) indicated that the program was a specialty track, and the remainder described the program as a component of another nursing track.

Some oncology nurse educators advocate the oncology track; yet the 1979 NLN *Characteristics of Graduate Education in Nursing Leading to the Master's Degree* specified that areas of clinical study should reflect societal needs for nursing service and be sufficiently broad in scope to enable persons to prepare to serve in a variety of settings and locales (National League for Nursing, 1979). The dilemma was approached more definitively at the First National Invitational Conference on "The Oncology Nurse Specialist: Role Analysis and Future Projections" (Donoghue & Spross, 1985). The report of this meeting indicated less concern among educators regarding the placement of the major and more concern with the details of curriculum, faculty preparation, availability of preceptors, and role socialization within the program.

The issue of clinical specialization also raises the question of the validity of the clinical nurse specialist role components. The role components of the oncology clinical nurse specialist identified in the ACS-ONS *The Master's Degree with a Specialty in Oncology Nursing: Role Definition and Curriculum Guide* (1988) included teacher, clinician, researcher, consultant, and change agent. Expertise in each of these subroles is not feasible; therefore, the issue to be addressed is the relative importance of the subroles with respect to the individual oncology clinical nurse specialist and the goals of the employing agency. One oncology clinical nurse specialist (Welch-McCaffrey, 1986, p. 250) proposed that the role components of teacher, researcher, and consultant are "important vehicles in establishing competence and credibility" in practice. A modified Delphi survey of competencies of the oncology clinical nurse specialist as identified by oncology nurses, administrators, and educators indicated that the roles of consultant and direct care provider were ranked higher than the educator, manager, and researcher role components in terms of importance to successful functioning (McGee, Powell, Broadwell, & Clark, 1987).

The role of the clinical nurse specialist is to improve the quality of nursing care and to advance the profession of nursing, yet the discussion of the role components attests to the diffuse nature of the role. Further research is needed to minimize role ambiguity and role conflict (Edlund & Hodges, 1983; Starck, 1983).

Outcome Behaviors Related to Graduate Research

Nursing educators concur that the educational outcomes related to research at the baccalaureate level should be to prepare consumers of research. The outcome at the doctoral level differs with the clinical or research doctorates, but the independent researcher is a minimal expectation. The outcome at the master's level is less well delineated. The primary issue at the master's level is whether graduates should be independent researchers. The American Association of Colleges of Nursing (AACN) recommended teaching master's students the research knowledge and skills necessary to understand how investigative studies are conducted, to participate in research programs, and to begin to use research findings (Copp, Felton, & Hawken, 1981), but it stopped short of recommending that master's level research courses teach students to be independent researchers. The AACN position statement is compatible with the recommendations of the ANA's Commission on Nursing Research (Fontes, 1986).

In terms of teaching research, the other issue is whether to require completion of a thesis. Fontes (1986) proposed that the distinction between clinical problem solving and research may help make the distinction between master's and doctorally prepared nurse researchers. Proponents of the clinical problem-solving goal may require a clinical paper, rather than a thesis.

However, some oncology clinical nurse specialists propose that the primary mark of professionalism in practice is the development of a scientific rationale for nursing practice (Siehl, 1982). A review of the credentials of authors in the *Oncology Nursing Forum* and *Cancer Nursing* indicates that a relatively high percentage of these articles are authored by master's prepared nurses. Master's papers also constitute a large proportion of the papers presented at the annual ONS congresses. With the limited number of doctorally prepared nurses in the specialty, the nurse with a master's degree will probably continue to contribute significantly to the body of oncology knowledge through independent and joint research. The strategies to achieve these outcomes were the topic of discussion at the annual meeting of oncology nurse educators at the 1987 ONS congress. Strategies varied from the thesis requirement to clinical papers to simulations.

CURRICULUM IMPLEMENTATION

Multistrategy Approaches

Historically, the education of nurses in general and oncology nurses in particular has occurred using traditional medical model strategies, including lecture, case studies, clinical rounds, and seminars. As the diversity of doctorates among nursing faculty has increased, teaching methodologies have been expanded.

Modules

A module is a self-directed learning package that has a single topic or concept focus and limited, but well-developed, learning objectives. In the 1970s faculty from M.D. Anderson Hospital developed a series of self-paced learning modules on the psychosocial and rehabilitative aspects of cancer care. The ACS also developed learning objectives, content outlines, teaching strategies, and evaluation techniques for site-specific cancers to be used in both undergraduate and continuing education nursing programs.

Nursing journals, such as the *American Journal of Nursing* and *Cancer Nursing*, published learning modules on cancer nursing updates, chemotherapy, radiation therapy, immunology, and immunotherapy during the late 1970s and early 1980s. In addition, Yasko was instrumental in the development of a series of modules on nutrition, treatment modalities of radiation therapy and chemotherapy, and management of side effects of radiation therapy and chemotherapy (Brager & Yasko, 1984; Donoghue, Nunnally, & Yasko, 1982; Yasko, 1982).

Case Studies and Clinical Rounds

The case study method has been a viable strategy for teaching the interdisciplinary approach to the management of clients with cancer and their families. Student team members have an opportunity to develop collegial relationships with other professionals and to examine how each discipline contributes to cancer care. Similar collaborative experiences have been developed within the context of clinical rounds (Itano, Gwern, Oki, & Noboru, 1983).

Simulations

Simulations in health education serve to provide the student opportunities to interact in clinical situations that are not commonly found in clinical practice or that require advanced expertise, yet ensure patient safety. The use of simulations in nursing education has increased as attention has focused on evaluating higher-level cognitive, psychomotor, and affective competencies.

Kramer (1984) described the development of a microcomputer clinical simulation to allow students to synthesize and apply theoretically based knowledge to a case study of a pediatric patient with leukemia. Preliminary evaluation indicated that the program was a time and cost-effective teaching strategy.

Media

The use of media in oncology, including pamphlets, books, photographs, posters, audiotapes, slides, sound and slide programs, 16-mm movies, video tapes, and video discs to convey concepts, situations, and procedures amenable to a lecture or discussion format has increased. The ACS was instrumental in the development of media for cancer nursing education. Early media were focused on the detection and treatment of site-specific cancers. As early as 1950, *A Cancer Source Book for Nurses* (American Cancer Society, 1981) was published by the ACS and was reported to be the most frequently used cancer text in undergraduate schools of nursing (Brown, Johnson, & Groenwald, 1983). The expansion of media focused on oncology nursing care and roles was supported by the ACS, individual schools of nursing, the NCI, M.D. Anderson Hospital, Memorial-Sloan Kettering, and St. Jude's Children's Hospital. Media interviews with children, adults, families, and health care professionals provided insights into the psychosocial aspects of patient and family coping. The proliferation of printed materials from the NCI during the 1980s provided additional site-specific and issue-specific information for both undergraduate and graduate nursing programs. In addition, the ONS provides a forum for sharing both written and audiovisual educational materials at the annual congresses.

In spite of the proliferation of written and audiovisual materials for undergraduate and graduate nursing education, limited systematic evaluation of content, technical quality, and effectiveness of oncology media in meeting specific learning objectives has occurred. Critique of content, appropriate audience, and technical quality of selected written and audiovisual materials related to oncology care may be found in oncology nursing publications, such as the reviews section of the *Oncology Nursing Forum* and *Cancer Nursing*. An additional concern related to oncology media is the rapidity with which content and practice change, which necessitates the development of formats that can be revised easily.

Computer-Assisted Instruction

The introduction of computer technology has resulted in the "information revolution." Through the use of computers, knowledge development and dissemination have increased. Computers have been identified as the single most important development affecting the teaching and learning process today (Brose, 1984).

In spite of the purported advantages of using computer instruction in nursing and the increasing use of computer technology in the health care system, limited integration in the traditional nursing curricula has occurred because of three factors: lack of computer resources in education and service settings, lack of computer literacy among nurses, and lack of knowledge of health care among computer specialists (Ziemer, 1984).

Even faculty members who are prepared to integrate computer technology find limited software programs available to meet specific objectives in nursing. Ziemer (1984) cited several factors that contribute to the lack of nursing-specific software: (1) insufficient computer expertise among nursing experts, (2) high cost of development, (3) lack of incentives related to promotion or tenure for development of course materials, (4) lack of distribution sources, and (5) incompatibility among computers.

In recent years, suppliers of oncology drugs and equipment have developed software programs for oncology nurses. Topics focus on diagnosis and treatment of selected site-specific cancers, effects of cancer on nutrition, and handling antineoplastic agents. However, these programs have not been widely distributed within schools of nursing or health care agencies.

Strategies to increase the number of computer-assisted learning programs available specifically related to oncology nursing are to create a demand for such programs from nursing education and service and to provide nurse experts as content specialists. Another source of collaborative efforts for software development in nursing is the private sector. In the Southeast, the Health Sciences Consortium offers design and technical assistance to faculty in the development of clinical nursing simulations. Relying on faculty for content, this group will provide critique of proposals for software development.

Independent Study

Historically, independent study was the learning strategy used by many nurses in practice and education to gain knowledge, skills, and attitudes required in oncology nursing. Articles in the literature and abstracts from the ONS annual congresses attest to creative learning plans designed by nurses in oncology. For students in graduate programs, the independent study option allows students in other clinical majors an opportunity to focus on the special needs of clients and families facing cancer. Cancer nursing concepts are germain to many clinical specialties, including pediatrics, gerontology, rehabilitation, and critical care. For students in undergraduate programs, the independent study option allows similar exploration of concepts of care, research, or career paths available in oncology nursing.

Role Practicum

Throughout the history of nursing education, clinical practicum and internships have been popular teaching strategies for role socialization. The integration of a role practicum experience within undergraduate curricula gained support in the 1970s as a method to augment clinical experience. The closing of diploma schools of nursing and the limited clinical time allotted in baccalaureate programs forced educators to evaluate strategies to teach clinical competencies needed by novice nurses. Thus the role practicum gained popularity as a method for developing clinical skills and decreasing reality shock.

Role practicum has had a positive effect on the number of students choosing oncology nursing as a career. Through the practicum experience, students evaluate the demands, responsibilities, and satisfactions of caring for patients and families facing cancer. Exposure to oncology nursing while still in the protected environment of the educational program may decrease anxiety about working with cancer patients and form the basis for socialization into oncology nursing. Because many students choose to remain in the agency and specialty area of the role practicum experience, agencies frequently request students for practicum experiences as a recruiting strategy.

In summary, the teaching methods of oncology nursing education today are a kaleidoscope of time-proven methods of the past and technologies of the future. Educators of the future, particularly in service professions, must incorporate technologies that enhance the science of the profession yet preserve the humanistic component of the profession.

CURRICULUM EVALUATION

In times of increased accountability in nursing, evaluation of nursing education programs has become a key issue facing nursing educators in the 1990s. Unfortunately, many nursing program evaluations have focused on components of the programs, such as achievement of objectives, curriculum content, or clinical experiences, more than on the program as a whole. Factors that have contributed to inadequate evaluation include lack of consistent evaluation criteria; lack of operational definitions of knowledge, skills, attitudes, and human traits necessary to perform at the generalist or specialist level; lack of valid, reliable, and practical measurement instruments; and lack of consensus on desired outcomes of undergraduate and graduate nursing education. In addition, variability in prerequisites, length of programs, curricula, and terminal objectives in nursing programs at undergraduate and graduate levels have made evaluation across programs virtually impossible.

Using a systems approach, various evaluation models are available to guide program evaluation (Stake, 1967; Stufflebeam et al., 1971; Waltz & McGurn, 1983). In addition, the NLN provides guidance through publication of characteristics of baccalaureate and graduate education in nursing and program evaluation monographs.

To evaluate oncology nursing content at the undergraduate level, Brown, Johnson, and Groenwald (1983) conducted a mail survey of 982 diploma, associate degree, and baccalaureate degree schools of nursing accredited by the NLN. Responses were received from 672 schools (68 per cent) from 48 states. The most frequent amount of time spent on oncology nursing content in the curriculum was 14.5 hours. The majority of that time was spent on the pathophysiology of cancer, and the least amount was devoted to cancer nursing practice. Schools most commonly used general medical-surgical and pediatric textbooks for oncology nursing content. Only 18 per cent of schools used *A Cancer Source Book for Nurses* published by the ACS. Only 41 per cent of the faculty reported graduate preparation in oncology nursing. Most of those faculty were in baccalaureate programs.

Evaluation of oncology nursing programs at the graduate level is somewhat easier than at the undergraduate level, because the ONS, the APON, and the ACS have developed education standards at the generalist and advanced practice levels, core curriculum for oncology nursing, standards of practice, outcome standards of care, and curriculum guidelines for master's education in oncology to assist faculty in oncology nursing program development and evaluation. How-

ever, the extent to which these guidelines are implemented varies.

A final issue in evaluation of oncology programs in general is the lack of valid, reliable, and practical instruments. Education abstracts appearing in recent *Proceedings of the Oncology Nursing Society Congress* describe instrument development to evaluate oncology content in an undergraduate program (Longman & Verran, 1987) and to evaluate changes in knowledge, skills, and attitudes of students enrolled in a postmaster's fellowship program in oncology nursing education (Holcombe, Henderson, & Jackson, 1984). In addition, Piper, Moore, and Dodd (1984) reported the use of the ONS conceptual framework and *Outcome Standards for Oncology Nursing Education: Fundamental Level* as the basis to develop, test, and revise curriculum evaluation instruments and the program of study in oncology nursing at the graduate level. Presentations and publications related to evaluation and instrument development contribute to a more systematic and standardized evaluation.

FUTURE OF ONCOLOGY NURSING EDUCATION

Why would one speculate on the future of a field of specialty education, when Naisbitt (1982) in *Megatrends* declared that 5 years after a specialist graduates, 40 per cent of the acquired knowledge and 50 per cent of the technical equipment used is obsolete? The "why" is answered by the fact that a failure to speculate precludes the possibility of planned change.

Recruitment to Oncology

The nursing shortage highlights the concern regarding adequate recruitment to a field of care that is known to evoke fear and pessimism. This concern is compounded by the public fear of acquired immune deficiency syndrome (AIDS) and the increasing link of AIDS and oncology. Recruitment can be enhanced by oncology nurses capitalizing on opportunities to speak on talk shows, publish in lay magazines, or consult with program producers to ensure that the positive aspects of oncology nursing are communicated. Without a sweeping change in societal values that results in compensation of service professionals commensurate with educational preparation and professional responsibility, academic counselors will continue to hesitate to advise males and highly successful females to enter nursing. Therefore, oncology nurses must be the primary recruiters to the specialty profession.

Strategies to limit attrition must have a high priority as well. Research is needed to determine the characteristics of dropouts versus graduates. Studies of personality characteristics of nurses of the 1980s (Hafer & Ambrose, 1983; Little & Brain, 1982), if replicated, could serve as a basis for career counseling to find the most suitable role for the respective nurse.

Scientific and Technologic Advances: Impact on Curriculum

The United States Department of Health and Human Services (1981) defined emerging technologies as ones under development that appear likely to be used in practice within 5 years. The categories of technologies described by McCormick (1983) should be considered in oncology nursing education. Endorphins, infusion pumps, hyperthermia, and other technologies listed are not foreign to most oncology nurses. Does this mean that oncology nurses are on the "cutting edge," and, if so, what are the technologies and sciences of the future needed to retain this edge?

Monitoring the science courses taught traditionally in nursing will ensure that the courses are adequate for a nursing model and for what is now known about cancer. Educators must consider the need for knowledge of physics to understand monitoring devices, the use of principles of genetics for risk appraisal, and the application of principles of logic in decision analysis models for planning cancer prevention and control programs. The answer is not to lengthen the curriculum, but to give up the "sacred cow" content and to be responsive to a changing health care environment.

Focus or Direction of Knowledge

McCormick (1983) noted the change in focus from the cell to society. In oncology, the direction is more likely to be the application of knowledge at the cellular and subcellular level to meet societal needs as effectively as possible within the constraints of societal resources and values. Again the task is to question tradition and to heed the admonishments of innovative thinkers, such as Benner (1984), who contends that the essence of nursing can be revealed in the study of clinical nursing practice. If nurses can extrapolate the "excellence and power" Benner described as imbedded in practice, then the future can be anticipated with greater assurance and nurses can make a contribution to issues that will affect cancer morbidity and mortality in the future, such as nuclear accidents, chemical warfare, or potential hazards of space travel, while continuing to address the present day problems of oncology care.

Professional Conditions and Controls

Control implies insight and motivation to act. The ONS, APON, ANA, and ACS have worked jointly to provide the documents and standards to assist nursing leaders to control the quality of oncology nursing education and practice. The oncology literature reflects some potential changes in oncology specialization that may follow from the changes discussed previously. For example, the high technology of treatment may result in more nurses entering treatment-related specialization tracks, such as radiation oncology or biologic response modifier therapy. The problems of intense treatment protocols and long-term survivorship may result in a critical care oncology specialization. Other options may be symptom-related specialists, such as in pain control or skin care. The professional responsibility is to prevent a proliferation of specialization without long-term planning. Oncology as a specialty may not be appropriate in the foreseeable future. After all, this designation of specialization focuses on the disease rather than on the response to or risk of the disease.

SUMMARY

Oncology nursing education has a rich history, and the events of the past have provided a strong basis for the present. The ONS has been commended for launching an extensive strategic planning program while at a pinnacle of functioning, rather than waiting for a crisis to initiate proactive planning. Oncology educators have the same opportunity. Unresolved issues merit attention, and the realm of possible educational strategies deserve the imagination of all nurses involved in cancer care.

References

American Cancer Society. (1986, June). *Special report on cancer in the economically disadvantaged*. New York: Author.

American Cancer Society. (1981). *A cancer source book for nurses*. New York: Author.

American Cancer Society/Oncology Nursing Society. (1988). *The masters' degree with a specialty in oncology nursing: Role definition and curriculum guide*. New York: Author.

Benner, P. E. (1984). *Novice to expert: Excellence and power in clinical nursing practice*. Menlow Park, CA: Addison-Wesley Publishing Co.

Benoliel, J. Q. (1983). The historical development of cancer nursing research in the United States. *Cancer Nursing, 6*, 261–268.

Brager, B. L., & Yasko, J. M. (1984). *Care of the client receiving chemotherapy: A self-learning module for the nurse caring for the client with cancer*. Reston, VA: Reston Publishing Co.

Brose, C. H. (1984). Computer technology in nursing: Revolution or renaissance. *Nursing and Health Care, 5*, 531–534.

Brown, J. K., Johnson, J. L., & Groenwald, S. L. (1983). Survey of cancer nursing in U.S. schools of nursing. *Oncology Nursing Forum, 10*(4), 82–83.

Copp, L., Felton, G., & Hawken, P. (1981). *Position on nursing research* (draft 4). American Association of Colleges of Nursing, Washington, DC.

Corless, I. B. (1983). Models of hospice care. In N. Chaska (Ed.), *The nursing profession: A time to speak* (pp. 540–550). New York: McGraw-Hill Book Co.

Craytor, J. K. (1985). Highlights in education for cancer nursing. *Oncology Nursing Forum, 12* (1, Suppl.), 19–27.

Davis, A. (1983). Ethics and nursing administration. In N. Chaska (Ed.), *The nursing profession: A time to speak* (pp. 650–658). New York: McGraw-Hill Book Co.

Donoghue, M., Nunnally, C., & Yasko, J. M. (1982). *Nutritional aspects of cancer care: A self-learning module for the nurse caring for the client with cancer*. Reston, VA: Reston Publishing Co.

Donoghue, M., & Spross, J. A. (1985). A report from the First National Invitational Conference. The oncology nurse specialist: Role analysis and future projections. *Oncology Nursing Forum, 12*(2), 35–36.

Edlund, B., & Hodges, L. (1983). Preparing and using the clinical nurse specialist. *Nursing Clinics of North America, 18*, 499–507.

Fanslow, J. (1985). Attitudes of nurses toward cancer and cancer therapies. *Oncology Nursing Forum, 12*(1), 43–47.

Fontes, H. (1986). Stratifying research curricula—the logical next step. *Nursing and Health Care, 7*, 259–262.

Grant, M. M., & Padilla, G. U. (1985). An overview of cancer nursing research. *Oncology Nursing Forum, 12*(1, Suppl.), 28–39.

Hafer, J. C., & Ambrose, D. M. (1983). Psychographic analysis of nursing students: Implications for the marketing and development of the nursing profession. *Health Care Management Review, 8*(3), 69–76.

Hilkemeyer, R. (1985). A historical perspective. *Oncology Nursing Forum, 12*(1, Suppl.), 6–15.

Hinds, P. (1989). Survey of graduate programs in cancer nursing. *Oncology Nursing Forum, 16*, 881–887.

Holcombe, J. K., Henderson, B. R., & Jackson, J. (1984). Development of program evaluation instruments for the post-masters' fellowship program in oncology nursing education. Proceedings of the 9th Annual Congress. *Oncology Nursing Forum, 11*(2), 115. (Abstract)

Hunkins, F. P. (1980). *Curriculum development: Program improvement*. Columbus, OH: Charles E. Merrill Publishing Co.

Institute of Medicine, Division of Health Care Services. (1983). *Nursing and nursing education: Public policies and private actions*. Washington, DC: National Academy Press.

Itano, J. K., Gwern, S. F., Oki, B., & Noboru, O. (1983). Interdisciplinary oncology student health teams. Proceedings of the 8th Annual Congress. *Oncology Nursing Forum, 10*(2), 48. (Abstract)

Kramer, R. (1984). Microcomputer clinical simulations: New developments in oncology nursing education. Proceedings of the 9th Annual Congress, *Oncology Nursing Forum, 11*(2), 85. (Abstract)

Kruse, L. C. (1986). Undergraduate cancer nursing education. In R. McCorkle & G. Hongladaron (Eds.), *Issues and topics in cancer nursing* (pp. 65–75). Norwalk, CT: Appleton-Century-Crofts.

Little, M., & Brain, S. (1982). The challengers, interactors, and mainstreamers: Second step education and nursing roles. *Nursing Research, 31*, 239–245.

Longman, A., & Verran, J. A. (1987). Testing oncology nursing content in an undergraduate program. Proceedings from the 12th Annual Congress. *Oncology Nursing Forum, 14*(2), 125.

Louie, K. (1985). Transcending cultural bias: The literature speaks. *Topics in Clinical Nursing, 7*(3), 78–84.

Mast, M. E., & Van Atta, M. J. (1986). Applying adult learning principles in instructional module design. *Nurse Educator, 11*(1), 35–39.

McCabe, S. (1982). An overview of hospice care. *Cancer Nursing, 5*, 103–108.

McCorkle, R., & Germino, B. M. (1984). What makes nurses need to know about home care. *Oncology Nursing Forum, 11*(6), 63–69.

McCormick, K. A. (1983). Preparing nurses for the technological future. *Nursing and Health Care, 4*, 379–382.

McGee, R. F., Powell, M. L., Broadwell, D., & Clark, J. (1987). A Delphi survey of oncology clinical nurse specialist competencies. *Oncology Nursing Forum, 14*(2), 29–33.

Miller, S., & Herbst, S. (1978). Summary of the ONS membership survey. *Oncology Nursing Forum, 5*(3), 22–23.

Naisbitt, J. (1982). *Megatrends: Ten new directions transforming our lives*. New York: Warner Books.

National League for Nursing. (1977). *Cultural dimensions in the baccalaureate nursing curriculum* (NLN Pub. No. 15–1662). New York: Author.

National League for Nursing. (1979). *Characteristics of graduate education in nursing leading to the master's degree* (NLN Pub. No. 15–1759). New York: Author.

National League for Nursing. (1985). *Master's education in nursing: Route to opportunities in contemporary nursing* (NLN Pub. No. 15–1312). New York: Author.

Norris, C. M. (1985). The PhD in nursing program: A five year projection. *Nurse Educator, 10*(2), 6–11.

Oncology Nursing Society. (1982). *Outcome standards for cancer nursing education: Fundamental level*. Pittsburgh: Author.

Oncology Nursing Society. (1989). *Standards of oncology nursing education: Generalist and advanced practice levels*. Pittsburgh: Author.

Pennington, E. A. (1986). The integrated curriculum: A 15-year perspective. In E. A. Pennington (Ed.), *Curriculum revisited: An update of curriculum design* (NLN Pub. No. 15–2165) (pp. 37–38). New York: National League for Nursing.

Piemme, J. A. (1985). Oncology clinical nurse specialist education. *Oncology Nursing Forum, 12*(2), 45–48.

Piper, B. F., Moore, I. M., & Dodd, M. J. (1984). Using the O.N.S. conceptual framework for graduate curriculum development and evaluation. Proceedings of the 9th Annual Congress. *Oncology Nursing Forum, 11*(2), 113. (Abstract)

Piper, B. F., Moore, I. M., & Dodd, M. (1985). Changes in cancer-related knowledge and attitudes: One graduate curriculum's experience. *Cancer Nursing, 8*, 272–277.

Reed, S., & Hoffman, S. E. (1986). The enigma of graduate education: Advanced generalist? Specialist? *Nursing and Health Care, 7*, 43–49.

Siehl, S. (1982). The clinical nurse specialist in oncology. *Nursing Clinics of North America, 17*, 753–761.

Stake, R. E. (Ed). (1967). Curriculum evaluation. *AERA Monograph Series on Evaluation* (No. 1). Chicago: Rand McNally.

Starck, P. (1983). Factors influencing the role of the oncology clinical nurse specialist. *Oncology Nursing Forum, 10*(4), 54–59.

Stufflebeam, D. L., Foley, W. J., Gephart, W. J., Guba, E. G., Hammond, R. L., Merriman, H. O., & Drovus, M. M. (1971). *Educational evaluation and decision-making*. Itasca, IL: Peacock Publishers.

Torres, G. (1974). Educational trends in the integrated curriculum approach in nursing. In National League for Nursing. Faculty-curriculum development: Unifying the curriculum—the integrated approach (Part 4) (NLN Pub. No. 15–1522) (pp. 1–6). New York: National League for Nursing.

U.S. Department of Health and Human Services, Office of Health Research, Statistics and Technology. (1981, August). *1980–1981 list of emerging health care technologies*. Washington, DC: The National Center for Health Care Technology.

Waltz, C. F., & McGurn, W. C. (1983). An approach to the assessment of programs in nursing education. *Nursing and Health Care, 4*, 576–582.

Weinrich, S. P., & Nussbaum, J. (1984). Cancer in the elderly: Early detection. *Cancer Nursing, 7*, 475–482.

Welch-McCaffrey, D. (1986). Role performance issues for oncology nurse specialists. *Cancer Nursing, 9*, 287–294.

Werley, H., & Newcomb, B. J. (1983). The research mentor: A missing element in nursing? In N. Chaska (Ed.), *The nursing profession: A time to speak* (pp. 202–215). New York: McGraw-Hill Book Co.

Whelan, J. (1984). Oncology nurses' attitudes toward cancer treatment and survival. *Cancer Nursing, 7*, 375–383.

Yasko, J. M. (1982). *Care of the client receiving external radiation therapy: A self-learning module for the nurse caring for the client with cancer*. Reston, VA: Reston Publishing.

Yasko, J. M. (1983). A survey of oncology nurse specialists. *Oncology Nursing Forum, 10*(1), 25–30.

Ziegfeld, C. R. (1987). Preface. In C. R. Ziegfeld (Ed.), *Core curriculum for oncology nursing*. Philadelphia: W. B. Saunders Co.

Ziemer, M. M. (1984). Issues of computer literacy in nursing education. *Nursing and Health Care, 5*, 537–542.

CHAPTER 66

Marketing Cancer Nursing

DOROTHY J. DEL BUENO

DEVELOPING THE IDEA
MARKET RESEARCH
    Needs, Wants, and Demands
    Market Populations
    Forecasting
SELLING STRATEGIES

Identifying Benefits
Advertising and Publicity
CREDIBILITY AND PACKAGING
Pricing Tactics
SUMMARY

Until recently nurses rarely talked about marketing their services. If they thought about marketing at all, the perception was that marketing was something commercial, possibly even suspect, and done only by *Fortune* 500 companies or advertising agencies. One explanation for nurses' lack of interest in marketing is that in the past nursing schools, hospitals, and ambulatory services had easy access to customers and resources. Changes in reimbursement, tax laws, capitation, and consumer awareness have created a more competitive environment in which the business of nursing education and practice is conducted. Cancer nursing, like any commodity or product, must now compete with both similar and different services for limited customers and resources. Schools offering a cancer nursing curriculum for graduate students, acute care facilities wishing to expand inpatient clinical facilities, or individual nurses offering home-based hospice services all need more than honest intentions and a good idea to attract, capture, and keep the customers and resources needed for business success.

Successful businesses and individuals develop and implement a marketing plan. This plan may be formal and complex or informal and simple. In either case the plan—a constellation of activities intended to achieve a specific purpose—includes the following components: market research, goals and objectives, advertising and publicity, selling strategies, pricing tactics, and financing.

DEVELOPING THE IDEA

Every successful business venture begins with an idea or concept for a new commodity or product, for a different way of doing business, or for an expansion of current services. A good idea is one that both works and is worth the time, energy, and commitment needed to make it successful. To evaluate the worthiness of a new or different idea, the following questions need to be answered.

What Exactly Will Be Offered or Sold? For instance,

several community health nurses with extensive experience coordinating cancer care for patients and families decide they want to launch a teaching-consulting business. These nurses believe they can improve the quality of care and satisfaction of homebound cancer patients if they provide opportunities for families, patients, and physicians to learn current techniques of pain management. Is their new business an interpersonal consultation service, a product such as education materials, a hands-on direct patient service, all of these, a combination of these, or none of the above? Ideally any new business idea should be both sufficiently specific to target market research activities and sufficiently ambiguous to allow revision, adaptation, or modification after analysis of research data.

Is the Idea Simple Enough or Clear Enough for Others to Understand? Nurses have a proclivity to make the simple complex and to use jargon to express themselves. If venture success depends on nonnurses or lay persons, the idea must be described in everyday language. The idea must be practical and compatible with buyers' or users' values and attitudes. If the idea is too exotic, bizarre, or incompatible with ordinary life styles, needs, wants, or demands, it will have a limited market appeal.

Will the Idea Work? It must be both feasible and timely. The potential customer must be able and willing to pay for it. In 1978, I offered workshops to nurses on persuasion and selling strategies. These workshops were only marginally successful. Nurses were not receptive to these ideas then, because the competitive environment had not yet become a reality in health care. Similar workshops now attract nurses from both education and service settings.

MARKET RESEARCH

After the idea is conceived and formulated, market research is done to answer questions and validate hunches or hypotheses related to who will buy, for what reason, at what price, when, how often, and for how long. These questions need to be answered before, during, and after launching the idea. Markets, buyers, and the conditions in which buying is done can change rapidly, particularly when technology and scientific research affect the way health care is both perceived and practiced. Nurses have begun to recognize, as have others in health care administration, that the use of marketing concepts can provide a sound basis for planning future directions (Adams, Hockema, & Ware, 1988).

Needs, Wants, and Demands

Nurses are educated to believe that they are prepared to meet patient or family needs, which are defined as gaps or deficiency between what is and what could or should be. Common examples are the need a person has for relief when in pain or the need of a mother, newly diagnosed with cancer, for education when she is ignorant about how to both take care of her family and conserve her own energy.

It is important to explore the factors that motivate customer behavior because, unfortunately, individuals may not want what they need, or they may not perceive the need and its fulfillment as a priority. Wants are defined as those services, products, or opportunities that individuals desire or yearn for, put on their wish list, or fantasize about. Unfortunately, wants are sometimes incompatible with needs, good health, long life, or the good of society. There is no guarantee that individuals will do what it takes to achieve, acquire, or possess what they want or what they need. More often people only fantasize, dream about, or continue to want. For example, smokers at risk for lung cancer want the satisfaction or release offered by the cigarette, even if it causes disease or death, more than they want to reduce the risk by stopping smoking.

Demands are those needs or wants that individuals *are* willing to do anything to acquire or meet regardless of expense or risk. The microwave oven is an example of a want converted to a demand. People do not *need* microwave ovens because food can be cooked by other means, yet housewives and working people buy them because they perceive the needs for convenience and timesaving a priority for which they are willing to pay. Demands are not fixed or the same for everyone.

Chaney (1986) describes several demand states. *No demand* exists when a potential market shows no interest or is indifferent. *Negative demand* exists when potential customers dislike the service or product so much that they ignore it, delay using it, or pay a price to avoid it. Seat belts and proctoscopies are examples of a negative demand. *Under demand* exists when a previously popular service or product loses its appeal. *Over demand* exists when there are more buyers for the product or service than can be accommodated. This last condition sounds highly desirable but can be undesirable if it results in frustrated customers who turn to other providers to satisfy their demands.

Some marketing experts believe demands can be created; through advertising or selling strategies, individuals or groups can be persuaded or motivated to convert a need or want into a demand. Two market research approaches are used relative to demand: mirror marketing and window marketing. Mirror marketing determines the extent of an already defined demand, such as how great the demand is for aspirin-free analgesics. Window marketing determines what demands exist currently that have not been satisfied yet or even defined; for example, is there a demand for a home Papanicolaou test that would be easy to use? Or, using the previous hypothetic situation of the nurses who wanted to start a teaching-consulting pain management business, one market research activity would be to use a physician-focus group to gather data on their acceptance and interest in printed materials and individual consultation on pain management. Conversely, the nurses could use a questionnaire and telephone survey to query patients with cancer and their families about their greatest concerns related to pain. A group of nurse practitioners used this approach to determine the market for their services (Shamansky, Schilling, & Holbrook, 1985) (Box 66–1). The survey approach, intended to identify needs, wants, or demands, is a window approach, whereas contacting the physician-focus group is compatible with mirror marketing. Whichever market research approach is used, nurses cannot presume to know clients' needs, wants, or demands. It is naive and foolish to proceed on what nurses think people will buy or use without validation or clarification of those assumptions.

Market Populations

Who will buy? A potential market includes every individual, group, or organization that could possibly use the service, product, or idea. The actual market is composed of those highly likely to become buyers or users. Accurate determination of the actual market is the goal of market research. Within the actual market are segments or portions that include both present customers and individuals most likely to become customers. A variety of theories, techniques, and strategies are used to determine market segments in nursing (Andreoli, Carollo, & Poltage, 1988; Auttonberry, 1988; Freitag, 1988; Johnson et al., 1987; Stanton & Stanton, 1988). Generally market research collects data about the demographics of both one-time buyers and repeaters: age, income, gender, geographic location, marital status, ethnicity, and religious affiliation of the buyers. It is more difficult, of course, to predict future buyers or who might be motivated to become repeat buyers.

One market approach attempts to determine the values of buyers and life styles, commonly referred to as VALS ("Use Demographics Include," 1985). Potential customers have been segmented into eight VALS categories. Belongers, who account for 33 per cent of the population, are outer-directed individuals who have stable traditional values. Achievers, also outer-directed, are materialistic, usually middle-aged, and make up 25 per cent of the population. Emulators, or

---

Box 66–1. DETERMINING THE MARKET FOR NURSE PRACTITIONER SERVICE

To market new products effectively, the needs of consumers must be understood, and the factors influencing purchase decisions must be identified. To determine the market for nurse practitioner services in New Haven, Connecticut, a study was undertaken examining factors associated with the intent to use nurse practitioner services. Using a descriptive, cross-sectional design, 600 names of individuals were drawn from telephone directories. Because Connecticut has a high rate of telephone coverage for its residents (98 per cent), the telephone was viewed as an appropriate mode for data collection. Letters explaining the study were sent to potential respondents 1 week before telephone contact. The interviews required between 15 and 20 min to complete. Each phone number was called up to three times at different hours to maximize contact. A 55 per cent response rate was achieved. The 71-item survey investigated the significance of selected socioeconomic, attitudinal, cognitive, and health care use characteristics known to influence choices consumers make about provider and service. Results indicate that 62 per cent of study respondents would use nurse practitioner services. Dissatisfaction with present health care services, family size, and age were statistically the best predicators of respondents' intent to use practitioner services. Respondents demonstrated concern about the issues of availability and cost of care. They indicated they would seek nurse practitioner care if it were covered by insurance and cost less than physician care. Although the study has limitations in its reliance on participants with telephones and no follow-up of nonrespondents, the study is a good example of one form of a marketing needs assessment. Although the *intent to use* practitioner services rather than *actual use* was measured, those factors influencing the intent were identified (Shamansky et al., 1985).

---

ambitious newcomers, make up 10 per cent of a market population. The remaining 32 per cent of the population are distributed among the inner-directed, socially conscious do-gooders (9 per cent) and experimenters (7 per cent), the need-driven sustainers who are resentful about not making it (7 per cent), the impulsive narcissists (5 per cent), and the poor, hopeless need-driven survivors (4 per cent). According to VALS theorists, internal values dictate overt buying behavior. Determination of these values is done by focus groups, surveys, questionnaires, and other data collection methodologies.

Predicting buying behavior even with reliable data is difficult because of the irrational nature of human behavior. People do not always act from logic or in congruence with their values. Many services and products have been enormously successful, at least for a brief time, because of their illogical appeal: pet rocks, the Hollywood diet, eyeline tattooing, video arcades, and the hula hoop. These fads, although short lived, were extremely popular and made large profits for their creators and providers. It is not always easy to determine whether a product or service will be a momentary fad or a long-lasting trend. The latter continue to sell because of both appeal and practical utility.

Forecasting

The purpose of collecting either demographic or lifestyle data is to predict or forecast the extent to which the market can be penetrated. For example, will the nurses who intend to develop a pain management service be able to capture 10, 20, or 50 per cent of the market of identified physicians, patients with cancer, or families of these patients? Forecasting, like any other prediction, is fraught with risk. The database on which the forecast is made may be faulty, conditions and environments can change, or other competing providers can enter a market suddenly.

Rarely is an idea, concept, or product so unique or

unusual that it is totally new. Most innovative products and services are variations on a theme or reconfigurations of previous concepts. For example, primary nursing is a variation on the case management method used by social workers, public health, and private duty nurses. Thus in most cases, the innovation must replace, substitute, or supplement an already existing product or service and is, therefore, in competition with it. Even a truly unique product or service that becomes successful will ultimately become the competitive target of other imitative products and services.

To compete successfully it is necessary to know who and how strong the competition is and what market niche it serves (Gardner & Weinrauch, 1988). For example, an oncology nurse with many years of experience caring for debilitated, terminally ill patients has developed a skin care product to prevent and treat decubitus ulcers. The nurse has used the product on a large group of patients, has obtained excellent results, and now wants to bring the product to market either independently or by selling the formula to a reputable manufacturer. Before attempting to sell the formula or go into business, the nurse will need to answer the following questions: how many similar products are currently on the market, who buys those products, in what volume, how are they sold (e.g., by direct mail, through sales' or manufacturers' representatives, or by wholesale houses), at what price, how long have the competitors been in business, and what are their reputations?

Obviously, it is easier to replace a service or product that is not well established or that is overpriced, has a poor reputation, or is limited in its distribution. Imagine how difficult it would be, however, to capture any segment of successfully entrenched markets, such as the soft drink or automobile market. However, market research or creative thinking can uncover market segments and demands that are not being serviced or met. Referring back to the example of the new skin product, perhaps all the other similar products are sold primarily to long-term facilities and rehabilitation centers. Because cancer affects all age groups, the nurse could target this product to pediatric oncology units, hospices, ambulatory treatment centers, or by direct mail to the families of patients with cancer, markets previously unsolicited or approached.

Another variable affecting the reliability of forecasting is environmental volatility. Economic, legislative, and demographic conditions can and do change. Much has been written about the effects of diagnosis-related groups and prospective payment systems on health care providers and payers. These effects are still creating and diminishing markets (Krampitz & Coleman, 1985). No one predicted the surplus of nurses in 1984 to 1985 that created demands for job placement, counseling, and voluntary time off while decreasing demand for nurse recruiters and orientation programs. Although this condition lasted only 18 to 24 months, it changed market conditions during that period from a seller- to a buyer-driven market. The current problem with the acquired immune deficiency syndrome (AIDS), a condition reaching epidemic proportions that no one had predicted, is another example of an external force that affects health care markets. Although it is unlikely that even the best and most extensive market research will uncover all relevant data, it is still a useful and necessary process, because opportunity and demand are always present for new and different ideas. However, even good concepts, products, and services still have to be sold.

SELLING STRATEGIES

Selling—a win-win strategy—persuades individuals to part with some limited resource, such as time, money, energy, or pleasure, in return for something perceived as a benefit. People buy benefits, not features. For example, Mercedes Benz buyers may claim to buy these automobiles because of fine engineering, but in reality most owners purchase them because of their snob appeal, expense, image and self-esteem enhancement value, or ability to make others envious. Identifying a product's or service's benefit is essential before attempting to sell it.

Identifying Benefits

Successful sellers ask "what's in it" for the buyers? What will make buyers part with limited resources for this particular product or service? Convincing people to buy requires that the seller identify benefits from the buyer's perspective. Nurses are sometimes naive about why patients, families, and clients *should* buy nursing services and products. Therefore, they are puzzled or frustrated when their offer is not accepted immediately. They sometimes are also naive about the difference between *buyers,* who pay for services or products, and *consumers,* who use them. For example, inpatient services are paid for primarily by employers who give hospitalization insurance to employees and by governments that support state and federal programs. In some instances, of course, the buyer and the consumer are the same customer. Whether the same or different, successful sellers are prepared to identify and promote benefits for their customers.

Some benefits are obvious. For example, the benefits of a pain management program are the elimination of pain, ability to continue activities of daily living, and psychological relief from anxiety about pain. Pain management program consumers would certainly perceive these as worthwhile benefits for which they may be personally willing and able to pay. However, there are additional less obvious benefits for which customers also may be willing to pay. Family members may pay for the benefit of a peaceful night's sleep or the release from undesired feelings of guilt, anger, or hostility toward the patient or the pain. Physicians may be willing to make referrals to a pain management program to realize the benefit of reducing their frustration in trying to manage the patient's pain.

It is not as easy to identify the benefits of other products and services. For example, what perceived benefit will be sufficient to persuade potential graduate students to pay time, energy, and money (or debt) for a degree in oncology nursing? Are opportunities for career advancement, increased ability to manage patients' problems, credibility with professional colleagues, or job security persuasive enough to sell graduate oncology programs? Or will a personal need to serve be more persuasive? Market research can identify the benefits perceived by past and current customers of graduate and continuing oncology nursing programs. These identified benefits can be used to raise the awareness of potential or future customers.

Advertising and Publicity

Advertising is one of the best ways to be visible and capture the buyer's attention. The primary purposes of advertising are to raise or maintain customer awareness, to get or keep customers' attention, and to create a desire to buy. Effective advertising depends on the targeted buyer or market and on the nature of the specific product (Johnson et al., 1987). Professional journals or displays and handouts at professional meetings may be best for therapeutic products targeted at physicians and nurses. A mass medium, such as television, may be best for broad-based consumer items. Personal contacts and word of mouth may be best for low-volume but high-priced complex services, such as management information systems. Nurses at the Maine Medical Center, seeing an opportunity to promote the services of their resource people to other providers, used a poster to visualize their services (Brocker, 1988) (Box 66–2). Whatever the method, advertising and publicity campaigns should be focused on the previously identified benefits to past, current, and potential buyers.

CREDIBILITY AND PACKAGING

The seller's credibility is extremely important for success. Nurses wishing to sell their services, products,

---

Box 66–2. PROMOTING NURSE RESOURCES THROUGH ADVERTISING

Nurses at the Maine Medical Center in Portland recognized that they had resources and services to offer nurses outside their regional treatment center. Through reorganization of the Department of Nursing, a Division of Nursing Resources was formed that consolidated staff development instructors, patient educators, clinical nurse specialists, and outreach education nurses. To promote their resources both within the medical center and to outside facilities, an 11-inch by 14-inch poster was created that described how the Division of Nursing Resources could be used and contacted. Photographs of each nurse expert along with areas of expertise and telephone numbers were included. These posters with appropriate cover letters were mailed to directors of nursing in all hospitals, nursing homes, and community health agencies in the state. The response was favorable and included inquiries for new consultation, which were prompted by an increased awareness of the expertise available to provide information and to help solve problems (Brocker, 1988).

---

or ideas must have a proven track record, credentials, and positive image in the buyer's eyes. Successful sellers speak the language of the buyer and are both confident and enthusiastic about what they are selling.

Although repeat buying or customer loyalty depends on buyers' satisfaction with promised benefits, awareness, attention, and desire to buy are created by the presentation or packaging of what is being sold. Packaging is a part of advertising; therefore, it is essential to package the product or service attractively. Intangible products or services, such as education, consulting, or health care, are particularly difficult to package, because they are concepts or abstractions that cannot be touched, felt, or tried out in advance of need. What is packaged and advertised usually are surrogates or symbols of the service. Therefore, descriptive materials, brochures, or handouts must be done professionally. Sellers should look professional and act in a businesslike manner. This does not necessarily mean wearing a navy blue suit. The hypothetical nurses who want to sell the pain management program may project a more credible image to physicians and families if they wear a traditional uniform or white coat, particularly if they are selling to *belongers* and *achievers*.

Advertising and packaging can be an expensive process. Therefore, any free visibility and publicity are highly desirable. Public service announcements, mention in newsletters, alumni bulletins, or feature stories in local newspapers are all useful sources of free advertising. If the product or service is dramatic enough to capture national attention, appearances on talk shows can be worth many thousands of dollars. Another powerful free advertising source are testimonials from previous or current customers, particularly if those customers are credible or well known. Whatever the nature or cost of the advertising, it is a necessary part of successful marketing.

Pricing Tactics

No price is too great if the perceived benefits are worth it. Conversely, no price is low enough if the potential buyer sees no benefit. Sometimes people will not "buy" even when what is offered is free. An example is the staff education program that no one attends in spite of their presumed need or assessed want.

Some pricing strategies that help sell a product or service, particularly a new one attempting to capture a share of a highly competitive market, include free trial offers, loss leaders, and value enhancement. Opportunity to try out a service or product without charge enables a reluctant customer to realize benefits without risks. Obviously, the customer still has to perceive a benefit to be willing to try.

The loss leader is a selling and pricing strategy in which an unfamiliar service or product is introduced or offered in conjunction with an already established product that is priced lower than usual. Supermarkets use this tactic when they offer a bargain price on popular items to bring customers into the store, where, management hopes, they will purchase other regular-priced items. This same tactic could be used by faculty who offer a low-priced oncology nursing continuing education program in hopes of interesting participants in a more extensive graduate oncology degree program.

Value enhancement tactics offer customers an opportunity to use a new service or product and thus maintain buyer loyalty. Inpatient cancer units could offer the pain management program to those physicians who refer or admit their patients to the unit. In turn, these physicians may be willing to recommend the program to other physicians. Each of these pricing tactics is risky for the seller, who assumes both the cost and the possibility that the tactics may not succeed.

The price charged for a service or product should have some relationship to the cost of producing and delivering it. The hypothetic nurses who want to provide a pain management service to cancer patients need to estimate all direct costs of advertising and packaging; cost of actual time spent in providing and selling the service; costs of services of secretaries, lawyers, and accountants; and any travel or delivery costs. Indirect costs include opportunities lost by engaging in this business rather than some other income-producing venture, taxes, and benefits previously paid by employers that now must be assumed by the entrepreneurs. The price paid by subsequent customers must be equal to or greater than these costs unless, of course, the service is subsidized or the nurses have another source of income.

SUMMARY

Marketing is a planned set of activities designed to achieve specific predetermined goals and objectives.

These may include financial gain, personal satisfaction, improved health status of patients, organizational or behavioral changes, buyer satisfaction or well-being, and professional status achievement. These goals and objectives need definition to serve as a guide for action. They also need to be continuously refined and revised based on success or lack of achievement. Concomitant with implementation of the marketing plan is the willingness and ability to take both personal and financial risks. Success in any business venture is not simply a matter of having good luck and a great idea, product, or service. Successful marketing of cancer nursing will require credibility, a well thought-out plan, hard work, commitment, and perseverance.

References

Adams, G. A., Hockema, M. L., & Ware, L. (1988). Integrating marketing into nursing service. *Nursing Management, 19*(9), 30–34.

Andreoli, K. G., Carollo, J. R., & Poltage, M. W. (1988). Marketing strategies: Projecting an image of nursing that reflects achievement. *Nursing Administration Quarterly, 12*(4), 5–14.

Auttonberry, D. S. (1988). The emerging role of the master's-prepared nurse in marketing. *Nursing Management, 19*(19), 40–42.

Brocker, C. A. (1988). Promoting nursing resources. *Journal of Nursing Administration, 18*(3), 38.

Chaney, H. S. (1986). Practical approaches to marketing. *Journal of Nursing Administration, 16*(9), 33–38.

Freitag, E. M. (1988). Marketing in home health care: A practical approach. *Nursing Clinics of North America, 23*, 415–429.

Gardner, K. L., & Weinrauch, D. (1988). Marketing strategies for nurse entrepreneurs. *Nurse Practitioner, 13*(5), 46–49.

Johnson, J. E., Arevidson, A. C., Costa, L. L., Hekhuis, F. M., Lennox, L. A., Marshall, S. B., & Moran, M. J. (1987). Marketing your nursing product line: Reaping the benefits. *Journal of Nursing Administration, 17*(11), 29–33.

Krampitz, S. D., & Coleman, J. R. (1985). Marketing—a must in a competitive health care system. *Nursing Economics, 3*, 286–294.

Shamansky, S. L., Schilling, L. S., & Holbrook, T. L. (1985). Determining the market for nurse practitioner services: The New Haven experience. *Nursing Research, 34*, 242–247.

Stanton, M., & Stanton, G. W. (1988). Marketing nursing: A model for success. *Nursing Management, 19*(9), 36–38.

Use demographics include data on volumes and life styles. (1985). *Hospitals, 59*, 43.

THE DELIVERY OF CANCER CARE SERVICES: RESOURCES AND REFERRAL SYSTEMS

CHAPTER **67**

The Organization of Cancer Service Settings

JEROME W. YATES
CATHERINE LYONS

The microenvironment of cancer service settings (office, clinic, hospital, and community) is influenced strongly by the various resources in the macroenvironment (technology, manpower, and economics). Canadian cancer care, as planned by the provincial governments, falls into both center and community-dominated systems (Rusthoven, Wodinsky, & Osoba, 1986). In the United States, system variation is greater because multiple reimbursement pressures influence existing health care delivery. Governmental agencies, employers, and third-party payors become active participants in health care availability and delivery systems and can be expected to further transform American medicine (Winkenwerder & Ball, 1988).

The continuum from idea generation through application to the transfer of technology is quite dynamic as the world continually improves technology and develops new expertise. Innovative proposals from academic cancer centers, confirmatory studies carried out by cooperative clinical trials groups, and economic policies set by the government all influence and control the public's knowledge, access, and utilization of health care services. They contribute to the framework for our present cancer care settings. Even in today's climate of cost containment, new and expensive techno-logic developments (such as magnetic resonance imaging), which appear to provide a contribution toward the best patient management, gain rapid acceptance. Efficacy and revenue generation, balanced with cost, have become an expected part of today's emerging technologies. Economic constraints have forced the research community to consider costs as it designs clinical trials and anticipates the retrospective review of the data by those responsible for setting reimbursement policy.

HISTORICAL PERSPECTIVE

The historical emergence of the three major treatment methods (surgery, radiation therapy, and chemo/biologic) has influenced the organization of cancer services to the greatest degree. As each method evolved, concurrent support services developed, assuming the characteristics of the principal method.

Surgery

Until the mid-twentieth century, surgery was generally considered the only effective treatment that could lead to a cure for cancer. Studies of patient response to surgical treatment were largely nonsystematic aggregates of anecdotal information. Initial descriptive reports of procedures carried out in selected patients were generally enthusiastic, only to be followed by confirmatory studies that usually yielded fewer favorable responses. Encumbered by a long tradition of cancer management conducted by general surgeons, academic surgical oncology has begun only recently to emerge as a specialty with cancer interests that extend beyond surgical technique (Lawrence, 1982; Rosenberg, 1984; Wilson, 1984).

Radiation Therapy

Although radiation therapy was introduced in the nineteenth century, it was not until after World War II that radiation training programs and routine management of cancer using this method developed (Rubin, 1985). Radiation therapy developed as an offshoot of diagnostic radiology. With more rigorous requirements for expertise, radiation therapy became recognized as a distinct department in most academic institutions. Paralleling the advances from the application of local radium, orthovoltage, cobalt, and subsequently other high energy forms of radiation was the accumulation of curative results after radiation therapy for primary cancers of the skin, oral cavity, larynx, breast, uterine cervix, and rectum. As radiation therapists gained experience using various doses and schedules, it became apparent that surgical intervention alone often resulted in local recurrences. Radiation therapy was added to surgery in an attempt to improve treatment results through better regional control.

Chemotherapy

Because of the systemic nature of acute leukemia, surgery and radiation therapy were not even considered as treatment options with curative potential for this disease. In the late 1940s aminopterin was first used by Farber to treat childhood acute lymphocytic leukemia (Farber, Diamond, Mercer, Sylvester, & Wolff, 1948). Encouraged by the induction of the first partial remissions (based on laboratory evidence of neoplastic cell differences in folic acid metabolism), cancer treatment with chemotherapeutic agents gained momentum. The hematologic malignancies contributed to the training of a cadre of investigators in programs maintained in an academic atmosphere of clinical investigation (Kennedy, 1986; Kennedy, Calabresi, Clarkson, & Frenkel, 1986). Hematologists began to specialize in the chemotherapeutic treatment of the leukemias and lymphomas as successful management appeared possible. The paucity of childhood leukemia patients forged the formation of multi-institutional collaborative clinical research efforts among these pioneers in chemotherapy. Immunotherapy and cytokine therapy have been tested in the clinic using methods and expertise gained in chemotherapy research.

Emergence of Clinical Trials

Protocol-driven collaborative studies were extended to involve many institutions to ensure adequate accrual for studies of the leukemias and lymphomas. Protocols guaranteed greater specificity in the descriptions of treatment regimens and outcome variables. Comparability of data gathered from many investigators and institutions was a major achievement and continues to receive attention in the drive toward optimal management (Horiot et al., 1986). Surgeons and radiation therapists studied the common cancers (lung, colon, and breast) in single institutions, because they were able to accrue sufficient numbers of patients for their descriptive reports. The lack of interinstitutional collaboration and cross criticism among surgeons and radiation therapists delayed their appreciation of the benefit derived from common definitions. This led to some confusion and noncomparability of published reports. One of the best examples is the continuing confusion in the surgical literature because of the different "Dukes" staging systems used for colorectal cancer (Hamilton, 1986).

Collaborative Practice

Administering chemotherapy and collecting data for clinical trials are labor-intensive efforts. As a result, teamwork to develop collaborative clinical research involving both the medical oncologist and the oncology nurse evolved. These relationships are somewhat different from those developed in surgery and radiation therapy. Because chemotherapeutic regimens are labor intensive and morbidity is often chronic, there is an increased need for patient-caregiver education. Historically nurses have assumed this key role. The interactions between nurses and surgical and radiation therapy patients at the time of treatment delivery tends to be minimal, whereas the opposite is true throughout the administration of chemotherapy. Nursing support during the late nineteenth and early twentieth century for office-based surgery was displaced when general anesthesia became more sophisticated and surgery moved to the hospital. With greater emphasis on outpatient endoscopy and ambulatory surgery, the important role of today's outpatient surgical nurse has emerged again. Nurses provide critical education for the anxious patient about to undergo a biopsy or endoscopy. Interactions between radiation therapists and their patients in the United States are often temporary and technical, because usually the referring physician maintains the continuing primary care role. Radiation therapy technologists are major providers of educational and psychosocial support in this setting, and nursing is less represented in most radiation therapy departments.

Improvement in cancer management has affected the evolution of both the delivery system and the conduct of clinical research. Clinical research participation is a foundation that facilitates continuing education for all involved professionals. As cancer management and clinical research achieve greater sophistication and productivity, a new level of cooperation between the oncology nurse and various medical specialties can be expected.

MULTI-INSTITUTIONAL COOPERATIVE CLINICAL TRIALS GROUPS

Dr. James Ewing in 1929 made a number of observations that are critical to the subsequent successful development of the systematic clinical investigation of cancer (Holleb, 1980). He noted the importance of precision in the diagnosis and the classification of various types of cancer. He demeaned the "unattached physician without experience and equipment" and extolled the importance of colleagial advice in attempting to identify solutions to the "life and death of the patient." These were the conceptual beginnings of cancer centers, hospital tumor boards, and the clinical trials groups. Ewing felt that progress in the management of cancer would come if the appropriate environment was operational. He was an early believer in cancer centers and also an optimist about available interventions as reflected in his statement: "It would be desirable to establish a limited number of broadly organized, fully equipped cancer institutes, covering every arm of the service. . . . there is hardly a stage of cancer that you can't do something for" (Holleb, 1980).

With greater specialization in the management of cancer, it became apparent that an understanding of the biology of the cancer as well as the factors influencing host reactions to treatment were important. Pathologists have improved our understanding of cancer biology, whereas clinicians have focused on diagnosis and treatment. Karnofsky and Burchenal (1948) provided one of the first reliable categorizations of patient performance status, a contribution whose importance took almost 25 years to become fully appreciated. Performance status has proved subsequently to be an important variable in the stratification of patients in prospective trials and also an important measure of comparison between patient groups in retrospective analyses. The development of the randomized trial to minimize the probability of selection bias provided the "gold standard" for credible clinical research. Additional costs of randomized trials were incurred by the increased need for patient and family education to ensure accrual and compliance as well as to educate participants in the course of the study and ensure the informed consent process.

Early cancer treatment with single-method therapy had known limitations. Local recurrence following cancer resection led surgeons to consider the addition of regional radiation therapy following surgery. The appearance of leukemia in sanctuary sites in children who were otherwise in hematologic remission stimulated the use of regional radiation therapy, and this led to the first significant numbers of cures in children with acute lymphocytic leukemia.

In an effort to control recurrent and systemic disease following local surgical resection for breast and colorectal cancer, surgeons and their colleagues explored the use of adjuvant chemotherapy. The logic of multidisciplinary planning in the early management of cancer, particularly in those patients having a poor prognosis after single-method treatment, stimulated collaboration among consultants in the most respected hospitals. Documented benefits through multimodality management encouraged new research. Recognizing the benefit of such collaboration, the American College of Surgeons required multidisciplinary tumor boards to be recognized as possessing a hospital cancer program (Gross, 1987; Henson et al., 1988). These meetings have become an important contribution to local professional education.

Tumor boards were one of the first organized attempts at quality assurance. Open discussion of patient management was accomplished when previously none would have occurred. Their use as a local educational vehicle became commonplace with both patient-focused discussions and lectures as the usual formats. Even today, these meetings are often the only regularly scheduled educational conferences held in small and midsize community hospitals. Varied opinions related to diagnoses, treatment options, potential morbidity, and expected outcome provide the basis for stimulating discussions involving consultants and staff physicians.

In all treatment methods, advancement of technology and knowledge supports more aggressive and accurate treatment. The result has included ancillary advances in supportive care aimed at decreasing morbidity and mortality, blood product transfusions, safer anesthesia, improved nutritional support, effective antibiotics, and specialized nursing care. All have facilitated the implementation of more aggressive surgical management of cancer. Improved imaging for port definition, treatment simulation, and sophisticated equipment for delivery of radiation therapy have enhanced this modality. The development of laboratory techniques critical to understanding pharmacokinetics and pharmacodynamics, animal models and tissue culture methods for testing drug sensitivity, and the elucidation of prognostic factors that are important in assessing the efficacy of chemotherapy have all promoted the growth of medical oncology. Refinements in pathologic diagnoses, staging to assess the extent of disease, and imposition of statistical standards in the interpretation of clinical trial outcomes have intensified the teamwork and facilitated the expansion of the multidisciplinary clinical trials groups. Refinements in all of these areas provided the basis for protocol-driven studies that embraced more precise classifications of patients, treatment interventions, and outcome assessments, leading to a better understanding of the biology and course of treated cancer.

The development of acceptable standards for collecting, managing, and subsequently analyzing data is a major byproduct of the multi-institutional cancer trials funded by the National Cancer Institute (NCI). In the small early trials, the critical review for quality was often missing. Data were collected and often managed haphazardly by attending physicians, medical students, resident trainees, and fellows. As quality control received much needed attention from a group of frustrated clinical trials statisticians, the members of the cooperative groups gave data management increased attention. Issues such as patient recruitment, protocol adherence, data management, and periodic reports joined the pursuit of science in the list of priorities.

Nurses became the linchpins for the successful conduct of many clinical trials in their supervision of the data management, treatment delivery, and provision of patient education. Physicians found the oncology nurse indispensable to ensuring both adequate study accrual and necessary patient follow-up. Nurses became more specialized, developing an in-depth knowledge of the course of cancer, the required nursing care, the available anticancer and supportive care treatments, the active research studies, the protocol requirements, and the data management techniques. They provided a level of continuing and supportive care not always available from attending physicians and almost never from the rotating house staff at institutions involved in clinical trials. Often their responsibility for the administration of chemotherapy provided a timely opportunity for patient education. Psychosocial tasks that involve labor-intensive interventions aimed at recognizing changes in disease status, treatment toxicity, and symptom control (e.g., nausea, pain) and that provide psychosocial support to patients and assistance to families in their negotiation of the health care system are now routine efforts assumed largely by oncology nurses. As multi-institutional clinical trial groups expand beyond treatment into other areas of cancer control, they will be even more dependent on the coordinating role of the nurse as a prime member of the team. All indicators suggest the extent of their presence and responsibilities in the oncologic research environment will expand even more over the next decade.

In summary, the success of multi-institutional clinical trials has been dependent on the sufficient accruals of informed and educated patients, maintenance of data in a logical and organized fashion, and systematic follow-up. The role of oncology nurses in this endeavor is, perhaps, the best example of collaborative practice models in clinical research and health care.

CANCER RESEARCH AND THE ORGANIZATION OF CARE DELIVERY

Cancer care may be provided independently or in conjunction with clinical research in cancer centers. The centers stress research interests but are also expected to provide exemplary patient care. In the community, the emphasis has been on the delivery of care; however, with the influx of trained oncologists into outlying hospitals, interest in clinical research has expanded. Rapid communications, available expertise, and access through improved transportation has decreased the difference between the clinical research capabilities of the cancer centers and their community counterparts. Currently, only phase I (toxicity) pharmacologic studies remain restricted to the cancer cen-

ters. Competition for patients has led to a decrease in accruals to center trials and increased patient accrual from community facilities to cooperative group efforts. Community physicians have demonstrated their ability to provide the best cancer care and also participate in clinical research comparable to that conducted in major cancer centers.

Cancer Centers

The classification of cancer centers by the NCI includes (1) comprehensive, (2) clinical, (3) basic science, and (4) consortium. Competitive providers interested in marketing their services often use labels to extol the comprehensiveness of their services and their self-sufficiency by calling themselves "free-standing." They characterize their geographic importance and influence through descriptive terms such as *regional* or *metropolitan*. The NCI restricts the use of the term *NCI-designated* to those centers that have been successful in competition for funding through a core grant award. This designation attempts to counteract the efforts of some community hospitals to perpetuate confusion among the public and signifies that such a center has a high level of peer-reviewed research excellence.

The four types of NCI centers are similar in that all have a foundation of peer-reviewed research support even though they represent a wide spectrum of research and provider activities. Basic science centers are involved primarily in "wet-bench" laboratory research only (animal or cell studies); clinical centers conduct both basic laboratory and clinical research (human trials); comprehensive centers pursue research in laboratories, cancer control and clinical areas, while conducting other cancer control activities; and consortium centers are involved generally in both clinical and cancer control research and also cancer control activities.

Cancer control research is defined as "the reduction of incidence, morbidity, and mortality through an orderly sequence from research on interventions and their impact in defined populations to the broad systematic application of the research results" (Greenwald & Cullen, 1984). Cancer control activities are those interventions that are applied but not fully evaluated. In the mid 1970s the designation of comprehensiveness was conferred by the National Cancer Advisory Board on those qualified clinical centers that assumed regional responsibility for cancer control also. After the successful defense of a separate application for comprehensive status, they were designated as comprehensive centers.

The comprehensive designation, originally intended to identify the premier cancer centers, has lost some of its original luster. In 1990 the NCI revived reviews for comprehensive status and hopes to develop a set of goals that centers, particularly those with comprehensive status, will pursue. There is a great overlap between comprehensive and clinical centers in the breadth of cancer control research done by each type of center. Some comprehensive centers have minimal cancer control research, whereas selected clinical centers conduct large cancer control programs. Reviews of comprehensive status will renew interest in regional responsibilities for some centers.

The lay public generally thinks of cancer centers as centers of excellence in the diagnosis and management of cancer with or without ongoing research. Cancer centers designated by the NCI as holders of center core grants comprise a select group of 50 distinguished research institutions. The core grant funding they receive provides support for (1) shared resources (e.g., animal facilities, a data management office, large pieces of equipment), (2) leadership for research programs (affinity groups that include participants from many departments), (3) administrative leadership, and (4) developmental funding (small start-up grants reviewed and awarded largely to young center investigators, or for new major program development). Private practitioners located in the area of many cancer centers view them as research institutions acting primarily as a site for laboratory and clinical research. Often regional providers feel that centers render somewhat depersonalized care for patients while offering few management advantages over that available in the community.

Cancer centers can and do have an environment enabling the conduct of efficient and synergistic research. Administrative and programmatic leadership, availability of shared resources, and flexible developmental funding all contribute to their success. However, the impact of these centers on regional cancer care is highly variable because of self-defined research, variations in cancer control interests, and constraints imposed by the existing health care system. Most centers are located in medical schools that historically have been somewhat introspective. These institutions often behave as if their only regional obligation is to ensure good care through their undergraduate, graduate, and continuing medical education programs. Because "wet-bench" laboratory research is a major focus of most cancer centers, there has been less interest in studying the application of new results (e.g., cancer control) that go beyond convenient educational programs. The effect of competition for patients has strained relationships among regional providers, further distancing some centers from their local medical communities.

Cooperative Clinical Trials Groups

The naming of the cooperative clinical trials groups arose in several ways: the descriptions of their regional coverage, the specialty of the membership, or the scope of their target cancer. A few examples of these groups include those named after a specific group of diseases being studied (e.g., Acute Leukemia Group B, now called CALGB), a geographic area of the country from which the member institutions were drawn (e.g., Eastern Cooperative Oncology Group, or ECOG), a specialty group (e.g., Pediatric Oncology Group, called POG, or the Radiation Therapy Oncology Group,

RTOG), and collaborative groups involving participants from two or more major clinical trials groups. Approximately 25,000 patients per year participate in clinical trials supported by the NCI with participating investigators coming from almost all areas of the country. Although the primary goal of the groups is to conduct clinical research, the groups have also developed into one of the largest ongoing systems of expert scientific peer review and continuing medical education. They have provided a fertile ground for refining the talents of researchers involved in drug investigation, clinical trials statistics, data management, cancer nursing, cancer control, and many other related disciplines.

With the increasing participation in the last decade from community physicians in cooperative groups, the influence of this continuing educational aspect extends to most of the major communities in North America. This system serves as a vehicle for academically developed pilot studies to be carried to confirmation, community physician participation in clinical research, and exposure of patients to a reliable source of the most current management information. Vigorous exchange during study development provides a level of internal peer review seldom available in most other medical specialties conducting clinical research. Cooperative groups contribute to the training of young and established oncologic specialists through their meetings and conduct of protocol-driven research. Their innovation is often downplayed by some investigators, because group studies are confirmatory or extended explorations of previous reports. Some critics would say that the groups are too large and cumbersome in their deliberations, that their protocols have all of the shortcomings of research designed by a committee in response to the needs of the least skillful participant, and that innovative ideas seldom emerge as direct result of their massive deliberations. In keeping perspective, one must remember that the major contributions from the groups have been their accuracy in either sustaining or refuting promising results from single-institution studies. They provide a key control over early enthusiastic reports. Considering only their role in phase II (efficacy) and III (comparisons of treatments) studies, they are a definite success, but without an abundance of new ideas for testing, their sustenance is an expensive luxury. To date their contributions far outweigh the criticisms offered by detractors. They function as the greatest operational network of investigators capable of delivering a critical examination of promising preliminary clinical results.

Community-Based Oncology Service

As more medical oncologists were trained and left academic institutions in pursuit of community practice, a group of physicians capable of rigorous clinical research outside of the centers became available. Although they enjoy the autonomy of private practice, many wish to continue active participation in clinical research. By doing so they maintain their local identity as a research participant and ensure ongoing access to the latest disease management information. The National Surgical Adjuvant Breast Group (NSABP), with support from the NCI, stimulated collaboration between university and community physicians. Their success became a model for the generation of the Cooperative Group Outreach Program (CGOP) in 1976. This NCI effort supported the participation of community physicians in cooperative group studies. The success of this effort led to the subsequent funding of 61 Community Clinical Oncology Programs (CCOP) in 1983. Although both provide community support for study participation on a per patient basis, there is an annual expected accrual of 50 patients per year by each CCOP, and direct funding for the CCOP fosters a community identity as a clinical research resource. In many instances they have become the community cancer centers. By contrast, the usual contribution of patients per investigator in the CGOP is fewer than 10 patients per year, and this funding is controlled by the cooperative groups. Support is given to individual investigators, decreasing the opportunity for a community identity to develop around program participants.

One program that was not as successful as hoped was the Community Hospital Oncology Program, which sponsored the local development of patient management protocols in selected community hospitals. Developed in 1980, the original assumption was that local participation in the process of criteria development would enhance physician use and improve patient management through guideline compliance. The original assumption proved not to be true for these 17 selected hospitals for the most part, and the program was abandoned subsequently by the NCI (Ford, Hunter, Diehr, Frelick, & Yates, 1987).

Both the CGOP and the CCOP programs can be judged a success based on their increasing proportional patient accrual to the cooperative groups. Member institutions and cancer centers can no longer compete solely on their academic reputation to promote their superiority in providing cancer care. In fact, the ability of community physicians to contribute significantly to the clinical trials effort and to provide excellent patient care has received greater acceptance as a result of the reviews of these NCI-sponsored community programs.

With the advent of prospective reimbursement and the shift of patient management from the hospital to the ambulatory setting, dramatic changes have occurred in the delivery of cancer care. Large numbers of patients who were formerly referred to training institutions are being treated in the community settings, and this has had an adverse impact on oncology training programs. Leisurely teaching during ward rounds and treatment planning conferences are no longer possible as the "out quicker and sicker" syndrome comes to characterize the inpatient population. Special care units (such as adolescent facilities) are under pressures to maintain a high census (Delengowski & Dugan-Jordan, 1986). This has diminished the exposure of house staff to a wide variety of subacute and varied diagnostic patient problems. The system is pressuring a greater number of individual physicians to make decisions without seeking appropriate consultations. Patient management protocols provide some structured teaching in the clinic and, to a limited extent, blunt these changes in the health care system.

Another result has been the increasing dependence of cancer centers and large clinics on nurses to conduct patient education activities. Because of the time and economic pressures to see more patients more efficiently, and because of the labor intensity of house staff education, attending physicians no longer see themselves as the primary patient educator and have developed a greater reliance on nursing staff for routine patient education activities. Ensuring quality management of complicated cancer patients and keeping patients and their families informed requires professional knowledge, continuity of care, and availability of resources. Impending restrictions on physician house staff coverage will result in their replacement as the primary patient managers by nurse practitioners in some institutions. Nurses are expanding their roles as full research partners in many academic institutions.

FUTURE ISSUES

Cancer care was revolutionized in the 1980s through the development and use of highly technical and sophisticated equipment, procedures, and supportive care mechanisms. As health care consumes a larger percentage of the gross national product, issues such as availability and utilization of diminished resources become key issues for the 1990s.

The federal government is planning to extend prospective payment to the outpatient treatment centers and to intensify their efforts at cost containment. Monitoring the quality of care that is easily conducted in inpatient settings deserves comparable attention. Improved clinical efficiency, increased home care expertise, and pressure to ensure appropriate multidisciplinary management will be necessary if excellence in patient care is to be maintained.

Private insurance companies can be expected to review their payments for care and their support of the patient care aspects of clinical research in their efforts to remain competitive through rate reduction. They could refuse to support clinical investigation and developmental activity by deferring responsibility to the federal government. This possibility would have a major negative impact on clinical research, because insurers need to be convinced of the benefits of their continued reimbursement (Wittes, 1987). The cancer centers will have to change their present introspective attitude and develop networks with regional clinicians to encourage greater exchanges of patients and information. Nurses will develop expanded and extended roles in the conduct of clinical research with nurse practitioners and nurse specialists assuming increased responsibility for patient education. The movement toward the reduction of house staff hours to avoid excessive fatigue will increase the need for physician extenders in many teaching institutions. This will increase the demand for nurse practitioners and increase their salaries and may further aggravate the projected and actual nursing shortage in many areas of the country. The diminished supply of nursing resources at all levels must be anticipated, and concerted attempts must be made to provide career advancement and greater prestige to limit attrition and increase recruitment to the profession.

Community physicians will continue to manage most of their cancer patients except for treatment involving high technology, high-risk interventions, and for those patients who represent financial liabilities to community hospitals. Reasonable reimbursement to the cancer centers will have to be provided to ensure continued research progress in cancer management.

More NCI-directed intergroup studies will ensue because the existing groups are reluctant to give up their own initiatives to develop cooperation unless stimulated to do so. Greater speed in the conduct of confirmatory studies can be achieved with the stimulus of specific funding aimed at high priority studies. There will be an increasing reliance on cancer centers and an expectation that they will participate in regional cancer control efforts, including prevention, detection, and supportive care. Participation from nonphysician professionals in both cancer control research and activities will be expanded.

Computer communication for information exchange (PDQ) and data management will become the norm, and computer networking among investigators, hospitals, universities, cancer centers, and the NCI will become commonplace (Hubbard, Henney, & DeVita, 1987).

Integrated planning is necessary to ensure adequate research reimbursement to meet projected manpower needs to designate excellence in diagnostic and treatment centers and to systematically provide patient and public education. Without more integration among the various responsible agencies, redundancies and inadequacies in cancer management are likely to occur.

References

Delengowski, A., & Dugan-Jordan, M. (1986). Care of the adolescent cancer patient on an adult medical oncology unit. *Seminars in Oncology Nursing, 2*, 95–103.

Farber, S., Diamond, L. K., Mercer, R. D., Sylvester, R. F., Jr., & Wolff, J. A. (1948). Temporary remissions in acute leukemia in children produced by folic acid antagonist, 4-aminopteroylglutamic acid (Aminopterin). *New England Journal of Medicine, 238*, 787.

Ford, L. G., Hunter, C. P., Diehr, P., Frelick, R. W., & Yates, J. W. (1987). Effects of patient management guidelines on physician practice patterns: The Community Hospital Oncology Program experience. *Journal of Clinical Oncology, 5*, 504–511.

Greenwald, P., & Cullen, J. W. (1984). The scientific approach to cancer control. *CA: A Journal for Clinicians, 34*, 328–334.

Gross, G. E. (1987). The role of the tumor board in a community hospital. *Cancer, 2*, 88–92.

Hamilton, S. R. (1986). Pathologic diagnosis of colorectal and anal malignancies: Classification and prognostic features of pathologic findings. In O. H. Beahrs, G. A. Higgins, & J. J. Weinstein (Eds.), *Colorectal tumors* (pp. 107–112). Philadelphia: J. B. Lippincott Co.

Henson, D. E., Frelick, R. W., Ford, L. G., Smart, C. R., Winchester, D., Mettlin, C., & Yates, J. W. (1988). *Characteristics of hospital tumor conferences. Results of a national survey.* Manuscript submitted for publication.

Holleb, A. I. (1980). *The many faces of surgical oncology.* Paper presented at the James Ewing Lecture, meeting of the Society of Surgical Oncology, San Francisco, CA.

Horiot, J. C., Johansson, K. A., Gonzalez, D. G., van der Schueren, E., van den Bogaert, W., & Notter, G. (1986). Quality assurance control in the EORTC cooperative group of radiotherapy staff and equipment. *Radiotherapy and Oncology, 6[4]*, 275–284.

Hubbard, S. M., Henney, J. E., & DeVita, V. T., Jr. (1987). A computer data base for information on cancer treatment. *New England Journal of Medicine, 5*, 315–318.

Karnofsky, D. A., & Burchenal, J. H. (1949). The clinical evaluation of chemo therapeutic agents in cancer. In C. M. Macleod (Ed.), *Evaluation of chemo therapeutic agents.* New York: Columbia Univ. Press.

Kennedy, B. J. (1986). Medical oncology manpower supply. *Medical and Pediatric Oncology, 14*, 195–201.

Kennedy, B. J., Calabresi, P., Clarkson, B., & Frenkel E. (1986). Letter to the editor. *Annals of Internal Medicine, 104*, 279.

Lawrence, W., Jr. (1982). Oncology: General considerations. The scope of surgical oncology. *Australian and New Zealand Journal of Surgery, 52*, 325–330.

Rosenberg, S. A. (1984). The organization of surgical oncology in university departments of surgery. *Surgery, 95*, 632–634.

Rubin, F. (1985). The emergence of radiation oncology as a distinct medical specialty. *International Journal of Radiation Oncology, Biology, Physics, 2*, 1247–1270.

Rusthoven, J. J., Wodinsky, H., & Osoba, D. (1986). Canadian cancer care: Organizational models. *Annals of Internal Medicine, 105*, 932–936.

Wilson, R. E. (1984). Surgical oncology. *Cancer, 54*, 2595–2598.

Winkenwerder, W., & Ball, J. R. (1988). Transformation of American health care. The role of the medical profession. *The New England Journal of Medicine, 318*, 317–319.

Wittes, R. E. (1987). Paying for patient care in treatment research—who is responsible? *Cancer Treatment Reports, 71*, 107–113.

68

Continuity of Care and Discharge Planning

GERALDINE PADILLA

TERRI KIRSHNER

This chapter describes the function of discharge planning in promoting continuity of care for patients with cancer as they leave the hospital environment to return home or to enter another health care facility. "Discharge Planning is defined as the process of activities that involve the patient and a team of individuals from various disciplines working together to facilitate the transition of that patient from one environment to another" (Shine, 1983). Continuity of care is a process of providing arrangements that facilitate the smooth transfer of the patient; the information that is communicated between hospital staff, patient, and family or other caregivers to ensure that the patient is ready to leave the hospital; and the information that is communicated to outside agencies so the agency is ready to receive the patient. This chapter includes a discussion of hospital-to-home transition systems, cancer as a chronic disease, the discharge planning team, the discharge plan, coordination of care, and quality assurance as related to discharge planning.

HOSPITAL-TO-HOME TRANSITION SYSTEMS

Systems for transition from hospital to home were formalized in 1905 at the time social work was integrated into general hospitals (Rossen, 1984). Discharge planning is the commonly used means of promoting continuity of care from hospital to home. Highly sophisticated, computerized approaches to discharge care planning are available, as in the case of the National Institutes of Health Clinical Center. The system implemented by the center includes computer printouts of discharge nursing care plans and multidisciplinary outcome summaries that contain the patient data necessary for continuity of care from hospital to home, from referring physician to the community (Romano, 1984).

The team approach to discharge planning has been identified as an important vehicle for providing a smooth transition from the hospital to the home setting (Dwyer & Held, 1982). It is further recommended that some member of the discharge team, such as the social worker or home health care coordinator, visit the home to gather objective data on how the patient's needs might be met in the home environment. However, the most common approach to discharge planning involves a single health care professional as discharge planner rather than a team (Henry & Subcommittee on Discharge Planning, 1981).

The discharge planner is generally an employee of the hospital, not of the home care agency staff. Predictions of home care requirements are based on an acute care viewpoint. Further, when discharge planning is the sole responsibility of a non-nurse, the patient may be at a disadvantage, because a non-nurse is unlikely to be able to predict or to communicate to the home care agency nurse the complex nursing care and medical treatment needs of the patient with cancer. However, a nurse with an understanding of home care requirements, a commitment to the home care agency, and an opportunity to assess home care needs while the patient is still in the hospital would be the most qualified to assess home nursing care needs of patients with cancer (Tulga, 1981). The liaison nurse role fits these characteristics (Hospital Home Health Care Agency job description). The role serves as a communication link between agencies and between patient and health care professionals. Patient and family concerns in the treatment phase include lack of communication with health team members, such as the physician and nurse (Northhouse, 1984). The use of a nurse as the communication link is accepted by the patient, family, and home health service (Tulga, 1981).

Hospital-to-home transition systems can be characterized by their level of integration. Criteria for defining the level of system integration include organization and fiscal arrangements; information exchange arrangements involving professional roles, patient conferences, and access to data bases; and geographic proximity of hospital and home care agencies and departments.

Various hospital-to-home transition systems are currently in effect and cover a wide range of models with greater or lesser integration between hospital and home care agencies. At one end of the continuum is the institution that provides a fully integrated range of services, including inpatient care, discharge planning, outpatient clinics, and home care. In this type of system, discharge planners are responsible for a specific cluster of patients in relation to screening, assessment, planning, and follow-up. Knowledge about the home care needs of patients is maximized during the transition.

Several types of partially integrated systems have been implemented. Partially integrated systems are labeled as such because they provide a link between the hospital and home care experiences of the patient. For example, the Oncology Transition Services Cancer Program provides six oncology clinical nurse specialists trained at the master's level to operate in the community at large, following patients from diagnosis to terminal stage (McCorkle & Germino, 1984; Tornberg, McGrath, & Benoliel, 1984). The direct services provided by these clinical specialists include management of crises, management of treatment protocols, care of the patient with special needs, and management of symptoms, as well as ongoing assessment of the patient to provide current responsive care and individualized care for these patients. The nurse provides the primary physician with ongoing information about the patient that is invaluable to the medical treatment plan.

Another partially integrated system model involves an area-wide oncology nurse coordinator, who operates primarily as a consultant-practitioner (May, Oleske, Justo-Ober, & Heide, 1982). The nurse coordinator makes a joint visit with the agency nurse; assesses the patient, family, and environment; and develops a nursing care plan. After the initial visit, the coordinator communicates with the primary agency nurse by telephone or through face-to-face consultation and is updated on the progress of the patient. However, it is the agency nurse who remains responsible for communicating specific problems to the physician and for requesting medical orders.

Another partially integrated system model is that developed by the Hospital Home Health Care Agency and its ten member hospitals and other affiliated hospitals (Tatge, 1984). This model uses a liaison nurse who works with a specific member hospital or hospitals on a continuous basis. The liaison nurse, who is paid by the home care agency but functions in the hospital as defined by hospital policy, may then review referral patients' charts and see patients and their families before discharge. The liaison nurse initiates the home care intake form, using the available hospital information on patients' skilled care requirements. The liaison nurse adds a further dimension of continuity of care in the discharge planning program of the hospital

and provides feedback to discharge planners and hospital and home care staff concerning patient care plans, progress, and final disposition.

At the other extreme of the continuum are the completely nonintegrated systems that represent the most common types of structures. In these systems there is no formal link between the hospital and home care agencies, which are completely independent of one another.

The comparative value of each of these systems in meeting the complex home care requirements of patients has not been tested. However, it seems logical to predict that the fully and partially integrated hospital-to-home transition systems, with their built-in emphasis on coordination of care, would provide greater continuity of care and thus would result in more positive outcomes for patients. Further, it seems reasonable to conclude that a partially integrated system based on the liaison nurse role offers the most promise as a mechanism for improving continuity of care. Although no data are available, the liaison nurse role is (1) simpler and more economical to implement than a series of fully integrated systems, because one liaison nurse works with a home care agency servicing patients from more than one hospital (Tatge, 1984); (2) more likely to promote continuity of care than the area-wide nurse coordination mechanism (May et al., 1982) or nonintegrated systems, because the liaison nurse works for a home care agency while having formal commitments to specific affiliated hospitals (Tatge, 1984); and (3) more cost effective than the community oncology clinical specialists' approach (McCorkle & Germino, 1984; Tornberg et al., 1984), because liaison nurses are not required to be specialists.

A significant aspect of a hospital-to-home transition system that affects continuity of care and ultimately patient outcomes is the skill of the health care professionals involved in providing high-technology care, preparing the patient for discharge, coordinating hospital-to-home care, and promoting self-care in the home. Patients discharged home with a need for high-technology care require educational activities that start in the hospital and continue in the home so that patients and families can be responsible and competent in giving needed care. Discharge planning should involve the patients and families in making decisions about long-term care (Coulton, Dunkle, Goode, & MacKintosh, 1982).

Oberst and James (1985) found that following cancer surgery, care given in the hospital matches closely the need for care. After discharge, care given in the home drops sharply, yet patients perceive an increased need for care. This need may exceed that which the family caregivers can provide. Moreover, patients and particularly spouses experience emotional distress that accompanies ineffective coping with life's daily hassles. This problem indicates the need for better discharge planning that includes the family caregiver as well as the patient. The discharge plan can be more effective if it stresses the usual time frame for common postdischarge occurrences. These occurrences include lifestyle disruptions; physical care difficulties; symptom distress; uncertainty; emotional distress; problems with roles, identity, and stigma; and acquisition of information about the health care system and finances (Oberst & James, 1985). A few well-planned home visits provided at the most critical periods, immediately after hospital discharge and 30 to 60 days later, may greatly improve the postdischarge recovery trajectory for both patients and family caregivers.

Hospital-to-home transition systems are in a critical state of change (Wood, 1985). As hospitals progress toward early discharge of patients who require complex care, home care agencies are admitting more acutely ill patients. The importance of continuity of care increases as the complexity of home care increases, because lack of continuity is more likely to have a deleterious effect on patient outcomes with more complex care. As these system changes occur, it is recommended that investigators examine the role of the discharge planner within various transition systems and the impact of the role of continuity of care and patient outcomes.

THE DISCHARGE PLANNING PROCESS

The Discharge Planning Team

For discharge planning to be successful for the patient with cancer, a multidisciplinary team is needed (Table 68–1). The most important member of the team changes, depending on each patient's particular problem or need. For the hematology patient who needs frequent transfusions, the social worker may be the team member who interacts the most with the patient, arranging for transportation. For a surgical patient recovering from abdominal surgery with nutritional deficits, the dietitian may be the team member most involved.

One effective way to coordinate discharge plans is for the team to hold discharge planning rounds or discharge planning conferences once a week at a specified time. These meetings must be well structured, with the discharge planning nurse acting as coordinator. The discharge planning team should agree on what information should be given, and the team should provide that information as succinctly as possible. The team may elect to discuss only those patients who will be discharged in the coming week. However, because the date of the patient's discharge is not always known, it is dangerous to exclude any patient from discussion. Continuity of care is jeopardized when a patient's needs have not been addressed before an unanticipated discharge.

Information exchanged in the discharge planning conference includes the patient's name, room number, diagnosis, treatment plan, family and psychosocial resources, expected discharge date, and continued care needs. The discussion of each discipline represented at the conference should focus on the patient's continued care needs and should explain the role of each discipline in following up on identified problems during the posthospitalization period.

Table 68–1. DISCHARGE PLANNING TEAM RESPONSIBILITIES

Role	Responsibility
Physician	Establishes a medical plan (Marcus, 1987).
Staff Nurse	Communicates the collaborative plan of care to the multidisciplinary team; ensures that the patient has received discharge instructions (Connolly, 1981; Knight, 1985; Romano, 1984).
Social Worker	Presents information on the patient's psychosocial makeup and family's resources; assesses the patient's value system and offers advice on community programs and support groups for physical care, psychological assistance, or both.
Dietitian	Monitors pre- and postoperation diet, weight, protein, serum albumin, enteral nutrition regime; designs and individualizes a diet plan (e.g., for dysphagia, physical changes, anorexia, side effects of chemotherapy, radiation therapy, and disease process).
Pharmacist	Provides information on drugs; participates in plans for hospital and home hyperalimentation, enteral nutrition, and parenteral analgesia; provides community or home care pharmacy continuity on hyperalimentation additives and lipids under the direction of a physician.
Discharge Planner	Moves the patient from the hospital to the community with little disruption; ensures continuity in the quality of care in the community; coordinates and collaborates with the multidisciplinary team to bridge distance and community services; plans, intervenes in, and evaluates the patient's care, based on a good understanding of the patient's needs; counsels, interprets available financial resources, solves problems, and sets priorities; implements the discharge plan (City of Hope, 1987).
Physical Therapist	Provides information on the strength of the patient's lower extremities; recommends safety devices needed at home; writes a plan for continuity of care if the patient will be seeing a therapist in the community (e.g., amputation, with use of prosthesis).
Occupational Therapist	Provides information on the strength of the patient's upper extremities; recommends safety devices for the bathroom and kitchen; instructs in swallowing training after debilitating head and neck surgery; writes a plan for continuity of care if the patient is to be followed in the community.
Speech Therapist	Works with patients who have had head and neck surgery and have had alterations in their patterns of speech.

It is important that every discipline be represented at the discharge planning conference, but the most important participant is the staff nurse who will be working with the patient (Connolly, 1981). The conference should be held at a time and place that will allow the nurse, or a representative of the nurse from the unit, to attend. Because the staff nurse is responsible for preparing the patient to go home, this nurse must know what has been discussed at the discharge planning meeting. As the discharge plan is developed during the patient's hospitalization, it is the responsibility of the staff nurse and the discharge planner to record the plan on the patient's Kardex or care plan, which allows all shifts of nurses who care for the patient to be oriented to the discharge needs of the patient.

The discharge planning conference should not be used as a patient care conference and should last no longer than 1 hour. If the meetings are longer, extraneous information is introduced and team members will need to leave and not be committed to attending the meetings. Patient care conferences should be held separately but may include the discharge planning needs of a particular patient.

At a patient care conference the focus is on the hospitalized patient and the plan of care for that patient. The conference may center on problems that the nursing staff and others have encountered in meeting goals set for the patient. This is usually an informal meeting of the personnel who deal directly with the patient. At the discharge planning conference, responsibility for planning ways to meet a patient's specific needs may be assigned to the appropriate team member. An example of this may be planning how to accomplish payment for a prosthetic limb. If the rehabilitation department is handling these matters, the social worker may not have to be involved. However, if this need is not being addressed, the social worker must help locate financial assistance. With good communication and succinct information, the discharge planning conference allows a coordinated plan to develop. A good plan clarifies the responsibility of each member, hence decreasing the likelihood of confusion and increasing the team's coordination and goal orientation in helping the patient leave the hospital. It is a recognized fact that nurses have an advocacy role in the health care of patients (*Koenigner v. Eckrich,* 1988). Nurses have a duty to attempt to delay a patient's discharge if the patient's condition warrants continued hospitalization.

Case Study

J. B. was prepared to be discharged on the weekend after a lengthy recovery period from major head and neck surgery. J. B.'s disabilities included a tracheostomy with a communicating salivary-to-skin fistula. Flap closure failure had produced a neck wound that was open and deep, necessitating carotid precautions. J. B.'s wife had begun to learn the wound care of the neck and was to have been the caretaker under the supervision of a home care nurse. J. B.'s wife displayed anxiety during the teaching sessions with the nurse, many times not arriving at all for the teaching session. At other times she voiced disgust and dismay at the responsibility; however, because there was no other identified caregiver, plans proceeded for J. B.'s wife to assume this responsibility at discharge. On Saturday, the identified discharge day, J. B.'s wife never arrived to pick him up to transport him home. Instead, she had taken her children and moved out of the home. J. B. was upset and wanted desperately to leave the hospital, but

because of the wound placement it was felt that this was an unsafe plan. Even though, by utilization review standards, payment may have been cut off, the nurses could not allow this patient to leave the hospital.

It is important to recognize that the discharge plan concerns not only the patient, but also the family and outside regulators. The development of a properly balanced plan must be suitable to all concerned.

The Discharge Plan

Assessment of Patient Needs

The chronic aspects of cancer (McCorkle & Germino, 1984), the use of high-technology treatments (Holmes, 1985; Hughes et al., 1985; Knollmueller, 1985; Louden, 1985; Millman, 1985; Sumser, 1985; Turner, 1985), and the rise of hospital costs (Halamandaris, 1984) have resulted in the expeditious discharge of patients with complex posthospitalization care requirements (Rogatz, 1983, 1985). These requirements include peripheral and central intravenous lines to administer fluids, chemotherapy, antibiotic therapy, analgesics, and parenteral nutrition; daily intravenous catheter and surgical wound dressings and enteral nutrition administration; power spray administration; and daily management of ostomies, radiation and chemotherapy side effects (such as nausea, vomiting, and skin desquamation), and complications from disease and treatment.

The increased use of high-technology posthospitalization cancer care requirements has been identified in anecdotal reports and small-scale studies. In Pennsylvania, visiting nurses provide skilled nursing care for hyperalimentation in the home; intravenous therapy, such as parenteral fluid administration for dehydrated patients; and chemotherapy in the hospital environment (Hunter & Johnson, 1980). In Seattle, visiting nurse services include complex skilled nursing care provided by oncology clinical specialists shortly after diagnosis, during and after treatment, and in the terminal stage (McCorkle & Germino, 1984). Other studies report needs for special equipment and pain management, sleep and elimination management, ostomy care, nutritional supplementation, radiation and chemotherapy preparation, side effects management, catheter care, injections, nasogastric tube care, dressing changes, and blood sample collection (Googe & Varricchio, 1981; May et al., 1982; Oleske, Hauck, & Heide, 1983).

Assessment of the complex posthospitalization needs of patients is most successful if done by an experienced oncology nurse. Although it is a multidisciplinary team that creates the plan, it is the discharge planner who has primary responsibility for orchestrating the patient's exit from the hospital. By basing the discharge plan on outcome criteria (what the patient is able to do) rather than on process criteria (what the nurse tells the patient), the nurse can better prepare the patient to continue care after discharge from the hospital (Mezzanotte, 1980).

All patients should be evaluated for discharge needs. The level of the patient's disease will have an impact on the complexity of the discharge plan. A patient who is discharged after a local excision of a melanoma may only require instruction on the care of the wound site, activity level, and in some cases, life-style changes. On the other hand, a new laryngectomy patient will require, in addition to the aforementioned instructions, teaching on complex procedures, such as how to suction and how to change the laryngectomy tube. Further, the patient will need to learn how to care for a suction machine at home.

Patients should be assessed using patient criteria as discussed in the section on quality assessment later. If any biopsychosocial problems exist, the patient must be evaluated for a discharge plan that is sensitive to that patient's individualized needs. Biologic problems that should be evaluated in the cancer patient can include alterations in comfort, such as chills, conjunctivitis, photophobia, diarrhea, fever, nausea and vomiting, and pruritus. Additional biologic problems are weight gain or loss, bowel and bladder dysfunction, self-care limitations, and functional limitations, as well as the cleansing, packing, and dressing of body cavities and wounds. Psychosocial problems that require assessment and planning for discharge can include anxiety, depression, family responsibilities, financial concerns, and transportation needs.

Complex nursing needs can result from any of the previously mentioned problems. Patients may need to be discharged from the hospital with leaking fistulas, nephrostomy tubes, biliary stints, and drainage tubes. Careful evaluation must be made regarding the patient's ability to handle this type of care. In some cases, it will be impossible for the patient to perform the procedure because of the placement of the drains and tubes. A caretaker must be identified and then trained by the nursing staff. If a caretaker is not available, alternative arrangements need to be made, such as referral to a home care agency. A home health referral may be required to continue the teaching of a caretaker or the patient. With the proliferation of home care providers, the discharge planner may have a variety of options in assisting a cancer patient to go home. Alternatives must be explored carefully, taking into consideration the patient's insurance coverage for services at home, his or her ability to pay for services and supplies, and the ability of the agency or pharmacy to coordinate its services with those of the hospital. Many home care agencies and pharmacies have contracted services from each other, making the services more specific to the needs of the patient. Patients who require the services of home care agencies and pharmacies are those receiving posthospitalization hyperalimentation, enteral nutrition, or antibiotic therapy.

Assessment of Caregiver Needs

More and more family members or significant others are being called on to perform health care skills of a complex nature. Patients who may have once been independent now must rely on a caregiver. Feelings of depression, anger, and withdrawal are not uncommon. The patient's resentment of this dependence may be projected onto the loved ones or caregivers. In addition to the change in family relationships, the caregiver may have to adjust to around-the-clock responsibility. Will the loved one or significant other be able to handle this stress? What about a potential patient crisis? Even if the caregiver has been instructed well, the feeling of responsibility can be overwhelming (Feuer, 1987).

The discharge planner must discuss all aspects of the patient's care with the primary caregiver. Home caregivers must know what to expect given the patient's condition, as well as what specific treatments and procedures need to be done. A supportive working environment can be created with the caregiver by providing names and phone numbers of community services that might assist the patient at home. A home care agency referral may be appropriate to facilitate the transition between hospital and home. Also, it is important for home caregivers to be prepared for their own feelings of depression and hostility that can develop as time wears on and the patient's needs are constantly placed before the caregiver's needs. Feuer (1987) has developed a list of key issues and questions to be addressed by the discharge planner in assessing home caregiver needs (Table 68–2).

Congruity Between Patient and Professional Goals

Exploring the values of the patient and any family member close to the patient is of prime importance when the discharge plan is being formulated. Each person, both health care professional and patient, has

---

Table 68–2. ISSUES TO BE ADDRESSED WITH THE HOME CAREGIVER

- Age
- Mental and physical condition in relationship to responsibility
- Living accommodations
- Relief time
- Patient's medical condition
- Instructions on administering medications and watching for side effects
- Expected course of treatment
- Anticipated changes in patient's condition
- Name of physician directing home care plan
- Name of agency providing care (i.e., home care agency, infusion company)
- Name of company providing medical equipment
- List of telephone numbers (e.g., emergency, physician, home care agency, equipment supplier, family members)
- Follow-up appointments for patient
- Functional abilities and disabilities
- Funds for filling prescriptions
- Questions regarding financial matters and home care needs
- Person to notify if caregiver can no longer provide care
- Medications that must be given in the first 24 hours
- Appropriate support groups in the community
- Discharge planner's name and phone number
- Educational material regarding patient's diagnosis
- Questions regarding any problems

(Developed by Feuer, L. C. [1987]. Discharge planning: Home caregivers need your support, too. *Nursing Management, 18*(4), 58–59.)

personal and cultural values. It is important that the discharge plan center around the patient's values, not those of the professional or the institution. The values of the patient, professional, and institution may sometimes conflict with one another. When conflict occurs, a realistic plan is needed that considers institutional constraints as well as the safety and care of the patient. The discharge planner and the multidisciplinary team must choose the plan that will work best for all parties concerned (Blumenfield & Lowe, 1987).

Discharge planning for the terminally ill can be an unhappy occasion for everyone concerned when it involves the transfer of a patient who is awaiting death. Families become upset by the need to focus their attention on suitable arrangements for care, rather than on the dying person (Lind, 1984). Families are made to feel that the·health care system is only interested in making money. Often, a close relationship has developed among the physician, the family, and the patient. A change to a lower level of care can be particularly devastating for all involved. For the patient and family, it may mean the loss of the physician who has seen the patient through the course of the illness. For the physician, it may be painful to witness the patient's transition to terminal care.

In the practice of oncology nursing, conflicting needs are encountered frequently. A patient may refuse to accept a deterioration in condition and may refuse to be discharged to a lower level of care. A patient may refuse to go to a skilled nursing facility but want, instead, to return to a less than adequate living environment. Family members may understand the importance of home health care and may need the reinforcement and support of outside professionals, yet the patient may refuse to have strangers in the home. When conflict occurs, it is necessary to gather pertinent information from the weekly discharge planning conferences and patient and family conferences. Compromises by all parties may be required as a way out of the dilemma. If a patient experiences a measure of control in the development of the discharge plan, then the patient may be motivated to make it a success. However, there will be times when a discharge planner will have doubts about the outcome of a plan. The discharge planner and other team members should take pride in the fact that the best was done with the resources available to them and to the patient (Blumenfield & Lowe, 1987).

COORDINATION OF CARE WITH HEALTH PROFESSIONALS OUTSIDE THE HOSPITAL

For a discharge planner to be successful, continuous contact with the community is critical. This process allows the discharge planning nurse to know what resources and services are available and to choose the most appropriate for each patient. Community programs may include home care agencies, support groups, homemaker services, nutritional services, hospices, or clinic-based services. Problems that require management include lack of psychological support, anorexia, nausea and vomiting, stomatitis, constipation, diarrhea, alopecia, impaired mobility, pain, and wound care (Brown, Kiss, Outlaw, & Viamontes, 1986).

The appropriateness of a clinic-based service is dependent on the client's needs and the goals of the care plan (Elkins, 1984). Patients can benefit from sharing problems, providing mutual support, and learning from one another. Usually, oncology clinics are part of a major cancer center, or they can be part of an oncologist's private practice.

Home care for the homebound patient can be offered in conjunction with clinic services. Those patients eligible for home care require intermittent services and cannot leave their home without a great deal of difficulty. Programs vary regarding the services that are offered and the payment that is required. Therefore, it is important for the discharge planner to know the agency that is accepting the patient for care and to know that the agency understands all the patient's needs. Extended hours of nursing care may be required for support of the terminally ill or as respite for the caregivers. Many home care agencies now offer extended hours of care as well as intermittent care.

Hospice care is characterized by care of the terminally ill patient at home with medical, nursing, psychosocial, and spiritual support. The care given is symptom management, both physical and emotional. This service is available 24 hours a day, 7 days a week, and emphasizes the quality of life for both patient and family. A team approach is used to provide care. Specially trained volunteers are used to provide support. The bereaved family is supported after the patient dies (Elkins, 1984).

Some patients may require skilled nursing care in a nursing home. It is important that the discharge planner closely evaluate the level of care the nursing home can provide before transferring the patient. A complete report of the patient's care needs and goals must be well understood *before* the patient is discharged from the acute care setting. Patients can have widely diverse skilled nursing needs and physical care requirements. Not all skilled nursing facilities are equipped to care for patients with cancer; therefore, careful evaluation is in the best interest of the patient.

Coordination of the discharge plan with other agencies and resources is usually the responsibility of the discharge planning nurse. The discharge planner makes sure that the plan is complete and that all aspects of the plan are conveyed to the responsible parties outside of the hospital. Good communication is the only way to implement a discharge plan properly.

The goal of discharge planning is to move patients from one hospital to another or from the hospital to the community with as much continuity of care and as little disruption as possible. At the time of discharge, information should be recorded on a patient transfer and referral form. Information on this form includes data related to demographics, transition process, and medical care. Demographic information includes name, sex, marital status, religion, address, birth date, and age. Transition information includes hospital number; hospital admission date; hospital discharge date; type of transportation; insurance information; social security number (or other identifying information); nearest relatives or friends and their addresses and phone numbers; physician in charge of the patient's care along with his or her address and phone number; physician who will be caring for the patient in the transferring facility; names of recent nursing home, home care agency, or acute care hospital (give dates of care, if known); agency transferred to; agency transferred from; possessions that accompany the patient; languages spoken and understood; and time of the last meal. Medical care information includes primary diagnosis; secondary diagnosis; rehabilitation potential; medical orders for continued care, including medications, treatments, diet, activities, and procedures to be taught; home health services needed and how often needed; level of self-care; pressure areas or decubitus ulcers; current medications; a report by the hospital nurse; and a report by the multidisciplinary team, if appropriate. Appendix 68–1 is a sample form used by the City of Hope National Medical Center.

In addition to sending a written record of the patient's present care plan, a telephone call to the referral hospital or agency does much to ensure continuity and timely follow-up. If the patient is being transferred to a nursing home or home health agency, it is important to inform the facility or agency of the long-term goals for the patient. If the patient is being transferred to another hospital for continued cancer treatment, it is important to communicate both past medical information and present treatment modalities to the receiving institution. This process needs to take place from physician to physician and from nurse to nurse. If it is not possible to talk to a nurse at the accepting hospital because a bed assignment has not been made, the information can be given to the admitting office, or the name and telephone number of the person completing the transfer form can be left with instructions to call. Because a written record does take time to get to a home health agency or other community program, it is important that all information be communicated by phone with the written record following close behind or faxed.

QUALITY ASSESSMENT AND DISCHARGE PLANNING

Criteria must be established and used by the discharge planner and multidisciplinary team to ensure a quality program. Patients who meet any one of the established discharge planning criteria should be assessed by the multidisciplinary team. Criteria can be clustered in four categories: diagnostic, psychosocial, teaching needs, and physical functional limitations (Table 68–3). The City of Hope National Medical Center Discharge Planning Quality Assessment Worksheet is an example of this discharge planning criteria (Appendix 68–2). Once the plan has been established, based on the patient's needs, the discharge planner should

Table 68–3. DISCHARGE PLANNING CRITERIA

Diagnosis	Psychosocial	Special Teaching Needs	Physical or Functional Limitations
Metastatic disease End-stage disease Extensive head and neck cancer Congestive heart failure or chronic obstructive pulmonary disease in addition to cancer New amputation Leukemia or lymphoma Any surgical procedure Bowel obstruction Multiple myeloma	Altered body image Older than 65 yr Living alone No support system Poor coping skills Limited economic resources Currently seen by home health care agency or transferred from extended care facility	Tracheostomy Feeding tube Oxygen Ostomies Drains (e.g., T tube, nephrostomy, Foley catheter) Open wounds or decubitus ulcers New right atrial catheter Complex medication regime Total parenteral nutrition Chemotherapy Nutrition	Need for rehabilitative service (e.g., of occupational therapist, registered physical therapist, speech therapist) Bowel or bladder problems Mental confusion Pain Poor nutrition Need for durable medical equipment

refer the patient to appropriate community resources when acute level of care is no longer needed.

Evaluating the outcome of the patient's discharge plan should be a part of the discharge planning department's quality assurance program. There are different ways of ensuring the effectiveness of the discharge plan. Sometimes a phone call to the patient several days after discharge can be made to assess compliance or to reinforce teaching that was done in the hospital. A phone call to the referral agency will give the discharge planner information on the effectiveness of the discharge plan. Contacting the private physician or clinic that is managing the follow-up will reveal whether the physician feels the patient's needs at home are being met (Kanar, 1987).

In addition to the aforementioned measures, another good way to evaluate the overall discharge planning program in the hospital objectively is to track admissions and flag all cases that are readmitted for the same problem. On an intermittent basis, these charts can be reviewed by the multidisciplinary team, and a judgment can be made on the quality, appropriateness, and resolution of the problems identified during the discharge planning process.

Charts of patients readmitted to the hospital within 15 days of discharge can be reviewed for appropriateness of discharge management, medical stability at time of discharge, and quality of the hospital care provided. This peer review can be done on a monthly basis, using a multidisciplinary approach. A review worksheet, similar to the one in Appendix 68–2, can be completed by the team member on each chart reviewed. The findings from these chart reviews can be compiled by the department director, who is responsible for the overall management of the discharge planning program. The findings should be analyzed and reported to the quality assurance committee as well as to the chairperson of the utilization review committee. The department responsible for the discharge plan can then identify weaknessness in its plan, the departments involved, the action taken, and the resolution of those problems.

Discharge planning is a function that involves all of the patient care departments. The assessment of discharge planning outcomes must include all disciplines involved and must have the support of those individuals who head those departments. With cooperation comes a commitment from all patient care departments to provide the best possible discharge planning for patients.

References

Blumenfield, S., & Lowe, J. I. (1987). A template for analyzing ethical dilemmas in discharge planning. *Health and Social Work, 12,* 47–56.

Brown, M. H., Kiss, M. E., Outlaw, E. M., & Viamontes, C. M. (1986). *Standards of oncology nursing practice.* New York: John Wiley and Sons.

City of Hope National Medical Center. (1987). *Position description.* Duarte, CA: Author.

Connolly, M. L. (1981). Organize your workday for more effective discharge planning. *Nursing, 11*(7), 44–47.

Coulton, C. J., Dunkle, R. E., Goode, R. A., & MacKintosh, J. (1982). Discharge planning and decision making. *Health and Social Work, 7,* 253–261.

Dwyer, J. E., & Held, D. M. (1982). Home management of the adult patient with leukemia. *Nursing Clinics of North America, 17,* 665–675.

Elkins, C. P. (1984). Part III: Approaches in implementing community health nursing services. *Community health nursing skills and strategies* (pp. 231–279). Bowie, MD: Robert J Brady Co.

Feuer, L. C. (1987). Discharge planning: Home caregivers need your support, too. *Nursing Management, 18*(4), 58–59.

Googe, M. C., & Varricchio, C. G. (1981). A pilot investigation of home health care needs of cancer patients and their families. *Oncology Nursing Forum, 8*(4), 24–28.

Halamandaris, V. J. (1984). President's page. *Caring, 3,* 112.

Henry, R., & Subcommittee on Discharge Planning, Southern California Chapter of the Society for Hospital Work Directors. (1981). *Status of discharge planning in southern California.* Unpublished report.

Holmes, W. (1985). Subcutaneous chemotherapy at home. *American Journal of Nursing, 85,* 168–169.

Hughes, C., Knapp, J., & Redden, C. (1985). Caring for ventilation dependent patients. *Caring, 4,* 4–6.

Hunter, G., & Johnson, S. H. (1980). Physical support systems for the homebound oncology patient. *Oncology Nursing Forum, 7*(3), 21–23.

Kanar, R. J. (1987). Standards of nursing practice assessed through the application of the nursing process. *Journal of Nursing Quality Assurance, 1*(2), 72–78.

Knight, C. (1985). Staff nurses doing discharge planning—but they need help. *Journal of Nursing Administration, 15*(12), 15, 30, 37.

Knollmueller, R. N. (1985). The growth and development of home care: From no-tech to high tech. *Caring, 4,* 3–4, 6–8.

Koenigner v. Eckrich, 422 N. W. 2d 600, S. D. (1988).

Lind, S. E. (1984). Transferring the terminally ill. *New England Journal of Medicine, 311,* 1181–1182.

Louden, T. L. (1985). Planning your niche in the "high tech" home care market. *Caring, 4,* 21–22, 24–25.

Marcus, L. J. (1987). Discharge planning: An organizational perspective. *Health and Social Work, 12,* 39–46.

May, D. M., Oleske, D., Justo-Ober, P. K., & Heide, E. (1982). The role of the area-wide oncology nurse coordinator in the home care of cancer patients. *Oncology Nursing Forum, 9*(4), 39–43.

McCorkle, R., & Germino, B. (1984). What nurses need to know about home care. *Oncology Nursing Forum, 11*(6), 63–69.

Mezzanotte, E. J. (1980). A checklist for better discharge planning. *Nursing, 10*(11), 64.

Millman, D. S. (1985). Advances in medical technology: Legal problems and approaches . . . Health care financing administration. *Caring, 4,* 11–12, 14, 16–18.

Northhouse, L. (1984). The impact of cancer on the family: An overview. *International Journal of Psychiatry in Medicine, 14*(3), 87–114.

Oberst, M. T., & James, R. H. (1985, April). Going home: Patient and spouse adjustment following cancer surgery. *Topics in Clinical Nursing,* pp. 46–57.

Oleske, D., Hauck, W., & Heide, E. (1983). Characteristics of cancer patient referrals to home care: A regional perspective. *American Journal of Public Health, 73,* 678–682.

Rogatz, P. (1983). What's behind the changes in today's hospital service? *Trustee, 36,* 17–19.

Rogatz, P. (1985). Home health care: Some social and economic considerations. *Home Health Care Nurse, 3,* 38–43.

Romano, C. A. (1984). A computerized approach to discharge care planning. *Nursing Outlook, 32,* 23–25.

Rossen, S. (1984). Adapting discharge planning to prospective pricing. Prompting efficient use of resources and enhancing continuity of care. *Hospitals, 58*(5), 71, 75, 79.

Shine, M. S. (1983). Discharge planning for the elderly patient in the acute care setting. *Nursing Clinics of North America, 18,* 403–410.

Sumser, S. S. (1985). Creating a safe environment for high tech home care. *Caring, 4,* 47–50.

Tatge, M. (1984). Home care agency adjusts to competing interests of hospitals. *Modern Health Care, 14,* 31–34, 38.

Tornberg, M. J., McGrath, B. B., & Benoliel, J. Q. (1984). Oncology transition services: Partnerships of nurses and families. *Cancer Nursing, 7,* 131–137.

Tulga, G. (1981). A community approach to cancer control. Bridging the gap between hospital and home. *Family Community Health, 4,* 57–60.

Turner, N. C. (1985). Nutritional support at home: Parenteral and enteral hyperalimention. *Caring, 3*(11), 21–22.

Wood, J. B. (1985). Home care agencies and health care competition. *Home Health Care Nurse, 3,* 22–24.

ADMINISTRATIVE INFORMATION

Patient			Sex	Marital Status S M W D SEP	Relig.

Address			City		Phone

Birth Date	Age	Hosp. No.	Adm. Date	Disch. Date	Type of Transportation ☐ Amb. ☐ Other

Medicare No. | Soc. Security No.
Medi-Cal No. | Other (Identify)

Nearest Relative or Friend/Address | Relationship | Phone | Home | Bus.

Physician in Charge at Time of Transfer or Discharge | Address | Phone

Will this Physician Continue to Care for Patient? ☐ Yes ☐ No
If No, Physician for Continued Care | Address | Phone

Name of Prior Nursing Home, Hospital, or Home Health Service. If Known, Include Admission and Discharge Date(s)

MEDICAL INFORMATION

Report of Physician: Include Surgical Procedures and Dates

Primary Diagnosis (Onset)

Secondary Diagnosis (Onset)

Rehab. Potential
Patient Knows Diagnosis and Prognosis ☐ Yes ☐ No

Medical Orders for Continued Care: Include Medications, Treatments, Diet, Activities and Procedures to Be Taught, Home Health Services/Frequency.

_____   _____
Date   Physician Signature

Transferred to | Address | Phone

Transferred from | Address | Phone | Discharge Coordinator

NURSING INFORMATION

	Indep.	Assist.	Unable		Usually	Occ.	Rarely
Bathe				Able to Communicate			
Dress				Motivated to Self Care			
Eating				Follows Directions			
Personal Hygiene				Bowel Control (Date Last BM)			
Transfers				Bladder Control (Date Cath. Inserted)			
Ambulate				Restraints			

Amb Cane ☐ Crutch ☐ Walker ☐ Alert ☐ Confused ☐ Forgetful ☐ Noisy ☐ Wanders ☐

Pressure Areas (Describe)

Decubitus Ulcers

Languages Spoken and Understood

Equipment & Supplies (Indicate)   Diet   Time of Previous Meal
Sent with Patient ☐ Needed ☐

Patient Possessions Transferred (Dentures, Hearing Aid, Glasses, Money, Prosthesis, Jewelry, Other Valuables) | Current Medications. Include Date and Time Last Dose

Report of Hospital Nurse: (Allergies, Observations, Instructions Given, Continuing Teaching Needed, Unique Approaches Used, Nursing Care Plan, Goals)

_____
Date   Signature   R.N.

OTHER PERTINENT INFORMATION (Therapists, Dietitian, Social Service, etc.)

_____
Date   Signature   Phone

_____
                                                             Phone

ADDITIONAL NURSING CARE INFORMATION

REHABILITATION INFORMATION	SOCIAL INFORMATION
(adjustment to disability, motivation for self-care, special equipment needs, rehabilitation potential, etc.)	(family/other support systems, socializing ability, financial problems, emotional status, etc.)

APPENDIX 68–2

DISCHARGE PLANNING DEPARTMENT QUALITY ASSURANCE WORKSHEET
READMISSIONS WITHIN 15 DAYS OF DISCHARGE

Total Admissions	Yes	No
Readmitted Within 15 Days of Discharge	Yes	No
Length of Stay	Yes	No
Surgical Procedures Performed	Yes	No
Abnormal Lab Results	Yes	No
Abnormal Lab Results Not Addressed in Progress Record	Yes	No
Wound Drainage Present	Yes	No
Seen by Rehabilitation	Yes	No
Rehabilitation Follow-Up Plan	Yes	No
Rehabilitation Discharge Follow-Up	Yes	No
Seen by Dietitian	Yes	No
Dietary Follow-Up Plan	Yes	No
Dietary Discharge Follow-Up	Yes	No
Seen by Social Service	Yes	No
Social Service Follow-Up Plan	Yes	No
Social Service Discharge Plan	Yes	No
Seen by Discharge Planning	Yes	No
Discharge Planning Follow-Up Plan	Yes	No
Discharge Follow-Up Needed	Yes	No
Discharge Vital Signs Recorded	Yes	No
Temperature Over 38° C on Day of Discharge	Yes	No
Pulse Over 120 or Less Than 50 on Day of Discharge	Yes	No
Systolic BP on Day Before or Day of Discharge = <85 or >175	Yes	No
Diastolic BP on Day Before or Day of Discharge = <50 or >110	Yes	No
IV Medications Day of Discharge	Yes	No
IV's Day of Discharge	Yes	No
Wound Drainage Documented	Yes	No
Present 48 Hours Prior to Discharge	Yes	No
Any Change at Time of Discharge	Yes	No
Teaching Needs Identified	Yes	No
Person To Be Taught Identified	Yes	No
Evaluation of Teaching	Yes	No
Patient Level of Independence Apparent	Yes	No
Discharge Instructions Written	Yes	No
Discharge Instructions Legible	Yes	No
Discharge Instructions Complete	Yes	No
Discharge Instructions Appropriate	Yes	No
Could Readmission Have Been Prevented	Yes	No
Service Discharging Patient	Yes	No

CHAPTER 69

Ambulatory Care Services

BARBARA A. FARLEY

HISTORICAL PERSPECTIVE

Ambulatory oncology care, as it is known today, has been slow in emerging as a distinct specialty area. Before the mid 1970s, most "clinic" nurses were seen and utilized as assistants to physicians and coordinators of patient flow. Patients came to the clinic or physician's office for evaluation of initial symptoms and for postoperative follow-up, such as suture removal, dressing changes, and the like, but the bulk of care was delivered on an inpatient basis.

Evolution as a Distinct Area of Health Care

There are several reasons why ambulatory care was seen as the stepchild of health care and nonessential. The period from post–World War II through the mid 1970s was a period of uninterrupted growth in health care facilities, mainly inpatient facilities. Bed shortages were nonexistent. Consequently, little incentive existed to look for alternate care delivery sites. In addition, inpatient care was generally covered by insurance, whereas ambulatory care often was not. In oncology the scientific advancements that led to a new specialty—medical oncology—did not provide major treatment options outside of research settings until the publication of the article by DeVita and colleagues (1970) on combination chemotherapy. Following that landmark publication, the world of cancer care saw the

rapid emergence of medical oncologic expertise and the use of multimodality therapy. Technical advances to complement this scientific explosion began to emerge also, such as autoinfusion pumps and various venous access devices.

This same time period was also the beginning of consumer awareness in health care. Although the 1960s are generally accepted as the beginning of the consumer movement, it was in the 1970s that the consumer movement had its greatest impact on oncology care. Public involvement in the issues surrounding death and dying broadened gradually to encompass quality of life in all stages of illness. The person with cancer became acutely aware of that precious item called time. When faced with the possibility of decreased quantity of time, quality of time became essential. Cancer patients and their families forced the development of alternatives to hospitalization to help them maximize the quality of their remaining time together.

The scientific and technical advances combined with the consumer demands of the 1970s were major influences on the development of ambulatory care as a distinct component of oncology health care. By the late 1970s, the American Hospital Association statistics showed that bed occupancy rates in hospitals were falling, whereas the number of ambulatory visits was starting to climb (Aiken, 1977). The impact of these advances on oncology care and oncology nursing has been profound. The entire March 1980 issue of *Seminars in Oncology* documents this fact with remarkable clarity. This issue described the evolution and nature of a wide variety of nursing roles in cancer care and research. In cancer centers throughout the country, ambulatory services gradually shifted focus from primarily surgical follow-up visits, and expanded to include medical oncology programs. With increasing oncology nursing skill available, the safe delivery of complex chemotherapy also moved to these settings. Several models of ambulatory oncology care began to appear.

Development of Ambulatory Settings

One response to alternative care delivery has been regional oncology centers. Isler (1977) described a regional ambulatory cancer center in Boise, Idaho, that was established in 1968. The center provided multidisciplinary expertise to patients and their families that included evaluation, therapeutic recommendations, as well as actual delivery of cancer therapy. The regional center was able to centralize high-quality care until patients could be referred back to their home communities—some as far as 150 miles away (Isler, 1977). The regional centers served also as a resource to health professionals in the area. The 1980's version of the early regional programs was described in a 1985 issue of *Hospitals*. Several companies, such as Salick Health Care, Inc., and others, are developing networks of outpatient cancer centers that will offer a full range of cancer care, including cancer screening, diagnostic work-up, outpatient surgery, chemotherapy, radiation, rehabilitation therapy, immunotherapy, as well as patient education and counseling. The networks will also link the oncology centers to tertiary care facilities ("Management Rounds," 1985). This decade has seen ambulatory cancer care come of age; it has also seen it become big business.

In 1979 Memorial Sloan-Kettering Cancer Center published an article about treating adolescent patients with osteogenic sarcoma using aggressive chemotherapy in a day hospital setting. This pediatric ambulatory care program was open from 8 A.M. to 6 P.M., Monday through Friday, and was designed to allow young patients "to live as normal a life as possible" (Nirenberg & Rosen, 1979). The concept of a day hospital was a radical change in the ambulatory practice of the time, and nursing and medical professionals used the model to change ambulatory care delivery in their respective settings around the country. Today, the day hospital concept has been incorporated into many cancer centers and community settings. It is being scrutinized presently for economic feasibility as an alternative to full hospitalization (Clark, 1986). The day hospital raises issues of changing hospital case mix and cost effectiveness, because highly skilled nursing is required. Studies addressing these issues are now emerging. The most recent pilot was a prospective random-assignment trial that compared outcomes for inpatient versus medical adult day hospital (ADH) care. More than 400 patients were randomly assigned to the ADH or the hospital inpatient facility. Medical outcomes, psychosocial results, and cost were evaluated. The study found no difference in therapeutic outcomes for patients assigned to the ADH or the inpatient facility, and there was a high level of patient and family acceptance of the ADH. Cost, however, was shown to be significantly lower in the ADH (Gralla et al., 1987).

Rising hospital costs have certainly influenced a shift toward ambulatory care. One response was the emergence of health maintenance organizations (HMOs). The Health Maintenance Act of 1973 encouraged the establishment of private prepaid health programs. The concept of prepaid medical care first came to the attention of many through the efforts of the industrialist Henry J. Kaiser. Today's HMOs' prepayment mechanisms provide physicians with incentives to manage medical care in a cost-conscious manner. "Research supports the contention that prepaid medical care achieves cost savings by reducing the use of services, particularly hospitalization" (Reisler, 1985). However, this development has raised a new concern. Does cost containment in this setting affect timely access to care for patients with cancer? In a study by Greenwald (1987) of patients with newly diagnosed cancer, findings suggest that patients with copayment policies and those enrolled in HMOs experience more delay in the initiation of treatment than those with fully financed fee-for-service coverage. Because oncology care is both cost and labor intensive, the specialty has presented a challenge to many health maintenance programs. They do provide another option in ambulatory-focused care, however.

An often overlooked ambulatory setting is the physician's office. Understanding the role and contribution of the oncology nurse in an office setting has been slow. This is at least partially caused by limited publication about the private practice setting. However, Schulmeister (1987) has reported that recognition of this role as a distinct subspecialty is increasing. Indeed, *The Role of The Oncology Nurse in the Office Setting* (Baird, Hartigan, & Holton-Smith, 1987) not only is an excellent reference for the office (ambulatory) nurse but also should serve to bridge the informational gap. It is worth noting that office setting issues have been included in the Oncology Nursing Society (ONS) congress programs since 1986. The unique contributions and experience of the office nurse, not infrequently the patient's first contact with health care personnel, will benefit all involved in ambulatory care delivery.

AMBULATORY ONCOLOGY NURSING ROLE DEVELOPMENT

Evolution from Research To University and Community Settings

Oncology nursing as a specialty began in centers dedicated to cancer care. Nurses learned from experience, and early knowledge focused on surgical management and care. With the advent of medical oncology, new nursing knowledge and skill regarding chemotherapy developed rapidly. As described by Henke (1980), the first expanded nursing role in oncology was associated with the development of clinical trials. This nursing role began as data collector, expanded to include skilled administration and monitoring of experimental drugs, and finally included involvement in protocol design. The growth of clinical trials took place in the 1960s and resulted in a unique medical-nursing collaborative practice. As these early medical oncologists left research facilities for community practice, they realized the need for the same skilled nursing knowledge in the community setting. Some physicians took experienced nurses with them, whereas others educated new nurses to care for oncology patients. Thus began the expansion of oncology nursing (see also Chapter 2).

To the surprise of no one, patients and families much prefer to receive care in ambulatory settings and avoid hospitalization. Finding ways of adapting schedules to meet patients' attempts to maintain the most normal life style possible is a deserving challenge for all involved in oncology care. Nursing's response to this has been positive and significant. As nursing knowledge grew, it became possible to administer chemotherapy safely on an outpatient basis. This made ambulatory treatment an option not previously available. That fact, combined with all the reasons stated earlier, resulted in the transference of a major portion of oncology care to the ambulatory setting, and thus began the evolution of the ambulatory oncology nursing role.

Early Expanded Roles

There were two early expanded ambulatory nursing roles that deserve special mention, because in many instances they were pacesetters: the enterostomal therapist and the nurse practitioner.

Enterostomal Therapist

Hilkemeyer (1982) and Jackson (1980) have outlined the development of the enterostomal therapist. Both researchers suggest that the need for this type of patient support dates to 1958 and was initiated by Dr. Rupert Turnbull at the Cleveland Clinic. Although ostomies can result from the treatment of many different diseases, the early surgical treatment of bowel and bladder cancer resulted in large numbers of oncology patients with ostomy care needs. Many nurses at the bedside learned how to care for draining wounds and ostomies from an enterostomal therapy nurse. This group was also instrumental in the development of better products to support care needs. The care of these patients certainly extended beyond hospitalization, and thus the enterostomal therapists found themselves early deliverers of ambulatory care.

Nurse Practitioner

The role of the nurse practitioner in oncology practice is perhaps best known in pediatrics. The role of the adult oncology nurse practitioner is not well doc-

umented. Two early articles described individual accounts of role development (Maxwell, 1979; Van Scoy-Mosher, 1978). These accounts pointed out that the practitioner role crossed inpatient, outpatient, and home settings frequently. However, it is safe to say that the common focal point of practice has been the ambulatory setting. Although the role of the nurse practitioner is acknowledged to be one of the early examples of an expanded nursing role, it is also clear that many ambulatory oncology nurses, with or without practitioner skills, have incorporated many of the advanced role functions first described by practitioners into present practice. These nurses have served as role models for many in ambulatory oncology nursing.

Ambulatory Role Distinction

Who is the ambulatory oncology nurse and how does the ambulatory role differ, if at all, from the role of colleagues in the inpatient and community settings? There are at least three elements that make this role unique: the scope of practice, the ambulatory nurse's role in continuity, and the importance of telephone use in care delivery.

Scope of Practice

By definition, the ambulatory nurse bridges the gap between the acute care setting and the home. To do this effectively requires a broad knowledge base. Ambulatory practice commonly spans care focused on prevention and detection at one end of the spectrum, to symptom management in terminal care at the other. The knowledge base of the nurse must include the following: the pathophysiology and treatment of various cancers, a working knowledge of research application and protocol development, safe chemotherapy administration, management of treatment side effects, symptom control (i.e., pain management), and a working knowledge of both hospital and community resources available. In addition to excellent observational and assessment skills, the ambulatory nurse also must be committed to patient education. The patient and nurse must be partners in developing a self-care plan. To accomplish this, ambulatory patients must know as much as the professional about their cancer and its treatment if they are able and wish to do so; if not, a family member must be educated at this level. The educational process fosters informed self-care, which results in safe care. Patient education is incorporated into every interaction and activity. Other knowledge needs of the ambulatory nurse include nutritional support measures, rehabilitation nursing skills, the ability to assess and work with families, and techniques to provide emotional support. Finally, it is the ability to communicate well with colleagues in other disciplines and with professionals in a variety of settings that allows for effective coordination of the many facets of care required. Skilled interpersonal communication in this role is a must.

The hallmark of an outstanding nurse in any setting

is the ability to anticipate and intervene to avoid unnecessary problems. This is particularly true in ambulatory care. The task is slightly more difficult, however, because contact with the patient is limited. The inpatient nurse has a defined number of days in which to accomplish care goals. Whether that happens to be 2 days or 20 days, it is a definable amount of continuous time. The ambulatory nurse, on the other hand, deals with episodes of care, generally known as visits. Despite preplanning and protocol schema, ambulatory care is unpredictable. High patient acuity, which results in unplanned visits; increasing numbers of patients, which may limit patient-nurse interaction; and even transportation problems frequently combine (often all on the same day) to make goal achievement seem beyond reach. Learning to anticipate in the ambulatory setting must become à finely honed skill. It is a challenge to be sure.

Although many of the nursing skills identified are also necessary in the acute and community settings, it is the in-depth juggling of all on a daily basis that makes ambulatory practice unique. Thus the ideal ambulatory oncology nurse is one who has had the opportunity to work in the acute setting and has acquired knowledge of the major cancers, their treatment, and nursing care required in the acute phase of illness and is ready to build on that base to provide a broader scope of care.

Continuity

In most instances, cancer is a chronic illness with occasional acute episodes. Because of bed and economic constraints, hospital beds are used for only the most acute episodes of illness. This is usually for diagnosis and initial treatment, at the time of recurrence or an oncologic emergency, for complex therapy that cannot be done on an ambulatory basis, and occasionally for death. Consequently, the major portion of treatment is delivered in the ambulatory setting, allowing the ambulatory nurse to follow patients for long periods of time—months or years rather than weeks. This fact gives the ambulatory oncology nurse the opportunity to act as a liaison between hospital and home. Because hospitalization is utilized for acute episodes and home care is often required for limited periods of time, it is the ambulatory nurse who most frequently maintains the continuity with patient and family. When patients are doing well they are still seen for follow-up visits in ambulatory care; if patients relapse or if problems surface, they usually re-enter the system via ambulatory care or a physician's office. This liaison role demands that the ambulatory nurse become an expert communicator. One of the more important nursing role functions is to bridge the information gap for colleagues in the hospital or home care agency when a patient's status changes.

In many teaching and community hospitals the physicians (residents or fellows) rotate frequently, and it is the nurse who often becomes the consistent caretaker. Patients have taught us the importance of continuity in providing care. Although this is a responsibility belonging to nurses in all settings, it is the ambulatory nurse who is best placed to "pull it all together." Consequently, the task of providing continuity of care weighs more heavily on the ambulatory oncology nurse.

Telephone Care

The third unique feature of ambulatory practice is the amount of time spent on the telephone. Little has been written about this important function, but any ambulatory nurse will tell you that the telephone is one of the most, if not the most, important pieces of equipment in ambulatory care. In support of this observation, ambulatory oncology nurses have begun to document relevant issues related to telephone use. A study by Nail and colleagues (1989) on the delivery of nursing care by telephone reported findings on 1844 patient calls over a 6-month period (Box 69–1). Telephone triage in any ambulatory setting is vital. In a published monograph on oncology office practice, Hartigan (1987) outlined this function in detail and stated that "the skills necessary for phone triage include expert assessment, proficient communication (speaking and listening) and phone etiquette." In a university ambulatory setting, Medvec and Calzone (1989) utilized protocols developed by a primary nurse-physician team to handle a nurse-managed telephone triage system. These authors raised several issues regarding telephone care, such as the legalities of telephone advice, adequate documentation, referral support, as well as the positive outcomes relative to patient satisfaction.

No matter how carefully patient and family education is carried out, issues may arise at home that generate questions and increase anxiety. The nurse who answers questions knowledgeably and shares with the patient in decision making is able to diffuse unnecessary fears and, at the same time, anticipate problems and intervene appropriately. Frequently this process limits unnecessary emergency visits to the hospital as well. For example, the patient whose blood counts are about to nadir following chemotherapy and who develops a fever will be advised to come in and be seen, whereas the patient with normal counts whose children have the flu, and who develops muscle aches and a slight fever, will probably be managed by telephone and given reassurance.

The telephone is also used for follow-up. Calling a patient the day after a treatment or a procedure gives the nurse the opportunity not only to reinforce instructions, but also to evaluate the patient's status and suggest appropriate changes. Not infrequently, patients are reluctant to call with questions, even if they have been encouraged to do so. By taking the initiative in this instance, the ambulatory oncology nurse is frequently able to avert problems.

Monitoring symptom control is another area in which the telephone offers major assistance. Coyle and co-workers (1986) described their experience treating patients with chronic pain by utilizing continuous subcutaneous infusions. Treatment was initiated and the drug was titrated while the patient was hospitalized. After discharge, these patients were followed by the supportive care pain management team, which included a nurse clinician in daily telephone contact with the patient or a responsible family member.

It is well known that patients perceive calls from a consistent caretaker to be positive and supportive. Synonyms for the word *support* in the *American Heritage Dictionary* include "uphold," "sustain," "maintain," "advocate," and "champion." Ambulatory oncology patients need all of the aforementioned, but they do not have the consistent presence of a professional available to fill the role. The use of the telephone is the best method of rendering support in its broadest sense. For the patient, it will frequently mean the difference between a night's sleep and no sleep at all.

An additional benefit to using the telephone in ambulatory care is the credibility gained by the nurse. Nurses are seen as valued and knowledgeable members of the team. Another benefit described by Hartigan (1987) is that "patients gain confidence in their self-care abilities by the support they receive during these conversations."

The importance of this often-neglected management tool cannot be overstated. Some researchers have begun to look at the impact that telephone use in ambulatory practice has had on both program productivity and nursing workload (Medvec & Calzone, 1989; Nail et al., 1989). Future studies in this area are critical, because findings have the potential to validate a unique role component and to support the need for additional oncology nursing staff in ambulatory settings.

MODELS OF AMBULATORY CARE DELIVERY

Role Evolution

We have established that the role of the ambulatory oncology nurse, in most cases, did not come packaged as a defined entity but rather has evolved. Knowing that fact, it is easy to understand why there are almost as many models of care delivery as there are care delivery settings. Another fact affecting the nursing role in care delivery is the complexity of care requirements now seen in ambulatory oncology settings.

Care Complexity

Care associated with inpatient settings just a few years ago is now handled routinely in ambulatory care. The availability of venous access devices along with advances in infusion pump technology has facilitated the move to ambulatory care. This technology has made continuous infusion a safe option in the ambulatory setting. The use of this technique to deliver continuous chemotherapy or nutritional support is well documented in the literature (Quebbeman, 1985). A published report regarding the use of ambulatory hepatic artery infusion for liver disease (although still somewhat controversial) is an excellent example of the complexity of care experienced in ambulatory oncology (Thirlwell, 1986). Similarly, an ONS congress abstract described the outpatient management of bone marrow transplant (BMT) patients (Nims, Buchsel, & Jacom, 1985). Delineating the nursing role for the care of these patients was the focus of that abstract.

Drugs, such as etoposide (VP-16) and cisplatin, originally thought to require hospitalization, are now commonly given in ambulatory settings (Brock & Alberts, 1986). It is of interest that at least two medical investigators mention the importance of nursing involvement. Evans (1986) listed "experienced nursing personnel" as one factor necessary for safe care delivery, and Slater and colleagues (1985) spoke to the need for a nursing specialist to be a consistent part of the team. In addition to chemotherapy administration, new approaches to symptom control, such as pain control (previously described), and management of such complications as pleural effusions have also found their way to the ambulatory setting (Avery, 1986).

Multidisciplinary Teams

Given the level of care required by this patient population, it is clear that no one person, or indeed one discipline, can meet all potential needs, even with the help of high-technology devices. To address patient and family needs in the ambulatory setting requires a multidisciplinary team. The composition of the team is not nearly as important as the team's ability to work collaboratively. It is safe to say that in successful settings collaboration and respect among disciplines are earned, although often not easily. Ryan, Edwards, and Rickles (1980) described at length the importance of collaboration and collegial relationships in their article on joint practice. The teams that are successful at achieving true collaborative practice commonly experience role overlap.

There are two additional factors in successful care delivery. First, no matter what the model design, it must include consistency. Ambulatory patients are followed over long periods of time; thus to provide effective, safe, and satisfying care (for patient and caretaker) demands that *someone* be consistent. Second, the model must meet the needs of the particular setting. It is hopeless to attempt adapting a setting to a model; rather, the model should be adapted to the setting.

Although nursing literature on ambulatory care is just coming of age, evidence of ambulatory program and model development dates back to the 1970s (Buchanan, 1977; Kepnes, 1984). Subsequently, Brosnan and Johnston (1980) described a matrix-team concept developed at Children's Hospital of Los Angeles. In this review much attention was focused on the nursing role development. At present, the literature dealing specifically with ambulatory oncology models is sparse. Belis and colleagues (1980) described a primary care model that included nurse practitioners and chemotherapy nurses, as well as representatives from other disciplines. In this model the medical oncologist is responsible for the organization and coordination of all team members. Ryan and co-workers (1980) described a joint practice model between an oncology nurse practitioner and a physician at a Veterans' Administration Center in Connecticut. Farley (1981) described a primary nursing model developed at a university teaching hospital in Boston. Tighe and co-investigators (1985) studied oncology ambulatory nurses and nononcology ambulatory nurses in the same facility to compare role activities of each group.

Primary Nursing

Nursing has struggled long and hard to find a care delivery model that would ensure high-quality care and at the same time allow nurses to realize high levels of professional satisfaction. Primary nursing was developed in the late 1960s in response to staff dissatisfaction and patient complaints resulting from the fragmentation of care inherent in team nursing. Manthey (1980) first described four elements necessary for primary nursing: "allocation and acceptance of individual responsibility for decision-making to one individual; assignments of daily care by case method; direct person-to-person communication; and one person operationally responsible for the quality of care administered to patients (on a unit) twenty-four hours a day, 7 days a week." Since Manthey and the staff at the University of Minnesota first implemented primary nursing on the inpatient units in 1969, the model has been adapted and implemented in many settings, some with success, some without.

Because primary nursing is a professional practice model that "demands accountability for coordinating a comprehensive plan of care that can be constantly reassessed, evaluated, modified, and carried out by a consistent caretaker, it is a care delivery system tailor-made for the cancer patient" (Farley, 1981). However, primary nursing is not without controversy. Although Brown (1985) agrees that primary nursing is the "best approach to providing optimal nursing care currently available," she also states that because of the nature of ambulatory care, it is difficult to implement in that setting. Indeed, we know that today's realities of ambulatory care include high patient to low staff ratios in a sophisticated and complex care environment. Many ask if it is possible to practice primary nursing in ambulatory care. The answer is a firm yes! The following section discusses the practical issues involved.

Elements Necessary to Accomplish Primary Nursing

First, by definition primary nursing requires a decentralized system in which responsibility and authority are given back to the caretaker (primary nurse). This requirement is met easily in ambulatory oncology if staff selection has been done based on role requirements rather than on the old seniority method. Given the nature of ambulatory care today, the nurse in that setting must be qualified to deal with complex care (as described earlier) and also able to function comfortably in an expanded, independent role. With the proper staff in place, management must then give the authority to the staff selected. The manager becomes a facilitator, a resource, a teacher, and a validator of decision making.

Second, other resources must be in place throughout the system for the primary nurse to utilize. Although routinely put in place for inpatient primary nursing practice, they frequently have to be negotiated for availability in ambulatory care. If the ambulatory nurse is expected to deliver comprehensive care and initiate referrals when appropriate, experts must be available for consultation and referrals. Usually this requires negotiation on the part of management and cannot be assumed to exist.

Third, adequate staffing is necessary to provide quality care. The word *adequate* is used deliberately because the "ideal" is a myth almost never obtained, although it must always be the goal. It is rare to find an ambulatory oncology setting in which volumes are not steadily increasing. That fact alone, coupled with the increased acuity of patients, can be used successfully to justify increased staffing. In some settings nursing charges have been negotiated with the hospital administrator and state rate-setting commissions; that income then pays for the additional staff required. To accomplish any staff increase, nursing management must be able to articulate exactly what it is the nurse does. This is often easier in ambulatory practice, in which nurses are running prevention and detection clinics, giving chemotherapy, and performing other complex activities.

Another reality of today's practice in all settings, including ambulatory care, is the possible need to change the staff mix. The old tasks of managing patient flow, assisting physicians, and putting patients in rooms no longer have to be done by a nurse. Well-trained nursing assistants are quite capable of taking over these functions. When increasing staff, decisions must be made concerning whether to add a nurse or a nursing assistant, and what functions the nursing staff is willing to share and supervise. Scheduling, a task long given to clerks on inpatient units, is still done by ambulatory nurses in some settings. Collaboration between nurses and all ancillary personnel will relieve the nurse of many routine tasks and allow concentration on care delivery.

Examples of Primary Nursing

The question as to whether primary nursing can be done in high-volume settings is yes. This affirmation can perhaps best be illustrated by using an actual example—the National Cancer Institute (NCI) ambulatory settings. The NCI has four clinical branches that have established ambulatory care: pediatrics, medical oncology, surgical oncology, and radiation oncology. In addition, the breast clinic, although technically a part of the radiation branch, schedules patients in a separate ambulatory setting 1 day per week. Dermatology is also a separate service with a generally low volume, and immunology schedules oncology patients in the surgical outpatient setting. The patient volume in each area varies considerably. The medicine branch has a high volume: 50 to 70 visits per day, 5 days per week; patients are also scheduled on Saturday and Sunday to cover necessary daily treatment and emergencies. Pediatrics, however, has a low volume, with approximately 20 patients per day, and surgery has a moderate volume, with an average of 30 patients per day.

In discussing the implementation of primary nursing in a high-volume setting, the medicine branch will be used as an example. In 1984, the nursing staff consisted of four R.N.s and two nursing assistants. After a 6-month period of assessment, a fifth R.N. was added. There were two unit clerks to manage appointment scheduling and a stock clerk to order and replenish supplies. Patient acuity was extremely high, as would be true in any major research setting involved in phase I and II trials. It was not uncommon to admit at least two patients a week directly to an intensive care unit from the medicine branch clinic at that point.

The staff in place were trying valiantly to practice primary nursing, but some adaptation was desperately needed. As volumes rose, the staff workload became impossible. Over the next year several changes were made to civilize the approach and allow for quality care through primary nursing.

To begin with, scheduling had to be adjusted, because the starting time for seeing patients was 1:00 P.M.; needless to say, working until 7:00 P.M. became commonplace but unacceptable. Negotiations began with the Branch Chief to allow for an all-day schedule. Because the physicians (fellows) had inpatient and conference obligations in the morning, such a schedule was difficult to arrange. The solution was to allow an agreed-on patient population to be seen by nurses only in the morning. These included patients scheduled for day 8 or day 15 treatments, patients on protocol who required pretesting or hydration, 5-day treatment patients, and patients who required transfusions. Medical consultation was available by page or telephone, but independent decision making by nursing was supported. This change made the afternoon schedule almost manageable.

Second, a primary nursing plan had to be agreed on. Should nurses follow patients on specific protocols or be paired with specific physicians? The fellows had specific ambulatory days, either Monday and Wednesday, or Tuesday and Thursday. The nurses chose to work with specific physicians consistently and were paired with two to three physicians from each group. The nurse to patient ratio remained high.

Third, nurses looked at categories of patient visits to determine nursing requirements. These categories are described in detail by Hastings, Costa, and Farley (1985) and included the following: (1) new or screening visits, (2) consultation visits, (3) active protocol visits, (4) long-term follow-up visits, and (5) urgent or emergency visits. Similar categories are built into most ambulatory settings even if they are labeled differently or not labeled at all.

If it were true that the primary nurses could not see all patients with present staffing, where should they concentrate efforts? The obvious choices were new patients and those in active treatment. Active treatment patients were in fact the only ones being consistently seen at that beginning point. An agreement was reached with physicians to introduce the primary nurse to new patients even if time for a nurse visit was not possible. If it was known that the patient would return for treatment, the patient was scheduled for a nurse visit (morning) for teaching purposes and initial assessment. This visit was frequently on or before the first day of treatment, depending on patient and nurse schedule. Of the other categories, consultation was handled by the physician alone unless there were specific nursing needs. For the long-term follow-up patients, nurses always found time to say hello if not to do an updated assessment. Collaboration with physicians developed to the point that physicians sought out the primary nurse to discuss the patients that nurses frequently knew better (had known longer) than the physician. If all else failed, patients *always* found their primary nurse! Emergency visits were handled by the appropriate primary nurse, who often utilized an associate nurse to assist with the scheduled primary patients.

At the same time, it was agreed that because physicians had a printed schedule of visits, they could put their own patients in rooms without assistance. If help was required, the nursing assistant was available. Over time two additional adaptations made this system work. The physician and the primary nurse met at the beginning of each session to share information and agree on a plan. For some this took 2 min and for others it took as long as 10 min. It saved hours of duplicated effort and confusion.

After observing primary nursing in action, the unit clerks asked to become primary clerks. They were then assigned to schedule for specific physicians on a regular basis. This decreased confusion immediately while assisting communication and collaboration. Primary nursing is not perfect in this high-volume setting, but it is well implemented as evidenced by patient, nurse, and physician satisfaction. Quality care is provided on a consistent basis.

In contrast, each of the other branches elected to implement primary nursing in slightly different ways. It is the adaptability of this care delivery system that makes it the system of choice for ambulatory care. To achieve the right adaptation for a particular setting, creativity should be encouraged and risks allowed.

Summary

There are risks and benefits to any system, and primary nursing is no exception. The risks include exposing one's nursing practice to patients, peers, managers, and other health professionals. There is risk of isolation because of involvement in one's own patient panel. Managers must work with staff to balance this. Because *the essence of primary nursing is the relationship between the patient and the primary nurse,* there is always the potential for overinvolvement. This concern is not new to oncology nursing and is overcome as a nurse matures and learns to utilize resources for patients and for self.

The benefits are many. New peer relationships are developed, and it is possible to realize collaborative practice with other professionals; both increase professional satisfaction. Growing respect for one another enhances the ability of staff to work together. And, of course, the special relationships that are developed with patients and families over time cannot be quantified but are cherished.

During the present nursing shortage, achieving professional practice in ambulatory care may be a major challenge. However, this is exactly the time to utilize every resource available to preserve professional practice. If it is lost now, it may be lost forever. An encouraging finding from The National Survey of Salary, Staffing, and Professional Practice Patterns in Oncology Nursing (ONS, 1989) is that most respondents (47.33%) reported practicing primary nursing in their oncology settings. Data specific to ambulatory care were not obtained in this survey. Utilizing the principles of primary nursing can help to accomplish the task of providing quality care while enhancing professional satisfaction. It is a delivery model worthy of all ambulatory oncology nurses committed to consistent, quality care.

NURSING OPPORTUNITIES PRESENTED BY AMBULATORY CARE

Patient and Family Issues

Education

The need for and the how to of patient and family education are addressed in detail in Unit IX of this book. However, the importance of maximizing self-care in the oncology ambulatory population cannot be overemphasized.

As pointed out by both Smith (1977) and Dodd (1982), patients frequently do not perceive nurses as a major source of information. Ambulatory oncology nurses have an opportunity to change that perception. It is known that informational needs change over time in the chronically ill patient, certainly in the oncology patient. We also know that a variety of factors, such as anxiety level, make it necessary to repeat information. One of the real advantages of primary nursing in ambulatory oncology care is the continuity that allows the primary nurse to know the patient well. This relationship facilitates well-planned, well-received, and most important, effective teaching. Teich and Raia (1984) have outlined the role of the primary nurse in a successful ambulatory oncology structured teaching program. The complex therapy being delivered in ambulatory oncology today demands that nurses find time to teach self-care. For the patient receiving chemotherapy, one-to-one patient-nurse time is available. If possible, patient teaching visits should be considered. Patient teaching should be accepted as a valid reason for a nurse visit in the oncology setting. A well-informed patient is less dependent, has more control, and makes better decisions, all of which give the nurse time to spend with the next patient and family.

Waiting Time

What do we know of the patient perspective of the ambulatory experience? Two excellent articles, one by Gardner (1980) and the other by Welch (1981), give us some clues that the professional and the patient perceptions may be quite different. Both articles, one written by the wife of a patient receiving radiation therapy and the other by a professional (oncology nurse), challenge us to do better, especially during periods of waiting. Some amount of waiting is a reality, but the fact remains that waiting increases anxiety. Nurses could influence scheduling to decrease waiting and could have an impact on this time in other positive ways. Patients are a captive audience in the ambulatory setting, and this time can be used for structured programs. One method of providing information, as well as distraction, is short teaching sessions utilizing homemade or commercial videotapes. Small gestures, such as greeting patients and families, sitting in the waiting room with them for 1 to 2 min, and giving explanations of delays and procedures, are all things some take for granted, but judging by the literature and personal observation, nurses should not. It is not unusual for patients and families to develop supportive waiting room relationships. Open-ended support groups facilitated by a psychiatric clinical nurse specialist, social worker, or staff psychologist is another approach used in some settings to make better use of this time. The opportunities are there; we must do better at using them.

Collaboration and Communication

Another golden opportunity built into ambulatory practice is the chance to excel in the area of communication. Keeping colleagues (nursing, medical, and social service) informed is a major task that indeed takes time. If it is done well, it actually saves time. Often it is assumed that colleagues know of changes in patient status or treatment decisions. Instead, we should use the telephone to call the visiting nurse or hospice nurse, write a note for the inpatient nurse, and call the social worker to keep them up to date on the latest problem or to say that all is well. Weekly multidisciplinary rounds, although often difficult to arrange in ambulatory care, are an excellent method of sharing information and enhancing communication. Good communication is a cornerstone of collaborative practice (Baird, 1987).

Staff Support

Stress and support issues have been addressed at length elsewhere in this text. Most of the areas noted are applicable to all areas of oncology nursing. If there is one factor with significance for the ambulatory nurse it is the longevity of the patient-nurse relationship. For the primary nurse who follows patients for months to years, a relapse, recurrence, or loss of one of these patients is particularly painful. It is important for nursing administration in ambulatory areas to be cognizant of this fact and to build in appropriate support systems. Certainly part of a manager's function is to assist staff in developing their own support mechanisms. In addition, support should be built into the system. Unit-based support groups in which staff meet regularly with a psychiatric clinical nurse specialist are just one example. Nurses must first learn to take care of themselves so that they can better support one another.

ISSUES FOR THE 1990s

Classification and Quality Assurance

Patient classification has long been a way of life for inpatient care. Establishing classification for outpatient care is a challenge still to be met. Verran (1981)

published a taxonomy of ambulatory care nursing. This study was meant to define ambulatory nursing practice and thus provide a framework for a "variety of management tools" to support ambulatory practice. In 1986, Verran described the components of ambulatory classification instruments and emphasized the potential role of classification in clinical and managerial decisions, including budgetary decisions. Tighe and colleagues (1985) expanded the Verran taxonomy to include three additional areas of indirect ambulatory nursing responsibility: communication, documentation, and planning. This study looked also at the role of the oncology nurse compared with nononcology nurses in the ambulatory setting. These investigators provide an excellent base for building a valid classification, and ultimately, quality assurance programs, applicable to ambulatory oncology practice—not an easy task.

As we know, quality assurance methods and tools have been developed for inpatient services in which each patient episode has a beginning and end point. Ambulatory care lacks these clear criteria in most instances, certainly in oncology practice. O'Neal (1978) and Dorsey and Hussa (1979) published early efforts to focus attention on ambulatory practice evaluation. More recently the actual task of adapting accepted criteria toward the development of an ambulatory quality assurance program was well presented by Hastings (1987). The situation presented is for a nononcology specialty area but could serve easily as a model for oncology.

The key to any process of evaluation is accurate quality documentation. The documentation dilemma in ambulatory care is well known to oncology nurses. The time required to record information on large numbers of patients and the lack of chart availability are just two barriers nurses face when attempting to document. To overcome these and other problems, it is generally accepted that each setting must define appropriate standards that nurses can follow. One possible solution presented at the 1989 Oncology Nursing Society Congress utilizes flow sheets to decrease narrative notes and improve the quality of documentation (Moore & Knobf, 1989) (Box 69–2).

In this era of increasingly complex ambulatory care delivery and diminishing human and economic resources, the need to define oncology ambulatory practice and to develop appropriate tools to justify and measure that practice is imperative. Henninger and Dailey (1983) present one approach used to measure nursing workload in an oncology center outpatient department. The intent was to measure actual practice rather than tasks. This measure was then used to predict staffing needs with some accuracy and to form the basis for a future system of nursing charges.

The topic of ambulatory patient classification is increasing slowly in the literature (Hoffman & Wakefield, 1986). Defining and quantifying ambulatory practice is a tool that can be used to support the nursing skill level required in oncology care. The task need not be made overly complex. There is evidence in the literature of several good beginnings. For those who have yet to address this issue, the time is now.

Box 69–2. DOCUMENTATION IN AMBULATORY ONCOLOGY—USE OF A NURSING CARE FLOW SHEET

The volume and complexity of patients in ambulatory oncology demands creative approaches to documentation. The use of flow sheets has been recognized as an efficient and practical way to follow physical problems. Using the Oncology Nursing Society–American Nurses' Association outcome standards, we developed a documentation tool that clearly and concisely identifies current nursing problems, eliminates most narrative notes, and has potential for computerization. A nursing care flow sheet was developed that outlined nursing problems related to ventilation, nutrition, elimination, mobility, sexuality, comfort, and coping. Vascular access device maintenance, vesicant administration, patient education, and home care were also addressed. For each problem, a graded scale (flow sheet key) was established. This allowed the nurse to quantify the problem and to follow it over time. Relief measures are rated on a likert-type scale. Adjustment to the flow sheet key required minimal extra nursing time initially. Flow sheet use improved quality and efficiency of nursing documentation. Patient care is enhanced by providing easily located, objective data to evaluate active nursing problems and resolution. Primary nurses and associates are able to identify in seconds the patient's clinical status and quickly focus their assessment using the flow sheet. This tool may assist administrators analyzing nurse workloads by identifying areas requiring concentrated nursing time in primary nurse caseloads.

(From Moore, J., and Knobf, T. [1989]. Documentation in ambulatory oncology—use of a nursing care flow sheet. *Oncology Nursing Forum, 16* (Suppl.). (Abstract No. 293A). Reproduced by permission.)

Reimbursement

A related issue requiring attention is the costing of ambulatory nursing services. Griffith (1986) notes that 25 states have legislation providing third-party reimbursement for either specific groups of nurses or all nurses. It is hard to determine whether that fact has helped nursing to realize the actual costing of services. The literature does establish two facts. First, most costing mechanisms are based on some type of classification, and second, the focus is on inpatient costing for nursing rather than outpatient. McCloskey, Gardner, and Johnson (1987) have published an annotated bibliography on the subject, and of the 68 articles reviewed only one mentions ambulatory care in the title or in the summary.

Concern with costing appears to parallel the implementation of diagnosis-related groups (DRGs) on the inpatient side. In assessing the topic for ambulatory practice, one could certainly ask why bother in a climate of prospective payment. One answer is that it would help physicians, hospital administrators, patients, and families to understand the value of nursing provided. In this health care climate, value has a definite economic component. Should ambulatory oncology nursing, skilled as it is, not be unbundled and recognized as a separate entity? It is a question those of us in ambulatory practice will be called on to answer. As attempts are made to cut staffing in an area in which acuity is rising, reimbursement for nursing care delivered may be one answer.

Payment for ambulatory services is of concern to both patient and caretakers. What will the government do? The Omnibus Reconciliation Budget Act of 1986 included a provision to begin looking at ambulatory services to find a method, other than DRGs, of paying for care. The Health Care Financing Administration (HCFA), charged with this task, is just beginning to collect and analyze data. The goal of these present pilot studies is to identify patterns and predict cost. Under the same act, a report on payment for day surgery was due to Congress by April 1989, and the HCFA is required to submit a report on how to pay for ambulatory care, other than what is currently paid, by January 1991 (C. Booth, Director of Office of Reimbursement Policy, HCFA, personal communication, February 1988).

The dilemma of establishing reasonable coverage for increasingly complex ambulatory care will not be solved in the immediate future. Knowing this can be a major advantage to a specialty group. It gives us a window of time in which to collect data and justify nursing's role in oncology ambulatory practice. We know that nursing makes a significant contribution, but we must be ready to support this knowledge with solid facts and figures. Oncology ambulatory nurses have a tremendous opportunity to work together to accomplish many positive outcomes for nursing and for patients. If the classification of ambulatory oncology patients and the resulting nursing care required are firmly established, charging for those services will be easier to justify and may in fact help to clarify for the HCFA what reasonable cost and coverage should be. Of course, it is only one component of a complicated picture, but it is clearly an important one.

Occupational Hazards

Safe Handling—Antineoplastic Agents

Another area demanding oncology nursing attention is that of occupational hazards. Two major issues come to mind: safe handling of antineoplastic agents and blood and body fluid precautions. Barry and Booher (1985) published a comprehensive review of what was then known regarding the hazards of handling antineoplastic agents. At that time the Occupational Safety and Health Administration (OSHA) had not set guidelines for safe handling of antineoplastic agents; however, the ONS had published guidelines for safe handling in 1984. The investigators acknowledged that the entire topic of hazards related to handling antineoplastic agents was still controversial, but they were concerned about the safety of personnel involved with these drugs as well as the potential hazards to the community and environment. Of the 16 facilities surveyed in this study, only two reported having any written guidelines. Wearing gloves during drug preparation was the most common practice reported. Prompted by the increased use of ambulatory settings as the care delivery site for cancer patients, these authors presented guidelines for the preparation, administration, and disposal of parenteral antineoplastic agents in the community setting. They also strongly recommended inservice education programs on a regular basis to keep staff current regarding these issues. In January 1986, OSHA did issue guidelines for protection in handling antineoplastic agents (OSHA, 1986).

Despite a growing body of knowledge, there is concern that practice lags behind current recommendations. Valanis and Shortridge (1987) studied nurses' utilization of protective measures in a variety of work settings and determined when and for what reasons protective measures were not used. The sample included more than 600 ONS members. Although data supported an increase in the use of protective measures in general, it also raised major concerns. "Nurses working in physicians' offices reported the least use of protection" despite the fact that they report handling higher volumes than nurses in other settings. Perhaps most distressing were the reasons given for not using protection. The principal reasons cited were "inconvenience (33 per cent); don't believe there is danger (25 per cent); not available (14 per cent); and use is deemed inappropriate (12 per cent) (Valanis & Shortridge, 1987). One has to wonder with Baird (1987) why we err not on the side of caution. One must also ask what price we will pay if we fail to do so.

Because of the volume of drugs given in all ambulatory settings and the mounting data to support the use of protective measures, all ambulatory oncology nursing administrators should consider themselves ethically and legally bound to establish protective measures in their settings. The ONS has published guidelines specific to ambulatory care, and they were presented at the national congress in May 1988 (Oncology Nursing Society, 1988). The new guidelines should assist those who have not had access to earlier material. An additional resource is presented in Gullo's (1988) detailed summary of information on safe handling.

Protective Guidelines—Blood and Body Fluids

The issue of protective guidelines for the prevention of human immunodeficiency virus (HIV) transmission has essentially been settled by the Centers for Disease Control (CDC) recommendations published in August 1987. These state clearly that blood and body fluid precautions be used consistently for *all* patients. Oncology patients are not only a frequently transfused patient population, but current care necessitates frequent exposure of staff to patients' blood and body fluids. This is true in all oncology settings. In brief, the CDC recommendations include routine use of appropriate barrier precautions to prevent skin and mucous membrane exposure; thorough handwashing procedures; precautions against injuries due to needles, scalpels, and other sharp instruments; and availability of mouthpieces, resuscitation bags, and other ventilation devices for use in emergency situations. The CDC recommends also that staff with exudative lesions or weeping dermatitis should refrain from direct care until the condition resolves, and that pregnant health care workers should be familiar with and strictly adhere to the aforementioned precautions.

These recommendations undoubtedly will increase supply budgets; however, the issue is no longer one of luxury but one of necessity. As oncology nurses we must support these recommendations to protect both ourselves and our patients.

What will the 1990s bring? There is no doubt that care changed with the emergence of chemotherapy. Advances in the use of biologic agents, lymphokines, monoclonal antibodies (especially those associated with toxins or radioisotopes), and other immunologically based agents and the introduction of chemopreventive protocols will also affect ambulatory oncology nursing practice. Recent history has shown that we are capable of rising to the challenge. Undoubtedly, ambulatory oncology nurses not only will continue to progress but also will do so in a manner that preserves professional practice despite nursing shortages and economic constraints.

References

Aiken, L. (1977). Primary care: The challenge for nursing. *American Journal of Nursing, 77*, 1828–1832.

Avery, J. (1986). Outpatient management of CA pleural effusion (case presentation). *Hospital Practice, 21*(4), 64A.

Baird, S. B. (1987). Until the answers are in (editorial). *Oncology Nursing Forum, 14*(3), 9.

Baird, S. B., Hartigan, K., & Holton-Smith, D. (Eds.). (1987). *The role of the oncology nurse in the office setting*. Ohio: Adria Laboratories.

Barry, L. K., & Booher, R. B. (1985). Promoting the responsible handling of antineoplastic agents in the community. *Oncology Nursing Forum, 12*(5), 41–46.

Belis, L., Weiss, R., & Trush, D. (1980). The oncology clinic: A primary care facility. *Cancer Nursing, 3*, 47–52.

Brock, J., & Alberts, D. (1986). Safe, rapid administration of cisplatin in the outpatient clinic. *Cancer Treatment Reports, 70*, 1409–1414.

Brosnan, J., & Johnston, M. (1980). Stressed but satisfied: Organizational change in ambulatory care. *Journal of Nursing Organization, 10*(11), 43–46.

Brown, J. K. (1985). Ambulatory services: The mainstay of cancer nursing care. *Oncology Nursing Forum, 12*(1), 57–59.

Buchanan, G. (1977). Development of a program for ambulatory nursing care. *Nursing Clinics of North America, 12*, 543–551.

Centers for Disease Control. (1987). Recommendations for prevention of HIV transmission in health-care settings. *Morbidity and Mortality Weekly Report, 36*(Suppl. 2S).

Clark, M. (1986). A day hospital for cancer patients: Clinical and economic feasibility. *Oncology Nursing Forum, 13*(6), 41–45.

Coyle, N., Mauskop, A., Maggard, J., & Foley, K. (1986). Continuous subcutaneous infusions of opiates in cancer patients with pain. *Oncology Nursing Forum, 13*(4), 53–57.

DeVita, V. T., Jr., Serpick, A. A., & Carbone, P. P. (1970).

Combination chemotherapy in the treatment of advanced Hodgkin's disease. *Annals of Internal Medicine, 73,* 881–895.

Dodd, M. (1982). Assessing patient self-care for side effects of cancer chemotherapy—Part I. *Cancer Nursing, 5,* 447–451.

Dorsey, B., & Hussa, R. (1979). Evaluating ambulatory care: Three approaches. *Journal of Nursing Administration, 9*(1), 34–43.

Evans, T. (1986). Outpatient administration of VP-16 and cisplatin. *Seminars in Oncology, 13*(3, Suppl. 3), 79–82.

Farley, B. (1981). Primary nursing in the oncology ambulatory setting. *Nursing Administration Quarterly, 5*(4), 44–53.

Gardner, M. E. (1980). Notes from a waiting room. *American Journal of Nursing, 80,* 86–89.

Gralla, R. J., Stalker, M. Z., Mor, V., Sher, H. I., Park, D., Marks, P., & Oettgen, H. F. (1987). A medical adult day hospital (ADH) as an alternative to inpatient care: Results of a prospective random-assignment trial. *Proceedings of the American Society of Clinical Oncology.* (Abstract No. 1009)

Greenwald, H. (1987). HMO Membership, copayment, and initiation of care for cancer: A study of working adults. *American Journal of Public Health, 77,* 461–466.

Griffith, H. (1986). Implementation of direct third party reimbursement legislation for nursing services. *Nursing Economics, 4*(6), 299–304.

Gullo, S. (1988). Safe handling of antineoplastic drugs: Translating the recommendations into practice. *Oncology Nursing Forum, 15,* 595–601.

Hartigan, K. (1987). Administrative issues for the oncology nurse in the office setting. In S. Baird (Ed.), *The role of the oncology nurse in the office setting* (pp. 9–16). Ohio: Adria Laboratories.

Hastings, C. E. (1987). Measuring quality in ambulatory care nursing. *Journal of Nursing Administration, 17*(4), 12–20.

Hastings, C. E., Costa, L., & Farley, B. (1985). Developing professional practice in ambulatory care: Issues for the middle manager. *Ambulatory Nursing Administration, 7*(5), 1–3.

Henke, C. (1980). Emerging roles of the nurse in oncology. *Seminars in Oncology, 7,* 4–8.

Henninger, D., & Dailey, C. (1983). Measuring nursing workload in an outpatient department. *Journal of Nursing Administration, 13*(9), 20–23.

Hilkemeyer, R. (1982). A historical perspective in cancer nursing. *Oncology Nursing Forum, 9*(2), 47–56.

Hoffman, F., & Wakefield, D. (1986). Ambulatory care patient classification. *Journal of Nursing Administration, 16*(4), 23–30.

Isler, C. (1977). Emerging in cancer care: The regional ambulatory center. *R.N., 40*(2), 33–46.

Jackson, B. (1980). The growing role of nurses in enterostomal therapy. *Seminars in Oncology, 7,* 48–55.

Kepnes, L. (1984). Professional nursing practice in ambulatory care. *Nursing Management, 15*(5), 28–30.

Management rounds: Outpatient cancer centers begin to gain attention. (1985). *Hospitals, 59*(18), 54.

Manthey, M. (1980). *The practice of primary nursing.* Boston: Blackwell Scientific Publications.

Maxwell, M. B. (1979). Nurse practitioner chemotherapy clinic. *Cancer Nursing, 2,* 211–218.

McCloskey, J. C., Gardner, D. L., & Johnson, M. R. (1987). Costing out nursing services: An annotated bibliography. *Nursing Economics, 5,* 245–253.

Medvec, B., & Calzone, K. (1989). Effective ambulatory oncology nursing: Winning the telephone management war. *Oncology Nursing Forum, 16* (Suppl.). (Abstract No. 141A)

Moore, J., & Knobf, T. (1989). Documentation in ambulatory oncology—use of a nursing care flow sheet. *Oncology Nursing Forum, 16* (Suppl.). (Abstract No. 293A)

Nail, L., Greene, D., Jones, L., & Flannery, M. (1989). Nursing care by telephone: Describing practice in an ambulatory oncology center. *Oncology Nursing Forum, 16,* 387–395.

Nims, J., Buchsel, P., & Jacom, J. (1985). Outpatient management of the bone marrow transplant (BMT) patient: A nursing perspective. *Oncology Nursing Forum, 12* (Suppl.). (Abstract No. 56)

Nirenberg, A., & Rosen, G. (1979). The day hospital: Ambulatory care. *American Journal of Nursing, 79,* 500–504.

Oncology Nursing Society. (1984). *Cancer chemotherapy: Guidelines and recommendations for nursing education and practice.* Pittsburgh: Author.

Oncology Nursing Society. (1988). *Cancer chemotherapy guidelines: Module III—recommendations for nursing practice in the outpatient setting.* Pittsburgh: Author.

O'Neal, E. A. (1978). A framework for ambulatory care evaluation. *Journal of Nursing Administration, 8*(7), 15–20.

OSHA. (1986, January 29). *Work practice guidelines for personnel dealing with cytotoxic (antineoplastic) drugs* (OSHA Instruction Pub. 8-1.1). Washington, DC: Office of Occupational Medicine, OSHA.

Quebbeman, E., Ausman, R., Hansen, R., Becker, T., Caballero, G., Ritch, P., Jenkins, D., Blake, D., Tangen, L., & Schulte, W. (1985). Long-term ambulatory treatment of metastatic colorectal adenocarcinoma by continuous intravenous infusion of 5-fluorouracil. *Journal of Surgical Oncology, 30,* 60–65.

Reisler, M. (1985). Business in Richmond attacks health care costs. *Harvard Business Review, 63,* 145–155.

Ryan, L., Edwards, R., & Rickles, F. (1980). A joint practice approach to the care of persons with cancer. *Oncology Nursing Forum, 7*(1), 8–11.

Schulmeister, L. (1987). Trends in health care delivery: Their impact on oncology nurses in the office setting. In S. Baird (Ed.), *The role of the oncology nurse in the office setting* (pp. 3–8). Ohio: Adria Laboratories.

Slater, H., Goldfarb, I. W., Jacob, H., Hill, J., & Srodes, C. (1985). Experience with long-term outpatient venous access utilizing percutaneously placed silicone elastomer catheters. *Cancer, 56,* 2074–2077.

Smith, C. (1977). Patient education in ambulatory care. *Nursing Clinics of North America, 12,* 595–608.

Teich, C. J., & Raia, K. (1984). Teaching strategies for an ambulatory chemotherapy program. *Oncology Nursing Forum, 11*(5), 24–28.

Thirlwell, M., Hollingsworth, L., Herba, M., Boileau, G., Boos, G., & MacFarlane, J. (1986). Ambulatory hepatic artery infusion chemotherapy for cancer of the liver. *The American Journal of Surgery, 151,* 585–589.

Tighe, M. G., Fisher, S. G., Hastings, C., & Heller, B. (1985). A study of the oncology nurse role in ambulatory care. *Oncology Nursing Forum, 12*(6), 23–27.

Valanis, B., & Shortridge, L. (1987). Self protective practices of nurses handling antineoplastic drugs. *Oncology Nursing Forum, 14*(3), 23–27.

Van Scoy-Mosher, C. (1978). The oncology nurse in independent professional practice. *Cancer Nursing, 1,* 21–28.

Verran, J. A. (1981). Delineation of ambulatory nursing practice. *The Journal of Ambulatory Care Management, 4,* 1–10.

Welch, D. A. (1981). Waiting, worry and the cancer experience. *Oncology Nursing Forum, 8*(2), 14–18.

70

Home Care Services

MARILYN D. HARRIS
CAROL ANN PARENTE

In the "good old days," the sick were cared for at home. There were no sophisticated health care facilities available. It was a natural occurrence to have family, neighbors, and friends provide assistance in times of need. Adequate help was available to do the housework, take care of the children, prepare meals, and care for the sick person. Many times families lived together or near one another. Wives or mothers were home to care for the sick family member and the children.

Today home care services are dramatically different. These changes are due to many factors, including changes in demographics, family structure, and reimbursement and technologic advances.

HOME CARE—THE PRESENT

The American Nurses' Association (1978) states that "home care services are mobile, decentralized, and able to be dispersed over a geographical area." The services are designed to assist the patient to assume responsibility for his or her own care. Home health care services are provided to individuals and families in their places of residence for the purpose of preventing illness; promoting, maintaining, or restoring health; or minimizing the effects of illness and disability (Box 70–1).

The National Association for Home Care (1988, p. 10) states that "home care is a service to the recovering, disabled or clinically ill person providing for treatment and/or effective functioning in the home environment. Generally home care is appropriate whenever a person needs assistance that cannot be easily or effectively provided only by a family member or friend on an ongoing basis for a short or long period of time."

REFERRALS TO HOME CARE

Referrals to home care can be made by physicians, nurses, hospital social workers and discharge planners, patients and families, or neighbors and friends (Lucas & Pancoast, 1988). The referral process will vary with a specific agency, but in general, the process should follow the scenario in Figure 70–1.

The selection of a home health care agency is important to the patient and family and physician. Certain questions should be asked when making a decision on a home care agency that will be best for everyone involved. A list of these questions as suggested by the National Association for Home Care (1984) is found in Table 70–1. Additional consumer guides are found in Table 70–2.

STAFF AND SERVICES

An adequate and qualified staff is essential to the delivery of health care services in the home. The Medicare Conditions of Participation (COP) (Federal Register, 1989) are used as a reference for describing home care services recognized for reimbursement under this program, because many other insurers follow the same guidelines.

Home care services are provided by a highly professional staff consisting of representatives of many disciplines and support personnel. The Medicare program provides for reimbursement for six services.

Nursing Care

Highly skilled registered nurses can be of immense help in speeding patients' recovery after operations or

---

Box 70–1. A RANDOMIZED CLINICAL TRIAL OF HOME NURSING CARE FOR LUNG CANCER PATIENTS

A randomized clinical trial was conducted to assess the effects of home nursing care for patients with progressive lung cancer. One hundred and sixty-six patients were assigned to an oncology home care group (OHC) that received care from oncology home care nurses, a standard home care group (SHC) that received care from regular home care nurses, or an office care group (OC) that received whatever care they needed except for home care. Patients were entered into the study 2 months after diagnosis and followed for 6 months. Patients were interviewed at 6-week intervals across five occasions. At the end of the study, there were no differences in pain, mood disturbance, and concerns among the three groups. There were significant differences in symptom distress, enforced social dependency, and health perceptions. The two home nursing care groups had less distress and greater independence 6 weeks longer than the office care group. In addition, the two home nursing care groups reported steadily worse health perceptions over time. Thus it was remarkable that the office care group, which indicated more symptom distress and social dependency with time, also indicated perceptions of improved health with time. These results suggest that home nursing care assists patients with forestalling distress from symptoms and maintaining their independence longer than no home nursing care. Home care may also include assisting patients in acknowledging the reality of their situation.

(From McCorkle, R., Benoliel, J. Q., Donaldson, G., Georgiadou, F., Moinpour, C., & Goodell, B. [1989]. A randomized clinical trial of home nursing care for lung cancer patients. *Cancer, 64*[6], 1375–1382.)

---

illness and can provide ongoing care to the aged or chronically ill. Often with the help of a visiting nurse, lengthy hospital stays and burdens on family members can be avoided. Following consultation with the physician, the nurse performs specific tasks, which include instructing families on the care of acutely ill patients, dressing surgical wounds, supervising treatment and diet, providing instruction and supervision of medication, providing intravenous or chemotherapy, and offering health counseling and physical care. Staff assist patients and their families with crisis intervention, such as obtaining hospice care or monitoring life-threatening illness.

Physical Therapy

Physical therapy can help a patient regain the use of impaired muscles, increase joint motion, control pain, or perform activities of daily living. Physical therapists plan physical rehabilitation programs for patients.

Occupational Therapy

Following an accident or illness, a patient may have to relearn physical and general awareness skills. An occupational therapist assesses the patient's abilities and works out a comprehensive, individualized program that helps the patient regain many skills. With instruction, and sometimes with an adaptive device, a person can begin to do more things without help and thus become more independent.

Speech Pathologist

A speech pathologist helps the patient learn how to communicate after an accident or illness or because of a learning disability. The pathologist evaluates the patient's needs and then carries out specific programs of instruction and exercise that help the patient regain speech.

Medical Social Service

On occasion, professional help is indicated when a patient finds it difficult to cope with the emotional and social stresses of illness or an accident. A medical social worker studies the patient's situation and works toward resolving problems. This problem-solving process entails such things as finding housing and financial relief, intervening in family relationships, or correcting environmental problems. The social workers provide support and encouragement to both the patient and the family.

Home Health Aides

Under the supervision of the professional staff, home health aides help patients follow regimens prescribed by physicians, help in personal care (such as bathing and exercises), and perform light housekeeping tasks and errands.

Additional home care services may include one or more of the following:

- nutritional support
- durable medical equipment
- laboratory studies
- radiographs
- portable electrocardiograms
- medical supplies, such as catheters and dressings
- transportation
- emergency alert system
- Meals-on-Wheels (home delivered meals)
- telephone reassurance

Additional personnel may also be involved in providing home care services: homemaker-attendant care that provides help with shopping and doing household

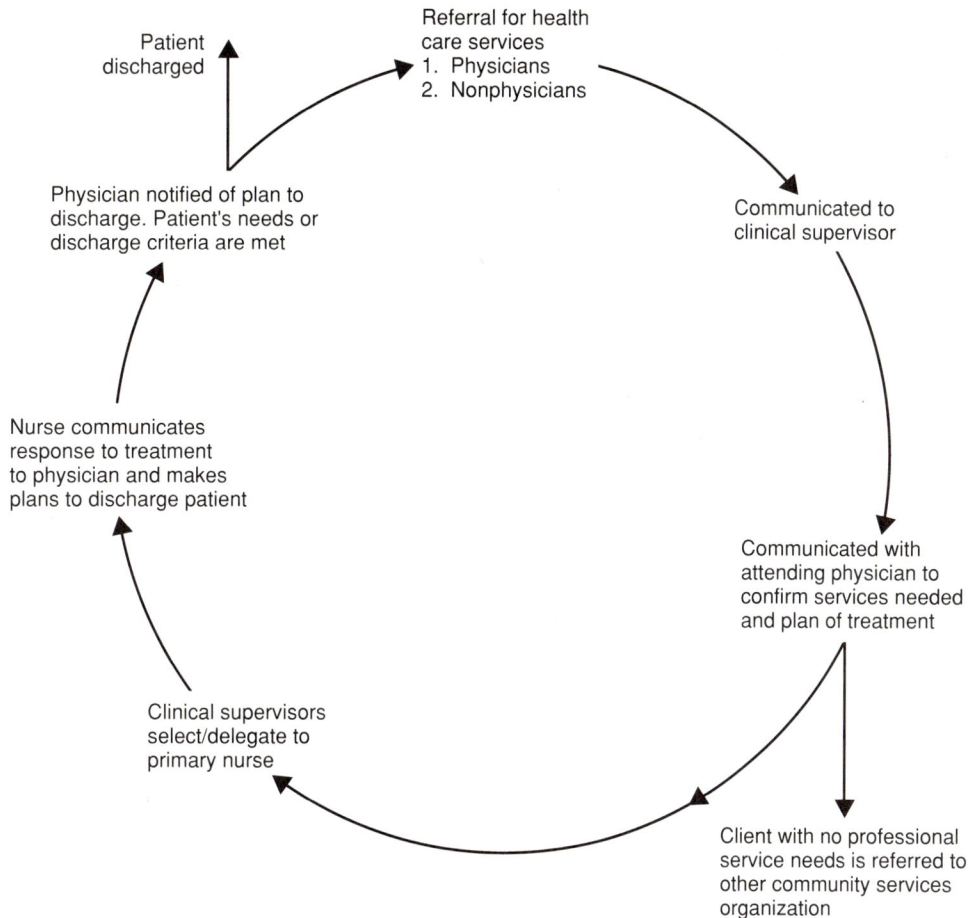

Figure 70–1. Home care referral flow chart.

chores that enables individuals to remain in their homes; volunteers; dentists; clergy; physicians; and ophthalmologists.

A case study description illustrates a coordinated home health team approach for the management of a patient with an inoperable brain tumor.

Case Study

Bob A. was a 56-year-old male who presented to his family physician in May 1989 with ataxia and headaches. A neurologic work-up, including a computed tomographic (CT) scan, showed no significant findings. The symptoms persisted, and a subsequent magnetic resonance image (MRI) showed a lesion on the brain.

The patient's care was shifted to a university medical center for treatment, including chemotherapy and radiation. The patient's symptoms lessened, and he was able to maintain his functional status, including a part-time job as a maintenance man.

Bob lived with his wife, Pat, in a small one-story house. Their grown son lived nearby with his family. As Bob's condition worsened, Bob and Pat asked his recently widowed mother to move from the Midwest to assist with Bob's care, because Pat worked full time to maintain their income.

The referral for home care was initiated by Pat. Her call to the Visiting Nurse Association (VNA) was prompted by a sharp decline in the patient's abilities during a vacation cruise. The patient developed left-sided hemiparesis, required moderate to maximum help with his activities of daily living, and was incontinent of urine. Bob was scheduled for chemotherapy at the university hospital the following week, but it was clear to Pat that his response to treatment was lessening. She wished to explore home care options before this hospitalization to have services and equipment ready for Bob on discharge.

Bob was admitted to VNA services the following day, and the initial nursing assessment showed the following problems: alteration in urinary elimination, incontinence; impaired mobility; knowledge deficit related to management of dexamethasone (Decadron)-induced diabetes; and self-care deficit.

The following week the patient was admitted as scheduled for his chemotherapy. During that hospital stay, he developed a deep vein thrombophlebitis in his left leg with further weakness and increased difficulty in transfers. At discharge from the hospital, Bob and Pat made a decision for "no more chemotherapy." The physicians agreed that palliative care was most appropriate, and the VNA hospice team was notified.

On readmission to the VNA facility, the patient's mobility was of prime concern, because he was experiencing left-sided hemiplegia, and at 6 feet 2 inches in height and 200 pounds in weight he was quite a challenge to move from bed to chair. Physical therapy referral was initiated for instruction in transfers and range of motion exercises.

An occupational therapist was requested to instruct the patient and the family in adaptations of activities of daily living to promote Bob's independence. He was instructed

Table 70–1. HOW TO CHOOSE A HOME CARE AGENCY

Finding the best home care agency for your needs requires research, but it is time well spent. Quality of care and caliber of personnel will be overriding factors, of course. Fortunately, in most communities families have a wide choice of agencies from which to choose. Some offer sliding-scale fee schedules. Some will accept indigent patients.

Here are some questions to consider when making a decision on what home care agency is best for you:

1. How long has the agency been serving the community?
2. Does my physician know the reputation of the agency?
3. Is it certified by Medicare? Even if your care will not be paid for by Medicare, the fact that an agency is Medicare-certified is one measure of quality. It means that the agency has met certain minimum requirements in financial management and patient care.
4. Is the agency licensed? In most states a home care agency must be licensed by the state, usually by the state health department.
5. Does the agency provide written statements describing its services, eligibility requirements, fees, and funding sources? Often an annual report will offer helpful guidance on the agency.
6. How does an agency choose its employees? Does it protect its workers with written personnel policies, benefit packages, and malpractice insurance?
7. Does a nurse or therapist conduct an evaluation of your needs in the home? What is included—consultations with family members? with the patient's physician? with other health professionals?
8. Is the plan of care written out? Does it include the specific duties to be performed, by whom, at what intervals, and for how long? Can you review the plan?
9. Does the plan provide for the family to undertake as much of the care as is deemed practical?
10. What are the financial arrangements? Can you get them in writing, including any minimum hour or day requirements the agency may have and any extra charges to be involved in the care program.
11. Does the professional supervising your home care plan visit your home regularly? Are your questions followed up and resolved?
12. What arrangements are made for emergencies?
13. What arrangements are made to ensure patient confidentiality?
14. Will the agency continue service if Medicare or other reimbursement sources are exhausted?
15. Some people feel that accreditation assures quality of service. Accreditation is a voluntary process conducted by nonprofit professional organizations. Visiting nurse associations and other community nursing groups are accredited by the Community Health Accreditation Program (CHAP). The Joint Commission on Accreditation of Hospitals accredits hospitals and their affiliate agencies. And the National HomeCaring Council accredits homemaker-home health aide services.

To locate home care agencies in your community, you might start by asking your doctor, or consult with the hospital discharge planner, if home care will follow hospitalization. Agencies will be listed in the yellow pages under any of several health-related headings. Your county or city will have listings of publicly funded services. If your community has an information and referral service, check with it. Often Information and Referrals (I&Rs) are affiliated with the local United Way (sometimes called United Fund).

Most states have state home care associations that can help you locate a good agency. The National Association for Home Care (NAHC) can help you contact your state association. Their address is 519 C Street, N.E., Stanton Park, Washington, DC 20002.

(National Association for Home Care. [1984]. How to choose a home care agency. Washington, DC: Author. Reproduced by permission.)

in the use of a sling, hand splint, and adaptive eating devices.

Over the course of the next few weeks, Bob's speech deteriorated and his conversations were marked with rage and frustration with his expressive aphasia. Speech therapy assisted the patient and his family with communications, including refining a picture board Pat had devised.

Table 70–2. CONSUMER GUIDES

A Consumer's Guide to Home Health Care (1985)
National Consumer League
600 Maryland Avenue, S.W., Suite 202 West
Washington, DC 20024
A Guide to Home Health Care (1982), A. E. Nourse, M.D.
Upjohn Health Care Services
3651 Van Rick Drive
Kalamazoo, MI 49002
A Handbook about Care in the Home (1982)
American Association of Retired Persons
1909 K Street, N.W.
Washington, DC 20049
All about Home Care: A Consumer's Guide (1982)
National Home Caring Council and the Better Business Bureau
of Metropolitan New York, Inc.
235 Park Avenue South
New York, NY 10003
Home Care (1984)
National Association for Home Care
519 C Street, N.E.
Washington, DC 20002
*Home Health Care: A Complete Guide for Patients and Their
Families* (1986), JoAnn Friedman
New York: W. W. Norton
The Home Health Care Solution (1985), Janet Zhun Nassif
New York: Harper & Row

Home health aides visited Bob to assist in personal care needs, including transfers to the tub for a shower. Visits were initially three times each week and increased as Bob's status declined.

Nursing activities included instruction, assessment of diabetes management, and insulin administration. Control of Bob's urinary incontinence became more difficult. Various external devices were tried and found to be ineffective for him, and skin deterioration necessitated a Foley catheter.

A hospice volunteer was assigned to provide companionship and respite for Bob's mother, who was far from her own circle of friends in the Midwest. Volunteers also provided transportation for Bob's mother for her own health appointments and made extended visits to Bob when she was recovering from cataract surgery and was unable to provide direct care to Bob.

The chaplain visited the family at regular intervals to offer spiritual support, sometimes praying with the patient and sometimes just listening.

The social worker secured added caregiving support for Bob from a county program as he declined and his care became more difficult for his mother to manage. The social worker also focused on emotional support for Bob and his family.

In October 1989, the patient developed increased difficulty swallowing, increased aphasia, and weakness in all extremities. His wife was determined to keep Bob at home, and when he could no longer swallow, private duty nurses (also covered by his insurance plan) were provided to administer parenteral anticonvulsants.

Bob died at home 214 days after his initial VNA evaluation. The integration of multidisciplinary services offered Bob and his family the care needed to keep him at home during the terminal phase of his illness.

ROLE OF THE CANCER NURSE IN HOME CARE

The home care nurse today faces an often overwhelming onslaught of problems in the care of oncology (and other) patients in the community. Reimbursement forces in both acute care settings and in home care dramatically influence the kind of patient seen by the home care staff nurse.

Length of stay for many hospitalized patients has been shortened. Patients are now being discharged "quicker and sicker." Recovery periods for many take place now at home rather than in acute care beds. In addition, most high-technology care equipment (e.g., intravenous lines and pumps, feeding tubes, tracheostomy tubes or trachs, and ventilators) can accompany patients to their homes. When hospital stays are shortened, patients' families and caregivers do not always have time to receive the teaching they need to manage equipment and procedures at home. The patient's situation at home may be very confused, with many questions not yet answered, symptoms not totally controlled, and stressed family members who need help themselves.

Enter the home care nurse. Most agencies require the beginning community health nurse to have a B.S.N. degree or to be working toward a nursing degree (Yuan, 1988). Although the community nurse may be a specialist in home care, traditionally the role is one of a generalist. The typical home care nurse carries a caseload of five to seven adult patients per day with a variety of diagnoses and needs. The nurse's assessment and intervention skills must be equally well honed for a cardiac, diabetic, or oncology patient. The nursing role is independent, challenging, and frustrating when the nurse confronts the complexities of the home care patient and his or her family.

In most home care agencies, the patients with cancer represent a sizable portion of the patient population. Figures from the Pennsylvania Department of Health, Division of Primary Care and Home Health Licensing Survey (1987) of 299 home health agencies indicate neoplasms as the second most frequently occurring diagnoses, following diseases of the circulatory system. Visit statistics from the Visiting Nurse Association of Eastern Montgomery County (1987) reflect the state figures with the top five diagnoses for patients seen in 1987 as follows: (1) diseases of the circulatory system, (2) neoplasms, (3) respiratory diseases, (4) accidents, and (5) skin and subcutaneous tissue damage.

Patient care procedures that may be commonplace in the acute care setting occur with less regularity in the home. Although ventilators are possible at home, only two or three individuals of a home care agency population may have them at any one time. Intravenous therapy, home chemotherapy, feeding tubes, and associated pumps may be more commonplace in the community health setting, but they still occur with relative infrequency in any one home care nurse's caseload. The infrequency of practice of many highly technical procedures contributes to concern among supervisory and nursing staffs about the provision of safe, quality patient care.

Symptom management and patient family education play a vital part in the home care management of all patients. Oncology symptoms may present challenges to home care nurses who have a general knowledge of oncology patients from their educational and clinical background. The oncology patient population in home care may range from the newly diagnosed patient who has just had surgery, to the patient who may need chemotherapy at home, to the hospice patient. As patients with cancer at home move through different stages, their needs may vary widely, and many of their problems may be managed directly by home care nursing activities. Nutrition, activities of daily living, pain, and safety issues through oncologic emergencies may be evaluated and treated initially by the home care nurse. Other members of the home care team (e.g., home health aide; physical, occupational, and speech therapists; medical social worker; and dietitian) may all be involved to further assist with symptom management. Coordination of the multidisciplinary team efforts is done by the nurse in accordance with the Medicare conditions of participation (Department of Health Education and Welfare, 1973).

Numbers of visits alloted by third-party reimbursement regulations may further compound the home care efforts for the oncology patient. Visit patterns are preset or limited to a certain schedule by some insurers. Denial of payment by Medicare for home visits already made is now a fact of life for the home care agency and its staff. The home care staff must be aware of Medicare and other reimburser guidelines. For example, determination of "skilled nursing" services is often more difficult than one would first imagine. Emphasis is placed on assessment and instruction and involvement of family or other caregivers toward the goal of self care (Della Monica, 1988), rather than on provision of maintenance level or long-term care.

Need for Specialization

Shortened acute care stays, technology advances, varied patient needs, and time constraints all have an impact on the care of patients at home. To meet the needs of both patient and nursing staffs, some agencies have established high-technology teams (Weisslein, 1984). Although some agencies utilize specialty teams (e.g., intravenous care teams and respiratory care teams), others may also employ nurse practitioners, both pediatric and adult, and clinical nurse specialists (e.g., geriatric and oncologic specialists). These advanced nurse clinicians may all be employed by an agency to assist visiting and supervisory staffs in the management of complex or specialized patients. The role of the oncology clinical nurse specialist (OCNS) may be practiced fully in the home care setting. As clinician, educator, consultant, researcher, and change agent, the specialist may be a valuable asset to the home care agency and to the community being served.

Oncology Clinical Nurse Specialist

The growth of diagnosis-related groups (DRGs) and prospective payment systems, increasing technology in cancer care, and increasing need for symptom management will have an impact on the role of the OCNS in the next 10 years (Donoghue & Spross, 1985). Paulen (1985) also sees the growth of the home care market as an option for the OCNS as consumers and reimbursers become more health-cost conscious.

Clinical Competency

To fill the role of a clinical nurse specialist most effectively, the nurse must maintain clinical competence in the practice field. This may be realized for the OCNS in home care in a variety of ways. The OCNS may choose to carry a caseload of patients with intense, multifaceted problems. In this scenario, the OCNS manages the patients' care needs totally, assessing, planning, implementing, and evaluating care for the patient and family at home.

Another mechanism to allow the OCNS to provide direct care to the patient is in a consultative role to the visiting staff. In this instance, the OCNS may visit patients on an "as needed" basis at the request of supervisory or field staff. The OCNS may make home visits alone or with the primary nurse, depending on the nature of the problem. Requests for visits to patients with complex problems may be for symptom management, for specialized instruction of the patient or family or visiting staff, or for specific procedures (e.g., chemotherapy). Solo visits by the OCNS offer home care patients several unique opportunities. The specialist brings expanded preparation and experience into the patient's home. Because specialists usually make fewer visits per day than staff, the OCNS is not as constrained by time limits, and the extended home visit allows the opportunity to explore the patient's problem in some depth. Several home visits by the OCNS may be helpful to provide follow-up evaluation of the specialist's nursing interventions, but subsequent home visits may or may not be needed. Following a home visit, the OCNS may offer assistance to the primary home care nurse in problem solving and patient care management through both postvisit conferences and careful documentation of the consultation visit (McCorkle & Germino, 1984).

Joint visits with the visiting staff offer the opportunity for the OCNS to provide both patient and staff teaching during the same interval. This mechanism for visiting is particularly helpful if the field staff is uncertain or inexperienced in certain assessment skills or procedures.

Staff Teaching

Staff teaching is another focus of practice for the OCNS in a home care or community agency. Maintaining proficiency in myriad diagnoses is difficult for the home care nurse. Becoming well versed in a specialty such as oncology in the generalist practice base of home care is even more difficult. The presence of an OCNS in a home care agency setting provides a resource for staff in the formal education process, such as staff development or inservice programs, and in informal settings, such as patient care or team conferences.

Staff Consultation

Staff consultations with or without home visits provide yet another area of OCNS home care practice. Here the clinical specialist offers a resource in trouble shooting and problem solving to the field staff. Frequently consultation centers on symptom management choices, for example, selecting an appropriate bowel regime for an oncology patient who is on narcotics for pain management. Professional support offered by the OCNS through consultation and education is invaluable in the community setting, where nursing practice is usually a solo venture.

Research

Research in a home care setting is an integral part of the OCNS role also. Practice and symptom management issues that have been well explored in the acute care setting may change as the variables of home and nonprofessional (family) caregivers enter the scene. The opportunities for research in home-based nursing are many and varied. In addition to the clinical issues, the OCNS may contribute to administrative research efforts. As reimbursement policies continue to influence practice dramatically, research, such as evaluation of costs, will shape future practice and policies (Harris, Peters, Parente, & Smith, 1986). Development and evaluation of nursing strategies, for example, teaching tools and standardized care plans, specific to the agency and its population may be yet another facet of the OCNS role.

Program Development

Opportunities for program development in the home care field are also available to the OCNS as agencies seek to diversify to maintain a competitive edge in the growing market. Wellness seminars for patients, nutrition hints, makeup and hair care, sexuality discussions, adult day care for patients, cancer support groups for patients and families, and hospice and bereavement programs are all within range of the home care agency (Harris, 1988). The OCNS may be instrumental in developing and participating in any of these programs.

Outside Consultant

The OCNS may also participate in activities related to home care practice as an external consultant. Consultation may be offered to both hospital and long-term care facilities to assist with patient care management or home care planning. Staff education in other facilities or in continuing education programs enhances a home care agency's network in the community. Education programs may be related directly to home care programs (e.g., hospice) or to common patient management problems (e.g., pain or anorexia). Co-operative exchange or information between inpatient and home care may at times be facilitated by the OCNS, who may be called on to evaluate the patient in the inpatient facility and learn specifics about the patient's problems or highly technical procedures. This transfer of "first-hand" information may soothe the transition of patient to home for both client and staff, particularly when there are complex patient problems.

Education programs for the public in association with the American Cancer Society or local community groups also strengthen the home care agency's community ties. Topics may include cancer prevention, early detection, treatment of symptoms, and identification and utilization of community resources.

Potential and Challenges

For the OCNS, the expanding home care market represents an area of career growth. The tradition of nursing independence in the home setting lends itself to the OCNS role. Changes in the home care field that demand highly technical skills and reimbursement restrictions may also encourage the use of nurse specialists, thus maximizing the expertise available to patients at home. As consumers and third-party payors focus on the home care environment, the use of OCNS in the field may strengthen an agency's delivery of quality patient care services.

High-technology care in the home continues to grow as a result of technologic advances and shortened hospital stays. For a home care agency seeking to develop a high-technology practice base, the clinical nurse specialist may provide one option: alone, as part of the agency's high-technology team, or in alliance with a high-technology agency. Home chemotherapy and pain and symptom management are just two areas that could require the use of high-technology equipment and advanced nursing skills.

For both OCNS and the home care agency, many challenges are inherent to the OCNS role. In describing administrative support issues for the acute care OCNS, Baird (1985) raises ideas that may be applied to the home care arena as well. Where does the OCNS fit into the organizational structure—if not staff or supervisor, then what? In an age of cost consciousness, can a home care agency afford to support an OCNS position? How will the staff receive the OCNS role?

The astute home care administrator and OCNS may use the same strategies espoused by Baird: emphasize clinical competence, document outcomes, and publish. Clinical competence for the OCNS in the specialty area as the home care staff nurse may be difficult to maintain, depending on the size of the agency and its oncology population. Once again, cooperative efforts

between local acute care and home care settings may benefit all concerned.

Because the OCNS may be "one of a kind" in an agency, peer support and continuing education for the OCNS through professional organizations and colleagues will be imperative. Administrative support in resources, office space, and availability will help ease the way for development of the OCNS role in home care. Staff, particularly the independent, experienced home care nurse, may have some difficulty accepting the OCNS role. Awareness of staff perceptions and sensitivity to their needs and expertise will help the OCNS in the home care setting as well as in the inpatient area. Oncology nursing practice will continue to grow in the home care field, and the role of an OCNS in home care can have a dynamic, positive impact on patients, staff, agency, and the community.

LEGISLATIVE AND REGULATORY ISSUES

The major change that affected the delivery of home health services was the enactment of the Medicare legislation in 1965. Between 1965 and 1988, an increasing number of legislative acts and regulations have had a major impact on the delivery of home health services. The major issues in the 1980s, their intent, and the impact that they have had on home care services and staff are presented in Table 70–3.

Each year the National Association for Home Care (NAHC) (1988) prepares and publishes a NAHC Blueprint for Action. The 1988 blueprint addressed three major issues: (1) making home care more readily available to those who need it, (2) preserving the present home care benefits, and (3) improving quality of care and public awareness. The goal is to have Congress enact legislation that will improve the quality of life for millions of Americans who must turn to others for their help and protection.

In addition to national issues, some individual state issues are of concern to home care nurses. One such issue is the pronouncement of death by nurses. Laws in different states vary in this area. Many states still require that a person's death be pronounced by a physician.

Reimbursement

Funding for home care services is a complex and dynamic process. Some of the specific stipulations that are important for nurses to understand are summarized here. Medicare legislation was signed into law by President Lyndon B. Johnson in 1965. It provides for payment for home care services for individuals who are older than 65 years or who are disabled. Specific criteria must be met: the patient must be homebound; he or she must require skilled, intermittent services; and the services must be ordered by a physician. The Medicare program provides for covered services described earlier in this chapter. In 1989, an additional restriction of prepayment review was initiated. Medi-

Table 70–3. LEGISLATIVE OR REGULATORY ISSUES THAT AFFECT HOME CARE

Issue	Date	Intent	Impact
Tax Equity and Fiscal Responsibility Act (TEFRA)	1982	Mandate the prospective payment system in acute care hospitals	Patients were discharged from hospitals in the acute or early recovery phase of an illness; the need for more intensive home care services increased
Peer Review Improvement Act	1982	Review care provided to Medicare patients in acute care settings	
Section 9353 (e) of Omnibus Budget Reconciliation Act (OBRA)	1986	Extend peer review organizations' (PRO) regulations to home health agencies and skilled nursing facilities Use generic screen to review complaints	Records that are requested by PRO must be copied and returned within specified time period Increased workload for office and professional staff
PL 97-248 Hospice Medicare Benefit	1982	Provide expanded home health services to terminally ill patients who elect this benefit in lieu of the traditional Medicare benefit	Per diem (rather than per visit) rate for services
Budget Reconciliation Act	1986		Selected care services must be provided by staff (not contract) Hospice must provide interdisciplinary team management and inpatient management and must assume responsibility for care of the patient until death
Social Security Amendments, Diagnosis-Related Groups (DRGs)	1983	Provide hospital payment for specific illness groups	Discharge of more acutely ill patients following a shorter length of stay in acute care facility
Omnibus Deficit Reduction Act	1984	Authorize Secretary of Health and Human Services to deem national accrediting bodies: Community Health Accreditation Program of the National League for Nursing and Joint Commission on the Accreditation of Healthcare Organization	Decision of these accrediting bodies would determine whether a provider meets requirements for Medicare participation (Not implemented as of 7/90)
Omnibus Deficit Reduction Act	1984	Reduce the number of fiscal intermediaries (FI) to 10 regional FIs	All agencies that are not now with one of the 10 FIs had to transfer, beginning in late 1988
Balanced Budget and Emergency Deficit Act (Gramm-Rudman-Hollings)	1985	Balance the federal budget by 1991 through annual reductions in the deficit	Automatic cuts to the Medicare program of 1% in the first year and 2% in subsequent years Home care, as a cost reimbursed program, was reimbursed at 1% and 2% below costs
Home and Community-Based Services for the Elderly Act	1985	Establish a block grant program to provide services similar to those demonstrated under waiver programs	Make additional service available to eligible patients
Use of standardized plan of care (POC) forms: 485-6-7-8	1985 1988 (revised)	Standardize POCs throughout the United States	Increased costs for home health agencies (HHA) HHA experienced Medicare and technical denials after the new POCs were initiated Financial crisis for HHA Poor morale for staff and administrators Potential for decreased service to patients
Omnibus Budget Reconciliation Act	1987	Mandate a prospective payment demonstration project to be implemented in 1990; reports are due in 1992	Payment methods for service will include per episode, per visit, and per case basis
Medicare Catastrophic Protection Act	1988	Expansion of Medicare program to cover catastrophic health expenses	Extended waiver of liability
Long-Term Care Assistance Act	1988	Provide long-term home health and nursing home insurance	Requirement for skilled services, homebound status, and intermittent care would no longer apply
Omnibus Budget Reconciliation Act Section 1819 (f) and 1919 (f) of the Social Security Act	1987	Direct the secretary to establish requirements for the approval of nurse aide training and competency evaluation programs plus other related matters no later than September 1, 1988	There is more demand for the home health aide level of worker in home care than there are aides available The increased cost of meeting the increased training and continuing education requirements will have a financial impact on HHA
Section 4062 of P.L. 100–203 Omnibus Reconciliation Act	1987	Require that payment for DME furnished under the Part A home health benefit and Part B DME, orthotic and prosthetic devices, be made on the basis of a fee schedule	Certain home health benefits that were previously billed under supplies are required to be billed as prosthetic and and orthotic devices; this requires a change in billing procedures and includes a copayment by patients (Rescinded)

Table 70–4. ORGANIZATIONAL STANDARDS

Standard	Credential
Community Health Accreditation Program (CHAP) of the National League for Nursing	Accreditation
Joint Commission on the Accreditation of Healthcare Organizations (JCAHO)—home health; hospice	Accreditation
Medicare conditions of participation (COP) for home health agencies	Certification
Medicare COP for hospice	Certification
State licensure laws	Licensure

caid funding provides coverage for individuals who meet specific income levels. Reimbursement varies from state to state (e.g., cost versus a flat fee for service).

Private insurance coverage for home care services varies with the carrier. Individuals should become aware of the options included in their individual insurance policy. Private pay service is available through some agencies. Also, service agencies may adjust fees to the individual's ability to pay. Other funding sources include the Older Americans Act—Title III, Title XX, the Veterans' Administration, worker's compensation, health maintenance organizations and preferred provider organizations.

QUALITY ASSURANCE

The assurance of quality care is an ongoing challenge. Because of the elusive nature of quality, the difficulty in reaching a consensus on a definition of quality, and the inherent problem in measuring quality, consumers, third-party payors, physicians, regulatory agencies, professional review organizations, professionals, and home health agencies use different criteria to describe and evaluate quality.

Gould and Ruane (1988) state that a quality assurance program is designed to demonstrate and monitor the degree to which an organization's actual performance compares with expected outcomes. Although structure and process criteria are utilized to measure the quality of home care delivered to patients, the emphasis on outcome measures is increasing. Accrediting bodies such as the Joint Commission on Accreditation of Healthcare Organizations (JCAHO) and the National League for Nursing (NLN) stress the importance of evaluating patient outcomes and monitoring the outcomes of care provided to high-volume and high-risk cases.

Agency, professional, and individual standards are important to a quality assurance program. These include agency certification and accreditation standards (Federal Register, 1973; Joint Commission, 1988; Na-

Table 70–5. PROFESSIONAL STANDARDS

Organization	Credential
American Nurses' Association	Certification
Individual states	Certification Licensure
Professional associations (Fickerssen, 1985)	Certification

tional League for Nursing, 1987), professional standards from national organizations such as the American Nurses' Association (ANA) (American Nurses' Association, 1986a, 1986b), national and state trade organizations (National Association, 1986; Pennsylvania Association of Home Health Agencies, 1986), and individual licensure and certification (Fickerssen, 1985) (Tables 70–4 and 70–5). Administration and staff must be committed to the quality assurance program, which includes a commitment of time, money, and personnel to monitor progress toward established goals on an ongoing basis.

The report published by Arthur Anderson and Company and the American College of Health Care Executives (1987, p. 21) included some findings that must be considered when discussing quality assurance. Seventy-three per cent of the respondents agree that providers in 1995 will sacrifice quality of care for financial viability. Seventy-two per cent believe also that future capitation systems will sacrifice quality of care for financial viability.

In light of these projections, the quality issue and the agency's quality assurance program must receive high priority in the 1990s. The evaluation of quality must include both clinical and financial data related to patient care and patient outcomes. This is especially important, because the Omnibus Budget Reconciliation Act (OBRA) of 1987 mandated that a prospective payment demonstration project be implemented for home care services in mid 1988.

Tonges (1985) stated that in a cost-containment atmosphere, providers must either lower their standards or find ways to provide quality care more economically. The challenge in the 1990s is to provide quality care in a more economical manner, not to lower our standards of care.

References

American Nurses' Association. (1978, p. 6). *Health care at home: An essential component of a national health policy.* Kansas City, MO: Author.

American Nurses' Association. (1986a). *Standards—community health nursing practice.* Kansas City, MO: Author.

American Nurses' Association. (1986b). *Standards—home health nursing practice.* Kansas City, MO: Author.

Arthur Anderson and Company and the American College of Health Care Executives. (1987). *The future of healthcare, changes and choices.* American College of Health Care Executives.

Baird, S. B. (1985). Administration support issues and the oncology clinical nurse specialist. *Oncology Nursing Forum, 12*(2), 51–54.

Della Monica, E. (1988). Documentation. In M. Harris (Ed.), *Home health administration* (pp. 273–294). Owings Mills, MD: Rynd Communications.

Department of Health Education and Welfare. (1973). *Conditions of participation for home health agencies.* Washington, DC: U.S. Government Printing Office.

Department of Health and Human Services Health Care Financing Administration, Part II. 42 CFR Part 484 Medicare Program; Home Health Agencies: Condition of Participation and Reduction in Recordkeeping Requirements; Interim Final Rule. *Federal Register*, Monday, August 14, 1989.

Donoghue, M., & Spross, J. (1985). A report from the first national invitational conference: The oncology clinical nurse specialist role analyses and future projections. *Oncology Nursing Forum, 12*(2), 35–37.

Fickerssen, J. L. (1985). Getting certified. *American Journal of Nursing, 85*, 265–269.

Gould, J., & Ruane, N. (1988). Components of a quality assurance program. In M. Harris (Ed.), *Home health administration*. Owings Mills, MD: Rynd Communications.

Harris, M. (Ed.). (1988). *Home health administration*. Owings Mills, MD: Rynd Communications.

Harris, M., Peters, D., Parente, C., & Smith, J. (1986). *Cost of home care by nursing diagnoses*. Presented at Second National Nursing Symposium on Home Health Care. University of Michigan School of Nursing, Ann Arbor, MI.

Joint Commission on Accreditation of Health Organizations. (1988). *Home care standards and accreditation*. Chicago: Author.

Lucas, M., & Pancoast, L. (1988). Referral services. In M. Harris (Ed.), *Home health administration*. Owings Mills, MD: Rynd Communications.

McCorkle, R., Benoliel, J. Q., Donaldson, G., Georgiadou, F., Moinpour, C., & Goodell, B. (1989). A randomized clinical trial of home nursing care for lung cancer patients. *Cancer, 64*(6), 1375–1382.

McCorkle, R., & Germino, B. (1984). What nurses need to know about home care. *Oncology Nursing Forum, 11*, 63–69.

National Association for Home Care. (1984). *How to choose a home care agency*. Washington, DC: Author.

National Association for Home Care. (1986, August). *Code of ethics*. Washington, DC: Author.

National Association for Home Care. (1988). *NAHC-blueprint for action* (Vol. 4, pp. 1–16). Washington, DC: Author.

Out-patients are in. (1987, August 2). *New York Times*, sec. 3, p. 1.

Paulen, A. (1985). Practice issues for the oncology clinical nurse specialist. *Oncology Nursing Forum, 12*(2), 37–39.

Pennsylvania Association of Home Health Agencies. (1986, October). *Home health service provider standards*. Harrisburg, PA: Author.

Pennsylvania Department of Health. (1987). *Division of primary care and home health licensing survey*: Harrisburg, PA: Author.

Tonges, M. (1985). Quality with economy. Doing the right thing for less. *Nursing Economics, 3*, 205–211.

Visiting Nurse Association of Eastern Montgomery County. (1987). Visit statistics by diagnosis: Abington, PA: Author.

Weisslein, S. (1984). Home care today. *American Journal of Nursing, 84*, 341–345.

Yuan, J. (1988). Staff development in a home health agency. In M. Harris (Ed.), *Home health administration* (pp. 249–262). Owings Mills, MD: Rynd Communications.

CHAPTER 71

Hospice Services

MADALON AMENTA

THE PLACE OF HOSPICE CARE IN CANCER TREATMENT

The History of the Hospice Movement in the United States

Expansion of Technology and Denial of Death

During the period that began shortly after the end of World War II until the late 1960s there was a pervasive taboo against open acknowledgment of death in health care settings in the United States and Great Britain. Caregiving staff at all levels set the tone of denial, and patients and families went along by never mentioning what research was beginning to document: the point at which everyone knew that there was no realistic hope that the patient would recover or live much longer (Fiefel, 1959; Foster, Wald, & Wald, 1978; Glaser & Strauss, 1972; Hinton, 1972; Kalish & Reynolds, 1976; Kübler-Ross, 1971; Wald, 1981).

Brown (1978) was stunned while conducting a nationwide study of health care institutions and of education of nursing and medical students. The word *death* was almost never used. She found patients who had been on mechanical life support for many days characterized as "doing poorly." When patients finally died, it was said they had "expired" or "passed on." She noted also that the word *cancer* was never used in direct interaction with patients and families.

During this period the overriding objective of care was the application of high-technology "heroic" invasive measures to maintain physical function. This maintenance of biologic life was regarded by physicians not only as their professional obligation but also as evidence of their skill. The organizing principle of nursing care was the monitoring of machines, tubes, lines, and wires and the meticulous documentation of laboratory, pharmacologic, and radiologic data. "The patient as a person" was a concept taught in schools of nursing but one that was rarely observed in the real world of practice. Furthermore, dying patients who were *not* being maintained on mechanical life support tended to be neglected outright (Kastenbaum & Aisenberg, 1972; Quint, 1967) (Box 71–1).

The emotional, social, and financial implications of this "treat always and at any cost" philosophy were never questioned or examined. Patients and families were not regarded as people with significant needs other than medical ones, nor were their personally held values or the quality of their lives ever considered. Visiting hours were brief and rigidly maintained. When professionals knew patients' families at all, they knew them by sight and treated them formally and at best politely as guests, not as integral parts of the patient's life and recovery process.

Because the apparatus was more important than anything else in the care-giving mix, visiting family and friends were shooed out of the room to wait in the hall when a crisis did occur. Behind the closed door, the staff, unencumbered by the presence of laypersons, worked on both the apparatus and the patient. "When the miracle-working technology failed, the families were on their own. They signed the necessary forms, took the deceased's belongings, and left as quickly as possible. The modern hospital got right on with its proper function—curing" (Amenta & Bohnet, 1986, p. 2).

The 1960s and Social Change

By the mid 1960s, however, the social climate of the United States began to change. Antiauthoritarianism in the form of social protest found expression in the civil rights movement, women's liberation activity, and protest against the Vietnam War. The major themes and subliminal messages of these causes, thanks largely to television, spread throughout all socioeconomic levels of society.

The new antiauthoritarianism expressed itself in the health care sector as antiscience. People began to question the value of the application of an all-out life-saving technology in every instance, and they came to challenge the validity of physician-dominated policies in the organization of health care. Natural foods and natural remedies gained new interest and popularity. The option for natural or anesthesia-free childbirth became widely available also. The American Hospital Association began to take a formal interest in patients' rights, and new organizations such as the Society of Health and Human Values were founded (Amenta & Bohnet, 1986). The Hastings Institute, which studies emerging biomedical ethical issues, was founded in 1969.

The ancient common law precept of a person's primacy in the right to make decisions about his or her body was prominently revived with the women's movement's insistence that women be allowed to control their own bodies, especially in the area of reproductive health. New self-help groups like Make Today Count and Widow to Widow came into being. Awareness of the right to and the presumed healthiness of free and authentic communication was gaining ground at the same time that social science research was validating the need and desire of dying patients and families to be able to talk frankly about death and, later, bereavement (Fiefel, 1959; Raphael, 1977) (Box 71–2).

Evolution of a Science of Palliative Care

In the United States, where much of the research on attitudes about death, dying and bereavement, pain

---

Box 71–1. NURSING RESEARCH NOTE

Quint, J. (1967). *The nurse and the dying patient.* New York: Macmillan.

As an outgrowth of her work with B. Glaser and A. Strauss on a larger study of how hospital personnel gave care to dying patients (funded by a Public Health Service Grant from the Division of Nursing), the author concentrated on nursing education to discover what formal preparation students received in care of the dying. She was concerned particularly with communication skills in relation to the dying process.

Some of the research questions included the following:

- What are nursing students taught about death?
- In the course of the curricular progression, when is the material taught?
- What situations with dying patients give the students satisfaction?
- What situations with dying patients cause them difficulty?

Starting in 1961, data were collected from five schools of nursing in the San Francisco Bay area. One was a university school with both graduate and undergraduate programs. The other four were hospital schools selected for diversity of locale, organizational pattern, and type of facility.

Results indicated that nursing students (and by extension, graduates) found it difficult under most circumstances to communicate meaningfully with dying patients and their families. Only when the patient had already come to terms with death or was very old, or when the student could assure the patient that she or he would die easily, did the students find it professionally satisfying, or less difficult.

The author recommended increased work in the specifics of psychosocial support and communication skills in all elements of the curriculum. She particularly urged planned and organized faculty attention to and amplified and deepened student experiences in the care of the terminally ill.

Box 71–2. RESEARCH NOTE

Raphael, B. (1977). **Preventive intervention with the recently bereaved.** *Archives of General Psychiatry, 34,* 1450–1454.

Nonselected widows in a large urban area were contacted in the early weeks following their husbands' deaths and assessed for risk of poor bereavement outcome. In addition to a description of the course of the bereavement thus far, the semistructured, nondirective interview sought information about level of risk in terms of the preexisting relationship with the husband, the circumstances of the death, the presence of concurrent crises, and the griever's perception of availability of social support. Those who either ranked high on perception of nonsupportiveness of the social network or ranked somewhat lower but high on the other characteristics were considered to be at high risk. They were randomly assigned to intervention and nonintervention control groups.

The intervention consisted of supportive counseling that averaged four sessions of about 2 hr apiece in the widows' homes. The goals of the counseling were encouragement of the expression of grief, promotion of mourning, and direct discussion of the specific areas of risk for the particular widow. Interviews were recorded and rated by an independent evaluator for level of goal achievement. All subjects were contacted 13 months later and reevaluated on general health and adjustment dimensions.

At follow-up the high-risk subjects in the treatment group were significantly more likely to have had a good outcome than those who were not visited. Those at risk in the nontreatment group were worse off in terms of the health and adjustment scores than the non-high-risk controls, whereas the health of the intervention group approximated that of the non-high-risk subjects. Among the treatment subjects, those who had the highest scores for perception of lack of a supportive network were especially likely to have benefited from the intervention.

---

control, and effective communication techniques was being conducted, a body of knowledge was developing slowly about palliative—comfort, not curing—care. A persistent and growing concern with human and social values accompanied the increasing awareness that the organization of health care had a direct influence on patient outcomes. In addition, it was becoming apparent that to make organizational changes, caregivers themselves had to change their attitudes.

Questions of Costs of Care versus Quality of Life

In the meantime, the costs of care due to continuing advances in technology were escalating rapidly. A trend toward high costs of care in conventional settings, notably in the last year of life, first identified in studies published in the early 1970s, was solidly confirmed by later research (Mor & Masterson-Allen, 1987) (Table 71–1). Health care economists started to question the value of this highly intensive care in relation to quality of life, especially for very elderly people.

Influence of Saunders and Kübler-Ross

It was during these years that in London, England, Saunders was developing an organizational model of humane care for the dying (DuBoulay, 1984). Her synthesis of modern pharmacology to ease the pain of terminal illness with the historical religious-hospice functions of fastidious personal care, companionship, and spiritual support is generally accepted as the theoretical basis of modern hospice care. St. Christopher's, founded in 1967, is an inpatient facility with a home-like atmosphere where visiting schedules are flexible and families as well as patients are treated holistically and compassionately.

It was also during the 1960s in the United States that Dr. Elisabeth Kübler-Ross's work with dying patients resulted in her assertion that coping with death and dying can take place only in a climate that encourages and supports open communication. Her book, *On Death and Dying,* published in 1969, fostered a disseminated general interest in the subject.

In the 1960s both Kübler-Ross and Saunders spoke at seminars at Yale University, where a small group of clergy, nurses, physicians, students, and concerned laypersons were discussing the issues of mechanically and bureaucratically controlled death and dying. As a result of these sessions, the dean of the Yale School of Nursing, along with others, visited St. Christopher's to get a grounding in its organization and clinical practice.

There, Saunders was applying her theory that treating the whole person, rather than just the disease or the physical pain, brings beneficial results (DuBoulay, 1984). She and her staff had learned that pain is not just physical, but emotional, spiritual, and economic as well. By paying attention to the treatment of these other domains in a patient's and family's life, they found that the intensity of the patient's physical pain was often decreased. Over and over again, they were able to demonstrate that if patients perceived themselves to be heard and understood, physical pain was diminished.

Saunders and the Regular Giving of Pain Medication

The sensitively balanced and highly sophisticated pharmacologic pain control techniques developed by Saunders in her earlier research were also being systematically applied. Part of Saunders's innovative contribution to modern medicine was the regular giving of pain medication that she had observed during her student days in a nursing home. This system strives for prescribed medications, in whatever dosage or combination, to be given whenever possible by mouth on a

Table 71–1. SUMMARY OF STUDIES ON HEALTH COSTS IN LAST YEAR OF LIFE: TOTAL CHARGES AND PER CENT DISTRIBUTION OF CHARGES BY TYPE OF SERVICE

Study	Year	Sample	Total Cost/ Charge	Percent of Total			
				Hospital (%)	SNP (%)	MD & OPD (%)	Home Health (%)
Lubitz & Prihoda, 1984; Medicare Services in Last Year of Life	1978	All decedents n = 1,141,560	$4527 Medicare A and B	77	2	19	2
McCall, 1984; Medicare Cost in Last Year	1977–1978	Colorado decedents non-ESRD and disabled n = 9,971	$5955 Medicare A and B	80	1	15	1
Long et al., 1984; Blue Cross Cancer Beneficiary Last Year of Life Charges	1979 (1980$)	Michigan, Indiana, and Atlanta cancer decedents with high coverage plans n = 662	$21,219 all charges	73	—	24	—
Spector & Mor, 1984; Rhode Island Medicare and Blue Cross Last *Six Month* Charges for Cancer Decedents	1980–1981 (1980$)	Rhode Island cancer decedents with Medicare or Blue Cross n = 2,104	$10,548 Medicare A and B and Blue Cross–Blue Shield	84	3	10	2
Brooks & Smyth-Staruch, 1984; Last *Six Month* Medicare and Blue Cross for Cancer Decedents	1981	Cleveland nonhospice cancer decedents with Medicare or Blue Cross n = 1,397	$9362 Medicare A and B and Blue Cross–Blue Shield	94	2	3 Only OPD	1
Kidder, 1984; Medicare Costs in Last Year of Life	1980–1982 (1982$)	Nonhospice cancer hospital deaths n = 558	$14,799 Medicare Part A only	96	2	Not included	2

SNF, skilled nursing facility; OPD, outpatient department; ESRD, end stage renal disease.
(From Mor, V., & Masterson-Allen, S. [1987]. *Hospice care systems.* Heidelberg: Springer-Verlag. Reproduced by permission.)

regular schedule that anticipates the re-emergence of pain. If the patient requires 60 or 90 mg morphine every 2 hr because the pain has been documented to "bleed through" the analgesia barrier every 2 hr and 15 min, the patient gets it. Because this eliminates the anticipatory anxiety that enhances physical pain, the patient remains pain free.

The First American Hospice

Soon after visiting St. Christopher's, some of the New Haven study group, with the help of a small grant from the National Cancer Institute, mounted a demonstration of what the new system of care could accomplish (Brown, 1978). Although home care was not the emphasis of the St. Christopher's model, it became the most reasonable setting for the Connecticut project, because there was no physical structure available that would meet state building code standards as an inpatient facility, and also because there was no category in the licensure and reimbursement structures for hospice care. So in November 1971, Hospice, Inc., was incorporated as an independent, nonprofit organization to provide hospice services as a supplement to the services provided by home health agencies and

hospitals. Still later, in 1974, when a building was being planned, the organization changed its name to Connecticut Hospice, Inc., and in the fall of 1979 it opened its new 44-bed facility (Amenta & Bohnet, 1986).

In 1975 the second hospice program in the United States, the Hospice at St. Luke's, St. Luke's–Roosevelt Hospital in New York City, began offering services. This program, too, although housed in an acute care hospital, devised another uniquely American hospice care organizational variation, the scatter bed consultation model. Soon hospice planning groups sprang up all over the country, and the growth in the number of new operational hospices has been steady (Fig. 71–1). In fact, hospice care remains one of the most rapidly growing segments of the health care system ("NHO Reports," 1988).

CHARACTERISTICS OF THE MODERN AMERICAN HOSPICE

Philosophy

The contemporary American hospice—with several elements of care that distinguish it from traditional

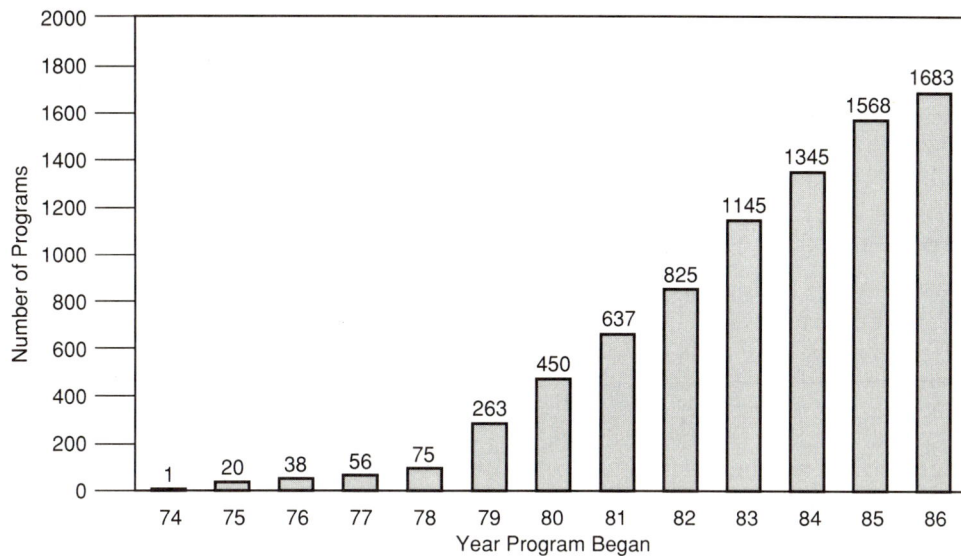

Figure 71–1. Growth of hospice in the United States. The first hospice in the United States was begun in 1974. (From *Hospice News*, February 1988, p. 1. National Hospice Organization. Redrawn with permission.)

care—is an array of services rooted in a holistic health care philosophy of living, dying, and living while dying (Amenta & Bohnet, 1986). It is a concept that unites treatment of terminally ill patients and their families, taken together as the unit of care, with modern science, belief, and caring. Its goal is the prolongation of meaningful life as the patient and family define it, not physiologic dying. As a general rule—and there are always exceptions in hospice care—no "active curative" measures or invasive diagnostic procedures are employed except for palliative or comfort-inducing reasons. For example, both radiation and chemotherapy may be used, not only for reduction of tumor size, but also for control of pain.

Program Elements

Pain and Symptom Control

The overall objective of pain and symptom control in hospice care is the balance of the potential side effects of palliative therapeutic treatments with the maintenance of an alert state in the patient. Ideally, patients should be as much like themselves as feasible, so that they can be in control of as much of the remaining time and as many of the remaining choices as possible.

Spiritual Support

A strong emphasis on spiritual support, individualized to meet patient and family needs, is another prominent characteristic of hospice care (Amenta & Bohnet, 1986). As patients and their families approach death in an open and forthright way in a freely communicating atmosphere, they should have the opportunity to examine the dimensions of meaning, relatedness, forgiveness, and transcendence if they wish, whether or not they are conventionally religious.

Home Care, Inpatient Care, and Bereavement Support

Hospice services are available in the home or inpatient facility when needed for stabilization of symptoms, development of pain control regimens, or brief periods of respite for the primary care giver. In addition to home and inpatient care, all bona fide hospice organizations must provide bereavement support also on a regular basis to selected, usually high-risk survivors.

The Interdisciplinary Team

All of these services are provided by an interdisciplinary team of nurses, physicians, social workers, counselors, and other therapists, clergy, and volunteers.

Volunteers

Volunteers play a major role in this country in the administration and delivery of all aspects of hospice care. Often bereavement components are managed completely by volunteers. Data compiled by the National Hospice Organization's (NHO) 1987 census showed that the average number of volunteers per hospice program in the United States was 52 ("NHO Reports," 1988). Reinforcing the significance of volunteers to hospice work is the finding of the NHO study that volunteers deliver 4.3 to 9 per cent of all home care hours (Mor & Masterson-Allen, 1987).

Staff Stress and Staff Support

Another hallmark of hospice care is support for staff to help them deal with the work-related stress many of them experience. Although some of the stress may be due to the wearing effect of losing one patient after another to death, more often it is team-related. A 1987 survey conducted by Dr. Dale Larson supports the findings of Vachon (Beresford, 1988; Vachon, 1987) (Box 71–3). The greatest impediments to effective hospice team functioning are the members' difficulty in openly and comfortably dealing with conflict and their lack of trust in the team.

Coordination of Care

The interdisciplinary team coordinates and supervises all hospice services 7 days a week, 24 hr a day. Careful monitoring of clinical care from one level to another is essential. There should be effective informal as well as formal two-way communication between the hospice organization and inpatient facilities, traditional home care agencies, physicians, and other community professionals, such as pharmacists, clergy, and funeral directors.

AVAILABILITY AND ORGANIZATION OF HOSPICE SERVICES IN THE UNITED STATES

Profile of Hospice Patients

Age

The average age of the American hospice patient is between 60 and 75 years (Mor & Masterson-Allen, 1987). There are slightly more women than men, and the vast majority are white. Approximately 1 per cent of all hospice patients are children ("NHO Reports," 1988).

Diagnostic Categories and Prognosis

Although few hospice programs reject applicants by disease category explicitly, slightly more than 90 per cent of all hospice patients have cancer (Mor & Masterson-Allen, 1987). In fact, in 1986 32.8 per cent of all Americans who died of cancer received hospice care ("NHO Reports," 1988). This is because more than 70 per cent of hospice programs have a 6 month or less prognosis as an admission requirement. This also reflects either the willingness or the ability of physicians to predict approximate time of death more accurately for advanced cancer than for other life-threatening diseases, such as hypertension, diabetes, end-stage renal disease, and amyotrophic lateral sclerosis. The major primary sites of the cancers in hospice patients are colon, lung, breast, and prostate (Mor & Masterson-Allen, 1987; "NHO Reports," 1988).

Persons with AIDS

The National Hospice Organization has called on hospices nationwide to serve the needs of persons with acquired immune deficiency syndrome (AIDS), their families, and significant others through existing hospice

---

Box 71–3. NURSING RESEARCH NOTE

Vachon, M. L. S. (1987). **Occupational stress in the care of the critically ill, the dying, and the bereaved.** Washington, DC: Hemisphere Publishing.

On the basis of what she had perceived in several years of providing staff support and consultation on team issues for workers in high-stress health care treatment centers—palliative care facilities, intensive care units, and chronic care hospitals—Vachon tried to validate her impressions systematically. She explored four questions about workplace-related stress:

- What were workers' perceptions of what caused them stress?
- How were these stresses affected by factors in their personal lives?
- How did these stresses manifest themselves?
- How did the workers cope with the stresses?

The author conducted unstructured interviews based on these questions with workers in oncology (25 per cent), palliative care (18 per cent), critical care (17 per cent), and other specialties in many parts of the world—Canada, the United States, Western Europe, Australia, India, South Africa, and the West Indies. Forty-nine per cent of the subjects were nurses, 24 per cent were physicians, and 71 per cent were women. Fifty-four per cent were clinicians, and another 21 per cent combined clinical work with teaching, research, or administrative activities. Fifty per cent were 30 to 45 years old, and 35 per cent were older than 45, thus increasing the likelihood that the group would have had experience in identifying and managing to cope with workplace-induced stresses.

There were 327 interviews with 600 caregivers, many in groups, that yielded a total of 8912 anecdotes, which were coded and analyzed. The anecdotes fell into four major categories: coping strategies (38 per cent), work environment stress (37 per cent), manifestations of stress (18 per cent), and personal mediating variables (7 per cent).

Of the anecdotes relating to stress in the work environment, 36 per cent dealt with the work setting itself, 26 per cent with occupational roles, and 23 per cent with issues connected with patients and families. Only 15 per cent were associated with patients' illnesses. The highest ranking item in this category was "problems with team communication," which had as the most frequently cited underlying source "control issues." Other work-setting stresses cited were nature of the unit, role ambiguity, role conflict, inadequate resources (staffing), and communication problems with others in the institution.

program structures. Of the estimated 13,971 people who died of AIDS in 1987, approximately 5,393 (38.6 per cent) received some hospice care (NHO Annual Report, 1988). This relatively small number may reflect certain problems inherent in the average American hospice's capacity to treat persons with AIDS.

A prominent deterrent lies with these patients themselves. Many do not want to forfeit the possible benefits of intensive technical care, nor are they prepared to abandon the goal of cure. They avidly and persistently seek out scientific as well as nontraditional therapies. A lucky few get the interferon injections or zidovudine provided by the scientific medical care establishment, but they, too, may drink herbal teas, take acupuncture treatments, go to faith healers, and consume large quantities of vitamin C, as do the majority who do not get the experimental treatments.

A second significant difficulty facing hospices in the care of persons with AIDS is that they require much more care and many more labor-intensive services for longer periods of time than the types of dying patients that have been traditionally served. The symptoms of AIDS are so severe, diverse, and unremitting and the downhill course is so rapidly progressive that treatment is extremely, arguably prohibitively, costly. There is a real fear among hospice administrators that just one too many of these patients might "break the bank."

The work-related group insurance of persons with AIDS is cancelled when they become too ill to continue at their jobs. Once out of a group plan, they cannot find individual coverage. Many of them do not live the 2 yr from diagnosis required to claim disability under Medicare, and because they are for the most part too young, they cannot claim the traditional Medicare benefits for those older than 65. One hope for relief of this situation is the growing number of states that are developing a new Medicaid hospice option benefit made possible by the 1986 Consolidated Omnibus Budget Reconciliation Act legislation (Beresford, 1988) (explained further in the section on "Reimbursement for Hospice Care").

Economic Considerations

The issue of cost savings for the total health care system through hospice care is not insignificant. Part of the reason for the great growth in the availability of the hospice option in the last decade has been the presumed cost effectiveness of hospice care through the substitution of home care days for inpatient days in acute care facilities during the last weeks of life (Mor & Masterson-Allen, 1987). In 1984 Lubitz and Prihoda (1984) found in an in-depth analysis of Medicare reimbursement statistics that 5.9 per cent of Medicare beneficiaries who had died within the year incurred 28 per cent of all Medicare expenditures. Those who died with cancer had the highest acute care hospital use and also the highest total Medicare reimbursements (see Table 71–1).

Organization

Hospice care is still so new that it is not yet standardized, and there is still considerable debate within the hospice and the health care communities about the impact of the various program types and about which type is the most effective clinically and fiscally (Kidder, 1987). The various shapes and sizes that hospice programs have assumed historically have depended more on the caregiving assets and the leadership structure of the communities in which they have developed than on rational planning and scientifically based needs assessments.

Generic Program Characteristics

Because organizational structure is related to both clinical and cost of care outcomes, it is important to know what hospice programs are like in general as well as the major administrative types in particular. Hospices are small, labor-intensive organizations. In 1988, the average hospice program had 13 full-time paid employees and treated 124 patients. The average length of stay was between 30 and 56 days (NHO Annual Report, 1988). Historically, hospices have treated an average of 10 to 20 patients a month (Kidder, 1987).

Program Availability

In its 1988 hospice census, the NHO identified 1700 programs in various stages of development, planning through fully operational, in all 50 states. One thousand six hundred and four were functioning at some level, and an estimated 1000 were providing a comprehensive set of services.

Ownership and Major Models

Of the 1604 operational programs identified in the 1988 NHO census, 42 per cent were independent, community-based organizations; 28 per cent were hospital-based; and 23 per cent were home health agency–based. The remaining 8 per cent were either coalition models or nursing home or long-term care facility–based programs.

Hospital-Based Hospices

Hospice programs based administratively in acute care hospitals enjoy the built-in advantage of having easy access to shared support services and various treatment specialties. There are three major types. The first is the discrete unit. In this type, from one to ten beds located together are designated for hospice care exclusively. The staff is specially trained and is assigned to the unit permanently. Characteristically, these units have nurse to patient ratios that are similar to those for acute and critical care levels.

In the second type of acute care hospital-based hospice, there is neither a designated contiguous group of beds nor a designated hospice team. In these programs, patients appropriate for hospice care are identified in all units of the institution and are treated palliatively through the existing caregiving structures.

The third type of acute care hospital-based hospice is what is known as the scatter bed model. In these programs an especially trained, designated hospice care team—at a minimum, a nurse, a physician, a social worker, and associated volunteers—sees appropriate patients anywhere in the hospital; rather than give direct care, they consult about palliative measures with the routine staff. In general, they do assessments, teach patients and families and unit staff, coordinate care, and act as patient advocates.

Long-Term Care, Facility-Based Hospices

Hospice programs in long-term care facilities have from one to four dedicated beds and may or may not have a specially trained, designated staff. For home care follow-up, they make arrangements with home health agencies or independent community-based hospices. Long-term care facilities that do not have hospice units but are sensitive to the needs of hospice patients and their families are important to the network of hospice caring institutions in any community. They are the facilities used most often for respite care by Medicare-certified hospices.

Community-Based Comprehensive Home Health Agency Hospices

There are two types of program organization in the community-based, home health agency–owned hospices. In the first type, there is a designated hospice care team, selected and trained for work with hospice patients and families exclusively. Because of the time involved in the care of hospice patients, these nurses on average see fewer patients and families per day than do regular home care nurses. Often three to five visits are all that can be managed realistically.

In other community-based comprehensive home health agencies that offer hospice services, the entire nursing staff, after appropriate orientation, carries one or two families in their districts as part of their generalized caseload. Usually there is ongoing education and consultation as well as staff support to help these nurses remain current in the hospice-specific aspects of care.

Independent Community-Based Hospices

Community-based independent hospice programs treat hospice patients and their families exclusively. Because many of these programs are also licensed and certified by Medicare as home health agencies, they may provide the full range of traditional home care services as well as the hospice-specific services arrayed above. Some supply only part of the home care and arrange with other comprehensive home health agencies to provide the rest. In addition to the Connecticut Hospice, 25 other programs reported themselves to the NHO as "freestanding" models (M. Duncan, personal communication, Coordinator of Membership Services, NHO, July 27, 1990). These independently managed hospices have their own inpatient care buildings as well as integrated home care services.

Coalition Hospices

Coalition hospices are also generally community-based and owned independently. Characteristically there is a small paid staff plus many volunteers who coordinate the traditional inpatient and home care received by patients and families and provide the hospice-specific services, such as pain and symptom control, spiritual care, bereavement support, social and volunteer services, and family and staff support, as well as community education.

In both the coalition and community-based independent models of hospice care, the primary responsibility for traditional services is assumed, for the most part, by the licensed and conventionally reimbursed agents of that care—the physician, the home health agency, and the hospital or long-term care facility. The hospice program coordinates these services across the various levels of care and supplies the hospice-specific services. These programs vary to the degree that they provide traditional care directly, rather than through referral or contract arrangements.

REIMBURSEMENT FOR HOSPICE SERVICES

Historical Aspects

Early in the history of the hospice movement in the United States, hospice services were reimbursed from many sources. Existing third-party payers covered the traditional medical, social, and nursing care charges generated by physicians, inpatient facilities, and home health agencies, but they did not pay for the hospice-specific elements of care (Amenta, 1985). The costs of managing extensive pain and symptom control consultation, volunteer components, family care, interdisciplinary team support, bereavement follow-up, and round-the-clock availability were met largely through donations and memorials, grants from foundations and philanthropic organizations, religious groups, and the United Way. In many instances, patients and families themselves paid out of pocket for these services. A small number of hospices had either state or federal funding for limited periods as pilot programs or research projects. Several local Blue Cross–Blue Shield organizations supported pilot projects, and although many did not acknowledge hospice programs officially, often they turned benign blind eyes and were frequently lenient in honoring claims.

Slowly and sporadically other insurance companies, industry, and unions began adopting hospice benefits not only as humane options for their beneficiaries but also as cost savers for their group plans. A deterrent to more rapid proliferation of reimbursement for hospice care as an alternative in the private sector was the lack of a legal definition of the nature and scope of hospice services as well a lack of generally accepted standards (Blum & Robbins, 1985).

The Medicare Hospice Benefit

In 1982, however, with the passage of the Medicare Hospice Benefit, an official definition of hospice as a discrete set of services was promulgated, federal regulations were established, and a steady stream of funding for hospice care became available (Cummings, 1985).

Scope of Services and Flow of Payment

Under the terms of this legislation, the qualified hospice program provides eligible beneficiaries with the following benefits: physician services; nursing care; medical social services; counseling; spiritual support; physical, occupational, and speech therapies; homemakers and home health aides; pharmaceutics and biologics required for the control of pain and other symptoms; medical equipment and supplies; and short-term inpatient care either for the management of acute or chronic symptoms or pain control or for respite for the patient's caregivers. The hospice program must provide continuous care in the home during periods of crisis, as well as bereavement counseling, volunteer services, and continuity of inpatient and home care. For every day the patient is enrolled, the hospice is reimbursed at a fixed rate for one of four levels of care. In turn, the hospice program pays for the services of all other agencies, professionals, and vendors.

Eligibility, Election, and Duration of Service

Eligibility is conferred on those entitled to Medicare Part A who are certified by an attending physician as terminally ill with a 6 month or less prognosis. The patient must sign an "election" statement indicating that she or he understands the palliative nature of the hospice program and that certain other traditional Medicare benefits, with the exception of the attending physician, who will continue to be reimbursed for services under Medicare Part B, will be waived.

There are three discrete benefit periods of 90, 90, and 30 days each, during which the patient may remain on the benefit as long as the diagnosis remains terminal illness and the prognosis is still short. During these benefit periods the patient may revoke the hospice option and resume traditional Medicare coverage. The patient may also reelect hospice care at any time.

Core Services and Hospice Program Hegemony

Those professionals providing the core services—medicine, nursing, medical social service, and counseling—must be employees of the hospice. The hospice is responsible for coordinating and controlling the quality of all other services. This makes the hospice organization responsible legally, clinically, and financially, for all care.

Availability of the Medicare Hospice Benefit

At the end of February 1989, the Government Accounting Office reported 609 hospices nationwide actually billing for hospice services under the Medicare benefit and an unknown number in the application process (GAO, 1989). The National Hospice Organization estimates that approximately 821 programs, or almost 50 per cent of the country's operational hospices, are involved to some degree with Medicare certification (M. Duncan, personal communication, Coordinator of Membership Services, NHO, July 27, 1990).

Other Public Sources of Reimbursement for Hospice Care

Traditional Medicare and Comprehensive Cancer Centers

In addition to the Hospice Medicare Benefit, other sources of reimbursement for hospice or hospice-like care exist in the wholly and partially publicly insured sector. Regular Medicare provides both inpatient and home care for indefinite periods, and many terminally ill patients and their families are satisfied with this traditional benefit. Patients and families are satisfied especially with the comprehensive cancer centers, where the strong commitment to patient and family psychosocial support from the day of diagnosis, the interdisciplinary team approach, and the integrated home care services are incorporated into total care (Beresford, 1988).

The Veterans Administration

A few Veterans Administration Hospitals have discrete hospice programs and others have "closet" hospices that provide palliative care (Knowles, 1985). Health maintenance organizations (HMOs) that participate in Medicare, although not required to provide "hands-on" hospice care to their Medicare enrollees, must inform them of the availability of local Medicare certified hospices.

Medicaid

As a result of the 1986 COBRA legislation, mentioned previously, 26 states—Arizona, California, Delaware, Florida, Georgia, Hawaii, Idaho, Illinois, Iowa, Kansas, Kentucky, Louisiana, Maryland, Massachusetts, Michigan, Minnesota, Missouri, New Mexico, New York, North Carolina, North Dakota, Ohio, Pennsylvania, Rhode Island, Vermont, and Wisconsin—are already paying for hospice care under Medicaid, and several others are developing a Medicaid hospice benefit to reimburse hospice care for low-income persons of any age (M. Duncan, personal communication, Coordinator of Membership Services, NHO, July 27, 1990). These Medicaid schemes essentially duplicate the structure of the Medicare benefit (Beresford, 1988).

Private Sources of Reimbursement for Hospice Care

The role of private insurers in funding hospice services has also grown with the establishment of hospice care as a discrete cluster of services. A 1978 survey found only 17 per cent of insurance companies offering coverage specifically designated for the terminally ill, and that coverage was limited to traditional medical and nursing care, not hospice specific services (Cummings, 1985). In 1985, the Washington Business Group on Health reported that 59 per cent of the *Fortune* 500 companies offered a hospice benefit to their employees (Freudenhaim, 1986). Presently, the National Hospice Organization reports that the majority of private insurance companies nationwide offer a hospice benefit, and over half of all American workers are now covered for hospice care. Blue Cross–Blue Shield at the national level has developed a model hospice benefit as a guide for affiliates, the majority of which now have a hospice benefit.

HOW TO FIND HOSPICE CARE

If hospice care is desired but not suggested at the time the patient is diagnosed with a terminal condition, the nurse or the family should know that there are several ways to find help. The National Hospice Organization publishes and sells an annual *Guide to the Nation's Hospices* that lists all known hospice organizations by state and town, contact person, phone number, type of hospice, operational status, scope of service, and counties served. The 1988 NHO Guide also lists the names, addresses, and phone numbers of the officers of the 43 state (plus District of Columbia) hospice organizations, most of which also maintain directories of hospices by location, contact person, and scope of services.

Other national organizations that assist families and professionals in the search for satisfactory hospice care through national telephone referral services are the Hospice Association of America (a subsidiary of the National Association for Homecare) and the National Institute for Jewish Hospice.

When choosing a hospice, the family should be alerted to standards of care expressed in national accreditation, certification, and state licensing credentials. In a state that licenses hospices, the state health department will have up-to-date lists of all caregiving organizations that meet this basic standard. The state health department will also have lists of all Medicare-certified hospices, and the Joint Commission on the Accreditation of Healthcare Organizations (JAHCO) lists all those that are accredited.* As a rule, a hospice will provide this information when contacted.

Some communities may have hospices at various levels of operation; some may be providing only referral, volunteer, and bereavement services, whereas others offer comprehensive programs fully certified, accredited, and licensed if applicable. The family should be assisted in making the decision, if there is a choice, based on their needs and their resources, human as well as financial.

References

Amenta, M. (1985). Hospice in the United States: Multiple models and varied programs. *Nursing Clinics of North America, 20,* 269–279.

Amenta, M., & Bohnet, N. (1986). *Nursing care of the terminally ill.* Boston: Little, Brown & Co.

Beresford, L. (Ed.). (1988, January). *Hospice Letter, 9,* 10 (Wall Township, NJ: Health Resources Publishing).

Blum, J., & Robbins, D. (1985). Considerations in licensure. In P. Torrens (Ed.), *Hospice programs and public policy* (pp. 73–79). Chicago: American Hospital Publishing.

Brown, E. (1978, May). Hospice in the United States—its origin and promise. In *Hospice as a social health care institution. Report of the pre-forum institute of the 105th annual forum of the National Conference of Social Welfare* (pp. 80–90). Los Angeles: Hillhaven Foundation.

Cummings, M. (1985). Current status of hospice financing. *In* P. Torrens (Ed.), *Hospice programs and public policy* (pp. 137–175). Chicago: American Hospital Publishing.

DuBoulay, S. (1984). *Cicely Saunders—founder of the modern hospice movement.* New York: The Amaryllis Press.

Fiefel, H. (1959). *The meaning of death.* New York: McGraw-Hill Book Co.

Foster, Z., Wald, F., & Wald, H. (1978). The hospice movement—a backward glance at its first two decades. *New Physician,* pp. 17–21.

Freudenhaim, M. (1986, February 12). Hospice care as an option. *New York Times,* p. 30.

General Accounting Office. (1989). *Report to the Subcommittee on Health, Committee of Ways and Means, House of Representatives. Medicare: Program Provisions and Payments Discourages Hospice Participation* (GAOHRD-89-111). Washington, D.C., United States General Accounting Office.

Glaser, B., & Strauss, A. (1965). *Awareness of dying.* Chicago: Aldine.

Hinton, J. (1972). *Dying.* Baltimore: Penguin.

Kalish, R., & Reynolds, D. (1976). *Death and ethnicity.* Los Angeles: University of Southern California Press.

Kastenbaum, R., & Aisenberg, R. (1972). *The psychology of death.* New York: Springer.

Kidder, D. (1987). *Medicare hospice benefit—program evaluation*

---

*Useful Addresses: National Hospice Organization, Membership Department, 1901 North Fort Myer Drive, Arlington, VA 22209, (703) 243-5900; Hospice Association of America, 210 7th Street, S.E., Washington, DC 20003, (202) 547-5263; Joint Commission on Accreditation of Healthcare Organizations, Hospice Programs, 875 North Michigan Avenue, Chicago, IL 60611, 800-621-8007; National Institute for Jewish Hospice, 6363 Wilshire Boulevard, Los Angeles, CA, 800-446-4448.

(HCFA Pub. No. 03248). Baltimore, MD: U.S. Department of Health and Human Services.

Knowles, C. (1985). Reimbursements and the Medicare certified hospice. *American Journal of Hospice Care, 2*(5), 15–21.

Kübler-Ross, E. (1969). *On death and dying.* New York: Macmillan.

Kübler-Ross, E. (1971). What is it like to be dying? *American Journal of Nursing, 71,* 54–59.

Lubitz, J., & Prihoda, R. (1984). The use and costs of Medicare services in the last 2 years of life. *Health Care Finance Review, 5,* 117–131.

Mor, V., & Masterson-Allen, S. (1987). *Hospice care systems.* New York: Springer.

NHO Annual Report. (1988).

NHO reports seven percent growth in hospice programs. (1988, February.) *Hospice News,* pp. 1–3.

Quint, J. (1967). *The nurse and the dying patient.* New York: Macmillan.

Raphael, B. (1977). Preventive intervention with the recently bereaved. *Archives of General Psychiatry, 34,* 1450–1454.

Vachon, M. (1987). *Occupational stress in the care of the critically ill, the dying, and the bereaved.* Washington, DC: Hemisphere Publishing.

Wald, F. (1981). Hospice care concepts. In *Hospice education program for nurses.* Hyattsville, MD: U.S. Department of Health and Human Services.

CHAPTER 72

Community Assessment: Congruence of Needs and Resources

JUDITH BAIGIS-SMITH
GLORIA A. HAGOPIAN

The community needs assessment is based on the premise that the community, not the individual, is the unit for study in any comprehensive plan to improve the community's health (Archer, 1985; Jarvis, 1985; Williams, 1984). Generally a community is viewed as having several elements: the people, the geographic area, the resources and services, and the relationships among them (Hanchett, 1979; Warren, 1969). Thus within the context of a community needs assessment, the idea of *community* need not be limited to a city or one of its census tracts but could be viewed as a cancer center, a nursing home, a factory, or the patients and staff of a teaching hospital's radiation oncology department.

Data from the needs assessment are utilized to make community-wide diagnoses (Clemen-Stone, Elasti, & McGuire, 1987). Therefore, the data collection and the resultant diagnoses focus on all of the people, services, and resources of a particular institution or area instead of a single patient and his or her disease. For example, instead of limiting oneself to caring for an individual with cancer in an institution such as a hospital or a community hospice, the oncology nurse is now being asked to think of both the sick *and* the healthy people in a particular community. The oncology nurse can draw on expertise in cancer care and can join with members of other disciplines who use the needs assessment techniques to diagnose the community's health and welfare status. Such expertise applied in this way can bring to the forefront such community ills as environmental risks or hazards (such as leaking dump sites or radiation hazards to hospital staff), identify groups in the community who are at risk for disease or who are already ill (promiscuous homosexual men, nurses administering neoplastic agents to patients, workers with asbestosis), and determine gaps in health and welfare services or resources (lack of transportation to treatment facilities, limited coverage by third-party payors for ambulatory clinic visits) (Box 72–1). Once community-wide diagnoses are made, they can be used to establish priorities for action that should improve the quality of life and health of the individuals living there. In short, adequate care and services for the *entire* community is viewed as taking priority over excellent care or services for just a few of its members (Box 72–2).

TYPES OF COMMUNITY NEEDS ASSESSMENTS

Fundamental to an accurate community diagnosis is the quality of the information on which this diagnosis rests. The information can be gathered by means of several methods that are outlined in the following paragraph. These methods of assessment can be used independently or as parts of an overall assessment program with each method being utilized sequentially.

The five methods for community needs assessments are summarized from the work of Warheit, Bell, and Schwab (1977): key informant, community forum, rates under treatment, social indicators, and field survey.

Key Informant

The key informant approach to needs assessment, viewed as simple to do and inexpensive, is based on

---

Box 72–1. NEEDS OF PERSONS WITH CANCER

Houts, P. H., Yasko, J. M., Kahn, S. B., Schelzel, G. W., & Marconi, K. M. (1986). **Unmet psychological, social, and economic needs of persons with cancer in Pennsylvania.** *Cancer, 8,* 2355–2361.

As one of the first steps in planning statewide cancer rehabilitation programs, the Cancer Control Advisory Board of the Pennsylvania Department of Health interviewed 629 persons with cancer, diagnosed within the year, and 397 support persons involved in their care to determine their unmet needs. In a telephone interview, respondents were asked about 67 types of psychological, social, and economic problems.

The findings indicated that approximately 21,300 persons reported unmet emotional, spiritual, social, and family needs. In this category, unmet emotional needs were reported by 14,000 people. Approximately 17,300 people reported unmet economic needs that included financial, insurance, or employment issues. Almost 10,000 persons had unmet needs that centered on information or treatment by the medical staff. Unmet community needs for transportation and home care were expressed by about 4400 people. Overall, it was estimated that approximately 33,000 people with cancer in the state had at least one unmet need, which represents approximately 59 per cent of the population.

The investigators recommended that priority should be given to planning several programs focusing on unmet emotional needs. Other needs, although less numerous, occurred with sufficient frequency to warrant attention. Periodic assessment of needs of persons with cancer was recommended to improve coping with the disease. The authors also recommended educational programs to alert professionals of the frequency of unmet needs and to inform them of the types of services available.

---

the assumption that the formal and informal leaders in the area or field chosen for study, for example, cancer care, know that area's or field's needs and can articulate them. Because, such individual perspectives may, in fact, be biased or incomplete, the key informants in an area such as cancer care should be chosen from a variety of fields, for example, public and private sector cancer service agencies, academic institutions, welfare organizations, the insurance industry, labor organizations, religious groups, politics, the media, and consumer groups.

Community Forum

The community forum approach to needs assessment is a variation of the town meeting idea. Public meetings are scheduled in strategic and well-publicized places so

that *all* persons interested in the topic to be discussed, such as cancer care or the local toxic waste dump site, can offer their opinions and share information about the community's needs. For best results, however, these meetings must be attended by a cross section of articulate, knowledgeable persons.

Rates under Treatment

In the rates-under-treatment approach to needs assessment, descriptive information from the records of persons who have received care from the local health and welfare agencies are used for insights into community needs. Directories of the types of health and welfare agencies in the community are generally available from the local community society or the equivalent of the United Way. Usually the directories list services

---

Box 72–2. UNMET NEEDS DURING TERMINAL CARE

Houts, P. H., Yasko, J. M., Harvey, H. A., Kahn, S. B., Hartz, A. J., Hermann, J. F., Schelzel, G. W., & Bartholomew, M. J. (1988). **Unmet needs of persons with cancer in Pennsylvania during the period of terminal care.** *Cancer, 62,* 627–634.

A second survey was commissioned by the Pennsylvania Department of Health to determine the unmet needs of patients with cancer during their last month of life. A sample of 433 randomly selected family members was interviewed.

The findings indicated that the most frequent unmet need was help with activities of daily living. This was indicated by 42 per cent of the respondents and involved approximately 11,000 persons. The second and third most frequent unmet needs were emotional and physical, estimated at 21 per cent. Insurance and financial needs were the next most frequent unmet needs at 19 and 15 per cent, respectively, followed by problems with medical staff. All other unmet needs were present in less than 15 per cent of the sample. Overall, 72 per cent of the respondents reported at least one unmet need during the terminal phase of illness.

The important consequence of this study and the one cited previously in Box 72–1 by the Pennsylvania Department of Health is that the findings have been a major stimulus for statewide programs to expand the use of existing support services. The Cancer Control Advisory Board has initiated a statewide program to educate nurses who work with patients with cancer to assist in obtaining necessary services. Consumer guides that describe services available in various geographic areas throughout the state have been distributed. Increasing the availability of home care services during the terminal period is a priority, as well as educating the health professional about the emotional problems that patients experience.

alphabetically and by category of service. They also include addresses, telephone numbers, services offered, catchment areas served, eligibility requirements for clients, and fees for service. The usual types of information collected in the rates-under-treatment approach include sociodemographic characteristics (age, sex, race, education, residence), presenting problems, types and frequency of care and services provided, source of referral, and treatment or service outcomes. This method bases its conclusions on data gathered from a sample of clients who seek such services and therefore could be quite narrow.

Social Indicators

The social indicators approach to a needs assessment is based on inferences drawn from the descriptive statistics of public records and reports, such as, census data, vital statistics, and government agency data. The data can be obtained from the United States Government Printing Office, the Department of Commerce, the Bureau of the Census, county health departments, county medical societies, what remains of the comprehensive health planning agencies, and local colleges and universities (Leahy, Cobb, & Jones, 1982). Such information includes, but is not limited to, morbidity and mortality rates, fertility rates, occupation, population characteristics (age, sex, race, national origin, marital status, religion, educational level), housing characteristics, income, and crime rates and arrest records. The underlying assumption is that it is possible to make useful estimates of the needs and social well-being of a community by analyzing statistics on factors found to be highly correlated with persons in need. For example, individuals who have low incomes and live in substandard housing generally have higher morbidity and mortality rates. Intervention should be directed then at all of the correlated events (housing, income and jobs, education, access to health care, health insurance coverage), not just at one or two of them. Because these are indirect indicators of need, in contrast to the key informant and community forum approaches, such data should be drawn from a wide variety of sources (Leahy et al., 1982, pp. 30–38).

Field Survey

In the field survey, information is collected from either a sample or the entire population of a community about such topics as health history and health status, use of health and welfare agencies, and social and health needs. Information-gathering approaches include telephone surveys, mailed questionnaires, and person-to-person interviews. Although this field survey method can be much more comprehensive than the others, it is also more expensive. In addition, because the targeted population does not consist of volunteers, a certain percentage of it generally refuses to give personal or family information, thereby limiting the representativeness of the groups surveyed.

THE PROCESS OF DATA COLLECTION AND ITS ANALYSIS

Selected components of the social indicators approach to a community needs assessment are outlined in more detail here because the information is available. (See Appendix 72–1 for a sample community assessment guide.) In making a community diagnosis within this context, information should be gathered about the following indicators, analyzed, and then the interrelationships among the items should be studied. In this section, examples of the type of information to be collected are presented, along with examples of the analysis, that is, what the data reveal.

Community Characteristics

The geographic boundaries of the community, its physical characteristics, and its climate and topography will suggest seasonal variation in the patterns of life as well as the kinds of illnesses likely to surface there. Thus three metropolitan cites—one in a subtropical area (Calcutta), one in a temperate climate (Philadelphia), and one in high desert (Santa Fe)—will have different personalities, life styles, and diseases that are influenced in part by their physical and spacial differences. As a result, different cancers may be more prevalent in one community than in another.

What form of government does the community have and what is its legislative process? What is its history? This kind of information defines the parameters of the community and serves to target political responsibilities for community-wide services. It can highlight the dysfunction in the organization and structure of government or the best methods to use to influence local policy in initiating cancer-related activities, for example.

Population Characteristics and Trends

The analysis of population characteristics and trends is a fundamental factor in guiding community development.

Numbers

How many people are living in the area of interest? Does this number represent an increase or decrease in size over the past decade? What is the rate of growth or of population decline? Do people with certain characteristics (similar income or race) tend to cluster in particular areas? If so, why? How mobile is the population? Knowledge of population trends is necessary in assessing needs for specific services and resources and other capital requirements. Analysis of population information helps decide the proper distribution of community facilities as diverse as clinics and transit lines. It is assumed that areas of greatest population increases will need most of the health and welfare services. However, trends in population decreases suggest that the monitoring of building activities is in order so that unneeded schools or hospitals are not begun. A decrease in the population signals a decrease also in the total tax base that is necessary for financing public services, such as transportation and clinics.

Age. What is the percentage of people in each age category? Has this percentage shifted over time? The age distribution within a community is an important determinant of need for goods and services in a population. A large infant and child population will have need for more schools, playgrounds, and pediatricians than one with a primarily elderly population that will have increased need for long-term care facilities or podiatry and dental services. In addition, communities with larger numbers of older people will have higher cancer rates, because the prevalence of cancer increases with age.

Race. What is the racial mix of the community? The need for certain kinds of goods and services are influenced by the racial makeup of the community. A large Asian population will want to have foods and condiments used in their native dishes available in the local supermarkets. Certain diseases are more prevalent among some racial groups, for example, breast cancer among black women and stomach cancer among the Japanese.

Sex. What is the distribution by sex in the community? The ratio of males to females in the population is viewed as a sign of the degree of stability in the population. For example, neighborhoods in flux tend to show a predominance of one sex over the other, but areas that have large female populations are generally more stable than areas with an overabundance of men.

Employment, Occupation and Place of Work. How many people are working, how do they earn their livings, and where do they work? What are the hazards of their work? Are there a high number of cancer-related occupational hazards? What are the work-related injuries and diseases? The percentage of people employed in managerial and professional positions as a percentage of the total number of people employed in an area is a good indicator of the area's economic status. An understanding of the numbers of people who have been disabled, who are at risk for work-related illnesses, or who live in the vicinity of an industry that places them at risk for diseases such as cancer can lead to monitoring and surveillance systems that may effectively reduce morbidity and mortality from such conditions. The nurse can play an important role in educating the community about these risks. Usually, the American Cancer Society participates in community activities that identify occupational risks of cancer.

Vital Statistics

The common vital statistics examined as part of a community assessment include the number of live births, neonatal and infant death rates, maternal deaths, and crude death rates. Incidence and prevalence rates for disease and disability should be examined along with the leading causes of death. What is the ratio of births to deaths? Such information gives insight into the growth patterns in the community. Comparison of these rates with those of other communities, the state, and the nation gives information about the local health problems and the effectiveness of local health services. Thus a community with a lung cancer mortality rate that is higher than that of surrounding communities, the state, and the nation alerts its citizens to the fact that they have a problem that needs to be addressed.

Health, Welfare, and Social Services

The adequacy of these services can be estimated by determining the number and distribution of such services and institutions in relation to the population to be served and the needs to be met. What are the number and types of hospitals, clinics, social service and welfare agencies, occupational health programs, insurance plans, and any other resource important to health and social welfare? What are the programs' purposes, types of services, numbers of beds, kind and number of personnel, and the relationships among these facilities (Tinkham, Voorhies, & McCarthy, 1984)?

To repeat, once the community assessment has been completed, the information can be analyzed critically. Strengths, weaknesses, and unmet needs will emerge. At this point, priorities and plans for action can be set. The needs of the community are assessed then by all of the aforementioned measures of its citizens' vital events and can be seen as equivalent to the individual's vital signs—temperature, pulse, respiration, and blood pressure. "Such statistical measures," to paraphrase Taylor in Mattison, 1968, "require a major conceptual shift in thinking. In clinical practice, for example, a woman is either pregnant or not pregnant; a community can be 3 per cent pregnant. A man may or may not have cancer; a community may always have cancer, though the rate may increase or decrease."

THE NEEDS OF PATIENTS WITH CANCER AND THEIR FAMILIES

An orientation to the health-related problems of the entire community contributes to the preparation of competent clinicians. A good clinician uses knowledge of demographic characteristics, seasonal variations in illness patterns, and knowledge of community resources, for example, in conjunction with his or her understanding of the natural history of disease, such as cancer, to provide the best possible service to the patient and his or her family. In addition to the analysis derived from community needs assessments, however, an analysis of the needs of patients and families who have to cope with particular diseases, such as cancer, must be undertaken. A number of studies have been carried out by nurses to identify the needs of patients with cancer and their families (Wright & Dyck, 1984; Rose, 1976; Edstrom & Miller, 1981; Welch, 1981; Stein, 1982). These studies indicate that patients and their families place a high value on receiving information. They want and need information on both medical and nonmedical aspects of their disease. Specifically, they want information on how to manage and deal with the symptoms and side effects of the disease; information on how to keep the patient comfortable; and the knowledge, skills, and procedures that are necessary to deal with day-to-day life. Patients and families also express a need to obtain information about the resources in the community that they could use. By having this information, family members can participate more fully in care, have a greater feeling of control, and improve the quality of life of the person with cancer. It is the nurse's responsibility to meet the needs that patients and their families have for information so that the goals of care can be achieved.

NEEDS ASSESSMENT IN PRACTICE

In addition to reviewing the literature to determine the needs of patients, the oncology nurse must do a needs assessment of patients and families encountered in clinical practice. Patients with cancer have many needs; those undergoing treatment have additional stresses, burdens, demands, and needs. To participate in treatment regimens, a number of social and emotional concerns must be addressed so that patients can take part in the treatment with a minimum amount of discomfort and disruption of their lives. Often the primary need is for information about the disease, the treatment, and its side effects. In a radiation therapy department, helping patients find answers to questions about medical problems, insurance, transportation, equipment, and using resources in the community are major concerns the nurse must deal with on the patient's behalf. Table 72–1 includes an assessment of major categories of needs.

Often the biggest problem is that of transportation. Patients undergoing radiation therapy must come to the department 5 days a week, Monday through Friday, over a 5- to 6-week period. The nurse should know the types of transportation services that are available, the costs, and the requirements for eligibility. Besides the usual medical transport companies, other organizations may have to be utilized, such as the American Cancer Society, union organizations, or volunteer ambulance services.

For example, consider an 84-year-old widow who has no family but needs radiation therapy over a 6-week period. Because she is over 65 years of age, she is ineligible for free transportation. However, she cannot afford the $7.00 per day for a cab, and public transportation, although inexpensive, requires two transfers and 1 hr of travel time each way. In this instance, a local taxi company that provides discounts to senior citizens and costs only $2.00 can be used.

Table 72–1. NEEDS ASSESSMENT OF PATIENT AND FAMILY

Category of Need	Factors to Assess
Knowledge	Information about disease
	Information about treatment
	Procedures and routines of department
	Side effects of treatment
	Self-care measures
Physical	Treatment
	Review of systems
	Symptom distress
	Side effects of treatment
	Strength, energy level, fatigue, sleep, rest
	Activities of daily living
	Medications
Socioeconomic	Family constellation
	Employment, finances, insurance
	Managing the household
	Knowledge and use of community resources
	Transportation
	Prosthesis—breast, wig, extremity, electronic larynx
	Equipment and supplies—cane, walker, wheelchair, commode, bed
	Peer support group
	Homemaker or home health aide
	Food—meals on wheels, food stamps
	Hospice
Emotional	Presence of anxiety, depression, anger, guilt, avoidance, denial
	Coping strategies used
	Communication patterns with family and friends
	Communication patterns with health care professionals
	Anticipation of future
	Spiritual concerns

RESPONSIBILITIES OF NURSES

Oncology nurses have a responsibility to assess and intervene at both the community and the patient and family level of practice (Box 72–3). At the community level, it is important that nurses know the community in which they work. Nurses should be alert to environmental risks and hazards in the community, serve on committees related to cancer, participate in cancer control programs, identify the availability and adequacy of community resources, and identify gaps in services. Nurses should promote the public's knowledge of cancer also and use the existing political methods to influence public policy as it relates to cancer. In the agencies in which they are employed, oncology nurses should serve on committees and practice safety procedures that provide protection against environmental hazards. They should participate in prevention and early detection programs in the workplace. At the family and individual level, assessment of needs and matching needs to available community resources is a priority.

The Outcome Standards for Public Cancer Education, Patient Education, and Nursing Practice deal explicitly with problem areas of communities, families, patients, and the responsibilities of oncology nurses (Oncology Nursing Society and American Nurses Association, 1979; Oncology Nursing Society Public Education Committee, 1982, 1983). The Standards for Public Cancer Information provide information and

---

options for prevention, early detection, rehabilitation, and living with cancer. The focus is on the community. The Standards for Patient Education were developed to identify the knowledge needed to maximize patients' ability to live with cancer. They can be used as guidelines to develop patient education strategies, to evaluate existing programs, and to assist patients in assessing financial factors related to the utilization of the health care system. The Standards for Nursing Practice emphasize patient and family functioning at an optimal level at any point on the health-illness continuum. The standards pertain to identification of community resources, prevention and early detection, information, coping, comfort, nutrition, protective mechanisms, mobility, elimination, sexuality, and ventilation. The standards should guide nursing practice in all areas of care and allow nurses to evaluate the effectiveness of their interventions.

IDENTIFYING RESOURCES FOR PATIENTS AND FAMILIES

Because the nursing literature indicates that patients and families need knowledge of resources in the community, it is imperative that nurses are knowledgeable about resources available at the local, state, and national levels. The American Cancer Society can assist with providing information about the services it offers, as well as referring patients and families to other resources. Another helpful source for identifying community resources is the Directory of Human Services. Usually these directories are published by the United Way and other community service groups and are available at nominal cost. One other source to learn about community services is the Cancer Information Service, a national telephone inquiry service that provides access to the latest information about cancer-related resources; it can be reached by a toll-free number, 1-800-4-CANCER. A detailed discussion of cancer resources can be found in other chapters in this unit.

Guidelines for Use of Community Resources

To effectively use the many different health, social, and welfare resources for the care of patients with cancer and their families, the information about these resources must be assembled carefully and organized for ready use by (1) locating the relevant resources, (2) knowing the scope and limitations of the services offered, (3) maintaining a file of resources, and (4) developing suitable referral procedures (Freeman, 1963).

Before referring the patient and family to a particular community resource, the nurse should talk with them to be sure that they see the need for the care and are ready to accept it. This preliminary step promotes optimal use of community resources (Oncology Nursing Society, Public Education Committee, 1983).

The patient and family should have the following information about the agency: (1) name, address, and phone number of a contact person, which assures accountability of a particular person at that agency for the patient's treatment (a visit to the agency to establish professional relations is always a good idea; along with meeting the staff and enlarging one's professional network, service delivery can be observed; if a visit cannot be made, the nurse should *always* make a phone call); (2) description of the agency's mission; (3) eligibility requirements; (4) services offered; (5) hours those services are provided; (6) fees for services and policies regarding insurances; (7) intake or admission procedures; (8) documents the patient must bring; (9) whether there is a waiting list; and (10) transportation routes to the agency. *The appropriate information about the patient must be received by the agency personnel before the patient's first visit.*

SUMMARY

Interest and skill in assessing the needs of both the *entire community* and people with cancer and their families means that the oncology nurse has yet another arena for participating in a variety of activities that can both prevent or ameliorate the occurrence of cancer and improve the quality of life for those who already have the disease. Diagnosis of the community's environmental cancer hazards via community needs assessments is well within the expertise of the oncology nurse. Community-wide planning and action committees can benefit from ideas and information brought from the "front lines" of oncology nursing practice. Both types of involvement (community diagnosis and clinical practice) can have an impact on public policy initiatives; both will raise the nurse's understanding of environmental and community health and their impact on the individuals being treated.

People with cancer and their families have many "needs" in common—needs for knowledge about the disease, coping strategies, pain management, and community resources, for example. Although the oncology nurse certainly has performed well in the clinical areas, methods for increasing effectiveness in addressing community-wide needs and utilizing community resources for better patient care have been presented here.

References

Archer, S. E. (1985). Selected concepts and processes for client-centered community health nursing. In S. E. Archer & R. P. Fleshman (Eds.), *Community health nursing* (3rd ed., pp. 96–130). Monterey, CA: Wadsworth Health Sciences.

Clemen-Stone, S., Eigsti, D. G., & McGuire, S. L. (1987). Community diagnosis for health planning. *Comprehensive family and community health nursing* (2nd ed., pp. 359–391). New York: McGraw-Hill Book Co.

Edstrom, S., & Miller, M. W. (1981). Preparing the family to care for the cancer patient at home. *Cancer nursing, 4,* 49–52.

Freeman, R. B. (1963). *Public health nursing practice* (3rd ed.). Philadelphia: W. B. Saunders Co.

Hanchett, E. S. (1979). *Community health assessment: A conceptual tool kit.* New York: John Wiley & Sons.

Jarvis, L. L. (1985). Population issues. *Community health nursing: Keeping the public healthy* (2nd ed., pp. 779–790). Philadelphia: F. A. Davis Co.

Leahy, K. M., Cobb, M. M., & Jones, M. C. (1982). *Community health nursing* (4th ed.). New York: McGraw-Hill Book Co.

Mattison, B. F. (1968). Community health planning and the health professions. *American Journal of Public Health, 58,* 1019.

Oncology Nursing Society and American Nurses' Association Division on Medical-Surgical Nursing Practice. (1979). *Outcome standards for cancer nursing practice.* Kansas City, MO: American Nurses' Association.

Oncology Nursing Society Education Committee. (1982). *Outcome standards for cancer patient education.* Pittsburgh: Oncology Nursing Society.

Oncology Nursing Society Education Committee. (1983). *Outcome standards for public cancer education.* Pittsburgh: Oncology Nursing Society.

Rose, M. A. (1976). Problems families face in home care. *American Journal of Nursing, 76,* 416–418.

Stein, K. Z. (1982). Classifying cancer client needs for community health nursing intervention. *Cancer Nursing, 5,* 283–286.

Tinkham, C. W., Voorhies, E. F., & McCarthy, N. C. (1984). *Community health nursing: Evolution and process in the family and community.* New York: Appleton-Century-Crofts.

Warheit, G. J., Bell, R. A., & Schwab, J. J. (1977). *Needs assessment approaches: Concepts and methods* (ADM–79–472). Washington, DC: U.S. Department of Health, Education and Welfare Publication.

Warren, R. L. (1969). *Studying your community.* New York: The Free Press.

Welch, D. (1981). Planning nursing interventions for family members of adult cancer patients. *Cancer Nursing, 4,* 365–370.

Williams, C. A. (1984). Population-focused practice. In M. Stanhope & J. Lancaster (Eds.), *Community health nursing: Process and practice for promoting health* (pp. 805–815). St. Louis: C. V. Mosby Co.

Wright, K., & Dyck, S. (1984). Expressed concerns of adult cancer patients family members. *Cancer Nursing, 7,* 371–374.

APPENDIX 72–1

COMMUNITY ASSESSMENT GUIDE*

Community _____ Date of Survey _____

I. THE COMMUNITY

A. Description: Include general identifying data, i.e., location, topography, climate, urban, rural.

B. Geographic Boundaries: Give specific boundaries surrounding study area. Include maps if necessary.

C. Type of government: (Mayor, City Manager, Board of Supervisors)

D. History: Include significant changes such as urban development, major highway construction, regionalization, shifts in industry.

*Adapted from Tinkham, C.W., Voorhies, E.F., & McCarthy, N.C. (1984). *Community health nursing: Evolution and process.* New York: Appleton-Century-Crofts.

Appendix continued on following page

II. POPULATION CHARACTERISTICS

A. Total population, 19___ (last census)
B. Population changes in last 10 years:
C. Population per square mile:
D. Mobility of population:
E. Population and age distribution:

CURRENT POPULATION 19___ AGE GROUP	COMMUNITY NUMBER/ PER CENT	STATE POPULATION NUMBER/PER CENT	NATIONAL POPULATION NUMBER/PER CENT
Under 5			
5–9			
10–14			
15–24			
25–34			
35–44			
45–54			
55–64			
65–74			
75–84			
85 +			

F. Race

Race	COMMUNITY NUMBER/PER CENT	STATE NUMBER/PER CENT	NATIONAL NUMBER/PER CENT

G. Sex Distribution

RACE	SEX	COMMUNITY NUMBER/PER CENT	STATE NUMBER/PER CENT	NATIONAL NUMBER/PER CENT
White	Female			
	Male			
Black	Female			
	Male			
Asian	Female			
	Male			
Other	Female			
	Male			

H. Nation of Origin:

Percent of total:

I. Marital Status

MARITAL STATUS	MALE			FEMALE		
	TOTAL	WHITE	NONWHITE	TOTAL	WHITE	NONWHITE
Single						
Married						
Separated						
Widowed						
Divorced						

J. Religion

RELIGION	COMMUNITY NUMBER/PER CENT	STATE NUMBER/PER CENT	NATIONAL NUMBER/PER CENT
Catholic			
Protestant			
Jewish			
Other			

K. Education Levels

EDUCATION	COMMUNITY NUMBER/PER CENT	STATE NUMBER/PER CENT	NATIONAL NUMBER/PER CENT
No Schooling			
Kindergarten			
Elementary (1–8 yr)			
High School (1–4 yr)			
College			
Median Years of Education			

L. Socioeconomic Characteristics

1. Income of Families, 19___

INCOME OF FAMILIES	COMMUNITY NUMBER/PER CENT	STATE NUMBER/PER CENT	NATIONAL NUMBER/PER CENT
Under $5,000			
$5,000–10,000			
$11,000–19,000			
$20,000 +			
$30,000 +			

2. Occupation, Employment

OCCUPATION	MALE %	FEMALE %
Professional/Technical		
Clerical		
Sales		
Craftspersons		
Operatives		
Private Household		
Service Workers (excluding private household)		
Laborers		
Others		

3. Leading Industries

4. Estimated level of unemployment

Community _____ State _____ National _____

III. HOUSING

A. Condition

CONDITION AND PLUMBING	COMMUNITY %	STATE %	NATIONAL %
Sound			
With All Facilities			
Lacking Facilities			
Deteriorating			
With All Facilities			
Lacking Facilities			
Dilapidated			

B. Ownership and Rental Status

Units owned % _____

Units rented % _____

IV. MORTALITY AND MORBIDITY DATA

A. Vital Statistics:

	COMMUNITY	STATE	NATIONAL
	NUMBER/PER CENT	NUMBER/PER CENT	NUMBER/PER CENT
Live Births			
Neonatal Deaths			
Infant Deaths			
Maternal Deaths			
Deaths			

B. Chronic Disease

	COMMUNITY	STATE	NATIONAL
DISEASE	NUMBER/PER CENT	NUMBER/PER CENT	NUMBER/PER CENT
Cardiovascular			
Cancer			
Diabetes			
Other Significant			

C. Leading Causes of Death

	COMMUNITY	STATE	NATIONAL
CAUSE OF DEATH	NUMBER/PER CENT	NUMBER/PER CENT	NUMBER/PER CENT
1.			
2.			
3.			
4.			
5.			
6.			
7.			
8.			
9.			
10.			

V. DEVIANCE: Number/Per cent

Substance Abuse
Out-of-Wedlock Births
Crime
Juvenile Delinquency
Other

VI. HEALTH, WELFARE, AND SOCIAL SERVICES

A. Major Facilities (types of services, number of beds, kind and number of personnel)

Hospitals

Clinics

Nursing Homes

Home Care Agencies

HMOs

Hospice Programs

Social Services

Welfare Services

Other

VII. MAJOR HEALTH PROBLEMS

VIII. PRIORITIES, NEEDS

73

The Development and Dissemination of Innovative Resources

MARY B. MAXWELL
BARBARA D. BLUMBERG

We all struggle with the numerous problems of patient care and seek creative solutions to them. On the one hand, we may decide that a certain need at our institution can be solved by new methods of care delivery, printed or visual materials to teach something, or novel ways to provide support to patients and families. When developed, the idea may become a valuable resource in our cancer care program. We may then wish to share the effective resource with others.

On the other hand, we may seek solutions to our vexing problems by constantly being on the lookout for innovative programs and materials developed and validated elsewhere that have the potential to be adopted in our setting. How can we be sure that the resource will "take" in the new locale? The purpose of this chapter is to explore the processes of resource development, dissemination, and adoption.

CANCER NURSING RESOURCES

A *resource* can be thought of as anything to which one turns for aid and assistance in time of need. In cancer nursing, important programs and materials that are used as resources have been developed over the years (Table 73–1). Sometimes the developmental processes are published. In terms of care delivery systems, these resources include oncology units, day treatment centers, cancer specialty clinics, and hospices. Successful approaches to support and education have included visitation programs such as Reach to Recovery and CanSurmount and groups such as TOUCH and I Can Cope. Cancer camps and lodges

and the Celebration of Cancer Survival are innovative resources that have spread to some areas. However, undoubtedly the resources most frequently developed and most often used by nurses are those involving the written or spoken word to communicate cancer information.

Booklets, audio tapes, pamphlets, video tapes, brochures, and handouts of all sizes, shapes, and colors

Table 73–1. EXAMPLES OF TYPES OF RESOURCES

Patient Education Materials and Programs
I Can Cope
"Chemotherapy and You," "Radiation Therapy and You," "Eating Hints," "Taking Time": Written materials developed by the National Cancer Institute
Patient Education products published bimonthly by *Oncology Nursing Forum*
Staff Education Materials
Guidelines for Cancer Nursing Practice
Cancer Chemotherapy: Guidelines and Recommendations for Nursing Education and Practice
Structured Emotional Support Programs
TOUCH
Make Today Count
Nursing Service Delivery Systems
Oncology units
Day treatment centers
Hospice units
Palliative care teams
Visitation Programs
Reach to Recovery
CanSurmount
Patient-to-patient volunteer program
Miscellaneous
We Can Weekend
Celebration of Cancer Survival
Cancer camp

are used daily by each of us in our practice to impart information. Some we may have put together ourselves, others may have come from the Patient Education section in *Oncology Nursing Forum* or from other hospitals, and still others were prepared by the American Cancer Society or National Cancer Institute. How were these last-named resources developed? Because there never seem to be enough resources to suit each of the varied community groups, oncology settings, and individualized needs of cancer patients and families, it is important to know how communication development techniques can be used successfully by others to adapt old informational resources or create new ones.

DEVELOPING CANCER INFORMATION RESOURCES: A PROCESS

Communicating information related to cancer effectively is a challenging task because such information is complex, technical, and subject to frequent revision. A key factor in the success of any communication about cancer concerns the extent to which it addresses the needs of its intended audience. Education and communications resources whose design is based on the needs and perceptions of the target audience are more apt to meet their goals and objectives than those designed in the absence of the target audience perspective (Blumberg, 1986). Audience research and careful subsequent planning are concomitants of effective resource design and production.

Social marketing, the theoretic base used in resource development, is drawn from commercial advertising and marketing (Bellinger, Bernhardt, & Goldstucker, 1976; Holbert, 1975; Lefebvre & Flora, 1988; McCall, 1975), which attributes successful ventures to providing products and services that meet consumer needs. This focus incorporates assessment of audience needs and perceptions at specified points in resource development and implementation. Although developing innovative resources aimed at communicating cancer information effectively is different from that of advertisement and marketing (they are selling consumer products), developers of health information have the similar goal of convincing a specific audience to use their product or resource.

Developing innovative resources can be viewed as a process that allocates time and resources efficiently to include concept, message, and resource development along with pretesting and evaluation research. For ease in explanation, the process is conceptualized in a six-part wheel (United States Department of Health and Human Services [USDHHS], 1984) (Fig. 73–1). Each section of the wheel represents a state in a circular process in which the last stage feeds back to the first one in a continuous loop of replanning and improvement.

THE KEY TO EFFECTIVE RESOURCE DEVELOPMENT: PRETESTING

The key to making this communication process work is pretesting, a qualitative research methodology car-

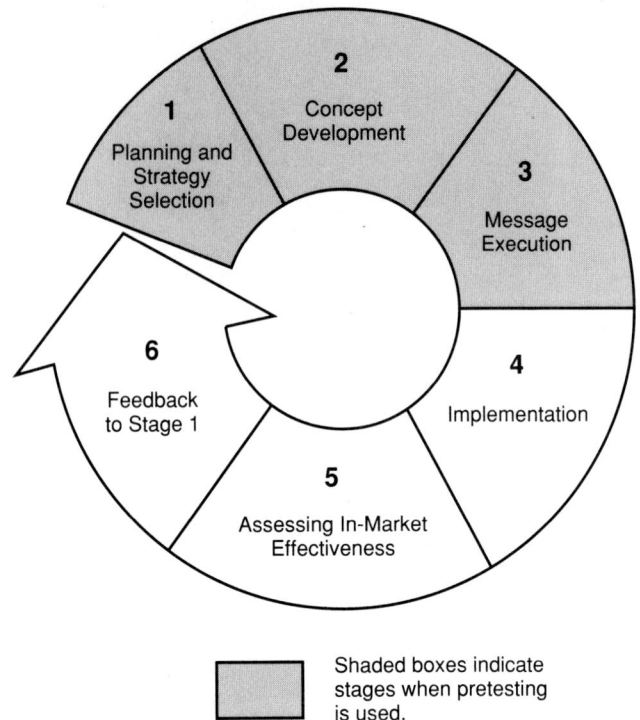

Figure 73–1. Stages in the development of innovative resources. (From U.S. Department of Health and Human Services. [1984]. *Pretesting in health communications* [NIH Publication No. 84-1493]. Washington, DC: U.S. Government Printing Office.)

ried out during the early stages of resource development (Bertrand, 1978). The purpose of pretesting is to gather target audience reactions to draft concepts and materials systematically before final production. Resources conducive to pretesting include pamphlets, booklets, teaching plans, audiovisual programs, and promotional materials. Pretesting is useful in determining which of several renditions of a message, concept, or material is most apt to meet stated objectives. In addition, the methodology can be used to identify strengths and weaknesses of draft materials successfully. In particular, pretesting is effective in qualitatively assessing the following message variables: awareness and interest, comprehension, relevance to needs, believability, acceptability, and short-term knowledge accrual.

Pretesting is appropriately included in many stages of the development of innovative messages and materials. The particular pretesting method employed depends on the audience, the message, and the amount of time and resources available. Diagnostic information derived from pretesting can lead to improvements in resources while revisions are still possible and affordable. However, it is essential to recognize that pretesting is qualitative and, therefore, does not yield results reportable in terms of their statistical significance. Results of a pretest do not absolutely predict success (or failure) of a message in terms of knowledge accrual, change in behavior, or any other relevant outcome measure. Rather, pretesting provides direction in the development of resources on the basis of perceptions and needs of representative members of the audience for whom the resource is intended.

Pretesting techniques appropriate for the development of innovative nursing resources include the following: readability testing, focus group interviews, individual in-depth interviews, self-administered questionnaires, and gatekeeper review. The particular technique chosen depends on the objectives of the resource being developed, the information that is needed from the pretest, the easiest method of access to members of the target audience, and the resources and time available for pretesting. Techniques are briefly described later; those recommended for use during a particular developmental stage are mentioned when that stage is discussed.

Readability testing is a simple technique employed to predict the level of reading comprehension a person needs to understand a given written document. After perusal of 12 selected formulas (USDHHS, 1984), the Office of Cancer Communications of the National Cancer Institute selected the SMOG grading formula for testing readability levels of its public and patient education materials (Bader, 1984). The SMOG formula was chosen because of its ease of use and accuracy in predicting readability. Readability testing considers the number of polysyllabic words included in a text to determine comprehension scores. Because variables such as organization of material, writing style, and content are not considered in readability testing, pretesting should also be carried out once the text is as "readable" as possible. Table 73–2 gives directions on how to apply this formula.

Focus group interviews are organized brainstorming sessions with discrete objectives that are carried out with a group of eight to ten persons sharing discrete target audience characteristics. Interviews are led by a facilitator who uses a list of open-ended questions to guide group discussion.

This technique, adapted by market researchers from group therapy, can be used for a variety of purposes. Focus group interviews are particularly useful in the concept development stage by providing insight into audience beliefs and perceptions. Focus group discussions encourage participants to converse around targeted subjects: they provide valuable information to resource developers for preparing materials in understandable language, using examples deemed relevant by the target audience. Perceptions of artwork and logos are also appropriate for focus group interviews. As with any qualitative research, however, focus group data should not be considered quantitatively. Focus group interviews should be regarded as valuable in terms of implications, suggestions, and directions for the resource under consideration.

Individual in-depth interviews are one-to-one discussions administered by an interviewer using a questionnaire consisting of both open-ended and closed-ended items. This technique is recommended when topics addressed are sensitive in nature or require in-depth probing. More commonly used are self-administered questionnaires that can be completed by subjects without the aid of an interviewer and consist primarily of closed-ended questions. Self-administered questionnaires can be either hand-carried to and retrieved from respondents or sent to them in the mail with a return envelope.

Frequently, resources reach their target audiences via a health professional or organization. These people, known as gatekeepers, determine whether the resource is actually distributed. As a result, the opinions of gatekeepers about a particular resource are crucial in the ultimate success of a resource. Review of draft materials by gatekeepers should be considered part of the formative review process. Although this stage of review should not be considered a replacement for either target audience pretesting or expert review for accuracy, this review step should not be overlooked. Gatekeeper review can be carried out through short self-administered questionnaires simultaneously with target audience review. If there is a discrepancy between the target audience and the gatekeepers, it is wise to err on the side of the former. When the resource is ultimately ready for gatekeeper distribution, gatekeepers should be sent a cover memo reflecting the fact that information included in the resource reflects the viewpoints of many individuals.

Planning and Strategy Selection

Developing innovative resources should begin with planning and strategy selection. During this period, the work of defining the problem to be addressed by the resource, setting subsequent communication objectives, identifying a discrete target audience, and deciding how the information should be communicated is determined. To facilitate planning and communication strategy selection, an informal needs assessment should be conducted by perusing the existing health literature that addresses topics related to the one in question as well as resources developed at other institutions. It may be necessary to conduct a more formal needs assessment with a select sample of the target audience to determine the exact nature of the information required as well as the most appropriate communications channel. For example, a formal needs assessment survey conducted with patients, family members, and health professionals participating in cancer clinical trials helped the staff charged with developing a resource for this audience determine that a booklet addressing specific issues would be useful to them (Blumberg & Nealon, 1984). Pretesting techniques that can be appropriately employed during this stage are in-depth interviews, focus group interviews, and small-scale surveys.

Message Content Development

During the next stage, draft resources are developed on the basis of those concepts deemed to have the most potential for communicating relevant messages. Drafts can range from typescript manuscripts with rough artwork to slides with dialogue read aloud to draft posters. During this message execution stage, it is important to conduct a formal pretest before pre-

Table 73–2. THE SMOG READABILITY FORMULA

To calculate the SMOG reading grade level, begin with the entire written work that is being assessed, and follow these 4 steps:

1. Count off ten consecutive sentences near the beginning, in the middle, and near the end of the text
2. From this sample of 30 sentences, circle all the words containing three or more syllables (polysyllabic), including repetitions of the same word, and total the number of words circled
3. Estimate the square root of the total number of polysyllabic words counted. This is done by finding the nearest perfect square and taking its square root
4. Finally, add a constant of 3 to the square root. This number gives the SMOG grade, or the reading grade level that a person must have reached if he or she is to understand fully the text being assessed

A few additional guidelines will help to clarify these directions:

A sentence is defined as a string of words punctuated with a period (.), an exclamation point (!), or a question mark (?)

Hyphenated words are considered as one word

Numbers that are written out should also be considered, and if in numeric form in the text, they should be pronounced to determine if they are polysyllabic

Proper nouns, if polysyllabic, should be counted, too

Abbreviations should be read as unabbreviated to determine if they are polysyllabic

Not all pamphlets, fact sheets, or other printed materials contain 30 sentences. To test a text that has fewer than 30 sentences:

1. Count all the polysyllabic words in the text
2. Count the number of sentences
3. Find the average number of polysyllabic words per sentence as follows:

$$\text{Average} = \frac{\text{total no. of polysyllabic words}}{\text{total no. of sentences}}$$

4. Multiply that average by the number of sentences *short of 30*
5. Add that figure on to the total number of polysyllabic words
6. Find the square root and add the constant of 3

Perhaps the quickest way to administer the SMOG grading test is by using the SMOG conversion table. Simply count the number of polysyllabic words in your chain of 30 sentences and look up the approximate grade level on the chart

SMOG Conversion Table*	
Total Polysyllabic Word Counts	**Approximate Grade Level (± 1.5 Grades)**
0–2	4
3–6	5
7–12	6
13–20	7
21–30	8
31–42	9
43–56	10
57–72	11
73–90	12
91–110	13
111–132	14
133–156	15
157–182	16
183–210	17
211–240	18

*Developed by Harold C. McGraw, Office of Educational Research, Baltimore County Schools, Towson, MD.

(From United States Department of Health and Human Services. [1984]. *Pretesting in health communications* [NIH Publication No. 84-1493]. Washington, DC: U.S. Government Printing Office.)

paring the resource in its final form. Gatekeeper review should also be employed during this stage to ensure that potential conduits for resource dissemination are in agreement. Self-administered questionnaires are most successfully used with members of the target audience during this stage. Message execution pretests should result in final revisions in resources before final production.

Implementation

The next stage involves resource implementation. During this stage, the resource is distributed in appropriate settings, and preliminary response to it is monitored. Using both informal comments and observations related to the use and usefulness of the product as well as more quantitative measures such as the numbers of copies distributed, a tentative assessment of success can be made. This informal gathering of initial reactions to the resource is called *process measurement* (Blumberg, 1981).

Assessing In-Market Effectiveness

The effectiveness of a resource in meeting the objectives stated during the planning and strategy selection stage is assessed during the next stage. Outcome evaluation is carried out to assess the results of resource implementation. Changes may have occurred in knowledge, attitudes, or reported behavior of target audience members. If this is the case, it is necessary to determine whether these changes can indeed be attributed to the resource or if other factors were responsible for the effect. Methodologies to assess in-market effectiveness of resources are beyond the scope of this chapter, but examples may be found elsewhere (Campbell & Stanley, 1966; Green, Kreuter, Deeds, & Partridge, 1980).

Back to Stage I

The final stage in the process of developing innovative resources involves analysis, for replanning purposes, of the information gathered during pretesting and other formative research and process and outcome evaluation. During this stage, problems incurred, along with strengths and weaknesses of the resource and its use, should be looked at in terms of opportunities for new or revised efforts. Now that the process has come full circle, how can maximum utilization of a new product be ensured?

RESOURCE DISSEMINATION AND ADOPTION

The prior section has focused on the techniques involved in resource development in the area of written or audiovisual products. We now turn to consideration of the idea of resources in more a broad perspective, as conceptualized in Table 73–1. Once a new resource has been successfully developed, tested, and found beneficial, be it printed material, an audiovisual product, a process or procedure, or a program of action, a major challenge must be confronted: its application into practice on a widespread basis.

At this point, the person or group that has developed the new resource probably imagines the following scenario: presentations are made at regional and national meetings communicating the new resource and how it was developed. Publications ensue. Soon, the originating group is beseiged by agencies from all over the United States with requests for assistance in establishing replicates in their own settings. In a brief period of time, the new resource has solved to a significant degree the problem it was designed to address. This fantasy, of course, is without basis in reality simply because the process of change does not proceed in such a simple, rational, spontaneous way. For this reason the special problems relating to the dynamics of dissemination, diffusion, adoption, and implementation of innovations are important.

Dissemination refers to a wide dispersal or spreading in various directions, often particularly in relation to knowledge. *Diffusion* is the deliberate spreading of either innovations or established processes or products from their sources of creation to their final users or adopters. *Adoption* is the initial decision to institute a particular change. Adoption itself is incomplete without *implementation,* the firm execution of the "adopted" program, process, product use, or applied idea into actual practice (Glaser, Abelson, & Garrison, 1983).

THE ADOPTION PROCESS

The adoption process is the mental stages or steps through which one passes from the time of first hearing of an innovation to its final adoption. Rogers (1962) conceptualizes five stages in the adoption process: awareness, interest, evaluation, trial, and adoption.

During the first stage, *awareness,* the individual is exposed to the innovation but is not yet motivated to seek further information. Although some see this exposure as a random event, it is unlikely that awareness will occur unless the individual has a problem or need that the innovation could solve. At the second stage of the adoption process, *interest,* the individual becomes interested in the innovation and actively seeks further information about it but has not yet made a judgment as to its efficacy in his or her own situation. At the third or *evaluation* stage, the individual mentally applies the innovation to a present and anticipated future situation to see if it will "fit." A decision is then made whether to try the innovation on the basis of weighing its advantages versus its disadvantages. The fourth or *trial* stage actually uses the innovation on a small scale to determine its utility in the individual's own situation so that a decision can be made about adoption. An innovation will usually not be adopted without first arranging for a trial on a probationary basis. At the fifth and final stage, *adoption,* a decision is made to continue full use of the innovation.

Of course, an innovation may also be rejected at any stage in the adoption process. As Fairweather and his colleagues (1974) discovered during their well-publicized attempts to spread the successful lodge program (a community mental health innovation in which clients lived in group homes rather than in institutions), experimenting with a new social treatment program is one thing; incorporating it into ongoing treatment programs is quite another. These innovators also found that when one is concerned with the adoption of a complex innovation, it cannot be assumed that adoption will automatically follow a decision to adopt. There is a big difference between positive attitudes toward a beneficial resource and actual behavior. They learned that perseverance in carrying out an implementation was a key factor in successful adoption completion. Of major importance were the principles of hard work and tolerance for confusion.

Many studies have demonstrated that impersonal, more cosmopolitan information sources are most important at the awareness stage of the adoption process, whereas personal and more local sources are most important at the evaluation stage (Rogers, 1962). It would appear, then, that oncology nurses might obtain initial awareness about new resources from journals and conferences such as those of the Oncology Nursing Society Congress, whereas experiences of friends or hometown colleagues might be influential in assisting in a decision to undertake a trial.

THE ADOPTION PERIOD

The adoption period is the length of time required to pass through the entire adoption process. It is a gestation period in which the new idea is fermenting in an individual or in group members' minds. To speed up the process, information can be communicated more adequately so that awareness occurs at an earlier date. Another method is to shorten the time required for adoption once an individual is aware of a new resource. However, it appears that it is not lack of knowledge about the innovations that delays their adoption. Nonadopters are often aware of an innovation but not motivated to try out and embrace it. Innovations with certain characteristics are generally adopted more quickly. Those that are relatively simple, divisible for preliminary trial, and compatible with previous experiences may have a shorter adoption period (Rogers, 1962). Changes that are inexpensive and can be accomplished with already existing materials, persons, and skills can be quickly introduced. As a rule, those that require large investments of time, money, and energy come more slowly.

Researchers have divided the total adoption period into two distinct times: (1) the *awareness-to-trial* period and (2) the *trial-to-adoption* period. For most innovations, the awareness-to-trial period is the longer of the two time periods. Because evidence suggests that the adoption stage directly follows the trial stage, efforts to encourage the preliminary trial of innovations may speed up the adoption process. For this reason, free samples of new products are often distributed. No matter how widely publicized positive tests of the product undertaken by the developer of the new resource are, individuals hesitate to adopt an innovation until it has been proved by their own cautious trials (Rogers, 1962).

CHARACTERISTICS OF THE INNOVATION

An important ingredient of the diffusion and adoption processes is the innovation itself. The characteristics of the new idea, as perceived by the individuals assessing it, affect its rate of adoption. Five characteristics of innovations have been summarized by Rogers (1962).

Relative advantage is the degree to which an innovation is superior to the situation currently in place. Cost-benefit is one aspect of relative advantage. *Com-patibility*, the second characteristic, is the degree to which an innovation is consistent with existing values and past experiences of the adopters. Perhaps one reason for the delay in hospice acceptance in the United States during the 1970s was the inconsistency of the hospice philosophy with our "high-tech" acute-care medical system. *Complexity*, the third characteristic of an innovation, is the degree to which it is difficult to understand and use. Fourth, *divisibility*, refers to the extent to which the innovation may be tried on a limited basis. New ideas that can be tried on the installment plan will usually be adopted more quickly. Earlier adopters may perceive divisibility as more important than later adopters because the more innovative individuals have no precedent to follow, whereas those who come later can draw on peers who have already accomplished the implementation. Last, *communicability* is the degree to which the results of an innovation may be diffused to others. Resources that are at a low level of abstraction, concrete, and easy to see spread more easily.

THE IMPORTANCE OF DISSEMINATION

Fairweather and Tornatzky (1977) liken the process of social innovation to a series of very expensive shops all inventing the same wagon wheel over and over again. They point out that many "new" innovations are not really new at all. A number of imaginative resources that one hears about have been tried before, found to be worthwhile in many cases, yet eventually faded from the scene because of a failure to disseminate them. Thus anyone who has developed a beneficial new resource in oncology nursing should plan a deliberate program of dissemination, including oral presentation at conferences and publication. The peer review quality control processes in place at professional conference and nursing journals will ensure that the most effective innovations receive priority in any dissemination effort. The successful dissemination of the I Can Cope program across the United States was due to its widespread initial presentation and publication

---

Box 73–1. I CAN COPE

I Can Cope is a structured patient education and group support program aimed at patients with all types of cancer. It was developed to include eight educational sessions over a 4-week period. Topics covered included (1) learning about the disease of cancer, (2) coping with daily health problems, (3) communicating with others, (4) liking yourself, (5) living with limits, and (6) helpful resources. Each session had goals, learning objectives, and study assignments. A learning resource center containing books, tapes, and games was available to all participants.

Developed to meet the requirements of a doctoral dissertation by Judy Johnson and implemented at the North Memorial Medical Center, Minneapolis, Minnesota, the success of the I Can Cope Program was first presented as a paper at the Oncology Nursing Society Congress in 1978. It was picked up by the Minnesota Division of the American Cancer Society, which made its materials available to interested institutions in Minnesota. As a result of the assertiveness of oncology nurses who had heard about it at Congress and wished to adopt it in other parts of the United States, the American Cancer Society decided to disseminate the program nationally. I Can Cope has thus been implemented in many locations, large and small, throughout the United States during the past years. It is soon to begin in Sweden.

The entire I Can Cope program has been published as a book and is available to patients and professionals for $9.00 at all commercial bookstores. (Johnson, J., & Klein, L. [1988]. *I Can Cope*. Minneapolis, MN: DCI Publishing.)

Table 73–3. A CHECKLIST FOR RESOURCE/INNOVATION ADOPTION

A—Ability

_____Are staff skills and knowledge appropriate to accommodate the new resource or innovation?

_____Are fiscal and physical resources adequate for change?

V—Values

_____Is the change consistent with the social, religious, political, and ethnic values of the beneficiaries?

_____Is the change consistent with the philosophies and policies of the program supporters?

_____Is the change consistent with the personal and professional values of the staff?

_____Is the top person in the organization in support of the desired resource?

_____Are the characteristics of the organization such as to make the innovation likely to succeed?

I—Information

_____Is information on the desired innovation clear?

_____Does information about the resource bear close relevance to the improvement needed?

_____Is the desired innovation one that is "tryable," observable, of demonstrated advantage, and so forth?

C—Circumstances

_____Are conditions at this setting similar to those where the resource was demonstrated to be effective?

_____Does the present situation seem to be conducive to successful adoption of this particular resource?

T—Timing

_____Is this a good time to implement this new idea?

_____Are other events going on or about to occur that could bear on the success of resource implementation?

O—Obligation

_____Has the need for this resource been ascertained through sound evaluation?

_____Has the need for this innovation been compared with other needs in the program?

R—Resistances

_____Have all reasons for _not_ adopting this resource been considered?

_____Has consideration been given to what may have to be abandoned if this resource is launched?

_____Has consideration been given to all who would lose in this change?

Y—Yield

_____Has the soundness of evidence about the benefits of this resource been carefully assessed?

_____Have possible indirect rewards for this change been examined?

(Adapted from Davis, H. R. [1971]. A checklist for change. In National Institute of Mental Health. _A manual for research utilization._ Washington, DC: U.S. Government Printing Office.)

and rapid diffusion by the American Cancer Society (Box 73–1).

Sometimes as the process of change progresses, further adoption of a new resource seems to become independent of intentional change agent activity. In other words, a "fad" effect occurs (Fairweather & Tornatzky, 1977).

HOW CAN THE INTRODUCTION OF A NEW RESOURCE BE EXAMINED ANALYTICALLY?

How can one know, in going through the mental stages of the adoption process while considering whether to introduce a new resource, if it will "take" in one's practice or institution? Various lists have been

developed of factors that determine the likelihood that a new resource will be used or an innovative program will be adopted in a given setting (Davis, 1971, 1973; Glaser, Abelson, & Garrison, 1983). The lists can be used as procedural tools for assessing an institution's readiness to adopt a proposed resource or change, identifying factors that affect successful adoption and may need to be attended to before any adoption attempt, and guiding the implementation process. Table 73–3 presents a checklist based on Davis's A Victory model for questions that can be applied to a possible change situation (Davis, 1971).

As might be expected, less radical changes are involved in borrowing an old idea or model for use in a new setting or activity than in introducing a completely new concept, procedure, or program. It should be kept in mind that utilization of an innovation is not necessarily adoption in toto but a process in which consensus on how the innovation can best be used in a given setting is gradually shaped. Adoption without some change in the innovation is rare; adaptation of the new resource to the new setting is frequent. The more simple the resource, however, the more likely that it will be adopted unchanged. For example, a brochure describing chemotherapy to patients can be introduced easily into a cancer clinic. The I Can Cope program, a more complex resource, has had many local adaptations as it spread from one part of the United States to the other. Table 73–4 lists factors to compare in thinking about transplanting a resource such as I Can Cope from one part of the United States to another.

Once a decision to adopt the new resource has been made, implementation begins. Depending on the complexity of the resource, planning processes are begun, including timing, budgets, staff preparation, and communication. Planning is simply a matter of determining where one is currently in terms of the resource and then deciding where one wishes to go and how to get there. An account of the activities involved in implementing a We Can Weekend (Johnson & Norby, 1981) in Cape Girardeau, Missouri, gives a fascinating behind-the-scenes glimpse of the hard work involved and many factors to be considered in introducing a complex resource (Lane & Davis, 1985) (Box 73–2). Planning began more than 15 months before the event and included five distinct phases: planning, publicity, training and organization, implementation, and evaluation.

Table 73–4. FACTORS TO CONSIDER AND COMPARE WHEN ADAPTING A RESOURCE FROM ONE SETTING TO ANOTHER

Locale
    Urban versus rural
Leadership/people
    Volunteers versus paid employees
    Professionals versus nonprofessionals
Availability of resources
    Money
    Space or facilities
    Materials
Recruitment of patients
Supporting organizations
From whom would permissions be needed?

Box 73–2. WE CAN WEEKEND

We Can Weekend is a family-centered education and support program developed in early 1980 at the North Memorial Medical Center, Minneapolis, Minnesota. The program was designed to (1) be flexible enough to include all ages of children, (2) be directive in discussing cancer and its ramifications, (3) provide a broad selection of educational activities to meet the varied interests of families, and (4) promote communication within the family about their feelings concerning cancer. The long-range goal was to help families use positive coping skills during the cancer experience.

The program was implemented as a weekend retreat in a rural Minnesota setting. The retreat site chosen offered classrooms, sleeping and eating facilities, a gymnasium, a swimming pool, and a large out-of-doors area for recreation. Families had the opportunity to learn together that cancer is a chronic illness, that resulting health problems can be managed, that diet and exercise are essential elements in treatment, and that expressing feelings helps in understanding one another. Art, movement, and music activities were integrated throughout the weekend to create group cohesiveness and sensitivity (Johnson & Norby, 1981).

Although information about the We Can Weekend was first published in *Cancer Nursing* in 1981, adoption was slow until an article in *Cope* magazine. Since then, 38 Weekend programs have been implemented around the United States. *Cope* is a relatively new commercial cancer-related magazine that is widely distributed nationally among all levels of oncology professionals.

The detailed implementation timetable developed by the organizers to guide their activities undoubtedly helped contribute to their successful implementation.

SUMMARY

It is too bad that people are frustrated and often defeated by difficulties for which someone else has found an effective remedy. The goal of this chapter has been to assist in solving problems by describing resource development and then illuminating the gap that often exists between the availability of the resource and the ability to put it to effective use.

The need for more promising ways to meet new or continuing challenges calls for the ongoing development of nursing resources, be they informational products or processes, demonstration projects, or validated exemplary programs. This development must be followed by the rapid diffusion of these resources. The potential benefits of nursing progress cannot be fully realized unless such knowledge is taken up and used by clinicians in ambulatory clinics, at the bedside, or in the patient's home.

References

Bader, L. A. (1984). *The SMOG readability formula*. Unpublished manuscript. Michigan State University, East Lansing.

Bellinger, D. N., Bernhardt, K. L., & Goldstucker, J. L. (1976). *Qualitative research in marketing*. Chicago: American Marketing Association, Monograph Series #3.

Bertrand, J. E. (1978). *Communications pretesting*. Chicago: Community and Family Study Center, University of Chicago, Media Monograph 6.

Blumberg, B. D. (1981). Evaluating patient education programs. *Oncology Nursing Forum, 8*(2), 29–31.

Blumberg, B. D. (1986, February). *Assessing and meeting the information needs of cancer patients and their families*. Paper presented at the South Florida Conference, Communicating with Patients, St. Petersburg Beach, FL.

Blumberg, B., & Nealon, E. (1984, May). *Educational needs of the patient considering clinical trials*. Paper presented at the Oncology Nursing Society Congress, Toronto, Canada.

Campbell, D. T., & Stanley, J. C. (1966). *Experimental and quasi-experimental designs for research*. Chicago: Rand McNally.

Davis, H. R. (1971). A checklist for change. In National Institute of Mental Health, *A manual for research utilization*. Washington, DC: U.S. Government Printing Office.

Davis, H. R. (1973). Change and innovation. In S. Feldman (Ed.), *Administration and mental health*. Springfield, IL: Charles C. Thomas.

Fairweather, G. W., Sanders, D. H., Tornatzky, L. G., & Harris, R. N. (1974). *Creating change in mental health organizations*. New York: Pergamon Press.

Fairweather, G. W., & Tornatzky, L. G. (1977). *Experimental methods for social policy research*. New York: Pergamon Press.

Glaser, E. M., Abelson, H. H., & Garrison, K. N. (1983). *Putting knowledge to use*. San Francisco: Jossey-Bass.

Green, L. W., Kreuter, M. W., Deeds, S. G., & Partridge, K. B. (1980). *Health education planning: a diagnostic approach*. Palo Alto, CA: Mayfield Publishing Co.

Holbert, N. (1975). *Advertising research*. Chicago: American Marketing Association, Monograph Series No. 1.

Johnson, J. L., & Norby, P. A. (1981). We can weekend: A program for cancer families. *Cancer Nursing, 2*, 23–27.

Lane, C. A., & Davis, A. W. (1985). Implementation: We can weekend in the rural setting. *Cancer Nursing, 8*, 323–328.

Lefebvre, R. C., & Flora, J. A. (1988). Social marketing and public health intervention. *Health Education Quarterly, 15*, 299–315.

McCall, D. B. (1975, August). What agency managers want from research. *Journal of Advertising Research*, pp. 7–10.

Rogers, E. M. (1962). *Diffusion of innovations*. New York: Free Press of Glencoe.

United States Department of Health and Human Services. (1984). *Pretesting in Health Communications* (NIH Publication No. 84-1493). Washington, DC: U.S. Government Printing Office.

PROFESSIONAL SUPPORT SYSTEMS

CHAPTER **74**

Social Support, Occupational Stressors, and Health in Cancer Nursing

MADELINE H. SCHMITT

The purpose of this chapter is to examine theory and research linking social support to occupational stress. The chapter begins with an examination of the multiple ways social support is defined. Next, stress is defined and linked to occupational stressors. In subsequent sections, research on the impact of social support on occupational stress is reviewed, looking separately at the effects of general social support and social support within the work situation. This general literature then is linked to the less abundant nursing literature on social support and occupational stress. Overall, the chapter provides a broad framework for the other chapters in this unit, which focus on stress in cancer nursing, strategies for taking care of oneself as a cancer nurse, and the rights of cancer nurses.

SOCIAL SUPPORT

Most globally, social support refers to some properties of human relationships that are purported to be health protective by theorists and researchers. The more specific definitions of social support reflect different theoretic ideas about which aspects of human relationships are the most important determinants of positive health outcomes. The specific definitions em-phasize three domains of social support, as shown in Table 74–1: social ties, social networks, and functional aspects of social support.

Social Ties

Social ties refers to the number of social relationships and the frequency of contact between an individual and family members, friends, and social organizations. Ideas about the health protective aspects of social ties have been around for a long time. At the turn of the century, the sociologist Émile Durkheim (1951) conducted ecologic research on suicide in which he linked greater social integration with lower suicide rates (Murawski, Penman, & Schmitt, 1978). Many subsequent ecologic and epidemiologic studies have examined the negative health impact of a lack of social ties that result from different social conditions, for example, geographic mobility. Research linking the lack of social

Table 74–1. DOMAINS OF SOCIAL SUPPORT

Social ties (general social support, companionship)
Social networks
Functional support (problem-focussed social
   support)

ties to the increased occurrence of physical illness and higher death rates has been reviewed by Berkman (1985) and by House and Kahn (1985). These studies consistently have shown patterns of higher mortality among those who "have been deprived of meaningful social contact" (Cassel, 1974). There is less agreement regarding the impact of social ties on the occurrence of physical illness. House and Kahn (1985) describe the research as providing convincing evidence of links between lack of social ties and increased morbidity, whereas Berkman (1985) and Cohen and Syme (1985) find the evidence a bit weaker. Other research reviews link the lack of social ties to poorer mental health (Cohen & Syme, 1985; House & Kahn, 1985; Kessler & McLeod, 1985).

Social Networks

A second set of indicators focuses on personal social networks, described variously as all the people with whom one has any sort of regular contact, personally important people that one feels close to, or those people from whom one obtains support (Wellman, 1981). The kind of information retrieved about social networks and how that information is interpreted may be powerfully affected by these different definitions of networks used by researchers. For example, defining the personal social network as those persons with whom an individual has any sort of regular contact allows for the study of supportive *and* unsupportive transactions, both of which may flow through some of the same persons. Networks that are defined in terms of those persons who are supportive eliminate this possibility. In the latter definition an assumption is made that support is a characteristic of a person and a relationship, rather than a dynamic variable that flows through a network or structure of relationships (Lieberman, 1986).

A variety of network properties may influence health. These properties include size, density, contact frequency, multiplexity, homogeneity, and duration (Mitchell, 1969; Mitchell & Trickett, 1980). Examination of these network properties ". . . focuses attention on how the properties of networks affect the flow of resources to focal individuals" (Hall & Wellman, 1985, p. 27). One example of a network property that has been positively associated with measures of health in research is network size (House & Kahn, 1985). A second network property, density, has a more complex relationship to health. Density refers to the number of people in a personal social network who know each other as a percentage of the total possible relationships. Networks with greater density are characterized by greater numbers of actual to potential relationships, whereas networks with less density have fewer network members acquainted with one another. The kind of ties associated with better health seems to depend on the context of relationships (House & Kahn, 1985). High-density networks have positive effects in situations of acute or chronic stress in which stress is not tied to an identity transition. In situations requiring

shifts in role identities, for example, widowhood or divorce (Hirsch, 1980, 1981), or job changes (Granovetter, 1973), less dense ties are more effective in connecting the focal person to needed resources for making an identity shift.

Functional Aspects of Social Support

A third domain of indicators of social support focuses on the functional aspects of social relationships. Caplan (1979, p. 111) describes social support from this perspective as ". . . an area of study dealing with hypothesized effects of behaviors intended to be helpful on the perceptions of such intention, on the feeling of being helped, and on the adaptation, adjustment, and well being of the target person." Various conceptualizations of these behaviors have been offered, including typologies by Caplan (1974), Kahn (1979), Weiss (1974), Gottlieb (1978), and Hirsch (1980). These typologies have been used to classify items used in surveys into categories of support and to develop instruments to measure various types of social support. This measurement usually includes an assessment of the amount of support, an estimate of its positiveness, and its source as well as the type(s) of support offered. Some consensus about the core content of categories in the typologies has been achieved, despite different labels across typologies (Mitchell & Trickett, 1980). Schaefer, Coyne and Lazarus (1981) have created a typology that reflects the categories of support most commonly examined in research: emotional support, informational support, and tangible aid (Box 74–1). Other categories are identified less frequently and depend on specific theoretical formulations, for example, House's (1981) addition of appraisal support and Hirsch's (1980) addition of social reinforcement and socializing.

Coping and Functional Aspects of Social Support

Coping is defined by Lazarus and Folkman (1984, p. 141) as "constantly changing cognitive and behavioral efforts to manage specific external and/or internal demands that are appraised as taxing or exceeding the resources of the person." Because seeking social support may be one coping response to stress, some theorists have integrated conceptualization and empirical study of social support with the study of coping. Lazarus and Folkman examine support from this frame of reference. In their instrument to assess ways of coping, one dimension assessed is seeking and using supportive others. Another formulation of this relationship is proposed by Thoits (1986). She argues that social support is coping assistance and that efforts an individual might undertake on his or her own behalf may also be sought from or offered by others. Consequently, problem-focused coping efforts such as altering the stressful situation directly, removing oneself from a stressful situation, or reinterpreting the situation so that it seems less threatening or distracting are

---

Box 74–1. HEALTH-RELATED FUNCTIONS OF SOCIAL SUPPORT

Social support research has been hampered by a lack of clarity both in the definitions of social support and in the conceptualization of its effects on health outcomes. The present study compared social network size and three types of perceived social support—tangible, emotional, and informational—in relation to stressful life events, psychological symptoms and morale, and physical health status in a sample of 100 persons 45 to 64 years old. Social network size was empirically separable from, although correlated with, perceived social support and had a weaker overall relationship to outcomes than did support. Low tangible support and emotional support, in addition to certain life events, were independently related to depression and negative morale; informational support was associated with positive morale. Neither social support nor stressful life events were associated with physical health. It was concluded that social support research would benefit from attention to the multidimensionality of support and greater specificity in hypotheses about the relationship between types of support and adaptational outcomes.

(Schaefer, C., Coyne, J. C., & Lazarus, R. S. [1981]. The health-related functions of social support. *Journal of Behavioral Medicine 4*, 381–405.)

---

efforts that can be enhanced or offered by others. Emotion-focused coping efforts such as use of mood modifiers (for example, drugs, alcohol); distress reduction practices, including meditation and self-hypnosis techniques; or reinterpreting mood states are also efforts that can be facilitated by others who believe such intervention to be helpful. Thoits argues that such support (coping assistance) is most acceptable and effective when it is offered by "socially similar others" who have encountered similar stressful experiences in their own lives. Her framework also makes clear the importance of distinguishing empirically between those actions that are intended to be helpful, those that are perceived as helpful, and those that ultimately have positive physical and emotional benefits. We need to know much more about the relative efficacy of various individual and network coping responses to perceived stressors.

Companionship versus Functional Aspects of Social Support

An important distinction has emerged in the literature as a consequence of increasing sophistication in theory and research on social support. This is the distinction between general social support and problem-focused support (House, 1981), or companionship versus social support (Rook, 1987). As described by Rook, companionship is interaction toward the positive expressive goal of mutual enjoyment. Social support, on the other hand, involves instrumental interactions directed toward the target person by others with the goal of addressing problems brought on by specific stressful situations. Although social support may serve primarily to restore disrupted functioning, companionship may provide continuing enhancement to the sense of well-being, regardless of the level of stress currently experienced. In several studies, Rook tested a series of hypotheses based on this theoretic argument. In a community sample, the psychological symptom-reducing effects of social support were limited to situations of reported high major life stress. Companionship, on the other hand, showed a general effect on reported symptoms regardless of major life stress level and also showed positive effects in situations of high minor life

stress. This finding is consistent with conclusions drawn by Cohen and Syme (1985) that studies in which social support has been measured using social tie indicators have shown a general or main effect on health (with the key contribution of social ties hypothesized by Rook to be the companionship that contributes to an overall sense of well-being and satisfaction), whereas studies that have employed functional social support indicators directed to specific needs and problems have shown effects primarily under situations of high life stress, that is, buffering effects. In further research, Rook found that companionship was more consistently associated with greater friendship satisfaction and less loneliness than were emotional or instrumental support. Satisfaction with family relationships primarily was associated with instrumental support.

THE STRESSFUL ASPECTS OF SOCIAL TIES AND SOCIAL NETWORKS

One of the common criticisms leveled against both the social tie and the social support network strategies for examining the general impact of social support is that these approaches equate the presence of social ties or a social network with the provision of support (Rook, 1984). Although lack of social ties has been identified as a psychosocial stressor linked to poorer physical and mental health, it does not logically follow that all social contacts are health protective. Early writers like Cassel (1974, p. 475) made it very clear that psychosocial processes were not ". . . unidimensional, stressor or not stressor, but rather . . . two dimensional, one category being stressors, and another being protective or beneficial." Later writers have reemphasized these two sides of human relationships in writing about social support (Coyne & De Longis, 1986; Fiore, Becker, & Coppel, 1983; Rook, 1984; Suls, 1982; Tilden & Galyen, 1987).

Little research in the social support literature focuses on the stress-producing qualities of ongoing social contacts. Exceptions occur. For example, in a sample of spouse caregivers of Alzheimer's patients, Fiore, Becker, and Coppel (1983) found that the extent of upset with the social network was the best predictor of depression, whereas the perceived supportiveness of the network was not associated with depression. On the basis of data gathered on a community sample of elderly women, Rook (1984) argued that the presence of problematic relationships may be a better predictor of general psychological well-being than the presence of supportive relationships.

HOW MUCH SOCIAL SUPPORT IS ENOUGH?

Just as it is erroneous to assume that all social contacts are positive, it may also be wrong to assume that the more social support, the better. How much companionship or support is enough is a question that has been raised by several researchers. Some have suggested that the availability of a single intimate confidant is the most essential part of social ties (Coyne & De Longis, 1986; Kahn & Antonucci, 1980). The demands of particular stress situations are thought to influence the types of network configurations that are most effective in reducing the health effects of the stress (Cohen & Syme, 1985; House & Kahn, 1985; Suls, 1982). Particular sources of support are relevant to specific crisis situations (Cohen & Syme, 1985), and it is not easy to compensate for their absence (Lieberman, 1986). How much support a person wants or is able to use during stressful situations may vary depending on personality and other social characteristics (Cohen & De Longis, 1986; Heller, 1979). Too much support, although well intended, may become stressful in itself, threaten self-reliance, or have the paradoxical effect of creating overdependency. This, too, is an area requiring considerable further research.

OCCUPATIONAL STRESSORS, SOCIAL SUPPORT, AND HEALTH

Definitions of Stress

Stress has been defined as an objective stressing stimulus (Holmes & Rahe, 1967) and as a situation perceived to be taxing and beyond the normal ability of the person to cope, which is threatening to the person's well-being (Lazarus & Folkman, 1984). The definition of stress as perceived stressors recognizes the fact that similar situations are not equally stressful to all individuals. The term also has been used to signify physiologic and psychological responses to stressors. Distinctions are sometimes made between short-term and long-term responses, with long-term responses often referred to as stress outcomes.

Certain events (objective social stressors) are of sufficient magnitude to produce stress reactions in many who are exposed. Following years of research focused on negative health outcomes related to different psychosocial stressors, Holmes and Rahe (1967, p. 217) published the Social Readjustment Rating Scale, a list of commonly experienced major life events re-

quiring ". . . a significant change in the ongoing life pattern of the individual" that was weighted for the potential magnitude of change likely to be required. These events included occurrences culturally evaluated as positive, for example, vacation, as well as those evaluated as negative, for example, death of a close friend. Subsequent research has established the greater negative health impact of negatively perceived events (Thoits, 1982, 1986).

There have been subsequent variations of the Holmes and Rahe scale, but, like the original scale, the new scales use a checklist of life events to gauge the amount of stressors in a person's recent experience. Scores on the scales are used in evaluating the role of social support in stress reduction and in examining health outcomes. Recognizing that not all stressors are associated with major life events, however, more recent models of stressors have added the concept of chronic strain (Pearlin, Lieberman, Menaghan, & Mullan, 1981). These models examine the impact of the life events on strains as well as the effects of both on health outcomes. The evaluation of the impact of social support in such models may focus on its ability to reduce perceived stressors, strain, or symptoms. A third concept of stressors has been the idea of daily hassles, ". . . the irritating, frustrating, distressing demands that . . . characterize everyday transactions . . ." (Kanner, Coyne, Schaefer, & Lazarus, 1981) (Box 74–2). In research comparing the ability of a major life events scale and a daily hassles scale to explain variance on psychological symptoms and negative moods, Kanner and colleagues demonstrated that the hassles scale was a stronger predictor. The three types of stressors that have been studied are summarized in Table 74–2.

Increasingly, researchers have recognized the limits of exploring generalized social support in situations of general life stress and have begun to explore the impact of different network configurations and different types and sources of support on particular life stressors, such as various stages of illness (Suls, 1982), specific illnesses such as cancer (Wortman, 1984) and psychiatric disorders (Hammer, 1981; Leavy, 1983), bereavement (O'Brien, 1987), pregnancy (Mercer & Ferketich, 1988), institutionalization in old age (Powers, 1988), and occupational stress, to name a few.

Occupational Stressors

House (1981) and Haw (1982) have concluded that a growing body of research links various forms of psychosocial stressors in the work situation to a broad array of negative physical and mental health outcomes. Occupational stressors have been considered among the categories of general life event stressors. In Holmes and Rahe's (1967) original Social Readjustment Rating Scale, seven of the 43 life events focused directly on occupational stressors. These stressors ranged from getting fired as the most stressful occupational event to changes in work hours or conditions and trouble with the boss, which were rated as the least stressful

---

Box 74–2. COMPARISON OF TWO MODES OF STRESS MEASUREMENT:
DAILY HASSLES AND UPLIFTS VERSUS MAJOR LIFE EVENTS

The standard life events methodology for the prediction of psychological symptoms was compared with one focussing on relatively minor events, namely, the hassles and uplifts of everyday life. Hassles and Uplifts Scales were constructed and administered once a month for 10 consecutive months to a community sample of middle-aged adults. It was found that the Hassles Scale was a better predictor of concurrent and subsequent psychological symptoms than were the life events scores, and that the scale shared most of the variance in symptoms accounted for by life events. When the effects of life event scores were removed, hassles and symptoms remained significantly correlated. Uplifts were positively related to symptoms for women but not for men. Hassles and uplifts were also shown to be related, although only modestly so, to positive and negative affect, thus providing discriminate validation for hassles and uplifts in comparison to measures of emotion. It was concluded that the assessment of daily hassles and uplifts may be a better approach to the prediction of adaptational outcomes than the usual life events approach.

(Kanner, A. D., Coyne, J. C., Schaefer, C., & Lazarus, R. S. [1981]. Comparison of two modes of stress measurement: Daily hassles and uplifts versus major life events. *Journal of Behavioral Medicine, 4,* 1–39.)

---

occupational life events (Holmes & Rahe, 1967). Some models of occupational stressors have separated objective stressors from perceived stressors or strain (Gore, 1978; LaRocco, House, & French, 1980). Some have incorporated the concept of chronic strain, focusing on the effects of job stress on a broad range of chronic life strains (Pearlin, et al., 1981). The measure of daily hassles emphasizes common stressful events related to daily work life, such as problems in getting along with fellow workers, concerns about job security, dislike of current work duties or fellow workers, and unchallenging work (Kanner, et al., 1981).

There seems to be considerable overlap in occupational experiences and events that are classified as stressors, strains, or hassles (Knapp, 1988). Categorically, some stressors apply generally to all employment experiences, for example, job loss. Others are viewed as endemic to certain kinds of occupations. For example, Greenberg and Valletutti (1980) argue that there are stressors unique to human services occupations. Chapters 75 and 76 identify some occupational stressors particularly relevant to nurses.

Social Ties, Occupational Stressors, and Health

Some studies of the effects of social support on the health outcomes of occupational stressors have looked primarily at the impact of social ties. Among these, some have focused specifically on the stressor of job loss (Gore, 1978; Pearlin, et al., 1981). For example, in a study that dealt with the effects of psychoemotional support received from spouse, friends, and relatives for 100 men after involuntary job loss through two plant closings, Gore (1978) found greater negative physical health (increased cholesterol levels and symptoms) and mental health (increased depression) out-

Table 74–2. TYPES OF STRESSORS

Life event stressors
Chronic strains
Daily hassles

comes in the unsupported group of men as compared with the supported group. She also found that, although lack of support was not related to the level of actual economic deprivation, it did increase perceptions of economic deprivation. Perceptions of economic deprivation, however, were not correlated with health outcomes. The pattern of findings led Gore to conclude that the amount of support available to individuals was a stable characteristic of the social environment. This was reflected in the measurement of social support, which heavily emphasized social ties. The effect of this support was to minimize negative health outcomes during the period of prolonged unemployment. On the other hand, the lack of supportive ties in the unemployment stress situation was an additional stressor that exacerbated negative health outcomes.

Using longitudinal data available on 1106 men and women from a study of 2300 subjects comprising a representative sample of the Chicago metropolitan area, Pearlin and colleagues (1981) found that involuntary job disruptions were significantly related to increases in depression. In exploring the mechanisms by which job disruptions increased depression, they found that the depression was intensified by chronic economic strain resulting from the job disruptions. Both the job disruption and the chronic strain led to decreases in self-esteem and mastery; the latter also contributed to overall depression. Both individual coping strategies and available social support were examined as mediators of the stress process. Overall, social support, as measured by a few items on marital status and availability of other confidants, was associated with reduced economic strain and a higher sense of mastery. More specifically, in the subsample of persons experiencing job disruption, social support significantly reduced the negative impact of the disruption on self-esteem and mastery, thereby reducing overall depression. These findings indicate that one way social support may reduce negative psychological outcomes is through reinforcement of a person's self-concept during stressful life events.

Using 1553 employed and unemployed husbands and wives from the same Chicago area database as that used by Pearlin and colleagues (1981), Vanfossen

(1986) examined sex differences in the effects of occupational stressors (personal relations on the job and feeling of job security) and economic strain (difficulties in meeting financial obligations) on mastery, self-esteem, and depression. Occupational stressors and economic strain had a significant negative effect on all three dependent variables for both sexes except for no effects of economic strain on the self-esteem of women. Vanfossen limited the study of the impact of social support to spouse support but used an expanded set of indicators of support that included emotional and instrumental support items (affirmation, affection, reciprocity, and helpfulness). Regardless of the overall level of occupational stressors and economic strain, spouse support had a powerful main effect, reducing levels of depression and enhancing mastery and self-esteem. Spouse support also was found to reduce the impact of occupational stress and economic strain on all three dependent variables for both sexes, with one exception. For unemployed men, available social support did not alter the high depression and low self-esteem associated with economic strain.

The most consistently important type of support identified for all subjects was affirmation. Intimacy was important for men, whereas reciprocity and helpfulness were important to employed wives. Women were somewhat less likely to receive support from their spouses, although, overall, employed men and women were equally likely to experience occupational stress. In general, men reported more negative impact from the stressors. The *most* negative outcomes, however, were experienced by unemployed housewives. Generally, employment enhanced women's mastery and self-esteem and reduced depression. The findings of this study add important information about women, social support, and occupational stress. Like other researchers (Gore, 1978; Rook, 1987), Vanfossen found that social support, especially affirmation, contributes to maintaining self-esteem and mastery and reducing depression in general and in stressful situations. In addition, however, specific types of support (helpfulness and reciprocity) between husbands and employed wives were important in reducing negative psychological effects related to occupational stressors for employed women. Vanfossen indicates that these factors are important in reducing the role overload employed wives experience because of their dual roles as employee and housekeeper.

Aneshensel (1986) studied more directly the interaction of marital and employment role strain, social support, and depression. Using a subsample of 490 women from a representative sample of 1003 Los Angeles county adults who participated in a 1-year panel design, she reported higher likelihood for depression among married women with high marital role strain and lower likelihood for depression among married women with low marital role strain. Unmarried women's depression scores fell between these two extremes. Looking at employment, women with low employment role strain had the least likelihood to be depressed and unemployed women the greatest likelihood to be depressed, and employed women with high employment role strain fell in between these extremes. The effects of the two types of strain were additive. The highest risk of depression was among unemployed women experiencing high marital role strain; the lowest risk of depression was among married, employed women with low marital and low employment role strain. Several items pertaining to emotional support and instrumental assistance were used as a measure of the impact of social support in reducing the depression associated with these strains. The findings suggested a main effect for support on depression, that is, regardless of level of marital or employment role strain, women with more support had less depression. There was no indication that social support buffered these strains, that is, reduced the overall effect of these strains. For employed women, high marital strain compounded occupational strain to increase levels of depression.

In summarizing the findings of these and other studies looking at the effects of social ties on health outcomes in situations of occupational stress, the literature suggests (1) that the support of intimates—spouses or other confidants—has a positive effect on mental and physical health; (2) that emotional support reduces depression through affirmation of a person's mastery and self-esteem; (3) that occupational stressors of various types have a negative effect on the psychological and physical health of both employed men and women, although the data linking occupational stressors to women's physical health is extremely limited (Haw, 1982); (4) that evidence of buffering effects of social ties in occupational stress situations is mixed; (5) that for employed women, reciprocity and helpfulness of the spouse are important types of support; and (6) that for employed women, marital role strain can compound the health effects of occupational role strain.

Work Supports, Occupational Stressors, and Health

Several surveys have examined the availability of social support in the work environment and its impact on occupational stressors and health outcomes. The specifics of most of these studies are not too helpful in looking at stress in cancer nursing for several reasons. They examine a diversity of occupations (sometimes in the same study) in which it is difficult to sort out the specific social support processes relevant to particular types of work settings (Kasl & Wells, 1985). Most of the settings studied involve managers or blue-collar workers in businesses in which there is production of goods, which are quite different from the complex human services organizations within which nurses work. Kasl and Wells (1985) also point out that the studies are cross-sectional in nature, preventing any analysis of the stress process. Furthermore, most of these studies use a few idiosyncratic items to measure social support, which may not sensitively represent the phenomenon. Most importantly, many of these studies either excluded women as subjects or did not analyze sex differences (Haw, 1982).

Nevertheless, some of the most consistent general findings from these studies are relevant to consider. These include the following (Kasl & Wells, 1985): (1) Occupational settings vary in overall availability of work-related support. (2) Support in the work setting is more important in dealing with occupational stressors than support from general social ties. Work sources of support include supervisors and co-workers. House's (1981) review of early work satisfaction studies makes the point that worker health, satisfaction, and productivity have been linked often to the interpersonal structure of the work setting—workers preferring to work cooperatively in the company of co-workers rather than in isolation. Early work by Cassel (1963) indicated that, for shift workers, cholesterol levels were related to whether their workmates were stable or constantly changing. (3) Work support and support from social ties is only moderately correlated (r of 0.30 or less). (4) Social support seems to have greater impact on psychological than physical health.

NURSING STRESSORS, SOCIAL SUPPORT, AND HEALTH

Chapter 75 systematically reviews the research literature on occupational stress and burnout in nursing with a special focus on cancer nursing. There is ample evidence presented that despite the many rewarding aspects of nursing, many aspects of nurses' work settings are stressful. Various individual coping and social support interventions are suggested in the nursing literature for dealing with work stress. However, the effects of each type of intervention have been poorly studied. Chapter 76 emphasizes the use of personal coping strategies; here the emphasis is on reporting work that illustrates the potential role of social support.

Norbeck (1985) tested the occupational stress–social support model developed by LaRocco, House, and French (1980) using a sample of 164 female critical care nurses from northern California hospitals. This model hypothesizes relationships among job stressors, perceived job strain, and health outcomes, with social support potentially having three main and three buffering effects on the three stressor variables, as shown in Figure 74–1. Job stressors examined were specific to critical care nursing. Job strain was defined as job dissatisfaction. The health outcome examined was psychological symptoms. The social support examined was instrumental and emotional support offered by subjects' social network, with two questions focussing on whether network members were responsive to work issues. The sum of responses for the two questions constituted a work support score.

Overall, nurses in this sample had clinical levels of psychological symptomatology. The results pertaining to the impact of social support were complicated. Nurses who reported higher overall support tended to report fewer job stressors, less job dissatisfaction, and fewer symptoms, although the effect of support on

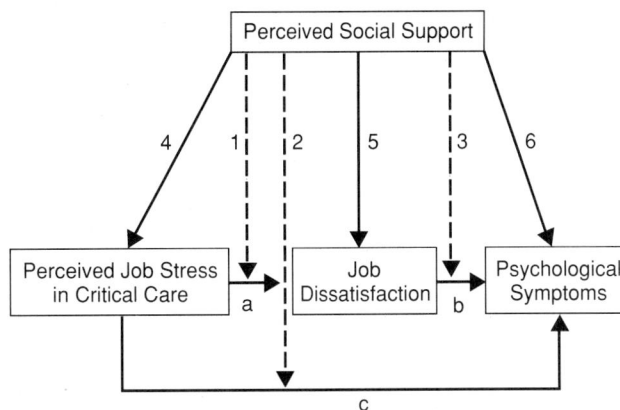

Figure 74–1. Model of relationships among study variables. Solid arrows indicate main effects; intermittent arrows signify interaction effects. (From Norbeck, J. S. [1985]. Types and sources of social support for managing job stress in critical care nursing. *Nursing Research, 34,* 225. Used with permission. All rights reserved. Adapted from LaRocco, J. M., House, J. S., & French, J. R. P., Jr. [1980]. Social support, occupational stress, and health. *Journal of Health and Social Behavior, 21,* 202–218.)

these variables was modest (5 per cent or less of the variance explained in each instance).

Separate analyses for married and unmarried subjects helped to sharpen the analysis. Key sources of support were different for the two groups. Married nurses received more support from relatives and spouse or partner; unmarried nurses received more support from friends. However, only relative support was significantly related to outcomes for unmarried nurses. Using support of all types from this source, social support accounted for 10 per cent and 12 per cent of the variance on job stressors and psychological symptoms, respectively. A buffering effect of social support under conditions of high job stressors was significant. Among married nurses, all sources of support were related to outcomes. Social support accounted for 14 per cent and 10 per cent of the variance explained in job stressors and psychological symptoms, respectively, in the homogeneous subsample. No buffering effects were found. When analysis was focused specifically on work support, the amount of variance explained on job stress rose to 24 per cent.

Overall, Norbeck concluded that the stress-reducing effects of social support are quite general, with weak evidence for buffering effects. These findings for critical care nurses are consistent with the previously reported findings of the general psychological health impact of supportive social ties. Norbeck's study suggests that when social ties can offer married nurses support that is work sensitive, job-related stress can be reduced; however, her study did not focus specifically on work-based sources of support.

The limitations of social ties as sources of support to nurses in occupational stress situations may be connected to a tendency to keep work networks and personal networks separate. In a study of nurse managers, Hirsch and David (1983) found work and nonwork social networks to be "almost totally segmented," that is, they reported work and nonwork network members did not know one another. This was unusual as compared with other human services workers. The nurses reported unusually high work pressure, and their negative mood scores were comparable to young widows. Hirsch and David argued that the network separation was defensive, to keep work stress from invading personal life. This separation is a self-care strategy also reported by staff nurses in other studies (Hutchinson, 1987; Vachon, 1987). Although this separation may be characteristic of some employed women's networks, Hirsch and David point out that it cuts off important support for work stress from the nonwork domain of social ties. They also point out that such restrictive ties may undermine nurses' ability to bring about changes in the work environment by limiting access to potential contacts through the broader network who may be used to change the work environment.

Two nursing studies have described work-related sources of support for nurses. These include intradisciplinary and interdisciplinary team relationships and support groups (Cox & Andrews, 1981; Vachon, 1987). Intraprofessional and interprofessional relationships also have been identified as a key source of stress (Steffen, 1980; Vachon, 1987), illustrating, in a nursing context, the ease with which some stressors and social support can be confounded. Despite the identified importance to nurses of interpersonal relations in the work setting, there has been an absence of systematic examination of the variations in intradisciplinary and interdisciplinary team dynamics—their relationships to social support, work stressors, and staff health outcomes (Schmitt, Farrell, & Heinemann, 1988).

Browner's (1987) report on job stressors, health, and the impact of team support focusses on 26 psychiatric technicians functioning in a state institutional work environment very similar to nurses' work settings. Although they worked with the severely and profoundedly mentally retarded who were often difficult management problems, the technicians did not cite patients as a major work stressor but rather as a major source of work satisfaction. This is similar to nurses who also report patient care more as a source of satisfaction than stress (Vachon, 1987). The exception was the technicians' fear of violent attack from a resident; the fear stemmed primarily from whether they could depend on co-workers for assistance in such an event. Lack of readily available team support was a stressor. Other major stressors were their lack of influence in planning treatment programs, in influencing institutional policies, and in managing the conditions of work, such as scheduling of work time and controlling paperwork. Although major stressors identified were similar across the four units studied, there was considerable variation in perceptions of social support. There was a significant difference in the illness symptoms reported by technicians on the most cohesive unit compared with the other three, where work-based social support was more limited. On these three units there was little common agreement about what work-based social support meant; work-related social support was minimally defined as assisting co-workers when they sought help. On the cohesive unit there was a common broad

definition of teamwork that included both emotional and instrumental support, resolution of unit-wide problems by the entire staff, excellent working relations with the supervisor, and out-of-work socializing and informal friendships among staff members.

Although Browner's (1987) research report emphasizes the importance of cohesive team relationships in reducing staff stress, other reports indicate positive interdisciplinary team relationships can directly affect patient outcomes (Feiger & Schmitt, 1979, Knaus, Draper, Wagner, & Zimmerman, 1985). However, there are also limits to the impact of highly cohesive work groups because priority given to maintaining good relations and a positive feeling can undermine the quality of the team's work effort through ignoring negative feedback about work effectiveness (Janis, 1972). Also, when small work groups such as teams are highly cohesive, integration of the work group into the larger organizational structure may be problematic, limiting the team's effectiveness and increasing job stress. A case-study report of work relations in a public psychiatric children's hospital by Judith Blau referred to by Granovetter (1982), in which treatment was difficult and outcomes often were uncertain, identified an extensive network of weak ties among staff members, with all 200 acquainted on a first-name basis, as a key factor in the prevention of low morale and staff turnover. Worker health was not examined. There were stable work groups such as programs, committees, and teams, but there was an absence of high cohesiveness, including an absence of strong friendship relations, that might undermine ties with individuals in other areas of the organization. Granovetter points out that such co-extensive weak ties may not be possible in larger organizations.

The report by Browner (1987) shares in common with reports on stressors among nurses that bureaucratic procedures are major stressors—lack of influence over policies and scheduling of work time and excessive paperwork. Although individual coping efforts are the most commonly reported (Vachon, 1987), these are not likely to make an impact on the potent organizational sources of work stress (Pearlin, et al., 1981). Using social support strategies to influence those aspects of the work environment that are changeable may make an important and unique contribution to reducing work stress. Hirsch and David (1983) descriptively report the use of "resource support groups" with nurse managers for emotional support, problem solving, and participatory decision making. Although such groups may have been stress-buffering in reducing the emotional consequences of work stressors, their major purpose was to develop programs and policies to enhance work life by reducing or eliminating work stressors. As the authors indicated, "we should exercise care so that emotional support is used to enhance empowerment, not to prevent it" (Hirsch & David, 1983, p. 498). Systemic studies are needed of the impact of such "resource support" groups.

One of the most frequently described sources of support, which, nevertheless, may not be commonly used (Vachon, 1987), is staff support groups (Baider

& Porath, 1981; Epting, 1981; Moynihan & Outlaw, 1984; Rosini, Howell, Todres, & Dorman, 1974; Skinner, 1980). Although the descriptive reports of staff support groups indicate the positive effects of this type of work-related support, some nurses have reported them as ineffective (Vachon, 1987). Careful reading of the reports suggests that groups that offer opportunities only for catharsis of emotions are not particularly helpful, and that active problem solving for work situations that are sources of stress is the main ingredient of successful groups.

The types of organizational changes that staff nurses perceive as positive in reducing work stress and the negative health consequences of nursing work situations are outlined in a report of the American Academy of Nursing (1983) and are in agreement with many of the organizational coping strategies reported by Vachon (1987) in her descriptive study of occupational stress and coping. These include institutional changes such as building effective intradisciplinary and interdisciplinary work groups, participatory management and policy setting, appropriate staffing and personnel policies, staff development and recognition programs, and provision for ongoing support in dealing with the daily stress of patient care.

SUMMARY

An examination of the current literature on social support, stressors, and health as it has been applied to the study of occupational stressors, and, particularly, stressors in nursing reveals the limitations of what we know currently about relationships among these phenomena. One key problem is differing general definitions of what a stressor is, which contributes to variations in definitions of stressors in occupational settings and in nursing specifically. Social support also is subject to varying definitions depending on whether the emphasis is on social ties, network configurations, or functional aspects of relationships. Outcomes most consistently studied have been psychological characteristics; long-term physical consequences of chronic stressors are harder to study because of the longitudinal designs required. One key problem when the effects of social support on occupational stressors are studied is examining separately general sources of support and work-related sources. A second major problem is sorting out main effects of social support, which act directly on the stressors, strains, and symptoms, from buffering effects, which reduce the negative impact of stressors after they have occurred.

Nursing is still a predominantly female occupation, and little of the social support and occupational stressor literature addresses the health effects for employed women. A very small amount of systematic nursing research has explored the relationships among all these variables. Because of the limited research, conclusions drawn about the relationship among social support, occupational stressors, and health in nursing remain tentative at this time. Hypothesized relationships that

may serve as a conceptual guide to future research are summarized in Figure 74–2 and include the following:

- Networks of social ties and networks of work relations are sources both of social support *and* of interpersonal stressors.
- Positive ties to family, friends, and community (companionship) are important in maintaining psychological health regardless of the type or level of work stress. Such ties also probably are important in maintaining physical health, but the mechanisms of effect are poorly understood. Among ideas that have been proposed are direct effects on neurochemical reactions, effects on health practices and health risk behaviors, and effects on resources needed for problem-solving situations affecting health (Lazarus & Folkman, 1984). On the other hand, interpersonal stressors have a direct negative effect on psychological and physical health.
- Occupational stressors have a negative impact on psychological and physical health. Although many occupational stressors are specific to the type of occupation, interpersonal relations are generally a potent source of work stress. The contribution of interpersonal stressors to occupational stressors is shown in Figure 74–2 via a dotted line.
- The most important sources of social support for work stressors are work specific; these support sources may vary by type of occupation. Work support operates both directly and indirectly (through reducing occupational stressors) to increase psychological and physical health. It may also buffer occupational stressors by reducing their negative consequences.
- Social ties (companionship) also may be a resource in reducing work stressors and their negative outcomes. The sources and types of ties that are helpful may differ whether the person is married or single, male or female. The degree of helpfulness of social ties also may depend on the type of occupational stressor, for example, job loss versus stressors related to the organization of the work environment.
- In effects on health, work stressors are additive with stressful interpersonal relations outside work, for example, marital role strain. The stress of nursing may encourage a segmentation of work relationships from the rest of one's social ties to prevent a negative feedback loop, with the goal of decreasing the stress on social ties emanating from the work environment. In Figure 74–2 this possible segmentation is represented by a question mark between the network of social ties and the network of work relationships. This defensive segmentation may undermine useful work support from a broader network of relationships.

There are several practical implications of these ideas for nurses' use of social support. Devoting time to building and maintaining positive primary relationships and to confronting negative relationships outside of work are important as overall life-style strategies. Negative primary relationships compound work stress.

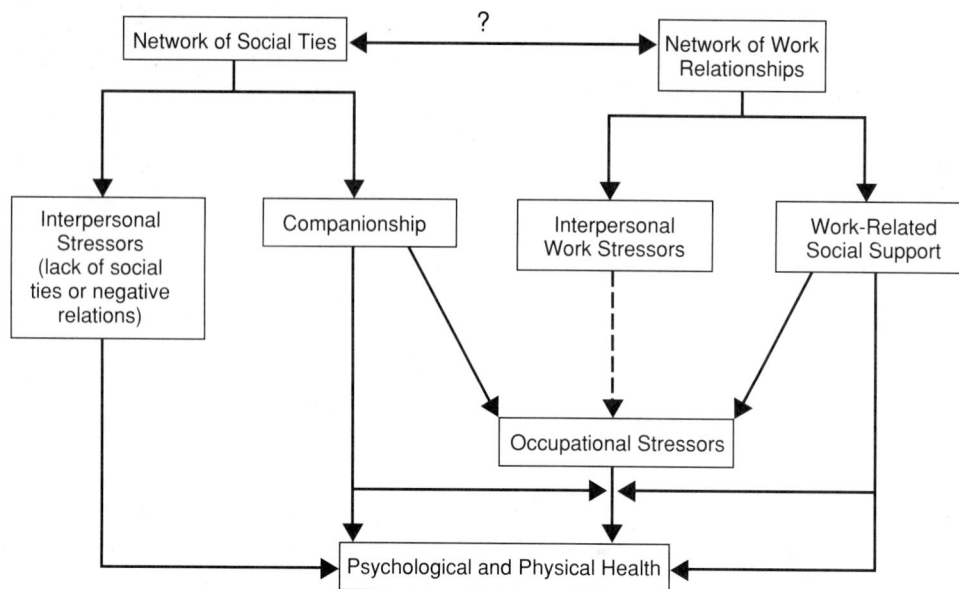

Figure 74–2. Hypothesized relationships among social supports, occupational stressors, and health.

Positive primary relationships generally help foster self-esteem and serve as an antidote against depression. They may be of some help for specific work stressors. However, it is important also to build appropriate work-based sources of support because these seem to be more potent reducers of occupational stressors. In nursing, the aim of work-based support most often should be institutional change rather than individual change, because many potent nursing stressors are organizational. Organizational sources of stress cannot be reduced or eliminated through individual coping efforts (although individual coping efforts may help reduce stress symptoms temporarily). Several kinds of networks of support seem important to develop in the work setting. First, fostering good relationships in intradisciplinary and interdisciplinary work groups facilitates both support and effective patient care. Second, support groups may be a useful additional type of support for difficult patient care situations. Third, developing networks of acquaintances in the larger organization provides a potential base of support and problem solving for addressing broader organizational sources of stress. Out of these, resource support groups may be formed as needed to address specific changes that are desired.

References

American Academy of Nursing, Task Force on Nursing Practice in Hospitals. (1983). *Magnet hospitals: Attraction and retention of professional nurses.* Kansas City, MO: American Nurses' Association.

Aneshensel, C. S. (1986). Marital and employment role strain, social support, and depression among adult women. In S. E. Hobfoll (Ed.), *Stress, social support, and women* (pp. 99–114). Washington: Hemisphere Publishing.

Baider, L., & Porath, S. (1981). Uncovering fear: Group experience of nurses in a cancer ward. *International Journal of Nursing Studies, 18,* 47–52.

Berkman, L. F. (1985). The relationship of social networks and social support to morbidity and mortality. In S. Cohen & S. L. Syme (Eds.), *Social support and health* (pp. 263–278). Orlando, FL: Academic Press, Inc.

Browner, C. H. (1987). Job stress and health: The role of social support at work. *Research in Nursing and Health, 10,* 93–100.

Caplan, G. (1974). *Supportive systems and community mental health.* New York: Behavioral Publications.

Caplan, R. D. (1979). Social support, person-environment fit, and coping. In L. A. Ferman & J. P. Gordus (Eds.), *Mental health and the economy* (pp. 89–137). Kalamazoo, MI: W.E. Upjohn Institute for Employment Research.

Cassel, J. C. (1963). The use of medical records: Opportunity for epidemiological studies. *Journal of Occupational Medicine, 5,* 185–190.

Cassel, J. C. (1974). Psychosocial processes and "stress": Theoretical formulation. *International Journal of Health Services, 4,* 471–481.

Cohen, S., & Syme, L. (1985). Issues in the study and application of social support. In S. Cohen & S. L. Syme (Eds.), *Social support and health* (pp. 3–22). Orlando, FL: Academic Press, Inc.

Cox, A., & Andrews, P. (1981). The development of support systems on oncology units. *Oncology Nursing Forum, 8*(3), 31–35.

Coyne, J. C., & De Longis, A. (1986). Going beyond social support: The role of social relations in adaptation. *Journal of Consulting and Clinical Psychology, 54,* 454–460.

Durkheim, E. (1951). *Suicide.* New York: The Free Press.

Epting, S. P. (1981). Coping with stress through peer support. *Topics in Clinical Nursing, 2,* 47–59.

Feiger, S. M., & Schmitt, M. H. (1979). Collegiality in interdisciplinary health teams: Its measurement and its effects. *Social Science and Medicine, 13A,* 217–229.

Fiore, J., Becker, J., & Coppel, D. B. (1983). Social network interactions: A buffer or a stress. *American Journal of Community Psychology, 11,* 423–439.

Gore, S. (1978). The effect of social support in moderating the health consequences of unemployment. *Journal of Health and Social Behavior, 19,* 157–165.

Gottlieb, B. H. (1978). The development and application of a classification scheme of informal helping behaviors. *Canadian Journal of Behavioral Science, 10,* 105–115.

Granovetter, M. S. (1973). The strength of weak ties. *American Journal of Sociology, 78,* 1360–1380.

Granovetter, M. S. (1982). The strength of weak ties: A network theory revisited. In P. V. Marsden & N. Lin (Eds.), *Social structure and network analysis* (pp. 105–130). Beverly Hills, CA: Sage Publications.

Greenberg, S. F., & Valletutti, P. J. (1980). *Stress and the helping professions.* Baltimore: Paul H. Brookes, Publishers.

Hall, A., & Wellman, B. (1985). Social networks and social support.

In S. Cohen & S. L. Syme (Eds.), *Social support and health* (pp. 23–41). Orlando, FL: Academic Press, Inc.

Hammer, M. (1981). Social supports, social networks and schizophrenia. *Schizophrenia Bulletin, 7,* 45–57.

Haw, M. A. (1982). Women, work, and stress. *Journal of Health and Social Behavior, 23,* 132–144.

Heller, K. (1979). The effects of social support: Prevention and treatment implications. In A. P. Goldstein & F. H. Kanfer (Eds.), *Maximizing treatment gains: Transfer enhancement in psychotherapy* (pp. 353–382). New York: Academic Press, Inc.

Hirsch, B. J. (1980). Natural support systems and coping with major life changes. *American Journal of Community Psychology, 8,* 159–172.

Hirsch, B. J. (1981). Social networks and the coping process: Creating personal communities. In B. H. Gottlieb (Ed.), *Social networks and social support* (pp. 149–170). Beverly Hills, CA: Sage Publications.

Hirsch, B. J., & David, T. G. (1983). Social networks and work/nonwork life: Action-research with nurse managers. *American Journal of Community Psychology, 11,* 493–507.

Holmes, T. H., & Rahe, R. H. (1967). The social readjustment rating scale. *Journal of Psychosomatic Research, 11,* 213–218.

House, J. S. (1981). *Work stress and social support.* Reading, MA: Addison-Wesley Publishing Co.

House, J. S., & Kahn, R. L. (1985). Measures and concepts of social support. In S. Cohen & S. L. Syme (Eds.), *Social support and health* (pp. 83–108). Orlando, FL: Academic Press, Inc.

Hutchinson, S. (1987). Self-care and job stress. *Image: Journal of Nursing Scholarship, 19,* 192–196.

Janis, I. L. (1972). *Victims of groupthink.* Boston: Houghton Mifflin Co.

Kahn, R. L. (1979). Aging and social support. In M. W. Riley (Ed.), *Aging from birth to death: Interdisciplinary perspectives* (pp. 77–91). Boulder, CO: Westview Press.

Kahn, R. L., & Antonucci, T. C. (1980). Convoys over the life course: Attachment, roles, and social support. In P. B. Baltes & O. Brim (Eds.), *Life span development and behavior, vol. 3* (pp. 253–286). New York: Academic Press, Inc.

Kanner, A. D., Coyne, J. C., Schaefer, C., & Lazarus, R. S. (1981). Comparison of two modes of stress measurement: Daily hassles and uplifts versus major life events. *Journal of Behavioral Medicine, 4,* 1–39.

Kasl, S. V., & Wells, J. A. (1985). Social support and health in the middle years: Work and the family. In S. Cohen & S. L. Syme (Eds.), *Social support and health* (pp. 175–198). Orlando, FL: Academic Press, Inc.

Kessler, R. C., & McLeod, J. D. (1983). Social support and mental health in community samples. In S. Cohen & S. L. Syme (Eds.), *Social support and health* (pp. 219–240). Orlando, FL: Academic Press, Inc.

Knapp, T. R. (1988). Stress versus strain: A methodological critique. *Nursing Research, 37,* 181–183.

Knaus, W. A., Draper, E. A., Wagner, D. P., & Zimmerman, J. E. (1985). An evaluation of outcome from intensive care in major medical centers. *Annals of Internal Medicine, 104,* 410–418.

LaRocco, J. M., House, J. S., & French, J. R. P., Jr. (1980). Social support, occupational stress, and health. *Journal of Health and Social Behavior, 21,* 202–218.

Lazarus, R. S., & Folkman, S. (1984). *Stress, appraisal, and coping.* New York: Springer Publishing Co.

Leavy, R. L. (1983). Social support and psychological disorder: A review. *Journal of Community Psychology, 11,* 133–143.

Lieberman, M. A. (1986). Social supports—the consequences of psychologizing: A commentary. *Journal of Consulting and Clinical Psychology, 54,* 461–465.

Mercer, R. T., & Ferketich, S. L. (1988). Stress and social support as predictors of anxiety and depression during pregnancy. *Advances in Nursing Science, 10,* 26–39.

Mitchell, J. C. (1969). The concept and use of social networks. In

J. C. Mitchell (Ed.), *Social networks in urban situations* (pp. 1–50). Bath, England: Manchester University Press.

Mitchell, R. E., & Trickett, E. J. (1980). Social networks as mediators of social support: An analysis of the effects and determinants of social networks. *Community Mental Health Journal, 16,* 27–44.

Moynihan, R. T., & Outlaw, E. (1984). Nursing support groups in a cancer center. *Journal of Psychosocial Oncology, 2,* 33–48.

Murawski, B. J., Penman, D., & Schmitt, M. H. (1978). Social support in health and illness: The concept and its measurement. *Cancer Nursing, 1,* 365–371.

Norbeck, J. S. (1985). Types and sources of social support for managing job stress in critical care nursing. *Nursing Research, 34,* 225–230.

O'Brien, R. A. (1987, November). *Role of social support in bereavement outcomes.* Paper presented at the annual meeting of the Gynecological Society of America, Washington, DC.

Pearlin, L. I., Lieberman, M. A., Menaghan, E. G., & Mullan, J. T. (1981). The stress process. *Journal of Health and Social Behavior, 22,* 337–356.

Powers, B. A. (1988). Social networks, social support, and elderly institutionalized people. *Advances in Nursing Science, 10,* 40–58.

Rook, K. S. (1984). The negative side of social interaction: Impact on psychological well being. *Journal of Personality and Social Psychology, 46,* 1097–1108.

Rook, K. S. (1987). Social support versus companionship: Effects on life stress, loneliness, and evaluation by others. *Journal of Personality and Social Psychology, 52,* 1132–1147.

Rosini, L. A., Howell, M. C., Todres, I. D., & Dorman, J. (1974). Group meetings in a pediatric intensive care unit. *Pediatrics, 53,* 371–374.

Schaefer, C., Coyne, J. C., & Lazarus, R. S. (1981). The health-related functions of social support. *Journal of Behavioral Medicine, 4,* 379–399.

Schmitt, M. H., Farrell, M. P., & Heinemann, G. D. (1988). Conceptual and methodological problems in studying the effects of interdisciplinary geriatric teams. *Gerontologist, 28,* 753–764.

Skinner, K. (1980). Support groups for ICU nurses. *Nursing Outlook, 28,* 296–299.

Steffen, S. M. (1980). Perceptions of stress: 1800 nurses tell their stories. In K. E. Klaus & J. T. Bailey (Eds.), *Living with stress and promoting well-being: A handbook for nurses* (pp. 38–58). St. Louis: C. V. Mosby Co.

Suls, J. (1982). Social support, interpersonal relations, and health: Benefits and liabilities. In G. S. Sanders & J. Suls (Eds.), *Social psychology of health and illness* (pp. 255–277). Hillsdale, NJ: Lawrence Erlbaum Associates, Publishers.

Thoits, P. A. (1982). Conceptual, methodological, and theoretical problems in studying social support as a buffer against life stress. *Journal of Health and Social Behavior, 23,* 145–159.

Thoits, P. A. (1986). Social support as coping assistance. *Journal of Consulting and Clinical Psychology, 54,* 416–423.

Tilden, V. P., & Galyen, R. D. (1987). Cost and conflict: The darker side of social support. *Western Journal of Nursing Research, 9,* 9–18.

Vachon, M. L. S. (1987). *Occupational stress in the care of the critically ill, the dying, and the bereaved.* Washington: Hemisphere Publishing.

Vanfossen, B. E. (1986). Sex differences in depression: The role of spouse support. In S. E. Hobfoll (Ed.), *Stress, social support, and women* (pp. 69–84). Washington: Hemisphere Publishing.

Weiss, R. S. (1974). The provisions of social relationships. In Z. Rubin (Ed.), *Doing unto others* (pp. 17–26). Englewood Cliffs, NJ: Prentice-Hall, Inc.

Wellman, B. (1981). Applying network analysis to the study of support. In B. H. Gottlieb (Ed.), *Social networks and social support* (pp. 171–200). Beverly Hills, CA: Sage Publications.

Wortman, C. B. (1984). Social support and the cancer patient. *Cancer, 53*(Suppl. 10), 2339–2360.

CHAPTER 75

The Generation of Stress in the Provision of Care

PATRICIA J. LARSON
BONNIE MOWINSKI JENNINGS

Perhaps more than any chronic disease other than acquired immune deficiency syndrome (AIDS), the diagnosis of cancer evokes a tremendous amount of fear. This fear may be based, in part, in the long history of negative connotations that surround cancer. These include visions of pain, disfigurement, helplessness, altered consciousness, financial distress, isolation, and death. As Schoenberg and Senescu (1970) asserted almost two decades ago, the word *cancer* stimulates thoughts of an eroding, devouring, and mutilating disease. Given this rather gruesome image of cancer as an illness, it is not surprising that individuals caring for patients with cancer are faced with a multitude of challenges and questions.

Caring—both the attitude and the activity—has been identified not only as the dominant theme of clinical nursing but also as a salient feature of cancer nursing (Larson, 1984; Styles, 1982). The demands facing nurses who care for patients with cancer are a complex composite of the patient's physical and psychosocial needs. Amid the flurry of checking doctors' orders, striving to control pain, writing myriad nursing notes, comforting families, making beds, formulating nursing diagnoses, and giving prescribed treatments, nurses must also confront personal issues concerning the care versus cure dichotomy and recognize their own mortality. These diverse and demanding responsibilities have generated a belief that nurses caring for patients with cancer experience a great deal of stress.

The purpose of this chapter is to examine the stress experienced by nurses in providing care to patients with cancer. This will be accomplished by reviewing stress research that pertains to nurses in general, evaluating empirical evidence of the stress of cancer nursing in particular, and examining how the patient's

cancer trajectory may influence the nurse's stress. To focus the discussion, a definition of stress and a brief mention of pertinent conceptual issues are offered.

THE MEANING OF STRESS

Defining stress is considerably more difficult than it may seem, because there is no agreed on definition. In fact, the concept is thickly veiled in conceptual confusion. Stress has been viewed as an antecedent or stimulus, a consequence or response, and an interactive process between the person and the environment (Lazarus & Launier, 1978; Mason, 1975). The last-mentioned perspective is particularly useful when considering stress in occupations as well as a more holistic view of individuals. Stress, then, occurs when there is a perceived imbalance between demands and abilities (Harrison, 1978).

In addition, there are two sides to stress; one is the positive, stimulating aspect, and the other is the negative, threatening component. The negative consequences of stress tend to receive more attention because they are more likely to lead to dysfunctional problems. Perhaps the most dangerous consequence is the potentially deleterious effect of stress on health (Holt, 1982; Pelletier, 1984). No one is immune from stress. It can affect both persons whose health is unimpaired as well as those whose health is compromised by disease.

The issue of perception and the subjective nature of stress must be emphasized. As Sutterley (1979, p. 8) articulates, "Stress lies in the perception of events, not in events themselves." Therefore, situations are not inherently stressful; rather, a dynamic process is involved. How one evaluates an occurrence—the event itself, the context in which it occurs, the circumstances preceding it, the incidents that are taking place concurrently—influences whether stress is evoked. Potential sources of stress range from demanding physical

The opinions or assertions in this chapter are the private views of the authors and are not to be construed as official or as reflecting the views of the Department of the Army or the Department of Defense.

activities; to draining emotional experiences, such as the death of a patient; to disturbing professional exchanges among persons with whom one works.

Stress, therefore, is a complex, ubiquitous phenomenon that is experienced by patients and nurses alike. The stresses experienced by the patient with cancer are many and varied and require study and interventions from a variety of health care professionals. The focus of this chapter, however, is on the stress generated by the nurse in the process of providing care.

STRESS IN NURSING

Despite its complexity, or perhaps because of it, stress in nursing has captured the interest of innumerable researchers dating back to 1960. It is useful to review the themes of these investigations as they have evolved over three decades to provide a background for more specifically evaluating stress generated by providing care to patients with cancer.

The 1960s

Menzies (1960) was the first investigator to examine stress in nursing. Data were collected over a 4-yr period in one British hospital using a participant observation approach. Although the actual number of observations was never presented, the findings suggested that nurses in this hospital experienced anxiety from four major sources: (1) caring for patients, (2) making decisions, (3) taking responsibility, and (4) dealing with change. The stress generated by patient care was a finding common to all accounts of stress in nursing that emerged in the 1960s (Cleland, 1965; Holsclaw, 1965; Jones, 1962; Kornfeld, Maxwell, & Momrow, 1968; Koumans, 1965; Strauss, 1968; Vreeland & Ellis, 1968).

With the exception of Cleland's (1965) experimental investigation of the effects of stress on medical-surgical nurses' job performance and ability to think, the understanding of stress in nursing generated during the 1960s was based on participant observations, case reports, and anecdotal accounts. Furthermore, these studies were conducted not only at the onset of the intensive care movement—which quickly narrowed the focus of most investigations to nurses in intensive care units (ICUs)—but also during the initial surge of nursing research. Although these classic works afford valuable insights into the demands of nursing, they must be appreciated for their heuristic value rather than for their scientific merit.

Nevertheless, the studies were the first to identify stresses experienced by nurses. The stressors, which were subsequently corroborated in ensuing decades, could be categorized by four themes: physical and emotional aspects of patient care, complexity of equipment used in providing patient care, inadequate staff support, and interpersonal relationships. Cleland's (1965) work departed from the trend of enumerating what factors evoked stress in nurses and instead con-

sidered the effects of stress. More precisely, Cleland demonstrated that nurses' ability to think deteriorated as the quantity of environmental stress increased. Table 75–1 depicts the major findings from the research on stress in nursing.

The 1970s

During the 1970s, the nursing unit of interest in studies of stress was almost exclusively some form of an ICU (Bilodeau, 1973; Cassem & Hackett, 1972; Huckabay & Jagla, 1979; Jacobson, 1978; Michaels, 1971; Olsen, 1977; Oskins, 1979). Although most studies were descriptive accounts of stressful experiences, the reports moved away from presenting anecdotal accounts to collecting data via interviews and questionnaires, with some semblance of validity and reliability testing evident in many of the questionnaires. Furthermore, although the number of participants remained low (n = 16 to 46) except in the case of Robinson's (1972) nationwide survey of 1111 directors of nursing, sample sizes were routinely reported.

The increased scientific merit of studies from this era corroborated the themes concerning nurses' stress that had emerged in the preceding decade (see Table 75–1). Patient care remained a potent source of stress. In addition, interpersonal relationships and the care environment were also stress producing. These stresses were experienced not only among adult care providers, but also among nurses working with critically ill neonates (Jacobson, 1978). The scope of interest also expanded to nurses in the operating room who listed missing and malfunctioning equipment and interpersonal relationships, rather than patients per se, as stress-producing irritants (Olsen, 1977).

In addition, three new ideas concerning stress among nurses emerged during the 1970s. First, positive aspects of nursing—particularly ICU nursing—were addressed by Michaels (Michaels, 1971). These included expanding one's knowledge, being closer to patients, and experiencing the exciting features of the work. In searching for sources of frustration and satisfaction in ICU nursing, Bilodeau (1973) identified a fascinating dichotomy: those things that frustrated the nurses—

Table 75–1. STRESS IN NURSING

1960s: First Studies of Stress among Nurses
  Identified sources of stress:
    Physical and emotional aspects of patient care
    Complex equipment
    Inadequate support for staff
    Interstaff relationships
1970s: New Dimensions of Stress in Nursing
  Inadequate knowledge and skills
  Sources of satisfaction
  Coping strategies
  Initial ICU/non-ICU comparison
1980s: Changing Trends in Nursing Stress Studies
  Renaissance of ICU/non-ICU comparisons
  Effects of personality
  Burnout
  Initial studies of stress in oncology nursing

ICU, intensive care unit.

patients, families, co-workers—were also the sources of satisfaction. For example, patient care was frustrating insofar as it involved repetitive routines, whereas it was satisfying when the pace quickened and crises occurred.

The second unique contribution of the 1970s was that coping strategies within the nurse's repertoire were also identified. Oskins (1979), in a study of 79 critical care nurses from five hospitals, discerned that nurses coped by talking with others, taking definite action, drawing on past experiences, and acknowledging their anxiety. This was an important beginning to the development of an understanding of what mechanisms protect nurses from succumbing to the deleterious effects of stress.

Finally, it was in the 1970s that the first comparison between ICU and non-ICU nurses was made. Gentry, Foster, and Froehling (1972) explored the emotional responses of 34 nurses working in three ICUs ($n = 26$) and one non-ICU ($n = 8$). This study came to be regarded as the hallmark report that established that ICU nurses were more stressed than their non-ICU colleagues. The caution with which these results should have been regarded, particularly with respect to the disproportionately small size of the non-ICU group, was not adequately communicated, thus giving rise to the myth that the ICU was the most stressful nursing environment.

The 1980s

Interest in studying stress in nurses burgeoned during the 1980s. The numerous descriptive studies from this decade continued the emphasis on ICU nursing and supported existing beliefs: the main stress experienced by nurses was related to patient care; inadequate knowledge and skills; interpersonal relations; and the environment, which included unit management (Anderson & Basteyns, 1981; Bailey, Steffen, & Grout, 1980; Kelly & Cross, 1985). Other themes that continued to prevail included appraising both stress and coping (Albrecht, 1982; Stockton, 1986), and corroborating that satisfaction was derived from the same features that provoked stress (Bargagliotti & Trygstad, 1987; Norbeck, 1985) (see Table 75–1).

The new ideas that emerged in the 1980s included considering how personality affected one's perception of stress (Ivancevich & Matteson, 1980; Keane, Du-Cette, & Adler, 1985; Maloney & Bartz, 1983; Numerof & Abrams, 1984; Rich & Rich, 1987) and examining an increasingly popular concept called *burnout* (Albrecht, 1982; Bartz & Maloney, 1986; Cronin-Stubbs & Rooks, 1985; Stone, Jebson, Walk, & Belsham, 1984). An important advance was that some investigators began to consider the need to view the pervasive stress phenomenon in relation to outcomes. In other words, given that the presence of stress had been repeatedly established, what were the effects of that stress? For example, stress was considered in regard to the way it affected job satisfaction (Norbeck,

1985) and produced psychological symptoms (Esteban, Ballesteros, & Caballero, 1983; Norbeck, 1985).

Perhaps the most significant contribution from the 1980s, however, was a renewal of curiosity regarding stress in ICU and non-ICU nursing environments. Repeated studies conducted in a variety of institutions consistently reported the same finding: there was no detectable difference in the stress experienced by ICU and non-ICU nurses (Albrecht, 1982; Fawsey, Wellisch, Pasnau, & Liebowitz, 1983; Maloney, 1982; Mohl, Denny, Mote, & Coldwater, 1982; Vincent & Coleman, 1986). Comparisons of ICU and non-ICU nurses in regard to job satisfaction (Nichols, Springford, & Searle, 1981) as well as personality (Jones, 1962; Maloney & Bartz, 1983) also indicated that nurses in general were more similar than they were different.

It was during this period of renewed interest in stress experienced by nurses outside the ICU setting that studies began to consider oncology units. Concomitantly, interest in oncology as a nursing specialty was escalating. Momentum had been building over several years, but in the 1980s oncology nursing gained a heightened prestige because of the unique talents and knowledge required to meet the challenge of caring for patients with cancer. The needs of these patients are complex and numerous; they cover all aspects of the psychological and physiologic spectra. As it became more evident that stress was indeed a common phenomenon among nurses and as the interest in oncology nursing grew, studies began to focus on the world of caring that is unique to cancer nurses.

STRESS IN CANCER NURSING

The premise underlying most studies of oncology nurses is that the prolonged exposure to very ill people and death puts them at particular risk for experiencing the negative effects of stress. In fact, Stockton's (1986) anecdotal account of burnout among oncology nurses refers to this syndrome as bereavement overload. However, as Vachon (1986) clearly conveys, some beliefs about oncology nursing appear to be more myth than fact when the empirical evidence is considered.

Although the essays by McElroy (1982) and Newlin and Wellisch (1978) are representative of the anecdotal accounts of the stress that is purported to exist in oncology nursing, a different impression is conveyed by the data-based studies that have evaluated the world of cancer nursing (Table 75–2). Overall, three approaches have prevailed in the study of stress experienced by oncology nurses. These are identification of the sources of stress, comparison of oncology nurses with nurses in other specialties, and evaluation of the extent of burnout experienced by oncology nurses.

Table 75–2. STRESS ISSUES AMONG CANCER NURSES

Inadequate staff support
Interpersonal interactions
Types of patient work environment
Questioning the reality of burnout

The sources of stress for oncology nurses have been studied less extensively than those for ICU nurses, which may account for the difficulty in discerning a pattern among the stressors. Donovan's (1981) study was designed to identify sources of stress among 22 oncology nurses—11 from an inpatient setting and 11 involved with home care. The stressors could be encompassed in three broad categories—work-related issues such as scheduling and paperwork, interpersonal encounters at work, and personal problems such as car trouble. Data from a study of three hospices evaluated the stressful events reported by 93 care providers, 70 of whom were nursing personnel (Yancik, 1984). The three major sources of stress among these individuals concerned lack of staff support, emotional issues arising from patient and family interactions, and frustrations with the disease process. Barstow (1980) examined stress in 26 hospice nursing personnel. The sources of stress were many and varied in intensity depending on the stage of the patient's illness.

Perhaps there is less consistency among sources of stress reported by oncology nurses because of the diverse settings in which care is delivered—hospitals, hospices, and homes. It may be that these settings are varied enough to preclude the discovery of a core of stressors among all cancer nurses. For example, Vachon (1986) found that the work environment and occupational role, not patients and families, were the dominant sources of stress among 100 hospice care providers. Furthermore, in the same study, it was reported that oncology nurses experienced more stress than nurses providing care in the hospice setting. Therefore, it may be that a complex combination of many factors contributes to stress rather than simply the fact of caring for persons with cancer.

Just as studies of ICU nurses have not, overall, demonstrated greater stress among critical care staff compared with other nurses, so too, it is difficult to demonstrate that oncology nurses experience greater stress than those in other nursing specialties (Fawsey et al., 1983; Stewart, Meyerowitz, Jackson, Yarkin, & Harvey, 1982; Vachon, 1986). In fact, in one study, oncology nurses not only displayed no greater stress than nurses in four other areas, but also noted considerable satisfaction with their jobs (Fawsey et al., 1983). Although this investigation was conducted in only one health care facility, thereby limiting the extent to which results can be generalized, it demonstrates that oncology may be no more stressful than other nursing specialties.

A particularly eloquent portrayal of the positive side of cancer care was reported by Trygstad (1986), who interviewed 17 oncology nurses. Koocher (1979) also elucidated a number of the rewards that may balance the demands of caring for persons with cancer. The positive aspects of working on a cancer unit were reflected in a study of 190 clinical staff members at a comprehensive cancer center (Box 75–1). The nurses in the study, like their physician and social work colleagues, uniformly rated their job satisfaction as high. Neither death itself or staff conflict were problems (Peteet et al., 1989).

Perhaps the concern over stress in oncology nursing has contributed to a narrow perspective that has failed to consider the benefits of oncology nursing. It may also be that the pessimistic attitudes that have prevailed among nurses in regard to caring for cancer patients have been modified by experience and education (Craytor, Brown, & Morrow, 1978; Craytor & Fass, 1982; Fanslow, 1985; Whelan, 1984).

Evaluating the extent of burnout is a strategy that is common in studies of stress in oncology nurses. This approach is not surprising, given the assumption that oncology nurses are particularly vulnerable to burnout because of the intense relationships with patients and families and the emotional stress of cancer. However, the presence of burnout has not been supported empirically.

Ogle (1983) studied 22 nurses from two hospitals with patient oncology units. Data were collected using the Maslach Burnout Inventory (Maslach & Jackson, 1986). Findings indicated some evidence of emotional exhaustion, the first stage of burnout, but even then scores were low compared with normative data. In a larger study based on a random sample of 152 Oncology Nursing Society members, burnout was measured with the Jones burnout scale (Jenkins & Ostchega, 1986). Here, too, burnout scores were lower than those reported by other nurses. Similarly, Yasko (1983) also found burnout to be minimal among 185 oncology clinical nurse specialists. Therefore, it appears that oncology nurses are not at greater risk for burnout, as some have surmised.

It is important to consider the degree to which support from staff members has been cited as a means of ameliorating burnout and other manifestations of stress (Barstow, 1980; Jenkins & Ostchega, 1986; Ogle, 1983; Yancik, 1984; Yasko, 1983). Although it may be that burnout is less prevalent than has previously been surmised, it is also possible that this conclusion reflects the way rewards, satisfaction, coping, and staff support attenuate the effects of stress and thwart the evolution of burnout. Also, because these nurses were all attracted to oncology, an alternate explanation is that they may be more resilient to the negative aspects of cancer care that could be deleterious to those not inclined to pursue this nursing specialty.

This assertion is defensible based on findings from two studies. Although burnout was low overall among nurses studied by Jenkins and Ostchega (1986), they found that as stressors, such as the number of deaths, escalated, levels of burnout increased. Concurrently, burnout was mitigated by satisfaction and support. Yasko (1983) also found that burnout was more intense among nurses who were dissatisfied with their role, under more stress, and not perceiving adequate psychological support.

Throughout the studies of oncology nurses, it is unclear to what extent patient care is a source of stress. As noted, patient care has both positive and negative aspects for nurses; patients are both a source of pride and reason for being a nurse as well as a key source of demands—the hard, physical care and the constant emotional bombardment that accompany involvement with persons

---

Box 75–1. JOB STRESS AND SATISFACTION

Peteet, J. R., Murray-Ross, D., Medeiros, C., Walsh-Burke, K., Rieker, P., & Finkelstein, D. (1989). **Job stress and satisfaction among the staff members at a cancer center.** *Cancer, 64,* 975–982.

The rewards and discomforts of working with cancer patients in a comprehensive cancer center was explored in a study of clinical staff that was composed of 94 registered nurses (RNs), 33 medical doctors (MDs), 11 social workers, and 45 allied health care workers. The dimensions of staff characteristics, patient care experience, and work environment on goal attainment and job satisfaction were examined. The study's conclusions were as follows:

- Helping patients was the most rewarding aspect of working in oncology for all subjects.
- RNs ranked emotional care as being their most valued goal. MDs selected treatment as their prime goal.
- Having high-technology procedures take precedence over patient comfort and experiencing ethical concerns over do-not-resuscitate status were the most discomforting for the RNs; inability to help patients was the most discomforting for the MDs.
- An interdisciplinary team approach was identified by both RNs and MDs as being most helpful in achieving goals.
- Job satisfaction was uniformly high (8.2 [SD = 1.9] on a scale of 1 to 10).

---

who face illnesses that are often the precursors to death. The studies to date have not adequately tapped the specifics of patient care that generate stress for nurses. The reports, especially those on oncology nurses, have not focused on specific aspects of patient care but rather have used a generalized approach and focused on the broad concept: the care of the patient with cancer. The reality of oncology is that nurses care for patients with a number of disease entities, each with its own trajectory of events, ranging from precancerous conditions to cure or to death. Larson (1987) contends that the cancer trajectory may help to explain why stress does indeed exist among oncology nurses and yet has not been found in previous inquiries.

THE CANCER TRAJECTORY

Larson asserts that each cancer disease and each patient's resulting illness experience has a unique trajectory that ranges from prevention through a number of possible outcomes that include cure or death. Each disease's trajectory, although unique, has common critical points, consisting of prevention, detection, diagnosis, treatment, remission, cure, relapse and treatment, or death (Fig. 75–1). Each of these trajectory points places different demands on the persons involved. The treatment and terminal care dimensions of the trajectory have the potential to be especially stressful for nurses. During these two points, nurses often have intense and involved interactions with patients and their families, who are also experiencing a period of high stress.

Research concerning the critical points of the trajectory has generally focused on patient needs. Examples of this are Stillman's (1977) work on health beliefs and breast self-examination, Dodd's and Larson's work on self-care and caring needs during treatment (Dodd, 1982, 1984a, 1984b; Larson, 1984), and Burns and Carney's (1986) focus on hospice costs. These studies, although not addressing the cancer trajectory perspective per se, do demonstrate that the various disease entities have a unique impact on the patient. It would

therefore seem reasonable to expect that each trajectory point for each disease entity would also place unique demands on those providing the care. This expectation is especially true for nurses, because they are the most consistent care providers throughout patients' illness experiences.

There are approximately 1,040,000 new cases of cancer diagnosed each year; all of these individuals will need nurses to help with their care (American Cancer Society, 1990). At the opposite end of the trajectory, more than 500,000 cancer-related deaths occur annually (American Cancer Society, 1990). Again, almost all of these individuals will have nurses provide care throughout the course of their dying. Many of the nurses providing care for the dying will be involved with more than one patient death; some nurses may experience more than 20 deaths per year. The magnitude of this death experience must surely have some effect on the nurses as they experience the process of attachment, loss, and mourning. In fact, Jenkins and Ostechega (1986) found that as patient deaths increased, nurses did indeed experience more stress.

In the middle of these extremes, the patients will encounter various modes of therapy. Surgical intervention, medical modalities, and radiation therapy can generate intense illness experiences for the patient. Again, nurses are the primary care providers during these times that require ingenious approaches to symptom control as well as emotional support for patients and their families (Lovejoy, 1986). Furthermore, interactions between patients and families may become so difficult that anger and rage provoked by the illness and all that it implies are turned on the nurse who is a convenient source on whom feelings can be released. Is it reasonable to believe that such emotional outpourings have no effect on the nurse?

Because the cancer trajectory is variable for each disease, nursing care may be provided intermittently or continuously. For example, the person with lung cancer or acute leukemia may have a shortened but almost continuous trajectory that is very intense, whereas someone with breast cancer or Hodgkin's

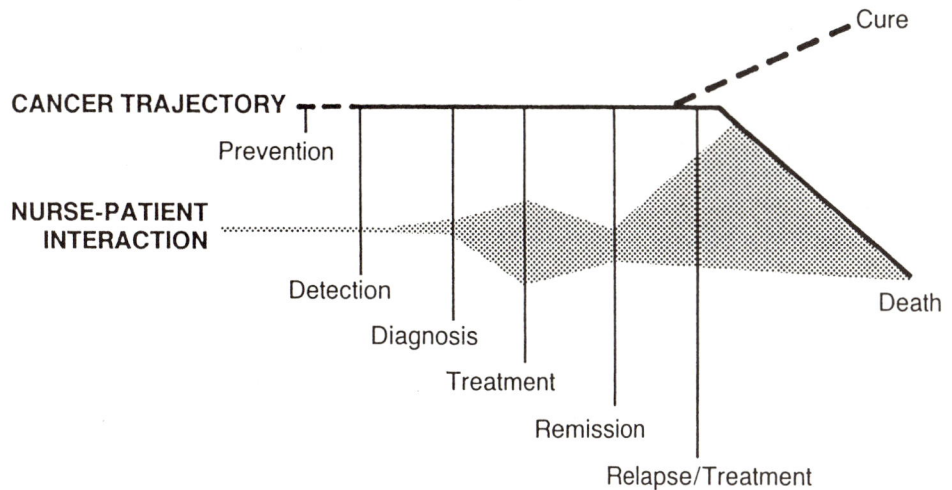

disease may have a lengthy intermittent trajectory that ultimately is marked only by sporadic follow-up care. These patients have very different nursing needs, but the needs are there nevertheless. Is it possible that nurses who have the difficult task of helping people deal with both dying and living are not affected by the intensity of the experience?

A final consideration is where the care is provided. It is unclear whether it is better to have persons with cancer scattered among other medical and surgical patients, on a special unit, or in a home care program (Cox & Andrews, 1981; Jones, 1981; Miller & Wegman, 1981; Tillman, 1984). It is important to consider who benefits from these care environments—the nurse or the patient—and how the different environments may affect the nurse's perception of stress from oncology care. However, with the increasing complexity and sophistication of cancer interventions, the professional imperative may mandate having a core nursing staff that is skilled in providing the special care needed by patients with cancer.

Consequently, as more oncology units evolve, it is possible that more nurses will be exposed to more intense patient relationships as they truly come to know patients as people. Trygstad (1986) referred to this process as being a "professional friend." Whatever the nomenclature, it seems feasible that as nurses have continued encounters with patients and come to know them better as people, a certain dread may be evoked when the patient reaches an unpromising point in the cancer trajectory. Just as the patient is traversing a course, so too the nurse is following a parallel process. The intensity of nurse-patient interactions is greatest for both nurses and patients during critical turning points. Is it possible that nurses are unaffected by these dynamics? Longitudinal studies could illuminate the processual dynamics of these relationships—the demands and the rewards.

In sum, the cancer trajectory, with its demanding critical points for patients, has the potential to place stresses on the nurses responsible for the varying treatment and management aspects required at each point. Empirically, little is known about how the cancer trajectory affects nurses. Clinically, it is evident that

nurses approach each point with different and varying skills and attitudes. It is therefore reasonable to expect that nurses would experience stress from a variety of sources, depending on where the care is delivered and at what point the patient is in his or her cancer trajectory.

SUMMARY

Stress engendered in the course of providing care to cancer patients is a topic that has intuitive appeal, especially for those nurses who have experienced the joys and the sorrows, the successes and the losses that are commonplace in working with oncology patients. It is startling to realize that empirical investigations only modestly support the notion that oncology nurses encounter stress. That is not to say that stress is absent but merely that it is an elusive phenomenon.

In oncology, it would appear that perhaps the approaches used in studying stress among nurses should be reconsidered. First, the sources of stress need to be better identified, with the understanding that the same issues—patients, for example—may represent both sources of satisfaction and frustration. Future research must also address the not yet identified sources of stress. Jennings's (1987) investigation of mental health in head nurses is a case in point. The study was conceptualized to include nonwork sources of stress as well as work-engendered stress in predicting mental health for a group of 300 head nurses.

Second, looking at the relationship between stress and outcome measures is important. As Norbeck (1985) noted, from a list of 16 stressors reported by critical care nurses, only seven were related to either job satisfaction or psychological symptoms. Previous research in oncology has taken outcomes into account; however, the focus has been almost exclusively on burnout. Would other outcome measures better demonstrate the effects of stress?

A third need is to move away from single point in time studies to better capture the dynamic process of stress. Clearly the cancer trajectory makes this need all the more compelling. Either longitudinal studies in the quantitative tradition or grounded theory or phenomenologic studies in the qualitative tradition would help to better address this process. Bargagliotti and Trygstad (1987) both studied work stress, but the former investigator used a quantitative approach and the latter researcher used a qualitative method. The findings, although not in conflict, were very different because the methodologies exposed varying facets of stress.

A fourth issue concerns coping. Although coping strategies have been identified, they have not been studied with regard to effectiveness. Albrecht (1982) noted that common suggestions for reducing burnout, such as taking time off or talking with individuals other than unit staff, did not in fact attenuate it. The need remains to explicate ways to moderate stress and to evaluate the actual effectiveness of these methods.

For nurses committed to the care of patients with cancer, several realities will continue. Cancer remains a leading cause of death, one that elicits many emotional and physical responses in the patient. Some cancers will race through the patient's body, causing a rapid downward course that quickly concludes in a fatal outcome. However, many cancers are being viewed as chronic diseases that, it is hoped, will allow the patient to have a longer but an ever-vigilant life. Curative-intent therapies will continue to be aggressive, demanding much from patients, families, and caregivers. Perhaps by taking a cue from the realities of oncology nursing, that the care of patients with cancer requires a fine balance between what is caring to patients—the competent know-how demonstrated in knowledgeable nursing actions—and what is caring to nurses—the personalized affective dimensions of talking, listening, and comforting (Larson, 1984, 1986; Mayer, 1987)—it may be possible to identify what is unique about oncology nurses and stress. Researchers will need to utilize old, new, and evolving methodologies to glean the aspects of oncology nursing that should remain unchanged and to delineate carefully those aspects that generate stress too burdensome for the nurse to remain a productive, caring, and vital person.

References

Albrecht, T. L. (1982). What job stress means for the staff nurse. *Nursing Administration Quarterly, 7*(1), 1–11.

American Cancer Society. (1990). *Cancer facts and figures—1990.* Atlanta: Author.

Anderson, C. A., & Basteyns, M. (1981). Stress and the critical care nurse reaffirmed. *Journal of Nursing Administration, 11*(1), 31–34.

Bailey, J. T., Steffen, S. M., & Grout, J. W. (1980). The stress audit: Identifying the stressors of ICU nursing. *Journal of Nursing Education, 19*(6), 15–25.

Bargagliotti, L. A., & Trygstad, L. N. (1987). Differences in stress and coping findings: A reflection of social realities or methodologies? *Nursing Research, 36,* 170–173.

Barstow, J. (1980). Stress variance in hospice nursing. *Nursing Outlook, 28,* 751–754.

Bartz, C., & Maloney, J. P. (1986). Burnout among intensive care nurses. *Research in Nursing and Health, 9,* 147–153.

Bilodeau, C. B. (1973). The nurse and her reactions to critical-care nursing. *Heart and Lung, 2,* 358–363.

Burns, N., & Carney, K. (1986). Patterns of hospice care—The RN role. *The Hospice Journal, 2*(1), 37–61.

Cassem, N. H., & Hackett, T. P. (1972). Sources of tension for the CCU nurse. *American Journal of Nursing, 72,* 1426–1430.

Cleland, V. S. (1965). The effect of stress on performance. *Nursing Research, 14,* 292–298.

Cox, A., & Andrews, P. (1981). The development of support systems on oncology units. *Oncology Nursing Forum, 8*(3), 31–35.

Cronin-Stubbs, D., & Rooks, C. A. (1985). The stress, social support, and burnout of critical care nurses: The results of research. *Heart and Lung, 14,* 31–39.

Craytor, J. K., Brown, J. K., & Morrow, G. R. (1978). Assessing learning needs of nurses who care for persons with cancer. *Cancer Nursing, 1,* 211–220.

Craytor, J. K., & Fass, M. L. (1982). Changing nurses' perceptions of cancer and cancer care. *Cancer Nursing, 5,* 43–49.

Dodd, M. J. (1982). Cancer patients' knowledge of chemotherapy: Assessment and informational interventions. *Oncology Nursing Forum, 9*(3), 39–44.

Dodd, M. J. (1984a). Patterns of self care in cancer patients receiving radiation therapy. *Oncology Nursing Forum, 11*(3), 23–27.

Dodd, M. J. (1984b). Self-care for patients with breast cancer to prevent side effects of chemotherapy: A concern for public health nursing. *Public Health Nursing, 1,* 202–209.

Donovan, M. I. (1981). Stress at work: Cancer nurses report. *Oncology Nursing Forum, 8*(2), 22–25.

Esteban, A., Ballesteros, P., & Caballero, J. (1983). Psychological evaluation of intensive care nurses. *Critical Care Medicine, 11,* 616–620.

Fanslow, J. (1985). Attitudes of nurses toward cancer and cancer therapies. *Oncology Nursing Forum, 12*(1), 43–47.

Fawsey, F. I., Wellisch, D. K., Pasnau, R. O., & Leibowitz, B. (1983). Preventing nursing burnout: A challenge for liaison psychiatry. *General Hospital Psychiatry, 5,* 141–149.

Gentry, W. D., Foster, S. B., & Froehling, S. (1972). Psychologic response to situational stress in intensive and nonintensive nursing. *Heart and Lung, 1,* 793–796.

Harrison, R. V. (1978). Person-environment fit and job stress. In C. L. Cooper & R. Payne (Eds.), *Stress at work* (pp. 175–205). New York: John Wiley & Sons.

Holsclaw, P. A. (1965). Nursing in high emotional risk areas. *Nursing Forum, 4*(4), 36–35.

Holt, R. R. (1982). Occupational stress. In L. Goldberger & S. Breznitz (Eds.), *Handbook of stress. Theoretical and clinical aspects* (pp. 419–444). New York: The Free Press.

Huckabay, L. M. D., & Jagla, B. (1979). Nurses' stress factors in the intensive care unit. *Journal of Nursing Administration, 9*(2), 21–26.

Ivancevich, J. M., & Matteson, M. T. (1980). Nurses and stress: Time to examine the potential problem. *Supervisor Nurse, 11*(6), 17–22.

Jacobson, S. P. (1978). Stressful situations for neonatal intensive care nurses. *Maternal Child Nursing Journal, 3,* 144–150.

Jenkins, J. F., & Ostchega, Y. (1986). Evaluation of burnout in oncology nurses. *Cancer Nursing, 9,* 108–116.

Jennings, B. M. (1987). *Stress, social support, and locus of control: Effects on head nurses' mental health.* Unpublished doctoral dissertation, University of California, San Francisco.

Jones, E. M. (1962). Who supports the nurse? *Nursing Outlook, 10,* 476–478.

Jones, L. S. (1981). I. A scattered-bed model for cancer inpatient care. [Organizing cancer inpatient care: Scattered-bed versus oncology unit approach]. *Oncology Nursing Forum, 8*(1), 31–34.

Keane, A., DuCette, J., & Adler, D. C. (1985). Stress in ICU and non-ICU nurses. *Nursing Research, 34,* 231–236.

Kelly, J. G., & Cross, D. G. (1985). Stress, coping behaviors, and recommendations for intensive care and medical surgical ward registered nurses. *Research in Nursing and Health, 8,* 321–328.

Koocher, G. P. (1979). Adjustment and coping strategies among the caretakers of cancer patients. *Social Work in Health, 5*(2), 145–150.

Kornfeld, D. S., Maxwell, T., & Momrow, D. (1968). Psychological hazards of the intensive care unit. *Nursing Clinics of North America, 3,* 41–51.

Koumans, A. J. R. (1965). Psychiatric consultation in an intensive care unit. *Journal of the American Medical Association, 194,* 633–637.

Larson, P. J. (1984). Important nurse caring behaviors perceived by patients with cancer. *Oncology Nursing Forum, 11*(6), 46–50.

Larson, P. J. (1986). Cancer nurses' perceptions of caring. *Cancer Nursing, 9,* 86–91.

Larson, P. J. (1987, May). *Patients and nursing stress: The paradox of cancer nursing.* Paper presented at the Twelfth Annual Congress, Oncology Nursing Society, Denver, CO.

Lazarus, R. S., & Launier, R. (1978). Stress-related transactions between person and environment. In L. A. Pervin & M. Lewis (Eds.), *Perspectives in interactional psychology* (pp. 287–327). New York: Plenum.

Lovejoy, N. (1986). Family responses to cancer hospitalizations. *Oncology Nursing Forum, 13*(2), 33–37.

Maloney, J. P. (1982). Job stress and its consequences on a group of intensive care and nonintensive care nurses. *Advances in Nursing Science, 4*(2), 31–42.

Maloney, J. P., & Bartz, C. (1983). Stress-tolerant people: Intensive care nurses compared with non-intensive care nurses. *Heart and Lung, 12,* 389–394.

Maslach, C., & Jackson, S. E. (1986). The Maslach Burnout Inventory (2nd ed). Palo Alto, CA: Consulting Psychologists Press.

Mason, J. W. (1975). A historical view of the stress filled. Part I. *Journal of Human Stress, 1*(1), 6–12.

Mayer, D. K. (1987). Oncology nurses' versus cancer patients' perceptions of nurse caring behavior: A replication study. *Oncology Nursing Forum, 14*(3), 48–52.

McElroy, A. M. (1982). Burnout—A review of the literature with application to cancer nursing. *Cancer Nursing, 5,* 211–217.

Menzies, I. E. P. (1960). Nurses under stress. *International Nursing Review, 7,* 9–16.

Michaels, D. R. (1971). Too much in need of support to give any? *American Journal of Nursing, 71,* 1932–1935.

Miller, N. J., & Wegman, J. A. (1981). II. The specialty unit approach to cancer care. [Organizing cancer inpatient care: Scattered-bed versus oncology unit approach]. *Oncology Nursing Forum, 8*(1), 35–37.

Mohl, P. C., Denny, N. R., Mote, T. A., & Coldwater, C. (1982). Hospital unit stressors that affect nurses: Primary task vs. social factors. *Psychosomatics, 23,* 366–374.

Newlin, N. J., & Wellisch, D. K. (1978). The oncology nurse: Life on an emotional roller coaster. *Cancer Nursing, 1,* 447–449.

Nichols, K. A., Springford, V., & Searle, J. (1981). An investigation of distress and discontent in various types of nursing. *Journal of Advanced Nursing, 6,* 311–318.

Norbeck, J. S. (1985). Perceived job stress, job satisfaction, and psychological symptoms in critical care nursing. *Research in Nursing and Health, 8,* 253–259.

Numerof, R. E., & Abrams, M. N. (1984). Sources of stress among nurses: An empirical investigation. *Journal of Human Stress, 10*(2), 88–100.

Ogle, M. E. (1983). Stages of burnout among oncology nurses in the hospital setting. *Oncology Nursing Forum, 10*(1), 31–34.

Olsen, M. (1977). OR nurses perception of stress. *AORN Journal, 25,* 43–48.

Oskins, S. L. (1979). Identification of situational stressors and coping methods by intensive care nurses. *Heart and Lung, 8,* 953–960.

Pelletier, K. (1984). *Healthy people in unhealthy places.* New York: Delacorte.

Peteet, J. R., Murray-Ross, D., Medeiros, C., Walsh-Burke, K., Riekeo, P., & Finkelstein, D. (1989). Job stress and satisfaction among the staff members at a cancer center. *Cancer, 64,* 975–982.

Rich, V. L., & Rich, A. R. (1987). Personality hardiness and burnout in female staff nurses. *Image, 19,* 63–66.

Robinson, A. M. (1972). Intensive care today—and tomorrow: A summing-up. *RN, 35*(9), 56–60.

Schoenberg, B., & Senescu, R. A. (1970). The patient's reaction to fatal illness. In B. Schoenberg, A. C. Carr, D. Peretz, & A. H. Kutscher (Eds.), *Loss and grief: Psychological management in medical practice.* New York: Columbia University Press.

Stewart, B. E., Meyerowitz, B. E., Jackson, L. E., Yarkin, K. L., & Harvey, J. H. (1982). Psychological stress associated with outpatient oncology nursing. *Cancer Nursing, 5,* 383–387.

Stillman, M. J. (1977). Women's health beliefs about breast cancer and breast self-examination. *Nursing Research, 26,* 121–127.

Stockton, M. V. (1986). Who's taking care of you? *Caring, 5*(10), 60–63.

Stone, G. L., Jebsen, P., Walk, P., & Belsham, R. (1984). Identification of stress and coping skills within a critical care setting. *Western Journal of Nursing, 6,* 201–211.

Strauss, A. (1968). The intensive care unit: Its characteristics and social relationships. *Nursing Clinics of North America, 3,* 7–15.

Styles, M. M. (1982). *On nursing. Toward a new endowment.* St. Louis: C. V. Mosby Co.

Sutterley, D. (1979). Stress and health: A survey of self-regulation modalities. *Topics in Clinical Nursing, 1*(1), 1–21.

Tillman, M. C. (1984). A comparison of nursing care requirements of patients on general medical-surgical units and on an oncology unit in a community hospital. *Oncology Nursing Forum, 11*(4), 42–45.

Trygstad, L. (1986). Professional friends. The inclusion of the personal into the professional. *Cancer Nursing, 9,* 326–332.

Vachon, M. L. S. (1986). Myths and realities in palliative/hospice care. *The Hospice Journal 2*(1), 63–79.

Vincent, P., & Coleman, W. F. (1986). Comparison of major stressors perceived by ICU and non-ICU nurses. *Critical Care Nurse, 6*(1), 64–69.

Vreeland, R., & Ellis, G. L. (1968). Stresses on the nurse in the intensive-care unit. *Journal of the American Medical Association, 208,* 332–334.

Whelan, J. (1984). Oncology nurses' attitudes toward cancer treatment and survival. *Cancer Nursing, 7,* 375–383.

Wolf, Z. R. (1986). Nurses' work: The sacred and the profane. *Holistic Nursing Practice, 1*(1), 29–35.

Yancik, R. (1984). Sources of work stress for hospice staff. *Journal of Psychosocial Oncology, 2*(1), 21–31.

Yasko, J. M. (1983). Variables which predict burnout experienced by oncology clinical nurse specialists. *Cancer Nursing, 6,* 109–116.

CHAPTER 76

Caring for the Caregiver: A Person-Centered Framework

MARY L. S. VACHON
STANLEY K. STYLIANOS

The care of persons with cancer confronts nurses with conflicting demands. Nurses are expected to be expert at the technologic aspects of caregiving aimed at cure yet must also convey the warmth and nurturing associated with "caring." They must be prepared to get involved but not too involved. They should be research-minded while remaining vigilant about clinical issues and the individuality of those in their care. They should be good team members yet ready to serve as patient advocates. They should be attentive to their own needs but willing to work an assigned time schedule and to conform to the norms of their work environment.

Oncology nurses work with a large number of people, some of whom they come to care for deeply over extended periods of treatment and follow-up. Despite treatment advances, many of these people will die, and these nurses will have to deal with grief, perhaps in a system that does not acknowledge that such feelings should exist or be problematic. Oncology settings are not necessarily "arid" or "malevolent climates" but may become so when they give rise to more threat than challenge and more stress than nourishment. How then does the nurse care for herself or himself in such environments?

Coping with stress in cancer nursing can be examined using a variety of different approaches that focus on the person, the environment, or both. Although managers of work environments in an ideal world have a responsibility to attend to employees' needs, the onus is often on the individual to be self-sustaining. At times the nurse may feel that he or she is fighting an uphill battle while trying to meet patient needs or existing in isolation, with little personal or professional support forthcoming from others in the work environment.

Recognizing that the individual does not always have the power to change the environment, the focus in this chapter is on some of the individual's inner resources and on finding some ways to cope and effectively survive in potentially difficult settings and situations. The chapter addresses issues such as appraisal of self, interaction with others, and involvement within the work environment to provide a means of enhancing personal satisfaction and professional efficacy. The chapter presents a preliminary framework that oncology nurses can use to evaluate their own coping efforts.

The perspective of the chapter is a person-centered approach derived from the person–environment fit model, coping theory, and interpersonal theory. Within this framework, stress and nourishment in the workplace derive from one's subjective evaluation of person-environment transactions. Individuals are viewed as being involved in ongoing, reciprocal interactions with the environments in which they are employed. Such environments are viewed as being interpersonal rather than simply being physical spaces in which person-environment transactions take place. In other words, one's sense of job satisfaction comes in part from being with others in the environment rather than simply from the physical environment; yet both can be important. If one enters into the workplace and no one acknowledges his or her presence, one can begin to feel like a nonperson or just another "cog in the wheel," even if the environment is quite pleasant. However, although colleagues may make one feel welcome in the work environment, the person may have great distress if there are not enough rubber gloves provided to give effective care to the persons with acquired immune deficiency syndrome (AIDS) with whom one will be working.

PERSON-ENVIRONMENT FIT

The person–environment fit model was developed by French, Rodgers, and Cobb (1974) to provide a quantitative measure of coping and environmental adaptation. The underlying principle of this model is that adaptation is a function of the "goodness of fit" between the characteristics of the person and the characteristics of work environment. "Fit" is assessed in terms of the mesh between the needs of the individual and the supplies or resources available within the environment, the abilities of the individual and the demands made by the work environment, or both. In part, fit is determined by the extent to which environmental supplies are available to meet individual needs and values; it is also determined by the ability of the person to manage the demands imposed by the environment (French, et al., 1974). For example, the new graduate may require a work environment in which mentors are readily available to help the nurse deal with difficult situations. If such a nurse is put into a situation in which he or she is expected to care for large numbers of very sick individuals and to make major decisions soon after starting a new job, the demands of the environment may well exceed the person's resources to perform the expected role.

Job satisfaction and occupational stress are the result of a dynamic interaction between the person holding a particular job and the environment in which he or she is employed (Rook, 1984). As noted by Harrison (1979, p. 178) "a job is stressful to the extent that it does not provide supplies to meet the individual's motives and to the extent that the ability of the individual falls below the demands of the job which are prerequisite to receiving supplies." Whether a poor person-environment fit is judged to be a consequence of a misfit between needs and supplies or demands and abilities is determined in part by the appraiser's perspective (Caplan, 1983). For example, the nurse in the aforementioned anecdote may decide that he or she is at fault for being unable to perform in the expected role. The nurse may feel inadequate, poorly educated, and incompetent to perform in the role of a professional nurse or, alternatively, the nurse may decide that the organization has completely unrealistic expectations of a new graduate and the fault is with the organization.

In assessing one's own goodness of fit within the work environment, it is important to be able to assess both self and work environment. Individuals need to have an accurate understanding of their own personal resources, values, and limitations as well as the resources available within the environment to meet their needs and to facilitate their being able to perform in their professional role. Although such assessments are apt to be subjective, with some experience the individual can develop the ability to judge the situation with some objectivity. It is worth noting, however, that there is some evidence that the individual's subjective assessment of both self and environment is more closely related to the occurrence of psychological and physical illness or well-being (Caplan, 1983).

STRESS, COPING, AND ADAPTATION

Stress has been defined in many ways. Antonovsky (1979) sees stress as evolving from exposure to stressors, which he differentiates from routine stimuli, and defines as being a demand made by the internal or external environment of the organism that upsets its homeostasis, restoration of which depends on a nonautomatic and not readily available energy-expending action. A routine stimuli may become a stressor under certain circumstances. It is not always possible to determine when and why this is happening. It must also be noted that one person's stressor may be another person's routine stimuli. Whether a given situation is perceived as being a stressor is dependent on the meaning of that stimulus to the person at that point in time and on the person's repertoire of coping mechanisms that are readily available.

Protection and enhancement of the self are considered basic to human functioning; mastery, the sense of being in control, and self-esteem, the assessment of one's worth, are resources that contribute strongly to the maintenance of one's identity (Pearlin, Lieberman, Menaghan, & Mullin, 1981; Pearlin & Schooler, 1978). The threat of a breakdown of one's sense of mastery and self-esteem may represent a common pathway to experiencing events as stressful.

Psychological distress derives from environmental circumstances that are perceived as threatening to self-esteem, personal effectiveness, or identity (Lazarus & Folkman, 1984; Pearlin, et al., 1981; Pearlin & Schooler, 1978). As noted by Lazarus and Folkman (1984, p. 19), psychological stress involves a relationship that occurs between the person and the environment that is "appraised by the person as taxing or exceeding his or her resources and endangering his or her well-being . . . appraisal is an evaluative process that determines why and to what extent a particular transaction or series of transactions between the person and environment are stressful."

The evaluation of transactions is accomplished through primary and secondary cognitive appraisal processes (Lazarus & Folkman, 1984). Through primary appraisal, events may be assessed as being irrelevant or benign with respect to well-being or as being potentially stressful, engendering loss, threat, or challenge to self. This process may involve an appraisal of damage or loss that has already been sustained. It may also entail the assessment of potential loss or threat and growth opportunities or challenge. Threat and challenge may be appraised concurrently and are not mutually exclusive. Both psychological and material coping resources are assessed through secondary appraisal. The evaluation of situational demands relative to a sense of control or "efficacy expectancy" are fundamental to this process (Folkman, 1984).

Appraisal processes are guided by commitment and belief (Lazarus & Folkman, 1984). Commitment represents the extent to which individuals are dedicated to particular choices, values, or goals and the extent to which they are invested in either their maintenance or achievement. Belief is defined through personal experience and cultural expectation and encompasses the preconceived "facts" about the environment. Commitments determine whether an individual will approach or avoid situations that are potentially stressful or challenging. Moreover, they influence a person's vigilance or attentiveness to particular aspects of the environment. Paradoxically, commitments can affect an appraisal so as both to enhance vulnerability to stress and to reduce threat (Lazarus & Folkman, 1984). Preoccupation with a prized goal can heighten sensitivity to environmental cues associated with a desired outcome, increasing the perception of threat. In contrast, strong commitments to valued principles or goals can facilitate effective coping, encouraging one to push forward in the face of adversity.

Beliefs about control and mastery are particularly influential in appraisal processes (Folkman, 1984; Lazarus & Folkman, 1984). The sense of being in control, as either a global or situation-specific perception, is related to outcome in stressful transactions; however, believing that one is in control can, in certain instances, augment feelings of threat (Folkman, 1984; Lazarus & Folkman, 1984). Thus secondary appraisals of stressful events as controllable do not always correlate positively with favorable outcomes. The relationship of control beliefs to evaluations of stressors as either challenging or threatening depends partly on the meaning of specific situations. It also depends on the ability of the individual to determine accurately the controllability of events in light of coping resources.

Antonovsky's (1979) sense of coherence contrasts with a sense of control. Coherence emphasizes the importance of predictability in both internal and external environments, coupled with the likelihood of things working out as well as can be expected. Antonovsky distinguishes between a sense of coherence and being in control, observing that coherence suggests that one has the ability to shape one's destiny, not that one is in control.

Coping comprises both behavioral and cognitive strategies aimed at managing the internal and external demands of stressful transactions (Lazarus & Folkman, 1984). These efforts, directed toward mastering, reducing, or tolerating demands, may be problem-focused or emotion-focused. Problem-focused mechanisms target the environment or self for direct intervention, whereas emotion-focused strategies target negative feelings arising from stressful episodes.

COPING AND INTERPERSONAL PROCESSES

Plas, Hoover-Dempsey, and Wallston (1985) have developed a conceptual framework that provides an overview of person-environment transactions. Their framework defines the environment as an "interpersonal field" in which stress and nourishment are the result of interactions with "support persons," "reference persons," and "persons-to-be-reckoned-with."

Support persons are identified as individuals who provide affective or instrumental aid. Reference per-

sons serve as a basis for personal and professional comparison; areas for personal comparison include interpersonal skills, personality, physical appearance, and life style, and professional reference items include competence, status, productivity, and professional style. Persons-to-be-reckoned-with are individuals who control needed resources and with whom one maintains obligatory, rather than voluntary, relationships.

Interpersonal theory is implicit in this model, which draws heavily on the work of Lewin (1935). As summarized by Kiesler (1982), interpersonal formulations emphasize that a sense of self derives primarily from social and interpersonal transactions as opposed to intrapsychic processes. Individuals develop recurrent patterns of interacting over time, and their social behaviors are a function of particular response predispositions, acting in concert with specific events. Situational factors of relevance to a person's behavior need to be subjectively appraised. Social exchanges between individuals are characterized as two-way interactions because participants in an interaction are both the causes and effects of each other's behavior. The framework of Plas and colleagues is noteworthy in its emphasis on the person-centered dimensions of environmental adaptation; in this context, stress and nourishment are the result of subjectively appraised person-environment transactions. Moreover, exchanges between the individual and his or her environment are largely interpersonal in nature; simply stated, the environment is made up of people who are simultaneously affecting and being affected by each other. The quality of both voluntary and obligatory relationships, as perceived by the individual, strongly contributes to individual adaptation in the work environment. The perspective of this chapter is that the individual is central to an understanding of work stressors and the coping process.

Ideally, the individual comes into the work situation with a well-established sense of self-esteem and self-efficacy, evolved through earlier life experiences. Interaction with others in the work environment should provide the requisite support and resources to define and carry out the nursing role effectively. If this "interpersonal space" is insufficiently supportive, or if access to resources is blocked, individual strategies should be available to reduce stressors directly or to elicit the support necessary to aid in coping.

COPING WITH STRESS IN ONCOLOGY

In a study of 581 professionals caring for the critically ill, dying, and bereaved, Vachon (1987a) found that caregivers were more apt to mention using personal coping mechanisms rather than using environmental coping mechanisms. The group as a whole was twice as likely to report personal coping strategies rather than environmental strategies as being helpful in dealing with and preventing occupational stress.

Personal Coping Strategies

On the basis of the findings of a subsample of 110 professionals in oncology who were part of the larger study previously cited, the most helpful personal coping strategies included developing a sense of competence, control, and pleasure from one's work; having control over aspects of one's practice; having a personal philosophy of illness, death, and one's professional role; managing one's life-style; and leaving the work situation.

Competence, Control, and Pleasure from One's Work

A sense of competence, control, and pleasure from one's work was the major coping strategy for the entire group as well as the major personal coping mechanism of those in oncology. In oncology this coping strategy involves coming to terms with the fact that one cannot control illness or death. Caregivers who have a sense of coherence come to believe that although they may not always succeed in saving people's lives, they have performed well both professionally and personally if they have done "as well as can be expected, given the circumstances" and if the person has had "a good enough" illness experience or death.

According to Antonovsky (1979) the sense of coherence is associated with the belief that power is appropriately vested in those who are capable of handling difficulties that might arise in the environment. Stress may be experienced if nurses believe that those in authority do not know what they are doing or are incapable of making important decisions.

The sense of competence, control, and pleasure in work was often associated with a sense of belonging to a team "that knew what it was doing." Through team affiliation one may derive an ongoing sense of personal worth that survives even though individual patients die. For caregivers who may not receive the validation they need through teamwork in their particular organization, the sense of belonging that may be associated with being a member of a professional interest group, such as the Oncology Nursing Society or the Canadian Association of Nurses in Oncology, may be very helpful.

The sense of competence was found to evolve through a series of stages that appeared to develop over time rather than being felt as soon as one graduated from a professional education program. Caregivers reported that they initially developed professional skills, learned to set goals for themselves, and had frequent tests of their competence. Once assured of a sense of competence through ongoing professional experiences, they could then share their expertise with others and bolster feelings of security in the work environment (Vachon, 1987a).

A sense of control was derived through secondary appraisal processes, including redefining particular situations as being a challenge instead of a threat, redefining one's role and involvement with people (e.g., "It is not my role to save people from their illness, rather it is my role to help people to lift the burden that is theirs"), developing more complex skills, and sharing decision making and control with patients.

A sense of pleasure in one's work evolved ". . . from one's work with individual patients, from pleasure in the utilization of professional skills, or satisfaction with the indirect impact that one's work can have on groups of patients and families that one might influence indirectly through teaching or administrative roles" (Vachon, 1987a, p. 188). Caregivers reported allowing themselves to feel pleasure at a job well done. This approach requires a certain maturity as well as an ability to distance oneself from the pain of others and to derive satisfaction objectively from one's role in helping to alleviate at least some of this suffering. Some caregivers have difficulty in distancing in this way and feel guilty if they experience a sense of satisfaction that is associated with the suffering of others.

Weisman (1981) speaks of the caregiver's tendency to identify with the patient's predicament. He notes that understanding the cancer patient involves being able to differentiate among the protocol (the treatment of the tumor), the plight of the patient (the nonmedical implications and ramifications of the disease), and the promise (the caregiver's view of the patient's predicament). He warns that caregivers can sometimes become more upset about the plight of their patients than the patients themselves. This may lead to a progressive demoralization and loss of self-esteem.

Weisman recommends that caregivers learn how to cope better with their own needs and know enough not to get caught in the subtle promises that are often made that "if only you take your treatment the way we prescribe, meditate on your white blood cells knocking out your cancer, and change your life style, all will be fine." He also recommends learning how to share one's concerns with colleagues, attempting to make a series of small contributions toward a patient's welfare rather than trying to be all things to all people. The ability to maintain realistic goals with the patients with whom one works allows caregivers to continue to experience pleasure even during many years of work in the field.

Caregivers also experienced pleasure when patients or families expressed their gratitude. Many took pleasure in keeping close at hand the letters or gifts patients had given them to express their appreciation (Vachon, 1987a). In a study of social workers, Davidson (1985) reported that patient responsiveness to help was a critical factor in the worker's experiencing satisfaction. In a qualitative study of 17 oncology nurses, Trygstad (1986) found that all nurses studied valued their relationships with patients (Box 76–1). Moreover, those who worked in settings with which they were dissatisfied found that their relationships with patients provided almost a refuge from an otherwise unrewarding job.

Control Over Aspects of One's Practice

This problem-focused coping strategy entailed setting limits on some aspect of one's practice and organizing work to give one a sense of personal satisfaction. For some this task was accomplished through the

---

Box 76–1. A QUALITATIVE STUDY OF 17 ONCOLOGY NURSES ASSESSED WORK EXPERIENCES AND WORK SATISFACTION

Although the work of oncology nurses is physically and emotionally demanding, this may not be perceived as the focus of oncology work by the nurses themselves. In a field study, 17 oncology nurses described a shift in work focus and redefinition of goals from quantitative progress to qualitative care. This created a new environment for nurse–patient interaction, in which the nurse perceived that nurse and patient were working together toward shared goals. The nurse's caring for the patient and family was a caring or connectedness with dimensions beyond that usually found in nursing work. The relationship remained professional but also went beyond that. These oncology nurses discussed the caring relationship aspect of their work and often called their work "real nursing." Those nurses who described the greatest overall satisfaction with their work also described a work environment that supported independence and was nourishing to the nurse. For those unhappy with their work setting, satisfaction with the nurse-patient relationship seemed as refuge from an otherwise unrewarding job. What these nurses seemed to receive from the nurse–patient exchange was a perception of self as a good person being a good nurse contributing to a worthwhile endeavor. The focus for these nurses was on having gained on two levels, that is, professional and personal. The impact from these two levels seemed to combine to have a positive impact on the nurses' lives extending beyond the work world.

(Trygstad, L. [1986]. Professional friends: The inclusion of the personal into the professional. *Cancer Nursing, 9,* 326–332.)

---

development of multiple roles that could bring special "treats" or rewards into one's practice. Oncology nurses have often developed multiple roles in the areas of clinical work, education, and research. Others have enriched their practice by participating in such diverse activities as running self-help groups, becoming involved with the American or Canadian Cancer Society, conducting cost-effectiveness studies of their roles, joining local or national oncology nursing organizations, becoming involved in decision making regarding the use of drugs and equipment, and writing brochures for their own patients. Such activities provide caregivers with opportunities for the enhancement of professional worth and effectiveness.

A Personal Philosophy

Although having a sense of competence, control, and pleasure from one's work and developing control over one's practice were seen to be important, the caregiver who is going to stay in the field for an extended period of time often feels the need for something "beyond" the present role. A personal philosophy of illness, death, and professional role was an important coping mechanism for many.

A personal philosophy takes considerable time and thought to develop. A philosophy that is helpful has been articulated by Weisman who said that when he sent young medical students to interview dying patients and they expressed their hesitancy to do so, he told them, "When you go to see these people don't feel guilty that they are dying and you are living. Remember, your time will come, and it may be sooner than you think. As you speak to these people ask yourself, 'What can I do now when it's not my turn that I hope someone else will do tomorrow when it may be' " (Vachon, 1987a, p. 195).

For some, a religious philosophy, centered around a commitment to serve others, may be both helpful and key to deriving a sense of meaning in difficult times. It may also be useful to assume the perspective that "it's not my fault that this person has the disease, but my responsibility is to do what I can to help to lift the burden." Consistent with this view, decision making is a shared responsibility. By participating in a collaborative relationship, caregivers can enable patients to heighten their sense of control through increased self-awareness and understanding of the disease process and treatment. This type of philosophy acknowledges what Martocchio (1987) refers to as authenticity, avoiding the paternalism that Gadow (1980, 1986) warns may be latent in all professionalism.

Inherent in a philosophy of practice is the right, and indeed obligation, to mourn for those who have died. Although not all patients will touch caregivers equally, in many situations patient deaths deserve recognition. Acknowledging the deaths of individual patients can enable practitioners to avoid the accumulation of grief that comes from repeated, unresolved losses (Mount, 1986). In addition, participating in a grief process can enable caregivers to assess gains that have been made, in a manner that may be helpful to future clinical practice (Vachon, 1986).

Life-Style Management

Although life-style management is certainly not a panacea for dealing with work stress, it enables one to have the energy to cope with stressors. It reflects an acknowledgment of an individual's need to learn his or her own body's response to stress to detect signals of significant overload. When one finds oneself experiencing symptoms of stress, such as headaches, gastric disturbances, increased infections, lack of pleasure in one's professional roles and responsibilities, or feeling overwhelmed by responsibilities, it is often time to take a break, before one develops more serious symptoms. This break may be a few hours away from one's desk to pursue another interest or a longer break of a few days or weeks.

Effective life-style management involves developing a balance between one's personal and professional lives. This can be very difficult, particularly for those who have developed multiple professional roles, such as clinician, researcher, and writer, while trying to maintain a healthy personal life. One technique for managing such role conflicts can be to use the "10-year rule." Ask yourself: "Ten years from now, which will matter more, that this article was a few days or weeks late or that I consistently sacrificed myself or members of my personal network for career goals, many of which may have been imposed by others?" Certainly there are times when career demands must take precedence, but if one always bows to career demands at personal sacrifice, one may need to do some looking at one's sense of self-esteem. Ask yourself: "Is my career more important to me than my own life?" For some people the answer is yes.

A physician spoke of being called in to see a dying patient in the middle of the night. As he was leaving at 4:00 A.M., a colleague was arriving for work. This overweight, diabetic physician was munching a chocolate bar. He had come to work to finish an article. The physician said to his colleague, "Are you crazy? You are going to kill yourself carrying on like this!"

His colleague's response was, "I'd rather be dead at 40 with 100 articles published than alive at 60 with only 40 articles to my name."

Practical care for one's body should be well understood by nurses but is often ignored. Despite shift rotations, it is necessary to maintain a healthful diet and obtain adequate amounts of sleep and exercise. Mount and Voyer (1980) have suggested several approaches to decreasing difficulty with shift rotation, including arranging important activities in their normal peak hours and using alcohol and food sparingly during the first 3 days of a new schedule. The use of alcohol, tranquilizers, and hypnotics should be monitored carefully because these agents are known to decrease rapid eye movement sleep and increase the risk of psychological disturbance.

"Decompression activities" can also aid in life-style management. This might consist of listening to music in the car, walking home, playing squash, or talking informally with colleagues before leaving work. The purpose of decompression activities is to establish a break between work and personal worlds.

Leaving the Work Situation

Vachon (1987a) has noted that many caregivers coped with persistent occupational stressors by leaving the workplace permanently. The turnover of newly hired nurses is estimated to be as high as 30 per cent. It has been suggested that the problem of turnover lies not in the motivation or characteristics of individual nurses but in the nature of hospital nursing jobs and incentive structures (Sanford, 1987).

Orsolits (1984) conducted a large study of oncology nurses who belonged to the Oncology Nursing Society. In contrast to published findings on nursing staff turnover, more than 80 per cent of those surveyed reported a high degree of decision making in the bureaucratic work settings in which they worked. Furthermore, 50 per cent intended to stay in their present position for the near future. The fact that these cancer nurses participated in decision making and did not intend to leave their present positions was again in contrast to published findings of staff turnover.

Orsolits's study sample had a larger proportion of subjects holding a bachelor's degree or higher and an unusually low rate of job change compared with subjects of other published studies. She suggests that the sample might differ from a random sample of nurses because cancer nursing is more highly specialized than general nursing. Moreover, her respondents were members of a professional organization, denoting a certain level of professional commitment, which may be commensurate with a high degree of assertiveness in claiming decision-making authority.

Nevertheless, Banning (1987) notes that it is not unusual for individuals to experience two or three careers in a lifetime and suggests that it is unrealistic to expect nurses to be any different. A relatively new phenomenon is for nurses to be employed continuously throughout their working years. Consistent with the view presented by Orsolits, Banning contends that hospital administrators may need to look at how to keep nurses satisfied and challenged over extended periods of time.

Environmental Coping Strategies

Although personal coping mechanisms are important, the work environment does have a role to play in helping caregivers provide effective care to those with cancer. The most important environmental coping strategy included in the top five was a sense of team philosophy, support, and team building (Vachon, 1987a). Although interpersonal transactions may be seen to engender negative as well as positive consequences (Rook, 1984), the development and maintenance of a supportive network is essential to assisting in the coping process. Within the work environment, the development of supportive, collaborative relationships may be fundamental to an enhancement of self-efficacy and self-esteem.

Pines, Aronson, and Kafry (1981) note that it is not sufficient for caregivers to have support from only members of their personal support system. They stress the need for support from professional colleagues who understand one's professional role and are thus able to provide technical support as well as technical challenge. In addition, nurses need resource people who share the social reality of the workplace. Such resource persons may be colleagues at work. Some nurses have also found it helpful to develop support networks of oncology nurses outside of their own work environment. These are colleagues who can share the reality of what it is like to be an oncology nurse while providing an outsider's perspective on how one might make the changes necessary in one's own work environment.

Team Relationships

In many ways, the interaction among team members can be seen as similar to exchanges among family members; each can be a source of great satisfaction or a major source of stress and pain (Vachon, 1987b). Although team building presupposes trust, trust may be difficult to cultivate in the context of intradisciplinary rivalries, interdisciplinary rivalries, or both (Mount & Voyer, 1980). In a study of social workers, however, Davidson (1985) found that the most important source of social support was their relationships with other staff in the hospital. Specific social work support groups and peer supervision did not provide the support that interaction with those from other disciplines did. Almost two thirds of the social workers studied reported that they frequently held discussions with colleagues from other disciplines. Other studies have also found that team relationships are a major source of support and that they enhance one's sense of self-esteem (Vachon, 1987b).

However, caregivers reported difficulty in the areas of developing trust within an interdisciplinary team, communicating information, dealing with power struggles, handling conflict, and ensuring team longevity (Vachon, 1987a). Some of these stressors are directly related to the perception of threat to self-esteem, personal effectiveness, and professional identity. For example, a nurse asked, "What do I do in a situation in which I have a good sense of self-esteem and make a suggestion to a physician who chooses to ignore me or to criticize the suggestions I make? You can take just so much of this before your sense of self-esteem begins to diminish."

With a good sense of self-esteem, one can attempt to clarify a contentious issue by consulting directly either with the physician involved or with co-workers. The latter approach can enable caregivers to identify coping strategies found helpful by others in similar situations. It can also provide insight into an individual's coping style. For example, was one being quite aggressive, defensive, or critical? Did one present the idea at an inappropriate time, for example, when the physician felt threatened because he or she was with colleagues or insecure because of uncertainty about how to proceed? Was one presenting the suggestion to someone thought to be a "support person," whose response was seen to be hurtful instead of comforting as expected? Was this person seen as a "reference person" whom the caregiver always respected and admired, and does the caregiver fear this person's censure? Or was this seen to be a "person-to-be-reckoned-with," who may now use this latest episode to discredit the caregiver in the eyes of colleagues?

Having developed some insight into the problem, a caregiver with good self-esteem can then decide how to handle this particular situation or to avoid such problems in the future. In the face of poor self-esteem, however, one may incorrectly assume responsibility for interpersonal problems and be prompted toward further self-denigration. Yet, even with a good sense of self-esteem, the presence of chronic team conflict or constant exposure to situations that threaten one's sense of competence or professional identity may seriously diminish one's sense of self-worth and self-efficacy, providing strong evidence of one's powerlessness to alter events (Pearlin, et al., 1981).

Schmalenberg and Kramer (1979) found that newly graduated nurses suffered an erosion of self-esteem if they felt incompetent in their new roles and received negative input from fellow staff members. Shaffer (1982, p. 153) has observed that "when people are happy and enjoy working together, the positive emotional climate generated by their interaction makes work pleasurable and satisfying. On the other hand, if there is an air of tension on the job, people sense it and begin to reflect that tension in their work or in their relationships with co-workers." Nason (1981) notes that team development always involves tension and conflict. This may be viewed as the result of competition, lack of role definition, or poor leadership, but it can also be viewed as a reflection of contradictory institutional goals. Team members may become entrapped in conflicting relationships through the interaction of limited resources, competing demands, and unrealistic institutional priorities and, as a consequence, come to represent differing value systems within the organization. For example, nurses and physicians may battle with one another about resource allocation when this issue is one about which their respective department heads are locked in combat.

In addition, team members may find themselves acting out the unconscious problems of patients or their families. For example, the senior author of this chapter has treated a number of women who have a diagnosis of breast cancer and whose mothers died of the same disease. The women's unresolved grief for their mothers, acting in concert with their disease, has triggered a regression in which these women became child-like and played off the "daddy" physician and the "mommy" nurse against one another. If team members are not clear on problem ownership, they can find themselves fighting one another instead of helping patients come to terms with their illness and its psychological sequelae.

Beckhard (1974) states that an effective team must have clarity of objectives, mission, and priorities that are shared by all team members. Role expectations should be realistic and well defined when they overlap. Effective decision-making and problem-solving processes should be in place to arrive at the "best" possible solution; environmental norms should exist that support the tasks of problem solving. There should be a concern for each other's needs and an opportunity for individuals to enlarge their roles and optimize their chances for personal growth.

Nason (1981) notes further that the movement from a multidisciplinary group to a well-functioning interdisciplinary team requires a means of bridging disciplines polarized by their respective frameworks so that tension and competition may be teased apart and the team refocused on patient issues.

Nurse-Nurse Collaborative Relationships

Some of the most common of the communication difficulties within the team are those that occur between nurses. Curtin and Flaherty (1986, p. 30) note that the nurse-nurse bond has been traditionally weak. They state " . . . nursing as a caring profession involves not only care for and of patients but also care for and of fellow nurses. It is on this base that the significance of the nurse–nurse relationship rests. . . . That nurses work collaboratively with members of other professions is obvious. What may be overlooked is the fact that nurses' professional interdependence demands special—even fraternal—relationships *among nurses.*" Curtin and Flaherty (1986) further suggest that one of the most effective means of promoting professional excellence and disseminating new information is for nurses to offer one another support and guidance. Failure to do so represents a breach of trust, not only with colleagues but also with patients, inasmuch as the quality of nursing care may be compromised.

In a discipline largely dominated by women, rivalry among women represents a potent barrier to relationship building among nurses. Madden (1987) notes that considerable conflict arises when women encounter other women in positions of authority. She suggests that part of this difficulty evolves from the fact that women come into the work force with a variety of motives, and these influence the ways in which women interact with one another. Many of the battles in which women engage in the work force can be seen as reflecting these conflicting motivations.

Madden notes that the concern over whether nursing is a job or a career, a profession or a technical skill, in part reflects the role conflict that nurses feel as they struggle to come to terms personally and professionally with these issues. It has been said that at an earlier stage in the profession's development some women chose to enter nursing because they saw it as a good preparation for marriage. It could be hypothesized that some nurses for whom this was true might not have married; others may have married but may feel that they are compelled by economic circumstances to work rather than having chosen to work because of the rewards inherent within the profession itself.

These nurses may have become ardent career women or may be struggling to balance personal and family commitments. These individuals may be working with other women who have always been career minded. Conflicts that ensue with regard to promotion, status, shift rotation, and paid maternity leave may reflect varying levels of professional commitment. Collaboration can be difficult when these dynamics exist. However, nurses can commit to the philosophy that all deserve the best possible care and that nurses from different belief systems can work together to achieve this end.

When conflict arises within the work situation, it is important to explore its possible sources and to develop ways of dealing with problematic issues. Lerner (1985) speaks of the dance of anger, noting that many individuals have particular patterns of expressing anger, which they tend to draw on in personal and work relationships. These response styles may be maladaptive, serving to maintain rather than resolve conflict.

When female nurses are able to overcome some of their natural reluctance to work together, their collaborative relationships can be quite effective in improving patient care and professional satisfaction. Malanka (1984) gives the example of developing a resource book of nurses and their specialties to facilitate the building of consultative relationships. This allows nurses to rely more heavily on one another rather than having to call on physicians to answer their questions. Collaborative research studies, or even books, written by nurses from a variety of settings can provide a great deal of satisfaction as well as enrichment. These projects can present a challenge that can increase self-esteem through personal accomplishment.

Interdisciplinary Collaboration

Nurses collaborate with individuals in various disciplines to ensure effective service delivery. Interdisciplinary collaboration is rife with the same communication difficulties inherent in nursing, but status issues may be particularly salient when nurses collaborate with groups that in the past have been seen to have "higher professional status." Sometimes members of the other discipline may "pull rank" around difficult decision making. However, nurses may all too readily defer to a higher status discipline or approach shared decision making with a defensive style that both anticipates and encourages rejection. Collaborative relationships have been described in the literature (Crowley & Wollner, 1987; Mioduszewski & McCray, 1985). They have been found to improve professional communication, trust, respect, and collegial relationships as well as to decrease interprofessional tensions, improve patient care, and improve staff retention and recruitment. Such collaboration, however, presupposes hospital environments that are receptive to change (Crowley & Wollner, 1987).

Education for collaborative practice has been started at various levels. Balassone (1981) describes one such program for nurse practitioner students and members of a variety of other professions. She notes the need for the students of each discipline to be able to define and defend their roles. She suggests that this requires baccalaureate preparation for nurses, undergraduate courses on ethics and philosophy for all professions that are not linked to the perspective of a particular discipline, personal attempts to articulate one's own professional position or philosophy, and interprofessional coursework beyond the level of basic clinical training.

Support Groups

Although support groups are recommended almost as a panacea for either team stress or problems with patients, they were found by Vachon (1987a) to be the least commonly mentioned organizational coping strategy. Furthermore, those using this coping strategy frequently found it ineffective. However, individuals may vary in their ability to develop supportive networks and mobilize help when confronted with stressful circumstances (Eckenrode, 1986). Moreover, Thoits's

(1986) conceptualization of social support as coping assistance is consistent with this observation because it emphasizes the role of the individual in eliciting helping behaviors in others.

Kanas (1986), in reviewing the literature on staff groups for mental-health trainees, found that the groups could be system oriented, involving team members from a particular unit who meet to solve the problems on that unit or to learn better ways of working together. They were also geared toward long-term membership, usually involving individuals from the same or similar professional backgrounds, who met to provide mutual support and to discuss ways of coping with job stress. Short-term groups that focus on the goal of providing support for job-related stress, to the relative exclusion of group process and personal issues, existed as well.

Despite differences in format, all groups have elements in common. Rosenberg (1984) states that the underlying goal in all cases is to alleviate stress through the sharing of individual experiences. Ventilation and problem solving may also occur in such groups. Typically, such groups address problems that are homogeneous in nature, involving similar classes of stressors. Moreover, participants are relatively healthy and able to share their experiences through a common, familiar language (Kanas, 1986).

SUMMARY

The framework detailed here has underscored the subjective dimensions of coping with occupational stressors in oncology. Cancer care settings are viewed most productively as interpersonal spaces, in which stress and nourishment arise through social transactions with both patients and co-workers. In part, individuals shape their work settings through personal and professional belief systems, preferred response styles, and the quality of their relationships. Coping and adaptation are processes guided by ongoing, subjective appraisals of the self in relation to the environment.

Vachon's empirical findings are compatible with a person-centered, phenomenologic perspective. Broadly among caregivers, the preferred coping strategies were personal rather than environmental and focused on bolstering feelings of competence, control, and pleasure. A sense of competence emerged gradually through repeated tests of professional effectiveness, beginning with skills acquisition and developing into global feelings of security in the work setting. A sense of control was derived largely from tasks related to occupational role definition. To an extent, this was accomplished through the development of multiple nursing roles to ensure professional rewards. A sense of control was also achieved by clearly establishing the limits of personal and professional ability and boundaries of responsibility. Control was related to Antonovsky's concept of coherence, that is, although events may not always be controllable, they are predictable. Feelings of pleasure or satisfaction in the workplace were closely intertwined with feelings of self-worth and self-efficacy.

The development of supportive and collaborative relationships within the work environment may be essential to the enhancement of self-esteem and professional effectiveness. Consistent with this view, the most important environmental coping strategy for oncology practitioners was the development of a sense of team philosophy, support, and team building.

Both intradisciplinary and interdisciplinary rivalries present formidable obstacles to team building and to the development of collegial relationships. From a historical standpoint, collaboration among nurses is poor; because nursing is a profession largely dominated by women, this difficulty may be a consequence of socialization. Encouraging cooperation within nursing and across other disciplines may require both a concerted individual effort and education specifically aimed at collaborative practice.

Support groups and supportive networks, both within and outside of the work environment, represent potentially significant but equivocal sources of coping assistance. Social support is viewed increasingly as a property of the individual, and, for this reason, general strategies for providing support are difficult to establish. The caregivers surveyed seldom reported drawing on support groups for aid in coping. However, little is understood about the ecology of naturally occurring supportive networks, and investigating these groups may provide important insights into the supportive elements of social relationships.

References

Antonovsky, A. (1979). *Health, stress and coping.* San Francisco: Jossey-Bass Publishers.

Balassone, P. D. (1981, April). Territorial issues in an interdisciplinary experience. *Nursing Outlook*, pp. 229–232.

Banning, J. A. (1987). Nursing for a lifetime? *Canadian Nurse, 83*(3), 3.

Beckhard, R. (1974). Organizational implications of team building. In H. Wise, R. Beckhard, I. Rubin, & A. L. Kyte (Eds.), *Making health teams work* (pp. 69–94). Cambridge: Ballinger.

Caplan, R. D. (1983). Person-environment fit: Past, present and future. In C. L. Cooper (Ed.), *Stress research. Issues for the eighties.* New York: John Wiley & Sons Ltd.

Crowley, S. A., & Wollner, I. S. (1987). Collaborative practice: A tool for change. *Oncology Nursing Forum, 14*(4), 59–63.

Curtin, L., & Flaherty, M. J. (1986). The nurse-nurse relationship. In R. McCorkle & G. Hongladarom (Eds.), *Issues and topics in cancer nursing* (pp. 29–40). Norwalk, CT: Appleton-Century-Crofts.

Davidson, K. W. (1985). Social work with cancer patients: Stresses and coping patterns. *Social Work in Health Care, 10*(4), 73–82.

Eckenrode, J. (1986). The mobilization of social supports: Some individual constraints. *American Journal of Community Psychology, 11*, 509–528.

Folkman, S. (1984). Personal control and stress and coping processes: A theoretical analysis. *Journal of Personality and Social Psychology, 46*, 839–852.

French, J. R. P., Rodgers, W., & Cobb, S. (1974). Adjustment as person-environment fit. In G. V. Coelho, D. A. Hamburg, & J. E. Adams (Eds.), *Coping and adaptation.* New York: Basic Books.

Gadow, S. (1980). Existential advocacy: Philosophical foundation of nursing. In S. F. Spicker & S. Gadow (Eds.), *Nursing: Images and ideals* (pp. 79–101). New York: Springer Publishing.

Gadow, S. (1986). Advocacy and paternalism in cancer nursing. In R. McCorkle & G. Hongladarom (Eds.), *Issues and topics in cancer nursing* (pp. 19–28). Norwalk, CT: Appleton-Century-Crofts.

Harrison, R. V. (1979). Person-environment fit and job stress. In C. L. Cooper & R. Payne (Eds.), *Stress at work* (pp. 175–205). Chichester: Wiley.

Hirsch, B. J., & David, T. G. (1983). Social networks and work/nonwork life: Action-research with nurse managers. *American Journal of Community Psychology, 11,* 493–507.

Holt, R. R. (1982). Occupational stress. In L. Goldberger & S. Breznitz (Eds.), *Handbook of stress. Theoretical and clinical aspects* (pp. 419–444). New York: The Free Press.

Kanas, N. (1986). Support groups for mental health staff and trainees. *International Journal of Group Psychotherapy, 36,* 279–296.

Kertesz, J. (1980). Permeability of individual boundaries: The critical factor for effective functioning of interdisciplinary health care teams. In D. C. Baldwin, M. A. Rowley, & B. A. Williams (Eds.), *Interdisciplinary health care teams in teaching and practice.* Proceedings of the First Annual Conference on Interdisciplinary Teams in Primary Care (pp. 23–27). Reno: University of Nevada Press.

Kiesler, D. J. (1982). Interpersonal theory for personality and psychotherapy. In J. C. Anchin & D. J. Kiesler (Eds.), *Handbook of interpersonal psychotherapy* (pp. 3–24). New York: Pergamon Press.

Larson, D. G. (1983). Developing effective hospice staff support groups: Pilot test of an innovative training program. *The Hospice Journal, 2*(2), 41–55.

Lazarus, R. S., & Folkman, S. (1984). *Stress, appraisal and coping.* New York: Springer Publishing.

Lerner, H. G. (1985). *The dance of anger.* New York: Harper & Row, Publishers.

Lewin, K. (1935). *A dynamic theory of personality.* New York: McGraw-Hill Book Co.

Madden, T. R. (1987). *Women vs. women: The uncivil business war.* New York: Amacom.

Malanka, P. (1984). Reaching for excellence: A look at what nursing can do. *Nursing Life, 4*(3), 41–46.

Martocchio, B. C. (1987). Authenticity, belonging, emotional closeness, and self representation. *Oncology Nursing Forum, 14*(4), 23–27.

McKegney, F. P., Visco, G., Yates, J., & Hughes, J. (1979). An exploration of cancer staff attitudes and values. *Medical and Pediatric Oncology, 6,* 325–337.

Mioduszewski, J., & McCray, N. (1985). The evolving role of the oncology nurse in managing cancer pain. *Seminars in Oncology Nursing, 1,* 123–125.

Mount, B. M. (1986). Dealing with our losses. *Journal of Clinical Oncology, 4,* 1127–1134.

Mount, B. M., & Voyer, J. (1980). Staff stress in palliative/hospice care. In I. Ajemian & B. M. Mount (Eds.), *The RVH manual on palliative/hospice care* (pp. 457–488). New York: ARNO.

Nason, F. (1981). Team tension as a vital sign. *General Hospital Psychiatry, 3,* 32–36.

Orsolits, M. (1984). Effects of organizational characteristics on the turnover in cancer nursing. *Oncology Nursing Forum, 11*(1), 59–63.

Pearlin, L. I., Lieberman, M. A., Menaghan, E. G., & Mullan, J. T. (1981). The stress process. *Journal of Health and Social Behavior, 22,* 337–356.

Pearlin, L. I., & Schooler, C. (1978). The structure of coping. *Journal of Health and Social Behavior, 19,* 2–21.

Pines, A., Aronson, E., & Kafry, D. (1981). *Burnout: From tedium to personal growth.* New York: The Free Press.

Plas, J. M., Hoover-Dempsey, K. V., & Wallston, B. S. (1985). A conceptualization of professional women's interpersonal fields: Social support, reference groups and persons-to-be-reckoned-with. In I. G. Sarason & B. R. Sarason (Eds.), *Social support: Theory, research and applications* (pp. 187–204). Dordrecht: The Netherlands: Martinus Nijhoff.

Rook, K. (1984). The negative side of social interaction: Impact on psychological well-being. *Journal of Personality and Social Psychology, 46,* 1097–1108.

Rosenberg, P. P. (1984). Support groups: A special therapeutic entity. *Small Group Behavior, 15,* 173–186.

Safran, J. D., & Greenberg, L. S. (1986). Hot cognition and psychotherapy process: An information-processing/ecological approach. *Advances in Cognitive-Behavioral Research, 5,* 143–178.

Sanford, R. C. (1987). Clinical ladders: Do they serve their purpose? *Journal of Nursing Administration, 17*(5), 34–37.

Schmalenberg, C., & Kramer, M. (1979). *Coping with reality shock: The voices of experience.* Wakefield, MA: Nursing Resources.

Shaffer, M. (1982). *Life after stress.* New York: Plenum.

Thoits, P. A. (1986). Social support as coping assistance. *Journal of Consulting and Clinical Psychology, 54,* 416–423.

Trygstad, L. (1986). Professional friends: The inclusion of the personal into the professional. *Cancer Nursing, 9,* 326–332.

Vachon, M. L. S. (1986). Losses and gains: A theoretical model of staff stress in oncology. In R. McCorkle & G. Hongladarom (Eds.), *Issues and topics in cancer nursing* (pp. 41–59). Norwalk, CT: Appleton-Century-Crofts.

Vachon, M. L. S. (1987a). *Occupational stress in the care of the critically ill, the dying and the bereaved.* Washington: Hemisphere Publishing.

Vachon, M. L. S. (1987b). Team stress in palliative/hospice care. *The Hospice Journal, 3*(2–3), 75–103.

Weisman, A. D. (1981). Understanding the cancer patient: The syndrome of caregiver plight. *Psychiatry, 44,* 161–168.

CHAPTER 77

Role Clarification: Rights and Responsibilities of Oncology Nurses

JEAN K. BROWN

Role clarification is a supportive strategy for managing stressors associated with the work environment. One facet of this process is to be cognizant of one's rights and responsibilities as a professional nurse and to apply them in practice. Knowledge of rights and responsibilities gives nurse clinicians at all levels of practice self-confidence regarding the scope of nursing practice, guidelines for dealing with role conflicts, and power to advocate for patients and negotiate changes in the work environment. Nurse managers use this knowledge to support their staff, evaluate performance, resolve conflicts, develop policies and procedures, negotiate with hospital administrators and representatives from other health care disciplines, meet regulatory standards, and ensure occupational safety. The purpose of this chapter is to provide an overview of responsibilities and rights of registered professional nurses that are particularly relevant to cancer nursing practice.

In many ways, the responsibilities and rights of professional nurses specializing in cancer care are similar to those of other nurses; however, there are significant differences in application. Many nursing specialties practice in areas in which procedures and treatment regimens are well-established and nursing responsibilities and rights are well understood and incorporated into practice. Cancer nurses, however,

often practice at the forefront of scientific knowledge and technology, where policies and procedures may not have been developed, and subsequently nursing responsibilities and rights may not have been fully incorporated into practice. Cancer nurse clinicians and managers must be highly vigilant regarding their practices to be sure that their actions are within their legal and professional responsibilities and that their rights are protected.

RIGHTS VERSUS RESPONSIBILITIES

Inherent in professionalism is the integral relationship between rights and responsibilities. Characteristics of professionalism include maximal competence in the service provided, provision of a service of significant value to society, and performing the service with a high degree of autonomy (Jameton, 1984). All of these imply that the professional is legally and ethically responsible for a level of performance that meets specified standards and societal expectations. In the United States, these responsibilities are defined by state law and by ethical codes and standards developed by professional societies.

Increased concern with human rights has contributed to society's changing view of the rights of persons in the helping professions such as nursing (Fagin, 1975). The nurse is an individual who has both individual and professional rights. Some of these rights are given by the law, for example, the right to express oneself freely

The author is the recipient of a National Research Service Award (#5F31NU05680) and an American Cancer Society Doctoral Scholarship in Cancer Nursing.

or refuse to carry out a physician's order that is contrary to acceptable nursing practice (Annas, Glantz, & Katz, 1981).

Other rights must be asserted or acted on by the individual nurse. "People seem to obtain rights by having an image of themselves as worthy of rights, through sharing positive information and publicity about themselves, through pressure, and through doing something for society which society values" (Fagin, 1975). For example, job satisfaction and professional growth are rights that cannot be given but require effort on the part of the individual. Job satisfaction requires a positive attitude about work, and professional growth requires learning. Neither can be given but must be acted on by the individual.

When functioning as a professional, the individual's rights and responsibilities must be considered together. The right to refuse a physician's order also has the responsibility to communicate with the physician about the order, take the matter to a higher authority if necessary, and document personal observations and responses of others in the manner in which institutional policy dictates (Annas, et al., 1981). Job satisfaction is a right that must be weighed against obligations for patient care. The dissatisfied nurse cannot walk away from responsibilities, leaving the patient without the care required (Creighton, 1986). The professional's individual rights must be considered within the framework of legal and ethical responsibilities.

RESPONSIBILITIES OF PROFESSIONAL NURSES

Legal Governance

Legislation regarding the practice of nursing occurs at the state level and consists of statutes enacted by the legislature as well as decisions and rulings of administrative agencies and common law. The statutes deal primarily with licensure and definitions of the scope of nursing practice. These vary from state to state. Individual nurses must be knowledgeable about the licensure and nurse practice laws in the state in which they practice.

Licensure statutes describe the criteria that must be met to be given and maintain the privilege of practicing nursing. Licensure can be mandatory or permissive (Creighton, 1986; Rhodes & Miller, 1984). Mandatory licensure requires that anyone practicing nursing must be licensed. Permissive licensure protects the title of registered nurse (RN) by allowing only licensed individuals to represent themselves as RNs; however, the practice of nursing by unlicensed individuals is not prohibited. Mandatory licensure exists in 48 states; permissive licensure exists in Oklahoma, Texas, and the District of Columbia (Creighton, 1986).

Nurse practice acts define nursing practice using three approaches (Rhodes & Miller 1984). The traditional approach uses the 1955 American Nurses' Association (ANA) definition.

The term "practice of professional nursing" means the performance, for compensation, of any acts in the observation, care, and counsel of the ill, injured, or infirm, or in the maintenance of health or prevention of illness in others or in the supervision and teaching of other personnel, or the administration of medications and treatments prescribed by a licensed physician or dentist, requiring substantial specialized judgment and skill and based on knowledge and application of the principles of biological, physical, and social science.

The second approach identifies specific acts that nurses may perform beyond the traditional definition and allows for nursing practice governed by standing physician orders (Rhodes & Miller, 1984). More modern, administrative approaches broaden the traditional definition to allow for expanded nursing roles and empower appropriate state regulatory agencies to authorize additions to nurse practice acts. An example of such a broad definition is the New York State Nurse Practice Act passed in 1972 and later adopted by the ANA. "Nursing is the diagnosis and treatment of human responses to actual or potential health problems" (American Nurses' Association [ANA], 1980).

State Boards of Nursing

The nurse practice acts create regulatory agencies—the state boards of nursing—to control licensure, develop rules and regulations, and deal with violations of rules or professional standards (Rhodes & Miller, 1984). Professional nurses need to be knowledgeable about the rules and regulations in their state as well as the statutes, or they may jeopardize their licenses unknowingly. For example, in the state of New York a nurse is reported to the State Board of Nursing if convicted of driving while intoxicated, which is a felony. Action taken by the State Board of Nursing ranges from censure and reprimand to revocation of license and permanent listing of the offense on the individual's professional record ("Nurses warned," 1987). The advice of an attorney should be obtained in such situations.

State Health Departments

The role of state health departments varies from state to state, but all are concerned with the health of the public. These agencies set standards that must be met by health care agencies, institutions, and professionals. In New York one of the duties of the state health department is the enforcement of the Patient Abuse Law. To accomplish the increasingly stricter enforcement of this law, the health department reviews all institutional and agency incident reports. Nurses responsible for an incident are advised of a health department hearing. No matter how minor the incident, the nurse should attend and may wish to seek legal counsel. Any nurse found guilty at such a hearing is guilty of malpractice and may be in danger of a reprimand or loss of license from the New York State Board of Nursing ("Nurses warned," 1987).

Other Regulatory Bodies

Two other regulatory bodies that have a great influence on the practice of nursing are the Joint Commission on Accreditation of Healthcare Organizations (JCAHO) and the Health Care Financing Administration (HCFA). The JCAHO accreditation is extremely important to hospitals because loss of accreditation may jeopardize reimbursement for services from health care insurance. Many standards set by JCAHO have a direct impact on nursing practice and also promote ANA standards of practice. For example, evidence of the nursing process must be documented in the medical record, and quality assurance studies must be done. Because JCAHO standards are usually incorporated into the policies and procedures of the hospital, nurses practicing in settings accredited by JCAHO are responsible for meeting these standards in their practice.

The HCFA is a federal agency responsible for overseeing the Medicare law and related prospective payment based on diagnosis-related groups (DRGs). Because cancer is a disease with a high incidence among elderly individuals, changes in the Medicare law have an influence on cancer nursing practice (Donley, 1984). The changes in reimbursement due to prospective payment based on DRGs have raised many economic issues and concerns among hospital administrators that have led to efforts for more cost-effective health care delivery. This has created both a threat to and a potential enhancement for nursing practice to which nurses have a responsibility to respond. Threats might include elimination of nursing positions to reduce costs. In this case, nurses, especially those in management, have a professional responsibility to ensure that the work environment is conducive to high-quality nursing care (ANA, 1985a). Potential enhancement of nursing practice includes an increased need and recognition of the positive results of high-quality nursing care in shortening hospital length of stay and providing high-quality ambulatory and home care. Nurses have a responsibility to clients and to the profession to develop and implement efficient, cost-effective approaches to high-quality nursing care; evaluate client outcomes to the use of these approaches; and publicize the outcomes to educate hospital administrators, other health care providers, and the public about the effectiveness of nursing care (Yasko & Meck, 1984).

Professional Standards and Guidelines

The ANA and the Oncology Nursing Society (ONS) have established professional standards and guidelines that are applicable to cancer nursing. These are developed for a variety of purposes. The most common is to define what the profession believes to be high-quality nursing practice and to provide a model for nurses in their practice. Legally, RNs must comply with the standard of care practiced by a reasonably prudent and competent RN, or they will be considered professionally negligent (Annas, et al., 1981). Professional standards provide a basis for legislation, court decisions, and rules adopted by state boards of nursing. An example of the latter is the adoption of the ANA's entry into practice resolution by the North Dakota State Board of Nursing in 1986 that requires registered professional nurses to have a baccalaureate degree. There are four documents describing professional standards and guidelines of particular relevance to the cancer nurse.

Code of Ethical Conduct

The ANA *Code for Nurses* (1985a) is a code of ethical conduct that delineates the primary goals and values of the profession of nursing (Table 77–1). There are four themes in this document: respect for human dignity and worth, safeguarding the client, responsibility for nursing practice, and responsibilities to nursing and society. Assistance in applying this code to specific situations can be obtained from the ANA.

Respect for human dignity and worth and safeguarding the client are two fundamental principles of nursing practice that have special significance in oncology. Nurses are obligated to protect and preserve human life as long as there is hope for recovery or benefit from treatment (ANA, 1985a). Self-determination is inherent in respect for human dignity and requires full involvement of clients in their health care. Thus the nurse is obligated to involve clients fully in their plan of care and its implementation and ensure informed consent. If a nurse is ethically opposed to specific procedures used in a client's care, refusal to participate

Table 77–1. AMERICAN NURSES' ASSOCIATION CODE FOR NURSES

The nurse provides services with respect for human dignity and the uniqueness of the client, unrestricted by considerations of social or economic status, personal attributes, or the nature of health problems.

The nurse safeguards the client's right to privacy by judiciously protecting information of a confidential nature.

The nurse acts to safeguard the client and the public when health care and safety are affected by the incompetent, unethical, or illegal practice of any person.

The nurse assumes responsibility and accountability for individual nursing judgments and actions.

The nurse maintains competence in nursing.

The nurse exercises informed judgment and uses individual competence and qualifications as criteria in seeking consultation, accepting responsibilities, and delegating nursing activities to others.

The nurse participates in activities that contribute to the ongoing development of the profession's body of knowledge.

The nurse participates in the profession's efforts to implement and improve standards of nursing.

The nurse participates in the profession's efforts to establish and maintain conditions of employment conducive to high quality nursing care.

The nurse participates in the profession's effort to protect the public from misinformation and misrepresentation and to maintain the integrity of nursing.

The nurse collaborates with members of the health professions and other citizens in promoting community and national efforts to meet the health needs of the public.

(Reprinted with permission from *Code for nurses with interpretive statements,* © 1985 [p. 1]. Kansas City, MO: American Nurses' Association).

is justified only if advance notice is given and other satisfactory arrangements are made for nursing care.

The *Code for Nurses* clearly indicates that nurses are responsible for their practice. They are answerable for their judgments and behaviors and are not relieved of this accountability by physician's orders or institutional policies. If unprepared to provide the nursing care needed because of lack of knowledge or experience, the nurse has the responsibility to seek consultation. Individual competency and experience must also be assessed in delegating responsibilities to others. Nurses are responsible for maintaining their own competence and should be open to peer review of their practice.

Nurses also have a responsibility to the profession of nursing and society to promote high-quality nursing care and health care of the public. All nurses have a role in the development of knowledge, whether as researchers, data collectors, subjects, or users of knowledge. The user of knowledge is as important as those involved in the research process because the clinical implementation and verification of knowledge generated by research are essential if the knowledge is to be useful.

Nurses are responsible to the public and the profession for the delivery of high-quality patient care. Knowledge, skills, and commitment essential to nursing practice must be demonstrated by those wishing to enter the profession. Nurse educators, in particular, have an obligation to ensure that their students demonstrate these qualities. Practicing nurses have the duty to implement and maintain standards of nursing care and to promote a practice and community environment in which these standards can be achieved.

Some institutions have developed a code of ethics for their health care providers. The University of Texas System Cancer Center became the first comprehensive cancer center to develop and adopt an ethical code. The purpose was "to help guide staff members in making professional decisions" ("University of Texas," 1984). Such action is highly relevant in a cancer treatment setting, where complex dilemmas and decision making are common.

Social Policy Statement

In 1980, the ANA published *Nursing: A Social Policy Statement,* which sought to clarify the evolving role of nursing. It was endorsed by the ONS in 1983 (Oncology Nursing Society [ONS], 1983). This statement deals with the social context of nursing, the nature and scope of nursing practice, and the issue of specialization. It is important to the clarification of nursing responsibilities because it is the most modern discussion of overall nursing practice obligations.

The core of nursing practice is the "diagnosis and treatment of human responses to actual or potential health problems" (ANA, 1980). This was reaffirmed and applied to the practice of the individual nurse in a report to the ANA House of Delegates in 1987. "The depth and breadth to which the individual nurse engages in the total scope of the clinical practice of nursing are defined by the knowledge base of the nurse, the role of the nurse and the nature of the client population within the practice environment" ("Report to house," 1987). Nursing functions include physical care, health teaching, anticipatory guidance, counseling, and other related activities. The method by which nursing is practiced is the nursing process.

The difference between generalists and specialists in nursing is also important in role clarification, especially since the public, other health professionals, and even some nurses are often confused about this. These roles were defined in *Nursing: A Social Policy Statement* and affirmed by the general membership of the ONS (ONS, 1983b). Generalists provide "a comprehensive approach to health care and can meet diversified health concerns of individuals, families, and communities" (ANA, 1980). The ONS gave cancer nurse generalists the title of "oncology nurse clinician"(ONS, 1983b).

Specialists "are experts in providing care focused on specific clusters of phenomena drawn from the range of general practice" (ANA, 1980). Specialists become expert in a specific clinical area through graduate study and supervised practice. The ONS (1983b) entitled the cancer nurse specialist role "oncology clinical nurse specialist" (OCNS). Because the role of the graduate prepared nurse specialist is relatively modern, having been conceptualized in the 1940s (Reiter, 1967) and debated through the 1970s, the ANA went on to define the functions of this role as follows:

- Identification of populations at risk
- Direct care of selected patients or clients in any setting, including private practice
- Intraprofessional consultation with nurse specialists in different clinical areas and with nurses in general practice
- Interprofessional consultation and collaboration in planning total patient care for individual and groups of patients, and in planning and evaluating health programs for population groups at risk related to the specialty or the public in general
- Contribution to the advancement of the profession as a whole and to the specialty field (ANA, 1980)

A national invitational conference held in 1984 analyzed the role of the OCNS and made recommendations for the future (Donoghue & Spross, 1985). This conference endorsed the aforementioned ANA-defined functions and described how the OCNS could accomplish these functions in regard to cost containment, consumerism, client populations, role development, type of practice, nontraditional settings, practice standards, and professional issues. A second invitational conference was held in 1990 to update recommendations.

Standards of Oncology Nursing Practice

The ONS, in collaboration with the ANA Council on Medical-Surgical Nursing Practice, developed practice standards intended for the oncology nurse clinician. These standards are focused on both professional practice and performance, with emphasis on 11 high-incidence problems common among individuals with cancer (Table 77–2). According to the ANA ethical code of conduct, it is the responsibility of oncology nurses to use these standards to guide practice.

In addition to the standards and their rationale, this document includes structure, process, and outcome criteria to assist in implementation and evaluate practice through quality assurance, peer review, or self-evaluation. The ONS has also published nursing practice guidelines that provide care plans for a large number of nursing diagnoses common to oncology nursing practice (McNally, Stair, & Somerville, 1985). For example, the guidelines provide the information needed by the nurse to assess and teach the individual who has a knowledge deficit related to the prevention and early detection of many forms of cancers.

Research Guidelines

Cancer nurses are frequently involved in caring for individuals participating in medical, pharmacologic, or nursing research or conducting research themselves. They are obligated to have a special concern and vigilance for human rights related to research as well as support the development of knowledge through research. The ANA's *Human Rights Guidelines for Nurses in Clinical and Other Research* (1985b) ad-

Table 77–2. STANDARDS OF ONCOLOGY NURSING PRACTICE

Professional Practice Standards

The oncology nurse applies theoretical concepts as a basis for decisions in practice.

The oncology nurse systematically and continually collects data regarding the health status of the client. The data are recorded, accessible, and communicated to the appropriate members of the multidisciplinary team.

The oncology nurse analyzes assessment data to formulate nursing diagnoses.

The oncology nurse develops an outcome-oriented care plan that is individualized and holistic. This plan is based on nursing diagnoses and incorporates preventive, therapeutic, rehabilitative, palliative, and comforting nursing actions.

The oncology nurse implements the nursing care plan to achieve the identified outcomes for the client.

The oncology nurse regularly and systematically evaluates the client's responses to intervention in order to determine progress toward achievement of outcomes and to revise the database, nursing diagnoses, and the plan of care.

Professional Performance Standards

The oncology nurse assumes responsibility for professional development and continuing education and contributes to the professional growth of others.

The oncology nurse collaborates with the multidisciplinary team in assessing, planning, implementing, and evaluating care.

The oncology nurse participates in peer review and interdisciplinary program evaluation to assure that high-quality nursing care is provided to clients.

The oncology nurse uses the code for nurses and "A Patient's Bill of Rights" as guides for ethical decision making in practice.

The oncology nurse contributes to the scientific base of nursing practice and the field of oncology through the review and application of research.

(Reprinted with permission from *Standards of oncology nursing practice,* © 1987 [pp. 6–20]. Kansas City, MO: American Nurses' Association).

dresses ethical guidelines, mechanisms for protecting rights, and responsibilities of nurses. Human rights refer to both research subjects and workers who are expected to participate in the research process. The protection of these rights includes the right to freedom from injury, right to privacy and dignity, and right to anonymity. Potential subjects must be informed about the degree of risk and benefits related to the study; be given full information about the study proposal, procedures, and instruments; and be assured of the confidentiality of their responses.

When nurses are involved in activities that are part of the research process, such as administering experimental cancer chemotherapeutic agents, their rights must be protected as well as those of the subjects. Informed consent applies to the nurse as well as the client. Nurses need to be informed in writing of the conditions of employment, expectations related to research studies, risks, and risk management.

There are three mechanisms for ensuring the protection of human rights: informed consent, institutional review boards (IRBs), and vigilant practicing professionals. Free and voluntary informed consent must be obtained from all potential research subjects before they participate in a research study. This requires:

. . . an explanation of the study and the procedures to be followed and their purposes; a description of physical risk or discomfort, any invasion of privacy, and any threat to dignity; and an explanation of the methods used to protect anonymity and ensure confidentiality. The subject should also receive a description of expected benefits to himself or to the development of new knowledge. In instances in which control groups are used and therapeutic measures such as drugs are withheld, appropriate alternative procedures that might be advantageous to the subject should be discussed. Also, subjects need to know they are free to discontinue participation in the study at any time without jeopardy (ANA, 1985b).

Institutions and agencies are responsible for establishing procedures to protect human rights and create IRBs to be responsible for this function. The IRBs should have representatives from all occupational groups, including nursing, that may conduct research or participate in the research process. The IRB must review all research proposals before data collection is initiated, and any problems occurring in the implementation of a study should be reported to the IRB.

In addition to the IRB review, many institutions have instituted a review by specialty groups for the purpose of preventing the overstudy of specific populations as well as ascertaining the scientific merit of the study. These groups should also consist of members from all occupations involved in conducting or participating in the research. In agencies with specialty review committees, research proposals must be approved by both review groups.

Practicing professional nurses must be vigilant regarding the protection of human rights. They often have much more contact with clients than investigators and may observe known or unknown violations of human rights. For example, an individual who is confused and unable to give true informed consent may be enrolled in a study. The nurse is responsible for notifying the investigator and being sure the situation in corrected. For situations in which notification or correction is not possible, a mechanism should be established in which nurses can report the violation of human rights and action be taken to deal with them.

RIGHTS OF PROFESSIONAL NURSES

Right to Practice Nursing

Defined Duties and Expectations

Nurses have a right to written job descriptions, policies, and procedures that describe their practices. This clarifies the nurse's role, gives direction for specific situations, and protects the nurse. This right is not always given and must be asserted by the nurses involved. For example, there are times in cancer nursing practice when a new procedure is implemented for which no written institutional procedures are developed. This problem frequently occurs when new technologies such as vascular access devices or implanted pumps become available and physicians are eager to use them in patient care. In these situations, nurses must insist on adequate training and preparation for all nurses involved so that safe nursing care can be given. Nurses should take the initiative in reviewing the literature, contacting other institutions that use the technology, and obtaining information from the company that makes the device to determine what constitutes optimal nursing practice. If nurses take these steps and incorporate their findings into practice, they will be practicing as reasonable and competent nurses; however, written policies and procedures should be developed as quickly as possible.

Cancer nurses practicing in ambulatory-care centers have special needs regarding the job description, policies, and procedures that guide their practice. Often these nurses have a great deal of autonomy, and their patient care functions occur in physician- and nurse-client visits as well as by telephone (Brown, 1985; Nail, Greene, Jones, & Flannery, 1989). Nurses functioning in this role have a right to a job description and policies that recognize the autonomy with which they are expected to function. It is also useful for them to have nursing protocols with physician standing orders, if needed, that can be used in the management of common patient problems and emergencies such as allergic reactions (Medvec, 1987). Often these rights are achieved by nursing management and clinicians working together to identify needs and develop the written, institutionally approved guidelines necessary.

Oncology clinical nurse specialists and nurse practitioners also have special problems in clarifying their roles with specific job descriptions. Of necessity, their job descriptions may be very broad. They may be establishing a new, incompletely defined role. A strategy that has been successful in this situation is to develop goals, objectives, and a plan of action that is mutually agreed on by the OCNS and employer that

guides the OCNS's or nurse practitioner's work ("Recommendations for administrative," 1985). This requires documentation of steps taken toward goal achievement and evaluation of outcomes. Over time this can contribute to the development of a clear, comprehensive job description.

Reasonable Time for Duties

Nurses have a right to a work environment that minimizes physical and emotional stress (Fagin, 1975) and should participate in efforts to create and maintain a work environment that is conducive to high-quality nursing care (ANA, 1985a). Legally, employers are responsible for providing sufficient nursing coverage to meet patients' needs (Creighton, 1986). Although nurses' rights and employer responsibilities are clear, nurse clinicians often believe that they do not have enough time to provide high-quality nursing care. As nursing shortages increase, these beliefs will become more prevalent.

A reasonable amount of time to perform one's duties is a right that may need to be asserted by sharing information with administrators and the public, using pressure, and having an image of oneself as being worthy of this right. Nurses may need to provide information and exert pressure on management by analyzing client needs with respect to nursing time required. They may also need to publicize their findings in their community. However, nurse clinicians and managers also need to examine their practice areas in terms of nursing care priorities and efficiency. Nursing care goals need to be reasonable with respect to the clients' length of stay and capabilities, and more efficient methods for routine aspects of nursing responsibilities may need to be developed and implemented. Job descriptions may need to be redefined to include fewer responsibilities. For example, in a new physician practice, a nurse may be hired to provide nursing care, administer chemotherapy, and collect and manage data for collaborative group studies. As the number of clients grows, the nurse may need to negotiate to have the job redefined to exclude data collection and management. Finally, if nurses believe they have exhausted their endurance and change strategies without establishing an environment in which they have a reasonable amount of time to perform their duties, their image of being worthy of this right could lead them to leave the position.

Autonomous Professional Role

Refusing Physician Orders. Nurses have the legal right to refuse physician orders that are believed to be contrary to good nursing practice (Annas, et al., 1981). Such an order might be the prescription of high-dose methotrexate without the essential order for leucovorin rescue. If this very dangerous order were followed, the nurse would be professionally negligent. When a nurse refuses an order, there is also the obligation for follow-up. The nurse should contact the physician and discuss concerns about the order. If unsatisfied with the outcome of the discussion with the physician, the nurse must report the matter to a higher authority, such as the nurse manager. For the nurse's and client's protection, complete documentation of the details observed and responses given by the physician and others should be done in the manner directed by the institution's policies.

Reporting Incompetent Conduct. Nurses have the right and obligation to report incompetent, illegal, and unethical conduct on the part of health-care providers, such as physicians, nurses, agencies, and institutions (ANA, 1985a; Annas, et al., 1981). When nurses become aware of such conduct, concern should be expressed to the individual or agency whose practice is being questioned, pointing out negative effects on the client. If the situation is not resolved in a satisfactory manner, it should be reported to a higher authority. The nurse must complete written documentation of the problem. There should be a mechanism for reporting incompetent, illegal, or unethical conduct in the institution or agency that protects the reporting individual from reprisals (ANA, 1985a).

In spite of the right and obligation to report professional wrongdoing, whistle-blowers take substantial risks in their actions and need to be aware of them (Bandman, 1985). Whistle blowing is often seen as evidence of disloyalty to the team or institution, and whistle-blowers often rightly fear retaliation. Nurses, however, need to take a broader moral and ethical point of view. Their primary responsibility as professionals is to respect human dignity and worth and to safeguard their clients. This clearly places their responsibility to clients at a higher level than their loyalty to professional colleagues and health care institutions.

There is no risk-free method for whistle blowing, but Bandman (1985) has identified some considerations that could improve effectiveness and safety based on the work of consumer rights activist Ralph Nader. First, one should identify the misconduct, the related threats to clients, and the amount of harm that could result from lack of disclosure. If the amount of harm is great, the likelihood of support for disclosure is greater. Second, one should be sure knowledge of the misconduct is accurate, have documentation of the misconduct, and obtain support from others. This action will allow the case to stand on its own merit even if the motives of the whistle-blower are questioned. Third, one should use nursing standards for practice, statutes, rules, and regulations to support the decision to disclose misconduct. Fourth, one should consider the responses of others and the risk to self in developing a plan of action. It is useful to exhaust all options within an agency or institution to remedy a situation, starting at the lowest levels and working up, before going to outside authorities. Anonymity in disclosure may also be a useful strategy for self-protection, but if used, it is imperative that the information disclosed can stand alone in evaluating the case. Finally, it would be helpful to locate a source of external support such as professional societies, legal counsel, state agencies, or special-interest groups.

Occupational Safety

As advances in cancer treatment have been made, occupational hazards to health care professionals providing cancer care have increased. Cancer nurses may be exposed to hazards such as radiation, antineoplastic drugs, and hepatitis B, and they have the right to protect themselves. Institutional policies and procedures for protection against hazards in the work environment should be consistent with those recommended by regulatory agencies such as the Occupational Safety and Health Administration (OSHA) or the National Council of Radiation Protection (NCRP).

Maximum permissible dose limits of radiation for occupational and general exposure have been established for many years by the NCRP (1976, 1977). Nurses may be in either the occupational or the general category depending on the nature of their position and the institution in which they are employed. Nurses working in a radiation treatment center or caring for patients receiving brachytherapy have the right to a radiation monitoring device, such as a film badge, provided by their employer. A written report of monthly exposure and a permanent cumulative record of exposure should be available to personnel. When filing any new application for radiation monitoring, the nurse should be sure to note previous radiation monitoring and the location of exposure records, so a cumulative lifetime exposure record can be maintained. Radiation safety procedures for nurses are described in Chapter 20.

The OSHA has developed guidelines for the safe mixing and administration of antineoplastic drugs, which are discussed in depth in Chapter 22. Compliance with these guidelines has varied according to the setting, with nurses working in physicians' offices handling more drugs and using fewer precautions than nurses in other settings (Valanis & Shortridge, 1987). Although it has been reported that the OSHA guidelines are not mandatory standards and that there are no penalties for noncompliance (Gullo, 1988), OSHA has cited and fined an oncology physician for failure to protect employees who were exposed to hazardous materials in his office ("Oregon physician," 1988). In this case, a ventilated hood for mixing antineoplastic drugs, separate refrigeration, and separate trash receptacles for needle disposal had not been provided. Although nurses are often sympathetic to the expense their employer must incur for employee protection (Barhamand, 1986), they have a right to this protection.

In 1983, OSHA identified nurses as high-risk employees in a hazard alert on hepatitis B (Richardson, 1987). Oncology nurses who administer chemotherapy should be considered especially at high risk. The OSHA recommended that nurses be vaccinated with hepatitis B vaccine and receive education and training in protective practices. The ANA, American Public Health Association, and several unions have urged OSHA to make this recommendation a standard and to mandate employers to provide the vaccine free of charge to high-risk employees (Richardson, 1987).

Job Satisfaction

There are both great satisfactions and emotional hazards for nurses practicing in the field of oncology. According to studies of oncology nurse clinicians and oncology clinical nurse specialists, the stressors encountered in cancer care are similar in quantity and character to those experienced in other specialties (Donovan, 1981; Jenkins & Ostchega, 1986; Yasko, 1983a). The major stressors for oncology nurse clinicians were identified as lack of psychological support, lack of work satisfaction, and high work stress (Donovan, 1981; Jenkins & Ostchega, 1986). Sources of stress for oncology clinical nurse specialists included lack of psychological support, complex bureaucratic organizational structures, and role development and expectations (Yasko, 1983a).

To minimize these stressors and enhance job satisfaction, nurses need to use strategies to cope with work stress effectively (Yasko, 1983b). "A good stress management plan has three objectives: eliminate those stressors you can eliminate, learn to master those situations which routinely produce stress, and develop a mechanism for relieving the residual stress response" (Donovan, 1981). At a personal level, training in time management, conflict resolution, and relaxation strategies are useful. At the management level, a commitment to providing adequate staffing for the workload, developing innovative strategies for recruitment and retention, and providing counseling for high-risk employees are needed to reduce employee work stress.

The development and maintenance of a professional support system is also helpful in decreasing stress and enhancing job satisfaction. Some institutions provide psychological support in formal support groups led by a trained group leader such as a psychologist. More often oncology nurses must develop their own support network. Professional colleagues are often able to be more supportive than family and friends because of their depth of understanding of the day-to-day experiences and stressors in cancer care. In some settings, oncology nurses may not have colleagues who are readily available to provide support. Oncology nurses may need to reach out to their local or regional community of nurses or other health care providers to identify a support system. In this case, nurses need to negotiate with their employer for time or make a personal time commitment to use their support system on a regular basis.

Professional Growth

Professional growth is both a right and a responsibility identified by the *Standards of Oncology Nursing Practice* (1987). Many opportunities for professional growth are available in oncology nursing. There are many continuing education opportunities provided by the ONS and American Cancer Society as well as a large number of journals in various disciplines that can be used for independent study and to keep current about research findings and new technology, treatment, and procedures. Another means for professional development is participation in professional and community organizations. This demonstrates professional responsibility, serves as a method for exchange of new knowledge among professional colleagues and the public, and provides a forum for heightening awareness of political, cultural, social, and ethical issues related to oncology.

Other mechanisms for professional growth are peer review and program evaluation. Although the primary goal of these activities is to ensure high-quality care of clients, a secondary outcome is self-evaluation. Critical evaluation of one's practice leads to the identification of factors critical to high-quality care and areas of needed growth that can contribute to improved practice.

Rights in the Nurse-Client Relationship

Communicating with Clients and Families

Answering Client Questions. The nurse has the right and obligation to answer clients' questions about their condition, treatment, and nursing care honestly, but there are limitations based on what would be expected of the reasonable and prudent nurse (Annas, et al., 1981; Payton, 1985). For example, the reasonable nurse would not advocate alternative treatments that were dangerous or ineffective. In fact, nurses are obligated by their professional code of ethics to advise clients against the use of such treatments.

The dilemma nurses often face is who should tell what (Payton, 1985). The best solution to this dilemma is multidisciplinary collaboration, especially between oncology nurses and physicians. The American Hospital Association's Patient's Bill of Rights (1975) affirms the right of patients to obtain current information regarding their diagnosis, treatment, and prognosis from their physician. If the physician appears reluctant to answer a client's question or the client does not understand the information provided by the physician, the nurse should discuss the situation with the physician, encourage an honest and clear discussion between physician and patient, and be sure that it takes place. Often it is helpful to the client for the nurse to be present when such a discussion occurs. When it is clear that clients have not received information they need and want, nurses have the right and obligation to ensure that the client receives that information (Payton, 1985).

In the case of Tuma v. Idaho Board of Nursing a significant legal decision about answering client questions was made that is relevant to cancer nursing (Annas, et al., 1981; Jameton, 1984). Ms. Tuma, a clinical nursing instructor, was assigned to a woman dying of myelogenous leukemia whose physician had told her that chemotherapy was her last hope. When Ms. Tuma approached the woman for the purpose of administering the chemotherapy and discussed the side effects, the woman was emotionally distraught and apprehensive about the treatment. She told the nurse that the leukemia had been controlled for 12 years by natural foods and that she believed God would cure her. Ms. Tuma then discussed several alternative cancer therapies with the woman and said they were not sanctioned by the medical profession. The family reported Ms. Tuma's actions to the physician, who reported them to the hospital. Action was taken against Ms. Tuma by the State Board of Nursing, and she was suspended from practice for 6 months for unprofessional conduct. The state nurses' association supported this action. Ms. Tuma appealed to the Idaho Supreme Court, and the decision was reversed. The basis for the reversal was that neither the licensing statute nor the state board regulations defined unprofessional conduct in such a way that forbade Ms. Tuma's actions. Because the court did not seek expert testimony, it is believed that there was concern about a nurse being disciplined for talking to a patient (Annas, et al., 1981). Although Ms. Tuma acted within her moral and ethical rights, it is reasonable to believe that the resulting disciplinary action could have been avoided if communication between the physician and Ms. Tuma had taken place (Jameton, 1984).

Disclosure to Families. The maintenance of confidentiality of client information is both a legal and an ethical obligation specifically identified in the ANA *Code for Nurses* (1985a). Disclosure to spouses is an area of legal controversy, with the American Medical Association contending that such disclosure is not a breach of confidentiality. Annas and colleagues (1981) advised that the best rule from the perspective of the rights of health care providers is that disclosures of confidential information to spouses and families should be made only with the client's express permission. Nurses should always determine and follow the client's wishes. When clients do not give permission for sharing of information with their spouse or family, the nurse has the right to discuss the family's need for information with the client and to promote open communication among family members.

Care of the Dying

Clients' Right to Know Their Condition. Clients have the right to know their prognosis, and they also have the right to refuse this knowledge. Because nurses' primary obligation is to their clients, physicians have no authority to order nurses to withhold information that the patient wishes to have (Annas, et al., 1981). Thus nurses have the right and obligation to answer client questions about prognosis honestly and openly. This information is important to the individual's ability to make informed decisions about consent or refusal of further treatment (Otte & Allen, 1987).

Honoring Client Refusal of Treatment. Competent adult patients have the right to refuse treatment, and health care providers have the right to honor a patient's refusal of treatment (Annas, et al., 1981). These rights have been consistently upheld in court and are perceived as an absolute constitutional right.

Dying individuals do not lose this right when they become incompetent. If they have made their wishes

known to refuse treatment before they became incompetent, health care providers have the right to honor these wishes. If individuals' wishes are not known, their right to accept or refuse treatment must be exercised for them by the next of kin, guardian, family members, physician, ethics committee, or court of law (Annas, et al., 1981). The decision is made on the basis of what most competent people would do and what decision the individual would make if able. A living will, discussed in Chapter 80, or another written document can be useful in communicating the incompetent individual's desires. This is especially true for individuals with cancer who may have the time to plan for this eventuality.

Ethics Committees. Institutional ethics committees have been initiated to deal with the dilemmas and resolve conflicts that often arise in caring for the dying. These committees usually have the following functions: policy development, education, and case consultation (Vaux & Savage, 1989). Committee members should be from a number of disciplines and should include nurse representatives. Nurses should have the right to bring cases to the committee for consultation.

Many ethics committees have been instrumental in developing do-not-resuscitate (DNR) policies. The JCAHO has mandated that hospitals have policies stating that DNR orders are permissible and describing exactly what these orders mean ("New policy," 1987). Advance discussion with the patient, family, and health care providers is needed to make DNR decisions. Nurses often initiate DNR discussions because they are frequently the health care providers that must begin resuscitation measures. Do-not-resuscitate orders should be written by the primary physician and communicated to all health care providers involved (Otte & Allen, 1987). If the patient improves or has a better prognosis, the DNR order should be reviewed. Also, DNR orders should not be automatically carried over from one hospitalization to another.

Rights Regarding Professional Liability and Compensation

Liability

A review of litigation involving oncology nurses indicated that the incidents involved medication discrepancies, incorrect follow-up or referral, and failure to provide reasonable care after chemotherapy extravasation (Schulmeister, 1987). Most nursing negligence falls under the rule of respondeat superior. This rule in essence states that employers are responsible for wrongful acts of their employees that occur in the course of performance of work duties. However, nurses are liable for patient injuries resulting from medication errors or not following the written policies and procedures of their hospital or agency (Hogue, 1986).

Nurses have a right to written policies and procedures that determine the standard of care in their workplace. They can reduce their liability by being sure that policies and procedures are comprehensive and cover all their responsibilities. If these are not complete, they can initiate and contribute to the development of those policies and procedures needed.

Many institutions have very specific guidelines for risk management. Familiarity with these guidelines can also be helpful in reducing liability. Guidelines for reporting and documenting patient injuries should be followed carefully.

Nurses also have a right to adequate liability insurance coverage. They should carefully investigate coverage provided by their employer and may need to engage their own attorney to understand these complex policies. Although many employers discourage nurses from carrying their own liability insurance, it is in the nurses' best interest to do so because they may be sued individually. Also, the employer's insurance company may seek restitution from the nurse if damages are paid (Schulmeister, 1987).

Adequate Compensation

Nurses have a right to adequate compensation, and the ANA has worked toward this goal through the legislative and legal systems since the 1950s and continues to do so. Although compensation has improved over this time period, many nurses believe they are undervalued. The ANA recommends four ways in which nurses can work to achieve pay equity: educate other nurses and the general public, pursue legal changes through the courts and government agencies, lobby for legislation, and use collective bargaining (Flanagan & Barnett, 1987).

As a result of a 1974 amendment to the National Labor Relations Act, employees of both profit and nonprofit hospitals and health care institutions have the right to be represented by unions (Annas, et al., 1981). They also have the right to strike and picket. However, they must give a 10-day advance notice so provisions can be made for continuity of health care. In some cases, unions bargain away the right to strike and substitute grievance and arbitration procedures. When returning to work after a strike, employees are entitled to return to their previous positions.

SUMMARY

The rights and responsibilities of professional nurses are very closely related. Having a clear understanding of these rights and responsibilities can assist nurses in clarifying their roles, enhancing their self-confidence in their practice, and providing the fortitude to assert their professional rights. Because oncology nurses often practice at the forefront of scientific knowledge and technology, these actions enhance high quality care for individuals with cancer and high standards for oncology nursing practice.

References

American Hospital Association. (1975). *A patient's bill of rights* (AHS Cat. No. 2415). Chicago: American Hospital Association.

American Nurses' Association. (1980). *Nursing: A social policy statement.* Kansas City, MO: Author.

American Nurses' Association. (1985a). *Code for nurses with interpretive statements.* Kansas City, MO: Author.

American Nurses' Association. (1985b). *Human rights guidelines for nurses in clinical and other research.* Kansas City, MO: Author.

American Nurses' Association & Oncology Nursing Society. (1987). *Standards of oncology nursing practice.* Kansas City, MO: American Nurses' Association.

ANA board approves a definition of nursing practice. (1955). *American Journal of Nursing, 55,* 1474.

Annas, G. J., Glantz, L. H., & Katz, B. F. (1981). *The rights of doctors, nurses and allied health professionals: A health law primer.* New York: Avon.

Bandman, E. (1985). Whistle-blowers take risk to halt wrongdoing. In American Nurses' Association Committee on Ethics, *Ethical dilemmas confronting nurses* (pp. 18–22). Kansas City, MO: American Nurses' Association.

Barhamand, B. A. (1986). Difficulties encountered in implementing guidelines for handling antineoplastics in the physician's office. *Cancer Nursing, 9,* 138–143.

Brown, J. K. (1985). Ambulatory services: The mainstay of cancer nursing care. *Oncology Nursing Forum, 12*(1), 57–59.

Creighton, H. (1986). *Law every nurse should know* (5th ed.). Philadelphia: W. B. Saunders Co.

Donley, S. R. (1984). The effects of changing health care policy on cancer nursing. *Oncology Nursing Forum, 11*(4), 64–66.

Donoghue, M., & Spross, J. A. (1985). A report from the first national invitational conference: The oncology clinical nurse specialist role analysis and future projections. *Oncology Nursing Forum, 12*(2), 35–73.

Donovan, M. (1981). Stress at work: Cancer nurses report. *Oncology Nursing Forum, 8*(2), 22–25.

Fagin, C. (1975). Nurses' rights. *American Journal of Nursing, 75,* 82–85.

Flanagan, L., & Barnett, E. (1987). Pay equity: What it means and how it affects nurses. Kansas City, MO: American Nurses' Association.

Gullo, S. M. (1988). Safe handling of antineoplastic drugs: Transplanting recommendations into practice. *Oncology Nursing Forum, 15,* 595–601.

Hogue, E. (1986). Lessons you can learn from court decisions. *Nursing 86, 16*(4), 45–47.

Jameton, A. (1984). *Nursing practice: The ethical issues.* Englewood Cliffs, NJ: Prentice-Hall, Inc.

Jenkins, J. F., & Ostchega, Y. (1986). Evaluation of burnout in oncology nurses. *Cancer Nursing, 9,* 108–116.

McNally, J. C., Stair, J. C., & Somerville, E. T. (1985). *Guidelines for cancer nursing practice.* New York: Grune & Stratton, Inc.

Medvec, B. R. (1987). Nursing protocols. *Outpatient Chemotherapy, 1*(4), 7.

Nail, L. M., Greene, D., Jones, L. S., & Flannery, M. (1989). Nursing care by telephone: Describing practice in an ambulatory oncology center. *Oncology Nursing Forum, 16,* 387–395.

National Council of Radiation Protection. (1976). *Radiation protection for medical and allied personnel* (NCRP Report No. 48). Washington, DC: U.S. Government Printing Office.

National Council of Radiation Protection. (1977). *Review of NCRP radiation dose limit for embryo and fetus in occupationally exposed women* (NCRP Publ. No. 53). Washington, DC: U.S. Government Printing Office.

New policy set on DNR orders. (1987). *Cope Magazine, 2*(1), 19.

Nurses warned that ignorance of law can jeopardize license to practice. (1987). *NYSNA Reports, 18*(1), 3.

Oncology Nursing Society. (1983a). Resolution to endorse *Nursing: A Social Policy Statement. Oncology Nursing Forum, 10*(3), 89–90.

Oncology Nursing Society. (1983b). Titles in oncology nursing practice. *Oncology Nursing Forum, 10*(3), 90.

Oregon physician cited for violations. (1988). *Cope Magazine, 2*(10), 38.

Otte, D. M., & Allen, K. S. (1987). Ethical principles in the nursing care of the terminally ill adult. *Oncology Nursing Forum, 14*(5), 87–91.

Payton, R. (1985). Truth essential for trust between nurse, patient. In American Nurses' Association Committee on Ethics, *Ethical dilemmas confronting nurses* (pp. 23–26). Kansas City, MO: American Nurses' Association.

Recommendations for administrative support of the oncology clinical nurse specialist. (1985). *Oncology Nursing Forum, 12*(2), 71–73.

Reiter, F. (1967). The nurse clinician. *American Journal of Nursing, 67,* 274–280.

Report to house outlines scope of nursing practice. (1987). *The American Nurse, 19*(6), 13–14.

Rhodes, A. M., & Miller, R. D. (1984). *Nursing & the law* (4th ed.). Rockville, MD: Aspen Publishers, Inc.

Richardson, D. (1987). Technology produces occupational hazards for nurses. *American Nurse, 19*(4), 7–8.

Schulmeister, L. (1987). Litigation involving oncology nurses. *Oncology Nursing Forum, 14*(2), 25–28.

University of Texas adopts formal code of ethics to help people. (1984). *Oncology Times, 6*(11), 12.

U.S. Department of Labor, Office of Occupational Medicine, Oc-cupational Safety and Health Administration. (1986). *Work practice guidelines for personnel dealing with cytotoxic (antineoplastic) drugs* (Publication No. 8-1.1). Washington, DC: Occupational Safety and Health Administration.

Valanis, B., & Shortridge, L. (1987). Self protective practices of nurses handling antineoplastic drugs. *Oncology Nursing Forum, 14,* 23–27.

Vaux, K. L., & Savage, T. A. (1989). Initiating and maintaining an ethics committee. *Seminars in Oncology Nursing, 5,* 82–88.

Yasko, J. M. (1983a). A survey of oncology clinical nurse specialists. *Oncology Nursing Forum, 10*(1), 25–30.

Yasko, J. M. (1983b). Burnout and oncology nursing. *Cancer Nursing, 6,* 109–116.

Yasko, J. M., & Fleck, A. (1984). Prospective payment (DRGs): What will be the impact on cancer care? *Oncology Nursing Forum, 11*(3), 63–72.

PUBLIC POLICY AND LEGISLATIVE ISSUES

CHAPTER 78

Introduction to Public Policy

DIANE O. McGIVERN

VALUE OF PUBLIC POLICY INVOLVEMENT
Social and Economic Policy
Public Policy Process
   Problem Identification
   Policy Formulation
   Policy Adoption
   Policy Implementation
   Policy Evaluation
Policy Participants
Public Policy, Health, and Nursing

Nurses as Participants in Public and Health
   Policy
Levels of Policy Participation
   Become Well Informed
   Discuss the Issues
   Participate Directly
   Engage in Policy Research
Outcomes of Policy Participation
Enhancing Opportunities
SUMMARY

VALUE OF PUBLIC POLICY INVOLVEMENT

Literature targeted to health professionals has insisted on attention to public policy, including the description of process and outcomes, and is designed to alert these professionals to the contributions they can make to policy development. It is hoped that this participation will produce public policy that is the result of a broader, more well-informed set of alternatives. The expanded participation of nurses and other providers and consumers will presumably encourage policymakers to be sensitive to this type of input for the improvement of cancer care. Thus nurses are hoping through their participation in the policy process to better define health and health care in the broadest sense for everyone, especially for persons at risk for and who have cancer.

On a different level, nursing is preoccupied with public policy participation insofar as the activity is a reflection of change in status. How far have nurses moved from the "slumbering giant of the health professions" (Aiken, 1981) to major league player position? Consideration of and participation in policy development is an opportunity for clinicians to expand their effectiveness as nurses, to relate clinical outcomes to social and economic programs in cancer care, and to widen the frame of reference for personal and professional satisfaction.

Social and Economic Policy

The world of policy is large, and the word *policy* is one we all use frequently. We often link policy to politics or political process or to the word *legislation*. However, policy is the broadest of the three because it encompasses "principles and courses of action (or inaction) adopted and pursued by established governments of societies as well as by various units within society" (Gil, 1981). Policies are designed to regulate social functioning, although they may influence other activities as an unintended effect. Policies do not need to be legislated, but in the United States they may be.

Two areas of public policy are social policy and economic policy; distinctions between the two are frequently difficult to make, however. Social policy can be considered broadly as all policy dealing with social issues or the social structure; it can be defined more narrowly in issues such as child care, education, divorce, or labor unions. Economic policy can also be defined broadly or narrowly, with a focus on such issues as unemployment, minimum wage, or price controls.

These distinctions become blurred when the examination of a social policy of nutrition programs for mothers and children evolves into an economic policy consideration of farm surplus and price supports. Antitrust policy is economic policy until it is examined as a social issue of discrimination against nurse midwives, osteopaths, or others who are denied hospital staff privileges (Boulding, 1981). Epstein's (1978) description of the United States Food and Drug Administration's proposed ban on saccharin as a potential carcinogen provides a good example of the breakdown in distinction between social and economic policies. The social policy intentions of the ban were counterbalanced by the economic considerations raised by the food and chemical industries.

A great deal is written about the boundaries of policy, the extent to which the examination of policy is defined by perspectives that reflect professional discipline, nationality, culture, economic climate, or religion. What is the value or liability of focusing too narrowly? Or too broadly? Although policy may be best served by the most inclusive approach, most policymakers are constrained by ability, time, or other factors in their efforts. The result of these constraints is that policy decisions are on occasion made with incomplete knowledge or conflicting motives or are the product of a compromise. This immediate, short-term approach is all too familiar. In fact, policy is developed on three wavelengths: short-term, incremental decision making; middle-range processes; and long-range trends (Crichton, 1981).

For health professionals and others, it is important to be aware of these two considerations of boundaries and process levels. Understanding how a policy issue is being defined and whether decisions are consistent with short-, mid-, or long-range processes are more accurate guidelines of what actions should be taken and provide a different yardstick to measure success.

Public Policy Process

The process by which certain problems or issues gain public and governmental attention is described by Jones (1977). Government, being largely reactive, is influenced by the perception of events and subsequent definition of the problem. A number of factors affect the routing of problems to the policy agenda. Jones notes that the precipitating event, degree of organizational response, access of groups, and relationship between affected groups and influential policymakers determine the attention a potential agenda item receives and reflect a potential bias in the system. Groups that want a response but lack resources to organize demonstrations, media events, and informational campaigns or lack entre to or identification with more powerful groups are less likely to stimulate action by government or other policymakers.

As an example of this inequality of resources, Rushefsky (1986) describes an attempt to counteract the decline in research support. Mary Lasker wanted a cancer cure to be on the national agenda. Aided by the 1968 publication of Solomon Gant's book *Care for Cancer: A National Goal,* Lasker organized a citizens' panel, which made the recommendation. This national agenda setting and the prepresidential election politics resulted in the National Cancer Act of 1971 and appropriations that grew from $233 million in 1971 to $815 million in 1977.

Policy formation has been described facetiously as four cars traveling at high speed into a four-way intersection and colliding. The resulting wreckage is

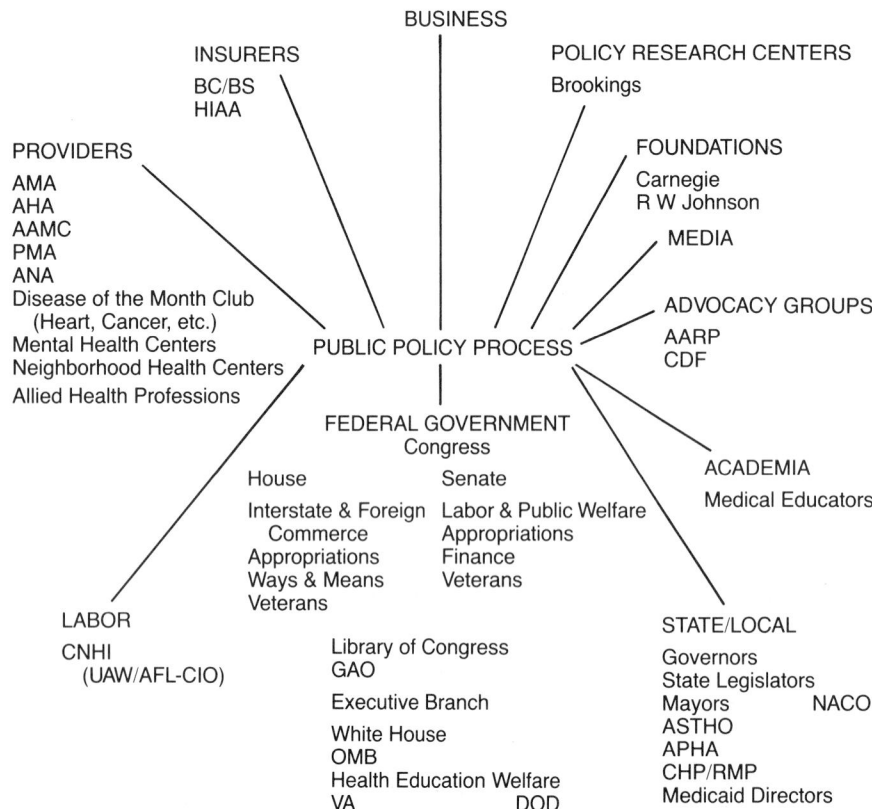

Figure 78–1. Public policy process for policy formation.

health policy. Random placement of bumpers, fenders, and other auto parts may seem an apt depiction of policy formation, but randomness and complexity are not quite the same. Policy development is a complex process because the issues are complicated, the input is large and diverse, and the process is slow. Wilbur Cohen, at the 1986 Medicare anniversary conference sponsored by the Leonard Davis Institute at the University of Pennsylvania, described the work that finally produced the Medicare legislation. In the 1930s Cohen became assistant to the director of the Committee on Economic Security. The work of that committee produced the provisions of the Social Security Act of 1935 but without the desired health insurance provision. By 1950, despite continued efforts, there was still no health insurance proposal, and Cohen was asked to develop one; he produced a memorandum that included the elements of Medicare. Subsequently, Cohen said he believed in the 30-year cycle of health policy achievements: 1935 Social Security, 1965 Medicare, and keep your eye on 1995!

The policy process outlined by Macrae and Wilde (1979), Litman and Robins (1984), and Lindblom (1980) and reflected on by Ferguson (1985) is a series of steps not unlike the nursing process: problem identification, policy formulation, adoption, implementation, and evaluation. These are deceivingly simple steps that translate into a fascinating, complicated, unpredictable, and frequently truncated process.

Problem Identification

Jones (1983) makes a distinction among events, public problems, issues, and issue areas that all may be labeled policy problems. Events are human or natural occurrences that affect the life of the population; problems, public or private, that require action; and issues or controversial public problems. The identification and definition of these can be subjective or objective and are made by individuals, agencies, corporations, or governments. Problem identification shapes the entire process; who defines the problem and how it is finally defined casts the outcome. For example, the high incidence of lung cancer in a particular county may be formulated as an environmental contamination problem, a politicoeconomic issue, or a problem of adequacy of long-term care services.

Policy Formulation

Policy formulation incorporates all the input of organizations, government agencies, informal constituency groups, and researchers. The diagram by Judy Miller Jones is useful in appreciating the number of inputs in policy formation (Fig. 78–1). In addition to the sheer numbers noted here and the ones readers can identify, each factor represents additional constraints. Each group or organization has one or more constituencies with priorities, preconceived notions or definitions of the problem, and sets of existing policies related in some way to the problem; in addition, the

organization's staff has its own view of the problem and solutions.

Alternate solutions are identified through available data, new research studies, discussion by experts, published viewpoints, and comparisons of different proposals. The interested parties know whom to influence and in turn are sources of information for public and health policymakers. Clinicians, professional lobbyists, and patient advocates not only serve as informational sources but also trade other groups' information as they go to a number of congressional and organizational offices. It is important to note that the outcome of the policymaking process may be that no solution is adopted and that the discussions may last for quite a period of time without resolution. Policy formulation affords participants various opportunities throughout the process to regain the advantage or become more persuasive (Jones, 1977).

The extent to which data supplied by clinicians, organizations, or research are influential in policy determination also depends on a variety of factors, including the degree to which experience or research data correspond to the desired policy outcomes of the other participants. Policy alternatives or proposed outcomes will also be selected depending on whether they promise greater benefits than other policies being considered.

Policy Adoption

Policy adoption can occur as an adoption of a course of action by an agency, through legislation, or as a result of a series of steps by a regulatory agency. Policy adoption has a number of sequelae; some groups claim victory, some claim it prematurely, others anticipate the effects of a policy, and some are affected by policy in an unintended manner.

Policy Implementation

Policy implementation is well described by Thompson (1981) in five case studies. In these examples and in his discussion he notes that legal errors, inefficiency, financing costs, lack of credibility, and timing shape the execution of the policy. Whether policy outcomes approximate the original intention is influenced by these factors and others that can be only partially anticipated and controlled at best.

Policy Evaluation

Policy evaluation is the study of the process by which policies were adopted as well as an examination of the policies once adopted and implemented. Evaluation is an ongoing aspect of the policy process because the analysis becomes refined as more information becomes available. Analysis of the intended and unintended effects also creates a biography of the issue and continues as long as the policy or legislation is in effect.

This brief description of the process makes one thing very clear: each step of the process requires informed, practical, and persevering participants. The process is frequently long, not well demarcated, and never assured. This reality is in direct opposition to our impression that a group lobbies for a particular bill, the bill is passed, and thus the group has been successful.

Policy Participants

The aforementioned description of the policy process suggests burgeoning numbers of policy participants. There is probably an inexhaustible list, but the dominant players come readily to mind: all branches of government, including the legislative, judicial, and executive, including regulatory agencies; the academic-professional community; consumer and environmental groups; and organized labor. Rushefsky (1986) refers to this as the "corporatist" model, which represents aggregated interests.

Legislative involvement frequently is emphasized to the exclusion of all other influences. Organizations identify key congressional members for their lobbying efforts, and daily media coverage emphasizes the congressional role. The core of the legislature's participation in the policy process is the committee system. Committees operate fairly independently and have jurisdictional control over the flow of legislation. Committee assignments are traditionally based on seniority, although tradition has been less important to some new members in recent years. Descriptions of the relevant committees can be found elsewhere; committee members and their staffs should be the object of long-term relationships by interested constituents. The legislatures play a balancing role with respect to the executive agenda.

The executive branch of government proposes an agenda of its own, lobbies vigorously for or against proposals offered by other branches of government or private organizations, and controls legislation by veto or by controlling funds through the Office of Management and Budget. The offices of the executive branch monitored by social and health policy observers include the Department of Health and Human Services, which in turn includes the Public Health Service, the Food and Drug Administration, the Centers for Disease Control, and the National Institutes of Health, particularly the National Cancer Institute. Agencies such as the Environmental Protection Agency, National Institute of Occupational Health and Safety, and Veterans Administration are only a few of the offices that engage in policy development important to clinicians (U.S. Department, 1986; Rosenthal, 1983).

Blank (1988), in discussing the courts as part of the policymaking process, notes that the complex problems of health and medical and nursing care are frequently referred to the courts because of the inability of the legislative and executive branches to make decisions on these matters. Issues such as termination of life, a patient's right to refuse treatment, and allocation of medical technologies are being determined by the legal system, which is creating policy by judicial decision. The judicial branch has more recently become the target of lobbying by special interest groups and other branches of government.

As Litman and Robins (1984) point out, the complex nature of public and health policy issues and the expanding governmental role in all aspects of life has been countered by increasingly well-organized special interest activity, which focuses on the key points in decision making and policy implementation and gives these groups and their constituencies a decided advantage.

Professionals and academicians have become increasingly prominent as participants with many and occasionally conflicting interests. According to Rushefsky (1986), the presumably neutral stance of science experts is altered by the fact that they represent their own profession's interest and may also be employed by many other groups. Some science experts have been advocates of cancer prevention policies, but others who work in industry are supportive of the corporate-industrial position. Scientists are being used by other interest groups to further their policy positions, which has led to the presentation of conflicting "scientific" evidence.

Increasing competition for resources and advancing technology stimulate more and more special interest group efforts, creating more factions with shifting alliances. The media, another special interest group, magnify the conflicts and demands of competing groups. Because of this, the agendas and activities of organized labor, environmentalists, and consumers are highly publicized and debated.

Nursing, for reasons not fully known, may not yet have achieved its potential for influencing the policy process. According to the "corporatist" model referred to earlier, nursing may not be clearly designated as academic-professional or organized labor. That lack of distinction may cause confusion among nurses about which participant role to play and may confuse other participants' reading of nursing's input.

Nursing's degree of appreciation for the four factors that influence agenda development—problem, degree of organization, access to influentials, and process—may stall participation. The definition of a policy problem is influenced by professional perspective, level of education, and status; agreement on problem definition may be difficult for a large and disparate group of professionals, such as nurses. The second factor—degree of organization and type of leadership—is a factor because of the range of general and specialty nursing groups and their resources. Access to influentials is determined by the degree of affinity and identification between constituents and policymakers. Nursing has considered itself strong in this area because many legislators are pleased to be identified with nurses and nursing. Lastly, the policy process is more responsive at times, an element that has to be gauged by policy activists.

Resources are necessary to organize activities that target the definition of policy problems and the selection and implementation of solutions. Nurses are not fully socialized in the importance of giving of time, money, or talent to improve their organizational representation.

Nursing's more powerful role in the policymaking process will come with the improving salary structure and the increased educational preparation of nurses today. If "organized" nursing chooses between an organized labor stance and an academic-professional identification and the majority of nurses follow suit, nurses' views will be more consistently formulated and problems and alternative solutions will be defined to match the good of the majority, the good of the profession, or both.

Public Policy, Health, and Nursing

The public policy arena as it relates to health is large, complex, and closely related to economics, social values, and the size and influence of the populations at risk. Health policy presents something of a problem for professionals who wish to become active participants and influential in this area. The difficulty relates to the potential scope of the issues and the investment required to select and become conversant with particular health policy issues.

Examination of health policy issues reinforces the difficulty in distinguishing between social and economic policy, the two categories of public policy. Health policy currently is a mixture of social and economic considerations, critics contending that health policy has become budget driven to the detriment of all.

Traditionally, public and health policy issues have been defined by the disciplines of medicine, epidemiology, health care economics, and law. Rarely have the issues been defined with nursing, social work, dentistry, or physical and occupational therapy in mind, as if these groups had nothing to do with the quality, outcomes, or cost of health care.

What are the public policy and health policy issues that nurses should be interested in and informed about? Broadly construed, they are all the issues important to health care, consumers, and nursing as a profession. These need not be totally congruent areas of interest. Rationalizing every policy and legislative effort in terms of "what's good for nursing is good for our clients" is unnecessary and misleading. However, the broad areas of public and health policy important to nursing make it difficult to identify specific areas of responsibility. The dilemma brings up two operating principles for all nurses who want to make a difference in influencing public policy: (1) nursing's effectiveness in the health policy arena depends on being versed in and verbal about a range of issues, not only subjects that are identified as "nursing issues"; and (2) no one can become equally conversant about all issues; nurses should strive to be informed on some issues and expert on others.

Health policy considerations have evolved over the years, beginning in the 1920s with topics that included maternal and child health; health care resources and financing; institutional infrastructure; and, more recently, cost constraints, rationing, and quality controls. Current health policy issues will remain in the forefront for some time: national health insurance or some form

of coverage for all (Freeman et al., 1987); long-term care for the elderly and chronically ill, including patients with cancer (Rothenberg et al., 1987; Shapiro, 1983) and acquired immune deficiency syndrome (AIDS); access to care for the uninsured (Report, 1985; Robinson, 1984); appropriate number, mix, and utilization of health care personnel; operational definitions of quality in health care; control of health professionals and their practice; and technology and ethics (Iglehart, 1987; Lewin, 1985). Within each of these policy areas are a large number of more detailed policy questions. Although these are contemporary issues, they all have significant legislative and political histories that help create the substance of the questions and color the discussions and resolutions. To learn the background and the players, some references are helpful, including Somers and Somers's *Health and Health Care; Policies in Perspective* (1977). This collection covers historical and contemporary public policy issues and the elements of modern health care, the historical development of the health care programs of the 1950s and 1960s, the intended and unintended effects of these well-intentioned programmatic efforts, and a proposed framework for future policies. An interesting book, *Shapers of American Health Care Policy,* gives a brief overview of the Committee on Costs of Medical Care; the Hill-Burton Act; the development of Medicare, Medicaid, and Blue Cross; and the evaluations of the American Hospital Association. It includes very brief biographies of the participants involved in these events. These are two of many books and journal articles that provide the critical background for policy participants who have more recently become involved in the issues.

For the broad prospective, nurses and other health professionals need exposure to participants, writers, analysts, and industry personnel. Information, personal views, and initiatives for action should be formed somewhat independently of the prescriptions formulated through more traditional nursing sources. Some of these sources are listed in *Integrating Public Policy into the Curriculum,* (Solomon & Roe, 1986); others may be gleaned from the *Political Action Handbook for Nurses* (Mason & Talbott, 1986). The conferences, publications, and materials from professional organizations of the health-related disciplines and government agencies are abundant and timely, and frequently they are the primary source for information incorporated into nursing publications.

It is possible that the health care cost-containment effort and the prospective reimbursement system can empower nurses and nursing to be vigorous participants in public and health policy development. The convergence of cost and quality-of-care issues, the beleaguered status of hospitals and health care professionals, and the impact of the nursing shortage have made government officials, hospital administrators, and others turn to nurses to protect patient care outcomes, to devise solutions for staff shortages, and to speak authoritatively on the broad spectrum of issues basic to these and related developments in the health care system.

The emergence of selected nurses and the nursing profession as policy participants is a development that can be sustained for several reasons. First, the pressure for advanced academic preparation, including grounding in research, policy, economics, and health care economics, will continue. Second, the increased percentage of women in the work force and their long-term career commitments help to sustain nursing's influence. Lastly, professions are being equalized to the extent that all health care providers feel they are currently at a disadvantage as targets of legislative, regulatory, and social changes.

Nurses as Participants in Public and Health Policy

Nurses can be important participants in the public and health policy debate; nurses are the largest group within the health provider sector, and they bring to policy discussions a unique and patient-oriented perspective. Nursing's greatest influence to date has been a result of its image as caregivers who are knowledgeable about health care problems and requirements. It is important to note, however, that two or more distinct groups contribute to public policy development: the knowledge makers and the policymakers. Clinicians are more frequently the individuals whose research, clinical practice, and consultations provide them with direct, experiential knowledge. Two steps are essential for clinicians to pass on their knowledge to policymakers. The first is to understand the legitimacy of their knowledge and their authority and expertise as licensed professionals. The second is to become skilled in packaging this knowledge so that it may become useful to policymakers.

The participation of nurses and nursing in policy development has been the object of the organized profession's promotion. In the last two decades, nurses individually and collectively have been urged to participate in legislative, political, and policy-related activities as both a right and a privilege of professional status. More recently, the effort has become institutionalized through the establishment of graduate nursing programs, nursing majors, and courses offered in public and health policy and the emphasis on preparation of the doctorally educated nurse researchers to contribute in this area. Groups such as the Nurses in Washington Roundtable have organized around the idea of nurses participating in health policy. National and state nurses' associations have identified subgroups and activities designed to involve members in policy and legislative issues.

Nurses as visible participants in mainstream policy discussions have emerged more recently, possessing credentials from academic preparation and direct and varied experiences in policy activities on boards, foundations, and commissions and in elected offices and relevant research activity. The constant theme of nursing's need to become active in the policy, political, and legislative arena and the more recent emergence of policy figures who are also nurses have created greater expectations of current clinicians.

Levels of Policy Participation

What are appropriate and useful expectations for nurses with respect to public policy? Have unrealistic examples of what nurses might do or how they might participate justified a lack of proactive involvement? There are four levels of policy participation that are realistic and serve nursing well. These levels represent a change in the traditional set of expectations and may be viewed by some as less visible or influential. How many clinicians have been put off by the admonition to become politically active, be prepared to testify before a legislative committee, or write a congressional representative immediately about an important issue? These expectations, which seem beyond the personal expectations of most, serve to excuse individuals who view these activities as beyond their ability, understanding, or level in the professional or organizational hierarchy. Therefore, a more appropriate set of expectations must be delineated that will enable and empower a greater number of nurses to become active in the public policy arena.

Become Well Informed

The first level of expectation for nursing and nurses is to become well informed. For nurses to become more knowledgeable, effective participants in policymaking they must understand process and content. High school civics is sufficiently removed either in time or in interest for the process of government to be familiar. Understanding the structure and function of the local, state, and federal governments provides a context for the issues and for ways to influence policy determinations. Although this information seems readily available, it is often presented in a diagrammatic, dogmatic way that does not convey the possibilities or potential excitement of playing the system.

Becoming conversant with the content of the issues is probably the single most important aspect of public policy participation. Understanding the issues means knowing the history of the problem, the proposed solutions, and the stakes of the other interested parties. What is necessary to achieve this first level of policy participation? Assuming that nurses' professional status carries the responsibility to expand individual knowledge and to contribute to the professional community, they must develop the following:

- an openness to reading about and discussing broadly defined health issues
- a willingness to read or learn about new issues
- a willingness to seek other opinions and points of view
- an access to literature broader than that found in traditional nursing sources to gain more varied definitions of the issue and perspectives of other disciplines, including economics, law, and ethics

Being well informed on issues and, conversely, knowing where the gaps in information are located makes the professional comfortable and able to discuss issues in a productive way.

Discuss the Issues

This second step of policy participation, discussing the issues, is necessary to gain exposure to different points of view and to give information to professional colleagues and others who seek data. The success of this step depends on

- initiating a discussion of policy issues with colleagues as a logical extension of the clinical practice, with patient-specific or professional association issues being frequently discussed
- practicing succinct logical presentations of issues so the listener recognizes the organization of thinking, the linkages developed, and the omissions
- a willingness to identify what is not known, is speculative, is clearly biased, or is an example of a special case. This step lends credibility to what is presented as factual
- an appreciation that direct clinical knowledge is unique and adds real evidence for the effects of a policy and may provide direction for policy development

This last point is the most underestimated by clinicians. Oncology nurses can draw on a wealth of direct patient care experience and work with patients' families and a knowledge of the impact of treatment, of reimbursement for various types of care, and of quality of life issues. This information is essential to the development of effective social and health policy but is not provided continually and systematically by those who know it best, clinicians in oncology.

Discussion with colleagues is good preparation for discussion of issues with broader segments of the nursing community, administrators, financial officers, and elected or appointed officials. Involvement with the nursing community through professional colleagues in practice, nursing specialty organizations, or national organizations adds strength to the individual clinician's point of view or the policy alternative being advanced. At this point in the development of policy, participants should identify the influential persons who should routinely receive information and well-considered views on nursing health care and related public policy issues.

Participate Directly

The next step in policy participation is the one frequently mentioned as the first activity: direct participation. The exhortations to run for office, participate in a political campaign, present testimony, or lobby for legislative proposals are premature without taking the steps to become well informed and skillful in discussing and outlining issues and policy directions. For the clinician who is interested in this level of policy

involvement, a variety of formal and informal opportunities exist to expand expertise.

Expert clinical opinion influences the formulation of policy and creates an environment for future policy modifications. Nurses identified as experts because of their research and training efforts in a specialty are called on by governmental agencies and professional organizations for testimony. Ruth McCorkle testified in the April 1988 National Cancer Advisory Board's public participation hearing on the importance of oncology education in the preparation and updating of new and experienced providers, citing a number of important education and research training programs.

Opportunities to take leadership positions in professional organizations' legislative and policy initiatives are always available. These committees or offices not only provide good experience for involvement in a range of issues but also afford access to a network of professionals interested in similar issues. Local and state officials and their staffs are always in need of information either on a particular issue or as part of an ongoing consultative process. State government is a particularly important target of policy and legislative activity for licensed professionals. State legislators' spheres of interest and influence are somewhat easier to identify than are those of legislators on the national scene, and the legislative and regulatory responsibility for licensed professionals, insurance, and implementation of many programs mandated nationally rest with these state officials.

The actual experience of working in the legislative, policy, and political arena is also available. Formal programs open to nurses and other professionals are listed in various places (Dicicco-Bloom, 1986; McGivern, 1986). For nurses constrained by time, obligations, or degree of interest, any number of informal arrangements may be made with organizations, legislative offices, or individual influentials. No one should be deterred by the lack of precedent for such participation in any office or organization; perhaps no one ever asked whether a particular experience could be arranged.

Engage in Policy Research

The fourth area of participation is policy research. Policy research is the "process of conducting research in a fundamental social problem in order to provide policy makers with pragmatic, action-oriented recommendations for alleviating the problem" (Majchrzak, 1984). The researcher identifies a problem of interest or imperative, such as health care for minorities, cancer incidence in health care workers, or depression in family caregivers, and through the research process identifies various actions or solutions. These policy alternatives become part of the basis of choice for policymakers and lawmakers (Davis, 1986). Policy research is different from policy analysis, which is the study of the process of policy selection and the effect of policies.

Hinshaw (1988) notes the importance of nursing research as a way to influence health policy at several levels and the relationship of the quality of doctoral programs to the preparation and socialization of researchers. Hinshaw makes important points about what doctoral programs need to incorporate to prepare effective policy researchers who will contribute to the solution of public and health care problems:

- Orientation toward use of data to affect health care policy to influence policymakers
- Responsibility for accurate and appropriate interpretation of research findings
- Ability to assess usefulness of micro- and macro-level studies
- Understanding the convergence of public policy needs and the nursing research perspective

Outcomes of Policy Participation

What are the expected outcomes of participation in the public policy arena? Given the complexity of policy development, no one should anticipate replicating Redman's experience in *The Dance of Legislation* (1973). Redman, as a college graduate and a junior staffer in Senator Warren Magnuson's office, spent two years drafting the National Health Service Bill and helped orchestrate for his senator the intricate maneuvers that culminated in the passage of this piece of legislation. His experience is exciting in the telling but certainly not typical of what intern, fellow staffer, or sometimes even congressional member experiences in a legislative lifetime. Realistically, health professionals should view policy participation as one set of professional responsibilities that can be personally and professionally satisfying.

A second outcome is the acknowledgment of the legitimate and authoritative viewpoint expressed by nurses and organized nursing. Nursing's perspective is an important part of the spectrum of information, analyses, and action necessary in every policy determination. The absence of nursing's contribution is detrimental to complete considerations of public policy questions.

Even when specific policy actions are not adopted and implemented, the dialogue created by active participation of many professionals produces an environment that sustains future consideration of policy questions. The participation itself clarifies the intricacies of the issues and stimulates examination of new options. The conventional wisdom describes policy development as incremental, and the increments can be small indeed. Success in the policy arena is not immediate or even visible at times.

Enhancing Opportunities

What can individual nurses and organized professional nursing do to enhance the opportunities for meaningful policy participation? First, it is helpful to recognize that nursing's traditional viewpoint has been strongly influenced by its history as a social reform movement. As such, the view of what is "right" as what ought to be done has framed many of organized nursing's responses to policy questions. The ability to deal only with the "right" point of view has kept the profession from appreciating the conflicting and competing interests of other interested parties. The essence of policy formulation is the balance of a spectrum of problem definitions, vested interests in desired outcomes, and capabilities of affecting the proposed solutions. Participants anticipating black and white problem identification and solutions will be ineffectual and quickly discouraged.

Preparation for policy interest can be enhanced by learning the content and language of the disciplines that influence the discussions. Economics, health care economics, health law, political science, and public administration are areas not strongly represented in our professional preparation. To the extent that an individual nurse or the nursing profession values public policy involvement, preparation in these and related areas is necessary. Nursing has taken two steps in this direction: the general acknowledgment of the importance of the profession's participation in policy and the beginning of educational programs that have begun to integrate relevant content.

SUMMARY

Nursing has an important contribution to make in identifying health and social problems and in formulating policy alternatives. The discipline's viewpoint is unique and authoritative because of the various roles nurses play, particularly the caregiver role. Most recently, preparation for nurses in policy, politics, legislation, and research has been made available through academic and continuing education programs, general nursing, and clinical specialty organization initiatives.

References

Aiken, L. H. (1981). The practice setting: An overview of health policy issues. In L. H. Aikin (Ed.), *Health policy and nursing practice* (p. 3). New York: McGraw-Hill Book Co.

Blank, R. (1988). *Life, death and public policy*. DeKalb, IL: Northern Illinois University Press.

Boulding, K. E. (1981). The boundaries of social policy. In A. Crichton (Ed.), *Health policy making* (pp. 31–38). Ann Arbor, MI: Health Administration Press.

Crichton, A. (1981). What is policy? In A. Crichton (Ed.), *Health policy making* (pp. 24–79). Ann Arbor, MI: Health Administration Press.

Davis, K. (1986). Research and policy formulation. In L. Aiken & D. Mechanic (Eds.), *Applications of social science to clinical medicine and health policy* (pp. 113–125). New Brunswick, NJ: Rutgers University Press.

Dicicco-Bloom, B. (1986). Legislative and political internships and fellowships. In D. J. Masson & S. W. Talbott (Eds.), *Political action handbook for nurses*. Menlo Park, CA: Addison-Wesley Publishing Co.

Epstein, S. S. (1978). *The politics of cancer* (pp. 189–207). San Francisco: Sierra Club Books.

Ferguson, V. (1985). Power, politics and policy in nursing. In R. R. Wieczorek (Ed.), *Power, politics, and policy in nursing* (p. 12). New York: Springer Publishing Co.

Freeman, H. E., Blendon, R., Aiken, L., Sudman, S., Mullinix, C., & Corey, C. (1987). Americans report on their access to health care. *Health affairs, 6*(1), 6–18.

Gil, D. H. (1981). A systematic approach to social policy analysis. In A. Crichton (Ed.), *Health policy making* (p. 48). Ann Arbor, MI: Health Administration Press.

Hinshaw, A. S. (1988). Using research to shape health policy. *Nursing Outlook, 36,* 21–28.

Iglehart, J. (Ed.). (1987). *Health affairs.* Milwood, VA: Project Hope.

Jones, O. (1977). *An introduction to the study of public policy* (2nd ed., p. 26). North Scituate, MA: Duxbury Press.

Lewin, M. E. (Ed.). (1985). *The health policy agenda.* Washington, DC: American Enterprise Institute for Public Policy Research.

Lindblom, C. (1980). *The policy making process.* Englewood Cliffs, NJ: Prentice-Hall, Inc.

Litman, J., & Robins, S. (1984). *Health politics and policy* (pp. 10–12). New York: John Wiley & Sons.

Macrae, D., Jr., & Wilde, J. (1979). *Policy analysis for public decisions.* Lanham, MD: University Press of America.

Majchrzak, A. (1984). *Methods for policy research* (p. 12). Beverly Hills, CA: Sage Publications.

Mason, D. J., & Talbott, S. W. (Eds.). (1986). *Political action handbook for nurses.* Menlo Park, CA: Addison-Wesley Publishing Co.

McGivern, D. O. (1986). Resources for teaching public policy. In S. B. Solomon & S. C. Roe (Eds.), *Integrating public policy into the curriculum* (pp. 77–100). New York: National League for Nursing.

Miller-Jones, J. National health policy forum. (1988).

Redman, E. (1973). *The dance of legislation.* New York: Simon & Schuster, Inc.

Report of the Secretary's Task Force on Black and Minority Health Department of Health and Human Services, August, 1985, Vol. 1. pp. 87–106.

Robinson, J. C. (1984). Racial equality and the probability of occupation related injury or illness. *Milbank Memorial Fund Quarterly: Health and Society, 62,* 567–590.

Rosenthal, G. (1983). The federal health structure. In D. Mechanic (Ed.), *Handbook of health, health care and the health professions.* New York: The Free Press.

Rothenberg, R., et al. (1987). Cancer. In R. Ambler & H. B. Dull (Eds.), *Closing the gap: The burden of unnecessary illness.* New York: Oxford University Press.

Rushefsky, M. E. (1986). *Making cancer policy.* Albany: State University of New York Press.

Shapiro, S. (1983). Epidemiology of ischemic heart disease and cancer. In D. Mechanic (Ed.), *Handbook of health, health care and the health professions.* New York: The Free Press.

Solomon, S. B., & Roe, S. C. (Eds.). (1986). *Integrating public policy into the curriculum.* New York: National League for Nursing.

Somers, A. R., & Somers, H. M. (Eds.). (1977). *Health and health care: Policies in perspective.* Germantown, MD: Aspen Systems.

Speeks, L. E., & Berman, H. J. (1985). *Shapers of American health care policy: An oral history.* Ann Arbor, MI: Health Administration Press.

Thompson, F. J. (1981). *Health policy and the bureaucracy* (pp. 252–282). Cambridge, MA: The MIT Press.

U.S. Department of Health and Human Services Task Force on Health Risk Assessment. (1986). *Determining risks to health.* Dover, MA: Auburn House Publishing Co.

CHAPTER 79

Understanding Cancer Reimbursement

LEE E. MORTENSON

Without question, reimbursement affects one's career in the health care professions. It determines whether facilities for work and research are open. It determines a hospital's ability to provide adequate care. It affects patient management and is likely to determine the settings in which a patient is treated. It affects research and availability of new therapies. In more and more cases, it may be a deciding factor in life and death resource judgments. Reimbursement, more than any other factor, artificially influences the ability to provide quality care to patients with cancer. The more that is known about it, the better it is possible to manage as a caregiver, a manager, or a researcher.

ANOTHER UNCONTROLLED GROWTH: HEALTH CARE EXPENDITURES

At the end of the 1980s, approximately 11 per cent of the annual United States gross national product was spent on health care. Few other industries can claim such a huge share of the economy. In fact, if another major segment of the economy was as large and growing, it would be called a major success with a robust future.

Instead, there are major economic concerns about the health care industry. Significant cutbacks are under way, and major political figures are stressing that they intend to find ways to trim health care expenditures. Hospitals are closing. Major layoffs of nursing person-

nel are taking place all over the country. Physicians are working for less money and are working longer hours. More patients are being treated under managed care plans—health maintenance organizations (HMOs), preferred provider organizations (PPOs), and independent practitioner associations (IPAs)—all of the time. And concern is real over the access of patients to health care and the creation of differing levels of care.

These seemingly contrasting pieces of information about the health care industry are both accurate. The costs of medical care have expanded radically since the federal government first began to underwrite the costs of the financially indigent (Medicaid) and of individuals older than 65 years of age (Medicare) in 1965. Over the following two and a half decades, health care costs have continued to increase as benefits have been extended to more people and as new, more expensive technology has been introduced. More individuals have access to care, and the care itself is more expensive.

The future is bleak for those who pay for health care. Over the next three decades, a greater percentage of the United States population will be older than 65, whereas the percentage of individuals younger than 65 who will pay for their care will drop. In the mid 1980s, 13 per cent of the United States population was older than 65; by 2030, more than 25 per cent will be in the Medicare-eligible age group. Moreover, the largest portion of this population will be older than 75, a group that typically includes a significant percentage of chronically impaired individuals and the frail elderly. Of course, this is also the population cohort with the highest incidence of cancer. With more people requiring care, fewer people contributing to the payment pool, and more high technology, it is not surprising that those responsible for paying for care are already trying to figure out where to get the money to pay the bills.

THE CHANGING FORMS OF REIMBURSEMENT: FROM RETROSPECTIVE TO PROSPECTIVE

Reimbursement is bewildering because it is done a variety of different ways through an ever-changing series of mechanisms. Moreover, reimbursement is in the midst of a major series of changes that began in the 1980s and will continue for the next decade.

The basic concept of health insurance was to provide financial coverage if an individual became ill. An insurance company pools together the premiums of a group of people, and actuaries compute the price of insurance based on the kinds of illnesses the group is statistically likely to have.

As individuals use physician and hospital services, they submit bills to their insurance companies, which, in turn, pay them. When insurance was first introduced, the patient selected the physician, and the physician selected the tests, the hospital, the consultants, the therapies, and the rest. Payment to all of these health care providers (physician, hospitals, etc.) was retrospective (after the fact) and based on the treatments given. Of course, layer on layer of bureaucracy and rules have complicated this simple concept.

Physician Reimbursement: A Continuing Series of Changes

To make certain that physicians do not charge whatever they please, insurance companies have developed profiles of charges by specialty, region of the country, and procedure. Now they issue checks based upon "usual and customary" fees and, in some cases, "prevailing" fees. *Usual and customary* relate to what the physician has charged in the past for the same procedure, so that he or she cannot suddenly increase the rates. *Prevailing* is used when a new physician tries to establish a payment schedule and the insurance companies want to make certain the charges remain close to the average profile.

Physicians have been restricted in a variety of ways over the past decade. Perhaps the most significant cost-containment step has been taken by the federal government, which pressured physicians to "take assignment." Fundamentally, this means that when a physician treats a Medicare patient, reimbursement will be made only for the amount allowed by Medicare. The physician cannot charge the patient more, even if the physician's usual fee is higher.

At the end of the 1980s, physician payment remained primarily retrospective, with few direct controls imposed on services provided on an outpatient basis except by insurance companies that indicated an unwillingness to pay for some procedures or drugs.

The dynamics of physician practice viability were significantly altered throughout the 1980s as a glut of physicians entered the marketplace. Although professional societies are attempting to cut back on the number of physicians in training by closing some weaker programs, younger physicians have encountered significant difficulties establishing a practice, given the large number of specialists now available in many communities. This glut of physicians also affects the viability of managed care plans, because many young physicians are willing to work longer hours for less pay with job security and a guaranteed income.

The federal government will implement a relative value scale in the early 1990s. This system will install regional and then national reimbursement profiles for each physician procedure and activity. The plan will put further pressure on physician incomes and if no adjustment is made for the higher costs of chemotherapy delivery in the office setting, it will create additional complications concerning where cancer patients can be viably managed.

Hospital Payment: Trying to Inspire Cost Consciousness by Direct Incentives

Initially, the federal government tried to pay hospitals on the basis of their charges (i.e., what they billed the patient). Looking at approximate hospital-wide costs, the federal government reimbursed hospitals at 70 to 80 per cent of charges, roughly what the federal government assumed were the actual, rough costs for delivering the care.

Under retrospective reimbursement, hospitals received a percentage of whatever they charged. If the patient's bill was $10,000 and the hospital was reimbursed for 70% of the charges (a rate that takes into account Medicare, overhead, charitable care, etc., by negotiated agreement with the federal government) the hospital received a check for $7000. If it charged $100,000, it received $70,000. No one asked if these charges had any basis in reality or any relation to the costs of providing the actual care. Both the federal government and hospitals were certain that no one had any idea what the actual costs of care were.

Indeed, hospitals are still having difficulty ascertaining their real costs, because most have been "cost shifting" from one department or procedure to another since the beginning of their operations. For example, the cost of a simple laboratory procedure may be only $0.13 but billed to the patient at $50.00; the actual cost of a room (overhead, facility, direct labor, etc.) may be $450.00 per day but billed at $250.00. When there is plenty of money, there is plenty of room for error. Hospitals had little incentive to cost account because the more they billed, the more they received.

The outcome of this system was the creation of a

series of incentives for hospitals to charge as much as possible, because this method would allow them to receive the maximum reimbursement and profit. There were no incentives to reduce charges to the end users, so the spiral of inflationary costs and inflationary insurance premiums continued.

FROM REGULATION TO COMPETITION

The first attempts to limit the costs of care were initiated in the early 1970s. The basic philosophy was to regulate the health care industry, especially the establishment of new, high-cost facilities (Feldstein, 1980). The federal government established a network of professional standards review organizations (PSROs) to issue certificates of need to hospitals that wished to build new buildings, buy major new equipment, or expand existing facilities. Local decisions were made by local appointees, and decisions could be appealed to statewide review organizations. As might be predicted, this approach was highly political. In the long run, almost all requests were approved.

One analysis by Salkever and Bice (1978) indicated that hospital investment was, at best, deflected to other facilities and services by the certificate of need process. Other analyses indicated that more than 90 per cent of the projects that were initially proposed were eventually allowed to go ahead. Indeed, delays caused by the lengthy political review process caused the costs of the facilities and equipment to increase substantially, thereby producing the opposite of the cost savings effect intended. The PSROs were widely criticized as restraints on the free market economy of health care. The bulk of opinion about ways to contain health care costs began to shift away from regulation and toward competition as the Reagan era of government began. In a 1980 article on "Fostering Competition in Health Care," Pollard said:

> Increasingly, policy makers are looking for answers to these questions that point to individual providers and consumers and away from federal and state regulators. Have they become more conservative, or have disappointing assessments of the performance of regulatory bodies such as Professional Standards Review Organizations (PSROs) and Health Systems Agencies (HSAs) simply undermined their faith in government-sponsored reforms? Perhaps they are simply embarrassed by the millions of dollars spent during the past ten years on regulatory programs that hospitals and physicians now claim have only served to escalate the inflationary spiral. While it may be impossible to pinpoint the reason why regulation and big government are unpopular, what really matters is the recognition that new methods for managing old problems are in order.

The total amount of federal and state commitment to health care rose precipitously from $5.7 billion in 1967 to $37.0 billion in 1977. Given this kind of environment, few hospitals could not make a profit. The rich got rich, and, with only a few exceptions, the poor got rich as well. At the same time, federal legislators began to realize the health care expenditures were growing at an incredible rate, one that could contribute to major national budgetary problems.

Prospective Reimbursement System Variations

In the early 1980s, Congress decided to take an entirely different approach to health care and switched strategies from regulation to competition as the major method of cost control. Before the Tax Equity and Fiscal Responsibility Act of 1982, it did not matter whether a hospital was efficient or inefficient. Almost all hospitals survived. Moreover, efficiency was not necessarily rewarded. The more a hospital charged, the more it was reimbursed. Congress figured that competition would drive out inefficient caregivers in favor of efficient ones and voted to establish a prospective payment system (PPS).

During the late 1970s and early 1980s, the federal government initiated a number of investigations into methods of cost containment that were not based on regulation. Several states were given the option to reimburse all of their Medicare patients with a single formula or to use some other mechanism. Waivers were granted to New York, New Jersey, and Maryland (Mortenson & Winn, 1983, 1984). New York and Maryland developed state rate review mechanisms. These rate reviews entailed the establishment of all-inclusive single-payment rates for each hospital that reflected all of their ongoing, approved activities.

The PPS was mandated by Congress in 1982. By 1983, the administration had selected diagnosis-related groups (DRGs) as the mechanism for prospective payment. The Health Care Financing Administration (HCFA) felt that it was a compromise between a retrospective system that had thousands of categories of payment and a form of prospective payment that had a single hospital rate system applied to each patient that allowed for very little case variation.

Work at Yale University in 1975 to develop a method for predicting the average length of stay for patients offered an interesting alternative, which was utilized by the state of New Jersey. Working with a large computer budget and medical faculty, the Yale research team developed a series of clinically cohesive groupings of length of stay. These DRGs pulled thousands of clinical diagnoses into 365 groups. These clusters were later refined into 470 DRGs by the federal government.

Length of stay is an important predictor of cost. Moreover, researchers determined that the groupings defined by the DRG system could be used to analyze current practice patterns and to assign average costs. Under a waiver from the federal HCFA, the state of New Jersey began to use these DRG categories as a method of reimbursing hospitals. Essentially the state took all reimbursement for patients in New Jersey for a year, determined which procedures (and billing) fell into which categories, and told hospitals that the state would reimburse the average of each category.

The theory was that hospitals regularly see cases

that cost more than the average and others that cost less than the average, but in the long run, these differences even out. At the same time, once the average reimbursement is established, hospitals have incentives to perform more and more efficiently in the delivery of care. Whenever a case falls below the average reimbursement, the hospital makes money. Whenever a case costs more than the average, the hospital loses money. Obviously there are significant incentives for the hospital to minimize costs for cases that are costing them more than the average. There are also incentives to avoid patients who are too costly and to seek "high-profit" patients.

The debate over which form of prospective payment as well as the entire concept of PPS raged during the later 1970s and the early 1980s. Pollard (1980) suggested that "The challenge for the future is to learn how to use competition to achieve a more efficient health care system without abandoning commitments to equity and access." As we shall see, this goal appears to be a significant challenge in the cancer care area.

Health Maintenance Organizations and Managed Care Plans

At the same time the federal government was changing from retrospective to prospective payment, it was also promoting competition by loosening up some of the rules for alternative delivery systems. When HMOs were first promoted in the 1970s, the federal government imposed a series of restrictions that forced them to take a balanced group of patients, not just those who were likely to want the fewest services.

To open competition, many of these restrictions were lifted. In the 1980s, HMOs and similar organizations began an enormous expansion. The two other HMO-type organizations are PPOs and IPAs. Although the classic HMO model has all of the health care resources necessary for care under central control, the new models piggyback on current provider resources and employ utilization review and discounts to lower their prices. All three types are collectively known as *managed care.* Managed care plans may restrict physician choice, hospital choice, tests, treatment, and other forms of care. All three types of organizations (HMOs, PPOs, and IPAs) guarantee lower costs through utilization review, preadmission review, and careful control of hospital and physician resources. Some also require that hospitals and physicians discount their usual fees 5 to 10 per cent or more. Health maintenance organizations receive a fixed cost per person, so there are very specific reasons to prevent disease and to minimize use of resources. Physicians usually work exclusively for the classic HMO at a very limited number of locations. Although PPOs and IPAs also work from a fixed cost per person, their physicians are usually independent contractors who work in their own office settings.

By the late 1980s, many hospitals found that 70 per cent of their reimbursement was coming from DRGs or managed care sources (some of which were also using the DRG format for reimbursement). The remaining 30 per cent came from retrospective reimbursement by companies and individuals who were willing to pay higher premiums to give their employees or themselves a choice of physicians and hospitals. Whatever costs were not paid through DRGs and managed care revenues were shifted to standard third-party insurance, making these plans less cost competitive.

Competitive Dynamics and Incentives

All of these competitive dynamics have caused great upheavals in care, some with special significance for cancer care providers. The following reviews the economic incentives of various groups in the health care system.

- *The federal government* has every incentive to keep increases in DRG payments as low as possible while shifting the burden of responsibility for selecting the right form of care to health care providers (e.g., the hospital, the physician, the nurse).
- *Hospitals* have significant incentives to shorten the length of stay, to minimize resource utilization, to attempt to attract patients who are economic "winners," and to avoid attracting "losers."
- *Businesses* have significant incentives to switch their employees to managed care plans and to continually shop around for the best-priced alternatives.
- *Third-party insurers* have major incentives to cut costs to compete with low-cost managed care plans and to gain more of a market share.
- *HMOs, PPOs, IPAs, and other managed care plans* have major incentives to contain costs, limit resource utilization, and select low-risk subscribers.

Some of these incentives are predictable and "good"; others are unintended consequences of the system and can be a cause for major problems or dysfunctions in it. For example, when it became apparent that managed care was likely to dominate the marketplace, many large hospitals launched managed care plans in an attempt to manage their own future. Unfortunately many of these met with rapid and significant losses.

Third-party insurers and managed care plans have both attempted to find new ways of cost cutting. Some of these have made the health care system more efficient, whereas others are threatening the quality of health care and the future of research.

Business and Health Care

Businesses have explored new ways to shop for insurance plans and to cut premium costs. Many larger businesses offer a menu of selections to employees, but more benefits are covered under the managed care plan choices. To lower costs, lower insurance plan overhead, and increase control, a major segment of business is turning to self-insurance. Although only 10 per cent of the market in the early 1980s, more than 40 per cent of the health insurance market was self-insured by the end of the 1980s. This form of insurance has the added benefit of being exempt from state laws governing insurance companies, so that some of the benefits required of insurance companies need not be offered.

Many businesses have hired third-party administrators to do their shopping and negotiating. These administrators assemble the menu for employees and work out arrangements for self-insured businesses to have regular insurance companies manage the details of their self-insured plans.

REIMBURSING CANCER CARE AND CANCER RESEARCH—THE CHALLENGES OF THE 1990s

A number of key factors about cancer care make it difficult to understand from a reimbursement perspective:

- All that is included in cancer care is impossible to lump together, although trying to do this is a common error. Cancer care involves hundreds of site and stage variations, uses many treatment methods, and includes a full spectrum of activities from prevention through terminal care. As a consequence, cancer patients are discharged under a wide spectrum of DRGs (Mortenson, 1985, 1986; Mortenson & Baum, 1985; Mortenson, Yarbro, Clarke, & Cahill, 1985; Mortenson, Young, & Ney, 1988; Young, Mortenson, & Ney, 1988), making it difficult for hospital administrators to know whether they are making or losing money on cancer patients.
- Cancer care is always changing as the national investment of more than $2 billion in research yields incremental changes in the way care is managed.
- Cancer care has a significant outpatient component but is also likely to remain an important portion of hospital inpatient revenues.
- Patients with cancer are chronically ill and require many admissions (Katterhagen, Clarke, & Mortenson, 1989) and long-term follow-up, with a significant secondary primary rate.
- Typically patients with cancer are managed in many facilities (on average, 1.5 to 1.8 hospitals)
- To advance cancer care, a large number of patients are annually enrolled in clinical research trials.
- Some types of cancer management are well established, whereas others are highly variable.
- Treatment patterns, reimbursement, and cooperative research group experience vary widely by region (Mortenson, Anderson, & Novak, 1986; Mortenson et al., 1988).

These factors cause confusion to health care policy-makers, providers, insurers, and hospital executives. Some of the problems that face each of these decision-making groups will be considered.

Hospital Cancer Programs: Defining the Cancer Program Product Line

Hospital administrators are often confused about the importance of patients with cancer to their hospital's survival. Much of this confusion stems from the diverse nature of cancer care. Over the past decade, hospitals have moved toward identifying three or four important diseases or services that they wish to emphasize. Cardiology, women's services, oncology, and trauma are examples of this concept (Mortenson & Yarbro, 1983; O'Leary, 1987). Unlike cardiology, however, cancer patients are discharged under a wide variety of DRGs.

Our research indicated that 40 DRGs include strictly cancer discharges, whereas 31 more have a significant proportion of cancer discharges but also include patients with other diagnoses (Mortenson et al., 1985). Yet, when patients with cancer are tracked over numerous admissions, records indicate that they are admitted under a wide variety of complications, making it exceedingly difficult to track their actual costs and reimbursement.

Non-small-cell lung cancer patients admitted to one midwestern medical facility were discharged under DRG 82 (Lung Cancer) and 28 other categories (Fig. 79–1) (Katterhagen et al., 1989). If a hospital administrator attempted to determine whether lung cancer was an economic "winner" by examining only the data from DRG 82, the administrator would see an incomplete picture of the revenues and costs generated.

Indeed, hospitals chronically underestimate the financial importance of their cancer programs, many by as much as 50 per cent. In tertiary care hospitals, it is not uncommon for cancer to account for 15 to 20 per cent of total gross revenues; however, in many cases, hospital administrators are unable to follow patients with cancer through their accounting systems across multiple admissions, and they lose track of a significant

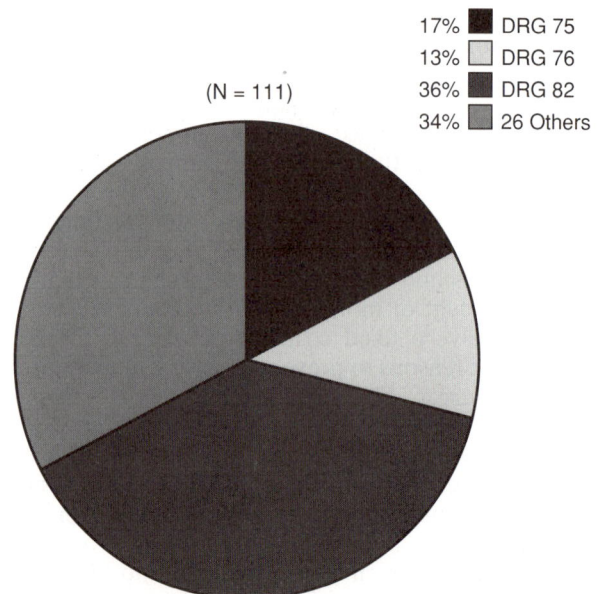

17%	DRG 75
13%	DRG 76
36%	DRG 82
34%	26 Others

(N = 111)

Figure 79–1. Frequency of non-small-cell lung cancer diagnosis-related groups (DRG).

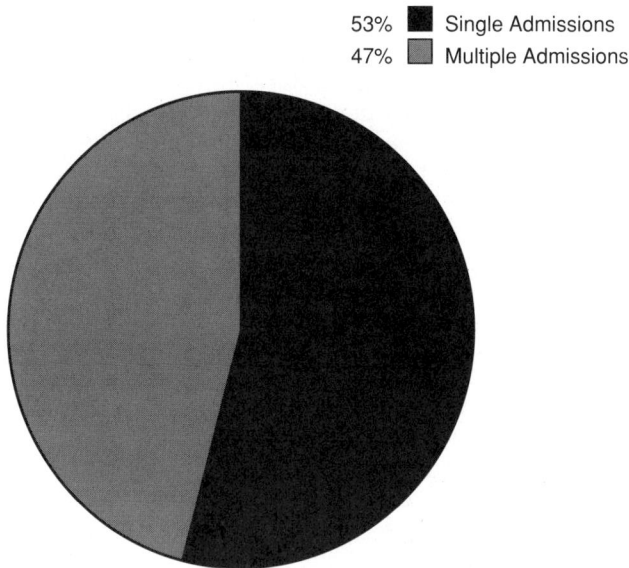

53% ■ Single Admissions
47% ■ Multiple Admissions

Figure 79–2. Percentage of different types of admissions.

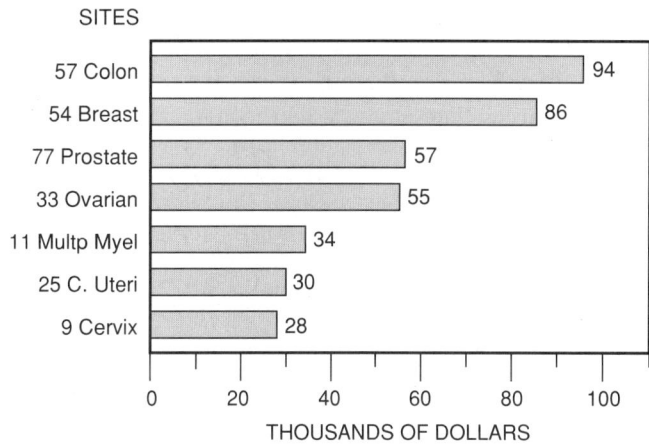

SITES

Figure 79–4. Diagnosis-related group major profit sites. *Multp. Myel.*, multiple myeloma; *C. Uteri.*, corpus uteri.

bone marrow transplant program. And they may wish to view the impact of the granulocyte colony stimulating factor (GCSF) on shortening hospital lengths of stay.

Figure 79–3 illustrates one facility's top DRG billings by cancer site. Although these sites have generated the highest volume of charges, they are not necessarily the most profitable. Figure 79–4 illustrates the most profitable cancer sites for this same facility, and Figure 79–5 illustrates the "losers."

It is important to note that even losers can be important to a facility's survival. When hospitals attempt to determine their costs of care, they develop a formula that is roughly half their fixed costs and half variable costs. A fixed cost is something that cannot be changed easily, such as the annual cost of maintaining the building itself and the amortized cost of construction. Therefore, half of the costs cannot be altered no matter what administrators do. The other half of hospital costs might be categorized into variable and semivariable costs. An example of a variable cost is the level of staffing of an oncology unit. An administrator can readily alter one or two positions up or

portion of their associated revenues. As Figure 79–2 illustrates, about half of the cancer patient admissions at one tertiary care facility (Katterhagen et al., 1989) came from patients who were admitted to the hospital only once, whereas the other half came from patients who were admitted many times. In this case (and in many similar cases), about three fourths of the patients generated half the admissions (those single admissions), whereas the other half of the admissions were generated by one quarter of the patients who returned to the facility a number of times. It is the patients who return to the facility many times who confuse the typical hospital accounting system and lower the estimates of the impact of cancer on hospital revenues.

In a few cases, hospital administrators have been able to track costs and are beginning to review subsets of patients with cancer and determine whether they are winners or losers. Thus, for example, administrators can determine whether they wish to offer low-cost mammography to increase breast cancer patient admissions. They may wish to look at patients with acute myelogenous leukemia and determine the value of a

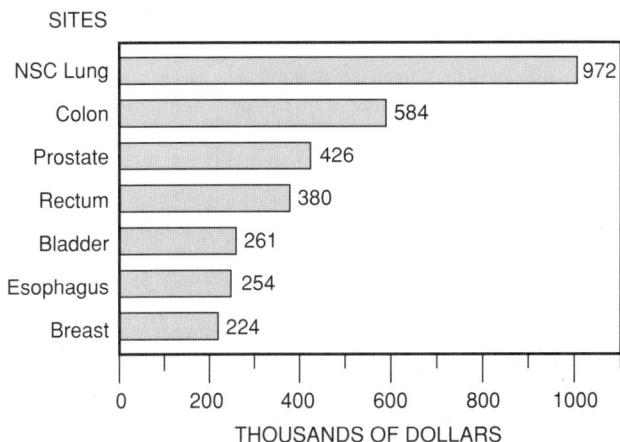

SITES

Figure 79–3. Top diagnosis-related group billings by cancer site. *NSC*, non-small-cell.

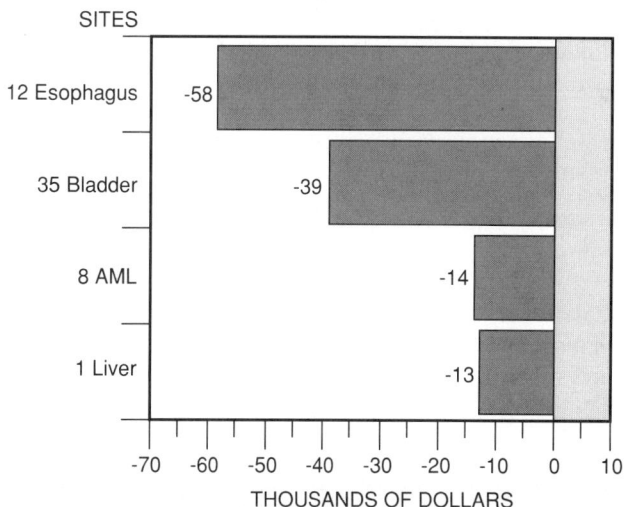

SITES

Figure 79–5. Diagnosis-related group major loss sites. *AML*, acute myelogenous leukemia.

down without too much difficulty. A semivariable cost might be the unit itself. Opening or closing a unit is a much bigger decision and has greater implications.

Discharges that generate high volume that are marginal losers can still be valuable to a hospital because they help to cover the fixed costs and assets that the administrator will have to pay for out of other patient revenues if not these cases. For example, non-small-cell lung cancer discharges may lose $16,000 on a volume of $1 million. This amount is still a vital part of the hospital's basic revenues, even if a small (marginal) amount is below costs. If these patients also contribute to semivariable and variable costs, they can be very valuable. Thus, for example, breast cancer at the facility reviewed earlier is valuable because of its high profit margin, whereas lung cancer is valuable for its high volume and contribution to overhead.

National Policy Setters: A Confusion of Goals and Values

The shift from retrospective to prospective and managed care reimbursement has had major implications for cancer care and research. Indeed, federal agencies have demonstrated a bewildering ability to head in more policy directions simultaneously than a confused hydra-headed monster.

Although the National Institutes of Health (NIH) is mandated to encourage research, technology transfer, and preventive care, the HCFA refuses to pay for patients on NIH experimental therapy (Wagner & Power, 1986), develops regulations that slow down the dissemination and use of new technologies, and does not pay for routine detection and prevention tests. Of course, all of these policies affect current and future cancer care.

Between 1982 and 1988, the NIH did not even acknowledge that there was a problem with reimbursement for patients who participate in formal clinical trials. But Medicare will not pay for the extra costs of patients in trials, and many insurance plans specifically exclude payment for such patients. Until the mid 1980s, this was not much of a problem because the policy was not generally enforced. As finances tightened, however, insurers began to identify patients in formal clinical research trials and to deny payment for tests, hospitalizations, and even physician fees (Antman, Schnipper, & Frei, 1988; Katterhagen & Mortenson, 1984; Lee & Mortenson, 1984; Mortenson, 1988c, 1989a; Wagner & Power, 1986; Yarbro & Mortenson, 1985).

Concern over the potential impact of fixed-price (DRG or capitated) reimbursement on cancer patient management and clinical research led to a series of investigations by the Association of Community Cancer Centers (ACCC). Two specific concerns emerge from the concept of a fixed-price system of reimbursement:

- Progress in management of patients with cancer depends on a significant number of research innovations. If innovative methods of care are more

expensive than the prevailing methods of care, there is little likelihood that the new methods will be adopted unless the fixed price shifts. In many cases, it seems likely that the more expensive forms of care will be foregone unless the therapeutic advantage is significant. Yet who is to determine what qualifies as a significant therapeutic advantage? Recently, one pharmaceutical company reported that reimbursement for a new form of therapy that extended the lives of patients with prostate cancer by 7 months was being refused by insurers despite the fact that it was lower in cost on a monthly basis than the prevailing forms of therapy (Mortenson, 1989a). The problem was that patients on the new therapy lived longer so the total cost of therapy was higher.

- If clinical research (vital to the development of new innovations) is more costly than conventional patient management, it is likely to be discouraged by hospital administrators or managed care executives who are trying to contain costs wherever possible (Yarbro & Mortenson, 1985). An overt federal policy that denies payment for patients in clinical trials and sets an example to other insurers is likely to lead to obstacles that stop all clinical research.

Problems with Reimbursement for Cancer Research

Before the introduction of PPS, there were already a large number of prohibitions on research on new drugs. In an article entitled "Federal Regulation and Pharmaceutical Innovation," the president of Pfizer noted that regulation was already shortening the effective patent life of a product from 13.8 years in 1966 to about 8.9 years in 1977, seriously affecting the viability of the American pharmaceutical industry and reducing the incentives for new drug development in the United States (Laubach, 1980). Recognizing these problems with the new PPS in 1982, the ACCC asked the Department of Health and Human Services (DHHS) to make some exceptions in the PPS law for cancer research.

Starting in 1982, the association and others began a series of studies aimed at determining the impact of DRG (fixed price) reimbursement on both treatment and clinical research (Katterhagen & Mortenson, 1984; Mortenson & Winn, 1984; Yarbro & Mortenson, 1985). Using this data, a case was then made to the Congress, the DHHS, the HCFA, and the NIH and the National Cancer Institute (NCI) regarding the difficulties uncovered.

Congress took several measures to ensure that innovation in health care would continue and that research in general, and cancer research in particular, would not be curtailed. One of the measures instructed the secretary of DHHS to exempt hospitals doing a considerable amount of cancer research and treatment from the new PPS. Another established the Prospective Payment Assessment Commission as an arm of the congressional Office of Technology Assessment and mandated that this new agency target required changes in the DRG (prospective pricing system) to ensure that quality of care is appropriately compensated and that innovation continues.

The Secretary of DHHS (then Margaret Heckler) and HCFA administrator Carolyn Davis recommended that nothing be done about providing extra compensation to hospitals engaged in research (Davis, 1985; Yarbro & Mortenson, 1985). Regulations formulated by DHHS required extremely high levels of cancer research for an institution to receive an exemption from PPS. Only five NCI-designated comprehensive cancer centers were declared exempt from PPS by the initial regulations.

After some pressure from Senator Robert Dole (then Chairman of the Health Appropriations Subcommittee), the secretary established a panel to review the potential problems; it met once and decided to take a "wait and see" attitude. Members of the panel from the ACCC, the American Medical Association, and other specialty societies argued that there were already concrete examples of innovations and research being halted when DRGs were in force. Yet other representatives of hospitals and medical schools remained publicly silent.

Members from the NIH, the NCI, the Assistant Secretary for Planning and Evaluation, the HCFA, and the DHHS secretary's office generally exhibited a "party line" approach to the problem during the commission meeting. However, at one point, the director of the NIH turned to the assistant secretary of DHHS and said, "I hope you are right about this policy because there is no way my budget can stand the stress of all the additional patient care costs of patients on research protocols." In the final analysis, however, the director of NIH said he perceived no problem. The DHHS secretary's office maintained that the "teaching supplement" provided to university medical schools for training was a proxy compensation for research activities and was sufficient to cover the extra costs of new research approaches.

Subsequent to the DHHS commission, only one adjustment was made to the regulations developed to compensate hospitals and centers that performed a great deal of cancer research. This was to drop the formula required to qualify for an exemption from the PPS from 75 per cent of all discharges to 50 per cent so that the M. D. Anderson Tumor Institute would qualify for an exemption and Congressman Jake Pickle would be satisfied. No other political accommodations were made, and only six university-based cancer institutes throughout the nation were declared exempt. Although the National Cancer Advisory Board issued a statement of concern that some hospitals and research institutions were in jeopardy, NCI officials publicly stated that they did not perceive a problem.

Studies initiated by the ACCC were followed by large-scale studies of cancer DRG reimbursement undertaken by the NCI to determine if any past change in reimbursement had affected research. Although critics suggested that the NCI studies were developed to serve as an apologist for the administration's position on DRGs, the Prospective Payment Assessment Commission (ProPAC) urged Congress to make several moves to compensate for new innovations and inadequacies in reimbursement for new innovations. The results of the NCI studies were never published.

Data developed by the ACCC were utilized by ProPAC as the basis for recommending that the reimbursement of leukemia patients be altered. The NCI and other research officials began to appraise the cost effectiveness of proposed new protocols to determine whether new institutions would be likely to undertake them.

Researchers at Johns Hopkins University issued research findings that pointed out that patients at organized cancer programs were more expensive to treat and that DRGs did not compensate for differences in severity (Horn & Sharkey, 1986; Mortenson, 1986b). Their data noted the significant disparities in funding for research patients that could be prohibitive.

Throughout the early 1980s, no public statement was made that departed from the policy expressed by HCFA Administrator Davis's article in the *Journal of the American Medical Association* (1985). In a response to an article in that journal by Yarbro and Mortenson (1985), Davis said that there was no cause for concern. Patient care costs of research patients were included in the national pool when the initial calculations of DRGs were made and thus they were covered by the PPS system.

As recently as 1986, two researchers from the Office of Technology Assessment reported " . . . cost-based payment permitted subsidy of some clinical research costs by Medicare, but the same data limitations that allowed such subsidies to occur also preclude accurate estimation of the magnitude of the subsidy. Yet, the impact of PPS on clinical research depends to a great extent on how large the subsidy was to begin with" (Wagner & Power, 1986). Noting that "it is not altogether clear at this time whether such 'fixes' are necessary or even desirable," the authors added the following:

The Association of Community Cancer Centers has suggested the establishment of a separate DRG for patients participating in research, and the National Cancer Advisory Board has suggested that research-related expenses for cancer patients be reimbursed as a cost pass-through. Of course, either of these alternatives requires official recognition of Medicare reimbursement for research-related costs. Since DHHS has interpreted the Medicare law as prohibiting payment for most kinds of research, these options are infeasible without regulatory or legislative changes.

Subsequently, federal and pharmaceutical research leaders have watched as clinical researchers report increasing difficulties in conducting their research trials. Medicare intermediaries are now denying all payments for research drugs even if they are commonly used for this indication. In many cases, individual physician fees and entire hospital stays are being denied on the basis that Medicare does not pay for research patients. Third parties are now denying payments for all of their clinical research patients. Clearly, the policy is having a major negative impact on NIH's mission. Yet it was not until 1988 that some leading NCI researchers broke ranks and began to discuss the problem in a series of federally sponsored forums.

Finally, late in 1988, the NCI and other NIH officials began a series of national meetings in an attempt to draw attention to the growing problems faced by the NIH. If the policy remains in effect, a great many innovations will be scrapped because they are too costly to test or appear initially to be more costly than the prevailing therapy. Of course, experience teaches that some higher-cost therapies are greatly reduced in price once in widespread use.

The HCFA is now suggesting that cost effectiveness be proved before a drug can be reimbursed. Because research methodologies for cost effectiveness are widely variable, significant problems in new drug approvals and reimbursements will occur.

The problems with health care policymaking are likely to continue. The HCFA's job is to contain costs. The NIH's job is to develop and promote the use of new technologies. National priorities in the 1990s will continue to focus on balancing the United States budget and reducing the budget deficit. These goals will require major economies in health care, and they are likely to take precedent over other priorities such as research. The best guess is that when clinical research is significantly crippled, some action will likely be taken to alleviate the problem.

Problems with Reimbursement for New Technologies

In addition to the problems with reimbursement for patients on clinical trials, reimbursement for the use of new technologies that have proved to be more effective has faced increasing obstacles as third-party intermediaries and other insurers attempt to find some uniform criteria for payment. These groups wish to establish Food and Drug Administration (FDA) labeling as the criteria for payment, which would cause a major problem for cancer care. To understand this problem, some knowledge about the drug approval process and the common use of drugs is necessary. Basically, the FDA has traditionally reviewed and approved new drugs, judging their safety and efficacy for a particular use or indication. This is a lengthy process, involving data analysis from highly controlled studies.

Once a drug is approved, pharmaceutical companies can market it for approved indications, and physicians can use it as they see fit. Of course, physicians who use drugs without regard to their scientific merit risk malpractice suits. Although pharmaceutical manufacturers cannot market their drugs outside of the approved FDA labeling, physicians and scientists have often used drugs for indications that were not listed on the label. In cancer, cooperative group research provides a strong basis for the use of chemotherapeutic and biologic agents, well beyond the indications approved by the labeling. In fact, my research indicates that approximately 47 per cent of all chemotherapy

use is outside of the approved labeling (Mortenson, 1988a, 1988b).

This finding is not unusual. In fact, three major reference compendia have been developed over the past several decades that include both FDA indications and other accepted uses of drugs. The U.S. Pharmacopeia's *Drug Information for the Health Care Professional,* the *AMA Drug Evaluations,* and the *American Hospital Formulary Service Drug Information* all involve scientists and clinicians in evaluations of the literature. All three compendia were cited in the ill fated federal Catastrophic Insurance Act as standard references. Data from the USPDI suggest that 25 per cent of the accepted indications are not on the FDA label. These other accepted indications could readily account for 40 to 50 per cent of all drug use.

If insurance companies force pharmaceutical and biotechnology manufacturers to seek FDA approval before they pay for every new use, proven technologies will take a great deal of time to gain widespread use. Indeed, physicians are reporting major difficulties in obtaining reimbursement for new cancer technologies and major increases in the administrative time required to cajole insurance companies into paying for new technology and care.

One three-member oncology group's experience may be indicative. Over the past 3 years, this group's members have seen a steady increase in the volume of patients they are managing; their total consultations and practice have increased by 30 per cent. Yet their revenues have remained the same, and they report an additional 20 per cent of their time is now being spent attempting to secure payment for drugs and agents for their patients. From a national policy standpoint, reimbursement for all current cancer therapy, all patients on clinical trials, and all new therapies would account for less than one tenth of 1 per cent of the national health care bill (Mortenson, 1989b), surely a good investment.

New Locations for Cancer Care

As patients with cancer have been removed from hospital settings, alternative delivery systems have sprung up. Freestanding cancer centers represent a move away from hospitals to outpatient centers. Although the primary method of care in many of these centers is radiation therapy, medical oncology and, in a few rare instances, outpatient surgical facilities are also included.

Home care is emerging as a major mechanism for delivery of chemotherapy because of the inability of hospitals to receive adequate reimbursement. Thus radiation therapy and chemotherapy have both moved away from the hospital setting to lower-cost outpatient settings. Yet new regulations from HCFA are proposing to end chemotherapy reimbursement in a home setting.

The Impact on Providers

As noted earlier, physicians are finding that setting up practice is more difficult, revenues are going down, patient load is going up, and more time is being spent on administration. Physicians are also faced with the reality of delivering very different levels of care to groups of patients. In some cases, HMOs and other managed care plans have indicated that they will not pay for the care of patients with cancers that have poor prognoses. Thus physicians may be restricted from providing the types of care that might ensure a small percentage of these patients longer survivals or remissions. Without a doubt, this consideration also adds to the stress of the job.

Medical oncologists and other physicians may find that additional restrictions are in the offing. Investments in any health care entity that they prefer are likely to be restricted by pending legislation. As more managed care plans appear, physicians' choices of caregiving locations, tests, and even treatments are going to be restricted. Indeed, I have suggested elsewhere that oncologists are being trained not to be innovators—a concept that has significant implications for future progress in cancer care.

The Future of Health Care Reimbursement

What do we face in the 1990s? All of the change in reimbursement schemes has a real impact on nurses, their patients, and the kind of care they can provide. It will also have an impact on the types of care that will be available in the future.

First, it should be noted that both Medicare and Medicaid are in significant financial trouble. Throughout the last half of the 1980s, a number of individuals have suggested that Medicare benefits would have to be cut. This problem has been exacerbated by the debate and repeal of the Catastrophic Insurance Act, which attempted to provide additional benefits to patients but which also increased the premiums required by individuals who are eligible for Medicare.

Medicaid is a major financial drain on the states, and talk of reform is just beginning. Given that AIDS patient management is approximately 40 per cent covered by Medicaid, many states are seeing their financial problems compounding rapidly. It is possible that several states will not be able to handle the burden of cost under the current system.

Second, as patients have been forced out or kept out of hospitals, outpatient costs have exploded. As the federal government attempts to deal with this growing problem, it is exploring systems such as ambulatory visit groups, which are similar to DRGs. Without question, the federal government will concentrate on categorizing outpatient care into some system with a limited number of options that will allow payment to be fixed to diagnoses and paid for on a fixed-price basis. The other alternative is to attempt to move a major portion of all health care into managed care plans.

Third, insurers are looking for ways to standardize approaches to care to minimize variations in costs and uncertainty. They are aware that 50 per cent of the average cost of care covers the last 6 months of life, and they often suggest that physicians and hospitals take too many measures that do not affect the ultimate outcome but do affect the cost. More and more insurers are attempting to cut costs by limiting the availability of care, restricting the use of new therapies, and insisting on a standardization of therapy. Using a variety of review mechanisms, patients are being kept out of high-cost settings (such as hospitals), discharged earlier, and provided with limited care whenever possible.

Fourth, as the costs of health care continue to rise inexorably as our population grows steadily older, as AIDS becomes more prevalent, and as new technology emerges, insurance plans of all types will be put under greater pressure. Of course, although federal and state governments pick up a major portion of the costs of care through Medicare and Medicaid, third-party insurance plans pick up a substantial portion of the total for industry. And industry has seen the costs of health care insurance skyrocketing. General Motors loudly complains that health care insurance absorbs more of the cost of its cars than steel. Industry leaders are eager to promote competition among health care providers and find alternative forms of care that are more cost effective. Insurance plans that provide consumers with options are likely to become less and less viable as cost shifting from fixed price and capitated systems to these patients continues.

Everyone involved in the competition to provide lower insurance premiums has been in a race since 1982. Each of the insurance companies and managed care plans has been trying to obtain the greatest possible market share (i.e., the percentage of consumers or businesses subscribing to their plan), pushing as many competitors out of the market as possible. At the same time that everyone was cutting prices to get more customers, new technology and other market forces continued to force up the costs of care. The result is that many hospital and private insurance plans have lost significant amounts of money. In 1988, the National Blue Cross and Blue Shield plans announced that they had lost $1 billion in the previous year (Mortenson, 1988d).

Fifth, hospitals have also had their reimbursement from the federal government radically cut as the DRG system starts to crank down the lid on variations. Initially hospital and regional variations in length of stay and practice were allowed, but the DRG system is now national and many hospitals that are used to operating with a profit margin will begin to operate below the break-even point. Many hospitals are experiencing losses now, and increasing numbers of them will fold (Mortenson, 1984). With tighter margins, hospitals will have to focus more attention on "winners" and on lowering the costs of care. They will have less funding for programs and new ventures and less funding for extras. This is likely to affect oncology units and their staffing, for example.

At the same time, some hospitals will build programs that stress "product lines" like oncology and will move to capture a major "market share" in inpatient, outpatient, and home care settings. Product lines are usually organized administrative units that focus the development, activities, and budgets of a particular cluster of services (two other examples are women's services and cardiology). Market share is the percentage of all patients in a region who go to a given hospital. If, for instance, the hospital sees 30 per cent of all of the cancer patients in its primary service area, it would have a 30 per cent market share.

Of course, not all of the news is bad. Many hospitals are still interested in supporting clinical research because they perceive it to be useful in positioning their cancer programs as superior. A whole new range of jobs has opened up in home health care. Some of the deinstitutionalization of patients has allowed them greater freedom, and new and innovative ways to deliver lower cost and ambulatory or outpatient therapies are constantly emerging.

New biotechnologies and pharmaceutical combinations are already in the pipeline, and many pharmaceutical companies are finding ways to support oncologists in their struggle to obtain reimbursement for their patients. National media attention on reimbursement problems is continuing and is likely to increase.

What Will Happen to the Insurance Industry?

In the 1990s, health insurance plans will continue to encounter major difficulties with survival. Self-insured companies will put increasing pressure on the current mechanisms of care, as will managed care organizations, both of which are steadily increasing their share of the marketplace.

Health insurance has often been considered to be the "loss leader" of the life insurance industry. During the late 1980s and the early 1990s, health insurance and life insurance companies have begun to divorce, weakening the base of major health insurance plans and causing higher premiums. The increasing number of patients with AIDS is also a major contributing factor. Smaller managed care plans, especially in medium-sized communities, will fail. As their reserves and margins go down, insurance plans will continue to cut services and restrict access to care while they attempt to force providers to maintain publicly acceptable quality standards (Futurist Predicts, 1988).

Unfortunately for patients with cancer, as with so many other aspects of the reimbursement system over the past decade, yesterday's good news is today's bad news. Because cancer was a life-threatening illness with no sure cure, insurance companies in the past allowed almost any cancer claim to be paid. Today, recognizing that many cancers are incurable and that the public perceives that cancer is most likely to be fatal, insurance companies are taking advantage and denying therapies and reimbursement. Only consumer or business pressure can force insurance companies to alter this trend, and the complexity of the issue militates against consumers understanding how their care is being manipulated and driven by inadequate reimbursement.

Concerns about Quality of Care

Entering the 1990s, increasing numbers of elderly, sick patients with significant health care problems are being seen on an inpatient basis. More patients will be seen as outpatients or at home. Care will be restricted. Different levels of care will be available to various patient groups.

Although a number of measures have been taken to cut costs, the federal government and insurers want to ensure that quality is not sacrificed. To force the industry to make a conscious effort, HCFA annually publishes mortality statistics for hospitals by categories, such as cardiology and oncology. Everyone, including the HCFA, agrees that the methodology that produces these statistics is terrible, but the press publishes the results, and the health care industry is scrambling to develop alternative measures of quality care. The Joint Commission on Accreditation of Healthcare Organizations is leading this charge, developing clinical indicators based on appropriate outcomes (Mortenson, Kerner, & Novak, 1987; O'Leary, 1987). Oncology clinical indicators were completed in 1989 and went into initial testing in 1989 and 1990. These clinical indicators are worthy of more discussion than can be managed here. However, it should be noted that clinical indicators are likely to be used by insurers to determine what they will pay for and where.

Although health care providers have classically disdained discussions of reimbursement, marketing, and advertising, they can no longer afford this luxury. Incentives drive the system. Quality care and research are directly affected by payment. Keeping up with these reimbursement and practice issues will help nurses understand the dynamics of cancer care and give them an opportunity to affect it by working within their professional organizations and the oncology community.

References

Antman, K., Schnipper, L., & Frei, E. (1988). The crisis in clinical cancer research: Third-party insurance and investigational therapy. *New England Journal of Medicine, 319,* 46.

Davis, C. (1985). The impact of prospective payment on clinical research progress. *Journal of the American Medical Association, 253,* 686–687.

Feldstein, P. J. (1980). The political environment of regulation. In A. Levin (Ed.), *Regulating health care: The struggle for control* (Proceedings of The Academy of Political Science), *33*(4).

Futurist predicts significant changes in health care. (1988). *Oncology Issues, 3,* 26.

Horn, S. D., & Sharkey, P. D. (1986). A study of patients in cancer-related DRGs. *Journal of Cancer Program Management, 1*(2), 8–14.

Katterhagen, J. G., Clarke, R. T., & Mortenson, L. E. (1989). Understanding the economics of inpatient cancer care. *Oncology Issues, 4,* 11–14.

Katterhagen, J. G., & Mortenson, L. E. (1984). Clinical research patients generate significant losses under diagnosis related groups (DRGs). *Seminars in Oncology, 11,* 330–331.

Laubach, G. D. (1980). Federal regulation and pharmaceutical innovation. In A. Levin (Ed.), *Regulating health care: The struggle for control* (Proceedings of The Academy of Political Science), *33*(4).

Lee, C., & Mortenson, L. E. (1984, August/September). Clinical research patients exceed costs of cancer patients within the same DRG category. *Cancer Program Bulletin*, pp. 6–7.

Mortenson, L. E. (1984). Can oncology nursing survive DRGs? *Journal of Oncology Nursing, 11*, 14–15.

Mortenson, L. E. (1985, September). *Cancer diagnosis related groups.* Washington, DC: Association of Community Cancer Centers.

Mortenson, L. E. (1986a). Cancer diagnosis related groups. In L. E. Mortenson, P. N. Anderson, & P. F. Engstrom (Eds.), *Advances in cancer control health care financing and research* (pp. 149–155). New York: Alan R. Liss, Inc.

Mortenson, L. E. (1986b). Without severity-adjusted DRGs, prospective payment may severely impair state-of-the art cancer care. *Journal of Cancer Program Management, 1*(2), 1.

Mortenson, L. E. (1988a). Audit indicates half of current chemotherapy users lack FDA approval. *Journal of Cancer Program Management, 3*(1), 21–26.

Mortenson, L. E. (1988b). Audit indicates many users of combination therapy are unlabeled. *Journal of Cancer Program Management, 3*(2), 33.

Mortenson, L. E. (1988c). The grocery store syndrome. *Oncology Nursing Forum, 15*, 545–546.

Mortenson, L. E. (1988d, May). The impact of reimbursement on quality cancer care. *Business and Health*, pp. 38–40.

Mortenson, L. E. (1989a). Starve them or shoot them. *Oncology Issues, 4*(1), 2.

Mortenson, L. E. (1989b, May 11). Tight-money casualties in the war on cancer: Insurers target chemotherapy payments. *Wall Street Journal*, p. A14.

Mortenson, L. E., Anderson, P. N., & Novak, C. (1986). What the research bases have to say about CCOPs. *Cancer Program Bulletin, 12*(1), 4–5.

Mortenson, L. E., & Baum, H. M. (1985, December). Cancer DRG's: 1985 analysis. *Cancer Program Bulletin*, pp. 7–11.

Mortenson, L. E., Kerner, J. F., & Novak, C. M. (1987). Striving for excellence: Evaluating quality of care in oncology. *Journal of Cancer Program Management, 2*(1), 21–29.

Mortenson, L. E., & Winn, R. (1983). The potential negative impact of prospective reimbursement on cancer treatment and clinical research progress. *Cancer Program Bulletin, 9*(3), 1–4.

Mortenson, L. E., & Winn, R. (1984). DRGs: How will they affect your practice—and cancer care. *Your Patient and Cancer, 4*(2), 28–38.

Mortenson, L. E., & Yarbro, J. W. (1983). Oncology DRG research produces key findings for cancer program managers and policy makers. *Journal of Cancer Program Management, 1*(2), 6–7.

Mortenson, L. E., Yarbro, J. W., Clarke, R. T., & Cahill, E. (1985, March). Conventional cancer patient management and DRG's: A first report of ACCC's DRG research program. *Cancer Program Bulletin, 11*, 3–5.

Mortenson, L. E., Young, J. L., Jr., & Ney, M. S. (1988). Variations in cancer DRG profit and loss by hospital size and region of the nation. *Journal of Cancer Program Management, 3*(4), 16–19.

O'Leary, D. S. (1987). Quality control challenges in the new competitive marketplace. *Journal of Cancer Program Management, 2*(1), 6–10.

Pollard, M. R. (1980). Fostering competition in health care. In A. Levin (Ed.), *Regulating health care: The struggle for control* (Proceedings of The Academy of Political Science) *33*(4).

Salkever, D., & Bice, T. (1978). Certificate-of-need legislation and hospital costs. In M. Zubkoff, I. Raskin, & R. Hanft (Eds.), *Hospital cost containment.* New York: PRODIST.

Wagner, J. L., & Power, E. (1986). Diagnosis-related groups (DRG) payment and clinical research: In search of the problem. *Cancer Investigation, 4*(1), 61–67.

Yarbro, J. W., & Mortenson, L. E. (1985). The need for DRG 471—protection for clinical research. *Journal of the American Medical Association, 253*, 684–685.

Young, J. L., Jr., Mortenson, L. E., & Ney, M. S. (1988). Hospital reimbursement, charges, and profit and loss for cancer and cancer-related DRGs. *Journal of Cancer Program Management, 3*(4), 9.

CHAPTER 80

Documentation of the Nursing Process in Cancer Nursing

CHRISTINE MIASKOWSKI
BEVERLY NIELSEN

Documentation of the nursing process is a critical part of professional nursing practice. The primary purpose of any documentation system is to ensure continuity of quality patient care (Morrissey-Koss, 1988). Most nurses, in all practice settings, see documentation as a time-consuming exercise that detracts from direct patient care activities rather than as an opportunity to communicate essential information about the patient's health status to other disciplines as well as document the essential contribution of professional nursing practice to the care of the patient.

The purpose of this chapter is to discuss the essential components of and present a framework for a nursing documentation system for the patient with cancer in the acute care setting. The chapter addresses the use of standards of care as part of a documentation system. The chapter concludes with a summary of legal issues involved in documentation and addresses issues related to computerization of the documentation process.

EXTERNAL STANDARDS AND THE DOCUMENTATION PROCESS

Documentation of nursing care is an essential component of the American Nurses' Association and the Oncology Nursing Society (ANA-ONS) *Standards of Oncology Nursing Practice* (1987), the ANA *Standards for Organized Nursing Services* (1988), and the Standards for Nursing Services developed by the Joint Commission for Accreditation of Health Care Organizations (JCAHO) (1987). All three standards focus on the nursing process as the essential framework for any documentation system. The nursing process represents a systematic method of providing care to patients (JCAHO, 1987). In the acute care setting, the nursing process begins the moment the patient enters the health care system and terminates when the patient

is discharged from the hospital. All three sets of standards concur that the essential elements of the nursing process are assessment, planning, implementation, and evaluation. These four components of the nursing process form the framework for all nursing activities. The nursing process itself (that is, nurse-patient interactions) is dynamic and ongoing; however, the various components of the process must be documented in the patient's record.

Although there are four essential steps in the nursing process, there are explicit substeps within each essential element. A schematic of the nursing process with its various subdivisions is illustrated in Figure 80–1. These substeps are usually documented in the patient record using (1) a formal assessment sheet; (2) a nursing care plan that includes nursing diagnoses or patient problems, patient outcome statements or goals, and nursing orders or interventions; and (3) flowsheets or progress notes to document implementation and evaluation of the plan of care.

The nursing service standards of the JCAHO (1987) provide guidance and direction on the key elements that should be included in documenting each specific portion of the nursing process. These standards, however, are a generic document that is meant to be used in a variety of patient care settings with a variety of patient populations. These standards should serve as the broad umbrella framework for designing any documentation system. The ANA-ONS standards (1987) were developed for use by oncology nurses. The standards can be used to develop patient assessment tools, formats for nursing care plans or standards of care for oncology patients, outcome evaluation criteria, and patient record systems specific to an oncology patient population. Integrating the essential elements of these two sets of standards will provide an excellent methodology for developing a clear and concise documentation system for use by oncology nurses caring for patients. The remainder of this chapter uses

I. ASSESSMENT

↓

IA. Initial data collection

↓

IB. Ongoing data collection

↓

IC. Formulation of nursing diagnoses

↓

II. PLANNING

↓

IIA. Outcome and goal setting

↓

IIB. Nursing orders and interventions

↓

III. IMPLEMENTATION

↓

IV. EVALUATION

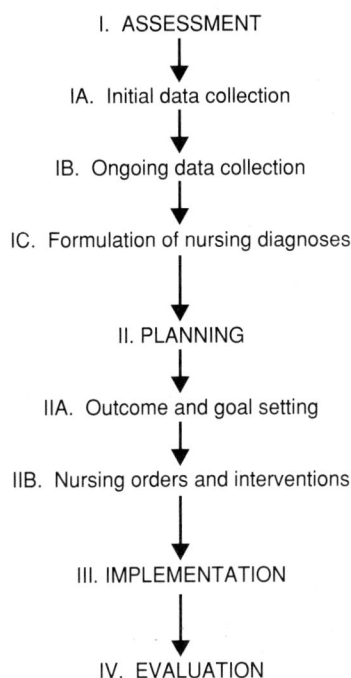

Figure 80–1. Steps in the nursing process. (From Miaskowski, C. [1985, August]. Nursing diagnosis within the context of the nursing process. *Occupational Health Nursing*, pp. 401–404. Adapted with permission.)

these two sets of standards in describing a clinically useful documentation system.

Documentation Process

Assessment

Assessment refers to the process of collecting information about a patient's health status. It is the most fundamental and critical portion of the nursing process because it provides the nurse with the essential data necessary to formulate nursing diagnoses and develop a plan of care (Miaskowski & Nielsen, 1985). The ANA-ONS standards (1987) mandate that "the oncology nurse systematically and continually collects data regarding the health status of the client." The JCAHO requires that each patient's nursing care needs be assessed by a registered professional nurse within 8 hours of admission to an acute care setting. Assessment parameters that should be included in the initial assessment are physical and functional characteristics, psychosocial characteristics, past and current medical history, current medications and treatments, patient and family educational needs, discharge planning needs, and environmental or equipment needs (JCAHO, 1987).

Several assessment tools designed for patients with cancer have been described (Dudjak, 1988; McCray, 1979; Miaskowski & Nielsen, 1985; Moritz, 1979; Welch, Follo & Nelson, 1982). The Cancer Nursing Assessment Tool, developed by Miaskowski and Nielsen (1985), has been revised (Nielsen & Miaskowski, 1987) and is presented in Appendix 80–1. This tool was developed on the basis of a review of the literature,

the personal experience of the authors, and the ANA-ONS *Standards of Oncology Nursing Practice* (1987). The aim of the tool was to create a clear and concise interview guide that optimized the collection of the initial assessment data. The 11 high incidence problem areas, common to patients, defined in the ANA-ONS standards became the framework for the tool's development (Table 80–1). By using an initial assessment tool that incorporates the ANA-ONS standards, the nurse is directed in gathering pertinent information that will enable the definition of actual or potential nursing diagnoses for persons with cancer. Specific sections devoted to the 11 high incidence problem areas allow for the gathering of systematic information on the most common problems experienced by patients with cancer.

Page 1 of the Cancer Nursing Assessment Tool is designed to gather demographic information and data on the patient's illness experience, including the presenting problem, the history of the cancer problem and the treatments employed, previous illnesses and hospitalizations, allergies, and medications. Also included in this portion of the assessment is information on expectations and concerns related to hospitalization and health maintenance habits. The instrument provides cues for the nurse to structure the interview. Data from this portion of the instrument can be used to formulate nursing diagnoses related to knowledge deficits about the disease and treatment as well as diagnoses related to potential or actual alterations in coping.

The remaining three pages of the instrument, entitled the Nursing Diagnosis Database, are structured around the 11 high incidence problem areas. Each section of the Nursing Diagnosis Database should be completed by first obtaining the information listed in the right-hand column of the tool. Then, using the cues listed in the left-hand column, the nurse should obtain additional information for the specific category. If there are no abnormalities within a specific category, the box next to the phrase "within normal limits" (WNL) should be checked.

This assessment tool is detailed and specific. It allows the nurse to collect *comprehensive baseline* data on the patient. By reviewing the database and evaluating those categories for which the box WNL is *not* checked,

Table 80–1. ELEVEN HIGH INCIDENCE PROBLEM AREAS IN ONCOLOGY

1. Prevention and early detection
2. Information
3. Coping
4. Comfort
5. Nutrition
6. Protective mechanisms
7. Mobility
8. Elimination
9. Sexuality
10. Ventilation
11. Circulation

(From American Nurses Association and Oncology Nursing Society. [1987]. *Standards of oncology nursing practice.* Kansas City, MO: American Nurses Association. Reprinted with permission.)

Table 80–2. INITIAL ASSESSMENT AND NURSING DIAGNOSIS FORMULATION

Mr. Jones is a 62-year-old man with a diagnosis of metastatic prostate cancer. Assessment of the comfort category reveals the following information:

Sleep pattern: For the past 3 weeks, awakens every 15–30 min during the night.

Pain description: Severe, continuous pain in back and legs of 3 weeks' duration. Pain is aggravated by any type of activity.

Pain severity: 9

Relief measures: Taking acetominophen with codeine every 3 hr without relief. "Nothing really helps."

Patient states that "the pain is unbearable. I can't go on like this anymore."

Nursing Diagnosis

Severe pain related to bony metastasis from prostate cancer.

the nurse is directed to formulate a nursing diagnosis related to that particular problem area. An example of how this process would occur is outlined in Table 80–2.

The final page of the assessment tool focuses on the assessment of the patient's coping abilities as well as social and economic supports. Emphasis is placed on performing a comprehensive assessment of the patient's family or significant others. This portion of the patient's admission assessment is critical because nurses must begin discharge planning on admission. In today's health care environment, with the early discharge of patients from the hospital, the family's strengths, weaknesses, and resources must be evaluated to determine their ability to serve as primary caregivers in the home. The social integrity, anticipated teaching needs, and discharge planning portions of the database provide cues for performing this portion of the assessment.

This type of initial assessment tool can be adapted to a variety of practice settings. The structure based on the ANA-ONS standards guides the nurse in performing a clear, concise, and structured interview that then enables him or her to formulate actual and potential nursing diagnoses easily and subsequently to develop a plan of care specific for the patient with cancer.

The process of patient assessment does not end with the initial interview. Data about the patient must be collected and recorded on an ongoing basis. These additional data are collected for the following purposes: (1) to complete the initial assessment, (2) to validate previous findings, or, most often, (3) to evaluate changes in the patient's clinical condition. Documentation of ongoing assessment data is best accomplished through the use of flowsheets. Information can be recorded on vital sign sheets, intake and output sheets, and temperature sheets. An example of a flowsheet that can be used to document the ongoing assessment of the oncology patient is illustrated in Appendix 80–2. This form allows the nurse on an 8-hour basis to document changes in the patient's condition in a clear, concise, and comprehensive manner. Again, the flowsheet is constructed around the 11 high incidence problem areas (ANA & ONS, 1987). The instrument requires simply checking the presence or absence of clinical signs and symptoms or simple doc-

umentation of pertinent information about the patient's condition or performance of activities of daily living by checking the appropriate box. The nurse may need to document more specific information on abnormal findings in the progress notes. In addition, this tool provides the nurse with a ready reference of the patient's status during the previous 24 hours.

Planning

Planning is the second step in the nursing process. The JCAHO requires that a registered professional nurse plan each patient's nursing care. The plan must be reviewed and revised as necessary. The plan must include (1) goals or outcomes that are realistic, measurable, and specific to the patient; (2) interventions that are specific to the patient and measurable; (3) evidence of patient and family involvement in the plan of care; and (4) discharge planning (JCAHO, 1987). The ANA-ONS standards (1987) state that the "oncology nurse develops an outcome-oriented care plan that is individualized and holistic. This plan is based on nursing diagnoses and incorporates preventive, therapeutic, rehabilitative, palliative, and comforting nursing actions." The purpose of developing a plan of care is to guide nursing interventions and facilitate the desired outcomes for the patient and the family.

The plan of care should be based on patient and family needs identified through assessment data. The ANA-ONS standards specify that patient needs should be described in terms of a nursing diagnosis. The diagnosis should be a statement of an actual or potential health problem that is amenable to nursing interventions. The diagnostic statement becomes the framework for the development of the nursing care plan. The diagnosis should be recorded and prioritized according to the actual or potential threat to the patient.

The process of developing a plan of care for each identified nursing diagnosis consists of two phases: (1) the formulation of goals or outcomes and (2) the determination of specific nursing orders or interventions to achieve the desired outcomes. Outcome statements must meet the criteria listed in Table 80–3. These outcome statements should be used to evaluate the patient's progress and the efficacy of the nursing interventions.

Nursing orders and interventions are designed to facilitate the medical care prescribed and to restore, maintain, or promote the patient's well-being. The

Table 80–3. CRITERIA FOR OUTCOME AND GOAL STATEMENTS

Outcome and goal statements for each nursing diagnosis are:
Developed with the patient to ensure individualization
Stated in realistic and measurable terms
Congruent with other planned therapies
Assigned a time period for achievement
Designed to maximize the patient's functional capabilities

(Adapted from *Hospital accreditation program scoring guidelines.* [1987]. Chicago: Joint Commission for Accreditation of Hospitals; and American Nurses Association & Oncology Nursing Society. [1987]. *Standards of oncology nursing practice.* Kansas City, MO: American Nurses Association.)

scope of the plan is determined by the patient's actual as well as anticipated needs (JCAHO, 1987). The plan should be developed on the basis of current scientific information and research findings (ANA & ONS, 1987). Individualized interventions should be designed to manage the following areas: (1) physical and functional factors, (2) psychosocial factors, (3) environmental factors, (4) patient and family education, and (5) discharge planning. A key element in documenting the plan of care in the patient's record is to provide evidence that the plan has been revised on the basis of the patient's progress or lack of progress toward goal achievement. Key aspects of planning care for patients, which have been identified in the ANA-ONS standards, are that the oncology nurse collaborates with appropriate members of the multidisciplinary team in planning the patient's treatment plan and that once the plan is formulated, the nurse is responsible for communicating the plan to the appropriate members of the multidisciplinary team.

Implementation

The third step in the nursing process is implementation. This is the action-oriented portion of the nursing process. Documentation of nursing interventions is again best accomplished through the use of flowsheets. These types of documentation tools should be designed to streamline the documentation of interventions. An example of one type of form for documenting nursing interventions is illustrated in Appendix 80–3. This tool has specific interventions frequently performed on an oncology unit preprinted on the form. The nurse simply indicates the frequency with which the interventions are performed and places the time the interventions were completed in the appropriate 8-hour interval. Additional interventions that are required for a particular patient can be added to the flowsheet.

Evaluation

The final step in the nursing process is evaluation. The ANA-ONS standards (1987) state that "the oncology nurse regularly and systematically evaluates the client's responses to interventions in order to determine progress toward achievement of outcomes and to revise the database, nursing diagnoses and the plan of care." The process of evaluation must be documented. It is not sufficient to record interventions. The nurse must document the patient's response to medical orders and the patient's response to the implementation of the individualized nursing care plan (JCAHO, 1987), which means that the patient's responses to nursing interventions must be reflected in the patient's record. This documentation is best accomplished in the progress notes. Nursing notes should not duplicate the information that has been recorded on flowsheets. The nursing note should address a specific patient problem and reflect whether or not the patient is progressing toward the desired outcome. If the patient's condition has deteriorated or remained unchanged, the nurse is obligated to evaluate the efficacy of the nursing care

plan and make the necessary revisions to promote the patient's optimal level of functioning. This evaluation and changes in the plan of care should be documented in the progress notes. The nurse can be guided in the evaluation process by asking the questions listed in Table 80–4.

USE OF STANDARDS OF CARE IN DOCUMENTATION

The development of patient care standards is an integral part of nursing practice and a major component of many nursing quality assurance programs. Standards of patient care are developed to guide nursing practice and to monitor and evaluate the quality of nursing care that the patient receives. Standards of care are working documents that need to be refined, modified, and revised on a continuous basis.

A system for integrating standards of patient care into a documentation system is illustrated in Appendix 80–4. The standard consists of the key components of the nursing care plan, that is, the nursing diagnosis, expected patient outcomes, and nursing orders. After the initial patient assessment, the appropriate standard of care for the particular patient is selected. The example provided in this chapter represents one of the 11 high incidence problem areas identified in the ANA-ONS standards, namely, infection. The standard of care must then be individualized for the patient. The nurse dates and initials the diagnostic statement and circles the appropriate etiology or etiologies for the patient. Selection of the etiology makes the diagnostic label highly specific and provides direction for determining the expected outcomes and choosing the nursing orders. The next step in the process is to delineate the expected outcomes for the patient. The outcomes, listed in this example, are directly from the ANA-ONS standards (1987). These outcome statements become the criteria by which the plan of care is evaluated. Following the establishment of patient-specific outcomes, the nurse dates and initials those nursing orders that must be done for the patient and specifies the frequency with which the interventions must be performed. The nurse individualizes the interventions for the patient and may add additional nursing orders as warranted by the patient's clinical condition. It should be noted that nursing protocols can be integrated into patient care standards. In this example, nursing order number 9 indicates that the neutropenia protocol is

Table 80–4. EVALUATION OF PLAN OF CARE

Is the patient/family making progress in achieving the established outcomes or goals?
If the outcomes or goals are not being achieved, why not?
Are the outcomes and goals realistic?
Do the outcomes and goals require more time to be achieved?
Are the nursing orders and interventions correct?
Do the frequency of any or all of the interventions need to be changed?
Are additional nursing orders and interventions required?
Is the nursing diagnosis incorrect, and must additional information be obtained and a new plan of care formulated?

instituted when the patient's neutrophil count falls below 1000. This is a convenient and efficient way to integrate nursing protocols and procedures into patient care standards.

This type of standard of care can become a permanent part of the patient's record. It serves multiple purposes. It establishes an expected level of performance for all nurses on the unit. It eliminates needless duplication of information from a reference manual. It can be individualized to each patient situation. It provides a place to document evidence of updating and revision of the plan of care. It serves as an excellent teaching tool for new staff in how to care for a patient, as in this example, with a potential for infection. This type of standard of care can also become computerized.

Nursing staff on an oncology unit should develop standards of care for the 11 high incidence problem areas listed in the ANA-ONS standards (1987) as well as patient care standards for their high volume patient populations. These types of patient care standards can be easily integrated into a nursing documentation system. They can streamline the documentation process, direct the nursing care provided to an oncology patient population, and serve as a tool to evaluate the quality of care that the patient receives.

LEGAL ISSUES IN DOCUMENTATION

It is beyond the scope of this chapter to document all the legal issues involved in documentation. Several points can be made, however, to ensure that progress notes reflect professional nursing practice, are truly reflective of the patient's condition, and are devoid of legal pitfalls. First, nurses must know the hospital's documentation policies and procedures. Charting of nursing assessments, interventions, and patient evaluations must be done on the correct forms and with the correct frequency. When flowsheets are used, they must be completed in total, including all required entries and without omitting information. Progress notes should describe all pertinent observations clearly and succinctly prior to the documentation of a conclusion. For example, a note should not state, "patient's abdominal wound is not healing." The more appropriate notation would be as follows: "patient's abdominal wound measures 2 × 10 cm. Wound is draining copious amounts of serous sanguinous fluid and necessitated dressing changes five times during the past 8 hours. No granulation tissue present. Patient complaining of pain around edges of the incision. Wound is not healing. Dr. Smith will evaluate the wound the next time the dressing is changed." A complete citation, like the latter example, including a specific description of the status of the wound, makes it easier to review the progress of the wound over time and to evaluate the efficacy of the treatment plan (Laros, 1987).

Another general rule of documentation is to avoid block charting. Progress notes should be dated, the specific time they are being written should be indicated. It is permissible to refer to specific times when documenting occurrences, within the body of the progress note, but do not make a rule of charting a note at the end of each shift stating "7:00 A.M. to 3:30 P.M." (Laros, 1987).

Another obvious rule about charting is never to obliterate an entry. Entries should not be inked out, covered with whiteout, or erased from a patient record. If a mistake is made, a single line should be drawn through the entry, it should be dated, and the error should be initialed. If a chart with an obliterated entry were subpoenaed in a lawsuit, the obliterated entry could be misconstrued to contain information that may have harmed the patient (Laros, 1987).

Another recommendation to help avoid legal problems if a chart were involved in litigation is not to try to insert a note in the body of the chart if it is not written at the time a specific incident occurred. Notes should be written in sequence, dated, and timed. If a late entry is required, an explanation of it should appear in the body of the note that this is a late entry (Laros, 1987).

Another rule about documentation is not to use abbreviations. Every hospital has a policy on acceptable abbreviation. If the acceptable list is not used, the meaning of the abbreviations in the progress note can be misconstrued and vital information can be misinterpreted. The record is the primary source of communication about the patient's progress among a variety of disciplines. Therefore, it is important to chart clearly and correctly. Progress notes should be grammatically correct, and correct spelling and punctuation should be used. Handwriting must be legible (Laros, 1987). As noted previously, documentation reflects professional nursing practice and serves as a record of the quality of care that the patient received; therefore, it must be done punctually, succinctly, and effectively.

COMPUTERIZATION AND DOCUMENTATION

In an excellent review of computerization in nursing, Staggers (1988) notes that computers "are fast becoming a part of nurses' everyday work settings." The direct benefits of computerized documentation systems are increased accountability and efficiency. Computers are designed to handle structured inputs. This type of format can improve the quality and accuracy of the patient's record by eliminating omission errors. Nurses are prompted, when using a computerized system, to complete specific items, which eliminates the need for recall of information (Staggers, 1988).

Another major advantage of a computerized documentation system is increased legibility of the patient's record. The typed record virtually eliminates transcription errors or misinterpretations of illegible notes. In addition, the information contained in the record is more accurate and timely (Staggers, 1988).

In terms of efficiency, computers benefit nursing by "decreasing the time spent in communicating, performing clerical activities, waiting for test results and reports, and duplicating data" (Staggers, 1988). Computers are designed to handle large amounts of information smoothly and efficiently. Data are readily accessible from other departments, such as the laboratory. There is no need to duplicate information that is already contained within the patient's database (Staggers, 1988).

The benefits of computerized documentation systems have not been fully appreciated at the present time because many institutions continue to use manual systems. However, nurses who are presently involved in developing documentation systems, for particular patient populations such as oncology, should design systems that are readily adaptable to computerization.

References

American Nurses Association. (1988). *Standards for organized nursing services and responsibilities of nurse administrators across all settings.* Kansas City, MO.

American Nurses Association & Oncology Nursing Society. (1987). *Standards of oncology nursing practice.* Kansas City, MO: American Nurses' Association.

Dudjak, L. (1988). Radiation therapy nursing care record: a tool for documentation. *Oncology Nursing Forum, 15*(6), 763–777.

Joint Commission for Accreditation of Hospitals. (1987). *Hospital accreditation program scoring guidelines.* Chicago.

Laros, P. (1987). Making the most of your charting time. *Nursing 87, 87*(5), 68–73.

McCray, N. D. (1979). Oncology patient assessment tool. *Oncology Nursing Forum, 6*(4), 15–18.

Miaskowski, C. (1985, August). Nursing diagnosis within the context of the nursing process. *Occupational Health Nursing,* pp. 401–404.

Miaskowski, C., & Nielsen, B. (1985). A cancer nursing assessment tool. *Oncology Nursing Forum, 12*(6), 37–42.

Moritz, D. A. (1979). Nursing histories—a guide yes, a form no→ *Oncology Nursing Forum, 6*(4), 18–19.

Morrissey-Ross, M. (1988). Documentation: If you haven't written it, you haven't done it. *Nursing Clinics of North America, 23*(2), 363–371.

Nielsen, B., & Miaskowski, C. (1987). Revision of a cancer nursing assessment tool. *Oncology Nursing Forum, 14*(2, Suppl.), 83.

Staggers, N. (1988). Using computers in nursing—documented benefits and needed studies. *Computers in Nursing, 6*(4), 164–170.

Welch, A., Follo, J., & Nelson, E. (1982). The development of a specialized nursing assessment tool for cancer patients. *Oncology Nursing Forum, 9*(1), 37–44.

APPENDIX 80–1

CANCER NURSING ASSESSMENT TOOL

Name _____

Address _____

_____

Phone _____ Age _____

Marital Status _____

Physician _____

Date	Time	From ☐ Home Other _____

Information From:

Via ☐ Ambulatory   ☐ Wheelchair   ☐ Stretcher

PRIMARY LANGUAGE	
PRESENTING PROBLEM (quote patient's chief complaint)	
HISTORY OF CANCER PROBLEM (description of chronology, duration of symptoms, understanding of conditions)	
PAST AND PRESENT CANCER TREATMENT SURGERY (type, date)	None ☐
RADIATION THERAPY (area radiated, number of courses)	None ☐
CHEMOTHERAPY (drugs, dose, routes, effects, schedule, access devices)	None ☐
OTHER THERAPIES (immunotherapy, hyperthermia, imagery, alternative therapies)	None ☐
OTHER ILLNESSES AND/OR HOSPITALIZATIONS (date and reason)	
FAMILY HISTORY OF CANCER	
EXPECTATIONS AND/OR CONCERNS ABOUT ILLNESS AT PRESENT TIME	
HEALTH MAINTENANCE HABITS (physical exam, exercise, BSE, Pap smear, proctoscopy, testicular exam, mammography, X-ray, dental exam, prostate exam, hemocult)	
ALLERGIES (food, drugs, other allergens and reactions)	None ☐
MEDICATIONS OTHER THAN CHEMOTHERAPY (name, dosages, frequency, home remedies, over-the-counter preparations)	None ☐
KNOWLEDGE OF MEDICATIONS	

NURSING DIAGNOSIS DATABASE—Complete all blank spaces in the right-hand column, then, using the cues in the left-hand column, make a statement in each category describing a deviation from normal; if no deviations, check the box stating "Within Normal Limits."

VENTILATORY INTEGRITY shortness of breath, dyspnea on exertion, paroxysmal nocturnal dyspnea, cyanosis, cough, sputum production, fatigue, tracheostomy, aids to breathing.	Respiratory Rate: Smoking: Breath Sounds: Category WNL ☐
CIRCULATORY INTEGRITY rhythm, pulse deficit, chest pain, palpitations, intermittent claudication, color of extremities, edema, neck veins (JVD), varicosities.	Blood Pressure: Pulse Category WNL ☐
NUTRITION Dysphagia, anorexia, changes in oral mucosa, nausea, vomiting, weight loss, changes in taste, food preferences, dietary patterns, nutritional supplements, feeding devices, hyperalimentation.	DIET: Food Preparation By: Food Intolerances: Height: Current Weight: Weight 6 mos. ago: Alcohol Intake: Dentures: Upper ☐ Lower ☐ Both ☐ None ☐ Oral Exam/Mucositis: Category WNL ☐
INTESTINAL INTEGRITY pain, constipation, diarrhea, distention, tarry stools, change in bowel habits, blood per rectum, hemorrhoids, colostomy, ileostomy, appliances, liver breadth, splenomegaly.	Normal Pattern: Last B.M.: Aids for Bowel Functioning: Hemoccult: Bowel Sounds: Category WNL ☐
RENAL-URINARY INTEGRITY frequency, burning, color, hematuria, nocturia, retention, polyuria, incontinence, flank pain, aids to urination, dialysis, appliances, catheter.	 Category WNL ☐
COMFORT Pain description—location, duration, periodicity, severity, aggravating factors. Relief measures—medication, biofeedback, meditation, TENS, visual imagery, diversional activity, music therapy	Sleep Pattern: Pain Description: Pain Severity (rate on scale of 1 to 10): 1 2 3 4 5 6 7 8 9 10 Relief Measures: Category WNL ☐

PROTECTIVE MECHANISMS Skin integrity—change in wart or mole, color, swelling, turgor, abrasions, petechiae, scars, ulcers, photosensitivity, pruritus, desquamation, temperature, extravasation.	 Category WNL ☐
Immune/Hematologic—chills, fever, rigors, petechiae, nosebleeds.	Temperature: Evidence of Bleeding: Evidence of Infection: Blood Values: Hct Hgb Platelets WBC: Category WNL ☐
SENSORY-PERCEPTUAL INTEGRITY—orientation, memory loss, personality changes, syncope, vertigo, convulsions, headache, numbness, tingling, alterations in heat and cold sensation.	Level of Consciousness: Pupils: Category WNL ☐
VISION—visual disturbances, diplopia, blurring, tearing.	Eye glasses? Yes ☐ No ☐ Contact Lenses? Yes ☐ No ☐ Glass Eye? Yes ☐ No ☐ Degree of Visual Acuity: Category WNL ☐
HEARING—tinnitus, vertigo, pain, discharge.	Hearing Aid? Yes ☐ No ☐ Degree of Hearing Loss: Category WNL ☐
SPEECH—language barrier, aphasia, dysarthria.	 Category WNL ☐
MOBILITY lethargy, gait, muscle weakness, paralysis, deformities, joint swelling, physical tolerance, muscle atrophy, tremors, range of motion, range of ambulation, fractures, set-up at home to assist mobility. **PERFORMANCE EVALUATION** Scale Score ☐	Muscle Strength: RUE LUE RLE LLE Level of Independence: Use of Aids: None ☐ Walker ☐ Cane ☐ Wheelchair ☐ Other: Category WNL ☐
SEXUAL INTEGRITY menses, contraception, pregnancies, breast changes, gynecomastia, impotence, changes in sexual activity, changes in sexual desire, changes in sexual performance.	LMP: Last Pap Smear: Breast Exam Findings: Testicular Exam Findings:

SUGGESTED QUESTIONS

Has having cancer (or its treatment) interfered with your being a mother (wife, husband, father)?

Has your cancer (or its treatment) changed the way you see yourself as a man (woman)?

Has your cancer (or its treatment) caused any change in your sexual functioning (sex life)?

Do you expect your sexual functioning (sex life) to be changed in any way after you leave the hospital?

COPING INTEGRITY
anxiety, anger, depression,
body image changes, affect,
self-esteem, stress, role changes,
communication patterns,
counseling
 	
SUGGESTED QUESTIONS
What do you think caused your
  illness?
Why do you think it started when
  it did?
What do you think your illness does
  to you? How does it work?
How severe is your illness? Does it
  have a long or short duration?
What kind of treatment do you think
  you should receive?
What are the most important results
  you hope to receive from this
  treatment?
What are the chief problems your
  illness has caused for you?
What do you fear most about your
  illness?
	Spirituality:
	Ethnic Background:
	
	Category WNL ☐

SOCIAL INTEGRITY	Occupation: Education: Family-Significant Other: With Whom Does Patient Live? Family Support Systems: Impact of Hospitalization on Family: Economic Resources: Previous Use of Community Agencies:
ANTICIPATED TEACHING NEEDS (Based on knowledge deficits assessed)	 None ☐
DISCHARGE PLAN	Anticipated Discharge to: Possible Need for Follow-Up Care (Check all that apply) ACS ☐ Hospice ☐ Reach to Recovery ☐ Ostomy Association ☐ Laryngectomy Association ☐ Social Service ☐ Counseling ☐ Other: Discharge Plan:

Signature _____ R.N.

APPENDIX 80–2

ONGOING NURSING ASSESSMENT TOOL

DATE _____

+ = present
− = absent
N/A = Not
    applicable

	*Check if patient is off unit and assessment is not done	*Check if patient is off unit and assessment is not done	*Check if patient is off unit and assessment is not done
	11 P.M.—7 A.M.	7 A.M.—3 P.M.	3 P.M.—11 P.M.
RESPIRATORY/ CIRCULATORY INTEGRITY	Breath Sounds: Normal___ N/A___ Abnormal___ Cough: +___ −___ Productive___ Nonproductive___ Rhythm: Regular___ Irregular___	Breath Sounds: Normal___ N/A___ Abnormal___ Cough: +___ −___ Productive___ Nonproductive___ Rhythm: Regular___ Irregular___ Edema: +___ −___	Breath Sounds: Normal___ N/A___ Abnormal___ Cough: +___ −___ Productive___ Nonproductive___ Rhythm: Regular___ Irregular___ Edema: +___ −___
SENSORY/ PERCEPTUAL INTEGRITY	Conscious___ Oriented × 3___ Unconscious___ Disoriented___	Conscious___ Oriented × 3___ Unconscious___ Disoriented___	Conscious___ Oriented × 3___ Unconscious___ Disoriented___
COMFORT	Pain severity score_____	Pain severity score_____	Pain severity score_____
SKIN INTEGRITY	Skin: Intact___ Not intact___ Intact Dressing: +___ −___ Drainage: +___ −___	Skin: Intact___ Not intact___ Intact Dressing: +___ −___ Drainage: +___ −___	Skin: Intact___ Not intact___ Intact Dressing: +___ −___ Drainage: +___ −___
FOOD AND FLUID INTAKE	Oral___ Tube Feeding___ NPO___ Parenteral___ N/A___ Supplemental Snacks: Taken___ Not taken___ N/A___	Weight:_____kg N/A___ Diet:_____ Oral___ Tube Feeding___ Parenteral___ Breakfast: Full___ Partial___ Refused___ NPO___ Lunch: Full___ Partial___ Refused___ NPO___ Supplemental Snacks: Taken___ Not taken___ N/A___	Diet: _____ Oral___ Tube Feeding___ Parenteral___ ___ Dinner: Full___ Partial___ Refused___ NPO___ Supplemental Snacks: Taken___ Not taken___ N/A___
MUCOUS MEMBRANES **RENAL/ INTESTINAL INTEGRITY**	Abdomen: Distended___ N/A___ Not distended___ Bowel Sounds: +___ −___ N/A___ Nausea___ Vomiting___ Diarrhea___ Voiding: Yes___ No___ Bowel Movement: Yes___ No___ Incontinent: Urine___ Stool___ Devices_____	Oral Exam Score_____ Abdomen: Distended___ N/A___ Not distended___ Bowel Sounds: +___ −___ N/A___ Nausea___ Vomiting___ Diarrhea___ Voiding: Yes___ No___ Bowel Movement: Yes___ No___ Incontinent: Urine___ Stool___ Devices_____	Abdomen: Distended___ N/A___ Not distended___ Bowel Sounds: +___ −___ N/A___ Nausea___ Vomiting___ Diarrhea___ Voiding: Yes___ No___ Bowel Movement: Yes___ No___ Incontinent: Urine___ Stool___ Devices_____
MOBILITY/ SLEEP-REST	Restraints: +___ −___ < 4 hours sleep___ > 4 hours sleep___ Restless___	Hygiene: Complete___ Partial___ Self-care___ OOB ad lib___ Bedrest___ ___Ambulated x_____ ___OOB to chair x_____ Restraints: +___ −___	PM Care: +___ −___ OOB ad lib___ Bedrest___ ___Ambulated x_____ ___OOB to chair x_____ Restraints: +___ −___
IMMUNE/ HEMATOLOGIC	Evidence of infection +___ −___ Evidence of bleeding +___ −___	Evidence of infection +___ −___ Evidence of bleeding +___ −___	Evidence of infection +___ −___ Evidence of bleeding +___ −___
R.N. Signature			

APPENDIX 80–3

TREATMENT SHEET

DATE _____

TREATMENTS	11 P.M.—7 A.M.	7 A.M.—3 P.M.	3 P.M.—11 P.M.
Cough and Deep Breathe q _____	N/A	N/A	N/A
Incentive Spirometer q _____	N/A	N/A	N/A
_____ Oxygen	N/A	N/A	N/A
TEDS ____ ACES ____ (Indicate hour removed)	N/A	N/A	N/A
Dressing # ____ (Indicate type of dressing, location, and frequency)	N/A	N/A	N/A
Dressing # ____ (Indicate type of dressing, location, and frequency)	N/A	N/A	N/A
IV Site Care	N/A	N/A	N/A
IV Tubing Change q _____	N/A	N/A	N/A
Access Device Care q _____	N/A	N/A	N/A
Stage _____ Oral Care q _____	N/A	N/A	N/A
Perineal Care	N/A	N/A	N/A
Granulocytopenia Protocol	N/A	N/A	N/A
Thrombocytopenia Protocol	N/A	N/A	N/A
Preventive Skin Care as per Standard	N/A	N/A	N/A
Stage _____ Decubitus Care as per Standard	N/A	N/A	N/A
N/G Tube Care as per Standard q _____	N/A	N/A	N/A
Safety Measures as per Standard	N/A	N/A	N/A
Capillary Blood Glucose Testing q _____	N/A	N/A	N/A

Initials   Signature   Initials   Signature

_____   _____   _____   _____

APPENDIX 80–4

NURSING CARE STANDARD FOR A PATIENT WITH A POTENTIAL FOR INFECTION

Date Initials	NURSING DIAGNOSIS	Date Initials	NURSING ORDERS	D/C date Initials
	1. Potential for infection related to:		1. Perform a skin assessment q _____	
	a. The disease _____		2. Perform a respiratory assessment q_____	
	b. Neutropenia secondary to chemotherapy,		3. Perform a nephro-urologic assessment q_____	
	steroids, radiation		4. Perform an oral assessment q_____	
	c. Malnutrition		5. Monitor for signs and symptoms of infection q_	
	d. A surgical or invasive procedure or an		including:	
	indwelling device		a. Temperature > 38°C	
	e. Antibiotic therapy		b. Shaking chills	
			c. Tenderness, redness, heat, or pain	
			d. Nonhealing, malodorous, draining wound	
			6. Monitor vital signs q_____	
	Expected Outcome(s): The patient will:		7. Monitor temperature q_____	
	1. List measure to prevent infection		8. Monitor WBC count and total neutrophic count	
	2. Identify the signs and symptoms of		q_____	
	infection		9. Institute neutropenia protocol for neutrophil count	
	3. Describe measures to manage infection		< 1000	
			10. Follow neutropenia teaching plan	

CHAPTER 81

Legal Responsibilities of the Nurse

TERRY CHAMORRO

It is evident that nursing as a profession has crossed the professional malpractice threshold to become legally accountable and self-reliant. The nurse, previously concealed within many layers of the health care community, was free from the realities of legal accountability. The public generally accepted its health management unaware of iatrogenic injury or negative outcomes, but the faith the public previously placed in its clinicians is disappearing. Consumers and their attorneys increasingly use malpractice claims as both a vehicle for compensation of injury and a mechanism for regulating quality of care (Marks, 1987).

Developments in diagnostic and therapeutic procedures in health care and rapid dissemination of information through the media have broadened the public's expectations of treatment outcomes when disease is personally encountered. This change is particularly true in cancer treatment. Increasing knowledge and consumer sophistication have changed the perspective with which the person views the nurse or physician. Opinions and conduct of the health care community are questioned. Greater accountability is now demanded of the professional in the field, and accountability carries with it a legal imperative.

PRACTICE DIMENSIONS IN CANCER NURSING

Competence in Nursing

Advancements in cancer treatment have dictated a reformulation of responsibilities among the various clinicians attending to this spectrum of diseases. The shift in responsibilities has expanded the scope of cancer nursing across all practice settings. Treatment advances demand change and extension of nurse competencies and skills. The oncology nurse undertakes more functions than before in administering treatment previously delivered solely by the physician (Lind & Bush, 1987). In addition to the physical care, the nurse now provides emotional support and teaching programs for patients undergoing complex cancer treatment that carries significant morbidity. Autonomy in the practice arena is becoming commonplace to many oncology nurses, especially in ambulatory and home care settings. The dimensions of cancer nursing have changed in conjunction with the whole of nursing, perhaps more so, in response to the rapid technologic changes in oncology treatment. Changes of this nature bring greater exposure in the legal arena, where the public will demand a remedy in event of an adverse outcome in health care.

Societal Expectations

Society expects of its professionals a standard of competence as persons possessing special skills and learning. This conduct, the duty of care, forms the basis for the professional's legal responsibilities (Northrop & Kelly, 1987). Legal obligations demanded of the oncology nurse in the various practice settings are not dictated solely by legal regulation. The complex of professional regulation, less direct in authority and obscure in nature, has powerful legal implications as well. Risk management in cancer nursing is based on understanding legal and professional regulations of practice plus recognition of potentially sensitive issues that may lead to liability exposure. In concert, legal and professional regulation determine the dimensions of nursing practice. This chapter addresses the essentials in defining legal responsibilities from the perspective of cancer nursing. It is meant to guide the nurse in instituting personal risk evaluation that can enhance professional security in the face of ever-changing conditions in cancer care.

Nurse Practice Acts

Competence in nursing is a reflection of decisions the nurse makes in practice. Many of those decisions are bound by public law, which is society's way of imposing its goals, compelling individuals and organizations to follow specified courses of actions. Statutory law, a variety of regulations enacted by legislative bodies, is the first legal boundary nurses should evaluate. A state's nurse practice act is statutory law that defines nursing performance in its most fundamental terms and exerts primary control over practice. Statutes vary in the language used to define the scope of professional nursing. Many practice acts stem from the model definition of nursing formulated by the American Nurses Association (ANA) in 1955. It contained a broadly constructed phrase stating that nursing practice is "acts based on knowledge and application of scientific principles." This phrase may not provide sufficient legal weight for the new tasks and functions nursing continually assumes as a result of scientific and technologic advances (Trandel-Korenchuk & Trandel-Korenchuk, 1980) or justify all facets of the expanding role of the oncology nurse.

Protocols for Complex Care

The statutes of many states recognize that greater interdependence in the position and role of nursing is important in modern health care and prepare for this by specifying the extent of physician involvement and supervision required as the role of the registered nurse expands. Specialization in any area of nursing denotes minimally acceptable conduct in the performance of professional services. Oncology nurses in independent situations must clearly interpret the limit of practice dimensions defined by regulatory statutes of their state. If they determine that the outer bounds of their practice extend beyond that of traditional nursing, it may be wise to consider placing on file written protocols and specific documentation attesting to their specialized skills and mode of acquisition.

Procedures that questionably exceed the scope of traditional nursing or overlap with medicine should be secured by a written protocol. Some statutes such as in California term these "standardized procedures." Written protocols may protect against claims of illegal practice of medicine in that they convey some authority for a nurse with appropriate skills and knowledge to undertake certain functions (Kelly & Garrick, 1984). The protocol should define the exact procedure and delineate circumstances that require a report or referral to the physician. Nurse practitioners have worked under such protocols for some time. Investigational cancer treatment may especially require protocols that define nurse-performed procedures. In other instances, oncology nurses may be delegated independent authority in cancer screening, physical assessment, or treatment.

A protocol is merely a guide that recommends an explicit set of actions. Instruction for some far-reaching function performed independently by the oncology nurse such as paracentesis may have been given by a collaborating physician. Documentation on file of a skills check by the supervising physician argues strongly as to nurse competency in these tasks if a challenge should occur on legal grounds. The relationship of protocols to law may be along the lines of "standing orders" (Greenfield, 1980). Because the protocol guides performance along a sequential decision-making process, it becomes a standard, outlining nursing practice and demanding a measure of competence. Nurses may overlook the value of a written protocol in planning a sound basis for legal protection or, in the busy workplace, may postpone the formality of writing one.

Certification

Many registered nurses have strengthened their professional positions by attaining certification. Certification requires testing for evidence of knowledge that other professionals consider essential and reflects a certain level of acumen and experience in the specialty. The process is standardized, and bias is diminished by use of a professional testing service. Fulfilling the criteria and passing the test for certification as an Oncology Certified Nurse is significant to a cancer nursing career. Legal connotations may be applied to the certification, however, if it is interpreted to attest to a specific level of competence in practice. Society will then hold the oncology nurse to the professional accountability denoted by the certification. Court opinion or rule has yet to test this premise, but the notion is suggestive that the information on which the nurse is tested may in fact imply the job description and responsibilities within that specialty. A lawyer in litigation involving a professionally certified nurse would be wise to use the implications of certification in attempting to prove or disprove the level of nurse competence and expectation of job-related functions.

Standards of Care

Defining Nursing Standards

The dimensions of nursing practice are defined by the accepted standards of care. Standards are in constant change as a result of influences such as the institution of new federal health care programs for a group of patients, consumer directives, new medical discoveries, or nurses' demands for greater involvement in health care decisions (Cantor, 1978). The decision on a malpractice suit is shaped by the arguments about standards of care. The outcome of litigation may, in turn, reshape nursing standards of practice. This becomes case law. *Standards of care* and *standards of practice* are interchangeable terms broadly interpreted as implying a level of performance. A health care facility may adopt written standards for governance of nursing practice, or there may be standards not specifically delineated but clearly operant in the setting. Sometimes, both exist and practice is found to deviate from the written standards or policies.

The Expert Witness

The standard of care is the measure on which malpractice law bases its decisions. Standards are established from evidence of usual and customary practice. In litigation, an attempt is made to define what the "reasonably prudent" professional would do under certain circumstances—what is common practice. Experts in the field express opinions as to generally accepted practice and actions appropriate to a situation. Both prosecution and defense will use the testimony of expert witnesses to help the court make an informed decision about particular issues of the litigation. Experts base their opinions on knowledge drawn from a variety of sources, experience being the most weighty. Experts cite facts of the case derived from medical documents and records placed in evidence. Testimony also introduces specialized literature, research and scientific inquiry, and general consensus on standards (Gosnell, 1987).

Community Standards

Standards of care, both written and implied, are the most important factor in molding the legal responsibilities of the nurse. Aside from explicit written standards, many people believe that professional nurses will be held to certain implicit standards that prevail in their community or locale. This is no longer true in matters under litigation. National and community standards are the same. The community cannot expect more or less than nationally accepted criteria in nursing practice (Fiesta, 1983). Nursing education and licensure are now standardized among all states through schools

accredited through the National League of Nurses and licensing examinations given concomitantly across the nation. Nursing journals and other media have eliminated the basis for variance in professional practice. In cancer nursing, information about practice is disseminated through several scholarly journals pertaining to the specialty. The most important tactic nurses can employ to avoid a legal encounter is to be aware of and to adhere to the standard of care generally applicable to the clinical situation (Northrup, 1986). The standard of care dictates the extent of the nurse's duty of care.

Professional Practice Standards

Written professional practice standards provide the foundation of nursing performance today. Beginning with the 1974 ANA *Standards: Medical–Surgical Nursing Practice*, professional organizations, especially specialty societies, have defined standards that represent current principles in nursing practice. The standard-bearer in cancer nursing is the *Outcome Standards for Cancer Nursing Practice* developed by the Oncology Nursing Society (ONS) (1979). These differ in format from ANA standards, which are arranged in the sequencing of steps in nursing "process." The ONS standards are product oriented rather than process oriented and delineate desired outcomes that patients may achieve with professional nursing planning and intervention. The ONS outcome standards and the ANA process standards are stated in broad terms. Both imply a sophisticated level of nursing. Some believe that the existence of practice standards in nursing specialties introduces potential legal exposure because they emphasize professionalism and set the groundwork for quality assurance evaluation (Marks, 1987). Knowledge of ONS professional practice standards is, therefore, of the greatest importance to the individual nurse in formulating the goals and purposes of patient care in cancer. Although not always explicitly stated, the standards imply the various activities and functions desired in meeting those goals. Familiarity with ANA medical-surgical standards and ONS outcome standards provides a strong armamentarium for nurses who wish to establish a sound practice that minimizes the risk of litigation. Furthermore, nurses should have a clear concept of the way they operationalize the standards in the course of daily practice.

Institutional Standards

Standards of nursing practice are shaped by agency policy, nursing procedure manuals, and job descriptions. These will be the first sources an attorney will refer to when challenging nursing performance in litigation. Probably the most important policies and procedures that influence cancer nursing practice are those pertaining to administration of chemotherapy and control of extravasation. Most facilities are sensitive to the potential for liability and have developed written guidelines for these treatments. Deviation from the prescribed guidelines invites challenge by attorneys if a situation of concern arises. Nurses must be cognizant of this governance because the court considers these documents as partial evidence of the standard of care. With continual advances and more efficacious ways of administering these treatments, the sophisticated nurse would be well advised to ensure that institutional policies are kept updated in conformity with state-of-the-art tactics outlined in professional texts and journals. Methodology outlined in the nurse's institutional policy, even though outdated in large measure, will likely prevail over techniques outlined in a recent journal.

Job descriptions also delineate nursing practice. Nurses often briefly review the facility's written job description when accepting employment but seldom refer to it thereafter. Nurses should periodically reread the job description to ensure that it matches the current performance of functions on the unit or area. As with other policies, these documents are infrequently upgraded in conformity to changing technologies and practice requisites. When confronted with litigation, the nurse using newer techniques that differ from the written policy or job description could be open to accusation of exceeding practice limits.

Another institutional standard affecting oncology nursing practice is that of certification. Nurses may be designated by the employment facility as "chemotherapy certified" on completion of certain didactic content and accompanying skills demonstration. This type of certification carries no distinction outside the facility. It is, however, among the battery of standards that will be used as evidence of the assumed level of nurse competence in a negligence charge. Ensuring that proper documents attesting to institutional certification standards are on file adds a measure of legal security to one's practice.

The Nurse in the Expanded Role

Extending Nursing Roles

A nursing role is profiled through its functions, and expanded nursing practice is an outgrowth of job responsibilities (Chamorro, 1979). Critical care nursing, now sanctioned by certification, is an example of an extension of job responsibilities dictated by need and advancing technology. Generally, the oncology nurse in an expanded role independently assumes some level of patient management in accordance with the medical regimen initiated by a physician, and certain aspects of diagnosis and prescription become a daily part of the nursing practice, particularly in the ambulatory setting where chemotherapy is administered (Chamorro, 1979). Many nurses carry out these activities autonomously without the supervision or support of even a junior physician on the premises. This may be true especially of nurses in research settings undertaking clinical trials (Johnson, 1986). Diagnosis of adverse effects from treatment may be made and medications prescribed by telephone under the general guidelines of the investigational study. In the event of

a patient injury and a resulting legal challenge, the question of nursing practice beyond the limits of the state practice act is in the hands of court opinion. Professional support for soundness of the procedure or skill of the individual nurse performing the procedure may be insufficient to influence the court's judgment to the contrary.

Collaborative Practice

Opportunity for the highest level of professional independence is offered to the nurse in collaborative practice with an oncologist in an office or clinic. The practice departs significantly from that of the staff nurse in that the nurse assumes considerable autonomy in decision making (Chamorro, 1979). Many nurses in this role may be prepared at the master's degree level as clinical specialists and possess considerable nursing skills in diagnosing or determining the importance of certain patient symptoms. Others may be specifically trained in the nurse practitioner role, in which the nurse legally can make certain diagnosis and treatment decisions. Nurse practitioners, and often other advanced-practice nurses, have formal status authorized under special laws by some states and under existing nurse practice acts in other states (Northrop & Kelly, 1987). Additional education is likely to be part of the criteria.

Some statutes allow prescriptive authority; others inferentially authorize nurses to prescribe (Rhodes & Miller, 1984). It is wise to base any collaborative practice on a collection of standing orders, standardized procedures, or protocols. The specific job description and responsibilities should be drafted, along with educational and specialty certification. The documents should demonstrate that any state statutory requirements have been met but need not be limited to the minimal requirements. Such a documentary packet proves that the nurse is serious in asserting professional status and the full accountability that goes with it.

LIABILITY ISSUES IN CANCER NURSING

Failures in Communication

Detection of Disease

Beyond the legal establishment of dimensions of practice, competence, and standards of care in cancer nursing, there are other relevant issues that impose a legal burden on the nurse. These are potential liability issues suggested by the needs and rights of patients with cancer in the continuum from diagnosis to the terminal phase. At the center of much health care litigation are failures in communication. If test results indicating a cancer diagnosis or recurrence are not communicated to appropriate persons and cause a delay in treatment, charges of negligence may be brought. Professional nurses in office settings are frequently the first line of contact with patients and their presenting symptoms. They are responsible for gathering test data or receiving calls from patients, which may require triage or referral. Staff nurses also bear a similar responsibility. Sound professional judgment is called for in determining abnormal laboratory and diagnostic results or interpreting symptoms reported by the patient.

Overlooking important data or misjudging the severity of patient complaints that require immediate physician attention may carry serious legal consequences for nurses. The value of delayed or missed opportunity for treatment has been contested in several cancer cases. The question of evaluating prospects for cure had earlier diagnosis allowed timely initiation of treatment is a difficult issue for the courts. Many times, juror sentiment and legal opinion have favored the plaintiff. For nurses in more independent roles, impeccable recordkeeping, particularly with respect to abnormal test findings, and intelligent judgment are mainstays in avoiding legal involvement in situations that have the potential for tragic outcomes (Gargaro, 1981, 1982).

Disclosure and Informed Decisions

Cancer carries such negative connotations that family members frequently enjoin the medical or nursing staff to conceal the diagnosis from the patient. A conspiracy of silence may ensue even though disclosure is desired by patients as well as mandated by law. Oncology nurses report being placed in this position especially when the patient is non-English-speaking and cultural overtones prevail. A conspiracy of silence is an ethical issue but becomes a legal issue under the doctrine of informed consent. This guarantees competent patients the right to receive sufficient information to make intelligent decisions about their care (Northrop & Kelly, 1987). The law requires that patients be told about risks of proposed treatment and additional options or alternative forms of treatment.

How much disclosure is required and whether the nurse as well as the treating physician has a duty to disclose are two important considerations. Extreme positions have been taken by courts across the United States regarding the scope of disclosure. Opinions vary from "reasonable" to "full and complete" disclosure. Increasingly, jurisdictions are adopting California law, which requires that a patient be advised of the risk of death or serious bodily harm plus recognized complications that might occur. Any other undisclosed information that reputable clinicians in the community would usually and customarily advise should also be discussed. The "informed consent" precept has now been extended to include what the court calls "informed refusal," in which the client is to be informed of risks or consequences inherent in refusing treatment or diagnostic tests. When cancer is in question, it is important for the oncology nurse to be knowledgeable of potentially adverse outcomes for the patient who refuses a diagnostic test or treatment.

To date, the clinician in charge of the treatment has been held responsible for obtaining informed consent. When nurses, because of their knowledge and exper-

tise, possess information that can improve a patient's ability to make rational decisions regarding treatment, the obligations of the nurse-patient relationship generally demand that the information be transmitted either directly by the nurse or by the physician through the nurse (Gargaro, 1978). A documented notation in the patient record regarding the nurse's assessment and advisement in informed consent or refusal is an important safeguard of the nurse.

Clearly, the oncology nurse must not support any misrepresentation of a procedure or treatment. In controversies, the nurse should first discuss the problem with the physician. If it is not resolved, the nursing supervisor should be notified or, finally, the matter brought to the attention of the patient, who may further pursue it. A well-known case, outlined in Box 81–1, involving the nurse-patient relationship and information regarding alternative treatment to proposed chemotherapy was of great interest to oncology nurses.

Encouraging informed decision making about treatment or care is part of the rationale for providing patient education. Oncology nurses have a special obligation to teach patients at the time of discharge to minimize any potential for injury when the patient assumes self-care. The merits of patient education as a quality assurance issue are well understood, and the legal foundation for patient teaching has been established as well by court opinion as early as 1944 (Creighton, 1985). Some believe that negligence in discharge instruction and health teaching will increase liability as nurses become legally accountable in more situations (Fiesta, 1983). Patient education, especially discharge teaching, should be documented in the medical record. In disputed testimony, reference to the written note overrides mere verbal confirmation.

Consent for Investigational Studies

Liability may be imposed when the nurse dispenses investigational or experimental drugs without ensuring that the hospital's procedure regarding protection of human subjects has been followed (Fiesta, 1983). The facility's institutional review board will approve an informed consent document relating to the specific clinical trial. A copy of this document bearing the patient's signature along with that of a witness should be in the medical record for verification by clinicians administering the treatment.

Confidentiality

Medical Record Disclosure

Confidentiality about the facts of a patient's case is a mandate well understood by most nurses in practice. Sensitivity issues associated with a diagnosis of cancer or acquired immune deficiency syndrome (AIDS) render a violation of confidence particularly grave. One frequently finds that patients prefer to keep a cancer diagnosis secret even from significant persons in their lives. This request should be documented in the record

---

Box 81–1. THE NURSE–PATIENT RELATIONSHIP IN INFORMED CONSENT

J. Tuma, while practicing as a licensed registered nurse in Twin Falls, Idaho, in 1976, was attending a patient, G. Wahlstrom, recently diagnosed with acute myelogenous leukemia. Chemotherapy was the treatment proposed by Ms. Wahlstrom's physician, who discussed the numerous side effects of the drugs in the presence of her family, explaining that they were potentially life-threatening. Dr. Desmond, the physician, testified that he obtained informed consent from the patient to receive this treatment. On the morning the chemotherapy was to be initiated, Ms. Tuma related that she found the patient in tears, stating that she was apprehensive about the drugs, although her son wanted her to take them. Nurse Tuma proceeded to advise the patient of the availability of alternative forms of treatments for her malignancy, such as herbs, natural foods, Laetrile and a form of massage, "reflexology." Although chemotherapy was begun, Ms. Wahlstrom expressed interest in the alternatives and requested Ms. Tuma to return that evening and repeat what she had said for the benefit of her son and daughter. Ms. Tuma, by her own admission, felt that her discussions were not "exactly legal" and requested that they not be discussed with the physician; however, Ms. Wahlstrom's daughter-in-law called Dr. Desmond and informed him of the earlier discussion. The physician did not interfere with the evening meeting, although he temporarily discontinued the chemotherapy. The family decision following the meeting was to continue chemotherapy. The patient expired 2 weeks later from her disease; she had experienced significant side effects from her drugs. Following a telephone complaint, the Board of Registered Nursing suspended Ms. Tuma's license on the grounds of "unprofessional conduct" in the interference of the physician–patient relationship. The Idaho Supreme Court later found in favor of Nurse Tuma, stating the term "unprofessional conduct" was vague and defied application of a standard of conduct by which the activity could be judged. The Tuma case has been widely discussed because it raised considerations about the nurse's right to inform in medical issues as well as legal and philosophical questions about nursing authority, responsibilities, and rights in the nurse–patient relationship.

---

and other members of the health team informed of the wishes. Such wishes must be honored to the limits feasible. Charges may be brought by patients and family against the indiscreet oncology nurse who shares this information inappropriately with a third party or to satisfy public curiosity. The law interprets this invasion as public disclosure of private facts (Fiesta, 1983).

Directives in Health Care

Wills

At times, nurses involved with patients experiencing progressive disease may likely encounter a request to draw up or witness a will. The nurse-patient relationship places a nurse in a good position to act as witness because of knowledge about the patient's physical and mental capacity at the time of the signing. If not a beneficiary, the nurse may witness a will but also has the equal right to refuse such a position without penalty. It is inappropriate, however, for the nurse to take part in drawing up a will because this may constitute the practice of law. The nurse may work through the facility's legal department to obtain legal assistance for the patient in constructing such a document (Northrop & Kelley, 1987).

Living Wills

The passage of so-called "right to die" laws allows competent persons in terminal illness to refuse the use of extreme life-sustaining procedures to remain alive. Several landmark cases have debated this issue. As a consequence, many states recognize a document known as a "living will," requesting the withholding or discontinuance of artificial measures when the patient's

lack of physical or mental competence prevents the specific expression of these wishes. A living will may have been executed at an earlier date, or some patients may request assistance in preparing one when disease progression is noted. It is the nurse's legal responsibility to bring a prepared living will to the attention of the attending physician and other health care personnel. Any nurse assisting a patient in preparing or witnessing a will needs some knowledge of statutory requirements of the particular jurisdiction involved (Bernzweig, 1987). Generally, the living will cannot take force until the patient has been examined and certified in writing by two physicians (one of whom is to be the attending physician) as to the terminal condition. Documentation of the patient's desires in these matters and any prepared living will should be prominent in the medical record.

Orders Not to Resuscitate

"Do not resuscitate" orders may be instituted based on a patient's expressed wishes even if they are not backed by a signed document. The physician must write the order and record a brief note regarding the circumstances. A frequent omission in caring for the patient is the failure to obtain the written order when circumstances dictate. An exception exists in facilities whose written policy allows the physician's telephone order to be enforced for a brief period until arrival on the premises to make written notation in the medical record. Under these specially defined conditions, the nurse accepting the verbal orders must execute care that the order is given directly by the physician, not his agent or other inappropriate individual. Failure to initiate resuscitation on the terminal patient without the written order may put the nurse in the legal position of practicing medicine without a license (Fiesta, 1983). Evaluating the patient and his or her desires regarding life-sustaining measures and preparing for the moment of death with appropriately written orders should be part of care planning by the professional nurse.

Durable Power of Attorney

The living will honors the patient's wishes in a serious illness but is limited in meeting all medical contingencies that may occur if the patient becomes incapacitated or incompetent. Some states have enacted the Uniform Durable Power of Attorney Act. A competent person may give a specified individual the *durable* power to act as his or her agent in medical decision making in the event he or she becomes incompetent to act in his or her own behalf. These decisions extend beyond life-sustaining procedures to include the power to select treatments, seek other therapeutic opinions and options, and remove physicians from the case (Bernzweig, 1987). The nurse is unlikely to become involved in the actual directives of the power of attorney but must understand that it is an acceptable legal mechanism in some jurisdictions. Health care workers are protected from liability when relying on this authority.

Negligence in Care

Adverse Outcomes of Treatment

Some oncology nurses have questioned whether liability exists if there is an adverse outcome of treatment that is otherwise expected to bring about a positive result. Battery can be claimed when medical treatment is performed without lawful authority or patient consent. The charge has no merit unless, as in the circumstances of "conspiracy of silence," the patient's implied consent does not even exist. A patient's severity of treatment side effects will not have legal consequence for any nurse, per se, unless negligence is charged because a nurse breaches the duty of care. In negligence, the plaintiff has several conditions to prove. If injury occurs because a nurse failed to enact the usual and customary set of actions consistent with the circumstance at hand, it could be proved that duty was breached. It must be clearly established, however, that the injury was a direct result of the deviation from duty.

Medication Errors

Medication injuries are frequently the cause of litigation. It is estimated that one out of every seven medication orders in hospitals is erroneously carried out (Bernzweig, 1987). One review of litigious actions against oncology nurses showed that administration of chemotherapy or narcotics to the wrong patient, in incorrect doses, or through the wrong route, or extravasation that caused tissue damage constituted 75 per cent of the cases (Schulmeister, 1987). Administering medications is considered the most potentially hazardous therapeutic activity nurses perform (Fiesta, 1983). Particular care must be taken in administering che-

motherapeutic agents because of their toxic effect. Double and triple checking of patient identification, physician orders, drug name, dose, and route cannot be overemphasized. Legal charges may be initiated, especially when a patient experiences life-threatening toxicities from administration of the wrong drug. In extravasation injuries, negligence may be proved if it is shown that the nurse failed to take due care in administering the drug or proper measures when infiltration of the vesicant was discovered. Aside from the pain and suffering associated with the injury, there may be a delay in reinstituting chemotherapy, leaving the nurse open to charges that the patient ostensibly is deprived of therapeutic benefit during postponement. Extravasation of drug is sometimes an unfortunate occurrence even with the nurse's impeccable technique.

In the event of an extravasation or an error in chemotherapy administration, immediate reporting and documentation of the event and the condition of the patient, following the facility's policy, become the immediate legal responsibilities of the nurse. Demonstration of a caring attitude to the patient is simply quality nursing care, but additionally it is often a successful strategy in the management of potentially litigious situations. Full disclosure of the event to appropriate supervisory persons and filing of an incident report in conformity with prescribed policy are also important tactics. Failure to do so may substantiate the court's opinion of negligence.

Reporting Patient's Condition

Failure to communicate the patient's condition to the physician is another breach of duty resulting in nurse liability. Management of specified patient complaints, a major component in oncology nursing, is especially common in office or clinic nursing. Advice about a symptom is given to the patient via telephone and then frequently dismissed from the nurse's mind in the busy office setting. Telephone instructions given to patients should be noted in the medical chart, no matter how minor the complaint. Astute nursing judgment is required to determine the significance of any complaint. For instance, a complaint of persistent nausea 1 week following chemotherapy may not be drug induced but may imply impending bowel obstruction. Failure to communicate essential data to the physician may result in delay in treatment and patient harm, leaving both physician and nurse liable.

Enacting Professional Judgment

Professional judgment is an obscure concept difficult to define out of specific context. Clinical judgment by a nurse is the outcome derived from the process of collecting and analyzing data about the patient for the purpose of determining nursing needs. Careful examination of most potentially litigious situations reveals frequent omissions or lack of competent judgment rather than commissions or errors in judgment. Professional judgment is demanded at every juncture of practice. Sound problem identification and reaffirmation of the desired outcomes for the patient are fundamental to professional nursing practice. The evidence of planned care for the patient is the stalwart providing the best defense against potential error and liability exposure.

Supervision

There is confusion among nurses about liability exposure when the professional nurse supervises nurse aides, vocational or practical nurses, or other registered nurses involved in direct patient care. The rule is that if the supervising nurse assigns duties to an otherwise competent nurse in conformity to his or her training and experience, the supervisor cannot be held liable for the subordinate's negligence. However, liability for negligence in supervision can be charged if the supervising nurse fails to determine the patient's needs adequately or fails to give closer personal attention to a subordinate who demonstrates need for such supervision (Bernzweig, 1987). The complexity of care required by patients with cancer may necessitate closer surveillance by supervising nurses than in other patient situations.

There is special concern about liability exposure should harm come to a patient when the oncology nurse is supervising students. The instructing nurse must take care to assign only tasks clearly within the student's capabilities or provide the extra measure of supervision and direction required of the situation. Orientation of new staff to the care of cancer patients is another area of concern in supervision. Orientation should be well planned and backed by documentation of completion of each new experience. Orienting to chemotherapy administration is an area requiring particularly close attention so that exposure is diminished for both preceptor and orientee. Consequently, there have been a number of institutional programs in chemotherapy certification established.

DEFENSIVE STRATEGIES FOR ONCOLOGY NURSES

Clinical Competence

Setting the Standards

Superior expertise in oncology nursing will diminish the likelihood of a malpractice claim against a nurse; however, real risk prevention is achieved by careful thought and a well-planned program. Many of the legal responsibilities a nurse may incur in the oncology setting have been previously defined and discussed. It is possible for the nurse to construct strategies that will improve the potential of remaining free from litigation during a professional career. In-depth knowledge of the standards of care is, perhaps, the prime defensive measure of all. The oncology nurse today has the advantages of journals and texts detailing guidelines for virtually every aspect in nursing care of patients with cancer, no matter what the site of malignancy or

clinical problem. Through association or active participation in local and national professional societies, the nurse has further access to advanced techniques and perspectives within the specialty. This is a primary tactic for amassing knowledge of nursing standards in oncology. Professional goals and purposes are defined by such a society, which helps the practicing nurse realize the standards of practice to which the professional will be held in a court of law. The ONS *Outcome Standards for Cancer Nursing Practice* (1979) delineates the specific goals in caring for the patient with cancer.

The oncology nurse is advised to take inventory of the myriad functions and activities encountered in the individual clinical setting. On the basis of this inventory, the nurse must determine if most activities are carried out in conformity to applicable policies and procedures or standards referenced in the literature of the specialty profession. In addition, the nurse might organize and collect references, maintaining a library of guidelines or care plans to upgrade and authenticate his or her practice. In the expanded role, the nurse engaging in more far-reaching procedures must ensure written standing orders and protocols for some diagnostic or treatment functions. These applications in essence define or set the standards commensurate with the characteristic practice of the nurse.

Job Description

Another strategy to establish competence is through the job description. The job outline may be either broad or specific in defining nurse activities. It is important that what the nurse actually does is contained and easily interpreted within the description. Scope of practice problems may continue to arise for nurses working in expanded or advanced roles, in which functions are traditionally viewed as within the domain of physicians or not generally recognized as legitimate nursing functions by an accredited professional organization (Bernzweig, 1987). Anticipating this, delineating the current scope of the job may diminish some legal exposure. Job descriptions should be updated as health care delivery continues to reorganize in cancer care.

Personal Risk Assessment

The judicious oncology nurse should make a personal risk assessment listing the parameters and all influencing factors on the individual nursing practice. Guidelines for making this personal assessment are outlined in Table 81–1.

Defensive Documentation

Comprehensive Documentation

The duty to keep accurate records of a patient's physical and mental status is one of the most fundamental of a nurse's legal responsibilities. It reflects the professional nurse's accountability for interpreting and

Table 81-1. PERSONAL RISK ASSESSMENT

Do you know the state Nurse Practice Act and its legal interpretation?

Do you have an expanded role in cancer nursing?

Do you have on file documents attesting to any of your specialized training?

Are standardized procedures required for your unique practice?

Are you certified in your area of expertise?

Have you identified the facility's policies most influential to your practice?

Is your job description up to date and accurate?

Are you familiar with written professional standards of care?

Have you operationalized the written standards in your practice?

Do the written standards dominate your practice framework?

Do you have guidelines for the significant activities of your practice?

Do you give proper attention to those you supervise?

Do you know your patients; are your assessments sharp?

Do you plan patient care and follow-up on the plan?

Is your documentation evaluative and interpretive?

Do you keep an open line of communication to patient, family, and team members?

Do you foster excellent public relations?

---

evaluating the patient's symptoms. Nurses often believe that charting is simply a function they perform as part of procedural rules. Many nurses have been taught to document only what was actually seen, not to interpret or diagnose. Frequently, the notion prevails that charting is done to "cover" oneself, to indicate that an activity was executed, no matter how well or poorly done or how successful the outcome. These are erroneous concepts. In litigation, testimony concerning the standards of care carries great weight, but the medical record notes of the nurse accused of negligence are the major chronicle of the situation. The nursing chart is the hard evidence that follows the jury into the deliberation room.

The best defense will lie not in flimsy documentation solely of what the nurse sees when delivering patient care but the interpretation and evaluation of that which is seen. This documentation provides the rationale or substantiation for activities the nurse subsequently carries out. As discussed previously, planned patient care by its very nature is activated by professional judgment. When clinical judgment is put into play, logic implies that this reflective approach will lead to a higher level of care and liability exposure potentially will be held in greater check.

Patient assessment is particularly important. In charting, common errors concern omissions of the observations of significance, what is selective and relevant in patient signs and symptoms in relationship to the medical problem or treatment. In assessment, positive or negative indicators associated with a particular problem should be emphasized. Nursing documentation must be continually reflective of the medical diagnosis because this will provide the experienced nurse with associated signs and symptoms for ongoing assessment. Nurses' notes devoid of comments about these anticipated symptoms will lead the court to form an unfavorable opinion about nursing competence.

Medical and Nursing Diagnoses

The use of nursing diagnoses has been avoided by some nurses or facilities for fear that "diagnosing" oversteps the bounds of nursing. However, there is the contrary opinion that the use of nursing diagnoses notably demonstrates a high level of professional functioning by meeting the nursing responsibility to interpret and evaluate assessment findings. Nursing diagnostic labels are a direct way to report not only patient symptoms but response and reactions to the nursing or medical regimen. The use of nursing diagnoses, furthermore, clearly indicates the planning activities the nurse applies to patient care. Nursing diagnoses are a defensible, even desirable, method of conveying information about the patient in the medical record. Their use leads to high-quality nursing by encouraging care on the basis of patient reactions and response. There is always greater legal protection in distinctive charting; a lawsuit may be avoided or won on the merits of nurses' notes. Unfortunately, there has not been wide acceptance of the use of nursing diagnoses by nurses in general and oncology nurses in particular; therefore, their application to cancer problems has been limited (Daeffler & Petrosino, 1989).

Public Relations

Harm Versus Mistreatment

The most important defensive strategy the nurse may undertake is the formation of a superior public relations stance. Anger breeds thoughts of legal recourse in patients and families who feel an affront by their health care provider. Often without justification, hurt feelings will occur through a lack of communication between nurse or physician and patient. The issue of mistreatment often surfaces, and the patient or family will threaten suit. This frightens the nurse, and further damage is potentially done to the relationship as the nurse reacts to the hostility. The nurse must clearly evaluate whether mistreatment has occurred or the more serious offense of *harm*. Basic to every nursing malpractice suit is a failure to meet the standard of care such that real harm or injury to the patient has occurred as a result of that failure.

The nurse must not compound the sensitive situation by retreating or covering up when confronted by a patient who has undergone actual or perceived mistreatment. Many malpractice suits involving nurses are traceable to the patient's psychological dissatisfaction with the nursing care. Nurturing patient relations is key in such instances. There is the belief that patients with cancer seldom initiate legal proceedings. This may be true because patients generally receive definitive psychological support from oncology nurses and physicians during the course of their health care. According to one authority, the success in preventing malpractice claims may lie in a patient-centered approach that encourages a more wholesome, therapeutic interaction between patient and nurse (Bernzweig, 1987).

Sensitivity to the Issues

The oncology nurse shoulders multiple legal responsibilities while providing complex care and maintaining sensitive patient interactions. It is difficult to anticipate every influencing factor in potentially litigious situations. The professional nurse meets this challenge by assembling an armamentarium consisting of discerning attention to the standards of care underlying a situation coupled with meticulous documentation of assessment, nursing care, and patient response. There must be judicious knowledge of the bounds of the traditional nursing role so that appropriate education and supporting policies or procedures are developed as nursing practice expands from advancing technology. Equally important is the nurse's regard for the powerful expectations the patient brings to the cancer treatment program. The greatest strategy for limiting liability exposure lies in sensitive communication and the establishment of sound nurse-patient relations.

References

American Nurses' Association. (1974). *Standards: medical-surgical nursing practice.* Kansas City, MO.

Bernzweig, E. P. (1987). *The nurse's liability for malpractice.* New York: McGraw-Hill.

Cantor, M. M. (1978). *Achieving nursing standards: internal and external* (pp. 3–15). Wakefield, MA: Nursing Resources, Inc.

Chamorro, T. (1979). The role of a nurse-clinician in joint practice with gynecologic oncologists. *Cancer, 48,* 622–631.

Creighton, H. (1985). Law for the nurse manager: Patient teaching. *Nursing Management, 16,* 12–18.

Daeffler, R., & Petrosino, B. (1989). *Manual of oncology nursing practice: Nursing diagnoses and care.* Rockville, MD: Aspen Publishers.

Fiesta, J. (1983). *The law and liability: A guide for nurses.* New York: John Wiley & Sons.

Gargaro, W. J. (1978). Informed consent: parts I, II, and III. *Cancer Nursing, 1*(1), 81–82; *1*(2), 167–172; *1*(3), 249–250; *1*(6), 467.

Gargaro, W. J. (1981 & 1982). Valuing the missed opportunity for treatment. *Cancer Nursing, 4*(6), 491–492; *5*(1), 65–66.

Gosnell, D. J. (1987). Acting as an expert witness: A professional responsibility. *Nursing Outlook, 35,* 102.

Greenfield, S. (1980). Protocols as analogs to standing orders. In B. Bullough (Ed.), *The law and the expanding nursing role* (pp. 186–202). Norwalk, CT: Appleton-Century-Crofts.

Johnson, J. M. (1986). Clinical trials: New responsibilities and roles for nurses. *Nursing Outlook, 34,* 149–152.

Kelly, M. E., & Garrick, T. R. (1984). Nursing negligence in collaborative practice: Legal liability in California. *Law, Medicine & Health Care, 12,* 260–267.

Lind, J., & Bush, N. J. (1987). Nursing's role in chemotherapy administration. *Seminars in Oncology Nursing, 3,* 83–86.

Marks, D. T. (1987). Legal implications of increased autonomy. *Journal of Gerontological Nursing, 13*(3), 26–31.

Northrop, C. (1986). Legal outlook: Malpractice and standards of care. *Nursing Outlook, 34,* 160.

Northrop, C., & Kelly, M. E. (1987). *Legal issues in nursing.* St. Louis: C. V. Mosby Co.

Oncology Nursing Society & American Nurses' Association. (1979) *Outcome standards for cancer nursing practice.* Kansas City, MO: American Nurses' Association.

Rhodes, A. M., & Miller, R. D. (1984). *Nursing and the law.* Rockville, MD: Aspen Publishers.

Schulmeister, L. (1987). Litigation involving oncology nurses. *Oncology Nursing Forum, 14*(2), 25–28.

Trandel-Korenchuk, D., & Trandel-Korenchuk, K. (1980). State nursing laws. *Nurse Practitioner, 5,* 39–41.

Tuma vs Board of Nursing (1979). 593 P. 2d711 (Supreme Court, Idaho, 1979).

CHAPTER 82

Cancer Legislation

MARY S. McCABE
JOAN A. PIEMME
MARGUERITE DONOGHUE

Nurses constitute the largest number of health care professionals in the United States, numbering approximately 2,033,000 registered nurses (ANA, personal communication, December 1989). Additionally, one in every 45 registered women voters is a registered nurse. To activate this political force, nurses must learn how to use and influence the legislative process effectively.

Nurses have the opportunity to take part in the legislative process in a multitude of ways at the local, state, and federal level—in their professional organization, workplace, or community. There is no question that nurses have recognized their professional responsibility and are interested in being politically informed and active, as evidenced by the number of Political Action Committees (PACs) at the district, state, and national levels of the American Nurses' Association (ANA). In addition, many nursing subspecialty organizations have legislative committees and are members of the National Federation of Nursing Subspecialty Organizations. In oncology nursing what is now the Government Relations Committee of the Oncology Nursing Society (ONS) began its legislative focus in 1980 and is represented by full-time legislative staff.

The nursing literature has devoted most of its attention to nursing's potential leverage at the federal or national level. Although this arena is important and powerful, nurses can "learn the ropes," gaining skill and confidence at the local level and progress with this political savvy to the state and national levels.

A voter exerts far more influence than a nonvoter. At the very basis of influence is the nurse's responsibility as a citizen to exercise the right to vote and to determine how tax dollars will be spent. To be able to tell an incumbent that an individual nurse or a nursing group was actively supportive in the last election commands attention from that candidate. As a group, nurses have become more sophisticated in the political process and are capable of exerting even more influence on the shaping and monitoring of policy affecting the public and the profession. For example, members of district and state PACs hold "meet the candidates" meetings and receptions to elicit the candidates' views on health care priorities as well as to communicate the nurses' views on health policy issues and priorities. Simply stated, "Those who produce the votes, contribute money, and communicate with their legislators develop political clout" (Vance, 1985).

HISTORICAL PERSPECTIVE

The history of the government's involvement in health care delivery dates back to the 1800s. Since that time, many milestones have occurred that have shaped the role and responsibility of the government today. The marriage of politics and health care in the United States has evolved as a major public policy issue; Table 82–1 clearly outlines some of the important legislative landmarks that established the government's role in health care.

In the early 1900s, the Sheppard-Towner Act, which established the government's role in providing funds to the states, was enacted and served as the model system for the funding of all programs through the Public Health Service. Within a few years after enactment of this law, the National Institutes of Health

Table 82–1. MAJOR LEGISLATIVE MILESTONES IN HEALTH CARE

1872	Establishment of the American Public Health Association
1898	Establishment of the U.S. Public Health Service and several PHS hospitals in East Coast seaports
1906	Legislation passed regulating the Food and Drug Industry
1912	Establishment of the Childrens' Bureau within the Department of Labor (forerunner of the Department of Health and Human Services)
1921	Enactment of the Sheppard-Towner Act (first legislation to provide federal financial aid to the states)
1930	Randall Act changed the Hygienic Laboratory on Staten Island, New York, into the first National Institute of Health
1935	Social Security Act (American Medical Association opposed Federal government's involvement in health care)
1946	Hill-Burton Hospital Construction Act
1956	Congress authorized student aid to public health schools
1963	Health Professions Educational Assistance Act
1964	The Nurse Training Act
1965	Title XVIII and XIX of the Social Security Act
1971	National Cancer Act
1971	Comprehensive Health Manpower Training Act
1973	Health Maintenance Organization Act
1974	Health Planning and Resources Development Act
1982	Tax Equity and Fiscal Responsibility Act
1986	Nurse Training Act
1988	Catastrophic Health Care Reform (repealed in 1989)

(NIH) was authorized under the Randall Act and established the role of government funding for research as a cornerstone to the improved health of the nation.

It is within the NIH that the National Cancer Institute (NCI) and the National Center for Nursing Research (NCNR) are located. These two NIH institutes are the source of federal funding for the National Cancer Program and provide much of the resources available to support nursing research.

Provision of services to the elderly and the indigent was brought under the purview of the government's responsibility by the passage of the Social Security Act of 1935, enacting Title XVIII and XIX programs—Medicare and Medicaid. As these populations have increased and the costs of technologies have skyrocketed, the government's share of health care has grown to be in excess of 11 per cent of the gross national product. As a result, efficiency of services, reimbursement, and cost containment have become the focus of the health care debate over the past 15 years. Many aspects of the reimbursement issue are thoroughly addressed in Chapter 79.

Cost containment promises to be the most significant single factor driving the health care system in the twenty-first century. It will be incumbent on the nursing profession to play a key role in the development of this system.

THE LEGISLATIVE PROCESS

To maximize the effectiveness of political action, one must know the process of making laws. When one knows the process, the commitment to become actively involved is more likely, and one is therefore more likely to be effective. According to Davis (1982), "By learning the art of politics, nurses can exert political influence and have a major effect on such health policy areas as nurses training, research, Medicaid and Medicare, and other legislation and regulations that affect both acute and long-term care agencies." First, one must know the legislative process.

Who Are the Players?

At the national level, the legislative process takes place in Washington, D.C. The task and responsibility of writing laws and regulating government operations lies in the Congress of the United States, "the people's branch" of the government. These 535 congressional lawmakers are the only federal officials elected directly by the people; even votes for the president are passed through the Electoral College. The authority to levy federal taxes and to decide how those revenues will be spent lies with Congress. Its members hold the "power of the purse." Although Congress is viewed as a "big spender," in only 3 of the last 37 years has Congress appropriated funds *above* the total figure recommended by the president. However, annually, Congress does take the liberty of redistributing the funding level proposed by the president.

Beginning with the process, it is important to understand the steps that bring an idea from its origins as a legislative proposal through to its enactment into law. This process certainly does not proceed in a vacuum. The work of making laws is complex, time-consuming, and overwhelming in detail. To give you an idea of the scope:

- Approximately 12,000 bills will cross a lawmaker's desk during a 2-year session.
- Congress has a budget of 1.6 billion dollars to accomplish its mission.
- There are 21,000 aides assisting and advising our congresspersons.
- There are 20,000 additional workers in supportive legislative agencies (Sheler, 1985).

What Are the Issues?

Where do the issues come from? Bills originate in many diverse quarters, and the sources of ideas are limitless. In the Burson-Marsteller Report (1981), Communications and Congress, Congressmen identified and rated their sources of information.

- The No. 1 source of ideas is *constituents*. This is reassuring because it tells us that what we say matters—constituents vote, and they have a voice.
- Rated No. 2 are *government employees,* including congressional aides, members of the administration, and other members of Congress.
- No. 3 and No. 4 are the *print media* and the *broadcast media,* respectively, which confirms the power of the communications industry and says that Congress gets its information the way we do, by

reading magazines and the daily newspaper and by watching the news on television.

- The No. 5 rated source is *special interest groups.* Special interests in the United States are very important and should not be underestimated.

These special interest groups are organized in a variety of ways. They include *coalitions* and *lobbying groups,* which exert a continuing influence on Congress. It is estimated there are more than 6500 registered lobbyists. In actuality, there are thought to be 15,000 persons involved in lobbying activities (Sheler, 1985).

How Do You Communicate?

Once the issue has been identified and developed, it is important to know how to communicate about the issue. Spontaneous, individually composed letters from constituents are the most effective way of communicating with congressional decision makers. These letters receive more attention than any other form of written communication, although orchestrated mail also receives high ratings. *An example of orchestrated mail* (an organized letter-writing effort) is the effort by the ONS to encourage Senators to support the Department of Transportation appropriations bill to ban smoking on commercial airlines.

Once the issue is identified and a communication route is established, it then becomes crucial to make contact with the appropriate individuals. It would seem most logical and beneficial to address the legislator directly, especially during visits. However, that is not necessarily the best way, because accompanying the rise of congressional power in the last decade has been the rise in power and influence of the congressional staff, commonly known as the legislative aides. The increasing complexity of issues with which Congress is concerned and the proliferation of legislative proposals have fostered a greater reliance among senators and representatives on their staffs for ideas, guidance, and, above all, information. It is both important and practical to realize that most congressional offices are organized so that the staff control the communication lines to and from the legislator. Some of the most experienced lobbyists value a 10-minute visit with a key staff person as much as equal time with a member of Congress.

By profile, this staff person is young and well educated. Unfortunately, only 20 per cent of these legislative aides are trained in any health profession. In addition, they handle at least four other issue areas and spend less than 10 hours weekly on health (Grupenhoff, 1983). These individuals are key to nurses in conveying ideas and registering support for the wide spectrum of health care issues.

What Is the Process of Lawmaking?

The work of Congress as defined by the "development of a bill" can be summarized in one important word—*compromise*. This point becomes obvious as a bill passes through the many groups and committees that have the opportunity to shape it (summarized in Fig. 82–1).

Bills can be proposed in either house of Congress, but the large majority of laws originate in the House of Representatives. In the House, a bill may be introduced at any time while the House is actually in session by simply placing it at the side of the clerk's desk in the House chamber. Permission is not required to introduce the measure or to make a statement at the time of introduction. The bill is then assigned its legislative number by the clerk and referred to the appropriate committees by the Speaker. In the Senate, a Senator usually introduces a bill or a resolution by presenting it to the clerk at the presiding officer's desk or by introducing it more formally on the floor of the Senate. It is then referred to the appropriate committee.

To follow subjects and topics of interest, one must know the labeling procedure designating a proposed piece of legislation. The abbreviation "H.R." denotes the House as the originator and "S" denotes the Senate. These abbreviations precede the bill number (e.g., H.R. 153.).

Most crucial and important to the legislative process is the action by the committees. It is here that the most intensive consideration is given to the proposed measures and at this point that citizens are given their opportunity to be heard. Each committee is responsible for certain subject matters of legislation and has jurisdiction over a particular area of the law. Most of the committees have two or more subcommittees that specialize in a particular class of bills. Each standing committee of the House, except the Committee on the Budget, must establish at least four subcommittees. In regard to health care issues, there are specific committees that initiate and review health legislation. It is these committees and their members that nurses want to access (Table 82–2). If the bill is important or controversial, the committee reviewing it will usually set a date for public hearings. Each hearing is required to be open to the public except when the testimony may endanger national security or defame or incriminate an individual (U.S. Government Printing Office, 1986). After hearings are completed, the bill will then go to a "mark-up" session. Here the legislators review both sides of the issue in detail and make amendments to the bill as introduced based on their discussion. At the conclusion of this deliberation, a vote is taken to determine the action of the subcommittee. The subcommittee may decide to report the bill favorably to the full committee, with or without amendment, or unfavorably, or to suggest that the committee table it, that is, postpone action indefinitely. Each member of the subcommittee has *one* vote, and if members are unable to attend the mark-up, the committee chairperson can have their "proxies"—or vote on their behalf. Mark-up of legislation must also be open to the public. The bill, with or without amendments, goes back to the full committee, which reports it to the entire membership with adequate opportunity for debate and proposing amendments.

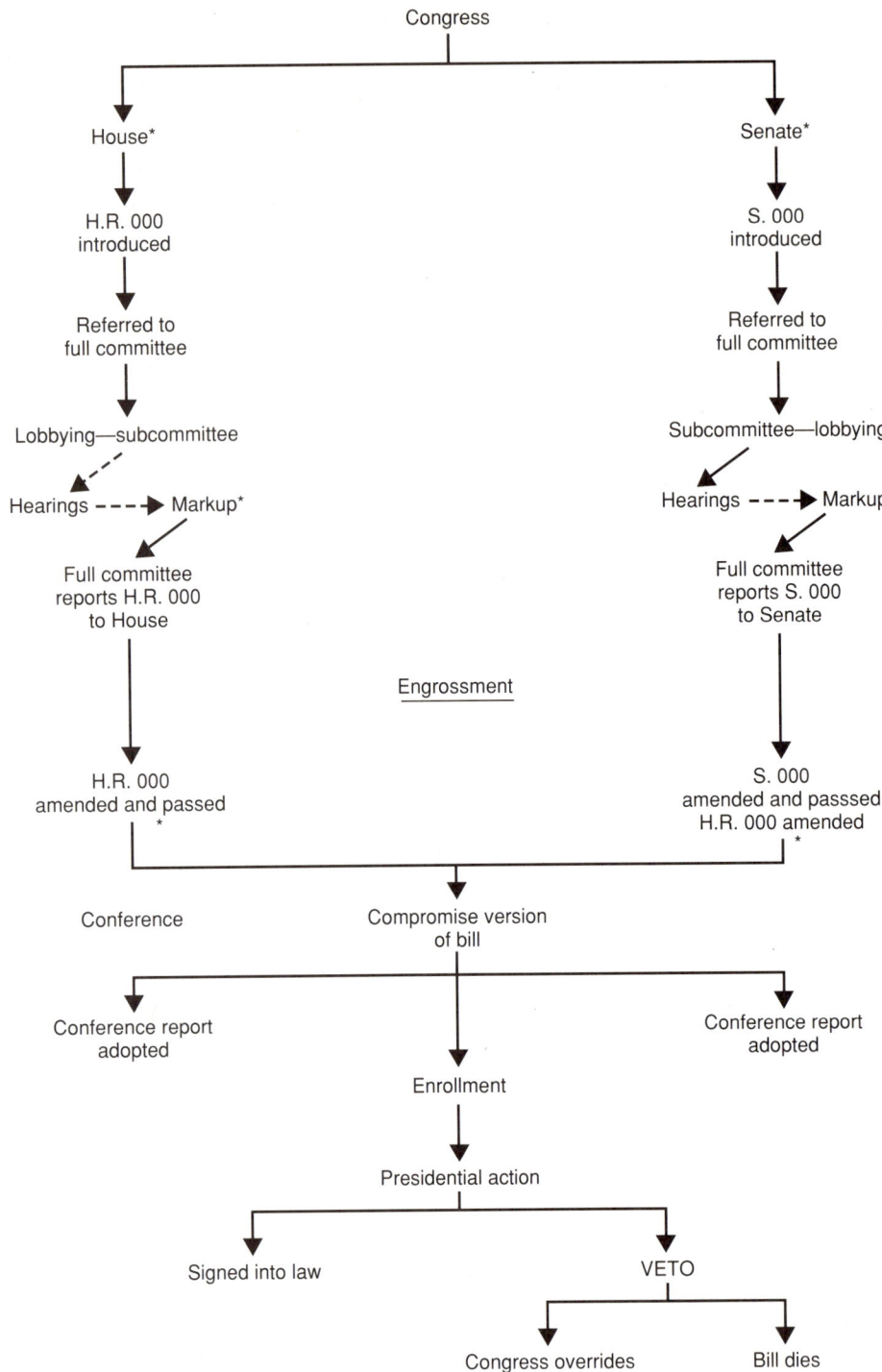

Figure 82–1. The making of a law.
* Lobbying efforts appropriate at these stages.

The Senate then receives a copy of the bill precisely as it passed the House. Then the Senate committees give the bill the same kind of detailed consideration it received in the House. After the Senate passes its version of the bill, a conference is called to resolve the differences between the two houses. When the conferees, by majority vote, have reached complete agreement, they prepare a report that must be signed by a majority of the conferees appointed by each body.

When the bill has been agreed to in identical form by both bodies in conference and passed on the floor of each chamber, a copy of the bill is enrolled for presentation (enrollment) to the president for signature or veto.

This general information of the legislative process can be directly related to health care and the action of nurses. The important points to remember as one gains expertise are the following:

• Develop the issue that is important
• Know the political process

Table 82–2. CONGRESSIONAL HEALTH COMMITTEES

Senate
Committee on Appropriations
  Subcommittee on Labor, Health and Human Services, Education
    and Related Agencies
Committee on the Budget
Committee on Finance
  Subcommittee on Health
Committee on Labor and Human Resources

House of Representatives
Committee on Appropriations
  Subcommittee on Labor, Health and Human Services, and
    Education
Committee on the Budget
  Task Force on Health
Committee on Ways and Means
  Subcommittee on Health
Committee on Energy and Commerce
  Subcommittee on Health and the Environment

- Cover the political territory where impact is most likely
- Respond and act when legislation is moving
- Gain support on the Hill for your issues

The success nursing has in understanding the legislative process will relate directly to its ability to participate.

USING THE LEGISLATIVE PROCESS

The notion of the legislative process most commonly brings to mind Washington, D.C. Although the Capitol is where a large part of political power and influence is located, it is often difficult for one or a few voices to be heard at this level. For nurses interested in becoming involved in the legislative process, it is wise to think of starting out at the local level, where the issues can be clearly identified and where it is more feasible to gather a ground swell to rally around an issue of importance in the community. To work and to be effective within this system, one must learn the system.

Local Government

Local governments are very involved in health care. Consider the concerns and services of agencies such as city-operated and county-operated hospitals, health departments, community service centers, consumer affairs departments, social service departments, and fire and rescue commissions, to name but a few. No matter what the particular interest of the nurse, there is an avenue for exploration and involvement at the local level of government. For example, an oncology nurse could be quite interested in determining from the Environmental Protection Agency how that agency oversees the disposal of hazardous waste. What procedures do hospitals, clinics, and physician's offices follow in disposing of chemotherapeutic drug waste? What are the safeguards? How is the compliance for these policies supervised?

Together with professional organizations (e.g., local American Cancer Society chapters), oncology nurses can raise the consciousness of local officials as to the prevalence of specific malignancies. In Washington, D.C., a multiorganizational effort was initiated to highlight the prevalence of colorectal cancer in the black population. In this endeavor, public and private health care agencies joined together to provide low-cost screening to residents for a designated period of time.

The nurse concerned about professional issues, quality of care, and public well-being needs to know the operational quirks of local government (Jordan, 1985). A city charter provides for one of three forms of city government: major-council (most common), commission, or council-manager (Jordan, 1985). The next level of local government is the county, which is the oldest form of local government in the United States. All states with the exception of Connecticut, Rhode Island, and Alaska are divided into counties.

An elected member of the District of Columbia city council had some very helpful advice for a group of local nurses. This councilwoman pointed out that the local medical society was "visible" to the members of city council (i.e., present at hearings, at open sessions of council) on a weekly basis, yet nurses were never seen. The point was also made that the physicians' presence was felt whether or not they were seeking support on a particular issue or piece of legislation. As a result of this observation, the nurses developed an action plan delegating responsibility for monitoring sessions of interest to nurses and ensuring a nursing presence as often as possible. After a period of increased visibility, nurses were requested to attend sessions to provide input and feedback to council members. Additionally, nurses realized the importance of being a visible presence and the long-term benefits that accrue from offering assistance to promote issues when nursing is *not* asking for something in return.

Reading the newspaper on a daily basis keeps the individual abreast of what is happening in the community. If the reader has unanswered questions about an issue, an effort needs to be made to become fully informed as quickly as possible. Resources for obtaining information, of course, vary depending on the area. After getting the necessary data, an individual nurse or a nursing group can write a letter to the newspaper editor or submit an entry to the opinion page or whatever avenue the newspaper may have. Often one letter will prompt another, or, if the letter was signed by an organized group, the organization may be contacted directly by interested parties.

The board of education is elected in many counties or appointed by the governor. A current interest of many pediatric and adult oncology nurses is the adoption by the board of education of policies regulating school attendance of children with acquired immune deficiency syndrome (AIDS). Because some children with human immunodeficiency virus (HIV) infection have been refused admission to schools, nurses interested in policy development can assume an active role in guaranteeing that the policy of the board of education reflects the most current information about the transmissibility of AIDS.

State Government

Nurses need to expand their understanding of state governments and increase their political power at the state level to influence health policy development and resource allocation as well as to ensure the proper state regulation of nursing practice (Long & Mason, 1985). The structures of state governments vary; therefore, as with local governmental structure, the first step is to learn the organization.

The legislative branch of the state government is similar to the structure on the federal level, with two houses composed of the Senate and the Assembly (or designated as House of Delegates or Representatives). The regular sessions of the legislature vary in length. Knowing the schedule is particularly important when planning nursing lobbying efforts.

It is instructive to realize that hundreds or perhaps more than a thousand bills will be introduced to a State Assembly or House and Senate during a session. Many of these bills will not be enacted into law but may be reintroduced at a subsequent session. To decrease one's frustration, it is helpful to look on the energy spent on efforts that may not have materialized into law as effective training and experience on which to build. Even though a bill may not be passed the first time it is introduced, it is also helpful to reflect on the "education" of the legislators that has occurred as a result of nursing's lobbying efforts. Some newspapers report the major bills in the state legislature, the action taken, and the current status of the bill. The vote of the legislator on a bill may be publicized or will be available through the legislator's office. Most elected officials send newsletters to voters indicating current issues and stands or votes taken on bills. Additionally, legislators hold periodic open forums to hear directly from constituents. It may be politically astute to write legislators a letter of appreciation acknowledging their stand on a specific issue.

The committee structure and function are of major importance because much of the legislative process occurs in committees. Each state capital or League of Women Voters can provide the name and domains of the state committees. In addition to committees dealing with health and welfare, the education committee concerns itself with professional practice, and the insurance committee often deals with reimbursement legislation (Long & Mason, 1985).

The executive branch, with the governor as the chief executive officer, relates to the two branches of state government. In many states, governors select health professionals as political appointees as well as for membership on commissions and task forces. This process provides a unique opportunity for nurses to become involved. Most often nurses gain attention through professional achievements or political or professional activities, or are recommended by professional organizations. When nurses have been ap-

pointed, it has provided an opportunity for nursing input into policy as well as a highly visible forum for nursing expertise and influence. It is becoming increasingly common for nurses to hold political office at the local and state levels (Table 82–3).

The regulatory process of state government under the secretary of state is as essential to monitor as the legislative process. The state board of nursing is accountable to the secretary of state. The education department frequently governs the certification of nursing education programs in the state (Long & Mason, 1985). Nurses need to become known to these department staff as knowledgeable and reliable sources of information. It is a good rule of thumb to build these relationships over time in an organized fashion, rather than becoming visible only during periods that are deemed critical for nursing.

Federal Government

At the federal level, the government is structured into three branches: the executive, the legislative, and the judicial. As on the state level, the legislative branch is the lawmaking body, the Congress. It is not realistic for each individual nurse to believe that a solitary voice can move legislative mountains on the federal level. Rather, the individual nurse can make the greatest contribution by maintaining frequent contact with the appropriate elected representatives and senators regarding issues as well as pending legislation that merit legislative action (Tables 82–4 and 82–5).

Much of the organized impact on the federal level will come about from the efforts that national nursing groups make through their legislative liaisons or lobbyists. Therefore, it is important not only to belong to the professional organizations but also to take an active role in helping to shape the priorities of those organizations (Table 82–6).

Table 82–3. NURSES HOLDING ELECTED OFFICE*

State-Wide Office

Iowa—1
Pennsylvania—1
Rhode island—1

**State Legislators
(Representatives, Senators, Assemblypersons, Delegates)**

Arizona—1	New Hampshire—10
Arkansas—1	North Carolina—1
California—1	North Dakota—2
Connecticut—2	Ohio—1
Hawaii—1	Oregon—1
Indiana—2	South Dakota—2
Kansas—4	Texas—2
Maine—3	Utah—1
Maryland—2	Vermont—1
Michigan—2	Washington—1
Minnesota—2	West Virginia—1
Mississippi—1	Wisconsin—2
Nevada—1	

Republican—22; Democratic—28;
Independent—1

*As of October 1989, American Nurses' Association, Inc.

Table 82–4. Activities for Individual Political Involvement

Vote at each election
Join organizations that will provide development, e.g., PAC,
  League of Women Voters
Secure accurate information on each issue
Become knowledgeable and conversant on issues
Demonstrate that an issue is important to the community—get a
  petition signed
Monitor meetings—city, council, school boards, commissions
Monitor officials' performance on health issues—voting record,
  public statements, news accounts
Testify—city council, public hearings on social, educational, or
  health-related topic
Know structure and function of health-related committees
Communicate with elected officials—telephone, telegram, letter,
  visit
Identify yourself as a nurse in verbal and written communications
Maintain contact with specific legislators, legislative aids, and staff
Have professional calling cards printed
Work on election campaign
Provide financial support to candidate of choice
Attend a fund-raising party for candiates running for office
Attend open forums sponsored by elected officials
Become a consultant on health care issues
Run for elected office

Nurses have various ways to keep informed about what is upcoming or the progress of key issues on the national level. The generic nursing journals (e.g., the *American Journal of Nursing* and *Nursing Outlook*) report on national legislative issues. *The American Nurse,* the monthly newsletter of the ANA sent to all ANA members, carries a "Capitol Commentary" column written by members of the ANA Washington office, the professional organization's lobbying group. Many national nursing organizations have newsletters, journals, or both that may carry legislative updates as a regular feature of issues of interest to the particular specialty. The *ONS News* carries a legislative update in its monthly publication, and a legislative summary is compiled by the Director of Government Relations.

Examples of publications that address legislative, nursing, and health policy issues of interest to nurses exclusively are the *Capitol Update,* published by the ANA Washington office and the *Legislative Network for Nurses,* published by LNN, Inc. A sampling of contacts that nurses will find useful is found in Table 82–7.

Table 82–5. GROUP POLITICAL ACTIVITIES

Monitor meetings to learn issues
Develop position statements on health issues
Monitor performance of official on health issues
Participate in election process—publicly endorse candidates,
  organize work banks for candidates, make financial contributions
  in key races
Propose member for seat on commission, task force, or board
Establish and join coalitions—nursing, women's political caucus,
  NOW, local political clubs
Mobilize group to lobby
Arrange for a social event for legislator and other key figures
Organize a telephone tree for member information or for political
  legislative action
Develop fact sheet about your professional organization—send to
  nurses and have available for legislative visits
Organize voter registration drives
Organize letter-writing campaign

**Table 82–6. HELPFUL HINTS FOR WRITING
YOUR LEGISLATOR**

Type letter—include home address on letter
Identify yourself as a nurse—in body of letter or with signature
Use own words—avoid form letters or modify model being
  circulated
Clearly and concisely state pro or con stand on issue or bill
Limit letter to one issue
If a bill has been introduced, know bill number. HR ___: S ___
Be proactive and positive; avoid harsh, negative statements
Enclose pertinent documentation for position
Offer assistance for providing additional information
Send copy of letter to nursing organization

The executive branch is responsible for administering the laws passed by Congress and may also appoint commissions to investigate areas of concern or interest, such as the Commission on Nursing (Table 82–8). For legislation supporting nursing education, the Department of Health and Human Services (DHHS) is responsible for implementing the legislation. This responsibility is further delegated to the NCNR at the NIH, the Division of Nursing of the Bureau of Health Professions of the Health Resources and Services Administration. The Division of Nursing is the operating program unit with knowledge and expertise in this area (Osgood & Elliot, 1985).

What is very clear in dealing with legislators at the federal level is that they and their staff have little first-hand knowledge of the health care delivery system and the complex issues with which health professionals deal on a daily basis. Yet, this is the group of policymakers that is responsible for shaping what the health care system of the next decade, and the next century, will look like.

One of the most vital roles that a nurse can assume from initial involvement in the legislative process is that of an educator. Nurses have tremendous knowledge, expertise, and understanding of the operations

Table 82–7. ACCESS TO CAPITOL HILL

Documents
Government Printing Office
  Superintendent of Documents
  U.S. Government Printing Office
  Washington, DC 20402
  (202) 275-3030

General Accounting Office Reports (GAO)
  U.S. General Accounting Office
  P.O. Box 6015
  Gaithersburg, MD 20877
  (202) 275–6241

Bills, Reports, and Public Laws
Senate Document Room
  Hart Senate Office Building, B-04
  Washington, D.C. 20510
  (202) 224-7860

Status of Bills "Legis" (202) 225-1772

Elected Officials
1. Office of the President (202) 456-1414
2. Capitol Switchboard (202) 224-3121
   Members of Congress
   Committees and Subcommittees
3. Supreme Court—Office of the Clerk (202) 479-3011

Table 82–8. COMMISSION ON NURSING RECOMMENDATIONS 1988

1. Preserve the time of the nurse for direct care of patients and families.
2. Adopt innovative nurse staffing patterns.
3. Sponsor further research to develop and use automated information systems.
4. Develop and implement better methods for costing, budgeting, reporting, and tracking nursing resource utilization.
5. Increase registered nurse compensation and improve long-term career orientation.
6. Government should reimburse at levels sufficient to allow organization to recruit and retain sufficient nurses.
7. Policymaking bodies should foster greater representation and participation of nurses in decision-making activities.
8. Employers of nurses should ensure their participation in the governance, administration, and management of their organizations.
9. Employers of nurses should recognize the appropriate clinical decision-making authority of nurses in relationship to other health care professionals.
10. Financial assistance to nursing students must be increased.
11. Nonfinancial barriers to nursing education must be minimized.
12. Nursing curricula must be relevant to contemporary and future practice settings.
13. The nursing profession must take responsibility for the promotion of positive images of the profession and the work of nurses.
14. The Department of Health and Human Services (DHHS) should create a commission to monitor the implementation of these recommendations.
15. The DHHS should support research and demonstrations on the effect of these recommendations on supply and demand, health care cost, and quality.
16. The federal government should develop the data necessary to assess nursing resources as they relate to health planning and manpower.

and realities of the health care system and what drives issues—access to care, availability of services, preventive health care. Through the professional nurses' expertise, legislators and their staff can gain pertinent insight and make informed policy decisions as they shape the government's continued role in the health and welfare of the United States.

What does the education have to look like? What nurses do on a daily basis with patients and families is easily transferred. New skills need not be developed; only the audience is different. When dealing with legislators, start with the basics and build on them. For instance, if a nurse is seeking the support of his or her legislator to expand federal funding of cancer prevention efforts, the following information would be useful to the legislator:

- What is cancer prevention?
- What types of cancer are prevalent in the legislator's district as evidenced by the nurse's experience in the workplace? How could prevention and education programs have an impact on this incidence of cancer?
- How would cancer prevention programs be made available? (Through the American Cancer Society, school programs, community outreach, hospital public information programs.)
- What role might the legislator play in the implementation of cancer prevention programs in his or her district? This could range from press coverage at the

time that federal funding is increased to encouraging constituents to participate in the program as a proactive health platform.

Although the benefit of this time-consuming investment may not be immediate, it will lay the groundwork for very important decisions in the future. A classic example of this long-term investment was experienced by the Pittsburgh Cancer Center, one of the NCI-funded cancer centers. Pennsylvania Republican Senator Arlen Specter, the ranking minority member of the Senate committee that funds the NCI, was invited to spend some time at the cancer center, touring it and meeting with the patients, researchers, nurses, and physicians. He came, saw, visited, and everyone wondered why they went to the effort—no promises to increase funding for cancer research were made. About 4 months later in a bipartisan meeting of the full Senate Appropriations Committee to decide how the budget for 1990 would be divided among the 13 different committees funding federal programs, Senator Specter put forth an amendment to return $379 million to health programs, including programs funded by the NCI, which was being diverted away in the allocation to the committees. His amendment lost 26 to 3, but at least he *tried*. And he tried because *one cancer center* thought enough of their work and his constituents to invite him to tour, and to learn, and to become a better Senator.

LEGISLATIVE INITIATIVES THAT HAVE SHAPED THE FACE OF ONCOLOGY NURSING

Education

Public Law 88–581, the Nurse Training Act of 1964, is the most significant federal legislation in support of nursing ever enacted in peacetime (Osgood & Elliot, 1985). This legislation postdated another significant peacetime law, the Health Amendment Act of 1956, which included a professional nurse traineeship program that provided funds for nurses pursuing leadership careers in teaching, administration, clinical practice, and public health (Miller, 1985).

Federal funds for nursing are often in jeopardy. Over the years, the percentage of allocation of the health care dollar for nursing has decreased. Nursing funds are for research and education primarily, with the greatest allocation for education. In the belief that education is a lifelong process and part of professional responsibility, nurses as individuals must assume responsibility for their continuing education. Institutions of employment or professional organizations and associations may assist with expenses for the benefit they derive, but federal monies cannot be expected to continue to support nursing education at previous levels. If nursing is going to continue to establish itself as a scientific discipline, nursing research is essential. Research studies are costly to conduct, and individual nursing researchers cannot afford the expense out of their department budgets alone or from their personal income. The institutions in which nursing research is conducted generally pick up some expense, if only some of the indirect costs.

It would be proactive for nursing to put forth this view rather than having a policy imposed through diminishing funding overall. A decrease in overall funding could limit initiatives in both education and research; affirmative action toward research efforts would help to establish professional priorities for federal support while providing concrete evidence that nursing understands the need to tighten the belt.

Research

For more than 100 years, since the NIH was established, research has received federal funding and therefore been an ever-present policy issue for presidents and elected officials to oversee and direct. It is frequently said that the way a nation allocates its budget reveals its true priorities. The decade of the 1980s has revealed research priorities of which no one should be proud and which everyone should work ardently in the close of this century to turn around.

In 1980, federal funding for research and development for defense and domestic programs was par. By 1989, the federal government was spending more in 24 months for defense research and development than had been spent for medical and nursing research in the 100 years' history of the NIH. For persons with cancer and the professionals who care for them, this shifting in priorities has meant that many important components of the NCI and the NCNR, have gone unfunded.

National Cancer Program

The legacy of our National Cancer Program began more than 50 years ago, when President Franklin D. Roosevelt signed into law the National Cancer Institute Act. This began a rich history of involvement by presidents and Congress in the growth and development of the current Cancer Program to "conduct research, investigations, experiments and studies relating to the cause, diagnosis and treatment of cancer."

In 1971, this effort was re-energized by the passage of the National Cancer Act, which was enacted as a result of the joint advocacy efforts of Congress, the scientific community, and, more important, "the people" (Table 82–9). The key supporters of this legislation, Mary Lasker and legislators Warren Magnuson, Claude Pepper, and Randolph Jennings, believed that the government had no direction or effective policy to manage this disease at the federal level.

The National Cancer Act codified their belief that special presidential authorities were necessary to manage this epidemic appropriately and that additional resources were necessary in the area of cancer control, basic and applied research, and outreach. Perhaps the single most important authority of this act is the bypass budget, a needs budget that is sent annually by the National Cancer Advisory Board directly to the

Table 82–9. AUTHORITIES OF THE NATIONAL CANCER ACT

Presidential Authorities
Bypass budget
Presidential appointment of Director, National Cancer Institute
Presidential appointment of National Cancer Advisory Board
President's Cancer Panel

Special Authorities
Special peer review authority for grants and contracts
Ability to establish cancer research centers and prevention and control programs
Ability to fund construction programs
Authority to train clinicians and researchers
Authorization to conduct research in foreign countries
Develop, support, and disseminate cancer education programs
Authority to convene experts, consultants, and special advisory groups

president and is not under the control or "editorial" licensure of any part of the administration. This legislation has also enabled the establishment of a nationwide network, which consists of cancer centers; community oncology programs; training for researchers, physicians and nurses; clinical cooperative groups; cancer prevention and control program; and cancer information systems.

National Center for Nursing Research

As the United States achieved worldwide preeminence in health, science, and technology, it became apparent to nurses within the government and in academia that nursing research needed to be expanded and that it merited federal support. In 1955, the Division of Nursing, an arm of the Public Health Service, was given the lead responsibility for developing a national program of nursing research and until 1987 was the sole source of federal funding for nursing research and education (Brown, 1985).

In 1983, an Institute of Medicine study recommended that a Center for Nursing Research was needed at a high level in the federal government to be a focal point for promoting the growth of quality research (Institute of Medicine, 1983). Based on recommendations of this report, Congressman Madigan (R-IL) introduced an amendment to the NIH Reauthorization Bill, H.R. 2350, to create an Institute for Nursing (Brown, 1985).

In the words of Congressman Madigan in his statement on the floor of the House of Representatives, "the purpose of the Institute is to conduct basic and clinical nursing research and training related to prevention of disease, health promotion and care of individuals and families with acute and chronic illness. This is a straightforward amendment that seeks to put nursing research into the mainstream of scientific investigations. . . . It is in our national interest for the Federal government to assume a major responsibility for developing the nursing leadership in the nation" (Madigan, 1983).

Although adoption of this amendment failed, the NCNR, as it is known today, was signed into law after a 3-year struggle and two presidential vetoes. It was a triumph of strong coalition building led by the Tri-council on Nursing, which includes the ANA, American Association of the Colleges of Nursing (AACN), and the National League for Nursing (NLN). The NCNR was authorized in 1985, under the Health Research Extension Act. Secretary Bowen, Department of Health and Human Services, announced its establishment as part of the NIH on April 18, 1986. Its broad purpose is to support a program of grants and awards promoting nursing research. The Division of Extramural Programs is the administrative branch of the NCNR responsible for program management of research and research training activities. The program is composed of four major branches:

- Health promotion and disease prevention
- Acute and chronic illness
- Nursing systems and special programs
- Research development and review (Merritt, 1986)

The realization of the NCNR provides the visibility and support that nursing research requires to meet the demands of the next century.

Clinical Practice

It is nearly impossible within the scope of this chapter to discuss all the state and federal legislation that has had an impact on the practice of oncology nursing. Any legislation that relates to patients and nurses, even in the general sense, may ultimately affect how oncology nurses care for their patients. Therefore, it is often important to have a broad interest in legislative issues related to health and not just those that are specifically related to cancer.

The general legislative headings that are of ongoing importance to oncology nursing are the nursing role, patient care services, and health care costs. These topics are discussed in detail elsewhere in this book as content areas of oncology nursing practice and are discussed here as issues in which elected officials share an interest with the nursing profession. It therefore becomes necessary that nurses join legislators in shaping the future health care delivery system and the role of the professionals who will deliver that care.

Nursing Role

The establishment of state nurse practice acts (see Chapter 81) set the historical standard that demonstrates how legislation can affect the professional practice of nursing. Legislation continues to address the advanced professional skills and the increasingly independent roles of nurses. The current focus of legislative proposals revising practice acts is the broadening of the nurse's role and the development of certification in nursing specialties. Both these issues are of importance to oncology nurses and require their involvement to direct the future definition and direction of nursing.

A critical nursing issue to be confronted at the state levels has been the American Medical Association's proposal for registered care technicians. This is an example of a generic nursing issue that certainly has the potential to affect clinical oncology nursing. It is most important for oncology nursing to join with the larger nursing community to thwart the initiation at the state level by working with the state nursing organizations. Campaigns have been successfully mounted in states such as Ohio and Alabama with the inclusion of oncology nurses.

Timely as well is the issue of reimbursement for nursing services. It is a topic to be addressed because bills are proposed for altering patterns of health care delivery. However, it must be addressed with the somber awareness that the health dollar is contracting and the number of groups seeking continued as well as expanded compensation for services is growing.

Patient Care Services

Since the implementation of prospective payment as the system for Medicare reimbursement for inpatient hospitalization, legislative initiatives have addressed the obvious movement of patient services to outpatient, home care, and hospice settings. Concern has been expressed over which services should be provided, who will provide them, and who will regulate them. Again, oncology nurses are intimately involved in the expansion of ambulatory services and should be involved in the legislative initiatives affecting the standards of care that they are committed to deliver.

Health Care Costs

Any discussion of patient care in the United States is overshadowed by the potential costs of such care. Never before has the issue of finances had such a great impact on the development of therapies and the treatment and care of patients. The problem of escalating health care costs cannot be ignored, and it has set into motion a continuing series of legislative and business initiatives focused on cost containment and not always focused on the resulting impact on the quality of care or the potential rationing of services.

At the federal level, diagnosis-related groups (DRGs) have become the accepted method of payment. States are moving to cut costs as well. For example, the state of Oregon has developed a Medicaid Priority-Setting Project, which is a priority-setting program regarding who should receive which program benefits.

Insurance companies now scrupulously review claims using technology assessment programs to determine if payment will be made for patient care services. At this time, even the type of insurance policies available are changing as enrollments from the traditional indemnity plans move to health maintenance organizations (HMOs) and preferred providers organizations (PPOs).

ISSUES AND ACTIONS

The Awakening of Oncology Nursing to Political Activity

There have always been individual oncology nurses who have participated in political activities at the local, state, and even national level. Now there are the strength and leadership of the ONS to support and encourage oncology nurses as they actively seek to have an impact on the health issues that affect them and their clients (Table 82–10).

Members are encouraged to recommend and submit issues to be considered as priorities by the ONS. The issues may have clinical, educational, or research relevance to oncology and nursing. Once approved by the board as a priority, activities may involve one or multiple approaches to action. These include mobilizing the corresponding members of the Government Relations Committee to take a specific stand (usually through a letter-writing campaign). It may involve joining an active coalition to bring together the voice of cancer nurses with multiple organizations such as the Nursing Coalition for Legislative Action. Alternatively, it may involve direct lobbying efforts orchestrated with the professional staff of ONS. One example of such an orchestrated activity is the concerted effort of ONS to support and ensure passage of antismoking legislation.

Smoking

The issue of smoking has had a long winding course through consumer awareness, concern by health care providers, and ultimately to legislative actions. In 1964, Surgeon General Luther Terry warned about the hazards of smoking, with the result that warning labels were placed on all packages of cigarettes. In the mid-1980s, the NCI adopted the elimination of smoking as one of its Year 2000 objectives to increase survival by 50 per cent, because it has been estimated that cigarette

smoking is responsible for 83 per cent of lung cancer cases (American Cancer Society, 1989).

The next significant step was to ban the advertising of all tobacco products on the electronic media. Over the past few years, many public facilities have adopted smoking restrictions, and for the past year, smoking has been prohibited in federal health care facilities. Many private health care facilities have followed suit, often at the behest of nurses.

The 101st Congress marked a significant milestone in extending the smoking ban on commercial flights in the United States from flights lasting less than 2 hours to flights lasting 6 hours or less. This affects virtually all domestic flights. We have come a long way from the time when minipacks of cigarettes were distributed on airlines.

At the state level, Minnesota is working toward being a banner state with an official policy of being smoke free by the year 2000. This could well be a model for other states and a project in which nurses are a natural for involvement.

Nurses, individually and collectively, have played a significant role in the drive toward a smoke-free society. First, they have frequently set the example by changing their own smoking habits. Additionally, nurses across the United States have supported such activities as the American Cancer Society's Great American Smokeout. The national meetings of ONS have been smoke free since 1985, and ONS has initiated a variety of collaborative efforts through its affiliation with the Coalition on Smoking OR Health.

The smoking issue serves as an effective model to demonstrate how the individual nurse and nursing organizations can work to bring significant and lasting changes. This issue will continue to require energetic leadership until there is truly a smoke-free society.

AIDS Legislation

Perhaps the most striking issue to affect political tides over the past decade has been the onset of the AIDS epidemic. The political momentum that has been mobilized in response to the epidemic has enabled a massive research, treatment, and civil rights program to chart the future of HIV infection in the United States. In fact, many believe that the AIDS epidemic will chart the course for how chronic and catastrophic diseases are reimbursed.

It is remarkable to realize that in the 9 years since the first case of HIV infection was recognized, our legislative process has accomplished the following:

- Established and funded programs that provide for AIDS research, education, and prevention; training of health professionals; and access to treatment that are *equal to* those for cancer research
- Convened and received the Report of the Presidential Commission on the Human Immunodeficiency Virus
- Mandated a Congressional AIDS Commission to work with Congress and the administration to carry

Table 82–10. DEVELOPMENT OF LEGISLATIVE ACTIVITY OF THE ONCOLOGY NURSING SOCIETY (ONS)

1980	Resolutions and legislation committee formed—the purpose was to "receive, determine appropriateness, clarify and respond to resolutions submitted by members."
1981	Meeting held to develop "legislative" focus.
1982–1983	Political-educational activities and priority setting of legislative issues began.
1984	Series of instructional sessions at Congress began. Participation in NFSNO–Nurse in Washington Internship initiated.
1985	Legislative training begun. Corresponding committee structure established. Board approval to track legislation and represent ONS in Washington. First lobbying efforts for Nurse Training Act and National Cancer Act. Letter-writing campaign to support appointment of a nurse to NCAB.
1986	ONS joined Coalition on Smoking or Health and Nurses Coalition for Legislative Action. Legislative column in ONS publications.
1987	Separate Government Relations Committee established.
1988	Political action workshop, Washington, DC. Professional "Director of Government Relations" hired—formal legislative priorities identified. "Legislative Summary" begins publication.
1989	Political activities expanded—include mammography, antismoking, reauthorization of National Cancer Act, reimbursement for clinical trials.

out the recommendations of the Presidential AIDS Commission
- Enacted in the closing session of the 100th Congress Public Law 100-607, a broad, comprehensive bill that dictates several of the key policy issues confronted by this epidemic (Table 82–11)

Many believe that the HIV epidemic has realized so many successes in such a short period of time because of one factor—grassroots support. Clearly the homosexual community—the community with the most significant rate of HIV infection—has put into operation a tremendously sophisticated network that has wielded substantial clout with policymakers. In essence, they have made the system work, as it should, in a way unequaled by any other constituency group in recent memory.

Mammography

Eleven national organizations have reached agreement on a mammography screening guideline. Women between the ages of 40 and 49 years should have mammograms every 1 to 2 years; women older than 50 years should be screened annually.

Mammography is of vital interest to oncology nursing because it is effective (90 per cent) for detecting breast cancer before palpable evidence of clinical disease. Despite this significant fact, coverage for this screening technology was initially negligible. The Medicare Catastrophic Coverage Act of 1988 (PL 100-360) providing for Medicare coverage for semiannual mammography for women older than 64 years was repealed. As of the close of 1989, 25 states have some form of legislation for mammography. Although this is a heartening trend, the inequity in coverage among states is significant (Thompson, 1989).

FUTURE

What issues are on the horizon? Where should nursing and particularly oncology nursing focus its

Table 82–11. KEY LEGISLATIVE ACHIEVEMENTS OF THE HEALTH OMNIBUS EXTENSION ACT OF 1988 IN AIDS PROGRAMS

Expediting grant and contract approval for AIDS
Twenty-one approve/disapprove by OMB for staff to implement government AIDS programs
Establishment of Clinical Research Review Committee
Expedited review of AIDS drugs by the FDA
Establishment of community-based clinical trials programs
Support for international research in AIDS
Establishment of AIDS Research Centers
Establishment of AIDS Data Bank
Establishment of National Blood Resource Education Program
Establishment of Research Training Programs
Authorized funding of federally supported home care programs for HIV-infected individuals
Authorized federal funding for education and prevention programs including a clearinghouse and toll-free hotline
Established a National Congressional Commission on AIDS

attention in an effort to influence health care policy, and thus patient care delivery, and the image of oncology nursing?

Dr. Louis Sullivan, Secretary of HHS, outlined five priorities of immediate concern: HIV infection, illicit drug use, health care for the poor and minorities, health care costs, and care for the elderly (Sullivan, 1989). These are not only concerns of today, but doubtless will be priorities through the decade of the 1990s. These issues are not separate entities, but rather inextricably interrelated and, in varying degrees, affect oncology nurses individually and collectively as a specialty group.

The HIV epidemic within the decade of the 1990s will involve an ever-increasing number of nurses. Although HIV infection is not a malignant disease in the classic sense, ONS has put forth the position for involvement and responsibility by oncology nurses. The ever-expanding problem of substance abuse is increasingly recognized as a health problem that affects nurses in every practice setting as an entity in and of itself or as a correlate to other health problems (e.g., HIV infection).

Health problems of the poor and minority groups seem never-ending, as does the continuing spiraling cost of health care. At the close of the 1980s more people were uninsured or underinsured than in any other time in the history of the United States. Today, in the United States 37 million people are uninsured and 20 to 25 million are underinsured. The question of health care as a right or privilege almost becomes moot except for philosophic discourse.

Cancer in the elderly has achieved more of a focus in oncology nursing recently and will command greater attention as the numbers of elderly increase. By the year 2030, 30 million more Americans will be over the age of 65.

Women's health has become a special focus in health care in the last decade and will continue to merit attention in the future. Nursing, primarily a women's health profession, should be a powerful lobbying force in advocating for legislation that affects women and their health, for example, efforts toward a smoke-free society in light of lung cancer being the number one cause of cancer deaths in women and greater allocation of the health care dollar to cancer screening measures such as mammography for earlier detection of the number one form of cancer in women. Although underrepresented in nursing, black and Hispanic women make up a significant population of the underserved, uninsured, and largely ignored health care consumer group.

How do these factors affect the practice of oncology nursing? The NCI's epidemiology program has released data demonstrating that the elderly and minorities do not survive cancer at the same rate as white middle-class Americans, and that in 1989, the incidence of cancer in women did exceed that of men. Clearly, these data give a mandate for oncology nurses.

The challenges are many and so are the opportunities. We have the chance to learn from the past and to shape tomorrow. It is only through a thoughtful and deliberate consideration of policy issues, as well as an understanding of how the system works and where we can and should have an impact, that nurses will realize their full potential, which could be substantial.

As Charles Francis Kettering stated, "We should all be concerned about the future because we will have to spend the rest of our lives there."

References

American Cancer Society. (1989) *Cancer Facts and Figures—1989.* Atlanta, GA.

Brown, B. J. (1985). Past and current status of nursing's role in influencing governmental policy for research and training in nursing. In J. C. McCloskey & H. K. Grace (Eds.), *Current issues in nursing* (2nd ed., pp. 697–712). Boston: Blackwell Scientific Publications.

Burson-Marsteller Report. (1981). *Communications and Congress.*

Davis, C. K., Oakley, D., & Sochalski, J. A. (1982). Leadership for expanding nursing influence on health policy. *Journal of Nursing Administration, 12,* 15–21.

Grupenhoff, J. T. (1983). Profile of congressional health legislative aides. *The Mount Sinai Journal of Medicine, 50*(1), 1–7.

Institute of Medicine. (1983). *Nursing and nursing education: Public policies and private actions.* Washington, DC: National Academy of Science Press.

Jordan, C. B. (1985). Local government. In D. J. Mason & S. W. Talbott (Eds.), *Political action handbook for nurses* (pp. 327–338). Menlo Park, CA: Addison-Wesley Publishing Co.

Long, M. N., & Mason, D. J. (1985). State government. In D. J. Mason & S. W. Talbott, (Eds.), *Political action handbook for nurses* (pp. 339–349). Menlo Park, CA: Addison-Wesley Publishing Co.

Madigan, E. R. (1983, November 17). House of Representatives. Congress of the United States.

Merritt, D. H. (1986). National Center for Nursing Research. *Image, 18*(3): 84–85.

Miller, P. G. (1985). The nurse training act: A historical perspective. *Advances in Nursing Science, 7*(2), 47–65.

Osgood, G. A., & Elliott, J. E. (1985). Federal government. In D. J. Mason & S. W. Talbott (Eds.), *Political action handbook for nurses* (pp. 350–358). Menlo Park, CA: Addison-Wesley Publishing Co.

Sheler, J. L. (1985, January 28). Congress: Proud protector of its independence. *U.S. News and World Report,* pp. 7–9.

Sullivan, L. W. (1989). Shattuck lecture—the health care priorities of the Bush Administration. *New England Journal of Medicine, 321,* 125–128.

Thompson, G. B., Kessler, L. G., & Boss, L. P. (1989). Breast cancer screening in the United States: A commentary. *American Journal of Public Health, 79,* 1541–1543.

U.S. Government Printing Office. (1986). *How our laws are made* (Rev. ed.). Washington, DC: Willett.

Vance, C. N. (1985). Political influence: Building effective interpersonal skills. In D. J. Mason & S. W. Talbott (Eds.). *Political action handbook for nurses* (p. 170). Menlo Park, CA: Addison-Wesley Publishing Co.

CHAPTER 83

Cancer Organizations

PATRICIA GREENE
TERESA ADES

Over the last two decades, since the identification of cancer by Congress as a national health problem, several organizations have been formed, ranging from professional societies to international agencies, all with a focus on some aspect of cancer care.

THE ROLE OF ORGANIZATIONS IN CANCER NURSING

Cancer organizations provide important functions for the health professional involved with caring for the patient with cancer. Although a number of organizations exist today with diverse purposes, each addresses two common objectives: (1) to generate new knowledge by providing education to both members and nonmembers and (2) to enhance the level of cancer care for a specific group of patients.

Two categories of cancer organizations exist: professional associations, which include both nursing and multidisciplinary groups, and voluntary health organizations. Professional associations have a common interest, are private, are nonprofit, and have a professional membership requirement. Unlike the professional association, a voluntary health agency is composed of both lay and professional persons and supported by voluntary contributions from the public. Voluntary organizations expend resources for education, research, and service programs relevant to a specified disease. Both types of organizations are dedicated to the prevention, alleviation, and cure of a particular disease or disability.

Several cancer organizations predate the National Cancer Act of 1971, including the American Cancer Society, which celebrated 75 years of service in 1988; the Leukemia Society of America, which dates back to 1949; and the International Union Against Cancer, founded in 1933. The long history of these organizations, with the current expansion of new organizations, points to the increased interest and growth occurring in the field of oncology. Nurses are challenged to assess the impact of these organizations on cancer health care.

The organizations are a primary source of reference for the nurse. See Appendix 83–1 for a summary list.

PROFESSIONAL ASSOCIATIONS

Nursing Associations

Association of Pediatric Oncology Nurses

The Association of Pediatric Oncology Nurses (APON), established in 1973, is a national specialty organization of nurses interested in the care of children with cancer. The objectives of the organization are to promote excellence in the specialty of pediatric oncology nursing, provide opportunities for communication among all nurses who work with children who have cancer, encourage dissemination of information among nurses about the medical and nursing care of pediatric oncology patients, encourage members to update professional and lay literature with regard to the care of children with cancer, and encourage and support research in the nursing care of children with cancer.

Organizational Structure. The activities of the association are conducted through the following committees: bylaws, membership, finance, publications, research, nominations, annual program, education, and local chapters (there are 14). A national board of directors serves as the executive body.

Membership. More than 900 registered professional nurses are members of APON. Membership is established and maintained with annual membership dues.

Publications. The organization's two periodicals are *The Journal of the Association of Pediatric Oncology Nursing* and *APON Newsletter*. The *Cancer Chemotherapy Booklet* (2nd ed., 1985) is a useful educational tool and reference guide for all pediatric nurses who work with cancer chemotherapy. In 1982, *Nursing Care of the Child with Cancer*, edited by Dianne Fochtman and Genevieve Foley, was published. This comprehensive textbook describes the diagnosis and treatment of childhood cancers and the physical and psychological care of the child and family. Chapters were contributed by APON members.

Programs and Services for Nurses. The resources of APON are valuable for nurses caring for children with cancer and those caring for adults who experienced cancer as children. An annual conference is held in the fall. The local chapters conduct regional conferences in collaboration with major institutions. A continuing education program, *Pediatric Nursing Update*, developed by APON, the National Association of Pediatric Nurse Associates and Practitioners (NAPNAP), and the National Association of School Nurses (NASN) is available for members. The home-administered program awards 26 contact hours.

International Association for Enterostomal Therapy

The International Association for Enterostomal Therapy, Inc. (IAET) is the professional organization for enterostomal therapy (ET) nurses. It was founded to represent and foster the membership of this nursing specialty established for the care of abdominal stomas. The purpose of IAET is to promote the education of patients, nurses, physicians, and allied health professionals in the biopsychosocial and sexual rehabilitation of persons with stomas, draining wounds, fistulas, pressure ulcers, vascular ulcers, and incontinence.

Organizational Structure. The Association was established in 1968. Regional groups, which operate on a portion of the annual dues, facilitate the objectives of the association.

Membership. Currently, there are more than 2000 members who actively participate in the functions of the association. Membership is available in three categories. Associate membership is extended to any health care professional or nursing student interested in the objectives of the corporation. These individuals enjoy all the privileges of membership except those of making motions, voting, and holding office. Active membership is open to graduates of an IAET-accredited ET nursing education program. Any health-related agency interested in the objectives of the association may join as an associate member.

Publications. On joining IAET, all members receive the *Journal of Enterostomal Therapy*, a bimonthly publication that contains articles related to enterostomal therapy, information on new products, and IAET news information. A *Reimbursement Resource Manual* is available that provides the ET nurse with valuable information on reimbursement, a description of reimbursement policies, and materials on ET nursing practice that support cost-effective ET nursing.

Programs and Serivces for Nurses. A national conference is held annually. Regional workshops and seminars contribute to promoting the association's emphasis on education and research.

Scholarships are made available through the ET Foundation by contributors. They are awarded three times each year. Recipients are chosen from individuals who meet specific eligibility criteria.

Board certification is a voluntary examination process available to ET nurses graduating from IAET-accredited education programs. This comprehensive examination, renewable every 5 years, indicates currency of knowledge in all areas of ET practice ("Enterostomal Therapy").

The International Society for Nurses in Cancer Care

The International Society for Nurses in Cancer Care (ISNCC) is a membership organization of cancer nurses worldwide that was established to enable the sharing of ideas and experiences complementary to the development of national or regional groups. The society was organized in 1984. The purpose of the organization is to advance the knowledge and understanding of cancer nursing and to foster the dissemination of this knowledge and understanding by

- Providing a communication network among national and regional oncology nursing societies
- Providing individual nurses in countries without an established national oncology nursing group with regular communication on developments in cancer nursing throughout the world
- Assisting nurses working in cancer care to establish national oncology nursing societies, preferably within their own national nursing organizations and, when appropriate, assisting in the development of regional organizations such as the European Oncology Nursing Society
- Supporting other international organizations such as the International Union Against Cancer and World Health Organization (WHO) by offering a valuable international resource of skilled nurses working in clinical practice, education, research, and management or administration to advise them on cancer nursing and the nurse's role in cancer care
- Serving as a link for other international, national, regional, and local organizations in promoting collaboration to achieve the society's goals
- Assuming responsibility for promoting the dissemination of advances in cancer care through the official

publication of the Society, *Cancer Nursing* (Ash, 1987)

Organizational Structure. The board of directors consists of 19 members: three members from five designated geographic areas (North America, Central and South America, Europe, Africa and the Middle East, and the Far East and Australia), three representatives from the editorial board of *Cancer Nursing*, and the most recent past president. The honorary president and vice-president are elected by and from the board of directors.

Membership. Membership in the society is open to an organization, institution, or agency involved or interested in cancer nursing. Membership dues are based on the size of the active membership of each member organization. For the purpose of the Society and its constitution, the following definitions of organization, institution, and agency apply:

- *Organization*—A group of individuals that has more or less constant membership, body of officers, purpose, and set of regulations. These groups may operate at international or national level (e.g., European Oncology Nursing Society, Veterans' Administration, national oncology nursing societies, national nursing associations)
- *Institution*—An association for the promotion of some learned or estimable cause or the welfare of some group that collectively constitutes a technical or professional authority in a given field (e.g., hospitals, schools of nursing, institutes for higher education, research institutes)
- *Agency*—An establishment in which business is done for others (e.g., cancer charities, journals)

Programs and Services for Nurses. The board of directors participates in planning international conferences on cancer nursing, which are held every 2 yr in the early fall. These conferences include updates in professional and technical knowledge and an opportunity for international networking.

Before the conference, workshops on primary health care for nurses from developing countries have been offered. Grants have been obtained to fund travel and accommodations for nurses attending those workshops.

The society supported the WHO's effort to promote the idea that cancer pain is not an inevitable part of cancer by participating in a survey and distributing the WHO publication, "Why Freedom from Cancer Pain?" An international directory of educational opportunities available to cancer nurses has been compiled and is available from the society.

Oncology Nursing Society

The Oncology Nursing Society (ONS) is a national specialty organization of registered nurses dedicated to excellence in patient care, teaching, research, and community service in the field of oncology. The mission of the society is to

- Promote the highest professional standards of oncology nursing
- Study, research, and exchange information, experiences, and ideas leading to improved oncology nursing
- Encourage nurses to specialize in the practice of oncology nursing
- Foster the professional development of oncology nurses, individually and collectively
- Maintain an organizational structure and function that is responsive to the changing needs of ONS members (ONS Fact Sheet, 1988)

Organizational Structure. The ONS was officially incorporated in 1975. Since the society was established, more than 100 local chapters have been formed to provide a network for education and peer support at the community level. Much of the work of the society is conducted by committees, which provide unlimited opportunities for volunteer involvement of members. These committees include bylaws and resolutions, chapters, clinical practice, congress, education, finance, member and public relations, legislation, nominating, nursing administration, research, *Oncology Nursing Forum*, and *ONS News*.

Membership. Registered professional nurses interested or involved in the care of patients with cancer are eligible for membership in ONS. An annual membership fee sustains membership. Since its inception in 1975, ONS has grown to include more than 15,000 members.

Publications. The society has developed numerous books and publications designed to help the professional nurse gain a foundation of knowledge about oncology nursing and remain up to date on developments in the field. Publications include

- *Oncology Nursing Forum*, the society's official journal
- *ONS News*, the society's newsletter
- *Outcome Standards for Cancer Nursing Practice, Cancer Nursing Education, Cancer Patient Education and Public Cancer Education*
- *Core Curriculum in Oncology Nursing*
- ONS consultant and research interest directories

Programs and Services for Nurses. An annual congress is held each spring. This congress is attended by several thousand nurses. It features precongress workshops; instructional, abstract, and poster sessions; roundtable discussions; and member and commercial exhibits. The society also sponsors or participates in numerous professional lectures, workshops, and meetings at local, national, and international levels. Additionally, ONS members provide continuing cancer education activities for other health care professionals, patients, and the general public.

In 1982, the Oncology Nursing Foundation, a sister organization of ONS, was established to enhance the quality of cancer nursing throughout the disease process. Annually, this national foundation awards nursing research grants, presents undergraduate and graduate scholarships, and funds public education projects. Additional awards include the Mara Mogensen Flaherty Memorial Lecture and the Pearl Moore Career Development Award.

In 1984, ONS established another sister organization, the Oncology Nursing Certification Corporation, whose purpose is to develop, administer, and evaluate a program for the certification of oncology nurses. The certification examination is aimed at testing the general oncology nursing knowledge base of the professional nurse. Testing is offered each year at the ONS Congress and at five different locations throughout the United States in the fall.

PROFESSIONAL ASSOCIATIONS

Multidisciplinary Associations

American Association for Cancer Education

The American Association for Cancer Education (AACE) is a not-for-profit educational and scientific organization incorporated in 1966. It includes individuals from all disciplines who are working to improve the quality of education in the field of oncology. The association provides a forum for those concerned with cancer education in a wide variety of areas, such as undergraduate, graduate, and continuing professional education; prevention, detection, treatment, and rehabilitation; training of paraprofessionals; and educational programs for the general public, populations at special risk, and patients.

Special sections of the association are charged with broadly advancing knowledge in related areas, such as the development and evaluation of new techniques and methods in education; the expansion of public education; the provision for international cooperative efforts in cancer education; the furtherance of education in cancer prevention; and the examination of educational objectives, courses, and evaluation instruments.

Organizational Structure. Standing committees meet the operational needs of the association. They are the advisory, bylaws, editorial, finance, local arrangements/public relations, membership, nominating, and program committees. Sections denoting special areas of interest have been established in a variety of disciplines, including nursing and psychosocial oncology.

Membership. Members are drawn from the faculties of schools of medicine, dentistry, osteopathy, nursing, education, public health, and social work as well as from research institutes, health agencies, and specialized institutions concerned with cancer.

All individuals engaged in any phase of cancer education are eligible for membership. Applications are made to the secretary on a prescribed form. Applications must be proposed by a voting member in good standing and seconded by another. They must be accompanied by a curriculum vitae and a list of publications. There are four categories of membership: active, corresponding, honorary, and senior.

Publications. The official journal of the association is the *Journal of Cancer Education*.

Programs and Services for Nurses. The association holds annual meetings in the fall of each year. Members are invited to present data on new and innovative techniques and programs in cancer education for students of the health professions, practicing health professionals, cancer patients, and the general public. Members also present data on the evaluation of cancer education–related materials such as films, slide-cassette presentations, texts, and computer-based education programs. Abstracts of the papers presented at the annual meeting are published.

Association of Community Cancer Centers

The Association of Community Cancer Centers (ACCC) was founded to provide a forum for the exchange of information among health care professionals who are committed to high-quality care for the patient with cancer who is treated in a community setting. Since 1974, the ACCC has been promoting quality cancer care at the community level.

The mission of ACCC is to provide advocacy for patients with cancer; to promote standards of excellence for high-quality cancer care; and to provide leadership to influence the political, cultural, and economic forces that affect cancer care. The association seeks to encourage a multidisciplinary approach to cancer treatment ("Leadership in Quality," 1988).

Membership. The unique membership that supports ACCC's mission includes all members of the cancer team: oncology nurses, oncology social workers, cancer program data managers, cancer program administrators, and medical directors as well as surgical, radiation, and medical oncologists.

Two types of membership are available: delegate and general. Delegate membership is restricted to institutions or organizations that have identified multidisciplinary cancer care as a major focus of their clinical program. Potential institutional members must meet specific criteria for membership. All applications are reviewed by the ACCC membership committee and approved by the ACCC board of trustees.

General membership is reserved for individuals or organizations that are interested in community cancer care and that do not otherwise meet the requirements for delegate membership. Current general members include various health care professionals, including tumor registrars, health care consultants, health care attorneys, medical supply and pharmaceutical manufacturers, health care insurers, government officials, physicians, and hospital administrators.

Publications. Each year, ACCC publishes the most recent comparative data on current cancer-related diagnosis-related groups. These reports contain analyses of average reimbursement, cost, profit and loss, and total reimbursement by hospital size and region.

A directory of ACCC members, both delegate and general, is published each year. The directory includes in-depth profiles of each delegate institution.

The association publishes a quarterly journal, *Oncology Issues: The Journal of Cancer Program Management*. This publication provides information on various health policy issues.

From time to time, the ACCC president will release special communiques to the ACCC membership regarding new initiatives, legislative issues, or other high-priority projects or concerns.

Programs and Services. Each spring, the ACCC holds its annual national meeting in Washington, D.C. A portion of this conference is dedicated to legislative initiatives and lobbying on Capitol Hill. One day is devoted to paper presentations on advances in cancer control, which are cosponsored by the National Cancer Institute and three other cancer associations. Another day features seminars designed to meet the needs of various special interests of the membership.

Each fall, the leadership conference is devoted to oncology economic topics. Nationally prominent researchers, health care policymakers, health care financing analysts, attorneys, clinicians, and other cancer care professionals participate in this national meeting.

Numerous initiatives have been developed to further the association's objectives. These initiatives include development of a self-assessment set of standards for cancer treatment, development of clinical indicators for more than a dozen cancer sites, and fostering the development of the National Cancer Institute's Community Clinical Oncology Program.

International Association of Psychosocial Rehabilitation Services

The purpose of the International Association of Psychosocial Rehabilitation Services (IAPSRS) is to help to advance the role, scope, and quality of services designed to facilitate the community adjustment of psychiatrically disabled persons. By helping the community bring together agencies and personnel devoted to this field, the association promotes the expansion and improvement of psychosocial rehabilitation services. The IAPSRS seeks to effect improved concepts, methods, and resources; to clarify and strengthen the role of community-oriented rehabilitation within mental health delivery systems; and to facilitate the coordination and continuity of programs within and among service providers (IAPSRS).

The IAPSRS was formed in response to increasing recognition by service providers of the need to improve community-oriented services for psychiatrically disabled individuals. As populations in institutions for the mentally ill have declined, as community mental health centers have developed, and as gaps in mental health delivery systems have become increasingly evident, the assurance of adequate psychosocial rehabilitation services for long-term mentally ill adults has become an urgent priority for planners, administrators, service providers, and advocates.

Membership. Membership in IAPSRS is available to both agencies and individuals. Agencies or facilities eligible for organizational membership include not-for-profit, community-oriented rehabilitation components of mental hospitals, community mental health centers, and other service organizations. Organizations that serve psychiatrically disabled adults and offer services in at least two of the following program areas are invited to apply for membership: (1) vocational, (2) residential, (3) social and recreational, and (4) educational. Individual memberships are available to interested practitioners and advocates in the field and to students preparing for professional practice.

Publications. The association has two publications issued to all members as a benefit: *IAPSRS Newsletter* and *Psychosocial Rehabilitation Journal*, both published quarterly. Other materials, such as legislative bulletins, documents, and congress reprints, are available.

Programs and Services. An annual congress is held each spring. Opportunities are available for members to participate in state and national conferences. Timely information is provided to members on the availability of federal grants and loans. Members have access to special training aids and technical assistance.

International Association for the Study of Pain

The International Association for the Study of Pain (IASP) was founded in May 1973, at the International Symposium on Pain held in Issaquah, Washington. The IASP was incorporated in May 1974, as a nonprofit international organization for the following purposes:

- To foster and encourage research of pain mechanisms and syndromes and to help improve the management of patients with pain by bringing together all health professionals who have interest in pain research and management
- To promote education and training in the field of pain
- To promote and facilitate the dissemination of new information in the field of pain
- To promote and sponsor a triennial world congress of the association and such other meetings as may be useful or desirable for the advancement of the purposes of the association
- To encourage the formation of national associations for the study and treatment of pain
- To encourage the adoption of a uniform classification, nomenclature, and definition regarding pain and pain syndromes
- To encourage the development of a national and international database and a uniform records system
- To inform the public of the results and implications of current research in the area
- To advise international, national, and regional agencies of standards relating to the use of drugs, appliances, and other procedures in the therapy of pain (IASP)

Organization. The IASP encourages the formation of national and regional chapters. At present, there are approximately 19 chapters, with several chapters in formation, located throughout the world. The American Pain Society (APS) is the United States chapter of IASP. The council, or board of directors, is the governing body of the association.

Membership. The IASP has a membership of more than 3500 persons, representing 70 countries and various specialty areas. Active membership is open to all scientists, physicians, dentists, psychologists, nurses, physical therapists, and other health professionals actively engaged in pain research and those who have a special interest in diagnosis and treatment of pain syndromes. Applicants must have sponsorship of two IASP members or of two persons senior to them. A copy of a curriculum vitae must accompany the application. Dues are on a sliding scale based on income.

A trainee membership is available for persons in training or within 3 years beyond completion of training.

Persons or organizations, including charitable foundations or business corporations, that are interested in furthering the purposes of the association and are not eligible for election as regular members may apply for contributing membership. Sponsorship by two IASP members is required.

Publications. The journal *Pain* is the official journal of IASP and is published monthly. The journal contains review articles, original research articles in both the clinical and the basic sciences, book reviews, letters to the editor, and a bibliography of recently published papers on pain. Special supplements are published periodically and have included abstracts of IASP world congresses.

Other publications include the *IASP Newsletter*, issued bimonthly as an insert to *Pain* to keep members abreast of ongoing association activities; *IASP Directory for Members: Curriculum on Pain for Medical Schools; Congress Proceedings;* and *Classification of Chronic Pain*, prepared by the IASP Subcommittee on Taxonomy.

Programs and Services. The IASP sponsors a world congress every 3 years, which is open to members and others in the field. The organization maintains a file of training opportunities for research on pain. Based on information submitted to IASP by universities, hospitals, and other institutes, this file lists the availability, location, duration, specialty area, sponsor, and special educational and other requirements of predoctoral and postdoctoral training programs.

International Psycho-Oncology Society

The International Psycho-Oncology Society (IPOS), founded in 1984, is a new international organization to further the development of the psychological and social aspects of cancer control and to study issues of quality of life of all persons with cancer. Specific objectives of the society are:

- To serve as an international forum for the dissemination of information about the psychological, psychosocial, psychiatric, social, psychobiologic, and behavioral aspects of oncology

- To serve as an international body that will encourage attention to the psychologic and social aspects of cancer
- To foster research and teaching in the areas of oncology within the speciality of psycho-oncology (psychological, psychiatric, social, and behavioral)
- To create, through the society's workshops, regional meetings and publications, a forum for the exchange of information among investigators engaged in this aspect of cancer care and research and those engaged in the psychological aspects of patient care.

Membership. The IPOS is not an exclusive organization. Membership is available to anyone caring for persons with cancer. Physicians, nurses, social workers, psychologists, epidemiologists, social scientists, and other profesionals at the master's or doctoral level or individuals with professional equivalence who have been actively engaged in research or clinical psychological aspects of cancer. Currently, there are approximately 105 members from 26 countries.

Several membership categories are available: active, associate, in-training for a student in any field of study, life members, honorary members, and organizational members. The membership fee is kept extremely low to encourage the involvement of individuals in as many countries as possible.

Publications. A newsletter, published quarterly, contains abstracts of recent papers, presentations, and books of importance to the field of psycho-oncology.

Programs and Services. Some of the services available for members include literary searches, reprints of articles, and bibliographies related to psycho-oncology as well as educational materials for patients. The society is presently developing a curriculum on psycho-oncology.

National Hospice Organization

The National Hospice Organization (NHO) is a nonprofit membership organization established in 1978 that promotes and maintains quality care for terminally ill individuals and their families. The organization is dedicated to integrating hospice in the United States health care system. As the representative of hospice providers and caregivers, NHO actively addresses areas of concern to established and newly forming hospices, including standards criteria, research and evaluation, reimbursement, licensure, professional liaison, ethics, public information, legislation affecting hospice, and education. The NHO is the only national association devoted exclusively to hospice ("About Hospice?" 1988).

Organizational Structure. The elected board of directors consists of 20 members: ten regional members representing each of the ten geographic regions, three members-at-large, and seven members appointed by the chairperson with approval by the board. Each member position is voluntary with the exception of president, which is a staff position.

The activities of the organization are conducted through four standing and ad hoc committees. The standing committees are nominating, finance, ethics, and standards and accreditation.

Membership. The NHO serves most of the nation's hospices and more than 1800 professional members. Any hospice staff and volunteer professional in the United States may join NHO as a professional member. Hospice providers may join under a separate provider membership category.

Publications. The *NHO Hospice News* is a monthly publication that provides the latest information on public policy issues, legislative updates, hospice management and reimbursement issues, symposiums, seminars, and publications. All members receive the publication as a member benefit. *The Annual Guide to the Nation's Hospices*, a national hospice directory, identifies all NHO provider members. *The Hospice Journal*, a quarterly publication, is designed to keep the members informed about the latest hospice research and state-of-the-art practice. Other publications include *The Hospice Quarterly, Annual Report*, special topic bulletins when needed, and technical assistance materials and monographs.

Programs and Services. The NHO provides educational programs through management and leadership conferences, annual meetings and symposiums, and seminars for hospice interdisciplinary teams. The organization serves its members with online technical support and publishes technical assistance bulletins. Advocacy and referral services are provided for the general public.

VOLUNTARY HEALTH ORGANIZATIONS

American Cancer Society

The American Cancer Society is the nationwide voluntary health agency dedicated to eliminating cancer as a major health problem by preventing cancer; saving lives from cancer; and diminishing suffering from cancer through research, education, and service.

Organizational Structure. The American Cancer Society is a nonprofit corporation with 57 affiliated divisions representing each of the 50 states, the District of Columbia, and Puerto Rico, plus five metropolitan centers such as New York City and Philadelphia. To carry out the society's programs locally, divisions are subdivided into more than 3000 units, many of which are organized by county. Each division participates in the affairs of the national society through elected delegate members who constitute the House of Delegates. The national board of directors, like the House of Delegates, is geographically representative of both the United States and the society's divisions. These bodies formulate the national policies of the society. Supplementary policies, necessary to govern local operations and programs, are developed by the division and unit boards of directors.

Membership. The society derives its strength from nearly 2.5 million volunteers, including nurses, who guide the development and implementation of its varied educational and service programs and actually deliver the programs at the local level.

Health professionals are very important American Cancer Society volunteers. Their knowledge, experience, and guidance help formulate the society's professional policies and programs. These volunteers also contribute their services in all the American Cancer Society programs. For example, they may join speakers' bureaus or appear on radio or television to discuss cancer. They often serve on committees, planning and conducting programs of public and professional education, service and rehabilitation, research, or fund raising. Although many volunteers are recruited by their friends and peers, any member of the health care team can become an American Cancer Society volunteer by contacting the nearest local or state American Cancer Society office and offer to help with the society's work. Addresses of division offices are listed in Appendix 83–2. There are no dues. The most important contributions of volunteers are background, training, expertise, interest in cancer control, and participation in programs ("American Cancer Society," 1987).

Financial Structure. Each year, volunteers participate in an educational and fund-raising crusade that provides support for developing and conducting the many activities of the society. Practically every home in the United States is reached, by word of mouth, the printed page, and radio and television, with the society's life-saving message on cancer prevention, early detection and diagnosis, and prompt treatment. Besides the annual crusade, other important sources of income are memorials and bequests.

Publications. The American Cancer Society publishes a wide variety of materials for public, patient, and professional education. *Ca : A Cancer Journal for Clinicians* is a bimonthly journal provided free through divisions. *Cancer* is a monthly technical journal for medical and scientific specialists.

Cancer Nursing News is a quarterly newsletter for nurses. It is provided free of charge through the national society to more than 90,000 nurses throughout the United States. It contains information about American Cancer Society programs and activities, continuing education programs, conferences and seminars, and new resources for professional education and patient care.

Through its local units and divisions, the society distributes thousands of publications and audiovisual materials to nurses each year. Many of these materials are distributed or loaned free of charge. *The Cancer Source Book for Nurses* is one of the society's most widely distributed publications.

Programs and Services for Nurses. Since its inception in 1913, the American Cancer Society has emphasized the importance of a sound professional education program using the talents of volunteers at the unit, division, and national levels. Two programs have contributed significantly to cancer nursing education: scholarships for master's degree and doctoral students in cancer nursing and professorships in oncology nursing. Each year stipends of $8000 per year for up to 2 yr of study are awarded to 20 master's degree students specializing in cancer nursing. Three new doctoral scholarships are awarded each year. These scholarships offer stipends of $8000 per year for up to 4 yr of study.

A program supporting professorships in oncology nursing was established to improve the quality of cancer nursing education and care of the cancer patient through emphasis on collaboration between the American Cancer Society and schools of nursing.

The grants for professorships in oncology nursing are provided by divisions. The applications are approved, first by an appropriate committee in the division, then by the national Subcommittee on Scholarships and Clinical Professorships in Oncology Nursing.

Each year thousands of nurses attend continuing education programs sponsored or cosponsored by the society. At the national level, national conferences on cancer nursing have been held every 2 to 4 yr. All the society's divisions, and many of its units, have professional education committees composed of physicians, nurses, and other health professionals. Also, many divisions and some units have nursing committees. These committees plan local programs to meet local needs.

Programs and Services for Patients. Service and rehabilitation programs provide direct assistance to cancer patients. Several types of services are available.

The *information and guidance services* of the society respond to patients' needs for information through referral to society services and community resources and by providing specific information about cancer.

Through the *home care items* service, the society provides necessary and useful home items for cancer patients; sickroom supplies and equipment; dressings; and gifts for the care, comfort, and recreation of cancer patients. Loan items range from small sickroom supplies to larger ones such as wheelchairs, beds, and bedside tables. Gift items cover an almost endless variety of articles, determined by the patient's needs.

The *transportation* service is rendered, as necessary, for diagnostic, treatment, and rehabilitation visits to the physician's office, hospital, or clinic. Requests for this service are made by the patient, physician, hospital, or community social worker. Road to Recovery, the American Cancer Society's volunteer transportation program, provides the mechanism to develop and maintain a volunteer driver program.

The society encourages *patient and family education* through the distribution and use of appropriate pamphlets, booklets, and audiovisual presentations to assist in the understanding of the disease and its management. Organized education programs such as I Can Cope provide information on cancer therapy, diet, resource availability, and other topics of interest to the patient with cancer and the family.

There are several *rehabilitation* programs designed to help patients with cancer return to their communities, occupations, and families and function, insofar as possible, as they did before diagnosis and treatment. Many of these programs also provide support to the patient's family.

The Reach to Recovery program is a comprehensive program for the rehabilitation of breast cancer patients. Volunteers, recovered from their own breast cancer, visit women undergoing treatment for the disease. The high quality of this program is ensured by uniform training under the direction of qualified professional advisers at the division and unit level. On the recommendation of the physician, the patient talks with another woman who has had the same surgery. Volunteers give practical information and advice and offer visible proof that after recovery the patient will be able to look as she did before surgery and return to her former activities. Visits and information are available for women seeking knowledge about breast reconstruction. Many volunteers are trained to make preoperative visits. As a result of new approaches in breast cancer management, specialized visitors are available in some units for visits to patients having lumpectomy, radiation, and adjuvant chemotherapy. An integral part of the program is assistance to the family, the husband and children, in understanding the disease and the needs of the patient.

Through the *Ostomy Rehabilitation Program*, volunteers of the American Cancer Society, in many instances working with volunteers of the United Ostomy Association, provide psychological reassurance for patients with ostomies. Again, careful selection of volunteers and high standards of training under professional supervision ensure high-quality assistance to the physician and the enterostomal therapist. The volunteer in the ostomy visitor program can provide the personalized assurance that no one else can give a patient.

The *Laryngectomy Patient Rehabilitation Program* is designed to assist the patient with a laryngectomy. Laryngectomy visitors provide preoperative and postoperative support to the new patient. Speech lessons may be included as part of the American Cancer Society program using trained lay teachers and speech pathologists. The rehabilitation clubs of the International Association of Laryngectomees play an important role in the rehabilitation of laryngectomy patients.

The *CanSurmount Program* is open to all cancer patients. This program provides the cancer patient with the one-to-one support of the trained CanSurmount visitor. All visitors are persons with cancer working under the direct supervision of a professional.

Self-help groups bring together individuals with advanced cancer and their families to share common problems resulting from the disease. They are given the opportunity and encouragement to discuss their mutual problems in a constructive manner and learn more about cancer and how to cope with it. The society also sponsors professionally directed support groups. It is hoped that association with these groups will enable patients and their families to conduct their lives as normally as possible.

Cooperative arrangements often exist between the society and local Candlelighter groups and other community organizations, agencies, and self-help groups that assist children, adolescents, and their families. A number of activities for children and families are carried out, including education and summer camps.

Programs and Services for the Public. The goal of the public education program is to inform people about cancer; tell them what they can do to protect themselves; and stress the importance of developing good health habits, including regular physical examinations. The emphasis of the educational effort is on those priority sites that offer the greatest opportunity for early detection and cure.

In the United States, priority sites include lung, breast, colon and rectum, uterine, skin, and oral cancer, with special attention given to the first four. For adults, programs are delivered at the workplace, clubs, home and neighborhood gatherings, and through other local health agencies. Youth audiences are reached in schools and colleges as well as outside the classroom through special educational activities.

The hallmark of public education program formats is people-to-people educational activities and two-way communication. This distinguishes them from those efforts that are largely informational, such as radio and television messages or literature distribution.

The Public Information Department uses the media to convey the society's message. Through news releases; television and radio spots; display materials, and millions of copies of flyers, pamphlets, and brochures, the public learns about the progress that has been made in the fight against cancer and the role that the American Cancer Society plays in that fight.

The public looks to the American Cancer Society as the authority on cancer and is better informed than ever before. Cancer has become a household word and a national issue.

The public issues program recommends policy regarding the society's official position on numerous issues, for example, carcinogens and other aspects of environmentally related cancer and all facets of governmental relations, including legislation. As federal and state governments have become more involved with legislation and funding of cancer control programs, the society both initiates and responds to government efforts.

Research. The key to attaining the American Cancer Society's long-range goal—total control of cancer—is research. Approximately 30 per cent of all society funds go directly into the national research program. Five categories of grants are awarded through this program.

Research and clinical investigation grants are intended to fit a variety of needs in scientific investigation related to cancer. A grant is generally made to cover the cost of such items as salaries for professional and technical assistance, equipment, animals, supplies, and other miscellaneous items required to conduct a proposed research project. Applications are reviewed by one of 11 scientific advisory committees. The recent establishment of a Scientific Advisory Committee on Psychosocial and Behavioral Research has provided opportunities for more nurse researchers. In evaluating the applications, reviewers consider the investigator's qualifications, productivity and experience in research; the facilities available; and the project's potential for controlling cancer or benefiting patients.

Institutional research grants are made to qualified institutions to foster meritorious cancer-related research that cannot readily be supported through other available sources. The primary purpose of these grants is to provide seed money to permit the initiation of promising new projects or novel ideas, especially by junior investigators. Because they are made to institutions as a whole, funds are available to support proposals from all schools and departments, including nursing.

Grants for support of personnel are divided into six types. These grants are designed to foster and support careers in cancer research for investigators at different stages in training and career development.

Research and development program grants allow rapid funding for a variety of critical and urgent needs.

Special institutional grants are designed to provide substantial, flexible, and relatively long-term support for interdisciplinary research programs concerned with cancer cause and prevention that cannot be feasibly supported through the society's other research grants.

The *Cancer Control Grant Program* is much smaller and separate from the research program. This program was established to fund meritorious cancer control projects that did not fall within the domain of the structured research program. Any institution or individual may apply for a 1-yr Cancer Control grant if the project meets the following criteria: (1) it is national in scope, (2) it is directed toward gaps or deficiencies in cancer control, (3) it is more appropriately funded by the society rather than by other sources, and (4) it requires seed money rather than long-term support. Through this mechanism the society has supported the establishment of enterostomal therapy training programs and the ONS survey of cancer content in undergraduate nursing education programs, among many other significant cancer control projects.

The society's diverse research program extends support to scientific activities in almost every state. It provides training for promising young investigators; support for established scientists; and fluid funds to stimulate exciting new ideas in cancer research in universities, research institutes, and teaching hospitals throughout the United States.

Leukemia Society of America

The Leukemia Society of America, Inc., is a national voluntary health agency dedicated solely to seeking the cause and eventual cure of leukemia and allied diseases. The society was established in 1949 as the de Villiers Foundation, named in memory of Robert Roesler de Villiers, a young man who died of leukemia. Renamed the Leukemia Society in 1954, the organization became the Leukemia Society of America, Inc., in 1967 in recognition of the increasing national awareness of the dangers of leukemia ("Facts about Leukemia" 1988).

Organizational Structure. The society, a single corporation licensed under New York state corporate laws, has 56 chapter offices located across the United

States. Activities are supervised and directed by a board of trustees and five standing committees: campaign, medical and scientific advisory, patient aid, professional education, public education and information.

Membership. Close to one million volunteers give generously of their time and talents to implement the society's programs. They provide professional guidance and help raise needed funds.

All local and national programs are supported by contributions from individuals, commerce and industry, unions and foundations, clubs and organizations, and bequests and memorials. Contributions are tax deductible.

Publications. Society publications include the following:

- *Leukemia*, a monthly scientific journal that brings the latest research and treatment advances information to the professional
- *Society News*, the bimonthly national newsletter
- *Leukemia Society of America, Annual Report*
- Numerous public education materials about various topics related to leukemia, such as "Making Intelligent Decisions," a brochure warning the public against relying on unproven methods of treatment

Programs and Services. The society supports five major programs: research, patient aid, public and professional education, and community service.

The *research program* is based on the belief that all medically sound approaches toward a cure or control of leukemia should be encouraged on a worldwide basis. Since its establishment, the society has awarded more than $50 million in research grants.

Research grants are overseen by the national Board of Trustees of the Leukemia Society of America. Grantees are selected by a subcommittee of the society's Medical and Scientific Committee, composed of leaders in the field of leukemia research, who carefully screen and evaluate all applications. Awards are made in three categories: scholarships, which are 5-yr grants totalling $200,000; special fellowships, which are 3-yr grants totalling $87,000; and fellowships, which are 3-yr grants totalling $70,500.

Supplementary financial assistance is provided to patients with leukemia, lymphoma, multiple myeloma, and preleukemia as well as referral services to other sources of help in the community through the society's *patient-aid program*. The program provides up to $750 per patient per year on an outpatient basis for (1) drugs used in treatment and control of the disease; (2) processing, typing, screening, and cross matching of blood components for transfusions; (3) transportation to and from a physician's office, hospital, or treatment center; and (4) initial induction x-ray therapy for patients with Hodgkin's disease and x-ray therapy for cranial radiation for acute leukemia.

The program is administered through the society's chapters. Assistance is available to all qualified patients without regard to sex, age, race, color, or creed. It begins on the date the application is received in the chapter office, provided the application is later approved by the chapter Patient-Aid Committee. Aid is limited in all cases to expenses not covered by other sources.

Through its *patient-aid program*, the society has developed local family support groups at a number of chapters throughout the United States. Guided by health professionals, each group is free of charge and open to patients, families, and friends. The groups are intended to provide information and support as well as encourage greater communication among patients, families, and medical personnel.

Through the *public health education program*, the society provides current information on leukemia and related diseases to the general public. It alerts the public to the disease and treatment through literature and posters, films and other audiovisual materials, speaking engagements, seminars and educational programs, news and feature releases, and public service advertising in all media.

Through seminars and symposia, audiovisual materials, and publications, the society's *professional education program* shares the latest research advances with physicians and health professionals. Symposiums are conducted locally and on the national level.

The *community service program* facilitates two-way communications with all social service agencies and treatment facilities in the area. Information is collected for the benefit of patients and families who may need to know about resources available to them. Chapters interact with all government health departments and many varied family assistance organizations.

International Union Against Cancer

The International Union Against Cancer (UICC) is a unique organization devoted to all aspects of the worldwide fight against cancer. Its objectives are to advance scientific and medical knowledge in research, diagnosis, treatment, and prevention of cancer and to promote all other aspects of the campaign against cancer throughout the world. Particular emphasis is placed on professional and public education (UICC, 1986).

Organization. Founded in 1933, the UICC is a nongovernmental, independent association, which today includes 254 member organizations in 84 countries, all working to control or eliminate cancer. The UICC is nonprofit, nonpolitical, and nonsectarian. Its headquarters are in Geneva, Switzerland. Democratically governed by its volunteer membership and administered by a professional staff, the UICC creates and carries out programs around the world. The UICC is supported by membership dues; by national subscriptions; by contracts and grants for specific programs and projects; and by donations from foundations, corporations, and individuals.

Membership. Membership is open to voluntary and professional cancer organizations, such as leagues and societies and cancer research and treatment centers.

Publications. The UICC publishes the *International*

Journal of Cancer, two volumes of six issues per year; *UICC Cancer Magazine*, four issues per year; an *International Calendar of Meetings on Cancer*, semiannually; and technical reports and monographs.

Programs and Services. Member organizations contribute expertise as well as logistic and financial support and also benefit from UICC expertise drawn from around the world. Each UICC program is coordinated by a program chairman. Within each program there are several projects each led by a project chairman together with a committee.

Current UICC programs are Committee on International Collaborative Activities (CICA); Campaign, Organization, and Public Education (COPE); Detection and Diagnosis; Epidemiology and Prevention; Fellowships and Personnel Exchange; Professional Education; Smoking and Cancer; Treatment and Rehabilitation; and Tumor Biology.

International cancer congresses are held every 4 yr. Periodic congresses, workshops, and conferences are also held.

THE FUTURE ROLE

As cancer organizations continue to generate new knowledge and enhance the level of care to patients, their responsibility to health care will become increasingly important. Research programs will continue to grow with more money allocated for support. Through collaborative efforts with nurses, these organizations can provide the leadership necessary to influence the political, cultural, and economic forces that affect cancer care.

References

About hospice. (1988). South Deerfield, MA: National Hospice Organization.

American Cancer Society factbook for health professionals. (1988). New York: American Cancer Society.

Ash, C. R. (1987). Editorial 1987. *Cancer Nursing, 10,* 1.

Enterostomal therapy nursing: ET nursing a specialty. (1988). Irving, CA: International Enterostomal Therapy, Inc.

Facts about the Leukemia Society of America. (1988). New York: Leukemia Society of America.

IAPSRS: International Association of Psychosocial Rehabilitation Service. (1988). U.S.A.: Author.

IASP: International Association for the Study of Pain. (1988). U.S.A.: Author.

Leadership in quality cancer care: Membership information. (1988). Rockville, MD: Association of Community Cancer Centers.

ONS fact sheet. (1988). Pittsburgh: Oncology Nursing Society.

UICC: International Union Against Cancer. (1986). Switzerland: Author.

APPENDIX 83–1

CANCER ORGANIZATIONS

NURSING ASSOCIATIONS

1. Association of Pediatric Oncology Nurses (APON)
   11508 Allecingie Parkway
   Suite C
   Richmond, VA 23235
   Telephone: (804) 379-5513

   A national specialty organization for nurses interested in the care of children with cancer.

   Membership dues: $55/yr U.S., $75/yr. foreign

2. International Association of Enterostomal Therapy (IAET)
   2081 Business Center Drive
   Suite 290
   Irvine, CA 92715
   Telephone: (714) 476-0268

   The professional organization for ET nurses and health care professionals involved in the care of patients with stomas, draining wounds, fistulas, pressure ulcers, or incontinence.

   Membership dues: $65/yr active, $60/yr associate, $32.50/yr retired

3. International Society for Nurses in Cancer Care (ISNCC)
   c/o Carol Reed-Ash, RN, EdD, Secretary-Treasurer
   Adelphi University
   School of Nursing
   Box 516
   Garden City, NY 11530
   Telephone: (516) 663-1001

   An organization of cancer nurses worldwide established to advance the knowledge and understanding of cancer nursing and to foster the dissemination of this knowledge.

   Membership dues: $100–250/yr based on size of organization

4. Oncology Nursing Society (ONS)
   1016 Greentree Road
   Suite 200
   Pittsburgh, PA 15220-3125
   Telephone: (412) 921-7373

   A national specialty organization of registered nurses dedicated to excellence in patient care, teaching, research, and community service in the field of oncology.

   Membership dues: $53/yr active, $26.50/yr student, $26.50/yr retired

MULTIDISCIPLINARY ASSOCIATIONS

1. American Association for Cancer Education (AACE)
   c/o C. Michael Brooks, EdD, Secretary
   401 Community Health Services Building
   Birmingham, AL 35294
   Telephone: (205) 934-3054

   An educational and scientific organization providing a forum for those concerned with cancer education.

   Membership dues: $75/yr

2. Association of Community Cancer Centers (ACCC)
   11600 Nebel Street
   Suite 201
   Rockville, MD 20852
   Telephone: (301) 984-9496

   An organization of health care professionals committed to high-quality care for the cancer patient treated in a community setting.

   Membership dues: $650/yr delegate, $100/yr general

3. International Association of Psychosocial Rehabilitation Services (IAPSRS)
   5550 Sterrett Place
   Suite 214
   Columbia, MD 21044
   (303) 730-7190

   An organization to help advance the role, scope, and quality of services designed to facilitate the community adjustment of psychiatrically disabled persons.

   Membership dues: $55/yr individual, $25/yr students; organization dues based on annual operating budget

4. International Association for the Study of Pain (IASP)
   909 N.E. 43rd Street
   Suite 306
   Seattle, WA 98105-6020
   Telephone: (206) 547-6409

APPENDIX 83–1

CANCER ORGANIZATIONS *Continued*

An international organization of health care professionals actively engaged in pain research and those who have a special interest in pain syndromes.

Membership dues: $55–110/yr regular, based on income; $55/yr trainee; $250/yr contributing affiliate; $1000/yr contributing support

5. International Psycho-Oncology Society (IPOS)
   c/o Anthony Marchini
   Executive Committee Assistant
   Memorial Sloan-Kettering Cancer Center
   1275 York Avenue
   New York, New York 10021
   Telephone: (212) 639-7051
   Telex: MSKCC NYKTLX 64-9169

An international organization to further the development of the psychological and social aspects of cancer control.

Membership dues: Extremely low to encourage membership from all parts of the world (approximately $20/yr)

6. The National Hospice Organization (NHO)
   1901 North Fort Myer Drive
   Suite 307
   Arlington, VA 22209
   Telephone: (703) 243-5900

A membership organization made up of hospice providers and professionals that promotes and maintains quality care for terminally ill individuals and their families.

Membership dues: $40/yr individuals; $200–500/yr hospice provider membership, based on number of patients served

VOLUNTARY HEALTH ORGANIZATIONS

1. American Cancer Society, Inc.
   1599 Clifton Road, N.E.
   Atlanta, GA 30329
   Telephone: (404) 320-3333

The nationwide voluntary health agency dedicated to eliminating cancer as a major health problem by preventing cancer, saving lives from cancer, and diminishing suffering from cancer through research, education, and service.

Membership dues: N/A

Each year, volunteers participate in an educational and fund-raising crusade that provides support for developing and conducting the many activities of the society.

2. Leukemia Society of America, Inc.
   National Headquarters
   733 Third Avenue
   New York, NY 10017
   Telephone: (212) 573-8484

A national voluntary health agency dedicated solely to seeking the cause and eventual cure of leukemia and allied diseases.

Membership dues: N/A

All programs are supported by contributions.

3. International Union Against Cancer (UICC)
   Rue du Conseil—General 3
   1205 Geneva, Switzerland
   Telephone: (41–22) 20 18 11

A unique organization of voluntary and professional cancer organizations devoted to all aspects of the worldwide fight against cancer.

Membership dues: $1000/yr or a share of a national subscription calculation based on WHO national assessments

APPENDIX 83–2

CHARTERED DIVISIONS OF THE AMERICAN CANCER SOCIETY

Alabama Division, Inc.
402 Office Park Drive
Suite 300
Birmingham, Alabama
35223
(205) 879-2242

Alaska Division, Inc.
406 West Fireweed Lane
Suite 204
Anchorage, Alaska 99503
(907) 277-8696

Arizona Division, Inc.
2929 East Thomas Road
Phoenix, Arizona 85016
(602) 224-0524

Arkansas Division, Inc.
P.O. Box 3822
Little Rock, Arkansas 72203
(501) 664-3480-1-2

California Division, Inc.
1710 Webster Street
P.O. Box 2061
Oakland, California 94612
(415) 893-7900

Colorado Division, Inc.
2255 South Oneida
Denver, Colorado 80224
(303) 758-2030

Connecticut Division, Inc.
Barnes Park South
14 Village Lane
Wallingford, Connecticut
06492
(203) 265-7161

Delaware Division, Inc.
1708 Lovering Avenue
Suite 202
Wilmington, Delaware
19806
(302) 654-6267

**District of Columbia
Division, Inc.**
Universal Building, South
1825 Connecticut Avenue,
N.W.
Suite 315
Washington, D.C. 20009
(202) 483-2600

Florida Division, Inc.
1001 South MacDill Avenue
Tampa, Florida 33629
(813) 253-0541

Georgia Division, Inc.
46 Fifth Street, NE
Atlanta, Georgia 30308
(404) 892-0026

**Hawaii Pacific Division,
Inc.**
Community Services Center
Bldg.
200 North Vineyard
Boulevard
Honolulu, Hawaii 96817
(808) 531-1662-3-4-5

Idaho Division, Inc.
1609 Abbs Street
P.O. Box 5386
Boise, Idaho 83705
(208) 343-4609

Illinois Division, Inc.
37 South Wabash Avenue
Chicago, Illinois 60603
(312) 372-0472

Indiana Division, Inc.
9575 N. Valparaiso Ct.
Indianapolis, Indiana 46268
(317) 872-4432

Iowa Division, Inc.
8364 Hickman Road,
Suite D
Des Moines, Iowa 50322
(515) 253-0147

Kansas Division, Inc.
3003 Van Buren Street
Topeka, Kansas 66611
(913) 267-0131

Kentucky Division, Inc.
Medical Arts Bldg.
1169 Eastern Parkway
Louisville, Kentucky 40217
(502) 459-1867

Louisiana Division, Inc.
Fidelity Homestead Bldg.
837 Gravier Street
Suite 700
New Orleans, Louisiana
70112-1509
(504) 523-4188

Maine Division, Inc.
52 Federal Street
Brunswick, Maine 04011
(207) 729-3339

Maryland Division, Inc.
8219 Town Center Drive
P.O. Box 82
White Marsh, Maryland
21162-0082
(301) 529-7272

Massachusetts Division, Inc.
247 Commonwealth Avenue
Boston, Massachusetts
02116
(617) 267-2650

Michigan Division, Inc.
1205 East Saginaw Street
Lansing, Michigan 48906
(517) 371-2920

Minnesota Division, Inc.
3316 West 66th Street
Minneapolis, Minnesota
55435
(612) 925-2772

Mississippi Division, Inc.
1380 Livingston Lane
Lakeover Office Park
Jackson, Mississippi 39213
(601) 362-8874

Missouri Division, Inc.
3322 American Avenue
Jefferson City, Missouri
65102
(314) 893-4800

Montana Division, Inc.
313 N. 32nd Street
Suite #1
Billings, Montana 59101
(406) 252-7111

Nebraska Division, Inc.
8502 West Center Road
Omaha, Nebraska
68124-5255
(402) 393-5800

Nevada Division, Inc.
1325 East Harmon
Las Vegas, Nevada 89119
(702) 798-6877

**New Hampshire Division,
Inc.***
360 Route 101, Unit 501
Bedford, New Hampshire
03102-6821
(603) 669-3270

New Jersey Division, Inc.
2600 Route 1, CNN 2201
North Brunswick,
New Jersey 08902
(201) 297-8000

New Mexico Division, Inc.
5800 Lomas Blvd., N.E.
Albuquerque, New Mexico
87110
(505) 262-2336

**New York State Division,
Inc.**
6725 Lyons Street
P.O. Box 7
East Syracuse, New York
13057
(315) 437-7025

☐ **Long Island Division, Inc.**
145 Pidgeon Hill Road
Huntington Station,
New York 11746
(516) 385-9100

☐ **New York City Division,
Inc.**
19 West 56th Street
New York, New York
10019
(212) 586-8700

☐ **Queens Division, Inc.**
112-25 Queens Boulevard
Forest Hills, New York
11375
(718) 263-2224

☐ **Westchester Division, Inc.**
30 Glenn St.
White Plains, New York
10603
(914) 949-4800

**North Carolina Division,
Inc.**
11 South Boylan Avenue
Suite 221
Raleigh, North Carolina
27603
(919) 834-8463

North Dakota Division, Inc.
Hotel Graver Annex Bldg.
123 Roberts Street
P.O. Box 426
Fargo, North Dakota 58107
(701) 232-1385

Ohio Divison, Inc.
5555 Frantz Road
Dublin, Ohio 43017
(614) 889-9565

Oklahoma Division, Inc.
3000 United Founders Blvd.
Suite 136
Oklahoma City, Oklahoma
73112
(405) 843-9888

Oregon Division, Inc.
0330 S.W. Curry
Portland, Oregon 97201
(503) 295-6422

Pennsylvania Division, Inc.
Route 422 & Sipe Avenue
P.O. Box 897
Hershey, Pennsylvania
17033-0897
(717) 533-6144

*New address effective April 15, 1989.

APPENDIX 83–2

CHARTERED DIVISIONS OF THE AMERICAN CANCER SOCIETY *Continued*

☐ **Philadelphia Division, Inc.**
1422 Chestnut Street
Philadelphia,
Pennsylvania 19102
(215) 665-2900

Puerto Rico Division, Inc.
Calle Alverio #577,
Esquina Sargento Medina,
Hato Rey, Puerto Rico
00918
(809) 764-2295

Rhode Island Division, Inc.
400 Main Street
Pawtucket, Rhode Island
02860
(401) 722-8480

South Carolina Division, Inc.
2214 Devine Street
Columbia, South Carolina
29205
(803) 256-0245

South Dakota Division, Inc.
4101 Carnegie Circle
Sioux Falls, South Dakota
57106-2322
(605) 361-8277

Tennessee Division, Inc.
1315 Eighth Avenue, South
Nashville, Tennessee 37203
(615) 255-1ACS

Texas Division, Inc.
P.O. Box 140435
Austin, Texas 78714-0435
(512) 928-2262

Utah Division, Inc.
610 East South Temple
Salt Lake City, Utah 84102
(801) 322-0431

Vermont Division, Inc.
13 Loomis Street, Drawer C
Montpelier, Vermont 05602
(802) 223-2348

Virginia Division, Inc.
4240 Park Place Court
Glen Allen, Virginia 23060
(804) 270-0142/
(800) 552-7996

Washington Division, Inc.
2120 First Avenue North
Seattle, Washington
98109-1140
(206) 283-1152

West Virginia Division, Inc.
2428 Kanawha Boulevard
East Charleston,
West Virginia 25311
(304) 344-3611

Wisconsin Division, Inc.
615 North Sherman Avenue
Madison, Wisconsin 53704
(608) 249-0487

Wyoming Division, Inc.
3109 Boxelder Drive
Cheyenne, Wyoming 82001
(307) 638-3331

Index

Page numbers in *italics* refer to illustrations; page numbers followed by b refer to boxed material and those followed by t refer to tables.

1177

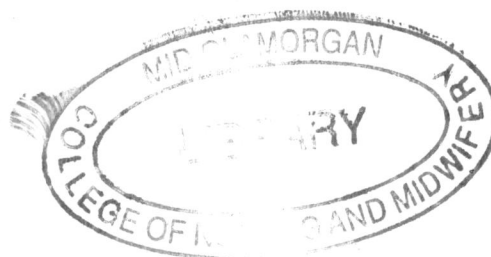